DRS. CRAVEN, ATKINS, LACY, WALLER
BELL, PROTHEROE & BAKER
NETTLEHAM MEDICAL PRACTICE
14 LODGE LANE, NETTLEHAM
LINCOLN LN2 2RS

CLINICAL ORTHOPAEDICS

section editors

Answorth A. Allen, MD

Oheneba Boachie-Adjei, MD

Robert L. Buly, MD

Frank P. Cammisa, Jr., MD

Denis R. Clohisy, MD

Michelle Gerwin, MD

Martin J. O'Malley, MD

Douglas E. Padgett, MD

Cathleen Raggio, MD

Bernard A. Rawlins, MD

Howard Anthony Rose, MD

CLINICAL ORTHOPAEDICS

Edward V. Craig, MD

The Hospital for Special Surgery
535 E. 70th Street
New York, New York

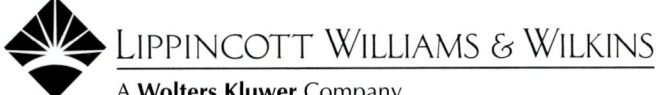

LIPPINCOTT WILLIAMS & WILKINS
A **Wolters Kluwer** Company
Philadelphia • Baltimore • New York • London
Buenos Aires • Hong Kong • Sydney • Tokyo

Acquisitions Editor: Danette Knopp
Developmental Editor: Keith Donnellan
Production Editor: Bill Cady
Marketing Manager: Diane Harnish
Design Coordinator: Mario Fernandez

351 West Camden Street
Baltimore, Maryland 21201–2436 USA

227 East Washington Square
Philadelphia, Pennsylvania 19106 USA

Printed in the United States of America

Library of Congress Cataloging-in-Publication Data
Clinical orthopaedics / Edward V. Craig. — 1st ed.
    p.   cm.
   Includes bibliographical references and index.
   ISBN 0-683-02180-X
   1. Orthopedic surgery. I. Craig, Edward V.
   [DNLM: 1. Orthopedics—methods.   2. Orthopedic procedures.
WE 168 C6406   1999]
RD731.C58   1999
617.4'7—DC21
DNLM/DLC
for Library of Congress   98-15922
                                      CIP

To purchase additional copies of this book, call our customer service department at (800) 638–3030 or fax orders to (301) 824–7390. International customers should call (301) 714–2324.

                       99 00 01 02
                   1 2 3 4 5 6 7 8 9 10

This work is dedicated to my father, Edward Vincent Craig,
a man who led by example and reinforced daily
the importance of hard work, education, and achievable goals.
His support, trust, encouragement, and confidence in me were unwavering.
Finally, he taught me the most invaluable lesson,
one that no one else could teach me, how to be a father.

preface

Clinical Orthopaedics, intended to fill the need for a comprehensive single-volume textbook of orthopaedic surgery, focuses on the clinical evaluation and management, both surgical and nonsurgical, of the vast array of conditions and problems faced by the practicing general orthopaedic surgeon and orthopaedic surgical resident. It is a general textbook that includes chapters on specialized topics written by specialists. The design, chapter organization, and choice of topics included provide the reader with a quick and practical guide to management and a road map to the variety of operative procedures faced by the general orthopaedist on any given day. Residents can use this single source to review the treatment, approach, and anatomical structures that will be encountered in a wide variety of procedures. Because of the textbook's single-source nature, it will also be useful to any practicing orthopaedic surgeon or practitioner dealing with a variety of musculoskeletal problems.

The book is presented in nine sections, covering the hand and wrist, shoulder and elbow, spine, hip, degenerative knee, athlete's knee, foot and ankle, common tumors, and pediatric orthopaedics. Each chapter begins with a clinical description of what is known about the pathomechanics of a condition and is followed by discussions of common patient complaints for the problem, the relevant physical findings, the most common imaging and ancillary studies used to arrive at a precise diagnosis, and the systematic approach to both the nonoperative and operative treatment and most commonly utilized operative approaches for each of the orthopaedic conditions. Accompanying nearly every chapter is a clinical table that, at a glance, presents the problem, indications for treatment, operative technique used for that condition, anatomy to be encountered, and the most common potential pitfalls of the surgery for that problem. These tables are for orthopaedists who need a quick refresher on what they are about to encounter in the operating room. Each chapter is organized in the same fashion, so that the reader can know precisely in which part of each chapter necessary information can be gleaned. The references and suggested readings are not exhaustive but contain the hallmark and landmark publications from which the treatment options identified in the chapter are based.

In summary, Clinical Orthopaedics provides the resident and general orthopaedist one manageable and comprehensive source of information, a companion to the ongoing education process that is a career in orthopaedic surgery.

Edward V. Craig, MD

acknowledgments

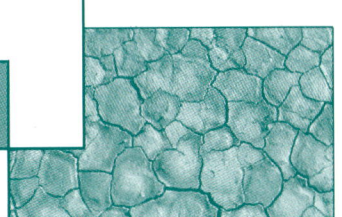

Numerous contributors, clinicians and nonclinicians alike, are responsible for bringing this book to publication. My heartfelt thanks go to each of the section editors and contributing authors for the preparation and review of the manuscripts, for the thought that went into trying to be concise yet thorough, and for following the guidelines and deadlines that inevitably accompany the preparation of manuscript.

Second, I would like to acknowledge the tremendous support given to me by the staff at Lippincott Williams & Wilkins, including Danette Knopp, Keith Donnellan, and Bill Cady, without whose persistence, dedication, and attention to detail this project would have stalled.

Finally, I would like to acknowledge, by this publication, the residents and postgraduate fellows who have contributed to this manuscript by their ongoing thirst for knowledge and who have indeed made the education process reciprocal between resident staff and contributors to this volume.

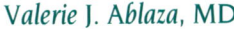
Valerie J. Ablaza, MD
The Plastic Surgery Group
Bloomfield, New Jersey

Answorth A. Allen, MD
Assistant Professor of Surgery (Orthopaedics)
Weill Medical College of Cornell University
Assistant Attending Physician
The Hospital for Special Surgery
New York, New York

Luis Alvarez, MD
Fundacion Jimenez Diaz
Servicio Dermatologia
Ciudad Universitaria
Madrid, Spain

Robert B. Anderson, MD
Miller Orthopaedic Clinic
Chief, Foot and Ankle Service
Carolinas Medical Center
Charlotte, North Carolina

Elizabeth A. Arendt, MD
Associate Professor, University of Minnesota
Director, Sports Medicine Institute
Medical Director, Men's and Women's Varsity Athletics
Team Physician, USA Hockey
Team Physician, USA Soccer
Minneapolis, Minnesota

Donna J. Astion, MD
Associate Chief of the Foot and Ankle Service
The Hospital for Joint Diseases
Orthopaedic Institute
New York, New York

Bernard R. Bach, Jr., MD
Associate Professor, Department of Orthopaedic Surgery
Director, Sports Medicine Section
Rush Medical College
Rush Presbyterian St. Luke's Medical Center
Chicago, Illinois

Craig S. Bartlett III, MD
Clinical Assistant Professor
University of Vermont
McClure Musculoskeletal Research Center
Burlington, Vermont

James E. Bates, MD
Orthopaedic Surgeon
Alvarado Orthopaedic Medical Group Inc.
San Diego, California

Michael Bednar, MD
Associate Professor of Orthopaedic Surgery
Loyola University Medical Center
Maywood, Illinois

Gloria M. Beim, MD
Director, Houghston Clinic of Colorado
Crested Butte, Colorado

John A. Bergfeld, MD
Medical Director
Cleveland Clinic, Sports Health
Team Physician, Cleveland Browns, NFL
Team Physician, Cleveland Cavaliers, NBA
Cleveland, Ohio

Leslie J. Bisson, MD
Orthopaedic Surgeon
Sports Medicine
Northtown Orthopaedic Group
East Amherst, New York

Oheneba Boachie-Adjei, MD
Chief, Scoliosis Service
Associate Orthopaedic Surgeon
The Hospital for Special Surgery
Attending Surgeon in Orthopaedics
The New York Hospital
Associate Clinical Professor in Orthopaedics
Cornell University Medical Center
Associate Attending Surgeon in Orthopaedics
Memorial Sloan-Kettering Cancer Center
New York, New York

Walther H. O. Bohne, MD
The Hospital for Special Surgery
New York, New York

Arthur L. Boland, MD
Assistant Clinical Professor of Orthopaedic Surgery
Harvard Medical School
Head Surgeon, Harvard Athletic Department
Chief of Orthopaedics
Harvard University Health Services
Boston, Massachusetts

James V. Bono, MD
Attending Surgeon
The New England Baptist Hospital
Assistant Clinical Professor of Surgery
Tufts University
Boston, Massachusetts

Joseph Borrelli, Jr., MD
Chief, Orthopaedic Trauma Service
Assistant Professor
Department of Orthopaedic Surgery
Washington University
St. Louis, Missouri

Mathias P. G. Bostrom, MD
Assistant Attending Orthopaedic Surgeon
Assistant Scientist, Division of Research
The Hospital for Special Surgery
Assisting Surgeon, Orthopaedics
New York Hospital
Instructor, Cornell University Medical College
New York, New York

Dahari Brooks, MD
The Hospital for Special Surgery
New York, New York

Robert L. Buly, MD
Assistant Professor of Orthopaedic Surgery
Cornell University Medical College
Assistant Attending Orthopaedic Surgeon
Surgical Arthritis Service
The Hospital for Special Surgery
Orthopaedic Trauma Service
New York Presbyterian Hospital
New York, New York

Frank P. Cammisa, Jr., MD
Associate Professor of Surgery
Weill Medical College of Cornell University
Chief, Spine Surgery
The Hospital for Special Surgery
New York, New York

Eric W. Carson, MD
Chief, Sports Medicine
LSU Medical Center, School of Medicine
Department of Orthopaedic Surgery
New Orleans, Louisiana

Richard A. Cautilli, Jr., MD
Thomas Jefferson University Affiliated Hospitals
Philadelphia, Pennsylvania

Wen Chao, MD
Assistant Attending, Department of Orthopaedics
St. Luke-Roosevelt Hospital Center
Presbyterian Hospital
Assistant Clinical Professor
Columbia University
Assistant Attending Orthopaedic Surgeon
New York Presbyterian Hospital
New York, New York

Edward Y. Cheng, MD
Associate Professor, Department of Orthopaedic Surgery
University of Minnesota
Minneapolis, Minnesota

Denis R. Clohisy, MD
Associate Professor, Department of Orthopaedic Surgery
University of Minnesota Hospital and Clinic
Minneapolis, Minnesota

Bruce E. Cohen, MD
Tallahassee Orthopaedic Clinic
Tallahassee, Florida

Charles N. Cornell, MD
Associate Professor of Surgery
Cornell University Medical College
Associate Attending Surgeon, Orthopaedics
New York Presbyterian Hospital
The Hospital for Special Surgery
New York, New York

Edward V. Craig, MD
Professor of Clinical Surgery
Weill Medical College of Cornell University
Attending Orthopaedic Surgeon
The Hospital for Special Surgery
New York, New York

Leigh Ann Curl, MD
Assistant Professor of Orthopaedic Surgery
University Sports Medicine
University of Maryland
Baltimore, Maryland

Jonathan T. Deland, MD.
Co-Director, Foot and Ankle Service
The Hospital for Special Surgery
Assistant Professor
Cornell University Medical College
Associate Editor, Foot and Ankle Journal
New York, New York

David M. Dines, MD
Associate Clinical Professor of Orthopaedic Surgery
Cornell University Medical College
Chairman, Department of Orthopaedic Surgery
Long Island Jewish Hospital
Attending Surgeon
The Hospital for Special Surgery
Sports and Shoulder Service
Consultant, New Jersey Devils Hockey Team
New York, New York

Daneca M. DiPaolo, MD
Clinical Assistant Professor of Orthopaedic Surgery
University of Medicine and Dentistry
Medical School of New Jersey
Newark, New Jersey
Director, Orthopaedic Hand Surgery
Vice-President and Clinical Director
Jersey City Medical Center
Jersey City, New Jersey
Associate Attending Surgeon
St. Barnabas Medical Center
Livingston, New Jersey

Jeffrey R. Dugas, MD
Resident in Orthopaedic Surgery
The Hospital for Special Surgery
New York, New York

Robert P. Dunbar, Jr., MD, LCDR, MC, USNR
Attending Orthopaedic Surgeon
U.S. Naval Hospital-Yokosuka
Yokosuka, Japan

Clive P. Duncan, MD, FRCS(C)
Professor & Chairman, Department of Orthopaedics
University of British Columbia
Chief, Department of Orthopaedics
Vancouver Hospital & Health Sciences Center
Vancouver, British Columbia, Canada

Cherise M. Dyal, MD
Assistant Professor of Orthopaedic Surgery
Albert Einstein College of Medicine
Chief, Foot and Ankle Service
Montefiore Medical Center
Bronx, New York

Dale J. Federico, MD
Assistant Professor of Orthopaedic Surgery
Section of Orthopaedic Sports Medicine and Rehabilitation
University of Chicago Sports Medicine
Chicago, Illinois

Mark P. Figgie, MD
Associate Attending Orthopaedic Surgeon
The Hospital for Special Surgery
Assistant Professor of Surgery
Weill Medical College of Cornell University
New York, New York

Marc J. Friedman, MD
Attending Physician
Southern California Orthopedic Institute
Van Nuys, California
Assistant Clinical Professor of Orthopaedic Surgery
UCLA School of Medicine
Los Angeles, California

John P. Fulkerson, MD
Clinical Professor
University of Connecticut Medical School
Orthopedic Associates of Hartford, P.C.
Farmington, Connecticut

Charles J. Gatt, Jr., MD
Clinical Assistant Professor of Surgery
Division of Orthopaedic Surgery
UMDNJ-Robert Wood Johnson Medical School
New Brunswick, New Jersey

Lloyd B. Gayle, MD, FACS
Assistant Professor of Clinical Surgery
Weill Medical College of Cornell University
Attending Surgeon, New York Presbyterian Hospital
New York, New York

Gaia Georgopoulos, MD
The Children's Hospital
Associate Professor, Orthopaedic Surgery
University of Colorado Health Sciences Center
Denver, Colorado

Michelle Gerwin, MD
Assistant Professor,
Weill Medical College of Cornell University
Assistant Attending Orthopaedic Surgeon
The Hospital for Special Surgery
New York, New York

Thomas J. Gilbert, MD, MPP
Center for Diagnostic Imaging
St. Louis Park, Minnesota

Federico P. Girardi, MD
Junior Attending Orthopaedic Surgeon
Spine and Scoliosis Service
The Hospital for Special Surgery
New York, New York

Steven B. Haas, MD
Orthopaedic Surgeon
The Hospital for Special Surgery
New York, New York

William G. Hamilton, MD
Clinical Professor of Orthopaedic Surgery
College of Physicians and Surgeons
Columbia University
Senior Attending Orthopaedic Surgeon
St. Luke's-Roosevelt Hospital Center
New York, New York

Jo A. Hannafin, MD, PhD
Assistant Attending Orthopaedic Surgeon
Associate Director, Laboratory for Soft Tissue Research
Orthopaedic Director, Women's Sports Medicine Center
The Hospital for Special Surgery
Assistant Attending Surgeon
New York Presbyterian Hospital
Assistant Professor of Surgery (Orthopaedics)
Weill Medical College of Cornell University
Team Physician, United States Rowing Team
New York, New York

Kenneth K. Hansraj, MD
Fellow
The Hospital for Special Surgery
New York, New York

Christopher D. Harner, MD
Blue Cross of Western Pennsylvania Professor of Orthopaedic
  Surgery
Chief, Division of Sports Medicine
University of Pittsburgh
Head Team Physician
Robert Morris College
Pittsburgh, Pennsylvania

Paul J. Hecht, MD
Assistant Professor, Orthopaedic Surgery
Associate Director, Foot & Ankle Center
MCP Hahnemann University
Philadelphia, Pennsylvania

David L. Helfet, MD
Director, Combined Orthopaedic Trauma Service
Attending Orthopaedic Surgeon
The Hospital for Special Surgery/New York Presbyterian Hospital
Professor, Orthopaedic Surgery
Weill Medical College of Cornell University
New York, New York

Haideh Hirmand, MD, MPA
Assistant Attending Plastic Surgeon
Manhattan Eye, Ear, and Throat Hospital
New York, New York

Lloyd A. Hoffman, MD, FACS
Associate Orthopaedic Surgeon
New York Presbyterian Hospital
New York, New York

Robert N. Hotchkiss, MD
Associate Attending Orthopaedic Surgeon
Chief of Hand Service
Director, Hand and Upper Extremity Fellowship
The Hospital for Special Surgery
Assistant Professor, Orthopaedic Surgery
Weill Medical College of Cornell University
New York, New York

Michael H. Huo, MD
Associate Professor
Department of Orthopaedic Surgery
Baylor College of Medicine
Houston, Texas

N. George Kasparyan, MD, PhD
Hand and Microvascular Surgery Fellow
The Hospital for Special Surgery
New York, New York
Hand and Orthopaedic Surgeon
Lahey Clinic
Burlington, Massachusetts

Paul K. Kosmatka, MD
Orthopaedic Surgeon
St. Cloud Orthopaedics and Associates
St. Cloud, Minnesota

Craig L. Levitz, MD
Director, Sports Medicine and Cartilage Repair
OCOA Orthopaedics
Rockville Center, New York

Jonathan D. Lewin, MD
Assistant Professor
Division of Spine Surgery
Montefiore Medical Center
Bronx, New York

Thomas N. Lindenfeld, MD
Associate Director, Cincinnati Sports Medicine and Orthopaedic
    Center
Deaconess Hospital
Cincinnati, Ohio

John C. L'Insalata, MD
Clinical Instructor in Surgery (Orthopaedic)
Cornell University Medical College
Assistant Attending Orthopaedic Surgeon
Bayley Seton Hospital
Lutheran Medical Center
The Hospital for Special Surgery
Active Attending Surgeon, Department of Orthopaedics
Staten Island University Hospital
New York, New York

Ferdinand J. Liotta, MD
Staff Orthopaedist
Valley View Hospital
Orthopaedic Associates of Aspen and Glenwood Springs
Glenwood Springs, Colorado

William A. Lohrer, MD
Associate Professor
Department of Orthopaedics
Rehabilitation College of Medicine
Pennsylvania State University
University Park, Pennsylvania

Baron S. Lonner, MD
Chief of Spine Service
Long Island Jewish Hospital
Manhasset, New York
Assistant Professor of Orthopaedic Surgery
Albert Einstein College of Medicine
New York, New York

Douglas J. Mackenzie, MD
Assistant Professor
Division of Plastic and Reconstructive Surgery
Oregon Health Sciences University
Portland, Oregon

Neil J. Macy, MD
Department of Orthopaedic Surgery
Montefiore Medical Center
Assistant Professor Orthopaedics
Assistant Professor Pediatrics
Albert Einstein College of Medicine of Yeshiva
    University
Bronx, New York

Joel W. Malin, MD
Fairfield Orthopaedic Associates
St. Vincent's Hospital
Bridgeport, Connecticut

Bassam A. Masri, MD, FRCS(C)
Clinical Associate Professor and Head
Division of Reconstructive Orthopaedics
University of British Columbia
Vancouver, British Columbia, Canada

Michael J. Maynard, MD
Assistant Attending Orthopaedic Surgeon
Sports Medicine and Shoulder Service
The Hospital for Special Surgery
Assistant Professor of Orthopaedic Surgery
Weill Medical College of Cornell University
Assistant Attending Orthopaedic Surgeon
New York Presbyterian Hospital
New York, New York

**John P. Mc Cabe, MD, MMSc, MCh, FRCS(I),
    FRCS(Orth)**
Consultant Orthopaedic Surgeon
Merlin Park Regional Hospital
Galway, Ireland

Richard R. McCormack, Jr., MD
Associate Attending Orthopaedic Surgeon
The Hospital for Special Surgery
Associate Attending Surgeon (Orthopaedic Surgery)
New York Presbyterian Hospital
Assistant Clinical Member (Affiliate)
Memorial Sloan-Kettering Cancer Center
Assistant Professor of Orthopaedic Surgery
Weill Medical College of Cornell University
New York, New York

Gregory S. McDowell, MD
Orthopedic Surgeons, PSC
Co-Director Northern Rockies Regional Spine Injury Center
Billings, Montana

Brian J. McGinley, MD
Orthopaedic Surgeon
Port Jefferson Specialty Associates
Mather/St. Charles Hospitals
Port Jefferson, New York

Brian E. McGrath, MD
Department of Orthopaedic Surgery
Buffalo General Hospital
Associate Clinical Professor
SUNY at Buffalo
Buffalo, New York

Elizabeth McLarney, MD, LCDR, MC, USNR
Department Head
Department of Orthopaedic Surgery
U.S. Naval Hospital-Yokosuka
Yokosuka, Japan

Louis S. Mezman, MD
Staff Surgeon
Holmes Regional Medical Center
Melbourne, Florida

Claude T. Moorman III, MD
Director, Sports Medicine
Assistant Professor, Orthopaedic Surgery
University Sports Medicine
University of Maryland Medical Center
Baltimore, Maryland

Bryan J. Nestor, MD
Assistant Professor of Orthopaedic Surgery
Weill Medical College of Cornell University
Assistant Attending Orthopaedic Surgeon
Assistant Attending Research Department
The Hospital for Special Surgery
New York, New York

Jeroen G. V. Neyt
Consultant Orthopaedic Surgeon
Chase Farm Hospitals
Enfield, England

Frank R. Noyes, MD
Director, Cincinnati Sports Medicine and Orthopaedic Center
Director, Cincinnati Sports Medicine Research and Education Foundation
Clinical Professor, Department of Orthopaedic Surgery
University of Cincinnati
Cincinnati, Ohio

Stephen J. O'Brien, MD
Associate Attending Orthopaedic Surgeon
The Hospital for Special Surgery
Associate Professor for Surgery (Orthopaedics)
Weill Medical College of Cornell University
Assistant Team Physician
New York Giants Football
New York, New York
Associate Attending Orthopaedic Surgeon
North Shore University Hospital
Glen Cove, New York

Enyi Okereke, PharmD, MD
Assistant Professor, Orthopaedics
Chief of the Foot and Ankle Service
Hospital of the University of Pennsylvania
Philadelphia, Pennsylvania

Patrick F. O'Leary, MD
Associate Professor of Surgery
Weill Medical College of Cornell University
Attending Orthopaedic Surgeon
The Hospital for Special Surgery
Chief, Spine Surgery
Lenox Hill Hospital
New York, New York

Martin J. O'Malley, MD
Assistant Attending Orthopaedic Surgeon
The Hospital for Special Surgery
Assistant Attending Surgeon (Orthopaedics)
New York Hospital
Assistant Professor of Surgery (Orthopaedics)
Weill Medical College of Cornell University
New York, New York
Provisional Active Attending Surgeon
New Milford Hospital
New Milford, Connecticut

Douglas E. Padgett, MD
Assistant Professor Orthopaedic Surgery
The Hospital for Special Surgery
Weill Medical College of Cornell
New York, New York

George A. Paletta, Jr., MD
Department of Orthopaedic Surgery
Washington University School of Medicine
Barnes Jewish Hospital
St. Louis, MO

Terrance D. Peabody, MD
Assistant Professor, Section of Orthopaedic Surgery
University of Chicago
Chicago, Illinois

Walter Pedowitz, MD
Associate Clinical Professor
Department of Orthopaedic Surgery
Columbia University
New York, New York
Union County Orthopaedic Group
Linden, New Jersey

Robert K. Peterson, MD
Davis Orthopaedics
Davis, California

Kevin D. Plancher, MD, MS
Assistant Professor
Albert Einstein College of Medicine
Attending, Montefiore Medical Center
Bronx, New York
Chief, Hand Service
Blythedale Children's Hospital
Plancher Hand and Sports Medicine
Stamford, Connecticut
Hand Consultant
Steadman Hawkins Clinic
Vail, Colorado

Cathleen Raggio, MD
Attending Orthopaedic Surgeon
The Hospital for Special Surgery
New York, New York

Bernard A. Rawlins, MD
Assistant Professor of Surgery (Orthopaedics)
Weill Medical College of Cornell University
Assistant Attending Surgeon
The Hospital for Special Surgery
The New York Hospital
New York, New York

Howard Anthony Rose, MD
Assistant Professor of Orthopaedic Surgery
Cornell University Medical College
New York, New York

Benjamin E. Rosenstadt, MD
Attending Orthopaedic Surgeon
C.V. Starr Hand Surgery Center
St. Luke's-Roosevelt Hospital
New York, New York

S. Robert Rozbruch, MD
Clinical Instructor of Orthopaedic Surgery
Weill Medical College of Cornell University
The Hospital for Special Surgery
New York, New York

Marc H. Rubman, MD
Northern New Jersey Orthopaedic Specialists
Madison, New Jersey

Marc R. Safran, MD
Director, Shoulder Services
Co-Director, Sports Medicine
Department of Orthopaedic Surgery
Kaiser Permanente, Orange County
Assistant Clinical Professor
University of California, Irvine
University of California, San Diego
Newport Beach, California

Matthew I. Samuelson, MD
Orthopaedic Surgeon
McHenry County Orthopaedics
Crystal Lake, Illinois

John F. Sarwark, MD
Associate Professor, Department of Orthopaedic Surgery
Northwestern University Medical School
Interim Division Head, Pediatric Orthopaedic Surgery
The Children's Memorial Hospital
Chicago, Illinois

Mark T. Scarborough, MD
Associate Professor and Chief
Division of Orthopaedic Oncology
Department of Orthopaedics
University of Florida
Gainesville, Florida

Wayne J. Sebastianelli, MD
Associate Professor
Department of Orthopaedics
Rehabilitation College of Medicine
Director of Athletic Medicine
Pennsylvania State University
University Park, Pennsylvania

Chester H. Sharps, MD
Orthopaedic Surgeon
Tuckahoe Orthopaedic Associates
Assistant Clinical Professor for Orthopaedic Surgery
Medical College of Virginia
Glen Allen, Virginia

K. Donald Shelbourne, MD
Clinical Associate Professor
Indiana University School of Medicine
Team Physician, Purdue University
Indianapolis, Indiana

Peter T. Simonian, MD
Associate Professor, Department of Orthopaedic Surgery
Chief, Sports Medicine Clinic
Director, Sports Medicine Research
University of Washington
Seattle, Washington

Domenick J. Sisto, MD
Sports Medicine Fellowship Director
Los Angeles Orthopaedic Institute
Sherman Oaks Hospital Medical Center
Sherman Oaks, California

Andrew V. Slucky, MD
Cervical Spine Surgeon
Pacific Orthopaedic Group
San Francisco, California

Stephen R. Southerland, MD, FRCS(C)
Fellow in Sports Medicine
Massachusetts General Hospital
Chestnut Hill, Massachusetts

Carl L. Stanitski, MD
Professor, Department of Orthopaedic Surgery
Medical University of South Carolina
Charleston, South Carolina

Steven H. Stern, MD
Associate Clinical Professor of Orthopaedic Surgery
Northwestern University School of Medicine
Attending Physician, Department of Orthopaedic Surgery
Northwestern Memorial Hospital
Chicago, Illinois

David B. Thordarson, MD
Associate Professor
Chief, Foot and Ankle Trauma and Reconstructive Surgery
University of Southern California Department of Orthopaedics
Los Angeles, California

Dwight Tyndall, MD
Orthopaedic Surgeon
Bone and Joint Surgeons Ltd.
Olympia Park, Illinois

Ann Van Heest, MD
Assistant Professor
Department of Orthopedic Surgery
University of Minnesota
Minneapolis, Minnesota

Barry J. Waldman, MD
Resident, Department of Orthopaedic Surgery
The Johns Hopkins School of Medicine
Baltimore, Maryland

Keith L. Wapner, MD
Professor, Orthopaedic Surgery
Director, Foot and Ankle Surgery
MCP Hahnemann Hospital
Philadelphia, Pennsylvania

Steven R. Wardell, MD
Adult Joint Reconstruction
Parkview Musculoskeletal Institute
Palos Heights, Illinois

Jon J. P. Warner, MD
Chief, Harvard Shoulder Service
Massachusetts General Hospital
Boston, Massachusetts

Russell F. Warren, MD
Professor of Surgery (Orthopaedics)
Chairman, Division of Orthopaedic Surgery
Weill Medical College of Cornell University
Surgeon-in-Chief
The Hospital for Special Surgery
New York, New York

Andrew J. Weiland, MD
Professor of Surgery, Orthopaedics and Plastic
Cornell University Medical College
Attending Surgeon
The Hospital for Special Surgery
New York, New York

Geoffrey H. Westrich, MD
Assistant Attending Orthopaedic Surgeon
Assistant Scientist
The Hospital for Special Surgery
Instructor in Surgery
Weill Medical College of Cornell University
New York, New York

Mark T. Wichman, MD
Orthopaedic Surgeon
Sports Medicine
Milwaukee Orthopaedic Specialists
Milwaukee, Wisconsin

Thomas L. Wickiewicz, MD, FACS
Chief, Sports Medicine and Shoulder Service
Associate Attending
The Hospital for Special Surgery
Associate Professor of Clinical Orthopaedic Surgery
Weill Medical College of Cornell University
New York, New York

Scott W. Wolfe, MD
Associate Professor
Director, Yale Hand and Upper Extremity Center
Yale Department of Orthopaedics and
    Rehabilitation
Yale School of Medicine
Yale University
New Haven, Connecticut

Christopher Wottowa, MD
Springfield Clinic
Springfield, Illinois

S. Steven Yang, MD, MPH
Assistant Adjunct, Department of Orthopaedic
    Surgery
Hand Surgery Service
The Lenox Hill Hospital
New York, New York

Alastair S. E. Younger, MBChB, FRCS(C)
Department of Orthopaedics
University of British Columbia
Vancouver, British Columbia, Canada

Stephen J. Zabinski, MD
Shore Orthopaedic University Associates
Summers Point, New Jersey

Lewis E. Zionts, MD
Associate Professor of Orthopaedics and Pediatrics
University of Southern California
Director, Pediatric Orthopaedic Service
Women's and Children's Hospital
Los Angeles County/University of Southern California Medical
    Center
Los Angeles, California

contents

section I   HAND AND WRIST

section editor: *Michelle Gerwin*

section II   SHOULDER AND ELBOW

section editor: *Answorth A. Allen*

section III ## SPINE

section editor: *Oheneba Boachie-Adjei, Frank P. Cammisa, Jr., and Bernard A. Rawlins*

section VII   FOOT AND ANKLE
section editor: *Martin J. O'Malley*

section VIII COMMON TUMORS
section editor: *Denis R. Clohisy*

section IX PEDIATRICS
section editor: *Cathleen Raggio*

HAND AND WRIST

1

Fractures of the Distal Radius

Fractures of the distal radius are among the most common injuries seen by the orthopaedic surgeon. Their reported incidence is approximately 1 in 500 persons, and they account for nearly one-sixth of all fractures seen in the emergency room. A bimodal age distribution exists, with one peak in early adolescence and the second in the older population. Reviews of these injuries have documented that fully 50% or greater are intra-articular injuries involving either the radiocarpal or distal radioulnar joints in addition to the radial metaphyseal fracture (1).

Unlike other periarticular and intra-articular fractures, however, the standard of treatment for the majority of the distal radius fractures has been closed reduction and immobilization. Colles' (2) often-quoted statement that deformity does not correlate with functional limitation has been entrenched in the orthopaedic mainstream. In addition, the predominance of injury to the elderly population—often with concomitant medical problems, perceived low functional demands, and significant osteoporosis—has helped further the establishment of closed treatment for the majority of these injuries.

Recently, there has been a dramatic improvement in our understanding of fracture patterns and the long-term effects of intra-articular and extra-articular malunion of the distal radius. The operative equipment and techniques necessary to successfully manage these injuries have been further studied and refined. This increased knowledge has led to a heightened interest in these injuries and to an appropriately more aggressive approach to their management.

This chapter reviews the anatomy and injury mechanisms pertinent to fractures of the distal radius. The most common and clinically useful classification schemes and the principles of clinical and radiographic evaluation are described. Finally, the indications, techniques, and pitfalls of both nonoperative and operative treatment of these injuries are discussed.

RELEVANT ANATOMY AND PATHOGENESIS

The distal radius serves two primary mechanical functions: It is a platform on which the hand and carpus rest and is the unit through which the hand and forearm rotate about the ulnar axis. These motions occur through distinct articulations with both the carpus and the ulna at its distal extent. The concave scaphoid and lunate articular fossae are separated by a central ridge and define distinct sites for articulation with the scaphoid and the lunate, respectively. The ulnar border consists of the concave sigmoid notch, which articulates with the ulnar head to form the distal radioulnar joint (the central axis for forearm rotation).

The palmar surface of the radius serves as the attachment site for the volar radiocarpal ligaments, which are the major supporting ligaments of the wrist. The surface is flat and covered broadly by the pronator quadratus muscle. The dorsal surface of the radius is the attachment site for the less well developed dorsal capsule and dorsal radiocarpal ligaments. It is convex and marked by a prominence (Lister's tubercle) that functions as a fulcrum for the extensor pollicis longus tendon. Six distinct extensor compartments overlay its surface.

The distal radioulnar joint is stabilized by the triangular fibrocartilage complex (TFCC), which also provides for ulnocarpal articulation and stability. The TFCC consists of a 1- to 2-mm-thick articular disk that attaches broadly at its periphery to the distal aspect of the sigmoid notch and the ulnar styloid base.

As discussed below, the normal distal radius slopes approximately 22° from the radial styloid tip to the ulnar aspect of the lunate fossa in the coronal plane. In the sagittal plane, the articular surface has a normal palmar tilt of approximately 11°. Ulnar variance (the relative lengths of the ulnar aspect of the lunate fossa and the ulnar head) is unique to the individual and should be compared to the

Figure 1.1. In Frykman's classification of distal radius fractures, types I and II are extra-articular, and types III to VIII involve the radiocarpal joint (types III and IV), the distal radioulnar joint (types V and VI), or both (types VII and VIII). Types II, IV, VI, and VIII are characterized by the presence of an ulnar styloid fracture. Modified from Palmer AK. Fractures of the distal radius. In: Green DP, ed. Operative hand surgery. New York: Churchill Livingstone, 1993.

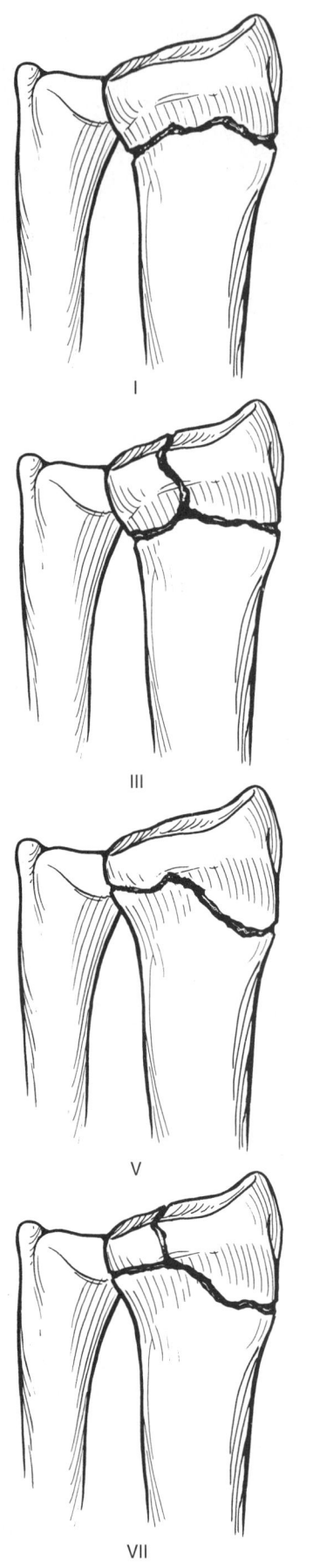
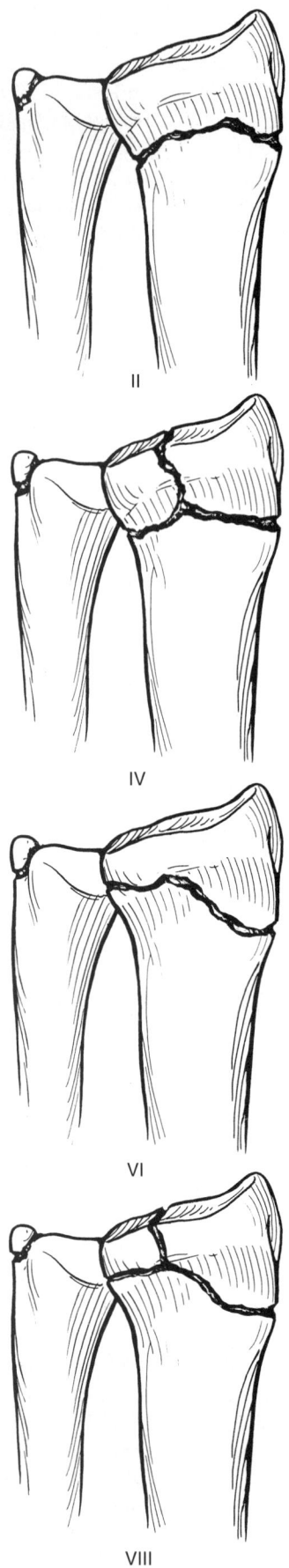

I   II

III   IV

V   VI

VII   VIII

opposite wrist. In most people, the ulna is shorter than the distal radius (ulnar negative).

The wrist is extremely mobile and is capable of up to 160° of flexion and extension and 180° of forearm rotation. Radial and ulnar deviation averages 50°. Approximately 80% of the load transmission across the wrist is through the radiocarpal articulation, and the remaining 20% is across the ulnocarpal articulation via the TFCC. Alterations in ulnar variance (as a result of anatomic variation or postfracture deformity) significantly alter this load transmission.

Mechanism of Injury

The majority of distal radius fractures result from a fall on an outstretched hand. Alternatively, these injuries may result from axial loads imposed during other events (most commonly motor vehicle accidents) or may be caused by direct blunt trauma with the hand in a fixed position.

Fernandez (3) advocated classifying distal radial fractures according to the mechanism of injury, believing that the methods of fracture reduction and fixation (open or closed) depend strictly on the forces at the time of injury. Type I fractures result from bending forces and represent extra-articular metaphyseal tensile failure (Colles' and Smith's fractures). Type II fractures result from shearing forces across the joint surface (Barton's and radial styloid fractures). Compression forces result in type III fractures, which involve impaction of subchondral and metaphyseal bone; several intra-articular fracture fragment patterns are possible (e.g., die-punch injuries). Type IV fractures result from avulsion forces and result in fracture at the site of ligament attachment. These injuries include a wide spectrum of radiocarpal sprains, subluxations, and dislocations. Finally, high-velocity injuries and combinations of other forces result in type V fractures, which are characterized by marked displacement, comminution, and instability.

Classification of Injury

The use of eponyms to describe various fracture patterns of the distal radius is imprecise and confusing. These limitations have led to the recent development of more specific classification schemes. The goal of these systems is to categorize fractures of the distal radius in a manner that will provide the orthopaedist with a guide to treatment options and expected outcome.

Since Gartland and Werley (4) first divided these injuries into extra-articular and intra-articular fractures, the majority of fracture classification schemes have been based on fracture anatomy. As methods of evaluating and treating these injuries have become more sophisticated, so too have the classification schemes become more complex. The Frykman classification is based on the involvement of the radiocarpal and/or distal radioulnar joint and the presence of an ulnar styloid fracture (Fig. 1.1). Despite its widespread use, this classification scheme does not include variables, such as direction and degree of displacement or comminution, that are vital in guiding fracture treatment and determining expected outcome.

Recent anatomic classifications have expanded the original Gartland and Werley scheme. McMurtry and Jupiter (5) retained the division between extra-articular and intra-articular injuries. Extra-articular injuries are further subdivided into stable and unstable fractures, based on the amount of comminution and angulation. Unstable injuries are characterized by extensive dorsal comminution, comminution extending volar to the midaxial plane of the radius, dorsal angulation of greater than 20°, and significant volar angulation. Intra-articular injuries are divided by the number of articular fracture fragments (Fig. 1.2): (a) two-part fractures, in which the opposite portion of the radiocarpal joint remains in continuity with the remainder of the radius (e.g., dorsal and volar Barton's, radial styloid, and isolated lunate fossa die-punch fractures); (b) three-part fractures, in which the intact lunate and scaphoid facets separate both from each other and from the radius; and (c) four-part fractures, in which the lunate fossa fragment of a three-part injury splits into dorsal and volar fragments. In addition, comminuted injuries (five or more parts), in which high-energy trauma completely disrupts the distal radius and its articulations, may occur.

Rayhack et al. (6) and Bradway et al. (7) have also stressed the importance of distinguishing between extra-articular and intra-articular injuries. Both classifications further classify distal radius fractures by the degree of displacement, reducibility, and stability after reduction.

Melone (8) classified four-part intra-articular fractures by the pattern of displacement. Type I fractures are minimally displaced. In type II fractures, dorsal or volar displacement of the lunate fossa fragments occurs as a unit, and the individual fragments are neither rotated nor widely separated. Recognizing fractures in which both the scaphoid and lunate impact the lunate fossa, Melone further divided these injuries into type IIa and type IIb. Closed reduction of these injuries will often fail if excessive dorsal or volar comminution occurs or if significant radiocarpal stepoff, shortening, or angulation exists. In type III fractures, displacement of the lunate fossa fragments is similar to that seen in type II injuries, but there is an associated metaphyseal spike (typically volar in dorsally displaced fractures), which further increases fracture instability and may create soft tissue complications. In type IV injuries, there is wide separation of the lunate fossa fragments; often, the rotation of the palmar medial fragment is as much as 180°. The type V, or explosion, fracture includes high-energy, highly comminuted injuries similar to McMurtry and Jupiter's five or more part class.

The most comprehensive, and perhaps cumbersome, anatomic classification scheme is the AO system (9). This system divides injuries into type A (extra-articular), type B (simple articular), and type C (complex articular). Within each type, fractures are further characterized by the pres-

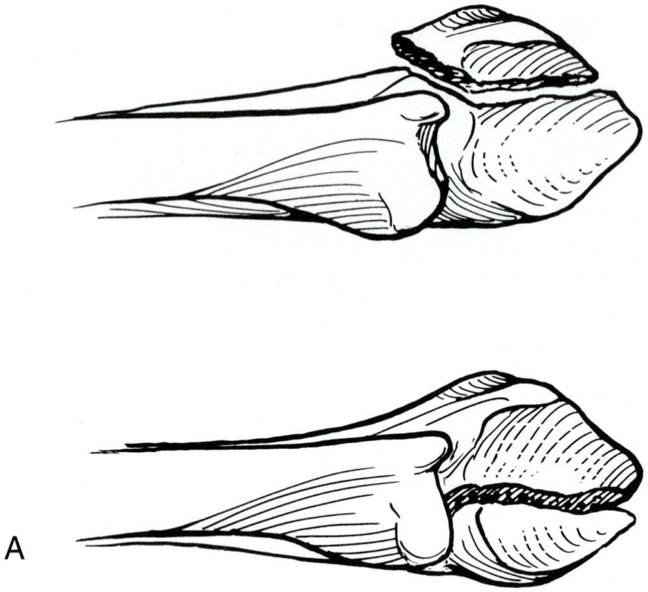

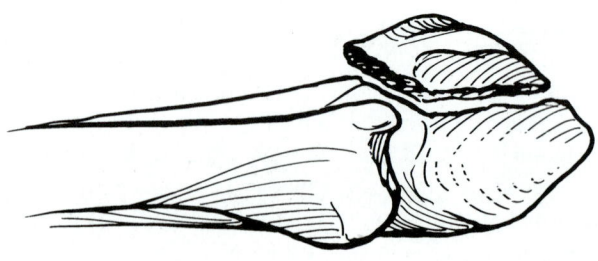

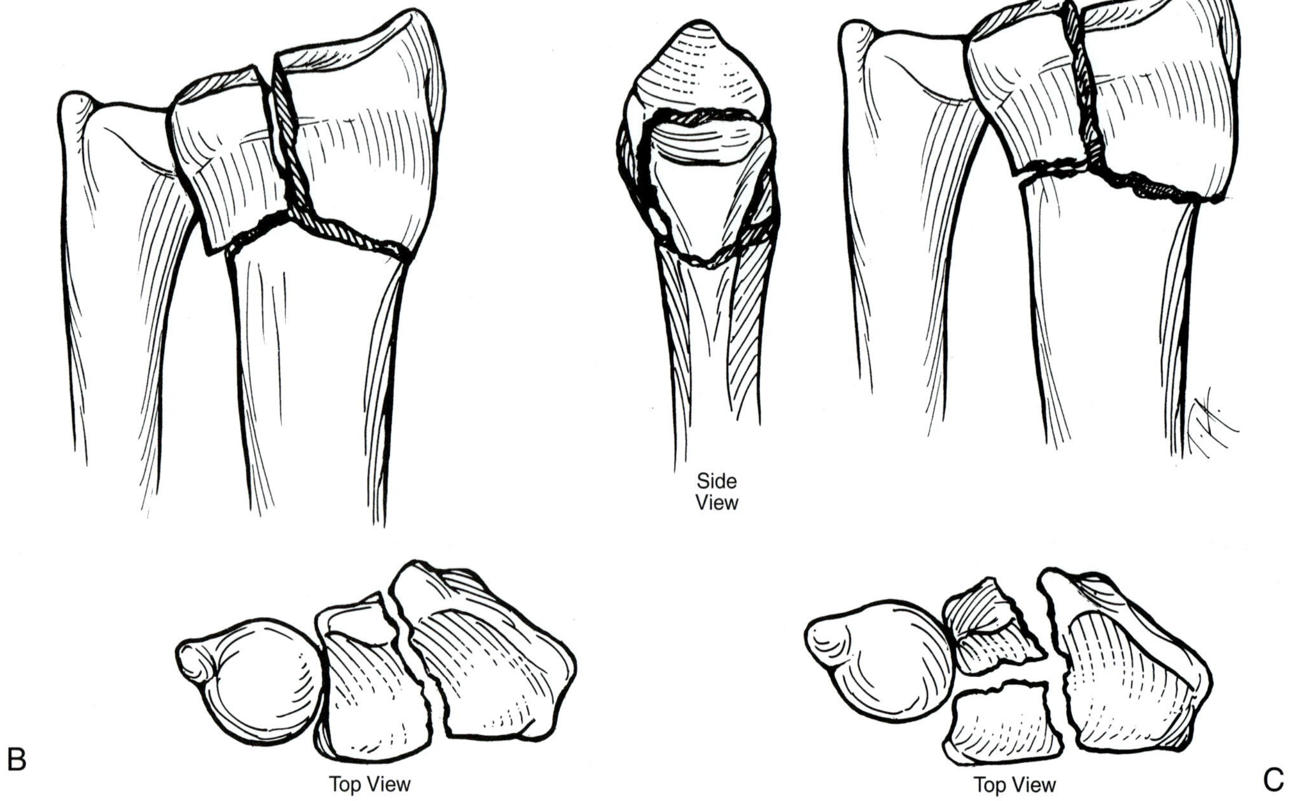

Figure 1.2. McMurtry and Jupiter's intra-articular fracture classification is based on the number of articular fragments. **A.** In two-part fractures, the dorsal or palmar articular fragment separates from the otherwise intact distal radius. **B.** In three part fractures, the articular surface splits into radial styloid and lunate fossa fragments. **C.** In four part fractures, the articular surface splits into radial styloid and dorsal palmar lunate fossa fragments. Modified from McMurtry RY, Jupiter JB. Fractures of the distal radius. In: Browner B, Jupiter JB, Levine A, et al., eds. Skeletal trauma. Philadelphia: Saunders, 1992.

A

Side View

B

Top View

Top View

C

ence and direction of displacement, the status of the ulna, and the presence and location of comminution. Using this system, the clinician can classify even the most complex distal radius injuries.

INITIAL FINDINGS, PHYSICAL EXAMINATION, AND DIAGNOSIS

As with most fractures, a systematic and thorough clinical evaluation of the patient's injury is vital before initiating treatment. The mechanism of injury is important in predicting the extent of injury and associated soft tissue damage. Falls from height and motor vehicle accidents are likely to result in more severe injury patterns than do other accidents. The position of the extremity and hand at the time of impact can also aid in understanding fracture mechanism and displacement patterns. In addition, it is important to assess whether the patient has any systemic (e.g., rheumatoid arthritis) or local (e.g., previous fracture) disease that may adversely affect outcome. Finally it is necessary to appreciate the socioeconomic importance of the injury to the individual patient. Did the injury occur in the dominant extremity? Does the patient engage in vocational or recreational activities that rely extensively on the wrist–hand unit that was injured? Is the patient willing or able to comply with treatment restrictions and rehabilitation?

After a physical exam for evidence of other bony injury, attention should be directed to the injured extremity. Careful palpation and passive range of motion of the ipsilateral shoulder, arm, elbow, forearm, and hand are vital to rule out associated skeletal injury. Particular attention should be directed to the elbow and carpus, where most associated fractures will occur. In Cooney et al.'s (10) review of 565 distal radius fractures, 4 scaphoid, 2 radial head, and 1 Bennett's fracture were unrecognized at the time of injury.

The examination must include an assessment of associated soft tissue injury, which is common. Although such injuries are usually closed, open fractures (especially in the setting of widely displaced or high-energy injuries) do occur; and therefore, skin integrity must be inspected and documented. Radial and ulnar pulses should be evaluated; and if absent despite fracture reduction, Doppler ultrasound evaluation is warranted. Although complete division of these structures is exceedingly rare, laceration or entrapment by fracture fragments can occur and is best managed by early repair or release.

A complete median, radial, and ulnar motor and sensory exam should also be part of the initial evaluation. The median nerve is the most commonly injured nerve after distal radius fractures. Neuropraxia secondary to contusion at the time of maximum fracture displacement and postinjury swelling remain the most common causes of

nerve dysfunction after injury; however, complete disruption of the median and ulnar nerves has been reported. Initial documentation of neurologic status is vital should neurologic sequelae develop later in treatment. In high-energy injuries or injuries in patients at risk (e.g., altered mental status secondary to head trauma), careful follow-up of swelling and neurologic function is vital to rule out a compartment syndrome.

Despite pain and swelling, tendon evaluation is also important; and with some gentle encouragement, a rapid evaluation of tendon function is easily performed. Although late attritional tendon rupture (usually the extensor pollicis longus) is most commonly seen, acute tendon laceration at the time of injury may occur. In injuries involving disruption of the distal radioulnar joint, extensor carpi ulnaris tendon entrapment may occur.

RADIOLOGIC STUDIES

Good quality PA, lateral, and oblique radiographs are sufficient in evaluating the majority of distal radius fractures. The PA view is facilitated by abducting the patient's humerus so that the elbow is at the same level as the shoulder, and the lateral is taken with the humerus adducted and the elbow flexed at 90°. The oblique view is obtained with the forearm supinated approximately 45°.

Three radiographic measurements are routinely recorded for injuries involving the displacement of the distal radius (Fig. 1.3). In the lateral view, the volar tilt of the distal radial articular surface should be measured. The

Figure 1.3. The radiographic evaluation of distal radius fracture displacement involves measuring volar tilt (normal value ≈ 11°) (A), radial length (normal value ≈ 11 mm) (B), and radial inclination (normal value ≈ 22°) (C). Modified from Metz VM, Gilula LA. Imaging techniques for distal radius fractures and related injuries. Orthop Clin North Am 1993;24(2):217–228.

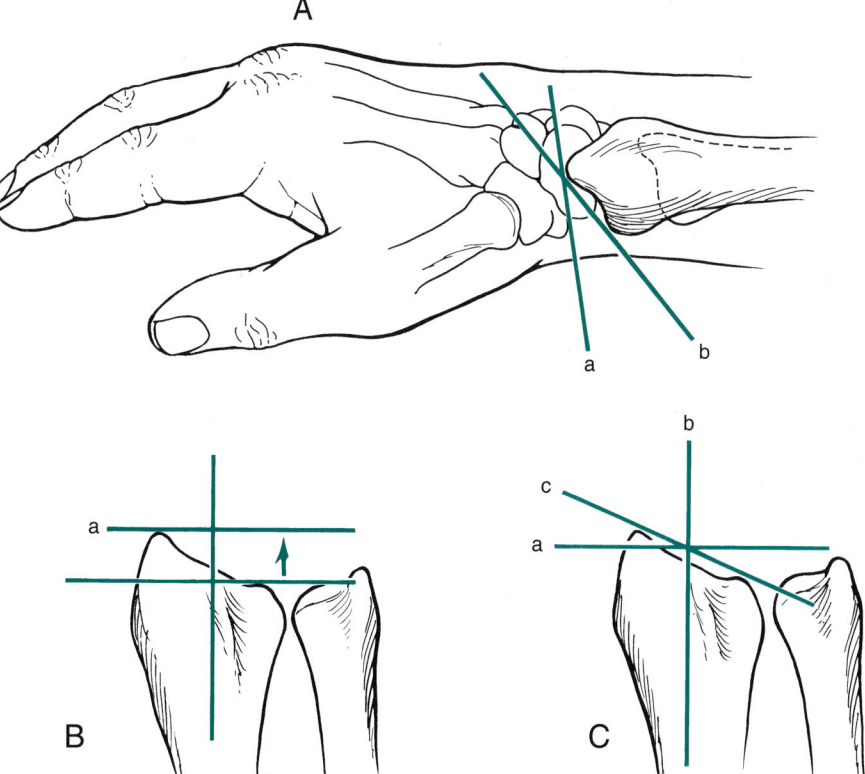

normal value is approximately 11°. In the PA view the radial length (or height), inclination, and width are routinely recorded. The radial length is measured as the distance between two lines perpendicular to the long axis of the radius, one drawn at the tip of the radial styloid and another drawn at the distal ulnar articular surface. The normal value is 11 to 12 mm. Alternatively, the radial length may be measured as the relative ulnar variance (vertical distance between the ulnar articular surface and the medial corner of the lunate facet) and compared to the opposite wrist. It has been suggested that this is a more accurate reflection of shortening, because this value is independent of alterations in the radial inclination. As ulnar variance changes with differing positions of pronation and supination, however, the views must be controlled for positional changes. Radial inclination is measured as the angle formed between a line drawn through the tip of the radial styloid and the medial corner of the lunate facet and a line perpendicular to the long axis of the radius. The normal value is 22° to 23°.

Additional factors should be considered when evaluating distal radius fractures. The degree and location of comminution is vital to predicting the outcome of management. Severe dorsal comminution is associated with shortening and redisplacement, whereas a volar butterfly fragment may be associated with median neuropraxia. It is also vital to access articular involvement and displacement, both for classifying these injuries and for making therapeutic decisions. Ulnar styloid fractures should be noted, as they suggest higher degrees of fracture displacement. Pogue et al. (11) could not produce dorsal angulation of greater than 15° or radial shortening of greater than 4 mm without fracturing the ulnar styloid. Carpal anatomy should be evaluated for evidence of fracture and for intercarpal ligament disruption.

Tomography and CT are occasionally indicated to evaluate the distal radioulnar joint and can assist in preoperative planning for complex, comminuted injuries. Splint materials and osteoporosis often make tomography difficult, however; and given its availability at most centers, CT scanning is now more commonly used in the evaluation of distal radius fractures. Scanning in 1- to 2-mm-thick sections in the axial, sagittal, and coronal planes is usually sufficient to define the relationships and integrity of the lunate and scaphoid facets, the congruity of the distal radioulnar joint, the degree of dorsal and/or palmar comminution, and the position and size of depressed articular fragments.

MRI does not offer the ability to define bony anatomy as well as does CT scanning; however, it does have a role in the management of some distal radius fractures. In patients with associated median neuropathy, rupture of flexor or extensor tendons, or carpal ligament disruption, MRI offers distinct advantages in further defining soft tissue injury. MRI has also been used extensively in recent years to evaluate the triangular fibrocartilage, which may be disrupted in a significant number of distal radial fractures.

TREATMENT

There are four principles in the treatment of distal radius fractures:

1. Restoration of articular congruity and axial alignment (reduction of fracture);
2. Maintenance of this reduction;
3. Achievement of bony union; and
4. Restoration of hand–wrist function.

These principles may be violated to some extent, depending on patient-specific variables. Factors such as low functional demand, significant medical illness, inability to comply with postoperative instructions, and previous fracture and deformity may justifiably lead to acceptance of less than anatomic results. It must be emphasized again, however, that chronological age does not correlate with functional age; and many of these fractures, even in older patients, will benefit from aggressive treatment.

Despite Colles' belief that deformity following distal radius fracture does not correlate with functional limitation, there has been dramatic evidence over the past 10 years that function is intimately related to form in regard to distal radial fractures. Both extra-articular and intra-articular malunion have been shown in the laboratory, as well as in clinical studies, to alter patients' function and their satisfaction with treatment outcome.

Extra-articular malunion relates primarily to three considerations: (a) the degree of dorsal or palmar angulation of the distal radial articular surface present in the sagittal plane, (b) the degree of radial inclination and radial shift present in the coronal plane, and (c) the shortening of the distal radius compared to the relative ulnar variance of the uninjured extremity. Cadaveric experiments using pressure-sensitive film have demonstrated that alterations in any of these anatomic values will alter loading patterns and concentration in the radiocarpal joint. Pogue et al. (11) found specifically that excessive dorsal or palmar angulation of the distal radius (greater than 30°) will result in increased forces at a position dorsal to their normal location in the radiocarpal joint. Loss of radial inclination beyond 10° resulted in increasing loads at the lunate fossa as did shortening the radius as little as 2 mm. Beyond 6 mm of shortening, triquetrolunate impingement occurred. Radial shortening and loss of radial inclination have also been shown to alter the kinematics of the distal radioulnar joint and to produce deformity within the triangular fibrocartilage (12). This may be related to the prevalence of distal radioulnar arthrosis after distal radial fracture. Similarly, Short et al. (13) observed that with a 45° dorsal articular angulation, 65% of the carpal loads are borne by the ulna (versus 20% in the normal wrist) and that the remainder of the loads are transmitted in high concentration dorsally in the scaphoid fossa.

A variety of clinical studies have confirmed laboratory data that correlate malunion with poor function. Pain, decreased range of motion, decreased grip strength, and poor patient function and satisfaction have been consistently associated with poor anatomic results after fracture (14–16). The position of the fracture at union, rather than the position at time of presentation, is highly correlated with long-term functional results. It appears that intra-articular fractures and dorsal articular angulation coincide with decreased range of motion, whereas radial shortening and shift are associated with decreased grip strength and pain. In regard to the magnitude of deformity seen after distal radius injury, McQueen and Caspers (16) have shown that patients with as little as 10° of dorsal angulation or 2 mm of radial shift are much more likely to experience pain, stiffness, weakness, and poor function at 4 years postfracture than do those patients with an anatomic reduction. In a 30-year follow-up of 29 extra-articular fractures, Kopylov et al. (17) found that shortening as little as 1 mm increases the risk of radiocarpal arthrosis by 20%. A shortening of 2 mm increased this risk to 50%. The patients with arthrosis frequently suffered pain and stiffness.

Dorsal articular angulation postfracture in young adults has been associated with dynamic midcarpal instability and pain, leading Taleisnik and Watson (18) to perform corrective osteotomy in nine patients. Correction of the extra-articular malunion resulted in relief of symptoms and restoration of carpal alignment in these patients. Bickerstaff and Bell (19) found that malunion with excessive dorsal angulation of the distal radius led to painful midcarpal instability and lower functional scores in patients who had sustained a distal radius fracture.

Intra-articular malunion has also been recognized as a factor in poor outcome in patients who suffer distal radius fractures. Kopylov et al. (17) reviewed 47 patients at 30 years post-intra-articular fracture and found that as little as 1 mm of joint incongruity significantly increased the risk of long-term degenerative changes, both in the radiocarpal and distal radioulnar joints. The presence of radiocarpal degenerative changes was strongly correlated with persistent symptoms of pain and motion loss. Knirk and Jupiter (20) concluded that failure to restore intra-articular anatomy is the most critical factor in patients who do poorly, even with adequate extra-articular restoration. In addition, soft tissue, intercarpal ligament and distal radioulnar joint disruption in these patients further worsens outcome. Although residual articular malalignment may be better tolerated in older patients who sustain lower-energy injuries, the longer life span and increased activity of our growing elderly population heightens the importance of anatomic articular restoration in this population as well.

Nonoperative Treatment

The initial step in the nonoperative treatment of all fractures of the distal radius is closed reduction. Reduction may be most easily attempted under local (hematoma block) anesthesia. After conducting the appropriate sterile preparation and draping, the clinician injects the fracture site with 5 to 10 mL lidocaine without epinephrine. Intravenous narcotics and sedation may be used as a supplement or as an alternative to the hematoma block; however, it is subsequently important to monitor the airway and vital signs in elderly patients. The use of a Bier block has been advocated by some authors; but because of its inherent risk for local anesthetic systemic toxicity, its use has been avoided by others.

Reduction should be achieved primarily by axial traction augmented by reduction of the specific deformity present through manual pressure over the fracture fragments. Excessive traction and gross exaggeration of the deformity have been associated with further soft tissue injury, and their use should be avoided. Although reduction may be accomplished by manual traction alone, at our institution most patients with displaced fractures of the distal radius are placed in finger traps and suspended with 4.5 kg (10 lb) of force to slowly distract the fracture fragments. Following 5 to 10 min of this gentle traction, the final reduction is achieved manually (Fig. 1.4).

Following reduction, the wrist must be immobilized. This may be accomplished through a sugar-tong plaster splint or a circumferential cast. It is important to remember, however, that if a circumferential cast is used, it should be split to allow for the significant soft tissue swelling that may occur within 24 to 48 h of injury. After immobilization, repeat biplanar x-rays should be obtained to allow for assessment of the adequacy of reduction.

Given recent evidence to support the role of anatomic reduction in improving functional results in these injuries, the following criteria for an acceptable reduction may be defined: (a) change in volar (palmar) tilt of no greater than 10° (i.e., neutral or 20° palmar slope), (b) radial shortening of no greater than 2 mm, and (c) change in radial inclination of no greater than 5°. In addition, when an intra-articular fracture is present, an articular stepoff of no greater than 1 to 2 mm should be accepted. If the fracture reduction does not meet these standards, then a repeat reduction should be attempted. If repeated attempts at reduction are unsuccessful, operative management with limited or formal open reduction and percutaneous, external, and/or internal fixation are indicated.

If fracture reduction is achieved, a reliable method of maintaining the reduction must be chosen. Initially, nondisplaced injuries are almost always amenable to closed treatment. Fractures that require reduction, however, must be further classified as stable or unstable. Stable fractures can be successfully held by closed means, whereas unstable fractures require external and/or internal fixation to maintain reduction.

Criteria for instability have been cited by a number of authors and include widely displaced intra-articular fractures, excessive dorsal or volar comminution, dorsal angulation of greater than 20°, and osteoporosis in elderly patients. Recent studies by Abbaszadegan et al. (21) and Jenkins (22) have shown that instability—defined as failure to maintain reduction by closed methods—most closely correlates with initial fracture displacement,

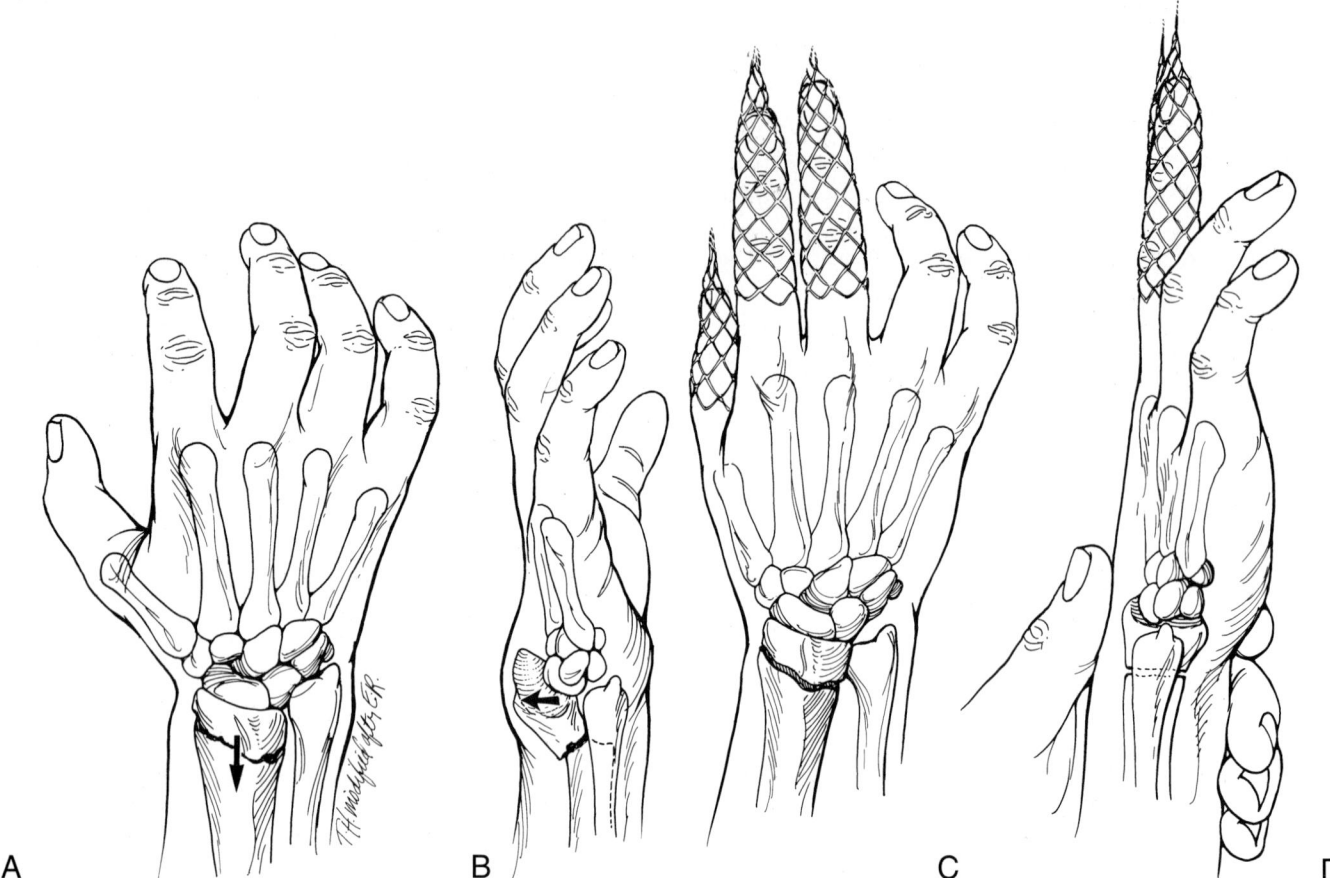

A   B   C   D

Figure 1.4. Manual reduction of distal radius fractures using finger trap traction. Reprinted with permission from AO classification system for distal radius fractures. In: Muller ME, Nazarian S, Koch P, et al., eds. The comprehensive classification of fractures of long bones. Berlin: Springer-Verlag, 1990:109.

specifically with shortening greater than 5 mm and dorsal comminution. Furthermore, articular margin injuries (Barton's and Chauffeur's fractures); palmarly displaced and comminuted extra-articular injuries (Smith's fractures); and high-energy, highly comminuted intra-articular injuries are often unstable and will fail nonoperative management.

Following acceptable closed reduction, cast immobilization is the method of choice for maintaining reduction during fracture healing for the majority of stable distal radius fractures. A well-molded sugar-tong splint may be changed to a short or long arm cast at the 1- or 2-week follow-up visit. Cast immobilization is typically maintained until fracture consolidation is complete at 6 to 8 weeks. A functional splint may be used for an additional 2 to 4 weeks, depending on the patient's comfort level and apprehension after cast removal.

Although commonly practiced at many centers in the United States, above-the-elbow immobilization has not been demonstrated to benefit fracture maintenance or functional outcome in any controlled study. The position of immobilization has also been widely debated. Although the Cotton–Loder position of extreme flexion and ulnar deviation has been abandoned because of median nerve complications, some degree of palmar flexion and ulnar

deviation is still used by most orthopaedists. A recent prospective comparison by Gupta (23), however, showed good anatomic and functional results through immobilization with the wrist in extension. He stressed that three-point molding at the fracture site is compatible with carpal dorsiflexion and that this not only uses the dorsal periosteal hinge but also places the hand and carpus in a functional position that will maintain reduction. In regard to forearm rotation, Sarmiento et al. (24) proposed that supination is superior to pronation because it negates the radial-displacing force of the brachioradialis and allows for greater functional recovery after a displaced fracture. Other authors have failed to document a benefit of either pronation or supination (25). The theoretical benefits of supination also extend to the maintenance of the distal radioulnar joint reduction following dorsal subluxation; and indeed in fractures involving disruption of this joint, it may be the position of choice. For the majority of distal radius fractures, however, forearm rotation does not appear to be important to final outcome.

A painless, functional wrist and hand can be expected in the majority of patients treated in a cast in whom the principles of maintaining acceptable alignment are followed. Loss of reduction is the most common pitfall of nonoperative treatment, and patients must be followed with weekly radiographs during the first 2 to 3 weeks of treatment to monitor the maintenance of the reduction. Early gross redisplacement of these injuries is less common than is the slow loss of reduction over the first 2 to 3 weeks of treatment (26). Redisplacement of fractures either in an acute or slowly progressive loss of reduction should be managed by relocation and maintenance of reduction through percutaneous pinning, external fixation, or internal fixation, not by repeated attempts at cast immobilization. Studies have shown that repeated attempts at nonoperative maintenance of reduction will meet with 50% or less satisfactory outcome (26).

A second major complication of nonoperative (and operative) management in these patients is loss of motion of the ipsilateral shoulder, elbow, and hand. Patients should be encouraged to perform shoulder elevation exercises as soon as possible after injury, and elbow motion should be started after the joint is no longer held in the immobilization device. In regard to the hand and digits, a precise casting technique that leaves the metacarpophalangeal joints free is vital for allowing full motion of these joints during the immobilization period. Early attention to edema control through elevation, use of a compressive glove, and daily digital tendon gliding exercises is also important for achieving full functional recovery in these patients. After immobilization is discontinued, all patients will need further instruction in regaining wrist motion and grip strength, which may be accomplished through either an outpatient occupational therapy center or a home-based therapy program.

Operative Treatment

The indications for operative management in fractures of the distal radius may be broadly grouped into three categories: (*a*) unreducible fractures, (*b*) unstable fractures (reduction cannot be held by closed means), and (*c*) fractures with associated soft tissue injury requiring treatment (open injuries; injuries with associated tendon, nerve, or vascular injury) (Clinical Table). A variety of operative techniques are available for treating these injuries. Among those most commonly used are percutaneous pinning, external fixation, and open reduction and internal fixation. It is important to note that there are limitations and complications inherent to each of these methods and, therefore, each is indicated for specific fracture patterns and contraindicated in others. Bone grafting, percutaneous or limited open fracture manipulation, and arthroscopy may be used in some cases as adjuncts to these techniques to achieve the goals of anatomic reduction and stable fixation.

PERCUTANEOUS PINNING

Indications and Contraindications

Percutaneous pinning is ideally suited for maintaining fracture sagittal alignment in unstable extra-articular injuries in which the volar cortex remains intact. It may also

be used for simple intra-articular injuries in which the articular surface is undisplaced or is in two large fragments. Percutaneous pinning will not reliably maintain fracture length when volar or bicortical comminution is present. Significant intra-articular displacement or comminution or inability to obtain closed reduction are also contraindications to the procedure.

Approach and Procedure

A variety of techniques of pin insertion have been described (Fig. 1.5). The most common is radial styloid pinning alone or in combination with dorsal radial pinning. Alternatively, pins may be passed through both the distal radius and the ulna (Rayhack's transulnar technique) or directly through the dorsal fracture line into the proximal fragment (Kapandji's intrafocal technique).

Regardless of which pin insertion technique is used, the procedure is performed in the operating room under regional or general anesthesia. Manual reduction is then

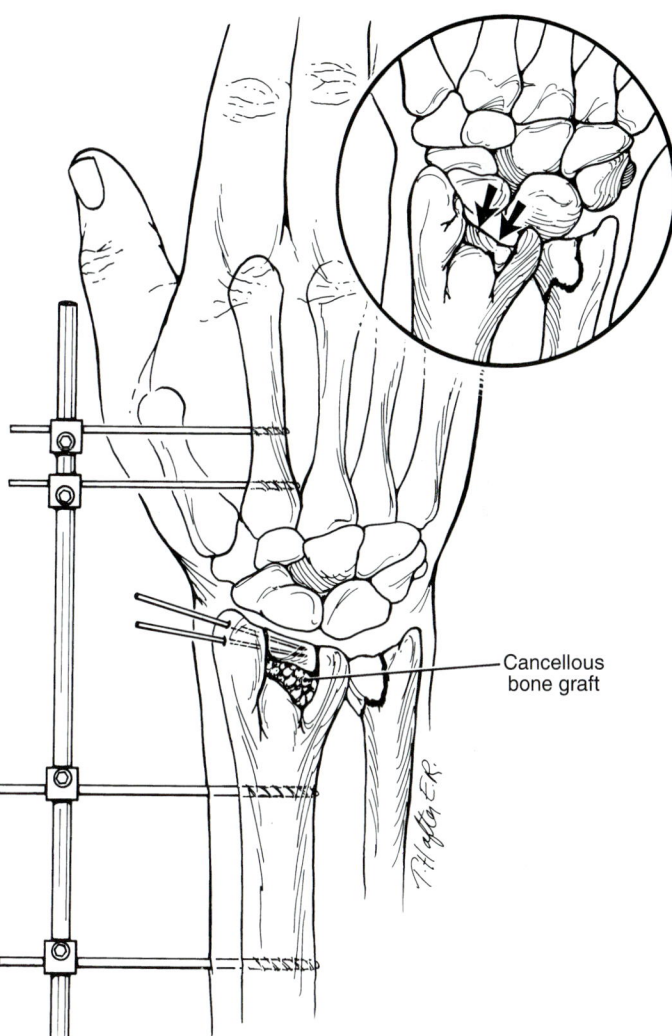

Cancellous bone graft

Figure 1.5. Intra-articular fracture of the distal radius treated with a combination of external fixation, limited open reduction with supplemental percutaneous pinning, and cancellous bone grafting. Modified from Palmer AK. Fractures of the distal radius. In: Green DP, ed. Operative hand surgery. New York: Churchill Livingstone, 1993.

Clinical Table: Fractures of the Distal Radius

Procedure	Indication	Technique	Anatomy	Pitfalls
Closed reduction and casting	• Nondisplacement fractures • Reducible, stable extra-articular fractures • Reducible, stable intra-articular fractures	• Hematoma block (or regional anesthesia) • Traction • Manipulative reduction • Splinting or casting	• No ideal immobilization position; avoid excessive wrist flexion • Some authors advocate above-elbow immobilization for first 2 weeks	• Inadequate reduction • Loss of reduction • Upper extremity disuse and stiffness
Percutaneous pinning	• Reducible, unstable extra-articular injuries with dorsal comminution • Reducible, simple intra-articular fractures	• Closed reduction • Pin insertion with fluoroscopic guidance • Cast or splint immobilization	• May use radial, transulnar, or intrafocal pinning techniques • Avoid tendons and superficial nerves during pin insertion	• Fracture redisplacement • Tendon or nerve injury by pins • Pin migration, breakage, or infection • Upper extremity disuse and stiffness
External fixation	• Unstable, extra-articular fractures with dorsal or bicortical comminution • Unstable, intra-articular fractures without volar fragment rotation • Fractures that have failed closed reduction and casting • Open fractures	• Pin insertion into index metacarpal and radius • Application of external fixator • Fracture reduction • Supplemental, limited open reduction; percutaneous pinning; and/or bone grafting for articular fragment reduction	• Extensor carpi radialis longus-brachioradialis interval for radial pins; avoid superficial radial nerve • Reflect first dorsal interosseous artery for metacarpal pin placement • Limited dorsal incision over compartment 3 for percutaneous reduction and bone grafting	• Failure to achieve anatomic reduction • Pin tract infection • Nerve or tendon injury at pin insertion • Upper extremity disuse and stiffness with or without associated median neuropathy or reflex sympathetic dystrophy
Open reduction and internal fixation	• Articular margin fractures • Comminuted unstable intra-articular fractures • Fractures with displaced volar cortical comminution • Fractures with metaphyseal-diaphyseal extension	• Dorsal, palmar, or combined approach, depending on fracture anatomy and soft tissue injury • Internal fixation choices included buttress plat, lag screws, and K wires • If highly comminuted or osteoporotic, combine with external fixation	• Dorsal exposure through or adjacent to extensor compartment 3 • Palmar exposure through the floor of the flexor carpi radialis or through the extended carpal tunnel approach (between the median nerve and flexor tendons)	• Iatrogenic nerve, vascular, or tendon injury • Failure of fixation with reduction loss • Inadequate reduction • Wound infection • Upper extremity disuse with or without associated median neuropathy or reflex sympathetic dystrophy

achieved as described above and confirmed by fluoroscopy. The reduction is then held by an assistant while the operating surgeon directs the Kirschner (K) wires. If no assistant is available, sterile finger traps may be used instead to help maintain the reduction

Most commonly, 0.0625 K wires are used. The first wire is introduced obliquely through the radial styloid and directed across the fracture until it engages the intact ulnar cortex of the radius. A second wire is then introduced into the dorsoulnar radius and directed proximally and volarly across the fracture site until it engages the volar cortex. In Kapandji's technique, the pins are directed into the fracture site and act as a buttress against displacement of the distal fragment. In Rayhack's technique, multiple 0.045 K wires are directed from the ulnar subcutaneous border across the distal radioulnar joint into the distal radial fracture fragments.

Results

Recent reports have clearly documented the superiority of percutaneous pinning to traditional casting techniques for unstable distal radius fractures in regard to both anatomic and functional results (27). Unfortunately, no study has compared the results of the different pinning techniques or pinning to external and internal fixation. Mah and Atkinson (28) reported 82% excellent anatomic and 100% excellent or good functional results with minimal complications using two radial styloid pins. Clancey (29) achieved excellent anatomic results in 90% of cases with radial styloid pinning combined with dorsal radial pinning. There were two cases of pin migration and one of tendon entrapment.

Rayhack et al. (6) reported that superior fixation is achieved by passing multiple small K wires across the ulna into the distal radius, allowing lightweight splinting at 3 weeks and avoiding risk to the radial sensory nerve. Although they report no long-term loss of pronation or supination, note that pin breakage, pin migration, and loss of reduction did occur in some patients. Finally, Greatting and Bishop (30) summarized the Mayo Clinic experience with Kapandji's intrafocal pinning technique, which is widely used in Europe and South America. Acceptable radiographic results were achieved in only 60% of patients older than 65; better anatomic but poorer functional results were seen in younger patients.

Pitfalls and Complications

Complications commonly reported with percutaneous pinning include fracture redisplacement, tendon or nerve injury, pin site infection, pin migration, pin breakage, and reflex sympathetic dystrophy. Careful attention to the indications and limitations of the technique, critical assessment of reduction and stability after pinning, and knowledge of local anatomy during pin placement minimize these complications. The use of polyglycolic acid rods in an attempt to do away with pin removal has been associated with soft tissue inflammation and osteolysis. Further study of this technique is required before it is put into widespread clinical use.

Rehabilitation

The standard of care, regardless of technique, after percutaneous pinning includes a variable period of supplemental immobilization with a cast or splint. When significant swelling or open wound care contraindicate a cast, external fixation should be used instead. Edema control, hand tendon gliding exercises, and therapeutic motion of the entire upper extremity are all vital to functional recovery. Pins are typically removed 6 to 8 weeks postsurgery, depending on fracture consolidation. Supplemental splinting may be continued for an additional 2 to 4 weeks, depending on healing and patient comfort.

EXTERNAL FIXATION

Indications and Contraindications

The commonly cited indications for external fixation of distal radius fractures include unstable extra-articular fractures with significant comminution, comminuted intra-articular fractures, fractures that have failed to maintain reduction with other treatment modalities, open fractures, and fractures in a multiply-injured patient. Volarly displaced and comminuted injuries usually require formal volar exposure and open reduction with internal fixation; however, external fixation is often used to augment stability when less-than-rigid fixation is achieved because of small bony fragments or osteoporosis.

To better understand the indications and limitations of external fixators it is vital to understand their biomechanical principles. External fixation devices provide fracture reduction and maintenance of that reduction through constant ligamentotaxis. Various fixator designs are available, and these vary greatly in their biomechanical properties and specific techniques. Advantages offered by more recent fixator designs include the ability to apply the fixator before fracture reduction, to control and adjust the traction force during the course of treatment, to apply the traction force in multiple planes, to place pins in a converging pattern, and to position the wrist in extension while maintaining fracture reduction.

Despite excellent reduction of radial length and inclination, it was evident from early reports that restoration of the palmar tilt of the distal radius and the anatomic reduction of the radiocarpal joint surface were often not achieved with external fixation. A study by Bartosh and Saldana (31) documented that during distraction, the dominant palmar ligaments become taut and limit radiocarpal distraction, while the weaker Z-shaped dorsal ligament complex has yet to reach maximum length. This prevents purely longitudinal traction from restoring palmar tilt. Similarly, reduction of the dorsomedial radiocarpal fragment is commonly not achieved.

Approach and Procedure

The precise operative procedure varies according to which of the many available fixators is being used. It is vital to understand the method of application and fracture reduction as outlined in the surgical technique literature that accompanies the device. There are, however, certain principles of exposure and application common to all fixators.

The first step in fixator application is to expose the index metacarpal and radius for pin placement. The longitudinal incision for the exposure of the radius is centered over its lateral surface approximately 10 cm proximal to the radial styloid. Branches of the lateral antebrachial cutaneous nerve may be encountered in the subcutaneous dissection. The forearm fascia is then incised in line with the skin incision. The radial sensory nerve must be identified, typically as it exits in the interval between the brachioradialis and the extensor carpi radialis longus, and protected. After developing this interval, the surgeon exposes the radial shaft subperiosteally. The dorsoradial shaft of the index metacarpal is then exposed through one or two longitudinal incisions. Small cutaneous branches of the radial nerve may be encountered subcutaneously. The first dorsal interosseous muscle should then be incised at its fascial aponeurosis along the radial aspect of the extensor mechanism. The muscle itself is then sharply and subperiosteally elevated off the metacarpal surface from its metaphyseal flare to its distal shaft (32).

All pins should be predrilled and placed in accordance with the specifications of the specific fixator being used. Correct pin positioning should be confirmed fluoroscopically. After pin placement, the wounds should be closed loosely, with no skin tension around the pins.

After securely placing the pins, the surgeon applies the external fixator device. Fracture reduction is subsequently achieved (either through manual traction and reduction or through distraction of the fixator itself) and the fixator is locked into place. Fluoroscopic views and/or hard copy radiographs should then be obtained to assess reduction. Near anatomic extra-articular anatomy (radial length, inclination, and volar tilt) should be successfully restored; if it is not, repeat reduction should be performed.

After restoration of the extra-articular anatomy, the intra-articular reduction should then be assessed. If a stable reduction with less than 1 to 2 mm of intra-articular incongruity is achieved, no further intervention is needed. If there is concern regarding the stability of the articular reduction (e.g., owing to significant underlying metaphyseal comminution) one or two 0.0625 K wires may be introduced through the radial styloid and/or dorsomedial lunate fossa fragment into the radial shaft to further secure the articular reduction.

If articular incongruity exceeds 1 to 2 mm, then reduction of this incongruity is indicated. Using a K wire as a joystick to effect reduction, the surgeon can perform percutaneous manipulation of the fracture fragments. Alternatively, limited open reduction though a small dorsal incision may be achieved (33,34). In this technique an elevator or similar device is introduced into the fracture site and used to directly elevate the fracture fragments. After achieving articular reduction, the fragments should be held by K wires and/or cancellous bone grafting of the metaphyseal bone defect through the dorsal incision. If these techniques fail to achieve an acceptable articular reduction, formal open reduction and internal fixation are indicated. In these instances the fixator is left in place to maintain extra-articular reduction.

Results

Several reviews have documented successful anatomic and functional outcome in 80 to 90% of patients treated with external fixation, despite high-energy comminuted injuries with few major complications (35–40). The choice of fixator is up to the individual surgeon, as no one device has been shown to be superior to the others. The use of dynamic external fixation of these injuries, however, should be avoided. These devices, which theoretically allow protected radiocarpal motion during treatment, have been shown to have a higher incidence of loss of reduction, more technical complications, and poorer functional outcome than do static fixators (41).

Pitfalls and Complications

There have been many complications with these devices, ranging from 15 to as high as 60% in early reports. These complications are related to achieving and maintaining reduction (failure to restore palmar tilt or radiocarpal alignment, overdistraction, late fracture displacement, and nonunion); to the use of the pins (pin tract infection, pin breakage, pin loosening, fracture through pin sites, and iatrogenic nerve and tendon injury); and to distal radius fractures in general, which may be affected by external fixation (median neuropathy, reflex sympathetic dystrophy, decreased motion, and grip strength).

Recent reports of the results of external fixation for distal radial fracture have shown a dramatic decrease in the complication rate owing to a greater appreciation of these potential problems. As stated above, the failure of longitudinal traction to restore palmar slope and radiocarpal alignment in some injuries must be recognized at the time of fixator placement. Agee (38) introduced the concept of triplanar ligamentotaxis with palmar translation of the carpus, which is used to achieve restoration of the palmar slope in response to this problem. Alternatively, limited open reduction techniques to correct both palmar slope and radiocarpal congruity may be used. As greater duration and magnitude of distraction force have been shown to be associated with posttreatment stiffness and decreased strength regardless of anatomic result (especially when associated with radiocarpal lengthening or positioning of the wrist in flexion during fixator treatment), care has been taken to limit radiocarpal distraction to 5 mm or less and to maintain the wrist in neutral or extension during the course of external fixation (42,43). The theoretical value of segmentally decreasing traction force after 3 weeks has not yet been specifically documented and has been associated with loss of reduction by some authors. Leung et al.

(44) have advocated cancellous bone grafting of the metaphyseal region to improve reduction and decrease the duration of external fixation to 3 weeks without this complication. Pin complications may be minimized by meticulous detail to identification of nerves and tendons, predrilling, appropriate pin sizing, and release of skin tension.

Rehabilitation

The importance of early aggressive treatment of pain, swelling, and limited motion cannot be overstated and includes organized and frequent occupational therapy, edema control, and adequate pain control. Early institution of tendon gliding exercises and therapeutic exercise of the entire upper extremity are vital to functional recovery.

The fixator is typically removed after 6 to 8 weeks, depending on fracture consolidation. As above, bone grafting may allow for earlier fixator removal. Supplemental splinting may be continued for an additional 2 to 4 weeks, depending on healing and patient comfort after fixator removal.

Pin care should consist of daily cleaning of the pin sites and of appropriate release of undue skin tension around the pins. Serous drainage and mild erythema may be treated with skin release and oral antibiotics. Pin site infection with loosening and bony erosion must be treated by pin removal and bony curettage followed by appropriate antibiotic therapy.

OPEN REDUCTION AND INTERNAL FIXATION

Indications and Contraindications

There are two primary indications for open reduction and internal fixation (ORIF). First are articular marginal injuries such as dorsal and volar lip fractures (Barton's fractures). These shearing fractures are often associated with carpal dislocation, intercarpal ligament injury, and carpal fractures. Although closed reduction may be possible, the articular surface is usually difficult to anatomically reduce; and because of muscle tension across the oblique fracture line, redisplacement is common. Radial styloid avulsion fractures may be managed by percutaneous pinning and cast treatment. However, when associated with perilunate dislocation (and scapholunate ligament disruption or scaphoid fracture) or when severe displacement or soft tissue interposition make closed reduction impossible, ORIF may be required.

The second major indication for ORIF is complex, comminuted intra-articular fractures. These represent a unique subset of distal radius injuries that are often the result of high-energy trauma, are associated with significant soft tissue and concomitant skeletal injuries, and have significant rotation and impaction of articular fragments. They include the Melone type 4 fractures, AO type C3 fractures,

and Fernandez combined injuries. Because of the underlying complexity of these injuries, ORIF has been increasingly combined with external fixation and bone grafting to achieve the goal of anatomic intra-articular and extra-articular reduction, which are vital to functional recovery.

Additional indications for primary or supplemental ORIF in distal radius fractures include associated distal ulnar shaft fractures, fractures with displaced volar cortical comminution, and fractures with metaphyseal–diaphyseal extension.

Approach and Procedure

Surgical exposure may be achieved through dorsal, palmar, or combined approaches. Choice of exposure is generally dictated by fracture anatomy and by the need for exploration and release of neurovascular structures. Dorsal exposure is gained through or on either side of the third extensor compartment; subperiosteal dissection both radially and ulnarly defines the dorsal articular margin. The extensor pollicis longus tendon is often transposed at closure. Palmar exposure may be through the floor of the flexor carpi radialis sheath or through an extended carpal tunnel incision with dissection between the median nerve and flexor tendons. The former exposure is relatively easy; whereas the latter exposure is more versatile because it allows for both median and ulnar neurovascular release, if needed, and greater exposure of the volar articular margin. Palmar lip fractures often may be reduced by aligning the metaphyseal surface of the fracture without violating the palmar carpal ligaments; however, in comminuted intra-articular fractures, capsular ligament incision and limited elevation may be required.

Choice of internal fixation includes buttress plate application, lag screw fixation and/or K wires. The 2.7-mm mini-fragment plates and screws may be used as alternatives to the 3.5-mm small fragment set. Owing to extensor tendon irritation and risk of attritional rupture, many authors recommend removing the dorsal plates. The lower profile of isolated lag screw(s) fixation is, therefore, attractive for fixation of radial styloid and dorsal lip fractures; however, small fragment size and regional osteoporosis limit their usefulness.

Results

Results of ORIF of articular marginal fractures have been generally excellent. Sprenger (45) reported on the treatment of 12 palmar marginal fractures managed with a buttress plate. Complications were few, and functional recovery was high. Pattee and Thompson (46) have shown, however, that when associated with carpal ligament injury or carpal fracture, the results of treatment will not be as rewarding. Careful evaluation for and appropriate treatment of associated carpal injuries are vital in the management of these fractures

Results of treatment of comminuted intra-articular fractures have been surprisingly good (47,48). Jupiter and Lipton (49) have shown that, despite the severity of these injuries, excellent anatomic results can be expected in greater than 85% of patients when preoperative planning, combined dorsal and palmar exposure (if needed), supplemental external fixation to neutralize compressive forces, and bone grafting are used. Trumble et al. (50) reported excellent anatomic and functional recovery in a majority of 43 patients with AO type C2 and C3 injuries who were treated with a similar combination of surgical procedures. Patients with residual articular stepoff, radial shortening, and a high number of initial fracture fragments fared the worst. At 3 years of follow-up, only 1 patient had developed symptomatic radiocarpal arthritis, and remarkably few had experienced difficulties during or after their treatment.

Pitfalls and Complications

The techniques described above are technically demanding and should be performed only by surgeons skilled both in the surgical exposure of the wrist and in the application of internal fixation devices. Iatrogenic nerve, vascular, or tendon injury may occur in inexperienced hands. In addition, inexperienced surgeons may achieve inadequate reduction and/or fixation, which will predispose to a poor result.

In the treatment of highly comminuted injuries, a variety of other complications may occur, including forearm compartment syndrome, median and ulnar neurovascular compromise, and wound infection. Early aggressive treatment of these problems, coupled with anatomic joint reduction, has been shown to result in greater than 80% successful outcome in most series.

Rehabilitation

The same rehabilitation principles of edema control, adequate pain relief, early institution of tendon gliding exercises, and therapeutic exercise of the entire upper extremity outlined above also apply to injuries in which open reduction and internal fixation have been performed. Supplemental splinting may be applied for a variable period of time, depending on patient comfort and subsequent fracture consolidation.

ARTHROSCOPY

Arthroscopy has been advocated by Cooney and Berger (51) and others as a minimally invasive means of assessing and facilitating intra-articular fracture reduction, thereby avoiding extensile exposure and palmar capsular incision. In addition, it serves as a means of identifying and potentially treating associated intercarpal ligament and triangular fibrocartilage lesions. Concerns in regard to arthroscopy include the extravasation of fluid into the forearm after acute fracture, limited ability of the arthroscope to accurately guide reduction, and the risks to displaced neurovascular structures. The true role of arthroscopy in the management of these injuries has yet to

be defined, and no prospective studies have demonstrated its efficacy or safety.

SUMMARY

Fractures of the distal radius remain among the most common of all injuries treated by the orthopaedic surgeon. The majority of these injuries result from a fall on an outstretched arm, although high-energy injury mechanisms may occur. After standard radiographic evaluation, each individual fracture is classified according to its displacement pattern, comminution, and articular involvement to assist in determining the prognosis and optimal treatment modality.

The goals of treatment are to achieve an anatomic reduction; to hold this reduction through the period of fracture healing; and most important, to restore function to the extremity. A variety of both nonoperative and operative methods exist for achieving these goals, and it is imperative that any orthopaedist treating these injuries be familiar with the indications, techniques, and potential pitfalls of each of these treatment modalities.

REFERENCES

1. Alffram PA, Bauer GCH. Epidemiology of fractures of the forearm. a biomechanical investigation of bone strength. J Bone Joint Surg 1962;44A:105–114.
2. Colles A. On the fracture of the carpal extremity of the radius. Edinburgh Med Surg J 1814;10:182–186.
3. Fernandez DL. Fractures of the distal radius: operative treatment. Instr Course Lect 1993;42:73–88.
4. Deleted in proof.
5. McMurtry RY, Jupiter JB. Fractures of the distal radius. In: Browner B, Jupiter JB, Levine A, et al., eds. Skeletal trauma. Philadelphia: Saunders, 1992.
6. Rayhack JM, Langworthy JN, Belsole RJ. Transulnar percutaneous pinning of displaced distal radial fractures: a preliminary report. J Orthop Trauma 1989;3(2):107–114.
7. Bradway JK, Amadio PC, Cooney WP. Open reduction and internal fixation of displaced, comminuted intra-articular fractures of the distal end of the radius. J Bone Joint Surg 1989;71A:839–847.
8. Melone CP. Distal radius fractures: patterns of articular fragmentation. Orthop Clin North Am 1993;24(2):239–253.
9. Muller ME, Nazarian S, Koch P. Classification AO des fractures. In: Les os longs. Berlin: Springer, 1987.
10. Cooney WP, Dobyns JH, et al. Complications of Colles fractures. J Bone Joint Surg 1980;62A(4):613–619.
11. Pogue DJ, Viegas SF, et al. Effects of distal radius fracture malunion on wrist joint mechanics. J Hand Surg 1990;15A:721–727.
12. Adams BD. Effects of radial deformity on distal radioulnar joint mechanics. J Hand Surg 1993;18A:492–498.
13. Short WH, Palmer AK, et al. A biomechanical study of distal radial fractures. J Hand Surg 1987;12A:529–534.
14. Jenkins NH, Mintowt-Czyz WJ. Mal-union and dysfunction in Colles' fracture. J Hand Surg 1988;13B:291–293.
15. Aro HT, Koivunen T. Minor axial shortening of the radius affects outcome of Colles' fracture treatment. J Hand Surg 1991;16A:392–398.
16. McQueen M, Caspers J. Colles' fracture: does the anatomic result affect the final function? J Bone Joint Surg 1988;70B:649–651.
17. Kopylov P, Johnell O, Redlund-Johnell L, Bengner U. Fractures of the distal end of the radius in young adults: a 30-year follow-up. J Hand Surg 1993;18B:45–49.

18. Taleisnik J, Watson HK. Midcarpal instability caused by malunited fractures of the distal radius. J Hand Surg 1984;9A:350–357.

19. Bickerstaff DR, Bell MJ. Carpal malalignment in Colles' fractures. J Hand Surg 1989;14B:155–160.

20. Knirk JL, Jupiter JB. Intra-articular fractures of the distal end of the radius in young adults. J Bone Joint Surg 1986;68A:647–659.

21. Abbaszadegan H, Jonsson U, Von Sivers K. Prediction of instability of Colles' fractures. Acta Orthop Scand 1989;60(6):646–650.

22. Jenkins NH. The unstable Colles' fracture. J Hand Surg 1989; 14B:149–154.

23. Gupta A. The treatment of Colles' fracture: immobilisation with the wrist dorsiflexed. Bone Joint Surg 1991;73B:312–315.

24. Sarmiento A, Zagorski JB, Sinclair WF. Functional bracing of Colles' fractures: a prospective study of immobilization in supination vs pronation. Clin Orthop 1980;146:175–183.

25. Van Der Linden W, Ericson R. Colles' fracture: how should its displacement be measured and how should it be immobilized? J Bone Joint Surg 1981;63A:1285–1288.

26. McQueen MM, MacLaren A, Chalmers J. The value of remanipulating Colles' fractures. J Bone Joint Surg 1986;68B:232–233.

27. Shankar NS, Craxford AD. Comminuted Colles' fracture: a prospective trial of management. J R Coll Surg Edinb 1992; 37:199–202.

28. Mah ET, Atkinson RN. Percutaneous Kirschner wire stabilization following closed reduction of Colles' fractures. J Hand Surg 1992; 17B:55–62.

29. Clancey GJ. Percutaneous Kirschner-wire fixation of Colles' fractures. J Bone Joint Surg 1984;66A:1008–1014.

30. Greatting MD, Bishop AT. Intrafocal (Kapandji) pinning of unstable fractures of the distal radius. Orthop Clin North Am 1993; 24(2):301–308.

31. Bartosh RA, Saldana MJ. Intra-articular fractures of the distal radius: a cadaveric study to determine if ligamentotaxis restores radiopalmar tilt. J Hand Surg 1990;15A:18–21.

32. Seitz WH, Putnam MD. Limited open surgical approach for external fixation of distal radius fractures. J Hand Surg 1990; 15A:288–293.

33. Axelrod T, Paley MD, et al. Limited open reduction of the lunate facet in comminuted intra-articular fractures of the distal radius. J Hand Surg 1988;13A:384–389.

34. Geissler WB, Fernandez DL. Percutaneous and limited open reduction of the articular surface of the distal radius. J Orthop Trauma 1991;5(3):255–264.

35. Abbaszadegan H, Jonsson U. External fixation or plaster cast for severely displaced Colles' fractures. Acta Orthop Scand 1990; 61(6):528–530.

36. Jenkins NH, Jones DG, et al. External fixation of Colles' fractures: an anatomical study. J Bone Joint Surg 1987;69B:208–211.

37. Howard PW, Stewart HD, et al. External fixation or plaster for severely displaced comminuted Colles' fractures? J Bone Joint Surg 1989;71B:68–73.

38. Agee JM. External fixation: technical advances based on multiplanar ligamentotaxis. Orthop Clin North Am 1993;24(2):265–274.

39. Edwards GS. Intra-articular fractures of the distal part of the radius treated with the small AO external fixator. J Bone Joint Surg 1991;73A:1241–1250.

40. Jakim I, Pieterese HS, Sweet MB. External fixation for intra-articular fractures of the distal radius. J Bone Joint Surg 1991; 73B:302–306.

41. Sommerkamp TG, Seeman M, et al. Dynamic external fixation of unstable fractures of the distal part of the radius. J Bone Joint Surg 1994;76A:1149–1160.

42. Kaempffe FA, Wheeler DR, et al. Severe fractures of the distal radius: effect of amount and duration of external fixator distraction on outcome. J Hand Surg 1993;18A:33–41.

43. Biyani A. Over-distraction of the radiocarpal and midcarpal joints following external fixation of comminuted distal radial fractures. J Hand Surg 1993;18B:506–510.

44. Leung KS, Shen WY, et al. An effective treatment of comminuted fractures of the distal radius. J Hand Surg 1990;15A:11–17.

45. Sprenger TR. Anterior margin articular fractures of the distal radius. J Orthop Trauma 1993;7(1):6–10.

46. Pattee GA, Thompson GH. Anterior and posterior marginal fracture-dislocations of the distal radius: an analysis of the results of treatment. Clin Orthop 1988;23:183–195.

47. Axelrod TS, McMurtry RY. Open reduction and internal fixation of comminuted, intra-articular fractures of the distal radius. J Hand Surg 1990;15A:1–11.

48. Porter ML, Tillman RM. Pilon fractures of the wrist. J Hand Surg 1992;17B:63–68.

49. Jupiter JB, Lipton H. The operative treatment of intra-articular fractures of the distal radius. Clin Orthop 1993;292:48–61.

50. Trumble TE, Schmitt SR, Vedder NB. Factors affecting functional outcome of displaced intra-articular distal radius fractures. J Hand Surg 1994;19A:325–340.

51. Cooney WP, Berger RA. Treatment of complex fractures of the distal radius: combined use of internal and external fixation and arthroscopic reduction. Hand Clin 1993;9(4):603–612.

chapter 2

Scott W. Wolfe and Elizabeth McLarney

Fractures and Dislocations of the Carpus

I Scaphoid Fractures and Nonunion

RELEVANT ANATOMY AND PATHOGENESIS

The scaphoid's unique position in the carpus makes it vulnerable to fracture and ligamentous injury. With full wrist extension, as generally occurs when falling on an outstretched wrist, the scaphoid extends until its long axis is nearly parallel to the long axis of the radius, and the proximal and distal poles become locked in position by the bony and ligamentous constraints of their respective carpal rows. Consequently, the compressive force of the fall is concentrated across its narrow, nonarticular waist; and failure occurs in a bending mode in the majority of cases. With increasing amounts of wrist extension, fractures occur farther proximally.

The blood supply of the scaphoid is tenuous. Vascular injection studies have documented two major vascular conduits: One supplies the scaphoid tubercle via perforators from the palmar branch of the radial artery, and the other perforates the nonarticular dorsal scaphoid ridge at its waist (1). Intraosseous flow is predominantly retrograde, and approximately 75% of the blood supply of the scaphoid emanates from the dorsal ridge perforators. Because of the retrograde blood supply, scaphoid fractures may be complicated by avascular necrosis of the proximal fragment, nonunion, and occasionally, collapse. The incidence of avascular necrosis of the scaphoid proximal fragment is inversely proportional to its size and approaches 20%.

The normal scaphoid functions to neutralize the compressive loads across the wrist, which, if unopposed, would drive the proximal and distal rows in opposite directions and produce a collapse deformity (dorsal interca-

lated segment instability). The scaphoid fracture site is subject to high shear stress, which is generated by these opposing rotational movements (Fig. 2.1). Failure to effectively neutralize these forces by appropriate casting or internal fixation leads to the eventual palmar collapse of the fracture site (the so-called humpback scaphoid) and a high rate of nonunion. Other factors that adversely affect scaphoid fracture healing include the intra-articular location of the fracture, the initial degree of displacement, the presence of comminution, and any associated ligamentous or bony injuries.

INITIAL FINDINGS: ACUTE FRACTURES

In the context of a hyperextension wrist injury, tenderness in the anatomic snuffbox connotes a scaphoid fracture, even in the presence of apparently normal radiographs. Pain and swelling may be minimal, and often patients do not present for treatment until weeks or months after the injury occurred. Tenderness over the proximal or distal poles and reduction in wrist range of motion are helpful clinical signs, and initial presentation overlaps with that of wrist ligamentous injury.

RADIOLOGIC STUDIES

Lateral, oblique, and PA wrist radiographs will adequately display a displaced scaphoid fracture. Normal standard views, in the context of an examination indicative of a scaphoid fracture, should prompt specialized radiographic views, including a PA x-ray with 30° of ulnar deviation (scaphoid view), and ulnar-deviated films with a 15° cranial tube angulation to profile the fracture site.

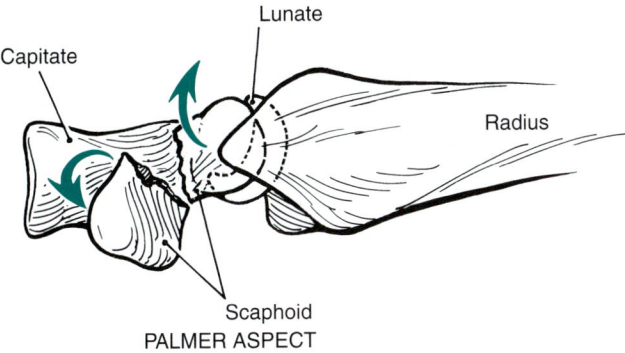

Figure 2.1. Effect of the opposing rotational movement of the proximal and distal carpal rows on the displaced scaphoid fracture, leading to dorsal intercalated segment instability.

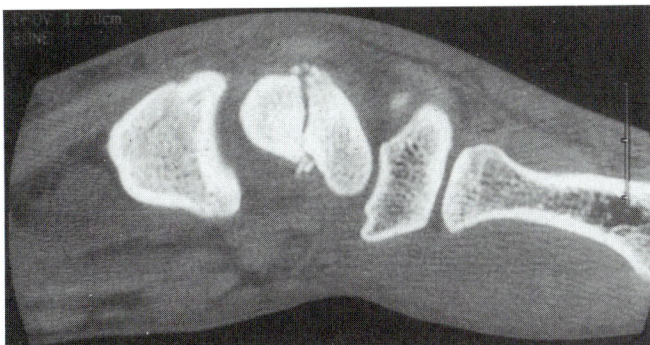

Figure 2.2. Computed tomography performed in 1.5-mm slices in the midaxial plane of the scaphoid gives unparalleled information about the status of union, alignment, comminution, and cystic change.

Increased angulation of the lunate on the lateral radiograph (more than a 15° dorsal tilt) is a poor prognostic sign, indicative of fracture angulation or concomitant scapholunate ligament disruption, both of which have a nonunion or malunion rate of 80% with cast treatment alone. Sclerosis, cyst formation, or a widened fracture gap in the context of an acute injury generally indicates disruption of a previously asymptomatic fibrous union; all are associated with a poor response to cast immobilization. Displacement of 1 mm or more on any radiograph is a poor prognostic sign for closed treatment. Of greatest prognostic significance is the fracture location; small proximal pole fragments are associated with the highest rate of avascular necrosis and nonunion.

Additional imaging studies are not generally indicated in the acute injury period. Repeat PA, lateral, and scaphoid radiographs after 10 to 14 days of cast immobilization will usually reveal an occult scaphoid fracture line as a result of bony resorption at the fracture site. A technetium bone scan will demonstrate increased uptake within 24 to 48 h of an acute fracture with 98% specificity and can obviate prophylactic casting for an active individual. CT scans in the midsagittal plane of the scaphoid are as accurate as the bone scan for the early detection of oc-

cult scaphoid fractures and provide an unparalleled demonstration of the fracture anatomy (2) (Fig. 2.2). MRI scans are best reserved for the evaluation of the vascular supply of the proximal pole and are not superior to CT scans for fracture detection or visualization.

TREATMENT

Nonoperative Treatment

Controversy abounds concerning the healing rate, duration of immobilization, type of cast, and position of immobilization necessary for closed treatment of scaphoid fractures. Indications for closed treatment include stable, nondisplaced fractures of the waist or distal pole, without associated bony or ligamentous injury. Relative contraindications for closed treatment include small proximal pole fractures, ipsilateral or contralateral fractures of the distal radius or elbow, polytrauma, subacute injuries (greater than 6 weeks), and lunate dorsal tilt. Absolute contraindications for closed treatment include irreducible displacement, marked angulation or lunate dorsal tilt, and associated perilunate or lunate dislocation.

In a randomized prospective trial, nondisplaced waist and proximal pole fractures treated with a long arm thumb spica cast for 6 weeks followed by a short arm thumb spica cast for 6 weeks showed higher and more rapid union rates than those treated with the short arm spica cast alone (3). A short arm cast is acceptable for distal pole fractures. Up to 6 months of immobilization may be required for proximal pole fractures, because of their intrinsic instability, altered vascular status, and intra-articular location.

AVASCULAR NECROSIS

Radiographic evidence of increased density of the proximal pole may be present as early as 4 weeks postinjury, but the predictive value of these radiographic changes for true avascular necrosis has been questioned by a number of authors. MRI studies may help confirm a clinical suspicion of osteonecrosis. Current recommendations are to treat acute nondisplaced fractures that demonstrate increased proximal pole density with 12 to 24 weeks of cast immobilization. A united fracture will generally progress to revascularization of the proximal pole and rarely to bony collapse.

Some authors have championed the use of adjuvant pulsed electromagnetic field (PEMF) stimulation for up to 9 months in undisplaced fractures with avascular proximal poles, citing initial healing rates of up to 89%. Long-term follow-up of avascular scaphoid nonunions initially determined to have healed with electrical stimulation demonstrated a substantial decline in healing rates over time (4).

Operative Treatment

Decisions regarding operative approach and type of fixation should be based on fracture location and degree of

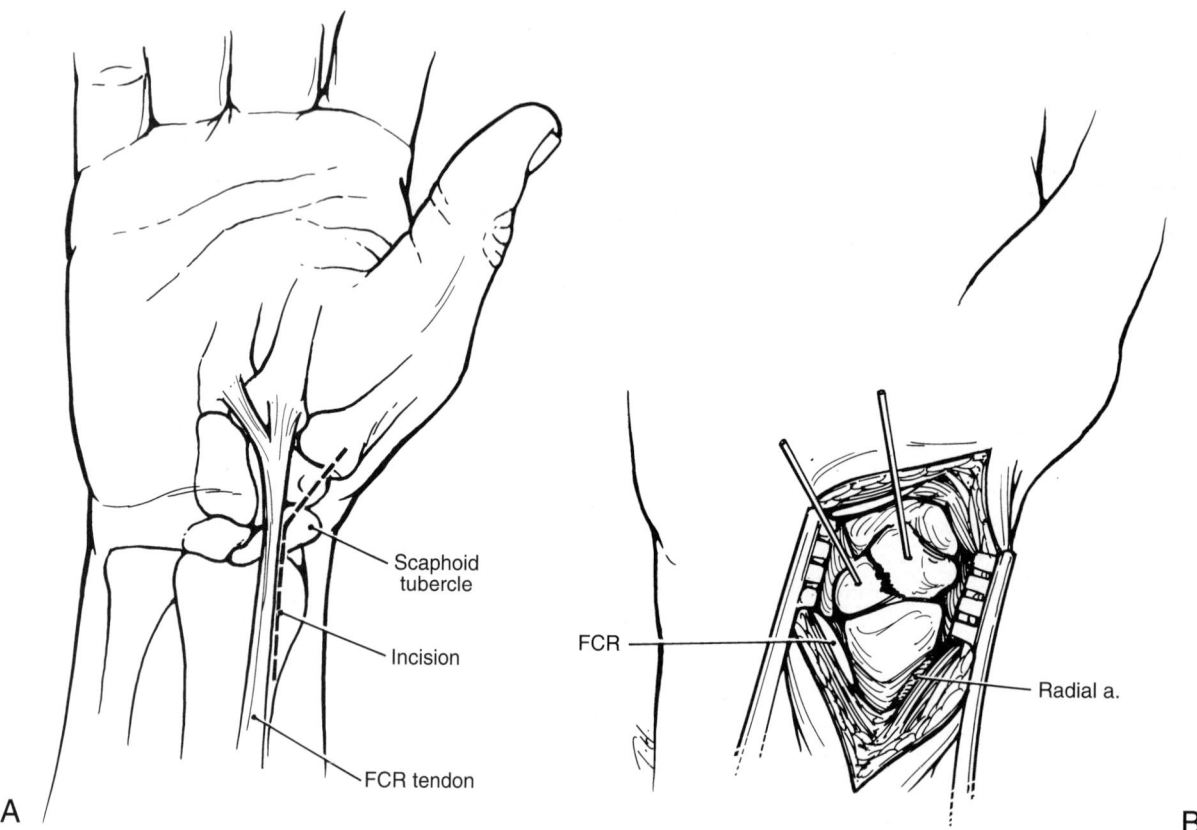

Figure 2.3. A. For the palmar approach to the scaphoid, a hockey stick–shaped skin incision is centered over the scaphoid tubercle. **B.** The fracture is exposed by the division and tagging of the palmar capsular ligaments.

displacement. In general, marked flexion of the scaphoid fragments indicates palmar comminution, which is best addressed via a palmar approach with bone grafting. Small proximal pole fragments should generally be internally fixed via a dorsal approach. Concomitant scapholunate ligament disruption or perilunate dislocation frequently mandates a combined dorsal and palmar approach.

PALMAR APPROACH

For the palmar approach, a C-arm image intensification or a small portable fluoroscopy unit is mandatory. A 5- to 7-cm hockey stick incision is centered over the scaphoid tubercle, running proximally over the subcutaneous flexor carpi radialis (FCR) tendon (Fig. 2.3). The FCR sheath is incised to retract the FCR tendon. The palmar branch of the radial artery may be ligated and divided. Exposure is continued through the floor of the FCR sheath to expose the palmar extrinsic ligaments. An incision is made along the long axis of the scaphoid through the wrist capsule and ligaments. A 4–0 Ethibond suture is used to tag both ends of the divided ligaments for later repair. The fracture is easily visualized and should be cleaned of clots and debris using irrigation and suction. To facilitate manipulation, 0.045 Kirschner (K) wires can be inserted into the proximal and distal poles and used as joysticks.

INTERNAL FIXATION

The choice of internal fixation is mandated in part by the inherent stability of the fracture and in part by the experience of the operating surgeon. Techniques of internal fixation have evolved from relatively simple K wire fixation to plate application and then to intermedullary fixation with standard and customized screws (Clinical Table: Scaphoid Fractures and Nonunion). The peculiar shape and oblique orientation of the scaphoid are formidable obstacles to the correct placement of an intermedullary device in the central axis of the bone. The alignment/compression device for inserting the Herbert screw addresses this problem; but there is a steep learning curve for the correct placement of the device. For optimal outcome, considerable practice on cadaveric wrists is recommended. Although technically the easiest method of internal fixation, K wire fixation is not sufficiently rigid to allow motion and must be supplemented with thumb spica cast immobilization until healing is evident on radiographs.

K Wire Fixation

K wire fixation is particularly useful when a rapid technique is need to allow the surgeon more time to address

Clinical Table: Scaphoid Fractures and Nonunion

Procedure	Indications	Technique	Anatomy	Pitfalls
Acute				
Palmar approach K wires	• Scaphoid fracture • Associated carpal or wrist fracture or dislocation	• Palmar ligament division open reduction • Percutaneous pinning	• Radial artery • Tubercle branches • Palmar cutaneous nerves	• Nonrigid fixation • No compression • Thumb spica cast
Herbert screws	• Displacement • Need for early mobility • Esp. simultaneous wrist fracture	• Scaphotrapezial joint exposed • Provisional K wire • Herbert compression jig	• Radial artery • Tubercle branches • Palmar cutaneous nerves • Radioscaphoid articular cartilage	• Steep learning curve • Perforation
Cannulated screws	• Displacement • Need for early mobility • Esp. simultaneous wrist fracture	• Scaphotrapezial joint exposed • Provisional K wire • Herbert compression jig • Fluoroscope guidewire insertion	• Radial artery • Tubercle branches • Palmar cutaneous nerves	• Wire breakage • Questions about burying screw head
Dorsal approach K wires	• Transscaphoid carpal dislocation • Wrist fracture	• Transverse or longitudinal incision over compartments two and three • T incision of capsule	• Radial sensory nerves; dorsal ridge artery	• Nonrigid fixation; questions about disrupting vascular supply
Herbert screws	• Small proximal pole • Transscaphoid carpal dislocation • Wrist fracture	• Transverse or longitudinal incision over compartments two and three • T incision of capsule • Freehand jig	• Radial sensory nerves; dorsal ridge artery	• Steep learning curve; no jig compression
Cannulated screws	• Small proximal pole • Transscaphoid carpal dislocation	• Transverse or longitudinal incision over compartments two and three • T incision of capsule • Provisional K wire	• Radial sensory nerves • Dorsal ridge artery	• Wire breakage
Nonunion				
Russe graft	• Undisplaced nonunion • No instability	• Palmar approach • Cavitate poles • Corticocancellous inlay	• Palmar radial articulation • Tubercle branches • Palmar cutaneous nerves • Articular cartilage	• No fixation • 4–6 months of healing
Matti (dorsal) graft	• Undisplaced nonunion • No instability	• Dorsal approach • Cavitate cancellous graft • Pin or screw	• Radial sensory nerves • Dorsal ridge artery	• Questions about devascularization of proximal pole • Cannot correct carpal instability or humpback

Continued

Clinical Table: Scaphoid Fractures and Nonunion (*continued*)

Procedure	Indications	Technique	Anatomy	Pitfalls
Palmar intercalated graft	• Humpback scaphoid • Carpal instability • *Early* degenerative changes	• Excise the nonunion • Iliac cortical wedge • Reduce lunate • Open reduction with internal fixation	• Radial sensory nerves (lunate transfixion wire)	• Increased nonunion rate • Technically challenging
Vascularized graft Zaidemberg et al. (5)	• Avascular proximal pole • Previous failed attempts	• Dorsal lateral approach • Vascular cortical-cancellous graft • K wires	• Radial sensory nerves • Ascending branch of the radial artery	• Loupes and micro-scope needed • Cannot correct carpal instability or humpback
Hori and Fernandez	• Avascular proximal pole • Previous radial bone graft	• Dorsal or combination approach • Transfer second metacarpal articular surface to proximal pole	• Radial sensory nerves • Dorsal second metacarpal artery	• Few reported series
Chronic Scapholunate Dissociation				
Scaphotrapezio-trapezoid arthrodesis	• SLD with early radioscaphoid DJD	• Radial styloidectomy • Reduce scaphoid • Decorticate STT • K wires, screws • Distal radial bone graft	• Radial sensory nerves • ECRB and ECRL tendons	• Overreduced scaphoid • Styloid impingement • Nonunion
Scaphocapitate arthrodesis	• SLD with early radioscaphoid and early midcarpal DJD	• Decorticate scaphoid and capitate • Preset wires in scaphoid	• ECRL and ECRB • Radial sensory nerve	• Overreduced scaphoid
Proximal row carpectomy	• SLAC wrist • No midcarpal DJD	• Dorsal incision • Divide scaphoid • Excise scaphoid, lunate, and triquetrum • Capsular closure • Early motion	• Dorsal sensory nerve • Palmar ligaments • Posterior interosseous nerves	• Preserve palmar ligaments • Minimal styloid resection • Stiffness from pro-longed immobilization
Scaphoid excision and four-corner (SLAC wrist) reconstruction	• SLAC wrist with midcarpal DJD	• Dorsal or paired transverse incision • Scaphoid excision • Radial bone graft • Wires and screws	• Dorsal sensory nerve • Posterior interosseous nerves • Palmar ligaments • Radial styloid	• Decreased range of motion • Silicone synovitis • Pseudarthrosis • Mechanical pain • Incomplete lunate reduction
Wrist arthrodesis	• Pan-carpal DJD • Failed previous surgeries	• Dorsal longitudinal incision • Decorticate carpus • Dorsal radial bone graft • Contoured plate	• Dorsal sensory nerve • Posterior interosseous nerves	• Index carpal-metacarpal DJD • Radioulnar DJD • Nonunion • Plate removal • Loss of motion

DJD, degenerative joint disease; *SLD*, scapholunate dissociation; *ECRB*, extensor carpi radialis brevis; *ECRL*, extensor carpi radialis longus; *ST-T*, scapho-trapeziotrapezoid; *SLAC*, scapholunate advanced collapse.

Figure 2.4. A. The surgeon's thumb compresses the fracture fragments with the barrel of the Herbert compression/alignment jig, while the scaphoid is elevated from the scaphotrapezial joint. Note the dorsal placement of the hook. **B.** A provisional wire holds the reduction while the device is applied. **C.** Healed scaphoid 3 months after the procedure. Note the partial excavation of the trapezium (*arrow*) to allow proper screw placement.

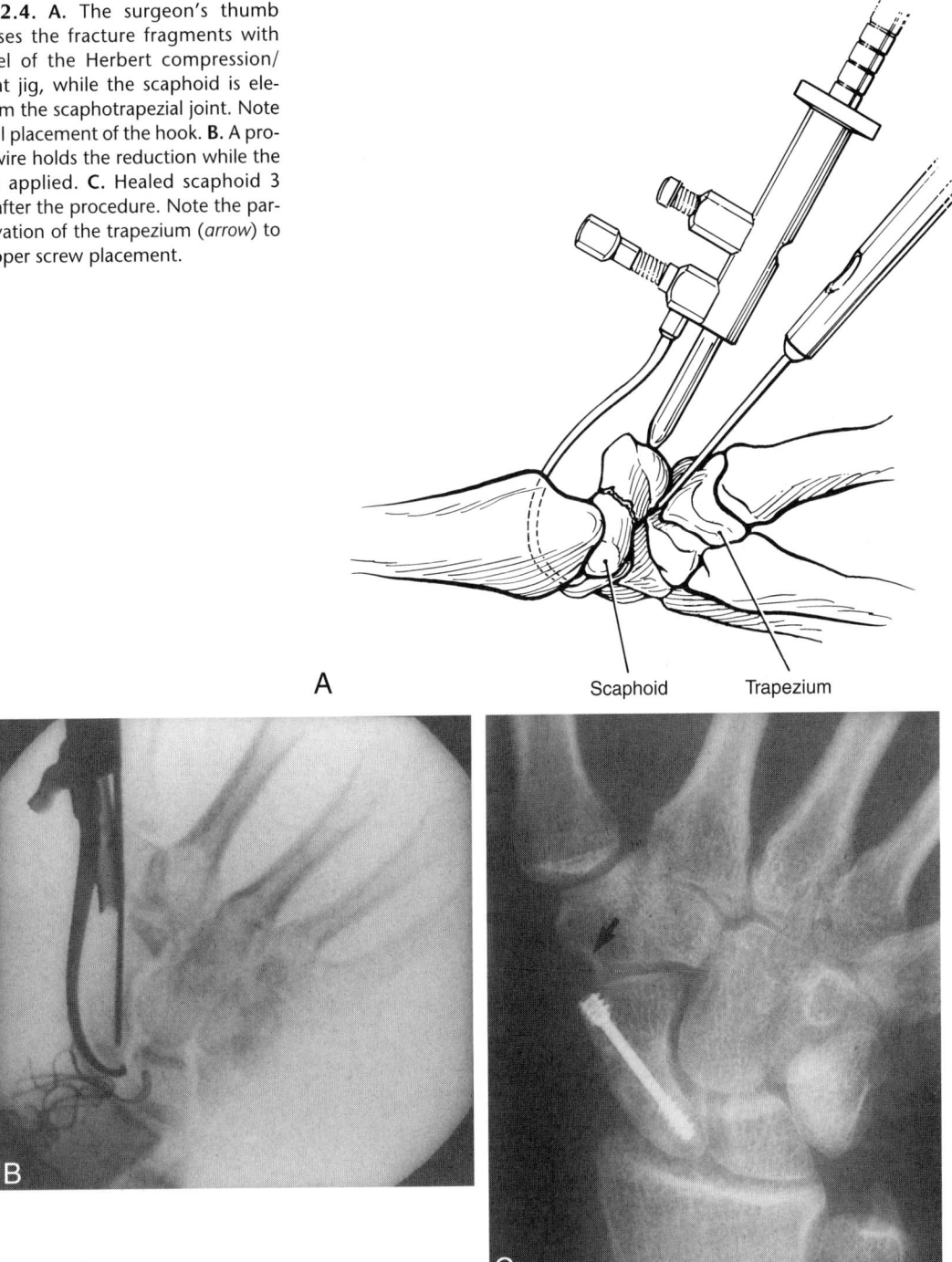

multiple ipsilateral injuries. A 14-gauge angiocatheter is used as a drill guide and soft tissue protector for the 0.045 K wires. The stylet is punctured through the thenar skin to engage the tubercle. Compression is applied while the surgeon drives the wires across the fracture site, aiming just dorsal to the scaphoid fossa of the distal radius. The position of the wire is checked with fluoroscopy, and a second wire is passed parallel to the first. Both wires are cut off beneath the thenar skin. Additional stability can be obtained at the discretion of the surgeon by fixing the distal pole to the capitate or by transfixing the lunate with a transstyloid pin. During closure, firm coaptation of the ra-

diocarpal ligaments must be performed with nonabsorbable sutures.

The arm is immobilized in a long arm cast for 6 weeks followed by a short arm cast until healing is complete. The pins are removed in the office when trabecular bridging is apparent on radiographs.

Herbert Screw

An intra-articular starting point at the scaphotrapezial (ST) joint is mandatory for the optimal positioning of the Herbert screw, an intramedullary device. The incision is extended longitudinally across the ST joint, and the capsule is reflected to allow mobilization of the distal pole. A small portion of the trapezium is excised with a rongeur for further exposure. The fracture is provisionally fixed with a K wire, which prevents the fragments from rotating when the screw is tightened. The alignment jig is checked for calibration before the surgeon proceeds. While an assistant distracts the radiocarpal joint by longitudinal traction on the thumb, the surgeon passes the alignment jig to the dorsal aspect of the proximal pole. Slight traction firmly seats the device. Next, the scaphoid distal pole is levered to the palmar aspect by inserting a thin elevator in the ST joint. The barrel of the alignment jig is slid into place, and the fracture is firmly compressed by the surgeon's thumb (Fig. 2.4). The length of the screw is read off of the barrel; and working through the alignment jig, the surgeon drills the distal and proximal poles and taps and places the screw. The final position of the screw is checked on multiple planes using image intensification before the jig is removed, and complete burial of the screw head is ensured with an extra turn of the screwdriver.

Capsular closure and ligament repair are protected for 4 weeks in a thumb spica cast. Depending on fracture stability, motion exercises may be initiated; but strengthening is deferred for at least 8 weeks.

Cannulated Screws

A number of cannulated screw systems, including a cannulated Herbert screw, are available, and the reader is referred to the manufacturer's guides for full technical details (Fig. 2.5).

DORSAL APPROACH

For the dorsal approach, a 3-cm transverse incision based 1 cm distal to the dorsal lip of the radius provides adequate exposure for simple proximal pole scaphoid fractures. Care is taken to identify and preserve the dorsal radial sensory nerve branches. The extensor retinaculum is partially divided over the second and third compartments to allow adequate retraction. Exposure of the fracture site may be best seen through an interval between the two radial wrist extensor tendons (6). The capsule is carefully reflected distally with an inverted T incision, avoiding the critical dorsal ridge vascular perforators.

Internal Fixation

For internal fixation, longitudinal K wires may be passed out the distal pole and pulled retrograde until the tips are buried beneath the articular cartilage. Pins are best clipped beneath the thenar skin. K wires are generally not adequate for fixation of small, unstable proximal pole fractures, and intramedullary screw fixation is generally recommended (Clinical Table: Scaphoid Fractures and Nonunion). The screw technique is similar to that used for palmar fixation, although the compression jigs cannot be used. The fracture is stabilized with a provisional wire, and a freehand jig may be used to allow manual compression of the fracture site during screw insertion.

INITIAL FINDINGS: SCAPHOID NONUNION

Differentiation of a scaphoid nonunion from an acute fracture may be difficult when a patient presents without precise recollection of trauma. Scaphoid nonunions may be relatively asymptomatic for several years and may become painful after a relatively trivial reinjury. Signs of sclerosis and secondary changes of carpal malalignment or degenerative change indicate a long-standing nonunion. Several long-term studies suggest that, over a 10-year pe-

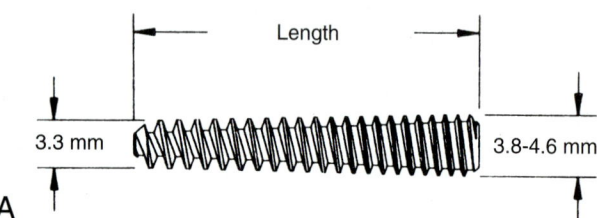
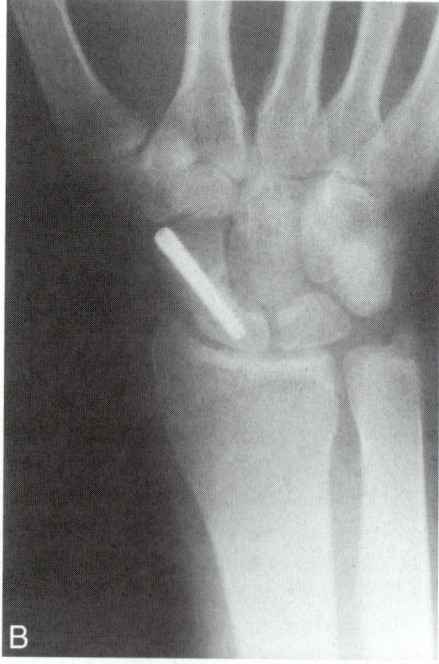

Figure 2.5. A. The Acutrak screw is a cannulated headless screw that has a tapered design and differential thread pitches for interfragmentary compression. Reprinted with permission from Acumed, Inc., Beaverton, OR. **B.** Navicular view of healed scaphoid following cannulated screw fixation.

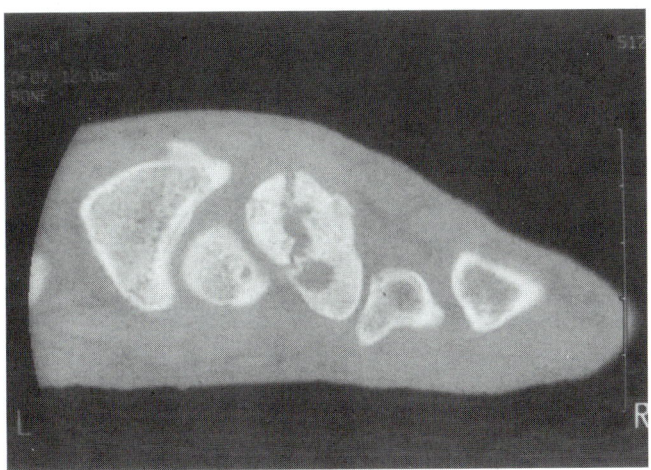

Figure 2.6. Sagittal CT image of scaphoid nonunion, demonstrating a humpback flexion deformity, cystic change, a radiodense proximal pole, and early degenerative changes.

riod, untreated scaphoid nonunions will progress to degenerative arthritis with a frequency approaching 100% (7).

Symptomatic scaphoid nonunions are associated with localized tenderness in the anatomic snuffbox, and a Watson's scaphoid shift test may produce fracture site crepitus and pain. Range of motion is usually limited by pain at the extremes of flexion and extension and radioulnar deviation. Depending on the duration of nonunion, swelling, synovitis, and midcarpal crepitus may be present.

RADIOLOGIC STUDIES

Although multiplanar tomography, arthrography, and MRI can all confirm nonunion, CT along the longitudinal axis of the scaphoid gives added information about alignment and rotation of the fracture fragments and may detect partial healing of a suspected nonunion (Fig. 2.6) (2).

Classification

Prognostic factors in the treatment of scaphoid nonunion include the duration of nonunion, degree of displacement, associated carpal instability, size and vascularity of the proximal pole, and secondary degenerative changes. Scaphoid nonunion leads to progressive carpal instability and degenerative change because the fragments behave as separate carpal bones and no longer link and coordinate synchronous carpal row motion. The opposing rotational movements of the proximal and distal carpal rows lead to an increasing flexion (humpback) deformity of the scaphoid, and the carpus assumes a dorsal intercalated segment instability (DISI) collapse deformity. Thus, because of a high association with carpal instability and secondary degenerative arthritis, duration of nonunion is perhaps the most important determinant of healing potential.

TREATMENT

In most cases, an attempt at reconstruction of the scaphoid nonunion is warranted, using a bone graft to reconstruct the deficiencies in palmar scaphoid integrity and as a stimulus to healing. Nonoperative treatment might be considered for an elderly patient with limited functional demands or a younger patient with moderate degenerative change who wishes to defer a salvage procedure, such as resection or partial arthrodesis. Since initial reports in the early 1960s, the Russe inlay bone graft has been a popular and straightforward treatment for the uncomplicated scaphoid nonunion.

Russe Bone Graft (Green Modification)

For the Green (8) modification of the Russe bone graft, the fracture site is exposed via a standard palmar approach. An oblong trough is created on either side of the fracture line, using sharp osteotomes and rongeurs, which is large enough to later admit two corticocancellous strips of inlay bone graft. Meticulous curettage of both proximal and distal poles is done by hand to avoid overheating the bone, which may occur when power instruments are used. Particular care must be exercised while excavating the often dense proximal pole to avoid fracturing the proximal fragment or perforating the articular cartilage. The viability of the proximal pole is assessed by noting the quality of the cancellous bone (soft, dense, sclerotic, marble) and the number of punctate bleeding points following curettage of the fracture surface. True avascular necrosis is quite rare, but it is associated with a 100% failure of this technique (8).

Two 16-mm corticocancellous strips are inserted into

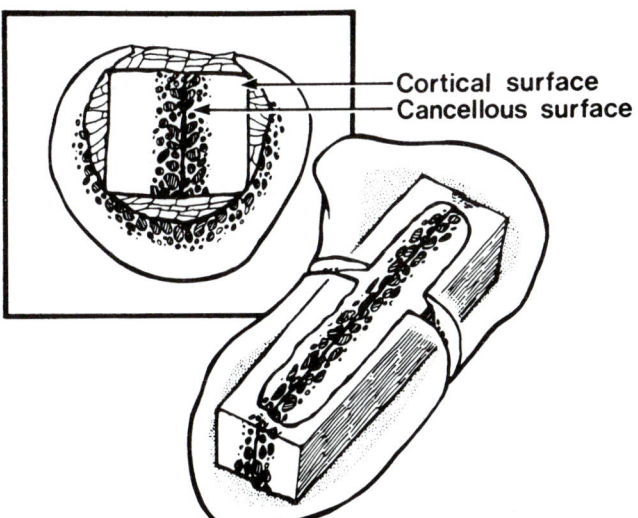

Cortical surface
Cancellous surface

Figure 2.7. Green's modification of Russe bone graft. Reprinted with permission from Green DP. The effect of avascular necrosis on Russe bone grafting for scaphoid nonunion. J Hand Surg 1985; 10A:597–605.

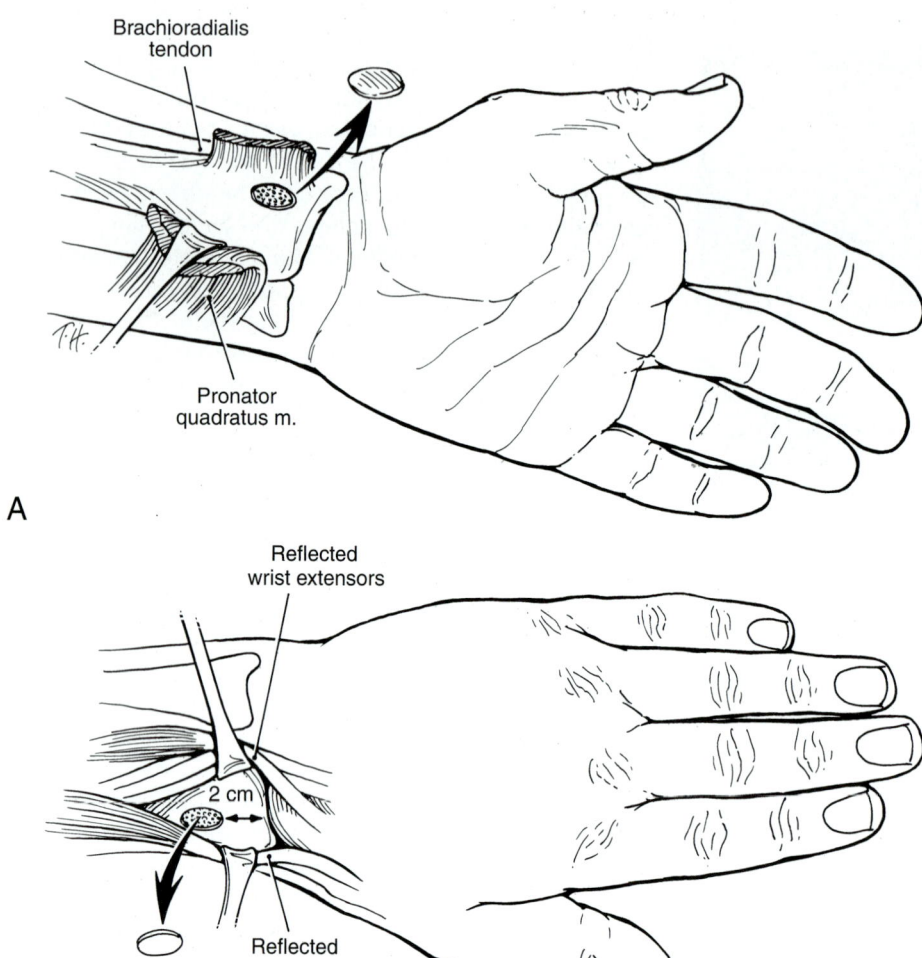

Brachioradialis
tendon

Pronator
quadratus m.

A

Reflected
wrist extensors

2 cm

Reflected
first dorsal
compartment

B

Figure 2.8. Palmar (**A**) and dorsal (**B**) approaches for a distal radius bone graft. The oval cortical window may be replaced following the graft harvest.

the cavity, with their cancellous surfaces apposed (Fig. 2.7). The distal radius graft is technically easier to obtain than is the iliac crest graft, and its decreased cortical thickness eases the sculpting process (Fig. 2.8). Supplemental cancellous chips are packed about the insert to fill the cavity and provide additional stability. If the cavity is solidly packed, internal or pin fixation is not necessary; and the wound is closed by firmly reapproximating the palmar capsular ligaments.

Immobilization in a long arm thumb spica cast for 8 weeks is followed by immobilization in a short arm thumb spica cast until healing is complete, which is generally 4 to 6 months with this approach.

Dorsal Bone Graft

The dorsal approach for treatment of scaphoid nonunions is favored by some surgeons because exposure is simple, the union rate is favorable, and there are few complications (6). It is particularly attractive for the small proximal pole fracture, maximizing exposure and fixation of the proximal fragment. A true humpback deformity with associated midcarpal instability cannot be adequately addressed with this approach.

The scaphoid is approached as detailed on page 23. K wire joysticks are placed in the proximal and distal poles. All fibrous tissue is removed from the nonunion site. A cavity is created in both proximal and distal poles, taking care to avoid intra-articular perforation. Viability of the fragments is assessed by observation of punctate bleeding points. A cancellous bone graft is packed tightly into the distal pole. Two double-ended 0.045 K wires are placed in the fracture site and driven through the distal pole to exit the thenar skin. The proximal pole is then packed with the remaining cancellous bone and toggled into anatomic alignment. If the lunate appears dorsally tilted by more than 10°, it must be manually reduced and pinned with a 0.062 transstyloid K wire. With the fragments aligned and held with manual compression, the surgeon can drive the previously placed wires antegrade into the subchondral bone of the proximal fragment. The positions of the pins are checked with fluoroscopy, and the pins are cut off below the thenar skin.

Immobilization in a long arm thumb spica cast is main-

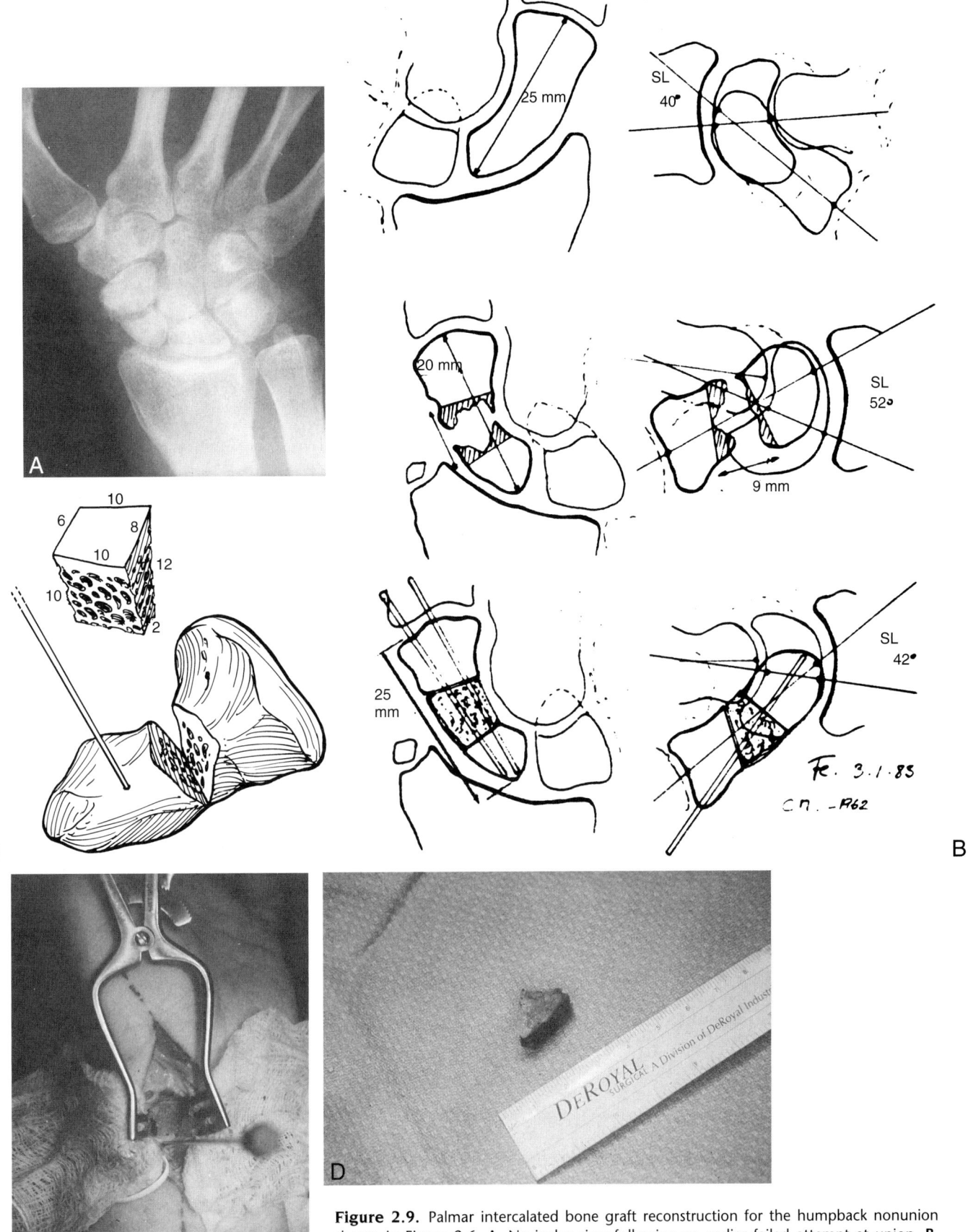

Figure 2.9. Palmar intercalated bone graft reconstruction for the humpback nonunion shown in Figure 2.6. **A.** Navicular view following an earlier failed attempt at union. **B.** Preoperative template of the bone graft size taken from radiographs of uninjured wrist. Reprinted with permission from Fernandez DL. A technique for anterior wedge-shaped grafts for scaphoid nonunions with carpal instability. J Hand Surg 1984;9A:733–737. **C.** Extended scaphoid following the excision of the sclerotic margins and curettage. The bone graft size is determined with osteotomes and a three-dimensional blueprint drawn to scale. **D.** Sculpted bicortical iliac crest bone graft. **E.** Bone graft wedged into position. Note the transfixion pin for the lunate. *(figure continues)*

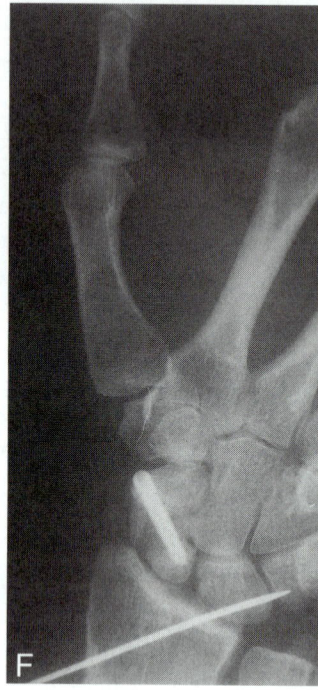

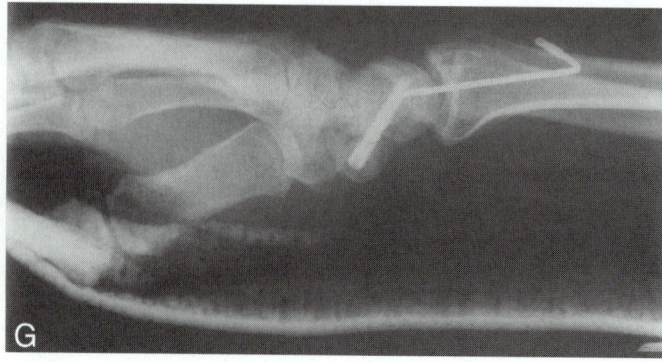

Figure 2.9 (continued). F and **G.** Navicular and lateral views following the lunate transfixion and internal fixation of the scaphoid.

tained for 6 weeks, at which time the lunate transfixion pin may be removed. The scaphoid pins may be removed at 8 to 12 weeks postsurgery. Immobilization is maintained until there is clinical and radiographic evidence of union, generally at 16 weeks.

We prefer the rigid internal fixation of the small proximal pole fragments using freehand Herbert or cannulated Acutrak (Acumed, Inc., Beaverton, OR) screws when using the dorsal approach.

Palmar Intercalated Bone Graft

For chronic nonunions with collapse deformity and secondary midcarpal instability, simple restitution of the union without reduction of the associated instability will not prevent degenerative change. Reconstruction of the scaphoid length and alignment via an opening wedge volar bone graft (9) is technically demanding and associated with a low union rate. Patients presenting with radiocarpal and midcarpal degenerative changes often have more symptoms from their arthritis than from the scaphoid nonunion, and serious consideration must be given to a salvage procedure (proximal row carpectomy versus partial wrist fusion).

Careful preoperative planning is crucial to a successful outcome. True PA, lateral, and navicular films of the normal wrist are obtained and used as templates for determining the graft dimensions (Fig. 2.9). A 1.5- to 2-cm cube of tricortical iliac crest graft is harvested based on preoperative measurements and kept in a moist saline sponge. The nonunion is exposed through a standard palmar approach, and K wires are inserted in the proximal and distal poles for manipulation. A microsagittal saw is used to create two flat surfaces for reconstruction. Cystic cavities are curetted to bleeding cancellous bone; and sclerotic, nonviable bone is removed from the proximal fragment with curettes and

gouges. It is neither necessary nor advantageous to cavitate either pole, as this will reduce the strength of the fixation.

Next, the lunate is reduced into a neutral or slightly flexed posture and held with a transstyloid 0.062 K wire. This rotates the attached proximal pole into proper alignment. Gentle extension of the wrist will now open the nonunion site for final calculation of the graft's dimensions, using small osteotomes as sizers. The surgeon must carefully sculpt the tricortical graft to fit the defect, using the microsagittal saw and rongeurs. The iliac inner table is generally the best match for the opposing capitate surface. Cavities in both poles are filled with cancellous bone. The graft is tapped snugly into place, and provisional fixation with a K wire is performed along one margin of the bone. Internal fixation with a Herbert screw or cannulated device is recommended for compression and long-term fixation until healing is complete. Protruding edges of the graft are smoothed with a rongeur or rasp, and radial styloidectomy is performed if degenerative changes are present. Careful capsular repair is performed, and postoperative care is dictated by the adequacy of internal fixation.

Salvage Procedures

A failed previous attempt at a nonunion repair, unequivocal radiographic, MRI evidence of avascular necrosis, and intraoperative confirmation of avascular marble bone without punctate bleeding are all poor prognostic signs for scaphoid union following standard bone grafting procedures. Techniques designed to revascularize an avascular proximal pole have been reported in a small series of patients and show promise in these difficult situations (5). Alternatively, serious consideration must be given to excision of the scaphoid fragment and partial wrist arthrodesis, proximal row carpectomy, or complete wrist fusion. These procedures are discussed in detail below.

SUMMARY

Acute scaphoid fractures are common and require careful evaluation and an often protracted course of treatment. Because of a relatively poor vascular supply, scaphoid fractures are intolerant of displacement or instability. Operative fixation is indicated in unstable or displaced fractures and presents several technical challenges. Scaphoid nonunion will predictably lead to de-generative change and, in most cases, should be treated aggressively to reconstruct scaphoid length and alignment and simultaneously restore normal carpal kinematics. Avascular necrosis of the scaphoid proximal pole may require special techniques such as vascularized bone grafting. Salvage procedures, including proximal row carpectomy and partial wrist arthrodesis, are indicated for progressive and symptomatic degenerative change.

II Carpal Dislocations

RELEVANT ANATOMY AND PATHOGENESIS

The complex motion of the carpus may be greatly simplified by grouping the carpals into proximal and distal rows. Dense ligamentous attachments anchor the distal carpal row (trapezium, trapezoid, capitate, and hamate) to the metacarpals, which collectively may be thought of as a single "hand" segment. Interposed between the hand segment and the radius and ulna (the "forearm" segment) is the "intercalated" segment, or proximal carpal row, composed of the scaphoid, lunate, and triquetrum (Fig. 2.10). In the uninjured state, the bones of the proximal carpal row rotate in a synchronous fashion; as the wrist extends or ulnar deviates, the scaphoid, lunate, and triquetrum extend. Conversely, as the wrist flexes or radial deviates, the scaphoid, lunate, and triquetrum flex. Unlike the distal carpal row, there is approximately 25° of motion between the bones of the proximal carpal row, limited by the constraints of the interosseous scapholunate and lunotriquetral (intrinsic) ligaments. Disruption of the intrinsic ligaments dissociates the proximal carpal row and creates abnormal kinematics, ultimately progressing to pain and degenerative arthritis.

The major extrinsic (capsular) ligaments span the carpal rows, restraining the motion between them (Fig. 2.11). Disruption of the extrinsic ligaments can, in isolation, lead to altered kinematics; but in combination with an intrinsic ligament injury, disruption will generally result in disabling destabilization of the entire carpus.

Progressive Perilunar Instability

In 1980, Mayfield et al. (10) described a cadaveric model of carpal ligament disruptions resulting from forced wrist hyperextension, ulnar deviation, and intercarpal supination termed progressive perilunar instability (PLI). A predictable sequence of ligamentous failures occurred, beginning with the scapholunate interosseous ligament (SLIL), coursing in a clockwise direction around the lunate, and culminating in complete lunate dislocation (Fig. 2.12). Perilunate dislocations (stage III) and lunate dislocation (stage IV) represent massive carpal ligamentous disruptions and demand prompt and aggressive treatment.

Patients with perilunate or lunate dislocations generally present with massive swelling, and radiographs reveal gross disruption of the normal architecture. Up to 25% of carpal dislocations are missed on initial presentation, and careful scrutiny of the radiographs is mandatory. An attempt at closed reduction, followed by operative repair of the torn intrinsic and extrinsic ligaments through a combined dorsovolar approach is recommended. The carpal bones are pinned in anatomic position for 4 to 6 weeks, followed by months of rehabilitation. Outcome is generally poor, because of the high energy of the injury and massive disruption of the carpal architecture.

INITIAL FINDINGS: SCAPHOLUNATE DISSOCIATION

Scapholunate dissociation, or disruption of the scapholunate interosseous ligament, is the most common wrist ligament injury. Diagnosis and management of this condition continue to be both challenging and controversial. Untreated scapholunate dissociation leads to abnormal flexion of the scaphoid and a compensatory zigzag collapse of the carpus (11). Abnormal carpal alignment leads to a reduction in the radioscaphoid contact area. Increased focal load on the articular cartilage will lead to a predictable pattern of increased wear and degenerative changes, termed scapholunate advanced collapse (SLAC) (12). Degenerative changes are at first confined to the ra-

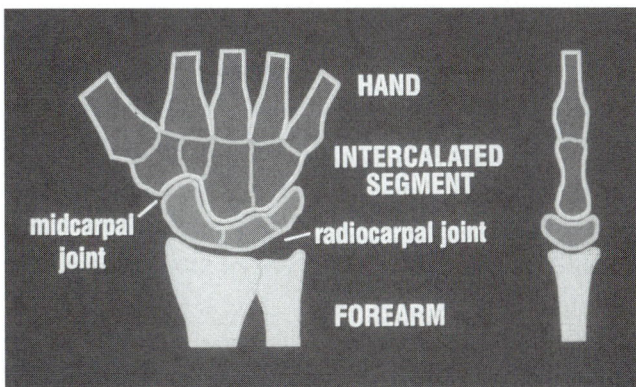

Figure 2.10. To simplify carpal kinematics, the proximal carpal row can be depicted as an intercalated segment situated between the fixed hand and forearm segments. The scaphoid, while not included in traditional descriptions of the proximal carpal row, behaves kinematically as a member of the proximal row.

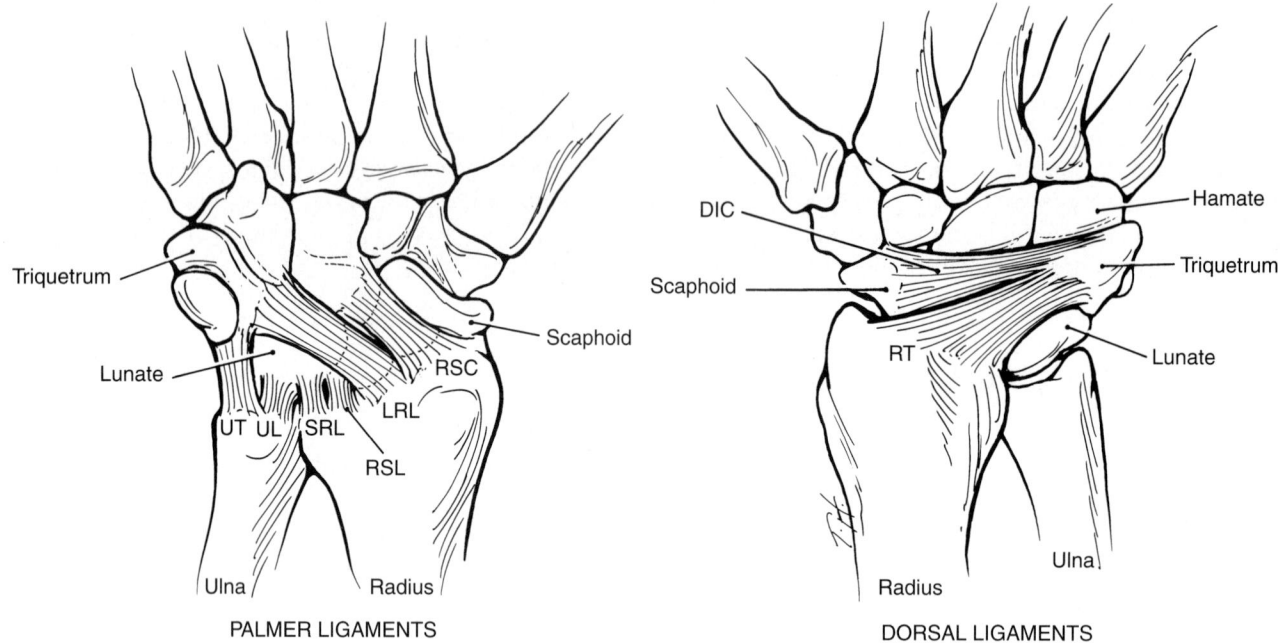

A
PALMER LIGAMENTS

B
DORSAL LIGAMENTS

Figure 2.11. Palmar and dorsal extrinsic ligaments. *RSC,* radioscaphocapitate; *LRL,* long radiolunate; *RSL,* radioscapholunate ligament; *SRL,* short radiolunate ligament; *UL,* ulnolunate ligament; *UT,* ulnotriquetral ligament; *DIC,* dorsal intercarpal ligament; *RT,* radiotriquetral ligament.

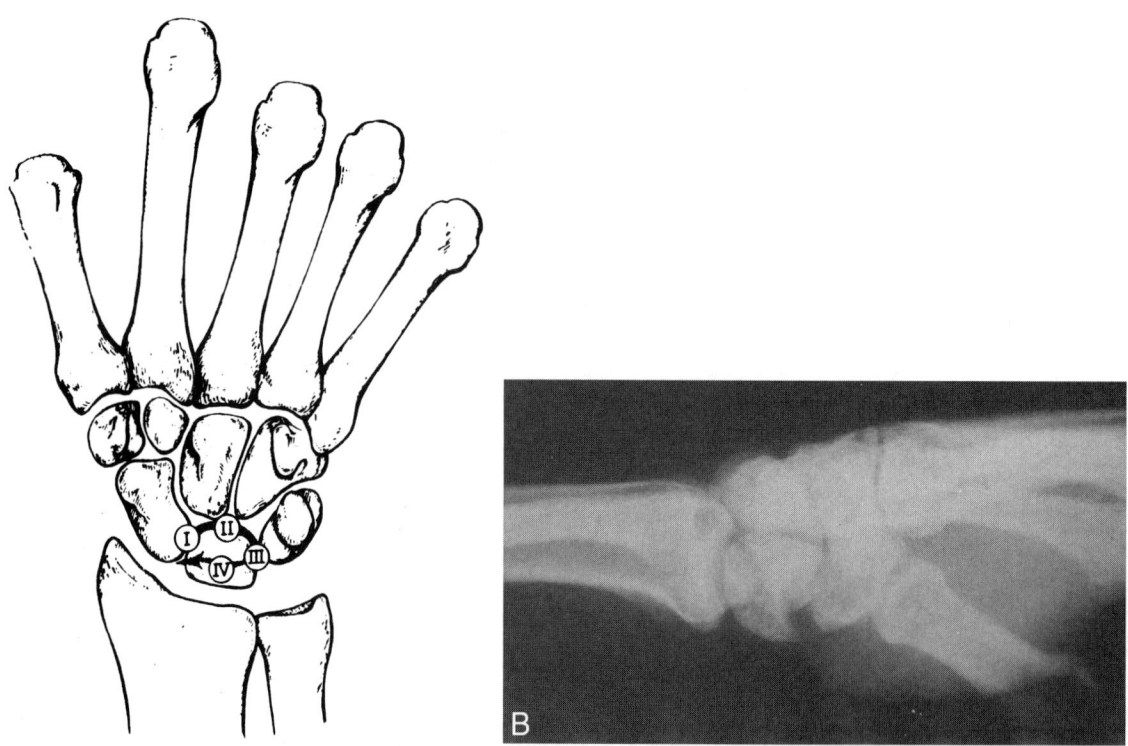

A

B

Figure 2.12. A. Stages (*I–IV*) of ligament disruption in progressive perilunar instability. Reprinted with permission from Mayfield JK. Wrist ligamentous anatomy and pathogenesis of carpal instability. *Orthop Clin North Am* 1984;15:209–216. **B.** Perilunate dislocation, or stage III PLI.

Figure 2.13. Three radiographic signs of scapholunate disruption: increased scapholunate interval (**A**), foreshortened scaphoid and cortical ring sign of superimposed scaphoid tubercle (**B**), and scaphoid and lunate malrotation with secondary DISI deformity (**C**).

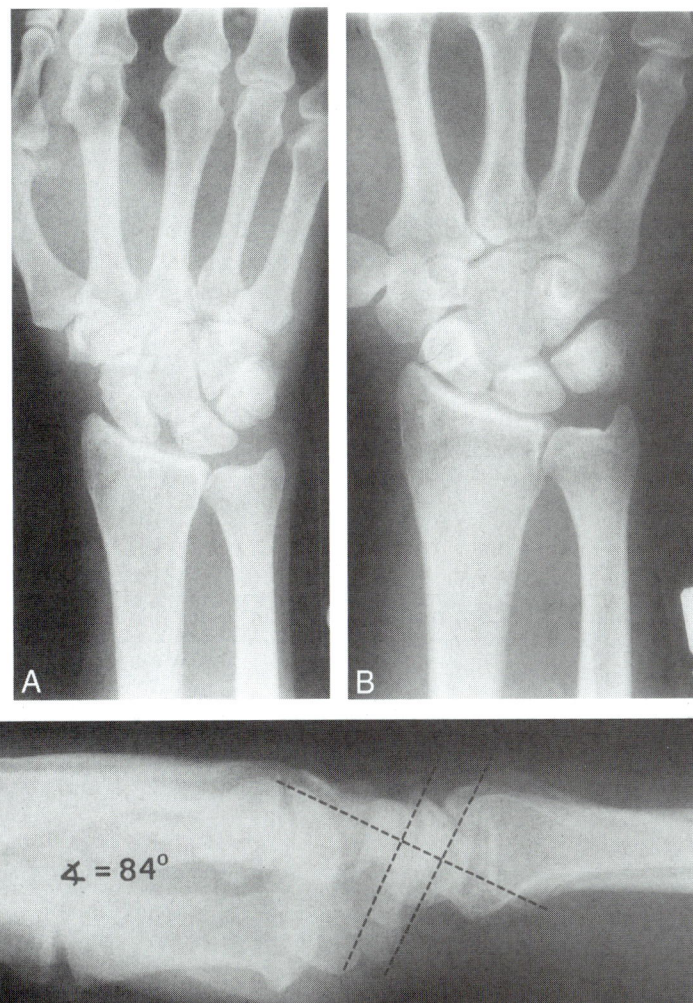

dioscaphoid joint but eventually involve the midcarpal joint as well.

The mechanism of injury in scapholunate dissociation is usually a fall with wrist hyperextension. Often patients with scapholunate dissociation relate only a distant history of a wrist sprain. In the rare acute presentation, wrist motion is limited, ecchymosis is usually present, and aspiration of a hemarthrosis is pathognomonic of a serious ligament injury. There is point tenderness over the scapholunate joint dorsally.

For patients presenting 6 weeks or more after injury, symptoms may include persistent pain and loss of motion. Exacerbation of pain with grip or activities and symptoms of "clunking," "popping," or "giving way" suggest SLIL injury. Watson's scaphoid shift test will usually be positive. To perform this test, the examiner applies a dorsally directed load to the scaphoid tubercle and palpates for painful subluxation of the scaphoid during ulnar to radial deviation. Patients with chronic injuries usually present with degenerative arthritis, severe loss of motion, and decreased scaphoid mobility during the scaphoid shift test.

RADIOLOGIC STUDIES

Specialized radiographic views should include a PA (supinated) clenched fist view, PA views in radial and ulnar deviation, and lateral views in flexion and extension. PA and lateral radiographs of the opposite wrist are recommended for comparison. A scapholunate gap of 1 to 2 mm greater than the opposite side on any view suggests a tear in the SLIL. Increased scaphoid flexion (rotatory subluxation) may accompany a SLIL tear and is demonstrated by a foreshortened scaphoid on the PA view. A so-called scaphoid ring sign may be seen on the PA view when the tubercle of the scaphoid is superimposed on its waist by increased flexion. Finally, a loss of the normal trapezoidal shape of the lunate is a subtle sign of abnormal lunate rotation and should alert the examiner to request further studies.

Rotatory subluxation of the scaphoid is best demonstrated on the lateral radiograph. A scapholunate angle greater than 70° indicates scapholunate dissociation (the normal angle is 30° to 60°) (11) (Fig. 2.13). The radiolunate angle quantifies the amount of dorsovolar tilt of the lunate, and if it is greater than 15° dorsal DISI is indicated.

Additional Studies

When plain and stress radiographs are normal, cineroentgenography may demonstrate an abrupt shift in carpal alignment during wrist motion or abnormal widening at the scapholunate (SL) interval. In most centers, MRI of ligaments is still considered investigational. Three-compartmental arthrography (radiocarpal, midcarpal, and radioulnar) is highly sensitive in identifying ligament defects; however, bilateral studies have shown a high prevalence of abnormal findings on the contralateral (asymptomatic) wrist. Arthroscopy is considered the gold standard for the diagnosis of carpal ligamentous pathologic states. Partial SLIL tears without associated carpal instability may be treated with limited débridement; acute injuries have been treated with arthroscopic-assisted K wire fixation.

TREATMENT

Treatment for scapholunate dissociation is based on time of diagnosis after injury and is directed at reversing abnormal kinematics and preventing further degenerative change. Acute treatment methods include closed reduction and casting, percutaneous pinning, open reduction and ligament repair, and ligament reconstruction (Clinical Table: Scapholunate Dissociation). Treatment for chronic scapholunate dissociation depends on the extent and location of the degenerative changes.

Clinical Table: Scapholunate Dissociation

Procedure	Indications	Technique	Anatomy	Pitfalls
Acute Scapholunate Dissociation				
Closed reduction				
Casting	• Acute injury • Reducible	• Reduction under fluoroscopy • Long arm cast		• Incomplete reduction or loss of reduction
Percutaneous pinning	• Acute injury • Reducible • Especially incomplete tears	• Reduction under fluoroscopy, with or without arthroscopy • Scapholunate and scaphocapitate K wires	• Radial sensory nerve • Radial artery • Extensor tendons	• Incomplete reduction or loss of reduction
Open scapholunate ligament repair	• Complete SLIL tear • Reducible • No DJD	• Dorsal incision • Transscaphoid direct repair • Scapholunate and scaphocapitate pinning • Dorsal capsulodesis	• Radial sensory nerve • Articular cartilage	• Irreducible scaphoid • Technically demanding • Stiffness
Capsulodesis				
Dorsal, from Blatt (13)	• Acute or subacute SLD • No fixed DISI • No DJD	• Radial-based capsular flap • Advance past scaphoid waist • K wires • Pullout sutures	• Dorsal scaphoid vascular supply • Radial sensory nerve	• Loss of flexion • Attenuation • Stiffness
Palmar	• Acute or subacute SLD	• Palmar approach • Debride the scapholunate interval • Imbricate the ligaments • K wire	• Median motor branch • Transverse carpal ligament • Radial sensory nerve	• Stiffness • Recurrent SLD • Pain
Four-bone ligament reconstruction	• Acute or subacute SLD	• Dorsal and palmar incisions • ECRB four-bone weave	• Median and radial sensory nerves	• Loss of reduction • Wire removal • Technically difficult
Scapholunate ligament reconstruction or augmentation	• Acute or subacute SLD	• Dorsal and palmar approach • Repair SLIL • ECRL transosseous augmentation	• Radial sensory and median nerves	• Attenuation • Kinematic alteration

Acute Treatment

A diagnosis of complete SLIL disruption should be treated with direct ligament repair. Casting may be adequate treatment for partial ligament injuries but will not prevent progression in complete SLIL disruptions. Some authors have advocated percutaneous pinning if adequate reduction can be obtained and documented fluoroscopically, but the disrupted ligaments may not adequately heal in their intrasynovial environment, particularly if 3 to 4 weeks have elapsed since injury.

SCAPHOLUNATE LIGAMENT REPAIR

Scapholunate ligament repair, while indicated for acute injuries, may also be effective in the subacute period if the scaphoid is reducible, there are no degenerative changes, and substantial remnants of the ligament remain (14). A 4-cm dorsal oblique incision is made just ulnar to Lister's tubercle. The third compartment is entered, and the extensor pollicis longus (EPL) is retracted. The dorsal wrist capsule is incised along the radial articular margin and extended in an inverted T along the axis of the capitate. K wires are placed in the scaphoid and lunate to use as joy-

Figure 2.14. A. Transosseous SLIL repair. Reprinted with permission from Lavernia CJ, Cohen MS, Taleisnik J. Treatment of scapholunate dissociation by ligamentous repair and capsulodesis. J Hand Surg 1992;17A:354–359. **B.** Operative view of the SLIL repair. Note the joysticks in the scaphoid and lunate. **C.** In the modified dorsal capsulodesis, the scaphoid-based flap of dorsal capsule is advanced proximally and sutured to anchors in the radius.

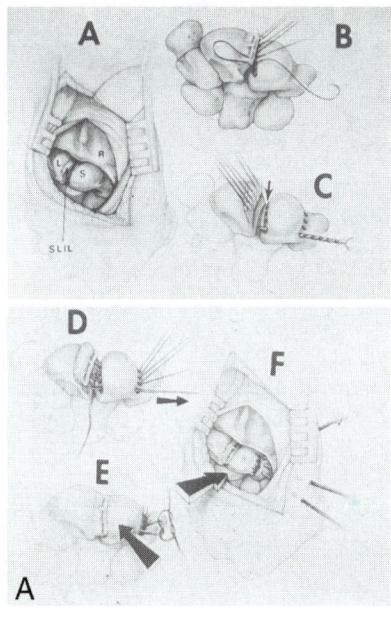

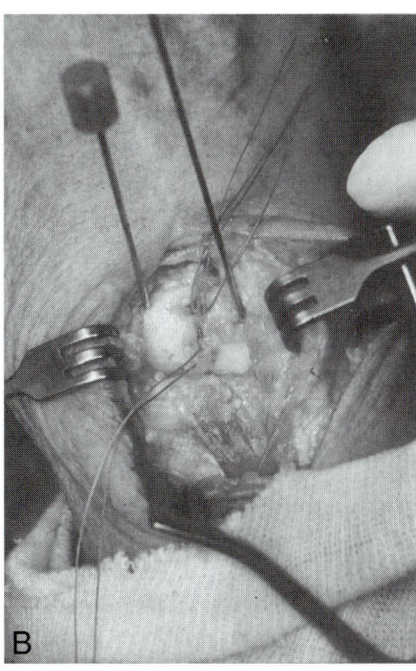

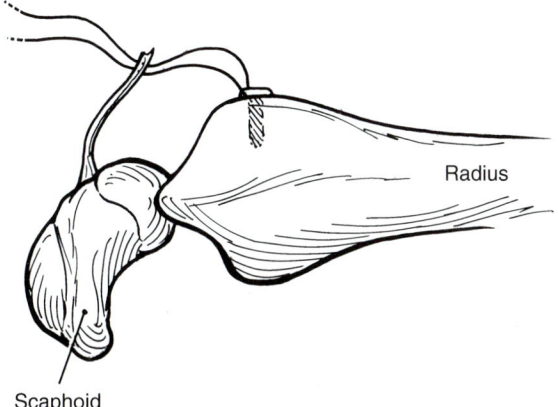

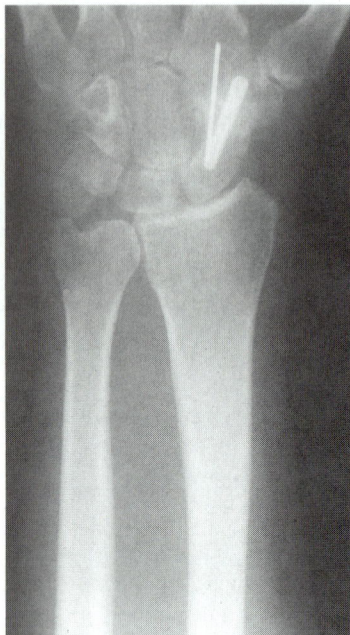

Figure 2.15. United STT fusion with a radial styloidectomy for rotatory subluxation.

sticks to assist with examination and reduction. Next, 3–0 nonabsorbable sutures are passed through the remnant of the interosseous ligament on the lunate. A burr is used to create a small trough in the lunate ridge of the scaphoid. Drill holes are then made through the scaphoid waist, exiting through the newly created trough; the lunate sutures are retrieved with Keith needles. The carpus is reduced, and the K wires are placed from the scaphoid to the lunate and from the scaphoid to the capitate. Overcorrection is recommended. Additional augmentation via a dorsal capsulodesis is recommended (Fig. 2.14).

Postsurgery, the wrist and the forearm are immobilized above the elbow for 4 weeks; then a short arm cast is used for 4 to 6 weeks more. The K wires are removed at 8 to 10 weeks, and protected mobilization is then begun. Strengthening begins at 3 to 4 months postsurgery.

DORSAL CAPSULODESIS

Blatt (13) advocates dorsal capsulodesis alone for patients who have a reducible scaphoid and no evidence of degenerative changes. The procedure creates a capsuloligamentous check rein distal to the midaxis of the scaphoid. The scaphoid is exposed through a dorsal incision, by raising a 1.5-cm-wide capsular flap based on the distal radius. Care is taken to avoid the dorsal vascular supply while raising the flap to the level of the scaphotrapeziotrapezoid (STT) joint. The scaphoid is manually reduced and held with a K wire, which is passed through the distal pole and into the capitate and middle metacarpal base. A burr is used to create a trough just proximal to the distal articular cartilage of the scaphoid for

the dorsal capsular insertion. The dorsal capsule is secured in its trough via a pullout 2–0 Prolene suture bought out over a button on the radial palmar surface.

Postsurgery, the patient is maintained in a short arm thumb spica cast for 2 months. At 2 months the patient is placed in a removable splint and started on range of motion exercises. The K wire is removed at 3 months. Activity is restricted for a total of 6 months. Blatt (13) reports a maximum deficit of 20° of flexion and a maximum loss of 20% of grip strength compared to the opposite side.

Chronic Treatment

A number of different ligament reconstructions have been attempted, yet none has proven as effective as primary repair of the injured ligament (Clinical Table: Scapholunate Dissociation). Simple passage of a tendon strip from lunate to scaphoid to recreate the interosseous ligament and the use of K wires or interosseous screws to create a scapholunate fibrous syndesmosis or arthrodesis have not worked well secondary to the high forces present between the scaphoid and lunate. For these reasons, we prefer one of several intercarpal fusions for the treatment of chronic fixed scapholunate subluxation without degenerative joint disease (DJD).

SCAPHOTRAPEZIOTRAPEZOID FUSION (TRISCAPHE FUSION)

Watson et al. (15) advocated the triscaphe arthrodesis to normalize load transmission across the chronically injured wrist. The STT joint is exposed through a dorsoradial transverse incision, by developing the interval between the radial wrist extensor tendons. Between 5 and 8 mm of the radial styloid is excised to increase exposure and prevent later impingement. The articular surfaces of the scaphoid, trapezium, and trapezoid are removed; and subcortical exposure of the distal scaphoid pole increases the cancellous fusion bed. Two K wires are preset in the trapezoid; they will later be drilled into the distal scaphoid pole. The bone graft is obtained from the distal radius through a separate incision and is packed into the excavated cavity. The scaphoid is held in the reduced position (50° radioscaphoid angle), and the preset K wires are passed into the bone (Fig. 2.15).

A long arm thumb spica cast that includes the index and long digits is worn for 4 weeks, followed by immobilization in a short arm cast for 4 weeks. At 8 weeks, the K wires are removed and range of motion exercises with removable splinting is started.

It is important to maintain the external dimensions of the three-bone unit during excision and grafting and to maintain the normal alignment of the three bones during reduction and pinning. Kleinman and Carroll (16) reported a 52% complication rate in 47 wrists treated with STT fusion for scaphoid instability; most of the complications were related to scaphoid malposition.

SCAPHOLUNATE ADVANCED COLLAPSE

Salvage procedures are indicated for chronic scaphoid instability associated with advanced degenerative disease and carpal collapse. Complete wrist arthrodesis is rarely indicated, as proximal row carpectomy, or scapholunate advanced collapse (SLAC), wrist reconstruction can generally restore a functional arc of motion and toleration of moderate manual loads (17). The proximal row carpectomy provides satisfactory pain relief and a large flexion–extension arc; is technically simple; and avoids the complications of nonunion, pin tract infection, and lengthy immobilization. SLAC wrist reconstruction may be best reserved for patients with capitolunate degenerative disease.

PROXIMAL ROW CARPECTOMY

For proximal row carpectomy, a 5-cm dorsal longitudinal incision is centered over the third extensor compartment, and a distal portion of the retinaculum is incised to retract the EPL tendon. The radiocarpal capsule is incised transversely, and the second and fourth extensor compartments may be retracted for exposure by limited subperiosteal dissection. The capsular incision is extended in an inverted T along the axis of the capitate. A threaded Steinmann pin is drilled into the scaphoid proximal pole to facilitate excision, and the scaphoid is divided at its waist with a saw or osteotome. Complete scaphoid excision requires careful circumferential dissection to avoid injury to the important palmar capsular ligaments. The lunate and triquetrum are excised in a similar fashion, using threaded Steinmann pins for leverage. A limited radial styloidectomy may be performed, but care should be taken to preserve the essential radioscaphocapitate ligament, preventing ulnar translation. The capitate is then settled into the lunate fossa (Fig. 2.16).

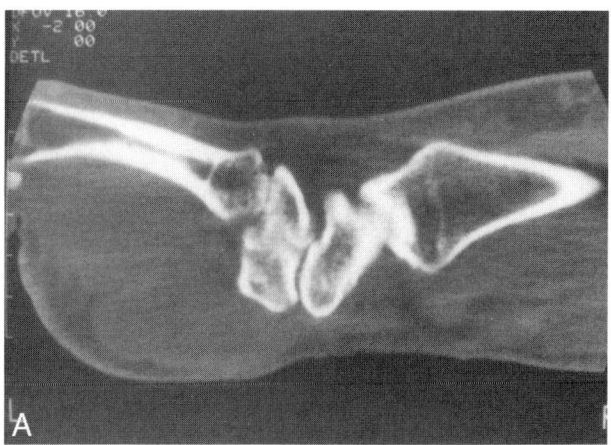

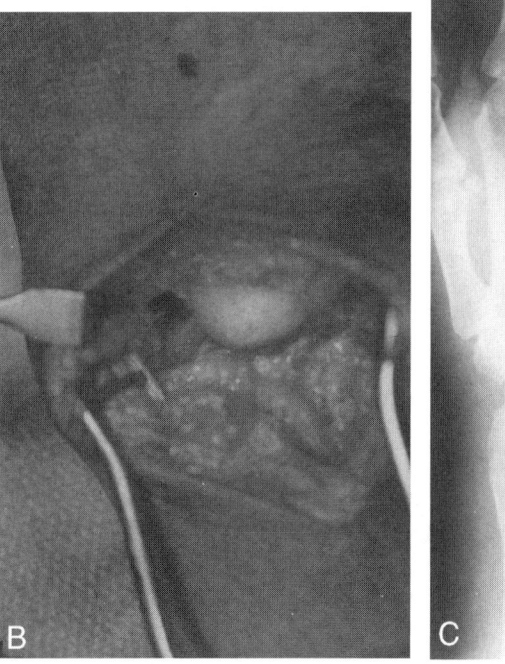
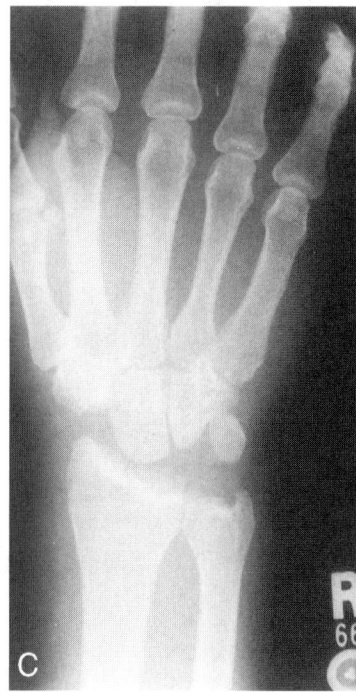

Figure 2.16. A. Chronic scapholunate dissociation with degenerative changes noted at the scaphoid proximal pole and dorsal pole of lunate. **B.** Following proximal row carpectomy, the capitate remains tethered by strong palmar ligaments. **C.** Postoperative appearance.

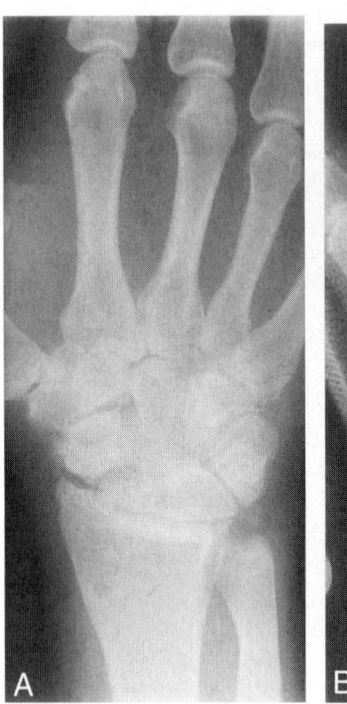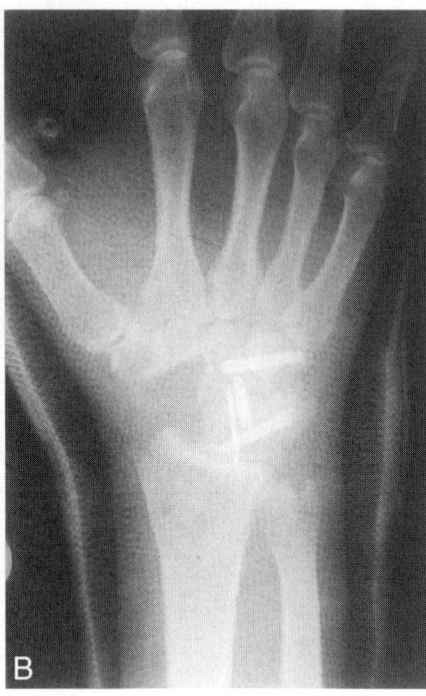

Figure 2.17. A. Chronic scaphoid nonunion with SLAC degenerative changes. **B.** Following scaphoid excision and capitolunotriquetrohamate fusion.

Postsurgery, the wrist is immobilized in 0° to 5° of extension for 3 weeks, and early range of motion exercises are begun. Although some patients return to heavy manual labor following this procedure, others report a lack of confidence in their repaired wrist. Grip strength and range of motion average 65 to 75% of the opposite side. Complications are few, and residual stiffness is related to excessive postoperative immobilization. While some authors have reported success using soft tissue interposition to modify this technique for patients with proximal capitate arthritis, most authors favor scaphoid excision and complete midcarpal fusion (SLAC wrist procedure) in these advanced cases.

SCAPHOID EXCISION AND FOUR-CORNER FUSION

The SLAC wrist reconstruction is designed to eliminate the arthritic scaphoid, stabilize the midcarpal joint, and transmit the load to the preserved radiolunate joint. The scaphoid is no longer replaced with silicone, because long-term follow-up demonstrated silicone fragmentation and synovitis.

The carpus is exposed through a dorsal longitudinal incision and inverted T capsular reflection, as described above. Limited subperiosteal dissection of the second and fourth extensor compartments increases exposure and provides a metaphyseal site for the bone graft. Complete scaphoid excision may be facilitated with a threaded Steinmann pin used as a joystick, and great care is taken to protect the palmar capsular ligaments. The articular surfaces of the lunate, capitate, hamate, and triquetrum are denuded; and the bone graft is packed in the intercarpal spaces. K wires or cannulated screws are used to fix the capitolunate, lunotriquetral, and capitohamate joints (Fig. 2.17).

Depending on the rigidity of fixation, the arm is immobilized for 4 weeks in a long arm cast and 2 to 4 weeks in a short arm thumb spica cast. Pin removal is performed at 6 to 8 weeks, when radiographs demonstrate crossing trabeculae.

WRIST ARTHRODESIS

Wrist arthrodesis restores a stable and high-demand platform for the hand at the expense of complete loss of wrist motion. It is best indicated for patients who have experienced several failed wrist procedures or who have advanced degenerative arthritis of the entire radiocarpal joint. Despite previous reports of high nonunion rates, recent techniques of dorsal wrist plating offer a 100% fusion rate with relatively few complications.

The entire carpus and distal radius are exposed through a long dorsal incision over the third extensor compartment. Wide subperiosteal exposure of the extensor tendons is performed after retraction of the EPL tendon, and Lister's tubercle is removed. The radiocarpal and all intercarpal joint spaces are exposed to bleeding cancellous bone. A local bone graft is obtained through a dorsal metaphyseal window, 3 cm proximal to the radial articular surface, and is packed into the excavated joint spaces. A precontoured plate (Synthes, USA) is fixed in compression, spanning the carpus from the radius to the middle metacarpal. Fusion of the index carpal–metacarpal (CMC) joint is optional. Excision of the distal ulna, if not performed primarily, may sometimes be required as a secondary procedure.

The patient is splinted postsurgery until the arthrodesis is solid (usually 6 to 8 weeks), and active light use of the hand and digits is encouraged in the postoperative period.

SUMMARY

Wrist hyperextension injuries, particularly in combination with ulnar deviation and intracarpal supination, cause a predictable and progressive disruption of the intrinsic and the extrinsic ligament that support the carpus. Perilunate dislocation and lunate dislocation present the most extreme form of carpal ligamentous injury; long-term outcome has been reported to be bleak, particularly in missed or neglected injuries. Far more commonly, the scapholunate interosseous ligament is disrupted, either alone or in combination with extrinsic wrist ligament injuries. Primary repair of the scapholunate interosseous ligament is indicated to prevent the otherwise inexorable progression to dorsal intercalated segment instability (DISI) and degenerative arthritis. Late cases of wrist collapse are best treated by partial intercarpal fusion, proximal row carpectomy, or complete wrist arthrodesis.

REFERENCES

1. Gelberman RH, Gross MS. The vascularity of the wrist: identification of arterial patterns at risk. Clin Orthop 1986;202:40–49.
2. Sanders WE. Evaluation of the humpback scaphoid by computed tomography in the longitudinal axial plane of the scaphoid. J Hand Surg 1988;13A:182–187.
3. Gellman H, Caputo RJ, Carter V, et al. Comparison of short and long thumb-spica casts for nondisplaced fractures of the carpal scaphoid. J Bone Joint Surg 1989;71A:354–357.
4. Adams BD, Frykman GK, Taleisnik J. Treatment of scaphoid nonunion with casting and pulsed electromagnetic fields: a study continuation. J Hand Surg 1992;17A:910–914.
5. Zaidemberg C, Siebert JW, Angrigiani C. A new vascularized bone graft for scaphoid nonunion. J Hand Surg 1991;16A:474–478.
6. Watson HK, Pitts EC, Ashmead D IV, et al. Dorsal approach to scaphoid nonunion. J Hand Surg 1993;18A:359–365.
7. Mack GR, Bosse MJ, Gelberman RH, Yu E. The natural history of scaphoid non-union. J Bone Joint Surg 1984;66A:504–509.
8. Green DP. The effect of avascular necrosis on Russe bone grafting for scaphoid nonunion. J Hand Surg 1985;10A:597–605.
9. Fernandez DL. A technique for anterior wedge-shaped grafts for scaphoid nonunions with carpal instability. J Hand Surg 1984;9A:733–737.
10. Mayfield JK, Johnson RP, Kilcoyne RK. Carpal dislocations: pathomechanics and progressive perilunar instability. J Hand Surg 1980;5A:226–241.
11. Linscheid RL, Dobyns JH, Beabout JW, Bryan RS. Traumatic instability of the wrist. J Bone Joint Surg 1972;54A:1262–1267.
12. Watson H, Ballet FL. The SLAC wrist: scapholunate advanced collapse pattern of degenerative arthritis. J Hand Surg 1984;9A:358–365.
13. Blatt G. Capsulodesis in reconstructive hand surgery. Dorsal capsulodesis for the unstable scaphoid and volar capsulodesis following excision of the distal ulna. Hand Clin 1987;3:81–102.
14. Lavernia CJ, Cohen MS, Taleisnik J. Treatment of scapholunate dissociation by ligamentous repair and capsulodesis. J Hand Surg 1992;17A:354–359.
15. Watson HK, Ryu J, Akelman E. Limited triscaphoid intercarpal arthrodesis for rotatory subluxation of the scaphoid. J Bone Joint Surg 1986;68A:345–349.
16. Kleinman WB, Carroll C IV. Scapho-trapezio-trapezoid arthrodesis for treatment of chronic static and dynamic scapho-lunate instability: a 10-year perspective on pitfalls and complications. J Hand Surg 1990;15A:408–414.
17. Wyrick JD, Stern PJ, Kiefhaber TR. Motion-preserving procedures in the treatment of scapholunate advanced collapse wrist: proximal row carpectomy versus four-corner arthrodesis. J Hand Surg 1995;6A:965–970.

c h a p t e r

S. Steven Yang

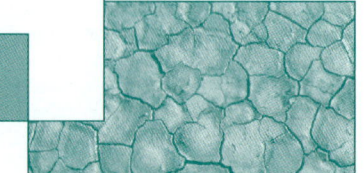

Fractures and Dislocations of the Hand

Skeletal injuries of the hand are extremely common because of the vulnerable exposure of the extremity in occupational and athletic activities. The hand is used defensively in falls and aggressively in altercations and is frequently damaged in gestures of frustration. A clear understanding of the complex anatomic relationship of the skeletal and soft tissue components of the hand is required to correct these injuries. Careful examination of the extremity will elucidate the exact nature of the injury. The treatment of metacarpal and phalangeal fractures or dislocations is directed at eliminating skeletal deformities and bony obstructions during healing while allowing early joint motion and tendon gliding to avoid contractures and adhesions. Although most hand fractures can be treated nonoperatively, advances in miniature internal and external fixation devices are broadening the indications for surgical interventions.

RELEVANT ANATOMY AND PATHOGENESIS

Fractures and dislocations of the hand require precise restoration of normal anatomy and attention to soft tissue injuries to avoid altering the functional unit. Fractures of the distal phalanx, for instance, are often associated with injuries to the specialized structures of the nail plate and bed. At the base of the distal phalanx are the insertions of the flexor digitorum profundus volarly and the terminal extensor tendon dorsally. Avulsion fractures of these tendons require specific attention.

The central slip of the extensor mechanism inserts at the dorsal proximal lip of the middle phalanx, whereas the flexor digitorum superficialis has a broad insertion along the volar shaft of the middle phalanx. The proximal phalanx is enveloped by the extensor hood dorsally. The interossei are palmar to the intermetacarpal ligaments and have insertions on the base of the proximal phalanx.

These relationships account for predictable patterns of displacement and angulation in hand fractures.

Proximal phalangeal fractures typically exhibit an apex palmar angulation as a result of an imbalance of forces generated by the flexor and extensor tendons (Fig. 3.1) (1). The interossei flex the proximal fragment, whereas the extensor hood acts to further shorten and angulate the bone. Progressive palmar angulation of the proximal phalanx effectively shortens the skeletal length (markedly dorsal), resulting in an incompetent extensor mechanism and an extensor lag. Angulation of middle phalangeal fractures depends on the location of the fracture (Fig. 3.2) (1). Fractures at the proximal one-fourth of the phalanx angulate with the apex dorsal as a result of the unbalanced pull of the central slip. Midshaft fractures can angulate dorsally or palmarly. Fractures at the distal one-fourth angulate with the apex palmar as a result of the strong flexion force of the superficialis on the proximal fragment.

Apex dorsal angulation of the shaft is typical in metacarpal fractures because of the pull of the interossei (Fig. 3.3). The border metacarpals (index and little) are more likely to shorten, since they do not have the suspensory effect of the adjacent metacarpals that act as a support through the intermetacarpal ligaments. Metacarpal and phalangeal shaft fractures can be classified by fracture pattern: transverse, oblique, spiral, and comminuted (Fig. 3.4). Axial loading forces generally result in transverse fractures. Torsional forces create either spiral or oblique patterns. Direct impact often causes comminuted and shortened fractures.

Because of the joint anatomy, the capsule and collateral ligaments of the metacarpophalangeal joint are in maximal tension in the fully flexed posture. Therefore, when splinted or cast, the metacarpophalangeal joints should be placed in flexion to avoid joint contractures. The interphalangeal joints are more likely to become

Figure 3.1. Typical apex volar angulation of a proximal phalanx shaft fracture. The proximal fragment is flexed by the bony insertion of the interossei into the base of the proximal phalanx. Collapse at the fracture site is aggravated by further pull on the extensor hood by the extrinsic tendons.

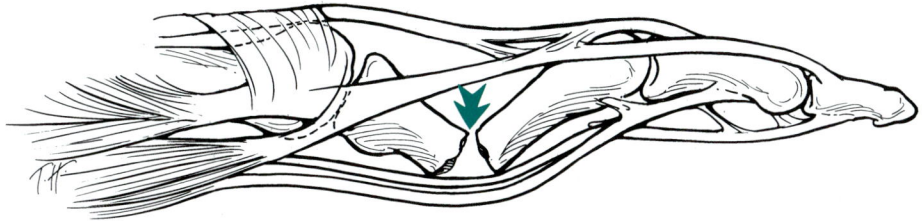

Figure 3.2. There is a broad insertion of the flexor superficialis along the shaft of the middle phalanx. Distal fractures are likely to have an apex volar angulation because of the strong pull of the superficialis tendon on the proximal fragment. Fractures through the base are more likely to angulate dorsally because of the extension force of the central slip on the proximal fragment and the flexion force on the distal fragment by the superficialis.

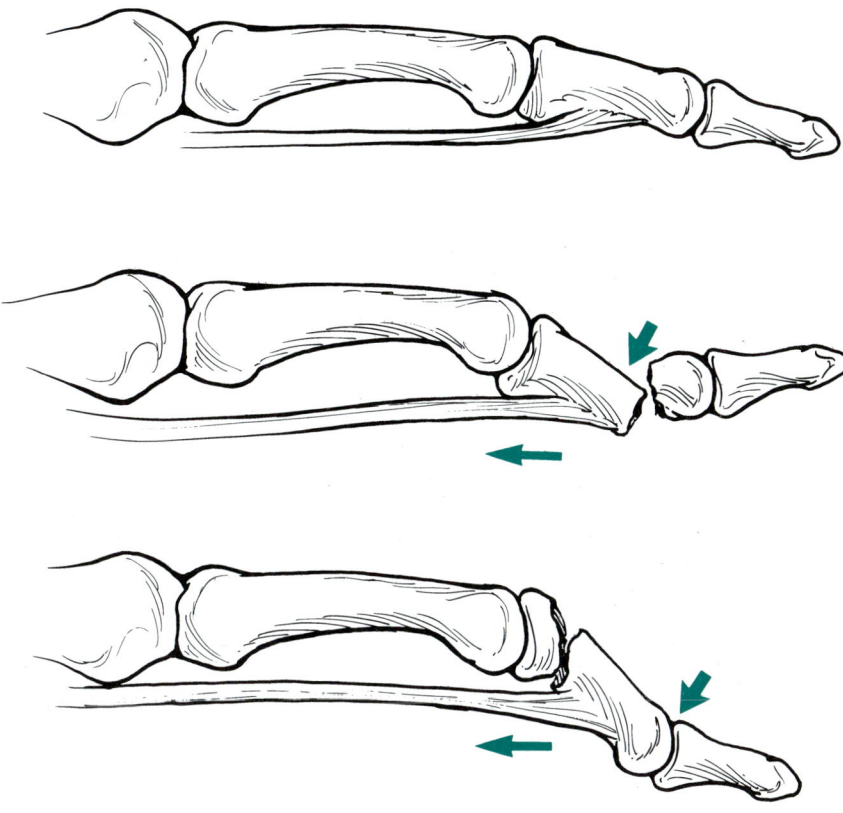

stiff in flexion; thus they should be immobilized in extension.

INITIAL FINDINGS, PHYSICAL EXAMINATION, AND DIAGNOSIS

A thorough history and physical examination are important in the evaluation of any fracture of the hand. A careful history elucidates the age and cause of the fracture or dislocation and alerts the physician to the likelihood of other injuries. Treatment choices may be affected by the patient's occupation, handedness, needs for use, and desired cosmesis.

Examination of the hand should identify the area of maximum tenderness, the location of any open wounds, the condition of all flexor and extensor tendons, and the neurovascular status. Evaluation of the digits for radial/ulnar deviation, volar/dorsal angulation, and length should be made both clinically and radiographically. Rotational alignment, must be assessed clinically, even when radiographs are taken. If the clinical examination is difficult because of pain, digital or wrist block anesthesia can be effective in allowing a full active and passive examination.

RADIOLOGIC STUDIES

Radiographs should always include true AP, lateral, and oblique views of the involved digit or metacarpal. For metacarpal fractures, 10° pronated and supinated views can help visualize the index and fifth metacarpals, respectively. Because of superimposition of the digits in a lateral view of the hand, a fan lateral is recommended in which the fingers are flexed an increasing amount from radial to ulnar, preventing overlap of the fingers. For intra-articular fractures, oblique and Brewerton views may help evaluate the articular surfaces. Occasionally CT scans or tomograms may be necessary to better visualize intra-articular injuries.

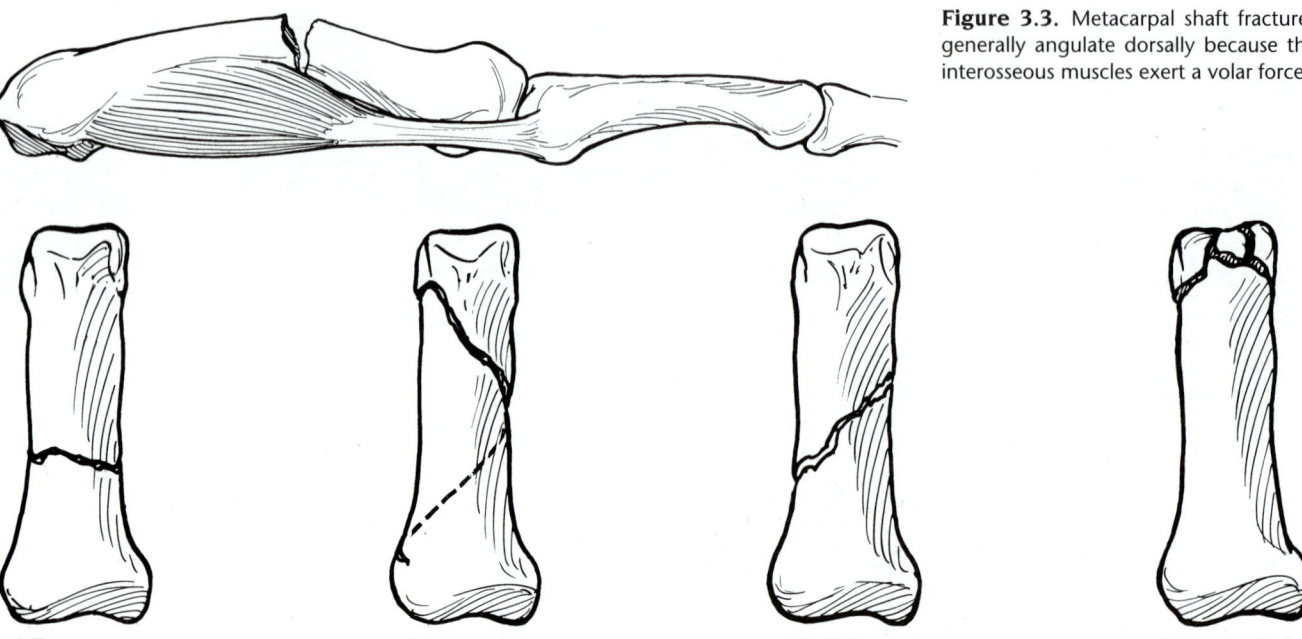

Figure 3.3. Metacarpal shaft fractures generally angulate dorsally because the interosseous muscles exert a volar force.

I. Transverse

II. Long spiral

III. Oblique

IV. Intra-articular

Figure 3.4. Phalangeal and metacarpal shaft fracture patterns.

TREATMENT

Phalangeal Fractures

NONOPERATIVE TREATMENT

Extra-articular distal phalangeal fractures are usually treated closed with protective splinting. The treatment of distal phalangeal fractures is straightforward; and any associated problems result from soft tissue injury, such as nail bed injuries, loss of tissue, and neuromas. In one study, more than 70% of patients at the 6-month follow-up continued to have functional impairment, pain, numbness, nail abnormalities, or less than 45° of active distal interphalangeal (DIP) joint flexion (2).

Mallet fractures are bony avulsions of the terminal extensor tendon insertion at the base of the distal phalanx. The majority of mallet fractures should be treated nonoperatively with extension splinting for 6 to 8 weeks. Conventionally, surgical treatment is reserved for mallet fractures that demonstrate subluxation of the DIP joint, although good results with conservative treatment have been reported regardless of joint subluxation or the size and amount of displacement of the bone fragment (3).

It is important to distinguish stable from unstable fracture patterns in the initial management of a phalangeal fracture. Nondisplaced fractures tend to be stable and can usually be immobilized for 3 weeks before beginning range of motion exercises. Occasionally, the fracture will slip and a repeat radiograph should be taken after several days and at weekly intervals to ensure maintenance of alignment.

Displaced fractures can be reduced under digital block anesthesia. No more than 10° of angulation in any plane of a proximal or middle phalangeal shaft fracture or any rotational malalignment should be accepted. The digit can be immobilized in malleable finger splints or in gutter splints or can be buddy taped to the adjacent finger if early motion can be safely initiated. Immobilization should hold the metacarpophalangeal (MP) joints in full flexion and the interphalangeal joints in extension to avoid capsular contractures. Active motion should begin no later than 4 weeks and preferably at 3 weeks, if clinical stability and healing permits (4). Radiographic signs of union lag behind clinical healing and should not be used as an indication for beginning range of motion exercises.

OPERATIVE TREATMENT

The treatment of choice for unstable phalangeal shaft fractures is fixation with smooth pins (Clinical Table). If open reduction is necessary, then rigid internal fixation is preferred, because it facilitates early active motion and improves the functional result. It has been demonstrated that internal fixation of hand fractures using lag screws, tension banding, or plate and screws reduced the incidence of joint stiffness and tendon adhesions (Fig. 3.5) (5). Both midaxial and straight dorsal extensor splitting approaches are possible.

External fixation offers advantages in the treatment of certain phalangeal fractures. Indications for external fixation include severely contaminated soft tissue trauma, gunshot wounds, severe intra-articular fractures, segmental bone loss, and highly comminuted fractures (6). Midlateral insertions are preferred, except in the proximal aspect of the proximal phalanx, where a dorsolateral in-

Clinical Table: Fractures and Dislocations of the Hand

Procedure	Indications	Technique	Anatomy	Pitfalls
Phalangeal internal fixation	• Mallet fractures with volar subluxation • Rotational, angular malalignment • Intra-articular fractures • Unstable fractures	• Percutaneous pinning • Interfragmentary screws • Plate and screws	• Terminal extensor tendon • Extensor hood • Neurovascular bundles	• Joint stiffness • Tendon adhesions • Malalignment
Phalangeal external fixation	• Segmental bone loss • Severe intra-articular comminution • Contaminated soft tissue injury	• Mini-external fixation	• Extensor hood • Neurovascular bundles	• Pin tract infection • Nonunion
Metacarpal internal fixation	• Unacceptable alignment • Multiple metacarpal fractures • Intra-articular fractures • Some severely angulated neck fractures • Unstable fractures	• Percutaneous pinning • Interfragmentary screws • Plate and screws	• Intermetacarpal ligaments • Extensor tendons	• Joint stiffness • Tendon adhesions • Malalignment
Metacarpal external fixation	• Segmental bone loss • Contaminated soft tissue injury	• Mini-external fixation	• Extensor tendons	• Nonunion • Pin tract infection
Volar plate arthroplasty	• Unstable proximal interphalangeal fracture dislocations	• Eaton-Littler	• Palmar plate • Central slip • Collateral ligaments	• Joint stiffness
Acute joint fusion	• Unsalvageable intra-articular fractures	• Crossed K wires • Herbert screw • 90–90 wire • Plate and screws	• Joint of function	• Failure of fusion
Metacarpo-phalangeal or proximal interphalangeal arthroplasty	• Unsalvageable intra-articular fractures	• Silastic arthroplasty	• Collateral ligaments	• Instability • Silicone synovitis • Fracture of implant

sertion is used because of space constraints. The final functional results depend on the severity of the initial injury (7). The advantages of mini-external fixation in finger fractures include minimal or no surgical exposure of the fracture site, adequate stability, and the ability to manipulate an inadequately reduced or secondarily displaced fracture.

Injuries of the Proximal Interphalangeal Joint

NONOPERATIVE TREATMENT

Pure dorsal dislocations of the proximal interphalangeal (PIP) joint are the most common articular injury in the hand. Interposition of the volar plate may infrequently necessitate open reduction. Once reduced, the PIP joint is usually stable and can be immediately mobilized with buddy taping to the adjacent digit. Development of a flexion contracture is the most common long-term sequela.

Palmar dislocations are a more rare and severe injury that sometimes include collateral ligament ruptures proximally and disruption of the central tendon. The lateral bands or central tendon often becomes interposed in the joint, blocking reduction. If full active extension of the PIP joint can be achieved after reduction, then early motion can be begun. If the patient cannot perform full active extension, then rupture of the central slip must have occurred and the PIP should be immobilized in full extension and treated as a closed boutonniere injury.

Fracture subluxations and dislocations at the PIP joint occur either dorsally with volar lip fractures or volarly with dorsal avulsion fractures at the insertion of the central slip. Dorsal fracture dislocations are usually axial compression injuries and can be comminuted, often involving a sub-

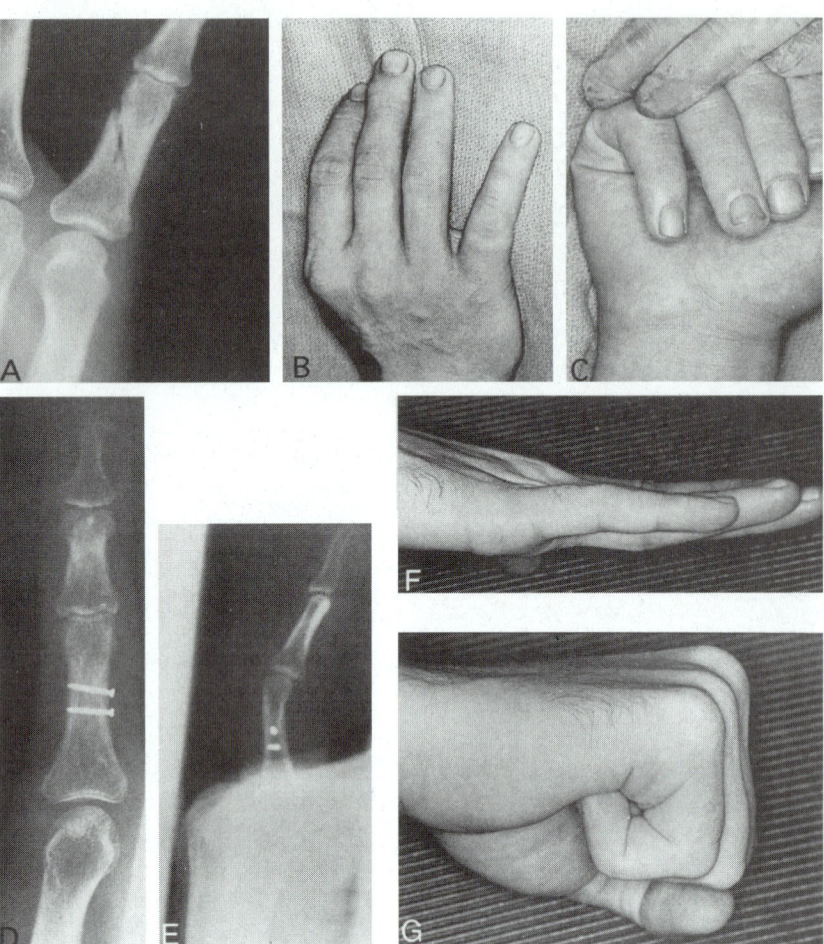

Figure 3.5. A. A minimally displaced spiral fracture of the proximal phalanx. **B** and **C.** Note the significant rotational deformity of the fifth finger. **D** and **E.** Open reduction and internal fixation with two 1.0-mm AO microscrews was performed. Immediate active and passive range of motion was practiced. **F** and **G.** Full range of motion was restored without rotatory deformity. Reprinted with permission from Orthopaedic knowledge updates: trauma. Rosemont, IL: American Academy of Orthopaedic Surgeons, 1996.

stantial portion of the volar articular surface. Reduction and extension block splinting in moderate flexion can usually maintain a reduced joint when less than 40% of the articular surface is fractured (8,9).

Volar fracture dislocations with central slip avulsions should be treated as a pure volar dislocation, and static splinting in full extension for the boutonniere component should be performed. Operative treatment should be considered only when a congruent joint reduction cannot be achieved or maintained.

OPERATIVE TREATMENT

When a congruent reduction cannot be maintained after reduction of a dorsal fracture dislocation, volar plate arthroplasty as described by Eaton and Malerich (8) or internal fixation of the fragment if it is large enough (9) should be considered (Fig. 3.6). Volar plate arthroplasty provides a volar restraint to dorsal subluxation and resurfaces an irregular and deficient volar articular surface.

Intra-articular fractures at the base of the middle phalanx unassociated with avulsions or dislocations can be treated with percutaneous Kirschner (K) wires or screws if the fragments are of sufficient size. Severe comminution or articular surface depression may necessitate static exter-

nal fixation, hinged external fixation, or dynamic traction splints. Both unicondylar and bicondylar fractures of the proximal phalanx are amenable to either K wire fixation or miniscrew and microscrew fixation. The minicondylar plate has also been used for intra-articular fractures.

Treatment alternatives for unsalvageable PIP joints are unattractive. Arthrodesis, silastic arthroplasty, and interpositional arthroplasty all restore length and stability but sacrifice much or all mobility. Swanson hinged implants used acutely for unsalvageable intra-articular fractures obtained an average active range of motion of only 29° in the PIP joint (10).

Metacarpal Fractures

NONOPERATIVE TREATMENT

Metacarpal neck fractures are the result of an axial load against a clenched fist and most commonly involve the ring and little fingers. Most authors would agree that any rotational or lateral deviation deformity of the metacarpal should be corrected; however, the amount of apex dorsal angulation (secondary to the pull of the interossei) that can be accepted varies. Less than 15° should be accepted in the index and long finger metacarpals because of their

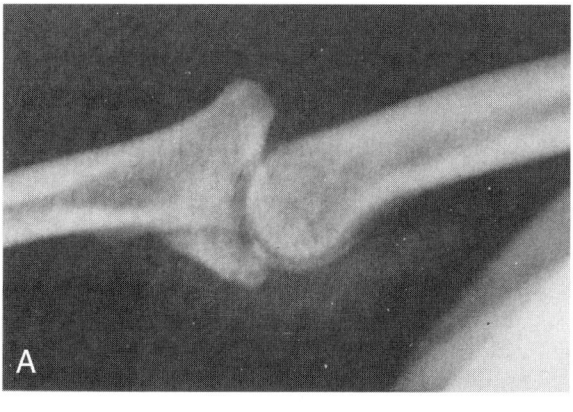
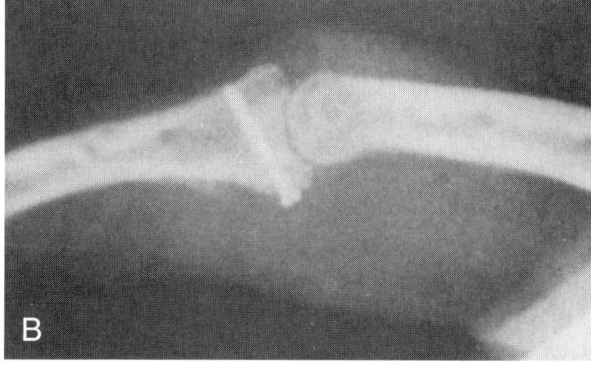
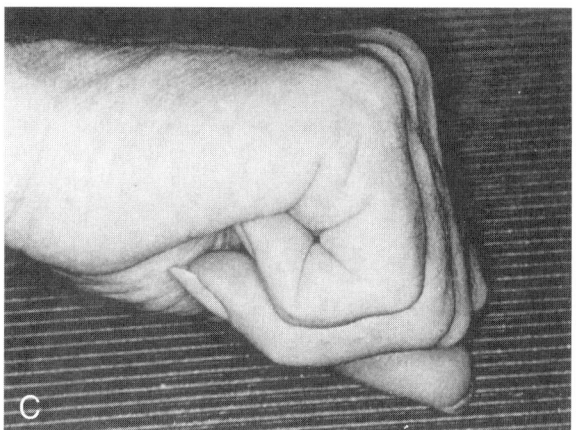
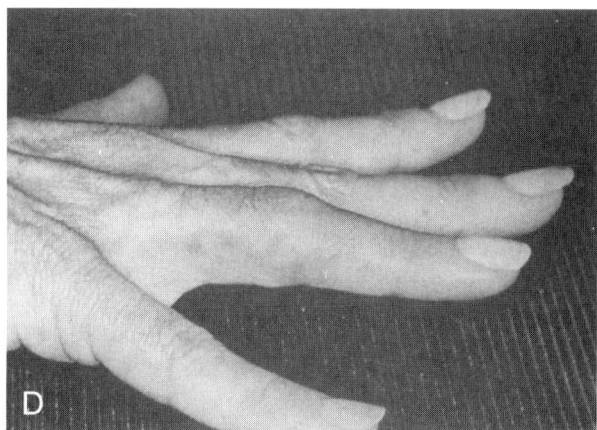

Figure 3.6. **A.** A dorsal fracture dislocation. **B.** Open reduction and internal fixation with a 1.0-mm microscrew and hinged external fixation for restoration of the articular surface and immediate range of motion were performed. **C** and **D.** Functional range of motion has been restored. Reprinted with permission from Orthopaedic knowledge updates: trauma. Rosemont, IL: American Academy of Orthopaedic Surgeons, 1996.

more rigid carpometacarpal (CMC) joints. In the more mobile ring and little fingers, up to 35° and 45° of dorsal angulation, respectively, can be accepted. However, even angular deformities of up to 70° degrees in the fifth metacarpal have been shown not to be associated with functional loss (11). Immobilization with splints, casts, and functional braces have been described.

The majority of metacarpal shaft fractures can be effectively treated with closed reduction and external splinting. Although angulation of metacarpal shaft fractures is generally well tolerated, reduction should be considered in fractures angulated in excess of 30° in the small finger, 20° in the ring finger, and any angulation in the middle and index fingers (12). Shortening of up to 0.5 cm in comminuted fractures does not affect function (13). Traditional treatment methods have always involved immobilization of the wrist and fingers or, as in phalangeal fractures, dorsal extension blocking splints to hold the wrist in extension and the MP joints in flexion.

OPERATIVE TREATMENT

Surgical treatment is recommended in metacarpal neck fractures for some open fractures, fractures with rotational or lateral malalignment, and fractures sufficiently angulated to produce a dorsal prominence and knuckle defor-

mity in patients who demand perfect cosmesis. In metacarpal shaft fractures, any rotational malalignment is not well tolerated. Only 5° of rotation causes 1.5 cm of finger overlap (14).

Open or percutaneous fixation of metacarpal shaft fractures is indicated for unstable fractures, displaced intraarticular fractures, displaced open fractures, multiple fractures, and fractures with segmental bone loss or concomitant soft tissue injury. Although the standard for fixation of metacarpal shaft fractures has been percutaneous fixation with K wires, open fixation with miniature AO internal fixation systems is increasingly used (Fig. 3.7) (15,16). Approximately 10% of metacarpal (and phalangeal) fractures are either irreducible by closed manipulation or unsuitable for percutaneous pinning and require open treatment (17). With new miniscrews and microscrews and plates, rigid fixation and early mobilization of the digit are possible. For open reduction, straight dorsal surgical approaches are recommended.

External fixation of the metacarpals is indicated for open fractures, severely comminuted fractures, and fractures with severe soft tissue injury or bone loss. The advantages and disadvantages are similar to those mentioned for external fixation of phalangeal fractures;

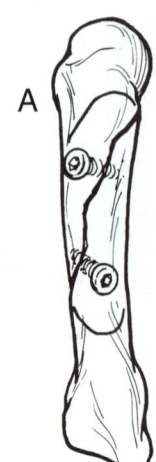
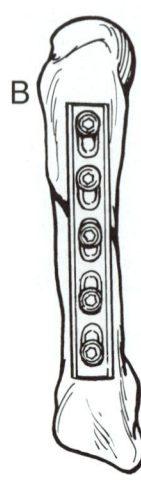
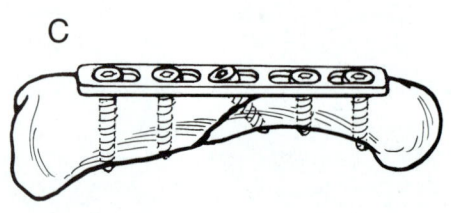
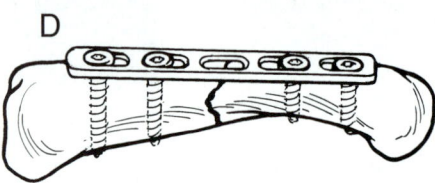

Figure 3.7. A. Lag screw fixation of a spiral metacarpal shaft fracture. **B.** Plate fixation of an oblique metacarpal shaft fracture with a separate lag screw across the fracture. **C.** Plate fixation of an oblique metacarpal shaft fracture with a lag screw across the fracture inserted through the plate. **D.** Plate fixation of a transverse metacarpal shaft fracture.

however, the functional results are generally better than in phalangeal fractures (18,19).

Fractures at the base of the metacarpals are relatively stable; however, even minor rotational malalignment at this level will be greatly magnified at the fingertips and will interfere with function. Fractures in this region are usually the result of crush injuries but may also be caused by avulsions of the extensor carpi radialis brevis or longus at the base of the middle and index metacarpals (20).

Articular Injuries of the MP and CMC Joints

Injuries of the metacarpophalangeal joint are less common than those of the proximal interphalangeal joint, but a poor outcome at this joint can have a profound effect on hand function. Intra-articular fractures with large articular fragments can be reduced open and fixed with K wires, minifragment or microfragment screws or minicondylar plates. Small ligamentous avulsions of bone can often be treated closed in the index through little fingers. Dislocations of the MP joint are typically dorsal. Simple dislocations can generally be reduced closed; however, complex dislocations resist reduction by traction and manipulation because of interposition of the volar plate and the noose effect of the lumbricals on one side and the flexor tendons on the other side of the metacarpal neck. For these irreducible dislocations, open reduction through a volar approach is recommended.

Fractures and dislocations of the carpometacarpal joints of the fingers are relatively rare and are often diagnosed late because of inadequate radiographs at the time of initial evaluation. They are usually the result of high-energy injuries. Swelling and local tenderness over the joints should raise the surgeon's suspicions. These dislocations can often be managed with closed reduction and percutaneous pinning; however, open reduction using a dorsal surgical approach may be necessary when there are interposed fracture fragments or ligamentous tissue (21,22).

Fractures and Dislocations of the Thumb

Fractures of the phalanges of the thumb should be evaluated and treated in the same way as are finger fractures. Fractures of the thumb metacarpal are, however, distinct from those of other metacarpals. Shaft fractures are rare because of the lack of structures fixing the proximal portion of the metacarpal. Forces are transmitted through the rigid diaphysis to the softer cancellous base, where metaphyseal or intra-articular fractures occur. Angulation of extra-articular base fractures of up to 30° is well tolerated because of the large compensatory motion available at the CMC joint. Excessive angulation, however, can result in adaptive hyperextension at the MP joint.

The carpometacarpal joint of the thumb is a highly specialized articulation designed to allow considerable motion required for pinch, grasp, and opposition while resisting joint compressive forces that are magnified more than 10-fold through the thumb metacarpal. Fractures and dislocations at the basilar joint of the thumb are caused by an axial force directed through a partially flexed metacarpal shaft. A Bennett's fracture is an intra-articular fracture with a small volar metacarpal fragment. A Rolando's fracture is essentially a T or Y intra-articular fracture that is often comminuted and results from a great injuring force. The volar fragments in both fracture configurations remain attached to the anterior oblique ligament, while the base of the shaft is displaced in a dorsal and radial direction by the pull of the abductor pollicis longus and the distal metacarpal is adducted by the adductor pollicis muscle.

Disagreement on the treatment of these fractures centers around the acceptable amount of intra-articular displacement. Follow-up studies of Bennett's and Rolando's fractures found no correlation between articular incongruity and symptomatic posttraumatic osteoarthritis (23,24). More recent reports advocate precise reconstitution of the articular surface by open reduction, if necessary (25).

Pure dislocations of the thumb carpometacarpal joint are rare. Although reduction of the joint is relatively simple, maintaining the reduction can be problematic. Immobilization in abduction, extension, and pronation best stabilizes the joint. Percutaneous pinning for 6 weeks may be necessary to maintain the reduction. Chronic instability of the thumb CMC joint may require stabilization with ligament reconstruction as described by Eaton and Littler (26).

Open Fractures and Infection

The abundant vascularity of the hand makes open fractures less susceptible to infection than are other open fractures; rates range from 6 to 11% (27,28). Infection rates are significantly increased in the presence of gross wound contamination, extensive soft tissue and skeletal crush injury, systemic illness, or a delay in treatment greater than 24 h (27). Nevertheless, delays in treatment of up to 12 h do not increase the incidence of infection or affect outcome (28). Infection rates are not increased by the presence of internal fixation; immediate wound closure; large wound size; or tendon, nerve, and vascular injuries. Delayed wound closure is still recommended for open injuries with gross contamination.

SUMMARY

The complex relationship of the anatomic components of the hand account for the predictable patterns of displacement and angulation in hand fractures. Knowledge of these factors during examination of the patient is required to successfully diagnose and treat these injuries. Fracture displacement, angulation, and shortening must be corrected, and articular congruity must be reestablished to restore normal function of the hand. Recent advances in the use of mini and micro screws and plates have enabled surgeons to perform accurate rigid internal fixation of fractures and facilitated earlier mobilization to avoid contractures and adhesions. New static and dynamic external fixation devices have been developed to better address highly comminuted or unstable intra-articular fractures of the hand.

REFERENCES

1. Agee J. Treatment principles for proximal and middle phalangeal fractures. Orthop Clin North Am 1992;23:35–40.
2. DaCruz DJ, Slade RJ, Malone W. Fractures of the distal phalanges. J Hand Surg 1988;13B:350–352.
3. Wehbe MA, Schneider LH. Mallet fractures. J Bone Joint Surg 1984; 66A:658–669.
4. Strickland JW, Steichen JB, Kleinman WB, et al. Phalangeal fractures: factors influencing digital performance. Orthop Rev 1982; 11:39–50.
5. Jabaley ME, Freeland AE. Rigid internal fixation in the hand: 104 cases. Plast Reconstr Surg 1986;77:288–297.
6. Nagy L. Static external fixation of finger fractures. Hand Clin 1993; 9:651–657.
7. Schuind F, Cooney WP, Burny F, An K. Small external fixation devices for the hand and wrist. Clin Orthop 1993;293:77–82.
8. Eaton RG, Malerich MM. Volar plate arthroplasty for the proximal interphalangeal joint: a ten year review. J Hand Surg 1980; 5A:260–268.
9. Durham-Smith G, MacCarten GM. Volar plate arthroplasty for closed proximal interphalangeal joint injuries. J Hand Surg 1992; 17B:422–428.
10. Nagle DJ, Ekenstam FW, Lister GD. Immediate silastic arthroplasty for non-salvageable intraarticular phalangeal fractures. Scand J Plast Reconstr Surg 1989;23:47–50.
11. Ford DJ, Ali MS, Steel WM. Fractures of the fifth metacarpal neck: is reduction or immobilisation necessary? J Hand Surg 1989; 14B:165–167.
12. Stern PJ. Fractures of the metacarpals and phalanges. In: Green DP, ed., Operative hand surgery. New York: Churchill Livingstone, 1993.
13. Burkhalter WE. Hand fractures. Instruct Course Lect 1990; 34:249–253.
14. Freeland AE, Jabaley ME, Hughs JL. Stable fixation of the hand and wrist. New York: Springer-Verlag, 1986.
15. Ford DJ, El-Haddidi S, Lunn PG, Burke FD. Fractures of the metacarpals: treatment by A.O. screw and plate fixation. J Hand Surg 1987;12B:34–37.
16. Bosscha K, Snellen JP. Internal fixation of metacarpal and phalangeal fractures with AO minifragment screws and plates: a prospective study. Injury 1993;24:166–168.
17. Melone CP. Rigid fixation of phalangeal and metacarpal fractures. Orthop Clin North Am 1986;17:421–435.
18. Shehadi SI. External fixation of metacarpal and phalangeal fractures. J Hand Surg 1991;16A:544–550.
19. Parsons SW, Fitzgerald JAW, Shearer JR. External fixation of unstable metacarpal and phalangeal fractures. J Hand Surg 1992; 17B:151–155.
20. Crichlow TPKR, Hoskinson J. Avulsion fracture of the index metacarpal base: three case reports. J Hand Surg 1988; 13B:212–214.
21. Gurland M. Carpometacarpal joint injuries of the fingers. Hand Clin 1992;8:733–744.
22. Lawlis JF, Gunther SF. Carpometacarpal dislocations: long-term follow-up. J Bone Joint Surg 1991;73A:52–58.
23. Cannon SR, Dowd GSE, Williams DH, Scott JM. A long-term study following Bennett's fracture. J Hand Surg 1986;11B:426–431.
24. Langhoff O, Andersen K, Kjaer-Petersen K. Rolando's fracture. J Hand Surg 1991;16B:454–459.
25. Kjaer-Petersen K, Langhoff O, Andersen K. Bennett's fracture. J Hand Surg 1990;15B:58–61.
26. Eaton RG, Littler JW. Ligament reconstruction for the painful thumb carpometacarpal joint. J Bone Joint Surg 1973; 55A:1655–1659.
27. Swanson TV, Szabo RM, Anderson DD. Open hand fractures: prognosis and classification. J Hand Surg 1991;16A:101–107.
28. McLain RF, Steyers C, Stoddard M. Infections in open fractures of the hand. J Hand Surg 1991;16A:109–112.

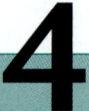
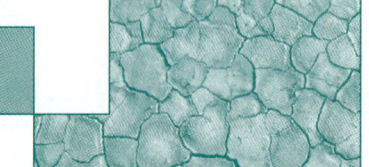

Arthroscopy of the Wrist

Arthroscopy of the wrist has become increasingly useful for both diagnosis and treatment of the painful wrist. Most technical advances in surgery begin with the simple notion of a better tool. As surgeons gain experience with the use and application of new technology, the basic concepts of how to treat the disorder are usually challenged and thus change. For instance, the initial goal of microsurgery was to permit the repair of small blood vessels; once this goal was met, the paradigm of wound treatment and soft tissue reconstruction was altered. Arthroscopy of the wrist began as an obvious technical expansion from the large joints. As technical proficiency advanced and the lesions of the wrist were more closely and completely observed, many concepts of anatomy, ligament injury, and pathology changed (1–3).

Using small arthroscopes, the surgeon can reliably inspect the painful wrist for ligament tears, osteochondral fractures, triangular fibrocartilage complex (TFCC) tears, and localized synovitis. Therapeutic wrist arthroscopy has also advanced. Smaller shavers and motorized burrs now make synovectomy, excision of small tears, and débridement of osteochondral defects relatively routine procedures. Surgeons are able to repair the TFCC by using a number of techniques that allow visualization for accurate placement of sutures (1,4–6).

This chapter reviews current techniques used for diagnostic and therapeutic arthroscopy of the wrist and provides practical and useful suggestions.

INDICATIONS

The indications for wrist arthroscopy generally fall into two categories. The first is to assess patients who have mechanical wrist pain that has not responded to nonoperative treatment. The second is to assess patients for whom a presumptive diagnosis has been made, such as a scapholunate ligament injury, triangular fibrocartilage tear, or osteochondral fracture. In the latter case, wrist arthroscopy is used to confirm the lesion, assess the ex-

tent of injury, and evaluate the possibility of arthroscopic treatment. If the lesion cannot be adequately addressed using arthroscopic techniques, the wrist can be treated by open surgery.

CLINICAL FINDINGS AND PHYSICAL EXAMINATION

Taking a careful history from the patient with wrist pain is crucial to successful treatment. The subject of wrist pain has been addressed in numerous texts and lies outside the more practical focus of this chapter. Every patient, however, must be carefully scrutinized and screened before any operative intervention can be considered.

A history of mechanical wrist pain usually begins with a specific injury or a repetitive mechanical stress, such as playing golf or tennis. The clinician should carefully retrace the onset of pain, its location, and its pattern of intensity, determine if there are provocative activities, and note whether the pain occurs at the time of use or at a later time. The clinician should record any clicks or clunks associated with the pain. In cases of significant ligament tears, such as scapholunate ligament injuries, patients may recall an initial serious fall with contemporaneous swelling. These injuries are often treated as a sprained wrist, and the more serious injury is not immediately discovered. The clinician should heed the adage: Beware of the sprained wrist.

The physical examination of the painful wrist is an art that should be constantly and progressively honed. The patient should be relaxed and sitting. The examiner should diligently search for a specific area of tenderness or signs of instability. The patient can usually localize or pinpoint the area of discomfort. In cases of instability, there may be a sense of weakness without a specific area of tenderness. An injection of lidocaine may help isolate the cause of pain to a particular location. If the patient has a generalized pattern of pain with poor temporal and anatomic specificity, the chances of a mechanical basis for the pain is low. The clinician should remember that patients with secondary gains might be influenced by their particular socioeconomic circumstances. Patients with, for example, workman's compensation or pending litigation should not be excluded from treatment solely on that basis.

RADIOLOGIC STUDIES

Imaging studies, beginning with plain x-rays in radial, ulnar deviation, and grip views, should be routine. A second tier of imaging studies should be considered if the diagnosis is not apparent. Technetium-99m bone scan, CT scans, and arthrography might also be indicated. Increasingly sophisticated software packages make MRI studies of the wrist a viable method of assessment, and arthrography has increasingly been shown to be of limited value (7). The quality of the magnet and the experience of the technical staff and radiologist are crucial to a useful and diagnostic MRI study of the wrist.

TREATMENT

Preparation for Arthroscopy

Before proceeding with arthroscopy, a presumptive diagnosis should be made, which provides two benefits. Surgeons enhance their skills of examination and overall evaluation by forcing themselves to make the diagnosis before looking. Second, surgeons should prepare the operating room and staff for possible repairs or reconstructive procedures that go beyond simple arthroscopic examination.

Many different operating room setups for arthroscopy of the wrist have been described. It is important to establish a consistent pattern so that the operating room personnel can anticipate what the surgeon will need. A list of equipment that is routinely used for arthroscopy of the wrist for diagnostic and a few specialized situations is shown in Table 4.1.

Axillary block anesthesia may be the preferred method of anesthetizing patients for two reasons. First, patients are generally comfortable with this kind of anesthesia and the recovery from it, when the technical expertise is available. Second, many patients appreciate the ability to view the video output while undergoing arthroscopy.

Technique

SETUP

A nonsterile tourniquet is applied to the upper arm before preparing the forearm, wrist, and hand. I prefer to use an arm board and simply affix the upper arm to the board with a nonsterile folded towel. The preparation and instrument setup are arranged so that no nonsterile component of the traction assembly is near the field. The surgeon must ensure that the entire field remains sterile in case

table	4.1	Routine Equipment for Arthroscopy of the Wrist

Diagnostic
  Short-barrel arthroscope (2.7 mm, 30°)
  Motorized shavers (full radius resector, burrs)
  Standard video setup (still-picture and video recorders)
  Finger-trap traction (overhead)
  Small wrist instruments (blunt nerve hook, blunt probes,
    basket forceps, curettes)
Specialized situations
  TFCC repair
    Suture passer (Tuohy needle)
    Wire loop suture grabber
    2–0 PDS suture
  Fracture pinning
    Small C-arm for imaging
    Kirschner wires (variety of types)
  Excision (radial styloid or wafer of distal ulna)
    Large burrs
    Small osteotomes

the arthroscopic procedure must be abandoned in favor of open surgery (e.g., for ligament reconstruction or triangular fibrocartilage repair).

The fingers are suspended by sterile finger-trap traction with approximately 3 kg (7 lb) of force (Fig. 4.1). There are several commercially available towers that perform the same function; however, I have not found these to be any better than the simple overhead traction bar.

With the upper arm affixed to the arm board, the forearm is free to rotate in pronation and supination. This flexibility is helpful when examining the distal radioulnar joint and the ulnar side of the wrist. The patient's forearm is placed in neutral rotation. The video monitor is set at the

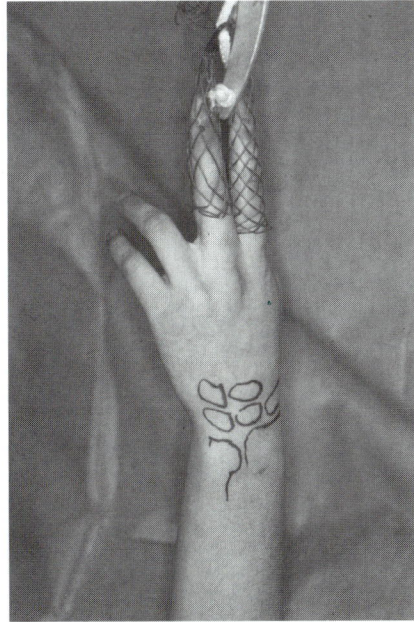

Figure 4.1. The index and long fingers are suspended in sterile finger traps.

foot of the table, and the primary surgeon sits facing the dorsal aspect of the wrist.

Once the hand is in the upright position, the forearm can be exsanguinated; the tourniquet is inflated to 333.25×10^2 Pa (250 mm Hg). I prefer to do the procedure under tourniquet, which avoids unnecessary bleeding both from the skin and from the débrided synovium.

INTRODUCTION OF THE ARTHROSCOPE

Before insufflating the wrist, the surgeon should identify the 3-4, the 4-5, 6U, and midcarpal portals (Fig. 4.2). The 3-4 portal is the first point of entry of the scope. To find the portal, the surgeon first locates Lister's tubercle, and then slides his or her thumb or finger into the soft spot just distal and slightly ulnar. After the 3-4 portal is identified, the surgeon should gently "tattoo" the site with a blunt trocar and mark the site with a pen (Fig. 4.3).

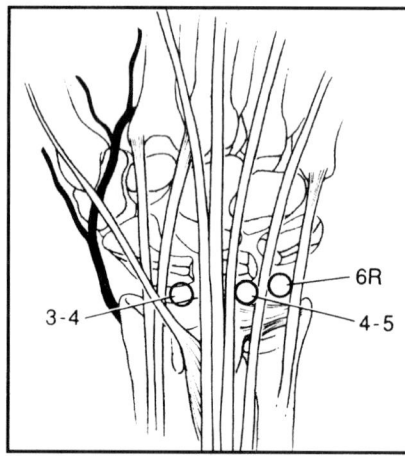

Figure 4.2. The locations of the 3-4, 4-5, and 6R portals are shown. The 6U portal is palmar to the extensor carpi ulnaris tendon.

The midcarpal portal is in the soft spot just distal to the 3-4 portal. This site is at the capitolunate joint just distal to the scapholunate interval. A common error is to mistake the midcarpal port for the 3-4 site. Remember that the 3-4 portal is roughly level with the ulnocarpal joint.

The 6U portal is used to insufflate the wrist with a sterile saline solution (Fig. 4.4). This is done with an 18-gauge needle or a small trocar placed just ulnar to the extensor carpi ulnaris. The angle of inclination for insertion is 20° to 30° distal to proximal. It is important to palpate the ulnar styloid and to be just volar to it; the surgeon must try to stay below the triquetrum but above the ulna.

Once the joint can be freely insufflated with saline solution, an incision through skin only is made over the 3-4 portal. The soft tissue is spread with a fine clamp down to the capsule. This step retracts small sensory nerves and extensor tendons.

At this point, I find it helpful to maximally insufflate the joint with saline solution to provide pressure against the capsule as the trocar enters the joint. Once the blunt trocar is introduced to the level of the capsule, the surgeon should gently twist the trocar down to the outer margin of the capsule; the surgeon may switch to a sharp trocar, if the exact location is carefully maintained. One gentle turn with carefully applied pressure will cut through the dorsal wrist capsule. It is important not to plunge into the wrist with a sharp trocar. Surgeons who are uncomfortable with this maneuver should begin with the blunt trocar.

Once a small rent is made in the capsule with a sharp trocar, a blunt trocar is reinserted into the cannula, which is introduced completely into the joint. A free flow of irrigant fluid should occur; if it does not, assume that the cannula is not in the wrist joint. It is sometimes possible to get into the midcarpal joint when first performing wrist arthroscopy.

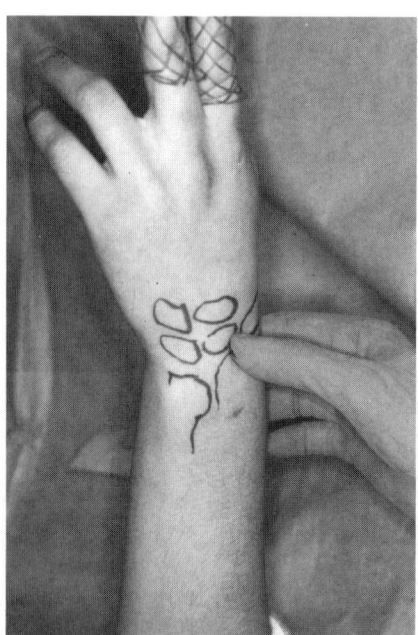

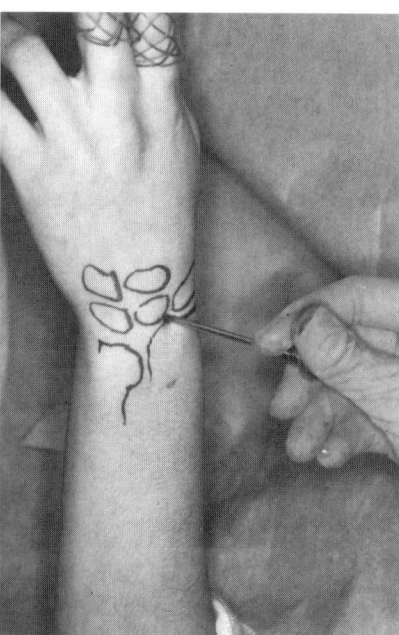

A

B

Figure 4.3. A. Use the thumb to palpate the soft spot of the 3-4 portal, which is distal to Lister's tubercle. **B.** Push a blunt trocar against the entry point for the 3-4 portal. *Arrow,* Lister's tubercle.

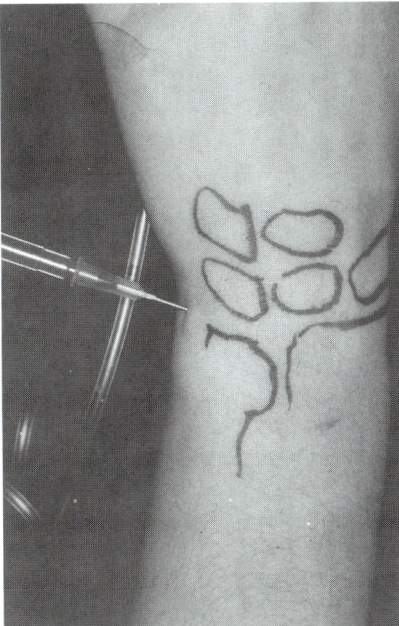

Figure 4.4. The joint is insufflated from the 6U portal. The scope will be introduced into the 3-4 portal.

table	4.2	Arthroscopic Examination of the Wrist Through the 3-4 Portal

Radial styloid recess
  Synovitis
  Styloid cartilage wear (early SLAC wrist)
Radioscaphoid joint
  State of the cartilage
Radiolunate joint
  State of the cartilage
TFCC and ulnocarpal joint (perhaps through the 6R portal)
  Synovitis
  TFCC tear
Volar extrinsic ligaments
  Radioscaphocapitate
  Long radiolunate
  Ulnocarpal ligaments
Intrinsic ligaments
  Scapholunate
  Lunotriquetral
Midcarpal joint (through a new portal)
  State of the cartilage
  Cartilage of the scaphotrapeziotrapezoid joint
  Intrinsic ligaments (scapholunate, lunotriquetral)
Distal radioulnar joint (through a new portal)
  Undersurface of the TFCC
  State of the cartilage

INSPECTION

Radiocarpal-Ulnocarpal Joint

Although a provisional diagnosis for the cause of the patient's wrist pain should have been made, the surgeon must not simply look in the area of suspicion but rather must perform a complete arthroscopic examination of the wrist, searching for any evidence of pathology that may be related to the patient's injury or condition.

Once the scope is introduced, it is important to have a systematic method of examination (Table 4.2) (Fig. 4.5). First begin on the radial aspect of the joint, at the radial styloid and distal radioscaphoid region. This region should be examined for the amount and character of the synovitis. Proliferative synovitis may reflect ongoing me-

chanical inflammation. Recently traumatized wrists often demonstrate a hemorrhagic synovitis.

As the scope is moved ulnarly across the joint, inspect the quality of the cartilage along the radius and matching surface of the scaphoid and lunate. Although the scapholunate ligament may be inspected at this point, I usually wait and return to this site after the more general inspection.

The TFCC and the ulnocarpal region are examined next. Frequently, synovitis and interposed soft tissue obscure the view of the entire TFCC. At this point, it may be necessary to use a motorized shaver (full-radius resector) to

Figure 4.5. The radioscaphoid-capitate (*RSC*), long radiolunate (*LRL*), ulnolunate (*UL*), and triangular fibrocartilage complex (*TFCC*) ligaments should be inspected.

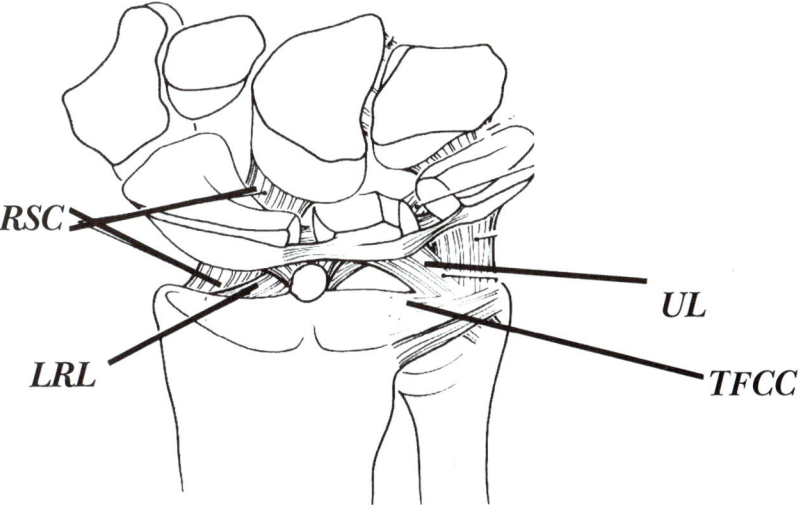

clear a better view. Occasionally, the scope itself should be moved to the 6R portal to obtain better visualization of this region. The next layer of inspection is at the volar extrinsic ligaments. Some wrist joints are relatively lax, and the scope can move easily to the volar edge of the radius as the scope is eased in a more palmar direction. Care should be taken not to scuff the cartilage.

The nomenclature varies depending on the author; I use Berger and Landsmeer's (8) system. In acute injuries with significant disruption, hemorrhage and tears can be seen in these ligaments. To evaluate fractures of the distal radius, the joint must be lavaged thoroughly to clear the hematoma (9). It is sometimes necessary to introduce a small shaver to help evacuate an organized hematoma.

Once the inspection of the volar carpal ligaments is made, the scope is moved ulnar to examine the TFCC. The area of the TFCC commonly displays synovial proliferation and/or synovitis. A complete inspection of the ulnar side of the wrist usually requires débridement of this synovium with a motorized shaver. The surgeon should inspect the entire area of the TFCC, being careful to assess both its radial and ulnar aspects. If there is any question that the periphery may be detached, it is necessary to introduce a motorized shaver to débride to the margin of the capsule.

Once the entire radial carpal and ulnar carpal ligament complexes and the TFCC are inspected, the surgeon should turn to the scapholunate and lunotriquetral ligaments. Relatively small tears in the scapholunate ligament may not be evident from the 3-4 portal; it may be necessary to inspect this ligament from the midcarpal joint. Nonetheless, it is helpful to introduce a blunt nerve hook through the 4-5 or the 6R portal to inspect the quality of the ligament and synovial material surrounding it.[a] The blunt nerve hook through this same portal can be used to test the resilience and mechanical behavior of the triangular fibrocartilage complex (5).

Midcarpal Joint

Although it is somewhat more difficult to introduce the 2.7-mm arthroscope into the midcarpal joint, a complete arthroscopic examination includes an inspection of the midcarpal joint for nearly all patients. The simplest way to find the point of entry between the lunate and the capitate is to mark the spot when first setting up to do the arthroscopy (Fig. 4.6). The area of the fossa (the so-called sulcus) is palpated at the radiocarpal joint, then the surgeon simply moves approximately 1 cm distally, palpating the lunate and capitate, while visualizing as best as possible the shape of the midcarpal joint. If necessary, a needle can be introduced near the triquetral hamate joint to insufflate the midcarpal joint; however, this is usually not necessary. If any instrumentation is to be introduced into the midcarpal joint, it is usually best done through this portal, at the intersection of the capitolunate and capitohamate joints (Figs. 4.6 and 4.7). It is helpful to angle the trocar slightly ulnar and slightly proximally when entering between the capitolunate interval.

Once the scope is introduced and the joint is insufflated sufficiently, an orderly inspection is undertaken. Examination begins with the scaphotrapezial region and gradually moves down to the scapholunate region. It is

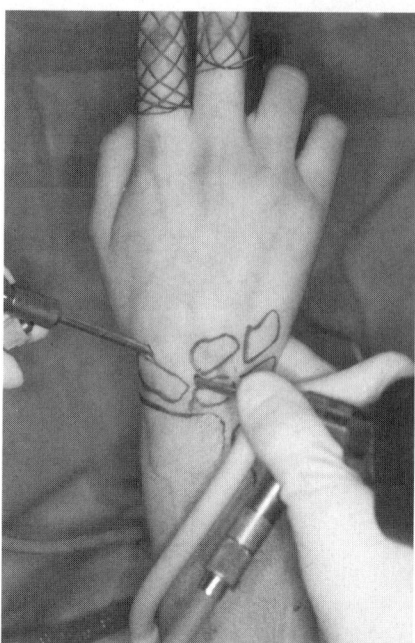

Figure 4.6. A cannula with a blunt trocar can be inserted in the midcarpal joint above the scapholunate interval.

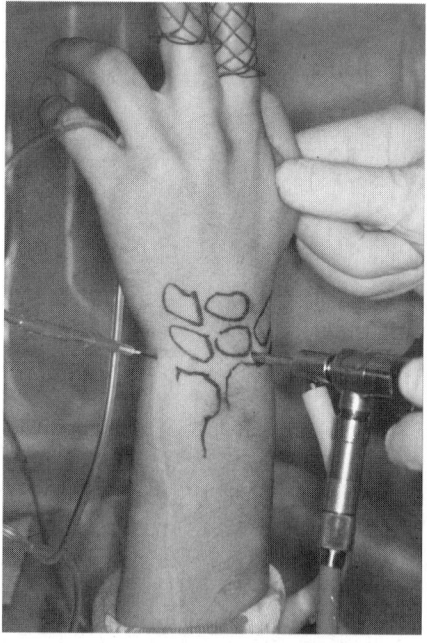

Figure 4.7. Instrumentation can be used by entering the radiocarpal joint.

[a]Note that the difference between the 4-5 and 6R portals may be one of semantics. The extensor digiti quinti tendon is difficult to palpate. As I enter the ulnocarpal joint ulnar to the fourth compartment, I prefer to remain slightly radial (the 4-5 portal) to avoid the ulnar sensory nerve, which may be located near the 6R portal.

easier to see the scapholunate region from this vantage point; the surgeon peers down proximally with the scope carefully rotated to maximize the downward (proximal) view of the scapholunate interval. If there is a great deal of play or gapping from this vantage point, the scapholunate ligament is usually torn. A more obvious separation, or the Grand Canyon sign, occurs when it seems as if the arthroscope could be pushed down through the scapholunate joint into the radial carpal joint from this position.

Once the scapholunate region is inspected from this vantage, the capitolunate and triquetral hamate joints are examined. The lunotriquetral joint may be inspected for laxity and instability. There is often more mobility between the lunate-triquetral region compared to the scapholunate region. A significant tear of the lunotriquetral ligament often permits visualization of the radius and TFCC from the midcarpal joint.

The distal radioulnar joint may also be inspected. Achieving visualization of this joint is more difficult than either the radiocarpal or the midcarpal joint. Nonetheless, there are instances when examination of this joint may be helpful. The trocar is best oriented distally with the starting point just proximal to the flare of the distal ulna.

Therapeutic Wrist Arthroscopy

Therapy beyond simple motorized débridement is beyond the scope of this chapter, and details are available in the literature. There are many possibilities for therapeutic wrist arthroscopy; new uses will become available as technological advances in arthroscopic instruments are made. Examples of procedures that can be performed with the assistance of the arthroscope are repair of the TFCC, manipulation and pinning of articular fractures of the distal radius, radial styloidectomy, excision of small ununited carpal fractures, and synovectomy.

REFERENCES

1. Nagle DJ, Benson LS. Wrist arthroscopy: indications and results. Arthroscopy 1992;8:198–203.
2. Hanker GJ. Diagnostic and operative arthroscopy of the wrist. Clin Orthop 1991;263:165–174.
3. Vanden Eynde S, De Smet L, Fabry G. Diagnostic value of arthrography and arthroscopy of the radiocarpal joint. Arthroscopy 1994; 10:50–53.
4. Rettig ME, Amadio PC. Wrist arthroscopy. Indications and clinical applications. J Hand Surg 1994;19B:774–777.
5. Whipple TL. The role of arthroscopy in treatment of wrist injuries in the athlete. Clin Sports 1997;11:327.
6. Peohling GG, Roth JH. Articular cartilage lesion of the wrist in operative arthroscopy. In: McGinty JB, et al., eds. Operative arthroscopy. New York: Raven, 1991.
7. Whipple TL. Arthroscopic surgery of the wrist. Philadelphia: Lippincott, 1992.
8. Berger RA, Landsmeer JM. The palmar radiocarpal ligaments: a study of adult and fetal human wrist joints. J Hand Surg 1990; 15A:847–854.
9. Abrams RA, Petersen M, Botte MJ. Arthroscopic portals of the wrist: an anatomic study. J Hand Surg 1994;19A:940–944.

Injury to the Distal Radioulnar Joint and Triangular Fibrocartilage Complex

Because both fine manipulation of the hand and activities that require strength of the hand are frequently complicated movements, including flexion, extension, pronation, and supination, injury to the distal radioulnar joint and triangular fibrocartilage complex can be particularly disabling. This type of injury may affect not only the recreational pursuits of patients but also both sedentary and more physical job activities. Injury to this area frequently will include both soft tissue and bony orthopaedic problems. Successful treatment of these conditions therefore requires accurate diagnosis, precisely identifying pathoanatomy by clinical and radiographic means, and recognition that the more specific the intervention, the more likely overall hand function will be improved. This complex anatomic area has been the subject of intense interest and scrutiny not only as clinical diagnosis becomes more precise but also as arthroscopic evaluation and treatment tend to become more of a reality in the wrist and become an important part of the armamentarium for treatment in this area.

RELEVANT ANATOMY AND PATHOGENESIS

The distal radioulnar joint consists of two articulations: The ulnar head articulates with the sigmoid notch of the radius to form the distal articulation of forearm rotation, and the distal ulnar articular surface interfaces with the ulnar carpus through the triangular fibrocartilage complex (TFCC). Werner et al. (1) have shown that approximately 20% of the force transmitted from the hand to the forearm goes through the ulnocarpal joint. This is irrespective of the ulnar variance, because the thickness of the TFCC is in-versely proportional to the amount of positive ulnar variance. However, if the ulnar variance is increased by 2 mm, as a result of either lengthening of the ulna or shortening of the radius, the force across the TFCC doubles.

Patients with a positive ulnar variance are more likely to develop problems on the ulnar side of the wrist (Fig. 5.1). When the ulnocarpal joint force increases significantly, a progression of problems develop. Palmer classified TFCC tears as traumatic (class 1) or degenerative (class 2). He further classified degenerative changes of the ulnocarpal joint into five subclasses (2). In class 2A injuries, a partial-thickness tear of the TFCC occurs. In class 2B tears, chondromalacia of the ulnar carpus and distal ulna are seen. Class 2C patients present with a full-thickness tear in the central portion of the TFCC. Class 2D injuries involve a tear of the lunotriquetral ligament. Class 2E changes show degenerative changes of the ulnar lunate, triquetrum, and distal ulna.

Clinically, all these patients present with pain on the ulnar side of the wrist. Pain is accentuated during activities that require ulnar deviation of the wrist. At times, the contact between the ulna and carpus can be so severe that the distal radioulnar joint becomes unstable. This collection of symptoms is called ulnocarpal impaction (or abutment) syndrome. This term is often confused with radioulnar impingement syndrome. The latter is abnormal contact between the radius and proximal stump of the distal ulna after ulnar head excision.

The distal radioulnar joint (DRUJ) is also subject to problems. This joint lacks congruity and, therefore, relies on soft tissue restraints for stability. The TFCC is the main stabilizer of the DRUJ. The TFCC consists of a number of

Figure 5.1. This patient has ulnocarpal abutment syndrome with a positive ulnar variance. Note the cystic and sclerotic changes in the lunate owing to the increased ulnocarpal joint force.

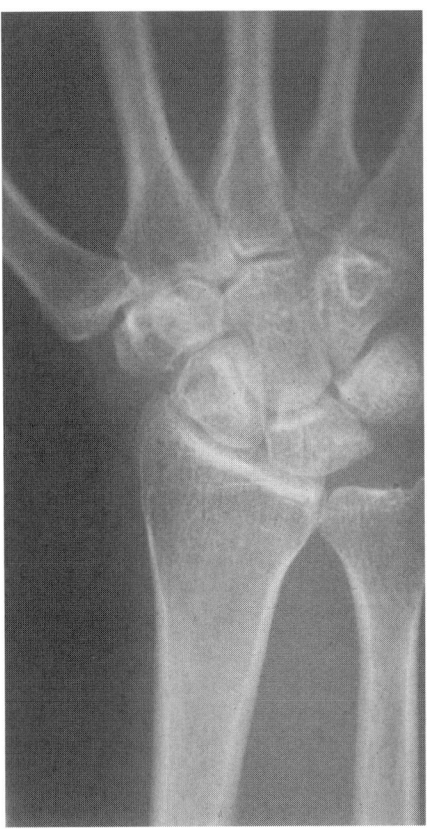

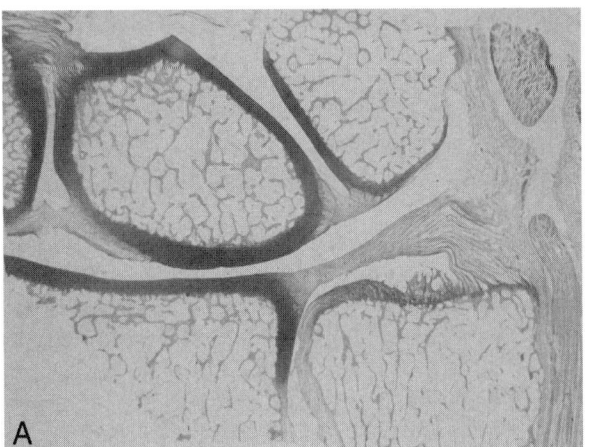

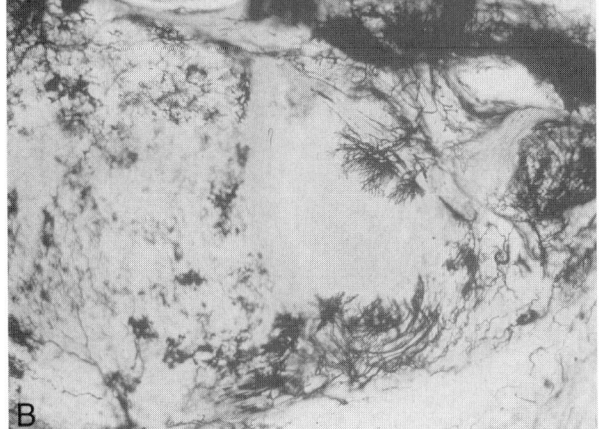

Figure 5.2. A. The histologic anatomy of the TFCC, which inserts into the fovea of the ulna and into the ulnar styloid. Studies of the vascular anatomy—axial (**B**) and coronal (**C**)—show that the peripheral 15 to 20% of the TFCC is vascularized and will heal if torn and repaired. There is no vascularity in the central attachment of the TFCC to the radius. Tears in this location are débrided.

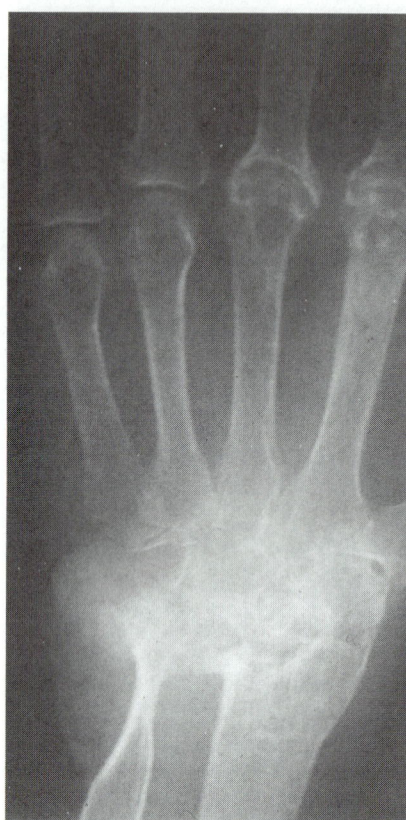

Figure 5.3. A patient with severe rheumatoid arthritis of the distal radioulnar joint. Pain, restricted range of motion, and digital extensor tendon ruptures are indications for surgical excision of the ulnar head.

soft tissue structures on the ulnar side of the wrist, including the articular disc, the dorsal and palmar ulnocarpal ligaments, the ulnotriquetral and ulnolunate ligaments, and the extensor carpi ulnaris sheath. The TFCC attaches to the ulnar fovea and styloid, the dorsal and palmar wrist capsule, and the distal rim of the sigmoid notch of the radius (Fig. 5.2). Similar to the knee meniscus, the peripheral 10 to 20% of the TFCC is vascularized (3).

Palmer (2) also classified traumatic tears of the TFCC. Class IA is a central perforation, which most commonly occurs 2 to 3 mm from the radial attachment of the TFCC and is directed palmar to dorsal. Since the inner portion of the TFCC is avascular, tears in this region are best treated with débridement. Class IB is an avulsion of the TFCC from its insertion into the distal ulna. Class IC is a peripheral tear of the TFCC. Since both of these tears occur in a vascularized region, repair of the perforation should be performed. Class ID is a traumatic avulsion of the TFCC from its attachment to the radius. Repair of tears from the sigmoid notch are currently an area of controversy. Repair of the dorsal or palmar radioulnar ligaments is indicated when the dorsal or palmar portions of the TFCC are injured. The central attachment of the TFCC can be repaired to the radius if the avascular tissue of the articular cartilage and subchondral bone are removed and the TFCC is inserted into the cancellous bone. It is unknown whether re-

pairs in the central portion provide better function than does débridement. When DRUJ stability cannot be achieved by a TFCC repair, various procedures have been designed to stabilize the joint and allow motion. These operations will not be discussed in this chapter.

In addition to problems at the ulnocarpal articulation, the DRUJ is also subject to traumatic, inflammatory, or degenerative arthritis at the sigmoid notch. Intra-articular fractures of the distal radius that extend through the sigmoid notch may lead to incongruity and posttraumatic arthritis. Even when the sigmoid notch is not involved in the fracture, incongruity between the sigmoid notch and distal ulna may occur if the radius is shortened and the articular surfaces are no longer in contact. The DRUJ is commonly affected in rheumatoid arthritis (Fig. 5.3). Erosions of the distal ulna from the pannus can lead to the development of a bone spur dorsally. As the forearm rotates, this spur moves across the extensor tendons, causing a sequential rupture of the individual finger extensor tendons from ulnar to radial.

PHYSICAL EXAMINATION

Patients with pain of the ulnar side of the wrist need to be carefully examined to determine the origin of the pain. The ulnar side of the wrist is best evaluated by having the examiner sit across an examining table from the patient. The patient's elbow is flexed and supported on a table, the fingers pointing toward the ceiling and the forearm in neutral rotation. The examiner should first exclude the extensor carpi ulnaris (ECU), flexor carpi ulnaris (FCU), the dorsal sensory branch of the ulnar nerve, and the pisotriquetral joint as potential sources of pain.

The stability of the DRUJ is tested by palmar and dorsal displacement of the distal ulna in neutral, pronation, and supination of the forearm. The piano key sign detects dorsal instability of the distal ulna in pronation. In this test, the palms are placed on the examining table with the forearms in pronation. The patient is asked to press the palms onto the table. Dorsal instability of the ulna is manifest by the ulna moving dorsal and palmar with this maneuver. Relative motion must be compared to the contralateral, normal side. The DRUJ is examined for crepitus. The wrist is then placed through a full range of motion. Pain with ulnar deviation suggests an ulnocarpal impaction syndrome. Point tenderness distal to the ulnar styloid between the ECU and FCU suggests that the pain is originating from the TFCC. Finally, instability of the lunotriquetral joint is tested by pushing the triquetrum dorsally by applying pressure on the pisiform while pushing the lunate palmar.

RADIOLOGIC STUDIES

Radiologic studies include AP and lateral views of the wrist in neutral forearm rotation (Fig. 5.4). The ulnar variance decreases as the forearm rotates from pronation to

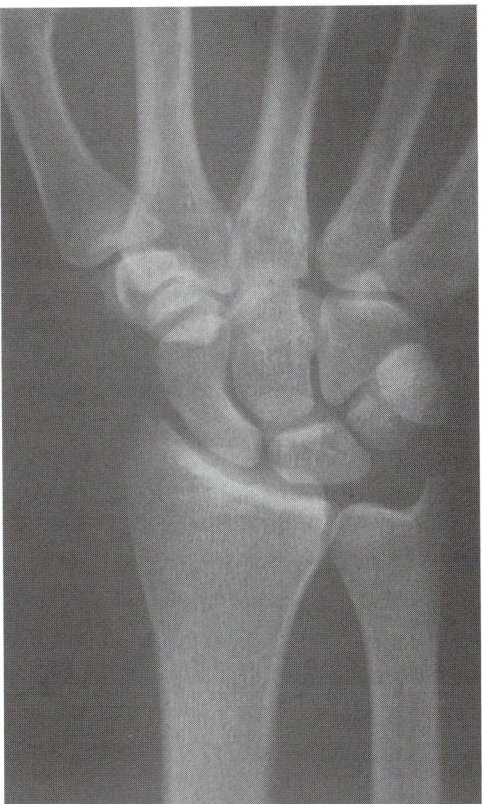

Figure 5.4. Since the ulnar variance changes with forearm rotation, ulnar variance can be measured only in neutral rotation. In an AP neutral rotation x-ray, the radial and ulnar styloids are see in profile on opposite sides of the wrist.

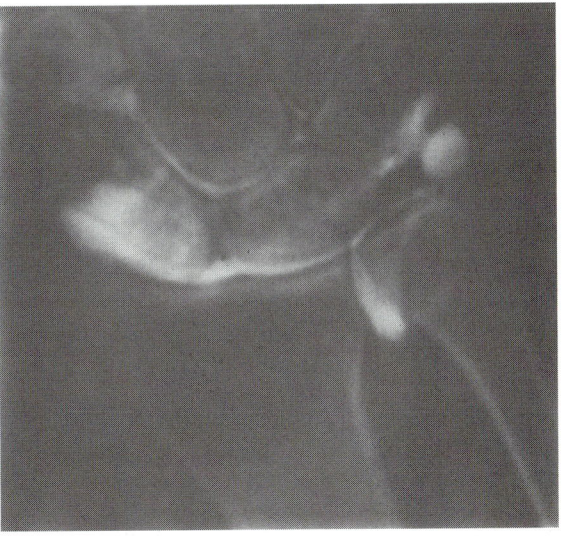

Figure 5.5. After being injected into the radiocarpal joint, the dye is seen leaking between the radius and ulna, indicating a TFCC tear, and into the midcarpal joint, indicating either a scapholunate or a lunotriquetral tear.

supination. When an x-ray is taken in neutral rotation, the radial and ulnar styloids are both seen in profile on opposite sides of the wrist. The DRUJ and ulnocarpal joints are inspected for degenerative changes. Nonunion of the ul-

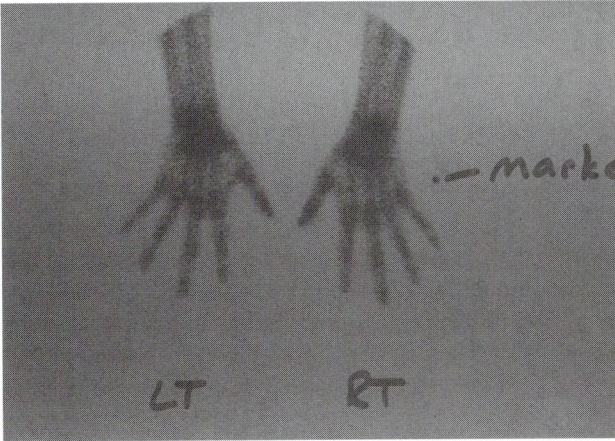

Figure 5.6. In a bone scan of the patient shown in Figure 5.1, increased uptake is seen at the ulnocarpal region of the right wrist. The scan confirms the diagnosis of an ulnocarpal abutment syndrome.

nar styloid may be seen following trauma. Although usually asymptomatic, the ununited ulnar styloid can occasionally be a source of pain. Fractures encompassing the entire styloid and a portion of the fovea may lead to TFCC instability.

The soft tissue elements, the scapholunate ligament, lunotriquetral ligament, and TFCC, can be assessed with a triple-injection arthrogram (Fig. 5.5). Dye is injected first into the radiocarpal joint. If the dye appears in the midcarpal joint, a perforation of the scapholunate or lunotriquetral ligament is presumed. If dye appears in the distal radioulnar joint, the cause is a perforation of the TFCC . Since a one-way valve may be present at an area of perforation, if no dye leakage is seen after the radiocarpal injection, the midcarpal and distal radioulnar joints are each separately injected. An arthrogram determines if a perforation is present, but it gives no information about the size of the perforation or whether the perforation is associated with intercarpal instability.

The soft tissue structures can also be visualized with MRI. The ability of an MRI study to precisely define wrist disease depends on the scanner, the sequences selected, and the interpretation of the radiologist. Bone scans can be helpful in identifying a source of pain in the wrist (Fig. 5.6). Pin et al. (4) have shown that radionucleotide scans of the wrist are valuable for detecting focal lesions in patients with hand and wrist pain.

TREATMENT

Nonoperative Treatment

Initial treatment of ulnar-sided wrist pain includes immobilization, nonsteroidal anti-inflammatory medications, and rest. If the pain is at the distal radioulnar joint, immobilization will require a long arm or sugar-tong splint to restrict forearm rotation. If symptoms are not relieved,

Clinical Table: Injuries of the Distal Radioulnar Joint and Triangular Fibrocartilage Complex

Procedure	Indications	Technique	Anatomy	Pitfalls
Hemiresection of the distal ulna	• Degeneration of the DRUJ • No ulnocarpal impaction	• Open	• DSBUN • ECU • EDQM • TFCC	• Injury to the DSBUN • Incomplete excision of the palmar ulna • Ulnocarpal impaction
Darrach's procedure	• Degeneration of the DRUJ • Ulnocarpal impaction • Incompetent TFCC	• Open	• DSBUN • ECU • EDQM • TFCC	• Injury to the DSBUN • Excessive excision of the ulna • Distal radioulnar impingement
Ulnar-shortening osteotomy	• Ulnocarpal impaction • No DRUJ arthritis	• Open	• DSBUN • ECU • FCU	• Injury to the DSBUN • Nonunion
Ulnar wafer procedure	• Ulnocarpal impaction • No DRUJ arthritis	• Open	• DSBUN • ECU • FCU	• Injury to the DSBUN • Restricted wrist motion
TFCC débridement	• Central TFCC tears	• Arthroscopic	• DSBUN • Dorsal extensor compartments	• Injury to the DSBUN • Injury to the articular cartilage
TFCC repair	• Peripheral TFCC tears • DRUJ instability	• Arthroscopic or open	• DSBUN • Dorsal extensor compartments	• Injury to the DSBUN • Continued DRUJ instability

DRUJ, distal radioulnar joint; *DSBUN*, dorsal sensory branch of the ulnar nerve; *ECU*, extensor carpi ulnaris; *EDQM*, extensor digiti quinti minimi; *TFCC*, triangular fibrocartilage complex, *FCU*, flexor carpi ulnaris.

the clinician may consider treating the joint with a cortisone injection.

Operative Treatment

Surgery is indicated when conservative measures fail. The type of operation depends on the residual signs and symptoms (Clinical Table). If pain and degenerative changes are seen in the DRUJ, excision of the articular surface of the ulna is required. This can be done with a hemiresection of the distal ulnar articular surface or a complete excision of the ulnar head (Darrach's procedure). The choice of procedure is often the surgeon's preference; but, in general, a hemiresection is favored when the TFCC is competent and contributes to stability of the DRUJ.

Treatment of the ulnocarpal joint is based on cause of injury. Traumatic tears of the TFCC are treated by débridement or repair, depending on their location and regional blood supply. Degenerative pathologic changes of the TFCC and ulnocarpal joint often reflect the relative length of the ulna. Patients with a negative or neutral ulnar variance are treated with a wrist arthroscopy and débridement of the TFCC. Patients with a positive ulnar variance are treated with an ulnar shortening osteotomy or an excision of the distal ulnar articular surface and subchondral bone (wafer procedure).

DORSAL APPROACH TO THE DISTAL RADIOULNAR JOINT

The operative approach to the DRUJ is dorsal. With the forearm in pronation, the ulnar head can be palpated between the ECU and the extensor digiti quinti minimi (EDQM). A 3-cm incision, angled radially at the distal end of the ulna, is made between these tendons over the distal ulna. Great care is taken to preserve the dorsal sensory branch of the ulnar nerve, which lies immediately ulnar to the incision, during the exposure. The proximal half of the extensor retinaculum is reflected from ulnar to the ECU to radial to the EDQM and is left attached to the septum between the EDQM and the extensor digitorum communis. The ECU will remain in its compartment, which is separate from the extensor retinaculum. Retraction of the EDQM will reveal the dorsal capsule of the DRUJ, which is longitudinally incised along its radial border, leaving a 2- to 3-mm cuff for reattachment. The capsule is then transversely cut at the proximal edge of the TFCC. As the capsule inserts ulnarly on the ulna, it can be subperiosteally elevated, with the ECU contained in its sheath, to give full exposure of the ulnar head.

ULNAR HEMIRESECTION

The undersurface of the TFCC can be inspected from this approach. If the TFCC is intact, a hemiresection of the

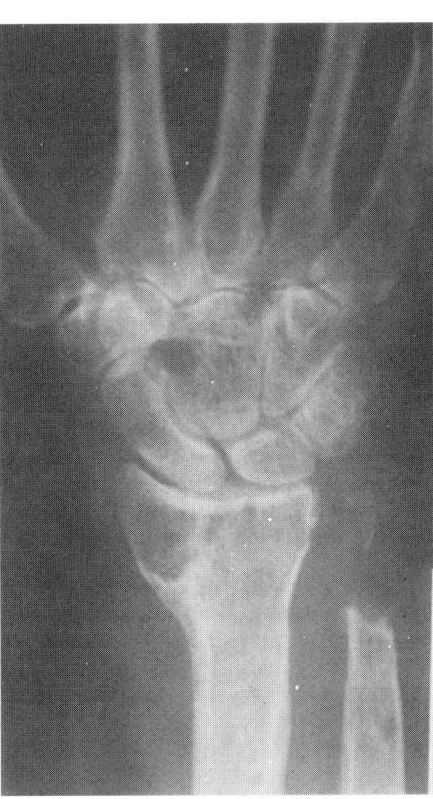

Figure 5.7. In Darrach's procedure, no more than the distal 2.5 cm of ulna should be removed. When more is excised, the ulna may become unstable, leading to an ulnar impingement syndrome.

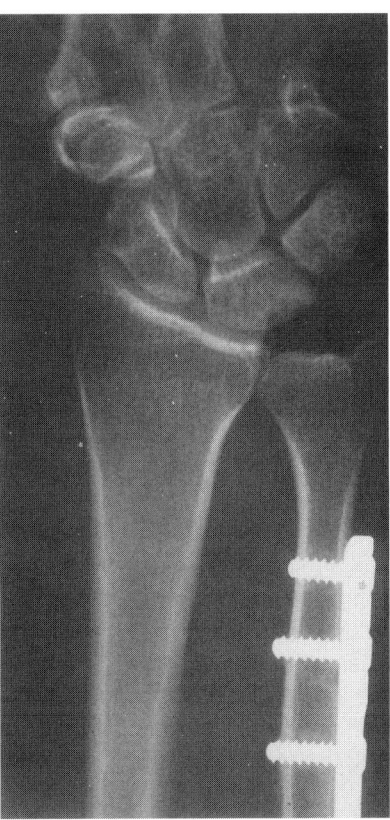

Figure 5.8. In the ulnar-shortening osteotomy, 2 to 3 mm of ulnar diaphyseal bone is usually excised. The osteotomy is held with a seven-hole dynamic compression plate and a lag screw across the osteotomy, as seen in the postoperative x-ray of the patient shown in Figure 5.1.

ulnar head will remove pathologic tissue and retain stability (5,6). The ulna is resected from proximal to the articular cartilage of the ulnar head to the ulnar styloid and the fovea distally, leaving a progressively narrowed end. Care must be taken to rotate the radius from pronation to supination to ensure that resection of the palmar ulna is complete. Once the ulnar head is resected, the styloid is able to move toward the midline, closer to the radius. As it does, the styloid may impact on the ulnar carpus. This is most likely to occur when the ulnar variance is positive. The newly occurring ulnar impaction syndrome can be treated by an ulnar-shortening osteotomy or by placing a tendinous spacer between the radius and ulna.

If no ulnar shortening was performed, the arm is placed into a short arm bulky dressing for 2 weeks, followed by the initiation of passive and active range of motion exercises and an interim splint for the ensuing 2 to 4 weeks. This is followed by unrestricted motion and strengthening. If an ulnar-shortening osteotomy was done, a short arm cast is placed until bony healing is evident, usually at 6 weeks, followed by range of motion and strengthening exercises.

DARRACH'S PROCEDURE

The most common indication for a Darrach resection is incompetence of the TFCC (e.g., in rheumatoid arthritis).

However, Darrach's procedure has been successfully used for years for the treatment of ulnar impaction syndrome following displaced distal radius fractures (7). After the distal ulna is approached dorsally, the ulna is transversely osteotomized at the level of the ulnar neck. No more than 2.5 cm of the distal ulna should be excised (Fig. 5.7). Resection of more bone may lead to distal radioulnar instability, a difficult problem to solve. A lesser degree of instability following a Darrach procedure causes rubbing between the radius and ulnar stump, the ulnar impingement syndrome. Recommendations for long arm casting postsurgery range from none to 6 weeks.

ULNAR-SHORTENING OSTEOTOMY

When the articular surface of the DRUJ is intact but ulnocarpal impaction is occurring, an ulnar-shortening osteotomy is effective (8,9) (Fig. 5.8). By preserving the DRUJ components, the potential complication of instability is avoided. Before performing shortening the ulna, a template of the new position of the ulna should be tested on the radius to ensure the area of contact at the joint will be sufficient. The approach to the ulna for an osteotomy is the plane between the flexor and extensor carpi ulnaris tendons. The dorsal sensory branch of the ulnar nerve often crosses from palmar to dorsal at the distal extent of the wound. The plate should be placed either palmar or ulnar.

The periosteum is stripped from the ulna along the length of the plate, usually a seven-hole, 3.5-mm dynamic compression plate. The plate is predrilled to the proximal side of the osteotomy site. The osteotomy, which is made at a 45° angle, can be cut freehand, by stacking a number of blades together to match the desired amount of bone to be removed, or can be cut by using a commercially available cutting jig. The osteotomy is begun on the side of the bone with the plate to allow greater compression during placement of the distal screws. A lag screw is placed in the middle hole of the plate across the osteotomy site.

The bulky dressing is removed at 2 weeks, and patients begin range of motion exercises when out of the splint. Strengthening is begun when the osteotomy is radiographically healed.

TFCC DÉBRIDEMENT AND REPAIR

Treatment of TFCC injuries depends on the location of the tear (2). Lesions in the avascular central portion may be treated with an arthroscopic débridement. The arthroscope is placed through the 3-4 portal, and the shaver or biter is placed through the 4-5 portal. The edges of the TFCC are débrided until a smooth edge is produced. Laboratory studies suggest that up to two-thirds of the central portion of the TFCC may be removed before instability of the DRUJ occurs. During débridement, care should be taken to avoid resection to the palmar or dorsal edges of the TFCC, which would injure the palmar or dorsal distal radioulnar ligaments. After débriding the TFCC, the surgeon should look for evidence of ulnar impaction syndrome by performing a careful arthroscopic inspection of the distal ulna, ulnar lunate, and triquetrum.

An alternative to an ulnar-shortening osteotomy in this instance can be an open or arthroscopic wafer procedure, in which only the distal ulnar articular cartilage and subchondral bone are removed (10). One advantage of the procedure is the fact that no plate is required. A disadvantage is that bleeding from the bone into the joint may prolong the rehabilitation of the wrist range of motion. When the wafer procedure is done arthroscopically, the distal ulna is approached through the débrided perforation in the center of the TFCC. With the open procedure, the approach is as described above. A 3- to 4-mm wafer of the distal ulnar is removed, with great care taken to remove bone from the palmar edge.

Peripheral tears of the TFCC may not be evident on arthrography. A normal arthrogram may be seen when scar from the vascularized tear prevents dye from crossing between the radiocarpal and distal radioulnar joints. Peripheral TFCC tears are best visualized arthroscopically. The TFCC is normally under tension, and when probed, the probe bounces off of the cartilage (the trampoline effect). Loss of the trampoline effect is pathognomonic of a TFCC tear. Another sign of loss of peripheral integrity is seen when the TFCC can be pulled radially with the probe, seeming to fold onto itself. Peripheral tears may be repaired either arthroscopically or open. When repaired

arthroscopically, the shaver, introduced through the 4-5 portal, débrides the torn edge of the cartilage. Two or three sutures are then placed percutaneously from proximal to distal through the torn edge of the TFCC. The sutures may be tied over a button, or an incision may be made and the sutures tied under the skin. Care must be taken to avoid injury to branches of the dorsal sensory branch of the ulnar nerve.

When an open approach to peripheral TFCC repair is used, the TFCC is approached dorsally (11). The TFCC is débrided of granulation and fibrous connective tissue and a trough is created in the fovea by curetting the ulna to cancellous bone. Drill holes are made through the fovea of the distal ulna and the TFCC is sutured to the ulna.

After peripheral TFCC repair with either the arthroscopic or open approach, the ulna and radius may be pinned in neutral rotation with two 0.0625 Kirschner (K) wires. The arm is kept in a long arm splint for 6 weeks, followed by K wire removal and short arm casting for an additional 6 weeks while the patient begins forearm rotation. At 12 weeks after surgery, range of motion and strengthening exercises for the hand and wrist are begun.

SUMMARY

The distal radioulnar joint is a complex structure. Selection of the proper operation for treatment of problems not improved with conservative care depends on the performance of a careful physical examination, critical interpretation of diagnostic studies, and consideration of the available surgical procedures.

REFERENCES

1. Werner FW, Palmer AK, Fortino MD, Short WH. Force transmission through the distal ulna: effect of ulnar variance, lunate fossa angulation, and radial and palmar tilt of the distal radius. J Hand Surg 1992;17A:423–428.
2. Palmer AK. Triangular fibrocartilage disorders: injury patterns and treatment. Arthroscopy 1990;6:125–132.
3. Bednar MS, Arnoczyk SP, Weiland AJ. The microvasculature of the triangular fibrocartilage complex: its clinical significance. J Hand Surg 1992;16A:1101–1105.
4. Pin PG, Semenkovich JW, Young VL, et al. Role of radionuclide imaging in the evaluation of wrist pain. J Hand Surg 1988;13A:810–814.
5. Bowers WH. Distal radioulnar joint arthroplasty: the hemiresection—interposition technique. J Hand Surg 1985;10A:169–178.
6. Watson HK, Ryu JY, Burgess RC. Matched distal ulnar resection. J Hand Surg 1986;11A:812–817.
7. Tulipan DJ, Eaton RG, Eberhart RE. The Darrach procedure defended: technique redefined and long-term follow-up. J Hand Surg 1991;16A:438–444.
8. Rayhack JM, Gasser SI, Latta LL, et al. Precision oblique osteotomy for shortening of the ulna. J Hand Surg 1993;18A:908–918.
9. Chun S, Palmer AK. The ulnar impaction syndrome: follow-up of ulnar shortening osteotomy. J Hand Surg 1993;18A:46–53.
10. Feldon P, Terrono AL, Belsky MR. The "wafer" procedure. Partial distal ulnar resection. Clin Orthop Res 1992;275:124–129.
11. Hermansdorfer JD, Kleinman WB. Management of chronic peripheral tears of the triangular fibrocartilage complex. J Hand Surg 1991;16A:341–349.

chapter 6

James E. Bates, Michelle Gerwin, Christopher Wottowa,
and Andrew J. Weiland

Avascular Necrosis of the Carpal Bones

Avascular necrosis of the bones of the carpus occurs most commonly in the proximal pole of the scaphoid and results from a fracture through the bone that interferes with its blood supply. Idiopathic forms of avascular necrosis of the carpal bones are unrelated and uncommon. The condition has, however, been thoroughly described in the lunate and reported in the scaphoid, capitate, hamate, and pisiform. This chapter concentrates on the diagnosis and treatment of idiopathic avascular necrosis of the lunate (Kienböck's disease) and briefly reviews the diagnosis and treatment of avascular necrosis of the scaphoid (Preiser's disease).

I | Avascular Necrosis of the Lunate (Kienböck's Disease)

In 1843, Peste (1) described the collapse of the lunate bone in cadaver dissections; he attributed the condition to be the result of traumatic fracture. The clinical diagnosis of lunate collapse did not gain popularity until 1910, when Kienböck (2,3) published his classic description of the x-ray changes and clinical symptoms associated with lunatomalacia; the disease is now associated with his name. Kienböck postulated that lunate collapse was related to avascular changes. The cause of Kienböck's disease has, however, remained a source of controversy. Other authors have cited fracture, with resultant traumatic disruption of the intraosseous or extraosseous blood supply, as the primary causal event (4,5).

In 1928, Hulten (4) reported the association of lunatomalacia with negative ulnar variance. Ulnar variance refers to the relative length of the ulna compared to the radius on standard AP radiographs of the wrist. Hulten found that in 78% of patients with Kienböck's disease the ulna was shorter than the radius (ulnar negative); thus he proposed radial shortening as a treatment (4,6). The concept of ulnar variance has since been brought into question (7–10), and current theory holds that negative ulnar variance is a predisposing factor for, but not the primary cause of, Kienböck's disease. Radial shortening, which decreases the forces across the lunate, remains a popular surgical treatment. Several other surgical procedures that focus on joint unloading have been developed, including ulnar lengthening (11) and capitate shortening (12). In addition, a variety of limited intercarpal fusions (9,11), fascial arthroplasties (13), and salvage procedures—such as proximal row carpectomy (14–17) and wrist arthrodesis (18,19)—have been recommended for the treatment of Kienböck's disease.

The cause of avascular necrosis of the lunate remains controversial. Some people may have lunates that are at risk for the disease: Lunates with limited vascularity are subjected to repetitive microtrauma as a result of anatomic and physiologic factors that create high loads across the bone.

Kienböck's disease classically progresses in stages from lunate collapse to intercarpal collapse and, ultimately, to degenerative arthritis of the wrist. The primary goal of treatment for Kienböck's disease has been to halt this progression. Treatment protocols, therefore, are based on the stage of the disease at diagnosis. A thorough understanding of the pathogenesis and clinical course of the disease is necessary to appreciate the methods and timing of surgical intervention.

RELEVANT ANATOMY AND PATHOGENESIS

The lunate, or semilunar bone, is named for its semicircular shape. It is positioned in the proximal carpal row of the wrist and articulates with the radius proximally and the capitate distally. The proximal and distal surfaces are completely covered by articular cartilage. The dorsal and volar radiolunate ligaments attach to the dorsal and volar surfaces of the lunate and carry the bone's blood supply (20). Injection studies of the extraosseous vascularity of the lunate have demonstrated a consistent volar blood supply and a frequent, but inconsistent, dorsal blood supply. Volarly, the radial, ulnar, and palmar branches of the anterior interosseous artery combine to form three transverse arches that supply the lunate. Dorsally, the radial, ulnar, and dorsal branches of the anterior interosseous artery also combine to form three arches. The dorsal blood supply of the lunate, when present, is derived from the proximal two of these transverse arches, which are located over the radiocarpal and intercarpal articulations (21,22).

A combined volar and dorsal blood supply has been demonstrated by studies of intraosseous vascularity in 75 to 100% of lunate bones (21,23,24). A single vascular supply is noted in 7% of lunates (25). Of those lunates with a dual blood supply, 31% have a single volar and dorsal vessel forming an anastomosis, 59% have a three-vessel anastomosis (two dorsal vessels and one volar, or two volar vessels and one dorsal), and 10% have a four-vessel anastomosis (two volar and two dorsal vessels) (21) (Fig. 6.1).

The pathogenesis of Kienböck's disease is intimately related to the vascular anatomy of the lunate. Disruption of the extraosseous blood supply is unlikely to cause osteonecrosis of the lunate because, as noted above, there are several volar and dorsal arches that contribute to its vascularity. Lunates with a single nutrient vessel, however, are subject to avascular necrosis of the entire bone if the vessel is compromised. Similarly, in single-vessel lunates, a coronal fracture could lead to avascularity of the opposite pole (volar or dorsal). Clinically, however, dorsal or volar avascularity is rare; more common is the avascularity of the proximal radial aspect of the lunate or the whole lunate. Thus intraosseous fracture is less likely to be a cause of avascularity than is disruption of the nutrient vessel in single-vessel lunates, which is the most probable cause of Kienböck's disease.

INITIAL FINDINGS, PHYSICAL EXAMINATION, AND DIAGNOSIS

The diagnosis of Kienböck's disease is suspected in the young adult (20 to 40 years old) who presents with the insidious onset of pain and stiffness of the dominant wrist, tenderness over the dorsal lunate, and decreased grip strength. Patients are typically heavy manual laborers. A history of trauma is frequently absent, although some patients will give a history of a recent hyperextension injury. The pain is usually aggravated by activity and partially relieved with rest and immobilization.

Physical examination may reveal a radiocarpal effusion, boggy synovitis of the radiocarpal joint, limited flexion and extension, and a decrease in grip strength (frequently to half that of the unaffected hand) (26).

RADIOLOGIC STUDIES

The diagnosis of Kienböck's disease is usually made by plain film radiography. A standardized technique of PA radiography should be employed to evaluate the condition of the lunate and its articulations and ulnar variance of the wrist. For the standardized radiograph, the shoulder is abducted 90°, the elbow flexed 90°, the forearm placed in neutral rotation, and the wrist held in neutral flexion/extension. An increase in the relative density of the lunate is the earliest sign of avascularity on plain radiographs. Radionuclide bone scan may be used to confirm the diagnosis if the plain radiographs are normal and clinical suspicion is high. Although there are reports of Kienböck's disease with negative initial bone scans but positive MRI studies (27), this has not been seen at our institution. Consequently, a bone scan is recommended as a relatively cost-effective first-line screening tool. MRI is more specific than the bone scan and may be used to confirm the diagnosis or determine the extent of avascularity for treatment purposes (28) (Fig. 6.2).

Classification

The classification system of Kienböck's disease was initially described by Stahl (29) and later modified by Lichtman et al. (30) (Fig. 6.3). It is based on the radiographic appearance of the lunate and its articulations and is a useful guide to gauge prognosis and select treatment options (Table 6.1). The prognosis is better for stages I and II disease than it is for stages II and IV disease; therefore, early diagnosis and treatment are important.

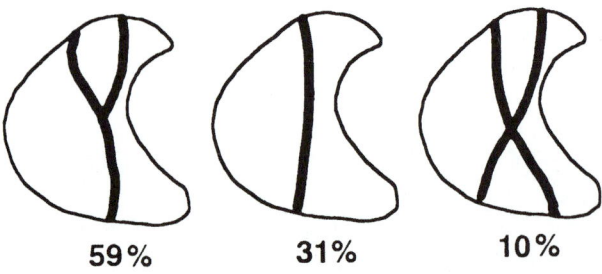

59%   **31%**   **10%**

Figure 6.1. The three patterns of intraosseous vascular anastomoses seen in lunates with an oval blood supply. The Y formation is most common; two dorsal or volar vessels anastomose with a single opposing vessel. Reprinted with permission from Williams CS, Gelberman RH. Vascularity of the lunate. Hand Clin 1993;9:395.

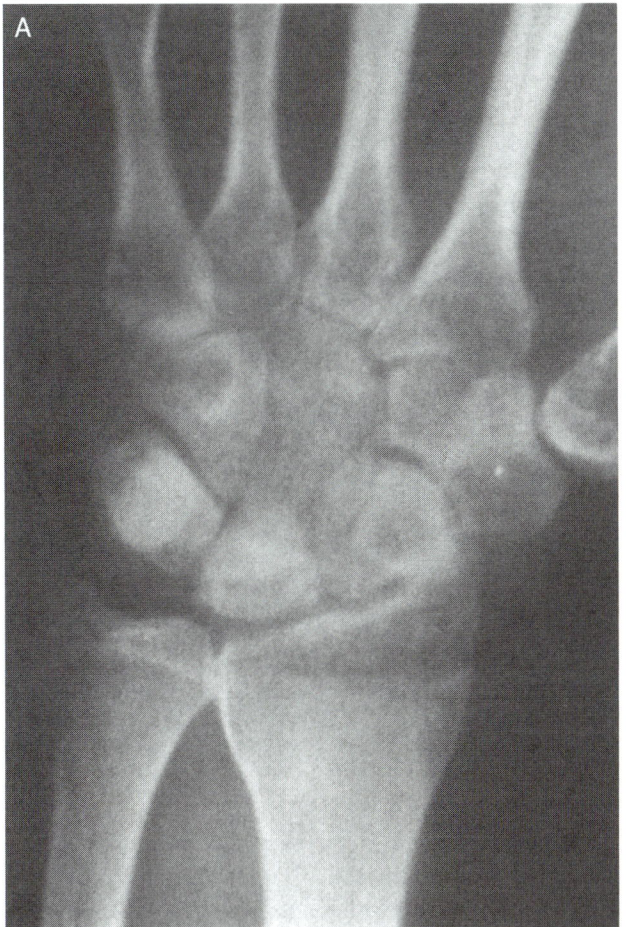

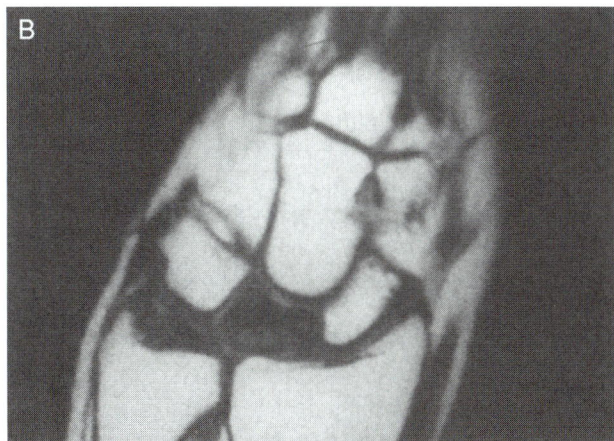

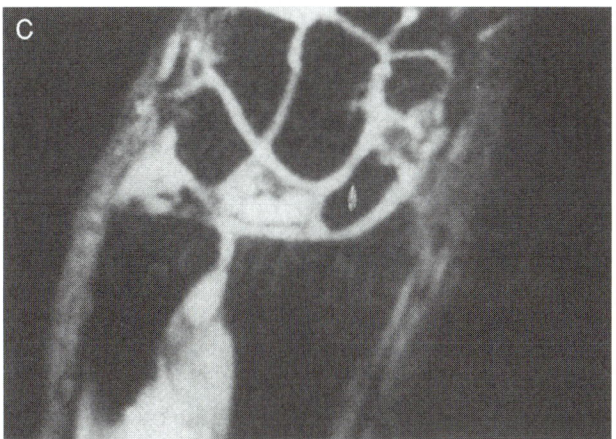

Figure 6.2. A. AP view showing state IIIA Kienböck's disease. T_1-weighted (**B**) and T_2-weighted (**C**) MRI studies showing low signal in the lunate. Reprinted with permission from Gerwin M, Weiland AJ. Avascular necrosis of the carpals. In: Peimer CA, ed. Surgery of the hand and upper extremity. New York: McGraw-Hill, 1996.

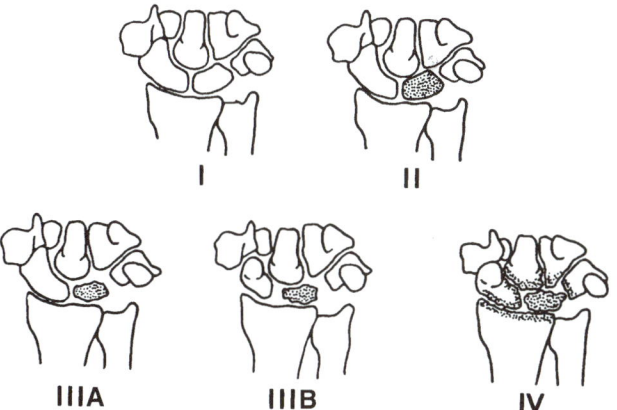

Figure 6.3. Lichtman et al.'s classification of Kienböck's disease. See text for details. Reprinted with permission from Weiss APC, Weiland AJ, Moore JR, Wilgis EFS. Radial shortening for Kienböck disease. J Bone Joint Surg 1991;73A:385–391.

STAGE I

In stage I disease, the lunate typically appears normal and shows no radiographic changes. Occasionally, small fracture lines are evident within the lunate on trispiral tomography. Diagnosis is usually made by radionuclide scan; increased uptake of the isotope is evident within the lunate. MRI may be useful if the diagnosis is suspected despite a negative bone scan. A decreased signal on both T_1- and T_2-weighted images suggests osteonecrosis (26).

STAGE II

In stage II Kienböck's disease, sclerosis is apparent in the lunate, but the size and shape of the bone remain unchanged. In addition, the intercarpal relationships remain unchanged; there is no evidence of carpal collapse. Late in stage II, some height may be lost on the radial side of the lunate. Pain and swelling in the wrist are the predominant clinical features during stage II.

table	6.1	Classification of Kienböck's Disease
Stage	**Characteristics**	
I	No radiographic change; bone scan or MRI positive	
II	Lunate sclerosis; no collapse	
IIIA	Lunate fragmentation or collapse; no carpal collapse	
IIIB	Lunate fragmentation or collapse; fixed rotary subluxation of the scaphoid	
IV	Degenerative changes	

STAGE III

Stage III disease is subdivided into two grades: stages IIIA and IIIB. Stage IIIA is characterized by the collapse of the bony architecture of the lunate, but there is no rotary subluxation of the scaphoid. Stage IIIB disease displays lunate and carpal collapse, which is associated with proximal migration of the capitate and fixed rotary subluxation of the scaphoid. In addition to pain and swelling, wrist stiffness becomes a significant symptom during this stage.

STAGE IV

In stage IV disease, degenerative changes occur in the radiolunate and adjacent intercarpal articulations. Subchondral sclerosis, joint space narrowing, osteophyte formation, and degenerative cysts occur within these articulations.

TREATMENT

Nonoperative Treatment

Immobilization has been advocated in all stages of Kienböck's disease but has not been shown to halt the progression of the disease or collapse of the bony architecture. Nonoperative treatment of Kienböck's disease has yielded poor results with greater than 50% of patients suffering daily symptoms (31). Initial treatment of stage I Kienböck's disease may include immobilization and anti-inflammatory medication. Often immobilization will produce a relative osteopenia of the surrounding carpal bones and make lunate sclerosis more apparent on plain film radiographs. When immobilization proves unsuccessful in alleviating symptoms, surgical intervention should be considered.

Operative Treatment

Many surgical options exist for the treatment of Kienböck's disease, including revascularization procedures, joint-leveling procedures, limited intercarpal fusion, and salvage procedures (e.g., proximal row carpectomy and wrist fusion). The type of surgical procedure chosen is based on the stage of the disease and the clinical picture (Clinical Table: Kienböck's Disease). Often there are several treatment options. Two major radiographic features affect the selection of the specific surgical treatment. The presence of wrist arthritis commits the surgeon to a salvage procedure, and the presence of positive ulnar variance prohibits the joint-leveling procedures of radial shortening and ulnar lengthening.

REVASCULARIZATION PROCEDURES

In stages I, II, and IIIA Kienböck's disease, it is possible for the lunate to reestablish blood supply and reconstitute. Revascularization by vascular bundle implantation or vascularized pedicle grafts have, therefore, been proposed as treatment options. Vascular bundle implantation relies on the principle that a significant amount of microcirculation exists between the artery and the vein in the bundle. With implantation of a vascular bundle, capillary beds proliferate and anastomose with the existing circulation to increase the delivery of osteogenic elements to the bone and accelerate the process of creeping substitution. Revascularization procedures can be used in stages I through IIIA, regardless of ulnar variance. Revascularization is contraindicated for stages IIIB and IV disease because carpal collapse and arthritis cannot be corrected. The technique of pedicled pronator quadratus muscle with radial bone has been described, and success at the 7-year follow-up has been reported (32). At our institution, the direct transplantation of a vascular bundle into the lunate as described by Hori et al. (33) is the preferred method.

Tamai et al. (34) reported their experience with 51 cases of vascular implantation followed for an average of 6 years. Of the 6 wrists with stage I or II disease, good results were obtained in 5 and fair results in 1. The results for stages III and IV disease were mixed, even though some patients had bone grafting or limited fusions at the time of revascularization. Good results were noted for 72% of all stage IIIA and IIIB wrists. On average, all patients reported improvement in range of motion and in grip strength.

Vascular Pedicle Transplantation

Before vascular pedicle transplantation surgery, the pulses of the second and third dorsal metacarpal arteries are confirmed with Doppler ultrasound, and the vessel with the stronger Doppler signal is selected as the donor pedicle. Under tourniquet control, a longitudinal incision is made on the dorsum of the hand from the second (or third) interdigital space to the wrist joint. The selected vascular bundle is dissected as a pedicle with the aid of microscope or loupe magnification. The vascular bundle is then ligated distally with an absorbable suture and cut at the level of the dorsal digital web space. It is important not to skeletonize the artery. The vascular bundle is then kept moist with 10% Xylocaine while the recipient bed is prepared.

The dorsal capsule is incised over the radiolunate joint, and the dorsal aspect of the lunate is exposed. A drill hole is made in the nonarticular portion of the lunate from dorsal to volar, and an 18-gauge needle is passed through it (Fig. 6.4). A small transverse volar wrist counterincision is then made while the flexor tendons and median nerve are retracted. A 21-gauge needle is inserted volar to dorsal into the 18-gauge needle, which should be visible through the volar cortex of the lunate; then the 18-gauge needle is withdrawn. The tagging suture on the end of the vascular bundle is passed through the 21-gauge needle from dorsal to volar to implant the bundle in the lunate, and the needle is withdrawn. The tagging suture is sutured to the volar capsule to hold the bundle in position within the lunate. There should be no tension on the pedicle.

For stage IIIA disease, all necrotic bone should be carefully removed with a burr or curette before the vascular bundle is implanted. Iliac crest or distal radius bone chips

Clinical Table: Kienböck's Disease

Procedure	Indications	Technique	Pitfalls
Nonoperative			
Immobilization	• Stage I disease	• Casting	• Progression
Revascularization			
Vascular pedicle transplantation	• Stage I–IIIA disease	• Dorsal 2nd or 3rd metacarpal artery or vein isolated as a vascular bundle	• Progression
Decompression, Joint Leveling			
Radial shortening	• Stages I–IIIA disease • Ulnar negative variance	• Volar approach • Shortening or wedge osteotomy	• Nonunion • Overshortening with ulnar impingement • Distal radioulnar joint incongruity
Ulnar lengthening	• Stages I–IIIA disease • Ulnar negative variance	• Ulnar approach • Dynamic compression plate	• Nonunion • Ulnar impingement • Graft site morbidity
Capitate shortening	• Stages I–IIIA disease • Ulnar negative variance	• Dorsal approach • Dynamic compression plate	• Violate capsule with decreased range of motion • Nonunion • Pin irritation
Limited Intercarpal Fusion			
Scaphotrapezio-trapezoid fusion	• Stage IIIB disease	• Dorsal approach	• Persistent pain • Nonunion
Scaphocapitate fusion	• Stage IIIB disease	• Dorsal approach	• Persistent pain • Nonunion
Salvage			
Proximal row carpectomy	• Stage IV disease	• Dorsal approach	• Weak grip
Wrist arthrodesis	• Stage IV disease	• Dorsal approach	• Nonunion • Loss of range of motion

may then be placed into the cavity. The vascularized pedicle graft should be transplanted through this.

The wrist is immobilized in some extension from the metacarpophalangeal (MP) joints to the elbow for 4 weeks postoperatively. The patient then begins gentle range of motion (ROM) exercises. A dorsal splint is worn for several more months to prevent wrist hyperextension.

JOINT-LEVELING PROCEDURES

Patients with negative ulnar variance may benefit from an equalization of the distal articular surfaces of the radius and ulna to reduce shear stress across the lunate. Results of these joint-leveling procedures, which include radial shortening and ulnar lengthening have been encouraging. Capitate shortening similarly reduces shear stresses across the lunate and is discussed below. These procedures are indicated in patients with stages I through IIIA Kienböck's disease. Ulnar negative variance is a prerequisite for radial shortening and ulnar lengthening.

Shortening the radius by 2 mm is enough to unload the lunate by 70%. This amount of shortening decreases the ra-

diolunate forces, increases the ulnolunate forces by 50%, and has no effect on the radioscaphoid forces (35,36). Radial displacement of the distal fragment along with shortening may help decrease the load across the distal radioulnar joint (39). A 4-year follow-up of radial shortening demonstrated an average increase of 30% in flexion and extension and a 50% increase in grip strength. Approximately 87% of patients experienced good to excellent results (37,38,40–47).

In patients with positive ulnar variance, a lateral closing or medial opening wedge osteotomy of the distal radius of 4° to 8° decreases the pressure load in the lunate fossa. In contrast, the reverse osteotomy increases radiolunate load (48). These changes have been confirmed by computer-generated models (49). At the 2-year follow-up of radial wedge osteotomy, 60% of patients reported good to excellent results (50). Even though these results are inferior to those of radial shortening (87 to 89%) (46,50), radial wedge osteotomy appears to be a good extra-articular treatment for ulnar-positive wrists and does not result in limited motion. In addition, radial wedge osteotomy does

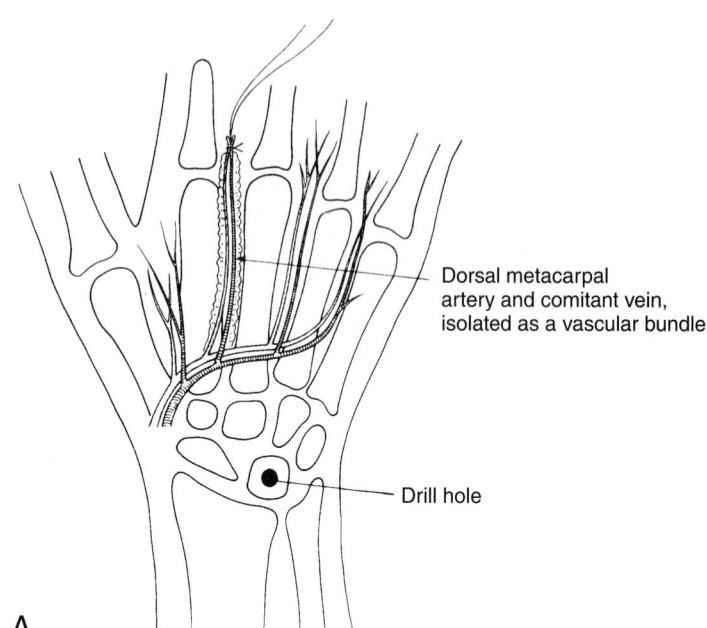

Figure 6.4. A. For a vascular pedicle transplantation, the second dorsal metacarpal artery and vein are isolated as a neurovascular pedicle. A drill hole is made in the lunate from dorsal to volar. **B.** The vascular pedicle is passed through the lunate from dorsal to volar with the assistance of a tagging suture and a 21-gauge needle. **C.** The vascular bundle is fixed to the volar capsule. Reprinted with permission from Tamai S, Yajima H, Ono H. Revascularization procedures in the treatment of Kienböck's disease. Hand Clin 1993;9:457.

Dorsal metacarpal
artery and comitant vein,
isolated as a vascular bundle

Drill hole

A

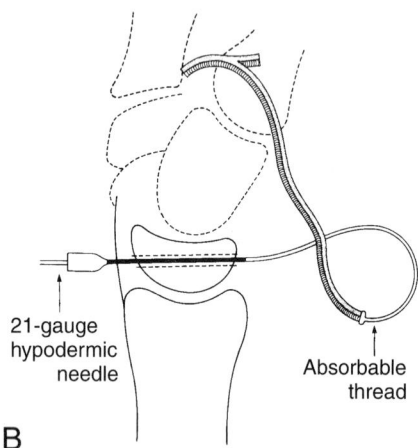

21-gauge
hypodermic
needle

Absorbable
thread

B

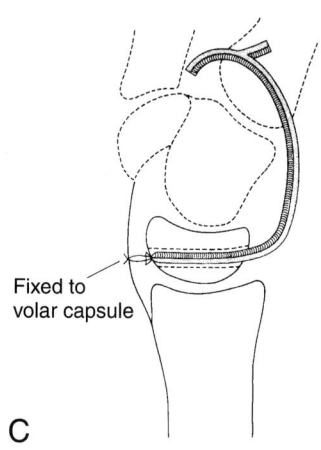

Fixed to
volar capsule

C

not preclude future options, including revascularization and limited wrist fusions, should they become necessary.

The ulnar-lengthening osteotomy accomplishes the same goal as radial-shortening osteotomy. Ulnar lengthening, however, produces an intercalary defect, which usually requires bone grafting. Drawbacks to ulnar lengthening include bone graft donor site morbidity and an increased risk of nonunion at the osteotomy site. The results of 60 patients treated with ulnar lengthening demonstrated 90% satisfaction rate at 7 years and pain relief in 86% of cases (51). Grip strength improved in most, whereas wrist motion remained essentially unchanged.

Capitate shortening has been shown to provide the greatest decrease in the compressive forces across the lunate (Fig. 6.5); however, it increases scaphotrapezial and triquetrohamate forces (52). The procedure may be performed in an ulnar-positive wrist. Because capitate shortening involves wrist capsulotomy, it may lead to more loss of wrist motion than will other joint-leveling procedures. Almquist (12) reported an 83% revascularization

rate of lunates after capitate shortening and capitohamate fusion.

Radial Shortening and Radial Wedge Osteotomy

The incision for radial shortening or radial wedge osteotomy is made under tourniquet control. A longitudinal incision of approximately 10 cm is made on the volar aspect of the forearm, over the flexor carpi radialis (FCR) tendon, extending proximally from the proximal wrist crease. The incision is carried down through subcutaneous tissue with sharp and blunt dissection. The radial artery is identified and retracted radially, and the FCR is retracted ulnarly. The deep aspect of the FCR sheath is incised, and the pronator quadratus muscle is exposed and elevated from the radial aspect of the radius; the surgeon should take care to leave a small radial portion intact for later reattachment over the plate. Subperiosteal stripping is carried proximally and distally to allow placement of the plate on the volar aspect of the radius. The volar radiocarpal ligaments should not be disturbed.

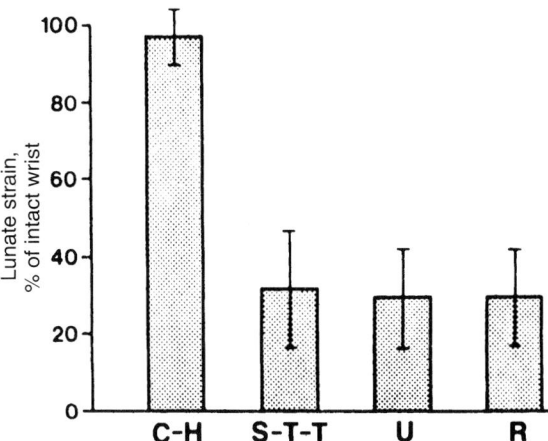

Figure 6.5. Lunate strain after simulated capitohamate fusion (*CH*), scaphotrapeziotrapezoid fusion (*S-T-T*), ulnar lengthening (*U*) by 3 mm, and radial shortening (*R*) by 3 mm in cadaver wrists. Reprinted with permission from Trumble T, Glisson RR, Seaber AV, et al. A biomechanical comparison of the methods for treating Kienböck's disease. J Hand Surg 1986;11A:88–93.

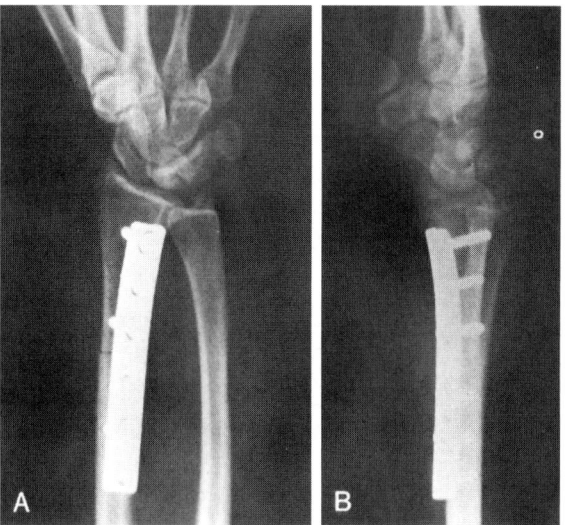

Figure 6.6. Radial shortening for Kienböck's disease, using a six-hole dynamic compression plate. Reprinted with permission from Weiss APC. Radial shortening. Hand Clin 1993;9:480.

A six-hole, 3.5-mm dynamic compression plate is contoured to the volar aspect of the radius as distally as possible to allow the osteotomy to be performed in the radial metaphysis. If the plate is placed too far distally, it will lie over the volar lip of the radius. The plate is fixed to the radius with a clamp, and the osteotomy site is marked on the radius at the midpoint of the plate (i.e., between the third and fourth holes). Next, two of the distal screw holes are drilled, tapped, and filled with 3.5-mm cortical screws in the usual neutral fashion. These two screws are removed, and the plate is temporarily removed.

The radial-shortening osteotomy is performed using an oscillating saw to remove a 2-mm segment of bone. Care must be taken not to remove too much radius. The thickness of the saw cut must be taken into account. This can be done in two ways: (*a*) A 2-mm osteotomy is marked out on the radius, and the saw cuts are made on the inner aspects of the mark to remove a wafer-thin slice of radius; or (*b*) two saw blades can be placed together (stacked) on the saw to cut a 2-mm osteotomy (this should be practiced before the surgery) (Fig. 6.6).

The lateral closing wedge osteotomy is performed as follows. A 2-mm radial-based wedge is resected by osteotomies that meet ulnarly. The distal osteotomy is begun first and almost fully completed. The second, more proximal osteotomy is then begun 2 mm proximal to the first and is aimed to intersect at the same point on the ulnar cortex. The osteotomies are then both completed (Fig. 6.7).

After either osteotomy, the dynamic compression plate is reattached to the distal radial fragment through the previously made screw holes. If possible, the radial fragment should be displaced slightly radially to reduce the forces on the distal radioulnar joint. The remaining screw holes are fastened proximally, using the dynamic compression aspect of the plate through two of the proximal holes. The

radial bone that was removed can be fragmented and used as bone graft in the osteotomy site.

Postsurgery, the wrist is immobilized for 2 weeks, at which time the sutures are removed and active-assisted range of motion (ROM) of the wrist, including pronation and supination, is begun. A removable protective wrist splint is worn full-time until union of the osteotomy is seen on radiographs.

Ulnar Lengthening

For ulnar lengthening, the involved extremity and the selected iliac crest site are prepared and draped (53,54). Under tourniquet control, a longitudinal incision is made over the ulnar aspect of the flexor carp ulnaris, extending proximally from the proximal wrist crease. By sharp and blunt dissection, the dorsal sensory branch of the ulnar nerve is identified and protected. The periosteum overlying the distal ulna is reflected. A four-hole dynamic compression plate is contoured to the volar aspect of the distal ulna. In heavier, larger individuals, the plate may be placed along the medial aspect of the ulna, although we prefer to use the volar surface, where the plate is less likely to be prominent. Two distal screw holes are drilled and filled with 3.5-mm cortical screws in the usual fashion. The osteotomy site is marked just between the third and fourth screw holes; the site is crosshatched to allow for proper rotational positioning after osteotomy. The previously placed screws and plate are temporarily removed.

The osteotomy is performed with an oscillating saw. Distraction of the osteotomy with a laminar spreader allows the surgeon to place a previously harvested 3-mm tricortical iliac crest graft. The plate is placed along the volar surface of the ulna, and the previously drilled screw holes are filled. Two proximal holes are drilled and filled for dynamic compression across the graft. The iliac crest graft is

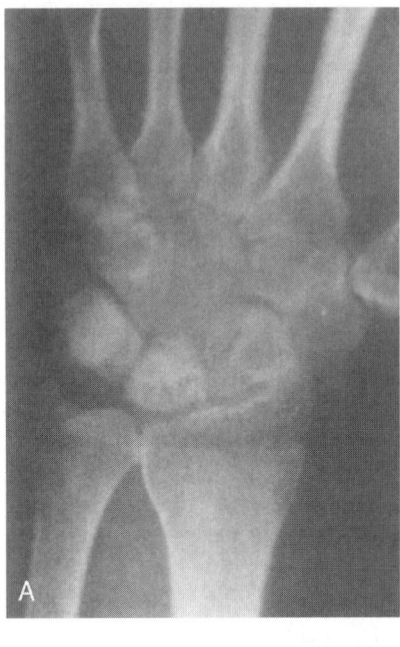

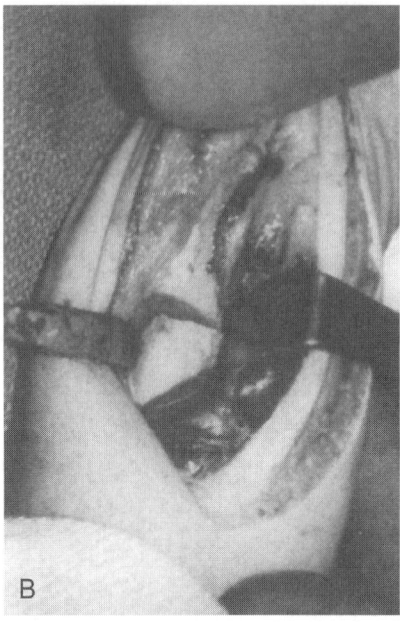

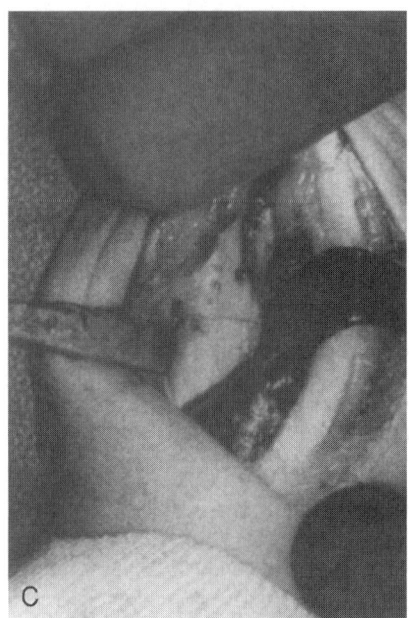

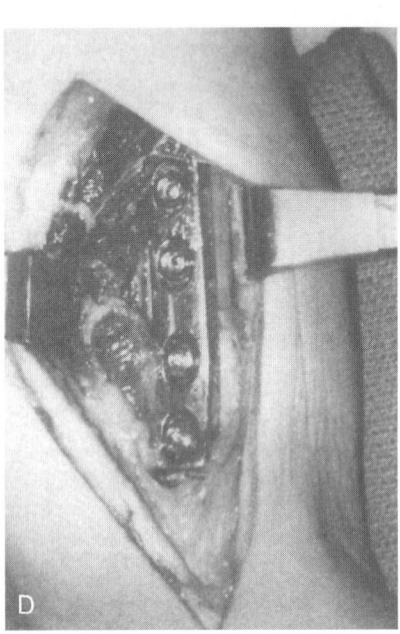

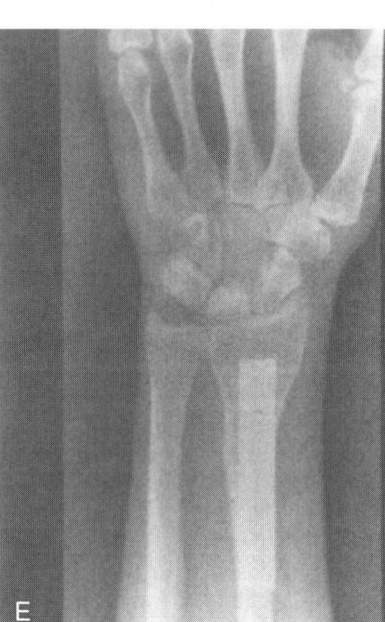

Figure 6.7. A. Preoperative view of an ulnar-positive wrist with stage IIIA Kienböck's disease that is a candidate for radial lateral closing wedge osteotomy. **B.** The lateral wedge osteotomy is resected. **C.** The osteotomy site is then closed. Note the distal predrilled screw hole. **D.** The dynamic compression plate is placed on the osteotomy site. **E.** Postoperative view showing ulnar neutral variance. Reprinted with permission from Gerwin M, Weiland AJ. Avascular necrosis of the carpals. In: Peimer CA, ed. Surgery of the hand and upper extremity. New York: McGraw-Hill, 1996.

then trimmed and smoothed to the existing ulna; additional cancellous bone graft is packed at the osteotomy site (Fig. 6.8).

Postsurgery, the patient is placed in a short arm splint with the wrist in 15° of extension for 6 to 8 weeks. A removable splint is worn until radiographic evidence of healing is present. Armistead et al. (53) recommend that the plate be removed 1 year after union to allow the grafted area to become stronger. We rarely remove forearm plates, but will if the patient complains of discomfort over the hardware.

Capitate Shortening

A straight dorsal longitudinal midline incision is used for the capitate shortening procedure. The extensor reti-naculum is opened through the fifth dorsal compartment, and the extensor digit quinti tendon is retracted ulnarly. Radial dissection of the extensor retinaculum is continued across to the radial aspect of the fourth dorsal compartment. The digital extensor tendons are retracted, and an incision is made in the dorsal wrist capsule to expose the capitate. The osteotomy of the capitate is begun with a thin osteotome at the distal margin of the dorsal articular surface of the scaphoid, but it is not yet carried to the volar cortex. The second cut is made 2 to 3 mm distal to the first. Both osteotomies are then continued simultaneously; the proximal osteotomy is completed first.

The volar capsule is kept intact, and the osteotomized wafer of capitate is removed. The capitate head is then held compressed to the distal pole of the capitate with an

Figure 6.8. Ulnar lengthening for stage III Kienböck's disease using a tricortical iliac crest graft. Positive ulnar variance is now +1 mm. Reprinted with permission from Quenzer DE, Linscheid RL. Ulnar lengthening procedures. Hand Clin 1993;9:469

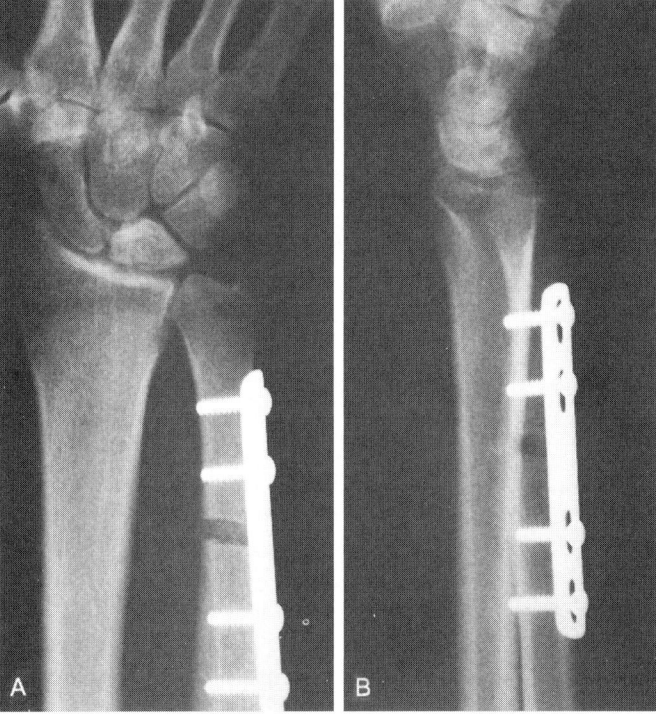

elevator, while crossed 1.55-mm (0.062-in.) Kirschner (K) wires are passed retrograde across the osteotomy site. Capitohamate fusion can be performed at this time, if desired, to increase the fusion mass. The dorsal two-thirds of the adjacent capitate and hamate joints are decorticated, and two more K wires are passed percutaneously through the hamate: One is passed through the proximal capitate and one through the distal pole (Fig. 6.9). Care is taken to avoid the dorsal branch of the ulnar nerve (which can be visualized through the skin flap). Bone resected from the capitate can be packed into the capitohamate fusion.

After surgery, the extremity is immobilized with a short arm splint with the wrist in a neutral position. At 10 days, the skin sutures are removed, and a short arm cast is placed on the extremity. At 8 weeks, the cast is removed, and if radiographs demonstrate early healing of the osteotomy site, the patient is placed in a removable wrist splint. When complete union is seen radiographically, the pins are removed. ROM exercises can begin when the removable splint is started, but the splint should be worn until revascularization of the lunate is seen radiographically.

RESECTION ARTHROPLASTY OF THE LUNATE

Long-term results of silicone lunate implantation have demonstrated that the incidence of silicone synovitis approaches 50%, and 80% of patients realize poor results owing to either silicone synovitis or dislocation of the prosthesis (55). Silicone synovitis may destroy joints that otherwise could have been salvaged with a different procedure. The typical Kienböck's disease patient is a young, active male who is ill-suited for silicone arthroplasty. No

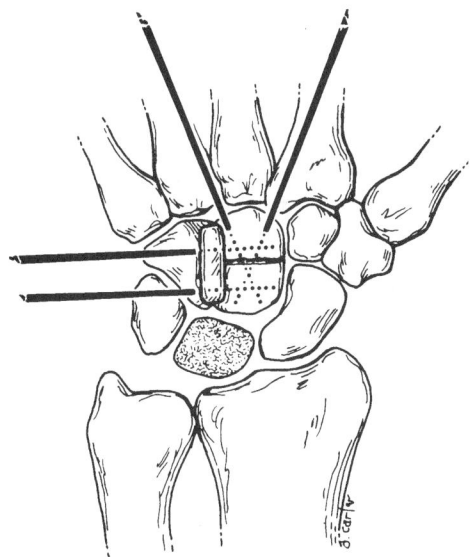

Figure 6.9. Adjacent surfaces of the hamate and capitate are decorticated and fixed with K wires along with the osteotomy of the capitate. Reprinted with permission from Almquist EA. Capitate shortening in the treatment of Kienböck's disease. Hand Clin 1993; 9:509.

long-term results of titanium lunate arthroplasty are available. At this time we do not see a place for silicone or titanium lunate arthroplasty in the treatment of Kienböck's disease.

Lunate resection and fascial or coiled tendon replacement have been unsuccessful owing to late carpal collapse and should be performed only in conjunction with a limited intercarpal fusion (13,56).

LIMITED INTERCARPAL FUSION

Scaphotrapeziotrapezoid (STT) and scaphocapitate (SC) fusions are good options for stage IIIB Kienböck's disease, especially in the presence of neutral or positive ulnar variance. Both procedures can address the rotary subluxation of the scaphoid and improve the pattern of carpal collapse, as well as unload the lunate. Scaphocapitate fusion is technically easier than scaphotrapeziotrapezoid fusion and, therefore, is usually the first choice for a limited intercarpal fusion. Scaphotrapeziotrapezoid and scaphocapitate arthrodeses have been shown to decrease lunate load an average of 70% compared to capitohamate arthrodesis and to be roughly equivalent to joint-leveling procedures (35,52). Fusion of the scaphoid in a neutral or extended position is important to reduce the load on the lunate, but it may increase load on the scaphoid and radioscaphoid joint (57). Capitohamate fusion does not decrease the load on the lunate experimentally, unless performed in conjunction with capitate shortening (35,52,57).

Experimental wrist kinematic studies have shown loss of motion after STT and SC fusion to be 15% of flexion/extension and 25% of radioulnar deviation (58). In vivo values would be expected to be different, secondary to early postoperative intra-articular fibrosis and, later, ligamentous stretching. Experimental studies have shown that the ideal radioscaphoid angle for maximal wrist motion after scaphotrapeziotrapezoid fusion is 41° to 60°; after scaphocapitate fusion, the angle is 30° to 57° (59).

On long-term (up to 5 years) follow-up of 35 STT arthrodeses, 80% of patients noted little or no rest pain, and 71% had no pain with activity (60). Approximately 82% of patients returned to their preoperative employment or activities, and grip strength was equal to 89% of the contralateral side. Average range of motion was 74° extension and 59° flexion.

Scaphotrapeziotrapezoid Arthrodesis

The incision for STT arthrodesis is done under tourniquet control. A transverse incision is made over the STT joint distal to the radial styloid and carried through subcutaneous tissues with blunt dissection to protect the branches of the superficial radial nerve and radial artery. The extensor retinaculum is opened over the extensor pollicis longus tendon, and the wrist is approached between the tendons of the extensor carpi radialis longus and brevis. The radioscaphoid joint should be inspected for the presence of arthritis, as this would preclude STT arthrodesis. Radial styloidectomy is typically performed by removing 5 mm of the styloid tip; this does not affect wrist motion but may lessen first extensor compartment symptoms. The STT joints are decorticated with a rongeur, saw, or burr. If a power burr or saw is used, the surgeon must be careful to prevent thermal necrosis of bone by using irrigation. The trapezium-trapezoid joint is decorticated proximally without disrupting the carpometacarpal joint distally. The lunate is inspected next; if it is fragmented, it is excised.

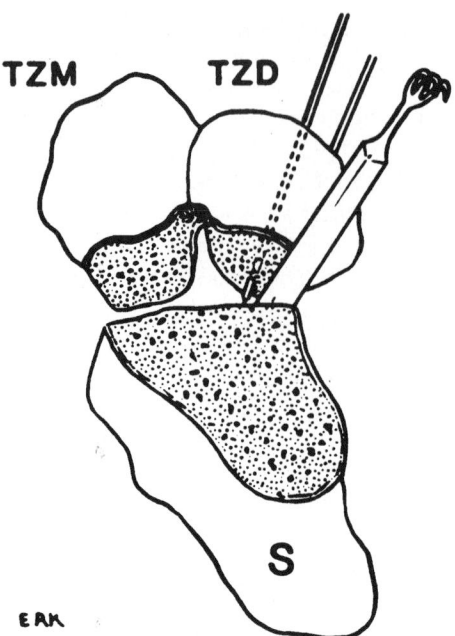

Figure 6.10. Adjacent surfaces of the scaphoid (*S*), trapezium (*TZM*) and trapezoid (*TZD*) are decorticated to cancellous bone. A 5-mm spacer is placed between the scaphoid and trapezoid, and two K wires are preloaded in the trapezoid. The wrist is then positioned in 25° of radial deviation, as the distal pole of the scaphoid is displaced dorsally as far as possible. The K wires are then driven retrograde across the scaphotrapezoid joint. Reprinted with permission from Watson HK, Pitts EC. Scapholunate dissociation: treatment by scaphotrapezio-trapezoid arthrodesis. Tech Orthop 1992;7:30.

A second transverse incision is made 2 cm proximal to the radial styloid, and subperiosteal dissection is performed under the first and second dorsal compartments. A cortical window is elevated from the radius, and a cancellous bone graft is harvested. The window is replaced and this wound is closed.

Two smooth K wires (1.13 or 1.55 mm; 0.045 or 0.062 in.) are preset in the trapezoid, and the scaphotrapezial joint is positioned as described by Watson et al. (60). A periosteal elevator is placed in the scaphotrapezial joint to create a 5-mm space, which prevents loss of carpal height owing to the decortication. The wrist is positioned in 25° of dorsiflexion and 20° of radial deviation. The scaphoid is then displaced as far as possible and the two K wires are driven retrograde across the scaphotrapezial joint (Fig. 6.10). This maneuver reduces the scaphoid to about 50° to 60° of volar flexion relative to the long axis of the radius. The previously harvested cancellous graft is then placed in the fusion site. Radiographs confirm bone and wire positions. The K wires are cut and buried beneath the skin, as they may need to remain in position for a long time.

Scaphocapitate Fusion

Under tourniquet control, a dorsal midline incision is made over the scaphocapitate region for the SC fusion. The third dorsal compartment is released longitudinally, and the extensor pollicis longus tendon is retracted. A longitudinal incision is made in the dorsal capsule, and the flaps are reflected. Cortical bone is removed from the dorsal two-thirds of the adjacent surfaces of the scaphoid and capitate. Retaining the palmar third of the cortical bone maintains carpal height. The decorticated area is filled with bone graft from either the radial styloid or the iliac crest, and multiple K wires are drilled across the fusion site. Care is taken to reduce the scaphoid to the capitate, and intraoperative radiographs should confirm acceptable alignment of scaphoid, capitate, radius, and lunate. When radial deviation past neutral is not possible intraoperatively, the scaphoid has probably been excessively dorsiflexed and needs to be repositioned.

Postsurgery, patients who have undergone STT and SC fusions are immobilized in long arm casts across the wrist and elbow with the forearm in neutral rotation, the thumb abducted, and the index and long finger in the intrinsic plus position. After 4 weeks, the long arm cast is replaced with a short arm thumb spica cast. At 6 weeks after surgery, radiographs should demonstrate healing. A CT scan aligned along the axis of the thumb may help asses the progression of the STT arthrodesis. Once arthrodesis is achieved, the pins are removed, and ROM exercises are begun.

WRIST DENERVATION

Buck-Gramcko (61,62) reported on wrist denervation alone as a treatment of Kienböck's disease. At the long-term (6.5 years) follow-up, 65% of patients had no pain or pain only with heavy activities. Results were unrelated to the stage of disease at time of surgery, suggesting that the procedure produced a true denervation effect. Progression of the lunate changes was seen radiographically in 50% of patients, but only five wrists showed progressive arthritic changes. Denervation alone is probably not sufficient treatment for Kienböck's disease, but resection of the terminal articular portion of the posterior interosseous nerve should be performed at the time of other procedures, if possible.

SALVAGE PROCEDURES

Treatment of stage IV Kienböck's disease requires a salvage procedure to preserve function and eliminate pain. The best options include proximal row carpectomy and wrist arthrodesis. Proximal row carpectomy is an alternative for wrists in which the articular surface of the lunate fossa of the radius and the head of the capitate are in good condition. It helps retain ROM; however, it does not provide for preservation of grip strength as does an arthrodesis. Patients who undergo a proximal row carpectomy may eventually need a wrist arthrodesis.

If there is articular loss on the head of the capitate or in the lunate fossa of the radius, distraction resection arthroplasty—in which the head of the capitate is excised, and the wrist is held distracted with K wires—has been proposed by some authors as a treatment alternative for patients who are not considered candidates for proximal row carpectomy because of joint degeneration. At our institu-

tion, this technique has not been used. Of 11 patients who underwent distraction resection arthroplasty for degenerative arthritis, 25% eventually required a wrist arthrodesis (63). Although arthrodesis eliminates motion, it ensures pain relief and good grip strength. The likelihood of needing subsequent procedures after arthrodesis is low.

After proximal row carpectomy, most patients gain approximately 30° of flexion and extension (14,15) and 50 to 80% of the contralateral grip strength (14,16,17). After wrist fusion, grip strength improves, but usually does not return to normal (18). Pseudarthrosis rates are less than 5% (18,19).

Proximal Row Carpectomy

For proximal row carpectomy, a dorsal longitudinal incision is preferred to a transverse incision, in case an arthrodesis is required later. The third dorsal compartment retinaculum is incised, and the extensor pollicis longus is retracted. The dorsal capsule is incised longitudinally and reflected subperiosteally from the radius and carpals to expose the scaphoid, lunate, and triquetrum. The articular surfaces are inspected. An acceptable articular surface on the lunate fossa and head of the capitate must be present. Threaded Steinmann pins or K wires can be placed in the scaphoid, lunate, and triquetrum and used as joysticks to provide leverage to facilitate removal of the bones.

Resection of the lunate is usually easiest and should be performed first. Care is taken to preserve the volar radio-carpal ligaments, as they will provide stability for the distal row. We also perform a moderate radial styloidectomy with a rongeur at this point, so that when the wrist is moved passively into radial deviation, there is no impingement of the trapezium on the radial styloid. If the volar ligaments are preserved, K wire fixation of the distal row to the radius is not necessary, even if the articulation feels loose (Fig. 6.11). Postoperative return of motor function will stabilize the articulation. The dorsal wrist capsule is repaired, as is the extensor retinaculum.

Postsurgery, the wrist is immobilized in a volar splint with the wrist in 15° of dorsiflexion. After 2 weeks, the sutures are removed, and a short arm cast is placed on the extremity when swelling decreases. Immobilization is continued for 1 month after surgery; then the patient is placed in a removable wrist splint and begins gentle active ROM exercises. When the patient feels no pain with motion, resistive exercises are begun. Manual laborers usually return to work by 6 months after surgery, but the return to peak power after proximal row carpectomy may take up to 1 year.

Wrist Arthrodesis

Under tourniquet control, a midline dorsal longitudinal incision is made for the wrist arthrodesis. The extensor retinaculum is divided over the third dorsal compartment, and the extensor pollicis longus tendon is retracted radially. Subperiosteal dissection is then performed radially and ulnarly to expose the distal radius, carpus, and base of the third metacarpal. The fourth dorsal compartment should

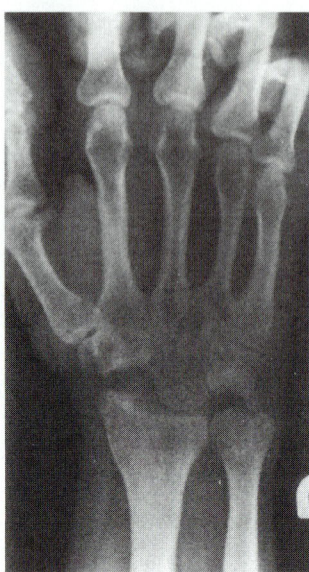

Figure 6.11. AP view showing a proximal row carpectomy. No postoperative fixation was necessary. Reprinted with permission from Gerwin M, Weiland AJ. Avascular necrosis of the carpals. In: Peimer CA, ed. Surgery of the hand and upper extremity. New York: McGraw-Hill, 1996.

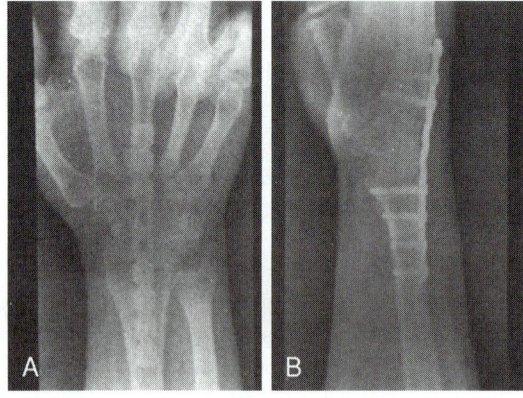

Figure 6.12. AP (**A**) and lateral (**B**) views of a wrist arthrodesis with a 3.5-mm reconstruction plate. Note the contouring of the plate. Reprinted with permission from Gerwin M, Weiland AJ. Avascular necrosis of the carpals. In: Peimer CA, ed. Surgery of the hand and upper extremity. New York: McGraw-Hill, 1996.

not be entered. Lister's tubercle is resected with a rongeur. A power burr is used to decorticate the distal radius, all of the carpal bones, and the third carpometacarpal joint. A 3.5-mm dynamic compression plate is then contoured to the distal radius, dorsum of the carpus, and base of third metacarpal. (A prefabricated wrist fusion plate may also be used.) Typically, an 8- to 10-hole plate is required to allow six cortices of purchase each in the distal radius and the third metacarpal (Fig. 6.12). The plate should be contoured to allow approximately 5° of wrist dorsiflexion. A cancellous iliac crest bone graft is packed between the carpal bones and beneath the plate. The retinaculum of the third dorsal compartment and the dorsal capsule are reapproximated

with nonabsorbable sutures. The extensor pollicis longus tendon is left superficial to the retinaculum. The skin is closed over a drain.

Postsurgery, the patient is placed in a volar splint. A removable splint is used 2 weeks after surgery, when the swelling decreases and the sutures are removed. Digital motion and forearm rotation are encouraged immediately postsurgery. Resistive strengthening exercises are delayed for 6 weeks until there is radiographic evidence of fusion.

COMPLICATIONS

There are three types of complications possible after distal radial shortening (18). Radial nonunion occurs in approximately 4% of cases and should be treated by repeat bone grafting after 5 to 6 months. Overshortening of the radius may lead to secondary ulnar impaction, which can be avoided by careful operative technique. The radius should be shortened only 2 mm for an ulnar-negative to ulnar-neutral wrist. Ulnar impingement at the distal radial ulnar joint can similarly result from excessive radial shortening and should be avoided.

With ulnar lengthening, complications occurred in 22% of patients (51): 14% of patients had a delayed union or nonunion, and 8% had symptoms of ulnocarpal impingement or impaction. Plate removal was necessary in 55% of patients. Five percent of patients needed a second operation because of nonunion. Approximately 7% of patients underwent additional procedures on the ulna to treat ulnar impaction. Although the ulnar lengthening was technically adequate, 11% of patients required additional surgery, which included limited intercarpal fusions and salvage procedures. No patients exhibited radiographic progression of the disease at follow-up.

After STT fusion, 30% of wrists may require late lunate excision secondary to pain. This, of course, assumes the lunate was not excised at the time of the initial procedure. If a nonunion occurs, it should be treated by repeat bone grafting at 3 to 4 months.

SUMMARY

Avascular necrosis of the lunate (Kienböck's disease) is generally a disease that occurs in the young laborer and may produce significant disability. The precise etiology of avascular necrosis of the lunate has not yet been established. Several theories have been proposed, but none has been universally accepted. The avascularity may be the result of a primary ischemic event, a traumatic vascular interuption, or a microfracture resulting in an intraosseous vascular interruption. Additionally, Kienböck's disease is a condition for which no consistently reliable treatment has been found. Nonoperative management is unsatisfactory in more than half the cases, and the disease may progress to lunate collapse and degenerative arthritis of the wrist joint. As a consequence, various surgical procedures that aim to correct one or more of the factors that may predispose to the disease or treat the lunate bone itself have been proposed as treatments in the early stages of the disease. Early results of revascularization of the lunate have been promising, but long-term follow-up is not available. More advanced disease at initial presentation portends a worse prognosis and frequently requires lunate excision, proximal row carpectomy, or some form of limited carpal or wrist joint fusion.

II Avascular Necrosis of the Scaphoid (Preiser's Disease)

Avascular necrosis of the scaphoid that occurs in the absence of fracture or trauma is rare. The avascular necrosis described by Preiser (64) probably occurred in fractured scaphoids (65). However, idiopathic avascular necrosis of the scaphoid (Preiser's disease) does occur. The etiology of this condition, as with Kienböck's disease, has yet to be determined. It is generally agreed that the scaphoid is at risk for avascularity because it only has one intraosseous vessel and no rich anastomotic system (66,67).

RELEVANT ANATOMY AND PATHOGENESIS

The scaphoid is an irregularly shaped bone that rests in a plane at approximately 45° to the longitudinal axis of the wrist. Eighty percent of the surface of the bone is covered by articular cartilage. The strong interosseous ligament secures the scaphoid to the lunate. The primary blood supply enters the scaphoid through the dorsal ligamentous structures. Studies have demonstrated that the major blood supply comes from the scaphoid branches of the radial artery, entering the dorsal ridge and supplying 70 to 80% of the bone, including the proximal pole (22,23). There is a second major group of vessels that enters the scaphoid tubercle, and this group perfuses the distal 30% of the bone.

INITIAL FINDINGS, PHYSICAL EXAMINATION, AND DIAGNOSIS

The patient with Preiser's disease typically relates a history of chronic or repetitive stress frequently related to occupational or recreational activity. Many patients have a history of steroid use. The dominant hand seems to be more frequently affected. Patients typically complain of local pain, tenderness, and decreased grip strength. Examination may reveal dorsal soft tissue swelling, scaphoid tenderness, and decreased range of motion. The etiology of Preiser's disease could very well be a fatigue fracture of the scaphoid. Radiographic evidence of sclerosis and fragmentation of the proximal pole of the scaphoid in the absence of a diagnosed fracture of the bone confirms the diagnosis.

RADIOLOGIC STUDIES

The initial radiographic appearance is characterized by cystic and sclerotic changes in the scaphoid that are followed by collapse and, in some instances, fracture, especially in the proximal portion of the bone. These findings typically resemble those of Kienböck's disease involving the lunate bone. Arthritic changes involving the articulations are seen in more advanced disease. MRI may be useful to diagnose the condition in very early stages of the disease. Ischemic necrosis is typically associated with loss of signal on T_1-weighted images.

TREATMENT

Treatment of avascular necrosis of the scaphoid has not been standardized. Current treatment recommendations include conservative management with immobilization, arthroscopic drilling of the lesion (68), revascularization

Clinical Table: Preiser's Disease

Procedure	Indications	Technique	Pitfalls
Immobilization	• Early stages	• Casting	• Progression • Persistent pain
Arthroscopic drilling	• Early disease prior to anatomic changes of the bone	• Wrist arthroscopy	• Progression
Revascularization	• Early disease prior to anatomic changes of the bone	• Pronator quadratus pedicle flap; vascularized distal radius graft; ulnar artery-based graft	• Failure • Progression
Scaphoid resection	• Advanced disease	• Excision ± interposition with soft tissue, or silicone prosthesis ± limited carpal arthrodesis	• Loss of range of motion • Persistent pain
Proximal row carpectomy	• Advanced disease	• Dorsal approach	• Weakness of grip
Wrist fusion	• Advanced disease	• Dorsal approach	• Nonunion • Loss of range of motion

procedures, scaphoid resection, interposition arthroplasty, proximal row carpectomy, scaphoid allograft, and fusion procedures (Clinical Table: Preiser's Disease). A vascularized bone graft is the procedure of choice if nonoperative methods (splint, rest, electrical stimulation) fail to resolve the problem in the early stages of the disease.

Four-Bone Fusion with Scaphoid Excision

For four-bone fusion with scaphoid excision, a dorsal midline longitudinal incision is preferred to allow for a secondary wrist arthrodesis, if necessary. The subcutaneous tissues are carefully dissected to avoid injury to the dorsal veins. The third compartment retinaculum is incised, and the extensor pollicis longus tendon is retracted. The dorsal capsule is incised longitudinally and subperiosteally reflected ulnarly and radially from the radius and carpal bones. Adjacent surfaces of the lunate, capitate, hamate, and triquetrum are decorticated. Longitudinal traction helps the surgeon visualize the joint surfaces. When the scaphoid is excised, the surgeon must be careful to not disrupt the volar ligaments. Bone graft may be obtained from the distal radius or iliac crest; it is packed into the intercarpal regions. The capitate and the lunate are aligned with the aid of fluoroscopy to prevent or correct a dorsal intercalated segment instability (DISI) deformity. Percutaneous K wires are passed from the capitate, triquetrum, and hamate into the lunate and from the triquetrum to the capitate. Radial styloidectomy is not necessarily performed with the four-bone fusion.

Postsurgery, the wrists are immobilized for 4 weeks with a long arm splint; then a cast is placed with the forearm in neutral rotation and the thumb free. Short arm cast immobilization is then continued until radiographs confirm healing at about 3 months. The pins are then removed and range of motion exercises begun. Resistive exercises are begun when radiographs demonstrate healing. Peak strength and range of motion is achieved at 8 to 12 months after surgery, and return to work depends on the type of employment.

COMPLICATIONS

Nonunion may occur and is usually recognized by 3 months postsurgery. Nonunion should be treated with repeat bone grafting.

Avascular necrosis of the capitate, hamate, and pisiform have been reported (70–73). Patients with avascular necrosis of the capitate present with stiff, painful wrists; and radiographs demonstrate avascular necrosis of the proximal pole of the capitate. Treatment has ranged from conservative immobilization, to proximal pole excision with palmaris longus interpositional arthroplasty, which has shown good short-term results. In theory, excision of the necrotic bone with midcarpal fusion is another option.

SUMMARY

Idiopathic avascular necrosis of the scaphoid (Preiser's disease) is a rare disease. The etiology of the condition, as well as the etiology of Kienböck's disease, has yet to be established. Initial management may include immobilization, but this is successful in only 20% of caes (69). Revascularization procedures are an attrractive option in early stages of the disease, but long-term outcomes are not available. Salvage procedures such as proximal row carpectomy, limited carpal arthrodesis, and wrist arthrodesis are options for advanced disease or for those failing other procedures, but they may be associated with complications and significant morbidity in this population. Further knowledge as to the cause of the avascularity in the carpal bones may lead to earlier diagnosis and better selection of treatment options.

REFERENCES

1. Peste JL. Discussion. Bull Soc Anat 1843;18:169.
2. Kienböck R. Über traumatische malazie des Mondbeins und ihre folgezustande: entartungsformen und kompressions frakturen. Fortschr Geb Rontgenstr Nuklearmed Erganzungsband 1910; 16:77.
3. Kienböck R. Concerning traumatic malacia of the lunate and its consequences: degeneration and compression fractures. Clin Orthop 1980;149:4–8.
4. Hulten O. Über anatomische der handgelenknochen. Acta Radiol 1928;9:155.
5. Muller W. Über die erweichung und verdichtung des os lunatum, eine typische erkrankung des handgelenks. Beitr Klin Chir 1920; 119:664.
6. Hulten O. Über die entstehung und behandlung der lunatummalazie (morbus Kienböck). Acta Chir Scand 1935;76:121.
7. Chen WS, Shih CH. Ulnar variance and Kienböck's disease. An investigation in Taiwan. Clin Orthop 1990;255:124–127.
8. Kristensen SS, Thomassen E, Christensen F. Ulnar variance in Kienböck's disease. J Hand Surg 1986;11B:258–260.
9. Nathan PA, Meadows KD. Ulna-minus variance and Kienböck's disease. J Hand Surg 1987;12A:777–788.
10. Chan KP, Huang P. Anatomic variations in radial and ulnar lengths in the wrists of Chinese. Clin Orthop 1971;80:17–20.
11. Persson M. Pathogenese und behandlung der Kienböckschen lunatum-malazie. Acta Chir Scand Suppl 1945:92.
12. Almquist EE. Capitate shortening in the treatment of Kienböck's disease. Hand Clin 1993;9:505–512.
13. Eaton RG. Excision and fascial interposition arthroplasty in the treatment of Kienböck's disease. Hand Clin 1993;9:513–516.
14. Imbriglia JE, Broudy AS, Hagberg WC, et al. Proximal row carpectomy: clinical evaluation. J Hand Surg 1990;15A:426–430.
15. White GM, Clark GL, Elias LS. Proximal row carpectomy for posttraumatic disorders of the wrist. J Hand Surg 1987;13A:310.
16. Ferlic DC, Clayton ML, Mills MF. Proximal row carpectomy: review of rheumatoid and nonrheumatoid wrists. J Hand Surg 1991; 16A:420–424.
17. Green DP. Proximal row carpectomy. Hand Clin 1987;3:163.
18. Wright CS, McMurtry RY. AO arthrodesis in the hand. J Hand Surg 1983;8A:932–935.
19. Larsson SE. Compression arthrodesis of the wrist: a consecutive series of 23 cases. Clin Orthop 1974;99:146–153.
20. Kaplan EB, Taleisnik J. The wrist. In: Spinner M, ed. Kaplan's functional and surgical anatomy of the hand. 3rd ed. 1984:156–159.
21. Gelberman RH, Bauman TD, Menon J, et al. The vascularity of the lunate bone and Kienböck's disease. J Hand Surg 1980; 5A:272–278.
22. Gelberman RH, Panagis JS, Taleisnik J, et al. The arterial anatomy of the human carpus. Part I: the extraosseous vascularity. J Hand Surg 1983;8A:367–375.
23. Lee MLH. The intraosseous arterial pattern of the carpal lunate bone and its relation to avascular necrosis. Acta Orthop Scand 1963;33:43–65.

24. Panagis JS, Gelberman RH, Taleisnik J, et al. The arterial anatomy of the human carpus. Part II: the intraosseous vascularity. J Hand Surg 1983;8A:375–382.

25. Williams CS, Gelberman RH. Vascularity of the lunate. Hand Clin 1993;9:391–398.

26. Beckenbaugh RD, Shives TC, Dobyns JH, et al. Kienböck's disease: the natural history of Kienböck's disease and consideration of the lunate fractures. Clin Orthop 19800;149:98–106.

27. Amadio PC, Hanssen AD, Berquist TH. The genesis of Kienböck's disease: evaluation of a case by magnetic resonance imaging. J Hand Surg 1987;12A:1044–1049.

28. Gerwin M, Potter H, Weiland AJ, et al. Use of magnetic resonance imaging in the evaluation of wrist disorders. Paper presented at the Annual Meeting of the American Society of Orthopaedic Surgeons, New Orleans, February 28, 1994.

29. Stahl F. On lunatomalacia (Kienböck's disease): a clinical and roentgenological study, especially on its pathogenesis ad the late results of immobilization treatment. Acta Chir Scand Suppl 1947; 95:3–73.

30. Lichtman DM, Mack GR, MacDonald RI, et al. Kienböck's disease: the role of silicone replacement arthroplasty. J Bone Joint Surg 1977;59A:899–908.

31. Mikkelsen SS, Gelineck J. Poor function after nonoperative treatment of Kienböck's disease. Acta Orthop Scand 1987;58:241.

32. Braun R. The pronator pedicle bone grafting in the forearm and proximal row. Paper presented at the 38th Annual Meeting of the American Society for Surgery of the Hand, March 1983.

33. Hori Y, Tomai S, Okuda H, et al. Blood vessel transplantation to bone. J Hand Surg 1979;4A:23–33.

34. Tamai S, Yajima H, Ono H. Revascularization procedures in the treatment of Kienböck's disease. Hand Clin 1993;9:455–466.

35. Trumble T, Glisson RR, Seaber AV, et al. A biomechanical comparison of the methods for treating Kienböck's disease. J Hand Surg 1986;11A:88–93.

36. Palmer A, Werner F. Biomechanics of the distal radioulnar joint. Clin Orthop 1984;187:26–35.

37. Nakamura R, Horii E, Imaeda T. Excessive radial shortening in Kienböck's disease. J Hand Surg 1990;15B:46–48.

38. Nakamura R, Imaeda T, Miura T. Radial shortening for Kienböck's disease: factors affecting the operative result. J Hand Surg 1990; 15B:40–45.

39. Werner FW, Murphy DJ, Palmer AK. Pressures in the distal radioulnar joint: effect of surgical procedures used for Kienböck's disease. J Orthop Res 1989;7:445–450.

40. Almquist EE, Burns JF Jr. Radial shortening for the treatment of Kienböck's disease. A 5 to 10 year follow-up. J Hand Surg 1982; 8A:348–352.

41. Eiken O, Niechajev I. Radius shortening in malacia of the lunate Scand J Plast Reconstr Surg Hand Surg 1980;14:191–196.

42. Grassi G, Santoro D, Coli G, et al. the surgical treatment of Kienböck's disease. Ital J Orthop Traumatol 1978;4:149–154.

43. Kinnard P, Tricoire JL, Basora J. Radial shortening for Kienböck's disease. Can J Surg 1983;26:261–262.

44. Ovesen J. Shortening of the radius in treatment of lunatomalacia. J Bone Joint Surg 1981;63B:231–232.

45. Schattenkerk ME, Nollen A, van Hussen F. The treatment of lunatomalacia. Radial shortening or ulnar lengthening. Acta Scand 1987;58:652–654.

46. Weiss APC, Weiland AJ, Moore JR, Wilgis EFS. Radial shortening for Kienböck disease. J Bone Joint Surg 1991;73A:384–391.

47. Weiss APC. Radial shortening. Hand Clin 1993;9:475.

48. Werner FW, Palmer AK, Utter RG. Distal radial osteotomy for the treatment of Kienböck's disease: a biomechanical study. Orthop Trans 1988;12:486–487.

49. Watanabe K, Nakamura R, Horii E, Miura T. Biomechanical analysis of radial wedge osteotomy for the treatment of Kienböck's disease. J Hand Surg 1986;18A:686–690.

50. Nakamura R, Kentaro W, Tsunoda K, Miura T. Radial osteotomy for Kienböck's disease evaluated by magnetic resonance imaging. Acta Othop Scand 1993;64:207.

51. Quenzer DE, Linscheid RL. Ulnar lengthening procedures. Hand Clin 1993;9:467–474.

52. Horii E, Garcia-Elias M, Bishop AT, et al. Effect on force transmission across the carpus in procedures used to treat Kienböck's disease. J Hand Surg 1990;15A:393–400.

53. Armistead RB, Linscheid RL, Dobyns JH, et al. Ulnar lengthening in the treatment of Kienböck's disease. J Bone Joint Surg 1992; 64A:170–178.

54. Sundberg SB, Linscheid RL. Kienböck's disease: results of treatment with ulnar lengthening. Clin Orthop 1984;187:43–51.

55. Alexander AH, Turner MA, Alexander CE, Lichtman DM. Lunate silicone replacement arthroplasty in Kienböck's disease: a long-term follow-up study. J Hand Surg 1990;15A:401–407.

56. Kato H, Usui M, Minami A. Long-term results of Kienböck's disease treated by excisional arthroplasty with a silicone implant or coiled palmaris longus tendon. J Hand Surg 1986;11A:645–653.

57. Short WH, Werner FW, Fortino MD, et al. Distribution of pressures and forces on the wrist after simulated intercarpal fusion and Kienböck's disease. J Hand Surg 1992;17A:443–449.

58. Garcia-Elias M, Cooney WP, Linscheid RL, et al. Wrist kinematics after limited intercarpal arthrodesis. J Hand Surg 1989; 14A:791–799.

59. Minamikawa Y, Peimer CA, Yamaguchi T, et al. Ideal scaphoid angle for intercarpal arthrodesis. J Hand Surg 1989;17A:370–375.

60. Watson HK, Fink JA, Monacelli DM. Use of the scaphotrapeziotrapezoid fusion in the treatment of Kienböck's disease. Hand Clin 1993;9:493–499.

61. Buck-Gramcko D. Denervation of the wrist joint. J Hand Surg 1977; 2A:54–61.

62. Buck-Gramcko D. Wrist denervation procedures in the treatment of Kienböck's disease. Hand Clin 1993;9:517–520.

63. Fitzgerald JP, Peimer CA, Smith RJ. Distraction resection arthroplasty of the wrist. J Hand Surg 1989;14A:774–781.

64. Preiser G. Zureine typische posttraumatische und zur spontanfraktur fuhrende ostitis des naviculare carpi. Fortschr Geb Rontgenstr Nuklearmed Erganzungsband 1910;15:189.

65. Ferlic DC, Morin P. Idiopathic avascular necrosis of the scaphoid: Preiser's disease? J Hand Surg 1989;14A:13–16.

66. Gelberman RH, Menon J. The vascularity of the scaphoid bone. J Hand Surg 1980;5A:508–513.

67. Taleisnik J, Kelly PJ. The extraosseous and intraosseous blood supply of the scaphoid bone. J Bone Joint Surg 1966; 8A:1125–1137.

68. Viegas SF. Arthroscopic treatment of osteochondritis dissecans of the scaphoid. Arthroscopy 1988;4:278–281.

69. Riley LH, Moore JR, Weiland AJ. Priser's disease: a report of ten cases. Paper presented at the 45th Annual Meeting of the American Society for Surgery of the Hand, Toronto, ON, Sept 1990.

70. Vander Grend R, Dell PC, Glowczewskie F, et al. Intraosseous blood supply of the capitate and its correlation with aseptic necrosis. J Hand Surg 1984;9A:677–683.

71. Rahme H. Idiopathic avascular necrosis of the capitate bone— case report. Hand 1983;15:274–275.

72. Van Demark RE, Parke WW. Avascular necrosis of the hamate: a case report with reference to the hamate blood supply. J Hand Surg 1992;17A:1086–1090.

73. Match RM. Nonspecific avascular necrosis of the pisiform bone: a case report. J Hand Surg 1980;5A:341–342.

Degenerative Arthropathy of the Hand and Wrist: Rheumatoid Involvement and Basal Joint Arthritis

In the evaluation and treatment of patients with rheumatoid arthritis the overall health of the patient and the degree of polyarticular involvement significantly influence the outcome of any treatment protocol. Treatment must be individualized to each patient. It is important for the patient and physician to understand the progression of the disease and to carefully evaluate the patient's functional ability. Treatment should commence only after appropriate goals have been set. Hand surgery makes up 25% of overall surgical intervention in the rheumatoid population (1). Surgery can be effective in relieving pain, improving function, and correcting deformity; however, it is not always as effective in restoring strength, motion, or dexterity (2–4). It must be kept in mind that range of motion and deformity do not always correlate with patient function.

With progression of disease, recurrence of pain or deformity may occur after any reconstructive procedure. As a result, the treatment of this disease is an ongoing process of evaluation and treatment. The hand surgeon should consult the rheumatologist, the orthopaedic surgeon, and the therapist to best provide a comprehensive treatment plan.

RELEVANT ANATOMY AND PATHOGENESIS

Rheumatoid arthritis affects primarily the synovium of joints. Soft tissue laxity, joint erosion, and deformity are a result of the effects of the chronically inflamed synovial tissue. Joint involvement is most significantly influenced by three factors: First, joints are designed for movement, which results in increased synovial cellularity. Second, they are a potential space lined by mesenchymal tissue. Third, the articular cartilage is a large area of avascular tissue, which allows for surface buildup of antigen–antibody complexes (5). It is the immune response to these complexes that leads to the destruction of the articular cartilage. Surrounding soft tissue support structures are stretched by the inflamed synovium, leading to increased joint laxity. This may result in altered force transmission across joints, allowing progressive deformity to occur. The synovial-lined flexor and extensor tendon sheaths may also be affected. The inflamed synovium of the tendon sheaths can cause painful swelling in addition to weakening of the tendon, which may result in tendon rupture.

Involvement of the wrist and hand in rheumatoid arthritis may result in derangement of the intricate architecture, which limits strength, motion, and function. Peripheral joints are involved 95% of cases; polyarthritis occurs in 25% of patients. The classic distal interphalangeal (DIP) joint involvement, including distal phalanx erosion, nail pitting, and onycholysis, occurs in 5% of patients. Fusiform swelling of the digits is generally the result of inflammation of periosteum, tendons, and tendon insertions. Psoriatic arthritis typically differs from rheumatoid arthritis in that it is associated with psoriatic skin lesions and involvement of the metacarpal–phalangeal (MP) joint results in extension contractures, not flexion contractures. Tenosynovectomy is usually not indicated (6).

Systemic lupus erythematosus–associated arthritis is

characterized primarily by ligamentous laxity. Clinically, symmetric joint swelling, pain, and decreased range of motion are common. Joints generally have a normal radiographic appearance. The absence of radiographic changes should not preclude arthrodesis, which is often the treatment of choice. Soft tissue procedures often fail owing to excessive laxity. Basal joint arthrodesis has been more effective than soft tissue reconstruction because of the recurrent deformity with the latter (7).

INITIAL FINDINGS, PHYSICAL EXAMINATION, AND DIAGNOSIS

Initial evaluation should include a thorough history of the patient's disease process, including other joints involved, previous and current treatment, functional limitations, and severity of pain. The entire upper extremity and cervical spine should be routinely examined. Joints are examined for all deformities, including malalignment, swelling, and nodule formation. Functional testing may include the ability to hold a pencil, grasp a cup, and button a shirt. Active and passive range of motion of the digits, wrist, forearm, elbow, shoulder, and cervical spine are recorded. Examination of the upper extremity includes evaluation for signs and symptoms of tenosynovitis, synovitis, instability, and nerve compression.

Tenosynovitis may occur in both the flexor and the extensor tendons. As they course under the extensor retinaculum, the extensor tendons are surrounded by tenosynovium, which ends at the base of the metacarpals. The flexor tendons are surrounded by tenosynovium as they course under the transverse carpal ligament. The flexor pollicis longus tendon continues in its synovial sheath to the thumb. As the finger flexors enter the carpal tunnel, a common tendon sheath forms that continues to the fifth digit. Separate tendon sheaths for the second, third, and fourth digits run from the level of the MP joint to the DIP joint.

Dorsal tenosynovitis may involve one or all of the extensor tendons. Swelling is prominent owing to the thin skin in this region. Often painless, it may progress to tendon rupture before the patient seeks treatment. The swollen area will usually move with extension of the digits. The most commonly ruptured tendons are the extensor digiti quinti (EDQ) and extensor digitorum communis (EDC) to the fourth and fifth digits and the extensor pollicis longus (EPL). The extensor tendons coursing over the distal ulna rupture as a result of the bony spurs and abrasion over the dorsally displaced ulna. The EPL tendon has a tenuous blood supply as it courses around Lister's tubercle, which may be further compromised by increased pressure owing to synovitis. If pain is associated with dorsal swelling, radiocarpal or radioulnar joint involvement should be considered.

Flexor tenosynovitis is less prominent owing to the thenar and hypothenar musculature. Carpal tunnel syndrome symptoms may be noted (8,9). The inflamed synovium degrades the outer portion of the tendons, fre-

quently causing intratendinous adhesions within the common flexor tendon sheath, which may result in decreased motion of the digits. The synovial tissue may also invade the tendon substance, eventually leading to tendon rupture. Chronic wear over scaphotrapezial joint osteophytes may result in flexor pollicis longus (FPL) rupture, known as the Mannerfelt lesion (10). The FPL is the most commonly ruptured flexor tendon, followed by the index flexor digitorum sublimis (FDS) and flexor digitorum profundus (FDP), which may also be caused by scaphotrapezial joint spurs.

Radioulnar synovitis leads to dorsal dislocation of the ulna, or caput ulna syndrome (11). The ligamentous complex of the distal radioulnar joint (DRUJ), including the triangular fibrocartilage complex (TFCC), is weakened by the synovitis, allowing for progressive supination of the carpus on the forearm and volar subluxation of the extensor carpi ulnaris (ECU) tendon (12,13). The synovitis and deformity may cause pain and weakness, with resulting instability and loss of forearm rotation.

Radiocarpal involvement leads to laxity of the dorsal and volar wrist ligaments. Resulting scaphoid instability allows the scaphoid to move into a volarly flexed position, exaggerating the supination of the carpus. Further collapse of the wrist causes an imbalance of the extensor tendons, resulting in a radial shift of the metacarpals and an ulnar deviation of the digits (14–16). The end result is a volarly dislocated wrist with dorsal dislocation of the ulna and destruction of the carpal bones.

The typical MP joint deformity is caused in part by the two planes of motion in this joint. The source of the classic volarly displaced and ulnarly deviated deformity remains controversial. Wrist deformity, laxity of the collateral ligaments, alteration of flexor and extensor tendon forces, intrinsic muscle imbalance, and gravitational force are significant factors causing the deformity (17,18).

The finger deformities seen in rheumatoid patients include swan-neck and boutonniere deformities, which are the result of muscular imbalance across the joints in the digit and soft tissue laxity surrounding the joints (Fig. 7.1). The swan-neck deformity results from an insufficiency of the volar plate of the proximal interphalangeal (PIP) joint, which leads to hyperextension of the PIP joint with compensatory DIP joint flexion (Fig. 7.2). The functional deficit is primarily owing to the loss of PIP motion. Four treatment groups are classified by the degree of loss of motion: no loss, partial loss, near total loss, and total loss (19,20).

Boutonniere deformity, like swan-neck deformity, is not specific to rheumatoid arthritis, although it does occurs frequently with this arthritis. Flexion of the PIP joint is the primary deformity, and there is secondary hyperextension of the DIP and MP joints (Fig. 7.3). Synovitis at the PIP joint attenuates the extensor mechanism, which can no longer provide full extension. The lateral bands slide volarly, contributing to flexion of the PIP joint. The oblique retinacular ligaments shorten, causing DIP hyperextension. Compensation of PIP joint flexion leads to MP hyperexten-

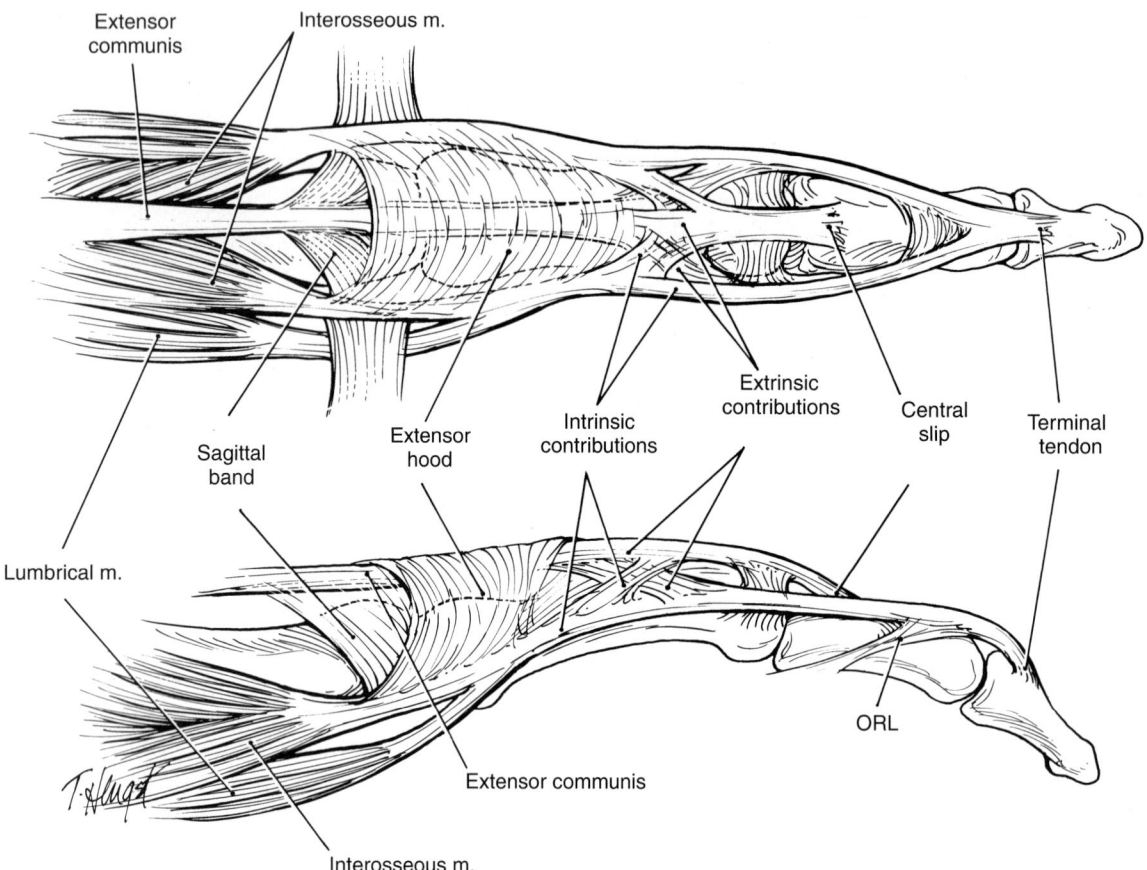

Figure 7.1. Dorsal and lateral views of the extensor mechanism. Note the extrinsic (extensor communis) and intrinsic (interosseous and lumbrical) contributions to the central slip and lateral bands.

Figure 7.2. Lateral view of the swan-neck deformity secondary to incompetence of the volar plate of the PIP joint. Dorsal displacement of the lateral bands causes hyperextension of the PIP joint and reciprocal flexion of the DIP joint. Modified from Littler J. The digital extensor-flexor system. In: Converse M, et al., eds. The hand and upper extremity. 2nd ed. Philadelphia: Saunders, 1977:3181.

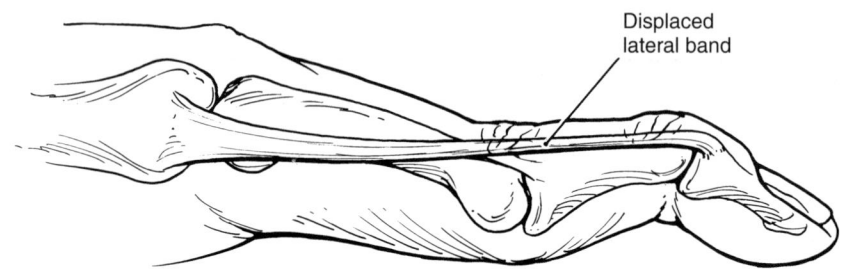

Figure 7.3. Lateral view of the boutonniere deformity. Attenuation or rupture of the central slip may allow the lateral bands to drop palmar to the PIP axis of rotation, causing flexion of the PIP joint and reciprocal extension of the DIP joint. Modified from Littler J. The digital extensor-flexor system. In: Converse M, et al., eds. The hand and upper extremity. 2nd ed. Philadelphia: Saunders, 1977:3176.

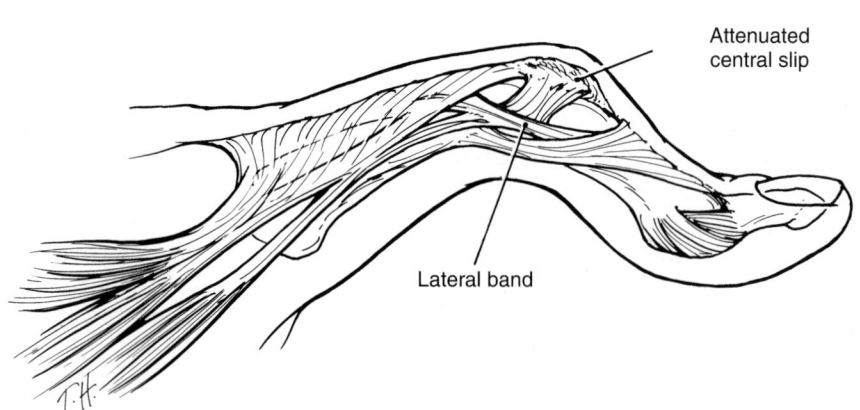

sion. Boutonniere deformities are also classified as mild, moderate, and severe, depending on PIP joint flexion, passive correction, and the PIP joint surface (19).

RADIOLOGIC STUDIES

Radiographic evaluation includes plain x-rays of the wrist and hand in the AP, lateral, and oblique planes. These should be evaluated for joint degradation, deformity, and subluxation. Involvement of the basal joint of the thumb may be staged with the Eaton classification (21), based on a true lateral x-ray of the basal joint. MRI and CT scan are rarely indicated.

TREATMENT

Nonoperative Treatment

Conservative treatment of rheumatoid arthritis involves a thorough evaluation of the patient and associated medical problems. Aspirin and nonsteroidal anti-inflammatory drugs (NSAIDs) have been the historic first-line drugs of choice. By inhibiting the chemical mediators of inflammation and controlling pain, NSAIDs may improve patient function. First-line drugs are used in conjunction with rest, splinting, and occasionally corticosteroid injection. Splinting is important and is usually helpful in relieving pain. It may also slow the progression of deformity, although it cannot reverse an existing deformity (22).

Second-line drugs include gold, penicillamine, and antimalarial drugs. These drugs require strict monitoring owing to their potential toxicity. Oral corticosteroids and cytotoxic drugs, such as methotrexate, are third-line drugs. The significant anti-inflammatory effects of oral corticosteroids must be weighed against the many undesirable side effects. Methotrexate acts by inhibiting DNA synthesis, thereby slowing cellular proliferation. The immunosuppressive effects of corticosteroids and methotrexate must also be monitored for the development of undesirable side effects.

Operative Treatment

Surgical intervention should be carefully planned, and realistic goals should be set. Alleviation of pain, improvement of function, slowing disease progression, and cosmesis are priorities of surgical treatment (Clinical Table). Certain principles should be kept in mind when planning surgery in the rheumatoid patient. Pain is the most important factor to be addressed. Carpal tunnel symptoms may be exacerbated by any surgery on the hand or wrist; therefore, carpal tunnel release should be considered when planning a procedure. Reconstruction of the MP joint should proceed PIP joint surgery. Flexor tendon function and wrist stability must be restored before MP joint arthroplasty. Shoulder and elbow reconstruction should gener-

ally be performed before wrist and hand surgery to enable adequate hand rehabilitation.

EXTENSOR TENOSYNOVECTOMY AND RECONSTRUCTION

Surgical technique for the extensor tenosynovectomy and reconstruction is important because of the frequent soft tissue problems seen with rheumatoid patients. Straight longitudinal incisions are recommended rather than zigzag or serpentine incisions, which increase the risk of skin necrosis. Thick skin flaps maintain superficial vasculature and nerves (23). The extensor retinaculum should be raised as radial- and ulnar-based flaps (Fig. 7.4). The posterior interosseous nerve lies under the fourth compartment and may be transected to denervate the wrist (24).

Extensor tenosynovectomy is performed through a straight longitudinal incision just ulnar of midline. The incision is carried down to the extensor retinaculum, and full-thickness skin flaps contain the superficial branches of the radial and ulnar nerves. The retinaculum is divided longitudinally over the fifth compartment. The retinaculum is reflected as radial and ulnar flaps. Each compartment is entered, and the synovitis is débrided while the flaps are reflected. The first dorsal compartment is not opened unless it is significantly involved. Attenuated tendons are imbricated; tendons with impending rupture are sutured to adjacent tendons (Fig. 7.5).

The distal radius and ulna are then evaluated for bony spicules, which should be removed. Dorsal dislocation or prominence of the distal ulna are indications for excision of the distal ulna. The radiocarpal joint must be evaluated for synovectomy at the same time. The extensor retinaculum is split transversely, and one leaf is placed below the tendons to allow smooth gliding and avoid abrasion. The other leaf is placed over the tendons to prevent bowstringing. If the retinaculum was split over the fourth compartment, a slip of the ulnar flap can be used to stabilize the ECU tendon to prevent volar subluxation.

The tourniquet should be released and homeostasis obtained before closure. Drains should be placed to prevent hematoma formation. A bulky dressing and volar splint with the wrist in neutral and fingers in extension are sufficient. Motion is started 24 to 48 h postsurgery. The most common complication is hematoma formation and skin slough.

Extensor tendon rupture is usually secondary to tenosynovitis associated with DRUJ synovitis and dorsal ulna prominence. An extensor tenosynovectomy is performed along with a resection of the distal ulna. The ruptured tendons are sutured to adjacent tendons at the appropriate tension to attain full finger extension with the wrist in flexion by the tenodesis effect. If the ruptured tendons do not have sufficient length for a side-to-side transfer, a transfer using the extensor indices proprius transfer is performed, frequently to the EDQ. Multiple extensor tendon ruptures require a transfer of the ring or long finger FDS. The flexor

Clinical Table: Degenerative Arthropathy of the Hand and Wrist: Rheumatoid Involvement and Basal Joint Arthritis

Procedure	Indications	Technique	Anatomy	Pitfalls
Tenosynovectomy	• Progressive synovitis	• Create retinacular flap	• Extensor retinaculum • Transverse carpal ligament	• Hematoma, skin slough
Tendon transfer	• Tendon ruptures • Wrist balancing	• EIP to EPL • FDS to FPL • ECRL to ECU		• Attenuated tendons
DRUJ reconstruction	• Dorsal ulnar subluxation • Caput ulna • Carpal translation	• Distal ulna excision (Darrach) • DRUJ fusion (Sauve-Kapandji) • Resect ulnar articular surface (hemiarthroplasty)	• Dorsal branch of the ulnar nerve • ECU tendon	• Ulnar stump instability • Painful forearm rotation
Wrist fusion	• Radiocarpal arthritis	• Dorsal approach • Excise distal ulna • Steinmann pin fixation	• Neutral to slight dorsiflexion	• Decreased motion • Painful forearm rotation • Skin slough • Avoid bilateral fusion
Wrist arthroplasty	• Low demand • Good extensor function • Bilateral involvement	• Dorsal approach • Silastic or total wrist • Proximal row carpectomy	• Extensor retinaculum	• Loosening • Poor long-term results
MP arthroplasty	• MP deformity • Subluxation	• Dorsal approach • Silastic implant • Reconstruct RCL	• Dorsal venous drainage • Extensor subluxation • Collateral ligaments	• May not show improved motion • Must correct wrist deformities • Consider index MP fusion
FDS tenodesis	• Type I swan neck	• Hemitenodesis of PIP joint with single slip of FDS	• Volar zigzag or midaxial approach	• PIP flexion contracture
Intrinsic release	• Type II swan neck	• Ulnar intrinsic resection with or without DIP fusion	• Ulnar lateral band	• Avoid radial lateral bands
Lateral band mobilization	• Type III swan neck	• Dorsal incision • Release adjacent to central slip	• Dorsally displaced lateral bands • Dorsal skin contracture	• Dorsal skin necrosis
PIP fusion	• Index and middle digits • Type IV swan neck • Stage III boutonniere	• Dorsal incision • Cut with saw • K wire fixation	• 25° flexion in index finger • 30° flexion in middle finger	• Dorsal skin necrosis
PIP arthroplasty	• Type IV swan neck	• Dorsal approach • Silicone implant • Ring and small digits	• Approach through ulnar side • Reconstruct collateral ligament	• Check for adequate flexor tendon excursion

EIP, extensor indicis proprius; *ECRL*, extensor carpi radialis longus; *RCL*, radial collateral ligament; *K*, Kirschner.

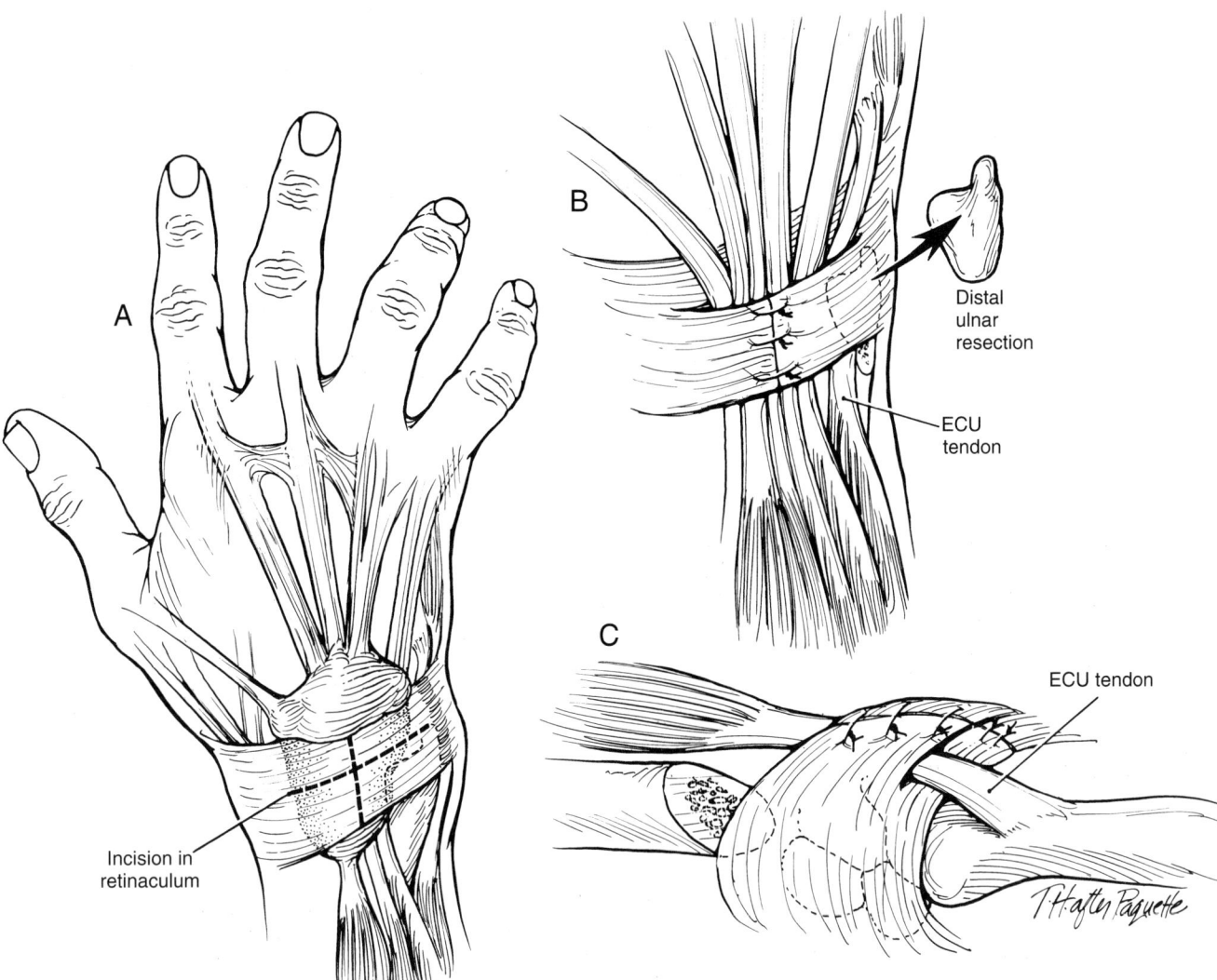

Figure 7.4. A. For a dorsal tenosynovectomy and excision of distal ulna, the extensor retinaculum is incised through the fourth compartment. Radial- and ulnar-based flaps are developed. **B.** The distal portion of retinaculum is repaired deep to the extensor tendons, reinforcing the dorsal capsular repair after distal ulna excision (the Darrach procedure). **C.** The ulnar aspect of the extensor retinaculum is left intact to prevent volar subluxation of ECU tendon. Modified from Blank J, Cassidy C. The distal radioulnar joint in rheumatoid arthritis. In: Ruby L, Cassidy C, eds. Hand clinics. Rheumatoid arthritis of the hand and wrist. Philadelphia: Saunders, 1996:532.

tendon is first evaluated for strength and excursion. The tendon is released at the A1 pulley region and withdrawn proximally through a separate volar forearm incision. The tendon may be passed through the interosseous membrane proximal to the pronator quadratus. It is then sutured to the ruptured extensor tendons, usually the EDC to the fourth and fifth digits and the EDQ. The EDC to second and third digits may be sutured to the adjacent intact extensor indicis proprius (EIP). Postoperatively, the patient is immobilized for 3 weeks in wrist extension, MP flexion, and digital extension.

Extensor pollicis longus tendon rupture occurs at Lister's tubercle. A transfer using the EIP tendon is performed. The EIP tendon is identified through a transverse incision at the MP joint and another at the wrist. The EIP muscle belly lies distal to that of the EDC tendons. The proprius tendons are found ulnar to their respective communis tendons. The EIP tendon is then divided at the MP joint and withdrawn proximally. A third incision is made over the MP joint of the thumb. The EIP tendon is passed subcutaneously into this incision. The tendon may be sutured through the extensor hood or directly repaired end to end. Tension allows thumb extension with wrist flexion and thumb to little finger approximation with wrist extension.

Postoperatively, the thumb is immobilized with the wrist in extension for 5 weeks (25).

FLEXOR TENOSYNOVECTOMY AND RECONSTRUCTION

Flexor tenosynovectomy is performed through a longitudinal incision parallel to the thenar crease. It may be extended across the wrist crease in a zigzag fashion. The pal-

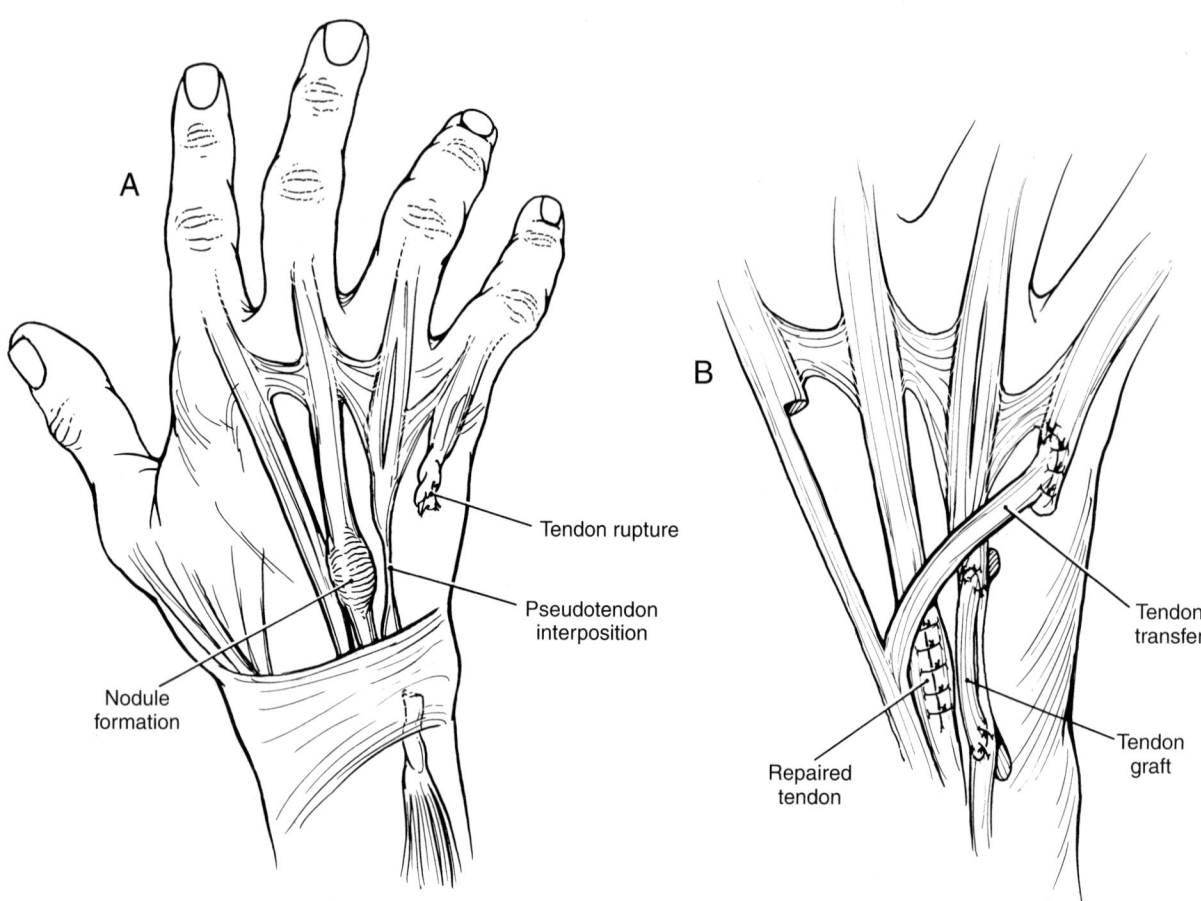

Figure 7.5. A. Rheumatoid disease may cause nodule formation, tendon rupture, or attenuation with pseudotendon interposition. **B.** Tendon nodules may be excised and repaired primarily. Tendon ruptures may be repaired with a transfer. Attenuated tendons may be re- paired with grafts. Modified from Wilson R, DeVio M. Extensor tendon problems in rheumatoid arthritis. In: Ruby L, Cassidy C, eds. Hand clinics. Rheumatoid arthritis of the hand and wrist. Philadelphia: Saunders, 1996:532.

mar cutaneous branch of the median nerve must be avoided. The palmar fascia is released in line with the ring finger to the transverse carpal ligament. The ligament is then incised to expose the carpal canal. The antebrachial fascia of the wrist and distal forearm is also released. The median nerve is dissected free, and its motor branch is traced to the thenar musculature. The tenosynovium is carefully excised. The flexor digitorum profundus tendons may be left bound together, if there is concern that a tear may be present and the tendons are pulling as a unit through scar. The superficial flexors are dissected free.

The floor of the carpal canal is then palpated for any bony spicules (particularly over the scaphoid), which must be removed. Exposed bony surfaces are covered by adjacent soft tissue. Excursion of the fingers is evaluated for catching or limited motion, which may indicate the presence of a nodule. Digital tenosynovectomy is carried out in any digit without smooth tendon motion. Zigzag incisions over the volar portion of the digit provide appropriate exposure (Fig. 7.6). The tenosynovium is excised, leaving as much of the pulleys as possible intact. A slip of the FDS tendon can be excised to further decompress the tendon

sheath to avoid excessive pulley resection. Tendon nodules are excised, and tendons are repaired with nylon sutures. Active and passive motion are tested. If active motion with traction on the tendons is not equal to passive motion, further tenosynovectomy is necessary. Range of motion exercises are started on the first postoperative day. Care is taken to range each joint individually to prevent superficial and deep tendon adhesion.

Flexor tendon ruptures occur by attrition or invasion. Attrition ruptures occur from abrasion over bony spicules, such as those seen with the FPL and index flexor tendons (Fig. 7.7). Ruptures from direct invasion may occur wherever tenosynovitis is present. The technique for flexor tendon reconstruction includes tenosynovectomy, as previously described. Bone spurs are removed, and the volar capsule and soft tissue are mobilized to cover any exposed bone. Primary repair is rarely an option because of attenuation or damage. FPL rupture may be treated with either a bridge graft, index FDS tendon transfer, or interphalangeal fusion. The palmaris longus tendon is the first choice for a bridge grafting. If this is not present, a portion of the flexor carpi radialis (FCR) tendon is suitable.

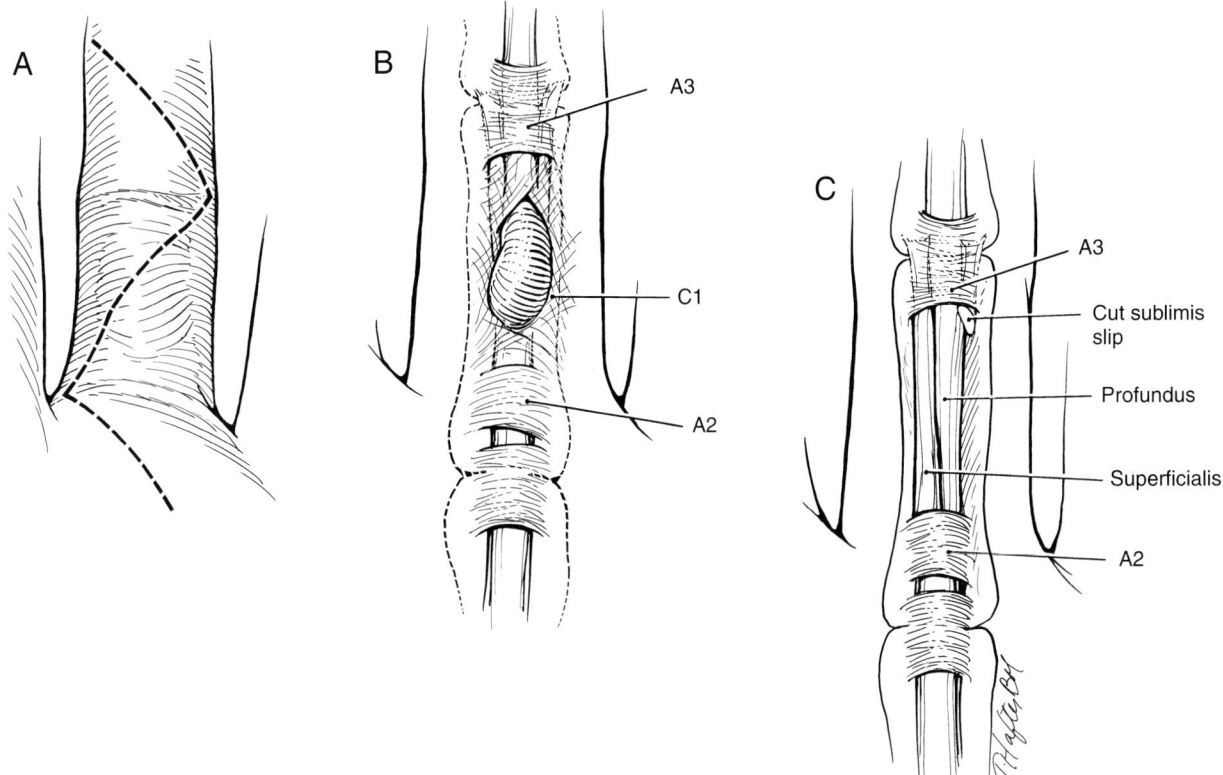

Figure 7.6. A. A volar zigzag incision is used for a tenosynovectomy at the digital flexors. **B.** The tenosynovium protrudes through the inner cruciate pulley. **C.** The tendon is debulked at flexor sheath by tenosynovectomy; an additional excision of one slip is made at the sublimis tendon. Modified from Feldon P, Millender L, Nalebuff E. Rheumatoid arthritis on the hand and wrist. In: Green D, ed. Operative hand surgery. New York: Churchill Livingstone, 1993:1611.

Transfer of the index FDS is performed by releasing the tendon in the distal palm and suturing it to the volar aspect of the thumb distal phalanx with a pullout suture. After surgery, the thumb is immobilized for 3 weeks. Then active motion is started.

Rupture of the deep flexor tendons can be compensated for by the superficial flexor or scarring to adjacent deep flexor tendons. The level of tendon rupture is important in planning treatment options (26). Ruptures occurring in the wrist or palm can often be sutured to adjacent deep tendons. Alternatively, the transfer of a superficial flexor to the distal profundus stump will provide digital flexion. If the rupture occurs within the fibroosseus sheath, a tenosynovectomy is performed with preservation of the FDS tendon.

THE DISTAL RADIOULNAR JOINT

The surgical options for distal radioulnar joint involvement include synovectomy, tendon transfer, hemiresection arthroplasty, ulnar pseudarthrosis, and distal ulna resection. Dorsal synovectomy is performed through a longitudinal incision, as described above. The DRUJ is exposed through a longitudinal capsular incision proximal to the TFCC, allowing the removal of synovium and bony spurs. The capsule is closed with nonabsorbable sutures with the forearm in supination. Balancing the wrist by ten-

don transfer can be performed by transferring the extensor carpi radialis longus (ECRL) tendon to the dorsally repositioned ECU tendon to prevent ulnar carpal volar subluxation. After surgery, the forearm is held in supination for 3 to 4 weeks.

Involvement of the DRUJ with dorsal prominence of the ulna has historically been treated with one of three procedures. Distal ulna excision and stabilization (the Darrach procedure) is performed through a straight dorsal longitudinal incision, and the DRUJ is approached through a capsular incision. The distal ulna is exposed subperiosteally and osteotomized at the sigmoid notch (more than 2 cm). The ECU tendon is identified and repositioned from the subluxed volar position to a dorsal position. It is then split from its insertion on the base of the fifth metacarpal to the musculotendinous junction proximally. A distally based ECU tendon slip is passed through a drill hole in the dorsal distal ulna and sutured on itself. The TFCC is sutured to the radius to correct carpal supination. The dorsal capsule is closed securely, and a retinacular flap is used to maintain the dorsal position of the ECU tendon.

The Sauve-Kapandji procedure involves arthrodesis of the DRUJ combined with resection of the ulna proximal to the fusion (27). This is done through the approach described above, followed by the removal of all soft tissue and articular cartilage in the DRUJ. The ulna is then reduced and fixed to the radius with screws through the

Figure 7.7. A. An FPL rupture secondary to scaphoid osteophyte. **B.** The osteophyte is excised, and the tendon is repaired with a graft. Capsular closure prevents further abrasion of tendon. Modified from Feldon P, Millender L, Nalebuff E. Rheumatoid arthritis on the hand and wrist. In: Green D, ed. Operative hand surgery. New York: Churchill Livingstone, 1993:1621.

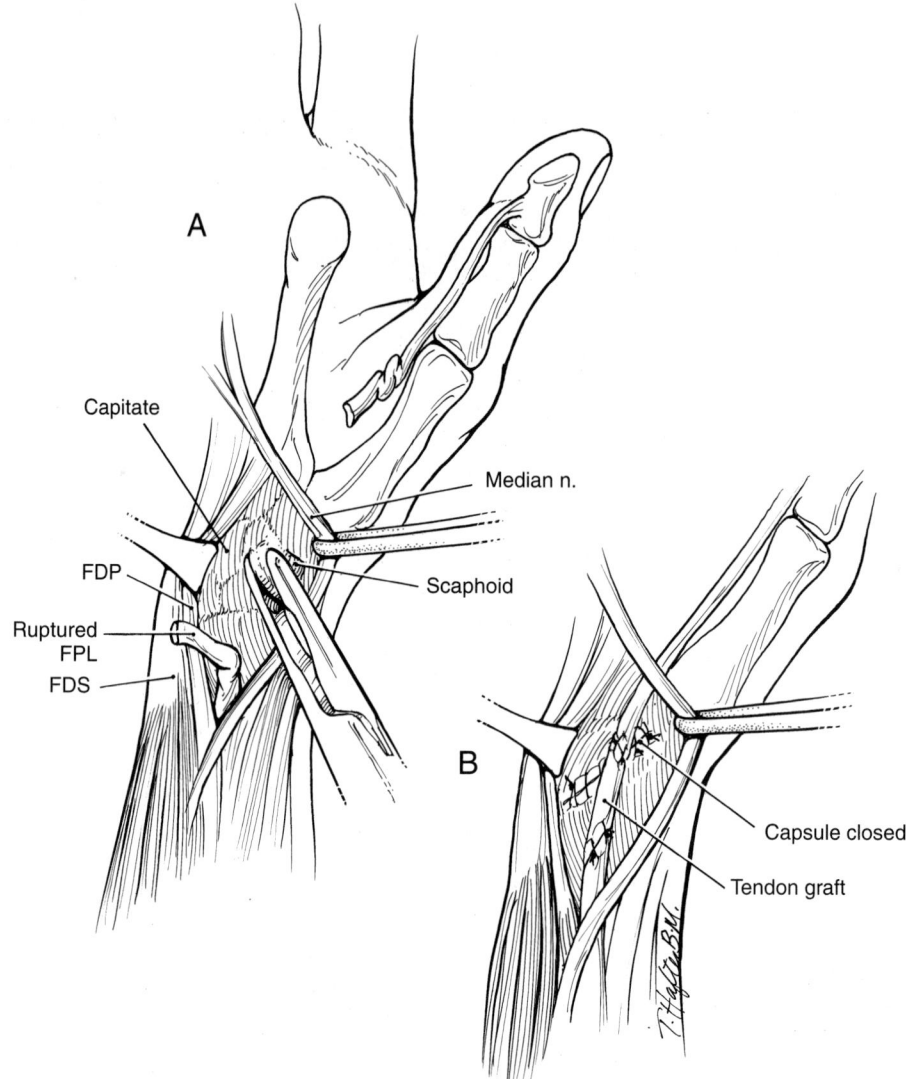

DRUJ. Between 2 and 3 cm of ulna, including the periosteum, proximal to the fusion are excised.

Hemiresection arthroplasty removes only the ulnar articular surface and subchondral bone through an oblique osteotomy. The ulna styloid, TFCC, and radioulnar and ulnocarpal ligaments are left intact. A capsular flap covering the osteotomy site is sutured volarly, adding stability to the ulna. Soft tissue balancing is performed as with distal ulna excision. Complications noted by Bowers include insufficient removal of bone, excess bone removal, and painful ECU tendon gliding (28).

THE RADIOCARPAL JOINT

Radiocarpal joint deformity and instability may be addressed by synovectomy, arthrodesis, or arthroplasty. Synovectomy is useful before radiographic evidence of joint degeneration. Synovectomy is performed through a straight dorsal longitudinal incision. The extensor compartments are evaluated for synovial masses, as described above. The capsule is reflected as a distally based flap.

Wrist-balancing tendon transfers are performed in conjunction with synovectomy to correct deformities.

Historically, arthrodesis has been the procedure of choice for the painful degenerative wrist. Arthrodesis is successful at relieving pain and correcting deformity. The resulting loss of motion may be an important consideration if the contralateral wrist is similarly involved. Arthrodesis is performed through the approach described above, with a distally based capsular flap. The distal ulna is exposed subperiosteally and excised. Synovectomy and removal of articular cartilage are performed. Removal of the carpal bone stock is limited to correct the deformity but maintain length. The radial intramedullary canal is prepared to accept one or two Steinmann pins. The Steinmann pins are placed dorsally in the second or third web space, avoiding the more volar neurovascular bundles. They are advanced across the carpus and into the intramedullary canal of the radius. The wrist is fused in neutral, although more palmar or dorsiflexion can be achieved using two smaller Steinmann pins. Placing a Steinmann pin down the shaft of the third metacarpal increases the stability of the fixation. The pin may be countersunk to allow for arthroplasties of the MP joints, which are often performed in conjunction with wrist arthrodesis to correct ulnar deviation of the digits. The wrist is immobilized for 4 to 6 weeks. Platform crutches can be used at 7 to 10 days. The pins can be removed after solid bony union is evident, usually at 4 to 6 months.

Partial arthrodesis is useful when the radiocarpal joint has been destroyed but the midcarpal joint is spared. This may be caused by the greater amount of ligamentous tissue at the radiocarpal joint, allowing for increased synovitis (29). Partial wrist arthrodesis usually involves fusion of the scaphoid and lunate to the radius. Leaving the midcarpal joints intact allows 20 to 50% of wrist motion. The evaluation for partial arthrodesis is done intraoperatively and depends on the bone stock and degeneration of the joints. The fusion can be stabilized by Kirschner (K) wires or Herbert screws.

Patients with bilateral shoulder and elbow involvement along with wrist involvement will require wrist motion. Silicone arthroplasty was introduced to maintain motion in patients with painful degenerative wrists. Despite good early results (30), longer-term studies have shown failure rates between 25 and 40% at 2.5 to 5 years (1,31). As a result, the indications for silicone wrist arthroplasty are limited to patients with low-demand wrist function, with intact extensor tendons, and good bone stock. The technique for silicon implant arthroplasty of the wrist is similar to that of arthrodesis. The preparation of the radius and carpus is more specific, maintaining subchondral bone of the radius to prevent settling. The scaphoid and lunate are removed, as are the proximal portions of the capitate and hamate. The radius, capitate, and third metacarpal are prepared for the implants. When using silicone implants, the goal is to limit the range of motion of 30° of flexion and extension to diminish stress on the prosthesis. Soft tissue balancing is important as well and may require tendon transfers or tendon and capsular tightening.

Total joint arthroplasty of the wrist is performed by a few centers in the United States. The rigidity of the components provides for a more stable construct and a fixed fulcrum for motion. Tension in the collapsed degenerative wrist with lax capsular ligaments and tendons may be restored by soft tissue distraction at the time of arthroplasty. Indications are rheumatoid arthritis patients over 50 years with intact extensor tendons and bilateral wrist degeneration. The complications of loosening in the constrained designs and balancing in the unconstrained design seem to have been improved with the semiconstrained design, which has reported satisfactory long-term follow up (19). Operative technique is similar to that for the silicone arthroplasty. Proper soft tissue tensioning is obtained with the use of trial components. The use of cement for prosthesis fixation depends on the fit and design of the prosthesis. The wrist is immobilized for 2 to 6 weeks postsurgery. A splint is worn for up to 12 weeks, while the patient undergoes range of motion therapy.

THE METACARPOPHALANGEAL JOINT

Involvement of the metacarpophalangeal joint results in volar subluxation and ulnar deviation. In the absence of deformity, synovectomy alone is controversial and rarely performed. Deformity and pain are effectively corrected with MP arthroplasty, and predictable and satisfactory long-term results are obtained. Good alignment and stability of the radiocarpal joint is necessary to prevent recurrent ulnar digital drift after MP joint arthroplasty. Wrist arthrodesis is often performed in combination with MP joint arthroplasty. Silicone implants are well tolerated in this location. Arthrodesis of the index MP joint may be indicated for younger, high-demand patients. The MP joints are approached through a dorsal transverse incision from the second to fifth MP joints. Care is taken to protect the dorsal veins and nerves. The extensor tendons are exposed; and the ulnar-sided sagittal band is incised, exposing the joint. Release of the ulnar intrinsic tendon at its insertion may be performed as necessary. The ulnar intrinsic mechanism to the index digit also provides a supinatory force and must be maintained if possible. The extensor mechanism is retracted radially, the capsule is opened, and synovectomy performed. The ulnar collateral ligament is released. The deep flexor tendon is exposed, and the tenosynovectomy performed while testing tendon excursion.

The joint is resected, and the ends of the bone are broached for the prosthesis. After the prosthesis is in place, soft tissue balancing is attained by tightening radial structures and releasing ulnar structures. After surgery, the MP joints are held in slight flexion and radial deviation; motion begins at 5 days. Splints and therapy are individualized and continue for 3 months.

THE DIGITS

Swan-neck deformities are divided into four types, depending on mobility and condition of the PIP joint. Flexible PIP joints (type I) can be treated by superficial flexor hemitenodesis to prevent hyperextension. Excessive flexion contracture must be avoided to prevent boutonniere deformity. Type II swan-neck deformities are caused by intrinsic tightness; there is limitation of PIP joint flexion when the MP joint is extended. Correction of the MP joint with intrinsic release is usually sufficient to correct the deformity. Fusion of the DIP joint may also be performed at the same time.

For type III deformities, PIP flexion is limited in all positions; however, the joint maintains a normal radiographic appearance. Again, correcting the MP joint deformity helps address the PIP joint stiffness. Flexion may be restored by freeing the dorsally displaced lateral bands from the central slip, allowing them to reduce volarly, followed by manipulation of the digit. The flexor tendons are also evaluated for possible adhesions or nodules limiting excursion. The dorsal skin incision is left open distally to maintain motion and prevent skin necrosis. After surgery, an extension blocking splint is used, and flexion therapy is started at 24 to 48 h. Splinting continues for 2 to 4 weeks.

Type IV deformities are characterized by stiff PIP joints and poor radiographic appearance; they may be treated with PIP arthrodesis or arthroplasty. Nalebuff (1) recommends fusion of the index and middle digits and arthroplasty of the ring and small digits. The index PIP joint is fixed at 25° of flexion; the middle PIP joint is fixed in slightly more flexion. Two K wires are sufficient for fixation, and the digits are splinted for 6 weeks. Arthroplasty of the ring and small digits is indicated if adjacent joints, soft tissues, and tendons are intact. A dorsal approach is used to expose the PIP joint. Collateral ligaments are preserved for reattachment at closure. Flexor tendon excursion must be evaluated, and dorsal skin releases performed if necessary. Postsurgery, the digits are splinted in slight flexion, and motion is started at 24 to 48 h.

The boutonniere deformity is a low priority for surgical correction owing to a low predictable surgical outcome. Nalebuff and Millender's (19) classification divides treatment into three stages based on range of motion. Stage I deformity is characterized by a mild extension lag and synovitis of the PIP joint. Hyperextension of the DIP joint may or may not be present. Treatment involves synovectomy and dorsal repositioning the lateral bands with or without distal tenotomy.

Stage II deformity shows a 30° to 40° PIP flexion deformity with an intact joint. Shortening the central slip and releasing the lateral bands combined with synovectomy and distal tenotomy are necessary to treat this deformity. The PIP joint is fixed in extension with a K wire and is maintained for 3 weeks.

In stage III, the PIP joint is stiff and cannot be passively corrected. Treatment options are arthrodesis or arthroplasty. Arthrodesis is performed as described for swanneck deformities, with PIP flexion increasing from 25° to 50° as you move from the index to the small digit. In the middle finger, PIP implant arthroplasty may be preferred. This may need to be coupled with reconstruction of the central tendon in the ring and small digits to provide motion for grasp.

Deformities of the thumb in rheumatoid arthritis are classified into five types. Type I, the most common, is the boutonniere thumb with MP flexion and IP hyperextension. The deformities are supple in the early stages and fixed in the later stages. Treatment depends on the status of the joints. If the joints are preserved, synovectomy with rerouting of the EPL to the MP joint capsule is preferred. More commonly, arthrodesis of the MP joint is performed. If, however, the condition of the IP joint necessitates fusion, then implant arthroplasty of the MP joint is preferred. Fusion of both MP and IP joints should be avoided if possible.

The swan-neck deformity (type III) is the next most common thumb deformity. This is primarily a result of involvement of the carpal–metacaparl (CMC) joint and is best treated with either hemiresection of the trapezium

(32) or complete trapezoidal excision (33). MP hyperextension is then addressed by either volar capsulodesis or arthrodesis, depending on the stability and degree of degeneration.

The gamekeeper's thumb (type IV deformity) is characterized by ulnar collateral ligament insufficiency with a resulting abduction deformity of the MP joint. An adduction contracture of the metacarpal may develop secondarily. In the early deformity, ulnar collateral ligament reconstruction may be performed. In later cases, MP fusion or arthroplasty is preferred.

The rare type II deformity is a combination of the boutonniere deformity with associated CMC joint involvement. This may be treated in the same manner as type I and III deformities. The type V deformity is a hyperextension deformity of the MP joint and is treated by either arthrodesis or volar capsulodesis.

OSTEOARTHRITIS OF THE BASAL JOINT OF THE THUMB

Primary osteoarthritis of the basal joint of the thumb most commonly involves the trapeziometacarpal (TM) joint and less frequently the scaphotrapezial (ST) joint. Staging of basal joint arthritis (Eaton classification) is based on radiographic changes demonstrated in a true lateral projection of the thumb. Stage I disease is characterized by normal radiographs in conjunction with painful synovitis and laxity of the trapeziometacarpal joint. Joint space widening as a result of synovitis may be noted on x-rays. Treatment at this stage consists of splinting and the use of anti-inflammatories. When nonoperative treatment is unsuccessful, volar ligament reconstruction, using a slip of flexor carpi radialis tendon, is recommended (32,34).

Stage II disease is characterized by early degeneration of the TM joint with osteophytes, cysts, or loose bodies that are smaller than 2 mm in size. Stage III is characterized by severe narrowing of the TM joint and joint debris greater than 2 mm. The scaphotrapezial joint remains uninvolved in both stages. Initial treatment is nonoperative. Hemiresection interposition arthroplasty (the Eaton procedure) or trapezial excision with ligament reconstruction (Burton LRTI) is recommended for those in whom nonoperative treatment is unsuccessful. Stage IV disease is characterized by significant narrowing of both the TM and ST joints and is generally treated with trapezial excision (LRTI).

SUMMARY

Rheumatoid arthritis of the hand is a common source of deformity and disability in the patient with polyarticular disease. Although surgical treatment may be effective in improving function, relieving pain, and correcting deformity, it must be recognized as a part of an overall treatment plan in the improved daily life of the patient with the chronic disease. Many patients have quite good function of the hand despite significant rheumatoid deformity and may not need any surgical treatment at all. Restoration of strength, motion, and dexterity, while important, is less predictable than improvement in pain and function. Quality of bone, other joint involvement, and inexact correlation between deformity and function are important factors that challenge the overall management of the rheumatoid hand.

REFERENCES

1. Nalebuff EA. Rheumatoid hand surgery update. J Hand Surg 1983; 8:673–682.
2. Flatt AE. The care of the rheumatoid hand. 3rd ed. St. Louis: Mosby, 1974.
3. Inglis AE. Rheumatoid arthritis of the hand. Am J Surg 1965; 109:368–374.
4. Millender LH, Nalebuff EA. Reconstructive surgery in the rheumatoid hand. Orthop Clin North Am 1975;6:709–732.
5. Harris ED. Pathogenesis of rheumatoid arthritis. In: Kelley WN, Harris ED, Ruddy S, Sledge CB, eds. Textbook of rheumatology. Philadelphia: Saunders, 1981:896–927.
6. Feldon P, Millender LH, Nalebuff EA. Rheumatoid arthritis in the hand and wrist. In: Green DP, ed. Operative hand surgery. New York: Churchill Livingstone, 1993:1587–1690.
7. Dray GJ. The hand in systemic lupus erythematosus. Hand Clin 1989;5:145–155.
8. Barnes CG, Currey HLF. Carpal tunnel syndrome in rheumatoid arthritis. Ann Rheum Dis 1967;26:226–233.
9. Vainio K. Carpal canal syndrome caused by tenosynovitis. Acta Rheum Scand 1957;4:22–27.
10. Mannerfelt L, Norman O. Attritional ruptures of flexor tendons in rheumatoid arthritis caused by bony spurs in the carpal canal. A clinical and radiographic study. J Bone Joint Surg 1969; 51B:270–277.
11. Blackdahl M. The caput ulnae syndrome in rheumatoid arthritis. Acta Rheum Scand 1963;5(Suppl):1–75.
12. Darrach W, Dwight K. Derangement of the inferior radioulnar articulation. Proc NY Acad Med 1915;87:78.
13. Swanson AB. The ulnar head syndrome and its treatment by implant resection arthroplasty. J Bone Joint Surg 1972;54A:906.
14. Taleisnik J. Rheumatoid arthritis of the hand. Hand Clin 1989; 5:257–278.
15. Taleisnik J. The wrist. New York: Churchill Livingstone, 1985.
16. Shapiro JS. A new factor in the etiology of ulnar drift. Clin Orthop 1970;68;32–43.
17. Flatt AE. Some pathomechanics of ulnar drift. Plast Reconstr Surg 1966;37:295–303.
18. Wilson RL, Carlbolm ER. The rheumatoid metacarpophalangeal joint. Hand Clin 1989;5:223–237.
19. Nalebuff EA, Millender LH. Surgical treatment of swan-neck deformity in rheumatoid arthritis. Orthop Clin North Am 1975; 6:733–752.
20. Welsh RP, Hastings DE. Swan-neck deformity in rheumatoid arthritis of the hand. Hand 1977;8:109–116.
21. Eaton RG, Glickel SZ. Trapeziometacarpal arthritis: staging as a rational for treatment. Hand Clinics 1987; (3)4:455-469.
22. Bennett R. Orthotic devices to prevent deformities of the hand in rheumatoid arthritis. Arthritis Rheum 1976;18:100.
23. Terrano AL, Feldon PG, Millender LH, Nalebuff EA. Evaluation and treatment of the rheumatoid wrist. J Bone Joint Surg 1995; 7:1116–1128.
24. Dellon Al. Partial dorsal denervation: resection of the posterior interosseous nerve. J Hand Surg 1985;10A:527–533.
25. Leslie BM. Rheumatoid extensor tendon ruptures. Hand Clin 1989;5:191–202.
26. Ertel AN. Flexor tendon ruptures in rheumatoid arthritis. Hand Clin 1989;5:177–190.
27. Sauve-Kapandji. Nouvelle technique de traitement chirurgical des luxations recidivantes isolees de l'extremite inferiure du cubitus. J Chir (Paris) 1936;47:589–594.
28. Bowers WH. Distal radioulnar joint arthroplasty: the hemiresection-interposition technique. J Hand Surg 1985;10A:169–178.
29. Taleisnik J. Wrist: anatomy, function and injury. Instruct Course Lect 1978;27:61–87.
30. Goodman MJ, Millender LH, Nalebuff EA, Phillips CA. Arthroplasty of the rheumatoid wrist with silicone rubber: an early evaluation. J Hand Surg 1980;5A:114–121.
31. Figgie MP, Ranawat CS, Inglis AE, et al. Trispherical total wrist arthroplasty in rheumatoid arthritis. J Hand Surg 1990; 15A:217–223.
32. Eaton RG, Littler JW. Ligament reconstruction for the painful thumb carpo-metacarpal joint. J Bone Joint Surg 1973; 55A:1655–1666.
33. Burton RI, Pellegrini VD Jr. Surgical management of basal arthritis of the thumb. Part II: ligament reconstruction with tendon interposition arthroplasty. J Hand Surg 1986;11A:324–332.
34. Eaton RG, Glickel SZ, Littler JW. Tendon interposition arthroplasty for degenerative arthritis of the trapeziometacarpal joint of the thumb. J Hand Surg 1985;10A:645–654.

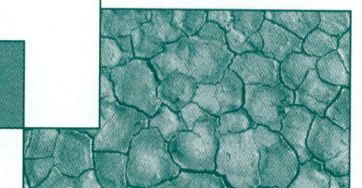

chapter 8

Valerie J. Ablaza, Douglas J. Mackenzie, Lloyd B. Gayle

Nerve Injury and Compression Neuropathy of the Hand and Forearm

Neuropathy and Nerve Injury

Valerie J. Ablaza, Douglas J. Mackenzie, Lloyd B. Gayle

RELEVANT ANATOMY AND PATHOGENESIS

The structural anatomy of the peripheral nerve must be clearly understood before nerve injuries can be managed. A peripheral nerve consists of both neural and connective tissues. A nerve cell, or neuron, consists of a cell body, nerve fiber (axon), and dendrites. The cell body of a motor nerve lies in the anterior horn of the spinal cord, whereas the cell body of the sensory nerve lies in the dorsal root ganglion. The axon is surrounded by Schwann cells, which may be myelinated. The macroscopic unit of a nerve is the fascicle, which consists of a group of axons.

The connective tissue components of nerves include the endoneurium, perineurium, and epineurium. These nonneural elements are not directly involved in impulse conduction but serve a supportive and nutritional role. The endoneurium is the fine connective tissue between nerve fibers. The perineurium, which consists of a multi-striated sheath of cells surrounding each fascicle, separates the internal and external environment of the nerve. The epineurium, made up of loosely attached sheets of laminated cells, has two components. The external epineurium surrounds the nerve perimeter; and the internal, or interfascicular, epineurium separates fascicles and is continuous with the external epineurium.

There are five basic fascicular patterns: monofascicular; oligofascicular, which has a few large fascicles; oligofascicular, which has more than five fascicles, polyfascicular, which is a group arrangement; and polyfascicular, which has no group arrangement. The difference between these patterns is important for surgical repair.

The vascular supply of peripheral nerves is via the arteriae nervorum. This vascular plexus consists of extrinsic blood vessels (extrinsic vascularity), which run between the grooves of fascicles, and interfascicular arterioles (internal vascularity), which supply the internal portions of the nerve and allow for safe elevation of the nerve from the tissue bed over a long distance.

Physiology

The membrane of a stimulated nerve undergoes a change in permeability to sodium and potassium ions, which leads to an action potential. The speed of conduction of an impulse through a nerve depends on the diameter of the nerve fiber and other membrane-proper ties. Myelinated nerve fibers conduct at a rapid rate, are relatively large in diameter, and are fairly sensitive to stimulation. Unmyelinated fibers are small in diameter, conduct slowly, and are generally associated with basal activity.

Innervation Patterns

The nerves of primary importance to the hand surgeon are the median, ulnar, and radial nerves, which originate in the brachial plexus. The median nerve innervates the forearm pronators; extrinsic flexors of the wrist, thumb, and finger thenar musculature; and the radial lumbricals. The sensory innervation involves the radial half of the palm and the palmar aspect of the thumb, index, and long finger and radial half of the ring finger. The ulnar nerve innervates the extrinsic wrist flexor, flexors of the ring and small fingers, interossei, ulnar lumbricals, hypothenar muscles, and thumb adductor and short flexor. The sensory pattern includes the ulnar aspect of the palm, ulnar half of the ring finger, and the small finger. The radial nerve primarily controls motor function and innervates the triceps and brachioradialis muscles and the muscles involved in supination and extension of the wrist, thumb, and fingers. The sensory area usually includes the dorsum of the hand and the thenar web space.

Nerve Injury

Damage caused by an object striking a nerve can be manifest as a blunt injury or as complete or partial transaction of the nerve. Nerves may also be stretched, torn, or twisted. Nerve injury leads to ultrastructural changes. For example, there is a reorganization of the somatosensory cortex, which decreases the area normally served by the injured nerve. The cell body metabolism accelerates, resulting in an increase in size and a change in production of materials, which persists during the period of axon regeneration. There is a threefold increase in cross-sectional area of the proximal nerve stump. Axons begin to sprout and divide at the site of injury. Schwann cell proliferation and axonal sprouting can occur as early as 48 h after injury. The distal nerve segment undergoes wallerian degeneration: Axons distal to the injury degenerate and die, and the more distal axons provide clean endoneurial tubes for the regenerating axons. If regeneration is delayed, the empty endoneurial tubes will shrink. Following degeneration, distal muscle fibers undergo atrophy, and eventually, it may not be possible to achieve functional recovery of a denervated muscle.

Classification

Seddon (1) proposed a classification of nerve injury that progresses from neurapraxia, which is the least severe injury, to neurotmesis, which is the most severe (Table 8.1). This system is based on the pathogenesis of neural degeneration and the time course of neural regeneration, but it does not take into account the complexity of nerve injury. Thus Sunderland (2) extended the classification to five grades. Mackinnon and Dellon's (3) mixed injury classification includes a sixth-degree injury, which combines various patterns of injury from fascicle to fascicle.

All these classification systems take into account that different degrees of nerve damage may occur; but unfortunately, none of these classifications is clinically meaningful, as it is impossible to determine exactly which structures have been disrupted. These schemes are, however, useful for predicting prognosis. It is important to emphasize that the degree of nerve damage may not be apparent at the time of injury, especially for crush and avulsion injuries.

INITIAL FINDINGS, PHYSICAL EXAMINATION, AND DIAGNOSIS

The diagnosis of most nerve injuries can be made on the basis of a thorough history and physical examination. The timing, site, and mechanism of injury, in addition to any preexisting conditions or injuries, are important elements of the history. Sensory and motor function in the median, ulnar, and radial nerves should be completely evaluated. Motor function is evaluated by manually testing individual muscles or groups of muscles and can be quantified by manual muscle grading or measuring grip or pinch strength (Table 8.2).

Because sensory territories are not rigidly fixed and commonly overlap, touch perception is most accurately evaluated in the autonomous zone of each peripheral nerve (Table 8.3). Specifically, the tip of the small finger is tested for the ulnar nerve, the tip of the index finger for the median nerve, and the dorsum of the thumb and first web space for the radial nerve. Sensory function may be quantified by determining innervation density (static or two-point discrimination), cutaneous pressure threshold (Semmes-Weinstein monofilaments), or cutaneous vibratory threshold (vibrometer).

The evaluation of both motor function and sensation may require electrodiagnostic testing if the patient is unconscious or uncooperative. When the motor or sensory examination is unreliable, surgical exploration of the wound in the operating room, especially for pediatric cases, may be required before a diagnosis can be made.

| table | 8.1 | Classification of Nerve Injury |

Classification System			
Seddon	Sunderland	Disruption	Prognosis
Neurapraxia	Grade 1	Myelin (conduction block)	Complete recovery (days to months)
Axonotmesis	Grade 2	Axon (wallerian degeneration)	Complete recovery (months)
Neurotmesis[a]	Grade 3	Axon (endoneurium)	Slow recovery (may be incomplete)
	Grade 4	Axon (endoneurium perineurium)	Moderate reduction in function; surgery required
	Grade 5	All structures	Marked reduction in function; no spontaneous recovery

[a]Seddon's neurotmesis subsumes Sunderland's grades 3–5.

table 8.2	Evaluation of Motor Recovery
Grade	Characteristic
M0	No contraction
M1	Return of perceptible contraction in proximal muscles
M2	Return of perceptible contraction in both proximal and distal muscles
M3	Return of function in both proximal and distal muscles to such a degree that all important muscles are sufficiently powerful to act against resistance
M4	Same as grade M3 plus all synergistic and independent movements are possible
M5	Complete recovery

table 8.3	Evaluation of Sensory Recovery
Grade	Characteristic
S0	Absence of sensibility in the autonomous area
S1	Recovery of deep cutaneous pain sensibility within the autonomous area of the nerve
S2	Return of some degree of superficial cutaneous pain and tactile sensitivity within the autonomous area of the nerve
S3	Return of superficial cutaneous pain and tactile sensibility throughout the autonomous area and disappearance of any previous overresponse.
S3+	Same as grade S3 plus some recovery of two-point discrimination within the autonomous area
S4	Complete recovery

RADIOLOGIC STUDIES

Frequently, nerve injuries are a part of an overall pattern of injury to the entire extremity. Appropriate radiologic studies will determine the extent of associated bone and joint abnormality. In addition, blunt trauma may reveal foreign bodies in the area of the injury to the nerve that may be associated with acute injury to the nerve. Relevant radiologic studies should be a routine part of the initial management and assessment of acute nerve injuries. Although most frequently plain radiologic studies are adequate, additional radiologic studies may be beneficial. For example, MRI scanning is an excellent technique of imaging all soft tissue. MRI may be able to identify the site of symptomatic neuroma formation and aid in exposure and surgical approach to this area.

TREATMENT

Nerve regeneration requires healing of both the proximal and the distal stumps and axonal sprouting that must connect the stumps. Thus the transacted nerve ends must be in close proximity. Ideally, nerve repair involves good alignment, minimal tension when the extremity is in a neutral position, and a well-vascularized bed. Concomitant tendon, bone, or joint injuries should be repaired before the nerve is repaired.

After identifying the nerve ends, the surgeon should prepare the stumps by performing partial resection of the damaged ends or interfascicular dissection. Then coaptation of the nerve stumps, fascicles, or groups of fascicles is performed. The standard method for maintaining coaptation in peripheral nerves is microscopic repair using 10–0 or 11–0 nylon sutures.

Operative Treatment

There are essentially three types of nerve repair; all attempt to align the fascicles accurately, but they differ in the location of suture placement (Clinical Table: Neuropathy and Nerve Injury). Comparative analyses have not demonstrated the superiority of one technique over the others. For external epineurial repair, the most commonly performed technique, the outer epineurium of each fascicle is coapted. This technique allows for maximal coaptation without extensive dissection and suturing and is easy to perform. Epineurial repair is a good technique for nerves less than 4 to 5 mm in diameter and is applicable to both primary and secondary repairs. This type of repair is carried out when the damaged fascicles have mixed sensory and motor functions and there are no well-defined groups of fascicles.

For fascicular repair, the fascicles are coapted on an individual basis by suturing the perineurium. It is more time-consuming and requires more surgical manipulation than standard techniques and has the potential for excessive fibrosis. This technique is important for repairing dissimilar fascicles (e.g., toe to hand transfers) and neurotized fascicles. Fascicular repair is the technique of choice for nerve grafting. This technique is used when fewer than five fascicles are present.

Group fascicular repair involves suturing around the perimeter of groups of fascicles to allow for better coaptation of the central nerve and thus better spatial alignment of the nerve. This repair is performed when a particular fascicle is recognized as mediating a specific function and is indicated for nerves in which there are a large number of central fascicles.

Although these three techniques rely on suture repair for restoring nerve continuity, there are a number of experimental and clinical studies that have demonstrated the efficacy of fibrin glue in peripheral nerve anastomoses, with or without the use of anchoring sutures (4).

NERVE GRAFTING

Nerve grafting is used to bridge the distance between nerve ends that may result from retraction or loss of sub-

Clinical Table: Neuropathy and Nerve Injury

Procedure	Indications	Technique	Anatomy	Pitfalls
External epineurial repair	• Transected nerve ends in close proximity	• Identify nerve ends • Prepare stump • Outer epineurium of each fascicle is coapted • Microscopic repair using 10–0 or 11–0 nylon sutures	• Epineurial sheath • Nerve fascicles	• Too much tension on nerve • Inadequate preparation of stump by not resecting damaged ends • Nonmaintenance of coaptation by failure to splint
Fascicular repair	• Transected nerve ends in close proximity	• Fascicles coapted on individual basis by suturing perineurium • This technique is important for repairing neurotized fascicles	• Epineurial sheath • Nerve fascicles	• Too much tension on nerve • Inadequate preparation of stump by not resecting damaged ends • Nonmaintenance of coaptation by failure to splint • Should not be used when more than five fascicles are present
Group fascicular repair	• Transected nerve ends in close proximity • Particular fascicle recognized as mediating specific function • Large number of central fascicles	• Suture around perimeter of groups of fascicles	• Epineurial sheath • Nerve fascicles	• Tension on nerve repair
Nerve grafting	• Retraction or loss of substance from injury or neuroma excision	• Identify and mobilize nerve ends • Cut back to viable tissue • Fascicles identified—proximal and distal • Cut grafts with joint in full extension, slightly longer • Minimal aligning of sutures	• Variable anatomy from donor site must be understood • Understand donor sensory deficit	• Donor site morbidity • Scarring at either end of nerve graft • Too few autograph

stance from injury or excision of a neuroma. Rather than acting as a substitute for the lost nerve segment, nerve grafts provide an environment that allows axons of the proximal stump to cross the defect.

Grafts were advocated and popularized in the modern era by Millesi et al. (6). The primary indication for the use of grafts is to span an excessive gap between nerve stumps, thus eliminating tension from the nerve repair. There are no specific distances that mandate the use of a nerve graft, because the location, level, and type of injury affect the decision. There are, however, certain guidelines that can aid in decision making. Most important, interposition grafts should be used when a tension-free repair is not possible.

When performing nerve grafting, the surgeon first identifies and mobilizes the nerve ends and cuts them back to viable tissue. Fascicles are identified at the proximal and distal stumps of the recipient nerve and aligned as well as possible. With the joints in full extension, the grafts are cut slightly longer than the defect to be bridged, and the minimal number of aligning sutures is used to maintain coaptation. According to Millesi (7), four or five autografts are necessary for the ulnar and radial nerves and five or six for the median nerve.

The disadvantages of nerve grafting with autogenous material include time to harvest and donor site morbidity. When nerve grafts are used, a donor sensory deficit is incurred. Furthermore, any nerve conduit requires two sites of coaptation and, therefore, two potential barriers to regenerating axons. The advantage of nerve grafts—to produce a tension-free repair—however, may outweigh all of the potential disadvantages.

The most common donor nerves are cutaneous nerves, including the sural nerve in the lower leg and the medial and lateral antebrachial cutaneous nerves of the forearm. Other donor nerves are the lateral femoral cutaneous nerve of the thigh and the superficial radial nerve and dorsal cutaneous branch of the ulnar nerve in the arm.

Free vascularized nerve grafts (8) may be useful when there is an adverse recipient bed or large nerve gaps and as carriers for nonvascularized nerve grafts (9), but the results and indications remain controversial. Other alternatives to standard nerve grafts include autogenous interpositional vein grafts (10) and interposition of a nonvital graft or type of tube as a pathway for neuromatous neurotization (11). Experimental work has been done using biodegradable polyglycolic acid conduits to manage short nerve gaps (12).

VARIABLES OF NERVE SURGERY

The many variables that influence the results of nerve repair can be divided into two groups. Variables not under the surgeon's control include age of patient, condition of the wound, and nerve gap. Variables under the control of the surgeon include type of repair and timing of repair, as well as the surgeon's skill.

Timing of Repair

The timing of nerve repairs is generally on a semielective basis; the surgeon judges the best time to establish the viability of the nerve ends. Primary repair is indicated when clinical and surgical conditions permit, e.g., when the nerves have been cleanly and sharply transected and when microinstrumentation and a skilled surgeon are available. The repair is best performed in a healthy patient who has no associated injuries that would compromise tissue viability or skin coverage. The advantages of primary repair include (a) less scarring with minimal dissection and (b) earlier recovery of function.

Delayed primary repair, or secondary repair, is indicated if clinical and surgical conditions are not met in the acute injury setting. Secondary neurorrhaphy under favorable conditions gives better results than does primary repair under unfavorable conditions. In cases in which the wound is débrided, the nerve stumps may be tagged or loosely approximated until definitive exploration and repair can be performed. Delayed repair is also indicated for nerves divided by crushing or traction injury or injured by high-velocity missile wounds, so that the extent of injury can be fully assessed and the level of viable nerve can be determined.

The upper limit between time of injury and time of repair that does not compromise return of sensation has not been clearly defined. Studies have not indicated a significant difference in recovery of functional sensation between acute and early secondary repair when the conditions are optimal (13).

Condition of the Wound

The recipient bed should be well vascularized; be free of infection, hematoma, and devitalized tissue; and have minimal scar tissue. Heavily contaminated wounds that carry the possibility of infection should undergo débridement with an open dressing for several days before nerve repair is conducted. The ideal conditions of the recipient bed are especially important for nerve grafting, because the graft undergoes wallerian degeneration upon removal and depends on revascularization at the recipient site.

Patient Age

Age of the patient correlates closely with the return of sensory function following nerve repair; younger patients experience better sensory return when other variables are the same. Young et al. (14) found that following digital nerve repair, 80% of patients under 20 years of age achieved useful two-point discrimination, whereas patients over 40 years achieved only protective sensation.

Nerve Gap

Recovery following nerve grafting is not as good as that following direct repairs with no tension, but it is superior to recovery from direct nerve repairs with tension. As a result, some surgeons prefer moderate joint flexion to nerve grafting if the nerve ends can be approximated without tension. Ways of decreasing the gap between two nerve stumps, other than nerve grafting, include extending the nerve to its original length to compensate for elastic retraction, transposing the nerve to a shorter route, and shortening adjacent bones.

REHABILITATION

Following surgical repair, immobilization should be continued for at least 10 days, and protective splinting should be maintained for several weeks more. A graded rehabilitation program is then begun to recover full range of motion of the joints. Once muscles have been reinnervated, muscle strengthening and coordination exercises are instituted. Direct muscle stimulation may be used to prevent muscle atrophy if it is anticipated that reinnervation will take more than 9 months.

Sensory reeducation is a structured program that assists patients in learning altered sense impulses. These techniques are associated with a high degree of patient compliance and have been established to maximize the functional level of sensory recovery. The appropriate timing for the institution of sensory retraining is when 256 cycles per second is perceived at the fingertips.

EVALUATION

The Tinel sign defines the level to which axons have regenerated and is demonstrated by paresthesias radiating distal to the site of nerve percussion (15). The Tinel sign advances along the course of the nerve at a rate of about 1 mm per day. It is not an absolute indicator of sensory function, but sensory recovery will rarely occur in the absence of a Tinel sign.

Two-point discrimination is generally accepted as the most reliable measure of sensory function. Static two-point discrimination is a measure of the minimum separation distance required to sense two points. The normal value is 2 to 5 mm at the fingertips. Moving two-point discrimination assesses the ability of the digits to detect movement and is thought to predict the return of normal hand function better than static traction. The normal threshold for detecting movement in the fingertips is 2 mm.

It is important to grade the return of function using a standard method. The most widely accepted classification of sensory recovery is that proposed by Highet and Sanders (16), which was later modified by the Nerve Committee of the British Medical Research Council. A grade of S4 for sensory recovery is considered normal and is equivalent to a static two-point discrimination of 6 mm or less (Table 8.3). Grade S3 or better is considered useful return of sensation and is equivalent to a static two-point discrimination of 15 mm.

It is important to note that sensory and motor recovery after peripheral nerve injury can continue to improve for more than 2 years after repair. The ultimate result after nerve repair cannot be accurately evaluated until 3 to 5 years postsurgery.

COMPLICATIONS

Regenerating axons may become entangled in a disorganized clump of scar tissue, known as a neuroma. Painful neuromas may form in an irreparable nerve stump. The preferred method of management involves en bloc relocation to an unscarred, protected site (17,18), although numerous physical and chemical alternatives have been described. Neuromas may also form at the site of a partial nerve transaction or other nerve trauma that has not been surgically explored. These cases of neuroma incontinuity may be managed by resection and repair, with or without a nerve graft, or merely with intraneural neurolysis if there is fascicular continuity (19).

If evidence of nerve regeneration is delayed beyond the time expected after neurorrhaphy, the patient should be observed for 6 weeks or more before electromyographic and nerve conduction velocity studies are performed. These results should be correlated with clinical serial examinations, including a Tinel test, to determine whether surgical exploration will be undertaken.

Reflex sympathetic dystrophy refers to a complex syndrome of posttraumatic pain (20). It remains an ill-defined disorder that is not well understood. It may be precipitated by a number of causes, including nerve and soft tissue injury in the hand. Treatment modalities include chemical and surgical sympathectomy, anti-inflammatory agents, psychotropic medications, transcutaneous electrical nerve stimulation (TENS), acupuncture, physical therapy, and psychotherapy (21). The most useful approach to this syndrome may be the institution of preventive measures.

SUMMARY

Compression neuropathies are a common source of upper extremity complaints and disability. Sensory or motor compression may produce a variety of clinical syndromes. Frequently, electrophysiology confirms the diagnosis. Adequate surgical release requires recognition of potential sites of compression along the entire course of the nerve.

 II   # Compression Neuropathies of the Upper Extremity

Douglas J. Mackenzie, Valerie Ablaza, Lloyd B. Gayle

Compression neuropathies are among the most common afflictions of the upper extremity. The incidence of compression neuropathies has been steadily increasing over the last two decades, likely owing to increased clinical awareness and more repetitive tasks at the workplace. Subjective symptoms may not readily correlate with objective findings, and added confusion may come into play from the varied interests of the patient, workers compensation boards, employers, and others.

RELEVANT ANATOMY AND PATHOGENESIS

Compression neuropathies, also known as entrapment neuropathics, generally occur at well-known anatomical sites in which the nerve passes through or adjacent to a rigid or semirigid structure. For example, the compression may be caused by a joint and its associated retinacular ligaments, a tendinous edge, an anomalous muscle belly, or the acute or chronic manifestations of musculoskeletal trauma. Otherwise subclinical levels of compression may manifest as compressive symptoms if the nerve is compressed at more than one level, the so-called double-crush syndrome (22,23). Associated systemic conditions may predispose a patient to compressive symptoms as well, particularly diabetes mellitus, hypothyroidism, collagen vascular disease, alcohol abuse, and possibly pyridoxine deficiency.

Nerve damage has been attributed to pressure-induced changes in blood flow, ion gradients, direct mechanical forces, or a combination of these. For example, the normal tissue pressure in the carpal tunnel is 7 to 8 mm Hg. In carpal tunnel syndrome, this may be increased to 30 and 90 mm Hg with wrist flexion and extension, respectively. Exceeding the normal capillary pressure of around 30 mm Hg produces ischemia and consequent symptoms of paresthesias and weakness (24,25).

Early nerve compression may occur only with wrist flexion or extension or with prolonged activity. Although blood–nerve barrier changes may result from the transient ischemia, histologic changes are absent. As the syndrome progresses and paresthesias become more constant, connective tissue changes occur; edema of the internal epineurium is followed by fibrosis and eventual degeneration of the perineurium. Focal nerve fiber damage follows, and changes include demyelination of large fibers and turnover of unmyelinated fibers with regeneration of smaller fibers. Variability of pathology among adjacent fascicles is seen, sometimes making the clinical findings confusing. Increasing duration and severity of compression leads to numbness, paralysis, muscle atrophy, and wallerian degeneration (22,25).

INITIAL FINDINGS, PHYSICAL EXAMINATION, AND DIAGNOSIS

A thorough history of the patient with compression neuropathy will benefit the clinical evaluation. The clinician should determine the duration and degree of pain, paresthesias, and weakness and understand the patient's provocative movements or activities. Distribution of discomfort must be carefully sought, because compression provokes symptoms along the distribution of the nerve or nerves in question, whereas peripheral polyneuropathies may cause distributions that are bilateral or that affect the lower extremity as well. Associated illnesses may be known or newly diagnosed and may predispose the patient to compression neuropathy. More proximal causes, such as thoracic outlet syndrome, may induce significant pain or contribute to a double-crush syndrome, confusing the diagnosis. Associated neck pain should be evaluated and imaged by a neurologist or neurosurgeon (22,26,27)

A complete physical examination of the upper extremity is performed, and the clinician should pay particular attention to motor and sensory nerve distributions. Strength is tested by the quantitative measurements of pinch and grip, and any atrophy is noted. Sensory testing begins with provocative tests, such as pressure over entrapment sites or by positioning of the extremity in flexion or extension. Sensory distributions are evaluated by threshold and innervation density testing. Cutaneous pressure and vibratory thresholds are tested with Semmes-Weinstein nylon monofilaments and a tuning fork or vibrometer, respectively. Innervation density is tested by static and moving two-point discrimination. Threshold changes always precede innervation density changes, which imply actual axonal loss (22,26).

ELECTRODIAGNOSIS AND RADIOLOGIC STUDIES

Electrophysiologic studies are useful adjuncts to the history and clinical examination, particularly when the diagnosis is difficult or a more objective evaluation is desired. Clinical correlation is necessary, because intervention would not be warranted in a situation in which abnormal electrophysiologic studies were associated with normal clinical findings. Patients with real symptoms may have normal studies if some fast-conducting fibers remain undamaged by the nerve compression. Routine nerve conduction studies evaluate the fastest-conducting myelinated fibers and may miss certain small fiber neuropathies. Anomalous innervation may also confuse the interpretation of electrophysiologic studies.

For compression neuropathics, the most important studies are the nerve conduction studies. Localizing the site of nerve compression can be demonstrated by focal slowing of the nerve conduction velocities. Polyneuropathies can be differentiated from compressive neuropathies via nerve conduction studies, and multiple and double-crush syndromes may be elucidated by a thorough evaluation over the entire course of the nerve. Electromyography in compression neuropathy is useful when severe compression has resulted in axonal loss and muscle fiber denervation. Muscle fiber denervation is best indicated by fibrillation potentials and positive sharp waves,

Reinnervation following nerve injury is indicated by decreasing fibrillation potentials and large polyphasic motor potentials (28,29).

Although a relatively new diagnostic modality for compression neuropathy, MRI has been advocated as a painless, noninvasive imaging technique for the carpal tunnel, capable of visualizing swelling or compression of the median nerve and differentiating space-occupying lesions from inflammatory conditions. MRI may also help in the postoperative evaluation of patients with persistent or recurrent symptoms (30).

SPECIFIC CONSIDERATIONS

Median Nerve

CARPAL TUNNEL SYNDROME

Symptomatic carpal tunnel syndrome frequently is successfully treated surgically by division of the transverse carpal ligament, effectively "unroofing" the median nerve. Traditionally, this has been done via an "open" technique, during which an incision is made and the ligament is divided under direct visualization while the contents of the canal are protected. In recent years, work has been done attempting to perfect an endoscopic technique of ligament release. There is some controversy over the best, safest, and most effective way to decompress the carpal canal. Advocates of open surgery point to the ability to divide and examine the contents of the carpal canal and the lower incidence of nerve injury as important reasons to perform the surgery this way. Advocates of endoscopic surgery release see decreased preoperative morbidity and pain as reasons favoring endoscopic surgery release (31,32). Perhaps on-going investigations and improved techniques will quell the controversy. Internal neurolysis is probably ineffective and unnecessary, although no definitive studies have yet been done (33). Continued or recurrent symptoms of carpal tunnel syndrome may indicate incomplete release of the transverse ligament, associated polyneuropathy, or a double-crush syndrome. Postoperative immobilization should be limited to 1 week, followed by range of motion exercises (Figs. 8.1 and 8.2).

PRONATOR SYNDROME

The hand symptoms of pronator syndrome may be similar to carpal tunnel syndrome; but in addition, the patient experiences pain with resisted forearm pronation and pain with resisted flexion of the proximal interphalangeal (PIP) joint of the long and ring fingers. There is a positive Tinel sign in the forearm (not at the wrist) and dysesthesia of the palmar triangle. Compression of the median nerve can be caused by the ligament of Struthers, lacertus fibrosis, pronator teres, or proximal arch of the flexor digitorum superficialis; and surgical exploration and release of these structures is effective when conservative measures fail (Figs. 8.3, 8.4, and 8.5).

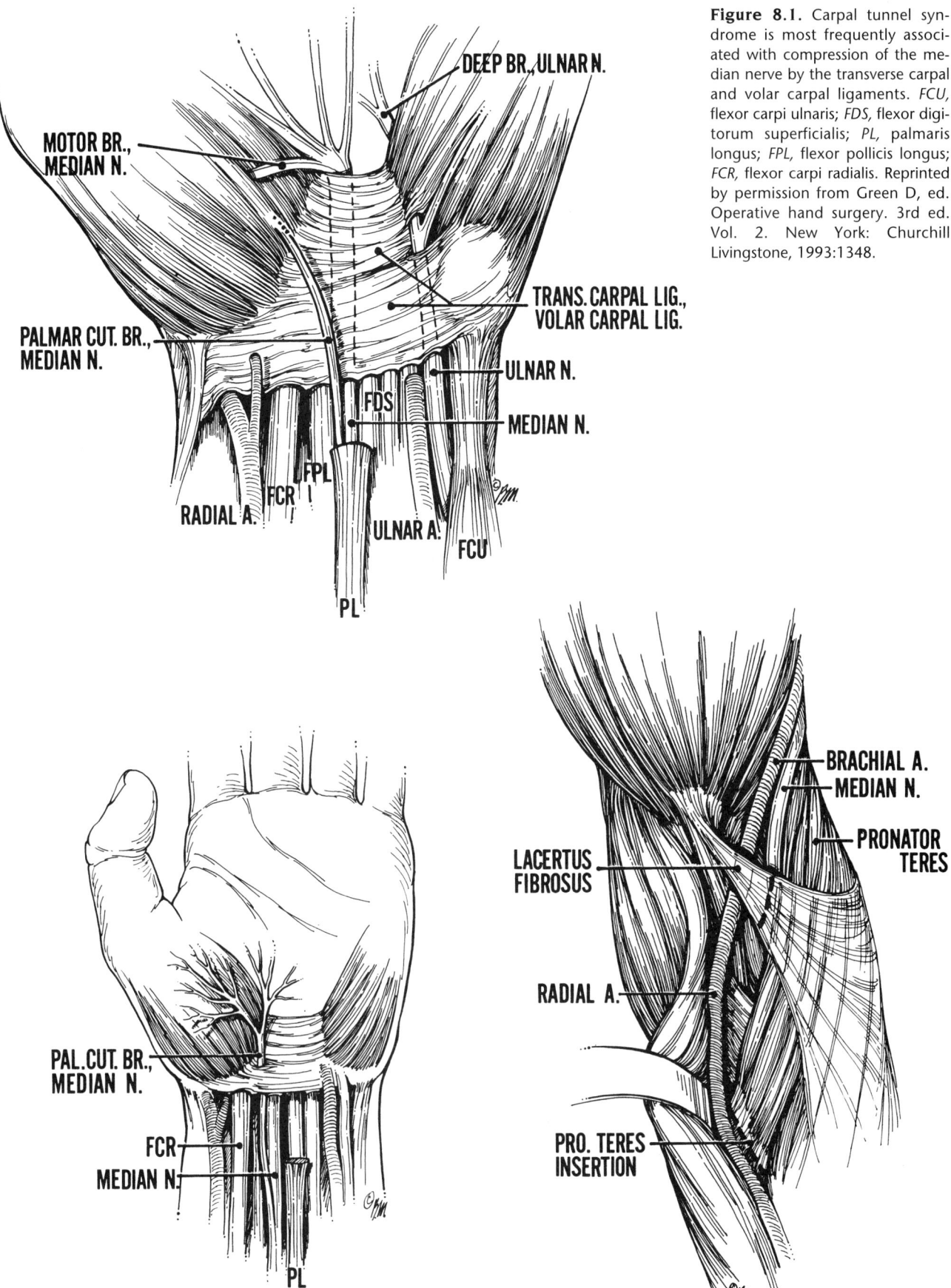

Figure 8.1. Carpal tunnel syndrome is most frequently associated with compression of the median nerve by the transverse carpal and volar carpal ligaments. *FCU,* flexor carpi ulnaris; *FDS,* flexor digitorum superficialis; *PL,* palmaris longus; *FPL,* flexor pollicis longus; *FCR,* flexor carpi radialis. Reprinted by permission from Green D, ed. Operative hand surgery. 3rd ed. Vol. 2. New York: Churchill Livingstone, 1993:1348.

DEEP BR., ULNAR N.

MOTOR BR., MEDIAN N.

PALMAR CUT. BR., MEDIAN N.

TRANS. CARPAL LIG., VOLAR CARPAL LIG.

ULNAR N.

MEDIAN N.

FDS

FPL

FCR

RADIAL A.

ULNAR A.

FCU

PL

PAL. CUT. BR., MEDIAN N.

FCR

MEDIAN N.

PL

BRACHIAL A.

MEDIAN N.

PRONATOR TERES

LACERTUS FIBROSUS

RADIAL A.

PRO. TERES INSERTION

Figure 8.2. The palmar cutaneous nerve is at risk during surgical approaches to the carpal canal, especially if the approach is too radial. *FCR,* flexor carpi radialis. Reprinted by permission from Green D, ed. Operative hand surgery. 3rd ed. Vol. 2. New York: Churchill Livingstone, 1993:1356.

Figure 8.3. Both the lacertus fibrosus and pronator teres muscles can compress the median nerve in the forearm. Reprinted by permission from Green D, ed. Operative hand surgery. 3rd ed. Vol. 2. New York: Churchill Livingstone, 1993:1345.

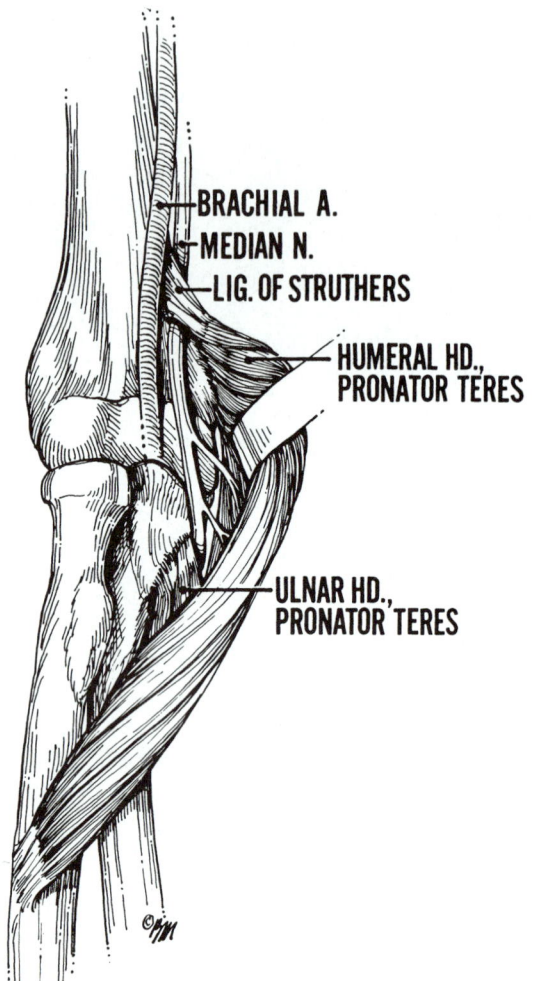

Figure 8.4. The median nerve can be entrapped by the supracondylar process and the ligament of Struthers, an accessory origin of the pronator teres. Reprinted by permission from Green D, ed. Operative hand surgery. 3rd ed. Vol. 2. New York: Churchill Livingstone, 1993:1343.

ANTERIOR INTEROSSEOUS SYNDROME

Forearm pain with exercise and weakness of pinch are typical symptoms of anterior interosseous syndrome. Although anomalous innervation patterns can confuse the diagnosis, paresis of the flexor pollicis longus, the flexor digitorum profundus to index and long fingers, and the pronator quadratus is classic (Fig. 8.6). Because the anterior interosseus is a motor nerve, sensory deficits are absent. The cause of this syndrome is usually tendinous bands in the proximal forearm from the deep head of the pronator teres or the arch of the flexor digitorum superficialis. Surgical exploration is indicated after confirmation by electrodiagnostic studies.

Ulnar Nerve

CUBITAL TUNNEL SYNDROME

Cubital tunnel syndrome is caused by compression of the ulnar nerve between the ulnar and humeral origins of the flexor carpi ulnaris at the elbow. Symptoms include

pain over the medial side of the proximal forearm, paresthesias of the ulnar innervated portion of the hand, and possible intrinsic atrophy. The syndrome may also be caused by other musculotendinous impingements, subluxation of the nerve at the elbow, osteophytes, or ganglia (Fig. 8.7). The physical examination reveals a positive elbow flexion test and Tinel sign over the cubital tunnel. Conservative treatment includes rest, avoidance of provocative activities, and extension splinting at night. Surgical options include decompression of the ulnar nerve at the elbow, anterior transposition of the ulnar nerve, and medial epicondylectomy.

ULNAR TUNNEL SYNDROME

Compression of the ulnar nerve in Guyon's canal may lead to pain, paresthesias, and intrinsic muscle weakness or atrophy. Causes include ganglia, blunt trauma, fractures, and ulnar artery thrombosis, making onset and progression of the symptoms swift. The sensory examination of the distribution of the dorsal sensory branch of the ulnar nerve is normal with isolated ulnar tunnel syndrome. A Tinel sign may be elicited over Guyon's canal, and an Allen test may suggest ulnar artery thrombosis. Surgical release divides the volar carpal ligament and pisohamate

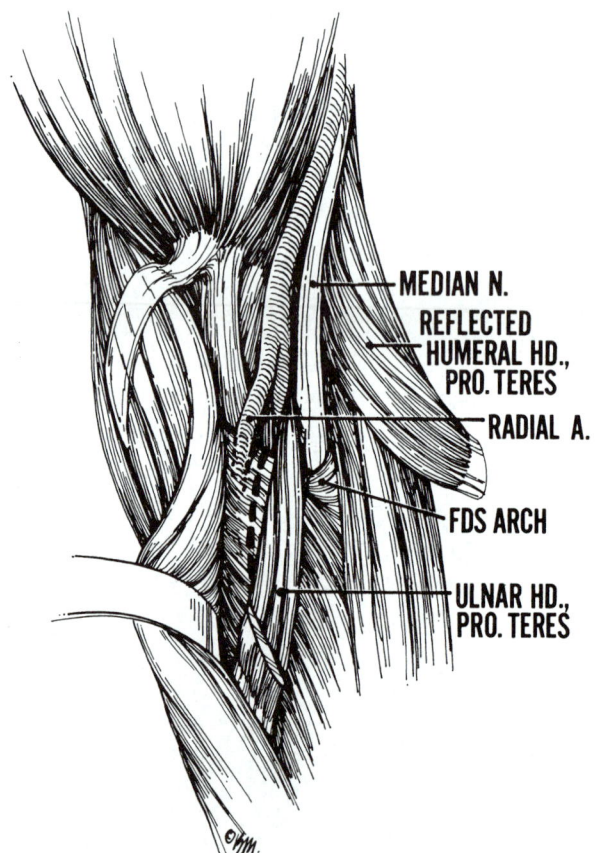

Figure 8.5. Compression of the median nerve can be caused by the arch of the flexor digitorum superficialis (FDS) muscle. Reprinted by permission from Green D, ed. Operative hand surgery. 3rd ed. Vol. 2. New York: Churchill Livingstone, 1993:1346.

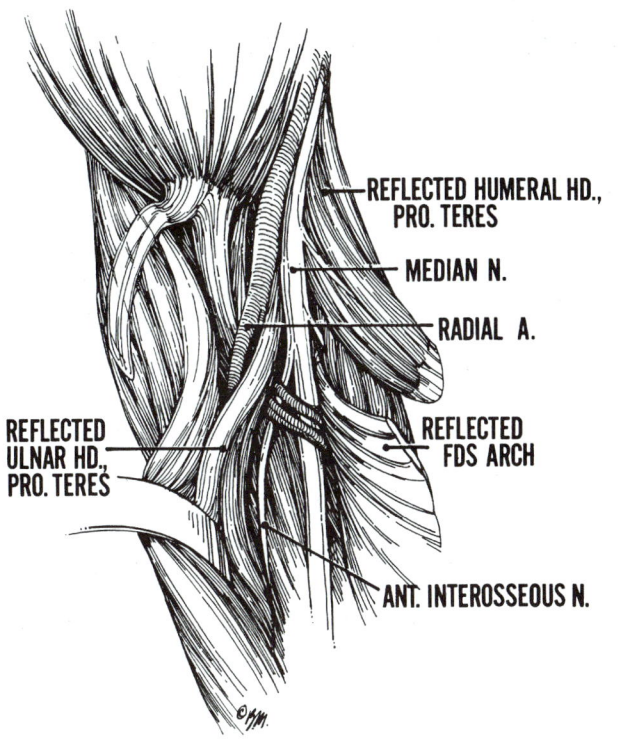

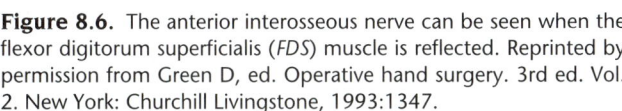

Figure 8.6. The anterior interosseous nerve can be seen when the flexor digitorum superficialis (*FDS*) muscle is reflected. Reprinted by permission from Green D, ed. Operative hand surgery. 3rd ed. Vol. 2. New York: Churchill Livingstone, 1993:1347.

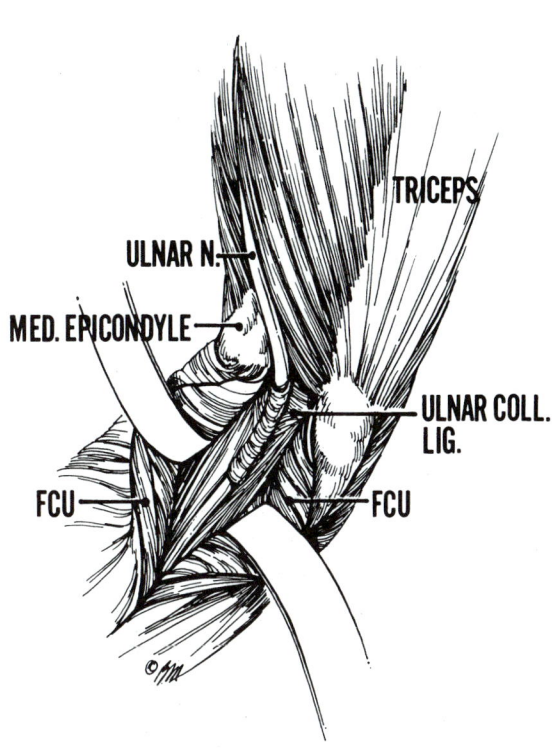

Figure 8.7. The ulnar nerve passes behind the medial epicondyle in the cubital tunnel before joining the two heads of the flexor carpal ulnaris (*FCU*). Reprinted by permission from Green D, ed. Operative hand surgery. 3rd ed. Vol. 2. New York: Churchill Livingstone, 1993:1357.

Clinical Table: Compression Neuropathies of the Upper Extremity

Procedure	Indications	Technique	Anatomy	Pitfalls
Carpal tunnel release	• Symptomatic carpal tunnel syndrome	• Expose transverse carpal ligament • Unroof median nerve • Open technique • Endoscopic technique	• Palmar cutaneous branch of median nerve • Motor branch of median nerve • Surrounding flexor tendons • Bony carpal canal	• Inadequate visualization • Division of palmar cutaneous branch • Division motor branch • Variable or anomalous motor branch
Flexor pronator release	• Proximal median nerve compression	• Open exploration of forearm median nerve	• Flexor pronator muscle • Brachial artery • Lacertus fibrosus • Radial artery	• Failure to recognize compression • Ligament of Struthers • Lacertus compression • Failure to recognize proximal arch or FDS
Anterior interosseous nerve release	• Forearm pain • Weakness of pinch secondary to anterior interosseous syndrome	• Explore forearm • Reflect humeral head pronator teres • Retract ulnar head pronator teres • Follow median nerve to anterior interosseous nerve	• Pronator teres • Radial artery • FDS arch • Main body of median nerve	• Inadequate release • Inexact or imprecise diagnosis
Cubital tunnel syndrome	• Symptomatic ulnar nerve compression behind medial epicondyle at cubital tunnel	• Incision of posterior elbow centered over cubital tunnel • Unroof cubital tunnel • Maintain vascularity • Decompose or transpose nerve • Minimal tension, flexion, and extension	• Flexor pronator origin/ulnar nerve • Articular branch • Branch to flexor	• Devascularization of nerve • Failure to recognize proximal compression • Transposition of nerve in excessive tension

Continued

Clinical Table: Compression Neuropathies of the Upper Extremity (continued)

Procedure	Indications	Technique	Anatomy	Pitfalls
Release ulnar tunnel	• Compression ulnar nerve Guyon's canal	• Open exploration of carpal and Guyon's canal • Divison of volar carpal ligament • Division of pisohemate ligament	• Median nerve • Ulnar narve • Palmar cutaneous branch • Motor branch/median nerve	• Associated ulnar artery thrombosis • Associated ganglia • Divison of dorsal branch ulnar nerve • Division of branch of median nerve
Radial nerve radial tunnel syndrome	• Pain from posterior interosseous • Radial tunnel syndrome symptomatic	• Explore radial nerve by anterior approach • Examine fibrous bands entrance to tunnel • Examine radial recurrent vessels • Examine tendinous margin of ECRB • Examine arcade of Frohse	• Extensor muscle of the forearm • Radial artery supinator muscle	• Inadequate examination of entire course of nerve • Tension and traction on nerve

FDS, flexor digitorum superficialis; ECRB, extensor carpi radialis brevis.

ligament and may be performed through a carpal tunnel incision during combined release.

Radial Nerve Radial Tunnel Syndrome

Often misdiagnosed as tennis elbow (lateral epicondylitis), radial tunnel syndrome is the most common entrapment neuropathy of the radial nerve and may coexist with lateral epicondylitis. Pain is experienced over the area of the extensor origin and is elicited with wrist flexion and pronation or wrist extension and forearm supination against resistance. Pain on resistance to middle finger extension is also seen. Failure of conservative therapy warrants surgery to explore the radial nerve and its four potential sites of compression in the radial tunnel: fibrous bands anterior to the radial head at the entrance to the radial tunnel; the radial recurrent vessels (the leash of Henry); the tendinous margin of the extensor carpi radians brevis; or (most common) the arcade of Frohse, which forms a ligamentous band over the deep radial nerve as it enters the supinator muscle.

SUMMARY

Much work in basic science and clinical neurology has improved our understanding of the way nerves are injured, regenerate, and function. Operative management of nerve injuries must take into consideration the basic biology of nerve repair to maximize the function when nerves are repaired or grafted (Clinical Table: Compression Neuropathies of the Upper Extremity).

REFERENCES

1. Seddon JH. A classification of nerve injuries. Br Med J 1942;2:237.
2. Sunderland S. Nerves and nerve injury. 2nd ed. London: Churchill Livingstone, 1978.
3. Mackinnon SE, Dellon AL. Surgery of the peripheral nerve. New York: Thieme, 1988.
4. Egloff DV, Narakas AO, Bonnard C. Results of nerve grafts with Tissucol (Tisseel) anastomosis. In: Schlag G, Redl H, eds. Fibrin sealant in operative medicine. Vol 2: Ophthalmology, neurosurgery. Berlin: Springer Verlag, 1986:181–185.
5. Huang TC, Blanks RH, Berns MW, Crumley RL. Laser vs. suture nerve anastomosis. Otoloaryngol Head Neck Surg 1992; 107:14–20.
6. Millesi H, Meissl G, Berger A. The interfascicular nerve-grafting of the median and ulnar nerves. J Bone Joint Surg 1972;54A:727–750.
7. Millesi H. Fascicular nerve repair and interfascicular nerve grafting. In: Daniel RK, Terzis JK, eds. Reconstructive microsurgery. Boston: Little, Brown, 1977:430–442.
8. Taylor GI, Ham FJ. The free vascularized nerve graft. Plast Reconstr Surg 1976;57:413–426.
9. Breidenbach W, Terzis JK. The anatomy of free vascularized nerve grafts. Clin Plast Surg 1984;11:65–71.
10. Chiu DT, Strauch B. A prospective clinical evaluation of autogenous vein grafts used as a nerve conduit for distal sensory defects of 3 cm or less. Plast Reconstr Surg 1990;86:928–934.
11. Glasby MA. Interposed muscle grafts in nerve repairs in the hand: an experimental basis for future clinical use. World J Surg 1991; 15:501–510.
12. Dellon AL, Mackinnon SE. An alternative to the classical nerve graft for the management of the short nerve gap. Plast Reconstr Surg 1988;82:849–856.
13. Onne L. Recovery of sensibility and sudomotor function in the hand after nerve suture. Acta Chir Scand 1962;Suppl 300:1.
14. Young L, Wray RC, Weeks PM. A randomized prospective comparison of fascicular and epineural digital nerve repairs. Plast Reconstr Surg 1981;68:89–93.
15. Tinel J. Le signe du "fourmillement" dans les lesion des nerfs peripheriques. Presse Med 1915;23:388.
16. Highet WB, Sanders FK. The effects of stretching nerves after suture. Br J Surg 1943;30:355.
17. Herndon JH, Eaton RG, Littler JW. Management of painful neuromas in the hand. J Bone Joint Surg 1976;58A:369–373.
18. Tupper JW, Booth DM. Treatment of painful neuromas of sensory nerves in the hand: a comparison of traditional and newer methods. J Hand Surg 1976;1A:144–151.
19. Daniel RK, Terzis JK. Reconstructive microsurgery. Boston: Little, Brown, 1977.
20. Amadio PC, Mackinnon SE, Merritt WH, et al. Reflex sympathetic dystrophy syndrome: consensus report of an ad hoc committee of the American Association for Hand Surgery on the definition of re-

flex sympathetic dystrophy syndrome. Plast Reconstr Surg 1991; 87:371–375.

21. Merritt WI. Reflex sympathetic dystrophy. In: May JW, Littler JW, eds. Plastic surgery: the hand. Philadelphia: Saunders, 1990:4884–4915.

22. Mackinnon SE. Double and multiple crush syndromes. Hand Clin 1992;8:369–390.

23. Upton ARM, McComas AJ. The double crush in nerve-entrapment syndromes. Lancet 1973;2:259–362.

24. Gelberman RH, Hergenroeder PT, Bargens AR, et al. The carpal tunnel syndrome—a study of carpal canal pressures. J Bone Joint Surg 1991;62A:380–383.

25. Rydevik B, Lundborg G. Permeability of intraneural microvessels and perineurium following acute, graded experimental nerve compression. Scand J Plast Reconstr Surg 1911;2:179–187.

26. Dellon AL. Patient evaluation and management considerations in nerve compression. Hand Clin 1992;8:229–239.

27. Reppel DM, Harrison RJ, Barnhart S. Work-related cumulative trauma disorders of the upper extremity. JAMA 1992;267:838–842.

28. Brumback RA, Bobele GB, Rayan GM. Electrodiagnosis of compressive nerve lesions. Hand Clin 1992;8:241–254.

29. Iyer VG. Understanding nerve conduction and electromyographic studies. Hand Clin 1993;9:273–287.

30. Mesgarzadeh M, Tfiolo J, Schneck CD. Carpal tunnel syndrome. NM imaging diagnosis. Magn Reson Imaging 1995;3:249–264.

31. Agee JM, McCarroll I-IR, Tortosa RD, et al. Endoscopic release of the carpal tunnel—a randomized prospective multicenter study. J Hand Surg 1992;17A:987–995.

32. Brown RA, Gelberman RH, Seiler JG, et al. Carpal tunnel release: a prospective randomized assessment of open and endoscopic methods. J Bone Joint Surg 1993;75A:1265–1275.

33. Gelberman RH, Pfeffer GB, Galbraith RT, et al. Results of treatment of severe carpal-tunnel syndrome without internal neurolysis of the median nerve. J Bone Joint Surg 1987;69A:896–903.

Flexor Tendon Injury and Tenosynovitis

Tendons are white, glistening fibrous cords, varying in length and thickness, sometimes round, sometimes flattened, of considerable strength, and devoid of elasticity. They consist almost entirely of white fibrous tissue, the fibrils of which have an undulating course parallel with each other and are firmly united together. They are very sparingly supplied with blood-vessels, the smaller tendons presenting in their interior not a trace of them. Nerves also are not present in smaller tendons.

—*Gray's Anatomy*

The primary function of a tendon is to glide, transferring the mechanical work of the muscle to the skeletal articulations and creating movement. The flexor tendons of the hand are crucially important, since loss or abnormalities of digital flexion are quite disabling. Treatment of pathologic conditions of the flexor tendon in the hand necessitates a clear understanding of the anatomy of the flexor tendon system.

I Flexor Tendon Injury

RELEVANT ANATOMY

The flexor digitorum superficialis (or flexor sublimis) originates from the medial epicondyle of the humerus, coronoid process of the ulna, and proximal radius. Its broad muscle fibers pass down the forearm and divide into two planes. The superficial plane of the muscle terminates as the flexor tendons to the middle and ring fingers, and the deep plane terminates as the flexor tendons to the index and small fingers. Thus as the superficialis flexor tendons pass into the carpal tunnel, they are arranged in pairs; the tendons to the long and ring fingers are located more volar or subcutaneous than are the tendons to the ring and small fingers (1). Once in the palm, the four tendons diverge, heading for their respective fingers. As each superficialis tendon approaches the proximal phalanx, it splits into two slips, which ultimately reunite when the tendon inserts onto the volar midaspect of the middle phalanx. Thus the flexor superficialis flexes the proximal interphalangeal joints of the fingers. It is innervated by the median nerve.

The flexor digitorum profundus also arises from the medial or ulnar side of the forearm, but immediately beneath the superficial flexors. Its origin is from the proximal ulna and the interosseous membrane of the forearm. It too passes down the forearm and divides into four tendons at the level of the distal forearm approaching the wrist. The profundus does not layer itself the way the superficialis does. Its unique aspect is that the portion of the muscle terminating in the tendon to the index finger is usually distinct or separate from the common muscle belly of the tendons to the long, ring, and small fingers (2). The surgeon must be aware of this common muscle belly arrangement when trying to determine isolated tendon injuries in the digits.

As the profundus tendons proceed distally in the palm, they pass through the split or branching of the superficialis tendon (chiasma of Camper) on their way to their insertions on the distal phalanges (Fig. 9.1). Thus, even though the profundus is the deep flexor tendon, based on its location in the forearm and wrist, it is actually the more vulnerable tendon once in the digit, because it is exposed

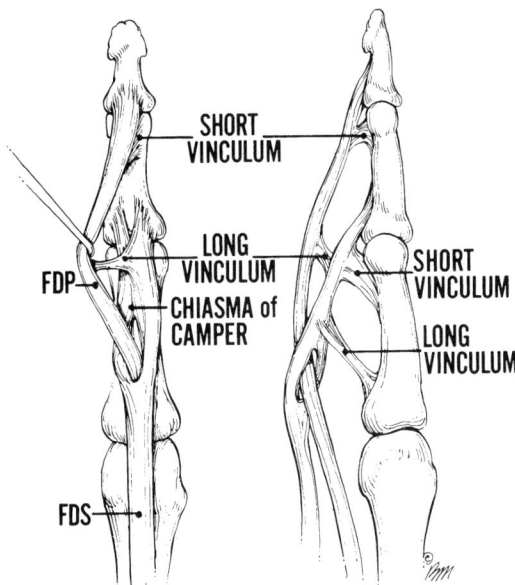

Figure 9.1. The chiasma of Camper is at the split in the sublimis through the profundus passes. *FDP,* flexor digitorum profundus; *FDS,* flexor digitorum superficialis. Reprinted with permission from Green DP, ed. Operative hand surgery. 3rd ed. New York: Churchill Livingstone, 1993.

along a greater length of the finger volarly. The profundus flexes the distal interphalangeal joints; the profundus to the ring and little fingers are innervated by the ulnar nerve, and the profundus to the index and long fingers are innervated by the median nerve.

The thumb has only one flexor tendon, the flexor pollicis longus. It originates from the coronoid process of the ulna and the middle third of the radius and adjacent interosseous membrane. It inserts onto the volar aspect of the distal phalanx. It flexes the distal interphalangeal joint of the thumb and is innervated by the median nerve.

In the palm, at the level of the metacarpal heads, the flexor tendons become enclosed within a synovial sheath. This sheath, or tunnel, is actually a tube that encloses both the superficialis and profundus tendons from the level of the metacarpal head to the terminal insertion at the distal phalanx. The sheath to the small finger communicates with the ulnar bursa in the palm. The sheath for the thumb communicates with the radial bursa in the palm. The sheath keeps the tendons located adjacent to the volar periosteum of the phalanges; hence, it is also known as the fibro-osseous tunnel. If the flexor tendons bowstring (bow) away from the bone with flexion of the digit, their muscle belly must exert a more forceful contraction to produce the same amount of motion than do tendons that remain adjacent to the bone (3). Through an igenious system of pulleys, the tunnel achieves its mechanical goal of keeping the flexor tendons adjacent to the bone without being so rigid that the flexibility of the digit is affected.

The pulley system of the flexor tendon sheath is actually a localized thickening and thinning of the sheath

(Fig. 9.2). The thickened areas of the sheath are called the annular pulleys and are the ones primarily responsible for preventing bowstringing (bowing), or movement of the tendons away from the bone. The cruciform pulleys are thin and pliable and allow the flexor tendon sheath to lengthen and shorten with excursion of the finger. There are four annular pulleys and three cruciform pulleys. The annular pulleys are designated Al through A4: A1 is located at the level of the metacarpal head; A2, at the base of the proximal phalanx; A3, at the head of the proximal phalanx; and A4, at the middle of the middle phalanx. The thumb has two annular and one oblique pulley (4). Thumb A1 is located at the metacarpal head; the oblique, at the midproximal phalanx; and thumb A2, at the interphalangeal joint. The A2 and A4 pulleys are primarily responsible for preventing bowstringing in the digits and thus should never be sacrificed. In fact, if they are absent they should be reconstructed. In the thumb, the oblique pulley is the most important and must be preserved.

In addition to its mechanical function, the sheath also plays a role in the nutrition of the tendons by bathing them in synovial fluid. The synovial fluid acts as a lubricant that is believed to be important in preserving the smooth, gliding function of the tendons. Within the sheath, the flexor superficialis and profundus are attached to each other by vincula, which are infoldings of the sheath (mesotendon) that receive end branches from the digital arteries, through which the flexor tendons are vascularized (5). They are located in the dorsal half of the tendons. Thus flexor tendons are nourished within the sheath by two mechanisms: vascular and synovial (6). Because of the poor and precarious vascularity of the flexor tendons, it was once thought that flexor tendons had no intrinsic capability of healing (7). This belief led to the view that adhesions within the flexor tendon sheath were necessary for the tendons to heal; i.e., the tendons required an extrinsic source of nourishment, supplied by scar adhesions between the tendon and the flexor sheath. It is now generally accepted that flexor tendons do have the intrinsic capability to heal and that adhesion formation not only is unnecessary but is, in fact, undesirable because it reduces mobility (8,9). Current surgical protocols for flexor tendon repair are designed to preserve vascularity and to prevent adhesions (10).

Because of the variability of the flexor tendon–sheath system throughout the wrist, palm, and fingers, researchers have classified the segments of the system based on contents in specific topographical areas. This labeling system facilitates communication between practitioners and gives an immediate visual representation of the levels of injury and their prognostic significance. The labeling system used is a modification of Verdan's zone system (6), which designated five zones (zone I is the most distal). Zone I is distal to the insertion of the superficialis at the mid-middle phalanx. Zone II is from the distal palmar crease to the insertion of the superficialis. Zone III is from the end of the carpal tunnel to the distal palmar

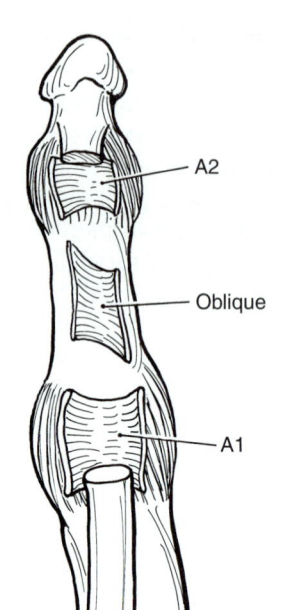

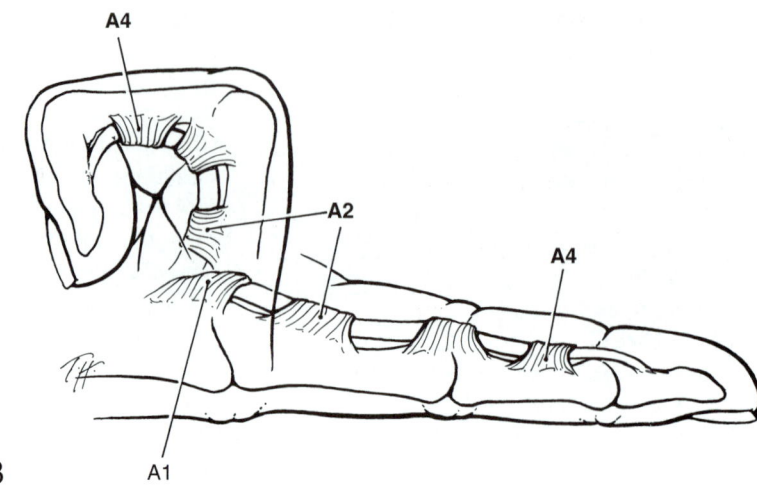

Figure 9.2. The oblique pulley of the thumb (**A**) and the A2 and A4 pulleys of the digits (**B**) prevent bowstringing of the tendons.

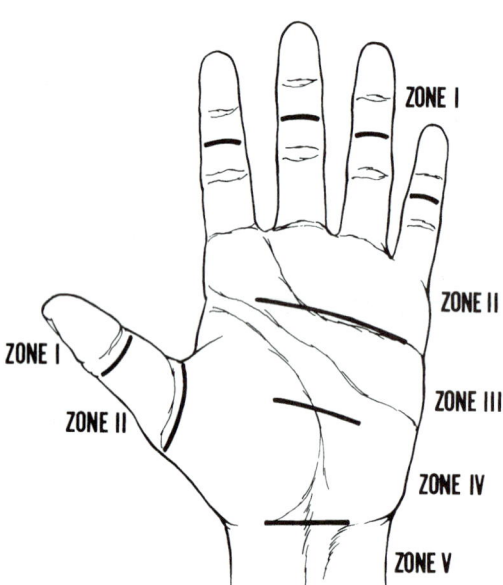

Figure 9.3. Zones of the wrist, palm, and fingers. Reprinted with permission from Green DP, ed. Operative hand surgery. 3rd ed. New York: Churchill Livingstone, 1993.

crease. Zone IV is the confines of the carpal tunnel. Zone V is the distal forearm, proximal to the carpal tunnel (Fig. 9.3).

From a prognostic viewpoint, zone II injuries are the worst. The sheath in zone II contains the two slips of the sublimis and the profundus tendon. The finite amount of space within the sheath in this area leaves little room for repair of these three tendon slips if they are lacerated. In

addition, any manipulations of the tendons can produce adhesions, which will limit the ability of the tendons to glide and produce independent proximal and distal interphalangeal motion. Because of the poor mobility that so often resulted from primary repairs in zone II, Bunnell called this area "no man's land," meaning no one should operate in this zone to perform primary repairs of lacerated flexor tendons (11,12). Before current surgical protocols, tendon lacerations in zone II were not repaired but were treated on a delayed basis with tendon grafts. In the 1960s Kleinert et al. (13) revolutionized hand surgery by obtaining good results with primary repairs in zone II (14). Their protocol emphasizes meticulous surgical technique in the operating room to maintain vascularity. By instituting an early range of motion protocol that protects the repair while allowing the tendon to glide, they were able to decrease the production of adhesions.

INITIAL FINDINGS, PHYSICAL EXAMINATION, AND DIAGNOSIS

Acute Flexor Tendon Injury

LACERATIONS

The volar or palmar aspect of the hand is vulnerable to injury. Lacerations are extremely common. Because of the subcutaneous location of vital structures, all palmar lacerations require thorough evaluation to rule out a tendon, nerve, or vascular injury.

As with any other medical condition, evaluation should begin with taking an accurate history. The time and mechanism of injury should be elicited. Lacerations that occur while the fingers are in a flexed position cause the distal edge of the tendon to be located distal to the skin wound (13). Assessment of any other associated injuries is important. Past medical history is reviewed along with any history of allergies. It is extremely important for the surgeon to ask about special interests or hobbies to determine if the patient has any particular special requirements. Occupation and handedness are also noted.

Examination of the injured area should be done gently and carefully. Exploration of wounds in the hand in the emergency room is not only futile but also counterproductive. Nothing loses a patient's confidence in his or her caretaker as quickly as undergoing the probing of a painful wound that results only in more bleeding and pain, with no gain in information. The wound should be covered lightly with sterile gauze. If bleeding is brisk, the hand should be elevated while gentle pressure is maintained over the laceration. Once brisk bleeding subsides, the hand may be lowered and an examination performed.

Examine the area distal to the wound to determine if any vital structures have been damaged. First, vascularity is assessed. Color, warmth, turgor, and capillary refill are noted. Next, sensory examination is performed by noting the presence or absence of light touch sensation on the radial and ulnar aspects of the digits. Range of motion testing is then performed. If the flexor profundus is intact, the patient should be able to actively flex the distal interphalangeal joint (DIP). The proximal interphalangeal joint (PIP) must be held in extension to isolate the function of the profundus. To test for superificialis function, the fingers not being tested must be held in extension by the examiner's hand while the patient actively flexes the PIP. Failure to do so may result in overlooking an isolated superficialis tendon laceration. Remember, the profundus has a common muscle belly, and contraction of the profundus will result in PIP and DIP flexion, since the profundus straddles both joints. The strength of flexion should be noted, because partial flexor tendon lacerations are possible. The character of the would should be classified. Highly contaminated wounds or wounds with tissue loss may need additional treatment, because a good soft tissue envelope is necessary for primary repair of the tendon.

Once a diagnosis is made, the wound should be gently cleansed and the laceration sutured. Even if operative repair is imminent, surgery can be delayed or canceled at the last moment, especially in busy trauma centers. If the wound has been closed in a timely fashion, operative repair can be safely carried out. If the wound is inadvertently left open for more than 12 h, then the risk of infection is increased and repair should be delayed 3 to 5 days until the wound declares itself. A light, nonconstrictive dressing should be applied, and the hand should be splinted both for comfort and to prevent further tendon retraction. Careful attention should be paid to the application of digital-based dressings, since they are often applied too tightly, especially by inexperienced staff. It is always wise to leave the pulp of the digit exposed in the dressing to allow for vascular checks. Tetanus prophylaxis should be given, depending on the immune status of the patient.

Range of motion testing and sensory examination may be difficult in a child or in an unconscious or uncooperative patient. Often, the diagnosis of flexor tendon laceration can be made just by observing the attitude of the fingers. If the profundus is cut, the normal cascade of the fingers is lost and the affected digit is in a relatively extended position at rest compared to the remaining fingers. With respect to sensation, noninnervated skin does not wrinkle when submerged in water. When a laceration is deep and located over vital structures, operative exploration should be performed if the physical examination is not clear.

RUPTURES AND AVULSIONS

Occasionally, tendon continuity may be disrupted from blunt trauma such as in a hyperextension injury. Ruptures differ from lacerations prognostically because the diagnosis is often delayed. Therefore, any finger "sprain" should be carefully evaluated for intactness of the flexor mechanism. This injury is particularly common in sporting events (known as *football jersey finger*) and usually occurs in the ring finger.

According to Leddy and Packer's (14) classification, the tendon retracts into the palm in type 1 injuries. Because of loss of its vincular blood supply and subsequent degeneration and muscle contracture, the tendon must be reinserted within 7 to 10 days. In type 2 injuries, the tendon retracts to the level of the PIP joint and reinsertion may be possible up to 6 weeks following injury. In type 3 injuries, a large bony fragment is avulsed off the distal phalanx and is trapped at the A4 pulley. Repair is accomplished via fracture fixation. Occasionally, the flexor digitorum profundus (FDP) may avulse separately from the fracture fragment (e.g., a bilevel injury) (15–17). If the delay in diagnosis exceeds 6 weeks, then primary repair is usually not feasible (18).

The most common location for flexor tendon rupture is of the profundus in zone I, although there have been reports of midsubstance rupture, ruptures in the palm, ruptures presenting on a delayed basis with hook of hamate fractures, and ruptures of the sublimis (19–24). The surgical repair for midsubstance ruptures is outlined below. At least 1 cm of the tendon must be available distally to do a midsubstance repair.

Chronic Flexor Tendon Injury

Flexor tendon lacerations and ruptures in the hand are major, serious injuries. Their diagnosis is sometimes difficult and, as outlined below, their treatment requires significant skill. If the diagnosis is made more than 6 weeks after injury, primary repair may not be possible and reconstruction with tendon grafts, either staged or primary, may be necessary. In addition, isolated pulley ruptures often go undetected. They present late as flexion contractures of the interphalangeal (IP) joints and bowstringing of the tendons (25).

RADIOLOGIC STUDIES

Obtaining an x-ray of the injured part should be the routine rather than the exception. Radiologic studies are important for excluding foreign bodies and associated fractures, especially if the mechanism of injury was one of crushing and cutting.

TREATMENT

Nonoperative Treatment and Indications for Surgery

All acute flexor tendon lacerations should be repaired primarily, unless the soft tissue envelope is inadequate either from tissue loss or infection. There is no role for nonoperative treatment. Rarely, the flexor tendon may be so mangled that primary repair will be obviously futile. Partial tendon lacerations should be repaired if they involve more than 50% of the tendon width (26,27).

Operative Treatment

Once the history and physical examination have been performed and acute care rendered, definitive treatment must be undertaken (Clinical Table). Associated injuries, such as nerve lacerations or fractures, do not preclude primary repair. If possible, fractures should be rigidly stabilized to allow for early range of motion. For complex wounds involving the dorsal and volar aspects of the digits, extensors and flexors may need to be fixed simultaneously. Preference is usually given to the rehabilitation of the flexor system, even if it means delaying reconstruction of the extensors. Primary or delayed primary repair should be performed as soon as possible and certainly within 7 to 10 days of the injury. The results of primary (within 24 h) and delayed primary repair are comparable (1). Emergent repair in the middle of the night is unnecessary unless there is concomitant vascular compromise of the digit.

Once treatment recommendations are made, it is extremely important to inform the patient, before surgery, about the nature of the injury and the treatment involved. A successful outcome requires a significant time commitment from and participation by the patient. It is often difficult for patients to understand that what seems like a relatively innocuous injury, based on the size of the wound, could precipitate such a lengthy and complicated treatment regimen. Ideally, the surgeon should describe the postoperative splint and exercise regimen before conducting the surgery. If time allows, a preoperative visit with the hand therapist is invaluable.

Surgical repair of the lacerated or ruptured flexor tendon may be performed under regional or general anesthesia. If general anesthesia is used, the anesthetist must be advised not to terminate it before the postoperative splint has been placed and hardened. Otherwise, invol-

untary muscular contractions during the reversal of the anesthesia may rupture the freshly repaired tendon. Surgery should be performed under tourniquet control in a bloodless field under magnification. The traumatic wounds need to be extended proximally and distally to avoid subsequent scar contracture (Fig. 9.4). Avoid making longitudinal incisions over the joint creases. Volar zigzag (Bruner type) incisions are most commonly used, although the midlateral approach is also useful. Surgical incisions should be planned so that islands of skin are not isolated, which would precipitate necrosis. If extension into the pulp of the finger is necessary, the incision should not cross the midline, avoiding denervation of the pulp skin. Atraumatic handling of the skin flaps is necessary. A 4-0 silk suture tagged with a hemostat is an atraumatic way to maintain retraction of skin flaps and facilitate exposure.

Once the skin is incised, blunt dissection is performed in the subcutaneous tissues. The flaps must be mobilized adequately so that the flexor tendon can be visualized. The stout dermal–fascial attachments must be released without damaging the digital neurovascular bundles. In palmar–forearm lacerations, dissection is performed around the major neurovascular structures (superficial palmar arch and median nerve). Associated injuries need to be recognized and treated. In the palm, hemorrhage often obscures the lacerated structures, and the FDP is recognized by its lumbrical attachment.

In digital injuries, the sheath is visualized in the midline. Hemorrhage is contained within it, and the traumatic puncture of the sheath is visualized. The severed tendon ends may be visualized within the field of exposure if retraction has not occurred. The sheath is sharply incised in an L-shaped fashion, ideally at the level of the traumatic puncture. The sheath must be opened in the cruciform pulley segments, not through the annular pulleys. The A2 and A4 pulleys of the digit and the oblique pulley of the thumb must be preserved.

Once the proximal severed tendon end is visualized, a 25-gauge needle may be used to tether the tendon within the sheath and prevent its retraction during suturing. If the proximal end cannot be visualized within the sheath, secondary incisions may be necessary in the palm or wrist to locate the retracted end. A catheter (pediatric feeding tube) can then be used to pass the retracted tendon through the sheath and deliver it distally to the repair site, avoiding large, unnecessary skin incisions and dissections. One or two gentle attempts may be made with a fine hemostat or forceps to retrieve the tendon from within the sheath if it has not retracted too far proximally. Remember, however, that each manipulation of the tendon and sheath will precipitate more scarring and adhesions. Distally exerted external pressure (milking of the forearm) with the wrist flexed may also help deliver the severed tendon to the repair site. The digit may have to be flexed to deliver the distal stump to the repair site and held in

Clinical Table: Flexor Tendon Injury and Tenosynovitis

Procedure	Indications	Technique	Anatomy	Pitfalls
Primary repair of laceration	• > 50% tendon involvement • Adequate soft tissue envelope	• Volar or midlateral • 4-0 nonabsorbable core suture with 6-0 epitendinous repair • Preserve A2 and A4 pulleys • Repair sheath, if possible	• Neurovascular bundles • Crucial pulleys • Tendon alignment in chiasm	• Inadequate exposure • Poor skin incision • Poor suture hold or technique • Gap at repair • Bulky repair • Poor suture material • Adjust rehabilitation for associated injuries
Primary repair of avulsion or rupture	• Loss of DIP flexion	• Volar or midlateral * 4-0 pullout suture	• Neurovascular bundles • Route tendon back under pulley	• Overadvancement or underadvancement • Inappropriate rehabilitation
Flexor tendon graft	• Delay in diagnosis • Supple finger • Rupture repair • Sensate finger	• Volar or midlateral • Free tendon donor • Pulvertaft weave	• Check for presence of donor tendon presurgery	• Inadequate sheath • Lack of pulley reconstruction • Poor proximal or distal junctures • Have silicone rods available as backup • Poor patient selection • One graft per finger
Staged tendon graft reconstruction	• Delay in diagnosis • Sensate finger • Compliant patient	• Volar or midlateral • Excise tendons • Implant silastic rods with distal attachment and free proximal end at wrist	• Rod placement through lumbrical canal	• Infection or inflammation of silastic • Rupture after second stage • Tendon adherence
Tenolysis	• Contracture with passive motion greater than active motion	• Volar or midlateral • Local anesthesia • Lyse adhesions	• Neurovascular bundles • Sheath and pulleys	• Rupture of repair • Unrecognized joint contracture • Need immediate postoperative motion • Adequate postoperative pain management
Trigger finger release open	• Triggering nonresponsive to conservative treatment	• Longitudinal or transverse incision at MC head in palm • Incise A1 pulley	• Digital nerves, especially radial digital nerve thumb	• Painful or adherent scar • Overrelease or underrelease of pulley • Overlook other hand pathologies
Percutaneous	• Triggering nonresponsive to conservative treatment	• 18-gauge needle	• Digital nerves	• Inadequate release • Tendon damage

flexion during the suturing, especially if the laceration is beneath a crucial pulley. Débridement of the tendon edges is rarely necessary. In fact, obliquity of the laceration may be helpful in obtaining the correct orientation of the tendon within the sheath. In addition, trimming the flexor tendon end may result in fraying and unnecessary manipulations.

Once the severed ends are delivered to the repair site in the digit or palm, suturing is performed with a 3-0 or 4-0 nonabsorbable suture, either braided polyester suture or monofilament. Monofilament may eventually stretch, resulting in gapping. The ideal suture material is flexible and strong and does not make bulky knots. The repair is performed using a modified Kessler core suture, which should be placed into the volar half of the tendon (Fig. 9.5). The excursion of the suture into the tendon should be about 1 cm. Two separate strands of suture for each side can be used (Tajima modification of the Kessler stitch) (28), which

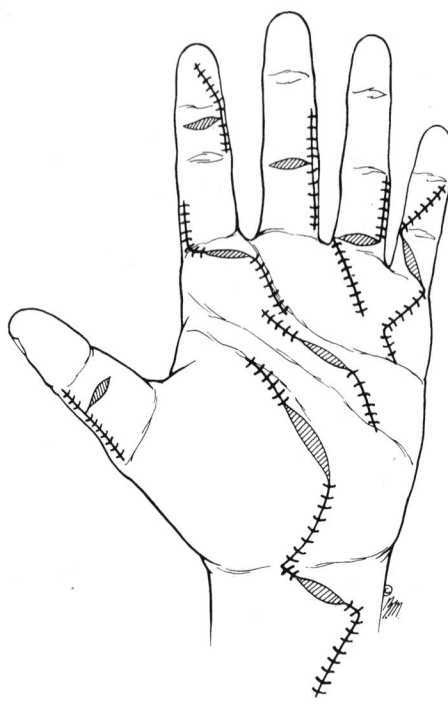

Figure 9.4. Extension of traumatic wounds. Reprinted with permission from Green DP, ed. Operative hand surgery. 3rd ed. New York: Churchill Livingstone, 1993.

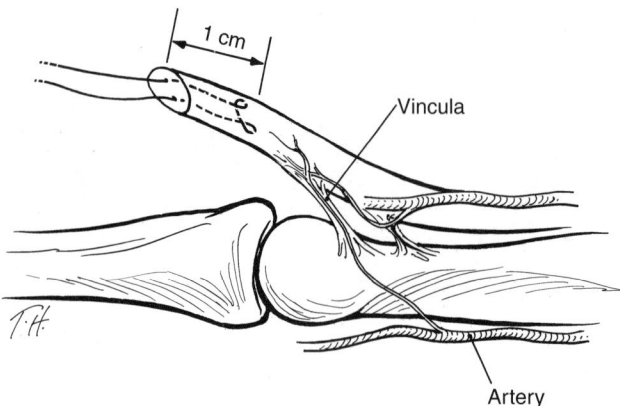

Figure 9.5. The modified Kessler core suture should be in the volar half of the tendon to avoid compromise of the vincular blood supply.

leaves two knots within the core of the tendon (Fig. 9.6). The benefit of this technique is that once a tendon end is visualized and retrieved, the suture can be loaded into the end, the needle can be cut off the suture, and the end can be tagged with a hemostat, eliminating further worries about reretraction of the tendon. This technique is especially useful when there are multiple fingers involved and many tendons to be tagged and sutured. The length of the suture bite into the tendon should be the same on each side of the repair; otherwise, when the tendon ends are brought together, there will be buckling. This buckling will increase the width of the tendon, which cannot then be tolerated in tight area of the fibro-osseous sheath, such as in zone II and the carpal tunnel. The tendon ends should be brought together without too much or too little tension. Gaps at the repair site may lead to rupture or poor healing.

Once the core suture is complete, a running epitendinous repair is performed with a 6-0 monofilament suture. The running suture is placed to cause inversion of the anastomosis, which not only tidies up the repair but adds considerable strength and resists gap formation during early range of motion protocols.

When the superficialis is lacerated in zone II, a core stitch cannot be used because of the tendon's flat configuration in this area. This injury must be repaired with a figure eight suture technique. Appropriate alignment of the superficialis can be determined by identifying the vincula, which is in the dorsal half of the tendon. Again, the repair must be kept neat and not bulky.

If the tendon has avulsed from the distal phalanx, it must be reattached to the bone via an intraosseous suture, which is tied dorsally on the finger over the nail plate (Fig. 9.7). The insertion site on the distal phalanx is roughened up to prepare a small trough into which the tendon is delivered. An alternative is to use a metallic suture anchor, but this may be difficult in small distal phalanges. If the tendon has been avulsed with a bony fragment, the fragment is usually too small to allow for osteosynthesis, although if feasible it certainly should be performed.

Postoperative care is the same as for lacerations, although rubber band traction is not recommended for zone I reinsertions (29) (Fig. 9.8). Early passive range of motion exercises for zone I injuries may increase gap formation and decrease eventual motion (30). In addition, since most ruptures involve only one of the two digital flexors, the incidence of adhesions should be lower.

Once the repair is complete, the sheath should be repaired if possible. Grafting of the sheath is not necessary as long as the digital A2 and A4 pulleys and thumb oblique pulley are maintained. If these pulleys have been irreversibly damaged, then primary pulley reconstruction with a tendon graft should be performed at the same time. A slip of the superficialis may be used or the palmaris, if it is present. Inspection of the repair site needs to be performed, and excursion should be tested intraoperatively to ensure that the repair is not catching on a leading edge of the sheath or triggering. If this is occurring, partial resection of the catching edge needs to be performed or the sheath should be closed. Nerve repairs should be performed now, though fractures should have been stabilized before the tendon repair. Any tension at the nerve repair must be noted, since it may affect the range of motion allowed in postoperative therapy. The tourniquet should be deflated and hemostasis obtained before skin closure. A 5-0 nylon suture is used for skin closure in the digits, and absorbable skin sutures should be used in children.

After application of a light dressing, a dorsal protective splint (Fig. 9.8A) should be applied in the operating room to protect the repair. The wrist should be immobilized in

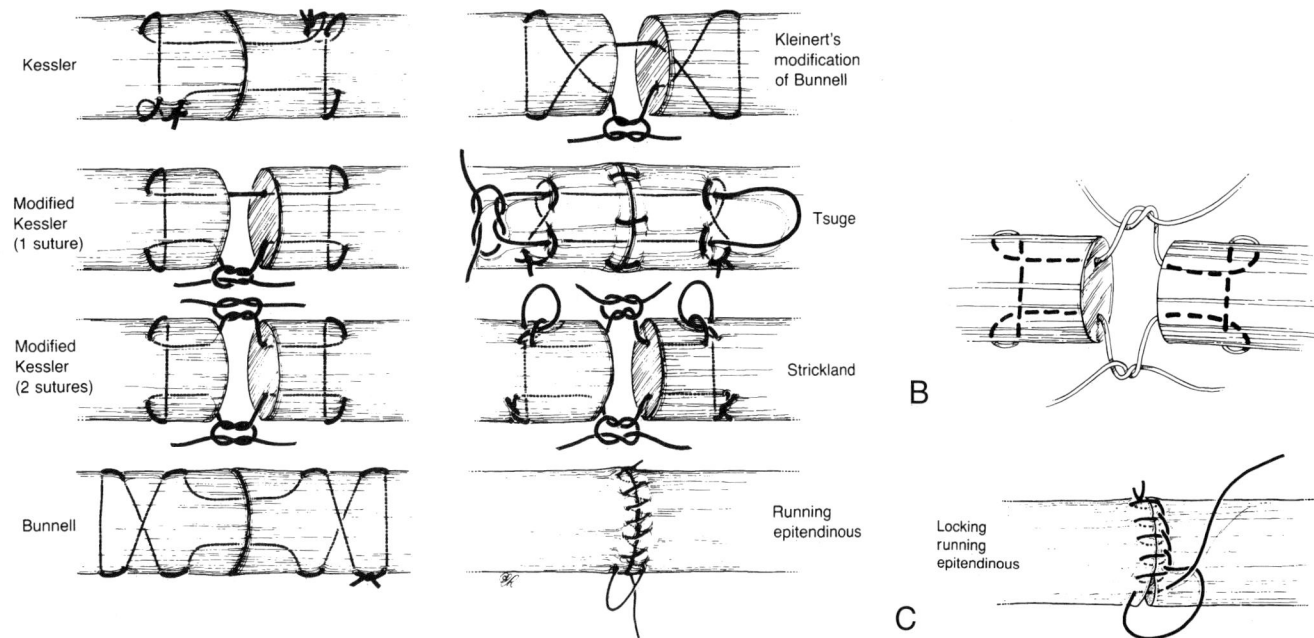

A
Figure 9.6. **A.** Tenorrhaphy suture techniques. **B.** Tajima modification of the Kessler stitch, with two knots in the central core. **C.** The join is finished with an epitendinous repair. Reprinted with permission from Green DP, ed. Operative hand surgery. 3rd ed. New York: Churchill Livingstone, 1993.

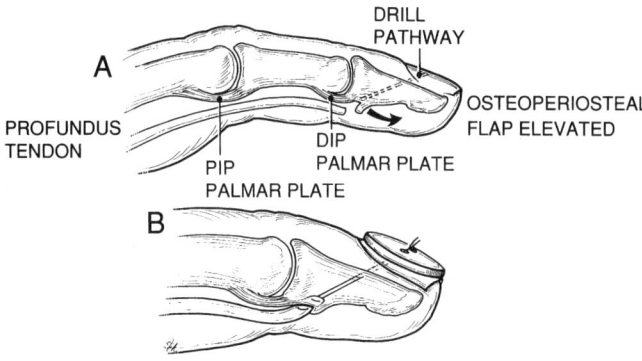

Figure 9.7. FDP reinsertion through an interosseous pullout suture at the distal phalanx. Reprinted with permission from Green DP, ed. Operative hand surgery. 3rd ed. New York: Churchill Livingstone, 1993.

30° of flexion; the metacarpal–phalangeal (MP) joints, in 60° to 70° of flexion; and the interphalangeal joints, in 0° of extension. For thumb injuries, the wrist and MP joint are similarly splinted in flexion (31). If passive rubber band traction is used for zone II digital injuries, a palmar pulley must be placed in the dressing to provide for enough DIP joint flexion. Rubber band traction is not recommended for zone I digital injuries or thumb injuries (31). The splint should be rigid enough to prevent inadvertent active wrist and finger extension, which would rupture the repair. In children, a long arm cast with a dorsal rigid extension to block finger extension is useful. The cast should be applied very carefully, since it must stay on for the duration of tendon healing. If there is concern regarding infection in a child, the cast must be changed under anesthesia, since an uncoop-

erative child may rupture the repair during a dressing change. Postoperative elevation should be maintained, and prophylactic antibiotics should be continued for 24 h.

FREE TENDON GRAFTS

It should not be advised unless the patient is determined to seek perfection and the surgeon is confident of his ability to offer a reasonable expectation of success without the risk of doing harm.

—G. Pulvertaft, 1960

In those instances when primary or delayed primary repair is not possible, consideration may be given to tendon grafting (32). Whether a free tendon graft or a staged reconstruction is used depends on the status of the finger, specifically the amount of scar.

The late treatment of a divided FDP with an intact flexor digitorum sublimis (FDS) is controversial (33). Caution should be observed, as noted by Pulvertaft (34). If special circumstances warrant—the age or occupation (musician, skilled technician)—of the patient, grafting through an intact sublimis may be indicated. If both flexors are divided, the decision to graft is less complicated. However, only one graft should be performed per finger (35).

Potential donor tendons, in order of preference, are the palmaris, long toe extensors, and plantaris. Contraindications to grafting (free or staged) are an insensate finger (at least one digital nerve must be intact), extremes of age (less than 3 years old or elderly), poor circulation, and excessive scarring. Tension of the graft intraoperatively should to have slightly more flexion than the normal resting digital cascade. The proximal juncture should be performed via a Pulvertaft weave (Fig. 9.9).

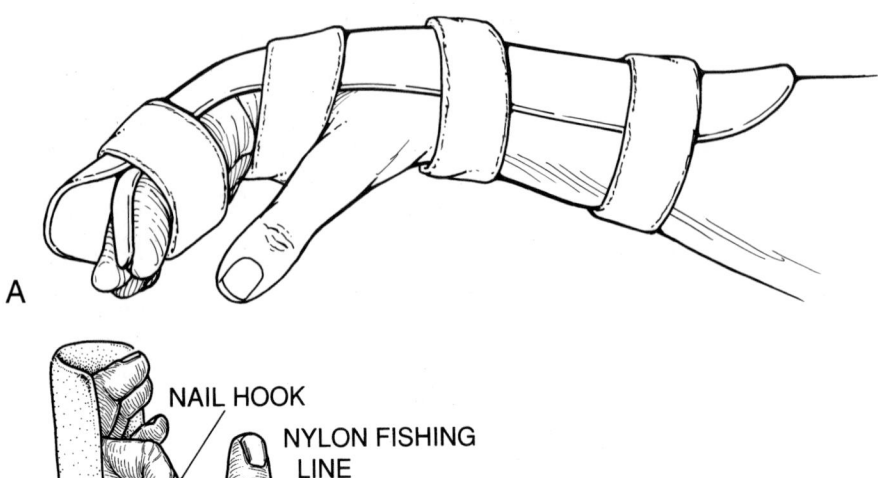

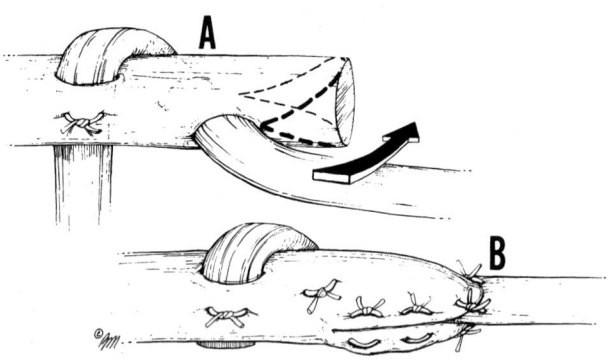

NAIL HOOK

NYLON FISHING
LINE

RUBBER BAND

B

Figure 9.8. **A.** Postoperative care of a zone I injury includes a static DIP flexion splint on the affected digit. **B.** For a zone II injury, a palmar pulley is used to increase dynamic DIP flexion. Reprinted with permission from Green DP, ed. Operative hand surgery. 3rd ed. New York: Churchill Livingstone, 1993.

Figure 9.9. The Pulvertaft-type weave technique is used for proximal anchoring of tendon grafts. Reprinted with permission from Green DP, ed. Operative hand surgery. 3rd ed. New York: Churchill Livingstone, 1993.

The repair site is immobilized for 3 weeks, and then a protected range of motion program is initiated (35). Tenolysis may be necessary on a delayed basis to obtain optimum motion. Silicone rods should be available during surgery in case there is more scar or sheath or pulley damage than had been anticipated presurgery.

STAGED RECONSTRUCTION OF CHRONIC FLEXOR TENDON INJURIES

Stage I involves removal of the scarred tendons and preservation of the sheath. If the pulleys are inadequate, they should be reconstructed at this stage. The excised unsalvageable tendons can be used to reconstruct the pulleys (36). A passive silicone tendon prosthesis (Hunter rod) should be inserted as a temporary spacer and su-

tured into the distal remnant of the tendon. At least 1 cm of the tendon insertion needs to be preserved to suture the prosthesis or graft into place. The silicone spacers are delivered proximally through the palm via the lumbrical canals. The proximal end of the prosthesis is left free in the distal forearm, proximal to the carpal tunnel.

After 3 weeks of immobilization in a dorsal protective splint, passive range of motion exercises are started. Radiographs are obtained 4 to 6 weeks postsurgery to confirm maintenance of the position of the implant and to determine if there is any bowstringing.

At 3 months postsurgery, the tendon grafts are inserted into the pseudosheaths formed by the silicone implants (36). The proximal end of the implant is located, and the graft is sutured to the implant. The distal juncture is then opened, the implant is used to pull the tendon into the sheath, and it is sutured into the distal juncture. The tendon grafts are immobilized for 3 weeks after the operation; then passive and active exercises are begun (37).

Complications of staged reconstructions include synovitis, infection, and contractures. The implants must be handled by a no-touch technique intraoperatively, since the silicone is electrostatic, absorbs foreign bodies easily, and is thus prone to infection. Early treatment of synovitis is immobilization to reduce the inflammation. If infection develops, the implants must be removed and intravenous antibiotics instituted. Contractures, if excessive, can be treated by releases of involved joints and tenolysis if passive motion exceeds active motion.

Active implants are also available on the market. They are made of silicone and dacron (38). Their distal juncture allows relatively rigid screw fixation into the distal phalanx. Their proximal end is fashioned into a loop, which is used as an anchor for a Pulvertaft weave into the proximal motor tendon. These implants are not designed to remain in the body indefinitely. Their advantage is to allow active flexion during stage 1 of the reconstructive process. However, their use is limited by ruptures and pullouts proximally and distally.

RECONSTRUCTION OF ISOLATED CHRONIC PULLEY RUPTURE

For patients with isolated pulley ruptures, local tissue is often inadequate for reconstruction. Free grafts may need to be taken. Postoperative treatment involves immobilization followed by hand therapy and external pulley support rings.

Postoperative Rehabilitation

To prevent rupture of the tendon repair, the hand must be splinted in a dorsal protective splint, as outlined above. The flexed position of the hand and wrist takes tension off the repair and prevents the patient from exerting a contraction forceful enough to rupture the repair. Without any digital motion of the splint, however, contracture, tendon adherence, and loss of motion occur. Several authors have documented the benefit of a postoperative controlled motion program that allows for some gliding of the tendons while protecting the repair. Currently, there is no controversy regarding the necessity of such a program, especially for zone II injuries (39); however, there are differing opinions about how this goal of protective motion should be achieved (40).

Lister et al. (41) introduced the concept of passive flexion–active extension into the rehabilitation protocol. In their protocol, a rubber band is attached to the fingertip to passively flex the digit into the palm. The rubber band may be attached to the dorsal aspect of the nail plate via a hook that is glued to the nail or via a suture placed through the fingertip. At rest, the rubber band keeps the finger passively flexed into the palm. Several times during the day (ideally hourly) the patient performs exercises that consist of active finger extension within the limits of the splint and against the pull of the rubber band. Lister et al. have shown that active extension of the finger relaxes the synergistic flexors, thus taking tension off the repair and allowing gliding of the tendon within the sheath.

Problems with this protocol include the development of flexion contractures of the interphalangeal joints, since the finger is maintained in a permanently flexed position except during the exercise intervals. In addition, the line of pull of the rubber band may be inadequate in providing for full DIP joint flexion and thus not produce as much tendon excursion as desired.

Modifications of the protocol exist. For example, placing a palmar pulley (i.e., having the rubber band pass under a pulley or safety pin located in the midpalm) will improve the line of pull of the passive flexion and provide for more DIP flexion and hence more tendon excursion (Fig. 9.8B). Also, removing the rubber band during nonexercise times or strapping the fingers into extension within the splint at night may help decrease the incidence of flexion contractures. Foam blocks placed at the dorsal surface of the proximal phalanx within the splint enhance the patient's ability to achieve full extension of the PIP joint during the active exercises. The rubber band should not be too stiff. Obviously, careful attention and meticulous technique are required in fabrication and use of the splint and this protocol. Patient understanding and compliance are crucial, as are the services of a skilled hand therapist.

Another protocol advocated for rehabilitation is the modified Duran technique. Passive range of motion exercises that produce 3 to 5 mm of tendon gliding are performed to mobilize the repair and prevent adhesions and joint contractures (28). This protocol uses a similar dorsal protective splint and immobilization position. However, no traction devices are used and the patient is instructed on passive range of motion exercises for flexion and extension of the digit within the confines of the splint. When the exercises are not being performed, the fingers are strapped into the splint at rest. The benefit of this protocol is that if the patient is noncompliant the interphalangeal joint contractures that develop will not be as severe. If the passive range of motion is not performed, however, then no tendon recursion will take place and the result will be akin to allowing healing with full-time immobilization.

Most clinicians use a combination or modification of these regimens (42,43). The best results reported in the literature are those of Chow's group who describe the "Washington regimen" (44–46). This regimen "incorporates the features of active extension against rubber passive flexion with those of therapist-assisted passive extension and passive flexion" (45). The controlled motion program consists of 6 weeks (divided into three phases) of immobilization in the dorsal protective splint with a palmar pulley. During the first 2 weeks, full passive flexion and extension exercises are performed by the therapist along with hourly exercises performed by the patient against the rubber band traction. By the 2nd week, full interphalangeal joint extension should be obtained, and the passive exercises are discontinued. Active exercises are continued during weeks 3 and 4. On day 28, the rubber band traction is discontinued; and during weeks 5 and 6, active flexion is begun within the limits of the splint along with the passive flexion exercises. Once the splint is discontinued, active wrist extension aids flexor tenodesis and rehabilitation.

Other authors recommend using place and hold exercises in addition to the standard protocols (47,48). This involves passive flexion of the digits fully into the palm and then an active contraction to hold the fingers flexed. This probably provides for the largest amount of tendon excursion within the sheath, though rupture rates may be higher (48–50). Unfortunately, current suture techniques are not strong enough to withstand unprotected motion (51).

Assessment of Results

Judging the quality of outcome of treatment of flexor tendon injury requires quantitative measurements of digital motion. Strickland's (54) total active motion criteria are the accepted standard. The total of the active flexion at the interphalangeal joints is added together (PIP + DIP flexion) minus the extension lag at these joints. This figure may be converted to a percentage of normal motion by dividing by 175° and multiplying by 100. Good to excellent results correlate with greater than 125° of motion (Table 9.2). Some authors use pulp to palm distance during fisting as a measurement tool, but this technique is not very accurate and reproducible. In addition to mobility, strength should be measured; grip, pinch and finger flexion strength may be reduced even after successful repair (55).

Complications

Joint contractures, rupture of the repair, and infection are complications associated with flexor tendon repair. The most common complication is interphalangeal flexion contracture, which results either from intrinsic joint contracture secondary to immobilization or from poor gliding of the tendons owing to adhesions within the flexor tendon sheath. Patients are generally dissatisfied with the results of repair if contractures are present, even if motion is within functional limits. If the soft tissue envelope is adequate and supple, then consideration may be given to tenolysis and contracture releases in a cooperative patient with access to good hand therapy. If passive motion exceeds active motion, then tenolysis may be indicated.

Tenolysis should be performed under local or regional anesthesia, which will allow the patient to flex intraoperatively, ensuring that all adhesions have been adequately lysed (56). Immediate postoperative therapy for active and passive range of motion must be instituted to prevent adhesions from reforming. To date, no chemical or pharmaceutical agents have been effective in preventing adhesion formation (57).

Rupture of the repair is a serious complication that needs to be addressed as soon as possible after diagnosis. The repair is at its weakest 7 to 10 days postsurgery, but ruptures can occur anytime during healing. They do tend to occur most commonly around postoperative week 5. The likelihood of rupture increases if there is gap formation at the repair, hence the importance of a good core suture and epitendinous repair. If the rupture is detected within 2 weeks of its occurrence, then secondary repair should be attempted. Allen et al. (58) noted that the results of prompt repair and rehabilitation with controlled motion exercises should give results comparable to an uncomplicated primary repair. If the rupture was not detected early enough or if the secondary repair could not be carried out, then tendon grafting is indicated (59).

For children, results are closely related to age (60). Good primary repair with adequate postoperative protection is crucial. Amadio et al. (61) documented a failure rate of 80% in children under 10 years of age undergoing staged reconstruction. Results of primary repairs are, on average, better in children older than 10 years and worse in those younger than 4 years. Absence of flexor tendon function also adversely affects digital growth (62).

table	9.1	Treatment Recommendations

Zone of Injury	Rehabilitation Protocol	Comments
I	Dorsal protective splint with additional static DIP flexion splint; no passive or active extension of DIP	These injuries have a tendency to stretch and have incomplete active DIP flexion, prompting avoidance of early range of motion exercises of just the DIP joint
II	Washington regimen: dorsal protective splint, rubber band traction with palmar pulley, place and hold exercises	These injuries require aggressive therapy because of they have a high incidence of adhesions
III	Modified Duran technique: dorsal protective splint, passive range of motion and place and hold exercises	There is more room for repair of these injuries because there is no tight fibro-osseous tunnel; but the tendons can still adhere, thus the use of place and hold exercises
IV	Modified Duran technique: dorsal protective splint, passive range of motion and place and hold exercises	There is more room for repair of these injuries because there is no tight fibro-osseous tunnel; but the tendons can still adhere, thus the use of place and hold exercises
V	Modified Duran technique: dorsal protective splint, passive range of motion exercise	These injuries may involves the musculotendinous junction, which does not hold sutures well; thus place and hold exercises are not recommended

table	9.2	Classification of Total Active Motion by the Strickland System	
Group		PIP + DIP Return (%)	PIP + DIP – Extensor Loss (°)
Excellent		85–100	150+
Good		70–84	125–149
Fair		50–69	90–124
Poor		50	90

Reprinted with permission from Strickland JW. Flexor tenolysis. Hand Clin 1985;1:121–132.

SUMMARY

In summary, the surgeon should use the protocol that he or she is most familiar with and that is best suited for a particular patient and repair (Table 9.1). Current research is emphasizing stronger repair techniques. No rehabilitation protocol can salvage a poorly repaired tendon, but it can help to maximize the potential motion obtained. At the minimum, all repairs should be protected for 4 to 6 weeks, and passive mobilization of the fingers should be performed during healing. The surgeon should give precise, clear instructions to the patient and therapist as to which ranges of motion are initially allowed. Tendon repairs in children need to be immobilized also. The younger the child, the less likely he or she will be able to participate in a complicated range-of-motion program (44). In children, the safest alternative is probably cast immobilization in the protected position up to the fingertips and passive mobilization. For best results, immobilization should not exceed 4 weeks in the child.

II   Tenosynovitis

RELEVANT ANATOMY

Inflammation of the tissue lining the flexor tendon sheaths commonly occurs. As the inflammation persists, the tissues of the sheath may actually thicken and become nodular. Pathologic examination of the abnormal pulley and sheath tissue has documented synovial proliferative changes and chondroblast formation. The thickening of the pulleys may progress to the point that they constrict the flexor tendon.

INITIAL FINDINGS, PHYSICAL EXAMINATION, AND DIAGNOSIS

Typically, the patient complains of soreness in the finger and palm that is worse in the morning. The thumb is most commonly involved, followed by the ring and long fingers (63). The index finger is rarely involved. Symptom onset is atraumatic and insidious. Women are more frequently affected than men, especially those with occupations involving repetitive use of the hand. This occupational relationship was established in the literature from the 1950s (64). The illness is most common in the fifth and sixth decades of life. As symptoms progress, snapping develops with range of motion, because a size discrepancy has developed between the stenotic sheath and nodular tendon. The patient experiences the snapping sensations at the level of the PIP joint in the fingers and IP joint of the thumb, although the pain localizes to the palm.

The actual pathologic process is at the level of the MP joint where the tendon is tethered at the A1 pulley (56).

Rarely, triggering may occur at the A2 level. A tender nodule may be palpated in this area, along with tenderness along the flexor tendon sheath. The nodule is actually an enlargement of the sheath. Snapping may progress to locking of the joint with the finger in flexion or extension. Differential diagnosis includes masses and tumors, foreign bodies, partial flexor tendon lacerations, rheumatoid arthritis, and locked MP joints (65,66). Locked MP joints are of sudden onset and are a separate clinical entity in which there is loss of extension, not flexion, and no abnormalities in IP joint range of motion (67).

RADIOLOGIC STUDIES

At least one series of baseline x-rays of the painful hand should be done, primarily to rule out other coexisting pathologies.

TREATMENT

Nonoperative Treatment and Indications for Surgery

Early cases of tenosynovitis should be treated nonoperatively with cortisone injections into the flexor tendon sheath (68). A 25-gauge needle is used to deliver 0.5 mL triamcinolone. Pain should decrease within 24 h, but snapping may be persist for several days after the injection. The efficacy of the injection in permanently alleviating symptoms depends on the severity of the inflammation at the time of presentation (69). Data in the literature support a 60 to 90% cure rate with injections. There are no adverse effects from the injection, though it should be used with caution in brittle diabetics, since it may affect their blood sugar level. Injection technique also plays a role in its success.

Operative Treatment

Patients who fail injection treatment or who present with fixed joint contractures should be considered surgical candidates (Clinical Table). Surgery is performed under local anesthesia and involves sectioning of the A1 pulley of the affected digit. For triggering at the A2 level, reduction flexor tenoplasty, not A2 release, is recommended (70). Surgical release may be performed using a standard open technique or percutaneously (71). For the open technique, longitudinal or horizontal incisions may be used (72). The proximal edges of the A1 pulleys of the ring and small fingers are located at the level of the distal palmar crease along the longitudinal axis of the fingers. In the long finger, the pulley edge is between the distal and proximal palmar creases. In the index finger, it is at the proximal palmar crease. In the thumb, it is located at the level of the MP joint crease. Staying in the midline of the sheath during pulley release prevents inadvertent damage to adjacent digital nerves. The radial digital nerve of the thumb is the most vulnerable to injury, since it is immediately subcutaneous, overlies the radial sesamoid, and can be lacerated during the transverse skin incision (73).

Postoperative management includes a light dressing for 48 h, followed by a bandage over the monofilament skin sutures. Range of motion exercises may begin immediately, and formal hand therapy is rarely necessary. The incision may remain sore to the touch for several weeks. Scar massage and desensitization can help alleviate this symptom.

Complications include digital nerve injuries, infection, stiffness, and scar sensitivity (74). Overzealous release of the pulley system with damage to the A2 pulley may result in bowstringing, which will decrease grip strength and limit digital extension (75).

Trigger Finger in Children

Congenital trigger finger most commonly affects the thumb. In newborns, observation is recommended since spontaneous resolution will occur by 1 year of age in 30% of children (76). Trigger thumbs diagnosed between 6 and 36 months of age should be observed for 6 months, since resolution will occur in 12% of patients. If the child is older than 3 years at diagnosis, surgery is recommended. Diagnosis is often delayed, since the problem may not be recognized because of the clenched fist attitude of the newborn. This entity should not be confused with congenital deficiencies in the extensor mechanism that result in MP joint flexion of the thumb. Trigger finger causes the IP joint of the thumb to be locked in flexion. In the remaining digits, trigger fingers diagnosed during childhood should also be treated operatively if they remain consistently symptomatic. The same surgical protocol is used in children as in adults, with the same precautions regarding potential complications.

SUMMARY

Treatment for stenosing tenosynovitis or trigger finger is not particularly difficult or complicated. However, care must still be rendered with attention to detail and anatomy to avoid complications. In addition, the presence or absence of interphalangeal flexion contracture must be noted, since this affects the ultimate prognosis.

REFERENCES

1. Hart RG, Kutz JE. Flexor tendon injuries of the hand. Emerg Clin North Am 1993;51:621–636.
2. Gray's anatomy. 15th ed. rev.
3. Lin GT, Amadio PC, An KN, Cooney WP. Functional anatomy of the human digital flexor pulley system. J Hand Surg 1989;14A:49–56.
4. Doyle JR, Blythe WF. Anatomy of the flexor tendon sheath and pulleys of the thumb. J Hand Surg 1977; 2A:149–151.
5. Kleinert HE, Schepel S, Gill T. Flexor tendon injuries. Surg Clin North Am 1981;61:267–286.
6. Strickland JW. Flexor tendon injuries, part 1. Orthop Rev 1986; 15:632–645.
7. Potenza AD. Tendon healing within the flexor digital sheath in the dog. J Bone Joint Surg 1962;44A:49–64.
8. Mass DP, Tuel RJ. Intrinsic healing of the laceration site in human superficialis flexor tendons in vitro. J Hand Surg 1991;16A:24–30.
9. Gelberman RH, VandeBerg JS, Lundborg GN, et al. Flexor tendon healing and restoration of the gliding surface. J Bone Joint Surg 1983;65A:70–80.
10. Strickland JS. Management of acute flexor tendon injuries. Orthop Clin North Am 1983;14:827–849.
11. Verdan CE. Half a century of flexor tendon surgery. J Bone Joint Surg 1972;54A:472–491.
12. Verdan CE. Primary repair of flexor tendons. J Bone Joint Surg 1960;42A:647–657.
13. Kleinert HE, Kutz JE, Atasoy E, Stormo A. Primary repair of flexor tendons. Orthop Clin North Am 1973;4:865–876.
14. Leddy JP, Packer JW. Avulsion of the profundus insertion in athletes. J Hand Surg 1977;2A:66–69.
15. Buscemi MJ, Page BJ. Flexor digitorum profundus avulsions with associated distal phalanx fractures. Am J Sports Med 1987; 15:366–370.
16. Eglesder WA, Russell JM. Type IV flexor digitorum profundus avulsion. J Hand Surg 1990;15A:735–739.
17. Ehlert KJ, Gould JS, Black KP. A simultaneous distal phalanx fracture with profundus tendon avulsion. Clin Orthop 1992; 283:265–269.
18. Trumble TE, Vedder NB, Benirschke SK. Misleading fractures after profundus tendon avulsions: a report of six cases. J Hand Surg 1992;17A:902–906.
19. Backe H, Posner MA. Simultaneous rupture of both flexor tendons in a finger. J Hand Surg 1994;19A:246–248.
20. Cheung KM, Chow SP. Closed avulsion of both flexor tendons of the ring finger. J Hand Surg 1995;20B:78–79.
21. De Roos WK, Zeeman RJ. A flexor tendon rupture in the palm of the hand. J Hand Surg 1991;16A:663–665.
22. Lanzetta M, Conolly WB. Closed rupture of both flexor tendons in the same digit. J Hand Surg 1992;17B:479–480.
23. Milek MA, Bouas HJ. Flexor tendon ruptures secondary to hamate hook fractures. J Hand Surg 1990;15A:740–744.

24. Naam NH. Intratendinous ruptures of the flexor digitorum profundus tendon in zones II and III. J Hand Surg 1995;20A:478–483.
25. Bowers WH, Kuzma GR, Bynum DK. Closed traumatic rupture of finger flexor pulleys. J Hand Surg 1994;19A:782–787.
26. Frewin PR, Scheker LR. Triggering secondary to an untreated partially-cut flexor tendon. J Hand Surg 1989;14B:419–421.
27. Schlenker JD, Lister GE, Kleinert HE. Three complications of untreated partial laceration of flexor tendon—entrapment, rupture, and triggering. J Hand Surg 1981;6A:392–398.
28. Strickland JS. Flexor tendon injuries, part 2. Flexor tendon repair. Orthop Rev 1986;15:701–721.
29. Gerbino PG, Saldana MJ, Westerbeck P, Schacherer TG. Complications experienced in the rehabilitation of zone I flexor tendon injuries with dynamic traction splinting. J Hand Surg 1991;16A:680–686.
30. Evans RB. A study of the zone I flexor tendon injury and implications for treatment. J Hand Ther 1990;3:133–148
31. Urbaniak JR: Repair of the flexor pollicis longus. Hand Clin 1985;1:69–76.
32. McClinton MA, Curtis RM, Wilgis EF. One hundred tendon grafts for isolated flexor digitorum profundus injuries. J Hand Surg 1982;7A:224–229.
33. Goldner JL, Coonrad RW. Tendon grafting of flexor profundus in presence of completely or partially intact flexor sublimis. J Bone Joint Surg 1969;51A:527–532.
34. Pulvertaft RG. The treatment of profundus division by free tendon graft. J Bone Joint Surg 1960;42A:1363–1380.
35. Strickland JW. Flexor tendon injuries, part 3. Free tendon grafts. Orthop Rev 1987;16:56–64.
36. Hunter JM. Staged flexor tendon reconstruction. J Hand Surg 1983;8A:789–793.
37. Chow JA, Thomes LJ, Dovelle S, et al. Controlled motion rehabilitation after flexor tendon repair and grafting. J Bone Joint Surg 1988;70B:591–595.
38. Hunter JM, Singer DI, Jaeger SH, Mackin EJ. Active tendon implants in flexor tendon reconstruction. J Hand Surg 1988;13A:849–859.
39. Strickland JS, Glogovac SV. Digital function following flexor tendon repair in zone II: a comparison of immobilization and controlled passive motion techniques. J Hand Surg 1980;5A:537–543.
40. May FJ, Silfverskiold KL, Sollerman CJ. Controlled mobilization after flexor tendon repair in zone II: a prospective comparison of three methods. J Hand Surg 1992;17A:942–952.
41. Lister GD, Kleinert HE, Kutz JE, Atasoy E. Primary flexor tendon repair followed by immediate controlled mobilization. J Hand Surg 1977;2A:441–451.
42. Edinburg M, Widgerow AD, Biddulph SL. Early postoperative mobilization of flexor tendon injuries using a modification of the Kleinert technique. J Hand Surg 1987;12A:34–38.
43. Werntz JR, Chesher SP, Breidenbach WC, et al. A new dynamic splint for postoperative treatment of flexor tendon injury. J Hand Surg 1989;14A:559–566.
44. Dovelle S, Heeter PK. The Washington regimen: rehabilitation of the hand following flexor tendon injuries. Phys Ther 1989;69:1034–1040.
45. Chow JA, Thomes LJ, Dovelle S, et al. A combined regimen of controlled motion following flexor tendon repair in "no man's land". Plast Reconstr Surg 1987;79:447–455.
46. Saldana MJ, Chow JA, Gerbino P, et al. Further experience in rehabilitation of zone II flexor tendon repair with dynamic traction splinting. Plast Reconstr Surg 1991;87:543–546.
47. Hagberg L, Selvik G. Tendon excursion and dehiscence during early controlled mobilization after flexor tendon repair in zone II. An x-ray stereophotogrammetric analysis. J Hand Surg 1991;16A:669–680.
48. Small JO, Brennen D, Colville J. Early active mobilization following flexor tendon repair in zone 2. J Hand Surg 1989;14B:383–391.
49. Bainbridge LC, Robertson C, Gillies D, Elliot D. A comparison of post-operative mobilization of flexor tendon repairs with "passive flexion–active extension" and "controlled motion" techniques. J Hand Surg 1994;19B:392–395.
50. Cullen KW, Tolhurst P, Lang D, Page RE. Flexor tendon repair in zone 2 followed by controlled active mobilization J Hand Surg 1989;14B:392–395.
51. Silfverskiold KL, May EJ. Flexor tendon repair in zone II with a new suture technique and an early mobilization program combining passive and active flexion. J Hand Surg 1994;19A:53–60.
52. Deleted in proof.
53. Deleted in proof.
54. Strickland JW. Results of flexor tendon surgery in zone II. Hand Clin 1985;1:167–179.
55. Gault DT. Reduction of grip strength, finger flexion pressure, finger pinch pressure and key pinch following flexor tendon repair. J Hand Surg 1987;12B:182–184.
56. Fahey JJ, Bolliner JA. Trigger finger in adults and children. J Bone Joint Surg 1954;36A:1210–1218.
57. Hagberg L. Exogenous hyaluronate as an adjunct in the prevention of adhesions after flexor tendon surgery: A controlled clinical trial. J Hand Surg 1992;17A:132–136.
58. Allen BN, Frykman GK, Unsell RS, Wood VE. Ruptured flexor tendon tenorrhaphies in zone II: repair and rehabilitation. J Hand Surg 1987;12A:18–21.
59. Wehbe MA, Hunter JH, Schneider LH, Goodwyn BL. Two-stage flexor tendon reconstruction. J Bone Joint Surg 1986;68A:752–763.
60. Berndtsson L, Ejeskar A. Zone II flexor tendon repairs in children. Scand J Plast Reconstr Hand Surg 1995;29:59–64.
61. Amadio PC, Wood MB, Cooney WP, Bogard SD. Staged flexor tendon reconstruction in the fingers and hand. J Hand Surg 1988;13A:559–562.
62. Cunningham MW, Yousif NJ, Matloub HS, et al. Retardation of finger growth after injury to the flexor tendons. J Hand Surg 1985;10A:115–117.
63. Bonnicci AV, Spencer JD. Survey of trigger finger in adults. J Hand Surg 1988;13B:202–203.
64. Conklin JE, White WL. Stenosing tenosynovitis. Surg Clin North Am 1960;40:531–540.
65. Laing PW. A tendon tumor presenting as a trigger finger. J Hand Surg 1986;11B:275.
66. Rankin EA, Reid BR. An unusual etiology of trigger finger: a case report. J Hand Surg 1985;10A:904–905.
67. Posner MA, Langa V, Green S. The locked metacarpophalangeal joint: diagnosis and treatment. J Hand Surg 1986;11A:249–253.
68. Freiberg A, Mulholland RS, Levine R. Nonoperative treatment of trigger fingers and thumbs. J Hand Surg 1989;14A:553–558
69. Marks MR, Gunther SF. Efficacy of cortisone injection in treatment of trigger fingers and thumbs. J Hand Surg 1989;14A:722–727.
70. Seradge H, Kleinert H. Reduction flexor tenoplasty. J Hand Surg 1981;6A:543–544.
71. Lorthioir J. Surgical treatment of trigger finger by a subcutaneous method. J Bone Joint Surg 1958;40A:793–795.
72. Stefanich RJ, Peimer CA. Longitudinal incision for trigger finger release. J Hand Surg 1989;14A:316–317.
73. Carrozella J, Stern PJ, Von Kuster LC. Transection of radial digital nerve of the thumb during trigger release. J Hand Surg 1989;14A:198–200.
74. Thorpe AP. Results of surgery for trigger finger. J Hand Surg 1988;13B:199–201.
75. Heithoff SJ, Millender LH, Helman J. Bowstringing as a complication of trigger finger release. J Hand Surg 1988;13A:567–570.
76. Dinham JM, Meggitt BF. Trigger thumbs in children. J Bone Joint Surg 1974;56B;153–155.

chapter 10

Kevin D. Plancher and Robert K. Peterson

Extensor Tendon Injuries and Common Tendinopathies

Extensor tendon injuries have long been regarded as simple problems solved by the reapproximation of defects. Recent studies, however, have shown that extensor tendon injuries may pose difficult problems for the physician and significant functional impairment for the patient. (1,2) The delicate, dynamic balance of the extensor mechanism demands that an exacting knowledge of its form and function be gained before it can be successfully treated.

This chapter provides an overview of the anatomy and pathomechanics of common acute and chronic extensor tendon injuries along with indications, techniques, pitfalls, and rehabilitation principles involved in treating these syndromes. Common extensor tendinopathies of the wrist and hand are also discussed.

RELEVANT ANATOMY

The extensor mechanism of the digits is known for its complexity, subtlety, and interdependence of structures. The mechanism is powered by two components: extrinsic, radially innervated musculature arising from the forearm or elbow and intrinsic, ulnar-median-innervated musculature arising within the hand.

The extrinsic muscles and tendons arise proximal to the hand and pass under the extensor retinaculum, which divides into six compartments dorsally (Fig. 10.1). The extensor pollicis brevis (EPB) and abductor pollicis longus (APL) pass through the first dorsal compartment, which is subdivided by one or more septa. The second compartment contains the extensor carpi radialis longus (ECRL) and extensor carpi radialis brevis (ECRB). The extensor pollicis longus (EPL) passes through the third compartment and around Lister's tubercle to the distal phalanx of the thumb. The fourth compartment contains the extensor digitorum communis (EDC) tendons to the four digit and the extensor indicis proprius (EIP), which lies ulnar to the

EDC on the index finger. The fifth compartment includes the extensor digiti minimi (EDM). The sixth compartment has a subsheath, below the extensor retinaculum, that holds the extensor carpi ulnaris (ECU) firmly against the ulna (Fig. 10.2).

The extensor retinaculum is a pulley that prevents bowstringing of the extensor tendons. The extensor tendons (fourth compartment) at the wrist are covered with tenosynovium and pass over the metacarpals. These tendons are connected by the juncturae tendinum. The juncturae are responsible for simultaneous and uniform finger extension (Fig. 10.3) and prevent tendon retraction after a laceration occurs over the dorsum of the hand.

The tendons to the digits cross the metacarpal–phalangeal (MP) joints and are held in place by the sagittal bands, which pass from the tendon to the volar plate of the proximal phalanx and prevent subluxation (Fig. 10.4). The intrinsic muscles lie volar to the axis of rotation and flex the MP joint. The extrinsic muscles and tendons remain dorsal and extend the MP joint. The extensor tendon trifurcates over the proximal phalanx to form the central slip and two lateral slips (Fig. 10.5). The lumbricals arise from the tendons of the flexor digitorum profundus (FDP) on the radial side of each digit. Distally, the lumbrical tendon remains volar to the deep transverse metacarpal ligament, passes radial to the MP joint, and divides to contribute to the central and lateral slips of the extensor mechanism (Fig. 10.6).

The three palmar interossei arise from the metacarpal shaft, pass dorsal to the deep transverse metacarpal ligament, and send one slip to the base of the proximal phalanx; the other slip mimics the insertion of the lumbrical. The four dorsal interossei arise from the two metacarpal shafts that border them. The dorsal interossei provide the same insertion pattern as the palmar interossei but pass above the MP axis. There is a considerable variation in the

Figure 10.1. Extensor retinaculum with the six dorsal compartments. *EPB,* extensor pollicis brevis; *APL,* abductor pollicis longus; *ECRL,* extensor carpi radialis longus; *ECRB,* extensor carpi radialis brevis; *EPL,* extensor pollicis longus; *ECU,* extensor carpi ulnaris; *EDM,* extensor digiti minimi; *EDC,* extensor digitorum communis; *EIP,* extensor indicis proprius.

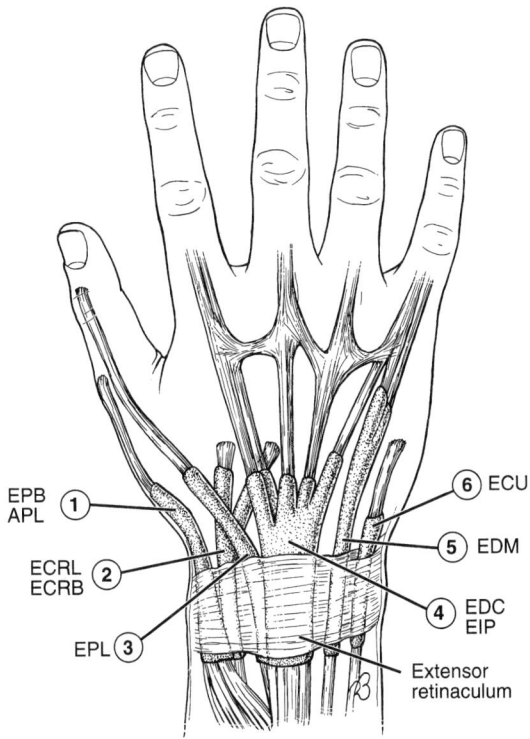

Figure 10.2. ECU and subsheath in a cadaveric dissection.

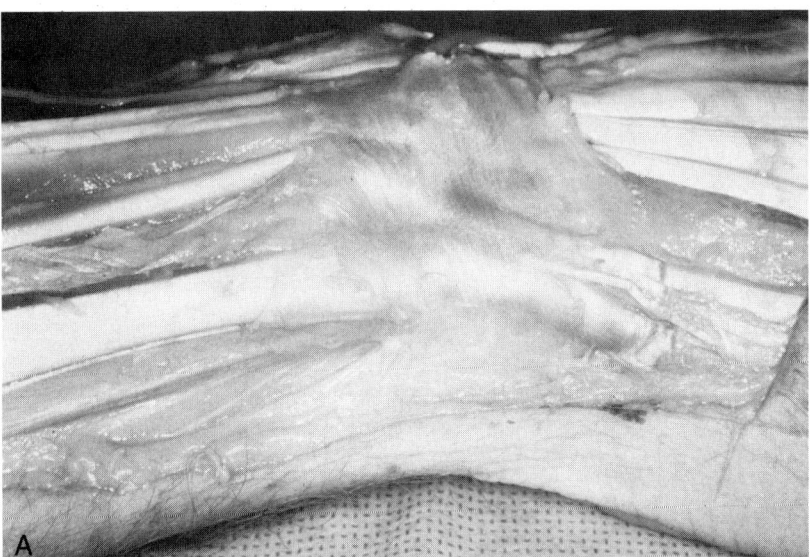

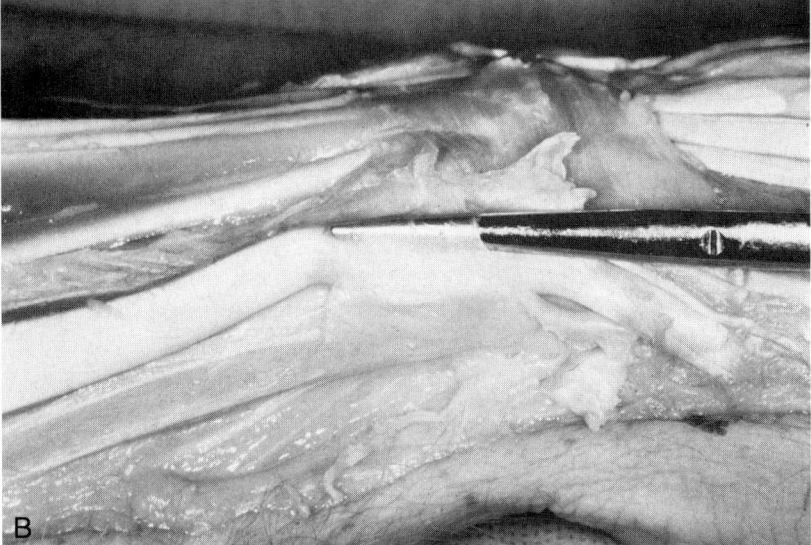

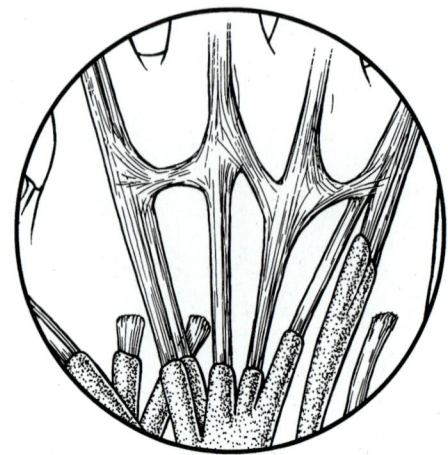

Figure 10.3. Juncturae of the wrist.

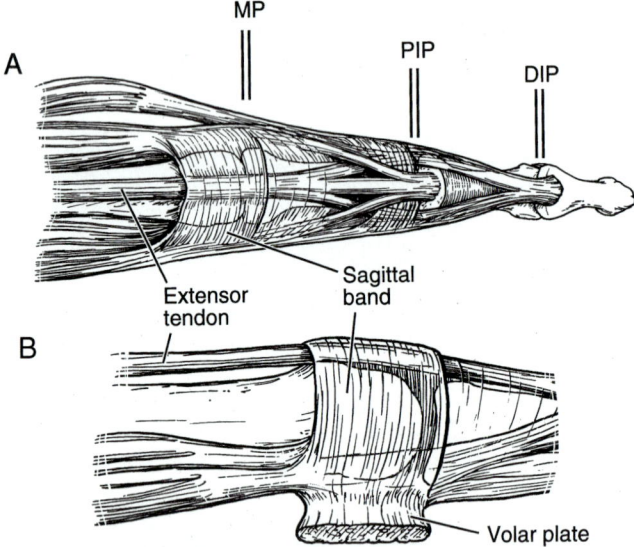

Figure 10.4. A. The sagittal band holds the extrinsic tendons in place at the MP joint. **B.** Lateral view of the sagittal band at the MP joint. *PIP,* proximal interphalangeal joint; *DIP,* distal interphalangeal joint.

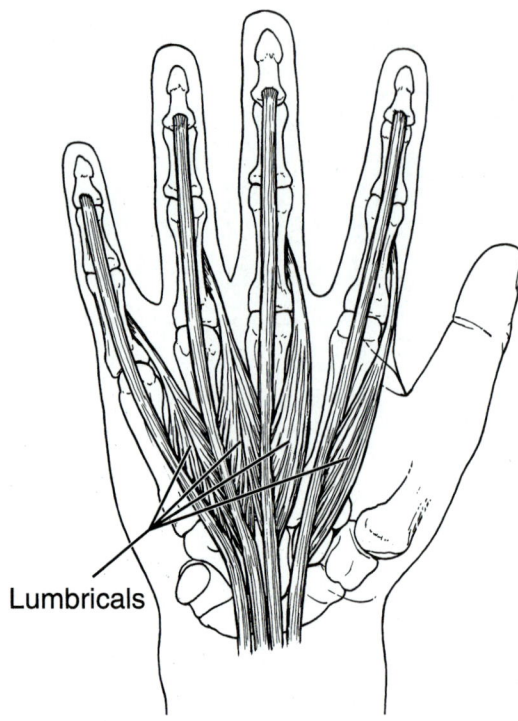

Figure 10.5. Lumbricals of the hand.

amount of insertion into the proximal phalanx or extensor mechanism between the digits (3) (Fig. 10.7). The functions of the dorsal and volar interossei are abduction and adduction, respectively.

On the dorsum of the proximal phalanx, the central slip is formed by the EDC and small contributions from the lumbrical and both interossei. These structures insert on to the base of the middle phalanx. The intrinsic tendons (lumbrical and interossei) form the lateral bands, which receive a small contribution of cross-over fibers from the central slip, e.g., the EDC. These lateral bands join on the dorsum of the middle phalanx to form the terminal tendon, which inserts onto the base of the distal phalanx (Fig. 10.5).

The extensor mechanism is stabilized by several accessory structures. The transverse retinacular ligament acts at the level of the proximal interphalangeal (PIP) joint to re-

strain dorsovolar translation of the lateral bands. More distally, the triangular ligament consists of transverse fibers holding the conjoined lateral bands together dorsally. It is these conjoined lateral bands that form the terminal extensor tendon. The oblique retinacular ligament runs from the flexor sheath, volar to the PIP joint to join the terminal tendon, inserting on the dorsal base of the distal phalanx. This ligament augments distal interphalangeal (DIP) extension with active extension of the PIP joint (4).

The extensor system of the thumb includes one muscle that inserts on each joint: the EPL inserts on the distal phalanx; EPB, on the proximal phalanx; and APL, on the base of the metacarpal. The extensor function of the thumb does not depend on the dynamic interrelationship of its components, though the dorsal hood does bear some resemblance to that of the finger.

The extensor mechanism has been divided into eight zones by Kleinert and Verdan (5). Disruption of the tendon at each level causes a different type of injury. The next section reviews injuries to zones I through VIII (Fig. 10.8).

ACUTE EXTENSOR TENDON INJURY

Zone I: Distal Interphalangeal Joint (Mallet Injuries)

Zone I extends from the most distal insertion of the extensor mechanism to the attachment of the central slip on the proximal end of the middle phalanx. Disruption of the terminal tendon or conjoined lateral bands at the DIP joint causes an extensor lag of the distal phalanx. This has been referred to as a drop, baseball, cricket, or (most com-

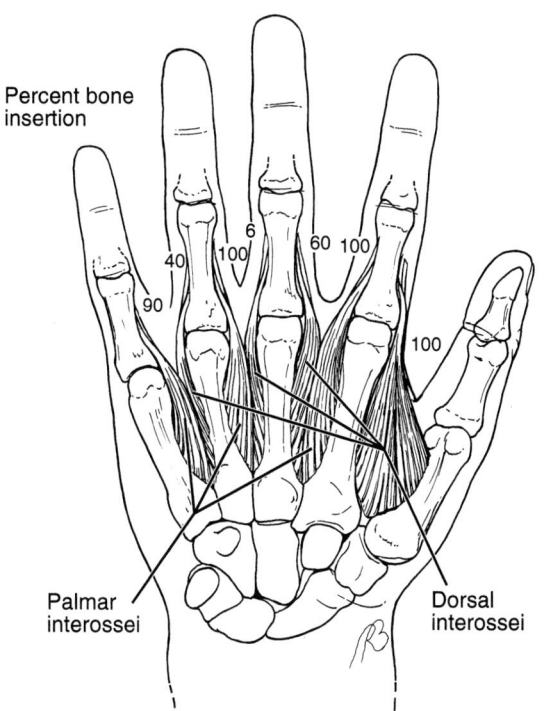

Figure 10.6. Dorsal and palmar interossei and the amount of insertion into the proximal phalanx or extensor mechanism.

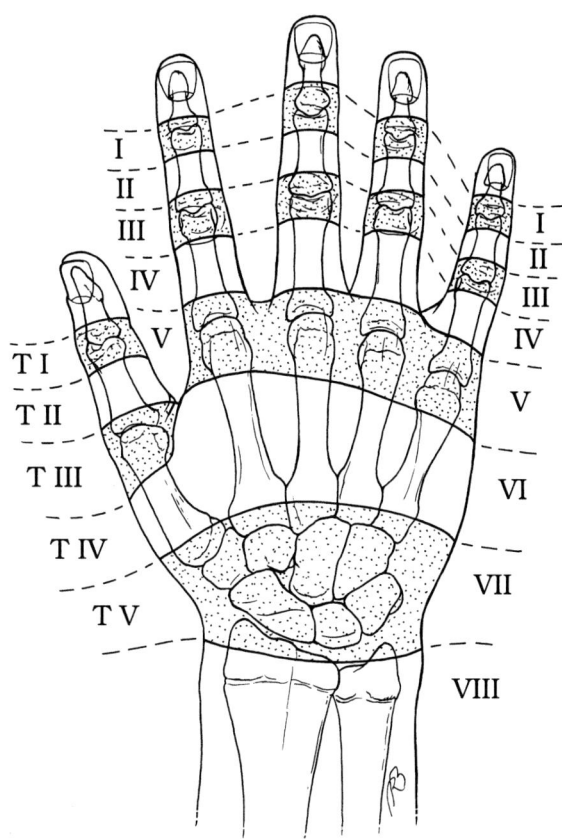

Figure 10.8. Zones of extensor tendon injuries.

Figure 10.7. AP (**A**) and lateral (**B**) views of the extensor mechanism of the digit. *PIP,* proximal interphalangeal joint; *DIP,* distal interphalangeal joint.

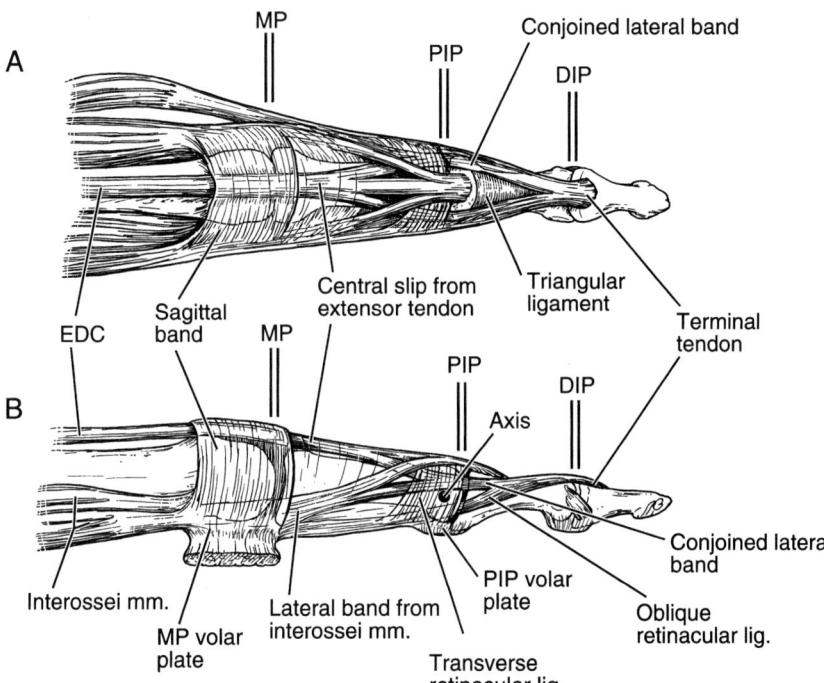

monly) mallet finger. This injury is seen in factory workers and as sports-related injuries. A mallet finger may occur spontaneously in a patient with rheumatoid arthritis or with minimal trauma to the digit (6). The mechanism of in-

jury involves a sudden flexion force on an extended digit. Less commonly, this injury may be produced by a hyperextension force, resulting in a dorsal fracture and subsequent mallet finger (Fig. 10.9).

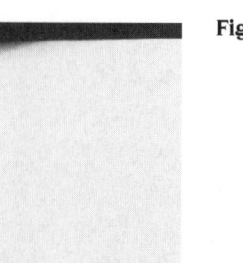

Figure 10.9. Dorsal mallet fracture.

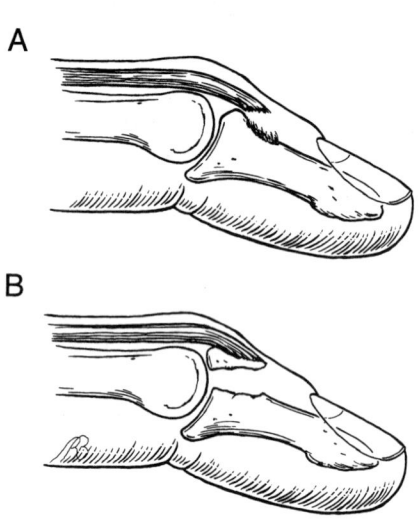

Figure 10.10. Hallmarks of a mallet finger.

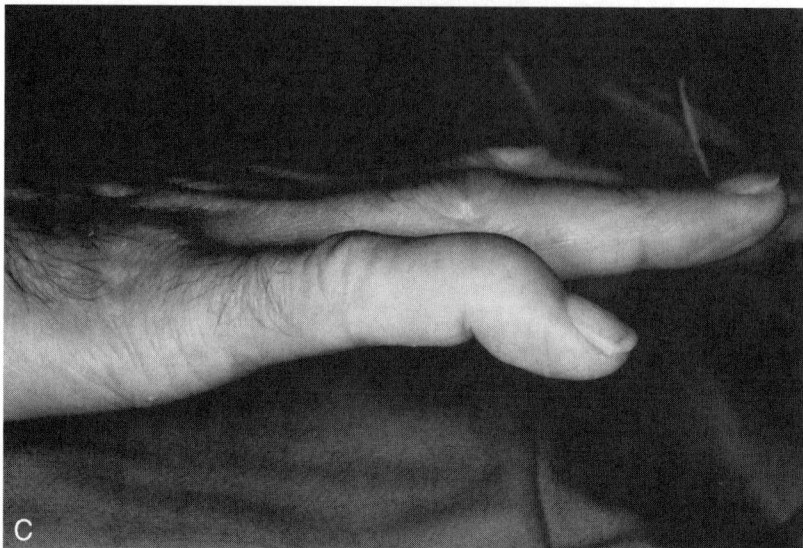

Warren et al. (7) localized an avascular critical zone at 11 to 16 mm from the insertion of the lateral bands, corresponding to an area of compression over the head of the middle phalanx when in flexion. These findings suggest that vascular compromise may also play a role in the cause of a mallet finger.

The hallmark finding of a mallet finger is the flexed posture of the DIP joint and loss of active terminal extension (Fig. 10.10). The degree of deformity can vary, and some authors (2,7) have noted that the appearance of the flexion deformity after trauma to the DIP joint may be delayed for several days. The chronic mallet finger has a flexion deformity at the DIP joint and hyperextension of the PIP joint. This is known as a secondary swan-neck deformity.

We recommend that radiographs be obtained with all acute and chronic mallet fingers. The lateral view can reveal a fracture fragment and joint subluxation. The AP view may show an associated collateral ligament injury (Fig. 10.11).

Doyle (2) classified mallet fingers into four types. A type I injury is caused by hyperflexion secondary to closed or blunt trauma. This injury involves disruption or stretching of the extensor tendon just proximal to its insertion and may or may not include a small avulsion fracture. A type II injury is a laceration that divides the terminal ten-

don. A type III mallet finger is characterized by a deep abrasion involving loss of the overlying soft tissue. Type IV injuries can be subdivided into three groups: (a) a transepiphyseal plate fracture in children, (b) a fracture involving 20 to 50% of the articular surface produced by a hyperflexion injury, and (c) a fracture produced by hyperextension that involves more than 50% of the articular surface and demonstrates volar subluxation of the distal phalanx (Fig. 10.12).

Closed acute mallet injuries are treated nonoperatively. The digit is immobilized with the DIP joint in extension by using a prefabricated plastic splint finger splint (8), a foam-padded aluminum splint, or a custom-made fingertip protector (Fig. 10.13). The splint should permit unrestricted motion of the PIP joint. Kaplan's (9) anatomic studies demonstrate relative relaxation of the extensor mechanism over all three joints when only the DIP joint was held in extension. More extensive splinting or Smillie's (10) serial casting method may be required for the active or uncooperative patient.

Treatment requires 6 to 8 weeks of continuous splinting, followed by 2 weeks of night splinting as the patient begins to resume flexion. The splint is applied during the weaning period if any recurrence or deformity is noted. We recommend that the splint be applied as soon as possible

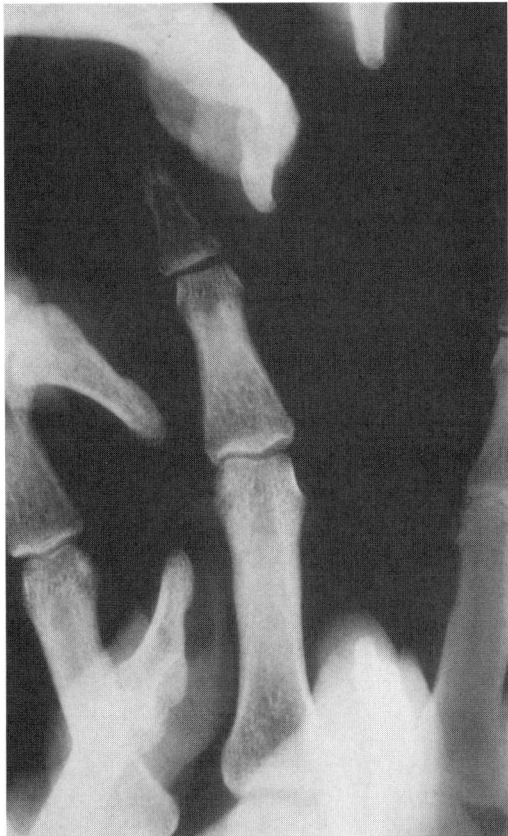

Figure 10.11. Stress radiograph showing injury to the collateral ligaments of the DIP joint.

A

B

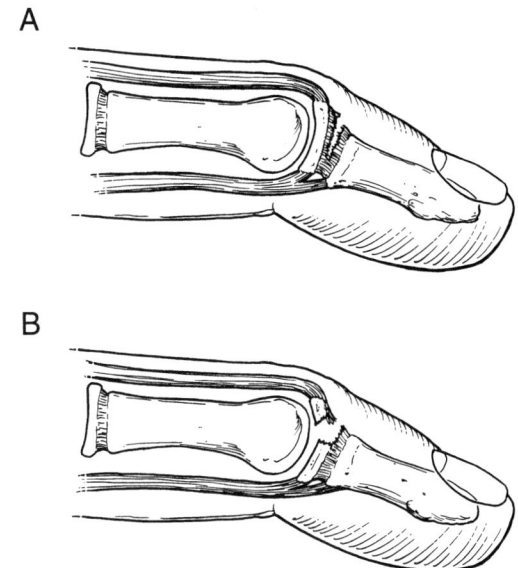

Figure 10.12. Transepiphyseal fracture in children, resulting in a mallet finger.

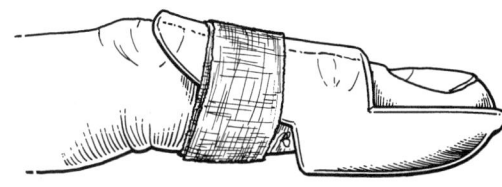

Figure 10.13. Custom-made fingertip protector for a mallet finger.

following the initial injury, although satisfactory results have been recorded with delays of 4 to 6 weeks. McFarlane and Hampole (11) found acceptable results up to 3 months postinjury, and Garberman et al. (12) showed good results in patients treated early and on a delayed basis.

The unusual transepiphyseal mallet fracture in children is caused by the attachment of the extensor tendon to the epiphysis of the distal phalanx. Treatment includes a closed reduction that extends the digit. The finger is placed in a splint for 3 to 4 weeks.

COMPLICATIONS

Complications with the use of a splint include ulceration and maceration of the skin. Extreme hyperextension and pressure over the dorsum of the joint must be avoided to prevent these complications. Patients are encouraged to keep the skin clean and the splint dry; but they must be warned to keep the DIP joint in extension when removing the splint.

OPERATIVE

Open repair of the closed injury is rarely necessary and has not been found to be efficacious, given the thin and tenuous nature of the extensor tendon at this level. Kirschner (K) wire fixation crossing the DIP obviates the need for an external splint and may be useful in patients

such as dentists, surgeons, and others whose daily activities do not allow wearing a splint (Clinical Table). The K wire is kept in for 6 weeks, after which motion is begun. Potential complications, such as a nail bed injury and osteomyelitis, must be explained to the patient before the K wire is used.

Open mallet finger injuries are treated by the reapproximation of the tissues, using the figure eight or roll suture technique. The DIP is splinted in extension postoperatively. Sutures are removed at 10 to 14 days, and splinting is continued as in a closed injury (Fig. 10.14). More significant open injuries with loss of skin and tendon require reconstructive procedures that will not be discussed here.

OUTCOME

The mallet finger with a small avulsion fragment can be treated in a closed fashion. Several authors have shown that the presence of this small piece of bone does not significantly affect the outcome of treatment (6,13,14). Wehbe and Schneider (14) recommend extensive splinting of all types of mallet fractures. They believe that joint congruity is not essential, since remodeling has been observed to lead to a functional and painless joint. Crawford (15) noted that splinting in hyperextension should be avoided in the presence of a significant fracture, as this may accentuate

Clinical Table: Extensor Tendon Injuries and Common Tendinopathies

Procedure	Indications	Technique	Anatomy	Pitfalls
Stack splint mallet repair	• Mallet finger (flexed DIP)	• Occupational therapy • Figure eight or roll suture or Kirschner wire repair	• Terminal tendon laceration	• Ulceration and maceration
Boutonniere repair	• Boutonniere PIP joint flexion with DIP joint hyperextension	• K-wire immobilization and primary repair central slip	• Discontinuity of the central slip vs. crush injury	• Stiff chronic boutonniere with missed diagnosis
Dislocated extrinsic extensor tendon repair	• Extensor tendon subluxation	• Splinting in extension vs. acute surgical repair	• Radial sagittal band	• Missed diagnosis
Extensor tendon laceration zone VI repair	• Extensor tendon laceration	• Tendon repair with non-absorbable sutures	• Extensor tendon and juncturae	• Failure of splinting to juncturae
Chronic mallet finger repair	• Flexed DIP • Fixed DIP contracture	• Tenodermodesis • K-wire immobilized arthrodesis PIP	• Repair of short-ened extensor mechanism • Degenerative DIP	• Wound breakdown • Infection
Littler reconstruction (24)	• Swan-neck deformity • Flexed DIP • Hyperextended PIP	• Reconstructing oblique retinacular ligament	• Fixed contracture and intrinsic tightness in the PIP	• Flexor tendon scarring and recurrence of deformity
Extensor tenolysis	• Fixed tendons with limited motion	• Release adhesions to skin, tendons, bones, and joints (26)	• Extensor tendons	• Rupture tendons or inadequate release
First dorsal compartment release	• De Quervain's tenosynovitis	• Surgical decompression of the first compartment	• APL • EPB	• Cut superficial radial nerve • Missed release • Independent septae

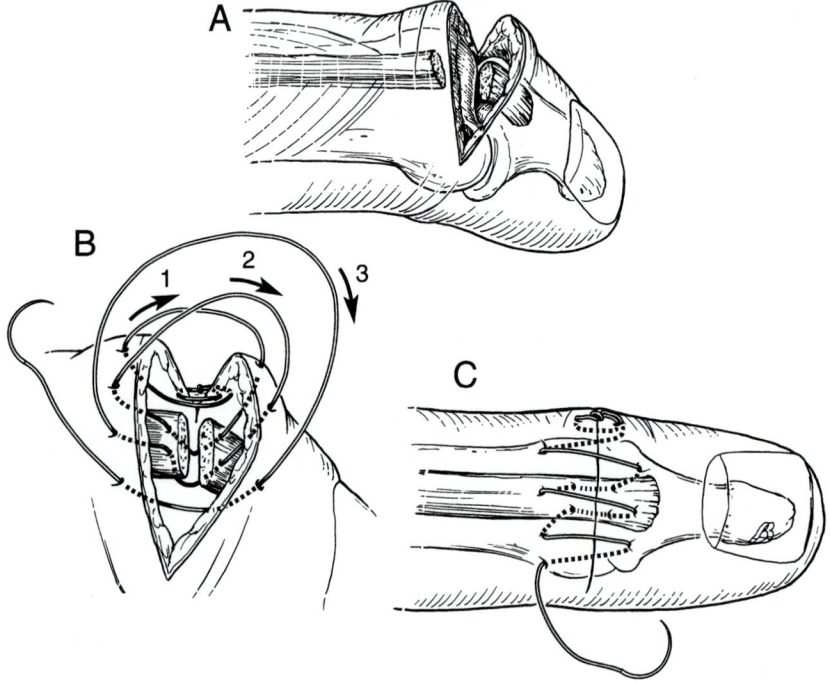

Figure 10.14. Roll suture technique for open mallet repair.

the subluxation. Some authors have recommended operative treatment for any fracture involving more than one-third of the articular surface. Most authors currently recommend open treatment to restore joint congruity only when joint subluxation has occurred (2,15,16).

If volar subluxation is present and the fracture is greater than 30%, the joint is exposed dorsally and a single K wire is placed longitudinally through the distal phalanx to reduce and hold the DIP joint. If the fracture fragment is not well apposed, a pullout suture or wire may be used and brought out over a button volarly (2,15,16). The DIP joint is then splinted for 6 weeks before the K wire is removed and rehabilitation begun.

Operative repair of mallet deformities can be challenging and often unnecessary. The surgeon must guard against comminution of the fracture fragment, resulting in an inability to reattach the extensor mechanism, skin necrosis, and a decrease in the range of motion at the DIP joint. Clement and Wray (17) reported a decrease in flexion of the PIP joint after DIP surgery. They also noted an incidence of cold intolerance and persistent pain.

Mallet thumb injuries are much less common than are mallet finger injuries, but the principles of treatment are similar. Though some surgeons recommend operative repair, Doyle (2) prefers splinting in extension for the closed injury. A laceration at the level of the interphalangeal joint lends itself to repair of the EPL tendon. A fracture through the joint with a pulloff of the EPL insertion requires operative reduction and internal fixation.

Zone II: Middle Phalanx

Zone II involves the middle phalanx. Lacerations at this level are seldom complete, owing to the width and curvature of the extensor mechanism. Zone II lacerations are treated similarly to zone I injuries, with figure eight or roll sutures and splinting of the DIP joint for 6 weeks. Lacerations of less than 50% do not require repair, and active motion may begin following wound healing with a frayed tendon program.

Zone III: PIP Joint (Boutonniere Injury)

PIP joint flexion with DIP joint hyperextension is the hallmark of the boutonniere deformity (Fig. 10.15). This results from discontinuity in the central slip of the extensor mechanism at the level of the PIP joint, with volar migration of the lateral bands. The injury is caused by laceration, forced flexion at the PIP joint, crush injuries, volar PIP dislocations, and synovitis from inflammatory arthritis.

Diagnosis in the acute setting may be difficult, and a high degree of suspicion is required. Suggestive findings include swelling and tenderness at the base of the dorsal middle phalanx with weak PIP joint extension against resistance. Volar dislocations of the PIP joint should alert the physician to the possibility of a late boutonniere injury. X-rays rarely show fracture fragments involving the dorsum of the middle phalanx. Acutely, the patient is often able to extend the PIP joint through the lateral bands. With continued use, the triangular ligament stretches and the transverse retinacular ligaments progressively contract. The lateral bands migrate volar to the axis of the PIP joint and begin to act as PIP flexors. This new alignment concentrates the force of the extensor mechanism at the DIP joint, which, along with the MP joint, begins to hyperextend. In a chronic boutonniere, the deformity becomes fixed secondary to contractures of the transverse retinacular, oblique retinacular, collateral ligaments, and volar plate. Fixed deformities are discussed later in this chapter.

The acute closed boutonniere deformity is treated with immobilization of the PIP joint in extension. This may be accomplished with a splint or a transarticular K wire. The PIP joint is immobilized and active flexion of the DIP joint is encouraged to prevent lateral band adhesions and contractures of the oblique retinacular ligament (18). The splint is worn for 6 weeks; active PIP flexion is begun, and the joint is protected in extension for 2 weeks more between exercises. Initially, some digits may not allow full extension, and serial splinting or casting may be required (2). The goal of treatment is to prevent a stiff, chronic boutonniere deformity.

Surgical treatment of an acute closed boutonniere deformity has been advocated for avulsion fracture, subacute boutonniere deformity in a young person (19), volar dislocation of the PIP joint, and lacerations across the PIP joint (20). Bony reattachment or excision of the fragment and central slip reattachment is the treatment of choice for an avulsion fracture (19). If no fracture is present, the central slip is explored and repaired, as are other structures requiring repair (20). In both circumstances a K wire is used to place the PIP joint in extension for 3 weeks.

Lacerations in the region of the PIP joint may be intra-articular and may require irrigation, débridement, and primary repair of the central slip and/or lateral bands with pullout sutures; K wire immobilization of the PIP joint in extension may also be necessary (Fig. 10.16). Several reconstructive procedures, using local tissues, are available to avoid a chronic deformity if there is tissue loss involving the extensor mechanism (2).

Zone IV: Proximal Phalanx

Lacerations in zone IV seldom result in complete transection, because of the broad, circumferential orientation of the extensor mechanism at this level. Partial lacerations are repaired primarily, and the patient is started on early range of motion protocols. Repairs involving the central slip are maintained in splints, with the PIP joint extended for 6 weeks to avoid lengthening of the central slip and developing a boutonniere-type deformity.

Zone V: MP Joint

The MP joint is a common location for abrasions and lacerations in the hand because of its prominence. A pen-

Figure 10.15. A. Hallmark of the boutonniere deformity. **B.** The lateral bands are subluxed in a boutonniere deformity.

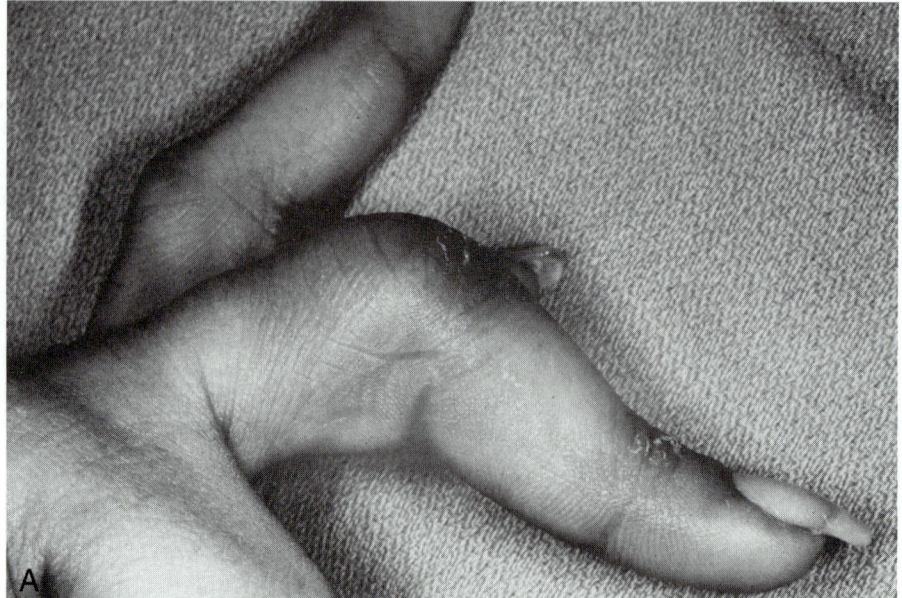

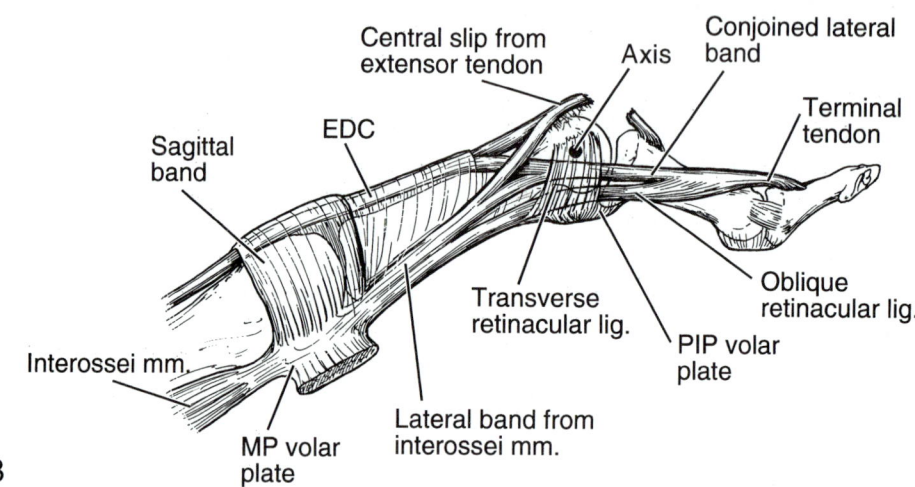

etrating injury at this level may affect the MP joint. All wounds must be inspected, cleaned, and débrided. Any small puncture wound in this location must be considered a human bite until proven otherwise. A human bite is a contaminated wound, usually polymicrobial involving gram-positive bacteria (streptococci, staphylococci) or gram-negative Eikenella. The wound should be extended, débrided, and irrigated. If the wound is identified within 6 h of injury, it may be closed; otherwise it is left open, and secondary tendon repair, if necessary, is planned for 4 to 7 days later. In simple, clean lacerations, the tendon is repaired primarily. Repair of the sagittal bands is performed to prevent subluxation of the extensor tendon. Dynamic splinting in an intrinsic-minus position and early motion are recommended after repair of the sagittal band.

Subluxation or dislocation of the extrinsic extensor tendon occurs at this level secondary to injury of the sagittal bands from a laceration, direct blow, or forceful flexion or extension stress. Most commonly seen in the middle finger, this involves a tear in the radial side of the sagittal

band and ulnar subluxation of the tendon. On examination, there is tenderness, swelling, and an inability to actively extend the MP joint. Ulnar deviation of the involved digit may be noted in flexion. If the extensor tendon is passively extended, the tendon will reduce, and the patient will then be able to actively maintain its position.

Initial treatment of a closed extensor tendon subluxation at the MP joint should consist of splinting in extension. Acute surgical repair of the radial sagittal band is preferred. Postsurgery, the MP joint is splinted in maximum extension for 4 weeks. Active motion of the PIP and DIP joints is begun at 2 weeks, with the MP extended.

Zone VI: Metacarpals

The extensor tendons over the dorsum of the hand are superficial and thus commonly injured. Prognosis after operative repair is good, but tendon lacerations associated with more severe injuries have an increased risk of adhesions. Tendons in this region may be repaired with nonabsorbable sutures and then splinted with the MP joint in neutral and the wrist slightly extended. Because of the juncturae, all the fingers should be splinted in EDC injuries. Dynamic splinting is started early, and protection is continued for 6 weeks.

Zone VII: Wrist

Treatment of extensor tendon injuries at the wrist is complicated by the presence of the extensor retinaculum. Tendon lacerations are routinely repaired using standard methods. Depending on the location of the repair, some portion of the extensor retinaculum must be excised to avoid impingement. Repair of the retinaculum proximal or distal to the tendon repair must remain intact to prevent bowstringing of the tendons. Dorsal lacerations may involve branches of the superficial radial or ulna nerve. These nerves should be repaired acutely at the time of tendon repair. Tendons often retract proximally after laceration at this level and may require longitudinal extension of the wound to identify the two cut ends.

After surgery, the surgeon must immobilize the wrist in extension and the MP joints in neutral. Multiple tendon injuries respond better to early motion, which promote excursion of the tendons beneath the retinaculum. Dynamic extension splinting is begun at 10 days. Protected range of motion exercises are begun between 4 and 6 weeks.

Zone VIII: Distal Forearm

Injuries to the distal forearm are caused by penetrating trauma. Deep penetration should caution the physician to perform a complete neurovascular examination. Diagnosis is confirmed with the loss of the tenodesis effect, causing digital extension of wrist flexion. Longitudinal extension of the wound and meticulous exploration are required to achieve satisfactory repair at this level. Injuries at the musculotendinous junction are repaired by approximating the tendon to the fibrous septa in the muscle belly. Intramuscular lacerations are reapposed using absorbable sutures. Postsurgery, the wrist is immobilized in extension, with the MP joints in slight flexion. The elbow is immobilized if the tendons involved have their origin proximal to the elbow. Protected range of motion is started at 4 weeks. The splint may be removed at 6 weeks.

EXTENSOR TENDON RECONSTRUCTION

Chronic Mallet Finger

An extensor lag at the DIP joint is treated with a splint up to 12 weeks postinjury, although the true limits of this time frame have yet to be established. Dysfunction with chronic mallet finger may be minimal and tolerable. Patients who have pain, deformity, and functional loss may desire surgical correction.

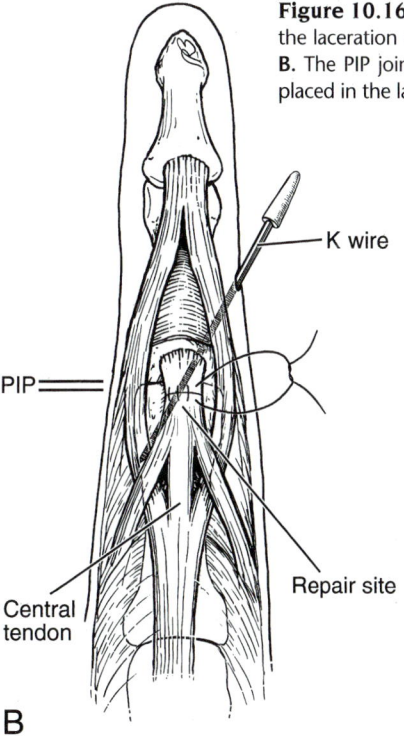

Figure 10.16. **A.** The K wire is in place, and the laceration of the central slip is visualized. **B.** The PIP joint is pinned, and the suture is placed in the lacerated extensor mechanism.

PIP

K wire

Repair site

Central tendon

B

A

Correction of a chronic mallet finger requires a repair that shortens the extensor mechanism. Through a dorsal approach to the DIP joint, this may be accomplished by three methods: (a) a segment of scar tissue may be resected, followed by end-to-end repair of the tendon; (b) the tendon may be imbricated on itself; and (c) the insertion of the scarred tendon may be divided, advanced, and reattached to bone (21). An alternative procedure is a tenodermodesis. The skin and extensor mechanism are excised in an elliptical fashion, and the edges are reapproximated as described by Iselin et al. (22). The joint is stabilized in extension with a longitudinal K wire and protected with a splint for 8 weeks.

Another technique used to treat chronic mallet fingers is the release of the central slip (23). Through a midlateral incision at the level of the PIP joint, the lateral band is identified; this structure and the entire extensor mechanism are elevated. The insertion of the central slip is released from the proximal middle phalanx. Postsurgery, the DIP joint is splinted in extension and the PIP joint is held at 30° flexion for 3 weeks, after which PIP motion is begun, with the DIP joint being held in extension for an additional 4 weeks. This procedure has the effect of moving the extensor mechanism proximal and tightening the lateral bands. It will also reduce tone at the PIP joint, avoiding hyperextension.

The procedures described all require a congruent and supple DIP joint. Chronic repair of the extensor mechanism, especially following mallet fractures, can be difficult and frustrating. The bony alignment may be restored; but contractures of the joint capsule, collateral ligaments, and volar plate may limit function. Fixed deformities, degenerative changes, and joint malalignment are all indications for arthrodesis of the DIP joint. We perform an arthrodesis with either K wires or a Herbert screw. An incision is made dorsally; and using a rongeur, the articular surface is removed. K wires are placed retrograde, whereas the Herbert screw may be placed antegrade under fluoroscopic guidance.

Swan-Neck Deformity

A swan-neck deformity is a flexed DIP joint with hyperextension at the PIP joint (Fig. 10.17). This deformity is caused by a dynamic imbalance that may be an interruption of the distal extensor mechanism, which focuses its force at the middle phalanx, or an incompetence of the volar plate at the PIP joint. The result is hyperextension of the PIP joint, leading to dorsal displacement of the lateral bands, which in effect lengthens the extensor mechanism. Factors leading to a swan-neck deformity include chronic mallet finger, fracture malunion, volar plate injury to the PIP joint, spasticity, rheumatoid arthritis, and ligamentous laxity.

Splinting and exercise may be used to relieve fixed contractures and intrinsic tightness, but they cannot correct a swan-neck deformity (21). Correction must limit hy-

perextension at the PIP joint and augment DIP extension. This is accomplished by constructing an oblique retinacular ligament analog and securing it in a volar position to prevent PIP hyperextension and create passive extension of the DIP joint as the PIP is actively extended.

The original technique described by Littler (24) made use of the lateral band. Thompson et al.'s (4) modification employs a free tendon graft. A dorsolateral approach is used to expose the lateral band. A hole is created in the anteroposterior direction at the base of the distal phalanx and transversely at the base of the proximal phalanx. An appropriate tendon graft (usually palmaris or plantaris) is secured through the distal phalanx using pullout sutures over a button or a mini-Mitek. The graft follows the course of the lateral band volarly and proximally across the middle phalanx. The graft passes deep to the neurovascular bundle to cross anteriorly to the opposite side of the proximal phalanx, where it is passed through the transverse hole and secured over a second button. Before securing the graft proximally, the surgeon sets the appropriate tension by pulling the graft until the DIP joint is in full extension and the PIP joint is held in approximately 20° of flexion. A K wire may be employed to hold the PIP joint in this position. K wires are removed at 4 weeks, and the finger is placed in a dorsal splint in the same position. Active flexion is also started. The splint is discontinued at 8 weeks, and active extension is begun. The patient is told not to attempt to stretch the PIP joint into full extension.

The major concern postoperatively is avoiding flexor tendon scarring and the recurrence of deformity (21). A well-supervised rehabilitation program is imperative. Preoperative patient selection is important. If the PIP joint is severely damaged, is deformed, or has a fixed contracture, the surgeon may wish to consider arthroplasty or an arthrodesis instead.

Chronic Boutonniere Deformity

Boutonniere deformities may lengthen the central slip, leading to increased volar migration and rigid fixation of the lateral bands. The deformity becomes fixed with a contracture of the transverse retinacular and oblique retinacular ligaments, the volar plate, and the collateral ligaments of the PIP joint. The treatment plan is determined by the PIP joint deformity and whether it is supple or fixed.

Many flexible boutonniere deformities will respond to splinting and therapeutic intervention (21). Active-assisted extension of the PIP will stretch volar structures and increase the tenodesis effect on the DIP joint. Active flexion of the DIP joint with the PIP joint held in extension will stretch the lateral bands and oblique retinacular ligaments.

The wide variety of procedures used to treat this deformity is a testament to the difficulty of successful treatment. Most of the procedures fall into one of four categories: anatomic repair of the central slip, reconstruction using the lateral bands or other local tissues, tendon graft,

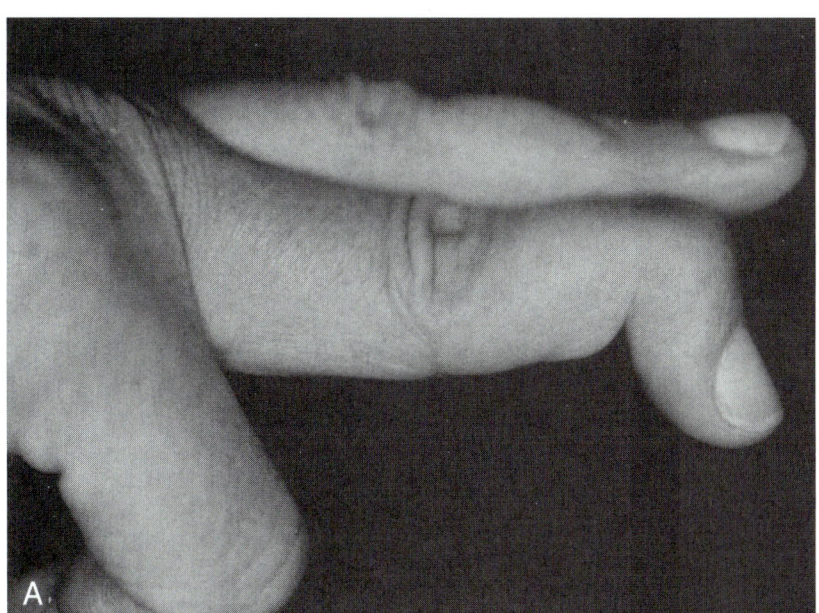

Figure 10.17. Hallmarks of the swan-neck deformity.

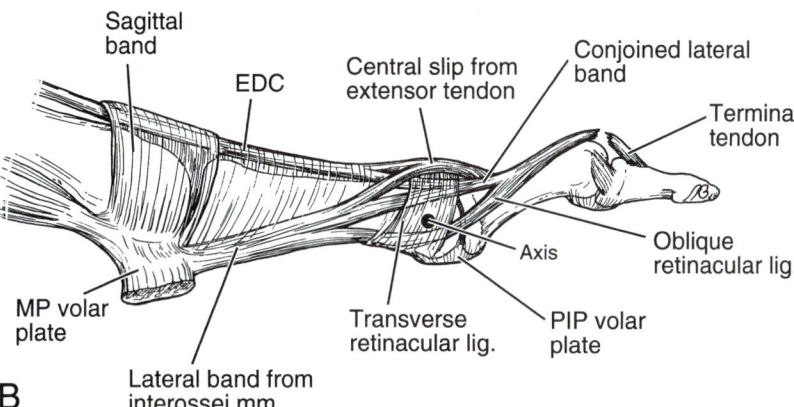

Sagittal band

EDC

Central slip from extensor tendon

Conjoined lateral band

Terminal tendon

Oblique retinacular lig.

Axis

MP volar plate

Transverse retinacular lig.

PIP volar plate

Lateral band from interossei mm.

B

or redistribution of joint forces. Burton (21) describes a procedure to realign joint forces. Using a dorsal bayonet incision centered over the PIP joint, the extensor tendon is divided over the proximal portion of the middle phalanx. This effectively lengthens the lateral bands, allowing proximal migration of the extensor mechanism, increasing tone in the central slip. The lateral bands maintain their dorsal positioning. Postsurgery, the PIP joint is splinted in extension, but active-assisted range of motion exercises continue. We perform the Elliott (25) repair for a flexible deformity (Fig. 10.18).

In a fixed deformity, the first priority is the reestablishment of passive motion. Dynamic or serial splinting and exercise may help. Operative release of the joint may become necessary, followed by staged reconstruction of the extensor mechanism. If there is evidence of degenerative changes or extensive fibrous ankylosis, we consider arthroplasty or arthrodesis.

Extensor Tenolysis

When extensor tendons become fixed at points other than the anatomic insertions (tenodesis), motion is limited. The simple release of extensor tendon adhesions (tenolysis) is the preferred procedure; but this may be inadequate if other anatomic structures are involved. Joint stiffness and contractures may necessitate capsule and collateral ligament release.

A technique of extensor tenolysis has been well described (26). We use a dorsal approach to the digit for maximal exposure. Adhesions between the skin and extensor tendon are lysed as the exposure is developed. Beginning with the proximal phalanx, the central and lateral slips are elevated, and the interval between the two is released at the level of the PIP joint. This provides access to the extensor mechanism and the dorsal capsule. The terminal extensor tendon is freed along its radial and ulnar borders to improve access to the dorsal capsule of the DIP joint (Fig. 10.19). If capsulotomies do not restore range of motion, collateral ligament release may be necessary. Partial collateral ligament release is preferred to preserve joint stability. Passive and active motion are tested before the completion of the soft tissue procedures.

Another approach to overcoming adhesions of the extensor mechanism is a tendon release. Extrinsic extensor tendon release is an attempt to separate the extrinsic and intrinsic systems. Excising the central portion of the extensor mechanism at the level of the proximal phalanx isolates the extrinsics as MP extensors and the intrinsics as interphalangeal extensors (21).

Full range of motion is started immediately postsurgery. Narcotic analgesia, indwelling catheters, and transcutaneous electrical nerve stimulation (TENS) are employed as required to reduce the pain of motion (27). Continuous passive motion (CPM) and dynamic splinting may assist with range of motion, but active use of the extensor tendons is essential. A well-supervised therapeutic regimen and a motivated patient are necessities.

Traumatic Tendon Subluxation at the MP Joint

Chronic extensor tendon subluxation causes impairment owing to the loss of active MP joint extension, ulnar drift of the involved digit, and secondary hyperextension of the PIP joint. Multiple operative techniques have been described to recentralize the extensor tendon (28). Most involve the creation of some type of check rein on the radial side of the tendon to resist dislocation in flexion. This is combined with limited ulnar-sided releases as needed. Postsurgery, the MP joint is splinted in extension for 4 weeks. PIP joint motion is allowed after wound healing to help with tendon excursion.

Proximal Reconstruction

Patients with a loss of MP joint or wrist extension display significant disability. Reconstructive procedures may be attempted to obtain a functional wrist. Direct delayed repair will be hampered by the presence of myotatic contractures. The options for reconstruction are tendon transfers and interpositional grafts. Transfers are generally preferred if a suitable donor exists. The patient's wrist is immobilized for 4 to 6 weeks before motion is started.

COMMON EXTENSOR TENDINOPATHIES

De Quervain's Tenosynovitis

De Quervain's tenosynovitis is a stenosing tenosynovitis of the first dorsal compartment. APL and EPB pass through a fibro-osseous tunnel formed by a groove in the radial styloid and the overlying retinaculum. Symptoms include pain over the radial styloid worsened with thumb or wrist motion, swelling, and occasional crepitus or triggering. A positive Finkelstein test (reproduction of pain with ulnar deviation of the wrist while the thumb is adducted) is typical but not pathognomonic (29,30) (Fig. 10.20).

Initial management includes thumb spica splinting, anti-inflammatory medication, and a corticosteroid injection into the first dorsal compartment (Fig. 10.21). If conservative care fails, surgical decompression of the first dor-

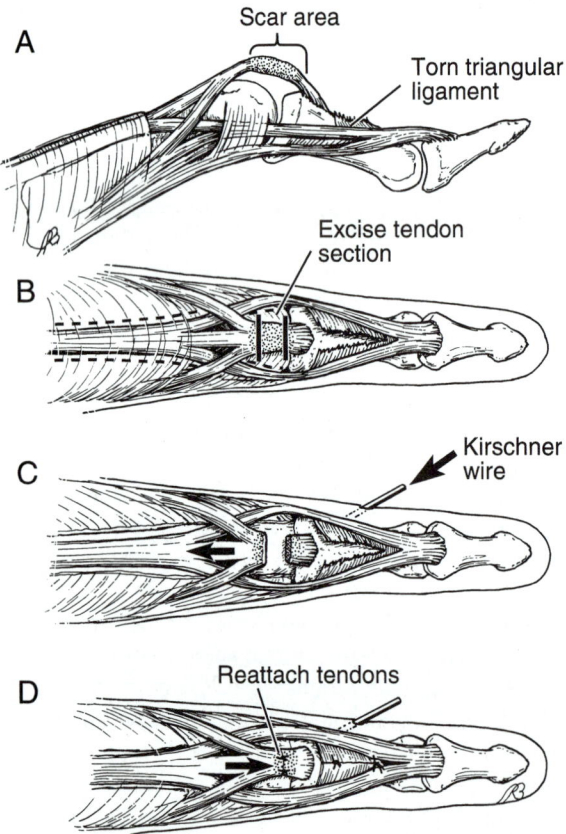

Figure 10.18. The Elliott repair of a chronic boutonniere deformity.

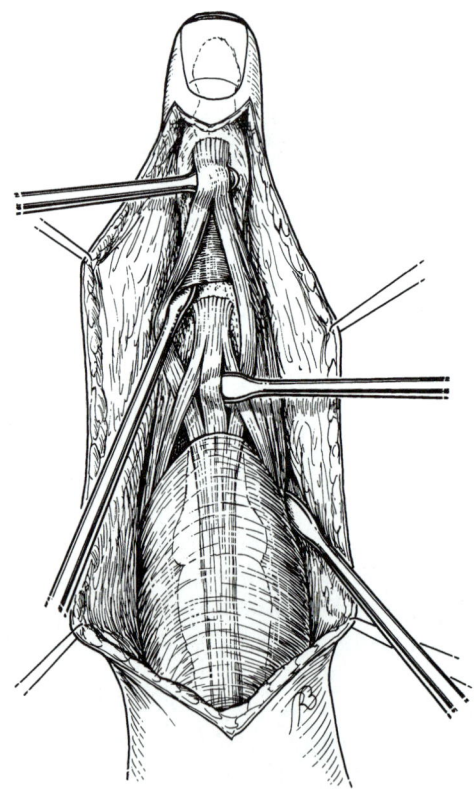

Figure 10.19. Surgical technique for an extensor tenolysis.

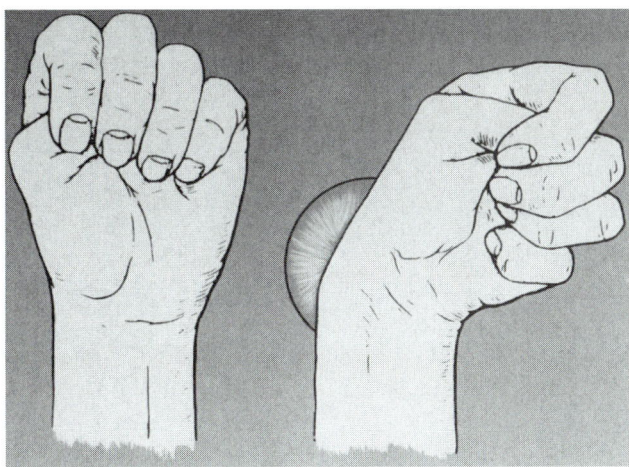

Figure 10.20. The Finkelstein test is used to diagnose de Quervain's tenosynovitis. Courtesy of Gary Schnitz, The Indiana Hand Center.

sal compartment is performed. Care is taken to divide any septa in the compartment, as anatomic studies have shown these are present in 20 to 30% of cases (29) (Fig. 10.22). Recognized complications include tendinous adhesions, volar tendon subluxation, superficial radial nerve injury, and persistence of symptoms.

Intersection Syndrome

Intersection syndrome is a tenosynovitis of the second dorsal compartment (31), commonly seen in athletes. The patient complains of swelling, tenderness, and crepitus 4 to 6 cm proximal to Lister's tubercle (Fig. 10.23). Conservative treatment is often successful (95%) and includes rest, a volar splint, anti-inflammatory medication, and a corticosteroid injection. If necessary, surgery will release the second dorsal compartment, with exploration of the zone of intersection between the radial wrist extensors

and APL and EPB. Any inflammatory or bursal tissue is removed, and the fascial sheaths of APL and EPB are released.

EPL Tendinitis

Originally described as "drummer boy palsy," EPL tendinitis is most commonly seen in patients with rheumatoid arthritis and those with a previous distal radius fracture. Patients complain of swelling, tenderness, and crepitus over the third dorsal compartment. Pain is aggravated by thumb motion. Initial treatment includes a thumb spica splint, rest, and anti-inflammatory medication. Corticosteroid injections are not recommended, because they increase local tissue pressure and may increase the risk of rupture (32). Surgical treatment involves the release of the third dorsal compartment, transposition of the EPL tendon to the radial side of Lister's tubercle, and closure of the retinaculum to prevent relocation (29) (Fig. 10.24).

EIP Syndrome

Irritation of EIP tendon may be precipitated by muscular hypertrophy or synovitis from overuse. The patient describes pain and swelling over the fourth dorsal compartment. Resisted extension of the index finger with the wrist extended is a reliable provocative test. Conservative treatment involves splinting of the wrist and metacarpal phalangeal joints, anti-inflammatory medication, and corticosteroid injections. If conservative therapy fails, the extensor retinaculum over the fourth dorsal compartment may be divided and a synovectomy performed.

EDM Tendinitis

Tenosynovitis of the fifth dorsal compartment is rare; it is associated with trauma, overuse, and anatomic anoma-

Figure 10.21. Corticosteroid injection into the first dorsal compartment.

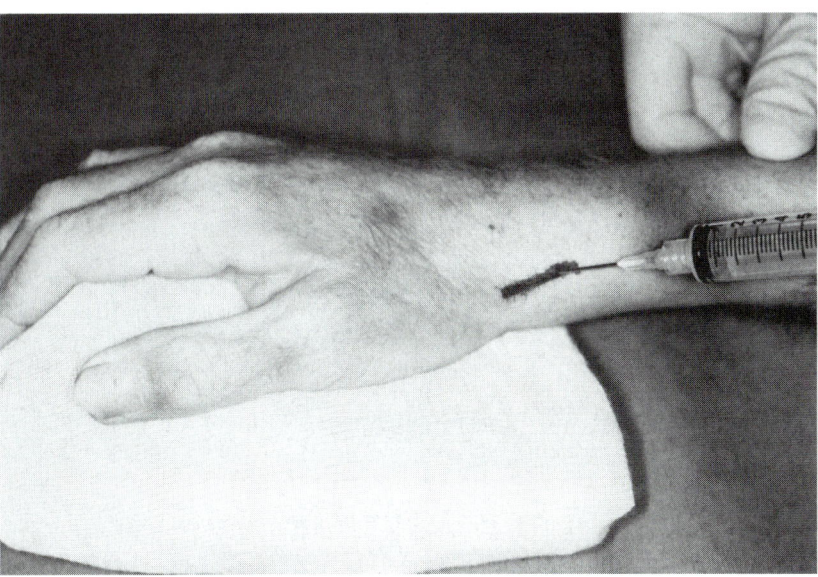

Figure 10.22. Anatomy of the first dorsal compartment and the septa sometimes seen between APL and EPB.

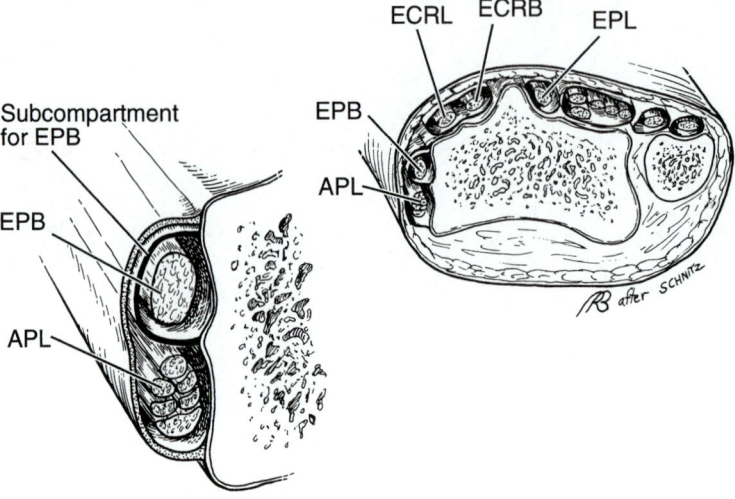

lies (30). Pain and swelling is detected just distal to the ulnar head. Standard conservative therapy includes an ulnar gutter splint. Surgical division of the retinaculum over the fifth dorsal compartment is required in resistant cases.

ECU Tendinitis

ECU tendinitis is the second most common stenosing tenosynovitis of the hand. Seen frequently as a sports injury, ECU tendinitis may be present from posttraumatic ECU subluxation. The ECU is unique because it passes through its own fibro-osseous tunnel, separate from the overlying extensor retinaculum (Fig. 10.2) (20). The fibrous subsheath overlying the ECU may rupture, even in the presence of an intact extensor retinaculum.

Patients with ECU tendinitis have pain and swelling distal to the ulnar head, exacerbated by resisted wrist extension and ulnar deviation. ECU subluxation may be elicited with supination and ulnar deviation, resulting in a painful snap of the dorsal wrist. If conservative therapy fails, Hajj and Wood (33) recommend a radial release of the fibro-osseous tunnel followed by repair of the extensor retinaculum. ECU subluxation may require a retinacular graft or sling to stabilize the tendon. After surgery the wrist is immobilized in pronation and slight dorsiflexion in a long arm cast.

SUMMARY

The complexity and interdependence of the various parts of the extensor mechanism make treatment of extensor tendon injuries and tendinopathies challenging. A thorough understanding of anatomy, pathomechanics, surgical technique, and rehabilitation is required to maximize

Figure 10.23. Anatomy of the intersection syndrome.

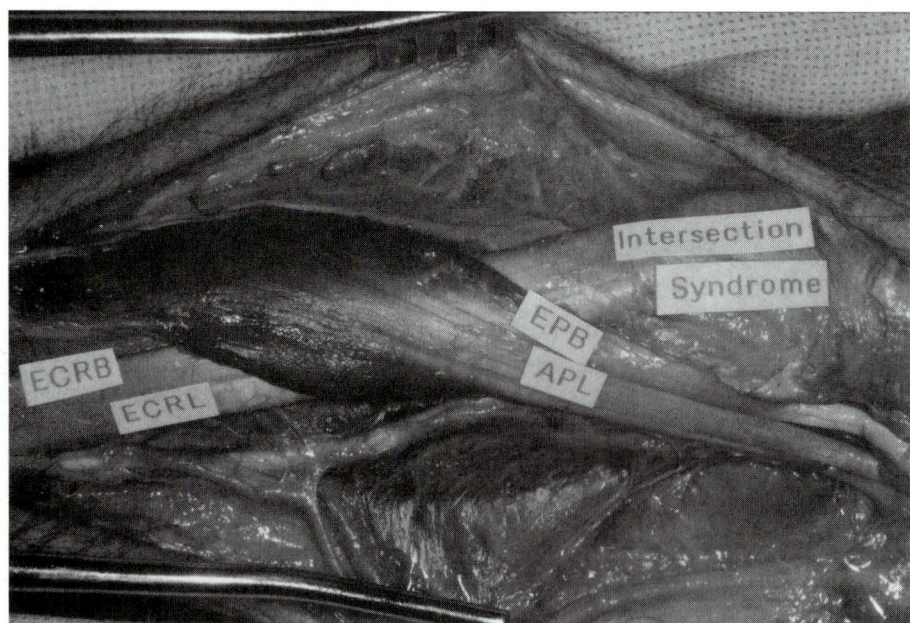

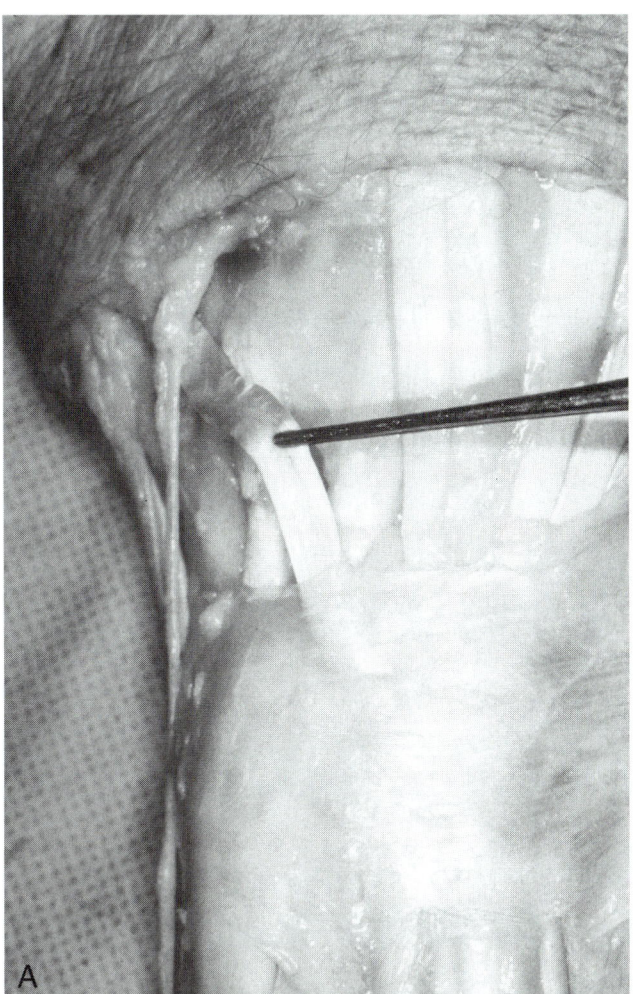
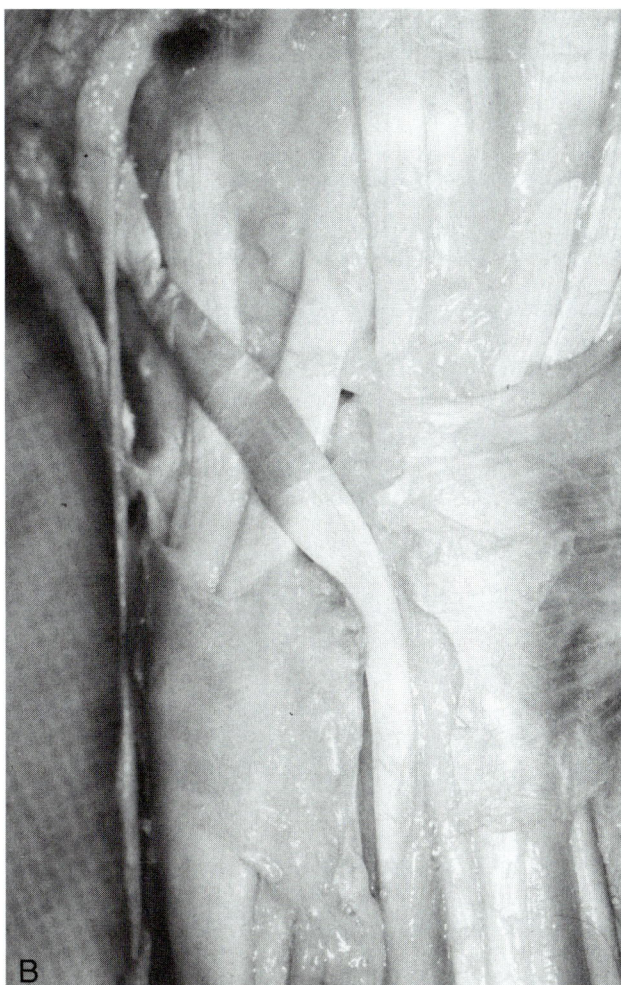

Figure 10.24. Release of the third dorsal compartment.

therapeutic outcome and avoid the many pitfalls inherent in extensor tendon surgery.

REFERENCES

1. Newport ML, Blair WF, Steyers CM Jr. Long term results of extensor tendon repair. J Hand Surg 1990;15A:961–966.
2. Doyle JR. Extensor tendons—acute injuries. In: Green DP, ed. Operative hand surgery. New York: Churchill Livingstone, 1992:1925–1954.
3. Eyler DL, Markee JE. J Bone Joint Surg 1954;36A:1.
4. Thompson JS, Littler JW, Upton J. The spiral oblique retinacular ligament (SORL). J Hand Surg 1978;3:482–487.
5. Kleinert HE, Verdan C. Report of the committee on tendon injuries. J Hand Surg 1983;8:794–798.
6. Abouna JM, Brown H. The treatment of mallet finger; the results in a series of 148 consecutive cases and a review of the literature. Br J Surg 1968;55:653–667.
7. Warren RA, Kay NRM, Norris SH. The microvascular anatomy of the distal digital extensor tendon. J Hand Surg 1988;13B:161–163.
8. Stack HG. A modified splint for mallet finger. J Hand Surg 1986;11B:263.
9. Kaplan EB. Anatomy, injuries, and treatment of the extensor apparatus of the hand and fingers. Clin Orthop 1959;13:24–41.
10. Smillie IS. Mallet finger. Br J Surg 1937;24:439–445.
11. McFarlane RM, Hampole MK. Treatment of extensor tendon injuries of the hand. Can J Surg 1973;16:366–375.
12. Garberman SF, Diao E, Peimer CA. Mallet finger: results of early versus delayed closed treatment. J Hand Surg 1994;19A:850–852.
13. Stark HH, Boyes JH, Wilson JN. Mallet finger. J Bone Joint Surg 1962;44A:1061–1068.
14. Wehbe MA, Schneider LH. Mallet fractures. J Bone Joint Surg 1984; 66A:658–669.
15. Crawford GP. The molded polyethylene splint for mallet finger deformities. J Hand Surg 1984;9A:231–237.
16. Lange RH, Engber WD. Hyperextension mallet finger. Orthopedics 1983;6:1426–1431.
17. Clement R, Wray RC Jr. Operative and nonoperative management of mallet finger. Ann Plast Surg 1986;16:136–141.
18. Coons MS, Green SM. Boutonniere deformity. Hand Clin 1995; 11:387–402.
19. Boyes JH. Bunnell's surgery of the hand. Philadelphia: Lippincott, 1970:439–442.
20. Spinner M. Choi BY. Anterior dislocation of the proximal interphalangeal joint, a cause of rupture of the central slip of the extensor mechanism. J Bone Joint Surg 1970;52A:1329–1336.
21. Burton RI. Extensor tendons—late reconstruction. In: Green DP, ed. Operative hand surgery. New York: Churchill Livingstone, 1992:1955–1988.
22. Iselin F, Levane J, Godoy J. A simplified technique for treating mallet fingers: tenodermodesis. J Hand Surg 1977;5:214.
23. Bowers WH, Hurst LC. Chronic mallet finger: the use of Fowler's central slip release. J Hand Surg 1978;3:373–376.
24. Littler JW. Restoration of the oblique retinacular ligament for cor-

rection of hyperextension deformity of the proximal interphalangeal joint. In: Fournice A, ed. La main theumatismale. Paris: Expansion Scientifique Francoise, 1966.

25. Elliott RA. Boutonniere deformity. Cramer LM, Chase RA, eds. Symposium on the hand. Vol. 3. St. Louis: Mosby, 1971:42–56.

26. Creighton JJ Jr, Steichen JB. Complications in phalangeal and metacarpal fracture, management result of extensor tenolysis. Hand Clin 1994;10:1.

27. Uhl RL. Salvage of extensor tendon function with tenolysis and joint release. Hand Clin 1995;3:461–470.

28. Vaccaro AR, Kupcha P, Schneider LH. The operative repair of chronic nontraumatic tensor tendon subluxations in the hand. Hand Clin 1995;11:431–440.

29. Froimson A. Tenosynovitis and tennis elbow. In: Green DP, ed. Operative hand surgery. New York: Churchill Livingstone, 1992:1989–2006.

30. Plancher KD, Peterson RK, Steichen JD. Compressive neuropathies and tendinopathies in the athletic elbow and wrist. Clin Sports Med 1996;15:331–370.

31. Grundberg AB, Reagan DS. Pathologic anatomy of the forearm intersection syndrome. J Hand Surg 1985;10:299–302.

32. Stern PJ. Tendinitis, overuse syndromes, and tendon injuries. Hand Clin 1990;6:467–476.

33. Hajj AA, Wood MB. Stenosing tenosynovitis of the extensor carpi ulnaris. J Hand Surg 1986;11:519–520.

chapter 11

Haideh Hirmand and Lloyd A. Hoffman

Dupuytren's Disease

Dupuytren's contracture is one of a group of fibromatoses of which the cause and exact mechanism of pathogenesis remain unclear. The first case of this condition was described by Plater in 1614. Dupuytren's, however, was the first (in 1831) to describe the anatomy. He localized the disease to the palmar fascia and recommended open fasciotomy as the definitive treatment (1). Hueston (2) introduced the term *Dupuytren's disease* to indicate a condition that could be more widespread than just contracture in the hands.

Dupuytren's disease is more common in people of northern European origin than in those of other ethnic backgrounds. The incidence varies among different populations and depends on the age and sex of the population in question. In a survey of 1227 patients in 12 countries, McFarlane (3) found that males were affected more than females (by 82:16) in all countries and races and 27% of patients had a positive family history. For the majority of patients (65%), the disease involved both hands; in more than one-third of the patients, the disease affected other areas: knuckle pads (22%), feet (10%), and penis (2%) (4).

Knuckle pads, Peyronie's disease, and plantar fibromatosis are frequently seen in association with Dupuytren's disease; knuckle pads are most common and Peyronie's disease is the least frequently seen. Other conditions that are seen in association with Dupuytren's disease include diabetes, epilepsy, alcoholism, and trauma to the hand.

RELATIVE ANATOMY AND PATHOGENESIS

Pathogenesis

The nodule is the center of the contracting process in Dupuytren's disease (5). Nodules are seen most frequently just proximal or just distal to the distal crease of the palm. They may be scattered in the palmar aponeurosis, at the level of the proximal interphalangeal (PIP) joint, at the base of the fifth digit, or at the base of the thumb.

Nodules can occasionally be seen at the level of distal interphalangeal (DIP) joint, especially in the fifth digit. Fibroblasts are most commonly found in early nodules, but myofibroblasts are thought to be involved in the contraction (6). Myofibroblasts have contractile properties and the ability to make collagen and elastin. Of note, the collagen found in the diseases fascia and the nodule of Dupuytren's disease is rich in types III and V and type I trimer collagen; this composition is similar to the collagen found in healing wounds and hypertrophic scars (7). The exact role of these biochemical characteristics in the pathogenesis of Dupuytren's disease is as yet unclear. Dupuytren's disease can be divided into three stages: early, active, and advanced (8,9).

In the early stage, there is thickening and nodularity in the palmar and digital fascia. Type III collagen is abundant, and fibroblasts predominate. In the active stage, nodules become large and contraction occurs. In this stage, types III and V collagen are abundant, and myofibroblasts predominate. The skin of the distal palm blanches with extension of the digits; it then adheres to the underlying fascia, following the attenuation of the subdermal fat pads. Palpable cords form proximal to the nodules in the palm or the digit and are responsible for the eventual joint contracture.

The mechanism of contraction is thought to involve both cellular and biomechanical forces. The cellular components are probably related to the contractile proteins of the myofibroblasts and the potential for synchronous contraction due to the cell-to-cell and cell-to-stroma junctions between the myofibrils (10,11). The biochemical component involves tissue remodeling resulting from the change in stress concentrations that accompanies adherence of diseased fascia to adjacent fascia and the overlying skin.

In the advanced stage, nodules are replaced by tendinous cords, and severe contracture of the joints occurs. As the nodules disappear, few cellular elements remain. These consist of the fibrocytes. Type I collagen is abundant, and type III collagen is present in smaller amounts. The collagen in the cords is oriented in a longitudinal fashion, contributing to the cords' architecture (12).

Anatomy: Normal and Pathologic

THE PALM

The palmar fascia has three components: natatory ligament, transverse fibers, and pretendinous bands of the palmar aponeurosis (Fig. 11.1). The natatory ligament and the pretendinous bands of the palmar aponeurosis are the two principal components of the diseased fascia. Normal fascia is differentiated from diseased fascia by referring to the former as bands and to the latter as cords (12).

The pretendinous bands are a common site of disease. They insert into the skin distal to the distal palmar crease. They also bifurcate and continue as spiral bands on either side of each digit. The pretendinous bands to thumb and the index finger may be missing. As the disease progresses, these bands become contracting cords and are responsible for the metacarpal–phalangeal (MP) joint contracture.

The natatory ligament extends across the distal palm, within each web space, and attaches to the surface of each flexor tendon sheath. It also sends fibers distally on either side of each digit to form the lateral digital bands. Disease in this structure is also common, leading to contracture in the digital web spaces, which brings the digits together and contributes to contracture at the PIP joints.

The transverse fibers of the palmar aponeurosis lie deep to the pretendinous bands at the level of the MP joints and are not generally involved in the disease process, although the fibers going to the base of the thumb may be affected (13).

THE THUMB AND FIRST WEB SPACE

There are three sources of fascia in the first web space: the pretendinous band to the thumb, the natatory ligament, and the transverse fibers of the palmar aponeurosis (14). These components can succumb to Dupuytren's disease individually or together; and one or two other components may result in MP and interphalangeal (IP) joint contractures and possible adduction contracture of the thumb. These fascial bands are all superficial to the neurovascular bundle to the thumb and the index finger (4). Disease in the thumb and the first web space, though common, usually does not cause severe contracture.

THE FINGER

To understand the disease process in the finger, it is important to be familiar with the normal fascial components of the digit (Fig. 11.2) (13). Cleland's ligament is a distinct fascial layer that extends from the side of the phalanges to the skin, passing dorsal to the neurovascular bundle. It is not involved in the Dupuytren's disease process.

Grayson's ligament is a less distinct fascial layer that extends from the tendon sheath to the lateral digital sheet, passing volar to the neurovascular bundle. It is located in

Figure 11.1. Components of the palmar fascia affected by Dupuytren's disease.

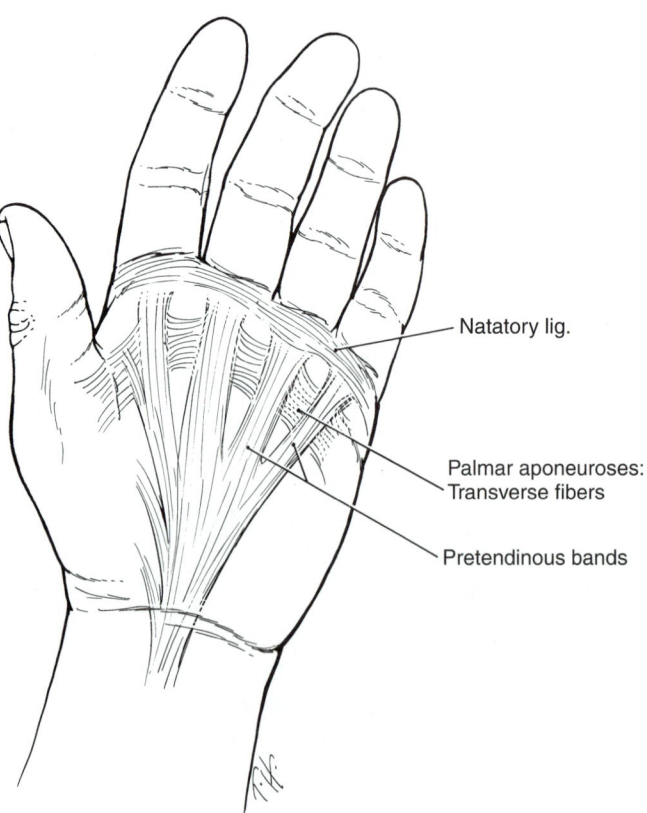

Natatory lig.

Palmar aponeuroses:
Transverse fibers

Pretendinous bands

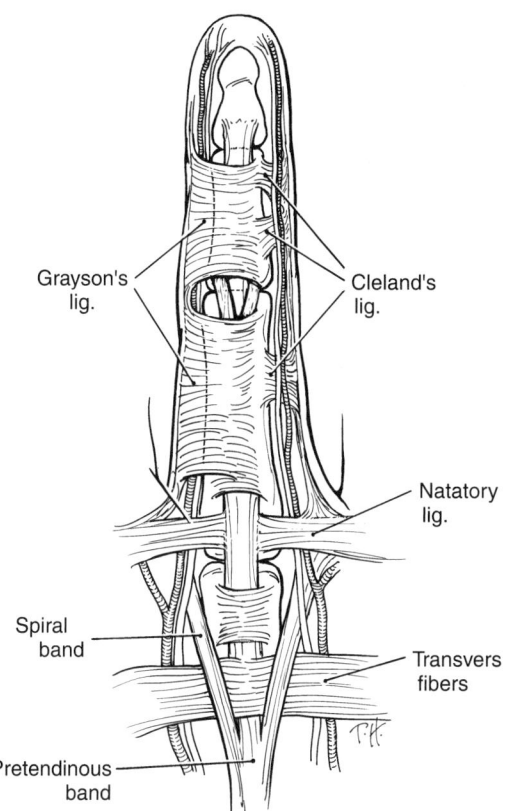

Figure 11.2. Normal fascial components of the digit. Modified from McFarlane RM. Patterns of the diseased fascia in the fingers in Dupuytren's contracture. Plast Reconstr Surg 1974;54:31.

the same plane as the natatory ligament and is often involved in the disease process. The lateral digital sheet is a longitudinal layer of superficial fascia on the lateral and media aspects of each digit. It receives fibers from the natatory ligament, spiral bands, and Grayson's and Cleland's ligaments.

The spiral bands are a continuation of the pretendinous bands of the palmar aponeurosis and are found on each side of the finger. These bands are deep to the neurovascular bundle as they enter the digit and then become superficial to it in the finger. These fascial structures contribute to the formation of the three cords that can cause PIP contracture in the digits (Fig. 11.3) (15). (*a*) The central cord is in continuity with the pretendinous cord and arises from the superficial fascial tissue between the neurovascular bundles. (*b*) The lateral cord arises from the lateral digital band and can adhere to the skin; it contributes little to PIP joint contracture (except in the fifth digit) but does contribute to DIP joint contracture. (*c*) The spiral cord arises from four components of normal fascia—pretendinous band, spiral band, lateral digital sheet, and Grayson's ligament (Fig. 11.4)—and inserts on the bone and tendon sheath of the middle phalanx. As the spiral cords contract, they displace the neurovascular bundle medially and superficially.

The retrovascular cord of Thomine (16) is a longitudinal fascial layer dorsal to the neurovascular bundle and palmar to Cleland's ligament. This structure originates from the lateral aspect of the proximal phalanx, passes close to

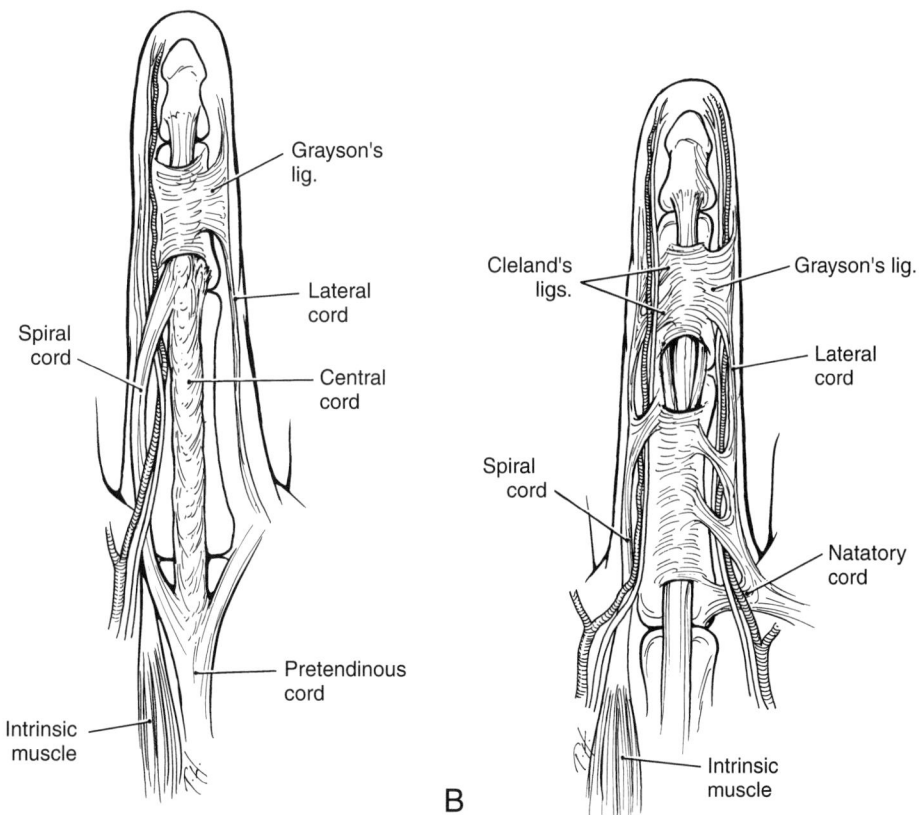

Figure 11.3. A. Diseased fascia associated with the pretendinous cord. **B.** Diseased fascia not associated with the pretendinous cord. Modified from McFarlane RM. Patterns of the diseased fascia in the fingers in Dupuytren's contracture. Plast Reconstr Surg 1974;54:31.

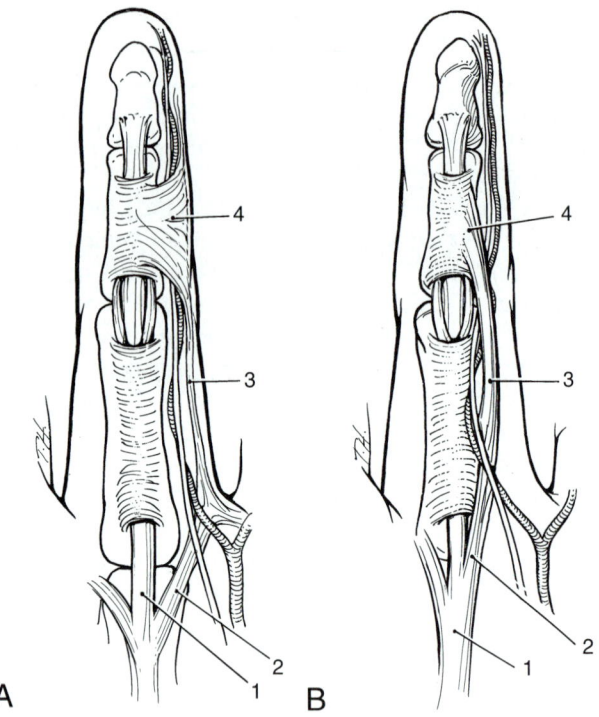

Figure 11.4. A. Components of normal fascia that produce the spiral cord. **B.** Note the medial displacement of the neurovascular bundle. *1,* Pretendinous band; *2,* spiral band; *3,* lateral digital sheet; *4,* Grayson's ligament. Modified from McFarlane RM. Patterns of the diseased fascia in the fingers in Dupuytren's contracture. Plast Reconstr Surg 1974;54:31.

the capsule of the PIP joint, and inserts on the lateral aspect of the distal phalanx. This fascial layer can form a diseased cord, which contributes to PIP and DIP joint contractures.

CLINICAL FINDINGS

The nodule is often the first clinical sign of Dupuytren's disease. Knuckle pads are seen in approximately 20% of patients. Both nodules and pads can become large and painful, but neither is an absolute indication for operative intervention. Local excision of either can lead to further activity in the area with recurrence and should be avoided if possible.

Joint contracture with functional limitation is the clinical finding used as an indication for surgery. Contracture at the MP joint can usually be corrected regardless of the severity and, 30° of contracture is disabling enough to justify an operation. Contracture at the PIP joint is more difficult to treat and often cannot be completely corrected. Some authors note the possibly greater effect of scar contracture on the PIP joint than on the MP joint. Operative treatment is thus recommended when there is any PIP joint contracture (17). Involvement of the distal palm and the formation of deep pits and folds and the subsequent maceration and infection from adduction contractures at

the web spaces are notable clinical findings and are considered relative indications for an operation.

RADIOLOGIC STUDIES

No particular radiographic changes have been directly attributed to Dupuytren's disease; however, x-ray studies are often obtained to evaluate the status of the bony structures and the limits of the involved areas.

TREATMENT

Nonoperative Alternatives

Presently, there are no proven nonoperative treatment alternatives. Steroid injection, oral vitamin E administration, and ultrasound application have been tried, but none has been proven effective in changing the disease process.

Operative Treatment

Definitive treatment for Dupuytren's disease is surgical. Several surgical techniques have been described, which fall into two main categories: fasciotomy and fasciectomy (Clinical Table).

FASCIOTOMY

In a fasciotomy, the diseased fascia is simply incised. Although fasciotomy is still cited as one of the treatment options, it is widely accepted that a high recurrence rate is associated with the procedure. Thus it is appropriate only for patients who cannot tolerate a more extensive excision of the fascia (17). Subcutaneous fasciotomy has been found to be more effective than palmar fasciotomy in treating MP joint contracture, because only the pretendinous cord needs to be incised. At the level of the PIP joint, more than one cord is involved; often these cannot all be incised safely because of the proximity of the neurovascular bundle (18).

FASCIECTOMY

The fasciectomy is based on the principle of excision of the diseased fascia. There are four types of fasciectomies (13).

Limited Fasciectomy

Gonzalez (19) described a procedure in which a portion of the diseased fascia was excised just enough to release the joint contracture in the palm and the fingers. The defect was closed with a split-thickness skin graft. Although the early results seemed to be good, there has been a high recurrence rate with the limited fasciectomy procedure.

Regional Fasciectomy

In the regional fasciectomy, only the diseased fascia is excised, which involves the diseased pretendinous cords

Clinical Table: Dupuytren's Disease

Procedure	Indications	Technique	Anatomy	Pitfalls
Fasciotomy	• Cannot tolerate extensive excision of fascia	• Incision of diseased fascia		• High rate of recurrence
Limited fasciectomy	• Release of joint contracture	• Limited excision of diseased fascia		• High rate of recurrence
Regional fasciectomy		• Complete excision of diseased fascia only	• Pretendinous cords in the palm • All fascial cords in the digits	• Residual disease in normal-appearing fascia
Extensive fasciectomy	• Extensive disease • Diathesis	• Excision of all normal and diseased fascia	• Palmar aponeurosis ligaments • All fascial bands in the digits	• Relative morbidity
Dermatofasciectomy	• Recurrent disease • Strong diathesis	• Excision of all fascia and overlying skin • Full-thickness skin graft		• High morbidity

and portions of the natatory ligament in the palm. In the digits, excision of only the diseased fascial cords is performed. All fascia that appears normal is left unexcised. It is known, however, that Dupuytren's disease may exist in normal-appearing fascia; thus good long-term results can be expected with the removal of all clinically involved fascia.

Extensive Fasciectomy

In extensive fasciectomy, all diseased and normal fascia is excised. This includes the palmar aponeurosis and the natatory ligaments in the palm and all of the fascial bands in the fingers. Extensive fasciectomy has been advocated in the fingers, where recurrent PIP joint contracture is common, whereas recurrence of MP contracture in the palm is uncommon. This procedure has also been advocated for patients with extensive involvement of the hand and those with a Dupuytren's diathesis. The operation is not popular, however, because of its associated morbidity.

Dermatofasciectomy

In dermatofasciectomy, the fascia is excised with the overlying skin, and coverage is accomplished by full-thickness skin grafting. The procedure is generally reserved for patients with recurrent disease and for those with a strong diathesis. Recurrence after this procedure is rare.

APPROACH: INCISIONS AND CLOSURE

Incisions of various forms have been used in the treatment of Dupuytren's disease and usually transverse or longitudinal. The type of operation affects the type of incision.

For access to a single digit, a midline longitudinal incision is used, extending from the proximal palm to the level of the DIP joint. At closure, Z-plasties are devised at each of proximal and distal finger creases and at the distal crease of the palm. A transverse incision at the level of the distal palmar crease can be used if more than one digit is involved. Longitudinal incisions, as described above, can be devised in conjunction; and the two incisions can be joined to access diseased fascia at the base of the fingers if necessary.

Alternatively, diseased fascia in the digits may be excised through multiple transverse incisions at the proximal and middle creases of the digits. Lazy S-type incisions have fallen out of favor because of high incidence of contraction. The Bruner zigzag incision is preferable because the sharp angles guard against scar contracture.

For exposure of the diseased fascia in the thumb, the best incision is a T-type one composed of a longitudinal incision along the axis of the thumb and a longitudinal incision along the thumb web space. These should be closed using Z-plasties (4,13).

Closure of the wound may be accomplished primarily by skin grafting, or the wound may be left open and allowed to close by secondary intention. Most wounds can be sutured without tension. Z-plasty or V–Y advancement modifications are occasionally used to help with the primary closure. If skin grafting is necessary, full-thickness grafts are preferable, because of the low incidence of wound contracture.

McCash (20) described an open palm technique that has since been advocated by some authors in both the fingers and the palm. As originally described, this technique consists of incisions in the transverse palmar and digital creases; removal of the diseased fascia; and closure of incisions, except the one along the distal palmar crease. A pressure dressing is applied, and motion is started at 1 week after the first dressing change. The open wound is allowed to heal by secondary intention with dressing changes.

Although the risk for postoperative wound necrosis and hematoma formation is thought to be minimal, long-term follow-up has not shown markedly improved results with this technique (21). In addition, results of the open palm technique are better at the MP joint than at the PIP joint, where full-thickness grafts yield the best result. Thus, in presence of PIP joint contracture, a combination of open palm technique and skin grafting in the affected digits can be used (13). As an alternative, full-thickness skin grafts can be used to close both the digits and the palm, giving satisfactory results (22).

PROCEDURE

The goal of an operation in Dupuytren's disease is to correct the contracture at the MP and PIP joints and to minimize the risk of recurrence. There are three basic components to the operative technique: exposure of fascia, identification of the neurovascular bundle, and excision of fascia (4,13).

The specific incision used is affected by the location of the disease, whether one or more rays are involved, and the surgeon's familiarity and experience with a particular type of incision. If more than one ray is involved, a transverse incision in the palm may be more desirable than a single longitudinal incision.

The exposure of fascia in the palm and the fingers is made easier by keeping a few key anatomic relationships in mind. In the proximal palm, there is a layer of subcutaneous tissue between the fascia and the overlying skin. The subcutaneous layer needs to be incised down to the fascia, and it is easy to develop a plane overlying the fascia in this area. Distally, the fascia becomes progressively closer to the skin; and at the level of the distal palmar crease, the fascia lies just under the skin. This relationship is preserved in the proximal digit. Distal to the middle crease of the finger, there is a subcutaneous layer between the skin and the fascia.

It is also important to note the relationship of the fascia to the flexor tendon sheath: In the palm, the fascia and the flexor tendon sheath are in close proximity; whereas in the proximal phalanx, there is a layer of areolar tissue separating the two. Distal to the PIP joint, the fascia adheres to the tendon sheath, and care must be taken during this part of the dissection to avoid injuring the sheath.

The dissection of the neurovascular bundle may be done distal or proximal or proximal to distal. With significant MP or PIP contracture, the neurovascular bundle may be easier to find proximally in the palm if less disease is present in this location. At the distal crease of the finger, the bundle is just deep to Grayson's ligament. The safest approach is blunt dissection and separation of the fascia

just millimeters at a time, as the bundle may be displaced by a spiral cord. Close to the MP joint, the neurovascular bundle should be followed and released proximally to the level of the MP joint, where it lies in a layer of loose areolar tissue. At this level, the bundle lies deep to the natatory ligament. In the presence of disease, the natatory cord is divided; and the bundle is followed to the level of the distal crease of the palm, where it lies deep to the transverse fibers of the palmar aponeurosis. It is usually sufficient to dissect and expose the neurovascular bundle to this level. The further exposure and excision of the diseased fascia in the palm is dictated by the location and extent of disease.

The excision of fascia can be started proximally or distally. McFarlane (3) advocates dividing the pretendinous cords in the palm as a first step, especially in patients with severe MP joint contracture. Straightening of the MP joint makes dissection in the finger easier. The excision of the diseased fascia is then performed starting distally at the distal crease of the finger. The diseased fascia in the finger is composed of the central, spiral, lateral, and retrovascular cords and is removed en bloc and in continuity with the pretendinous cords in the palm. In the finger, the fascia is meticulously dissected off each neurovascular bundle with slow proximal advancement.

Branches of the digital artery are cauterized with bipolar electrocautery. Some of the cutaneous branches of the digital nerve might need to be divided. At the proximal crease of the finger, the previously divided natatory ligament is excised with the neurovascular bundle exposed at all times. The excision continues into the palm, and all of the diseased pretendinous cords are removed. If any of the neurovascular bundles are injured, they should be repaired.

COMPLICATIONS

The estimates of overall complications have been as high as 20% (4). The most frequent complication is loss of flexion in the affected digit. Protecting against swelling and stiffness and early aggressive therapy help guard against this complication.

Reflex sympathetic dystrophy is the next most frequent postoperative complication; it is more common in women. Burning pain in the fingers and palm; swelling; and limitation of hand, elbow, or shoulder movement should raise the suspicion of this diagnosis, which if established requires prompt and aggressive treatment. Inadvertent division of the digital artery or nerve can be avoided by careful dissection and exposure of the neurovascular bundle. Division of the pretendinous cord and release of the MP contracture renders this dissection easier, as does placing the bundle on some tension by abducting the adjacent digits. In the event of injury to the nerve or the artery, repair should be undertaken.

Hematoma, infection, and skin loss are three common complications that are often inter-related. They are best avoided by taking preoperative and intraoperative precautions, such as cleansing and meticulous hemostasis and technique.

REHABILITATION

The goal of postoperative management in Dupuytren's disease is to maintain extension at the previously contracted joints while preserving flexion and restoring the overall function of the hand (13). Elevation of the hand is crucial during the first 24 to 48 h postsurgery. This decreases the risk of swelling, stiffness, and sympathetic dystrophy. A static splint is used during the immediate postoperative period to protect from scar contracture during the early healing process. The wrist is held in the neutral position, while the MP and the IP joints are held in extension. The splint is usually required for at least 3 months, but duration depends on the severity of the disease. The splint is worn around the clock for the first 2 weeks. After the 10th day postsurgery, the splint is removed for daily range of motion exercises, starting with passive and progressing to active exercises. It is sometimes beneficial to use the splint at night for an additional period of time.

Though postoperative loss of extension is uncommon at the MP joint, it is relatively common at the PIP joint, especially in the fifth digit. This is probably secondary to the attenuation of the central slip of the extensor mechanism, caused by prolonged flexion contracture. In such cases, a small splint can be devised for the little finger to keep the PIP in extension for an additional period of time.

Early mobilization is the key factor in preventing scar contracture. Range of motion exercises are best initiated early in the postoperative period, as described above. The frequency of these exercises is part of the postoperative rehabilitation regimen to help with restoration of hand function. Other useful modalities include heat therapy to help with early mobilization and pressure or silicone sheet therapy for scar management.

SPECIAL CONSIDERATIONS

Dupuytren's in the Fifth Digit

The fifth digit has special characteristics. In Dupuytren's disease, it is often more severely afflicted than the other digits, and the disease is usually more extensive on the ulnar side of the finger. Only in the little finger does the lateral cord cause severe PIP joint contracture. The lateral cord together with the spiral cord can severely distort the anatomy of the neurovascular bundle, making its dissection particularly difficult. Also of note is that the fascia distal to the DIP joint is often involved, even in the absence of DIP joint contracture. For this reason, it is best to extend the incision and dissection of the fifth digit beyond the DIP joint.

Like in the other digits, MP joint contracture can usually be corrected. In the fifth digit, more than in the other digits, PIP joint contracture can be improved but not completely corrected. McFarlane (13) reports a success rate of less of 20% for PIP joint contracture release. Application of a full-thickness skin graft is associated with the lowest postoperative contracture. A skin graft instead of primary suture closure is recommended in the presence of severe disease in the fifth digit or flexion contracture at the PIP joint in excess of 45°.

Knuckle Pads and Nodules

For a painful palmar nodule or knuckle pad, relief can be attempted by steroid injections. Repeated injections for palmar nodules have been advocated; but they are not recommended for knuckle pads, because of the risk of attenuation of the underlying extensor tendon and the overlying thin skin. For persistently painful nodules and knuckle pads, excision can be considered. In the case of palmar nodules, the associated pretendinous cord and the adjacent normal fascia should be excised with the nodule. This prevents recurrence of the nodule and disease in this area.

Knuckle pads are located just under the skin overlying the extensor tendon. They typically adhere to the extensor paratenon and must be dissected off carefully to avoid injuring the extensor tendon. They must be completely excised to minimize the chance of recurrence (13).

Recurrent Contracture

Recurrent disease usually consists of recurrent PIP contracture. The exact incidence is difficult to determine, but it has decreased with improving surgical techniques. Recurrences are mostly attributed to inadequate initial excision of fascia and a strong diathesis. Surgery for recurrent disease is made difficult by the presence of scar tissue, especially around the neurovascular bundles. It is important to assess the intactness of each neurovascular bundle before embarking on redissection.

McFarlane (13) recommends the following approach for recurrent disease (13): Completion fasciectomy is recommended when recurrent disease is thought to be caused by inadequate excision at the initial operation. Dermatofasciectomy is the best option when recurrence is the result of a strong diathesis and aggressive disease is present. For patients with multiple recurrences and fixed PIP contractures of 60° to 90°, PIP replacement arthroplasty or arthrodesis with bony shortening is recommended. With arthroplasty, there is usually a residual flexion contracture, but a range of movement of at least 40° can be achieved.

SUMMARY

The cause of Dupuytren's disease remains unclear. It is a potentially disabling condition that affects many patients each year. Operative intervention is the definitive treatment modality, and contractures at the MP joint are more amenable to complete correction than those at the PIP joint. Regional fasciectomy is the procedure of choice in most cases. To minimize the risk of recurrence in the fingers, extensive fasciectomy in these areas is recommended. The principles of postoperative management should be followed to promote wound healing and prevent possible complications.

REFERENCES

1. Dupuytren's G. De la retraction de doigts par suite d'une affection de l'apponeurose palmaire. J Univ Med Chir (Paris) 1831; 5:352.
2. Hueston JT. Dorsal Dupuytren's disease. J Hand Surg 1982; 7A:384–387.
3. McFarlane RM. The current status of Dupuytren's disease. J Hand Surg 1983;8A:703–708.
4. McFarlane RM. Dupuytren's disease. In: McCarthy JG, ed. Plastic surgery. Vol. 8: The hand. Philadelphia: Saunders, 1990: 5053–5085.
5. Luck JV. Dupuytren's contracture: a new concept of pathogenesis correlated with surgical management. J Bone Joint Surg 1959; 41A:635.
6. Ryan GB, Cliff WJ, Gabbiani G, et al. Myofibroblasts in human granulation tissue. Hum Pathol 1974;5:55–67.
7. Bailey AJ, Sims TJ, Gabbiani G, et al. Collagen of Dupuytren's disease. Clin Sci Mol Med 1977;53:499–502.
8. Chiu HF, McFarlane RM. Pathogenesis of Dupuytren's contracture: a correlative clinical-pathological study. J Hand Surg 1978;3A:1–10.
9. Gelberman RH, Amiel D, Rudolph MR, Vance RM. Dupuytren's contracture. An electron microscopic, biochemical, and clinical correlative study. J Bone Joint Surg 1980;62A:425–432.
10. Gabbiani G, Chapponier C, Huttner I. Cytoplasmic filaments and gap junctions in epithelial cells and myofibroblasts during wound healing. J Cell Biol 1978;76:561–568.
11. Tomasek JJ, Schultz RJ, Haaksma CJ. Extracellular matrix-cytoskeletal connections at the surface of the specialized contractile fibroblast (myofibroblast) in Dupuytren disease. J Bone Joint Surg 1987;69A:1400–1407.
12. Legge JW, Finlay JB, McFarlane RM. A study of Dupuytren's tissue with the scanning electron microscope. J Hand Surg 1981;5A: 482–492.
13. McFarlane RM. Dupuytren's contracture. In: Green DP, ed. Operative hand surgery. Vol. 1. New York: Churchill Livingstone, 1993:563–591.
14. Tubiana R, Simmons BP, Defrenne HA. Location of Dupuytren's disease on the radial aspect of the hand. Clin Orthop 1982; 168:222–229.
15. McFarlane RM. Patterns of the diseased fascia in the fingers in Dupuytren's contracture. Plast Reconstr Surg 1974;54:31–44.
16. Thomine JM. The development and anatomy of the digital fascia. In: Tubiana R, ed. Dupuytren's contracture. 2nd ed. Paris: Expansion Scientific Francais, 1972:3–12.
17. Colville J. Dupuytren's contracture—the role of fasciotomy. Hand 1983;15:162–166.
18. Rowley DI, Couch M, Chesney RB, Norris SH. Assessment of percutaneous fasciotomy in the management of Dupuytren's contracture. J Hand Surg 1984;9B:163–164.
19. Gonzalez RI. Dupuytren's contracture of the fingers: a simplified approach to surgical treatment. Calif Med 1971;115:25–31.
20. McCash CR. The open palm technique in Dupuytren's contracture. Br J Plast Surg 1964;17:271.
21. Schneider LH, Hankin FM, Eisenberg T. Surgery of Dupuytren's disease: a review of the open palm method. J Hand Surg 1986; 11A:23–27.
22. Ketchum LD, Hixson FP. Dermofasciectomy and full-thickness grafts in the treatment of Dupuytren's contracture. J Hand Surg 1987;12A:659–664.

Tumors of the Hand and Forearm

The incidence of true neoplasms of the hand and forearm is extremely small, and most masses seen in the hand would be better classified as tumor-like conditions. It is estimated that approximately 95% of all masses in the hand are reactive rather than true neoplasms (Table 12.1).

True neoplasms of the hand may be classified as benign, benign but aggressive, and malignant tumors. The incidence of benign lesions is much greater than is that of malignant ones. In fact, malignant tumors of the hand are so uncommon that there are few large series with enough data from which to make definitive statements about treatment and outcome. Much of the treatment of malignant tumors of the hand has been extrapolated from treatment of similar tumors arising elsewhere in the musculoskeletal system. The exception is malignant skin lesions (basal cell carcinoma, squamous carcinoma, and malignant melanoma), for which extrapolation from other areas is more applicable.

Since most of the tumors arising in the hand are not neoplasms and because the majority are benign, clinicians can become complacent regarding the diagnosis and treatment of tumors in this location. Of course, to regard a malignant tumor in the hand (as elsewhere) as benign and to treat it as such, with less than adequate surgical excision, is to complicate any further surgery and, in some cases, to preclude sparing of the extremity. The emphasis of this chapter is not only to present the common lesions seen in the hand and their treatment but also to sharpen the accuracy of the preoperative diagnosis to avoid missing and mistreating the statistically rare, but potentially life- and limb-threatening, malignant tumor. To quote a famous surgeon, "What your mind knows, your eye sees."

MEDICAL HISTORY

The medical history is extremely important in helping the clinician arrive at the correct diagnosis. The patient's age, sex, handedness, and occupation suggest certain diagnoses and rule out others. For example, a fibrous nodule arising in the palm of a child could be juvenile aponeurotic fibroma, an extremely aggressive lesion with a high likelihood of recurrence. That same lesion in a 65-year-old male would very likely be a Dupuytren's nodule, a benign condition that progresses slowly over a period of years.

The duration of symptoms can also help the physician with the differential diagnosis. Generally, lesions that have existed for many years are much less likely to be malignant than are those that arise over a short period of time. Exceptions to this rule exist, however; and it is not uncommon for some very malignant tumors to have been present for years before the current rapid growth is noted. Lesions that enlarge and then recede (e.g., ganglion, sebaceous cyst) are in all cases benign and usually imply a cystic lesion with changes in the content of the cyst. Inflammatory lesions (tenosynovitis) can also behave in this manner. Rapid rate of growth can imply a briskly dividing malignant tumor, but the common dorsal wrist ganglion can literally appear overnight, especially after vigorous physical activity (Fig. 12.1). Therefore, absolute conclusions based on the mass's rate of growth cannot be made.

The presence or absence of pain can help establish a working diagnosis. A ganglion, particularly when small, can elicit pain, often aggravated by activity. Enchondroma presenting as a pathologic fracture in a proximal phalanx, for

| table | 12.1 | Common Tumor-Like Conditions of the Hand |

Ganglion
Giant cell tumor of the tendon sheath (pigmented villonodular synovitis)
Dupuytren's nodule
Epidermoid inclusion cyst
Sebaceous cyst
Pyogenic granuloma
Fungal or tubercular infection

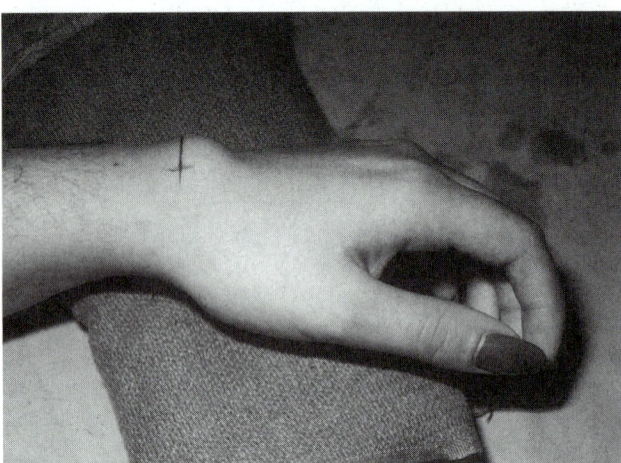

Figure 12.1. Clinical appearance of a dorsal wrist ganglion.

instance, is also painful. Generally, malignant lesions are not painful unless they cause pathologic fracture or invade bone, tendon, or nerve. Pain at night is a particularly ominous symptom in regard to malignancy, but it is also seen with infection.

A history of preexisting medical conditions, such as malignancies that are known to have a predilection for bony metastases (lung, kidney, thyroid, gastrointestinal, breast), can help the clinician assess destructive lesions in the bones of the hand (1). So-called acrometastases are often misdiagnosed as an infectious process. The patient's occupation can be important when it is possible that repeated trauma, actinic exposure, x-ray exposure, or chemical exposure is an inciting factor for malignant transformation, especially in the skin.

INITIAL FINDINGS, PHYSICAL EXAMINATION, AND DIAGNOSIS

The physical examination, in conjunction with the history, will probably yield the most information regarding the correct diagnosis. The location of the lesion is important, because some tumors occur in characteristic locations. Dorsal wrist ganglia nearly always arise from the dorsal portion of the scapholunate interosseous ligament. They emerge at the level of the radiocarpal joint between the third and fourth extensor compartments. Lipomas have a predilection for the first web space, although they can occur elsewhere in the palm and forearm. It is unusual to find them out in the fingers, where there is less fat to begin with. Although enchondroma can occur in any of the tubular bones of the hand, the proximal phalanx is most common location. Giant cell tumor of the tendon sheath (pigmented villonodular synovitis; PVNS) probably arises within the joint emerging at the vinculum of the flexor tendon sheath. As such, it is usually found eccentrically adjacent to the proximal interphalangeal (PIP) or the distal interphalangeal (DIP) joint if it extends subcutaneously. If a giant cell tumor is in the flexor sheath itself, it can extend proximally or distally, making complete excision difficult. Retinacular cysts (ganglions of the tendon sheath) arise in or near the A1 pulley. Nerve tumors, such as neurilemmoma or neurofibroma, are found along the course of the nerves. Malignant tumors, especially if they are large, tend to be found beyond their tissue of origin and do not respect normal boundaries.

The examining physician should measure the size of the tumor accurately (with a ruler, not an estimate) and record it in the patient's record. Certain lesions are characteristically small, such as the 2- to 3-mm retinacular cyst. Lipomas hidden in the first web space can grow to be quite large before being clinically noticeable. The prognosis for sarcomas bigger than 5 cm is significantly worse than for smaller tumors. Discoloration or pigmentation, particularly of skin and nail bed lesions, may suggest melanoma. Vascular tumors often appear bluish under the skin because of the Tindall effect.

Palpation of the mass yields additional information. Is it soft or firm? Mobile or fixed? What structures are affected? Sometimes the size of a mass can be estimated only by palpation, taking into account the thickness of the skin. It is extremely helpful to ascertain in what tissue plane the tumor resides. The physician should be able to determine if it is in the skin or the subcutaneous tissues; is attached to the palmar fascia, deep fascia, or retinaculum; involves the muscles or tendons, or is within bone or periosteum. If the clinician knows the anatomy in a given region, he or she should be able to localize the depth of a tumor and determine what structures are involved. Such information is important not only for diagnosis but also for staging. Palpation tests the tenderness of the mass. Inflammatory or infectious lesions are tender, whereas most neoplasms are not; ganglions can be tender to palpation. Through palpation, the clinician can often determine if the mass is solid or cystic. Pulsations suggest a vascular origin; however, arterial pulsations can be transmitted by other structures, especially those filled with a dense fluid, giving the erroneous impression of a pulsatile mass. Volar wrist ganglion adjacent to the radial artery can be misdiagnosed as an aneurysm.

Simple clinical tests can be performed to enhance diagnostic accuracy with minimal expense. Of these, the transillumination test is quite valuable. An otoscope with a black earpiece concentrates and specifically directs the light on the lesion with a minimum of scatter. Clinical testing of nerve function can identify nerve involvement by the tumor. Benign nerve tumors, particularly when small, do not cause nerve dysfunction; however, when large they may create sufficient pressure to alter function. Even lipomas in a confined space, such as Guyon's canal, can present with nerve dysfunction. Any malignant lesion invading a nerve causes pain and loss of function. Allen's test helps assess vascular compromise in the hand or wrist. Knowledge of vascular patency is important when planning surgical treatment, and Doppler ultrasound can help determine flow in vessels in which a pulse cannot be palpated. Finally, in cases for which the diagnosis is uncertain or a malignancy is suspected, clinical examination of regional lymph nodes (epitrochlear and axillary) assists in staging.

RADIOLOGIC STUDIES

The simplest and most convenient diagnostic study is plain radiography. For ganglions, retinacular cysts, and most skin lesions, radiography is unnecessary, although occasionally, dorsal wrist ganglion can have an intraosseous component that would be detected on radiographs. Plain film radiography can detect bony involvement and pathologic fracture and is diagnostic for enchondroma, osteochondroma, and hemangioma. Bony erosions are frequently seen with giant cell tumor of the tendon sheath. Calcifications may be seen not only in cartilage tumors but also in soft tissue tumors, such as synoviosarcoma. Depending on their substance, foreign bodies may be visible on plain radiographs.

Diagnostic ultrasound is most useful for distinguishing solid from cystic masses and is especially useful in making the diagnosis of occult dorsal wrist ganglion. It is good for establishing the location and depth of a mass but, with the exception of the dorsal wrist ganglion, is not helpful in establishing a diagnosis. Real-time ultrasonography can be used to visualize flexor tendons, and their excursion and will show lesions moving with the tendons. The simplest diagnostic test for lesions that transilluminate and seem to be cystic is aspiration (Fig. 12.2). For ganglions, aspiration may be therapeutic as well as diagnostic. A negative aspiration test implies a solid lesion; and biopsy, whether incisional or excisional, should be performed. Needle biopsy can be used to establish a histologic diagnosis of larger masses with suspected malignancy, although tumors in the hand are seldom large enough to recommend this.

Computed transaxial tomography (CTT) is of limited use in the evaluation of tumors of the hand and most helpful for bony lesions. For most cases, CTT has been replaced by MRI for evaluation of both the bony and soft tissue components of tumors. Some masses, such as ganglion, lipoma, hemangioma, and giant cell tumor of the tendon sheath, have characteristic signals that can assist in

the diagnosis. In addition, information about the extent of the mass and its proximity to important anatomical structures can be obtained, which helps in planning surgery. Magnetic resonance angiography (MRA) provides information about the vascularity of a mass; atypical vascularity or neovascularity suggests a malignant tumor.

TREATMENT

One of the simplest treatments for tumors of the hand is observation, which is reasonable if the diagnosis has been established. For other lesions, a finite period of observation, watching for change in size or other characteristics, may be recommended, provided that the patient is not lost to follow-up. If the mass regresses, it may have been infectious or inflammatory. Ganglia are well known to arise and disappear spontaneously. Masses that increase in size, with the exception of ganglions, should be excised or biopsied to establish a diagnosis. Observation is also appropriate treatment for small hemangiomas.

As discussed earlier, aspiration not only is helpful for diagnosis of ganglions but may also be therapeutic. Treatment by aspiration is really limited to ganglions, but it is useful when unsuccessful as a diagnostic test.

The importance of biopsying a potentially malignant tumor—even when the diagnosis is believed to be benign but is still not established—cannot be too heavily emphasized (2). Although most tumors found in the hand are benign, when the diagnosis is not certain, the surgeon should proceed with the assumption that it is malignant. Hand surgeons are fond of transverse or zigzag incisions, because they are cosmetically superior to straight longitudinal incisions and are designed to minimize scar contracture. The biopsy incision, however, is best designed as follows. Mark out the incision as if an en bloc resection of the tumor, with adequate margins, were to be done. Place the biopsy incision in the center of the proposed incision for definitive treatment. In nearly all cases, this will be a

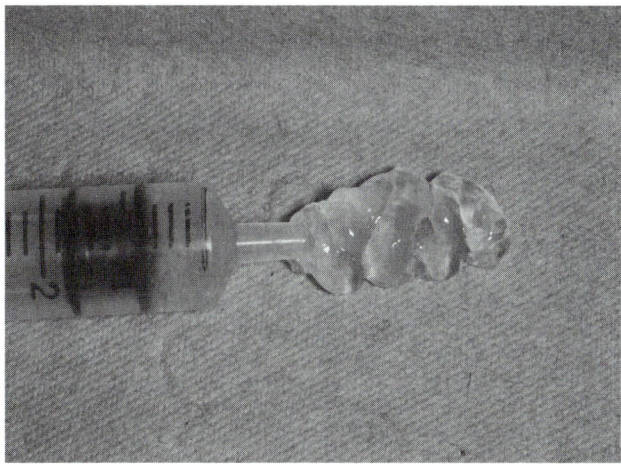

Figure 12.2. Characteristic mucinous material obtained at aspiration of a ganglion.

longitudinal incision aligned with the axis of the extremity. If additional surgery is required, the biopsy incision can be excised en bloc with the tumor mass via an elliptical incision.

Most small tumors in the hand can be treated by an excisional biopsy, which represents a marginal excision. If the lesion turns out to be benign, then no further surgery is likely to be necessary. If malignancy is suspected at the outset or if surgical exposure of the mass reveals atypical tissue, then an incisional biopsy can be performed. This technique has the advantage of not spreading tumor cells through the subcutaneous tissue planes and, if preoperative chemotherapy is used, leaves some tumor to follow clinically for therapeutic effect. In larger masses that are not located near important nerves or vessels, needle biopsy may be appropriate; however, it is seldom used in the hand.

Ganglion

The ganglion is the most common mass seen in the hand. Although it can present in any age group, it is most common in adolescents and young adults. It usually presents as a painless mass on the dorsum of the wrist overlying the scapholunate interval. It may seem to arise overnight; however, it is more likely that the appearance represents the mass making its way superficial to the extensor retinaculum. Often patients will have complained of dorsal wrist pain, aggravated by physical activity, before the onset of the mass. Pain on wrist dorsiflexion and the inability to do a pushup are characteristic symptoms and can be helpful in the diagnosis of the small, or occult, ganglion.

Ganglions may present in other locations besides the dorsum of the wrist, including—in order of frequency—at the volar radiocarpal joint, emerging adjacent to the radial artery; between the A1 and A2 pulleys in the finger, emerging at the digital palmar flexion crease (retinacular cyst); and at the DIP joint in an older individual (mucus cyst) related to early degenerative joint disease and always related to an intra-articular loose body. Ganglions arise as a mucoid degeneration of dense fibrous connective tissue and, therefore, can also arise in any joint capsule, ligament, tendon, and even bone (intraosseous ganglion). Another common location is on the first dorsal compartment associated with de Quervain's tenosynovitis.

On physical examination, ganglions may be hard or soft, large or small, fixed or mobile. Many feel clearly cystic in nature, but others may be tense and hard enough that they feel almost like bone. This finding is especially common at the first dorsal compartment. The diagnosis is easily made by the characteristic history and location and can be confirmed by the transillumination test. Difficulty arises with the small dorsal wrist ganglion, which is usually more painful than its larger counterpart, perhaps from pressure on the posterior interosseous nerve. The examination may be normal, except for a slight restriction of wrist dorsiflexion and tenderness to deep palpation over

the scapholunate interval. Compared to the opposite wrist, a small, firm, tender mass may be felt. The transillumination test is useless for an occult ganglion, and other imaging studies may be necessary to confirm the diagnosis.

Plain radiographs of the wrist are usually normal with the diagnosis of ganglion, but they help rule out other pathologic causes of wrist pain. Occasionally, an intra-osseous component may be seen on plain films, especially in the scaphoid or lunate, because the ganglion arises in a degenerated portion of the dorsal scapholunate interosseous ligament. Ultrasound is a sensitive, noninvasive diagnostic tool for the detection of occult ganglion. MRI is equally sensitive and far more specific, giving information about the ganglion and the surrounding ligaments, but at a far greater expense.

Treatment of ganglions runs the full spectrum from benign neglect to surgical excision. If the symptoms are minimal and the diagnosis is established with certainty, there is no reason to excise the mass. A reasonable plan of treatment is to aspirate the ganglion to confirm the diagnosis by obtaining the characteristic mucinous fluid, which will also make the cyst disappear, at least temporarily. The chance is better than even that it will return, but often the symptoms are less bothersome. If the ganglion returns and is symptomatic, then surgical excision is recommended. It does not make sense to repeatedly aspirate a ganglion. Special care must be taken when aspirating a volar wrist ganglion, because of the proximity of the radial artery and the size of the needle (18 gauge) required to aspirate the thick mucin. An occult dorsal wrist ganglion is usually impossible to aspirate because it is small and difficult to localize. They are usually more painful than the larger ganglions; so once confirmed by ultrasound or MRI, they are probably best dealt with by surgery (Fig. 12.3). Retinacular cysts, on the other hand, respond well to aspiration and usually do not recur.

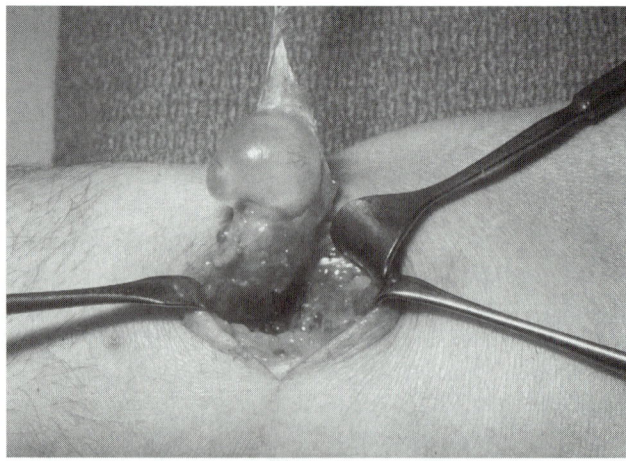

Figure 12.3. Intraoperative appearance of a dorsal wrist ganglion arising from the scapholunate joint.

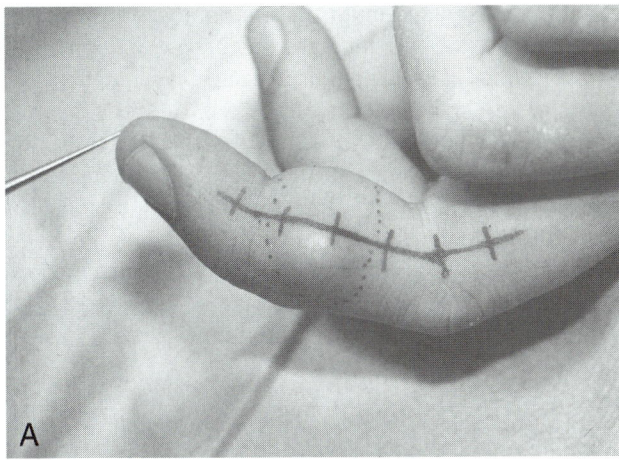

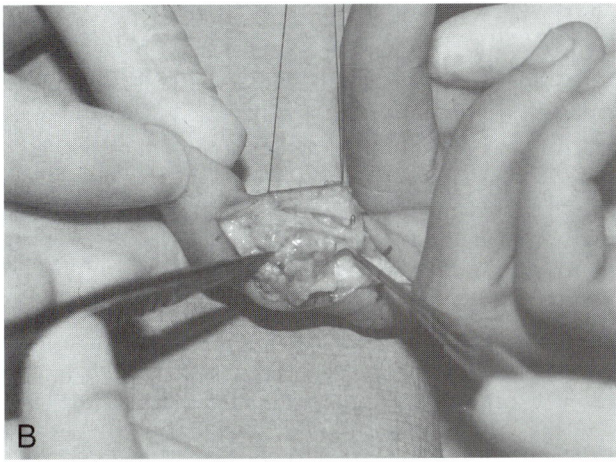

Figure 12.4. A. Clinical appearance of a GCT of the tendon sheath. **B.** Displacement of the neurovascular bundle by a GCT.

Giant Cell Tumor of the Tendon Sheath.

Giant cell tumor (GCT) of the tendon sheath (nodular tenosynovitis) presents as a painless, eccentric mass in the finger that has been present for several months to years and has been slowly enlarging (Fig. 12.4). Not seen in children, it is most common in the third through seventh decade, with a peak in the fourth decade. Histologically, the tumor is identical to PVNS as seen in larger joints. The term *xanthoma*, formerly used because of the tumor's yellow and brown appearance, is no longer correct and should be reserved for another lesion.

On examination, the mass is firm, rubbery, and nontender; it restricts joint motion only by virtue of its large size. The mass is located adjacent to the PIP or DIP joint and is fixed to the deep soft tissues (tendon sheath, joint capsule) but not to bone. They are most common (75%) on the volar side of the finger and can be traced back to the origin of the vincula or volar recess of the interphalangeal joint. Lesions found on the dorsum of the finger usually arise from one of the interphalangeal joints. The transillumination test is negative. Nerve deficit is unusual before surgical intervention. Arising from the joint near the vin-

cula, the tumor often follows the course of the branch to the vincula from the digital artery. This explains the eccentric location of the mass and its intimate attachment to the digital neurovascular bundle, often wrapping circumferentially around that structure.

The most helpful diagnostic studies are plain radiographs, which may show cortical erosion that is usually eccentric and retrocondylar. MRI studies can be particularly useful in difficult situations, not only because these images give information about the location of the tumor and its relationship to adjacent structures but also because hemosiderin (a ferromagnetic compound) displays a characteristic signal that can be diagnostic.

Treatment of GCT of the tendon sheath is by complete surgical excision. The characteristic gross appearance of the tumor—lipid-laden macrophages (yellow) and hemosiderin deposits (brown)—makes intraoperative diagnosis fairly accurate and frozen section unnecessary (Fig. 12.5). Careful marginal excision is probably curative, but intralesional excision results in recurrence. These tumors often extend proximally or distally in the tendon sheath, increasing the possibility that tumor will be left behind. They may also persist in the joint itself, resulting in intra-articular recurrence. DIP joint involvement may mimic a mucous cyst, but the transillumination test is negative. With primary, advanced joint involvement or recurrent tumor, especially with intra-articular involvement, arthrodesis of the joint may be necessary to control disease. The recurrence rate following surgery varies from 17 to 30%.

Enchondroma

Enchondroma is the most common tumor of bone arising in the hand. The usual presentation is pain from a pathologic fracture, usually from a minor traumatic incident (Fig. 12.6). Occasionally they will be discovered as an incidental finding on radiographs. They may present at

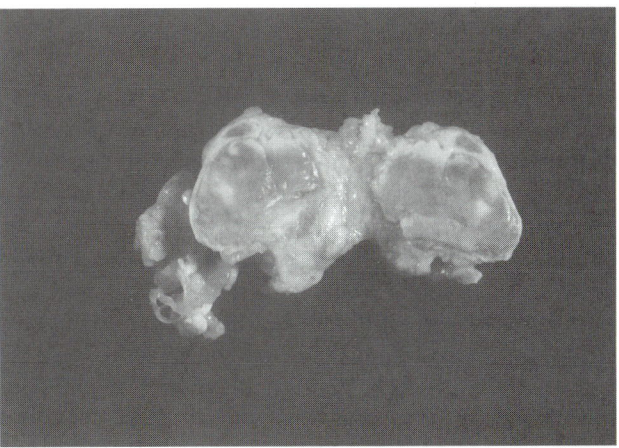

Figure 12.5. Gross appearance of the cut surface of a GCT, with xanthomatous and hemosiderin-pigmented areas.

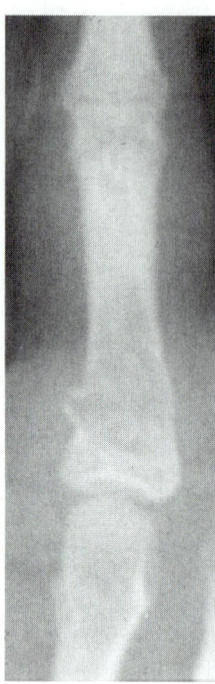

Figure 12.6. Pathologic fracture through an area of enchondroma in a proximal phalanx.

any age but usually appear after skeletal maturity. Lesions may present in several bones in Ollier's disease or Maffucci's syndrome, with multiple, localized bony expansions with or without pathologic fracture.

On examination, there is pain and swelling with ecchymosis, as seen with any fracture. The diagnosis is made radiographically at the time of fracture evaluation. More complex studies or imaging is unnecessary. In the hand, long bones with epiphyseal growth plates (metacarpals and phalanges) are involved, but not carpal bones. The base of the proximal phalanx is the most common location. Plain radiographic appearance of enchondroma is characterized by expansion of the cortex of the bone by a lytic, benign-appearing endosteal process. The cortical margin, although thinned, is always present and usually demonstrates a pathologic fracture. The lytic component has a ground glass appearance and may exhibit areas of punctate calcification within the cartilage matrix.

Treatment of enchondroma begins with treatment of the fracture. Because the energy required to fracture the expanded, weakened bone is minimal, the fracture is rarely badly displaced, as is often seen with traumatic phalangeal fractures. Transverse fracture configurations are also more common than spiral or oblique ones. Closed reduction and cast or splint immobilization are adequate for primary fracture healing. After 3 to 4 weeks, a sufficient callus has formed to lend stability to the fracture, and pain is diminished or absent. At this point, treatment of the enchondroma can be undertaken.

Thorough curettage of the lytic area and bone grafting with either autograft or allograft is the treatment of choice. Although the need for grafting has been questioned by some (3), most surgeons still use a bone graft, which not only assists in the healing of the fracture and lytic area but also, by virtue of its radiodense appearance, helps detect tumor recurrences. Following curettage and grafting, the operative site must be protected against refracture with a cast or removable splint. Recurrence in enchondroma is unusual and must raise suspicions about the biologic activity of the tumor. Low-grade chondrosarcoma has been reported in cases of previous histologically benign chondrosarcoma. In such cases, curettage and cryosurgery or amputation are necessary to control disease.

Nerve Tumors

Benign tumors of nerve sheath origin are not uncommon in the hand and fall into two major types: neurofibroma, arising from the cells responsible for the fibrous supporting structure of peripheral nerves (endoneurium and perineurium), and neurilemmoma, or Schwannoma, arising from the Schwann cells that produce the myelin axon sheaths (Fig. 12.7). These lesions are seldom seen in adults before the fourth decade. Being of nerve origin, they arise along the course of known peripheral nerves or their branches but may occasionally arise in small, unnamed branches. They present as a painless, slowly growing mass that may have been present for many years. Pain or neurologic dysfunction is usually not a presenting complaint, except for those tumors that have grown to a large size in a confined area, such as the carpal tunnel or Guyon's canal. In such cases, symptoms are those of a compressive neuropathy of the affected nerve. Significant pain (especially at night) or sensorimotor loss should raise the suspicion of malignancy.

On examination, a firm, mobile mass can be palpated in the subcutaneous plane along the course of a peripheral nerve. The mass is usually not tender. Deep tumors, such as in the palm, may be difficult to palpate or can grow to an extremely large size before causing symptoms. The tran-

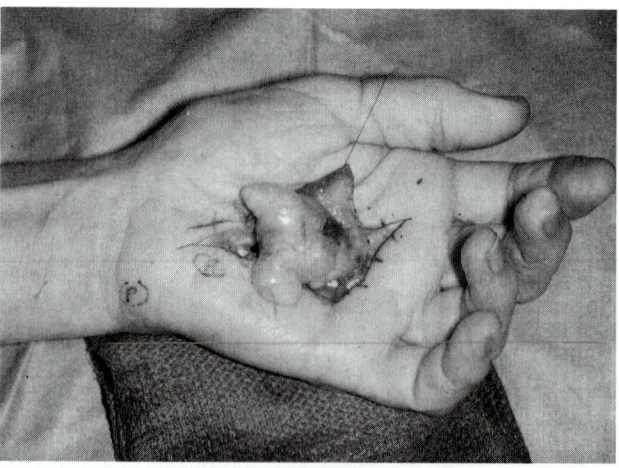

Figure 12.7. Large schwannoma arising from a small branch of the ulnar nerve deep in the palm. This patient presented with a low ulnar palsy from compression of the motor branch.

sillumination test indicates a solid tumor but may be equivocal in some Schwannomas because of the high lipid content. Although clinical nerve testing is certainly important as part of the preoperative assessment, it may not help make the diagnosis. It is necessary to document preoperative normal neurologic function, as it may change as a result of surgery. Nerve dysfunction, especially in those deep palmar tumors, can help localize the lesion (e.g., deep motor branch of the ulnar nerve).

For the superficial lesions, no further diagnostic workup is required before proceeding to surgical excision. For the deep palmar tumors, however, MRI is extremely useful for localizing the mass and its relationship to surrounding structures. Masses seen to arise within nerves on MRI scans suggest nerve sheath tumors. Neurilemmoma tends to be eccentric within the nerve, whereas neurofibroma has a more diffuse pattern. Neurofibroma of the median nerve has a characteristic magnetic resonance display: diffuse nerve involvement, dispersed fascicular bundles, and no suggestion of encapsulation. Neurilemmoma, on the other hand, has a more uniform, encapsulated appearance, with eccentric compression of the local neural tissue. These differences in internal nerve anatomy have significant implications for surgery, prognosis for recurrence, and postoperative neurologic deficit.

The treatment for these tumors is surgical excision. Although malignant nerve sheath tumors do exist (neurofibrosarcoma, malignant Schwannoma), they are rare, especially in the hand. The surgical approach to an unknown tumor in the palm, however, must take into account the possibility of malignancy, and incisions must be placed appropriately. Because of its encapsulated nature, neurilemmoma can usually be carefully dissected from the surrounding normal nerve tissue (marginal excision) with a minimum of postoperative neural deficit. The tumor is found to arise from a single small fascicle, which may need to be sacrificed during excision. Despite this, function usually remains unchanged from the preoperative state. Dissection of the tumor from the nerve is best performed with the operating microscope.

Excision of neurofibroma is a different situation because of the diffuse nature of the tumor within the nerve. An intralesional excision or a debulking procedure is normally done, which definitely requires the microscope. Complete nerve resection is necessary to completely excise the tumor, which can be done in conjunction with a nerve graft reconstruction. With a benign tumor, however, it is difficult to justify resecting the nerve, given its resultant disability. In most cases an intralesional excision is performed; the exception is a tumor arising in a small, purely sensory nerve that could be sacrificed with a minimal deficit. Unfortunately, neurofibroma seems to arise more commonly in a major peripheral mixed nerve. With incomplete excision, the patient must be cautioned about local recurrence (persistence).

There are many more kinds of benign tumors and tumor-like conditions that arise in the hand, and the diagnosis and treatment of all of them cannot be covered here. The examples given here illustrate principles of tumor diagnosis and treatment that can be applied to many different tumor types.

Malignant Tumors of the Hand

Although the diagnosis and treatment of malignant tumors in the hand that are extremely rare will not be discussed here, the important take-home lesson is to keep your index of suspicion high. Pain and rapid growth are unreliable indicators of malignancy. Epithelioid sarcoma, one of the most highly malignant lesions arising in the extremities, can be painless and slow growing and may have been present for several years before a diagnosis is made. In fact, its benign presentation can be extremely misleading, resulting in less than appropriately aggressive treatment. The comments earlier in this section regarding the biopsy of malignant tumors and the effect on the definitive surgery and outcome cannot be overstressed. It is an advantage for both the patient and the surgeon alike that malignant tumors of the hand are rare, but this fact does not excuse misdiagnosis and errors in treatment. If in doubt, refer the patient to someone familiar with these tumors.

SUMMARY

It is important for the clinician to be familiar with the characteristic clinical history, examination, and behavior of benign tumors and tumor-like conditions of the hand, since the majority of lesions in the hand are benign in nature. However, thorough recognition and understanding of the benign conditions serve an equally important purpose; i.e., that the more unusual tumor-like conditions of the hand can make the clinician more vigilant so that the rare malignant neoplasm is less likely to be overlooked, ignored, or not evaluated and worked up properly.

REFERENCES

1. Healy JH, Turnbull ADM, Miedema B, Lane JM. Acrometastases: a study of twenty-nine patients with osseous involvement of the hands and feet. J Bone Joint Surg 19866;8A:734.
2. Mankin H, Lange T, Spanier S. The hazards of biopsy in patients with malignant primary bone and soft tissue tumors. J Bone Joint Surg 1982;64A:1121–1127.
3. Hasselgren G, Forssblad P, Tornvall A. Bone grafting unnecessary in the treatment of enchondromas in the hand. J Hand Surg 1991;16A:139–142.

Selected Readings

Bogumill GB, Fleegler EJ, McFarland GB. Tumours of the hand and upper limb. (Hand & upper limb series no. 10). New York: Churchill Livingstone, 1993.

Diao E, Moy OJ. Common tumors. Orthop Clin North Am 1992; 23:187–196.

Mankin HJ. Principles of diagnosis and management of tumors of the hand. Hand Clin 1987;3:185–195.

Manske PR, ed. Hand surgery update. Park Ridge, IL: American Academy of Orthopaedic Surgeons, 1996.

Infections of the Hand and Wrist

Infections of the hand and wrist disseminate via anatomic compartments and planes and, therefore, may involve superficial skin, subcutaneous tissue, fascia, synovium, tendon sheaths, joints, and bone. The volar pulp of the finger pad and the perionychium of the nail are specialized compartments to the hand as well. This complex arrangement in tight quarters makes the hand susceptible to unique infectious processes (1).

PATHOGENESIS

Pathogens to the hand and wrist are introduced by direct penetration, are spread from local compartments, or are hematogenously disseminated. An understanding of the pathogenesis of typical hand infections is critical in making a timely diagnosis and instituting prompt treatment. The microorganisms most commonly found in pyogenic and cellulitis hand infections are *Staphylococcus aureus*, *Streptococcus* spp., and gram-negative bacteria. Numerous studies have shown that S. *aureus* is the principal pathogen in 50 to 80% of hand infections. Certain patterns of infectious processes are well described. Work-related and home-acquired injuries resulting in infection usually involve a single gram-positive organism. Infections secondary to intravenous drug use, farm- and soil-related injuries, bite wounds, and injuries in diabetics are often polymicrobial gram-positive, gram-negative, and anaerobic infections. α-Hemolytic *Streptococcus* and S. *aureus* are the most commonly found organisms in human bite infections; however, *Eikenella corrodens*, isolated in one-third of human bite infections, is more specific. *Pasteurella multocida* is the most common offending pathogen in infections from cat and dog bites and scratches. Unremitting and recalcitrant infections are often caused by atypical mycobacteria or fungi (1–3).

INITIAL FINDINGS, PHYSICAL EXAMINATION, AND DIAGNOSIS

As with all types of infections, the common initial findings in hand and wrist infections include edema, erythema, pain, and increase in warmth of the extremity. The presentation of the specific infections discussed below may be subtle, depending on the type of organism, route of administration, and specific anatomic location. To provide expeditious and optimal care, the physician must maintain a high index of suspicion and have an exacting understanding of the pathoanatomy. A thorough history and physical examination will usually allow the clinician to work through a differential algorithm and arrive at the likely source. Once the suspected source, route of administration, and probable organism are surmised, the culture and staining requests can be directed (1–3).

Physical examination should include evaluation for direct penetrating trauma or nidus; palpation for induration, fluctuance, and change in skin temperature; active and passive range of motion of each involved joint; and observation of hand posture, swelling, and color (1–3).

When specific bacterial, viral, or fungal microorganisms are suspected, the laboratory should be alerted to use specialized techniques. Standard aerobic and anaerobic cultures and Gram stain should always be performed. If atypical mycobacteria or *Nocardia* are suspected, Ziehl-Neelsen staining and cultures at 28° and 32°C in Lowenstein-Jensen medium must be performed. Examination for fungi uses a potassium hydroxide solution, Giemsa, or a silver stain. Herpes simplex virus may be identified with a Tzank smear of fluid from ruptured vesicles by demonstrating typical giant cells (1–3).

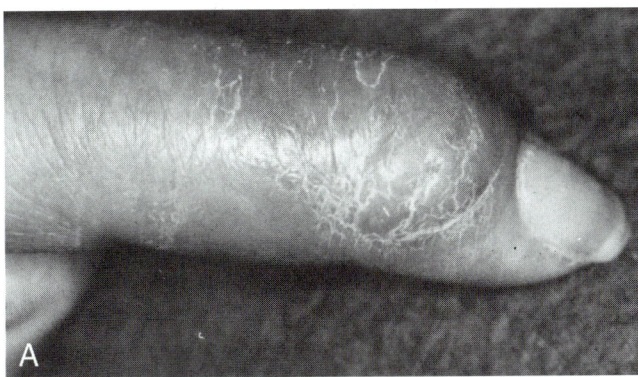

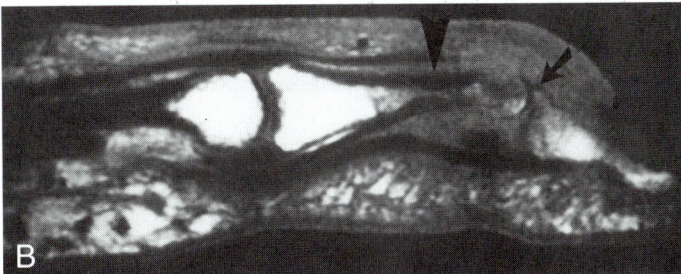

Figure 13.1. **A.** Index finger of a 50-year-old female 2 weeks after a dog bite. **B.** The sagittal MRI of the index finger demonstrates early onset of marrow edema of the middle phalanx (*arrowhead*) and a co-incident early involvement of the distal interphalangeal joint (*small arrow*), resulting in both osteomyelitis and septic arthritis.

RADIOLOGIC STUDIES

Plain films are useful for identifying a foreign body or nidus, bone lesions with a more advanced course of osteomyelitis, associated fractures, and the presence of gas formation in the soft tissues. Plain films in a minimum of two planes (90° to each other) should be the diagnostic standard when a hand or wrist infection is suspected.

A bone scan may find other distant foci of infection or multicentricity of disseminated hematogenous spread. The bone scan may be sensitive in defining an area of increased metabolic activity; yet this may not be specific for an infectious process. MRI is particularly useful for diagnosis of the earliest stage of osteomyelitis, before any plain x-ray changes are evident. MRI demonstrates the earliest changes in marrow edema that are consistent with osteomyelitis (Fig. 13.1). Although MRI is nearly 100% sensitive in delineating early osteomyelitis, it is far less specific. Marrow edema may be present in a number of disorders, as well as in postoperative healing tissues. The cost of these studies must always be weighed against the potential benefit to the patient in treatment alternatives. The clinician should always ask how the diagnostic test will affect the treatment plan (1–3).

GENERAL APPROACHES AND TREATMENT OPTIONS

A summary of the treatment approaches and options are outlined in Table 13.1 and the Clinical Table. Each type of hand infection has its own specific peculiarities; therefore, the approach must be individualized. Abrams and Botte (1) have reviewed the current thinking in the management of hand infections. Specific hand infections and their treatment are presented in the following section.

SPECIFIC INFECTIONS AND THEIR TREATMENT

Paronychia

Paronychia is an infection beneath the eponychial fold of the nail. A traumatic disruption of the tight seal between the nail plate and the eponychial fold allows a passageway for organisms. An abscess can form between the nail plate and the eponychial fold or may move more proximally and between the nail plate and nail matrix. Paronychia may be caused by nail biting, the stripping of the protective eponychial fold, poor nail hygiene and trimming, manicures, artificial nails, and chronic hangnails. The inciting organism is most commonly S. *aureus* (1,4,5) (Fig. 13.2).

Treatment is rarely adequate with oral antibiotics alone and usually requires appropriate drainage. Under sterile conditions, a digital block with 1 to 2% lidocaine without epinephrine will provide adequate anesthesia. A number 11 or 15 scalpel may be used to lift the eponychial fold off the nail plate, allowing the pus to be discharged. A small elevator or hemostat will aid in elevating the eponychial fold, and a small piece of gauze or sterile cotton will keep it open. If the clinician suspects that the abscess has tracked beneath the nail plate toward the matrix, the nail must be partially or completely removed (Fig. 13.3). This can be done atraumatically by placing a fine scissors di-

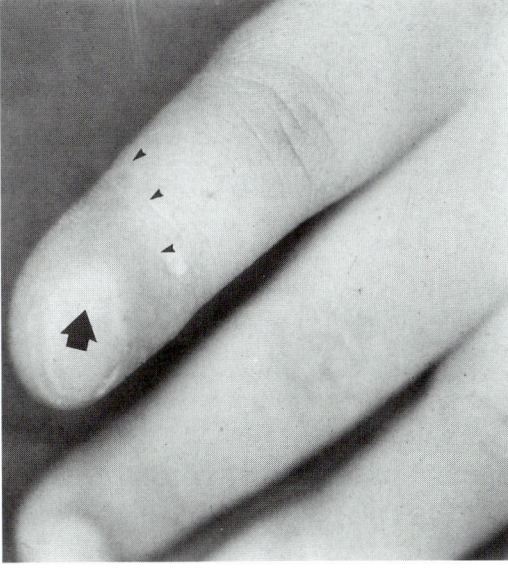

Figure 13.2. Middle finger of a 3-year-old boy with paronychia. The large *arrow* points to the localized collection of pus. The small *arrowheads* point to the extent of proximal migration dorsal to the infection.

| table | 13.1 | Empiric Antibiotic Recommendations for Hand Infections |

Infection	Possible Organisms	Antibiotic Dosage	Alternative Antibiotic Dosage
Felon, paronychia	S. *aureus*; oral anaerobes	Dicloxacillin, 250–500 mg PO q6h, *or* Nafcillin, 1–2 g IV q4–6h, *or* Clindamycin, 150–300 mg PO q6h	Cephalexin, 250–500 mg PO q6h *or* Cefazolin, 1 g IV q8h, *or* Erythromycin, 250–500 mg PO q6h
Flexor tenosynovitis	S. *aureus*; Streptococcus; gram-negative rods	Cefazolin, 1 g IV q8h	Nafcillin, 1–2 g IV q4–6h, or vancomycin, 1 g IV q12h, plus gentamicin,[a] *or* Imipenem, 0.5–1.0 g IV q6h
Herpetic whitlow	Herpes simplex virus	Consider acyclovir, 400 mg PO tid ×10 days	
Subcutaneous or deep-space abscess	S. *aureus*; anaerobes; gram-negative rods	Cefazolin, 1 g IV q8h, *or* Ampicillin-sulbactam, 1.5 mg IV q6h	Nafcillin, 1–2 g IV q4–6h, plus gentamicin,[a] *or* Imipenem, 0.5–1.0 g IV q6h
Cellulitis, lymphangitis	*Streptococcus, S. aureus*	Dicloxacillin, 250–500 mg PO q6h, *or* Nafcillin, 1–2 g IV q4–6h, *or* Cephalexin, 1 g IV q8h	Cephalexin, 250–500 mg PO q6h, *or* Erythromycin, 250–500 mg PO q6h
IV drug abuse–related	Gram positive, gram negative, or mixed, methicillin-resistant S. *aureus*	Nafcillin, 1–2 g IV q4–6h, plus gentamicin[a]	Vancomycin, 1 g IV q12h (for methicillin-resistant S. *aureus*), plus gentamicin[a] *or* Imipenem, 0.5–1.0 g IV q6h
Human bite	S. *aureus*; E. *corrodens*, Streptococcus, anaerobes	Cefazolin, 1 g IV q8h, plus penicillin, 2–4 million U IV q4–6h, *or* Clindamycin, 300 mg PO q6h, plus ciprofloxacin, 250–500 mg PO q12h, or trimethoprim-sulfamethoxazole (Septra DS) PO q12h	Nafcillin, 1–2 g, plus penicillin, 2–4 million U q4–6h, *or* Amoxicillin-clavulanate potassium, 250–500 mg PO q8h, *or* Ampicillin-sulbactam, 1.5 g IV q6h
Animal bite[b]	Gram-positive cocci; anaerobes; P. *multocida*	Cefazolin, 1 g IV q8h, plus penicillin, 2–4 million U IV q4–6h	Nafcillin, 1–2 g, plus penicillin, 2–4 million U q4–6h, *or* Amoxicillin-clavulanate potassium, 250–500 mg PO q8h, *or* Ampicillin-sulbactam, 1.5 g IV q6h
Diabetes related	Gram-positive cocci; gram-negative rods	Cefazolin, 1 g IV q8h, plus gentamicin[a]	Cefoxitin, 2 g IV q6h, *or* Ampicillin-sulbactam, 1.5 g IV q6h
Osteomyelitis	S. *aureus*, Streptococcus; (rarely) gram-negative rods	Cefazolin, 1 g IV q8h, plus gentamicin[a]	Nafcillin, 2 g IV q4h, *or* Vancomycin, 1 g IV q12h, *or* Clindamycin, 600–900 mg IV q8h, *or* Doxycycline, 100 mg PO q12h
Septic arthritis	S. *aureus*; Streptococcus (N. *gonorrhoeae*)	Cefazolin, 1 g IV q8h, *or* Ceftriaxone, 1 g IV q24h (for N. *gonorrhoeae*)	Nafcillin, 2 g IV q4h, *or* Vancomycin, 1 g IV q12h, *or* Clindamycin, 600–900 mg IV q8h, *or* Doxycycline, 100 mg PO q12h
Traumatic, contaminated woundc	S. *aureus*; Streptococcus; anaerobes; gram-negative rods	Imipenem, 0.5–1.0 g IV q6h	Cefazolin, 1 g IV q8h plus gentamicin[a]

Reprinted with permission from Abrams RA, Botte MJ. Hand infections. J Am Acad Orthop Surg 1996;4:220.
[a]Loading dose, 2 mg/kg body weight; then follow serum levels.
[b]Consider rabies prophylaxis.
[c]Consider tetanus prophylaxis.

Clinical Table: Infections of the Hand and Wrist

Infection	Procedure	Indications	Technique	Anatomy	Pitfalls
Felon	• I&D	• Abscess	• Midvolar • High lateral	• Pulp space	• Loculations
Paronychia	• I&D • Nail removal • Marsupialization	• Acute abscess beneath the eponychium • Chronic abscess	• 11-blade scissors • Freer 15-blade scissors	• Eponychium • Germinal and sterile matrix	• Injury to germinal matrix
Flexor tenosynovitis	• I&D	• Kanavel's four signs	• Proximal or distal incision • Catheter in sheath	• Flexor sheath	• Incomplete I&D
Herpetic whitlow	• None	• None	• None	• Paronychial vesicles	• Mistaken for paronychia
Subcutaneous abscess	• I&D	• Closed fluctuance	• Along skin lines	• Subcutaneous	• Early closure • Inadequate packing
Deep abscess	• I&D	• Dorsal subaponeurotic • Subfascial web • Midpalmar • Thenar • Parona's	• Second or fourth metacarpal • Volar or dorsal	• Interossei • Subfascial midpalm • Thenar muscles • Carpal canal	• Incisions on the tendon • Collar button • Tenosynovitis • Dumbbell • Median nerve compression
Cellulitis	• Observe	• Underlying infection	• None	• None	• Underlying abscess
IV drugs	• I&D	• Abscess	• Wide	• Dorsum hand	• Immuno-compromised • Rapid spread
Human bite	• I&D	• Suspicion	• Wide	• Dorsum metacarpo-phalangeals	• Improper I&D
Animal bite	• I&D	• Abscess	• Wide	• Local	• Rapid spread
Diabetes related	• I&D	• Abscess	• Wide	• Local	• Immuno-compromised
Osteomyelitis	• I&D of soft tissue and bone	• Positive radiograph	• Wide	• Bone	• Inadequate I&D
Septic arthritis	• I&D of the joint	• Positive aspiration • Pain on motion	• Arthrotomy	• Joint	• Inadequate I&D
Traumatic, contaminated	• I&D	• Open wound	• Wide	• Local	• Gangrene
Necrotizing fasciitis	• Emergent I&D	• Life threatening	• Wide	• Wide	• Delayed treatment
Mycobacteria	• I&D	• Chronic granuloma	• Local	• Local	• Missed history
Fungi	• I&D	• Chronic infection	• Local	• Local	• Incorrect treatment

I&D, incision and drainage.

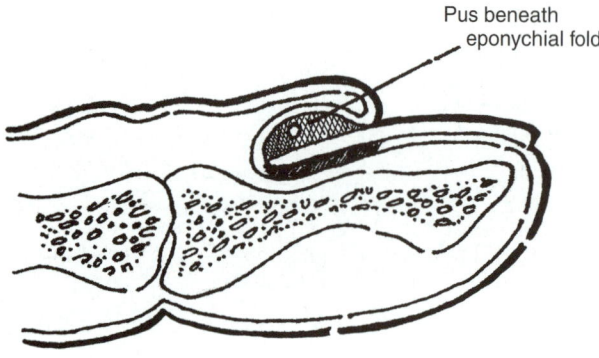

Figure 13.3. A sagittal section of the fingertip shows the collection of pus tracking beneath the eponychial fold and nail plate at the level of the germinal matrix.

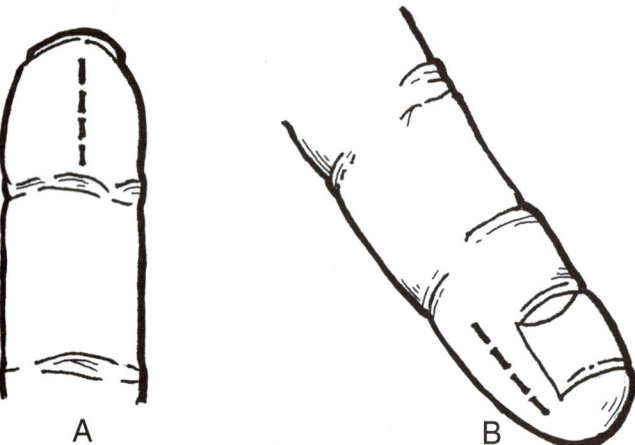

Figure 13.4. Midvolar (**A**) and midlateral (**B**) approaches for decompression of a felon.

rectly beneath the nail plate but above the nail matrix and advancing in a distal to proximal direction with gentle spreading. The nail is then cut longitudinally with scissors, and a portion of the nail is removed. The exposed matrix may be covered with a small piece of an adherent Adaptic gauze to allow a continued egress of the abscess. The eponychial fold should be stented open for at least 48 h with a fashioned piece of sterile plastic or foil. The dressing should be removed with a warm soak no later than 48 h and changed thereafter on a daily basis (1–5)

Chronic paronychia can be more difficult and is often recalcitrant to treatment. It presents with periods of intermittent cellulitis about the eponychium. The seal between the nail plate and eponychial fold becomes chronically separated; and fungi (specifically *Candida albicans*), atypical mycobacteria, and sometimes gram-negative organisms take hold. Treatment often includes full marsupialization of the eponychial fold and removal of the nail plate. Recent use of a topical corticosteroid antifungal ointment (3% clioquinol in a triamcinolone-nystatin mixture; mycol-

ogy) has been shown to be useful. It is vital to differentiate between an initial acute paronychia and a chronic unrelenting paronychia by history, since the offending pathogens and the appropriate surgical and antibiotic treatment are clearly different (1,5).

Felon

The volar soft pulp space of the finger pad is composed of a network of fascial septa, spanning from the distal phalanx to the skin. Felons occur as closed-space infections of this tissue, resulting in throbbing pain and severe edema of this compartment. The culprit is a penetrating injury with a resultant S. *aureus* infection. In the mild stage with minimal swelling and pain, treatment with elevation, soaks, and oral antibiotics is appropriate. Once a fluctuant abscess has formed, however, incision and drainage are critical. A poorly treated felon will lead to pulp space necrosis, osteomyelitis, and flexor tenosynovitis (1,5).

The approach to interventional treatment remains controversial. The U-shaped fish-mouth incision, advocated in the past, has recently fallen out of favor; the concern is compromised vascularity and subsequent poor healing in the fingertip. Presently, the high lateral or midvolar incision is usually used; the point of maximal fluctuance is the guide to placement of the incision. A high lateral incision on the ulnar aspect of the thumb and radial aspect of the index finger should be avoided, if possible, so fine pinch is not compromised (1,5) (Fig. 13.4).

Aftercare involves loose packing, dressing changes within 48 h, and empiric coverage of S. *aureus*. Continuation of warm soaks and dressing changes commonly leads to rapid resolution of the felon, once decompression has been performed (1,5)

Cellulitis

Cellulitis is a disseminated inflammatory process characterized by hyperemic tissue, white cell infiltration, and edema without the evidence of abscess formation. It may be accompanied by acute lymphangitis. It can be initiated by local skin penetration or a preexisting skin irritation. Cellulitis usually involves the skin and subcutaneous tissues but may involve deeper structures. The most common inciting organism is group A β-hemolytic *Streptococcus*. S. *aureus* cellulitis is less common and causes a less invasive infection (1,2).

Documentation of cellulitis is based purely on clinical examination. When a cellulitis is evident, it is crucial to rule out an underlying more extensive process such as a subcutaneous abscess, septic joint, or deep space infection before initiating antibiotics or operative intervention.

Specific treatment of early stages of cellulitis with oral antibiotics is appropriate. Close monitoring of resolution is important; and if resolution is not apparent between 24 and 48 h, initiating intravenous antibiotics may be indicated. Agents of choice orally include penicillin V and cephalexin. When the pathogen is unknown, coverage for both *Streptococcus* and S. *aureus* is fairly complete with cephalexin. Erythromycin is a reasonable alternative in cases of penicillin allergy (1,2).

Extensive or later-stage cellulitis requires starting intravenous antibiotics at the outset. Intravenous penicillin G and cefazolin are the drugs of choice; cephalosporin is preferred for empiric treatment. For patients with penicillin allergies, intravenous vancomycin is the first alternative and intravenous clindamycin as a second option. Inpatient observation for intravenous treatment is appropriate, followed by outpatient intravenous or oral treatment after significant improvement (1,2).

Subcutaneous Abscess

Unlike cellulitis, subcutaneous abscesses are commonly associated with a penetrating injury to the skin; S. *aureus* is the most common pathogen. Clinical examination often reveals a fluctuant mass with or without surrounding induration. Local regions of cellulitis and edema may border the central area of fluctuant mass. Specimen for culture and Gram stain may be obtained from the central area of fluctuance by sterile technique aspiration with a large-gauge needle in the emergency department or at the bedside. Depending on the anatomic site and its relation to more vital structures, incision and drainage may be carried out in the operating room setting. It is imperative that an adequate sample of purulence is appropriately harvested before starting any antibiotic therapy (1,2).

Postsurgery, the wound should be left open or partially open and packed with saline-soaked gauze dressings. Primary therapy may be started using a first-generation cephalosporin. If the injury is associated with soil, aerobic coverage with penicillin should be included. If the patient is an intravenous drug user or a diabetic, an amino glycoside should be added to the cephalosporin for coverage of gram-negative bacteria (1,2).

Suppurative Flexor Tenosynovitis

The flexor tendon sheath extends from the proximal margin of the A1 pulley to distal phalanx in the index, long, and ring fingers. The sheaths of the thumb and small finger are specialized; the thumb sheath is contiguous with radial bursa, and the small finger sheath is contiguous with the ulnar bursa. Both radial and ulnar bursa extend proximally to the level of the carpal tunnel, and in more than 50% of individuals the two bursa communicate (1,2,6,7) (Fig. 13.5).

A supportive flexor tenosynovitis is often a rapidly spreading bacterial infection within the sheath, usually resulting from penetrating trauma. S. *aureus* is the most common pathogen found; however *Streptococcus* and gram-negative organisms are not uncommon. A flexor tenosynovitis can originate from hematogenous spread of a gonococcal infection. Chronic infections may be the result of atypical mycobacteria with a characteristic proliferative tenosynovitis.

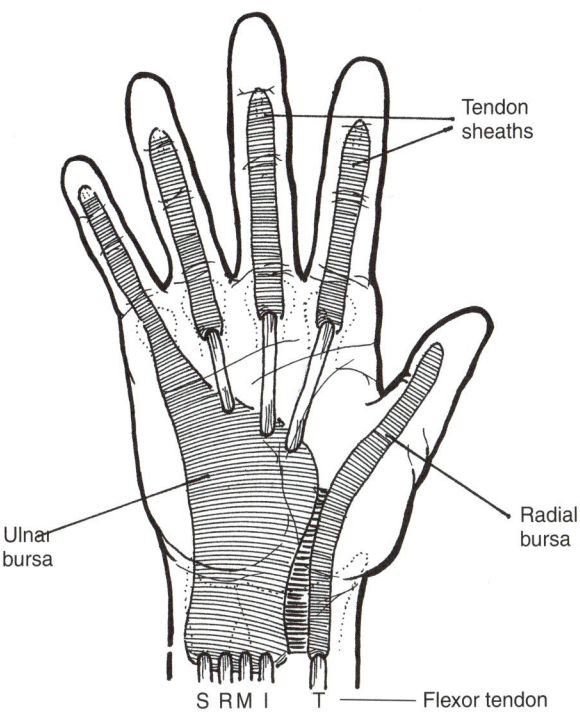

Figure 13.5. Communication and location of the flexor tendon sheaths and the bursa within the palm. Communication between the radial and ulnar palmar bursae occurs in 50 to 80% of individuals. *S,* small finger; *R,* ring finger; *M,* middle finger; *I,* index finger; *T,* thumb.

Kanavel's four cardinal signs remain the clinical hallmarks for rapid diagnosis: (*a*) a flexed posture of the involved digit, (*b*) tenderness along the flexor sheath, (*c*) diffuse circumferential swelling of the digit, and (*d*) exquisite pain on passive extension from the flexed position. One or all of the signs may be present, but early diagnosis and treatment is vital. Delay in treatment may result in adhesion formation and poor gliding of the tendons secondary to ischemia and necrosis (1,2,6,7). Treatment delay can also result in communication of the infection to other spaces. An infection in the substance of the small finger or thumb sheath may extend to the opposite side of the hand via communication of the ulnar and radial bursa, resulting in the characteristic horseshoe-shaped abscess in the hand. The infection may also spread more proximally, along the bursa to Parona's quadrilateral space at the wrist. Parona's space is bound by the pronator quadratus dorsally, the digital flexors, the flexor pollicis longus (FPL), and the flexor carpi ulnaris (FCU) tendons (1,2,6,7).

In very early cases or when diagnosis remains uncertain, the hand may be splinted and elevated with the simultaneous initiation of empiric intravenous antibiotics. If obvious improvement is not evident within 24 h, surgical treatment is necessary. Minimal incisions and catheter irrigation via the sheath limit the extent of dissection and help make a rapid recovery. A zigzag or oblique incision is made just proximal to the A1 pulley over the metacarpal head, and a midaxial or palmar transverse incision is made just proximal to the distal interphalangeal joint. A number 5 pediatric feeding tube or butterfly catheter can be inserted proximally or distally and sutured in place. The sheath is then copiously irrigated in the operating room, allowing a smooth uniform flow from both incisions.

The hand is then placed in a bulky absorptive dressing and splinted. A simple stop-cock system should be set up to allow house staff and nursing to easily irrigate the sheath three times a day. Dressings must be changed frequently to prevent skin breakdown. In 48 to 72 h, the catheter can be removed; hand therapy is started immediately to prevent stiffness. Whirlpool therapy may also be beneficial (1,2,6,7).

Infrequently, adequate irrigation and drainage cannot be completed by the limited-incision method. When this is the case, secondary to viscous purulence, the sheath must be opened fully. Experience has demonstrated that a full-length midaxial incision along the sheath may result in less postoperative morbidity than will a volar Bruner-type incision. Once appropriately decompressed, the midaxial incision can be closed loosely, without flap tip necrosis being a problem (1,2,6,7).

Deep Fascial Space Infections

The anatomy of the deep spaces of the hand is initially difficult to visualize. The spaces include the dorsal subaponeurotic space, the interdigital subfascial web space, the midpalmar space, the thenar space, and Parona's quadrilateral space. This set of closed compartments is prone to infection from penetrating trauma, spread from local compartments or hematogenous dissemination. The most common organisms are S. *aureus*, *Streptococcus* spp., and coliform pathogens (1,2,8).

The dorsal subaponeurotic space comprises the extensor tendons dorsally and the metacarpals and interossei volarly. An infection of this area presents with significant dorsal edema and may be difficult to discern from a subcutaneous abscess. The ideal method for decompression is by two longitudinal incisions, one centered over the second metacarpal and the other between the fourth and fifth metacarpal. Incisions directly over tendons should be avoided, if possible (1,2,8).

Subfascial web space infections often occur when palmar blisters or skin fissures become secondarily infected. Because of the adherence of the skin to the underlying fascia, purulence moves dorsally into the deep web space. This is contiguous with the dorsal subcutaneous interspace of the digits, thus forming an hourglass- or collar button-shaped abscess. The hourglass abscess can be differentiated from simple dorsal subcutaneous abscess by the characteristic abducted resting posture of the neighboring digits. Most authors favor both dorsal and volar incisions to decompress these infections (1,2,8).

The midpalmar space is bounded dorsally by the long and ring metacarpals and the second and third volar interossei, palmarly by the flexor tendons and lumbrical, ul-

narly by the hypothenar muscles, and radially by the midpalmar septum. Infection may be caused either by direct penetration or spread from the long and ring finger flexor tendon sheaths (rare). On clinical examination, the normal concavity of the palm is lost and the palm may appear full and convex, with marked tenderness to palpation. Drainage requires wide exposure with either an oblique or transverse palmar incision; the wound is packed loosely open with wet gauze. Dressing should be changed frequently (1,2,8).

The thenar space is bounded dorsally by the adductor pollicis; volarly by the index finger flexor profundus tendon; radially by the adductor pollicis insertion into the proximal phalanx and thenar muscle fascia; and ulnarly by the midpalmar septum, which extends from the middle finger metacarpal to the palmar fascia. This space can become infected from penetrating trauma or secondary infection from local spread of an index finger flexor tenosynovitis. The infection can migrate about the far edge of the adductor pollicis and the first dorsal interosseous muscles to involve the first dorsal web space. Thenar space infection should be suspected when there is an accumulation of pus adjacent to the first dorsal interosseous, resulting in the dumbbell or pantaloon effect (1,2,8).

Operative drainage of all of these deep space infections involves wide exposure with an oblique or transverse palmar incision (Figs. 13.6 and 13.7). The wound should be gently packed open; the hand, splinted; and the dressings, frequently changed.

Septic Arthritis

The most common organisms cultured from septic joints are S. *aureus* and *Streptococcus* spp. *Haemophilus influen-*

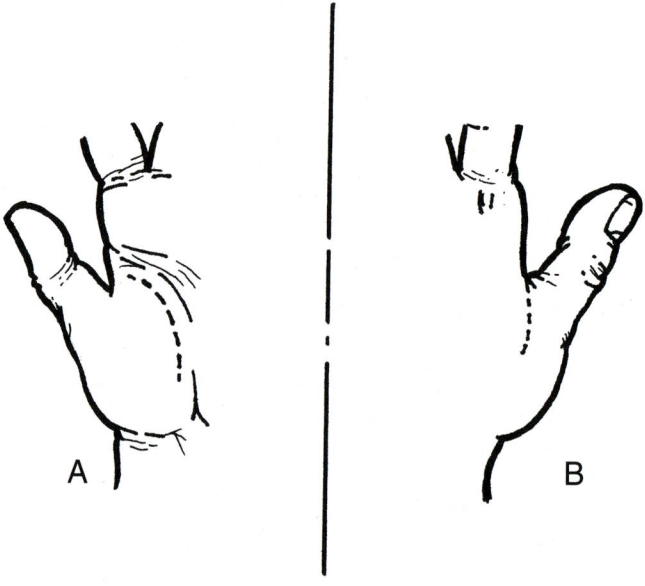

Figure 13.6. Preferred incisions for the decompression of thenar space infections. Both volar (**A**) and dorsal (**B**) incisions should be used to drain the entire extent of a thenar space abscess.

Figure 13.7. Incisions for draining deep palmar space infections: transverse (**A**); third lumbrical canal (**B**); combined longitudinal and transverse (**C**); and oblique (**D**).

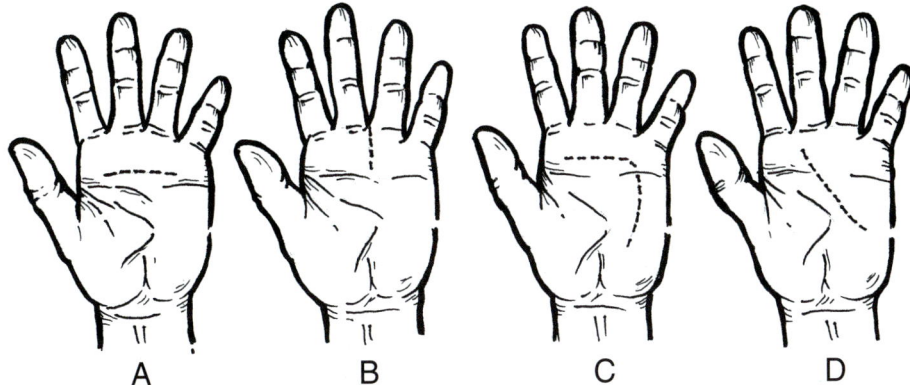

zae must be considered in young children, and gonococcal infection must be ruled out in young adults presenting with a monoarticular nontraumatic septic arthritis. A poor outcome can be predicted if cultures are positive for S. *aureus*, coliforms, gram-negative rods, anaerobes, polymicrobial infections, positive blood cultures, and associated osteomyelitis. Another key to outcome is duration of infection before adequate treatment was initiated (1–3,9).

The prevalent mechanisms of hand and wrist joint infections include direct penetrating trauma, local extension, and hematogenous spread. Damage to the joint cartilage is caused by bacterial toxins and proteolytic enzymes (as well as proteolytic enzymes of host cartilage origin), resulting in assisted autodestruction. As destruction increases, the intra-articular pressure rises, leading to tamponading of the blood supply to the synovial lining, causing further direct cartilage injury, capsule and bony erosion, sinus formation, and osteomyelitis (1,9).

On clinical examination the joint is painful, edematous, and erythematous and is held in a posture that increases volume within. There is often excruciating pain with motion and axial load. A joint aspiration should be performed to rule out crystal-producing arthropathies. Classical septic aspirate is characterized by a friable mucin clot; a white blood cell count greater than 50,000, of which 75% are polymorphonuclear leukocytes; and a low glucose level (1–3,9). Serial aspirations are usually not useful in the hand, and a definitive incision and drainage allows prompt evacuation of the pathogen and the pus. Once the necrotic debris has been decompressed, the joint pressure normalizes and the insult to the cartilage diminishes.

Incisions for septic joints should ideally be made straight. At the level of the wrist, a dorsal exposure between the third and fourth compartments is ideal. For the carpometacarpal joint, a dorsal approach on either side of the extensors is appropriate. In the metacarpophalangeal joints, a dorsal incision in the region of the proximal portion of the sagittal bands is best. In the digital interphalangeal joint and the thumb metacarpophalangeal joint, a midaxial approach between the accessory collateral ligament and the volar plate may yield the best result. The in-

cision may be left open for delayed primary closure or allowed to heal by secondary intention. When the joint is thought to be early in the septic process and extremely well irrigated, a drain or irrigation catheter may be left in place and the joint closed. The hand should be splinted for 2 to 3 days; then drains and catheters can be removed and early motion started (1–3,9).

The route of administration and length of the course of antibiotics remain controversial. The consensus is that intravenous antibiotics must be continued until local and systemic signs of infection have resolved. After which, intravenous or oral antibiotics are continued in the hospital or at home for another 2 to 4 weeks (1).

Osteomyelitis

Osteomyelitis in the hand most often occurs after open fractures or from secondary involvement of bone with local soft tissue infection. The infection rate in open fractures varies in the literature from 1 to 11%. Gustilo and Anderson type III fractures are more likely to become infected, because of gross contamination, soft tissue stripping, and high-energy skeletal trauma. Hematogenous spread is rare in osteomyelitis and much more common in children than in adults. S. *aureus* and *Streptococcus* are the most common pathogens. Patients that are immunocompromised, diabetic, or suffer mutilating severe injuries are more likely to acquire an infection from gram-negative, anaerobic, and polymicrobial organisms (1–3,9).

Clinical manifestations of osteomyelitis include pain, erythema, and edema. Generalized constitutional symptoms are uncommon, unless there is an associated septicemia. Recent studies have demonstrated that intraosseous and periosteal edema can be depicted by MRI at the earliest stage (Fig. 13.1B), followed closely by bone scan, before becoming evident on plain x-ray (Fig. 13.8). When radiographs become positive, early changes include local osteopenia and periosteal reaction. In the later phase, sequestrum and involucrum may be present radiographically. There should be a high index of suspicion that osteomyelitis is present when a soft tissue infection does

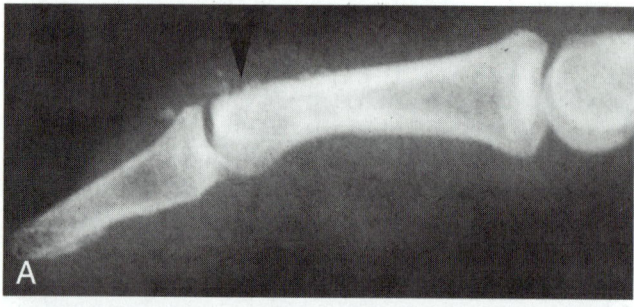

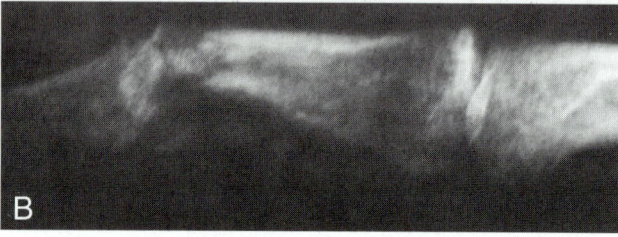

Figure 13.8. A. Lateral radiograph of a 50-year-old female with early osteomyelitis 2 weeks after injury. The *arrowhead* points to the periosteal elevation on the dorsal cortex. **B.** Same patient 4 weeks after injury. Note the marked destruction of the phalanges secondary to a staphylococcal infection.

not respond to appropriate local and antibiotic treatment or when such an infection resolves and returns persistently (1–3,9).

Open fractures that have become infected within 6 weeks of injury should have internal fixation retained for stability. If, however, union has not occurred by 6 weeks, internal fixation should be removed and replaced with new internal fixation, external fixation, or both.

Human Bites

In general, human bite wounds that present more than 24 h after injury should be assumed to be infected. Two basic types of injuries occur. Clenched-fist injuries to the dorsum of the metacarpal head of the middle and ring fingers caused by contacting the mouth are associated with the highest morbidity. Often, subcutaneous, subaponeurotic, joint, and tendon sheath may become involved in these injuries. The second type of injury is the true bite. Problems associated with these injuries arise because initially the wounds seem innocuous, as tendon and joint capsule injuries are not easily detectable in the multiple planes of tissue. In the clenched-fist position, the laceration of the skin, extensor tendon and join capsule are coincident. With extension of the digit, the extensor tendon migrates proximally and seals over the joint capsule laceration, preventing drainage and thereby causing a septic arthritis. Therefore, a wound on the dorsum of the metacarpophalangeal joints must be considered an open, intra-articular, clenched-fist bite injury until proven otherwise. The consequences of inadequate treatment can be catastrophic (1,10–12).

An analysis of human saliva has demonstrated 42 species of bacteria. The most prevalent in human bite infections are group A *Streptococcus*, *S. aureus*, and *E. corrodens*. Although *Staphylococcus* is more common in human bite infections, *E. corrodens* has variable susceptibility to cephalosporins but is not susceptible to penicillinase-resistant penicillins. *Bacteroides* is the most common anaerobe found in human bite infections and often is associated with polymicrobial cultures (1,10–12).

Standard care for noninfected bite wounds should include surgical extension of the wound, exploration, irrigation, and débridement. If the joint was entered, the patient should be admitted. The hand should be splinted and elevated, and the patient should be given intravenous antibiotics for 48 h. If there is no tendon or joint injury, treatment with débridement and antibiotics seems to provide better results than débridement alone (1,10–12).

Human bite wounds with obvious infection require formal irrigation and débridement, hospitalization, empiric parenteral antibiotic therapy with penicillin G, first-generation cephalosporin, and possibly an amino glycoside. A repeat débridement at 48 to 72 h should be considered, if necessary. Warm soaks in normal saline and wet to dry dressing changes should be started about 48 h after the initial incision and drainage. Wounds are allowed to heal before secondary granulation and tendon repairs are performed (1,10–12).

Animal Bites and Scratches

Animal bites can be the source of severe and disabling hand infections. They are most commonly inflicted by dogs, cats, and rodents, in decreasing order of prevalence. Snakebites, more common in the southwestern United States, should be considered a separate category, since they induce infection by the pathogen along with venom toxicity (1,2,13).

Studies differ in the incidence of infections caused by different animal bites. One study reported dog bites rarely becoming infected, whereas about 50% of cat bites and scratches become infected. The most common pathogen attributable to dog- and cat-induced infections is P. *multocida*. *Streptococcus*, *Staphylococcus*, and certain anaerobes are also common agents of infections (1,2,13).

Treatment for noninfected animal bites remains somewhat controversial. Careful topical cleaning and irrigation of the wound is prudent. Exploration of the wound is indicated, if there is suspicion of joint, bone, or tendon sheath penetration. Oral antibiotics are indicated as prophylactics for all but the most superficial wounds (1,2,13). Infected wounds commonly require formal incision and drainage with subsequent hospitalization and empiric parenteral antibiotic therapy. Therapy should include coverage for P. *multocida*, *Staphylococcus*, *Streptococcus*, and anaerobes with penicillin G and a first-generation cephalosporin (1,2,13).

Rabies infection deserves mention because of recent

sporadic outbreaks on the East Coast of the United States. An algorithm for prophylaxis has been put forth by the Centers for Disease Control and Prevention (Atlanta, GA). No treatment is required for bites inflicted by healthy dogs or cats that have been observed for 10 days. Individuals sustaining a bite from a skunk, bat, fox, coyote, raccoon, bobcat, or suspected domestic animal should be inoculated with human diploid cell vaccine and rabies immune globulin. Mice, rats, hamsters, rabbits, and squirrels should be considered on a case-by-case basis, but their bites rarely call for antirabies prophylaxis (1).

Snakebites are a complex problem; and debate continues about the appropriate treatment for severe snakebites with envenomation, toxemia, and associated infection. Southern states have the highest bite rates, resulting in 45,000 bites per year in the United States; 50% of those occur in the hand or upper extremity. Although snake venom plays a larger role in morbidity than does infection, most studies demonstrate that a superinfection results in 5 to 10% of snakebite wounds. The mouths of crotalids are colonized with multiple bacteria, and domesticated snakes have a wider range of pathogens, including *Proteus vulgaris*, E. *coli*, and *Corynebacterium diphtheria*. In general, hallmarks of care include a high index of suspicion for infection, culture of material, incision and drainage and/or débridement, fasciotomy (if necessary), and intravenous antibiotics. It is advisable to consult a poison center with expertise in snakebite treatment if there is no one with expertise at your medical center (1,2,13).

Necrotizing Fasciitis

Necrotizing fasciitis is truly a limb- and life-threatening emergency. A rapidly advancing and progressive soft tissue infection occurs most commonly, but not exclusively, in intravenous drug users. The extremities are usually the site of origin, secondary to contaminated needle tract infections. Immunocompromised hosts are also clearly more susceptible to this rapidly dissemination infection. The infection can be caused by a single pathogen, often group A β-hemolytic *Streptococcus*, *Staphylococcus*, and anaerobes (1,14,15).

The process is characterized by extreme pain, rapid advancement, cellulitis with poor margins, and tense swollen skin. In a matter of days, bullae and ecchymosis appear, followed by a classic elevation in white blood cell count but no other characteristic signs of infection. An inability to stabilize a patient's hemodynamics in the face of this superficial infection should strike an alarm to the possibility of necrotizing fasciitis (1,2,14,15).

Liquefaction of fat and fibrinous necrotic tissue, resulting in a foul-smelling "dish water" pus, is the surgical intervention hallmark of this infection. The pus is often accompanied by thrombosis of small subcutaneous vessels. Muscle is often spared. A complete débridement of involved tissue and skin is required (1,2,14,15).

Extremely rapid intervention must be started to save the host. Emergent initiation of penicillin G remains a standard first-line intervention; however, coverage for penicillinase-resistant S. *aureus* and an amino glycoside for the possibility of gram-negative pathogens is also essential. Poor prognostic factors include an age greater than 50 years old, underlying chronic illness, diabetes, and truncal spread. The single most important factor in recovery is early and thorough débridement (1,2,14,15).

Mycobacterial Infections

Infections of the hand and wrist caused by M*ycobacterium tuberculosis* are rare; however, infections secondary to atypical mycobacteria are not uncommon. M. *marinum* is the most commonly identified hand pathogen of this group. Other less common mycobacteria in hand infections include M. *kansasii*, M. *fortuitum*, and M. *chelonei*. Of infections caused by atypical mycobacteria, 75% involve the hand. Usually, these infections attack deep structures, resulting in delayed wound healing and poor hand function. Penetration usually occurs via contaminated swimming pools, fish tanks, piers, boats, fish bites, fish spines, or fins. The infection may result in superficial verrucae; subcutaneous granuloma; or deep penetration into tendon, bone, or joint. The clinical picture may appear as late as 6 months from the time of injury (1–3,16,17).

M. *marinum* inhabits both saltwater and freshwater. Appropriate diagnosis requires a high index of suspicion of these infections by taking a good history, with adequate tissue biopsy and correct culture. Skin testing is generally unreliable, and smears examined with acid fast stains are usually negative. M. *marinum* cultures must be incubated in Lowenstein-Jensen media at 30°C for up to 8 weeks. The histology demonstrates caseating and noncaseating granulomas. Systemic symptoms rarely occur. The white blood cell count and erythrocyte sedimentation rate (ESR) are often normal (1–3,16,17).

Treatment varies, depending on the severity of the clinical presentation. Superficial infection usually spontaneously resolves unless a subcutaneous lesion is present. A subcutaneous lesion must be débrided. Antibiotics are given for 8 to 26 weeks. Deeper infections may require tenosynovectomy, synovectomy, or decompression and débridement of the bone or joint infection; antibiotics are given from 16 weeks to 2 years (1–3,16,17).

A complete flexor tenosynovectomy with preservation of the annular pulleys must be performed in an M. *marinum* flexor tenosynovitis, A standard longitudinal approach can be made for extensor tenosynovitis, and an extensile carpal tunnel approach can be used for flexor tendon involvement at the wrist (1).

The present-day antibiotic of choice for these infections appears to be minocycline, because of its high efficacy and low incidence of side effects. Patients allergic to minocycline or who harbor resistant organisms may be treated with ethambutol and rifampin (1).

Fungal Infections

A fungal infection must be considered a high possibility in any chronic skin or nail infection of the hand. In the hand and upper extremities, fungal infections can occur as four subtypes: cutaneous, subcutaneous, deep, and systemic. The most common by far are cutaneous lesions involving the skin and nails. Dermatophytes are keratinophilic fungi that colonize glabrous skin, resulting in tinea corporis. They also settle in interdigital webs, causing tinea manuum, or in nails, resulting in onychomycosis with pitting and scaling. Definitive diagnosis can be made only by fungal cultures, but an early presumptive diagnosis can be made with potassium hydroxide preparations (1–3,18).

Simple skin infections can often be treated appropriately with over-the-counter antifungal creams, sprays, or powders containing miconazole or tolnaftate. One persistent and problematic infection is onychomycosis, which characteristically occurs in hands that remain moist. It begins as a minor paronychial infection that does not resolve and progresses to complete nail infection, with elevation, thickening, softening, and fissuring. These infections are resistant to treatment and have a high recurrence rate. Commonly, removal of the nail and administration of oral ketoconazole or griseofulvin are required; the best cure rates reported in the literature are 80% (1–3,18).

The most common subcutaneous fungal infection in North America is *Sporotrichosis*, a lymphocutaneous infection caused by the organism *Sporothrix schenckii*. It rarely causes a deep infection, but must be considered in cases of granulomatous synovitis. This pathogen is usually found in soil and plant materials. Exposure in florists via rose thorns, nursery workers, and farmers is not unusual. The infection occurs secondary to implantation of spores, after which a painless mass develops and subsequently ulcerates. Nodules can then begin to appear in cords along the lymphatics; the lesions heal and then recur unless treated. The treatment of choice is oral potassium iodide (1–3,18).

Deep fungal infections may result in significant morbidity involving tenosynovium, joints, or bones. A wide variety of opportunistic organisms such as mucormycosis, aspergillosis, and candida may occur in the immunocompromised host. More virulent organisms such as histoplasmosis, blastomycosis, and coccidioidomycosis may affect previously healthy patients with intact immune systems. Deep fungal infections are often introduced via the respiratory route and are disseminated into the upper extremity via hematogenous spread. The infections may present as flexor tenosynovitis, septic arthritis, or osteomyelitis. Coccidioidomycosis is endemic in the southwestern United States. Coccidioidomycosis arthritis is markedly resistant to treatment and can be managed only by amputation or arthrodesis. Blastomycosis and histoplasmosis are endemic in the Mississippi and Ohio River valleys. Treatment requires radical débridement and parenteral amphotericin B (1–3,18).

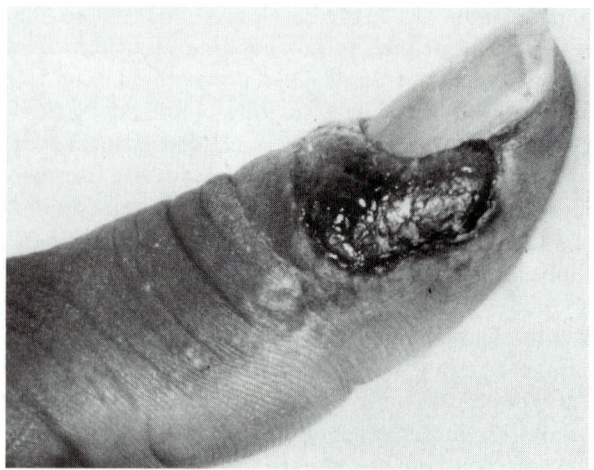

Figure 13.9. Herpetic whitlow caused by an HSV infection. Note the prominence of the vesicles with surrounded eschar.

Viral Infections

Viral infections in the hand occur infrequently, but the most common viral infection is the result of the herpes simplex virus (HSV), resulting in a cytolytic infection in the skin known as a herpetic whitlow (Fig. 13.9). The term *whitlow*, often used synonymously with *felon*, is neither a felon nor a paronychia. The herpetic whitlow usually occurs at the fingertip, but more proximal lesions have been reported. The lesion is self-limited; but as with all HSV lesions, it is believed to reside in its latent form in the neural ganglia, to be reactivated only by some form of stressor. In the past, these lesions were confused with both felons and paronychia and, as a result, were incised and drained. Surgical intervention of these lesions is contraindicated and should be avoided, because an incision may cause local tissue dissemination of the virus, with possible bacterial superinfection (1–3,19).

The pathogens are clinically indistinguishable forms of HSV types I and II. The virus is disseminated by direct contact, and health care workers are assumed to be at greater risk because of exposure to oral-tracheal secretions. The infections can also be passed via oral or genital lesions. A recent review found that only 14% of infections occurred in health care workers (1–3,19).

The infection begins with a painful cytolytic lesion 2 to 14 days after exposure. There is localized swelling and the appearance of clear vesicles. The vesicles can become turbid, mimicking a bacterial infection. Pain is often out of proportion to the lesion. During the subsequent 14 days, the vesicles mature and coalesce to unroof and form an ulcerated base. The ulcer gradually subsides over the next 2 to 4 weeks. Viral shedding may continue (infectious stage) until complete epithelialization of the lesion occurs. As the lesion subsides, the virus moves up the neural ganglia, avoiding the immune system to lie in its dormant state (1–3,19).

Diagnosis is usually made by eliciting a thorough history, including a work history, contacts, and recurrences. Physical findings of extreme pain, clear vesicles, and a soft pulp space aid in the presumptive diagnosis. Definitive diagnosis is made by viral cultures and Tzank smear (1).

Treatment involves recognition that a herpetic whitlow is not a felon or paronychia and must not be treated in the same way. Recent advances in the oral use of the antiviral drug acyclovir have demonstrated the ability to decrease the course of the infection and the number and duration of the recurrences. Topical acyclovir has not been shown to be helpful in treating acute lesions (1–3,19).

Gas-Forming Infections

Although rare, the morbidity and mortality (20%) of gas-forming infections can be devastating. Most often, these infections occur in an anaerobic environment, where open, soil-containing, mutilating injuries have occurred, such as in farming accidents. The most common offending pathogen in this scenario is *Clostridium perfringens*, a gram-positive anaerobic bacillus. Gas may not be present in the early stages of infection. Other organisms that produce gas include coliforms, anaerobic streptococci, and bacteroides (1–3).

The hallmarks of gas-forming infections are extreme pain from the gas production, rapidly dissemination, and progressive swelling of the soft tissues, skin dislocation, and a fetid odor of decaying tissue. This infection, like necrotizing fasciitis, is a limb- and life-threatening emergency that requires immediate radical débridement to remove devitalized tissue and expose the organisms to oxygen, high-dose intravenous penicillin, and hyperbaric oxygen when available (1,2).

THE IMMUNOCOMPROMISED PATIENT AND HIV

Immunocompromised patients have a greater susceptibility to viral, fungal, protozoal, and mycobacterial infections than the general population. Opportunistic organisms set down a foothold in the susceptible host. Infections of the hand may occur in the early prodromal part of the disease process. Glickel (20) reported on the most extensive series of HIV patients with hand infections. His work demonstrates that herpes infections are most common and often require antiviral medication for resolution. In general, infections of the hand in HIV patients are not more severe or more unusual, except for the slightly greater incidence of opportunistic organisms (3,20).

REHABILITATION OF THE INFECTED HAND

Mancini and Fort (21) nicely outlined the theory and treatment principles of postinfectious upper extremity rehabilitation. The theory involves aggressive medical management, followed by immediate mobilization on early resolution, and direct patient involvement. The early work centers around early incision and drainage, initiation of intravenous antibiotics, and close supervision (21,22). According to these authors, immediate mobilization should occur within 24 h of surgical intervention. The patient begins to work with the hand therapist and actively takes part in cleaning the wound and scrubbing necrotic debris. The theory is that the immediate involvement of the patient helps avert the dissociation of the patient from the infected appendage. The timing of immobilization and remobilization in hand infections remains controversial; however, if the patient becomes actively involved in the rehabilitation process, outcomes have been shown to be markedly improved (21,22).

SUMMARY

Infections of the hand are often complex and come in wide varieties. The orthopaedist needs to maintain a high index of suspicion for unusual types of infection related to specific mechanisms of injury. This chapter has detailed particularly troublesome processes that can occur and result in significant morbidity for the patient when misdiagnosed. Specific attention and focus on the patient's history and physical examination are critical when assessing benign-appearing injuries. Infections due to animal bites, human bites, and atypical organisms of fungal or macrobacterial nature can lead to catastrophic results when inappropriately treated. The basic tenet of early débridement of loculated contained infections followed by appropriate antibiotic treatment is vital for the patient's ability to maintain normal range of motion and function in the hand and wrist. The hallmarks of treatment in hand infections remain early diagnosis and rapid surgical or medical intervention. Once edema and erythema begin to resolve, rapid intervention with aggressive range of motion supervised by an appropriate hand therapist is critical to restoring the patient with a normal hand.

REFERENCES

1. Abrams RA, Botte MJ. Hand infections: treatment recommendations for specific types. J Am Acad Orthop Surg 1996;4:219–230.
2. Hausman MR, Lisser SP. Hand infections. Orthop Clin North Am 1992;23:171–185.
3. Bishop AT. Infections. In: Manske PR, ed. Hand surgery update. Rosemont, IL: American Society for Surgery of the Hand/American Academy of Orthopaedic Surgeons, 1996:395–404.
4. Canales FL, Newmeyer WL III, Kilgore ES Jr. The treatment of felons and paronychias. Hand Clin 1989;5:515–523.
5. Bednar MS, Lane LB. Eponychial marsupialization and nail removal for surgical treatment of chronic paronychia. J Hand Surg 1991;16A:314–317.
6. Neviaser RJ. Closed tendon sheath irrigation for pyogenic flexor tenosynovitis. J Hand Surg 1978;3A:462–466.
7. Neviaser RJ. Tenosynovitis. Hand Clin 1989;5:525–531.
8. Burkhalter WL. Deep space infections. Hand Clin 1989;5:533–552.
9. Freeland AE, Senter BS. Septic arthritis and osteomyelitis. Hand Clin 1989;5:533–552.

10. Coleman DA. Human bite wounds. Hand Clin 1989;5:561–570.
11. Patzakis MJ, Wilkins J, Bassett RL. Surgical findings in clenched-fist injuries. Clin Orthop 1987;220:237–240.
12. Chiunard RG, D'Ambrosia RD. Human bite infections of the hand. J Bone Joint Surg 1977:59A:416–418.
13. Snyder CC. Animal bite wounds. Hand Clin 1989;5:571–590.
14. Bisno AL, Stevens DL. Streptococcal infections of skin and soft tissues. N Engl J Med 1996;334:240–245.
15. Schecter W, Meyer A, Schecter G, et al. Necrotizing fasciitis of the upper extremity. J Hand Surg 1982;7A:15–19.
16. Bush D, Schneider L. Tuberculosis of the hand and wrist. J Hand Surg 1984;9A:391–398.
17. Gunther SS, Levy CS. Mycobacterial infections. Hand Clin 1989;5:591–598.
18. Hitchcock TF, Amadio PC. Fungal infections. Hand Clin 1989;5:599–612.
19. Fowler JR. Viral infections. Hand Clin 1989;5:613–628.
20. Louis DS, Silva J Jr. Herpetic whitlow: herpetic infections of the digits. J Hand Surg 1979;4A:90–94.
21. Mancini LH, Fort LK. Rehabilitation of the infected hand. Hand Clin 1989;5:635–644.
22. Glass KD. Factors related to the resolution of treated hand infections. J Hand Surg 1982;7A:388–394.

SHOULDER AND ELBOW

chapter 14

Leigh Ann Curl and Edward V. Craig

Fractures and Nonunions of the Proximal Humerus

I Fractures of the Proximal Humerus

Fractures of the proximal humerus make up 5 to 7% of all fractures and roughly 50% of all humeral fractures. Epidemiologic data show that the incidence of these fractures is on the rise, as an increasing percentage of the population reaches the age of osteopenic-related fractures. In fact, there is a strong similarity between the incidence and pattern of proximal humeral and proximal femoral fractures. Compared with distal humeral fractures, proximal humeral fractures occur with less trauma, in older patients, and more often in females than in males (1).

Proximal humeral fractures do not pose a diagnostic dilemma but are frequently difficult to treat because distorted bony anatomy reflects disordered rotator cuff anatomy, disrupted function, and lengthy immobilization, which can result in marked limitation of shoulder flexibility and strength. In addition, bone quality frequently makes rigid internal fixation challenging. Moreover, hovering over many of these fractures is the specter of an interrupted blood supply to the humeral head, which threatens humeral head viability, possibly leading to the late sequela of posttraumatic osteonecrosis.

Although many proximal humeral fractures can be treated nonoperatively, treatment of the soft tissues of the shoulder is as important as treatment of the skeletal tissues. A healed proximal humeral fracture can result in dramatic limitation of function and comfort if the clinician fails to recognize the importance of related soft tissue injuries. Hence a thorough understanding of the functional anatomy of the shoulder assists in the evaluation and management of these injuries.

RELEVANT ANATOMY AND PATHOGENESIS

Smooth and fluid motion with normal flexibility and strength is the result of the unique architecture of the shoulder. The humeral head rests along the articular surface of the glenoid and is stabilized and moved by the surrounding soft tissue. The articular surface area of the humeral head is approximately four times the surface area of the glenoid, so that at any time and in any position, only a portion of the available humeral head articular surface is in contact with the glenoid. As the arm is elevated, the humeral head–glenoid contact is maintained, while the scapula rotates on the chest wall, thus reinforcing the important contribution of both glenohumeral and scapulothoracic motion.

The important bony landmarks for understanding proximal humeral fractures are the tuberosities, the anatomic neck, the surgical neck, the bicipital groove, and the remaining humeral shaft. The greater tuberosity is the bony prominence to which the supraspinatus, infraspinatus, and teres minor of the rotator cuff attach; and it is these tendons that are responsible for displacement of the greater tuberosity, if this should occur, with a proximal humeral fracture. The lesser tuberosity is the smaller bony prominence to which the subscapularis attaches; and the tuberosities are joined to one another through the bicipital groove on the anterior humeral cortex, which is the anterior location for the long head of the biceps tendon. The anatomic neck is at the juncture of the articular cartilage and the top of the tuberosities, and the surgical neck lies below the greater and lesser tuberosities at their junction with the shaft.

Normal shoulder motion is provided by the interaction of the two main muscle groups responsible for shoulder strength: the deltoid and the rotator cuff. The four rotator cuff muscles function together to rotate, stabilize, and center the humeral head so that the deltoid can supply the power to elevate the arm. A poorly functioning or scarred rotator cuff can dramatically alter shoulder function and negate the effects of the powerful deltoid muscle. In addition, when a fracture occurs, the cuff attachments determine the displacement of the bony segments. For example, the greater tuberosity, when displaced, is pulled superiorly by the supraspinatus or posteriorly by the infraspinatus–teres minor combination; and these muscle forces must be neutralized for proper reduction and fixation of the fracture. The lesser tuberosity, when displaced, is pulled medially by the pull of the subscapularis. Because the long head of biceps is located midway between the greater and lesser tuberosities, it tends to get caught among the bony fragments after fractures of the tuberosities or surgical neck, preventing reduction. In addition, the muscle attachments to the humeral shaft tend to displace the shaft medially relative to the humeral head and tuberosity segments.

The rotator cuff is ordinarily covered by a thin film of tissue, the subacromial bursa, which facilitates the gliding of the cuff within the coracoacromial arch. Alternation of this bursa owing to hemorrhage or scarring can be a factor in painful limitation of shoulder motion.

The coracoacromial arch is composed of the anterior portion of the acromion and the coracoacromial ligament. The rotator cuff and bursa glide beneath the acromion as the arm is elevated overhead. The normal coracoacromial space is 0.5 to 1 cm wide. Malunion or nonunion of the proximal humeral segment can impinge on the available space under the coracoacromial arch, limiting the smooth movement and function of the shoulder. In fact, the goal of aggressive management of proximal humeral fractures is the maintenance or repair of the normal anatomic spaces and gliding surfaces.

Classification

The Neer classification of proximal humeral fractures is the most widely used and accepted today (Fig. 14.1). The system is based on an observation made by Codman in 1934 that when the proximal humerus is fractured, it tends to break along epiphyseal lines, resulting in four main segments—the anatomical head, the greater tuberosity, the lesser tuberosity, and the humeral shaft.

Neer recognized that the segments were displaced by the pull of the attached cuff and shaft muscles, resulting in predictable patterns of displacement, which, if significant,

result in marked functional limitation. He devised the four-segment classification based on the location and position of each displaced segment and on the number of displaced segments (not the number of fracture lines). A segment is considered displaced if it has moved at least 1 cm or is angled at least 45° (Fig. 14.2). This is independent of the number of fracture lines or degree of comminution present. The essence of the Neer classification is that if

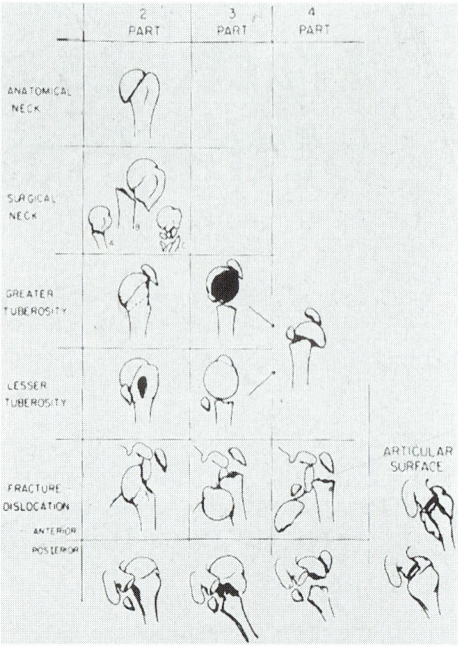

Figure 14.1. The Neer classification of proximal humeral fractures is based on the number of displaced segments.

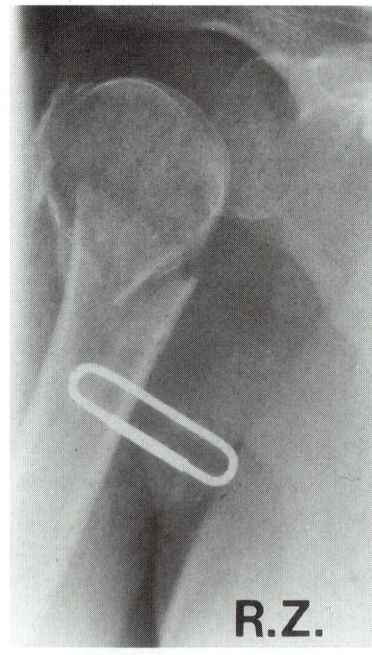

Figure 14.2. This 1-part comminuted fracture is considered nondisplaced according to the Neer system because none of the segments is displaced more than 1 cm.

proper x-rays are obtained and interpreted correctly, all proximal humeral fractures can be classified according to the number of displaced parts. A 2-part fracture has one part (either the greater tuberosity, lesser tuberosity, humeral head, or humeral shaft) displaced from the other three. A 3-part fracture has three displaced segments, not only from each other but from the intact segments. A 4-part fracture has all segments displaced from each other. Once the segments are localized radiographically, the fracture can be classified and appropriate treatment instituted. The Neer classification requires no memorization; however, good-quality x-rays in multiple planes are essential.

Blood Supply

The blood supply to the humeral head is through branches of the anterior circumflex, the posterior circumflex, and the tendon–bone attachment of the rotator cuff. Interruption of the vascular supply to the humeral head, either by interruption from the fracture line or by extensive dissection during internal fixation, may lead to avascular necrosis, late collapse of the humeral head, and (ultimately) loss of joint congruity.

INITIAL FINDINGS, PHYSICAL EXAMINATION, AND DIAGNOSIS

The most common mechanism of a proximal humeral fracture is a fall on an outstretched hand, although a direct blow to the shoulder can also produce this injury, particularly in osteopenic bone. If the arm is excessively rotated, such as may occur with a hyperabducted position, a dislocation can also occur, compounding the extent of the fracture injury and resulting in significantly more bone and soft tissue trauma than occurs with a proximal humeral fracture without a dislocation.

As with most fractures, the most common presentation is pain, swelling, tenderness, and limitation of active and passive range of motion. Tenderness over the fracture site is frequently accompanied by bony crepitation on range of motion. Any attempt to move the extremity is met with resistance. The soft tissue swelling, particularly in a muscular person, may obscure humeral head and an associated dislocation. Ecchymosis can be dramatic and extend down the entire arm to the chest wall and even to the flank, as these are the dependent body portions available for dissecting blood under loose areolar tissue.

Neurovascular injuries are not common but may be overlooked, so careful neurologic and vascular examinations are mandatory. Peripheral pulses should be checked, and a rapidly expanding hematoma or diminished pulse should alert the examiner to a possible associated vascular injury. The neurologic check should include all peripheral nerves in the upper extremity but should predominately focus on testing axillary and muscu-

locutaneous nerve function, since these are the two most commonly injured nerves, particularly in the presence of a shoulder dislocation. Sensory examination of the two peripheral nerves may be unreliable, particularly in the presence of a painful fracture. Palpation of a contracting deltoid or biceps muscle can be done isometrically with the patient's arm in a sling and is enough to ensure the function of these two nerves.

RADIOLOGIC STUDIES

Since proper classification and treatment critically depend on the accurate identification and position of the fracture fragments, good-quality x-rays in multiple planes are essential. A trauma series allows reliable evaluation of the proximal humerus and can be done with the patient in or out of a sling, standing or supine. The series consists of a true AP view of the glenohumeral joint (Fig. 14.3), a true lateral view of the scapula, and an axillary view (Fig. 14.4). The axillary view is the best means of assessing the true relationship of the humeral head to the glenoid and can often reveal dislocations not seen on other views.

If the precise position of the greater tuberosity is difficult to ascertain by plain x-ray, a CT scan should be considered. CT studies give precise information about any abnormal position of the greater tuberosity, lesser tuberosity, or humeral head and allows visualization of the glenoid (Fig. 14.5). They are less helpful for detecting surgical neck fractures. MRI studies provide information

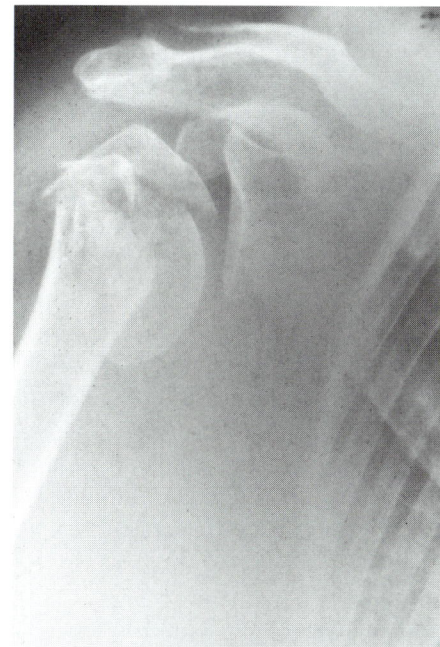

Figure 14.3. True AP view of the glenohumeral joint showing a fracture through the surgical neck and a comminuted fracture of the greater tuberosity.

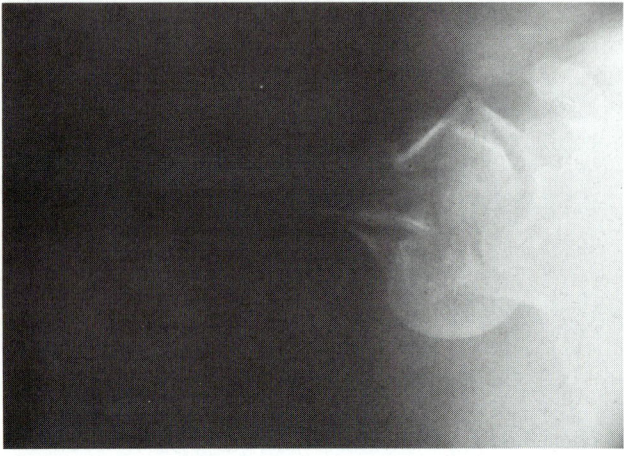

Figure 14.4. Axillary view showing a locked posterior dislocation of the humeral head behind the glenoid.

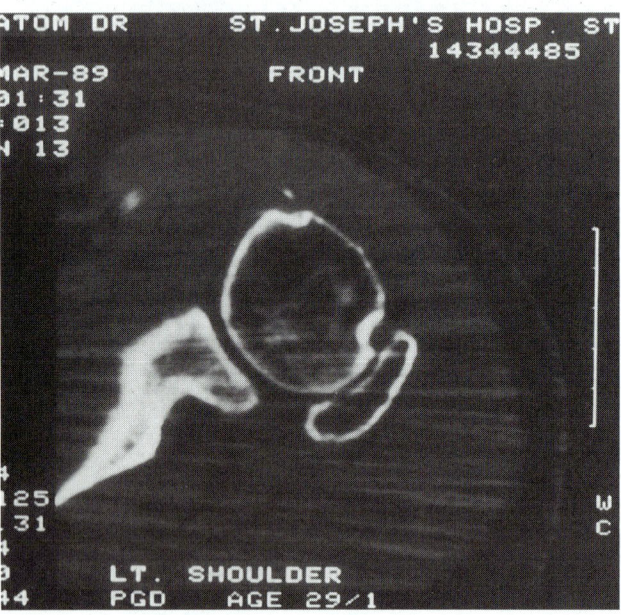

Figure 14.5. CT scan showing a posteriorly displaced greater tuberosity.

about the rotator cuff, head viability, and tuberosity position but do not reveal bony details as clearly as CT scans.

Three-dimensional reconstruction of CT images in complex, multiplane, or comminuted proximal humeral fractures—particularly those associated with glenoid, acromial, or clavicular fractures—can add information about the position of the segments and degree of comminution. They can be used for planning the approach or internal fixation of the fracture.

An electromyogram (EMG) should be considered if neurologic damage is suspected in a proximal humeral fracture. If injury is suspected, it is wise to document the presence and extent of nerve injury before manipulation or operative internal fixation.

TREATMENT

Nonoperative Treatment

Patients with nondisplaced proximal humeral fractures can usually be treated nonoperatively with expectations of a good outcome. This is independent of the number of fracture lines and degree of comminution. For example, a patient with nondisplaced fractures of the greater tuberosity, lesser tuberosity, and surgical neck with comminution can be treated exactly as a patient with a nondisplaced isolated greater tuberosity fracture. A possible exception is an isolated greater tuberosity fracture with superior displacement less than 1 cm. In this fracture, small degrees of superior displacement may lead to late subacromial space impingement; thus consideration should be given for early aggressive restoration of the normal anatomy in this fracture.

The arm is placed in a sling for comfort. When the initial discomfort has receded, gentle range of motion exercises are started that concentrate on forward flexion, external rotation, and internal rotation. In addition, isometric exercises for the cuff and deltoid can be begun when comfort permits. Resistive strengthening exercises are best left until radiographic union of the fracture occurs, usually at 6 to 8 weeks after injury. The fracture should be stable and move the entire extremity as a unit before exercises are begun. The best way to determine whether the humerus moves as a unit is by palpation of the greater tuberosity with one hand while the other hand provides gentle rotation of the distal humerus. If the tuberosity moves beneath the fingers as the humerus rotates, the humerus can be considered to be moving as a unit.

In addition, nonoperative treatment might be considered in patients who have displaced fractures of the proximal humerus who are willing to accept a limited range of motion and function. Consider treating a displaced fracture nonoperatively if the patient is elderly, the fracture involves a nondominant arm, the bone is quite osteopenic, or medical problems exist that may be associated with significant morbidity from operative fixation. Remember to treat the patient first, not the fracture.

Operative Treatment

The operative treatment of proximal humeral fractures depends not only on the fracture anatomy but also on the needs and goals of the patient and the skills of the surgeon. Various techniques are available, and treatment is best addressed according to each individual fracture; generalizations are difficult when applying criteria for internal fixation (Clinical Table).

SURGICAL NECK FRACTURE

Fractures that occur below the level of the tuberosities involve the surgical neck of the humerus. The humeral shaft is frequently displaced medially by the pull of the

Clinical Table: Fractures and Nounions of the Proximal Humerus

Procedure	Indications	Technique	Anatomy	Pitfalls
ORIF: 2-part surgical neck fractures	• Displaced fracture through the surgical neck	• Long deltopectoral approach • Secure the humeral head to shaft • Tension band • Fixation	• Deltopectoral location • Rotator cuff • Biceps tendon	• Soft tissue interposition (biceps tendon) • Insecure fixation in osteopenic bone • Rod backout if intramedullary rods used
ORIF: 2-part greater or lesser tuberosity fractures	• Displaced greater or lesser tuberosity segment	• Anterior and superior approach • Deltoid split • Identify the biceps tendon as a guide to the displaced tuberosity segment • Secure the fragment with tension band or screw • Repair rotator cuff deficit	• Terminal branch of the axillary nerve • Biceps tendon • Cuff tendon attached to displaced tuberosity segment	• Insecure fixation in osteopenic bone, particularly if screws are used • Nonanatomic greater tuberosity repair, leading to late impingement
ORIF: 3-part fractures with displacement	• Displaced 3-part humeral fracture	• Long deltopectoral approach • Secure the displaced tuberosity to the head–intact tuberosity fragment • Secure the head–tuberosity fragment to the shaft • Bone graft juncture • Figure eight tension band	• Biceps tendon • Rotator cuff • Head rotated by intact tuberosity • Head may be in varus or valgus position	• Tuberosity repositioning too high • Top of humeral head 3 mm above top of greater tuberosity • Inadequate fixation; use tension band • Superior prominence borders if plate is used
Prosthetic replacement	• 4-part, head split • 3-part fracture in osteopenic bone	• Long deltopectoral incision • Find the biceps tendon • Tag and identify the tuberosity fragments • Prepare the humerus for the prosthesis • Place the prosthesis in proper version with proper height • Secure the tuberosity to both humeral prosthesis and humeral shaft	• Biceps tendon is guide to displaced tuberosity segments • Axillary nerve near the subscapularis musculotendinous junction	• Prosthesis placed too high or too low in humeral shaft • Failure to place proper soft tissue tension • Prosthesis with improper version; retroversion should be 30–40 • Failure to secure greater tuberosity to humerus (bone graft) • Rigid fixation of tuberosity to humeral shaft and implant
ORIF or hemiarthroplasty of nonunions	• Symptomatic nonunions of the proximal humerus	• Technique depends on the condition of the glenohumeral joint • Bone graft at the nonunion site	• Axillary nerve • Rotator cuff	• Insufficient soft tissues and capsular releases to restore shoulder motion • Osteopenic bone and inadequate fixation • Too early return of motion, leading to persistent nonunion • Failure to use bone graft

pectoralis major and other large muscle groups that insert on the shaft of the humerus. The head and greater tuberosity segment may be in a neutral position or may be in slight abduction. Some displaced surgical neck fractures are amenable to closed manipulation, whereas others require percutaneous pin fixation or formal open reduction and internal fixation (ORIF) (Fig. 14.6).

Closed manipulation may be considered in some surgical neck fractures. The goal is to position the shaft under the head–tuberosity segment, impacting it in that position; thus gentle traction and abduction to relax the pectoralis major usually results in satisfactory positioning of the humeral shaft under the tuberosity. Once the muscles are relaxed and the shaft is repositioned under the tuberosity–head segment, the shaft can be impacted into the cancellous area of the fracture. The fracture is usually stabilized at this point. If the fracture remains stable and reduction is not lost, the patient is kept in a sling until early healing occurs and range of motion exercises are begun.

If the fracture is either irreducible or reducible and unstable (the reduction cannot be maintained), the fracture must be stabilized. If the fracture cannot be reduced, there is frequently soft tissue interposition (from the biceps or capsule), and the surgeon should proceed to ORIF. If the fracture is reducible but stability is lost, the fracture should be stabilized by percutaneous pin fixation or ORIF. Closed reduction and percutaneous pin fixation is a good technique to use if the neck fracture can be reduced but is unstable. In osteopenic bone, adequate purchase may preclude successful use of this technique. Once the fracture is stabilized, early exercises for range of motion and strength can be performed.

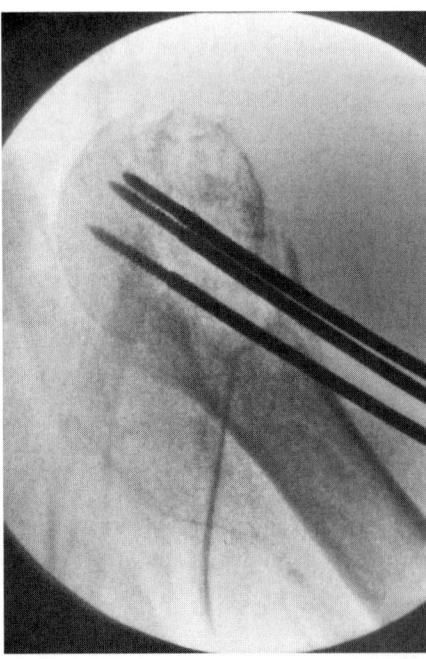

Figure 14.6. A displaced 2-part surgical neck fracture may be treated by closed reduction and stabilized by percutaneous pins, which are placed under fluoroscopic control.

The technique for percutaneous pin fixation is as follows. Under image intensification, two AO threaded tip pins are placed in the humeral shaft at or near the deltoid insertion to control the shaft segment. One pin is placed superiorly to inferiorly in the greater tuberosity and a second pin is placed horizontally to serve as joysticks to manipulate the head segment and the shaft together. Once the shaft is reduced under the head segment, the greater tuberosity pin can be advanced from superior to inferior to secure the head segment to the shaft. Once the cortex is penetrated, the lateral humeral pins can be angled and redirected into the head of the humerus. Care must be taken to achieve adequate visualization on the image intensifier so that penetration of the humeral articular surface does not occur. If this technique is used, the pins can be removed in about 3 weeks, at which time the fracture is usually stable enough that the segments will no longer displace.

ORIF is reserved primarily for irreducible fractures, severely osteopenic bone, or a muscular or heavy arm; intra-articular percutaneous purchase of pins in bony segments cannot be obtained. A number of techniques for ORIF are available, including minimal pin internal fixation, intramedullary rod fixation, plate fixation, tension banding, and combinations of these.

In recent years, minimal internal fixation has become a popular method. This technique involves minimal stripping of the fracture site in an effort to save the vascularity of humeral head and to encourage healing. Because the exposure of the fracture fragments is limited with this technique, rigid internal fixation is sacrificed. Multiple pins are used to provide fixation enough to stabilize the fracture without the extensive dissection frequently needed for formal ORIF with a plate and screws.

If rigid internal fixation is to be attempted, the fracture is exposed through a deltopectoral approach. The deltoid and pectoralis are retracted, the biceps and pectoralis major are identified, and the fracture is identified. Any interposed soft tissue is removed, and the fracture is reduced. A drill hole is made in the lateral humeral cortex, and either heavy-gauge wire or heavy nonabsorbable suture (number 5) is passed through a drill hole in the humerus. This suture is then passed through the rotator cuff at the tuberosity–cuff junction and tightened in a figure eight fashion. A figure eight tension band technique can be combined with an intramedullary rod (such as a Rush rod). Because intramedullary devices can lose their purchase and back out of the cuff superiorly, causing late rotator cuff problems, it is more desirable to approach this fracture using a figure eight wire or suture alone.

TWO-PART GREATER TUBEROSITY FRACTURE

The 2-part greater tuberosity fracture is frequently associated with anterior dislocations of the shoulder. When displaced, the greater tuberosity segment is pulled superiorly and posteriorly (Fig. 14.7). If the fracture is permitted to heal in this position, external rotation and abduction will be blocked and motion will be extremely limited. Thus it is important to achieve near anatomic restoration

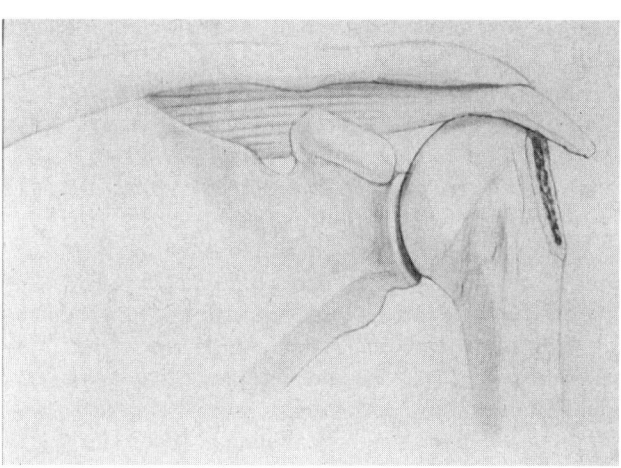

Figure 14.7. A 2-part greater tuberosity fracture is displaced superiorly by the pull of the supraspinatus.

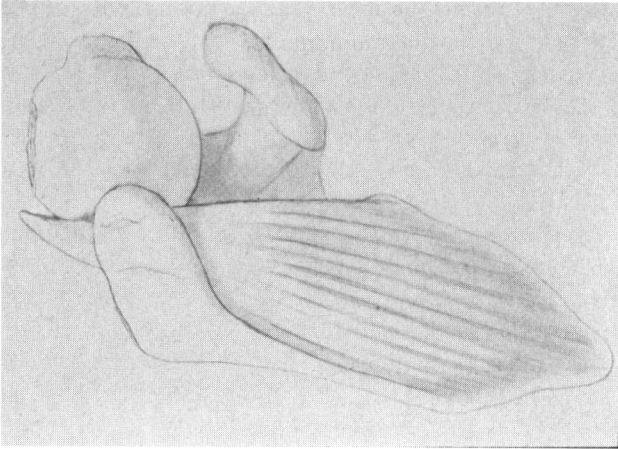

Figure 14.8. A 2-part greater tuberosity fracture displaced posteriorly, pulling all external rotators.

of the greater tuberosity segment. Although the Neer definition of displacement is 1 cm, smaller degrees of superior displacement of the greater tuberosity may result in significantly diminished function.

Closed reduction of a 2-part greater tuberosity fracture is difficult if the greater tuberosity is significantly displaced posteriorly or superiorly. Some authors have advocated percutaneous pinning of the greater tuberosity segment and manipulating it back into place, but this frequently compromises the anatomic restoration of the tuberosity.

However, when accompanied by an anterior dislocation, the greater tuberosity may be maintained at a near anatomic location. Once the humeral head is relocated, the tuberosity may be in an acceptable position and early rehabilitation may be begun. If the greater tuberosity is displaced once the humeral head is relocated, however, reduction via internal fixation should be performed. Because late displacement of the tuberosity segment may occur, sequential x-rays should be performed to assess its position.

Greater tuberosity displacement implies a tear in the rotator cuff, usually at the interval between the supraspinatus and the subscapularis. If the greater tuberosity is anatomic once the fracture is reduced, the rotator interval may heal. If the greater tuberosity is not anatomic, a defect in the rotator interval persists. If the greater tuberosity is internally fixed, the rotator interval tear should be closed at that time (Fig. 14.8).

ORIF should be performed when the greater tuberosity segment is displaced significantly posteriorly or superiorly to avoid the sequela of tuberosity malunion or nonunion. The fracture is approached through a superior incision. The deltoid muscle is split, taking care not to extend the split beyond 5 cm from the deltoid origin on the acromion to minimize the chance of injury to the terminal branches of the axillary nerve. With the deltoid muscle retracted, the long head of biceps is located and followed up to the area of the rotator interval (the biceps is a good

guide to the position of the greater and lesser tuberosities). The greater tuberosity with attached rotator cuff is posterior to the long head of biceps. Several stay sutures are placed in the rotator cuff, and the greater tuberosity can be manipulated back to its donor site.

The two most effective means of internal fixation are use of a screw (with a washer) and a figure eight tension band with heavy nonabsorbable suture. A screw and washer are usually satisfactory for internal fixation when the bone is not osteopenic; moving the screw can get purchase on the medial cortex and avoid intra-articular penetration. If a tension band is to be used, heavy nonabsorbable suture is passed through the greater tuberosity and through the humeral shaft; a figure eight technique secures the greater tuberosity tightly to the donor site on the humeral shaft. Once greater tuberosity fixation is anatomic, the rotator cuff tear can be repaired by closure of the rotator interval.

TWO-PART LESSER TUBEROSITY FRACTURE

The 2-part lesser tuberosity fracture is much less common than the greater tuberosity fracture. When displaced, the lesser tuberosity is pulled medially by the subscapularis muscle. Some displacement of this fragment is acceptable, because late impingement is not common. A lesser tuberosity fracture may be accompanied by a posterior dislocation, and the position of the lesser tuberosity may be identified once relocation of the humeral head has been performed.

If ORIF is performed, the surgical approach is similar to that described for a greater tuberosity fracture. If the lesser tuberosity piece is quite small and comminuted and if purchase is difficult on the segment, the bony fragment can be excised, and the subscapularis tendons can be sutured directly to the donor site adjacent to the bicipital groove.

THREE-PART FRACTURE

Three-part fractures of the proximal humerus are among the most difficult fractures to treat. These injuries include a fracture through the surgical neck, and the pull of the pectoralis major displaces the shaft medially. Either the greater or the lesser tuberosity is also fractured and displaced, and the remaining intact tuberosity rotates the articular surface either posteriorly (if the lesser tuberosity is intact) or anteriorly (if the greater tuberosity is intact) (Fig. 14.9). It is the rotational deformity combined with the shaft displacement that makes evaluation and anatomic restoration difficult. These fractures tend to occur in osteopenic bone and occur frequently in elderly patients; thus the clinician must decide whether to attempt restoration of the anatomy or to replace the humeral head surface with a prosthetic device. In addition, there are some patients in whom marked fracture deformity with its attended limitations may be acceptable if other circumstances surrounding the patient make this the better option (such as medical risk).

Closed reduction of a 3-part fracture is particularly difficult because the intact tuberosity rotates the humeral head through the surgical neck fracture. The surgical neck fracture makes positioning the arm precisely under the rotated head and the tuberosity segment nearly impossible. Some authors advocate using temporary pins in the intact tuberosity–head segment as joysticks to manipulate the segment into place. This, however, is an extremely technically demanding procedure, as reduction must be accomplished in multiple planes with pins that are placed through quite osteopenic bone. There is a marked tendency for the fracture fragments to displace.

ORIF is by far the most common method of treating a 3-part fracture. The displaced tuberosity segment is aligned with the intact head–tuberosity segment and then secured to the shaft of the humerus. For some patients, particularly if there is a marked comminution or osteopenic bone, the surgeon may decide to sacrifice the humeral head and reconstruct both tuberosities to a prosthetic hemiarthroplasty. This may permit early rehabilitation and return of range of motion. In a young patient with good-quality bone, ORIF is probably a better choice.

Many techniques for ORIF of 3-part fractures have been described, including the use of plate and screws, intramedullary rods, staples, and wires. The most popular method was described by Hawkins et al. (2). With a tension band, either of wire or heavy nonabsorbable suture, the surgeon reduces the fracture by securing the displaced greater tuberosity to the head and intact tuberosity segment, thus derotating the humeral head. Once the humeral head is derotated, the head segment can be joined to the humeral shaft segment.

In this technique, the shoulder is approached via long deltopectoral incision. Once the clavipectoral fascia has been incised, hematoma, bone fragments, and debris are removed. Next, the long head of biceps is identified, and the tendon is followed superiorly to the rotator interval as a guide to the position of the greater and lesser tuberosities. Stay sutures are placed in the two tuberosity–cuff segments; and the tuberosities are reduced to one another, which derotates the head. Using a colpotomy needle or a large Intracath needle, the surgeon passes heavy gauge wire or nonabsorbable suture through both tuberosity segments. When these are secured and tightened, the wire or suture is passed through drill holes in the lateral humeral shaft, and a figure eight tension band secures the two tuberosities to the lateral shaft of the humerus.

For patients with marked comminution of a greater or lesser tuberosity segment and those with osteopenic bone that make internal fixation difficult, it is probably better to consider prosthetic arthroplasty and repair of the tuberosities around the implant and to the shaft directly. The technique of prosthetic insertion for a 3-part fracture is identical to that described for a 4-part displacement (below).

FOUR-PART AND HEAD-SPLIT FRACTURES

In 4-part fractures, both tuberosities are fractured and displaced from one another, the shaft is displaced, and the articular surface is separated from both tuberosity segments (Fig. 14.10). Usually the only soft tissue attachment to the humeral head is residual capsular tissue. Because the humeral head is separated from its blood supply, there is concern about the viability of the humeral head and late avascular necrosis (Fig. 14.11). Thus, although saving the humeral head has been advocated by some authors, particularly if the fracture occurs in a young person, it is probable that prosthetic arthroplasty offers the best chance for long-term pain relief, restoration of function, and early rehabilitation. Other fractures in which a humeral head arthroplasty may be considered are the head-split fracture, some 3-part fractures, fractures in elderly or osteopenic patients, and fractures involving a fixed dislocation of the humeral head in which more than 40% of the articular surface is destroyed.

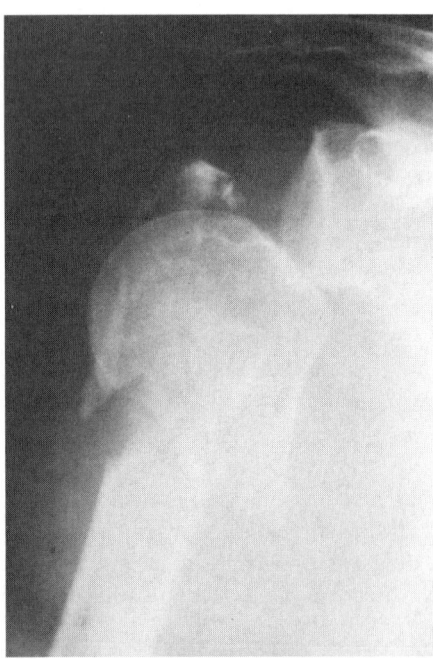

Figure 14.9. AP view showing a 3-part fracture. The articular surface is rotated by intact lesser tuberosity. The greater tuberosity is displaced superiorly.

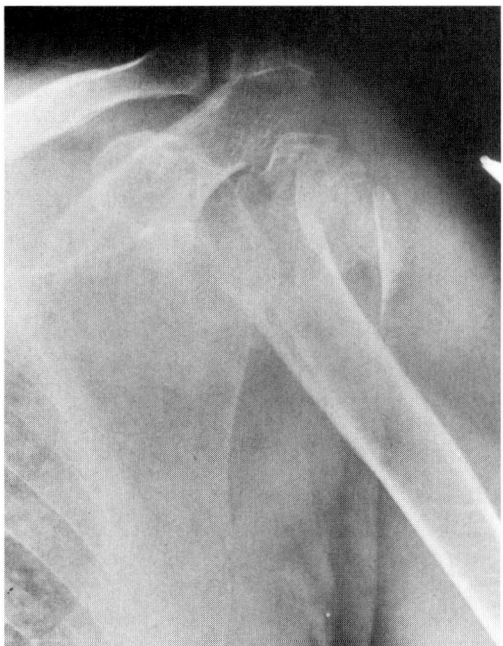

Figure 14.10. X-ray of 4-part fracture-dislocation.

marked degenerative changes and cartilage loss have occurred, consideration is given to resurfacing the glenoid as well. The humeral head fragment is preserved for later bone grafting. Next, the exposed proximal shaft is delivered into the wound for preparation.

The humeral shaft is prepared to accept an appropriately sized implant. Since the tuberosities will be reconstructed around the implant, the difficult intraoperative decision making revolves around precise implant positioning, specifically the superior and inferior depth to which the prosthesis should be inserted in the humeral canal and the degree of retroversion. If the implant is inserted too deeply, prominence of the tuberosity along with late impingement or laxity of the soft tissue surrounding the implant along with instability can result. If the implant is too proud, a high degree of tension can exist in the soft tissue around the implant, limiting the range of motion and causing pain. So proper superior and inferior implant depth is critical. One way to measure the proper depth of the implant is through the tension of the biceps tendon. If the biceps tendon around the implant is too taut, the humeral head will probably be too proud, or prominent. Likewise, if the biceps tendon is slack, the humeral head is probably too low.

The surgeon should attempt to reproduce the normal humeral head retroversion of approximately 30° to 40°. Retroversion can be estimated by the prosthetic device's position relative to the transverse axis of the elbow or can be precisely measured with a commercial guide.

Once the soft tissue is under the proper tension and the position of the implant has been determined relative to the humeral shaft, the tuberosities are brought to the anatomic position around the implant. Most humeral components are cemented, since stability is lost once the tuberosities are fractured. Since the greater and lesser tuberosities will be secured to the humeral shaft, drill

The technique of humeral head replacement has become well established. The approach is through a long deltopectoral incision. The deltoid and pectoralis are retracted, the clavipectoral fascia is incised up to the level of the coracoacromial ligament, and the conjoined tendon is retracted medially. The biceps is identified and followed to the area of the rotator interval. The rotator interval is released, and stay sutures are placed around the subscapularis and supraspinatus tendons for control of both tuberosity segments. Hematoma, bony debris, and fibrous tissue are removed, and the joint is examined. Usually, the glenoid cartilage is satisfactory and can be left alone. If

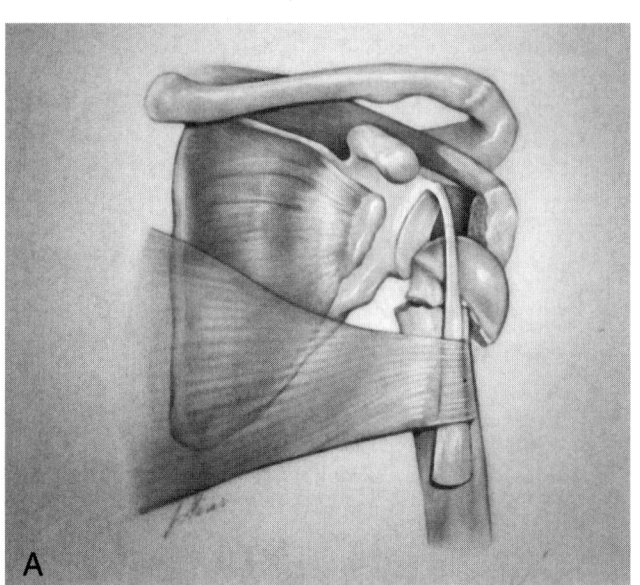
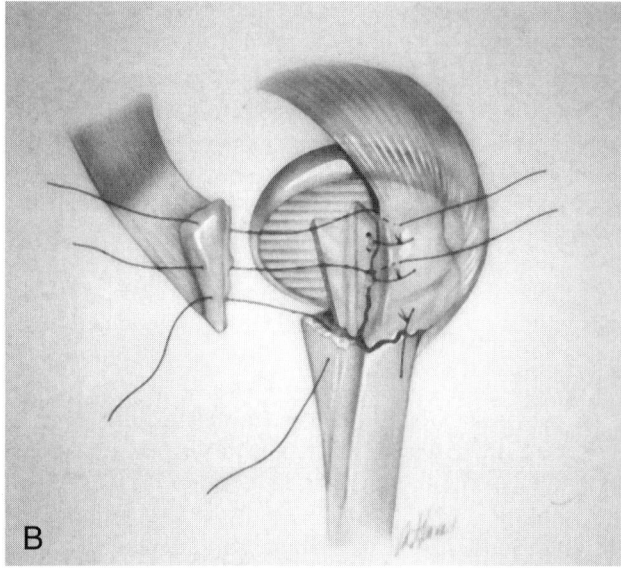

Figure 14.11. A. A 4-part fracture. All segments are displaced from one another. **B.** For hemi-arthroplasty, tuberosity segments are secured to implant, to each other, and to shaft.

holes in the shaft are made, and nonabsorbable suture is passed through the holes before the implant is cemented.

Once the hemiarthroplasty is cemented into place, the greater and lesser tuberosities are secured via sutures both to the implant and to the shaft of the humerus. The tuberosity–shaft junction is filled with bone graft harvested from the removed humeral head. It is the healing of the tuberosity to the shaft that determines the degree of power and function, since the rotator cuff transmits its forces from the greater and lesser tuberosities to the shaft. Once the tuberosity is anchored into place, the rotator interval is closed, and the wound is closed in layers. Passive range of motion is begun soon after surgery, but active range of motion is not permitted until there is radiographic union of the tuberosity segments to the shaft.

PITFALLS AND COMMON MISTAKES

Two-Part Fractures

One pitfall of ORIF of 2-part surgical neck fractures is hardware failure. If insecure, Rush rods and other intramedullary fixation devices may back out through the rotator cuff and become prominent. If they interfere with cuff function, they need to be removed. Secure plate fixation in osteopenic bone may be difficult, particularly if an inadequate number of screws are used. Furthermore, it is difficult to secure the greater tuberosity to the shaft with just one screw. Although a washer may help, a second screw and washer and bone graft should be considered. A tension band may be the better choice for reconstructing osteopenic bone.

When repairing displaced greater and lesser tuberosity fragments, the surgeon can damage the deltoid. If it is split past 4 or 5 cm from its origin, the terminal branches of the axillary nerve may be injured, which in turn denervate the deltoid muscle.

Nonanatomic reduction of the tuberosity leads to late cuff dysfunction and impingement and eventually may necessitate an osteotomy. To minimize a nonanatomic relocation of the tuberosity segment, the greater and lesser tuberosities should be placed precisely in the donor defect. In addition, if a reduction and internal fixation of the greater tuberosity is done, consideration for an adjunctive anterior acromioplasty should be given to provide more room in a subacromial space.

Three-Part Fractures

Hardware failure is a pitfall of ORIF of 3-part fractures. A common mistake is to extend the plate too far superior to the greater tuberosity, which interferes with subacromial motion. The internal fixation purchase may be compromised in osteopenic bone, necessitating a long rehabilitation rather than early mobilization. Hemiarthroplasty should be considered for osteopenic patients.

If the head is not derotated and positioned anatomically relative to the tuberosities, the tuberosities may be too prominent. Care should be taken to make certain that the greater tuberosities are positioned beneath the humeral head. Normally, the top of the humeral head is 3 to 4 mm above the top of the greater tuberosity.

Four-Part Fractures

Proper implant placement is important with hemiarthroplasty. If the humeral head is too high, an overly tight shoulder with secondary glenoid pain may occur. If the humeral head is positioned too low, prominence of the greater tuberosity and laxity and instability of the implant often occur. The tension in the biceps tendon is a useful guide for correct superior and inferior positioning of the humeral head.

If there is a loss of greater tuberosity fixation and adequate healing of the greater tuberosity does not occur, the rotator cuff cannot transmit its power to the shaft of the humerus, making it impossible to position the arm and limiting range of motion. Attention should be paid to secure fixation of the greater tuberosity not only to the humeral replacement but also to the humeral shaft. Bone graft should be used at the greater tuberosity–shaft junction.

SUMMARY

Fractures of the proximal humerus are extremely common and occur throughout a variety of age groups. Their successful treatment, whether closed or open, must take into account associated injury, subsequent deforming forces, and impact on the musculotendinous rotator cuff and pectoralis major. Successful closed treatment requires neutralization of these deforming forces. Successful operative treatment requires recognition that repair and rehabilitation are equally important for the associated soft tissue injury as for the bony injury.

II Nonunions of the Proximal Humerus

Nonunions of the proximal humerus can be broadly categorized as those resulting from general medical conditions inhibiting healing and those relating to specific features of the anatomy, biomechanics, and fracture treatment. Hypertension, alcoholism, diabetes, and obstructive lung disease are associated with an increased incidence of humeral nonunion, just as they are associated with delayed or inadequate healing of all fractures. Soft tissue interposition, particularly of the deltoid muscle, biceps tendon, and shoulder capsule, can contribute to the development of proximal humeral nonunion, especially with fractures involving the surgical neck. Insecure immobilization, particularly if it contributes to fracture distraction (e.g., with a hanging cast), is thought to interfere with the healing process.

Fracture biology may also contribute to nonunion development in the proximal humerus. Many fractures that result in nonunion are intra-articular. Joint fluid contains proteolytic enzymes that may alter the environment for healing, particularly in fractures involving the surgical and anatomic necks. In addition, operative internal fixation, especially in osteopenic bone, can contribute to nonunion via fracture distraction, operative infection, or devascularization of fragments. A false sense of security may lead to overly aggressive postoperative therapy, which can cause movement through the fracture site, resulting in nonunion.

INITIAL FINDINGS, PHYSICAL EXAMINATION, AND DIAGNOSIS

The most common complaints with a symptomatic nonunion of a proximal humerus fracture are pain and stiffness. The stiffness is often present in both the shoulder and elbow and is often related to extended immobilization associated with the fracture treatment (3). Stiffness is common with nonunions involving one or both tuberosities. With a surgical neck nonunion, gross motion is often present through the fracture site, and the motion of the humeral head is not transmitted to the rest of the extremity. Such patients generally complain of weakness or loss of control of the extremity, since the rotator cuff has lost its ability to center, rotate, and position the upper extremity (4).

On clinical examination, poorly localized tenderness, with or without crepitus at the fracture site, may be present. With displaced tuberosity nonunions, a bony block to active and passive range of motion is often present. A displaced greater tuberosity may block external rotation and abduction, whereas a displaced lesser tuberosity may block internal rotation. With surgical neck nonunions, passive range of motion is difficult to estimate because of the gross motion at the nonunion site and the pain produced by this movement. A particularly common clinical sign is loss of rotatory control: If the extremity is positioned at the side and is passively externally rotated, the patient is unable to maintain the position because the external rotators are not able to control the entire humeral shaft through the nonunion. Active elevation of the arm is limited because while the humeral head may be elevated, the shaft is not.

If the nonunion is associated with prior internal fixation, consideration should be given to the possible presence of underlying infection. A history of initial postoperative wound drainage or infection or postoperative fever and persistent pain should be sought. Blood work, radioisotope scanning, and even site aspiration and culture should be considered.

RADIOLOGIC STUDIES

Plain radiographs, including the trauma series, should be the initial step in the evaluation of a suspected nonunion. X-rays not only will confirm the presence of a nonunion but can be used to assess the condition of the glenohumeral joint and to estimate the bone quality and degree of osteopenia. In long-standing surgical neck nonunions, constant motion at the neck shaft junction can lead to resorption of a substantial volume of soft cancellous bone of the humeral head. If this has occurred, primary reduction and internal fixation with bone grafting may be impossible because of limited bone stock. In this case, arthroplasty rather than nonunion repair is considered.

If plain x-rays leave doubt about the existence of a nonunion, CT studies usually establish the diagnosis. For complex nonunions, which involve not only the surgical neck but also the tuberosities, CT scans, with or without three-dimensional reconstruction, help visualize the pathologic anatomy.

TREATMENT

Two-Part Surgical Neck Nonunion

The 2-part surgical neck nonunion is the most common proximal humeral nonunion encountered in daily orthopaedic practice. Not all surgical nonunions require operative intervention. Some patients experience little pain and minimal functional limitations and, therefore, can be managed nonoperatively. For patients with severe underlying medical conditions, the risk of operative intervention may be too great. Operative intervention should be considered for the majority of symptomatic patients.

Operative management of a surgical neck nonunion depends on the particular fracture anatomy, the presence of associated injuries, the neurovascular status of the extremity, the quality of the bone, and the demands and needs of the patient. Surgical treatment involves either preservation of the humeral head and fixation with grafts or a humeral head replacement. If there is adequate bone stock present and the glenoid is not arthritic, an attempt is made to proceed with reduction and fixation.

A number of different techniques have been used to address the internal fixation of surgical neck nonunions (4). The presence of osteopenic bone, capsular intended contracture, and extra-articular adhesions must all be considered. If there is little capsular and glenoidal joint stiffness, if the proximal fragment seems to be mobile enough to maintain postoperative motion, and if the bone quality is good, an attempt is made to perform internal fixation.

If, however, marked stiffness exists in the glenohumeral joint (common with long-standing nonunions), the surgeon should consider a two-stage approach to surgical fixation. In stage one, the nonunion is taken down and internal fixation with bone grafting is done. The patient is then immobilized for a period of time without any attempt at motion to maximize the chance at obtaining fracture union. Once union has been obtained, the second stage consists of removing hardware and adhesions, releasing the contracted tissue, and early mobilization.

The same principles of fracture reduction and fixation that apply to acute 2-part surgical neck fractures apply to this situation. The use of tension band techniques alone or in conjunction with intramedullary devices help control the rotational torque supplied by the rotator cuff muscles on the proximal humeral fragment. Furthermore, tension band sutures or wires can incorporate the cuff tissue and give improved fixation in soft bone of the humeral head. Regardless of which fixation technique is chosen, bone grafting of the nonunion site is important.

In patients with glenohumeral arthrosis or severely osteopenic bone, humeral arthroplasty should be considered. In the presence of joint degeneration, internal fixation, even if successful, may lead to a high failure rate because of the persistence of postoperative pain and restricted joint motion. The use of primary humeral head arthroplasty, with or without bone grafting of the nonunion site, provides immediate stability and offers the chance for a relatively rapid postoperative rehabilitation.

Greater Tuberosity Nonunion

Tuberosity nonunions are rare in clinical practice; although greater tuberosity nonunions are much more common than lesser tuberosity nonunions. Greater tuberosity nonunion usually presents with pain and loss of abduction; and the majority of motion loss results from a mechanical block, as the tuberosity displaces posterosuperiorly into the subacromial space. The lesser tuberosity may displace medially, restricting internal rotation. These nonunions usually result from failure to recognize displacement at the time of the initial injury or during follow-up evaluation.

Most tuberosity nonunions are amenable to treatment by open ORIF, even in the presence of significant osteoporosis. Only in the presence of advanced osteoarthritis should the surgeon consider arthroplasty as a treatment option. This typically does not occur with isolated tuberosity nonunion, but it may occur with complex combined tuberosity and neck nonunions (3- and 4-part fractures).

Symptoms of greater tuberosity nonunion are related to the loss of cuff function and the mechanical obstruction of the displaced fragment into the subacromial space. Thus the primary complaints are difficulty with external rotation and abduction, and the predominant symptoms are related to the position of the displaced fragment. On physical examination, a mechanical block to active and passive abduction may be present, and the presence of a block to external rotation when the arm is maximally abducted should raise suspicions for this pathology. With posterior displacement of the tuberosity, the patient tends to have marked weakness to external rotation, and the clinician may sense a mechanical block to passive external rotation with the humeral head tending to lever against the glenoid.

At the time of evaluation it is critical to obtain AP, lateral, and axillary views of the affected shoulder. The axillary view will often identify tuberosity displacement not appreciated on the AP or lateral views. A CT scan can be obtained to clarify fracture anatomy if needed. Small, comminuted, partially resorbed displaced greater tuberosity fragments in the subacromial space have occasionally been confused with chronic calcific tendonitis.

Treatment of greater tuberosity nonunion is difficult, in part because the long-standing fixed displacement results in fixed contracture and shortening of the rotator cuff and capsule; the cuff must be released before the fragment can be adequately repositioned. Most tuberosity nonunions are amenable to ORIF, even in the presence of significant osteoporosis.

The greater tuberosity nonunion is best approached through a standard deltopectoral incision. This gives maximum flexibility for mobilization of the fragment and release of contracted soft tissues. Acromioplasty is frequently done, particularly in older patients and those whose radiographs reveal anterior acromial spurs. The greater tuberosity fragments should be identified, attached scar and fibrous tissue released, and the fragments advanced to the original donor position. It may be necessary to release the posterior and superior capsule at the glenoid margin so that adequate restoration of the tuberosity to its natural site can be achieved. Once the fragment is reduced, it is secured to the proximal humerus with nonabsorbable suture.

Lesser Tuberosity Nonunion

Lesser tuberosity nonunions, as with lesser tuberosity fractures, are much less common than either surgical neck or greater tuberosity nonunions. They generally occur in conjunction with posterior dislocation of the shoulder. If there is not much displacement, the injury is better tolerated than is greater tuberosity displacement, even if nonunion develops. There are two reasons for this: The lesser tuberosity does not impinge in the subacromial space, and the other internal rotators of the shoulder (pectoralis, teres major, latissimus dorsi) may compensate for any strength deficits. Clinical symptoms, if they occur, may be mechanical (blocks to internal rotation) in nature or related to weakness.

Rarely will lesser tuberosity nonunions be symptomatic enough to warrant surgical intervention. If symptoms are significant, however, a surgical subscapularis repair to the donor site should be attempted. Because the lesser tuberosity segment itself is usually quite small, it is often possible to simply excise the fragment. Other, less practical options include performing internal fixation with a bone graft. Capsular release at the glenoid neck may be required to achieve appropriate length and avoid internal rotation contracture.

Anatomic Neck Nonunion

The anatomic neck fracture passes from superolateral to inferomedial on the humeral head, separating the articular surface of the humeral head from the surrounding bone. Because the blood supply to the humeral head comes mainly from the circumflex artery, fractures of the anatomic neck often devascularize the articular fragment, resulting in avascular necrosis. Isolated anatomic neck fractures are rare and are most commonly seen in younger patients. The true incidence of nonunion is unknown. Most anatomic nonunions are seen as late sequela to 4-part humeral fractures, which by definition have an anatomic neck fracture as one component.

The treatment of surgical neck nonunion is typically humeral head arthroplasty. ORIF does not have a role in the management of this injury because options for secure fixation are limited and vascular considerations make the odds of successful union slim. Surgical exposure and manipulation of the articular fragment subject it to further devascularization.

Postoperative Management

For both ORIF and glenohumeral arthroplasty, intraoperative fixation should be secure enough to allow for immediate postoperative passive range of motion. Complete postoperative immobilization should not routinely be used to compensate for poor surgical fixation. Immobilization will lead to loss of postoperative range of motion and increase the odds of obtaining a poor result. The only exception to this situation is when a 2-stage approach to surgical neck nonunion is undertaken.

Once fracture healing has occurred, typically within 6 to 8 weeks, gentle assisted active motion is started. This is continued and progressed over the following 4 to 6 weeks. At that time fracture healing should be far enough along so that resistive exercises may be begun. A rehabilitation course that progresses too quickly before healing is complete may lead to recurrence or persistence of the nonunion.

SUMMARY

Although malunion and nonunion of the proximal humerus are uncommon, they are a frequent cause of late pain, stiffness, loss of function, and deformity following a shoulder fracture period. Successful operative treatment of this requires recognition of the dual impact of bone deformity and soft tissue scarring; contracture and dysfunction must be evaluated, corrected, and rehabilitated.

REFERENCES

1. Kristiansen D, Bredensen J, Erin-Madsen J, et al. Epidemiology of proximal humeral fractures. Act Orthop Scand 1987;58:75–77.
2. Hawkins RJ, Bell RH, Gurr K. The three-part fracture of the proximal part of the humerus. Operative treatment. J Bone Joint Surg 1986;68A:1410–1414.
3. Beredjiklian PK, Iannotti JP, Norris TP, et al. Operative treatment of malunion of a fracture of the proximal aspect of the humerus. J Bone Joint Surg 1998;88A:1484–1497.
4. Healy WL, Jupiter JB, Kristiansen TK, et al. Non-union of the proximal humerus. J Orthop Trauma 1990;4:424–431.

Michael J. Maynard

Acromioclavicular Joint Injury and Repair

The acromioclavicular (AC) joint is the most peripheral component of the upper extremity appendicular linkage, which also includes the clavicle and the sternoclavicular joint. Together, these components provide the direct mechanical connection of the upper extremity to the axial skeleton. All significant mechanical forces applied directly to or through the upper extremity are ultimately transmitted across this linkage. The acromioclavicular joint complex includes the acromion, the coracoid, the distal clavicle, the acromioclavicular ligaments (AC joint capsule), the coracoclavicular ligaments (conoid and trapezoid), and the deltoid and trapezius muscles.

Large and/or rapidly applied forces may exceed the mechanical strength parameters of the linkage components, resulting in injuries such as damage to the acromioclavicular joint, fracture of the clavicle, damage to the sternoclavicular joint, and damage to nearby soft tissues (including the brachial plexus and nearby vascular structures). Therefore, although the focus of this chapter is on the recognition and treatment of acromioclavicular joint linkage, it is important to keep in mind local neurovascular structures, supporting muscular, and other soft tissues when assessing and treating injury to the AC joint.

INITIAL FINDINGS, PHYSICAL EXAMINATION, AND DIAGNOSIS

Injury to the acromioclavicular joint is commonly referred to as AC separation or shoulder separation. The two most common settings for AC joint injury are athletics and motor vehicle accidents. Specifically, the most common precipitating event is a force application directly onto the lateral edge of the acromion (1). Rockwood and Young's (2) classification system of AC joint injuries is well accepted and comprises six grades of injury (Fig. 15.1).

A grade 1 injury is a mild sprain of the acromioclavicular and coracoclavicular ligaments, without significant disruption of the joint. Clinical findings include point tenderness over the AC joint and minor joint irritation on adduction of the arm across the chest. Radiographs are normal. After several hours, subcutaneous edema may develop around the joint.

A grade 2 injury involves the partial upward displacement of the distal clavicle relative to the acromion (less than the width of the clavicle), as seen on stress radiographs. This injury represents a second-degree sprain of the acromioclavicular and coracoclavicular ligaments. On clinical exam there is tenderness of the AC joint and a palpable step-off between the distal clavicle and the acromion. Abduction and adduction are uncomfortable. Several minutes to hours after injury, subcutaneous edema is usually present in the tissues overlying the joint.

A grade 3 injury involves the complete upward dislocation of the distal clavicle relative to the acromion (greater than the width of the clavicle), with complete rupture of the acromioclavicular and coracoclavicular ligaments. These findings are usually obvious on both clinical examination and radiographs. This injury is accompanied by severe pain and restriction of motion at the shoulder and AC joint. Tenderness is present immediately; and within several minutes, edema develops in the tissues surrounding the joint and in the interval between the coracoid and the clavicle.

Posterior dislocation of the clavicle relative to the acromion is a grade 4 injury. The distal clavicle may be displaced into or through the trapezius muscle. The acromioclavicular ligaments are ruptured. The coracoclavicular ligaments may be fully ruptured, partially ruptured, or "stretched." Clinically, there is severe pain and restriction of motion at the shoulder and AC joints. The coracoid process may appear abnormally prominent because of the relative posterior displacement of the clavicle. Tenderness and edema develop rapidly in the tissues surrounding the joint.

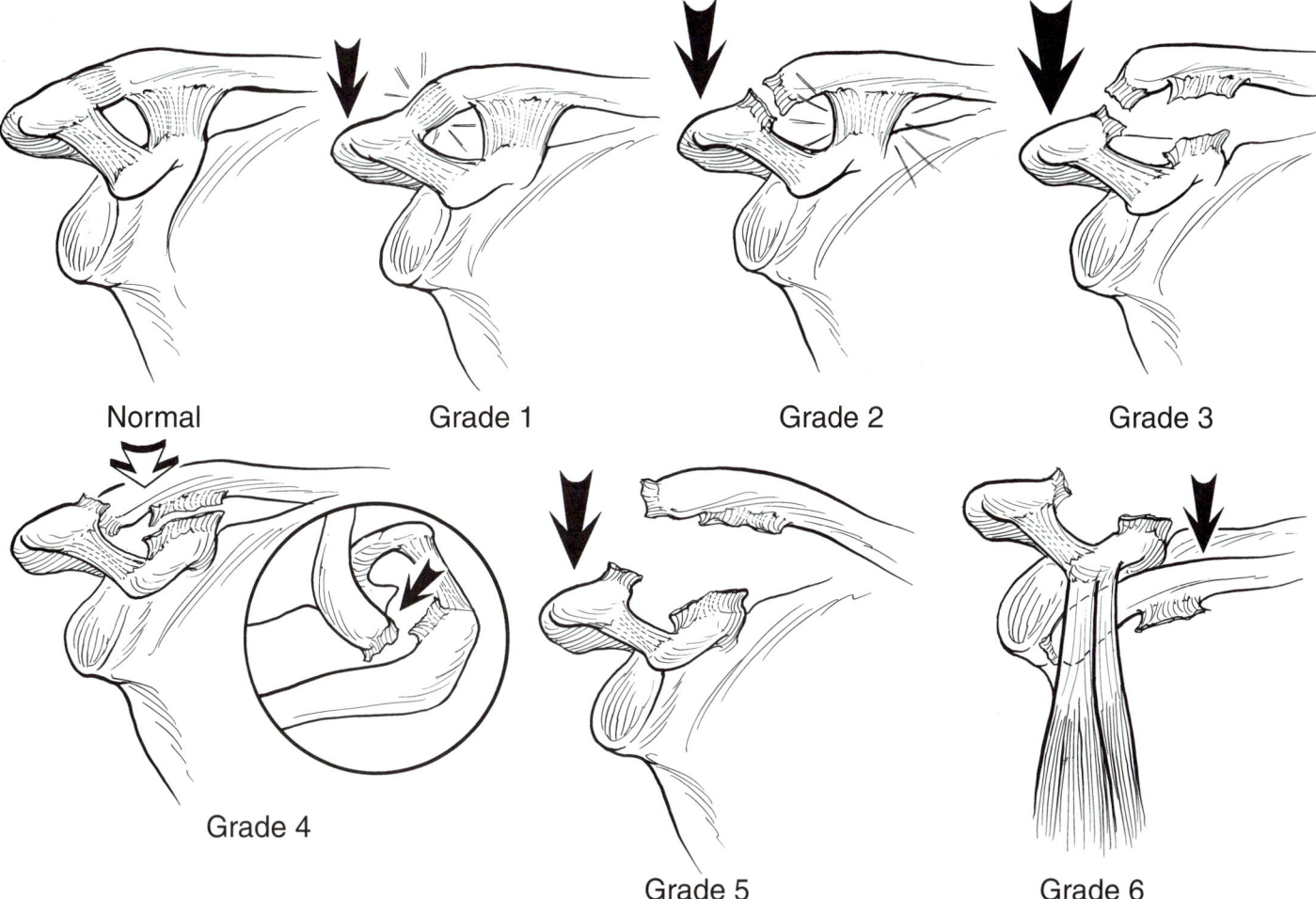

Normal   Grade 1   Grade 2   Grade 3

Grade 4

Grade 5   Grade 6

Figure 15.1. Acromioclavicular joint injuries. Modified from Rockwood CA Jr, Young DC. Disorders of the acromioclavicular joint. In: Rockwood CA Jr, Matsen FA III, eds. The shoulder. Philadelphia: Saunders, 1990:413–476.

A grade 5 injury is a severe upward dislocation of the distal clavicle relative to the acromion, with complete destruction of the acromioclavicular and coracoclavicular ligaments and disruption of the deltoid and trapezius muscle attachments to the clavicle. The clavicle may pierce the muscle and even the skin, in some cases. Tenderness is present immediately, and edema develops rapidly in the tissues surrounding the joint and in the interval between the coracoid and the clavicle.

Inferior dislocation of the clavicle underneath the coracoid is a grade 6 injury. This occurs after the application of a tremendous deforming force and indicates complete acromioclavicular and coracoclavicular ligament rupture. The most common setting is severe trauma, as is seen in motor vehicle accidents. Injury to the underlying neurovascular structures is likely and should be thoroughly investigated and treated as appropriate.

RADIOLOGIC STUDIES

AP radiographs of both the involved and the uninvolved AC joints under normal and weighted conditions are useful for differentiating grades 1, 2, and 3 injuries. The

status of the AC joint is most clearly demonstrated on a Zanca view, which is an AP projection with a cephalic tilt, as described by Rockwood and Matsen (3) (Fig. 15.2). To obtain stress views, a 4.5-kg (10-lb) weight should be hung passively from both of the patient's wrists, not held in the hands, to allow relaxation of the shoulder musculature for a true representation of the ligament integrity. In the case of a suspected grade 4 injury, an axillary view is necessary. Grade 5 and 6 injuries are usually obvious on clinical examination and plain AP radiographs. Therefore, stress views are not necessary or advisable.

TREATMENT

Grade 1 and 2 injuries are best treated symptomatically with ice, rest, and anti-inflammatory medication. For grade 1 injuries, a sling may be used for comfort. If return to athletics is contemplated, the area can be padded as necessary. For grade 2 injuries, a sling is usually required to relieve the discomfort imposed by traction from the weight of the arm. I have not found the use of special braces or slings designed to reduce the AC joint to be of consistent

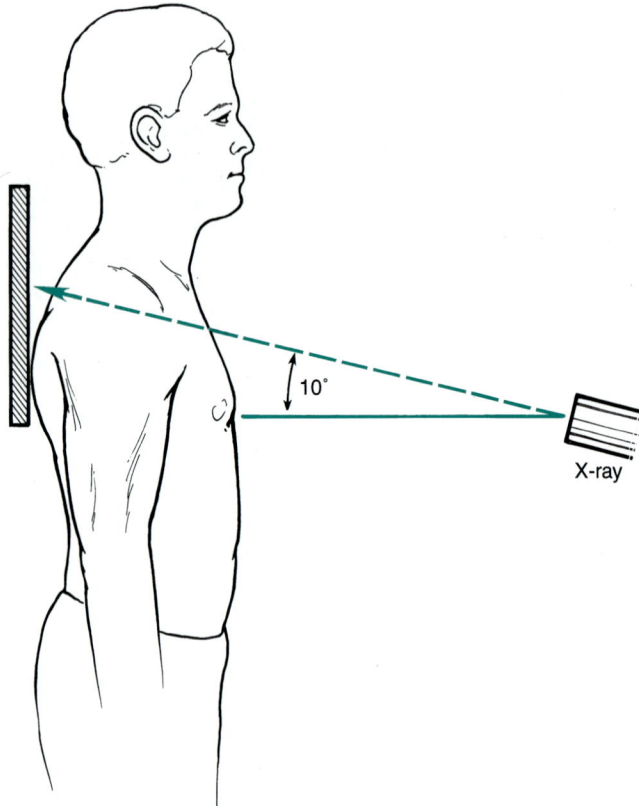

Figure 15.2. Radiographic technique for obtaining the Zanca view. Modified from Rockwood CA Jr, Young DC. Disorders of the acromio-clavicular joint. In: Rockwood CA Jr, Matsen FA III, eds. The shoulder. Philadelphia: Saunders, 1990:413–476.

benefit. Return to physical activity may proceed as pain resolution allows.

Grade 3 injuries present a treatment dilemma. Considerable controversy exists among orthopaedic surgeons concerning the selection of conservative versus acute surgical treatment for grade 3 injuries. My preferred approach has been to treat all grade 3 injuries initially with rest, ice, anti-inflammatory medication, and a sling for 3 weeks. This is followed by a 6- to 10-week course of physical therapy aimed at eliminating pain and restoring shoulder function. If the patient is unhappy with the shoulder after this approach, I will perform constructive surgery of the coracoclavicular ligaments (described below).

Grade 4, 5, and 6 injuries usually require surgical reduction and stabilization, with repair of all soft tissue injuries, in the acute setting (Clinical Table).

Surgery for AC Joint Injuries

Numerous surgical procedures have been advocated for the treatment of AC joint injuries (4,5). Procedures that involve the use of metallic internal fixation (e.g., transfixation pins or a clavicle-to-coracoid screw) have had significant complication rates caused by the hardware (6,7). Procedures that involve the use of synthetic grafts have

shown a significant incidence of symptomatic bony erosion (8).

I prefer the use of autogenous grafts to address coracoclavicular ligament reconstruction in most acute and chronic AC joint injuries. Autogenous grafts may be fashioned locally from coracoacromial ligament or conjoined tendon or harvested distantly from hamstring tendon. At surgery, I also place a synthetic graft of absorbable suture material to augment and protect the autogenous graft during the early postoperative period. This procedure, which is a variation of Weaver and Dunn's (9), is outlined below.

Coracoclavicular Ligament Reconstruction

To prepare for making the skin incision, palpate the bony landmarks and indicate their contours on the skin with a marking pen. If desired, the exact location of the AC joint may be ascertained by palpation with a spinal needle along the anterior surface of the acromion until it plunges off the medial edge into the joint. Before making the skin incision, infiltration of the local subcutaneous tissues with a dilute solution of epinephrine and saline is used to aid hemostasis.

The skin incision is placed in Langer's lines directly over the AC joint. Dissection is carried out carefully through the subcutaneous tissues to expose the fascia in the region of the AC joint. The skin incision and subcutaneous dissection should be extended anteriorly enough to eventually allow easy visualization of the tip of the coracoid process and the most proximal portion of the conjoined tendon. It should extend posteriorly enough to allow easy access to the posterior border of the distal clavicle. Subcutaneous dissection laterally should expose the entire deltoid insertion on the anterior border of the acromion. Medially, the clavicle should be visible out to about 2 cm medial to a vertical line drawn from the medial border of the coracoid process.

Deeper bony exposure is initiated with the incision of fascia and periosteum down to bone along the axis of the distal clavicle, across the AC joint, and onto the acromion. The distal clavicle should be fully exposed first. Care should be exercised to identify and release the fascial attachments of the deltoid and trapezius muscles from the distal clavicle and AC joint in a manner appropriate to their late repair. This exposure should extend medially at least 1 cm past a vertical line erected from the medial border of the coracoid process. Next, retract the deltoid anteriorly and inferiorly from the clavicle. Where the deltoid crosses the AC joint, develop a plane within the fibers of the muscle to expose the tip of the coracoid process and the proximal portion of the conjoined tendon. Through this interval, identify the coracoacromial ligament where it inserts on the coracoid, and develop the plane between it and the under surface of the deltoid up to its insertion on the acromion. Then, with a periosteal elevator or other instrument protecting the coracoacromial ligament, carefully elevate the deltoid off of the anterior acromion, working in a medial to lateral direction.

Clinical Table: Acromioclavicular Joint Injury and Repair

Procedure	Indications	Technique	Anatomy	Pitfalls
Coracoclavicular ligament reconstruction	• Acute grade 4, 5, and 6 injuries • Some grade 3 injuries • Late reconstruction	• Superior push to AC joint • Detach coracoacromial ligament from undersurface of acromion and transfer to exposed distal clavicle that has been resected • Reconstruct coracoclavicular ligaments • Braided suture or tape looped around clavicle	• Trapezius insertion • Deltoid origin • Coracoid process • Musculocutaneous nerve • Rotator cuff	• Loss of reduction • Injury to musculocutaneous nerve
Transacromial intermedullary device	• Acute grade 4, 5, and 6 injuries • Some grade 3 injuries • Late reconstruction	• Reduce AC joint • Drill device from posterolateral corner of acromion down into medullary canal of clavicle	• Trapezius fascia • Deltoid origin • Distal clavicle • Acromion	• Penetration of the subacromial space • Loss of reduction • Hardware breakage
Resection of distal clavicle	• Rarely acutely • Late reconstruction • Late injury • No symptomatic instability	• Anterior superior approach • Elevate split deltoid muscle, split trapezius fascia • Subperiosteal elevation in exposition of distal clavicle • Remove traumatized disc • Resect distal 2 cm of clavicle	• Trapezius and attachment • Deltoid origin • Distal clavicle	• Too little resection • Too much resection • Continued instability from lack of reduction

With the coracoacromial ligament thus exposed, detach it carefully from the acromion. Some surgeons prefer to use an oscillating saw or an osteotome to detach the ligament along with a small piece of bone from the acromion. Next, obtain control of the acromial end of the ligament with sutures. Then, while applying firm longitudinal traction on the ligament, free the ligament of all soft tissue attachments, working back toward the coracoid. Take care to avoid injury to the coracoid attachment.

Next, resect the distal clavicle at a point just medial to a line drawn vertically from the coracoid origin of the acromioclavicular ligament. This osteotomy may be angled slightly in a posteromedial and inferomedial direction, if desired. Then, depress the distal end of the clavicle down into a reduced position while drawing the coracoacromial ligament up across the anterior surface of the clavicle, directly over the inferior edge of the osteotomy. In this position, measure the length of the ligament from the point at which it crosses the inferior cortex of the clavicle to its acromial end. This measurement represents the amount of ligament available for drawing up into the medullary canal of the clavicle. If necessary, trim the ligament so that 5 to 8 mm will be drawn up into the clavicle.

Complete the preparation of the ligament graft by first placing at least two number 1 nonabsorbable sutures for firm control at the free end. Some surgeons prefer to gain further control of the graft by using a number 1 or 2 non-absorbable suture in a Bunnell fashion. This is accomplished by weaving two limbs of each suture in a crisscross pattern up from the coracoid base of the ligament and out the acromial end; this may be repeated with two or more sutures. You should end up with an even number of suture

ends, which may be divided into two equal groups for securing the graft to the clavicle.

Complete the preparation of the clavicle by cleaning out the medullary canal for a distance of at least 10 to 12 mm. Then place two drill holes through the superior cortex

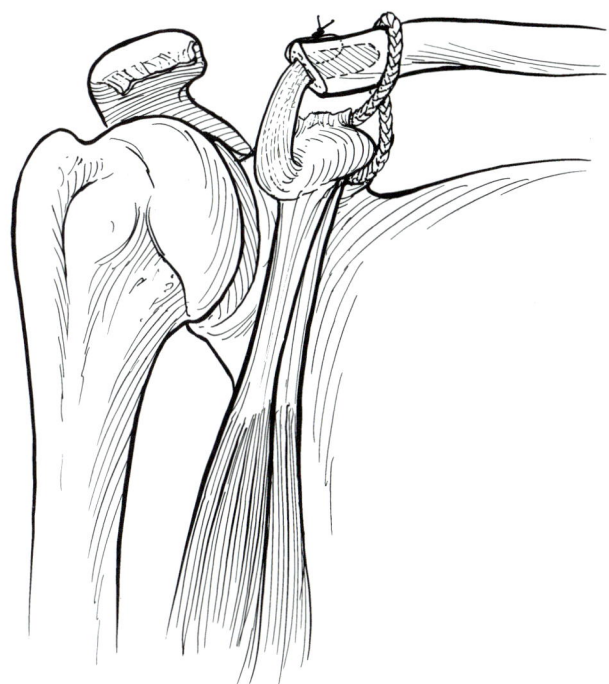

Figure 15.3. Coracoclavicular ligament reconstruction using a coracoacromial ligament graft and absorbable suture braid augmentation.

of the clavicle into the medial end of the cleaned-out portion of medullary canal. Offset the holes from each other slightly along the longitudinal axis of the clavicle to avoid forming a stress riser, which might lead to fracture. Then place a loop of surgical steel wire, or other suture retrieval device, through each drill hole and out the lateral end of the clavicle for later use in leading the graft.

Débride the soft tissues of the AC joint, taking care to preserve the fascial attachments of the deltoid and trapezius for their later repair over the region. Inspect the acromion. Perform an acromioplasty as appropriate. A bursectomy may also be performed, if necessary.

Prepare a 20-cm braid of polydioxanone (PDS) using three pairs of number 1 suture material. Use a loop of surgical steel, or other suture retrieval device, to lead this braid around the coracoid process, just underneath the conjoined tendon. Care must be exercised during this process to avoid entrapment or other injury to the musculocutaneous nerve. This is accomplished by staying close to bone on the coracoid at all times. Once the braid has been placed around the coracoid, draw the lateral limb of the braid beneath the clavicle, medial to the coracoclavicular ligament graft, and through the trapezius fascia at the posterior border of the clavicle. Secure the two ends of the braid together with a clamp for later use.

Once the braid has been positioned, use the previously placed suture retrieval devices to draw the graft-controlling sutures into the canal of the clavicle and out the drill holes. While an assistant depresses the distal clavicle into a reduced position (within 3 to 5 mm of the coracoid process), draw the ligament graft into the medullary canal. Make sure that the graft end passes freely into the canal by making any necessary adjustments to the graft or the medullary canal. Finally, with the bone held in a reduced position and the graft drawn taut, tie the graft sutures securely over the bone. Release the reducing force on the clavicle and assess the stability of the construct. If it is too loose, first check that the graft is fully seated in the medullary canal of the clavicle. If the effective length of the graft appears to be excessive, make adjustments as necessary to remedy this situation. This may require trimming the graft and replacing the sutures in the graft. If the construct is satisfactory, tie the PDS braid securely over the bone (Fig. 15.3) to act as a reinforcement for the graft during the early healing period. After tying, this now can be slid anteriorly off the bone to rest in the interval between the clavicle and coracoid.

Irrigate the wound and place a drain in the AC joint if deemed appropriate. Reattach the deltoid to the acromion using heavy nonabsorbable sutures through drill holes in the acromion. Take care to incorporate both the superficial and deep layers of the deltoid fascia in the repair. Repair the fascia of the trapezius and the deltoid to each other over the distal clavicle and AC joint with absorbable or nonabsorbable sutures. Irrigate again and close the subcutaneous tissues and skin as desired.

Postoperative Rehabilitation

If present, the drain is removed within 24 h. The wound is kept clean and dry until the sutures are removed in 7 to 10 days. The arm is supported in a sling at all times, except when exercising, for 6 weeks. The sling is removed twice daily for Codman's exercises starting on postoperative day 1 and continuing for 3 weeks. At the 3-week point, physical therapy is initiated, but activities are kept below shoulder height. No carrying, lifting, or other activity that places distal traction on the upper extremity is allowed. The patient is frequently reminded that any significant carrying or traction on the arm will directly stress the reconstruction. These restrictions are strictly enforced until 6 weeks after the surgery. At 6 weeks, physical therapy is advanced to achieve full range of motion and improve strength. The sling is discounted. Lifting, carrying, and traction on the arm are limited to 2.3 to 4.5 kg (5 to 10 lb) maximum for another 6 weeks. At 3 months postsurgery the patient is usually released to return to normal activities as tolerated.

Transacromial Internal Fixation

As an alternative to coracoclavicular ligament reconstruction with some acute high-grade AC injuries, a transacromial internal fixation with either a Kirschner wire or a specialized pin can reduce the acute grade 3 injury and permit healing of the ligaments.

If this is to be performed, a longitudinal or horizontal incision is made centered over the area of the AC joint. The rent in the trapezius fascia is identified, the area of the AC joint is identified, and an incision is made centered over the AC joint. The disc material, which is frequently disrupted, is removed, and the clavicle is reduced adjacent to the acromion. An intermedullary device such as a Kirschner wire, Knowles pin, or Hagie pin is used next. The pin is drilled from the posterolateral aspect of the acromion through the AC joint and into the medullary canal of the clavicle. The pin is cut off beneath the skin for ease of removal at a later time. Care must be taken to make certain that the pin is not penetrating into the subacromial space and that the joint is adequately reduced.

Coracoacromial ligament transfer may be added at this time, and this internal fixation can be supplemented with traditional coracoclavicular fixation methods such as braided suture, Mersilene tape, or hamstring tendon. The potential benefit of using an intermedullary fixation device is that by reducing the clavicle first and holding with a intermedullary device, overreduction and overtightening are prevented when the coracoclavicular reconstruction is performed. In addition, the device acts as a belt and suspenders to protect the coracoclavicular reconstruction from stretching out. Likewise, if pin tract difficulties ensue before the hardware is to be removed, then the coracoclavicular ligament reconstruction acts as a backup to this fixation method.

Ordinarily the hardware is removed in 4 to 6 weeks.

Distal Clavicle Excision

Occasionally following AC joint injuries, distal clavicle excision alone may be considered without coracoclavicular reconstruction. In the older, more sedentary population whose predominant problem is the bump over the AC joint and pain, rather than AC joint instability and the pain associated with chronic instability of the joint, then distal clavicle excision alone might be considered.

If an isolated distal clavicle excision (Mumford procedure) is to be considered, the AC joint is approached via a superior incision, and the trapezoideltoid interval is divided. The deltoid muscle is split in line with its fibers, and the distal clavicle is exposed periosteally. The distal 2 cm of clavicle are then resected by using an oscillating saw or a rib cutter. The deltoid and trapezius can then be closed.

SUMMARY

The treatment of high-grade AC injuries has often been controversial. In general, there is little argument that the low-grade AC joint injuries, grades 1 and 2, can be treated initially nonoperatively. If late problems occur with low-grade AC joint injuries, since instability is not involved, then distal clavicle excision alone is a good late choice. There is also little controversy that highest grade AC joint injuries, grades 4, 5, and 6, should be treated operatively, particularly in the active patient population. These injuries are often associated with significant soft tissue trauma and have irreducible clavicular position through a ruptured trapezius muscle and fascia. Good internal fixation methods exist to treat this problem.

The controversy continues to center around the appropriate treatment of grade 3 AC joint injuries. Nonoperative management of many of these injuries is certainly satisfactory, and some clinicians have achieved good results with braces to reduce the grade of the injury, and surgeons have had good surgical results with operative treatment of grade 3 injuries. It appears that decision making regarding the appropriate treatment of the high-grade AC injuries depends on the age of the patient, dominance of the arm, activity level of the patient, and willingness of the patient to accept the prominence of an unreduced AC joint injury. If surgical treatment is chosen, the hallmark of operative treatment of this injury is to reduce the high-degree AC joint injury and maintain the reduction either with fixation that traverses the acromion and goes down the intramedullary canal of the clavicle or with one that attempts to repair and reconstruct the injured coracoclavicular ligaments.

REFERENCES

1. Rockwood CA Jr. Injuries to the acromioclavicular joint. In: Rockwood CA Jr, Green DP, eds. Fractures in adults. Philadelphia: Lippincott, 1984:860–910.
2. Rockwood CA Jr, Young DC. Disorders of the acromioclavicular joint. In: Rockwood CA Jr, Matsen FA III, eds. The shoulder. Philadelphia: Saunders, 1990:413-476.
3. Smith M, Stewart M. Acute acromioclavicular separations. Am J Sports Med 1979;7:62–71.
4. Bundens W Jr, Cook J. Repair of acromioclavicular separations by deltoid-trapezius imbrications. Clin Orthop 1961;20:109–114.
5. Bosworth B. Acromioclavicular separation: new method of repair. Surg Gynecol Obstet 1941;73:866–871.
6. Kennedy J. Complete dislocation of the acromioclavicular joint: 14 years later. J Trauma 1968;8:311–318.
7. Bearden J, Hughston J, Whatley C. Acromioclavicular dislocation: method of treatment. J Sports Med 1973;1:5–17.
8. Mumford E. Acromioclavicular dislocation. J Bone Joint Surg 1941; 23:799–802.
9. Weaver J, Dunn H. Treatment of acromioclavicular injuries, especially complete acromioclavicular separation. J Bone Joint Surg 1972;54A:1187–1197.

Suggested Readings

Bailey R. A dynamic repair for complete acromioclavicular joint dislocation. J Bone Joint Surg 1965;47A:858.

Dahl E. Follow-up after coracoclavicular ligament prosthesis for acromioclavicular joint dislocation. Acta Chir Scand 1981; 506(Suppl):96.

Lindsey R, Gutowski W. The migration of a broken pin following fixation of the acromioclavicular joint: a case report and review for the literature. Orthopedics 1986;9:413–416.

Mazet R. Migration of a Kirschner wire from the shoulder region into the lung: report of two cases. J Bone Joint Surg 1943;25A:477–483.

Norrell H, Llewellyn R. Migration of a threaded Steinmann pin from an acromioclavicular joint into the spinal canal: a case report. J Bone Joint Surg 1965;47A:1024–1026.

chapter

16

Charles N. Cornell

Fractures and Nonunions of the Clavicle

The clavicle is among the most frequently fractured bones, accounting for 5 to 10% of adult skeletal injuries. The majority of clavicle fractures heal uneventfully, and many nonunions are sufficiently asymptomatic to not require surgical repair. A subset of these injuries, however, are characterized by significant shortening or angulation of the clavicle and are debilitating secondary to pain and impairment of shoulder function. The fractures and nonunions of this type benefit from surgical repair. Because of the unique anatomic features of the clavicle and the technical difficulty encountered in achieving secure fixation, treatment of clavicle fractures and nonunions is a major challenge for the orthopaedic surgeon (1).

RELEVANT ANATOMY AND BIOMECHANICS

The clavicle has a unique S-shape with two major curves (Fig. 16.1). There is a convex anterior curve medially and a convex posterior curve laterally. The clavicle is held at the ends by the acromioclavicular and sternoclavicular joints. There are numerous muscle insertions along the medial and lateral thirds and relatively little soft tissue coverage over the middle third. In cross section, the ends of the clavicle flatten and flare with the cancellous bone structure as the end joints are approached. The middle third of the clavicle is made up of tubular dense cortical bone. The central third of the clavicle, with its sparse soft tissue coverage and lack of medullary bone, is the site of the majority of clavicular nonunions.

Functionally, the clavicle acts as a cantilevered support that links the chest with the upper limb and contributes power and stability to the extremity, especially in overhead activities (2). The clavicle also transmits the pull of the trapezius to the scapula through the coracoclavicular ligaments.

During elevation of the arm in forward flexion and abduction, the trapezius elevates the clavicle approximately 30° through the sternoclavicular joint. When the coracoclavicular ligaments are intact, this clavicular elevation is accompanied by scapular rotation during protraction, retraction, and elevation of the shoulder. The scapular has an excursion of up to 50° of rotation and elevation with respect to the sternoclavicular joint. The clavicle moves to transmit and support these motions. In the maximal elevation of the arm, the clavicle elevates 30°, angles posteriorly 35°, and rotates 50° around its axis. The shape and structure of the bone are crucial to these movements. Significant deformity of or loss of continuity in the clavicle compromises these movements and adversely affects shoulder girdle strength and movement. Clavicle deformity can also cause compression of underlying neurovascular structures when shoulder elevation is attempted. It is imperative that reconstruction of the clavicle restores the S-shaped curve accurately to ensure proper and complete restoration of shoulder girdle movement and function (1,3).

INITIAL FINDINGS, PHYSICAL EXAMINATION, AND DIAGNOSIS

Patients with clavicle fractures present with acute pain and inability to move the affected limb, usually following a direct blow or fall onto the affected shoulder. Visual inspection of the shoulder girdle often suffices to confirm the diagnosis. Palpation of the clavicle, which is facilitated by its subcutaneous position, helps pinpoint the exact location and displacement of the fracture. The examination should strive to rule out open wounds, perforation of muscle leading to soft tissue interposition, and any neurovascular injury. Brachial plexus injury is heralded by paresthesias and loss of motor function distally in the extremity.

Figure 16.1. The clavicle's S-shape must be maintained when it is reconstructed.

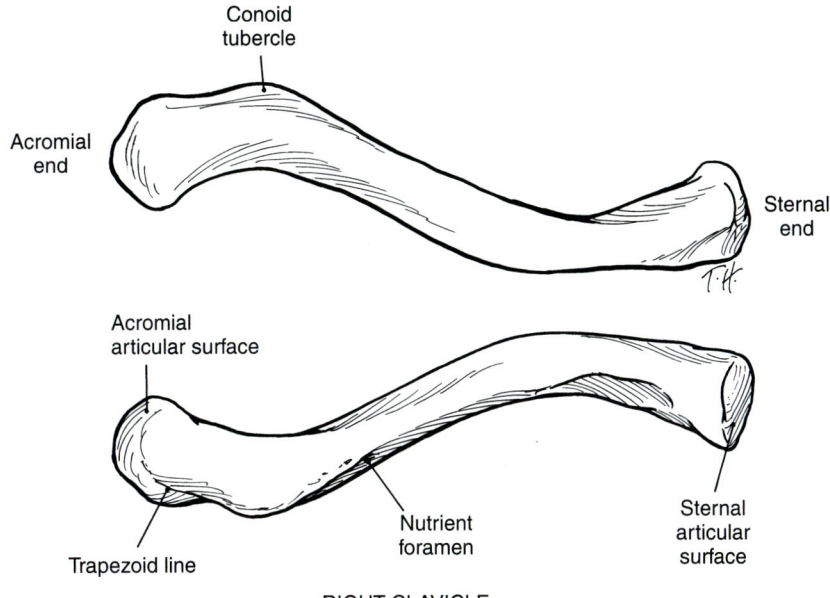

RIGHT CLAVICLE

Brachial and axillary artery injury usually present with hypotension, paresthesias in the limb, expanding hematoma, and a probable diminished radial pulse. It is possible through collateral circulation to have a palatable pulse with complete occlusion of the axillary artery; but parerethises, significant swelling and hematoma, and pulse asymmetry are usually present.

RADIOLOGIC STUDIES AND CLASSIFICATION

Routine plain radiographs of the shoulder usually suffice to identify clavicle fractures and determine their severity. The classification described by Allman (4) is well accepted and delineates the basic fracture patterns encountered. The classification recognizes three basic groups according to the anatomic location of the fracture: Grade I fractures involve the middle third and account for 80% of all clavicle fractures. Grade 2 fractures involve the lateral third and account for 10 to 15% of all clavicle fractures. Grade 3 fractures involve the medial third of the clavicle and are rare.

Neer further subclassified grade 2 fractures on the basis of the relationship of the fracture to the coracoclavicular ligaments (5) (Table 16.1). Neer (6) argued that frac-

table	**16.1**	Fractures of Distal End of Clavicle: Neer Classification

Type	Injury Pattern	Surgery
I	Fractures lateral to coracoclavicular ligament	No
II	Fracture dislocation; acromioclavicular joint intact; coracoclavicular ligament avulsed	Yes
III	Intra-articular fractures; coracoclavicular ligament intact	No

tures of the distal clavicle accompanied by rupture of the coracoclavicular ligaments usually heal poorly when treated conservatively. When the coracoclavicular is ruptured, the fracture displaces as a result of muscle forces and the weight of the arm. These grade 2 injuries benefit from open reduction and internal fixation (ORIF).

TREATMENT

Nonoperative Treatment

As mentioned, the majority of clavicle fractures should be managed by closed means (Clinical Table) (Fig. 16.2). Although the incidence of nonunion has been previously underestimated, it is difficult to predict which closed injuries will fail to unite. Furthermore, the results of delayed surgical treatment are as good as early treatment, justifying an attempt at closed management (7). In addition, most surgical series cite a 10% complication rate, which is daunting and argues for an attempt at closed reduction. Concomitant brachial plexus injury by itself is not a reason to proceed surgically, since 60% of patients recover with closed treatment (8).

Closed treatment attempts to achieve reduction of the fracture with sufficient comfort and stability to allow early range of motion and light functional use of the arm. The figure eight bandage is a standard means of treatment. The bandage indirectly reduces the fracture by encouraging the patient's shoulders to be held in the military position. When applied correctly, the figure eight bandage decreases fracture pain and holds the fracture position enough to allow some functional use of the arm. An alternative to the figure eight bandage is a sling or sling and swathe, which merely immobilize the shoulder. White et al. (9) found the figure eight bandage to be superior in a

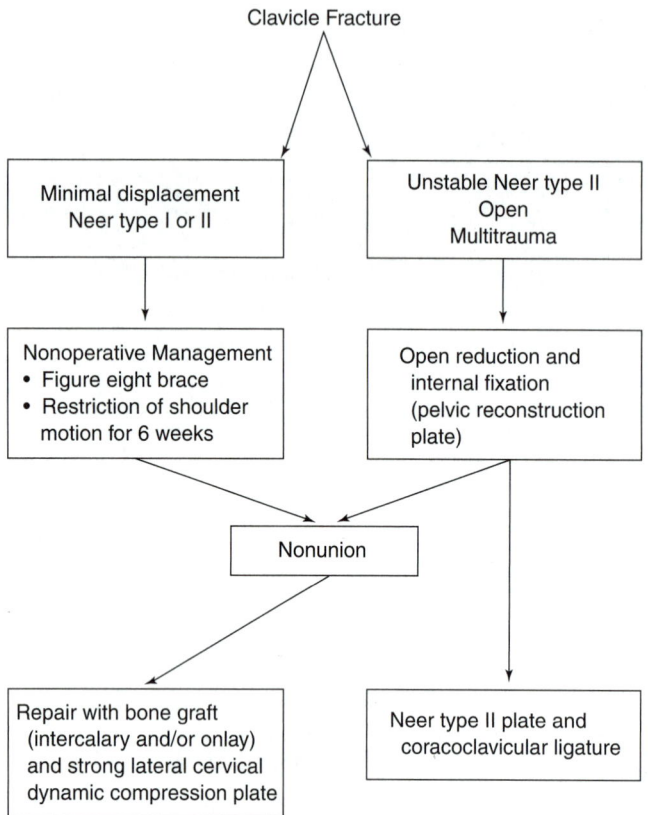

Figure 16.2. Treatment of clavicle fractures.

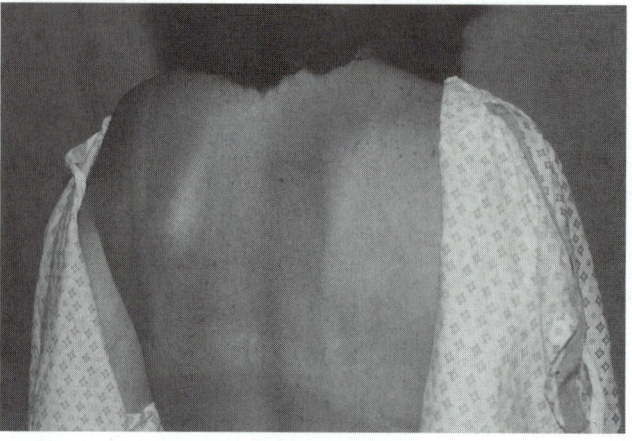

Figure 16.3. Example of scapular winging in a patient with a shortened clavicular fracture, resulting in ptosis of the shoulder.

can then be performed. Return to active supports with unrestricted use of the arm is generally safe after 3 months. Reinjury before 3 months should be avoided, as this commonly leads to nonunion.

Operative Treatment

INDICATIONS

Acute fractures that should be considered for open reduction include refractures, open fractures, fractures with obvious soft tissue interposition, and fractures with shortening or angulation significant enough to lead to obvious ptosis of the shoulder or winging of the scapula. *Ptosis* is a term used by Jupiter and Leffert (1) to describe the forward rotation of the scapula that occurs following loss of clavicular support. It is most easily recognized on physical examination by the presence of winging of the body of the scapula off the chest wall (Fig. 16.3). Ptosis should be corrected, as it compromises shoulder rotation and strength in overhead activities.

small series, whereas Andersen et al. (10) found no difference in outcome if a simple sling was used. I favor the figure eight bandage but realize that it must be applied correctly and that the patient must adjust it daily. I see no reason to use shoulder spica casts. If a fracture is unstable enough to require plaster immobilization, it should undergo ORIF to allow early functional shoulder motion.

Most clavicle fractures heal sufficiently to discontinue the bandage or sling in 6 weeks. Active overhead exercises

Clinical Table: Fractures of the Clavicle

Procedure	Indications	Technique	Anatomy
Midshaft	• Closed treatment in majority of cases • ORIF (open fracture, soft tissue interposition, shoulder ptosis)	• Sling • Figure eight strap • Contoured pelvic reconstruction plate	• Nonunion or malunion • Excessive shortening or angulation leading to ptosis • Visible scar • Prominent hardware • Need for hardware removal
Distal clavicle			
Neer I	• Closed management	• Sling	• Few
Neer II	• Requires ORIF	• Plate and coracoclavicular ligature	• Few
Neer III	• Closed management	• Sling	• Few
Nonunion	• Repair with bone graft intercalary or onlay graft	• Reinforced reconstruction or LC-DCP	• Need to reconstruct clavicular length and contour

LC-DCP, lateral cervical dynamic compression plate.

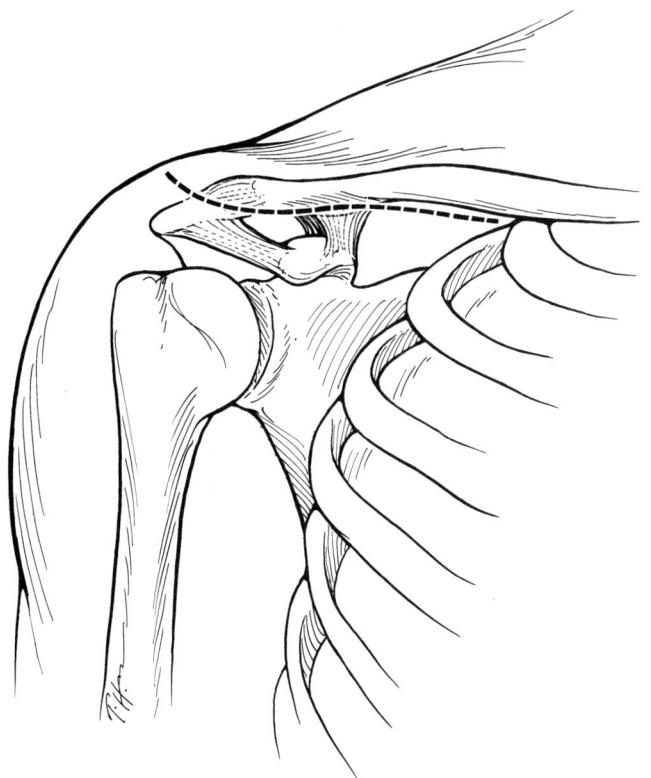

Figure 16.4. The skin incision used for exposure of the clavicle follows Langer's lines and provides an acceptable cosmetic healing.

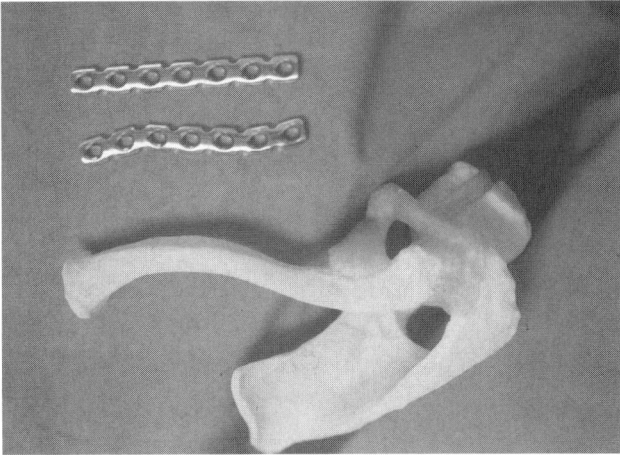

Figure 16.5. The 3.5-mm reconstruction plate can be contoured before surgery against a dry skeletal specimen.

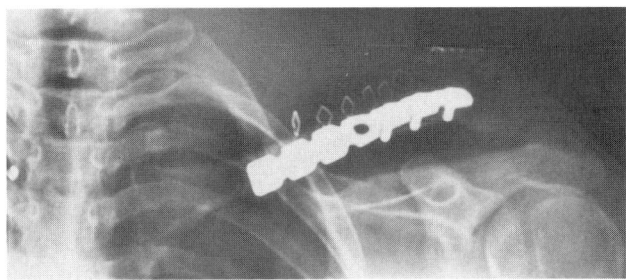

Figure 16.6. Well-done plating of a clavicular fracture.

Open reduction should also be employed in the multiple trauma patient with a closed head injury or seizures and when bone fragments tent the skin, threatening an inside-out puncture. Combination injuries to the shoulder girdle that involve a fracture of the scapular neck and clavicle resulting in a floating glenoid are best managed by ORIF. ORIF of the clavicle is usually sufficient to stabilize the scapular neck fracture, restoring stability to the shoulder girdle (11). Likewise, repair of the clavicle generally restores stability to the upper limb after scapulothoracic dissociation.

OPEN REDUCTION AND INTERNAL FIXATION

General anesthesia is usually required for exposure and stabilization of clavicle fractures, because of the need for medial dissection close to the sternoclavicular joint. The patient is positioned in the beach chair position with the head upright, which allows easy, direct visualization of the superior aspect of the shoulder and clavicle. A towel should be placed in the interscapular area to encourage extension of the shoulder and scapular. The entire extremity should be draped free, and a bone graft donor site should be prepared when needed.

The skin incision is placed directly over the fracture site and extends from posterolateral to anterior medial, following Langer's lines as closely as possible (Fig. 16.4). The incision is extended through the platysma; and using subperiosteal dissection, the surgeon exposes the clavicle. In acute fractures, care should be taken to limit soft tissue dissection of the fracture and comminuted fragments. By limiting the exposure to only that needed for application of the plate, the surgeon preserves the blood supply needed for rapid healing.

Fixation of the clavicle can be obtained by intramedullary pin fixation or by plate and screw fixation. Although intramedullary pin fixation (12) has its proponents, I believe that plate fixation is more secure and allows more accurate anatomical restoration. For fixation of acute clavicle fractures, a 3.5-mm reconstruction plate, or lateral cervical dynamic compression plate (LC-DCP), should be used (13) (Fig. 16.5). The plate should be carefully contoured to re-create the S-shaped curve of the clavicle. The plate can be contoured before surgery to match a skeletal specimen and is fine-tuned during surgery. The plate is then fixed to the medial fragment, and the lateral fragment is reduced to the plate screws. The surgeon should strive to place a cortical lag screw though the plate. By limiting dissection, this technique can achieve indirect reduction of comminuted fragments and encourage rapid healing with a periosteal callus.

An optimal fixation would place six cortices on each side of the fracture with a lag screw (Fig. 16.6); occasionally, however, only four cortices can be used for lateral fractures. In fractures that are lateral enough to involve or have an associated rupture of the coracoclavicular ligaments, a braid of reabsorbable suture can be passed around the

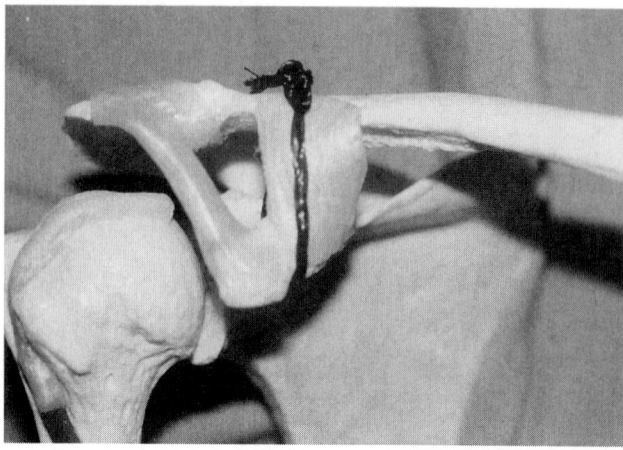

Figure 16.7. A distal clavicle fracture fixation can be supplemented by a resorbable braid that cerclages the clavicle to the coracoid.

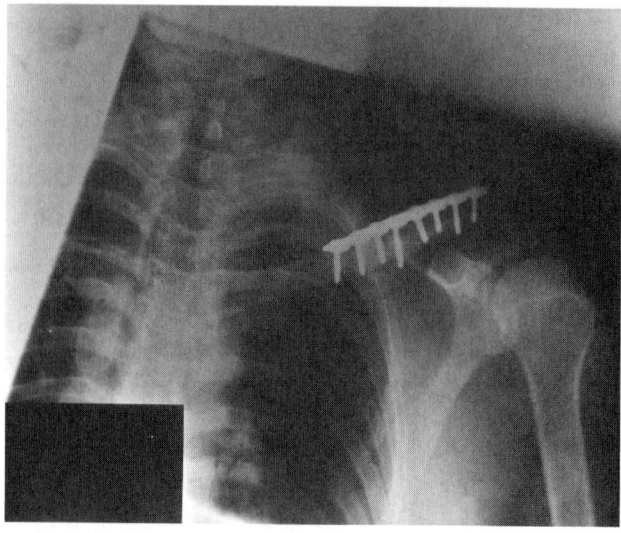

Figure 16.8. Reconstruction of a clavicular nonunion using a plate and corticocancellous bone graft.

clavicle and coracoid as a suture ligature to help secure the proximal fragment (Fig. 16.7). This technique can be used alone or in conjunction with plate fixation.

REPAIR OF CLAVICULAR NONUNIONS

Fixation of clavicular nonunions poses several technical problems not usually encountered in acute fracture fixation. The nonunion usually leads to clavicular shortening as a result of an overlap of the fracture ends and bony reabsorption of the ends of the fracture. This shortening must be corrected to restore normal length and position. Failure to do this leaves the patient with an adducted scapula, which restricts shoulder motion and leads to chronic pain in the periscapular musculature. Bone grafting is a necessary step in the reconstruction of a shortened clavicle. The technique described by Jupiter and Leffert should be considered (1).

As with acute fractures, careful preoperative planning is needed. An appropriately sized 3.5-mm LC-DCP should be precontoured using a skeletal specimen or by extrapolating from the mirror image of the patient's contralateral clavicle. A 3.5-mm pelvic reconstruction plate can be used in a small patient; but the stress across chronic nonunions often bends the plate, causing loss of correction of deformity. The stiff LC-DCP is the implant of choice in chronic nonunions.

After exposure of the clavicle, extensive dissection may be required to mobilize the ends of the nonunion. The pseudarthrosis should be resected, and excessive bulk should be débrided. Great care must be taken when dissecting beneath the clavicle, because of the proximity of neurovascular structures. A corticocancellous bone graft is harvested and contoured to fit precisely into the gap created by mobilizing the clavicle to its appropriate length. The precontoured plate is a useful template to help guide the surgeon in judging adequate length. The medial frag-

ment is usually superior to the distal fragment. Fixation of the plate to the medial fragment allows the lateral fragment to be elevated to the plate, correcting the scapular malposition and clavicular shortening. The distal fragment is held to the plate with a reduction forceps. The contoured graft is then placed into the gap. A slightly long graft (1 to 2 mm) creates compression with the host bone (Fig. 16.8). Rose petaling of the nonunion ends and opening the medullary canals before insertion of the graft may promote healing. Secure plate fixation is needed, including six cortices on each side of the nonunion if possible. Braided resorbable suture ligature replacement of the coracoclavicular ligament is recommended for small distal fragments. An alternative to plate fixation that uses threaded intramedullary Steinmann pins has been noted to have good results (11).

REHABILITATION

Following fixation of the clavicle, restriction of overhead activities of the arm should be observed for 4 to 6 weeks or until secure healing of the clavicle is noted. Motion of the arm up to 90° of flexion or abduction can occur with little motion of the clavicle. Codman-type pendulum and active range of motion exercises of the elbow, wrist, and hand should be performed for 4 to 6 weeks. Thereafter, a full shoulder and upper extremity program can be begun.

Full unrestricted use of the arm should be withheld for 3 months or until bridging callous and recortication of the fracture or nonunion is seen on x-ray. I consider hardware removal only after 1 year postsurgery to allow adequate remodeling and consolidation of the fracture site.

With careful surgical management, treatment of clavicle fractures and nonunions is predictably excellent. Plate fixation with corticocancellous grafting in nonunions has had excellent results in most reported series.

SUMMARY

Operative management of clavicle fractures and nonunions is rarely needed. Nonetheless, patients presenting with significant clavicular shorting or angular deformity benefit from reconstruction with relief of pain and improved shoulder girdle power when clavicular anatomy is restored. Jupiter and Leffert (1) achieved success in 92% of cases with excellent relief of pain and restoration of function in all cases. Their review documents similar results in smaller series. Although the union rate with intramedullary pin fixation is similar to that of Jupiter and Leffert, reports of technical problems are more frequent with this technique. Most cases of pin fixation require hardware removal, and a few cases of hardware migration have been noted.

ORIF with reconstruction plates allows precise reconstruction. Corticocancellous sculpted bone grafts are needed to restore length in nonunions. Healing rates are outstanding and are accompanied by excellent clinical improvement.

REFERENCES

1. Jupiter JB, Leffert RD. Non union of the clavicle: associated complications and surgical management. J Bone Joint Surg 1987; 69A:753–760.
2. Abbott LC, Lucas DB. The function of the clavicle: its surgical significance. Ann Surg 1954;140:583–599.
3. Simpson NS, Jupiter JB. Clavicular nonunion and malunion: evaluation and surgical management. J Am Acad Orthop Surg 1996; 4:1–8.
4. Allman FL Jr. Fractures and ligamentous injuries of the clavicle and its articulation. J Bone Joint Surg 1967;49A:774–784.
5. Craig EV. Fractures of the clavicle. In: Rockwood CA Jr, Matsen FA III, eds. The shoulder. Vol. 1. Philadelphia: Saunders, 1990:367–412.
6. Neer CS. Fractures of the distal one third of the clavicle. Clin Orthop 1968;58:43–50.
7. Neer CS II. Nonunion of the clavicle. JAMA 1960;172:1006–1011.
8. Sturm JT, Perry JF. Brachial plexus injuries from blunt trauma—a harbinger of vascular and thoracic injury. Ann Emerg Med 1987; 16:404–406.
9. White RR, Anson DS, Kristainsen T, Healy W. Adult clavicle fractures: the relationship between mechanism of injury and healing. Orthop Trans 1988.
10. Andersen K, Jersen PO, Lauritzen J. Treatment of clavicular fractures. Figure-of-eight bandage versus a simple sling. Acta Orthop Scand 1987;58:71–74.
11. Rikli D, Regazzoni P, Renner N. The unstable shoulder girdle: early functional treatment utilizing open reduction and internal fixation. J Orthop Trauma 1995;9:93–97.
12. Capicotto PN, Heiple KG, Wilbur JH. Midshaft clavicle nonunions treated with intramedullary Steinmann pin fixation and onlay bone graft. J Orthop Trauma 1994;8:88–93.
13. Mullaji AB, Jupiter JB. Low contact compression plating of the clavicle. Injury 1994;25:41–45.

chapter

17

Answorth A. Allen, Stephen J. O'Brien, and Dahari Brooks

Anterior Shoulder Instability: Open and Arthroscopic Repair

The glenohumeral joint is the joint with the greatest degree of mobility in the human body. Unlike the hip joint, which derives its stability primarily from the osseous anatomy, shoulder stability depends not only on articular congruence but on the supporting soft tissue structures, such as the glenoid labrum, the joint capsule, the glenohumeral ligaments, and the rotator cuff. Dynamic stability is accomplished by the action of muscular contractions across the joint, which directs the humeral head into the glenoid fossa and creates a concavity-compression fit of the joint surfaces. Static stability depends on the labrum, the joint capsule, and the glenohumeral ligaments. Controlled coordinated motion, therefore, depends on both dynamic and static stability (1–3).

In general, glenohumeral instability is the result of inadequacy of the dynamic and/or static stabilizers of the shoulder. Increased translation of the humeral head relative to the glenoid may produce the clinical signs and symptoms of shoulder instability. The spectrum of clinical presentations ranges from glenohumeral subluxation (symptomatic translation of the humeral head relative to the glenoid articular surface) to glenohumeral dislocation (complete separation of the articular surfaces). Anterior glenohumeral instability problems can pose significant diagnostic and therapeutic dilemmas for the clinician. In general, no one procedure or therapeutic regimen should be used for the management of anterior shoulder instability. This chapter outlines our approach to the evaluation, diagnosis, and treatment of anterior shoulder instability.

RELEVANT ANATOMY AND PATHOGENESIS

The traditional classification of glenohumeral instability is based on the degree, direction, frequency, and cause of shoulder instability (Table 17.1). Anterior shoulder instability is the most common instability pattern observed in both the general and the athletic patient populations. Acute traumatic anterior shoulder dislocations usually occur from a macrotraumatic event during the second decade. An indirect force that causes excessive abduction, external rotation, and extension of the arm is the most common mechanism for this injury. Rarely, a direct force to the posterior or posterolateral aspect of the shoulder will cause an anterior dislocation.

The anterior capsulolabral structures are often stripped from the anterior-inferior glenoid rim after anterior dislocations (Bankart lesion). Although it was initially believed that the Bankart lesion was the essential lesion in traumatic anterior shoulder dislocations (4,5), recent studies have shown that the presence of a Bankart lesion in the absence of capsular injury is not enough to cause an anterior dislocation of the glenohumeral joint (6,7). The pathologic process of anterior shoulder instability includes capsulolabral injuries (Bankart lesion), posterior humeral head defects (Hill-Sachs lesion), bony glenoid injuries, rotator cuff injuries, tuberosities, and surgical neck fractures. Rotator cuff tears can occur after an acute anterior dislocation, and the incidence increases significantly in patients over the age of 40. Acute subscapularis tendon tears can occur with forced abduction and external rotation of the shoulder and may cause anterior shoulder instability.

The most common type of anterior dislocation is the subcoracoid dislocation. The humeral head is forced anterior to the glenoid and inferior to the coracoid process. Other types of traumatic anterior dislocations include subclavicular (the humeral head is medial to the coracoid process), subglenoid (the humeral head is anterior and inferior to the glenoid cavity), and intrathoracic (the humeral

184

table	17.1	Shoulder Instability Classification

Frequency	Acute Recurrent Fixed (chronic)
Cause	Traumatic (macrotrauma) Atraumatic (voluntary, involuntary) Microtrauma Congenital Neuromuscular (Erb's palsy, cerebral palsy, seizures)
Direction	Anterior Posterior Inferior Multidirectional
Degree	Dislocation Subluxation Micro (transient)

head is fixed between the ribs and the thoracic cavity). The latter is often associated with major traumatic events such as motor vehicular accidents. There may be associated life-threatening injuries, such as pneumothorax, hemothorax, or vascular injuries (8).

Chronic recurrent anterior shoulder dislocations usually occur in the setting of untreated or conservatively treated traumatic anterior shoulder dislocations. The redislocation rate may be as high as 90% in the athletic population (9), and the patient's age at the time of the initial dislocation appears to be the most significant factor influencing the redislocation rate.

Chronic locked anterior dislocations are less common than locked posterior dislocations. The former can occur after seizures. In debilitated or confused patients, an acute dislocation may not be recognized and the shoulder may remain dislocated.

Anterior shoulder subluxation may occur after a macrotraumatic episode to the shoulder in which the shoulder dislocates and reduces spontaneously or from a capsulolabral injury that is not sufficient to cause a complete separation (dislocation) of the articular surfaces (10). The labrum can tear and become interposed between the humerus and the glenoid, resulting in functional instability. These patients may present with a painful pseudolocking of the glenohumeral joint. Repetitive microtrauma from overhead sports, such as tennis or swimming, can lead to excessive capsular laxity and glenohumeral joint instability. Recurrent anterior subluxation is manifested by shoulder pain during overhead activities; a sensation of the glenohumeral joint slipping with the arm in certain positions; and the "dead arm" syndrome, which includes numbness, tingling, and a transient loss of sensation in the upper extremity after certain provocative maneuvers.

INITIAL FINDINGS, PHYSICAL EXAMINATION, AND DIAGNOSIS

The initial step in the evaluation and treatment of anterior glenohumeral instability is an accurate and detailed history. The clinical presentation can vary from a painful, deformed shoulder after an acute traumatic anterior shoulder dislocation to the relatively vague sensations of pain or mild discomfort, neurologic symptoms, and a sense of instability with maneuvers associated with glenohumeral subluxation. The circumstances surrounding the index dislocation episode should be determined, including documentation of the dislocation and the need for reduction. The patient should be questioned about the arm positions or activities that aggravate their symptoms. A detailed history of prior therapeutic interventions should also be elicited. For athletic patients, the type of sports and position played and the frequency and duration of involvement are important factors that can aid in the proper diagnosis and treatment. Patients will often avoid the activities and arm positions that put them at risk for instability episodes, specifically overhead activities with the arm in external rotation and abduction.

Some patients with recurrent subluxation of the shoulder will complain that the shoulder feels "loose," and they may have a sense that the shoulder joint "slips" with contact and overhead activities. Secondary nonoutlet impingement may result from inflammation and tendinitis of the rotator cuff, which may result in a confusing clinical presentation. One must be careful not to confuse the diagnosis of instability with primary outlet impingement syndrome. Others may present with vague neurologic symptoms, such as paresthesias and neuropraxia, which may be secondary to traction on the brachial plexus from anterior-inferior subluxation of the humeral head. The physical examination is used to confirm the predominant direction and type of instability pattern.

The physical examination should be directed and is used to clarify the nature and scope of the problem. A systematic approach to the shoulder examination should include inspection, palpitation, range of motion, strength testing, neurovascular examination, and provocative testing. Both shoulders should be examined. We prefer to examine the uninvolved shoulder first.

On inspection, the presence of asymmetry, deformity, and muscle atrophy should be noted. The patient with an acute anteriorly dislocated shoulder will typically present in intense pain from muscle spasms and will hold the affected arm in slight abduction and internal rotation. In addition, the humeral head may be visibly displaced anteriorly and the patient may be reluctant to move the shoulder. The range of motion may be relatively normal in most patients with chronic shoulder instability. In the acute situation, strength may be diminished because of pain.

The neurovascular status should be carefully documented, especially after an acute dislocation. The incidence of nerve injuries can be as high as 35%, and the axillary nerve is most often involved. Skin sensation in the distribution of the axillary and lateral antebrachial cutaneous nerves should be assessed and documented (11). Vascular injuries are rare but can occur in the older patient population.

Laxity is defined as the amount of asymptomatic passive translation of the humeral head relative to the glenoid during the physical examination. Since inherent capsular laxity is a contributing factor to shoulder instability, the degree of generalized ligamentous laxity should be determined. Thumb hyperabduction, index metacarpal hyperextention, and elbow and knee hyperextension should be assessed (12).

The key to the physical diagnosis of anterior glenohumeral instability is provocative testing. The patient will often demonstrate apprehension (i.e., pain and anxiety) when the arm is placed in abduction and external rotation (Fig. 17.1). A positive relocation test may also be helpful. This is demonstrated by reducing the subluxed humeral head with a posteriorly directed force. Drawer testing is used to assess the degree of humeral head translation relative to the glenoid and is performed with the patient in the supine position. The arm is placed in abduction and external rotation, and an axial load is applied to the humerus. The humeral head is forcibly translated relative to the glenoid, and the amount of translation with the arm in different positions is graded and compared to the unaffected shoulder. The sulcus sign is elicited by standing in front of the patient and placing traction on the wrist in an inferior direction on both arms simultaneously. If there is inferior instability, a sulcus will develop between the lateral border of the acromion and the humeral head (13–15).

RADIOLOGIC STUDIES

Routine radiographic evaluation of patients with suspected anterior instability includes an AP view with the arm in internal rotation, a Stryker notch view, and a West Point axillary view (16). The latter allows examination of the anterior glenoid rim to rule out a bony Bankart lesion and calcification of the glenoid rim. The Stryker notch view and the internally rotated AP views help demonstrate the presence of a Hill-Sachs lesion. In older patients with traumatic injuries, tuberosity fractures and subtle proximal humeral fractures may be present (17).

In the past, we used the CT arthrogram as the ancillary study of choice to assess the degree of capsulolabral involvement, to detect chondral injuries, and to assess glenoid version. Today, we use MRI, when indicated, for similar purposes. The MRI is extremely sensitive; is noninvasive; and can be used to assess other structures, such as the labrum, cartilage, and rotator cuff.

TREATMENT

Nonoperative Treatment

For most patients who present with acute anterior dislocation of the shoulder, radiographs are obtained to document the direction of dislocation and to rule out any associated fractures. Subtle proximal humeral fractures may be present in the older patients that may be displaced by the reduction maneuver; thus we prefer to take radiographs before the reduction is attempted. When the dislocation was witnessed (e.g., during an athletic event), reduction without radiographs may be appropriate.

There are a number of different techniques that can be used to reduce the anteriorly dislocated shoulder. Irrespective of the technique used, it is important that the patient be relaxed before the reduction is attempted. The reduction maneuver we prefer in the acute situation is gentle longitudinal traction on the humerus with gradual forward flexion and internal derotation of the arm (Row maneuver) (Fig. 17.2). If this fails, the patient is placed in a controlled environment, and muscle relaxation and pain relief are obtained with intravenous sedation or an intraarticular injection of a local anesthetic. The patient is placed in the prone position, and the arm is allowed to hang in a dependent position off the edge of the table. The scapula can be manipulated or a 2.3-kg (5-lb) weight can be hung from the arm to facilitate the reduction (Stimson's technique). Other reduction maneuvers include the Kocher technique and the technique described by Cooper.

Radiographic confirmation of the reduction should be obtained. A thorough neurovascular examination should

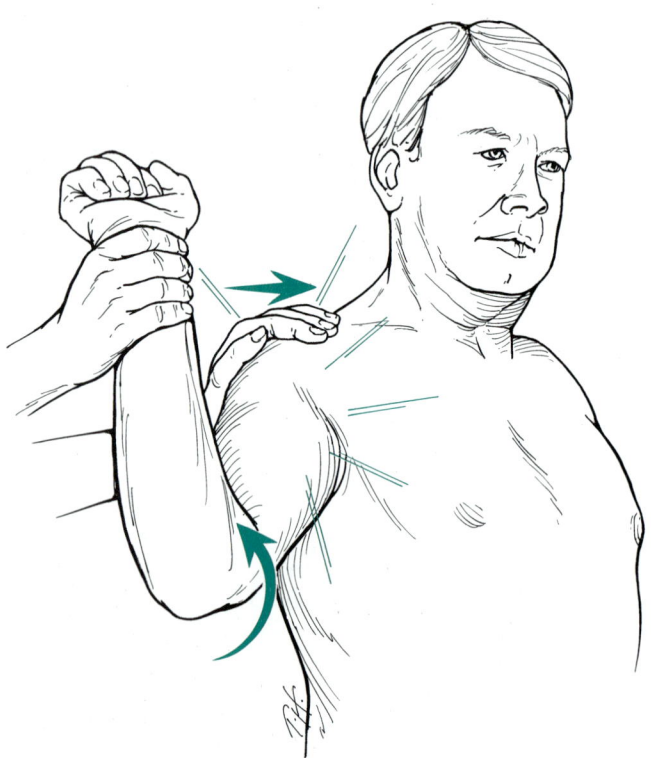

Figure 17.1. Apprehension test for shoulder dislocation.

Figure 17.2. Closed reduction (Rowe) maneuver for anterior shoulder dislocation.

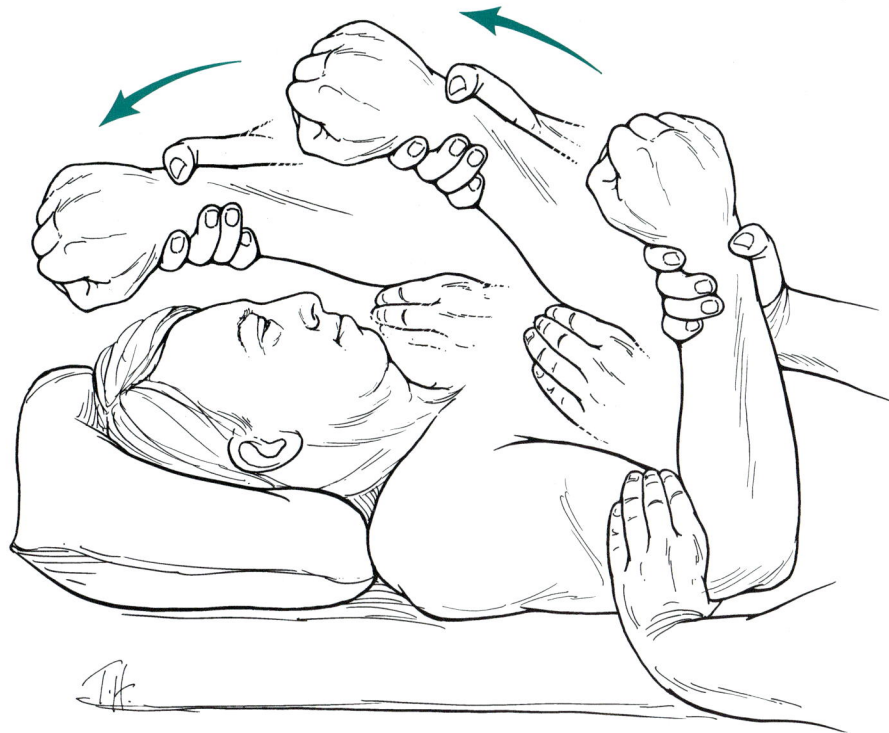

be performed before and after relocation of the shoulder. The arm should be immobilized in a sling and swathe.

Several studies have shown that despite the duration of immobilization—typically 2 to 6 weeks—the recurrence rates for anterior shoulder dislocations can be very high (18). The patient's age at the time of the index dislocation appears to be the most significant factor, and there is a precipitous drop in the redislocation rates in patients over the age of 40 years (10 to 15%). Rehabilitation of the shoulder should focus on rotator cuff and periscapular muscle strengthening to improve dynamic stability. Patients will often avoid activities and provocative maneuvers that put them at risk for instability episodes.

A supervised rehabilitation program is used to strengthen the dynamic stabilizers in patients with recurrent anterior shoulder subluxation. The individual rotator cuff muscles are strengthened with a combination of isometric and isokinetic exercises. In patients with anterior and inferior instability, supervised rehabilitation is recommended for at least 3 months before surgery is even considered (19).

Operative Treatment

In general, no one surgical procedure should be used for the operative management of shoulder instability. The procedure used should be tailored to address the specific pathologic process present and the functional demands of the patient (Clinical Table). The indications for operative treatment include (*a*) recurrent anterior instability and/or pain, despite supervised physical therapy, and (*b*) shoulder instability in the presence of a full-thickness rotator cuff tear. There may be a role for arthroscopic

stabilization in the patient with a first-time dislocation, especially if the patient is an athlete who engages in overhead motion.

The operative management of anterior instability has a rich and storied history. The surgical techniques have evolved from nonanatomic reconstructions, which attempted to correct the instability not by addressing the specific problem but by altering the secondary restraints, to more anatomic reconstructions, in which there is definitive correction of the underlying problem. Many of these patients developed recurrent shoulder instability; and in some cases, when the joint was stable it was frequently overconstrained, resulting in alteration of the joint biomechanics and the subsequent development of arthritis of instability (20,21).

In more recent surgical series, good to excellent results have been reported with the anatomic approach. The detached capsulolabral complex is repaired to the glenoid (4,22), and the capsule is shifted or plicated as needed to reduce capsular laxity (23,24). If the patient has recurrent anterior subluxation, a capsular shift only is performed. The degree of capsular shift should be based the amount of capsular laxity and the functional demands of the patient. Although most of these patients will have a stable shoulder, they will often sacrifice some degree of shoulder mobility, which can have disastrous consequences in the competitive overhead athlete and may preclude premorbid sports participation.

SURGICAL TECHNIQUE

We prefer to use an interscalene block with or without a general anesthetic. A general anesthetic is preferred in muscular individuals, in whom it is difficult to achieve re-

Clinical Table: Anterior Shoulder Instability

Procedure	Indications	Technique	Anatomy	Pitfalls
Bankart repair	• Capsulolabral injury	• Suture anchors	• Bankart lesion	• Failure to identify lesion • Medial shortening of capsul
Inferior capsular shift	• Anterior-inferior instability	• Laterally based T capsulotomy • Inferior flap shifted first	• Axillary nerve • Capsular redundancy • Labral injury	• Axillary nerve injury • Overcorrection leading to osteoarthritis • Limitation of external rotation
T capsulotomy	• Anterior-inferior instability	• Medially based T capsulotomy	• Axillary nerve • Capsular redundancy • Labral injury	• Axillary nerve injury • Overcorrection leading to osteoarthritis • Limitation of external rotation
Anterior capsulolabral reconstruction	• Throwing athlete	• Subscapularis muscle split • Arm in relative abduction and external rotation	• Capsular redundancy • Labral injury	• Limitation of external rotation
Bristow procedure	• Anterior instability	• Coracoid process transfer • Screw fixation	• Musculocutaneous nerve	• Musculocutaneous nerve injury • Recurrent instability • Loss of motion
Putti-Plat	• Anterior instability	• Plication subscapular tendon		• Loss of motion • Recurrent instability • Arthritis of instability
Magnuson-Stack	• Anterior instability	• Subscapular tendon transfer to greater tuberosity		• Loss of motion • Recurrent instability • Arthritis of instability

laxation of the pectoralis major. The examination under anesthesia is performed to confirm the direction and degree of instability. Emphasis is placed on drawer testing, and the direction and degree of instability are graded and recorded presurgery. The patient is placed in the modified beach-chair position on the operating table to allow exposure of the anterior and posterior aspects of the glenohumeral joint. A sterile articulated arm holder (McConnell shoulder holder; McConnell Orthopaedic Manufacturing Co., Greenville, TX) is placed on the side of the operating table and is used to accurately position the arm during the capsular repair and to allow the procedure to be performed with only one assistant.

A standard anterior deltopectoral approach is used, and the skin incision is placed in the axillary fold along the relaxed skin tension for better cosmesis. The deltopectoral interval is developed, and the cephalic vein is dissected and retracted laterally with the deltoid. The clavipectoral fascia is incised laterally to expose the conjoined tendon, which is retracted medially. If the exposure is less than adequate, a transverse relaxing incision is made in the conjoined tendon just distal to the tip of coracoid process. The leading edge of the coracoacromial ligament is resected, and a retractor is placed to allow exposure of the superior capsule. The circumflex vessels are identified along the inferior aspect of the subscapularis

tendon and are preserved or ligated. The axillary nerve is always palpated but is usually not visualized.

The subscapularis tendon is released from the anterior capsule in the coronal plane using a needle tip electrocautery. The arm is placed in adduction and external rotation, to tension the subscapularis tendon and to allow the axillary nerve to fall away from the capsule. The dissection begins 1 to 1.5 cm medial to the lesser tuberosity, and tagging sutures are placed in the edge of the tendon. The capsule is inspected for the presence and size of a rotator interval defect and the degree of capsular laxity. If there is no significant rotator interval capsular defect, a T-shaped capsulotomy incision is made; the vertical limb is along the humeral head and a cuff of capsular tissue is left for the repair. The horizontal limb extends toward the equator of the glenoid.

The degree of capsular laxity can be assessed intraoperatively by placing the finger in the axillary pouch. The inferior extension of the vertical capsulotomy can be carried to the 6- or 8-o'clock position on the humeral neck, depending on the degree of capsular laxity. The superior limb of the capsule is extended to the edge of the supraspinatus tendon. Tagging sutures are placed in the edges of the capsular tissue to facilitate retraction.

The humeral head is then retracted, and the joint and the anterior labral attachment to the capsule are inspected. Chondral lesions and loose bodies may also be present in the joint. If a Bankart lesion is present, it is enlarged by stripping the capsulolabral attachments farther medially off the scapular neck. The anterior scapular neck is decorticated with a small burr or osteotome; and suture anchors, loaded with a single number 1 Ethibond suture, are then placed in the bone of the articular margin of the glenoid at the 6-, 4-, and 2-o'clock positions (for a right shoulder). The sutures are placed through the capsule from inside out and tightened over the capsule, while the subscapularis muscle is retracted medially. The Bankart lesion is repaired anatomically, without shortening the capsule in a medial direction. No attempt is made to shift the capsule during this part of the procedure (Fig. 17.3).

The shoulder position for the repair is determined on an individual basis, depending on the patient's needs and hand dominance. For example, a throwing athlete with instability of the dominant shoulder will need a fair amount of abduction and external rotation, whereas a lower extremity athlete with nondominant shoulder involvement can get away with less abduction and external rotation. The arm is usually positioned between 45° to 60° of abduction, 25° to 45° of external rotation, and 10° of forward flexion. The surgeon should ensure that the humeral head is reduced into the glenoid fossa before the capsular shift is performed. The inferior capsule is shifted superiorly and laterally and repaired to the cuff of capsular tissue on the humeral head. Occasionally, if there is less than adequate lateral capsular tissue for the repair, soft tissue anchors are placed in the humeral neck to secure the repair. The arm is then positioned in 0° of abduction and the appropriate amount of external rotation (25° to 45°), and the superior capsular flap is sutured inferiorly and laterally over the inferior flap. Sutures in the horizontal limb of the inferior flap are repaired to the superior flap in a pants-over-vest fashion.

A large rotator interval defect can be incorporated into the capsulotomy incision as a horizontal limb, making an upside-down L-shaped capsulotomy. In this case, the inferior capsule is repaired as previously described, and the superior capsule is tensioned by bringing the horizontal portion of the inferior flap over the superior capsule, with the arm in 0° abduction and the appropriate amount of external rotation (25° to 45°) (Fig. 17.4).

When the capsular repair is completed, range of motion and laxity are retested. It should be possible to abduct the arm to approximately 90° in the scapular plane and externally rotate the arm between 25° and 45° before the capsule experiences tension. A similar amount of external rotation should be possible when the arm is at the side. Drawer testing should be performed carefully and should demonstrate an anterior and posterior drawer of not more than 1+ with the arm in 45° of abduction and neutral rotation but should decrease to 0° when the arm is externally rotated and further abducted. The inferior drawer should be 0 to 1+ with the arm adducted. The subscapularis tendon is then repaired anatomically and the deltoid–pectoral interval is reapproximated. The skin is closed with subcuticular sutures.

Postsurgery, the arm is maintained in a sling and swath for 4 weeks. Depending on the patient's demand and the nature of the repair, elbow flexion and extension and grip strengthening are permitted, but shoulder motion is limited to approximately 25° of abduction and the arm is kept in internal rotation to allow access to the axilla for washing. The sling is removed at 4 weeks, and active-assisted range of motion exercise is initiated. External rotation is usually limited to the degree of external rotation at which the capsule is repaired for approximately 6 weeks, so the subscapularis repair is not stressed. Isometric strengthening is begun for external rotation, flexion extension, and abduction of the arm; but internal rotation strengthening is delayed until the subscapularis tendon heals. At 8 weeks, isotonic strengthening is instituted using the Thera-Band system. At 4 months, the patient is permitted to swim and begin tossing a ball or hitting ground strokes in tennis. At 4 to 6 months postsurgery, the patient is permitted to begin throwing with more force. Contact sports are usually allowed after 6 to 8 months, depending on the progress with physical therapy.

Recurrent Anterior Subluxation

Surgical stabilization may be indicated in patients who fail a supervised rehabilitation program and those with recurrent anterior subluxation that affects their activities of daily living and sports performance. In most cases, there is excessive laxity of the joint capsule, and the capsular redundancy must be addressed at the time of surgery. Most authors recommended an open approach; but there is a risk of shoulder stiffness, especially in the throwing athlete. Some authors have used subscapularis muscle splitting and tensioned the shoulder with the arm in relative abduction and external rotation to minimize the risk of shoulder stiffness.

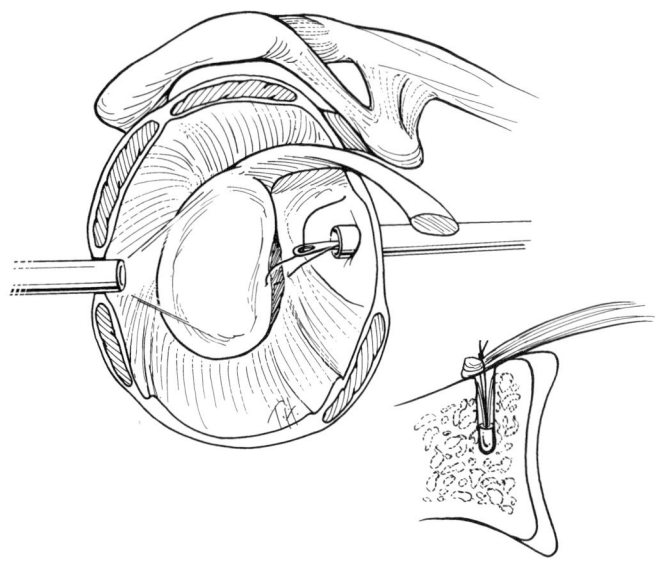

Figure 17.3. For the Bankart repair, suture anchors are placed in the anterior glenoid rim.

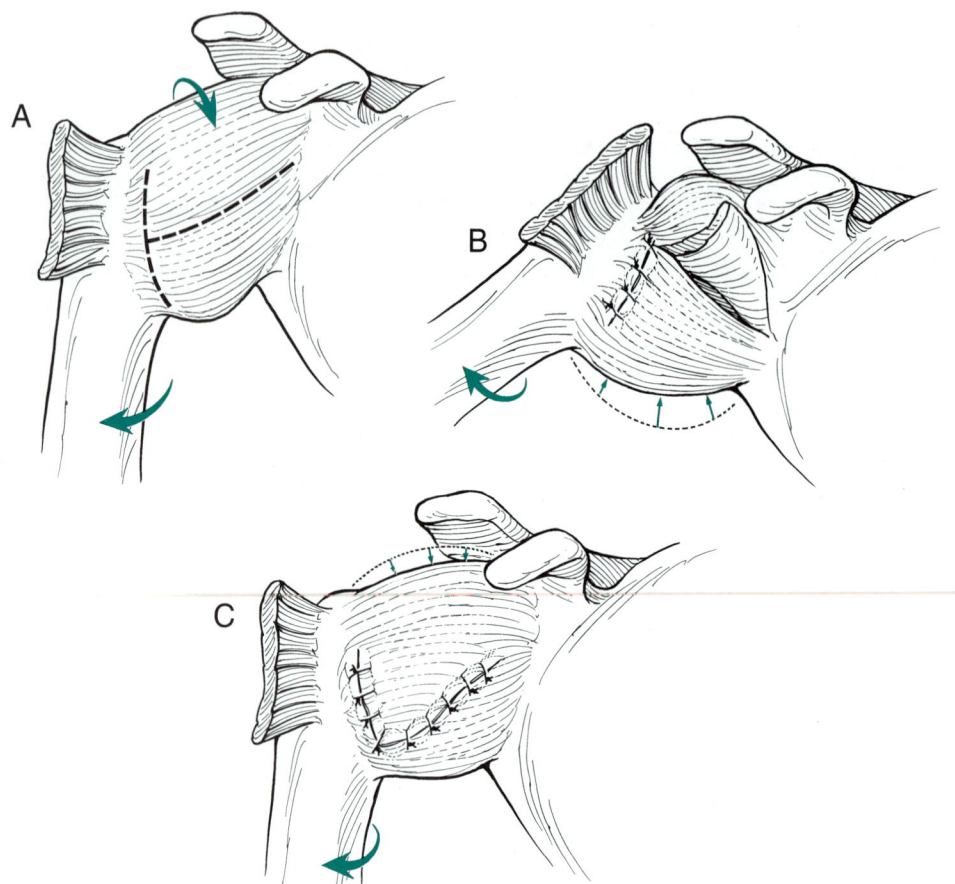

Figure 17.4. Capsular plication in the selective capsular shift.

Our preference is to perform a variation of the selective capsular shift, with the arm tensioned in more abduction and external rotation than that indicated for the individual patient or capsular plication through a subscapularis muscle-splitting approach.

Arthroscopic Shoulder Stabilization

The role of shoulder arthroscopy in patients with glenohumeral instability is evolving. The arthroscope can be used to diagnose and treat suspected glenohumeral instability. The theoretical advantage of the arthroscope is that it is a less invasive approach, with minimal distortion of normal anatomy. Arthroscopic stabilization is indicated primarily in patients with recurrent posttraumatic unidirectional anterior instability. The detached anterior labrum is reattached, and the inferior glenohumeral ligament complex is retensioned.

The various techniques developed for arthroscopic stabilization of the glenohumeral joint have used staples, sutures, and plastic and bioabsorbable fixation devices. Significant complications have been related to the use of metallic implants, including loosening, recurrent instability, and the destruction of the articular surface. Complications related to the use of traditional arthroscopic suture techniques include inadequate fixation and suprascapular nerve injury from transglenoid drilling. With the recent development of intra-articular knot-tying

techniques, these issues are less of a problem and the use of modern suture techniques appears promising.

Presently, our preference is to use a biodegradable cannulated tack system (Suretac; Acufex Microsurgical, Inc., Mansfield, MA) that allows good initial tissue fixation without the risks of hardware complications or transglenoid drilling (25) (Fig. 17.5). Disadvantages of this technique are that it allows only limited shifting of the capsule and does not allow closure of the rotator interval.

We reserve this procedure for patients with recurrent posttraumatic unidirectional anterior instability. The preoperative decision-making process is crucial to determining which patients will have a good result with arthroscopic stabilization using the Suretac device. In our experience, arthroscopic stabilization with the Suretac device is relatively contraindicated in patients involved in contact sports, who may be at a higher risk for redislocation. The final decision is made at the time of arthroscopy and is based on the presence of a Bankart lesion and well-developed inferior glenohumeral ligaments.

Arthroscopy has developed into a valuable diagnostic and therapeutic instrument. Patients typically have shorter hospital stays, less postoperative pain, and more cosmetically favorable results than those who undergo open surgery. Arthroscopic shoulder stabilization can be technically demanding; and generally, the re-

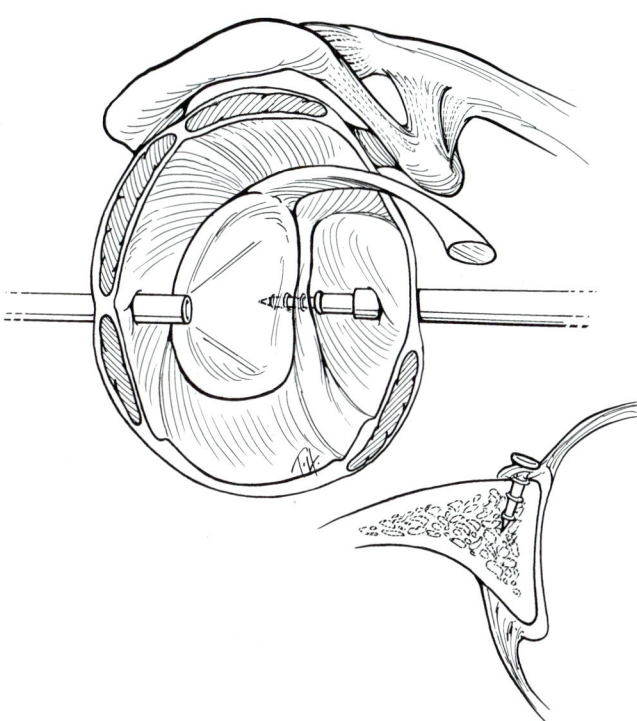

Figure 17.5. Anterior shoulder stabilization with the Suretac device.

currence rates appear to be higher than with open stabilization.

SUMMARY

Anterior shoulder instability is one of the most common disorders in the shoulder. It represents a spectrum of disorders, ranging from shoulder subluxation to shoulder dislocation. The initial challenge for the practitioner is to make the correct diagnosis by understanding and recognizing the instability pattern. A detailed history and physical examination are essential, and advanced imaging studies are rarely indicated. Most patients are treated initially with a supervised rehabilitation program, but initial arthroscopic surgical management of first-time dislocators is becoming more common. The surgical treatment is based on an anatomic approach; the anterior labral lesion is repaired and capsular laxity is reduced. Most cases of recurrent anterior subluxation will respond to an aggressive rehabilitation. If surgery is indicated in the throwing athlete, the surgical approach should not compromise mobility for stability.

REFERENCES

1. Blasier RB, Goldberg RE, Tothman ED. Anterior shoulder stability: contributions of rotator cuff forces and the capsular ligaments in a cadaveric model. J Shoulder Elbow Surg 1992;1:40–150.
2. O'Brien SJ, Neves MC, Arnoczky SJ, et al. The anatomy and the histology of the inferior glenohumeral ligament complex of the shoulder. Am J Sports Med 1990;18:449–456.
3. O'Connell PW, Nuber GW, Mileski RA, Lautenschlager E. The con-
tribution of the glenohumeral ligaments to anterior stability of the shoulder joint. Am J Sports Med 1990;18:579–589.
4. Bankart ASB. The pathology and treatment of recurrent dislocation of the shoulder joint. Br J Surg 1938;26:23–29.
5. Bost FC, Inman VC. The pathological changes in recurrent dislocation of the shoulder: a report of Bankart's operative procedure. J Bone Joint Surg 1942;23A:596–613.
6. Bigliani LU, Pollack RG, Soslowski LJ, et al. Tensile properties of the glenohumeral ligament. J Orthop Res 1992;10:187–197.
7. Speer KP, Deng X, Torzilli PA, Altchek DW. A biomechanical evaluation of the Bankart lesion. Trans Orthop Res Soc 1988;39:315.
8. Patel MR, Pordee ML, Sincerman RC. Intrathoracic dislocation of the head of the humerus. J Bone Joint Surg 1963;45A:1712–1714.
9. Rowe CR. Prognosis in dislocations of the shoulder. J Bone Joint Surg 1956;38A:957–977.
10. Rowe CR, Zarins B. Recurrent transient subluxation of the shoulder. J Bone Joint Surg 1981;63A:863–872.
11. Blom S, Dahlback CO. Nerve injuries in dislocations of the shoulder joint and fractures of the neck of the humerus: a clinical and electromyographic study. Acta Chir Scand 1970;136:461–466.
12. Harryman D, Sidles J, Harris S, Matsen F. Role of the rotator interval capsule in passive motion and stability of the shoulder. J Bone Joint Surg 1992;72A:53–66.
13. Cofield RH, Irving JF. Evaluation and classification of shoulder instability: with reference to examination under anesthesia. Clin Orthop 1987;223:32–36.
14. Cofield RH, Kavanaugh BF, Frassica FJ. Anterior shoulder instability. Instr Course Lect 1972;21:42–52.
15. Gerber C, Ganz R. Clinical assessment of instability of the shoulder (with special reference to anterior and posterior drawer tests). J Bone Joint Surg 1984;66B:551–556.
16. Roukos J, Feagin J, Abbott H. Modified axillary roentgenogram: a useful adjunct in the diagnosis of recurrent instability of the shoulder. Clin Orthop 1972;82:84–86.
17. Hall R, Issac F, Booth C. Dislocations of the shoulder with special reference to accompanying small fractures. J Bone Joint Surg 1959;41A:489–494.
18. Emery RJH, Mullaji MD. Glenohumeral joint instability in normal adolescents. Incidence and significance. J Bone Joint Surg 1991; 73B:406–408.
19. Burkhead W, Rockwood C. Treatment of instability of the shoulder with an exercise program. J Bone Joint Surg 1992; 74A:890–896.
20. Hawkins R, Kunkel S, Nayak N. Inferior capsular shift for multidirectional instability of the shoulder: 2–5 year follow-up. Orthop Trans 1991;15:765.
21. Lusardi DA, Wirth MA, Wurtz D, Rockwood DA Jr. Loss of external rotation following anterior capsulorrhaphy of the shoulder. J Bone Joint Surg 1993;75A:1185–1192.
22. Rowe CR, Patel D, Southmayd WW. The Bankart procedure; a long-term end result study. J Bone Joint Surg 1978;60A:1–16.
23. Neer CS II, Foster CR. Inferior capsular shift for involuntary inferior and multidirectional instability of the shoulder. J Bone Joint Surg 1980;2A:897–907.
24. Altchek DW, Warren RF, Skyhar MJ, Ortiz, G. T-plasty modification of the Bankart procedure for multidirectional instability of the anterior and inferior types. J Bone Joint Surg 1991;73A: 105–112.
25. Warner JJP, Warren RF. Arthroscopic Bankart repair using a cannulated, absorbable fixation device. Oper Tech Orthop 1991; 1:192–197.

Suggested Readings

Morgan C, Bodenstab A. Arthroscopic transglenoid Bankart suture repair. Oper Tech Orthop 1991;1:117.
Warner JJP, Johnson D, Miller MD, Caborn DNM. The concept of a "selective capsular shift" for treatment of anterior-inferior shoulder instability. Paper presented at the Annual Meeting of the American Shoulder and Elbow Surgeons, New Orleans, February 21, 1994.

chapter 18

Gloria M. Beim and Jon J. P. Warner

Posterior Instability of the Shoulder

Posterior dislocation of the shoulder has been described since the early 1800s. Although it has been considered a rare occurrence, more recent reports in the literature indicate that it is more prevalent than was previously appreciated. Traumatic posterior dislocations represent less than 4% of all shoulder dislocations in most series reported in the literature (1–3). Recurrent posterior instability, especially when manifesting as subluxation, is a diagnostic and therapeutic challenge. The symptoms may mimic other disorders; and because complete dislocation does not always occur, the diagnosis may be difficult to confirm with radiographs. Interpretation of the literature is also unclear because of the poorly defined criteria for the diagnosis; some authors have used the terms subluxation and dislocation interchangeably. The recurrence rate for subluxation remains unspecified but is probably higher than that for posterior dislocation.

Posterior subluxation is increasingly recognized in the athlete. True posterior dislocation in athletes is rare, and most such dislocations spontaneously reduce. Posterior instability, when it occurs, is more typically recurrent subluxation rather than dislocation. In this setting, the diagnosis may be subtle, because patients often present with pain rather than instability.

In cases of recognized traumatic posterior dislocation, a supervised physical therapy program is usually instituted after a period of shoulder immobilization. The program generally consists of strengthening the dynamic stabilizers of the shoulder and avoiding exercises that place the arm in a flexed, relatively adducted position. When nonoperative treatment is unsuccessful and the instability is disabling, most authors recommend operative stabilization. Because of the variable experience with posterior capsulolabral repair, there has been no consensus on the optimal method of operative stabilization.

The surgical treatment protocols for posterior disloca-

tion and subluxation can be divided into two groups. One group addresses soft tissue abnormalities, such as capsular detachment or laxity. The other group addresses bony pathology through osteotomy or bone block procedures.

RELEVANT ANATOMY AND PATHOGENESIS

The shoulder is the most mobile joint in the body; and unlike other large joints, such as the hip, it has little inherent stability from articular and bony anatomy. Therefore, the surrounding soft tissue envelope of the capsule, ligaments, and rotator cuff muscles functions as the primary stabilizer of the shoulder joint. Furthermore, to allow for multiplanar motion in this joint, the capsule and ligaments are relatively lax but are also passive static restraints to excessive translation and rotation of the humeral head on the glenoid at the end ranges of rotation. Stability against posterior translation is principally maintained by articular congruence, glenoid version, humeral torsion, capsulolabral integrity, and normal function of the rotator cuff and extrinsic shoulder muscles.

The posterior capsule is posterior and superior to the posterior band of the inferior glenohumeral ligament complex (IGHLC). It represents the thinnest region of the joint capsule, with a normal thickness of less than 1 mm (4). It is the primary static restraint to posterior translation when the shoulder is forward flexed, adducted, and internally rotated (1). The rotator interval region is the anterior-superior portion of the shoulder capsule between the subscapularis and supraspinatus tendons. Its major components are the superior glenohumeral and coracohumeral ligaments. When the shoulder is flexed, adducted, and internally rotated, these ligaments tighten and act as secondary static restraints to posterior translation of the humeral head (5). Thus both the anterior and the posterior capsule contribute to posterior stability of the glenohumeral joint when the shoulder is flexed, adducted, and internally rotated. Furthermore, when the shoulder is abducted in the plane of the scapula, both the anterior and the posterior portions of the inferior glenohumeral ligament complex contribute to posterior stability. In a position of abduction, this structure supports the humeral head in the glenoid in a "hammock" (6).

The rotator cuff complex encircles the humeral head and is intricately conjoined with the underlying joint capsule. These structures contribute to the stability of the glenohumeral joint dynamically through two mechanisms. First, the combined action of these muscles results in joint compression, creating a concavity compression fit of the articular surfaces (1). Second, synchronous and coordinated contraction of these muscle units maintains stability by steering the humeral head into the glenoid cavity during shoulder motion.

Although there has been some controversy about the cause of posterior instability, most shoulder surgeons believe the primary lesion is posterior capsular laxity (7,8). In some cases of traumatic injury, a posterior Bankart lesion may be created; but in all cases, capsular laxity must be addressed. In rare cases, congenital retroversion or dysplasia of the glenoid may be a factor, but articular abnormalities are usually acquired from injury to the posterior glenoid (9,10). Some surgeons (11) have suggested that humeral retroversion is a factor; this is not a common opinion in North America.

CLASSIFICATION

In general, a classification of shoulder instability is based on four factors: the degree of instability, the frequency of occurrence, the direction, and the cause of the instability. First one must distinguish between laxity and instability. Instability is defined as excessive, symptomatic translation of the humeral head on the glenoid during active shoulder motion. Laxity is defined as the amount of passive, asymptomatic translation of the humeral head on the glenoid as determined by clinical examination. Such a distinction is important, since some young athletic individuals may have significant laxity or looseness of the shoulder when examined under anesthesia and yet have not symptoms. Conversely, a less lax shoulder may actually be found in an individual with symptomatic instability.

The classification of posterior instability is organized in a way that gives insight into the pathology and natural history of the problem (Table 18.1). For example, an individual with recurrent posterior subluxation may be amenable to therapy; if this fails, surgery will usually be required to treat posterior capsular laxity. Conversely, an individual with voluntary instability and the ability to put the shoulder "out the back" with muscle contraction will not be a suitable operative candidate (12). In the case of a chronic, locked posterior dislocation, the size of the reverse Hill-Sachs lesion and the chronicity of the dislocation have a direct bearing on the method of treatment employed. In

table	18.1	Classification of Posterior Instability of the Shoulder

Type	Description
1	Traumatic, acute dislocation; recurrent dislocation
2	Traumatic, acute subluxation; recurrent subluxation
3	Voluntary (atraumatic) subluxation or dislocation
a	Positional type
b	Muscular type
4	Involuntary (atraumatic) subluxation or dislocation
5	Posterior type with anterior or inferior instability
6	Chronic, locked dislocation
a	Size of reverse Hill-Sachs lesion: <25% of the articular surface
b	Size of reverse Hill-Sachs lesion: 25–40% of the articular surface
c	Size of reverse Hill-Sachs lesion: >40% of the articular surface

the case of multidirectional instability, it is important to recognize all directions of symptomatic instability so that a global capsular tightening procedure can be performed, sometimes through a combined anterior and posterior approach, if necessary (13).

INITIAL FINDINGS, PHYSICAL EXAMINATION, AND DIAGNOSIS

Posterior dislocations of the shoulder may be missed at the time of initial presentation in 50 to 80% of patients (3). The key to diagnosing posterior instability is an appropriate level of suspicion and a careful history and physical examination. A history of electrical shock or seizure should give the surgeon a high index of suspicion for posterior instability. Posterior dislocations or subluxations usually spontaneously reduce, and the patient presents with only pain. Sometimes individuals have a sense of posterior movement of the humeral head when the shoulder is placed in certain positions. The patient should be carefully evaluated for posterior subluxation as the arm is forward flexed. An alcoholic or demented patient who presents with pain and limited external rotation should be suspected to have a locked, chronic posterior dislocation.

Typically, a patient with recurrent posterior subluxation complains of pain or a sensation of shoulder instability when performing activities that place the arm in the forward flexed and adducted position with the shoulder internally rotated. These activities include rowing; bench pressing; swimming, particularly during the pull-through phase of specific strokes; and pitching, particularly during the follow-through phase. Pain is usually limited to the episodes of instability. The location of pain is variable and can be about the posterior shoulder, over the biceps tendon, or about the superior rotator cuff and is similar to the pain felt with impingement syndrome. Some patients may complain of persistent pain, although this is not a common presentation. Frequently, pain or the sensation of instability develops over a period of several months. Initially it may be associated with specific sports activities but then may occur with routine use of the arm.

It is important to determine whether the instability is voluntary or involuntary. Posterior voluntary instability can be divided into two forms: muscular and positional. Patients in the latter group have muscular control of their instability; and with in this group is a subgroup of patients with significant emotional and character problems who use their disability for secondary gain. Patients in this subgroup should receive psychiatric counseling not surgical treatment. Most patients with positional control of their posterior instability have an involuntary component as well. If these patients are disabled and do not respond to a directed therapy program of rotator cuff strengthening, they may be candidates for surgical repair.

A significant finding on physical examination of a patient with a posterior dislocation is the arm position of internal rotation with limited external rotation. There may be a fullness in the posterior shoulder region and a prominent coracoid process anteriorly.

A patient with recurrent posterior subluxation may have subtle physical findings, although several special tests can be helpful. There will be no obvious asymmetry on inspection. Posterior joint line tenderness may be present. Crepitus in the region of the posterior joint line may represent labral or chondral injury. Pain may be elicited by placing the arm in forward flexion to 90° and then internally rotating it while directing a compression force axially down the humeral shaft; this is the posterior stress test (2). The jerk test is also useful: The arm is placed in a position of flexion, and a posterior force is applied down the shaft of the humerus by pushing on the flexed elbow. The shoulder is then slowly brought into extension behind the plane of the scapula. A palpable, often painful, and audible shift will occur as the humeral head reduces over the glenoid rim and into the glenoid fossa from its subluxated position.

In most patients, range of motion is normal. Strength may be diminished secondary to discomfort. Patients with painful posterior instability on one side may have demonstrable but painless laxity in the same direction in the opposite shoulder. Comparison is important in the assessment of generalized laxity but does not prove whether the pain on the involved side is caused by instability. Other causes of shoulder pain must be ruled out before the diagnosis of symptomatic instability is entertained.

One of the most important findings in voluntary subluxators is their ability to reproduce the subluxation episode. Basically, these individuals perform a voluntary jerk test: The patient initiates forward elevation with the arm in a somewhat internally rotated position. The subluxation takes place between 90° and 120° of forward elevation. The humeral head will spontaneously reduce between 120° and 180° of forward elevation as abduction is added to the movement. This is the positional-type voluntary instability. Individuals with the muscle-type voluntary instability can subluxate their shoulder with their arm at their side.

A sulcus sign may also be present in patients with posterior instability. This is demonstrated by pulling downward on the adducted arm. The presence of the sulcus inferior to the acromion suggests an inferior component to the instability. If the degree of the sulcus decreases with external rotation of the arm, it may be deemed a physiologic sulcus sign, which should be compared to the noninvolved shoulder.

Congenital hyperlaxity is important when diagnosing the patient with a suspected posterior instability. It is assessed by detecting the presence of recurvatum at the elbow, hyperextensibility at the thumb metacarpophalangeal joint, genu recurvatum, and hyperextensibility at the proximal interphalangeal joints of the hand.

Any multidirectional component of the instability must be recognized before a plan of treatment is made (13). Failure to do so may result in an asymmetric capsular repair, which causes the humeral head to subluxate in the opposite direction. The consequences of this condition may be degenerative arthritis from fixed incongruity of the joint surfaces.

RADIOLOGIC STUDIES

Radiographic evaluation of patients with posterior subluxation should include the standard views taken for patients with suspected anterior instability: an AP view with the arm in internal rotation, a West Point axillary view, and a Stryker notch view (14). Together these views are sensitive for Bankart and Hill-Sachs lesions. For detection of posterior instability, a good axillary view is crucial to attempt to demonstrate subtle static posterior subluxation, bony reaction along the posterior glenoid rim, articular erosion, arthritis, fracture, and reverse Hill-Sachs lesion. Sometimes a patient may actually demonstrate posterior subluxation by positioning the arm during the radiographic imaging.

Ancillary three-dimensional imaging may be very helpful. A CT arthrogram may demonstrate excessive retroversion of the glenoid, glenoid fracture, posterior articular loss, posterior Bankart lesion, and reverse Hill-Sachs lesion. We usually employ double-contrast CT arthrograms but reserve such studies for cases in which we suspect Bankart and reverse Hill-Sachs lesions and thus need more quantitative information on which to base our treatment plans. MRI is used less frequently, and we do not believe it is cost-effective or sensitive for posterior instability with these lesions.

TREATMENT

Nonoperative Treatment

Nonoperative treatment of posterior glenohumeral instability is the recommended initial treatment of many authors. Rockwood et al. (15) found that patients with posterior instability, whether of traumatic or atraumatic origin, did better with rehabilitative exercises than did patients with primary anterior instability. Furthermore, Huber and Gerber (16) found that adolescents with voluntary posterior instability fared better with nonoperative treatment than with operative treatment. On long-term evaluation, patients who did not have surgery tended to experience few episodes of instability and did not have any disability. Conversely, those who had surgical repairs had relatively more disability and pain, which were believed to be sequelae of that form of treatment.

Conservative treatment of shoulder instability generally involves strengthening the dynamic muscular stabilizers of the glenohumeral joint to compensate for deficient or damaged static structures, such as the labrum and capsuloligamentous complex surrounding the joint. Specifically, the exercises must target the rotator cuff, long head of the biceps, and the periscapular muscles (serratus anterior, trapezius, rhomboids) to restore effective scapulohumeral motion. Furthermore, exercises that place the arm in a flexed, relatively adducted position, such as the bench press, should be avoided.

Most patients with acute posterior dislocations have a spontaneous reduction. If a patient presents with an acute posterior dislocation, a locked dislocation must be ruled out before a reduction attempt is made. If reduction is attempted, this must be done cautiously and preferably in the operating room with the patient under anesthesia. If a locked dislocation is encountered, the surgeon must be prepared to perform an anterior approach for open reduction. Once the shoulder is reduced, whether closed or open, the shoulder should be immobilized in a brace that maintains the shoulder in neutral flexion-extension, internal-external rotation, and slight abduction. In this position, the posterior capsule is lax and can heal with little chance of elongation or stretching.

The surgeon should also rule out associated medical conditions that might have played a causative role in the dislocation. Such conditions include seizure and electrical shock. Other medical conditions may also be involved, some of which may need urgent treatment.

Operative Treatment

The indications for operative treatment include recurrent pain and/or instability despite supervised physical therapy; and acute, irreducible locked posterior dislocation (Clinical Table). Surgical repair of posterior instability has given fair to poor results compared to surgical repair of anterior instability (2).

Some surgeons have suggested an anterior approach and capsular shift as the best form of treatment. This philosophy basically treats posterior instability as a variant of multidirectional instability and thus prescribes a global capsular shift. Most recent surgical series, however, report good reliability with posterior repair using a capsular shift technique (7,8). These surgeons recognize the need to

shift and reinforce the posterior capsule, which is lax. Prior approaches that employed modifications of the Bankart repair, Putti-Platt, and capsular stapling were often unsuccessful because they ignored the capsular laxity (17,18). Some European surgeons have suggested routinely performing a posterior glenoid opening wedge osteotomy or a rotational osteotomy of the humerus (9–11). In North America, however, these procedures are not generally employed; most surgeons believe that only rare cases have excessive glenoid retroversion or femoral retroversion that requires correction.

Contraindications to posterior-inferior capsular shift include voluntary (muscular-type) instability, true multidirectional instability with a significant anterior component, significant bone loss, and significant glenoid retroversion. In the last three conditions, additional procedures may be required, which will be described below.

SURGICAL TREATMENT OF SPECIFIC CONDITIONS

Within the diagnosis of posterior instability there are seven conditions that may require surgical repair: (a) chronic, locked dislocation; (b) recurrent, posttraumatic subluxation; (c) involuntary, recurrent, atraumatic subluxation; (d) posterior instability in combination with anterior instability; (e) fixed subluxation with posterior articular loss; (f) articular loss in combination with posterior instability; and (g) glenoid retroversion (dysplasia).

Chronic, Locked Posterior Dislocation

Operative treatment of chronic, locked posterior dislocations vary, depending on the chronicity, the age of the patient, and the size of the humeral head defect. Initially, associated conditions, such as seizure disorders, dementia, psychiatric disorders, or brachial plexopathies, must be ruled out. The chronicity of the dislocation is important, because dislocations that have been unreduced for more than 6 months may not have viable articular cartilage, and osteoporosis of the humeral head may be extreme. These conditions may render the articular surfaces unable to withstand the normal forces in the shoulder once reduced. Furthermore, closed reduction in these cases risks fracture of the humeral head through the reverse Hill-Sachs lesion.

The treatment approach is also based on the size of the reverse Hill-Sachs lesion. If the patient is young and the reverse Hill-Sachs lesion is less than 40% of the articular surface, the surgical options include humeral head osteotomy, transfer of the lesser tuberosity and subscapularis tendon into the humeral head defect (the McLaughlin procedure), bone graft into the defect, and osteochondral allograft reconstruction of the articular surface (9). If the patient is older or if more than 40% of the articular surface is involved, a hemiarthroplasty replacement of the humeral head may be the best treatment option.

Recurrent, Posttraumatic Subluxation

For recurrent, posttraumatic subluxation, posterior capsular laxity with or without a Bankart lesion is the main problem to address (1,7,19). Our preferred approach to

Clinical Table: Posterior Shoulder Instability

Procedure	Indications	Technique	Anatomy	Pitfalls
Reverse Bankart repair	• Posterior labral injury	• Suture anchors		• Failure to identify redundant capsular tissue
Posteroinferior capsular shift	• Posterior instability	• T-capsular incision • Inferior flap shifted first	• Axillary nerve • Suprascapular nerve	• Failure to repair reverse Bankart lesion • Overlooked MDI • Overcorrection, leading to osteoarthritis
Capsular shift with bone block	• Posterior instability with either —Deficient osseous rim posterior glenoid —Pronounced attenuation of the capsule during the shift	• Bone block from the iliac crest • Internal fixation with hardware • Capsular repair done before bone graft placement	• Axillary nerve • Suprascapular nerve	• Same as in shift without bone block • Glenoid articular penetration
Open wedge glenoid osteotomy	• Excessive glenoid retroversion	• Osteotomy made >1 cm from the glenoid articular surface • Iliac crest bone graft into wedge	• Plane of the glenoid	• Avoid glenoid fracture • Glenoid penetration can cause OA • Glenoid AVN • Undercorrection • Failure to identify capsular redundancy
Humeral rotational osteotomy	• Excessive humeral retroversion	• Deltopectoral approach • Osteotomy as close to humeral head as possible AO T-plate	• Deltopectoral approach • Pectoralis major insertion	• Undercorrection • Pseudarthrosis • Hardware failure • Instability in more than one plane

MDI, multidirectional instability; *OA,* osteoarthritis; *AVN,* avascular necrosis.

patients with refractory chronic posterior instability who have failed an intense rehabilitation program is a posterior capsular shift. In rare cases, some patients may have glenoid dysplasia or excessive retroversion. If this can be documented on a CT arthrogram, it must also be addressed by either an opening wedge osteotomy or a bone block procedure to augment a deficient posterior glenoid articular surface.

Recent clinical experience with posterior capsular shift has been good. Fronek et al. (7) reported the results of 27 patients with posterior subluxation. A total of 16 patients noted no major single causative traumatic event and were successfully treated with rehabilitation alone. The other 11 patients experienced a traumatic episode or major disability caused by instability and were treated surgically with a posteroinferior T-plasty capsular shift based along the glenoid. They reported a 91% successful outcome. Bone block procedures were rarely necessary, and the ability to voluntarily subluxate the shoulder by positioning it did not affect the result.

Bigliani et al. (8) reported similar results for a posteroinferior capsular shift based along the humeral side to address posterior and inferior capsular redundancy. The

outcome was good to excellent in 23 of the 24 shoulders that underwent a superior shift of the posteroinferior aspect of the capsule as the initial repair.

A posteroinferior capsular shift can be combined with a labral repair when there is a concomitant reverse Bankart lesion. Augmentation with a bone graft harvested from the scapular spine is used only in rare cases, for example, when significant glenoid hypoplasia is present or when there is frank loss of the posterior glenoid surface.

Our method of the posteroinferior capsular shift is similar to that described by Fronek et al. (7) and Bigliani et al. (19). Once the diagnosis of posterior instability is confirmed with an examination under anesthesia, the patient is positioned on a deflatable beanbag in the lateral decubitus position with the involved side up (Fig. 18.1A). Muscle paralysis is instituted by anesthesia, all bony prominences are carefully padded, and intravenous antibiotics are administered before the skin incision is made. The involved arm is prepped and draped free, and a special arm holder with a sterile articulated ball joint is used to support and position the arm (McConnell Orthopaedic Manufacturing Co., Greenville, TX).

The procedure is performed through a cosmetic skin incision centered over the posterior aspect of the gleno-humeral joint and in Langer's lines. The layer of subcutaneous tissue is dissected to permit retraction of the skin and to permit visualization of the deltoid muscle fibers. The deltoid muscle is then split in line with its fibers at the level of the palpable posterior joint line, beginning at the scapular spine and extending distally 5 to 6 cm (Fig. 18.1B). Care is taken to avoid splitting the deltoid muscle distally beyond the teres minor muscle, because this might injure the axillary nerve.

The infraspinatus is identified and then split bluntly in line with its fibers at the level of the glenoid equator. The layer between the infraspinatus and capsule is then carefully developed, and a 2-cm portion of the infraspinatus insertion is then divided off the greater tuberosity (Fig. 18.1C). The capsule is opened horizontally, beginning at the equator of the glenoid; and a vertical paraglenoid incision is made both inferiorly and superiorly to develop two capsular flaps, which will be shifted along the glenoid (Fig. 18.1D). Sutures are placed in each capsular flap so they can be reflected, and then a humeral head retractor is inserted into the joint to displace the humeral head anteriorly.

The posterior aspect of the joint is then inspected. Degenerative changes in the articular cartilage and vertical clefts in the posterior part of the labrum are frequently seen as a result of repeated subluxation. An extensive Bankart lesion of the labrum, as often seen with anterior instability, is rarely found posteriorly. If, however, the posterior aspect of the labrum is found to be completely detached, it is repaired before the capsule is shifted. The insertion site of the labrum on the glenoid is roughened with a curet; and the labrum, together with the capsule medially, is reattached to the osseous rim with suture anchors and nonabsorbable, braided suture material of at least 1 gauge. The inferior capsular flap is shifted superiorly to obliterate the inferior pouch and is reattached with suture anchors (Fig. 18.1E). The superior flap is shifted inferiorly to reinforce the repair (Fig. 18.1F).

During closure of the inferior and superior capsular flaps, the shoulder is positioned in 20° of abduction and neutral rotation. The infraspinatus deltoid muscle splits are reapproximated with 2–0 absorbable suture. The subcutaneous layer is closed, and a subcuticular skin closure with absorbable suture is performed. Postoperatively, the patient is placed in a prefabricated gunslinger brace with the shoulder positioned in neutral rotation with 10° of abduction and 10° of extension. The brace is worn full-time for 6 weeks.

Over the past 5 years, one of us (Warner) has surgically treated 36 cases of recurrent posterior subluxation using this technique. Good to excellent results were achieved in 33 patients, which included several collegiate football players, wrestlers, and recreational racquet sport athletes. There was 1 case of recurrent instability, and 2 developed shoulder stiffness that required treatment.

POSTERIOR CAPSULAR SHIFT WITH BONE BLOCK

Bone block is indicated in cases for which there is actual loss of the posterior glenoid articular surface (3). It is combined with a capsular shift as an extra-articular extension of the glenoid. It functions mechanically to extend the glenoid surface contour posteriorly rather than to block posterior luxation of the humeral head. Placement of the bone block in a too prominent position may result in its fracture if the humeral head impinges against it; placement in a recessed location medial to the glenoid will result in its resorption since there will be no stress on it (Fig. 18.2).

POSTERIOR OPENING WEDGE GLENOID OSTEOTOMY

The posterior opening wedge glenoid osteotomy is indicated in only rare cases, such as atraumatic posterior instability with glenoid dysplasia and traumatic loss of the posterior glenoid articular surface, resulting in acquired retroversion. In each case, retroversion should exceed 20°, as lesser amounts may be within the range of normal and may not be biomechanically important. One us (Warner) has seen six cases of traumatic articular loss of the posterior glenoid in which the loss of articular cartilage of the posterior half of the glenoid resulted in an increased articular retroversion of 16° to 30° as measured by CT arthrography.

The operative setup and initial dissection are the same as described above for the posteroinferior capsular shift (9) (Fig. 18.3). Once the capsule is exposed, a vertical capsulotomy is made 1 cm lateral to the glenoid rim; and the medial capsule is detached sharply from the posterior aspect of the glenoid. The labrum is left attached to the posterior rim of the glenoid.

A humeral head retractor is placed into the joint, and the humeral head is displaced anteriorly. This gives an unobstructed view of the glenoid surface, allowing visualization and orientation of the plane of the glenoid. The line of the osteotomy is marked 1 cm medial to the glenoid, and drill holes are made through both the anterior and the posterior cortices. The location of the suprascapular neurovascular pedicle is about 2 cm from the posterior glenoid rim (20).

A depth gauge is used to measure the anteroposterior depth of the glenoid neck. The saw blade is marked with the glenoid depth, thus eliminating the potential for creating a free-floating glenoid fragment by transecting both the anterior and posterior cortices. When the osteotomy is complete, a 2.5-cm osteotome is gently tapped into place, and the osteotomy is opened by gently levering with the osteotome. Alternatively, several broad, flat osteotomes can be inserted into the osteotomy site one after the other, gradually wedging it open. Care must be taken to avoid interarticular penetration, glenoid fracture, and over-anteversion of the glenoid (Fig. 18.4) (10). A tricortical piece of bone is harvested from the iliac crest and placed

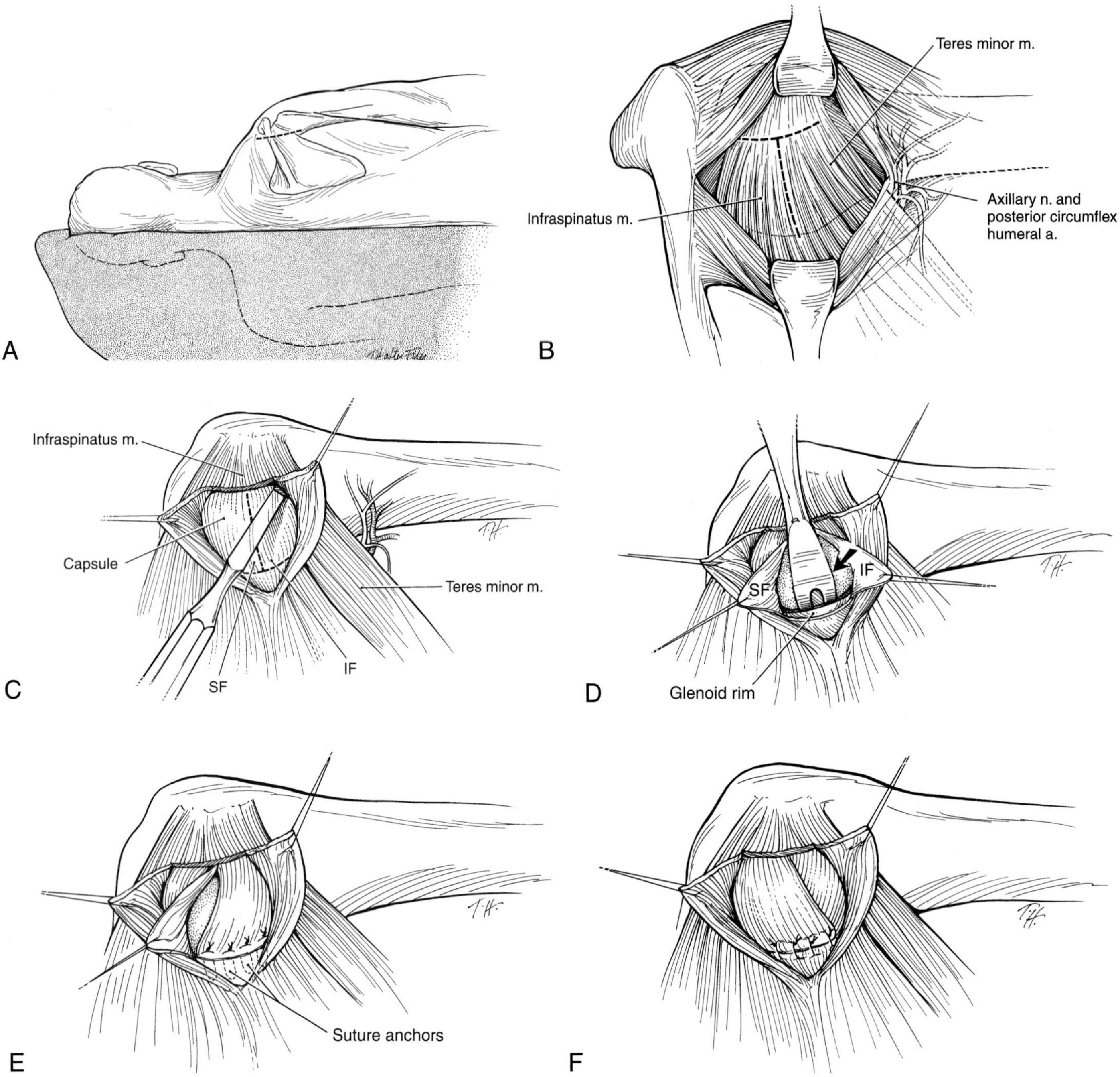

Figure 18.1. A. The patient is placed in the lateral decubitus position on a long beanbag. **B.** The deltoid muscle is split longitudinally over the joint line, and retractors are placed in the subdeltoid interval. The infraspinatus and teres minor are exposed. **C.** The infraspinatus muscle is split in line with its fibers at the equator of the joint. Dissection is from medial to lateral; the muscle is then detached from its insertion for a distance of 1 cm both inferiorly and superiorly. An elevator facilitates the dissection between the tendon and the un-derlying capsule. **D.** The infraspinatus has been reflected, and the underlying capsule has been opened to create inferior and superior flaps with a T-shaped incision along the glenoid rim. **E.** First, the inferior flap of the capsule is shifted superiorly and medially; then the superior flap is shifted over the inferior flap. **F.** After the capsular shift has been performed, the posterior capsule is reinforced by the flaps, which are overlapped. *SF,* superior flap; *IF,* inferior flap.

into the osteotomy. If there is a good interference wedge fit of the graft within the osteotomy site, screw fixation is not needed to keep the graft in place. A capsular shift is then performed as described above. Postoperative treatment is as described above for the posterior capsular shift procedure alone.

POSTOPERATIVE REHABILITATION

The postoperative rehabilitation program is similar for the posteroinferior capsular shift, the capsular shift with bone block, and the open wedge glenoid osteotomy. After 6 weeks of immobilization, the gunslinger brace is removed and a program of rehabilitation begins, which in-

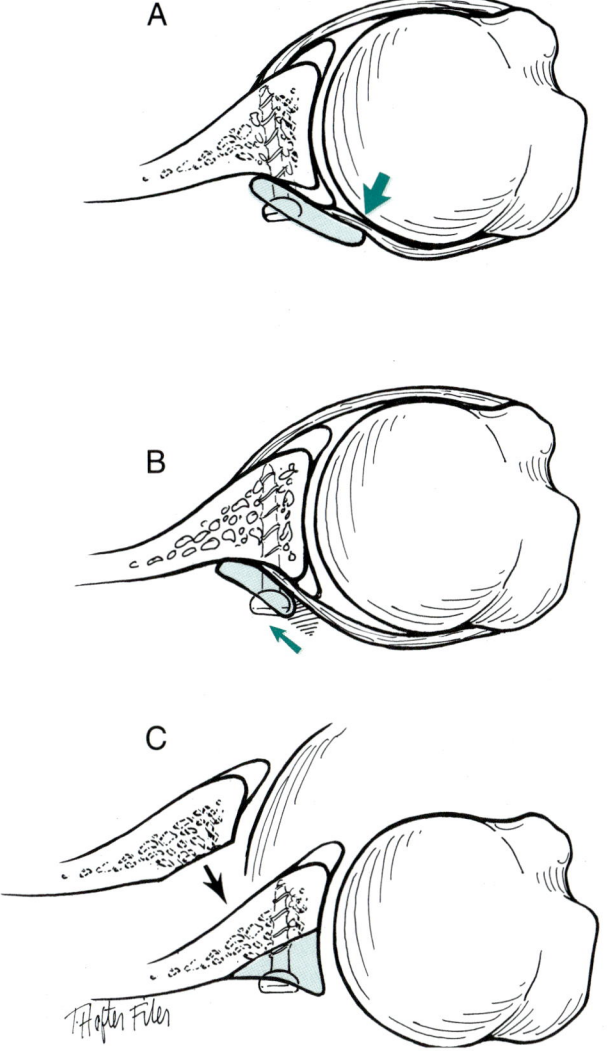

Figure 18.2. A. A posterior bone block placed too laterally creates impingement on the humeral head (*arrow*). **B.** A posterior bone block placed too medially (*arrow*) is unloaded and will thus resorb over time. **C.** A correctly placed posterior bone block extends the deficient glenoid surface and supports the humeral head.

cludes range of motion and muscle strengthening exercises. Emphasis must be placed on strengthening the rotator cuff musculature, especially the external rotators. The initial program consists of active range of motion without strengthening. Internal and external rotation isometric and isotonic exercises are begun 12 weeks postsurgery, which will have allowed for secure healing of the posterior rotator cuff and deltoid. Exercise with light free weights can be started 4 months after surgery. Noncontact and nonthrowing sports may be resumed at 6 months, and throwing or racquet sports are begun after 9 months.

ROTATIONAL OSTEOTOMY OF THE HUMERUS

The rotational osteotomy of the humerus is reserved for individuals with documented excessive retrotorsion or those who have a large reverse Hill-Sachs lesion that is contributing to recurrent instability (11). Some authors have hypothesized that any procedure that restricts the active internal rotation of the humeral head in the scapulohumeral joint may also resolve the posterior instability. During the osteotomy, the posterior portion of the humeral head is rotated anteriorly relative to the humeral shaft. In this position, it cannot slip over the rim of the glenoid during internal rotation of the arm. The external rotation of the humeral head during the operation also stretches the anterior portion of the joint capsule. After the operation, the tightened joint capsule prevents additional posterior sliding of the humeral head.

Surin et al. (11) reported their experience of humeral osteotomy in 10 patients (12 shoulders) with a follow-up between 2 and 12 years. The patients rated the result as excellent or good in 10 of 12 shoulders; and using objective measures, the authors reported only 2 as fair and the remaining 10 as excellent or good. Of the 5 shoulders that had not had a previous operation, 3 had more than 75% of normal external rotation; of the 7 shoulders that had had a previous operation, none achieved more than 70% of normal external rotation.

Surgical Technique

The surgical approach is through a standard deltopectoral incision with the patient in the supine position. The humeral shaft and the lateral aspect of the humeral metaphysis proximal to the insertion of the pectoralis major are exposed subperiosteally. The site of the osteotomy should be as close to the humeral head as possible to allow enough space for three screws to be placed in the head through the transverse arm of an AO T-plate (AO humeral plate). The transverse arm of the T-plate is applied and fixed to the humeral head by the screws.

While the forearm is held perpendicular to the table, two 5-mm guidepins are inserted in the humerus parallel to the forearm, one proximal and the other distal to the planned osteotomy site. After the osteotomy has been completed, the surgeon externally rotates the humeral head 30°, using the guidepins as levers. The osteotomy site is then compressed, and the screws are inserted in the distal part of the plate.

Instability in more than one plane is a contraindication to rotational osteotomy of the humerus. Surin et al. (11) noted only one patient who had painful recurrent posterior subluxation postosteotomy without a previous traumatic dislocation. This patient had undergone two unsuccessful anterior bone block procedures before the humeral osteotomy; in retrospect the patient is believed to have had multidirectional instability.

Postoperative Rehabilitation

Postsurgery, the shoulder is maintained in a stockinette for 4 weeks before active exercises are begun. Sports activities are permitted 12 to 16 weeks postsurgery, when radiographs show evidence of healing at the osteotomy site. The plate is usually removed after 1 year.

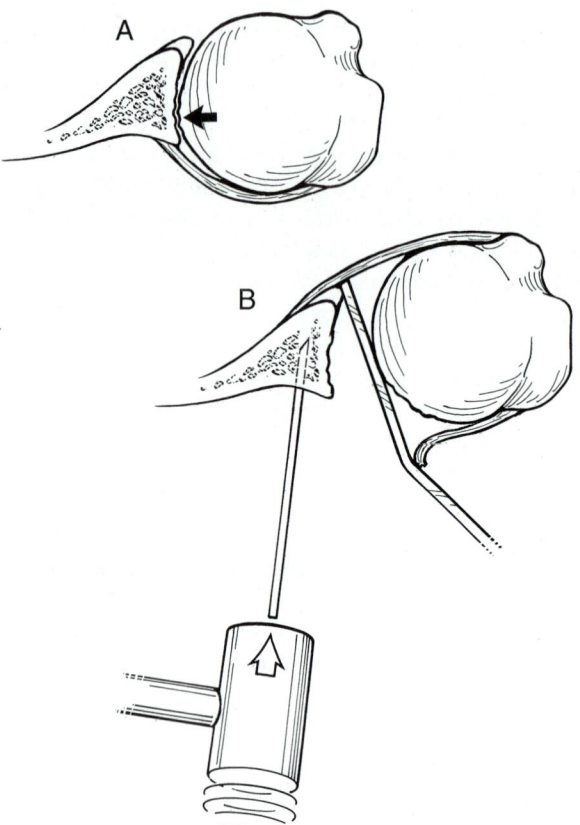

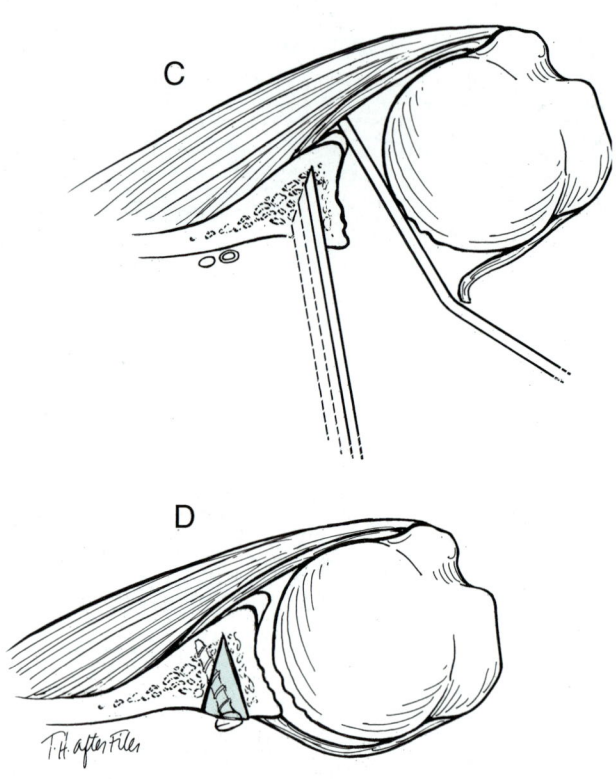

Figure 18.3. Posterior opening wedge glenoid osteotomy. **A.** Fixed posterior humeral head subluxation may lead to posterior glenoid wear and aquired retroversion. **B.** Opening wedge os-teotomy may restore normal version. **C.** Gradual opening of wedge osteotomy is performed while joint surface is visualized. **D.** Triangular bone graft is inserted into opening wedge osteotomy.

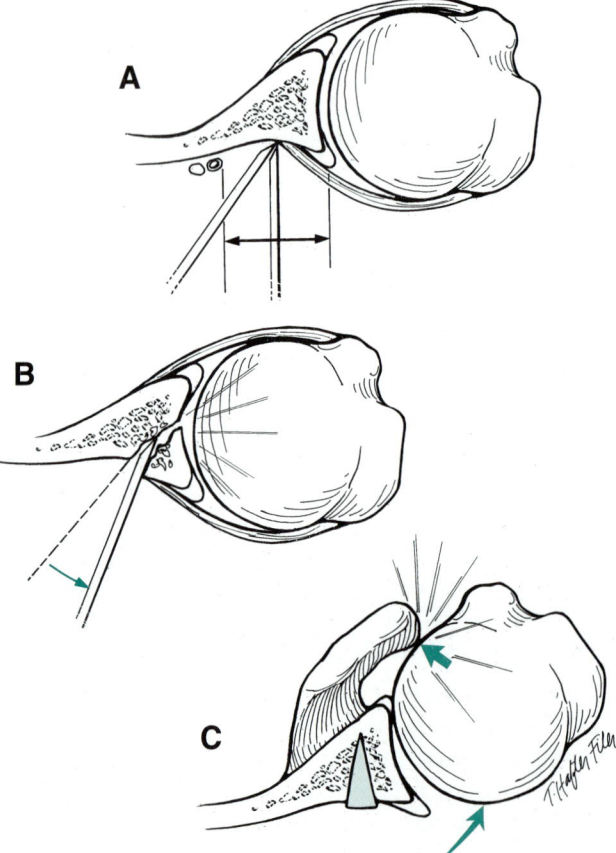

Figure 18.4. Errors in glenoid osteotomy. **A.** Osteotome orientation toward glenoid. **B.** Intra-articular fracture. **C.** Overcorrection increases anteversion and causes subcoracoid impingement *(arrow)*.

CHRONIC, LOCKED POSTERIOR DISLOCATION

In cases of chronic, locked posterior dislocation, the initial history must rule out associated conditions, such as seizure, electrical shock, intoxication, or other reason for altered mental state. We usually reduce these in the operating room setting, although if there is any question about the chronicity of the condition, the size of the reverse Hill-Sachs impaction fracture, associated fractures, or articular condition, a CT scan is obtained before any manipulation or operative intervention is conducted. There may be significant risk of fracturing the humeral head through the Hill-Sachs lesion if excessive force is used, especially in the case of a chronic dislocation. Furthermore, long-standing cases of locked dislocation are often associated with significant osteopenia of the humeral head, which also renders it susceptible to fracture from manipulation.

In the case of a reverse Hill-Sachs impaction defect involving less than 25% of the articular surface, the approach is as follows. An open reduction is performed through an anterior deltopectoral approach. This is done by osteotomizing a portion of the lesser tuberosity along with the subscapularis and then gently reducing the humeral head into the glenoid by lateral traction on the arm. In acute or subacute cases in which the articular surface is depressed but not destroyed, a small extra-articular tunnel can be made to the level of the subchondral bone and the depressed defect is then elevated. The bone graft is then packed underneath the elevated articular surface. If the articular surface is destroyed by the impaction fracture, the lesser tuberosity and subscapularis are transferred into it and fixed in place using transosseous sutures. The shoulder is immobilized in a gunslinger brace, as described above.

When the humeral head defect involves 25 to 40% of the articular surface, the chronicity of the dislocation and quality of the remaining humeral head articular cartilage and bone determine the treatment. In cases in which there is severe osteopenia and the articular cartilage is destroyed, a hemiarthroplasty is the best form of treatment. If the individual is young and if the bone and articular cartilage of the humeral head are of good quality, the treatment options include rotational osteotomy or articular reconstruction with bone graft. The preferred technique for one of us (Warner) is articular reconstruction using matched osteochondral allograft. This re-establishes normal anatomy and allows for a full arc or rotation after graft fixation.

In cases in which the reverse Hill-Sachs impaction fracture involves more than 40% of the articular surface, the only alternative is hemiarthroplasty reconstruction.

COMBINED ANTERIOR AND POSTERIOR INSTABILITY

Patients who have symptoms of instability in both an anterior and a posterior direction are rarely encountered. These individuals also have inferior instability. Neer and Foster (21) described this condition but did not elaborate on its treatment other than to suggest it could usually be handled through an anterior approach. In our experience,

individuals who have a shoulder that can be dislocated in more than one direction will require soft-tissue stabilization from both those directions. It is extremely important in such cases to rule out connective tissue diseases such as Ehlers-Danlos syndrome or Marfan's disease, and these individuals may also have varying degrees of dysplasia and ligamentous laxity. When these conditions are ruled out, we enter the shoulder first through a posterior approach and perform a capsular shift. If there is still marked laxity in an anterior direction, a capsular shift is performed from that direction. The shoulder is then immobilized in a brace for 6 weeks, and the rehabilitation program is cautiously followed over the course of the following year.

Arthroscopy

Arthroscopy is not routinely performed in the treatment of posterior shoulder instability. Most diagnoses of posterior instability can be obtained by the history, physical examination, and special diagnostic tests, as previously discussed. There are no arthroscopic techniques at this time that have been established to treat posterior instability. Therefore, there is an argument against an arthroscopic evaluation before the definitive open procedure owing to the added cost and operative time.

SUMMARY

Our current understanding of posterior instability is based on a classification system that recognizes the different pathologic lesions that can cause this condition. Furthermore, the natural history may be quite different in each case. Posterior subluxation of the glenohumeral joint is a distinct entity that is more common than posterior dislocation. Clinically, posterior subluxation is more often associated with pain than with instability symptoms, yet both may be present. Physical findings may be more subtle for these patients than for patients with anterior instability; radiographic studies are often normal. Thus it is necessary for the physician to have a high level of suspicion to make the diagnosis of posterior instability. A good history is also important for the elucidation of this diagnosis.

Nonoperative treatment is the recommended initial treatment; however, if patients do not respond to an aggressive rehabilitation program, surgical intervention may be necessary. In these cases, the critical element of any surgical repair is reduction of the capsular laxity and reinforcement of the posterior capsule. Rarely are bony procedures needed in addition to the soft tissue repair. Patients with voluntary instability are generally managed best with nonoperative courses of treatment, and the prognosis in these cases is good.

For cases of locked, posterior dislocation, the chronicity of the dislocation and size of the humeral head defect determine the form of treatment best suited to each patient. Treatment options for this kind of instability include rotational osteotomy of the humerus, subscapularis and lesser tuberosity transfer into the humeral head defect, osteochondral allograft reconstruction of the articular surface, and humeral head replacement. In all of these forms of posterior instability, surgical treatment usually results in improved motion, stability, and pain relief.

REFERENCES

1. Warner JJP, Schulte KR, Imhoff AB. Current concepts in shoulder instability. Adv Oper Orthop 1995;3:217–248.
2. Pollock RG, Bigliani LU. Recurrent posterior shoulder instability. Diagnosis and treatment. Clin Orthop 1993;291:85–96.
3. Bowen MK, Warren RF. Surgical approaches to posterior instability of the shoulder. Oper Technol Sports Med 1993;1:301–310.
4. Mow VC, Bigliani LU, Flatow EL, et al. Material properties of the inferior glenohumeral ligament and the glenohumeral articular cartilage. In: Matsen FA III, Fu FH, Hawkins RJ, eds. The shoulder: a balance of mobility and stability. Rosemont, IL: American Academy of Orthopaedic Surgeons, 1994:29–67.
5. Schwartz R, O'Brien SJ, Warren RF, et al. Capsular restraints to anterior-posterior motion of the abducted shoulder. Orthop Trans 1988;12:727.
6. O'Brien SJ, Neeves MC, Arnoczky SJ, et al. The anatomy and histology of the inferior glenohumeral ligament complex of the shoulder. Am J Sports Med 1990;18:449–456.
7. Fronek J, Warren RF, Bowen M. Posterior subluxation of the glenohumeral joint. J Bone Joint Surg 1989;71A:205–216.
8. Bigliani LU, Pollock RG, McIlveen SJ, et al. Shift of the posteroinferior aspect of the capsule for recurrent posterior glenohumeral instability. J Bone Joint Surg 1995;77A:1011–1020.
9. Bell RH, Noble JS. An appreciation of posterior instability of the shoulder. Clin Sports Med 1991;10:887–899.
10. Johnston GH, Hawkins RJ, Hadda R, Fowle PJ. A complication of posterior glenoid osteotomy for recurrent posterior shoulder instability. Clin Orthop 1984;187:147–149.
11. Surin V, Blader S, Markhede G, Sundholm K. Rotational osteotomy of the humerus for posterior instability of the shoulder. J Bone Joint Surg 1990;72A:181–186.
12. Gerber C, Ganz R. Clinical assessment of instability of the shoulder (with special reference to anterior and posterior drawer tests). J Bone Joint Surg 1984;66B:551–556.
13. Neer CS II. Shoulder reconstruction. Philadelphia: Saunders, 1990.
14. Pavlov H, Warren RF Weiss C, et al. The roentgenographic evaluation of certain surgical conditions. Clin Orthop 1985;184:153–158.
15. Rockwood CA Jr, Burkhead WZ Jr, Brna J. Subluxation of the glenohumeral joint: response to rehabilitative exercise, traumatic vs. atraumatic instability. Orthop Trans 1986;10:220–226.
16. Huber H, Gerber C. Voluntary subluxation of the shoulder in children. A long-term follow-up study of 36 shoulders. J Bone Joint Surg 1994;76B:118–122.
17. Hawkins RJ, Kopper G, Johnson G. Recurrent posterior instability (subluxation) of the shoulder. J Bone Joint Surg 1984;66A:169.
18. Tibone J, Ting A. Capsulorrhaphy with a staple for recurrent posterior subluxation of the shoulder. J Bone Joint Surg 1990;72A:999–1002.
19. Bigliani L U, Endrizzi DP, McIlveen SJ, et al. Operative management of posterior shoulder instability. Orthop Trans 1989;13:232.
20. Warner JJP, Krushell RJ, Masquelet A, et al. Anatomy and relationships of the suprascapular nerve: anatomical constraints to mobilization of the supraspinatus and infraspinatus muscles in the management of massive rotator cuff tears. J Bone Joint Surg 1992; 74A:36–45.
21. Neer CS II, Foster CR. Inferior capsular shift for involuntary inferior and multidirectional instability of the shoulder: a preliminary report. J Bone Joint Surg 1980;62A:897–908.

Eric W. Carson and Russell F. Warren

Multidirectional Instability: Diagnosis and Management

Much has been written about the diagnosis and management of anterior shoulder instability. The term *multidirectional instability* of the shoulder was introduced by Neer and Foster (1) in 1980. Since then, multidirectional instability, once considered rare, has increasingly been recognized as an important subtype of shoulder instability. If the subtle signs and symptoms of multidirectional instability go unrecognized, the clinician cannot fully address the pathologic shoulder. Indeed, undetected multidirectional instability is one of the two most frequently cited reasons for failed shoulder stabilization procedures. At present, the condition is difficult both to diagnosis and to manage.

Simply stated, multidirectional instability presents as recurrent shoulder instability in more than one direction and has a component of inferior instability. This definition is, however, an oversimplification. Neer and Foster (1) described three types of multidirectional instability: (*a*) anterior-inferior dislocation with postsubluxation (type 1), (*b*) posterior-inferior dislocation with anterior subluxation (type 2), and (*c*) global dislocation (type 3). Noting the complexity of classifying shoulder instability, particularly multidirectional instability, Hawkins and Mohtadi (2) proposed a more complex system based on five questions (Table 19.1):

- What is the frequency of the instability?
- What is the relationship of the instability to trauma?
- Is the instability voluntary or involuntary?
- What is the degree of instability?
- What is the primary direction of the instability or is it multidirectional?

RELEVANT ANATOMY AND PATHOGENESIS

The primary pathologic syndrome in the shoulder with multidirectional instability is a loose, redundant capsule, particularly in the inferior pouch, that extends both anteri-orly and posteriorly. The goal of surgery is to reduce the capsular volume on all three sides while maintaining a functional range of motion.

The cause of the redundant capsule is multifactorial, including biochemical collagen abnormalities, muscular imbalance of the rotator cuff and scapular stabilizers, deficiency of capsuloligamentous supports, and structural changes of the glenoid and labrum. A thorough understanding of the capsuloligamentous structures—in particular the superior glenohumeral ligament (SGHL), middle glenohumeral ligament (MGHL), the anterior and posterior bands of the inferior glenohumeral ligament (IGHL), and the rotator interval (RI)—is of the utmost importance in understanding the pathoanatomy of multidirectional instability (Table 19.2).

INITIAL FINDINGS, PHYSICAL EXAMINATION, AND DIAGNOSIS

Thomas and Matsen (6) introduced a classification of shoulder instability that describes clinical presentation, pathoanatomy, prognosis, and treatment. The first group is characterized by *t*raumatic instability that is *u*nidirectional, that usually includes a Bankart lesion, and that requires *s*urgery for successful resolution (TUBS). The second group is characterized by *a*traumatic instability that is *m*ultidirectional and often *b*ilateral; that usually responds favorably to a *r*ehabilitation program; and that, when surgery is required, is best addressed with an *i*nferior capsular shift (AMBRI). Although this system is useful for distinguishing between two distinct patterns of shoulder instability, not all patients, especially those with multidirectional instability, can be easily placed into one group. As Hawkins and Mohtadi (2) noted, "the terms traumatic and atraumatic are a great oversimplification," which can cause an error in diagnosis. This is particularly true with multidirectional instability, which can involve a spectrum of injury patterns and symptoms.

Classic multidirectional instability is typically found in young, sedentary patients who have generalized ligamentous laxity. These patients have a long history of shoulder symptoms that began in childhood with episodes of subluxation or dislocation that were the result of minimal or no trauma. Dislocations in these patients are frequent and transient; reduction can usually be achieved without the assistance of a physician. Often both shoulders display symptoms.

Patients may develop acquired multidirectional instability after sustaining a frank dislocation with Bankart lesion. Athletes who engage in overhead activities (e.g., baseball players, swimmers, gymnasts) sustain repetitive microtraumatic injury to the capsuloligament structure of the shoulder, which causes the shoulder capsule to stretch out, increasing the glenohumeral joint volume and ultimately leading to multidirectional instability. Patients with acquired multidirectional instability tend to have a milder generalized joint laxity than do patients with classic instability.

The most useful method of diagnosing multidirectional instability is to conduct a thorough history and physical examination. Symptoms described by the patient may suggest the direction of the instability involved. Patients with anterior instability describe symptoms that occur during overhead activities, with the shoulder in an abducted, externally rotated position. Patients with posterior instability report pain when punching open a heavy door with the arm in a forward flexed, internally rotated position. Patients with inferior instability have pain when carrying a heavy suitcase or bags. In addition to the inferior translation of the shoulder associated with such activities, some patients complain of traction paresthesias or dysesthesias in the upper extremity.

Most patients with multidirectional instability describe a feeling of looseness in the shoulder and note that their shoulder "slips out of place." Patients often complain that subluxations or dislocations occur throughout each day and often during the night. This results in a continuous vague ache, with a feeling of heaviness throughout the entire upper extremity. In contrast, patients with unidirectional instability typically experience infrequent but more intense episodes of pain associated with dislocations or subluxations.

Physical examination may demonstrate evidence of generalized ligamentous laxity (such as hypertension of elbows, knees, and metacarpophalangeal joints), patellar femoral subluxation, and the ability to approximate the thumb to forearm. These findings are more common in patients with classic multidirectional instability than in those with the acquired variant. Provocative tests that can determine the specific direction of instability include the anterior and posterior load and shift test, the anterior and posterior apprehension test, the fulcrum test, the relocation test, Fukuda's test, the push-pull stress test, and most important, the sulcus test. Many clinicians believe the mere presence of a sulcus sign, which is indicative of inferior instability, is pathognomonic for multidirectional instability. To be truly positive and diagnostic for multidirectional instability, however, the sulcus test not only should be palpable and visible but should reproduce the patient's symptoms (pain and discomfort). Rotator cuff and deltoid strength and range of motion are typically normal.

Other conditions may mimic the symptoms of multidirectional instability or may occur concomitantly, overshadowing the problem. Many patients with multidirectional instability present with signs and symptoms consistent with impingement of the rotator cuff. This may be sec-

table	19.1	Classification of Shoulder Instability

Frequency	Degree
Acute	Dislocation
Recurrent	Subluxation
Fixed	
	Direction
Onset	Anterior
Traumatic	Posterior
Atraumatic	Multidirectional
Overuse	Anterior-inferior
	Posterior-inferior
Volition	Anterior-posterior
Voluntary	Global
Involuntary	

Data are from Hawkins RJ, Mohtadi NGH. Clinical evaluation of shoulder instability. Clin Sports Med 1991;1: 59–64.

table	19.2	Capsuloligaments of the Shoulder

Primary Restraint of	Capsuloligament	Pathoanatomy	Reference
Anterior instability	Anterior band of the IGHL at 90° of abduction; the MGHL at 60–90° of abduction; the SGHL at <60° of abduction	To re-create an anterior dislocation requires permanent deformation of the IGHL with or without Bankart lesion	3
Posterior instability	Posterior capsule and RI; posterior band of the IGHL at 90°	To re-create a posterior instability requires an incision of the posterior capsule and RI	4
Inferior instability	The SGHL and RI in adduction; the IGHL at 45° of abduction	To re-create an inferior instability requies an incision of the RI (which increases the inferior translation by >100%)	5

ondary to the increased translation of the shoulder that occurs with multidirectional instability, particularly in the superior direction, causing symptoms within the rotator cuff or biceps tendon.

As previously mentioned, patients with a significant inferior laxity may present with paresthesias and dysesthesias. These findings can easily be confused with thoracic outlet syndrome, cervical radicular–type symptoms, and possibly nerve entrapment and may ultimately mask the primary diagnosis of multidirectional instability. Other diagnoses that must be entertained include a hypermobile or arthritic acromioclavicular joint and sternoclavicular joint.

Addressing the specific shoulder instability related to the multidirectional instability is the treatment of choice. Recognizing the correct diagnosis can avoid such surgical errors as biceps tenodesis or anterior acromioplasty.

RADIOLOGIC STUDIES

A plain radiograph shoulder series for instability (including AP views in internal and external rotation, axillary, Stryker notch, and apical oblique views) are generally normal in patients with multidirectional instability. Plain radiographs must, however, be closely scrutinized, because patients with acquired multidirectional instability may also have either humeral head lesions (Hill-Sachs) or Bankart lesions. It is important to recognize such lesions before surgery, especially Bankart lesions, which must be addressed at the time of surgery for optimal results.

The axillary view must be closely examined to detect any developmental abnormalities of the glenoid, such as glenoid hypoplasia or aplasia or excessive glenoid version. Such patients often present with similar symptoms as do patients with multidirectional instability. Both conditions are poorly treated with instability procedures. Stress radiographs can demonstrate laxity, especially inferior subluxation, but are not generally necessary.

Additional imaging modalities include double-contrast CT arthrograms and MRI with intra-articular gadolinium. Both imaging techniques have the ability to demonstrate the increased capsular volume associated with multidirectional instability. MRI, however, has a distinct advantage because it can demonstrate the redundant capsuloligament of the shoulder in multidirectional instability and expose labral lesions and rotator cuff disease. Both techniques have reported a degree of accuracy that approaches 95%.

TREATMENT

Nonoperative Treatment

Once the diagnosis of multidirectional instability has been established, a prolonged course of rehabilitation—lasting from 6 to 12 months—is instituted before any surgical intervention is undertaken. A review of the literature

shows that this approach is effective. Cooper and Brems (7) treated less than 16% of their multidirectional instability patients by surgical intervention. Similar results were reported by Burkhead and Rockwood (8), who studied 140 unstable shoulders in 115 patients who were treated with a specific physician-directed rehabilitation program. Poor results were noted in patients with traumatic instability, whereas 80% of patients with atraumatic instability realized good to excellent results.

The nonoperative therapy for multidirectional instability involves strengthening the rotator cuff and deltoid, education, and modification of activities and occupation. An attempt may be made to change the mechanics of a throwing athlete. The emphasis should be placed on strengthening the muscles on the side of the joint with greatest instability: the internal rotators should be strengthened when the greatest instability is anterior and inferior and the external rotators should be strengthened when the greatest instability is posterior and inferior. In the rare patient with global instability, both the internal and external rotators should be strengthened.

The benefit of a lengthy preoperative conservative treatment program is its proven effectiveness for most multidirectional instability patients; it also allows the physician an opportunity to evaluate the patient's motivation. In addition, the physician can identify patients with secondary gain (workers' compensation), voluntary dislocators with possible psychologic impairment, and patients with unrealistic goals who have been shown to respond poorly to surgery.

Operative Treatment

In the surgical management of multidirectional instability, patient selection is of the utmost importance. Patients with symptomatic multidirectional instability, who have failed a 6- to 12-month physician-directed rehabilitation program aimed at strengthening the rotator cuff, deltoid, and scapular stabilizer are considered candidates for surgery. Patients with recurrent instability secondary to a failed shift procedure and those with recurrent instability who had unrecognized multidirectional instability and underwent a traditional unidirectional procedure may also be considered candidates for surgery.

The primary goal of all operative procedures for multidirectional instability is to create a stable joint by reducing the capsular volume of the glenohumeral joint while maintaining a full functional range of motion (Clinical Table). Generally, the surgical approach should be made on the side associated with the greatest amount of clinical instability. This can be difficult to determine owing to secondary voluntary guarding by the patient who tries to protect the shoulder from pain. Through repeated examination, the physician can gain the trust of the patient so that he or she can relax and the physician can better assess the pattern of instability.

Clinical Table: Multidirectional Instability: Diagnosis and Management

Procedure	Indications	Technique	Anatomy	Pitfalls
Anterior-inferior capsular shift	• Multidirectional instability, predominantly anterior and inferior direction	• Examination under anesthesia • Deltopectoral interval • Divide subscapularis • Capsulotomy • Mobilize inferior flap for control of posterior capsule • Inferior capsular shift superiorly • Crisscross superior flap and close rotator interval	• Subscapularis • Glenohumeral ligament • Rotator interval • Axillary nerve • Musculocutaneous nerve	• Incomplete correction of global instability • Inadequate reduction of capsular volume • Nerve injury • Overtightening exacerbating contralateral instability
Posterior-inferior capsular shift	• Multidirectional instability, predominantly posterior direction	• Examination under anesthesia • Deltoid split • Interval between infraspinatus and teres minor • Capsulotomy • Inferior capsular mobilization • Capsular tightening	• Posterior deltoid • Safe interval between infraspinatus and teres minor • Axillary nerve • Suprascapular nerve • Posterior circumflex artery	• Rotator cuff weakness • Incomplete correction • Overtightening posterior • Axillary nerve injury • Suprascapular nerve injury
Combined anterior and posterior approach	• Incomplete correction of global instability after unilateral approach	• Sequential anterior and then posterior approach as above	• Same as anterior and posterior approaches above	• Overtightening joint • Nerve injury
Arthroscopic capsular shift	• Multidirectional instability • Strong arthroscopic skills	• Divide anterior and inferior capsule • Proper glenoid preparation • Mobilize capsular sutures • Planned glenoid drill holes	• Glenohumeral ligaments • Axillary nerve • Suprascapular nerve	• Incomplete correction • Nerve injury • Inadequate arthroscopic portals

In most cases, the anterior approach can accomplish global tightening of the entire shoulder capsule and can even be used in patients with moderate posterior laxity (Table 19.3). Imbrication or closure of the rotation interval and shifting of the anterior, inferior, and posterior capsule can stabilize most shoulders with posterior laxity. In rare instances both an anterior and a posterior approach may be necessary.

Before the reconstructive procedure, the patient should be examined under either general or regional anesthesia. Such an examination can confirm the direction of greatest instability or subtle laxity not appreciated on preoperative examination. In some cases, an arthroscopic examination may aid in the decision-making process. This allows for the identification of a Bankart lesion, which may require repair and treatment of associated abnormality, including partial rotator cuff tears or labral tears opposite the side of the approach.

ANTERIOR APPROACH

Neer and Foster (1) proposed that the inferior capsular shift procedure be the means of surgical treatment to address the primary pathology of multidirectional instability: redundant inferior capsule.

After administration of regional or general anesthesia with adequate relaxation, the patient is positioned supine with the head elevated 20° and the arm draped free for full manipulation. A standard anterior incision is made along Langer's lines, extending from the coracoid process into the anterior axillary fold (Fig. 19.1).

Dissection proceeds through subcutaneous tissue to identify the deltopectoral interval. The cephalic vein can be noted coursing along the deltopectoral interval and crossing the incision in a diagonal fashion. The cephalic vein is carefully preserved and retracted laterally with the deltoid. Blunt dissection helps develop the deltopectoral interval from the coracoid down to the pectoralis major tendon. Releasing the proximal 1 to 2 cm of the pectoralis major tendon can aid in the visualization of the inferior

table	19.3	Indications for Approach		
Approach	Anterior Signs		Posterior Signs	
Anterior	Subluxation	+	Stable or subluxation	
	Dislocation	+	Subluxation or dislocation	
Posterior	Stable	+	Subluxation or dislocation	
	Subluxation	+	Dislocation	

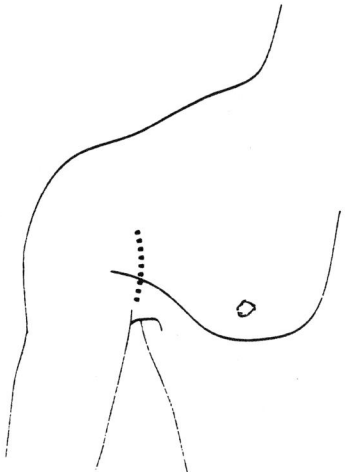

Figure 19.1. Anterior axillary approach to the shoulder.

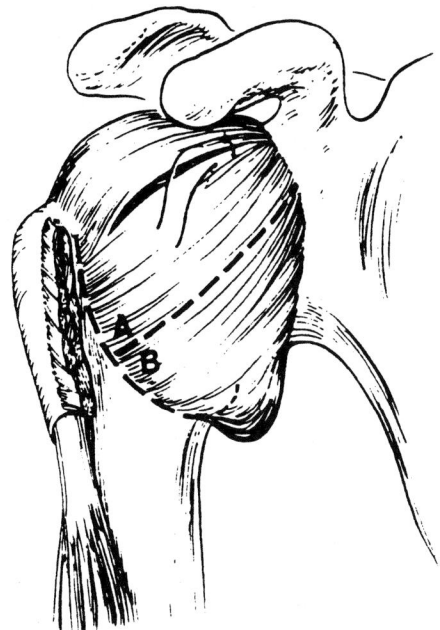

Figure 19.2. Modified T capsulotomy.

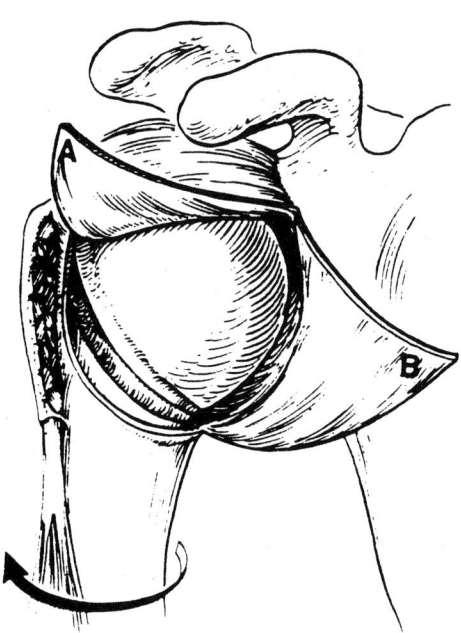

Figure 19.3. Humeral electroresection to expose inferior capsule. Creation of superior flap (A) and inferior flap (B).

capsule. The clavipectoral fascia overlying the conjoined tendon is divided just laterally and carried proximal to the coracoacromial ligament. Use extreme caution with retraction under the conjoined tendon, because the musculocutaneous nerve courses beneath it; vigorous retraction puts the nerve at risk.

The arm is then placed in a slight external rotation to facilitate identification of the superior and inferior borders of the subscapularis. The subscapularis tendon is incised 1.5 to 2 cm medial to its insertion on the lesser tuberosity. Care is taken to avoid penetrating the underlying anterior capsule while separating the subscapularis from the adherent capsule. At the inferior aspect, the anterior humeral circumflex vessels are identified and cauterized to prevent bleeding and to allow further release of the muscular portion of the subscapularis. Stay sutures are placed into the subscapular tendon and retracted medially and into the RI for repair after completing the capsular shift. The capsule is then incised in a longitudinal fashion 5 mm medial to its humeral insertion (Fig. 19.2). A finger may be placed in the inferior pouch to assess its size and the amount of redundant capsule that must be released from the humerus to obtain an adequate shift. The modified T capsulotomy is completed laterally with release of the capsule along the humeral neck. The humerus is externally rotated even more and flexed to expose the inferior and posterior capsule for release (Fig. 19.3). This maneuver also protects the axillary nerve from injury, since it passes along the humeral neck.

A Fukuda ring retractor is then placed into the joint, and the joint is inspected carefully for a possible Bankart lesion. If present, the Bankart lesion must be repaired with suture anchors or drill holes at this time.

The arm is then positioned in 15° to 20° of abduction and 25° of external rotation. The position of the arm can be modified, particularly for overhead throwing athletes who may require more abduction and external rotation. The inferior capsule flap is mobilized and shifted superiorly to the lateral capsule flap, obliterating the inferior redundant pouch. The amount of capsular advancement depends on the individual patient and depends on the overall laxity of the capsule present and the degree of instability. The RI is then closed from medial to lateral. The superior flap is advanced inferiorly in a similar manner to reinforce the advanced inferior capsule flap (Fig. 19.4). Finally, the subscapularis tendon is reattached to its anatomic insertion.

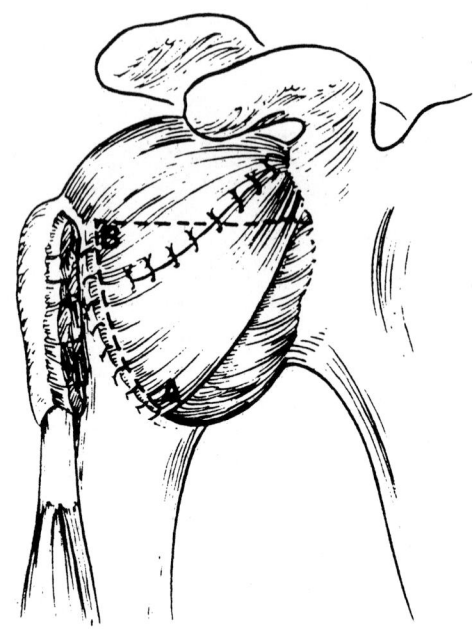

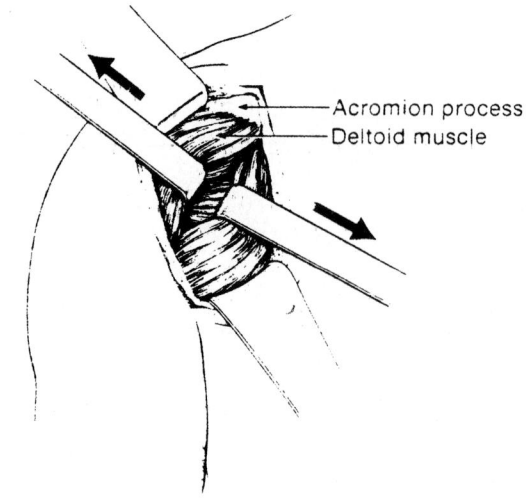

Figure 19.6. Split the deltoid muscle to expose the infraspinatus.

Figure 19.4. The inferior flap *(B)* is shifted superiorly while the superior flap *(A)* is shifted inferiorly in a pants-over-vest fashion.

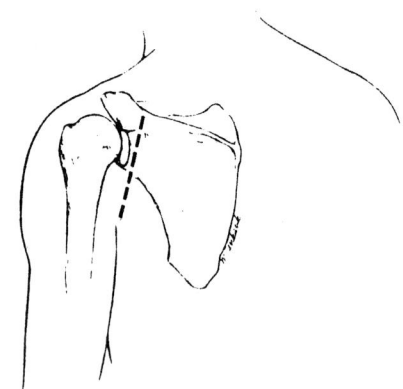

Figure 19.5. Posterior approach to the shoulder.

POSTERIOR APPROACH

The posterior approach is used less frequently than is the anterior approach. Many cases of posterior instability can be addressed from an anterior approach, as noted earlier; however, if the primary direction of instability is posterior, the posterior approach is used.

The patient can be positioned in either a lateral decubitus or a beach chair position, depending on the surgeon's preference. A vertical incision centered over the posterior glenohumeral joint is made just medial to the posterolateral corner of the acromion and extends distally toward the axilla (Fig. 19.5). Dissection proceeds down through the subcutaneous tissue to the deltoid fascia. The fascia overlying the deltoid is then sharply dissected (Fig. 19.6). The deltoid is split in line with its fibers 4 to 5 cm from the posterior tip of the acromion. Deep retractors are placed to expose the infraspinatus. If additional exposure

is needed, 1 to 2 cm of the posterior deltoid can be removed from the posterior lateral tip of the acromion; this does not significantly weaken the deltoid and can be easily repaired. The infraspinatus is then split along its fibers to expose the posterior capsule (Fig. 19.7). The dissection should not be carried too far medially to avoid injury to the suprascapular nerve.

A periosteal elevator is used to develop the plane between the infraspinatus and capsule. The capsule is incised vertically 0.5 to 1 cm from its insertion on the greater tuberosity, starting superiorly and working distally (Fig. 19.8). Care must be taken to leave enough capsular tissue on the humerus for reattachment. As the capsule is incised inferiorly, the arm should be internally rotated and extended to expose the inferior pouch. The capsule should be removed from the humeral neck with great care to avoid injury to the axillary nerve. The horizontal component of the capsulotomy is made at the level of the midglenoid. The joint is then inspected for any evidence of detachment of the posterior labrum, which must be repaired before the shift is undertaken (Fig. 19.9).

The posterior capsular shift is slightly different from the anterior shift: The superior capsule flap is first shifted inferiorly (Figs. 19.10 and 19.11), and then the inferior capsular flap is shifted superiorly, obliterating the inferior redundant pouch. If the quality of the posterior capsule is poor, the shift may be augmented with the infraspinatus.

ARTHROSCOPIC CAPSULAR SHIFT

Arthroscopic capsular shift was first described by Duncan and Savoie (9). The patient is positioned in a beach chair or lateral decubitus position, and a diagnostic shoulder arthroscopy is performed through the standard anterior and posterior portals. The entire anterior and inferior capsule is divided with an end-cutting shaver, beginning at the 1-o'clock position (SGHL) of the glenoid face and continuing inferiorly (MGHL) and around the pos-

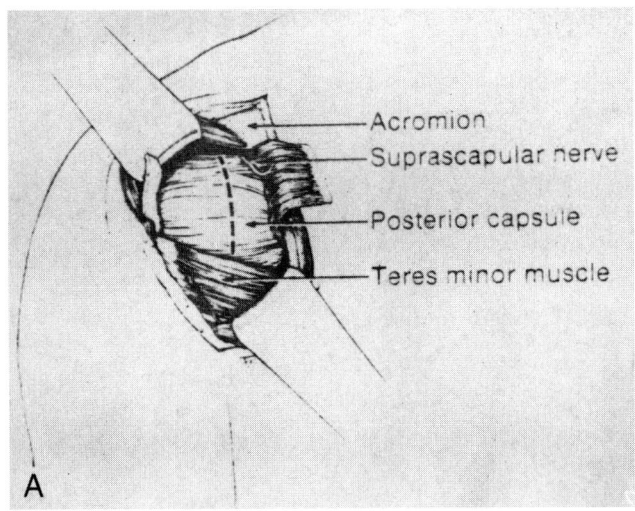

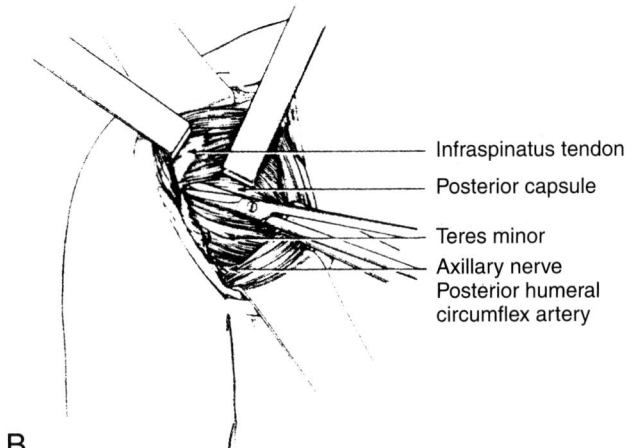

Figure 19.7. Split the infraspinatus to expose the posterior capsule.

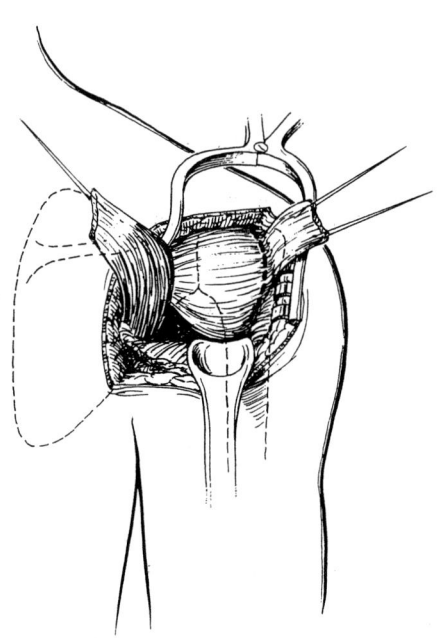

Figure 19.8. Exposure of the posterior capsule.

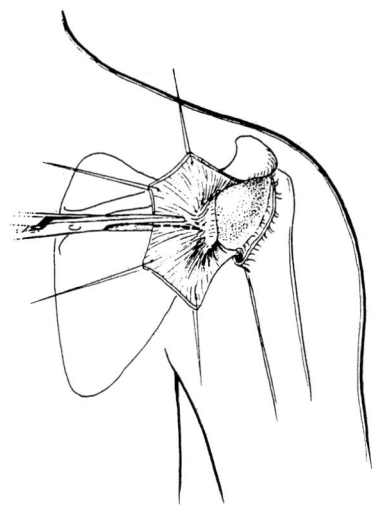

Figure 19.9. Posterior capsule released from the humeral neck.

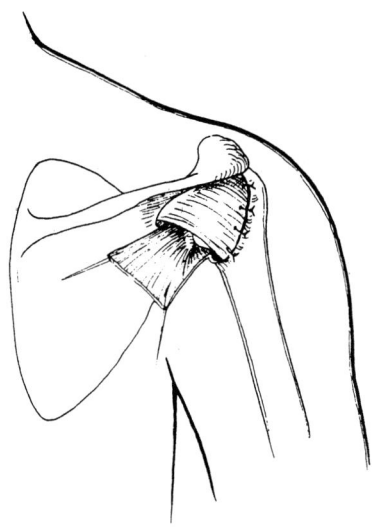

Figure 19.10. Shifting the inferior flap inferiorly.

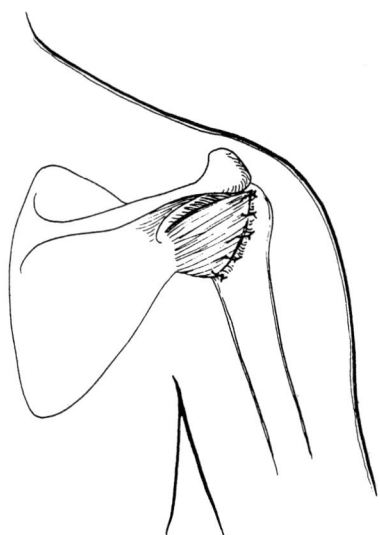

Figure 19.11. Shifting the inferior flap superiorly in a pants-over-vest fashion.

teroinferior aspect of the glenoid at the 6-o'clock position (posterior band of the IGHL) (Fig. 19.12).

The glenoid neck is prepared with a rasp or arthroscopic burr (Fig. 19.13). Sutures are sequentially placed in the posterior band of the IGHL, anterior band of the IGHL, MGHL, and the SGHL with a suture punch (Fig. 19.14). The multiple sutures are then passed through the anterior portal to assess the shift arthroscopically. If the shift is inadequate, additional inferior capsule can be released posteriorly. Next, a transglenoid drill hole is placed at the 1-o'clock position; the hole is oriented so it exits inferiorly and posteriorly on the scapula (Fig. 19.15). The multiple sutures are passed with a Beath pin, and the shift is reevaluated (Fig. 19.16). If shift is adequate, the sutures are tied with the arm in an adducted, internally rotated position.

The patient is protected in a shoulder immobilizer for 4 to 6 weeks.

Preliminary results have been reviewed for 10 patients with multidirectional instability. Follow-up ranged from 1 to 3 years, and satisfactory results were noted in all 10 patients, with no recurrent instability. Longer follow-up and larger numbers of patients must be examined to better assess the procedure's efficacy in the management of multidirectional instability.

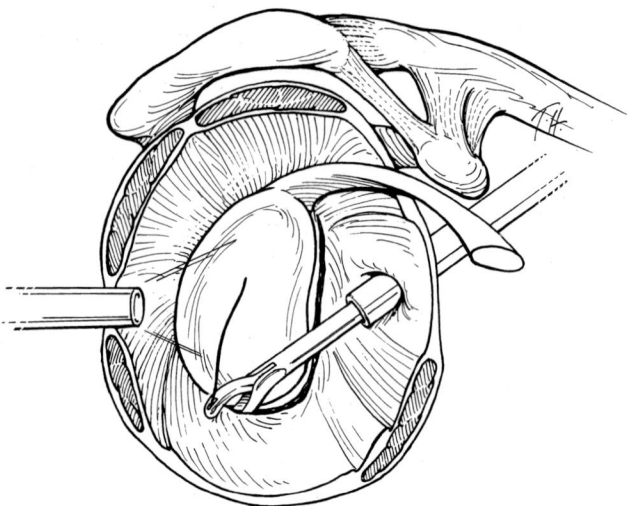

Figure 19.14. Placement of sutures into the capsule with a suture punch.

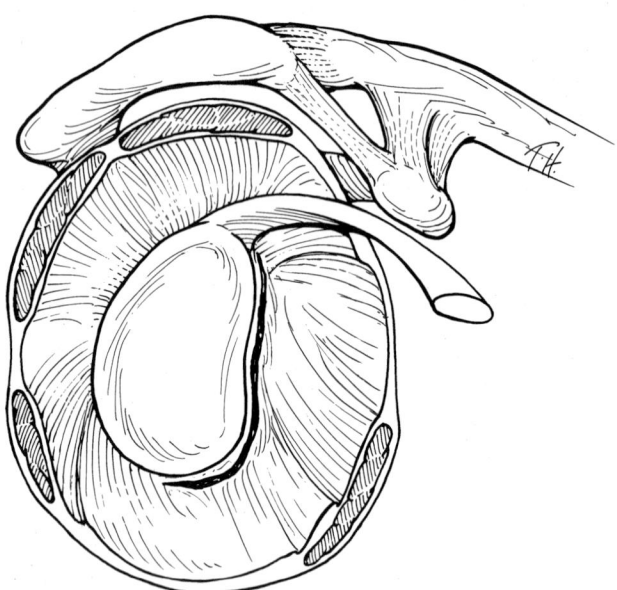

Figure 19.12. Release of the anterior and inferior capsules.

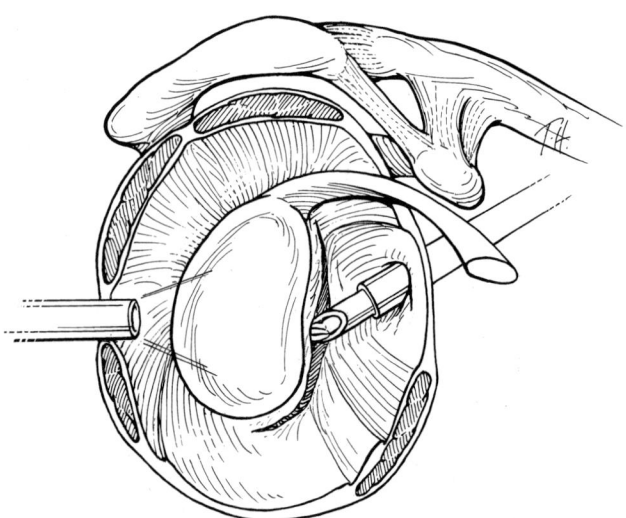

Figure 19.13. Preparation of the glenoid neck with an arthroscopic burr.

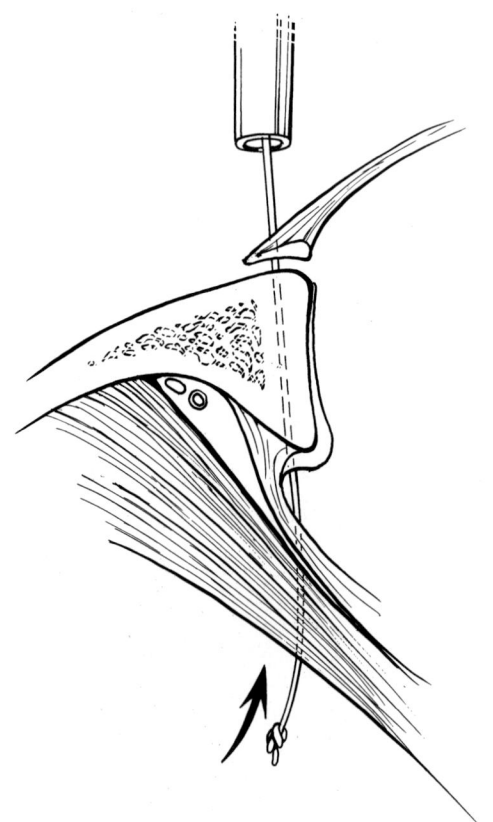

Figure 19.15. Transglenoid Beath pin.

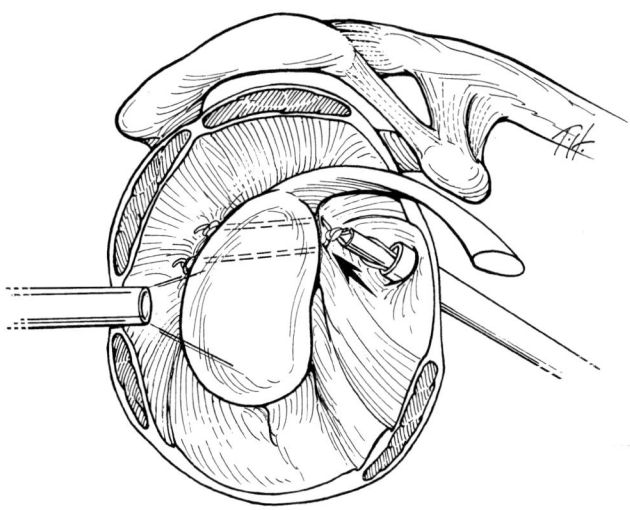

Figure 19.16. Evaluate shift. The sutures are secured over the posterior glenoid.

POSTOPERATIVE TREATMENT

The goal of a rehabilitation program following a multidirectional instability procedure is to regain the functional range of motion while maintaining stability. Rapid progression or overly aggressive rehabilitation defeats this goal and ultimately leads to recurrent instability. There is no routine postoperative management for multidirectional instability; each program must be geared to the individual patient.

Anterior Instability

Following surgery for anterior instability, the patient is placed in a shoulder immobilizer in a neutral position. Patients requiring revision surgery are best protected in a prefabricated shoulder orthotic brace that supports the elbow in a cephalad direction, preventing any stretching or stress on the inferior capsule during the healing phase. The shoulder is immobilized for 4 to 6 weeks, during which time only gentle isometric exercises are allowed with supervised elbow range of motion. The shoulder immobilizer may then be discontinued, and range of motion is gradually increased, particularly external rotation and forward flexion. At 12 weeks, strengthening with resistive exercises is begun and the range of motion continues to be increased. Return to strenuous exercise or contact sports is generally restricted for 9 to 12 months.

Posterior Instability

The postsurgical rehabilitation for posterior instability is similar to that of anterior instability, except for immobilization. A brace is generally recommended for posterior repairs, owing to the fragility and poor quality of the posterior capsule. The arm is positioned in a slight external rotation to prevent stress on the posterior capsule during the healing phase. Immobilization is usually required for a minimum of 6 weeks, at which time range of motion exercises concentrating on forward elevation and external rotation are prescribed. Internal rotation and adduction should be avoided during the early postoperative period. Isometric exercises are started and progressed, as tolerated, to full strengthening exercises. Full forward elevation after a posterior repair is often difficult to achieve during the first 12 months.

Results of Surgery

Neer and Foster (1) were the first to report results on the inferior capsular shift procedure for the treatment of multidirectional instability. They reported on 40 shoulders in 36 patients who underwent surgery during a 5-year period. All 36 patients had some degree of inferior laxity on examination; 5 were found to have a Bankart lesion at the time of surgery. A total of 35 patients experienced satisfactory results; 1 patient noted subluxation after 7 months.

Cooper and Brems (7) reported similar results with 43 shoulders in 38 patients treated over a 6-year period with a minimum 2-year follow-up. A total of 28 patients had laxity in the opposite shoulder and 20 had generalized ligament laxity. After surgery, 39 (91%) shoulders were rated satisfactory by the patients, who noted no recurrent instability. Postoperative recurrent symptomatic instability developed in 4 (11%) patients. Cooper and Brems concluded that the inferior capsular shift procedure provided satisfactory objective and subjective results and that failure with subsequent recurrent symptomatic instability generally occurred in the early postoperative period.

Bigliani et al. (3) reported the results of the inferior capsular shift procedure for classic multidirectional instability (anterior, posterior, and inferior) in 52 shoulders; 36 shoulders were treated with an anterior surgical approach and 16 with a posterior approach. Satisfactory results were achieved in 94% of cases.

Altchek et al. (10) reported the results of a T-plasty modification of the Bankart procedure in 40 patients with acquired multidirectional instability. A total of 39 patients suffered a traumatic onset; 36 of which suffered a frank dislocation. There was no evidence of laxity in the opposite shoulder in 28 patients, and 20 had no evidence of generalized laxity. In all, 38 shoulders had a Bankart lesion and 24 had a Hill-Sachs lesion, noted at during surgery. Patient satisfaction was rated as excellent for 95% of the shoulders.

PITFALLS

To avoid neurovascular injury, the surgeon must make careful identification and have an in-depth understanding of the anatomy. For both the anterior and the posterior capsular shifts, avoid excessive retraction beneath the conjoined tendon to avoid injuring the musculocutaneous nerve and stay close to the humeral neck to avoid injuring the axillary nerve. Sensory neuropraxias are relatively common, and motor neuropraxias are relatively rare.

Excessive tightening of the anterior capsule can result in loss of external rotation. Before leaving the operating room, the surgeon should be able to obtain 25° to 30° of passive external rotation.

Recurrent multidirectional instability can occur when the capsular shift was inadequate, Bankart lesions were not repaired, and the RI was not closed or imbricated. Inadequate immobilization prevents soft tissue healing.

Posterior instability is the result of excessive tightening of the anterior capsule, which causes posterior displacement of the humeral head.

FUTURE DIRECTIONS

Other procedures have been proposed to address the complexity of multidirectional instability, including isolated closure of the RI, glenoid osteotomy to correct inferior inclination of the glenoid, and a capsular shrinkage procedure that uses lasers to decrease capsular volume. These procedures are considered experimental and require further examination to assess their efficacy in the management of multidirectional instability.

SUMMARY

Multidirectional instability of the shoulder is a complex, multifactorial problem. A high index of suspicion is necessary for a correct diagnosis. The standard operation for unidirectional traumatic instability fails to correct the primary abnormality of multidirectional instability: a loose redundant capsule. The clinician must be able to differentiate between classic multidirectional instability and acquired multidirectional instability.

Most patients with multidirectional instability respond well to a nonoperative physician-directed program involving strengthening the deltoid, rotator cuff muscle group, and scapular stabilizers of the shoulder. Some patients, however, fail this regimen and are considered candidates for surgical intervention. These patients must be screened carefully to confirm the diagnosis of multidirectional instability and to assess their motivation. Once these rigid criteria have been met, surgery can be proposed.

Surgical results of the inferior capsular shift have uniformly been good to excellent in more than 90% of patients. Attention to detail can result in a restoration of patients' full functional range of motion and a stable shoulder.

REFERENCES

1. Neer CS, Foster CR. Inferior capsular shift for involuntary inferior and multidirectional instability of the shoulder. J Bone Joint Surg 1980;62A:897–908.
2. Hawkins RJ, Mohtadi NGH. Clinical evaluation of shoulder instability. Clin Sports Med 1991;1:59–64.
3. Bigliani LU, Pollock RG, Owens JM. The inferior capsular shift procedure for multidirectional instability of the shoulder. Orthop Trans 1994;17:576.
4. Schwartz E, Warren RF, O'Brien SJ. Posterior shoulder instability. Orthop Clin North Am 1987;18:409–419.
5. Harryman DT, Sidles JA, Harris SL, Matsen FA. The role of the rotator interval capsule in passive motion and stability of the shoulder. J Bone Joint Surg 1992;74A:53–66.
6. Thomas SC, Matsen FA III. An approach to the repair of the glenohumeral ligaments in the management of traumatic anterior glenohumeral instability. J Bone Joint Surg 1989;71A:506–513.
7. Cooper RA, Brems JJ. The inferior capsular-shift procedure for multidirectional instability of the shoulder. J Bone Joint Surg 1992; 74A:1516.
8. Burkhead WZ, Rockwood CA. Treatment of instability of the shoulder with an exercise program. J. Bone Joint Surg 1992; 74A:890–896.
9. Duncan R, Savoie FH. Arthroscopic inferior capsular shift for multidirectional instability of the shoulder: a preliminary report. Arthroscopy 1993;9:24–27.
10. Altchek DW, Warren RF, Skyhar MJ, Ortiz G. T-plasty modification of the Bankart procedure for multidirectional instability of the anterior and inferior types. J. Bone Joint Surg 1991;73A:105–112.

Suggested Readings

Arendt EA. Multidirectional shoulder instability. Orthopedics 1988; 11:113–120.

Mallon W, Speer K. Multidirectional instability: current concepts. J Shoulder Elbow Surg 1995;4:54–64.

Warner J, Caborn D, Berger R, et al. Dynamic capsuloligamentous anatomy of the glenohumeral joint. J Shoulder Elbow Surg 1993; 2:115–133.

Yamaguchi K, Flatow E. Management of multidirectional instability. Clin Sports Med 1995;14:885–901.

chapter 20

Edward V. Craig

Impingement and Rotator Cuff Tear: Treatment by Anterior Acromioplasty and Repair

Rotator cuff disease and subacromial space dysfunction are generally considered to be the most common causes of shoulder pain in the world. The spectrum of causes in this areas is broad and encompasses combinations of extrinsic compression of the rotator cuff, intrinsic degeneration of the rotator cuff, instability of the shoulder joint, and both microtraumatic and macrotraumatic injury to the shoulder.

Although this area of pain is extremely common, much has been learned about the successful treatment of rotator cuff pathology over the past half century. Anterior acromioplasty and repair of disease, damage, and torn tendon are important answers to this frequent area of shoulder disability.

RELEVANT ANATOMY AND PATHOGENESIS

The tendons of the rotator cuff have several critical functions for normal use of the shoulder. They provide a stabilizing effect against shoulder dislocation and subluxation, both through their anatomic location relative to humeral head and through their action to compress the humeral head against the glenoid, which helps the articular surfaces resist translational loads. The cuff tendons depress and center the humeral head on the glenoid, providing an important fulcrum for the deltoid to elevate the arm. They supply 90% of the power for the external rotation of the humeral head in the glenoid, a critical motion for overhead use of the extremity. Finally, by providing a watertight compartment, they also are important in maintaining nourishment of the articular cartilage surfaces via the joint fluid.

Anatomically, the rotator cuff inserts on the greater and lesser tuberosities of the humerus, passing underneath the relatively fixed coracoacromial arch formed by the an-

terior acromion and coracoacromial ligament. In addition, the supraspinatus passes directly beneath the undersurface of the acromioclavicular (AC) joint. The subdeltoid bursa helps provide a smooth gliding surface for the cuff moving beneath these structures.

Rotator cuff tears are caused by both intrinsic factors (e.g., normal aging) and extrinsic factors (e.g., morphology of the coracoacromial arch). In addition, tendon vascularity, healing potential, and trauma seem to affect the pathogenesis of cuff tears. Ordinarily, there are several millimeters of clearance beneath the coracoacromial arch for the rotator cuff and overlying bursa as they pass toward the greater tuberosity; however, aging and muscle deconditioning can alter the spatial relationships to the surrounding local anatomy. This space may be narrowed by changes in the acromion's shape, thickening of the tendon or overlying bursa, proliferative spurs on the undersurface of the AC joint, or cuff weakness that makes the head depressant activity ineffective. As a result of these alterations in anatomy, the rotator cuff and, in particular, the supraspinatus tendon, may undergo mechanical compression by the relatively fixed coracoacromial arch. This compression, or impingement, puts direct external pressure on the tendon and may result in the clinical syndrome of subacromial impingement, in which shoulder pain is produced via direct external pressure on the cuff. Eventually, this external pressure may lead to tendon wear, fraying, and ultimately fiber failure: a rotator cuff tear. Clearly, subacromial impingement is an important etiologic factor of cuff tears.

The degree of trauma to which the cuff is subjected to over a lifetime and the way in which the rotator cuff is used on a daily basis also affect the integrity of the rotator cuff. Vascular factors contribute to rotator cuff degeneration:

The distal 2 cm of the supraspinatus, the site of most rotator cuff tears, has a diminished blood supply and a thus poor potential for healing relative to the rest of the rotator cuff. As the patient ages, the tendon degenerates because the collagen loses its normal organized structure, cellularity and compliance. Once the tear begins, the adjacent tendon fibers are loaded and the tearing of the cuff becomes progressive. The course of rotator cuff failure begins with tendon inflammation and advances to fraying, wearing, and ultimately partial- and full-thickness tearing.

INITIAL FINDINGS, PHYSICAL EXAMINATION, AND DIAGNOSIS

The clinical signs of the patient with subacromial impingement usually reflect the pathogenesis of rotator cuff disease. There is typically pain with overhead use of the arm as the rotator cuff passes beneath the coracoacromial arch. Although the pain initially occurs only with use, it can become constant and occur at rest, particularly if the rotator cuff tears completely. The pain most commonly radi-

ates down the outer portion of the arm toward the deltoid insertion but may radiate into the scapula as well. There may be a sensation of clicking and popping as the associated thickened subacromial bursa or a leading edge of the torn tendon passes beneath the coracoacromial ligament. The patient may notice weakness in the arm. Activities commonly affected include reaching above shoulder level, tucking in a shirt or blouse behind the back, and using the arm away from the side of the body (Fig. 20.1).

The physical findings often include painful subacromial crepitus and a painful arc as the arm is lowered from 120° to 70° of elevation. There may be tenderness of the AC joint, since associated AC disease is not uncommon. There may be changes in the biceps tendon, ranging from an inflammatory reaction and local tenderness to frank rupture of the tendon itself. Although passive range of motion may be normal, it is often slightly decreased, particularly with internal rotation and forward elevation. A positive impingement sign is evoked by reproducing the pain with forced forward elevation of the arm on a stabilized scapula (Fig. 20.2). With the arm elevated to 90° in the scapular plane, slight internal rotation often duplicates the pain of impingement. Pain is frequently elicited by external rotation or abduction against resistance.

Perhaps the most important diagnostic clinical test is the impingement injection test (Fig. 20.3). After receiving an injection of 12 mL 1% Xylocaine into the subacromial space, which effectively numbs the superficial surface of the tendon and subacromial bursa, the patient should experience reduced pain when performing the maneuvers noted above.

The hallmark clinical finding of a full-thickness rotator cuff tear is weakness of external rotation with the arm near the side of the body. There may, in addition, be a dis-

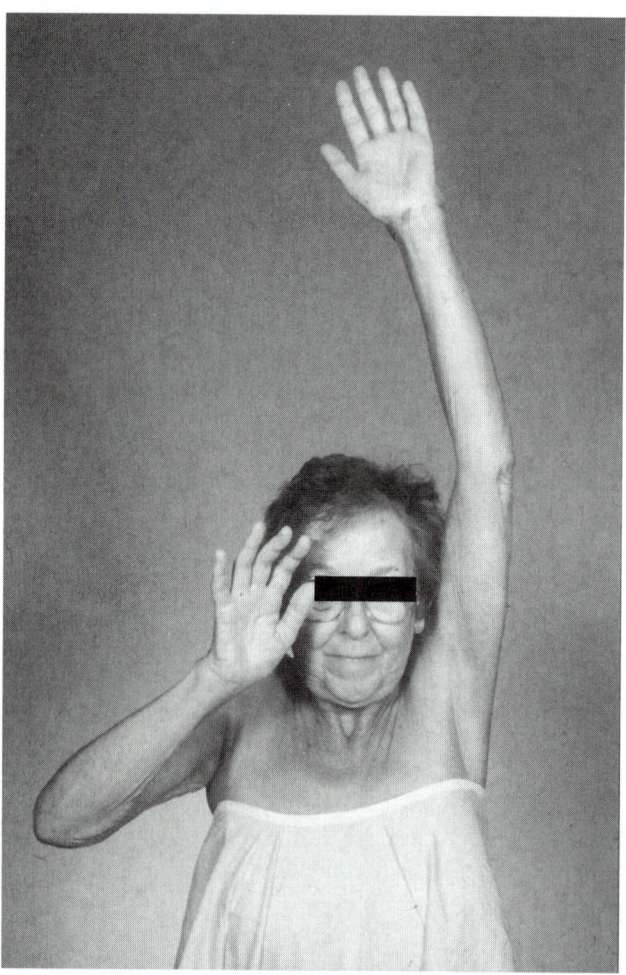

Figure 20.1. A 72-year-old woman with a large rotator cuff tear. She has marked weakness and is unable to abduct and forward elevate her arm.

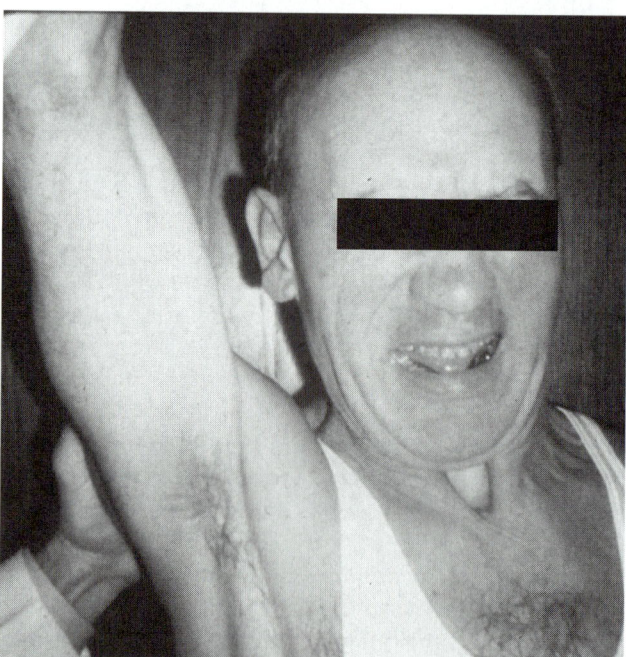

Figure 20.2. Positive impingement sign.

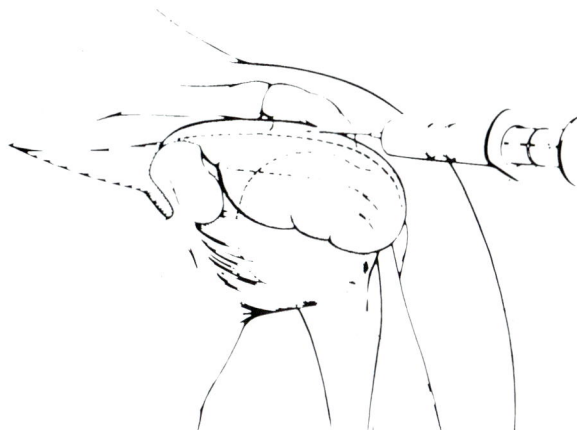

Figure 20.3. Impingement injection test.

crepancy between active and passive motion because of cuff weakness. When the tear is large enough to prevent the rotator cuff from stabilizing the humeral head, the shoulder may actually appear to shrug as the deltoid pulls the humeral head superiorly and the scapula attempts to contribute to arm elevation. With long-standing cuff ruptures, there is often associated supraspinatus and infraspinatus fossa atrophy.

RADIOLOGIC STUDIES

The shoulder x-ray of patients with impingement syndrome may be normal. X-ray studies typically ordered are AP, lateral outlet view (a lateral view of the scapula taken with a 10° caudal tilt of the beam), and axillary views. Plain radiographic findings, if present, include cystic changes or reactive bone changes on the greater tuberosity at the insertion site of the supraspinatus and a subacromial traction spur at the location of the insertion of the coracoacromial ligament. The lateral view may show an increased curve in the anterior acromion or sclerotic changes on the undersurface of the acromion (Fig. 20.4). Degenerative changes of the AC joint, including an inferior osteophyte, may be present. Radiographs of large tears in which humeral head depression activity in the rotator cuff is lost may reveal a diminution in the acromiohumeral interval. Long-standing, extremely large cuff tears may produce arthritic changes in the glenohumeral joint, a condition known as cuff tear arthropathy.

Standard radiologic studies that have been effective in assessing rotator cuff integrity are arthrography, ultrasonography, and MRI. Arthrograms of a torn cuff reveal contrast material in both the glenohumeral joint and the subacromial space, with communication through the tear (Fig. 20.5). Sonographic findings of a cuff tear include absence of the rotator cuff layer, increased echogenicity in the rotator cuff, and interruption of the homogenous layer of the supraspinatus between the deltoid and humeral head.

MRI findings include changes in the AC joint, acromion, and humeral head; however, the hallmark of a rotator cuff tear is an increased signal in both T_1- and T_2-weighted images (Fig. 20.6). MRI studies are able to reveal partial-thickness tears of the rotator cuff and may help assess muscle atrophy or irreversible scarring in the cuff muscle, which may have prognostic implications regarding the surgical restoration of arm strength.

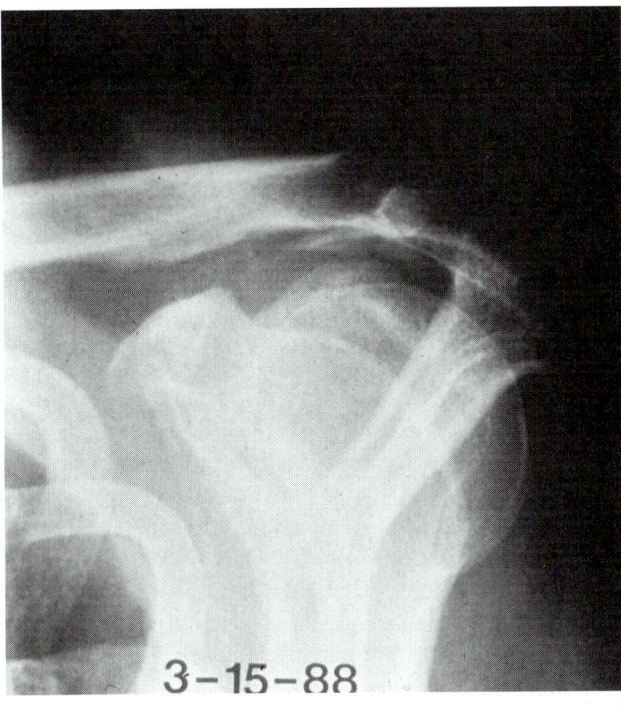

Figure 20.4. Lateral view showing a subacromial spur tracking into the substance of the coracoacromial ligament.

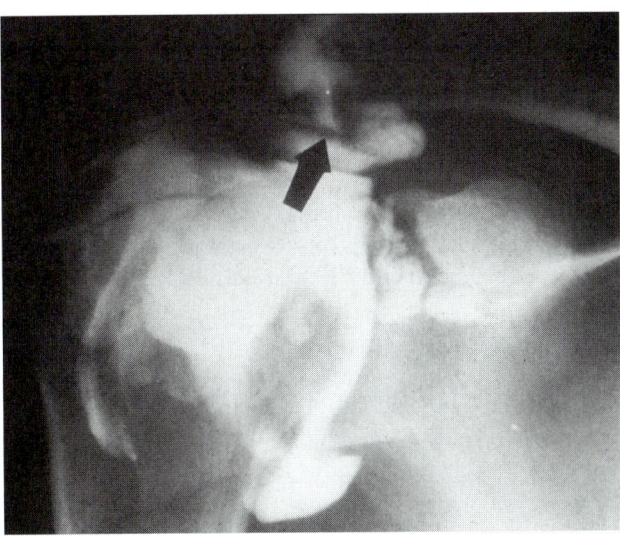

Figure 20.5. Positive arthrogram of a patient with a full-thickness rotator cuff tear (*arrow*). Note the dye in the glenohumeral joint, in the subacromial space, and even in the AC joint.

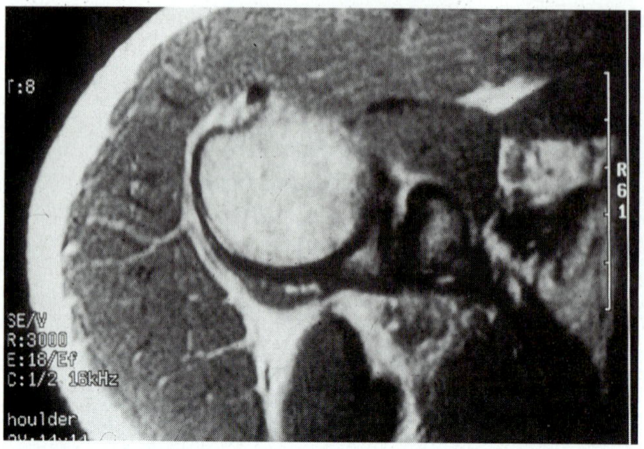

Figure 20.6. Axial view MRI study showing a posteriorly intact infraspinatus, an anterior subscapular rupture, and a biceps tendon in the tuberosity.

TREATMENT

Nonoperative Treatment

The nonoperative approach to the impingement syndrome is intended to reverse the external mechanical compression of the rotator cuff, which is caused by altered coracoacromial arch anatomy, cuff dysfunction, or inflammation. Nonsteroidal anti-inflammatory drugs (NSAIDs) may eliminate tendon or bursal inflammation.

Exercises and physical therapy focus on flexibility and strength. Range of motion exercises are intended to restore the normal joint flexibility, as restrictions in glenohumeral motion increase with the symptoms of impingement. Internal and external rotation strengthening exercises, either isometric or isokinetic, are invaluable; these exercises are performed with the arm near the side. It is hoped that the recovery of cuff strength will reestablish the centering mechanism of the humeral head, eliminating the superior migration of the head and effectively producing dynamic restoration of the subacromial space. A limited number of subacromial injections of cortisone may help the treatment of this disease, if the potential deleterious local effects of cortisone on tendons are recognized.

These therapies do not play a role in the rehabilitation of patients with full-thickness tears. In fact, exercise may increase the patient's discomfort. Subacromial injections are not used for full-thickness rotator cuff tears, unless the patient has a medical condition that precludes tendon repair.

Operative Treatment

The general indications for surgical treatment of the impingement syndrome and rotator cuff tear include (*a*) failure of a 6-month nonoperative treatment program, (*b*) documented presence of a symptomatic full-thickness tear, and (*c*) sufficient pain to warrant the risks of surgery (Clinical Table). Surgery for weakness in the absence of pain should be approached with caution, because restoration of strength depends on many factors besides suc-

cessful tendon reattachment. The surgical procedure consists of anterior acromioplasty that is designed to decompress the coracoacromial arch, creating more space for the repaired tendons to pass; repair of any full-thickness tendon tears; and resection of the portion of the distal clavicle that is contributing to external impingement.

ARTHROSCOPIC ACROMIOPLASTY

Anterior acromioplasty, the surgical reshaping of the anterior acromial edge and the removal of protruding osteophytes, can be accomplished either by arthroscopic or open surgery (1). The general indications for arthroscopic anterior acromioplasty are a documented subacromial impingement syndrome that includes a hook or down sloping of the anterior acromion and a partial-thickness tear of the rotator cuff that can be débrided to stimulate healing. Arthroscopy can be performed during an open rotator cuff surgical repair (a mini open technique) and be used when the surgeon elects only to débride the rotator cuff and not to attempt a surgical repair (rare).

The contraindications to an arthroscopic approach to the impingement syndrome include shoulder pain not secondary to mechanical impingement and impingement secondary to other disease processes (e.g., shoulder instability, scapula dysfunction, and nerve injury). A relative contraindication to arthroscopic acromioplasty alone is the presence of a repairable full-thickness tear, as published results of anterior acromioplasty and cuff repair are far superior to those of anterior acromioplasty alone in the presence of a full-thickness tear.

Technique

The patient can be positioned either in the decubitus position with the arm suspended or in a sitting position with the arm at the side. There are three standard operating arthroscopic portals: the posterior or posterolateral portal, the anterior portal, and the lateral portal. The posterior portal is placed 2 cm inferior and 2 cm medial to the posterolateral corner of the acromion or the posterolateral portal is placed 2 cm lateral to the posterolateral corner of the acromion. The anterior portal is located 2 cm medial and 1 cm inferior to the anterolateral edge of the acromion but lateral to the coracoid process. The lateral portal is usually 2 cm lateral to the lateral edge of the acromion. The AP position of the lateral portal varies, depending on surgical preference. In addition to standard arthroscopic instrumentation, a pump and electrocautery are helpful.

The operation begins with an arthroscopic examination of the glenohumeral joint. The arthroscope is introduced through the posterior portal, and the anterior portal may be used for outflow, problems, or surgical instruments. A careful examination of the glenohumeral joint includes assessing the status of the articular cartilage, glenohumeral ligaments, biceps anchor attachment, anterior and posterior capsular tissue, deep surface of the rotator cuff, and intra-articular portion of biceps tendon. An additional amount of biceps may be visualized by inserting a probe

Clinical Table: Impingement and Rotator Cuff Tear: Treatment by Anterior Acromioplasty and Repair

Procedure	Indications	Technique	Anatomy	Pitfalls
Open acromioplasty and cuff repair	• Impingement syndrome • Cuff tear	• Anterior supraspinatus • Detach deltoid • Acromioplasty • AC repair with number 1 suture	• Deltoid • Axillary nerve • Acromial branch of the thoracoacromial trunk	• Irregular design • Insecure repair
Arthroscopic acromioplasty	• Impingement syndrome		• Acromion • Bones • Coracoacromial ligament • AC joint	• Irregular design • Acromial fracture debris
Mini open repair	• Small cuff tear • Impingement syndrome		• Deltoid	• Irregular for repair

superior to the biceps tendon and pulling inferior, while the bicipital groove area is visualized. Gentle abduction of the arm may increase the ability to visualize the deep surface of the rotator cuff near its insertion on the greater tuberosity. Examination of the glenohumeral joint may reveal deep surface tearing of the rotator cuff; partial tearing of the biceps; and abnormalities of the glenoid labrum, such as superior labrum anterior and posterior lesions, cracking, or fraying. The surgeon may consider débridement or repair of any associated intra-articular lesions.

For the subacromial decompression, the arthroscope is introduced into the subacromial space through the posterior or posterolateral portal (Fig. 20.7). The trocar may initially be used to break up any subacromial adhesions and to create a more optimal space for visualization. The operating instrument is introduced via the lateral portal. It is essential to maintain proper orientation of the acromion, coracoacromial arch, superficial surface of the cuff, and AC joint. Orientation may be aided by maintaining visualization of the medial and lateral borders of the anterior acromion and the attached coracoacromial ligament. Spinal needles on the medial and lateral borders of the coracoacromial ligament help outline its margins and maintain the orientation. The coracoacromial ligament is then resected, from medial to lateral, with cautery. As the ligament is removed from the acromial attachment, the reddish deep fibers of the deltoid are identified above the deep deltoid fascia.

The anterior undersurface of the acromion is then outlined; and any remaining soft tissue, ligaments, and periosteal attachments are removed, giving clear exposure of the entire bony anterior acromion. The amount of acromial bone to be removed is confirmed (a preoperative lateral acromial x-ray may assist in this), making certain that proper orientation is maintained throughout the acromioplasty. The extents of the medial to lateral excision and the anterior posterior excision are plotted.

The anterior acromioplasty is performed by removing a wedge of bone that tapers from anterior to posterior toward the midportion of acromion and extends completely from the anteromedial to the anterolateral edges of acromion. Using either a round or oval burr or full-radius synovial resector, the surgeon contours the undersurface of acromion, producing a "flat" surface. The acromioplasty is begun laterally, and the bone can be removed by an AP sweeping motion; the acromioplasty is completed from the lateral to medial direction. At the conclusion of the acromioplasty, the curved or overhanging undersurface of the acromion should have been converted to a flat area. The surgeon can gauge his or her success by introducing the arthroscope into the lateral portal and examining the undersurface of the acromion. The surgical instruments can be placed through the posterior portal, and any remaining smoothing can be accomplished in this fashion with a bone shaver or rasp.

If a portion of the undersurface of clavicle is to be removed or if a complete distal clavicle excision is to be done independently of the acromioplasty, the arthro-

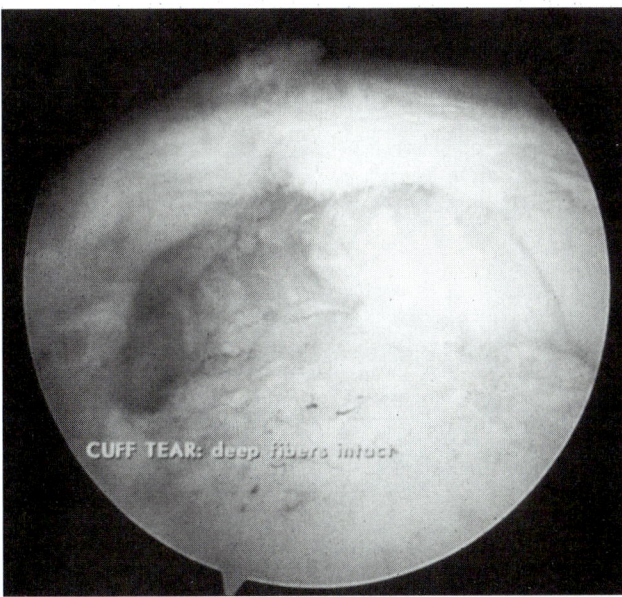

Figure 20.7. Arthroscopic view of the subacromial space showing a bursa side tear of the rotator cuff. Note the extensive bursal side erosion, although the deepest portion of the supraspinatus attachment remains intact.

scope is replaced in the posterior portal, and the initial clavicle excision is begun through the lateral portal. When enough space is obtained, the distal clavicle excision is completed by placing the arthroscope in the lateral portal and the surgical instruments though the anterior portal. Once the bony resection is completed, the thick, abnormal bursa can be removed, and any irregular or frayed surgical cuff fibers can be débrided.

OPEN ANTERIOR ACROMIOPLASTY AND ROTATOR CUFF REPAIR

An open anterior acromioplasty may be performed either as an isolated procedure to treat a mechanical subacromial impingement or in conjunction with a repair of the rotator cuff (2,3). The aims of an open anterior acromioplasty are identical to those of an arthroscopic acromioplasty, i.e., to remove the anterior acromial overhang and to produce a flat undersurface to the acromion. Open anterior acromioplasty is performed as an adjunctive procedure to an open rotator cuff repair; as revision surgery, in which arthroscopic visualization may be difficult; and when the surgeon's arthroscopic experience precludes predictable and precise removal of acromial bone. Although the skin incision and the addition of dissection trauma to the deltoid muscle may be disadvantages of the open anterior acromioplasty, the degree of predictability of bone removal via direct visualization of the acromion and rotator cuff is an important advantage of the procedure.

Technique

With the patient positioned in a semi–beach chair position, an anterior superior oblique incision is made. The subcutaneous tissue is divided down to the deltoid fascia. The deltoid muscle may be split beginning at the AC joint; and if needed, a small amount of anterior deltoid may be detached. The deltoid should be kept as an intact muscular sleeve, with both the superior and the inferior deltoid fascias preserved, to help secure the deltoid repair and reattachment. With the deltoid reflected, the coracoacromial ligament can be directly visualized and removed. Manual release of the subdeltoid adhesions may aid in restoration of the deltoid muscle, allowing the undersurface of the anterior acromion to be directly visualized.

During arthroscopic acromioplasty, a wedge of the anterior undersurface of acromion is removed. In its thickest portion, the wedge is usually 0.6 to 0.8 cm, but it rapidly tapers to the midportion of acromion. The anterior acromioplasty is completed from the most anterolateral corner of the acromion to the anteromedial edge of acromion and often includes the acromial facet of AC joint. At the conclusion of the anterior acromioplasty, direct visualization of the flattened undersurface of the anterior acromion may be done by placing a flat retractor under the acromion and levering down on the humeral head (Fig. 20.8).

At this point, the rotator cuff is examined and the extent of the tear is identified. The supraspinatus may be retracted medially by the pull of the coracohumeral liga-

ment and superior capsule. Release of the coracohumeral ligament and rotator interval between the supraspinatus and subscapularis aids tendon mobilization. The infraspinatus is often pulled inferiorly by the teres minor. If a subscapularis tear is present, there may be a concomitant medial dislocation of the biceps tendon (Fig. 20.9).

Once the extent of the tendon is identified, the tendon may be mobilized by the release of the extra-articular and intra-articular adhesions. Nonabsorbable stay sutures through the tendon edge permit traction to be placed on the tendon during mobilization. Additional techniques of cuff mobilization include a capsulotomy within the joint and muscle tendon slides. The reattachment site for the rotator cuff on the greater or lesser tuberosity (if the subscapularis is torn) is identified. The bone is prepared so that the reattachment site is relatively viable bleeding bone (Fig. 20.10). The edge of the torn retracted tendon is freshened to augment tendon to bone healing. The rotator cuff is usually reattached with nonabsorbable sutures through drill holes in the greater tuberosity (Fig. 20.11).

Occasionally, there may be a role for a suture anchor reattachment of the rotator cuff, particularly to augment the drill hole technique. Osteopenic bone, however, may diminish the effectiveness of the suture anchor. In many

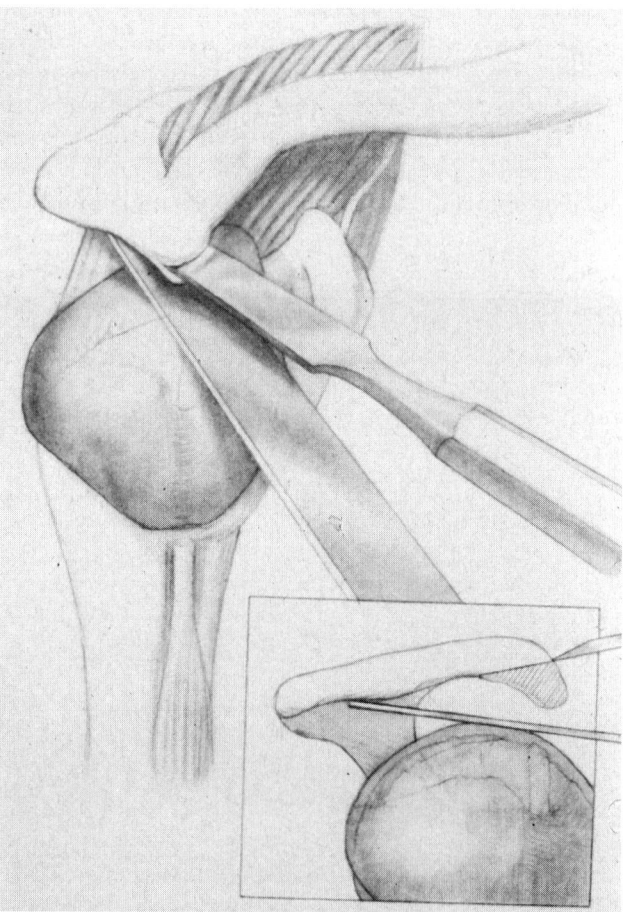

Figure 20.8. For an anterior acromioplasty, part of the anterior inferior undersurface of the acromion is removed to create more room for the repaired supraspinatus.

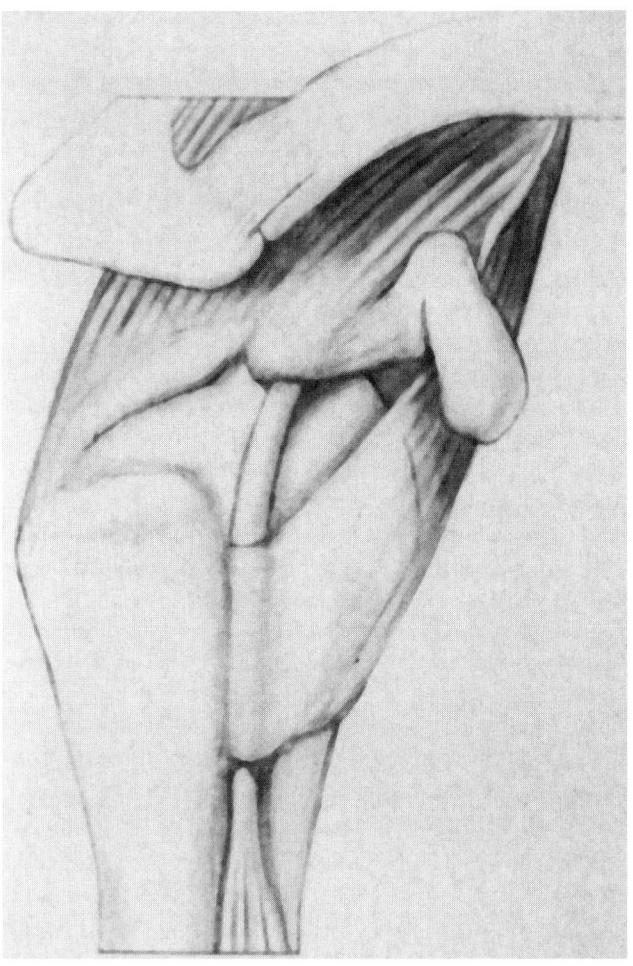

Figure 20.9. Full-thickness tear of the rotator cuff with detachment of the supraspinatus from the greater tuberosity.

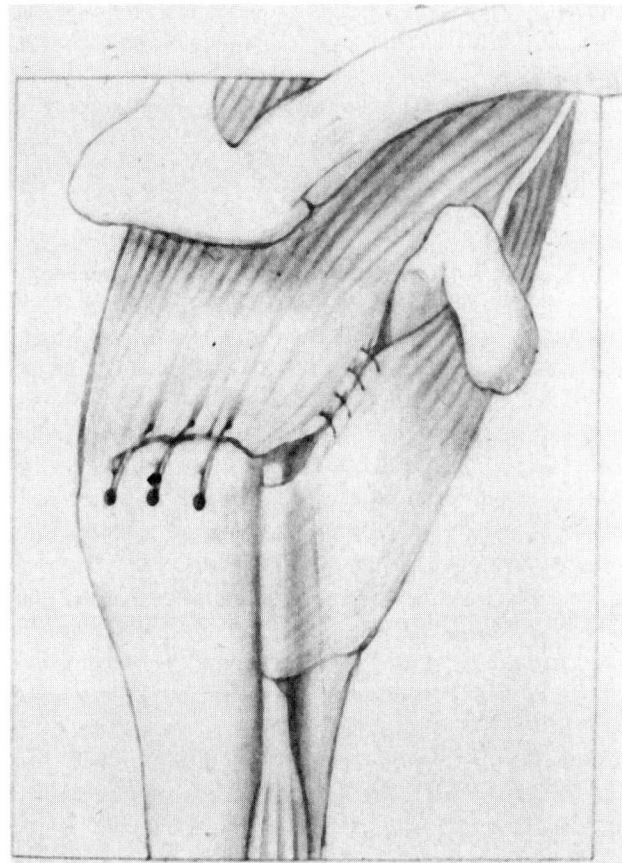

Figure 20.11. Completed rotator cuff tear repair. The supraspinatus has been reattached to the greater tuberosity with nonabsorbable sutures.

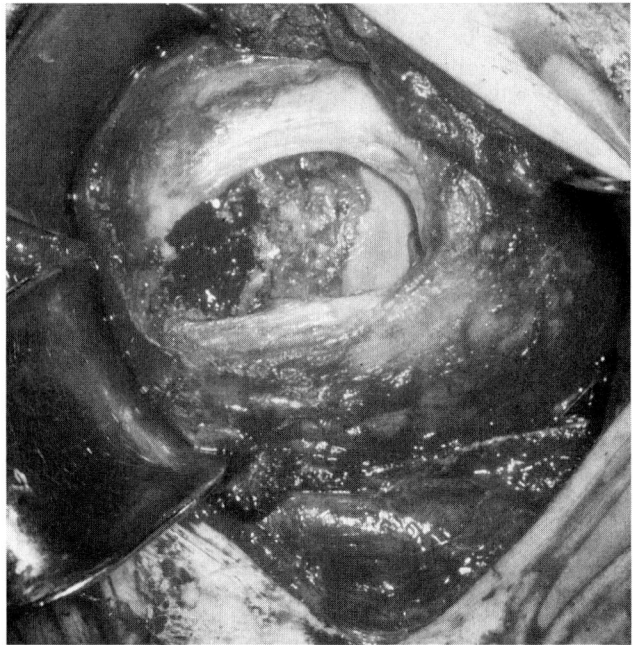

Figure 20.10. Intraoperative view of a patient with a clavicle full-thickness tear of the rotator cuff.

older patients, the degree of osteopenia precludes effective and secured suture anchor repair of the tendon.

Once the tendon is reattached to bleeding bone with nonabsorbable sutures, the arm is ranged into forward elevation, external rotation, and internal rotation to ensure clearance under the anterior acromion. The biceps tendon is usually left intact during cuff repair; however, if it is diseased or torn or if it will be used in the tendon repair, it may be tenodised in its groove. Any thickened or fibrotic subacromial bursa is removed before the rotator cuff repair is completed. After the rotator cuff has been securely reattached, the deltoid muscle, if it has been detached, is repaired. It is securely reattached to the AC joint capsule, the deltoid tendon origin, and the trapezius insertion with nonabsorbable sutures. Any split in the deltoid is then closed, and layered closure of the skin and subcutaneous tissues is performed.

MINI OPEN REPAIR

A mini open repair combines arthroscopic subacromial decompression with a limited exposure of the rotator cuff to effect a rotator cuff repair without extensive deltoid dissection (4). In general, the indications for a mini open repair are (*a*) a documented full-thickness tear of the rotator cuff that is small and does not require extensive mobilization and (b) an acromion that is amenable to an arthroscopic decompression. The surgeon must have the skills to expeditiously perform an arthroscopic anterior acromioplasty.

Technique

The patient is positioned as described for arthroscopic subacromial decompression, and the same portal sites are used. An expeditious arthroscopic anterior acromioplasty is performed in the same fashion as outlined above. At the conclusion of the arthroscopic decompression, the lateral portal site is extended proximally and distally for a distance of 3 cm. The deltoid muscle, which has been violated by the arthroscopy portal site, is split to the level of the anterior lateral acromion and retracted. It is beneficial to either directly visualize or to palpate the adequacy of the arthroscopic subacromial decompression; if necessary, it can be modified at the time. Once the adequacy of the anterior acromioplasty is confirmed, the abnormal bursa covering the rotator cuff is removed. With the deltoid retracted, rotation of the humerus permits direct visualization of the cuff defect. The most frequent location of the cuff tear, the supraspinatus insertion, is usually readily seen by this method. Nonabsorbable sutures bring the tendon defect back to the prepared bone, as outlined above.

One advantage of the mini open repair is less deltoid dissection; its disadvantages include limits on exposure and alterations of the normal external anatomic landmarks, particularly if much time is spent performing the arthroscopic subacromial decompression.

PITFALLS AND COMMON MISTAKES

Arthroscopic Subacromial Decompression

Portal problems. If the posterior portal is too inferior, visualization in the subacromial space may be difficult because the arthroscope must come over the humeral head. If the lateral portal is too superior, use of surgical instruments in the subacromial space may be difficult and may make introduction and use of the electrocautery (which is quite flexible) impossible. On the other hand, if the lateral portal is too inferior, the branches of the axillary nerve may be damaged. If the anterior portal is too medial, the musculocutaneous nerve may be injured.

Bleeding problems. Bleeding problems can be burdensome, particularly from the acromial branch of the thoracoacromial trunk as the coracoacromial ligament is resected. Bleeding may be controlled by maintaining epinephrine in the solution, by liberally using electrocauterization, by using an arthroscopic pump, and by keeping the patient's blood pressure low. Uncontrolled bleeding makes visualization difficult.

Inappropriate removal of acromial bone. Bone may be removed from the acromion that is inappropriate in location or in amount. Excessive removal of acromion can lead to

acromial fracture or nonunion and weakening of the deltoid origin. If too little acromial bone is removed, the patient may experience continued subacromial impingement. Jagged edges and bone debris left in the subacromial space may lead to calcification.

Open Anterior Acromioplasty and Rotator Cuff Repair

Axillary nerve injury. Damage to the terminal branches of the axillary nerve may be caused by splitting the deltoid muscle more than 4 to 5 cm from its origin. Damage can be avoided by taking care to limit the deltoid split and by using a stay suture in the distal portion of the split.

Excessive deltoid detachment or insecure repair. If damage to the deltoid origin is left unrepaired or is insecurely repaired, the arm may be permanently weakened. Care must be taken during deltoid detachment to limit the amount of muscle removed and to securely reattach it either to the tendinous origin and AC joint capsule or through drill holes in the acromion.

Inadequate acromioplasty. Inadequate acromioplasty may lead to continued impingement. The entire undersurface should be removed, leaving a flat surface.

Insecure repair of the rotator cuff tendon. An insecure repair of the rotator cuff can lead to rerupture of the tendon, inadequate healing, and continued pain and weakness. To minimize complications, the tendon should be securely repaired through drill holes in the bone and with nonabsorbable sutures. Postsurgery, the repair should be protected.

Mini Open Repair

The pitfalls of the mini open repair include all those of both the arthroscopic acromioplasty and the open rotator cuff repair. In addition, if the arthroscopic part of the operation takes excessively long, swelling and distention of the soft tissues in the skin, subcutaneous tissue, and deltoid muscle can obscure the bony landmarks, make the deltoid and subdeltoid dissection extremely difficult, and limit the exposure and ability to effectively repair the rotator cuff tear.

Rehabilitation

The challenge of postoperative rehabilitation is to establish early motion, so that stiffness does not adversely affect the surgical result, while protecting the tendon and deltoid muscle repairs. In general, the postoperative rehabilitation from an arthroscopic anterior acromioplasty without a rotator cuff repair does not require protection of the deltoid and rotator cuff. Early range of motion can include both passive and active motion. Beginning in the immediate postoperative period, the patient may begin passive and assistive exercises aimed at restoring forward elevation in the plane of the scapula, external rotation, and internal rotation. The patient performs a series of assistive exercises with or without the direct supervision of a physical therapist.

After a full-thickness rotator cuff tear repair, a mini open repair, or an open anterior acromioplasty in which the deltoid was detached and resutured, early range of motion is essential; however, the tendon repair must be protected. The tension on the operative repair should be observed intraoperatively by bringing the arm into full elevation, external rotation, and internal rotation. Early postoperative range of motion concentrates on forward flexion and external rotation and is begun on the postoperative day 1; the tendon repair is protected by limiting exercises to either passive range of motion (done by a physical therapist, trainer, or family member) or assistive exercises (the motion is supplied by the extremity not operated on).

When tendon healing has occurred (6 to 8 weeks), the patient may begin to use the arm for light activity, and rehabilitation may include isometric exercises in a submaximal fashion. At 3 months, the patient may begin resistive exercises to restore the strength of the deltoid muscle and rotator cuff.

Results

Anterior acromioplasty with rotator cuff repair has an established history of surgical success for rotator cuff disease produced by the subacromial impingement syndrome. Whether the anterior acromioplasty is performed by an arthroscopic or open technique, the surgical success in terms of relieving the patient's impingement pain is 85 to 90% in most series (5).

The surgical repair of a concomitant full-thickness tear increases the success of the outcome. For patients with a full-thickness tear, particularly if the tear is large, pain relief is probably a more predictable result than is complete restoration of strength. Muscle strength is ordinarily improved by the addition of a tendon repair; however, because many variables are involved (quality of the tissue, size of the tear, ability of the patient to perform rehabilitation safely, avoidance of reinjury), the degree of improvement is unpredictable.

Although impingement pain is often gone quite soon after surgery, the total rehabilitation time following an anterior acromioplasty and rotator cuff repair can be surprisingly long, often taking 6 to 12 months. Nevertheless, large series have noted that patients with an impingement syndrome who underwent acromioplasty report satisfying results.

SUMMARY

The association of problems in the acromial and coracoacromial arch with rotator cuff disease and pain has long been recognized. Success in the recognition, identification, and management of disorders of the coracoacromial arch, subacromial space, and rotator cuff, whether by nonoperative, arthroscopic, or open operative methods, continues to be high.

REFERENCES

1. Ellman H, Kay SP. Arthroscopic subacromial decompression for chronic impingement. Two-to five-year results. J Bone Joint Surg 1991;73B:395–398.
2. Neer CS II. Impingement lesions. Clin Orthop 1983;173:73–77.
3. Craig EV. Anterior acromioplasty and rotator cuff repair. In: Craig EV, ed. The shoulder. New York: Raven Press, 1995.
4. Paulos LE, Kody MH. Arthroscopically enhanced "mini approach to rotator cuff repair." Am J Sports Med 1994;22:19–25.
5. Cofield RH. Rotator cuff disease of the shoulder. J Bone Joint Surg 1985;67A:974–979.

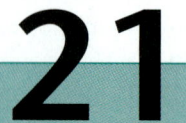

chapter 21

Leslie J. Bisson and David M. Dines

Total Shoulder Arthroplasty

Total shoulder arthroplasty (TSA) is the treatment of choice for painful, destructive processes of the glenohumeral joint. In 1994 more than 14,000 shoulder arthroplasties were performed in the United States, a substantial increase from the 6,000 that were inserted in 1990. The significant increase in arthroplasties over the last several years is the result of several factors, including improved understanding of the functional anatomy and pathophysiology of the shoulder, the availability of improved prostheses, and advances in surgical technique.

The first recorded TSA was carried out in 1892, when Pean inserted a platinum and rubber prosthesis into a shoulder infected with tuberculosis (1). It was removed 1 year later because of recurrent infection. The modern era of shoulder arthroplasty began in 1952, when Neer successfully implanted stemmed metal implants to replace the humeral head. Neer later introduced an unconstrained polyethylene glenoid component in an attempt to improve the results of shoulder arthroplasty in patients with osteoarthritis. As the indications for TSA were expanded, constrained implants were developed for use in rotator cuff-deficient shoulders. The results of these prostheses were poor, owing to high rates of glenoid loosening and mechanical failure.

Modular implants were introduced in 1985 in an effort to improve soft tissue balancing and reproduction of the normal anatomy. Modular prostheses also offered the ability to deal with specific pathologic processes more efficiently. Bone and soft tissue loss seen in traumatic arthritis could be addressed using modular components. A large-size humeral head component could be used in cases of rotator cuff insufficiency, cuff tear arthropathy, and severe rheumatoid arthritis. Finally, the ability to remove the humeral head allowed better access to the glenoid without the need to remove a well-fixed humeral component in revision cases.

The most common indication for TSA is painful glenohumeral incongruity owing to osteoarthritis, rheumatoid arthritis, avascular necrosis, posttraumatic arthritis, and ro-

tator cuff arthropathy. The unique characteristics of each of these disease processes require selective surgical consideration for each situation.

RELEVANT ANATOMY

To perform a successful arthroplasty of the shoulder, it is imperative for the surgeon to understand the vascular, neurologic, and osseous anatomy of the shoulder region and the relevant biomechanics of the glenohumeral joint.

Vascular Anatomy

The main blood supply of the shoulder region is via the axillary artery, with the exception of the suprascapular artery from the thyrocervical trunk (2). The third part of the axillary artery (that portion distal to the pectoralis minor) and its branches are the relevant vascular structures involved in TSA.

The third part of the axillary artery has three branches: the subscapular artery and the anterior and posterior humeral circumflex arteries. The subscapular artery descends along the lateral border of the subscapularis muscle and divides into the circumflex scapular artery and the thoracodorsal arteries. The anterior and posterior humeral circumflex arteries pass around the surgical neck of the humerus; the ascending branch of the anterior humeral circumflex supplies the majority of the humeral head via the ascending branch of Laing (3,4). The blood supply to the humeral head can be disrupted in fractures of the proximal humerus with separation of the head from the shaft and tuberosities.

Neuroanatomy

The axillary, musculocutaneous, and suprascapular nerves are in close proximity to the surgical field during TSA. A thorough knowledge of the location of these nerves is imperative for avoiding their injury, either directly or via the injudicious placement or overzealous use of retractors.

The axillary nerve, a large terminal branch of the posterior cord of the brachial plexus, crosses the anteroinferior and then the lateral border of the subscapularis muscle, joins the posterior humeral circumflex artery, and exits the quadrangular space. It splits into two trunks: the posterior trunk, which supplies the teres minor and posterior deltoid before terminating as the superior lateral cutaneous nerve of the arm, and the anterior trunk, which supplies the middle and anterior portions of the deltoid (5–7) Burkhead et al. (8) detailed the significant variations in the course and position of the axillary nerve. It is in greatest danger during dissection along the inferior rim of the glenoid and along the inferior humeral neck. The axillary nerve may be difficult to identify during revision surgery and may be buried in scar tissue or contracted.

The musculocutaneous nerve is a terminal branch of the lateral cord of the brachial plexus. This nerve enters the deep surface of the coracobrachialis muscle from 3.1 to 8.2 cm distal to the tip of the coracoid (9) and innervates the biceps, brachialis, and coracobrachialis muscles before it becomes the lateral antebrachial cutaneous nerve. Vigorous retraction of the conjoint tendon medially can result in a traction injury to this nerve.

The suprascapular nerve arises from the upper trunk of the brachial plexus and passes through the suprascapular notch in the scapula. It supplies the supraspinatus muscle and then proceeds through the spinoglenoid notch to supply the infraspinatus muscle. Injury to the nerve can result from careless dissection posterior to the glenoid, and the position of the nerve limits the mobilization of the infraspinatus.

Osseous Anatomy

The scapula (and, therefore, the glenoid) is inclined on the posterior chest wall 30° to 40° anterior to the coronal plane of the body (10,11); and the humeral head and its articular surface are retroverted a corresponding amount, allowing the two articular surfaces to line up (12). The proximal humerus is retroverted 12° to 36° (12–16); the neck-shaft angle is 115° to 129° (13,17). The humeral head is significantly larger than the glenoid fossa, and the glenoid covers approximately 75% of the humeral head in the vertical plane and 57% in the transverse plane (12).

The glenoid fossa is pear shaped, becoming narrow superiorly with the supraglenoid tubercle at its upper border. A small amount of cancellous bone is available in the glenoid vault for prosthetic fixation. The long-axis dimension of the glenoid averages 3.5 to 4 cm, and the depth in the sagittal plane is 2.5 to 3 cm (18). The mean glenoid version varies from slightly anteverted to slightly retroverted (19,20).

Biomechanics

Elevation of the arm is the result of both glenohumeral and scapulothoracic motion, which has been termed scapulothoracic rhythm. The overall ratio of glenohumeral to scapulothoracic motion during the entire arc of arm elevation is approximately 2:1; the greatest variability occurs at the extremes of motion. Greater motion occurs at the glenohumeral joint during the first 30° of abduction, and the last 60° of elevation are owing to almost equal contributions of glenohumeral and scapulothoracic motion.

The center of rotation of the glenohumeral joint has been defined as a group of points situated within 6 mm of the anatomic center of the humeral head (21). This suggests that only a small amount of translation occurs at this joint. Joint reaction forces of the glenohumeral joint are approximately 0.4 times body weight at 60° of abduction, increasing to 0.9 times body weight at 90° of abduction (21). At 0° of abduction, the glenohumeral resultant force is directed below the glenoid center. From 30° to 60° of abduction, the resultant force is directed above the glenoid center; and above 60° of abduction, the resultant force is directed at the glenoid center (22,23).

PATHOGENESIS AND PATHOANATOMY

As was mentioned earlier, each disease process affecting the glenohumeral joint has unique characteristics that must be recognized by the surgeon and specifically addressed during the shoulder arthroplasty.

Osteoarthritis

The main characteristics of osteoarthritis are remarkably consistent among patients (Fig. 21.1). The rotator cuff and deltoid muscles usually retain satisfactory function, and rotator cuff tears are the rare exception in 1 to 5% (24). In long-standing cases, a large anterior-inferior osteophyte on the neck of the humerus is often accompanied by a loss of subscapularis excursion (with corresponding loss in external rotation) and an inferior capsular contracture (24–26). This osteophyte must be removed to facilitate the surgical exposure and allow proper placement of the humeral prosthesis. The loss of articular cartilage is most severe when contact between the humeral head and the glenoid occurs at the highest joint reaction force, i.e., 60° to 100° of abduction (27). The glenoid frequently demonstrates posterior erosion, flattening, and marginal osteophytes (24); and if the erosion is not recognized before surgery, then improper placement of the glenoid may occur.

Rheumatoid Arthritis

Patients with rheumatoid arthritis (RA) typically have a much more challenging pathoanatomy than those with osteoarthritis (Fig. 21.2) (28,29). Some of the changes in these patients are owing to the disease process itself,

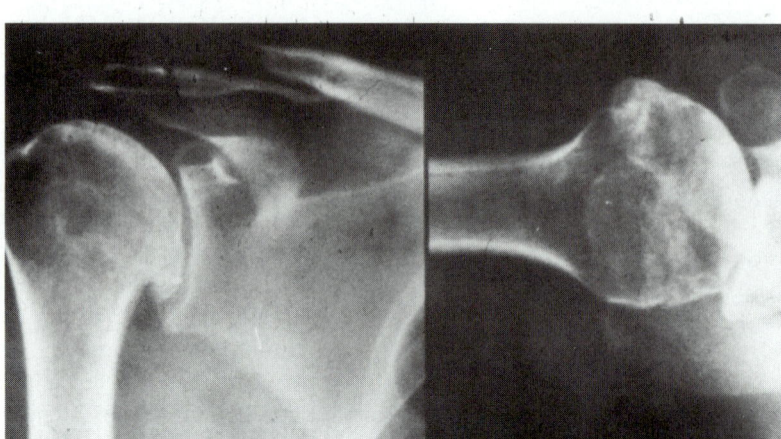

Figure 21.1. Shoulder afflicted with osteoarthritis.

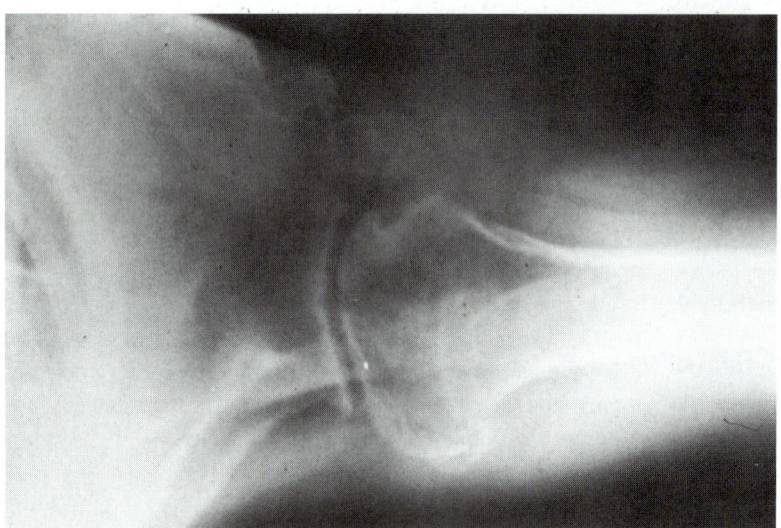

Figure 21.2. Axillary view of a shoulder afflicted with rheumatoid arthritis. Note the severe bone loss and medial erosion of glenoid.

whereas others are secondary to medications required to treat the process. These patients usually have atrophic skin; thus the planning of incisions and the handling of the skin are critical. They also have osteopenic bone as a result of inflammation, disuse, and corticosteroids and may have significant bone loss and destruction. Both the humeral head and glenoid may have large cysts filled with granulation tissue, leading to compromised fixation. Glenoid erosions in rheumatoid patients tend to be anterior and central (26,30) rather than posterior as in osteoarthritis. Medial erosion may be severe enough to completely remove the base of the coracoid and preclude placement of a glenoid component. Finally and perhaps most important, there is often attrition or complete rupture of the rotator cuff (26,31,32).

Rotator cuff tears seen by arthrography occur in 46% of patients with RA (32), and attenuation not visible arthrographically occurs in many more patients (33). In many of these cases, hemiarthroplasty as a salvage procedure is necessary to relieve pain; limited functional goals are the expectation. Earlier treatment of the rheumatoid shoulder (before significant bone loss and irreparable rotator cuff

degeneration occur) may allow better restoration of normal anatomy and improved results of arthroplasty.

Avascular Necrosis

Avascular necrosis of the humeral head can be related to traumatic conditions or to various disease processes. Conditions associated with necrosis of bone include, but are not limited to, systemic corticosteroid use, alcoholism, dysbaric phenomena, Cushing's syndrome, Gaucher's disease, hemoglobinopathies, irradiation, and thermal injuries (34,35). Systemic conditions may affect the condition of the soft tissues around the glenohumeral joint, and these need to be individually addressed.

The decision to resurface the glenoid needs to be made at the time of surgery. If a hemiarthroplasty is done, the humeral replacement may eventually erode the glenoid cartilage and necessitate subsequent conversion to a total shoulder arthroplasty (36). For this reason, a modular total shoulder replacement system may be preferred in these individuals. A second consideration is the quality of avascular bone. Several series have shown decreased longevity of both uncemented and cemented hip prosthesis in patients with avascular necrosis (37,38). It is not currently known whether this is also the case in the shoulder.

Posttraumatic Degenerative Joint Disease

Chronic fractures of the proximal humerus require special consideration (Fig. 21.3) (39). The surgery in cases of proximal humeral malunion with degenerative joint disease (DJD) is technically demanding because of distortion of the bony anatomy and soft tissue scarring; there is greater blood loss, higher complications, and less predictable results after surgery than in cases without DJD (40,41). Appropriate preoperative assessment of the soft tissue and bony anatomy is mandatory and may require special studies, such as CT scanning to ascertain tuberosity position and MRI to evaluate the condition of the rotator cuff. Often previous scars need to be considered. Malposition of the greater and lesser tuberosities may require osteotomy and repositioning of the respective tuberosity to prevent impingement or instability (39,42–44). Scanograms may also be necessary in these cases to ensure reconstruction of appropriate humeral height and re-creation of the correct deltoid length and tension (39,42,43). Bone graft augmentation of humeral length is often necessary (39,42,43,45).

Rotator Cuff Arthropathy

Degenerative arthritis associated with a massive defect of the rotator cuff is a complex problem (Fig. 21.4). Such patients, by definition, have a large defect of the rotator cuff, which is often irreparable. They also frequently have significant osteopenia of the proximal humerus, with collapse of the humeral head and superior and anterior dislocation of the glenohumeral joint (46). Associated features are glenoid erosions, a rounding off of the greater tuberosity, and a shortened acromiohumeral distance with acromial and acromioclavicular joint erosion (46). Resurfacing of the

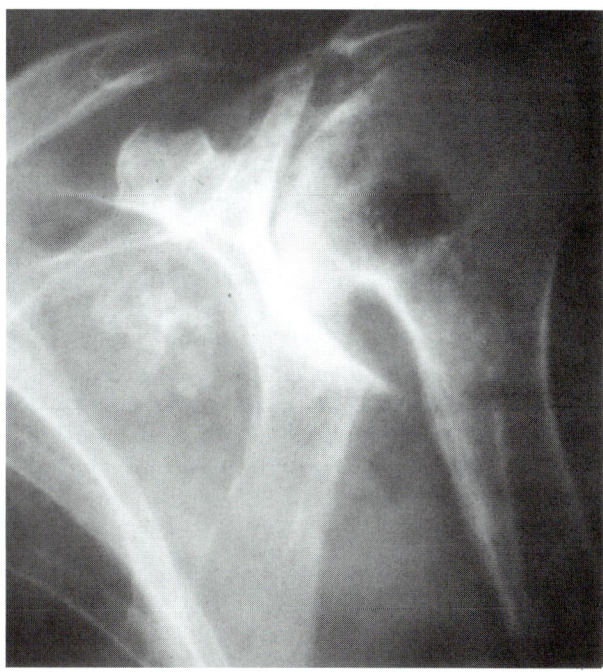

Figure 21.4. AP view of a shoulder afflicted with rotator cuff arthropathy.

glenoid in these cases often leads to loosening of the glenoid component (47). It is believed that the absence of a rotator cuff allows superior translation of the humeral head during initiation of abduction, causing edge loading of the glenoid component and a rocking-horse effect. It is important to preserve the coracoacromial ligament during the surgery, with the expectation that this will help prevent superior migration of the prosthesis (48,49).

INITIAL FINDINGS, PHYSICAL EXAMINATION, AND DIAGNOSIS

Osteoarthritis

Osteoarthritis is characterized by a gradual loss of range of motion in the glenohumeral joint associated with increasing pain. The patient may complain of catching in the joint, difficulty sleeping on the affected side, and impairment of activities of daily living. On physical examination, the clinician may find some atrophy of the deltoid and rotator cuff muscles, but strength is generally good. There is tenderness at the posterior joint line and decreased active and passive range of motion, especially internal and external rotation in abduction. The examiner may be able to detect posterior subluxation of the glenohumeral joint with flexion as the humeral head slides backward on the eburnated posterior surface of the glenoid (44). It is not uncommon to have coexistent acromioclavicular joint and subacromial abnormalities, and diagnostic injections are often useful in determining the primary source of pathologic changes. It is important to assess the cervical spine in these patients (and all patients with shoulder complaints),

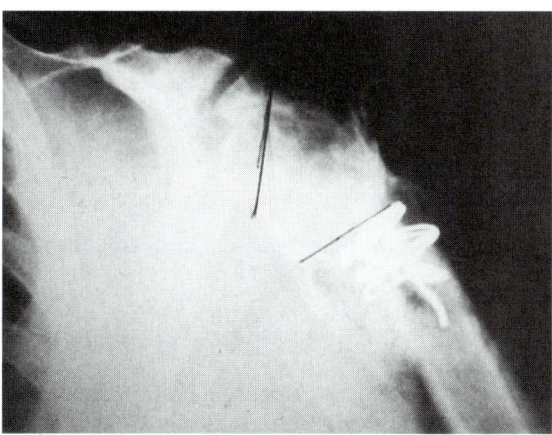

Figure 21.3. AP view of a shoulder afflicted with posttraumatic arthritis.

because arthritic degeneration of this region may occur as a concomitant condition.

Rheumatoid Arthritis

Rheumatoid arthritis of the glenohumeral joint may eventually be present in 50 to 60% of persons with polyarticular disease (50,51). The course of rheumatoid arthritis of the glenohumeral joint is characterized by insidious onset and progression of pain, punctuated by acute exacerbations that leave the patient with further shoulder stiffness. The pain is often poorly localized, radiating into the neck and scapula and down the arm to the elbow. Often, sleeping habits are altered because of the pain. On physical examination, cervical myelopathy and peripheral neuropathy must be ruled out. The shoulder joint should be assessed for muscle atrophy, swelling, synovial thickening, tenderness, and warmth. The range of motion should be documented, noting that glenohumeral motion tends to be lost in preference to scapulothoracic motion (52). Between 30 and 40% of patients will have rotator cuff tears, and many more will have attenuation of the rotator cuff (31,44).

Avascular Necrosis

The clinical findings in osteonecrosis of the humeral head are related to the cause of the necrosis; however, some generalizations are possible. In patients with early stages of the disease, when the glenoid cartilage is preserved, the predominant finding is pain, with loss of active motion greater than passive motion (53). Strength is generally quite good, and the rotator cuff is usually intact. When the disease has advanced enough to include involvement of the glenoid cartilage, the findings resemble those of primary osteoarthritis.

Posttraumatic Arthritis

Patients with degenerative joint disease of the glenohumeral joint following trauma often have significant pain, soft tissue scarring from previous surgery, and markedly limited active and passive range of motion secondary to malposition of the tuberosities and capsular scarring. It is imperative to search for and document, before surgery, any neurologic deficit that may be present.

Rotator Cuff Arthropathy

Individuals with massive rotator cuff tear and glenohumeral arthritis have painful loss of shoulder motion. The pain is worse with activity and interferes with sleep. The symptoms have often been present for many years. The patients are typically elderly and female, and they frequently have discomfort in the contralateral shoulder (46). Many patients will have a history of receiving multiple corticosteroid injections into their shoulder, but the injec-

tions do not seem to be an etiologic factor (46). On physical examination, there is atrophy of the supraspinatus and infraspinatus muscles and weakness of flexion, external rotation, and abduction. Many individuals have recurrent swelling in the shoulder region (46).

RADIOLOGIC STUDIES

Routine preoperative evaluation should include an AP view of the shoulder in internal rotation, a true AP view of the glenohumeral joint in external rotation, and an axillary view (54). The AP view in internal rotation shows the rounded contour of the humeral head, whereas the external rotation view shows the greater tuberosity in profile. The true AP view of the glenohumeral joint allows assessment of the amount of joint space narrowing. The axillary view enables one to assess the amount of glenoid erosion and is often the most sensitive view for discerning early loss of cartilage. If the cervical spine, acromioclavicular joint, or subacromial space is clinically symptomatic, then appropriate views of that region should be obtained as well.

CT scanning helps the surgeon assess the preoperative shoulder, especially with respect to glenoid bone stock in cases of glenoid erosion. This technique provides an image in the axial plane, provides excellent spatial resolution, and shows the cortical outlines better than does MRI. CT scanning is also used to evaluate the position of the tuberosities in cases of chronic trauma.

MRI is used to evaluate the rotator cuff in patients thought to have clinical evidence of rotator cuff dysfunction. It can be used to examine the glenoid surface in individuals suspected of having glenoid erosion. Imaging of the shoulder is usually done in axial, coronal oblique, and sagittal oblique planes.

TREATMENT

Nonoperative management of painful degeneration of the glenohumeral joint includes systemic medications—such as nonsteroidal anti-inflammatory drugs and antirheumatic agents (in the case of rheumatoid arthritis)—and local measures—such as the judicious use of intra-articular steroid injections. Other local modalities such as ultrasound, thermal measures, and gentle physical therapy may serve to delay the need for surgery.

Indications for Surgery

The primary indication for prosthetic shoulder arthroplasty in any of these disorders is disabling pain associated with the loss of articular cartilage when nonoperative management has failed. A secondary indication is a severe limitation of the range of motion with significant functional impairment (Clinical Table).

Contraindications to prosthetic shoulder arthroplasty include recent sepsis of the glenohumeral joint, paralysis of the shoulder musculature with loss of deltoid function,

Clinical Table: Total Shoulder Arthroplasty

Procedure	Indications	Technique	Anatomy	Pitfalls
TSR	• Osteoarthritis	• Total shoulder replacement vs. hemiarthroplasty is controversial • Total shoulder replacement seems to yield best results • Glenoid component longevity a concern	• Good soft tissue, (rotator cuff, deltoid) • Must be aware of glenoid erosion and preoperatively determine whether subscapularis tendon lengthening is necessary to ensure good external rotation	• Unrecognized subscapularis contracture will lead to lack of external rotation • Unrecognized glenoid erosion will lead to malposition of glenoid component and possible instability of total shoulder replacement
	• Rheumatoid arthritis	• Total shoulder replacement with good glenoid bone stock and sufficient rotator cuff function • Hemiarthroplasty for cases of severe glenoid bone loss and/or severe rotator cuff insufficiency	• Often poor glenoid bone stock, often severe rotator cuff insufficiency • Often severe synovitis, possible severe multijoint involvement • Bone loss and tuberosity deformity • Assess for neurologic deficit and soft tissue contracture	• Avoid poor glenoid component fixation in cases of severe bone loss and rotator cuff insufficiency • Early and late rotator cuff insufficiency may lead to glenoid component loosening • Tuberosity impingement, humeral component malposition (height and version) leading to poor rotator cuff function or instability
	• Posttraumatic osteoarthritis/malunion	• May require tuberosity osteotomy to produce premorbid anatomy • Hemiarthroplasty in cases of normal glenoid • Total shoulder replacements in cases where glenoid arthrosis exists • Must place humeral component at the right height and version • Careful preoperative assessment is necessary (CT scans, multiple plain x-ray views)		
	• Postinstability arthropathy	• Lengthen subscapularis • Correct glenoid deformity • Total shoulder replacement	• Anterior contractures • Secondary posterior glenoid erosion may be severe	• Component instability due to failure to recognize glenoid erosion/deformity or to lengthen subscapularis
	• Cuff tear arthropathy	• Hemiarthroplasty utilizes head size to produce stable glenohumeral articulation • Attempt to repair subscapularis and infraspinatus tendon for stability • Do not replace glenoid	• No reparable rotator cuff, secondary bone changes with flattening of the glenoid, usually severe • Must save coracoacromial ligament and subacromial support for stability	• Results fair in this salvaged procedure • Must be stable and in anterior, posterior plane • Must have a suitable subacromial arch for superior support • If coracoacromial ligament is absent, do not do the procedure because of devastating instability complications

the presence of a painless arthrodesis or resection arthroplasty, severely compromised bone stock, neuropathic joint degeneration, alcoholism (because of anecdotal reports of increased instability), and severe skin contracture. Severe medical infirmity and the inability to cooperate with the rehabilitation program are other contraindications. Remote sepsis of the glenohumeral joint is a relative contraindication. The inability to reconstruct a functional rotator cuff is believed to be a relative contraindication to resurfacing of the glenoid (47).

Resurfacing of the Glenoid

There are arguments both for and against resurfacing the glenoid in the case of glenoid arthritis. The advantage of more predictable pain relief when the glenoid is resurfaced must be balanced against the potential for loosening. Resurfacing of the glenoid also improves stability, lowers friction, and increases the mechanical advantage of the deltoid and rotator cuff mechanism by moving the proximal humerus laterally (47). The decision to leave the glenoid unresurfaced makes the surgery technically easier; spares bone; and avoids complications, such as glenoid loosening and polyethylene wear (55). Problems such as prosthetic humeral head erosion of the native glenoid and incomplete pain relief, however, remain disadvantages (55). Patients with inflammatory arthritis appear to have better pain relief, range of motion, and satisfaction when the glenoid has been resurfaced (55,56), but this has not been shown in a prospective, randomized study.

Cofield et al. (57) used humeral head replacement alone in a group of 67 shoulders (35 with osteoarthritis, 32 with RA). At the 9.3-year follow-up, 66% had variable pain relief and 18% needed revision surgery. Of these patients, 51% were rated as being unsatisfactory.

Torchia et al. (58) reviewed 113 shoulders in 100 patients who had total shoulder arthroplasty with the Neer prosthesis. At the 12-year follow-up, 82% of the patients had relief of pain. Although 44% of the glenoid components were radiographically loose, only 5.6% of patients needed glenoid revision.

The presence and development of radiolucent lines at the bone–cement interface of glenoid components are of uncertain significance. Brems (59) reviewed the literature regarding the glenoid component and found that 38.6% of 1413 total shoulders had lucent lines, 2.9% of 1413 total shoulders needed glenoid revision, and 7.7% of 546 total shoulders had glenoid lucencies requiring revision.

It thus appears that total shoulder arthroplasty produces fairly consistent relief of pain and patient satisfaction in individuals with osteoarthritis and rheumatoid arthritis. It is true that cemented glenoid components loosen, but revision surgery for symptomatic glenoid loosening is uncommon (33,58,59).

We would continue to recommend humeral head resurfacing as the best option in cases of rotator cuff arthropathy, acute trauma, and early stages of avascular necrosis. We favor total shoulder arthroplasty for cases of osteoarthritis, rheumatoid arthritis, chronic trauma, and late stages of avascular necrosis with involvement of the glenoid.

Choice of Implant

There are three principal types of implants available, each offering variable amounts of constraint to compensate for deficiencies in the soft tissue envelope around the shoulder. Constrained prostheses are characterized by a connection between the glenoid and humeral components that is designed to prevent their separation. These prostheses are used as salvage devices in patients with disabling pain whose deltoid, rotator cuff, and capsule are ineffective in maintaining shoulder stability (60–62). Problems with these prostheses have been component breakage, instability, loosening, and scapular fracture (62–64).

Semiconstrained total shoulder systems include a hooded glenoid component. The hood is designed to prevent superior subluxation of the humeral head in cases of irreparable tears of the rotator cuff. Concerns about increased force transmission to the glenoid bone–cement interface with subsequent glenoid loosening have limited the use of these implants. Increased incidence of loosening has indeed been seen with this type of implant, reaching 51% in one series (65).

Unconstrained implants of various designs are by far the most common type used in the United States. They generally consist of a metallic stemmed humeral component that is designed to articulate freely with a polyethylene glenoid component. Surgical technique is critical to the success of an unconstrained total shoulder arthroplasty. It is imperative that the capsule, rotator cuff, and deltoid muscle have the proper tension. It follows, therefore, that satisfactory deltoid and rotator cuff function is a prerequisite for optimal results using this type of prosthesis.

Unconstrained implants are available in both modular and nonmodular designs. The prototype of the nonmodular system is the Neer system, and more information is available in the orthopaedic literature on this system than on any other. Modularity in arthroplasty components was developed to improve our ability to create normal soft tissue tension. Modular humeral components allow the surgeon to reproduce the normal anatomy more accurately, to create the normal soft tissue tension around the shoulder in the capsule and the rotator cuff, and to upsize or downsize a component to deal with instability and/or a large soft tissue defect. The ability to remove the humeral head at a subsequent surgery allows easier revision or late resurfacing of the glenoid in the setting of a well-fixed humeral stem. Finally, in cases of instability, a modular system allows for the design of a custom humeral head component to incorporate the necessary amount of version: The surgeon simply changes the head. At our institution we prefer a modular system for both humeral head replacement and total shoulder arthroplasty because of the distinct advantages that exist in a modular system.

Fixation of the Prosthesis

Options for fixation of the implants include ingrowth components and those that use cement. The reported use of methylmethacrylate in the literature for humeral implants ranges from 0 to 100% (66–68). The incidence of radiolucent lines around humeral implants is approximately 12%, and the subsidence rate is 5 to 50% (66,69). There has recently been increased concern regarding late loosening of uncemented humeral stems, and some authors are currently recommending use of cement fixation in the humerus (70).

The majority of glenoid components reported in the English-language literature have been cemented, and this remains the method of fixation of choice at our institution. However, there is a high incidence of radiolucencies at the bone–cement interface (26,71), and late loosening of the glenoid with the need for revision remains a concern. To date, the need for revision of glenoid components owing to symptomatic loosening has remained reassuringly low (33).

Preoperative Planning

As in any reconstructive procedure, the preoperative plan is of paramount importance. Most implant systems have a variety of templates to allow preoperative approximation of implant size. The Bio-Modular system has templates for humeral sizing and the position of the osteotomy. It is necessary to determine of the amount of passive external rotation by examining the patient under anesthesia to decide whether lengthening of the subscapularis is needed at the time of arthroplasty.

Surgical Procedure

The anterior deltopectoral approach is used in the majority of cases. Important principles include preservation of the deltoid and protection of the axillary and musculocutaneous nerves.

The skin incision begins at the superior aspect of the clavicle over the acromioclavicular (AC) joint, passes over the coracoid process, and extends in a straight line to the insertion of the deltoid. The cephalic vein is identified in the deltopectoral interval, and we prefer to take the vein laterally with the deltoid muscle. A self-retaining shoulder retractor is used to retract the deltoid laterally and the pectoralis muscle medially. Additional exposure is provided by division of a portion of the pectoralis major insertion and is especially important in patients with a significant internal rotation contracture. Incision of the clavipectoral fascia just lateral to the short head of the biceps muscle allows access to the anterior humeral circumflex vessels and the subscapularis. We release a small portion of the coracoacromial ligament as well. If necessary, the origin of the conjoint tendon is partially divided 1 cm distal to the coracoid to allow gentle retraction of the short head of the biceps and coracobrachialis medially without excessive tension on the musculocutaneous nerve. The tendon is repaired at the completion of the procedure.

The axillary nerve may be palpated by sliding a finger down the anterior surface of the subscapularis tendon and hooking the nerve as it curves under the tendon. Identification of the nerve is especially important during revision procedures. The nerve must be carefully protected during release of the subscapularis tendon and inferior capsule. Before division of the inferior portion of the tendon and capsule, the anterior humeral circumflex ves-

sels are identified near the inferior border of the subscapularis and ligated.

At this time, the surgeon must decide whether lengthening of the subscapularis tendon is necessary. If adequate passive external rotation is present, the subscapularis tendon and the anterior shoulder capsule are divided approximately 1 cm medial to their insertion into the lesser tuberosity. If lengthening of the subscapularis is desired, the tendon and capsule are dissected subperiosteally from the lesser tuberosity as a unit and reattached to the humerus at the osteotomy site at the completion of the procedure (Fig. 21.5). This lengthens the tendon 2 to 3 cm and allows 20° to 30° of additional external rotation. The tendon is tagged with stay sutures and retracted medially.

The anterior inferior capsule is released to the 6-o'clock position with electrocautery or a number 15 blade, and care is taken to protect the axillary nerve at all times. External rotation, adduction, and extension of the arm will deliver the humeral head into the wound. If delivery of the head is difficult, it is probable that the inferior capsular release is incomplete.

The osteotomy of the humerus requires attention to detail (Fig. 21.6). In cases of osteoarthritis with significant osteophyte formation, it may be necessary to remove the osteophytes before making the cut to determine the true orientation of the articular surface. The ideal cut is made in

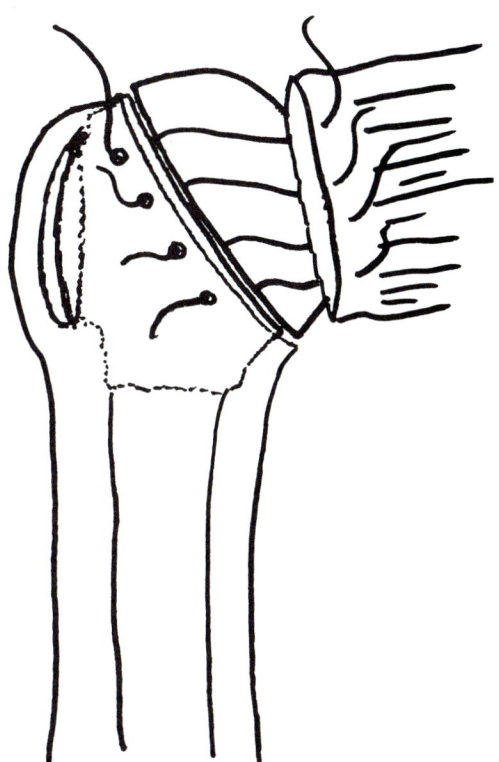

Figure 21.5. Procedure for lengthening the subscapularis tendon to improve external rotation: periosteal dissection of the subscapularis tendon off the lesser tuberosity and repair to the osteotomy site of humeral neck.

Figure 21.6. The technique of humeral osteotomy involves the use of a humeral resection guide in place with the arm externally rotated to the required retroversion.

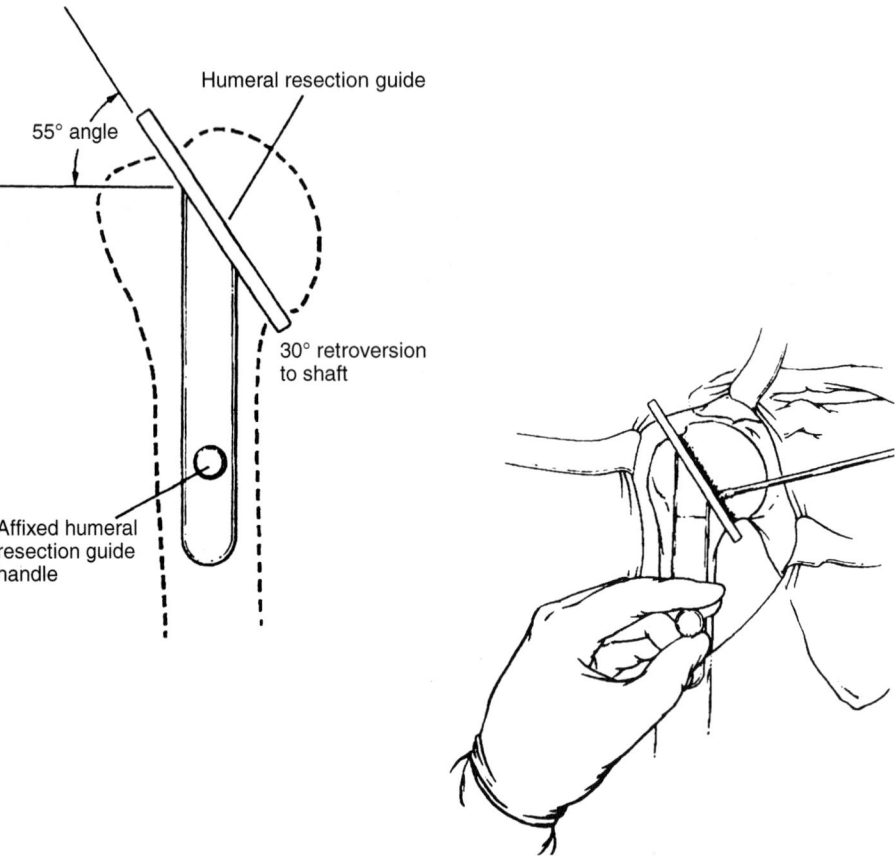

30° of retroversion, but this may vary significantly according to the specific pathologic process (72). The degree of the cut with respect to the humeral shaft must be matched to the prosthesis used; our prosthesis is equipped with a humeral head-cutting guide. The insertion of the rotator cuff into the greater tuberosity must be preserved. Often the amount of bone removed from the humeral head is surprisingly small. Once the head is removed, the rotator cuff is inspected, and any tears of the cuff are addressed. Every attempt must be made to repair a torn rotator cuff.

Excellent exposure of the glenoid cavity is afforded by the humeral head and osteophyte excision and capsular release. Successful glenoid resurfacing requires excellent exposure, normalization of the glenoid orientation, support of the glenoid component by bone rather than cement, secure fixation, and avoidance of overstuffing of the joint (Fig. 21.7). It is at this point that preoperative planning becomes quite important, because it is necessary to know whether the orientation of the glenoid is normal. CT scanning is invaluable in cases of glenoid erosion. When there are minor erosions, the glenoid face is burred on the high side to allow normal positioning of the component with respect to version. Severe cases of erosion require structural bone grafting of the defect (73).

We prefer to find the central canal of the glenoid with a high-speed burr. Placing a finger on the anterior glenoid neck helps define the limits of the glenoid vault. Concentric reaming of the glenoid surface to create a con-gruent fit between the glenoid and the back of the prosthesis is a critical part of glenoid preparation. A rasp is used to fine-tune the contour of the hole. A component is selected that covers the face of the glenoid with minimal overhang. A trial component is inserted and tested for stability to ensure that the prosthesis will be supported by bone. The bony surface is then irrigated and dried, and cement is pressurized digitally into the glenoid. The component is inserted and held with digital pressure while assistants remove any excess cement. When the cement has hardened, attention is turned to the proximal humerus.

To prepare the medullary canal of the humerus, begin with small-diameter reamers and progress to the size of the implant, taking care to avoid varus reaming and to protect the biceps tendon and rotator cuff. Rasps are used to prepare the proximal humerus for either a cemented or uncemented implant (Fig. 21.8). It is important to maintain the appropriate retroversion during humeral rasping. The flexed elbow and the biceps groove can be used as guides to the appropriate version of the prosthesis. A trial stem is inserted, and a modular head that reproduces the native head diameter and offset is selected. The shoulder is reduced, and stability and range of motion are assessed. We prefer a construct that allows 50% translation of the humeral head on the glenoid in the anteroposterior and superoinferior planes and 90° of abduction. It is important to ensure that adequate posterior laxity is present to allow 70° to 80° of internal rotation with the arm in 90° of abduction.

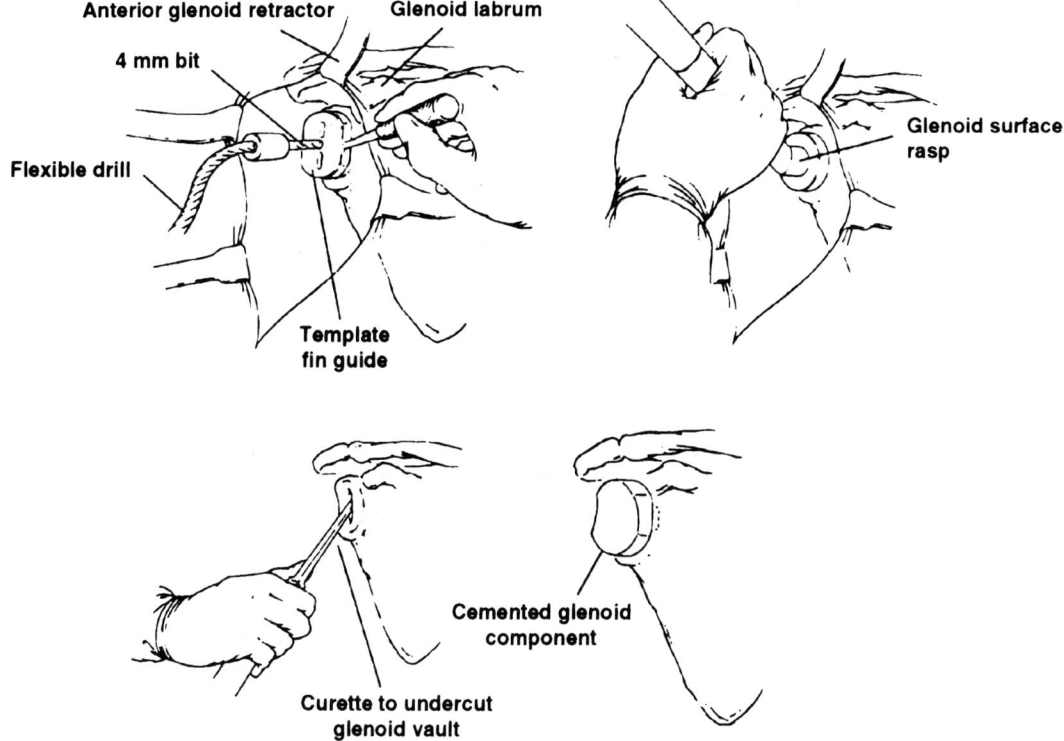

Figure 21.7. Preparing the glenoid for prosthesis insertion.

Figure 21.8. Preparing the humerus for prosthesis insertion.

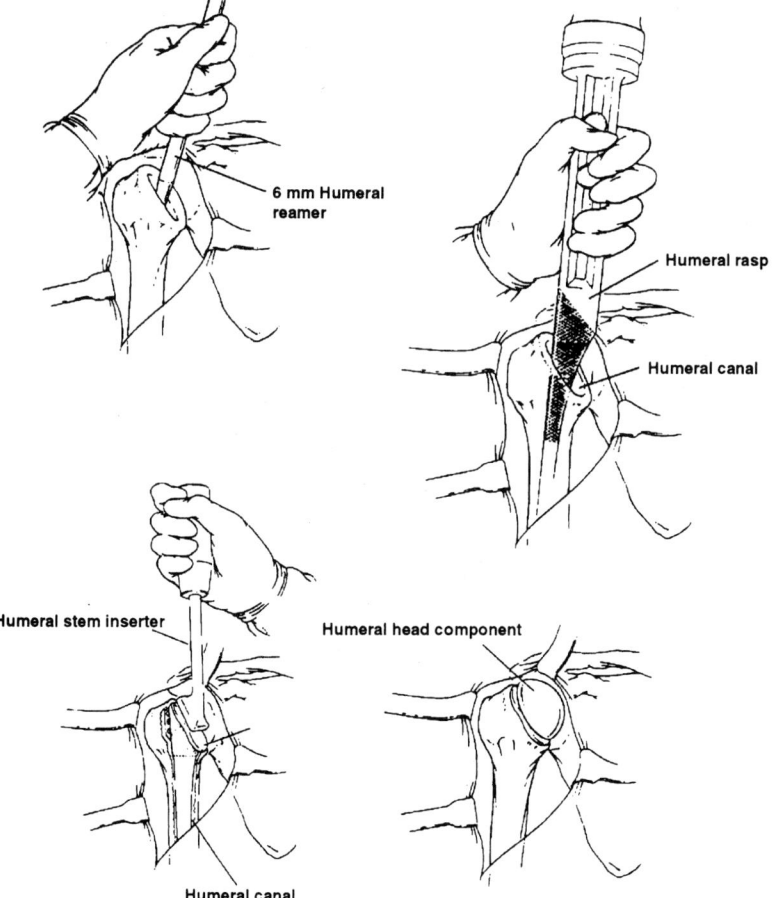

After insertion of the humeral prosthesis and impaction of the appropriate modular head, the subscapularis tendon is reapproximated using nonabsorbable sutures so that 40° of external rotation is possible. If lengthening was necessary, the tendon is reattached to the humerus at the site of the osteotomy. If preoperative external rotation was satisfactory, the tendon is reapproximated to its lateral stump. The wound is closed in layers over a suction drain and covered with sterile dressings (Fig. 21.9).

Surgical Pitfalls and Technical Mistakes

Prosthetic arthroplasty of the shoulder is a technically demanding procedure, and there are several pitfalls and technical mistakes that can lead to a suboptimal outcome (Fig. 21.10). The most common of these pitfalls are inadequate exposure, failure to address concomitant pathologies, improper osteotomy of the humerus, malposition of components, incorrect component size, and inadequate soft tissue tension.

Proper surgical exposure is a requirement of any operative procedure, and this is certainly the case for shoulder arthroplasty. Failure to adequately expose the glenoid and proximal humerus can lead to excessive retraction, with accompanying nerve and soft tissue injury, and increases the chance for fracture of the humerus during manipulation (74). It is important to use an incision that is long enough to allow tension-free retraction of soft tissues

and to release the pectoralis major from its insertion into the proximal humerus, if necessary. Damage to the musculocutaneous nerve can be avoided by the partial release of the conjoint tendon just distal to the coracoid process; exposure of the proximal humerus to facilitate osteotomy is aided by the complete release of a contracted inferior capsule, taking care to protect the axillary nerve.

It is necessary to appropriately address concomitant pathologies at the time of the shoulder arthroplasty. The preoperative examination—along with specific radiological studies, when indicated—makes the surgeon aware of coexisting rotator cuff and AC joint pathologies. The importance of an intact rotator cuff to the success of a shoulder arthroplasty cannot be overemphasized (29,69,75,76), and every attempt must be made to repair a torn cuff. Subacromial decompression should be done if impingement is noted following placement of the components. If significant symptoms seem to be arising from the AC joint as well as from the glenohumeral joint, then resection of the distal clavicle should be performed at the same time as the arthroplasty (56).

The position of the humeral osteotomy is critical to the success of the procedure. Too low an osteotomy carries the risk of transection of the insertion of the rotator cuff and may also damage the axillary nerve as it courses near the inferior capsule. It is often necessary to remove osteophytes along the inferior aspect of the humeral neck, which may mask the true size of the articular surface. The

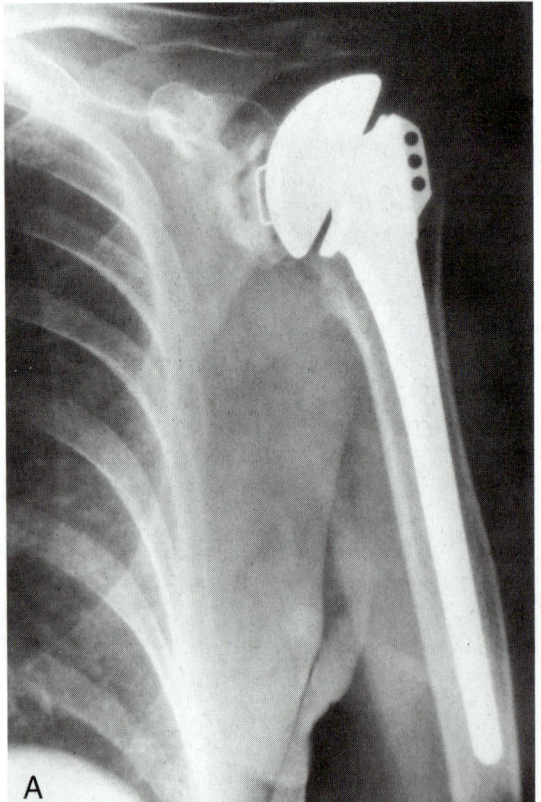
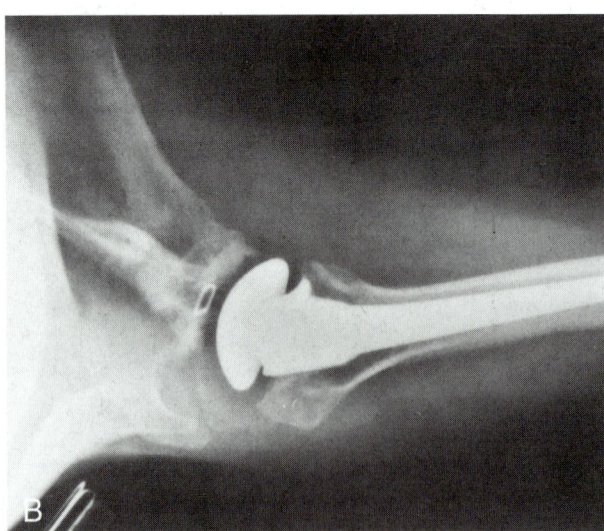

Figure 21.9. Total shoulder arthroplasty.

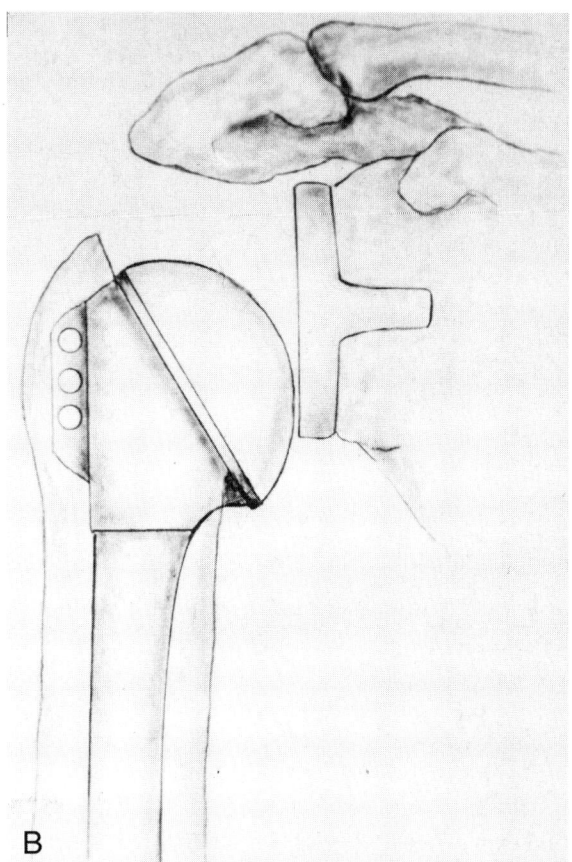

A

B

Figure 21.10. Common surgical pitfalls involve placing the humeral component in too superior of a position, leading to subacromial impingement (**A**); and placing the humeral component too low, causing instability (**B**). Reprinted with permission from Dines DM, Warren RF. Modular shoulder hemiarthroplasty for acute fractures: surgical considerations. Clin Orthop 1994;307:18–24.

humeral osteotomy also determines the version of the humeral component, the importance of which will be discussed shortly.

Both the humeral and glenoid component positions help determine the ultimate success of the shoulder arthroplasty. Malposition of the humeral component in the superoinferior plane can lead to pain and rotator cuff dysfunction if the prosthesis is too high and inadequate soft tissue tension and impingement of the greater tuberosity if the humerus is too low. The ideal height of the humerus is with the top of the head just above the top of the greater tuberosity. It is not uncommon for patients with acute and chronic trauma treated with hemiarthroplasty or TSA to have bone loss in the proximal humerus, which needs to be addressed by seating the prosthesis proud and using bone graft to restore the proper height. Positioning the head below the greater tuberosity leads to ineffective function of the rotator cuff and impingement of the greater tuberosity on the undersurface of the acromion. Rotational malposition of the humerus leads to instability; and excessive retroversion causes posterior instability and inadequate retroversion, leading to anterior instability. In certain circumstances (such as arthroplasty for osteoarthritis of recurrent instability), it may be desirable to vary the

version of the humeral component from the ideal of 30° of retroversion (72). Malposition of the glenoid component with respect to version can occur if there is unrecognized wear of the glenoid surface and may predispose to instability. It is again necessary to emphasize the need for adequate preoperative imaging studies. Poor fit of the glenoid on a strong bony base may also be associated with loosening of the glenoid component.

Selection of proper component size is important and helps avoid problems. The use of templates is necessary for selecting appropriate implant size. An uncemented humeral stem that is too large can, during insertion, fracture the humerus (74); when cement is used for fixation, a large humeral stem may produce a poor cement mantle. Too small a humeral stem leads to a poor press fit of an uncemented implant or to excessive cement when cement fixation is used. The ideal cement mantle is not known, but extrapolation from the hip and knee literature suggests that 2 to 3 mm is ideal (75,76). A glenoid component that is too thin may not give sufficient offset to provide optimal rotator cuff function and may, theoretically, lead to increased polyethylene wear. Excessive thickness of the glenoid component may overstuff the joint and cause pain and stiffness.

Finally, it is imperative to restore proper tissue tension in all planes. Restoration of proper humeral height allows the deltoid to function along its normal length–tension curve, and anatomic placement of the humerus and glenoid with respect to the tuberosities and rotator cuff muscles facilitates normal motion of the humerus on the glenoid. Inadequate rotator cuff function leads to superior translation of the humeral head and edge loading of the superior aspect of the glenoid, or the so-called rocking-horse glenoid (47) (Fig. 21.11); shortening of the subscapularis may cause excessive posterior translation of the humerus and edge loading of the posterior glenoid.

Rehabilitation

The specific rehabilitation program must be individualized for each patient and is critical to the results of the surgery. The passive range of motion of the shoulder is assessed at the completion of the surgery and is used to guide the therapist. The therapist is then instructed to lead the patient through passive range of motion of the shoulder, using the limits decided on by the surgeon, and to encourage active motion of the ipsilateral elbow, wrist, and hand. At 3 to 4 weeks, assisted pulley exercises are added; and by 4 to 6 weeks, isometric exercises can be started. Elastic resistance tubing strengthening exercises are added at 8 weeks, and gentle stretching is done as needed. Light weight-lifting may begin by 12 to 16 weeks following surgery.

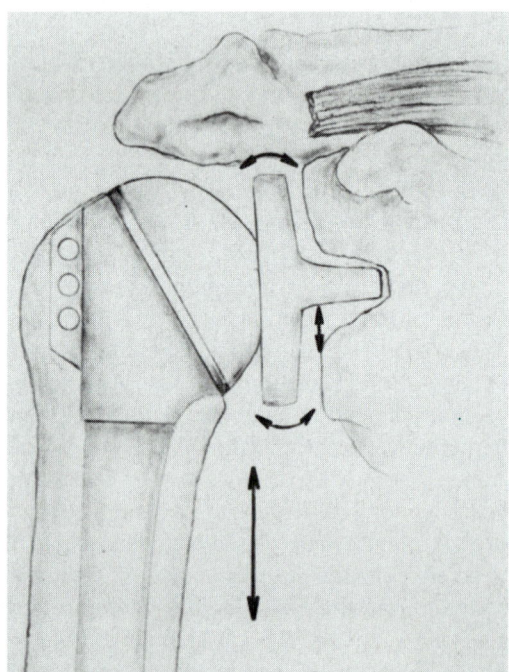

Figure 21.11. Glenoid resurfacing in the presence of rotator cuff insufficiency may lead to early glenoid loosening caused by edge loading of the superior part of the glenoid implant (the rocking-horse effect).

RESULTS

The overall results of shoulder arthroplasty are quite satisfying; pain relief occurs in 90 to 95% of patients (24,26,28–31,39,44,48,53,55,57,58,63,68,69,71,75,77–84). The return of motion varies and depends on the diagnosis, the degree of bone and soft tissue deficiencies (especially the rotator cuff), and the postoperative rehabilitation program. Generally, patients with osteoarthritis and avascular necrosis experience the greatest return of range of motion, followed by those with RA. Individuals with posttraumatic arthritis experience less return of motion, depending on the position of the tuberosities and the amount of soft tissue fibrosis (76). Radiolucent lines around the bone–cement interface of the glenoid component are quite common and range from 30 to 80% (29,44). However, revision of the glenoid for symptomatic loosening has been quite rare to date, at a rate of approximately 1% (33). One study quoted an overall survivorship of the Neer prosthesis of 74% at 11 years (85); another author reported a 9.6% chance of failure of an unconstrained TSA by 5 years (76).

Osteoarthritis

Results for TSA in osteoarthritis have been reported by several authors (24,26,44,75,77), and pain relief and ability to perform activities of daily living (ADLs) have been quite satisfactory. Improvement in range of motion is from 44° to 77° of flexion and from 32° to 51° of external rotation. The good return of strength and range of motion in the patients with osteoarthritis reflects the good quality of the rotator cuff.

We recently reviewed our experience with a modular system (Bio-Modular total shoulder system; Biomet Inc., Warsaw, IN) for osteoarthritis in a group of 70 patients with greater than 2 years of follow-up. A total of 94% of the patients had satisfactory results, and 80% scored good or excellent using the Hospital for Special Surgery score system. Use of the Bio-Modular total shoulder system was associated with a significant learning curve. All of the unsatisfactory and most of the fair results occurred in the first 30 patients. There were two subscapularis ruptures and two cases of instability, which were believed to be the result of improper head size. Glenoid lucency was seen in 33% but was greater than 2 mm in only 8%. Of the patients with significant glenoid lucencies, 2 had implantation of a metal-backed glenoid component, which has since been discontinued.

Rheumatoid Arthritis

Many authors have published the results of series involving cup arthroplasty, hemiarthroplasty, and TSA in rheumatoid patients (26,29,30,44,63,68,69,71,75,77,80,81). The most common prosthesis used today is an unconstrained one that resurfaces the glenoid and humerus. Patients have quite satisfactory pain relief and variable return of range of motion, strength, and ability to perform activities of daily living. The range of motion and ability to perform ADLs depend on the status of the rotator cuff, the ability of the surgeon to restore the patient's normal anatomy, and the systemic severity of the disease. When the rotator cuff can be repaired, pain relief and functional improvement are comparable to those obtained in patients with RA who have a normal or attenuated rotator cuff (31,80). Reported increases in range of motion are from 15° to 57° of forward flexion and from 13° to 60°of external rotation. These patients will often need a longer period of postoperative rehabilitation compared to other diagnoses (44). The reported survivorship of the Neer prosthesis in patients with RA is 92% at 11 years (85).

Avascular Necrosis

There are few series that deal specifically with the results of arthroplasty for avascular necrosis (AVN). Many of the larger series include patients with AVN, the results and complications of these patients are not reported separately from the general results. It appears, however, that these patients obtain excellent relief from pain and improvement in range of motion when treated with either hemiarthroplasty or TSA (53,79,82). The largest series of surgically treated individuals with AVN reported 94% pain relief when treated with hemiarthroplasty or total shoulder arthroplasty; postoperative range of motion averaged 161° of forward flexion and 77° of external rotation in the hemiarthroplasty group, and 150° of forward flexion and 67° of external rotation in the total shoulder arthroplasty group (82).

Posttraumatic Arthritis

The treatment of posttraumatic arthritis with either hemiarthroplasty or total shoulder arthroplasty has been reported, and relief of pain ranges from 88 to 98% (26,39,44,75,78). Increase in range of motion is from 12° to 50° of forward flexion and from 31° to 58° of external rotation. These patients may often need a limited goals-type of rehabilitation, depending on the status of the soft tissue (44).

We used modular prostheses to treat posttraumatic arthritis in 21 patients (39). Of these, 14 patients had hemiarthroplasty and 7 patients had total shoulder arthroplasty. Approximately 81% of patients had good to excellent results. Active elevation improved from 62° to 114°, external rotation improved 32°, and internal rotation averaged to L1. The patients who did not require tuberosity osteotomy had a significantly better result. Modular components significantly improved our ability to address bone and soft tissue defects.

Rotator Cuff Arthropathy

Several authors have summarized their results using hemiarthroplasty or total shoulder arthroplasty in patients with rotator cuff arthropathy (44,48,49,83). Pain relief oc-

curred in 83 to 92% of patients. Flexion increased from 43° to 50°, and external rotation increased by 10° to 15°. Pollock et al. (84) obtained better pain relief along with shorter operative time and hospital stay in a group of rotator cuff arthropathy patients treated with hemiarthroplasty compared to those treated with TSA. Neer et al. (44) recommended a limited goals-type of rehabilitation when treating these individuals with total shoulder arthroplasty.

We recently reported our results using large humeral head hemiarthroplasty for cuff tear arthropathy (86). We found that satisfactory pain relief but limited function could be expected in patients who did not have previous decompression acromioplasty. Patients with previous resection of the coracoacromial ligament all failed or had poor results.

COMPLICATIONS

Complications of prosthetic shoulder replacement can be divided into those occurring in hemiarthroplasty, nonconstrained total arthroplasty in nonrheumatoid patients, nonconstrained total arthroplasty in rheumatoid patients, constrained total arthroplasty in nonrheumatoid patients, and constrained total arthroplasty in rheumatoid patients (87). Overall, the most common complications requiring revision surgery are glenoid loosening and component instability. Constrained implants have a higher incidence of glenoid loosening (11.8%), dislocation (9.4%), and infection (3%), compared with unconstrained implants (64). The most common complications in unconstrained implants are glenoid loosening (4.7%), dislocation (2.7%), rotator cuff tear (2.2%), and subluxation (0.9%). Infection and nerve injury were relatively rare, occurring in 0.5 to 1% of patients (64,88).

Hemiarthroplasty

The most common complications of hemiarthroplasty are superior migration in 3.8% and component instability in 1% of patients. Less common complications are tuberosity nonunion in cases of acute and chronic trauma, postoperative fracture, and malposition of the humeral stem secondary to inadequate bone resection (87).

Unconstrained TSA

Complications occurring in nonconstrained total shoulder arthroplasties in nonrheumatoid patients include component instability in 3.5%, glenoid loosening in 2.7%, rotator cuff tear in 2.0%, and humeral loosening in 0.8% of patients (87). Nonconstrained implants in rheumatoid patients have a higher incidence of complications such as superior migration (9%), glenoid loosening (4.2%), intraoperative fracture (2.5%), component instability (1.6%), humeral subsidence (1.6%), rotator cuff tear (1.6%), infection (1%), humeral loosening (0.9%), and technical failure (0.9%) (87).

Constrained TSA

Constrained total shoulder arthroplasty also has a relatively high incidence of complications in both nonrheumatoid and rheumatoid patients. Complications in nonrheumatoid patients include instability in 10.2%, broken components in 9.4%, glenoid loosening in 6.3%, infection in 2.4%, and postoperative fracture in 2.4%. Complications in rheumatoid patients include glenoid loosening in 10.4%, instability in 5.2%, humeral loosening in 2.6%, infection in 2.0%, and postoperative fracture in 2.0%. It is clear that component loosening, breakage, and instability represent the majority of complications in constrained arthroplasties.

SUMMARY

Total shoulder replacement has become the procedure of choice for many disabling glenohumeral arthritides. In most cases, excellent long-term results can be achieved. Improved understanding of the pertinent pathologic anatomy, better surgical technique, and improved prosthetic options have led to these improved results.

The results of TSA are directly related to the surgeon's ability to deal with soft tissue repair and balancing, proper prosthetic placement and fixation, and a comprehensive rehabilitation program prescribed by the findings at surgery.

REFERENCES

1. Lugli T. Artificial shoulder joint by Pean (1893): the facts of an exceptional intervention and the prosthetic method. Clin Orthop 1978;133:215–218.
2. Moore KL. The upper limb. In: Moore KL, ed. Clinically oriented anatomy. Baltimore: Williams & Wilkins, 1985:651–654.
3. Laing PG. The arterial supply of the adult humerus. J Bone Joint Surg 1956;38A:1105–1116.
4. Gerber C, Schneeberger AG, Winh TS. The arterial vascularization of the humeral head. J Bone Joint Surg 1990;72A:1486–1494.
5. Hoppenfeld S, deBoer P. Surgical exposures in orthopaedics. The anatomic approach. 2nd ed. Philadelphia: Lippincott, 1994.
6. Abbott LC, Saunders JBM, Hogey H, et al. Surgical approaches to the shoulder joint. J Bone Joint Surg 1949;31A:235–244.
7. Linell EA. The distribution of nerves in the upper limb with reference to variabilities and their clinical significance. J Anat 1921;55:79–112.
8. Burkhead WZ, Scheinberg RR, Box G. Surgical anatomy of the axillary nerve. J Shoulder Elbow Surg 1992;1:31–36.
9. Flatow EL, Bigliani LU, April EW. An anatomical study of the musculocutaneous nerve and its relationship to the coracoid process. Clin Orthop 1989;244:166–171.
10. Johnston T. The movements of the shoulder joint. A plea for the use of the 'plane of the scapula' as the plane of reference for movements occurring at the humero-scapular joint. Br J Surg 1937;25:252–260.
11. Saha A. Mechanism of shoulder movements and a plea for the recognition of "zero position" of glenohumeral joint. Indian J Surg 1950;12:153–165.
12. Saha A. Dynamic stability of the glenohumeral joint. Acta Orthop Scand 1971;42:491–505.
13. Cyprine JM, Vasey HM, Burdet A, et al. Humeral retrotorsion and glenohumeral relationship in the normal shoulder and in recurrent anterior dislocation (scapulometry). Clin Orthop 1983;175:8.
14. Jones FW. Attainment of upright positions. Nature 1940;146:26.
15. Lewis WH. The development of the arm in man. Am J Anat 1902;1:145.
16. Watson DMS. The evolution of the tetrapod shoulder girdle and forelimb. J Anat 1918;52:1.
17. Gartsman GM, Becker DA. Shoulder: reconstruction. In: Orthopaedic knowledge update 4. Rosemont, IL: American Academy of Orthopaedic Surgeons, 1993:303.
18. Steindler A. Kinesiology of the human body under normal and pathological conditions. Springfield, IL: Thomas, 1955.
19. Friedman RJ. Biomechanics and design of shoulder arthroplasties. In: Friedman RJ, ed. Arthroplasty of the shoulder. New York: Thieme, 1994:27–40.
20. Friedman R, Hawthorne K, Genez B. The use of computerized tomography in the measurement of glenoid version. J Bone Joint Surg 1992;74A:1032–1037.
21. Poppen NK, Walker PS. Forces at the glenohumeral joint in abduction. Clin Orthop 1978;135:165–170.
22. Basmajian JV, Bazant FJ. Factors preventing downward dislocation of the shoulder joint. J Bone Joint Surg 1959;41A:1182.
23. Poppen NK, Walker PS. Normal and abnormal motion of the shoulder. J Bone Joint Surg 1976;58A:195–201.
24. Neer CS. Replacement arthroplasty for glenohumeral osteoarthritis. J Bone Joint Surg 1974;56A:1–13.
25. Dines DM, Altchek DW. Technical considerations in total shoulder arthroplasty. J Prof Sports Care 1993;4: 93–94.
26. Cofield RH. Total shoulder arthroplasty with the Neer prosthesis. J Bone Joint Surg 1984;66A:899–906.
27. Watson K. Glenohumeral osteoarthritis. In: Friedman RJ, ed. Arthroplasty of the shoulder. New York: Thieme, 1994:147.
28. Cofield RH. Degenerative and arthritic problems of the glenohumeral joint. In: Rockwood CA, Matsen FA, eds. The shoulder. Philadelphia: Saunders, 1990:678–749.
29. Kelly IG, Foster RS, Fisher WD. Neer total shoulder replacement in rheumatoid arthritis. J Bone Joint Surg 1987;69B:723–726
30. McCoy SR, Warren RF, Bade HA, et al. Total shoulder arthroplasty in rheumatoid arthritis. J Arthroplasty 1989;4:105–113.
31. Friedman RJ, Thornhill TS, Thomas WH, Sledge CB. Nonconstrained total shoulder replacement in patients who have rheumatoid arthritis and class-IV function. J Bone Joint Surg 1989;71A:494–498.
32. Ennevaara K. Painful shoulder joint in rheumatoid arthritis. Acta Rheumatol Scand 1967;11:1–116.
33. Neer CS. The shoulder. In: Kelly WN, Harris ED, Ruddy S, Sledge CB, eds. Textbook of rheumatology. 3rd ed. Philadelphia: Saunders, 1989:2013–2026.
34. Hungerford DS, Lennox DW. The importance of increased intraosseous pressure in the development of osteonecrosis of the femoral head: implications for treatment. Orthop Clin North Am 1985;16:635–654.
35. Jones JP Jr. Osteonecrosis. In: McCarty DJ, ed. Arthritis and allied conditions. Philadelphia: Lea & Febiger, 1985:1356–1373.
36. Cofield RH. Osteonecrosis. In: Friedman RJ, ed. Arthroplasty of the shoulder. New York: Thieme, 1994:170–182.
37. Salvati EA, Cornell CN. Long-term follow-up of total hip replacement in patients with avascular necrosis. Instr Course Lect 1988;37:67–73
38. Piston RW, Engh CA, DeCarvallio PI, Suthers K. Osteonecrosis of the femoral head treated with total hip arthroplasty without cement. J Bone Joint Surg 1994;76A:202–214.
39. Dines DM, Warren RF, Moeckel DM, Altchek D. Post-traumatic changes of the proximal humerus, malunion, osteonecrosis and non-union: treatment with modular hemiarthroplasty and total shoulder arthroplasty. J Shoulder Elbow Surg 1993;2:11–18.
40. Svend-Hansen H. Displaced proximal humeral fractures. A review of 49 patients. Acta Orthop Scand 1974;45:359–364.
41. Frich LH, Sojbjerg JO, Sneppen O. Shoulder arthroplasty in complex acute and chronic proximal humeral fractures. Orthopedics 1991;14:949–954.
42. Dines DM, Altchek D. Avoiding complications in hemiarthroplasty for fractures of the proximal humerus. Complications Orthop 1991;6:25–31.

43. Moeckel DM, Dines DM, Warren RF, Altchek D. Modular hemi-arthroplasty for acute fractures of the proximal humerus. J Bone Joint Surg 1992;74A:884–889.

44. Neer CS, Watson KC, Stanton FJ. Recent experience in total shoulder replacement. J Bone Joint Surg 1982;64A:319–337.

45. Neer CS. Glenohumeral arthroplasty. In: Neer CS, ed. Shoulder reconstruction. Philadelphia: Saunders, 1990.

46. Neer CS, Craig EV, Fukuda H. Cuff tear arthropathy. J Bone Joint Surg 1983;65A:1232–1244.

47. Franklin JL, Barrett WP, Jackins SE, Matsen FA. Glenoid loosening in total shoulder arthroplasty—association with rotator cuff deficiency. J Arthroplasty 1988;31:39–46.

48. Arntz CT, Jackins S, Matsen FA. Prosthetic replacement of the shoulder for the treatment of defects in the rotator cuff and the surface of the glenohumeral joint. J Bone Joint Surg 1993;75A:485–491.

49. Arntz CT, Matsen FA, Jackins S. Surgical management of complex irreparable rotator cuff deficiency. J Arthroplasty 1991;6:363–370.

50. Riordan J, Deippe P. Arthritis of the glenohumeral joint. Baillieres Clin Rheumatol 1989;3:607–625.

51. Souter WA. The surgical treatment of the rheumatoid shoulder. Ann Acad Med Singapore 1983;12:243–255.

52. Friedman R. Total shoulder biomechanics before and after total joint arthroplasty. Paper presented at the 17th SICOT Meeting, 1990.

53. Cruess RL. Steroid-induced avascular necrosis of the head of the humerus: natural history and management. J Bone Joint Surg 1976;58B:313–317.

54. Silvka J, Resnick D. An improved radiographic view of the glenohumeral joint. Can Assoc Radiol J 1979;30:83–85.

55. Boyd AJ, Thomas WH, Scott RD, et al. Total shoulder arthroplasty versus hemiarthroplasty. J Arthroplasty 1990;5:329–336.

56. Clayton ML, Ferlic DC, Jeffers PD. Prosthetic arthroplasties of the shoulder. Clin Orthop 1982;164:184–191.

57. Cofield RH, Frankle MA, Zuckerman JD. Humeral head replacement for glenohumeral arthritis. Semin Arthroplasty 1995;6:214–221.

58. Torchia ME, Cofield RH, Settergren CR. Total shoulder arthroplasty with the Neer prosthesis: long-term results. J Shoulder Elbow Surg 1997;6:495–505.

59. Brems J. The glenoid component in total shoulder arthroplasty. J Shoulder Elbow Surg 1993;2:47–54.

60. Post M. Constrained arthroplasty of the shoulder. Orthop Clin North Am 1987;18:455–462.

61. Post M. Shoulder arthroplasty and total shoulder replacement. In: Post M, ed. The shoulder. Philadelphia: Lea & Febiger, 1988:221–278.

62. Post M, Jablon M, Miller H, Singh M. Constrained total shoulder joint replacement: a critical review. Clin Orthop 1979;144:135–150.

63. Brostrom LB, Wallensten R, Olsson E, Anderson D. The Kessel prosthesis in total shoulder arthroplasty: a five year experience. Clin Orthop 1992;277:155–160.

64. Cofield RH, Edgerton BC. Total shoulder arthroplasty: complications and revision surgery. Instr Course Lect 1990;39:449–462.

65. Engelbrecht E, Heinert K. More than ten years' experience with unconstrained shoulder replacement. In: Kolbel R, Helbig B, Blauth W, eds. Shoulder replacement. Berlin: Springer-Verlag, 1987:85–91.

66. McElwain JP, English E. The early results of porous-coated total shoulder arthroplasty. Clin Orthop 1987;218:217–224.

67. Amstutz HC, Sew Hoy AL, Clarke IC. UCLA anatomic total shoulder arthroplasty. Clin Orthop 1981;155:7–20.

68. Figgie MP, Inglis AE, Figgie HE, et al. Custom total shoulder arthroplasty in inflammatory arthritis: preliminary results. J Arthroplasty 1992;7:1–6.

69. Barrett WP, Thornhill TS, Thomas WH, et al. Nonconstrained total shoulder arthroplasty in patients with polyarticular rheumatoid arthritis. J Arthroplasty 1989;4:91–96.

70. Torchia ME, Cofield RH. Long-term results of Neer shoulder arthroplasty. Orthop Trans 1995;18:977.

71. Figgie HE, Inglis AE, Goldberg VM, et al. An analysis of factors affecting the long-term results of total shoulder arthroplasty in inflammatory arthritis. J Arthroplasty 1988;3:123–130.

72. Pritchett JW, Clark JM. Prosthetic replacement for chronic unreduced dislocations of the shoulder. Clin Orthop 1987;216:89–93.

73. Neer CS, Morrison. Glenoid bone grafting in total shoulder replacement. J Bone Joint Surg 1988;70A:1154–1162.

74. Bonutti PM, Hawkins RJ. Fracture of the humeral shaft associated with total replacement arthroplasty of the shoulder: a case report. J Bone Joint Surg 1992;74A:617–618.

75. Barrett WP, Franklin JL, Jackins SE, et al. Total shoulder arthroplasty. J Bone Joint Surg 1987;69A:865–872.

76. Cofield RH. Unconstrained total shoulder prostheses. Clin Orthop 1983;173:97–108.

77. Hawkins RJ, Bell RH, Jallay B. Total shoulder arthroplasty. Clin Orthop 1989;242:188–194.

78. Tanner MW, Cofield RH. Prosthetic arthroplasty for fractures and fracture-dislocations of the proximal humerus. Clin Orthop 1983;179:116–128.

79. Kay SP, Amstutz HC. Shoulder hemiarthroplasty at UCLA. Clin Orthop 1988;228:42–48.

80. Petersson CJ. Shoulder surgery in rheumatoid arthritis. Acta Orthop Scand 1986;57:222–226.

81. Jonsson E, Egund N, Kelly I, et al. Cup arthroplasty of the rheumatoid shoulder. Acta Orthop Scand 1986;57:542–546.

82. Rutherford CS, Cofield RH. Osteonecrosis of the shoulder. Orthop Trans 1987;11:239.

83. Williams GR Jr. Glenohumeral acromial arthritis and severe cuff disease: management with hemiarthroplasty. Orthop Trans 1992;16:743.

84. Pollock RG, Deliz EB, McIlveen SJ, et al. Prosthetic replacement in rotator cuff deficient shoulders. J Shoulder Elbow Surg 1992;1:173–186.

85. Brennan, et al. Survivorship of unconstrained total shoulder replacement. J Bone Joint Surg 1989;71A:1289–1296.

86. Field LD, Dines DM, Zabinski SJ, Warren RF. Hemiarthroplasty of the shoulder for rotator cuff arthropathy. J Shoulder Elbow Surg 1997;6:18–23.

87. Silliman JF, Hawkins RJ. Complications following shoulder arthroplasty. In: Friedman RJ, ed. Arthroplasty of the shoulder. New York: Thieme, 1994:242–253.

88. Kalainov D, Bisson L, Brause B, et al. Management of infected shoulder arthroplasties. Paper presented at the Meeting of the Eastern Orthopaedic Association, Rome, Italy, 1995.

chapter 22

Jo A. Hannafin and Answorth A. Allen

Frozen Shoulder

The term *frozen shoulder* is a generic expression used to describe the pathologic loss of the normal mobility of the glenohumeral joint. It encompasses both primary adhesive capsulitis, which is characterized by idiopathic, progressive, and painful loss of active and passive shoulder motion; secondary adhesive capsulitis, which results from a known intrinsic or extrinsic cause; and secondary shoulder stiffness following surgical intervention. Evaluation and successful treatment of the stiff glenohumeral joint are critical to resumption of normal shoulder function and prevention of additional injury to the shoulder.

The absence of glenohumeral motion alters the normal kinematic relationship of the glenohumeral and scapulothoracic joints and can result in the development of secondary shoulder syndromes, including shoulder impingement and scapulothoracic pain. The management of primary and secondary adhesive capsulitis and secondary stiff shoulder is controversial. Treatment options documented in the literature include benign neglect, home-based therapy (1), supervised physical therapy (2,3), nonsteroidal anti-inflammatory medications (3,4), intra-articular injections (2,5), distension arthrography (6–8), closed manipulation (9,10), open surgical release (11), and more recently, arthroscopy and arthroscopic capsular release (12–16). This chapter summarizes our approach to the management of primary and secondary adhesive capsulitis of the shoulder; it does not address the problem of the iatrogenic stiff shoulder.

RELEVANT ANATOMY AND PATHOGENESIS

To formulate a logical approach to the treatment of primary and secondary adhesive capsulitis of the shoulder, it is necessary to understand the underlying structural and cellular pathophysiologic processes of this syndrome. A review of the literature reveals a multitude of strategies for the treatment of adhesive capsulitis that have given variable results. Neviaser and Neviaser (17,18) described the arthroscopic stages of adhesive capsulitis and stressed the importance of an individualized treatment plan based on the clinical stages of the syndrome. We believe that the inconsistency in the literature reflects a lack of understanding of the stages of adhesive capsulitis, which play a significant role in both diagnosis and treatment.

Adhesive capsulitis can be broken down into four stages, as originally described by Nevaiser (18). A correlation between the clinical presentation, examination under anesthesia, and histologic findings at biopsy is outlined in Table 22.1 for stages 1 to 3. In stage 1, patients present with pain, which is often described as achy at rest and sharp with extremes of motion. Symptoms have generally been present for less than 3 months; however, a steady progression in loss of motion is noted by the patient. Loss of extension and internal rotation and external rotation with the arm at the side is present along with a more subtle loss of forward flexion and abduction. A significantly improved range of motion is obtain after the glenohumeral joint is injected with a local anesthetic or after the patient is under anesthesia. Arthroscopic examination reveals a hypertrophic, vascular synovitis that coats the entire capsular lining but is most pronounced in the anterior-superior capsule. Biopsy of this material demonstrates an occasional lymphocytic infiltrate with a hypervascular synovitis and normal underlying capsular structure.

In stage 2 adhesive capsulitis, the patient has experienced symptoms for 3 to 9 months along with a progressive loss of motion and the persistence of the pain pattern described above. Examination following local anesthetic infiltration or a scalene block reveals relief of pain, without significant improvement in range of motion; thus the motion loss in stage 2 reflects a loss of capsular volume and flexibility, rather than a response to the painful synovitis. Arthroscopic examination reveals a dense, proliferative synovitis that remains hypervascular. Capsular biopsy is notable for a hypervascular synovitis with perivascular scar formation and a capsular fibroplasia with new deposition of disorganized collagen fibrils. No inflammatory infiltrates have been reported in stage 2.

| table | 22.1 | Clinical, Arthroscopic, and Histologic Stages of Adhesive Capsulitis of the Shoulder |

Stage	Clinical Examination	Examination under Anesthesia	Arthroscopic Examination	Histologic Examination
1	Painful limitation of glenohumeral motion	Full range of motion	Diffuse hypervascular synovitis	Hypervascular synovitis; normal underlying capsule
2	Painful limitation of glenohumeral motion	Limited range of motion	Diffuse pedunculated hypervascular synovitis	Hypervascular synovitis; proliferative fibroblastic capsular response; disorganized collagen
3	Mild or minimal pain at the end range of motion; significant loss of motion	Significant loss of motion	Minimal synovitis	Mild synovial hyperplasia; capsular fibroplasia with extensive scar formation in the underlying capsule

In stage 3, patients present with a history of painful stiffening of the shoulder and significant loss of range of motion. Symptoms have been present for 9 to 14 months and have been noted to change over time. The patients often recall an extremely painful phase that has resolved, leaving them with a relatively pain-free but stiff shoulder. Examination is unchanged by injection of local anesthetic or evaluation under anesthesia, reflecting the persistent loss of capsular volume and scarring of the glenohumeral joint capsule. Arthroscopic examination is generally unremarkable compared to stages 1 and 2. A residual filmy synovial layer is visible with patches of synovial thickening without hypervascularity. Capsular biopsy reveals a dense, hypercellular collagenous tissue.

Stage 4, or the thawing stage of adhesive capsulitis, is characterized by the slow, steady recovery of range of motion, resulting from capsular remodeling in response to use of the arm and shoulder. When examining a patient with a stiff or painful shoulder, it is helpful to remember that the clinical stage of the disease directs the treatment options.

INITIAL FINDINGS, PHYSICAL EXAMINATION, AND DIAGNOSIS

Primary and Secondary Adhesive Capsulitis

The diagnosis of primary adhesive capsulitis is made from the history and physical examination. This is an idiopathic condition and the diagnosis is made when other causes of pain and motion loss are eliminated. Primary adhesive capsulitis is more common in women than in men and is generally seen in patients aged 40 to 60 years. Approximately 30% of patients will report a history of mild trauma to the shoulder. Prolonged shoulder immobilization, radiation therapy following breast surgery, cervical spine disease, diabetes mellitus, and thyroid disease are reported risk factors for the development of primary adhesive capsulitis.

Secondary adhesive capsulitis occurs after rotator cuff trauma, shoulder or upper extremity fractures, and shoulder surgery. Secondary adhesive capsulitis is also seen concomitantly with impingement syndrome, calcific tendonitis, and glenohumeral arthritis.

The physical examination should always include an evaluation of the cervical spine and the shoulder. Although emphasis should be placed on both passive and active range of motion, passive motion loss is the key. The initial range of motion should be carefully documented to determine the efficacy of the treatment plan. Pure glenohumeral motion is measured while limiting scapulothoracic motion; *combined* motion includes glenohumeral and scapulothoracic motion. A series of measurements are taken to evaluate glenohumeral and total shoulder motion. Active and passive forward flexion, abduction, internal rotation (measured by having the patient place the thumb at the highest point possible on the spinous process) and external rotation in neutral abduction are measured and recorded with the patient standing. Passive glenohumeral motion is then measured with the patient supine and scapulothoracic motion constrained by manual pressure on the acromion and scapula. Measurements are made in the coronal plane instead of the scapular plane, because the anterior capsule is more lax in the scapular plane and hence gives the appearance of better range of motion. Measurements of supine passive internal and external rotation at 45° of glenohumeral abduction and maximal glenohumeral abduction are made and recorded.

An intra-articular injection can be extremely useful in primary and secondary adhesive capsulitis for diagnostic and therapeutic purposes. The injection of the glenohumeral joint in adhesive capsulitis is analogous to the Neer test for the impingement syndrome. Review of the stages, outlined above, provides the rationale for early intra-articular injection. Injection of a local anesthetic and corticosteroid in a patient with adhesive capsulitis is both diagnostic and therapeutic. Following injection, passive glenohumeral range of motion is reevaluated. Significant improvement in pain and range of motion confirms a stage 1 status. Significant improvement in pain with no significant improvement in range of motion characterizes stage 2 disease. Because of the lack of glenohumeral synovitis, there is no indication for glenohumeral injection in stages 3 and 4.

Secondary Shoulder Stiffness

The sine qua non of the secondary shoulder stiffness is the presence of an intrinsic shoulder abnormality, such as rotator cuff disease; postsurgical scarring; or trauma to the soft tissues, with or without a fracture, in the presence of prolonged immobilization. Systemic disorders, such as diabetes mellitus and other endocrine disorders, may also be contributory. These patients present with a discrete limitation of motion in specific planes, depending on what portion of the capsule is involved. For example, contractures in the anterior-superior capsular region (i.e., the rotator interval) limit external rotation of the adducted shoulder. Contracture of the anterior-inferior capsule results in loss of external rotation with the shoulder abducted. Scarring of the posterior capsule limits internal rotation in adduction and abduction and leads to loss of horizontal or cross-chest adduction. There is also an obligatory posterior-superior translation of the humeral head, which can result in secondary shoulder impingement.

The workup should include a careful history and examination. The surgical treatment of the secondary stiff shoulder is complicated by the sequelae of previous surgery, such as alteration of extra-articular tissue planes and iatrogenic contractures, and is not discussed here.

RADIOLOGIC STUDIES

Primary and Secondary Adhesive Capsulitis

Routine radiographic evaluation is recommended, including AP views in internal and external rotation, an axillary view, and an outlet view to rule out other causes for a stiff, painful shoulder (such as glenohumeral arthritis, calcific tendonitis, and long-standing rotator cuff disease). Radiographs are usually negative in patients with primary adhesive capsulitis, although there may be evidence of disuse osteopenia. Historically, arthrography was used for diagnostic purposes to demonstrate a decreased joint capacity (less than 5 to 10 mm) in stages 2 to 4; however, this is not used routinely. If the clinical diagnosis is unclear, MRI may be useful for evaluating the rotator cuff or labrum; but it is not routinely recommended.

Secondary Shoulder Stiffness

Routine radiographs provide information about joint congruity or fractures. An MRI scan provides information about the soft tissues, such as the rotator cuff.

TREATMENT

Nonoperative Treatment

PRIMARY AND SECONDARY ADHESIVE CAPSULITIS

Patients present in different stages of adhesive capsulitis, and management should be individualized to the given patient. There are, however, some basic principles that can be recommended. Patients who present with painful limitation of motion are placed on oral nonsteroidal anti-inflammatory drugs (NSAIDs), supplemented with narcotics as necessary. If a patient presents in stage 1 or 2, an intra-articular injection is performed. We prefer to start these patients on a supervised physical therapy program that emphasizes pendulums and gentle range of motion. The patient should be progressed from passive range of motion to active-assisted range of motion as tolerated. The patient is reevaluated after 2 weeks to determine the short-term response to the intra-articular injection. If the patient remains pain free there is no indication for a second intra-articular injection. Approximately 30% of patients in stages 1 and 2 require a second injection for full relief of the painful synovitis, which will often provide significant pain relief and allow more aggressive physical therapy.

Although most patients show significant improvement by 12 to 16 weeks, some patients do not improve and in fact will get worse. The options at this point include continued physical therapy or surgical intervention. Traditionally, the literature has recommended a prolonged course of physical therapy over many months. This may be extremely uncomfortable, and a subsection of patients are not able to tolerate this approach. Furthermore, there is the issue of the cost-effectiveness of a prolonged physical therapy program. At this point, the options of arthroscopic inspection, synovectomy, and closed manipulation are discussed with the patient. Rarely is surgical intervention indicated for stage 1 and early stage 2 adhesive capsulitis, because the painful synovitis can be well controlled with the use of intra-articular corticosteroid. The late stage 2 or stage 3 patient should be given the options of continued conservative treatment, arthroscopy, manipulation, and/or arthroscopic capsular release. The risks and benefits of these approaches should be discussed, including the risks of fracture, neurovascular injury, residual stiffness, instability, and infection.

SECONDARY SHOULDER STIFFNESS

Eccentric contracture of the joint capsule can have dire biomechanical consequences for the joint. For example, a tight anterior capsule can result in posterior subluxation of the humeral head relative to the glenoid, eccentric articular contact, and subsequent development of osteoarthritis. In general, an aggressive supervised therapy program is often ineffective in secondary shoulder stiffness. In these cases, it is important to decide if the cause of the limitation of motion is coming from an extra-articular or intra-articular source. The source will determine the best surgical approach to the management of this problem.

Operative Treatment

CLOSED MANIPULATION

Closed manipulation is contraindicated in patients with significant osteopenia or recent surgical repair of soft tissues about the shoulder; it is also contraindicated if there is any concern about fractures, disruption of the repair, nerve injuries, and instability. For shoulder manipulation to be successful, the patient must be well motivated and capable of performing the follow-up exercise program to maintain range of motion.

We prefer an arthroscopic examination of the glenohumeral joint before conducting closed or arthroscopically assisted manipulation. General or regional anesthesia can be used; however, our preference is to use an interscalene block with a long-acting agent, such as bupivacaine. The block can be performed with either a single percutaneous injection or through an indwelling interscalene catheter. The use of 0.5% bupivacaine will give about 12 h of anesthesia, which will reduce the patient's requirement for narcotics and increase his or her tolerance to physical therapy. The block can be repeated on the mornings of the 1st and 2nd postoperative days, if indicated based on the patient's pain tolerance. If the interscalene catheter is used, continuous bupivacaine infusion is administered for prolonged anesthesia.

ARTHROSCOPIC EVALUATION AND TREATMENT

Historically, arthroscopy has been of little diagnostic and therapeutic value in patients with adhesive capsulitis of the shoulder. It has been suggested, however, that the arthroscope may help delineate disease, document the result of closed manipulation, and treat concomitant intra-articular and subacromial disease (12–15). For these reasons, we are prepared to perform an arthroscopic capsular release if there are no suspected extra-articular factors contributing to the motion loss. The force of manual manipulation required to regain motion is greatly reduced by arthroscopically releasing the capsule before manipulating the shoulder.

SURGICAL TECHNIQUE

It is essential to document glenohumeral and total range of motion before initiating the surgical procedure. The timing of arthroscopy and manipulation remains controversial. Some surgeons prefer to manipulate the shoulder first and follow with the arthroscopic evaluation (12); however, rupture of the capsule with manipulation will greatly increase the risk of fluid extravasation in the soft tissues surrounding the shoulder joint and limit the surgeon's ability to perform a thorough synovectomy in stage 2. We prefer to perform a diagnostic arthroscopy and synovectomy before manipulating the shoulder, minimizing fluid extravasation into the soft tissues.

It may be difficult to insert the arthroscope into a stiff shoulder because of the capsular contracture and decreased joint volume (13,15); chondral damage is avoided by inserting the arthroscope over the humeral head. The capsule is more difficult to penetrate with the blunt trocar, because of the capsular fibrosis and thickening; and it is helpful to distend the capsule with fluid via a spinal needle before inserting the arthroscope. The smaller 3.8-mm arthroscope has been recommended (15), but we have routinely been able to use a standard arthroscope.

The arthroscopic appearance of the joint depends on the stage of adhesive capsulitis (as outlined previously). In stage 1, a diffuse hypervascular synovitis is noted, which may have areas of focal thickening in the anterior-superior capsule and along the proximal biceps tendon (Fig. 22.1). An arthroscopic cannula is inserted just underneath the biceps tendon, and this synovium is removed atraumatically with a 4.5-mm motorized shaver. It is important in stage 1 to perform a thorough synovectomy; thus it is necessary to view the shoulder from both anterior and posterior portals. An attempt should be made to resect any areas of synovitis in the inferior pouch. This is technically feasible in a stage 1 shoulder, but is often difficult in a stage 2 shoulder.

A capsular biopsy is routinely taken to confirm the histologic stage of the syndrome. In stage 2, the synovial lining remains hypervascular but is thicker and more pedunculated in appearance (Fig. 22.2). Again, a thorough synovectomy is indicated, and a capsular biopsy is obtained.

In stage 3, residual synovial thickening or scarring is noted, but the hypervascular appearance has generally resolved. The rotator interval region and the tendon of the subscapularis may be obscured by a sheet of capsular scar, which can be carefully débrided (Fig. 22.3).

At this point, the arthroscopic instruments are removed and a gentle manipulation is performed. In late stage 1 or early stage 2 disease with mild scarring and thickening of the capsule, a gentle manipulation will often regain full range of motion. We routinely perform the manipulation in the following order: forward flexion, extension, abduction, and internal and external rotation. In the early stages of adhesive capsulitis, a series of small pops are heard as the anterior and inferior capsule ruptures. If the arthroscope is

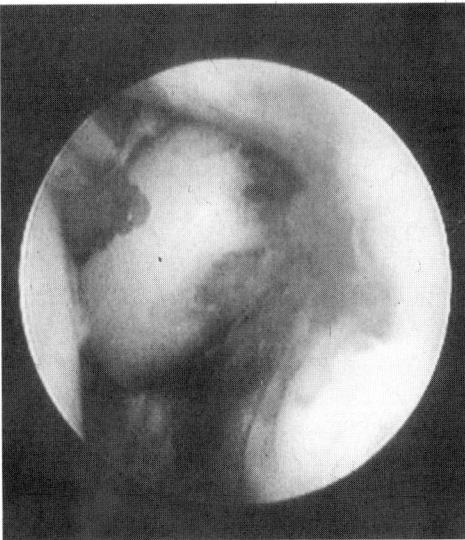

Figure 22.1. Arthroscopic appearance of stage 1 adhesive capsulitis of the shoulder. The thickened synovitis is most pronounced in the region of the rotator interval (demonstrated here) but is characteristically a diffuse process.

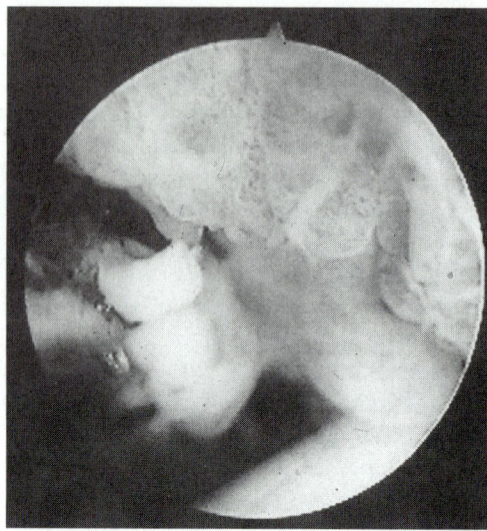

Figure 22.2. Arthroscopic appearance of stage 2 adhesive capsulitis. The synovium is pedunculated, which reflects the perivascular scar formation noted on histologic examination.

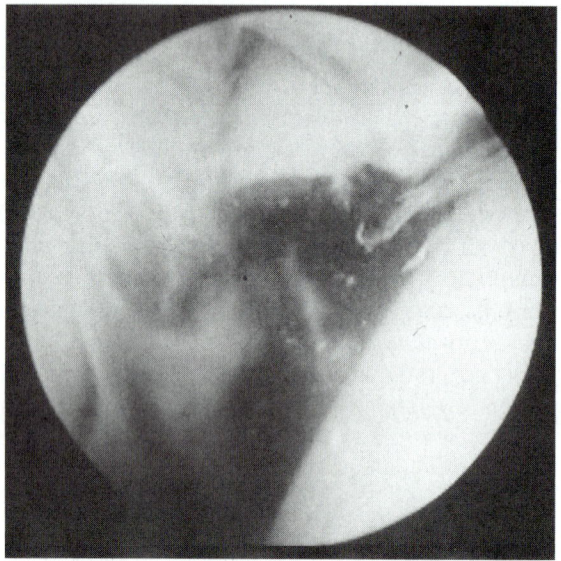

Figure 22.3. Arthroscopic appearance of stage 3 adhesive capsulitis. Minimal hyperemia is noted in the synovium, and wispy intra-articular adhesions and pericapsular scar can be visualized.

placed back into the shoulder, one can visualize a capsular tear that runs from approximately 2 to 6 o'clock then passes obliquely across the inferior axillary pouch.

In late stage 2 and stage 3 adhesive capsulitis, the capsular scarring is quite dense and may not respond to manipulation. An arthroscopic capsular release is then performed to facilitate manipulation under anesthesia. The capsular scar is divided using an electrocautery device and a motorized shaver. The capsular division begins superiorly from just anterior and inferior to the biceps tendon and continues inferiorly until the discrete upper edge of the subscapularis tendon is encountered (Fig. 22.4).

This constitutes a surgical release of the rotator interval region of the capsule (19).

Ozaki et al. (20) and Neer et al. (21) have pointed out that an open release of this area is usually successful in restoring external rotation in shoulders with refractory adhesive capsulitis. This thickened, scarred anterior-superior capsule will limit forward elevation and external rotation. As the capsule is released, the humeral head moves inferiorly and laterally, creating more room in the joint for the arthroscope to be moved into the anterior and inferior region of the joint. The capsular release is then continued inferiorly to 5 o'clock. We do not routinely attempt release of the inferior recess, because of risk to the underlying axillary nerve. Following the arthroscopic capsular release, the instrument is removed and a closed manipulation is performed. In most cases, external rotation in adduction is restored with almost no manipulation force. The shoulder can then be manipulated into other planes with minimal force and with audible and palpable yielding of tissue.

If the patient still lacks internal rotation in abduction, the arthroscope is reinserted into the joint via an anterior portal and a posterior capsular release is performed. We usually perform the release in the midcapsular region, and we have had no cases of axillary nerve injury with this technique.

If clinical evaluation warrants inspection of the subacromial space, this is undertaken following the manipulation. Subacromial bursal scarring and associated lesions, such as calcific tendonitis, acromioclavicular arthritis, and hypertrophy of the coracoacromial ligament, can then be treated (12).

Postoperative Management

Postoperative care must be individualized to the patient. Some patients can be successfully managed as outpatients, whereas others require admission for pain management. Outpatient therapy includes a daily visit with a physical therapist 5 days/week for the first 2 weeks. Patients are encouraged to use narcotic pain relievers for the physical therapy sessions during the first 2 weeks. The therapy sessions are then held 3 times/week for 6 to 8 weeks following surgical intervention. Patients are also taught a home program that focuses on passive or active-assisted range of motion.

A small subsection of patients require inpatient admission for management of postoperative pain. On the morning of the 1st postoperative day, a supervised physical therapy program is initiated. Adequate anesthesia is obtained from continuous bupivacaine infusion through the interscalene catheter or by repeating the block. Narcotic analgesia is used as necessary to supplement the interscalene block. Therapy is performed twice each day, in the morning and in the afternoon. Supervised therapy consists of an aggressive stretching program in all planes, and the patient is instructed in self-assisted stretching. Since the interscalene block usually results in only partial muscle

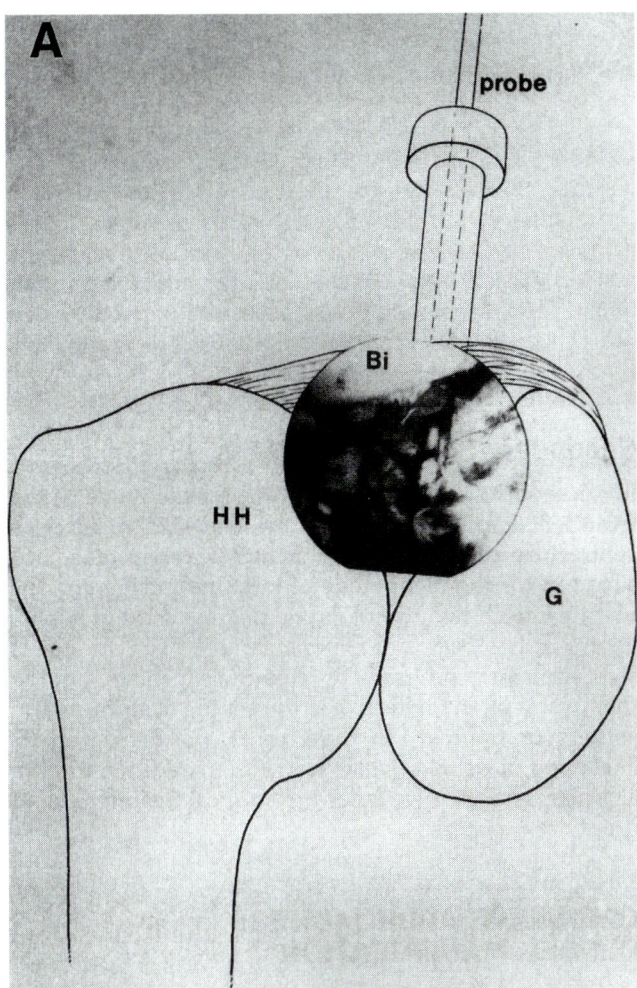
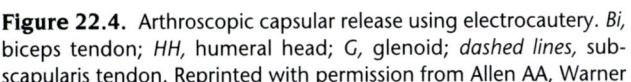
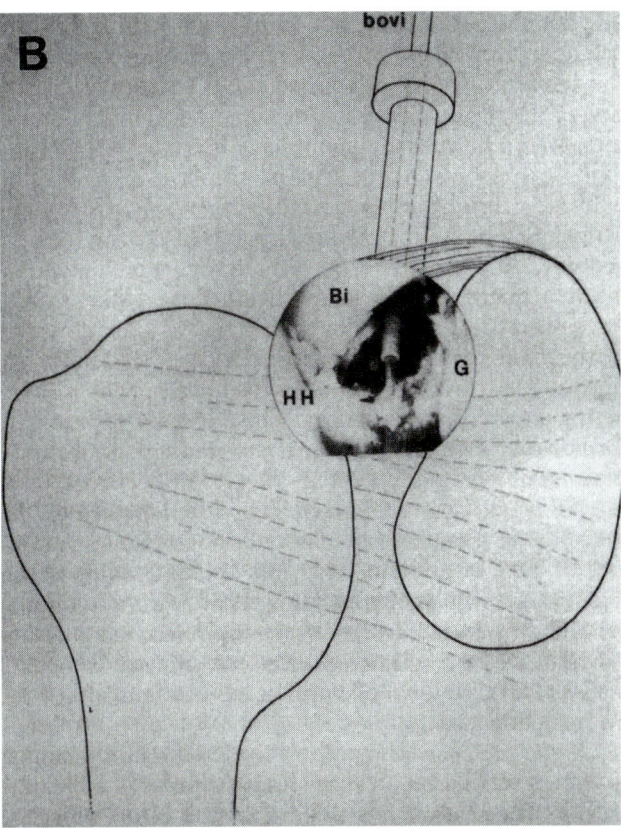

Figure 22.4. Arthroscopic capsular release using electrocautery. *Bi,* biceps tendon; *HH,* humeral head; *G, glenoid; dashed lines,* subscapularis tendon. Reprinted with permission from Allen AA, Warner JJP. Management of stiff shoulder. Oper Tech Orthop 1995; 5:238–247.

paralysis, the patient can perform some stretching by himself or herself.

No sling is used after surgery, and the patient is discharged on the 2nd postoperative day. He or she is encouraged to use the arm only for activities of daily living. The patient begins a home program with self-assisted stretching and a pulley device, in addition to a supervised physical therapy program on an outpatient basis, as described above. When full motion is achieved, the patient is progressed to a more aggressive strengthening program for the rotator cuff and scapular stabilizers, as significant weakness can be noted in patients with prolonged loss of normal range of motion of the shoulder.

SUMMARY

Treatment of adhesive capsulitis of the shoulder requires an individualized approach that takes into account the stage and natural history of the disease. In general, a conservative approach, including intra-articular corticosteroids, pain management, and a supervised physical therapy program, is the initial method of treatment. For cases that remain refractory to this approach, an arthroscopic evaluation and closed manipulation may be attempted. This will often be successful for patients with stage 2 adhesive capsulitis; however, some of these patients may continue to have motion loss.

In cases of late stage 2 and stage 3 adhesive capsulitis refractory to closed manipulation, an arthroscopic release technique may successfully restore motion. This technique is demanding, and proper patient selection, anesthesia, and postoperative analgesia are critical to its success. If a patient has a known extra-articular factor-limiting motion or if an arthroscopic approach fails, an open release can be performed along with a Z-plasty lengthening of the scarred subscapularis tendon and capsule. In these cases, the recovery may be slow because of need to protect the soft tissue repair.

REFERENCES

1. Miller MD, Rockwood CA. Thawing the frozen shoulder: the "patient" patient. Orthopedics 1996;19:849–853.

2. Bulgen DY, Binder AL, Hazelman BL, et al. Frozen shoulder: prospective clinical study with an evaluation of three treatment regimens. Ann Rheum Dis 1984;43:353–360.

3. Barry H, Fernandes I, Bloom B, et al. Clinical study comparing acupuncture, physiotherapy, injection and oral anti-inflammatory therapy in shoulder cuff lesions. Curr Med Res Opin 1980; 7:121–126.

4. Rhind V, Downie WW, Bird HA, et al. Naproxen and indomethacin in periarthritis of the shoulder. Rheumatol Rehabil 1982;21:51–53.

5. Quigley TB. Indications for manipulation and corticosteroids in the treatment of stiff shoulder. Surg Clin North Am 1975; 43:1715–1720.

6. Andren L, Lundberg BJ. Treatment of rigid shoulders by joint distention during arthrography. Acta Orthop Scand 1965;36:45–53.

7. Hsu SYC, Chan KM. Arthroscopic distension in the management of frozen shoulder. Int Orthop 1991;15:79–83.

8. Risk TE, Gavant ML, Pinals RS. Treatment of adhesive capsulitis with arthrographic capsular distention and rupture. Arch Phys Med Rehabil 1994;75:803–807.

9. Haines JF, Hargadon EJ. Manipulation as the primary treatment of frozen shoulder. J R Coll Surg Edinb 1982;27:5–8.

10. Thomas D, William RA, Smith DS. The frozen shoulder. A review of manipulative treatment. Rheumatol Rehabil 1980;19:173–179.

11. Kieras DM, Matsen FA III. Open release in the management of refractory frozen shoulder. Orthop Trans 1991;15:801–802.

12. Pollock RG, Duralde XA, Flatow EL, et al. The use of arthroscopy in treatment of resistant frozen shoulder. Clin Orthop 1994; 304:30–36.

13. Bradley JP: Arthroscopic treatment for frozen capsulitis. Oper Tech Orthop 1991;1:248–252.

14. Ogilvie-Harris DJ, Biggs DJ, Fitsialos DP, MacKay M. The resistant frozen shoulder: manipulation versus capsular release. Clin Orthop 1995;319:238–248.

15. Wiley AM. Arthroscopic appearance of frozen shoulder. Arthroscopy 1991;7:138–143.

16. Warner JJ, Allen A, Marks PH, Wong P. Arthroscopic release for chronic refractory adhesive capsulitis of the shoulder. J Bone Joint Surg 1996;78B:1808–1816.

17. Neviaser RJ, Neviaser TJ. The frozen shoulder. Diagnosis and management. Clin Orthop 1987;223:59–64.

18. Neviaser TJ. Adhesive capsulitis. Orthop Clin North Am 1987; 18:439–443.

19. Harryman DT III, Sidles JA, Harris SL, et al. The role of the rotator interval capsule in passive motion and stability of the shoulder. J Bone Joint Surg 1992;74A:53–66.

20. Ozaki J, Kakagawa Y, Sakurai G, et al. Recalcitrant chronic adhesive capsulitis of the shoulder: role of contracture of the coracohumeral ligament and rotator interval in pathogenesis and treatment. J Bone Joint Surg 1989;71A:1511.

21. Neer CS, Satterlee CC, Dalsey R, et al. The anatomy and potential effects of contracture of the coracohumeral ligament. Clin Orthop 1992;28:182–185.

chapter **23**

Joseph Borrelli, Jr., and Jeffrey R. Dugas

Humeral Shaft Fracture and Nonunion: Surgical Repair

Humeral diaphyseal fractures represent 1 to 2% of all fractures. This chapter reviews the anatomy, diagnosis, and treatment of humeral fractures and nonunions. Complications associated with the treatments will be discussed.

RELEVANT ANATOMY AND PATHOGENESIS

The humeral diaphysis, or shaft, extends from the proximal aspect of the pectoralis major insertion to the supracondylar ridge distally. Fractures of the humeral shaft are commonly described based on their location in the proximal, middle, or distal third of the bone. The routine description of these fractures includes the fracture pattern and degree of comminution. The clinician should note whether the fracture is open or closed. Although there is some discrepancy in the literature, approximately 50% of diaphyseal fractures occur within the middle third, 30% within the distal third, and 20% in the proximal third (1,2).

The proximal third extends from the superior aspect of the pectoralis major insertion to the proximal border of the deltoid insertion at the deltoid tuberosity. The major neurovascular structures in the proximal region include the brachial artery and vein; the radial, median, and ulnar nerves; and the basilic vein. These structures lie medial to the shaft, separated from it by the coracobrachialis muscle (Fig. 23.1). Muscles inserting into the proximal third include the pectoralis major (crest of the greater tuberosity), the latissimus dorsi (floor of the intertubercular groove), and the teres major (medial lip of the intertubercular groove). The lateral head of the triceps originates from the posterior surface of the humerus in this area.

Fractures of the proximal third, at or above the insertion of the pectoralis major, are characterized by abduction and external rotation of the proximal fragment, owing to the forces of the rotator cuff musculature. Fractures between the pectoralis insertion and the deltoid insertion are characterized by proximal and lateral displacement of the distal fragment with adduction of the proximal fragment, resulting in an overall shortening of the limb (Fig. 23.2).

The middle third of the humerus begins at the proximal deltoid insertion and extends down to the superior aspect of the origin of the brachioradialis muscle on the anteromedial surface. The bone in this region remains cylindrical and contains the deltoid tuberosity on the anterolateral surface. The medial and lateral intermuscular septa are prominent in this region and separate the anterior and posterior compartments of the arm. The major neurovascular structures remain on the medial side of the humerus throughout this region. The radial nerve is the exception; it travels from medial to lateral deep to the lateral head of the triceps and in close relation to the humerus posteriorly within the spiral groove. The radial nerve lies directly on the humerus only in the distal third of the humerus. Fractures distal to the deltoid insertion in the middle third are characterized by abduction of the proximal fragment (Fig. 23.2). Although compartment syndrome of the upper arm is uncommon, it is important to understand the location of the various neurovascular and muscular structures in relation to the bony anatomy.

In the distal third, the bone takes on a more triangular shape. The distal section extends from the superior border of the origin of the brachioradialis radialis muscle to the most proximal flaring of the supracondylar area. The majority of the neurovascular structures continue to lie medial to the shaft. The radial nerve crosses the lateral intermuscular septum in this region to lie in the anterior compartment between the brachioradialis and brachialis muscles (Fig. 23.1). Near the site where the nerve crosses the intermus-

245

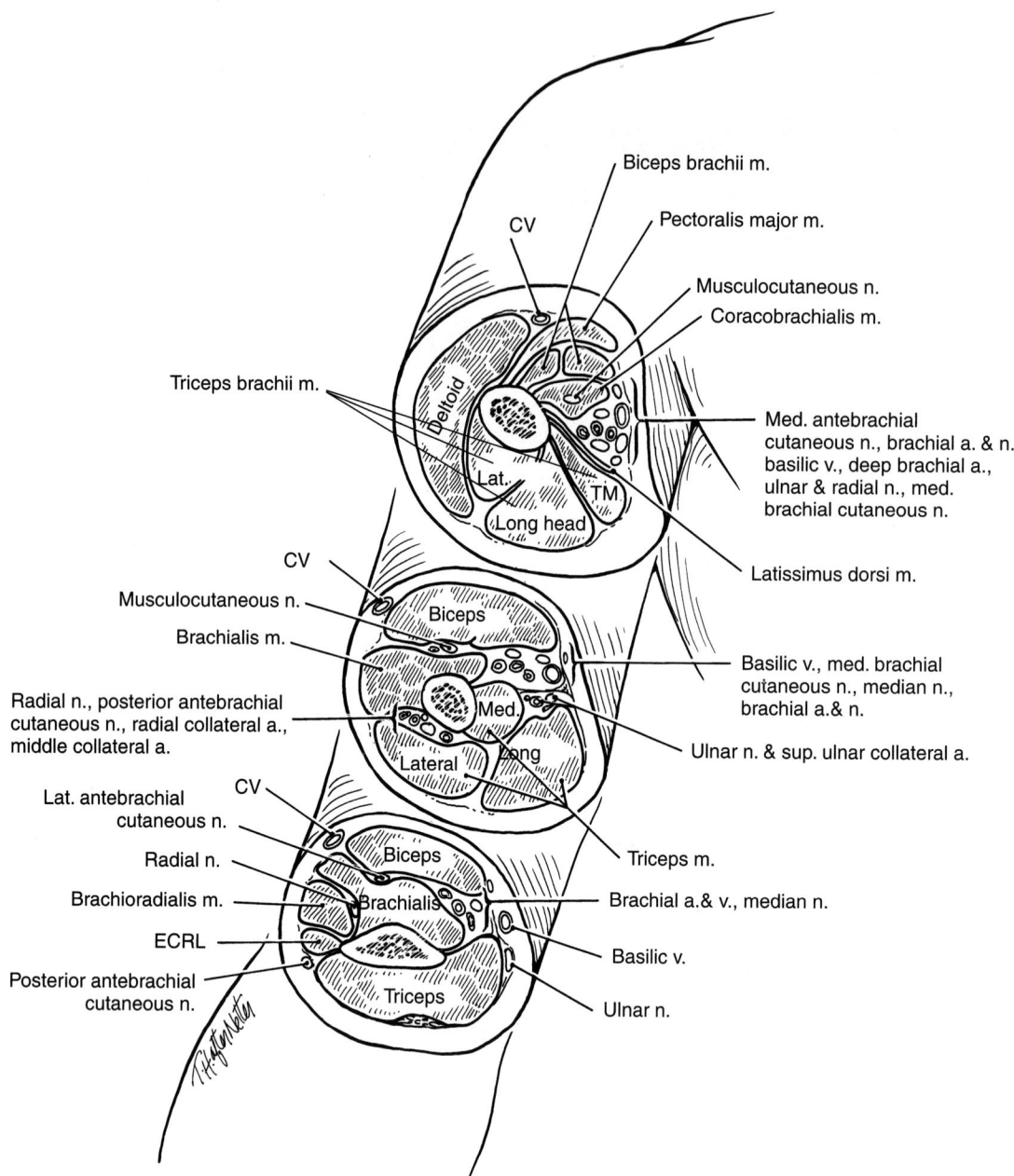

Figure 23.1. Cross-sectional anatomy of the upper, middle, and distal thirds of the upper arm. Note the location of the neurovascular structures in each section. *CV,* cephalic vein; *ECRL,* extensor carpi radialis longus.

cular septum, just above the supracondylar ridge, the nerve lies in direct contact with the humerus. This point is of clinical significance in that longitudinal fractures in the distal third have been shown to be associated with a relatively high incidence of radial nerve injury or entrapment (3). The blood supply to the humerus itself is from a branch of the brachial artery near the junction of the middle and distal thirds. In two-thirds of patients, this nutrient vessel then enters a foramen at the anteromedial aspect of the distal half of the middle third of the humerus. In the other third, the foramen is on the anterior or medial side. In general, fractures of the proximal half of the humerus do not jeopardize the blood supply to the bone (4,5).

Fractures of the humeral shaft commonly occur as a result of a direct blow to the arm, e.g., from motor vehicle accidents or falls. Other causes of humeral shaft fractures include pathologic fractures, child abuse, gunshot wounds, twisting injuries, and industrial accidents.

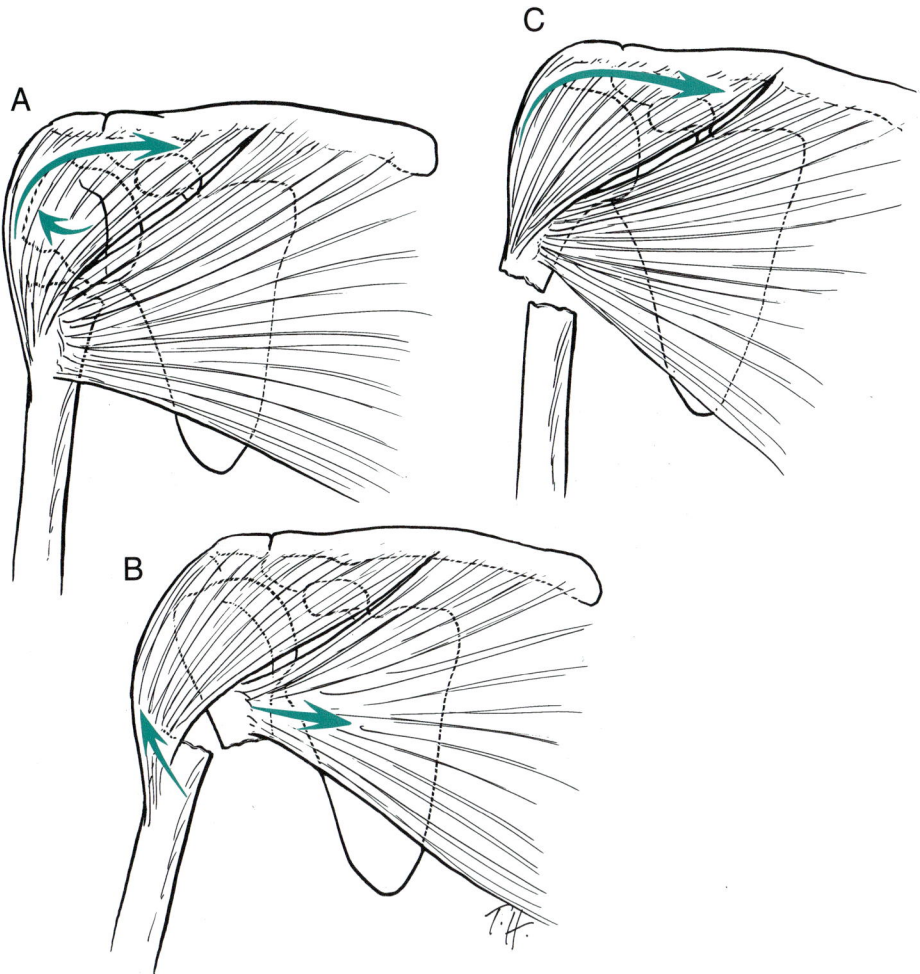

Figure 23.2. A. When the fracture is above the pectoralis major insertion, the proximal fragment is abducted and externally rotated (*arrows*). **B.** When the fracture is between the pectoralis major and deltoid insertions, the proximal fragment is adducted, and the distal fragment is displaced proximally and laterally (*arrows*). **C.** When the fracture is below the deltoid insertion, the proximal fragment is abducted (*arrow*).

INITIAL FINDINGS, PHYSICAL EXAMINATION, AND DIAGNOSIS

Patients with fracture of the humeral shaft present with pain in the arm that is often associated with swelling, deformity, crepitation, rotation, and shortening of the extremity (2). A comprehensive physical examination is necessary for all patients. The history should include the patient's age and the cause of injury; remember that the patient may have multiple injuries. The patient should be examined from the shoulder to the hand with the arm completely exposed. A thorough inspection of the overlying skin and soft tissues is necessary to diagnose an open humerus fracture, which requires emergent management.

The neurovascular examination should consist of palpating the distal radial and ulnar pulses and assessing sensory and motor function in the affected extremity. The nonaffected extremity should always be examined for comparison. Thorough documentation of normal and abnormal function is essential. Special attention should be paid to radial nerve function. Wrist and finger extension, specifically extension of the abductor pollicis longus, are

the simplest means of testing the motor function of the radial nerve. The sensory function is best tested on the dorsal surface of the hand in the web space between the thumb and index finger. In addition, the lower lateral brachial cutaneous branch of the radial nerve supplies the skin over the lateral supracondylar area.

Nonunion is the most common complication of both operative and nonoperative treatment of humerus fractures; it occurs in 2 to 8% of patients treated by nonoperative management and in up to 50% of patients treated with some types of intramedullary devices (2,6,7). Furthermore, delayed union has been demonstrated to occur in up to 15% of cases when conservative treatment is used (7). The Association for the Study of Internal Fixation (ASIF) defines *delayed union* as no evidence of a bridging callus at 4 months after the initiation of treatment. Studies have repeatedly shown that the average time to union of humeral diaphysis fractures ranges from 8 to 12 weeks. Thus we prefer to consider a nonunion as a fracture that demonstrates no evidence of bridging callus on three consecutive radiographs taken at 1-month intervals after the designated treatment.

Patients with nonunion of a humerus fracture typically present with persistent pain with motion at the fracture site and stiffness of the ipsilateral shoulder and elbow. Commonly patients who develop nonunion have associated comorbidities, including alcoholism, renal impairment, diabetes, and osteoporosis. Open fractures and fractures caused by high-energy injuries have an increased risk of nonunion owing to increased periosteal stripping and subsequent diminished vascularity of the fracture fragments. Operatively stabilized fractures may also go on to nonunion because of vascular compromise from excessive soft tissue or periosteal stripping, fixation instability, or infection. The anatomy of the fracture may also influence the development of a nonunion; short-oblique or transverse fractures of the middiaphysis have a higher incidence of nonunion owing to a decrease in the surface area of the bone fragments.

RADIOLOGIC STUDIES

Clinical suspicion of fracture or nonunion on the basis of history and physical examination warrants radiographic evaluation. The mainstay of the diagnosis of acute humerus fracture is the plain radiograph. Two views of the humerus should be obtained: an AP view, which includes the shoulder and elbow; and a lateral view (transthoracic view). The radiographs shown in Figure 23.3 are adequate because they show the fracture in two planes and include the joints above and below the fracture site. Plain radiographs of the ipsilateral shoulder and elbow should also be routinely obtained if these structures are not well visualized on the humerus films.

An isotope bone scan should be obtained for any patient in whom a nonunion is suspected but not clearly seen on the plain radiographs. An indium-labeled white blood cell scan can be helpful if infectious nonunion is suspected. CT and MRI studies rarely offer any additional clinical information in regard to altering the management of humerus fractures. An arteriogram is indicated if the patient has a pulseless, cool upper extremity at the time of examination.

Classification

The classification of humeral shaft fractures is commonly descriptive in nature and includes the location (proximal, middle, distal), the fracture pattern (transverse, oblique, spiral, segmental), and the degree of soft tissue injury (open, closed). Unfortunately, this approach cannot guide treatment or determine the prognosis at the time of injury, and it is inherently subjective.

The AO (Arbeitsgemeinschaft für Osteosynthesefragen) system is a precise classification scheme of long bone fractures that is gaining acceptance (Fig. 23.4). This is an alphanumeric coding system in which each long bone is identified first, followed by the portion of the bone involved in the fracture (thus two numbers). The fracture pattern is designated by an A, B, or C, depending on the complexity of the fracture, and by two more numbers further delineating the fracture morphology. Additional qualifiers can be added to more specifically classify the fracture. Although the AO system gives some insight into the severity of the fracture and, therefore, prognosis, it does have

Figure 23.3. AP (**A**) and lateral (**B**) views of a middiaphyseal humerus fracture, including joints above and joint below fracture.

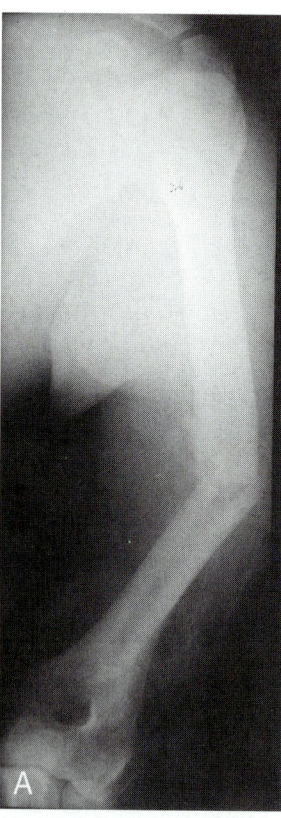
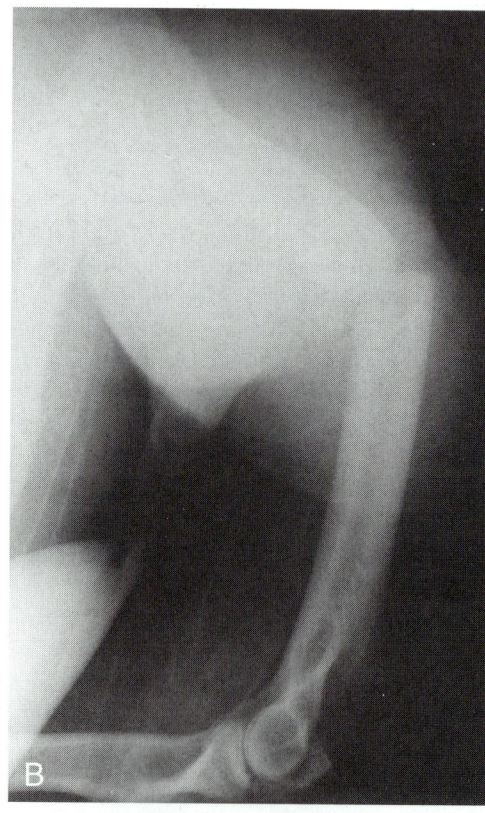

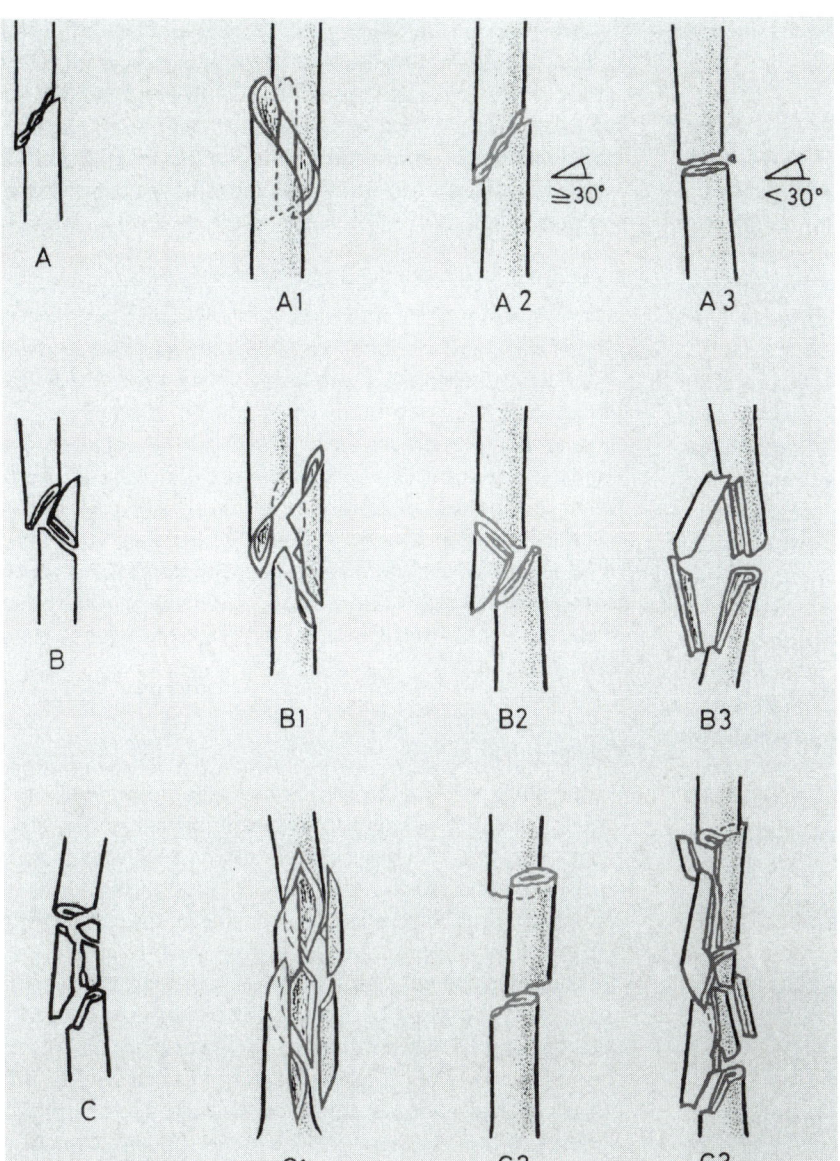

Figure 23.4. AO classification of diaphyseal fractures of the humerus. Reprinted with permission from Muller ME, Nazarian S, Koch P, Schatzker J. The comprehensive classification of fractures of long bones. Heidelberg: Springer-Verlag, 1990:67.

shortcomings in regard to guiding treatment, since it does not include clinically relevant information such as soft tissue injury, neurovascular injury, and associated injuries.

For fractures of the humeral diaphysis, the first number in the AO scheme is a 1, which signifies the humerus; the diaphysis is designated by a 2 (1 is used for the proximal metaphysis, and 3 for the distal metaphysis); and the letter identifies the fracture pattern (A for simple, B for wedge, and C for spiral fractures). Each fracture type can be subdivided to better describe the fracture pattern (8) (Fig. 23.4). Type A fractures are subdivided into simple spiral (A1), simple oblique (A2), and simple transverse (A3) fractures. Type B fractures are similarly subdivided into spiral wedge (B1), bending wedge (B2), and fragmented wedge (B3). Type C fractures are classified as complex spiral (C1), complex segmental (C2), and complex irregular (C3). These fractures can also be described by the number of bone fragments: C1.1 fractures have two intermediate fragments, C1.2 have three intermediate frag-

ments, and C1.3 have more than three intermediate fragments. Type C2.1 fractures have one intermediate segmental fragment, type C2.2 have one intermediate segmental fragment and additional wedge fragments, and type C2.3 have two intermediate segmental fragments. Type C3.1 fractures have two to three intermediate fragments, C3.2 have limited shattering (less than 5 cm), and C3.3 have extensive shattering (more than 5 cm).

TREATMENT

Nonoperative Treatment

Conservative methods have been the mainstay of treatment for humeral shaft fractures for many years. The rich blood supply and thick muscular coverage enhance the propensity for healing in these fractures. The excellent results obtained when using conservative management for diaphyseal humerus fractures have been borne out consistently in the literature for years; union rates range from 90 to 99% (1).

FRACTURE BRACING

One of the basic tenets of fracture care is to return the injured extremity to functional activity as soon as possible. The detrimental outcomes associated with immobilization (e.g., muscle atrophy, adhesive capsulitis, and disuse osteopenia) can be avoided by early return of motion. Fracture bracing of the humerus allows comfortable range of motion of both the shoulder and elbow. It also allows adequate hygiene about the arm and can be worn under most clothing (Fig. 23.5). The use of ready-made fracture braces for the treatment of isolated, closed humeral fractures has been associated with excellent results. Sarmiento et al. (1) successfully applied techniques of fracture bracing to both the lower and upper extremity and noted a nonunion rate of 2%. Similar results were obtained by Balfour et al. (9).

Fracture braces require an upright posture, and the patient should practice active flexion and extension of the elbow while wearing the brace. These braces are not as useful for comatose or bedridden patients, although they provide an excellent alternative to operative intervention. In general, the brace should be applied 7 to 10 days after injury, provided there is no prohibitive soft tissue swelling. Most authors advocate close follow-up after application of the brace to check the neurovascular status, proper fit of the brace, and fracture alignment.

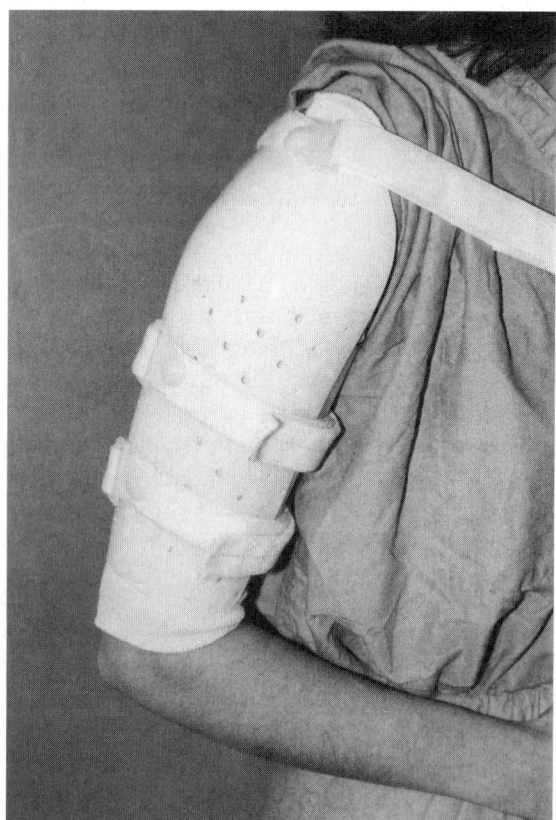

Figure 23.5. Sarmiento fracture brace.

Time to union averages 10 weeks. Documented nonunion rates are as low as 1 to 2% (1). In general, 20° of anteroposterior angulation and 30° of varus angulation have been associated with excellent cosmetic and functional results (2). Various end points of treatment with the brace have been reported, but most physicians recommend painless active abduction to 90°.

CUFF AND COLLAR OR HANGING ARM CAST

Application of a cuff-and-collar or hanging arm cast is simple, fast, and inexpensive. These devices can be used in the acute setting as a preliminary stabilizer before application of a fracture brace or as definitive management. As with fracture braces, these casts use gravity to help maintain the reduction of the humerus fracture; thus patients are instructed to remain in an upright position as much as possible. This is particularly important with short oblique, spiral, and transverse fracture patterns for which restoration of length is necessary. Union rates with the use of cuff-and-collar and hanging cast techniques range from 90 to 95% (10).

SLING-AND-SWATHE DEVICE WITH A VELPEAU DRESSING

The sling-and-swathe device with a Velpeau dressing is inexpensive and easily applied in the acute setting. The advantages of these devices over the hanging arm or cuff-and-collar casts are that they require less patient compliance and are more desirable in the comatose or elderly patient. The sling-and-swathe device with a Velpeau dressing is made out of soft material, which provides comfort and formability (Fig. 23.6). With the Velpeau dressing, pads are placed in the axilla proximally or more distally to control the angulation of the fracture site. Gravity is still beneficial, and patients should be instructed to be upright as much as can be tolerated. These devices are also often used as a temporary stabilization before application of a fracture brace or operative intervention. Reported union rates with these measures alone are approximately 90%.

COAPTATION SPLINT

The coaptation splint is a plaster sugar-tong-type splint that extends from the axilla medially, down around the elbow, and back up the lateral side of the arm and over the shoulder. As with other acute measures, this is a simple and inexpensive means of stabilizing the upper arm. Another benefit is that wrist motion is maintained, allowing more function of the ipsilateral hand. Disadvantages of the coaptation splint include irritation of the axilla and of the skin over the shoulder caused by the plaster. Angulation at the fracture site is common with this type of immobilization.

INDICATIONS FOR SURGERY

The indications for operative fixation of fractures of the humeral diaphysis can be divided into absolute and relative groups. Absolute indications include open fractures, fractures associated with radial nerve palsy that devel-

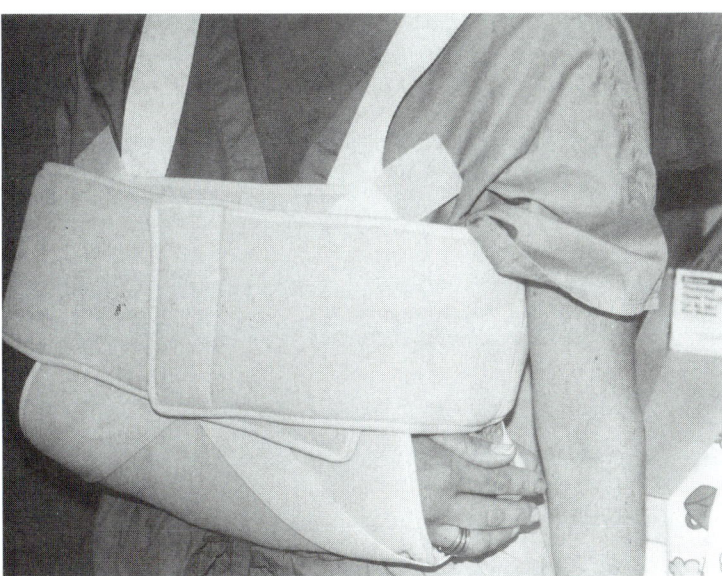

Figure 23.6. Sling-and-swathe device.

oped following manipulation, fractures associated with vascular injury, fractures associated multiple injuries or multiple long bone fractures, bilateral humerus fractures or ipsilateral forearm fractures (floating elbow), pathologic fractures, and nonunions. Relative indications include unstable transverse or short-oblique fractures, fractures in unreliable patients, and fractures associated concomitant diseases that make healing difficult (e.g., Parkinson disease).

Operative Treatment

Preoperative planning and a thorough knowledge of the anatomy of the upper extremity are essential in carrying out successful open reduction and internal fixation (ORIF) of fractures of the humeral diaphysis. The preoperative plan should be carefully drawn out using templates and plain radiographs to facilitate the operative procedure. The operative approach and choice of implant and stabilization technique are determined on the basis of fracture pattern and location, associated injuries, and the surgeon's experience (Clinical Table). ORIF using plates and screws allows anatomic reduction of the fracture fragments, whereas intramedullary nailing of diaphyseal fractures achieves stability via indirect reduction of the fracture fragments. Each approach has its own risks and benefits.

IMPLANTS

The choice of implants for operative stabilization of acute humerus fractures and humeral shaft nonunions include broad, large fragment dynamic compression plates and screws; locking intramedullary nails, typically placed in a reamed fashion; and unlocked flexible intramedullary (Ender) nails placed in a retrograde fashion, generally in the multiple-injured patient in emergent circumstances. Recently, plating of acutely fractured humeral shafts has become more popular than intramedullary rodding, owing to the high incidence of shoulder pain and loss of motion following antegrade intramedullary nailing.

Nonunions of the humeral shaft are generally treated with open reduction and internal fixation (broad, large fragment plates and screws) and iliac crest bone graft. Intramedullary rods are reserved for patients who may not tolerate the extension of the exposure for plating and for those who use their upper extremities for weight bearing, as this seems to aid in the development of a solid union.

ANTEROLATERAL APPROACH

The anterolateral, or Henri, approach is the preferred approach for internal fixation of fractures of the proximal third of the humerus. For this approach, the patient is positioned supine on the operating table with the arm abducted on an arm board; a tourniquet is not used. It is also possible to perform this approach with the patient in the lateral decubitus position with the arm draped free. The coracoid process of the scapula is palpated, as is the biceps tendon and muscle belly in the upper arm. The incision is started over the tip of the coracoid process, carried distally and laterally along the line of the deltopectoral groove, and continued distally along the lateral border of the biceps brachii muscle belly. The length of the incision is determined by the location of the fracture.

Under the skin, the subcutaneous fat overlies the deltopectoral fascia and should be incised in line with the skin incision. The cephalic vein will be prominent beneath the fascia and should be carefully dissected free and retracted laterally. The deltopectoral interval should then be developed from proximal to distal down to the insertion of the deltoid at the deltoid tuberosity and the insertion of the pectoralis major near the internal edge of the bicipital groove. This is an internervous plane: The deltoid is innervated by the axillary nerve, and the pectoralis major is innervated by the medial and lateral pec-

Clinical Table: Humeral Shaft Fracture and Nonunion: Surgical Repair

Procedure	Indications	Technique	Anatomy	Pitfalls
Open Reduction and Plate Osteosynthesis				
Fractures of the proximal third	• Need for open fixation • Oligotrophic and atrophic nonunion	• Anterolateral approach • Broad DCP • Bone graft for nonunion	• Cephalic vein • Axillary nerve • Anterior humeral circumflex vessels	• Leave cuff for subscapular repair • Radial nerve injury if dissection to spiral groove
Fractures of the distal two-thirds	• Need for open fixation • Oligotrophic and atrophic nonunion	• Posterior approach • Broad DCP • Bone graft for nonunion	• Radial nerve • Profunda brachii artery	• Ulnar nerve injury if overzealous on medial side
Fractures with neurovascular injury	• Medial soft tissue damage	• Medial approach	• Neurovascular bundle in field	• Injury to the neurovascular structures
Other Procedures				
Antegrade intramedullary statically locked nail	• Need for weight bearing on injured arm • Unstable closed fracture • Pathologic fracture • Hypertrophic nonunion	• Standard approach • Interlocking screws with soft tissue protection • Fluoroscopy	• Small longitudinal incision in deltoid and rotator cuff • Awl inserted lateral to articular surface	• Shoulder complaints • Neurovascular injury with screws • Nonunion
Retrograde flexible intramedullary nails	• Need for rapid stabilization in multitrauma patient	• Insert nails posteriorly just above the olecranon • Several nails are used to fit the canal	• Small incision through the distal triceps tendon	• Possibility of backout • Rotational instability • Elbow pain
External fixation	• Open fractures with segmental bone loss • Contaminated wound • Neurovascular compromise	• Two half-pins • Secure with unilateral frame • Fluoroscopy	• Improve rigidity by creating long lever arms • Bicortical purchase	• Pin tract infection • Possible contamination of the medullary canal (prevents later fixation) • Nonunion

DCP, dynamic compression plate.

toral nerves. The fascia overlying the biceps and the brachialis is incised in line with the skin incision to enable the development of this intermuscular interval if more distal exposure is necessary (Fig. 23.7). Access to the anatomic neck or head is obtained by dividing the tendon of the subscapularis muscle near its insertion. A 4- to 5-mm cuff of tendon should remain with the lesser tuberosity for later repair.

Structures at risk during this dissection include the axillary nerve, which lies on the under surface of the deltoid and can easily be damaged by overzealous retracting of the deltoid muscle. The anterior humeral circumflex artery and vein cross the operative field in the proximal exposure in the interval between the deltoid and the pectoralis major muscles. These vessels should be identified and ligated. The radial nerve is endangered if the exposure is continued distally to the level of the spiral groove.

POSTERIOR TRICEPS: SPLITTING APPROACH

The posterior approach is the preferred approach to fractures of the lower two-thirds of the humeral shaft. It can be performed with the patient in the prone position with the elbow flexed and the forearm hanging from the table or with the patient in the lateral decubitus position with the affected side up. Again, a preoperative plan and understanding of the anatomy are critical to success. The incision is made in the midline posteriorly beginning 8 cm distal to the acromion and proceeding distally along the midline toward the tip of the olecranon. The deep fascia is then divided in line with the skin incision.

Two heads of the triceps (the long and lateral heads) are exposed, and the interval between them is identified and developed. This is easiest to do proximally above the point at which the two heads join to form the triceps tendon. The tendon must be split in line with the interval to

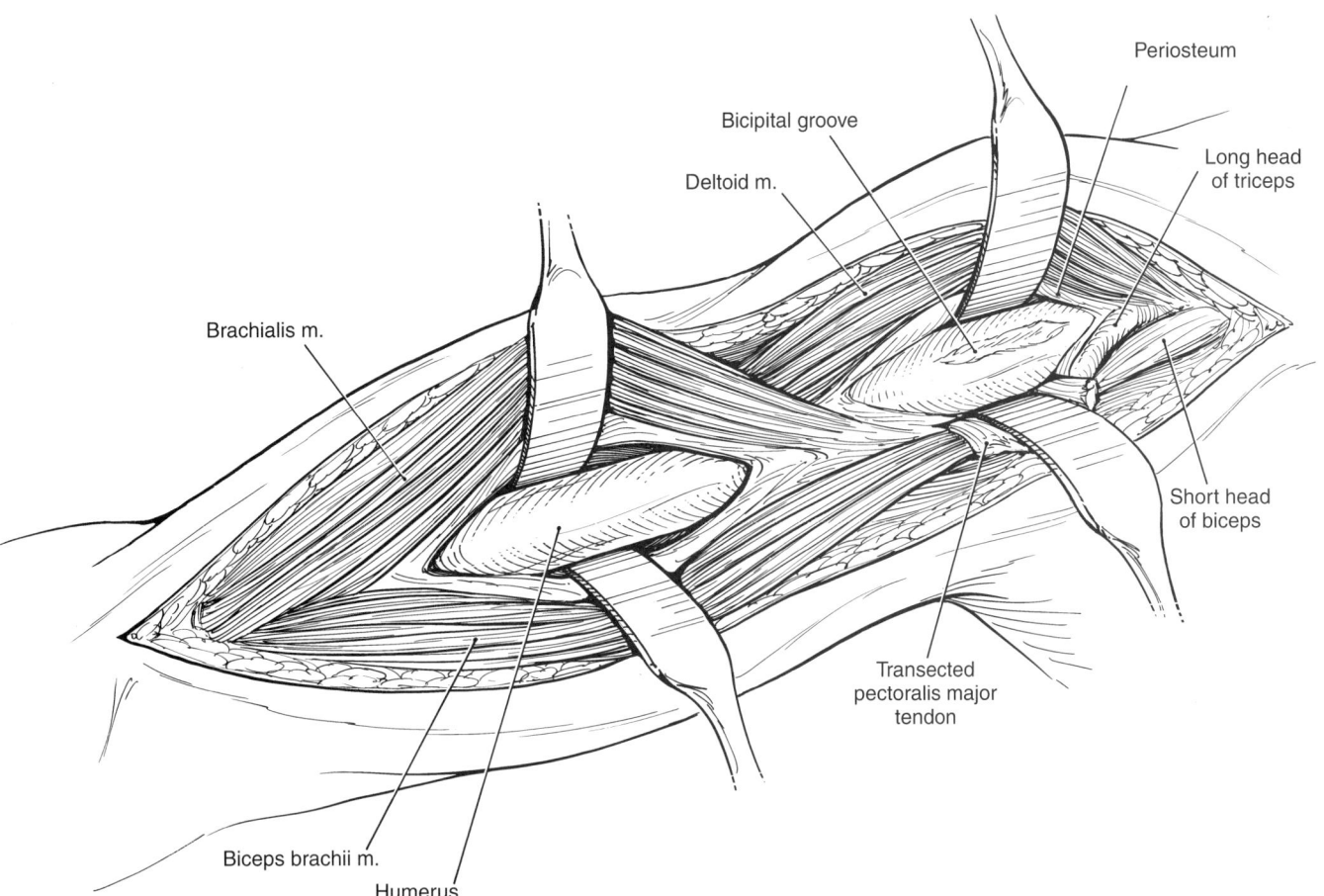

Figure 23.7. Using the anterolateral approach to humerus, the surgeon elevates the pectoralis major from the lesser tuberosity to expose the proximal humeral shaft and elevates the brachialis to expose the distal humeral shaft. Flexion at the elbow eases the elevation of the brachialis. Modified from Hoppenfeld S, deBoer P. Surgical exposures in orthopaedics. The anatomic approach. 2nd ed. Philadelphia: Lippincott, 1994.

gain exposure to the humeral shaft. Careful development of this interval allows identification of the medial head of the triceps, the radial nerve, and the profunda brachii artery (Fig. 23.8). The radial nerve and profunda brachii artery will be seen along the spiral groove passing from proximal medially to distal laterally. The medial head of the triceps originates just distal to the spiral groove. Once the radial nerve and artery are identified and safely retracted, the medial head of the triceps can be incised in the midline down through the periosteum of the humerus. The remainder of the dissection should be subperiosteal to protect the ulnar nerve as it courses from anterior to posterior through the intermuscular septum distally. Of course, soft tissue attachments to the fracture fragments should be maintained, minimizing periosteal stripping.

Structures at risk during this approach include the radial nerve, the profunda brachii artery, and the ulnar nerve. Extreme care and caution should be taken to identify, protect, and preserve them. In particular, deep dissection of the medial head of the triceps should not be attempted if the radial nerve has not been clearly identified and gently retracted.

MEDIAL APPROACH

The medial approach to the humerus has limited indications, which include fractures with neurovascular injury that requires medial exploration and repair. This approach is unfamiliar to many orthopaedists, and a thorough knowledge of the neurovascular anatomy is a strict prerequisite. This approach is performed with the patient supine and the affected arm draped free and abducted 90° on a hand table. A bump should be placed beneath the scapula, and a sterile tourniquet should be applied. The skin incision is started 5 cm distal to the axilla just over the brachial artery. The incision is then continued distally along the path of the brachial artery and finally across the antecubital fossa toward the lateral side of the elbow. The deep fascia is incised in line with the skin incision to expose the neurovascular bundle, which includes the brachial artery, the median nerve, and the ulnar nerve. The musculocutaneous nerve runs anterolateral to the bundle, emerging through the coracobrachialis muscle to lie on the brachialis. The median nerve, ulnar nerve, and brachial artery are retracted posteromedially, and the musculocutaneous nerve is identified. The branches of the musculocutaneous

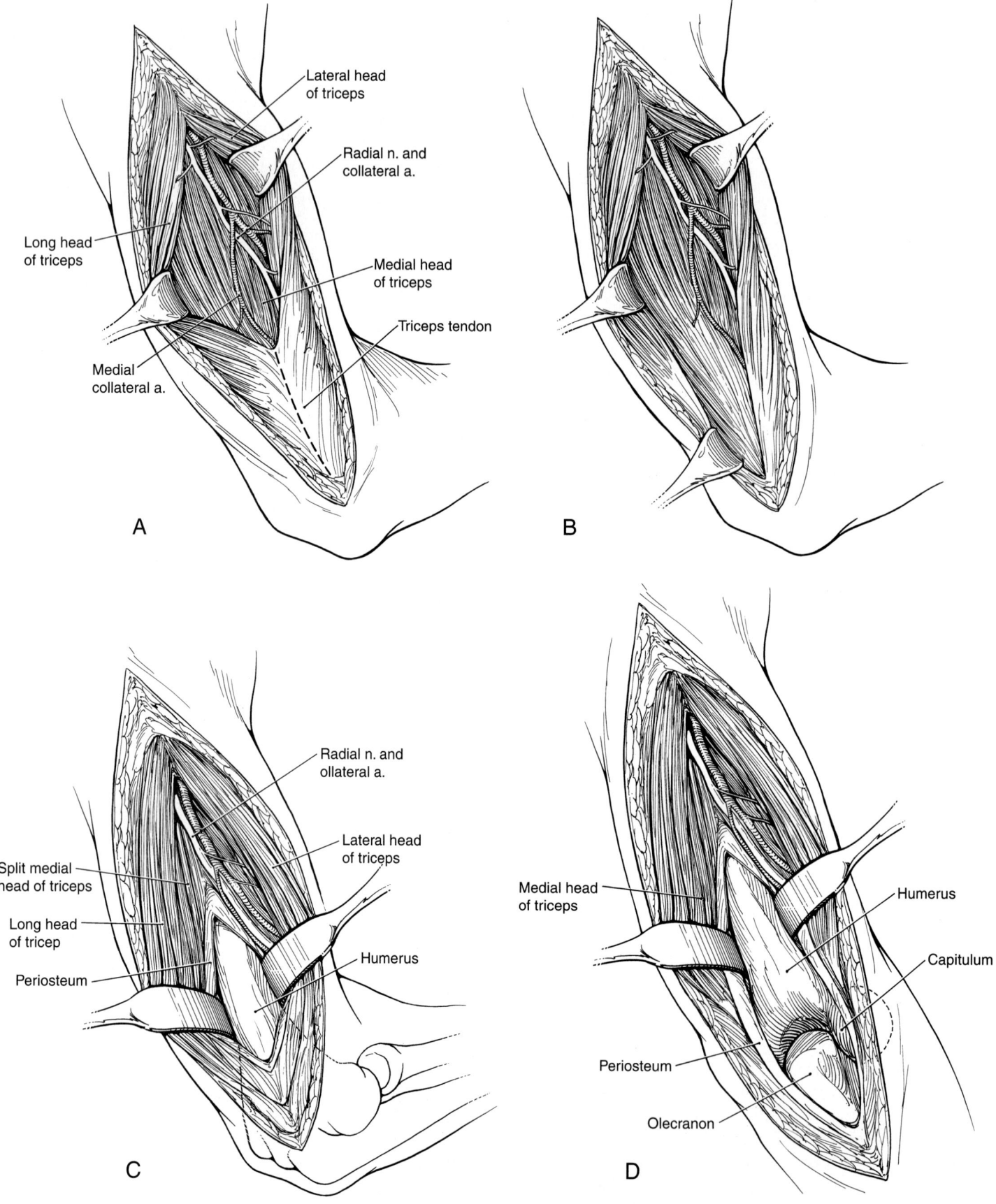

Figure 23.8. **A.** For the posterior triceps-splitting approach to the humerus, a plane is developed between the long and lateral heads of the triceps proximally. **B.** The common tendon is sharply split distally. **C.** The medial head of the triceps is split in the midline to expose the posterior periosteum of the humerus. **D.** Distal extension of the exposure can be obtained to gain access to the olecranon and elbow. Modified from Hoppenfeld S, deBoer P. Surgical exposures in orthopaedics. The anatomic approach. 2nd ed. Philadelphia: Lippincott, 1994.

nerve to the biceps and brachialis muscles are identified and preserved. While paying careful attention to these structures, the surgeon elevates the biceps and brachialis muscles from the anterior aspect of the humerus, exposing the shaft from the pectoralis insertion proximally to the coronoid fossa distally.

APPROACH FOR ANTEGRADE MEDULLARY FIXATION

For antegrade intramedullary fixation of humeral shaft fractures, the patient should be positioned either in the supine position with the operative-side scapula on a bump or in the lateral decubitus position with the operative side up. The head should be turned away from the operative field and gently held in place with tape; if general anesthesia is used, the endotracheal tube should be positioned away from the operative field. The shoulder and entire arm are draped free. A deltoid-splitting approach is used, and the incision extends from the most lateral border of the acromion for 3 to 4 cm distally toward the greater tuberosity (Fig. 23.9).

The deltoid fibers are split bluntly over the greater tuberosity, the subacromial bursa is identified and split, and the rotator cuff is exposed. A longitudinal incision in the rotator cuff should be made, and the leaflets of the cuff are retracted and protected. At this point, the proximal aspect of the humerus is exposed for insertion of the intramedullary device. The tip of the awl is placed just medial to the greater tuberosity in line with the medullary canal. Fluoroscopy is used to confirm the position of the awl, and the medullary canal is entered. Intramedullary rodding is performed with either reamed or unreamed

nails and locked according to the fracture pattern. We prefer locking intramedullary nails that have anterior to posterior distal locking screws; although they necessitate a freehand technique, they minimize the risk to the radial nerve during distal locking.

OPERATIVE STABILIZATION

Operative stabilization of acute humeral diaphyseal fractures is performed by external fixation, intramedullary rodding, or plate osteosynthesis. Each technique has its own indications and drawbacks.

External Fixation

External fixation of the humerus is generally reserved for multi-injured patients in whom rapid stabilization is required and/or for patients with grossly contaminated open humerus fractures with or without neurovascular injury or segmental bone loss. External fixation of an open humerus fracture is advantageous because it allows the fracture edges and surrounding soft tissues to be cleansed during serial irrigations and débridements. The fixator can also be extended to the distal forearm to temporarily stabilize concomitant fractures of the humerus, radius, and ulna (11–13).

The fixator is placed laterally with four 4- or 5-mm Schanz screws or half-pins. The pins should be placed about the fracture to maximize stability. Generally, a half-pin is placed as close as possible to the proximal and distal ends of the fracture site but still within viable soft tissue. The third and fourth pins are placed as far proximal

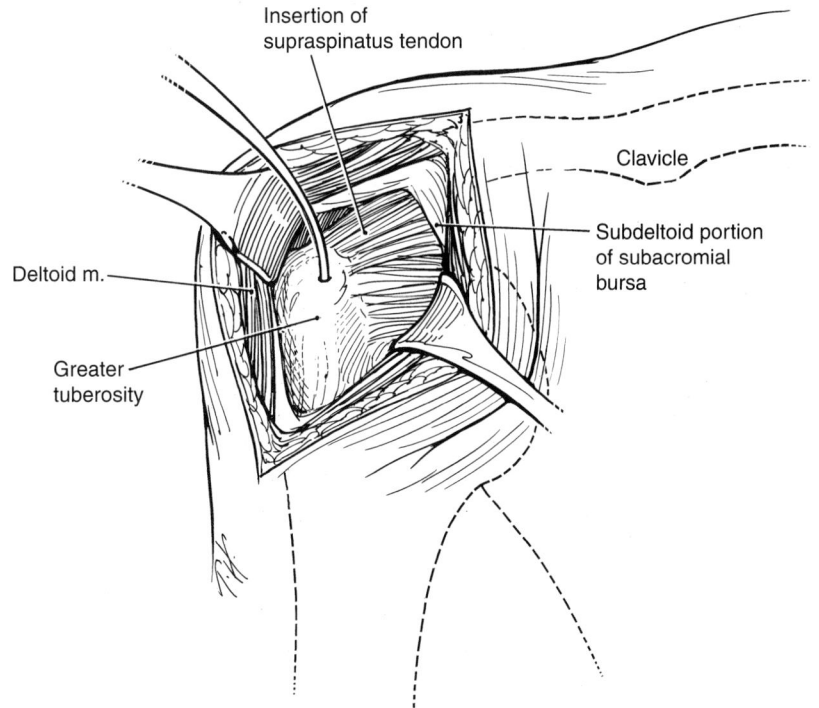

Insertion of
supraspinatus tendon

Clavicle

Subdeltoid portion
of subacromial
bursa

Deltoid m.

Greater
tuberosity

Figure 23.9. Approach for antegrade intramedullary nail fixation.

and distal in the humerus as possible to maximize the lever arm and thus the stability of the construct. Each pin should be placed through small incisions under direct visualization to prevent neurovascular injury.

The primary risks of using external fixation in the acute treatment of humerus fractures are the risk of injury to the neurovascular structures during pin placement (axillary and radial nerves); contamination of the medullary canal, which may prevent subsequent internal fixation; the development of malunions and nonunions; and associated pin tract complications. Even in light of these significant risks, external fixation is an extremely valuable tool and should be kept in the surgeons' armamentarium. When used temporarily, this technique allows the surgeon to gain control of the soft tissues before pin removal at the time of soft tissue closure or coverage and definitive fixation (14,15).

Intramedullary Nailing

There are two types of intramedullary devices that can be used to treat unstable fractures of the humeral diaphysis: less flexible, locking intramedullary nails (similar to those used in the tibia and femur) that are commonly placed in an antegrade fashion and flexible nails (Enders) that cannot be statically locked and are typically placed in a retrograde fashion.

Locked intramedullary nailing of the humerus has become common, although recent reports detailing the associated morbidity with this technique have dampened some of this enthusiasm. Intramedullary nailing is generally used for closed diaphyseal fractures that cannot be maintained in an acceptable alignment by closed techniques. They are also commonly used for the operative stabilization of impending and complete pathologic fractures; for hypertrophic nonunions; and for multi-injured patients, particularly for those with lower extremity fractures who will be using the upper extremities for weight-bearing. Contraindications include the presence of an associated neurologic deficit, open and grossly contaminated fractures, and atrophic or oligotrophic nonunions.

Flexible intramedullary nails are commonly used in the multitrauma patient, particularly for fractures above and below the elbow. They are generally placed in retrograde fashion from an entry point just above the olecranon fossa posteriorly. Several nails are placed tightly within the medullary canal to obtain an interference fit with the endosteum, providing some rotational and axial stability. The nails should be anchored distally; a screw can be placed through the distal eyelet or the ends of the nails can be wired together, to prevent backing out (16).

The benefits of intramedullary nailing of humeral shaft fractures include the use of a relatively small incision and approach; load sharing to promote healing; and rotational and axial stability, which are restored at the time of surgery because the nails can be statically locked. The major disadvantage of intramedullary nailing placed in antegrade fashion is the disruption of the rotator cuff and the morbidity associated with it (pain, impingement, stiffness). Distal locking from lateral to medial can be hazardous to the radial nerve, even with the use of a proximally based locking jig.

Flexible intramedullary nails provide an internal splint that helps maintain axial alignment, length, and rotation. This fixation is often used in conjunction with a functional brace. The major benefits of the retrograde nails is that they can be placed through an extension of the same incision used to operatively stabilize fractures of the elbow and forearm. This approach does not require disruption of the rotator cuff, but flexible nails have been known to backout and require removal.

Plate Osteosynthesis

ORIF is currently one of the most popular methods of treating unstable fractures of the humeral diaphysis. The implant of choice is a broad dynamic compression plate, which can be used for transverse fractures and oblique fractures, when the obliquity of the fracture is in the coronal plane (Fig. 23.10). In oblique fractures in the sagittal plane and in spiral fractures, lag screws placed outside the plate are used to achieve interfragmentary compression, and the plate is used to neutralize rotational forces. Past recommendations suggested that the plates be long enough to gain at least six cortices and preferably eight cortices above and below the fracture site. More recent investigations, however, have shown that the rigidity of the construct can be increased with longer plates and with the screws spread over a longer lever arm, which obviates the need to fill each hole in the plate or to necessarily gain purchase in eight cortices. This seems particularly true for strong cortical bone found in the typical trauma patient (17).

Plate osteosynthesis is recommended for the treatment of oligotrophic and atrophic nonunions of humeral fractures and failed plate osteosyntheses. In these situations, the open stabilization should be augmented with an autologous iliac crest bone graft.

The radial nerve and profundi brachial artery are at risk during the posterior triceps-splitting approach to the humerus. Extreme care should be taken to make sure the plate is not placed on top of the nerve and that the nerve does not get incarcerated within the fracture site.

Early range of motion of the shoulder and elbow are initiated on postoperative day 2. The arm is maintained in a sling, generally without any other form of immobilization. If the fixation is suspect or if the patient is likely to place demands on the humerus before complete healing has occurred, then a Sarmiento fracture brace should be used. At 6 to 8 weeks after surgery, active and active-assisted range of motion exercises of the shoulder, wrist, and elbow are started along with muscle strengthening.

Results

EXTERNAL FIXATION

External fixation of diaphyseal fractures is generally reserved for open, contaminated complex fractures and occasionally for segmental bone loss. Few studies are available that describe the results of humeral shaft fractures definitively treated with external fixation. External fixation of the humerus suffers from the same complications as external fixation of open tibia fractures. Malunion, nonunion, infection, and pin-tract infections are common. These are some of the reasons why external fixation of the humeral shaft is typically used as a temporary measure only. The fixators are applied acutely and are maintained until control of soft tissues is obtained; the fixators are then removed and internal fixation or intramedullary nailing is performed. Neumann et al. (16) reported a 93% union rate with a pin-tract infection rate of 7.5% in multitrauma patients with severe closed and open humerus fractures.

OPEN REDUCTION AND INTERNAL FIXATION

The results of ORIF using an AO technique are generally good to excellent, but not without risk (18–21). In some of the more recently published series, a combined union rate of 96% has been reported. Most common complications include radial nerve palsy (usually transient), infection, and loss of fixation (6,16,19–22).

INTRAMEDULLARY NAILING

Intramedullary fixation of humeral shaft fractures has been associated with good results. The use of flexible nails has been advocated as a means to provide an inter-

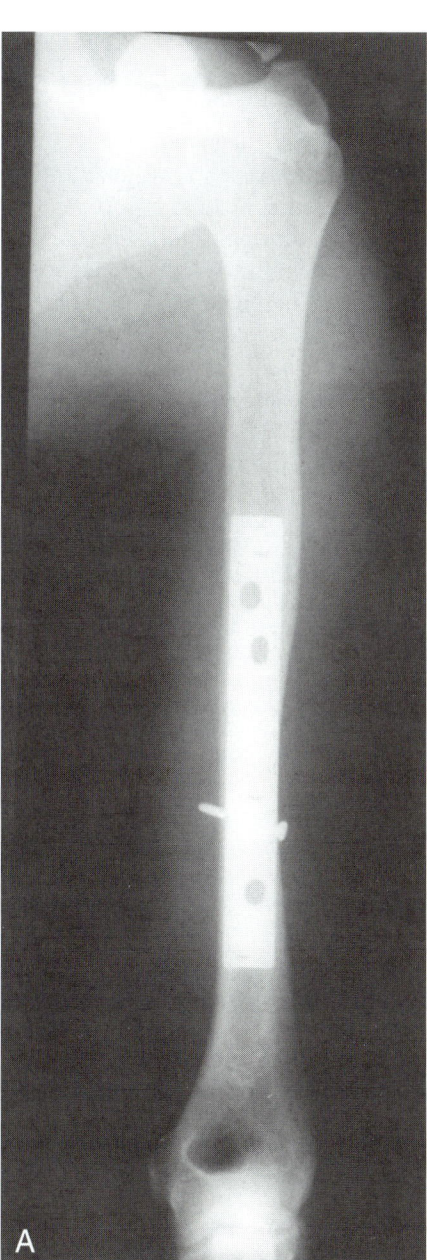
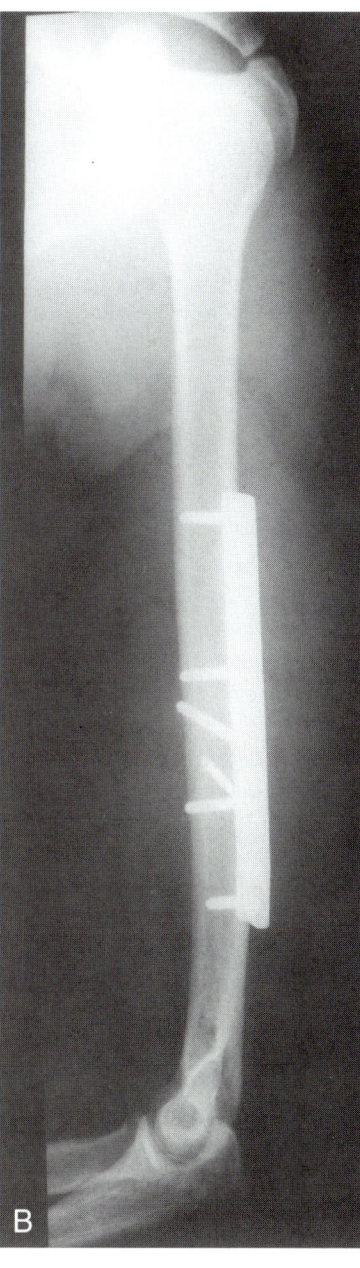

Figure 23.10. Postoperative AP (**A**) and lateral (**B**) views of the patient shown in Figure 23.3. The implant is a broad 4.5-mm dynamic compression plate fixed with interfragmentary lag screws.

nal splint. They can be inserted either antegrade or retrograde; the retrograde method is conveniently used in patients with multiple system injuries and/or multiple fractures. The union rate for humeral shaft fractures treated with flexible nails is believed to be in the range of 94 to 98%.

Locked reamed intramedullary nailing of humeral shaft fractures has become increasingly popular. Several methods of distal locking have been developed. Presently, the most commonly used nails are locked distally, and screws are placed lateral to medial or anterior to posterior. Results have been encouraging, although the union rates are not as reliable as those reported with AO plating techniques. Antegrade intramedullary nailing has been associated with nonunion, nerve injury, and common shoulder complaints (23–25).

Complications

MALUNIONS

Because of the wide range of motion of the glenohumeral joint, malunions of the humeral diaphysis are tolerated and not functionally problematic. Typically, up to 30° of angulation, 20° of rotation, and 3 cm of shortening are well tolerated. Osteotomy of the humerus with ORIF should be reserved for cases in which the malunion or accompanying deformities or limitations significantly alter function. In such cases, the osteotomy should be performed in the area of the greatest deformity and oriented to allow interfragmentary lag screw stabilization and neutralization plating.

NONUNIONS

Nonunions of humeral shaft fractures have been reported to occur in up to 5% of conservatively managed fractures and up to 25% in operatively treated humeral fractures (6,7,29). The nonunions may be atrophic, oligotrophic, or hypertrophic. The treatment of each must reflect the nature of the nonunion and surrounding environment. Atrophic nonunions are thought to require stimulation and revascularization to heal. Stimulation is often provided by resecting necrotic tissue; opening the medullary canal; adding autologous bone graft; and if the soft tissue envelop is severely compromised, supplying vascularized tissue in the form of rotational or free vascularized flaps.

Oligotrophic and hypertrophic nonunions are vascular but, owing to the unstable mechanical environment, fail to heal. ORIF or placement of a large-diameter, reamed intramedullary nail improves the stability of the nonunion site and commonly leads to union within 6 to 8 weeks. This improved stability is commonly augmented with an iliac crest bone graft to maximize the chances for union. Several articles have reported good success in the treatment of nonunions with ORIF when augmented with iliac crest bone graft (26–28).

RADIAL NERVE PALSY

Radial nerve palsy has been reported in the literature at rates of 1.8 to 18% (7,29). Radial nerve injury can range from complete or partial laceration, crush injury, entrapment in the fracture site or fracture callus, and perineural fibrosis. High-energy injuries in which the humerus is the only long bone fracture have a relatively high incidence of associated radial nerve palsy. Studies have shown that a longitudinal fracture in the distal third of the bone is also associated with a higher relative incidence of radial nerve injury or entrapment. Most radial nerve injury is transient; neuropraxia resolves spontaneously after 3 to 4 months. We believe that exploration of the radial nerve is indicated if there is an open fracture that requires open débridement, if the fracture is associated with penetrating trauma, and if radial nerve lesions develop secondary to manual manipulation or movement of the fracture site.

SUMMARY

Fractures of the humeral shaft are generally the result of high-energy trauma or low-energy rotational forces. Diagnosis is generally straightforward and based on physical examination and plain radiographs. Physical examination should include a thorough neurologic evaluation of the distal extremity, because of the risk of radial nerve injury following this fracture.

Treatment options include nonoperative and operative methods, each of which carries its own risks and benefits. In general, the union rate is good to excellent, and once union has occurred, functional rehabilitation of the extremity will often lead to restoration of normal function.

REFERENCES

1. Sarmiento A, Kinman PB, Galvin EG, et al. Functional bracing of fractures of the shaft of the humerus. J Bone Joint Surg 1977; 59A:596–601.
2. Klenerman L. Fractures of the shaft or the humerus. J Bone Joint Surg 1966;48B:105–111.
3. Bostman O, Bakalim G, Vainionpaa S, et al. Immediate radial nerve palsy complicating fracture of the shaft of the humerus: when is early exploration justified? Injury 1985;16:499–502.
4. Laing PG. The arterial supply of the adult humerus. J Bone Joint Surg 1956;38A:1105–1116.
5. Carroll SE. A study of the nutrient foramina of the humeral diaphysis. J Bone Joint Surg 1963;45B:176–181.
6. Foster RJ, Dixon GL Jr, Bach AW, et al. Internal fixation of fractures and non-unions of the humeral shaft. J Bone Joint Surg 1985; 67A:857–864.
7. Mast JW, Spiegel PG, Harvey JP Jr, Harrison C. Fractures of the humeral shaft. Clin Orthop 1985;12:254–262.
8. Miller ME, Allgower M, Schneider R, et al, eds. Manual of internal fixation. 3rd ed. Berlin: Springer-Verlag, 1991:118–150.
9. Balfour GW, Mooney V, Ashby ME. Diaphyseal fractures of the humerus treated with a ready-made fracture brace. J Bone Joint Surg 1982;64A:11–13.
10. Stewart MJ, Hundley JM. Fractures of the humerus—a compara-

tive study in methods of treatment. J Bone Joint Surg 1955; 37A:681–692.

11. Gerwin M, Hotchkiss, RN, Weiland AJ. Alternative operative exposures of the posterior aspect of the humeral diaphysis with reference to the radial nerve. J Bone Joint Surg 1996;78A,:1690–1694.

12. Green SA. Complications of external skeletal fixation. In: Uhthoft HK, ed. Current concepts of external fixation. Heidelberg: Springer-Verlag, 1982:43–52.

13. Costa P, Gancecchi F, Cavazzuti A, Tartaglia I. Internal and external fixation in complex diaphyseal and metaphyseal fixation of the humerus. Ital J Orthop Traumatol 1991;7:87–94.

14. Kim NH, Hahn SB, Park HW, Yang IH. The Orthofix external fixator for fractures of long bones. Int Orthop 1994;18:42–46.

15. Brumbeck RJ, Bosse MJ, Poka A, Burgess AR. Intramedullary stabilization of humeral shaft fractures in patients with multiple trauma J Bone Joint Surg 1986;68A:960–970.

16. Neumann HS, Brug E, Winckler S, et al. The surgical treatment of diaphyseal fractures of the humerus: stabilization with plate osteosynthesis, Hackethal nailing, locking nail and external fixation. Int J Orthop Trauma 1993;3(Suppl):25–28.

17. Hall RF Jr, Pankovich AM. Ender nailings of acute fractures of the humerus. A study of closed fixation by intramedullary nails without reaming. J Bone Joint Surg 1987;69A:558–567.

18. Bell MJ, Beauchamp CG, Kellam JK, et al. The results of plating humeral shaft fractures in patients with multiple injuries: the Sunnybrook experience. J Bone Joint Surg 1985;67B:293–296.

19. Heim D, Herbert F, Hess P et al. Surgical treatment of humeral shaft fractures: the Basel experience. J Trauma 1993;35:226–232.

20. Vander Griend R, Tomasin J, Ward EF. Open reduction and internal fixation of humeral shaft fractures. Results using AO plating techniques. J Bone Joint Surg 1986;68A:430–433.

21. Vander Griend RA, Ward EF, Tomasin J. Closed Küntscher nailing of humeral shaft fractures. J Trauma 1985;25:1167–1169.

22. Brooker AF, Edwards CC. External fixation—the current state of the art. Baltimore: Williams & Wilkins, 1979.

23. Watanabe RS. Intramedullary fixation of complicated fractures of the humeral shaft. Clin Orthop 1993;292:255–263.

24. Ingman AM, Waters DA. Locked intramedullary nailings of humeral shaft fractures: implant design, surgical technique, and clinical results. J Bone Joint Surg 1994;76B:23–29.

25. Healy WL, White GM, Mick CA, et al. Nonunion of the humeral shaft. Clin Orthop 1987;219:206–213.

26. Rosen H. The treatment of nonunions and pseudarthroses of the humeral shaft. Orthop Clin North Am 1990;21:725–742.

27. Barquet A, Fernandez A, Luvizio J, et al. A combined therapeutic protocol for aseptic nonunion of the humeral shaft: a report of 25 cases. J Trauma 1989;29:95–98.

28. Muller ME. Treatment of nonunions by comparison. Clin Orthop 1965;43:83.

29. Holstein A, Lewis GB. Fractures of the humerus with radial-nerve paralysis. J Bone Joint Surg 1963;45A:1382–1388.

Elbow Arthritis: Surgical Treatment

Bryan J. Nestor and Mark P. Figgie

The primary function of the upper extremity is to position the hand in space. A functioning elbow joint is essential for this task. A stiff shoulder or wrist can be accommodated, but loss of elbow motion results in a significant functional deficit for the upper extremity. Therefore, elbow arthritis with associated loss of functional motion can be quite debilitating.

The choice of treatment for the arthritic elbow largely depends on the pathogenesis, which can be broadly categorized into inflammatory arthritis, degenerative arthritis, and posttraumatic arthritis. In addition, the extent of joint destruction, age, and activity level of the patient influence the choice of treatment.

RELEVANT ANATOMY AND BIOMECHANICS

The elbow joint consists of three articulations: the proximal radioulnar, radiohumeral, and ulnohumeral joints. The elbow can be thought of as a trochoginglymoid joint, because of the combination of trochoid (rotational) motion at the proximal radiohumeral and radioulnar joints and ginglymoid (hinge-like) motion at the ulnohumeral joint (1). Although the elbow functions primarily as a hinge and allows for assumption of a fixed center of rotation, it is important to realize that some motion occurs out of plane (2–4). Relative to the humerus, the ulna moves from valgus (external) rotation in extension to varus (internal) rotation with flexion (3,4). The instant centers of rotation occupy a locus measuring 2×0.5 mm (4), which is located at the center of the arc formed by the articular surfaces of the capitellum and trochlea in the sagittal plane (2,3). This information is important in the design of prostheses and reconstructive procedures.

Elbow range of motion in the normal individual is from 0° to 145° of flexion, 75° of pronation, and 85° of supination. However, Morrey et al. (5) have shown that normal individuals use only 30° to 130° of flexion, 50° of pronation, and 50° of supination to accomplish most of the activities of daily living (5). This information is useful when trying to establish goals and assess surgical outcome in the treatment of the arthritic elbow.

The relative contributions of articulation and soft tissue to elbow joint stability have been studied extensively (1,6,7). There are four ligamentous structures that contribute to elbow stability: the medial collateral ligament (MCL); the lateral collateral ligament (LCL) complex, including the lateral ulnar collateral ligament (LUCL) (8,9) and the radial collateral ligament (RCL); and the annular ligament. The primary stabilizer to valgus stress is the anterior oblique portion of the MCL, particularly with flexion (6,10). Secondary stabilizers include the articular geometry of both the ulnohumeral and radiocapitellar joints and the anterior capsule. On the contrary, the primary stabilizer to varus stress is the ulnohumeral joint, in both flexion (75%) and extension (55%) (6). Secondary stabilizers include the anterior capsule in extension and, to a much lesser degree, the lateral collateral ligament (6).

The importance of the LCL complex, specifically the LUCL, in providing rotational stability of the elbow has only recently been recognized (11). Loss of functional integrity in the LUCL results in posterolateral rotatory instability of the elbow. An understanding of elbow stability in terms of normal anatomy and relative functional contributions of articular geometry and soft tissue (capsule, ligaments, and muscle) is important when considering reconstructive procedures for the elbow.

INITIAL FINDINGS, PHYSICAL EXAMINATION, AND DIAGNOSIS

Inflammatory Arthritis

Rheumatoid arthritis (RA) afflicts 1 to 2% of the general population (12) and affects the elbow in 20 to 50% of patients with RA (13,14). RA is the most common cause of elbow arthritis. The clinical presentation depends to some extent on the stage of disease, but pain and loss of functional motion are the most common complaints. In the early stages of disease, patients will often present with a warm, swollen, painful elbow with a flexion contracture and limitation of both pronation-supination and flexion-extension. Physical examination confirms an active synovitis. In later stages, painful limitation of elbow motion is present, but often without signs of active synovitis. In addition, up to 25% of patients may complain of instability with advanced joint destruction (15). Pain is present throughout the arc of motion and often with pronation and supination as well. Patients may also present with complaints consistent with an ulnar neuropathy. Most often this is the result of compression in the cubital tunnel from extension of the synovitis.

Osteoarthritis

Osteoarthritis of the elbow is uncommon, occurring in 1 to 2% of patients with degenerative arthritis (1). Although rare, the clinical presentation and radiographic features are consistent and predictable. Patients present with complaints of painful loss of motion (16). However, unlike rheumatoid arthritis, the arc of available motion is usually not painful. Pain occurs at the extremes of flexion and extension. The loss of motion is also characteristic, and the loss of extension is greater than the loss of flexion. Pronation and supination are generally not affected. This affliction is predominant in males and usually affects the dominant extremity (16–20). The clinician should also look for signs and symptoms of ulnar neuropathy. Osteophytes may encroach on the nerve in the cubital tunnel. Presence of loose bodies may result in mechanical symptoms of catching or locking.

Posttraumatic Arthritis

Patients with posttraumatic conditions of the elbow may present with pain, but almost universally they are affected by loss of motion (21,22). Many if not most patients have had one or more prior surgeries. Therefore, the possibility of concomitant infection must always be kept in mind. It is important to classify the posttraumatic loss of elbow motion in terms of the etiological factors involved (1,22). It is helpful to think in terms of extra-articular versus intra-articular and soft tissue versus osseous. An understanding of the pathologic process in terms of these factors is essential for selecting the proper choice of treatment.

The clinical presentation may be complicated by neural or vascular injuries incurred at the time of injury or subsequent treatment. The presentation may be further complicated by concomitant instability with chronic elbow subluxation or dislocation.

RADIOLOGIC STUDIES

Inflammatory Arthritis

Radiographic evaluation of the rheumatoid elbow should include AP and lateral views. These two views allow the surgeon to stage the extent of disease, using one of two common classification schemes: the Mayo classification and a modification of the Steinbrocker classification (23,24). According to the Hospital for Special Surgery modification of the Steinbrocker classification, stage 1 consists of a normal-appearing x-ray with mild to moderate synovitis clinically. Stage 2 disease consists of mild joint space narrowing on x-ray and active, recalcitrant synovitis. Stage 3a involves progression to complete loss of articular joint space on x-ray; clinically the synovitis may begin to resolve. Stage 3b disease is characterized by complete joint destruction with progressive loss of subchondral bone and obliteration of normal articular contour (Fig. 24.1A,B). By this stage of disease, the synovitis has often resolved. Patients with 3b disease may present with instability. Finally, stage 4 is characterized by bony ankylosis radiographically. Stage 4 is not a natural progression from stage 3; it is the end stage most typical of juvenile rheumatoid arthritis (JRA) and is occasionally found in other inflammatory arthritides (24).

Additional radiologic studies are not necessary as a rule. CT, however, may be used to accurately plan for custom prostheses sometimes necessary in patients with JRA.

Osteoarthritis

Osteoarthritis of the elbow has the following radiographic characteristics. On the AP view, there is usually preservation of articular joint space of both radiocapitellar and ulnohumeral joints and a characteristic ossification of the olecranon fossa (19). Peripheral osteophytes and/or loose bodies may be present medially and/or laterally. The lateral x-ray usually shows significant osteophyte formation involving both the coronoid and olecranon processes. The articular surface between the tip of the coronoid and the tip of the olecranon is usually preserved (Fig. 24.1C,D). This radiographic appearance is consistent with the clinical presentation of smooth, pain-free range of motion (ROM), except at the extremes of flexion and extension. In addition, the presence of loose bodies may be seen on the lateral x-ray. The radiocapitellar joint involvement is variable and usually mild to moderate, which is

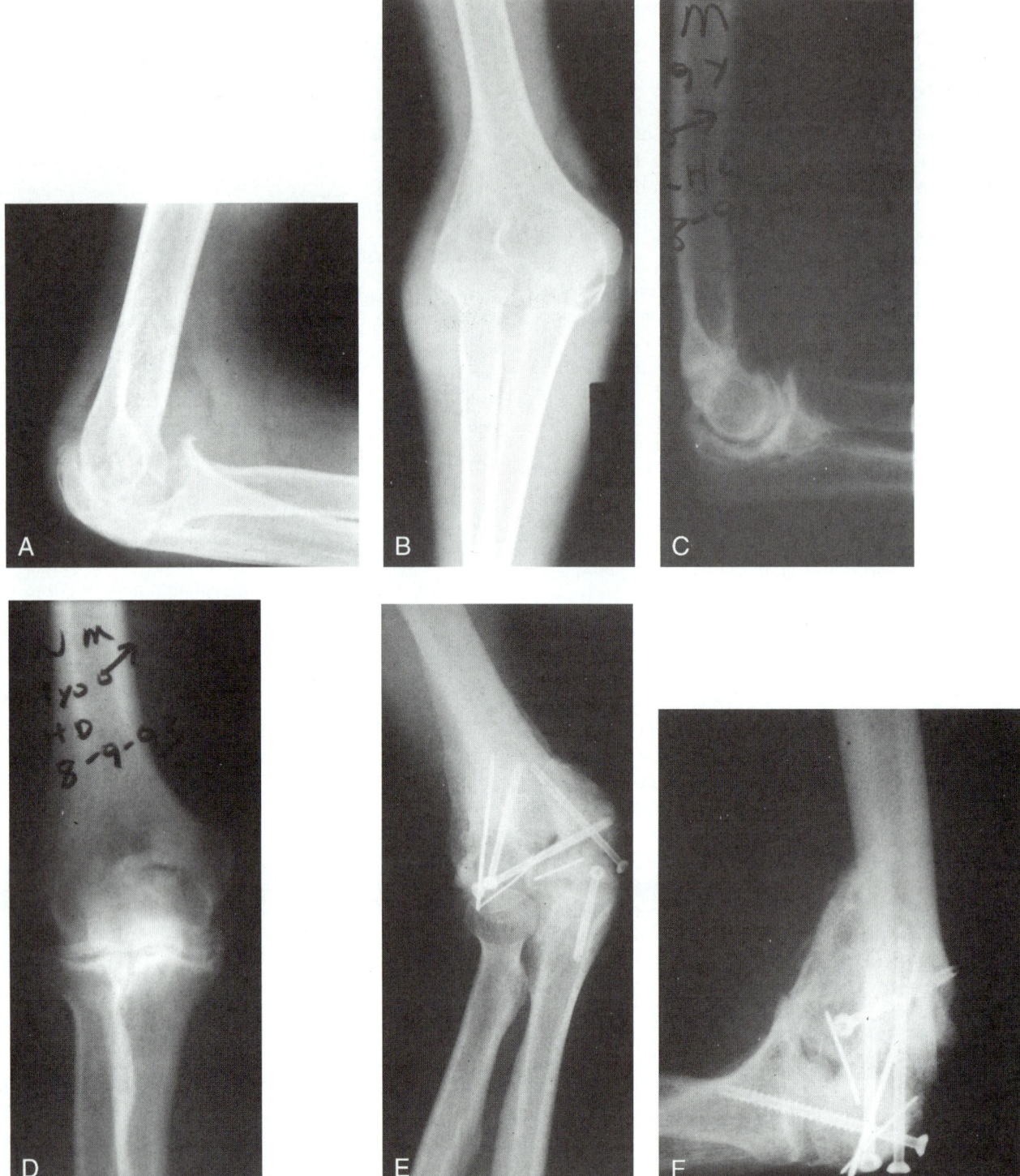

Figure 24.1. **A** and **B**. AP and lateral views of stage 3b rheumatoid arthritis. **C** and **D**. AP and lateral views of osteoarthritis. **E** and **F**. AP and lateral views of posttraumatic arthritis.

also consistent with the clinical absence of pain with pro-nation-supination.

Additional radiologic studies, such as tomography, arthrography, or CT, may be useful. Lateral tomography may be particularly helpful in identifying loose bodies and the presence of radiohumeral involvement (20).

Posttraumatic Arthritis

The initial evaluation of the stiff posttraumatic elbow begins with AP and lateral x-rays (Fig. 24.1E,F). Additional studies, particularly tomography, may be helpful. X-rays may reveal articular incongruity secondary to malunion or loss of articular cartilage, examples of intra-articular (intrinsic) lesions. Presence of heterotopic ossification, an extra-articular (extrinsic) osseous lesion, can also be determined. Absence of osseous lesions on x-ray allows the clinician to infer soft tissue contracture, which may be caused by intra-articular adhesions, extra-articular soft tissue contracture, or a combination of both. This combination of factors portends a poorer prognosis (1).

TREATMENT

Nonoperative Treatment and Surgical Indications

INFLAMMATORY ARTHRITIS

The choice of treatment for the rheumatoid elbow depends on the stage of disease. Synovectomy is a treatment option for patients with stage 1 or 2 disease (25–27). The primary indication for synovectomy is presence of painful synovitis, refractory to at least 6 months of optimal medical management. Synovectomy predictably relieves pain but does not predictably increase range of motion (25,26). Therefore, patients should have a functional range of motion before surgery. The other prerequisite for synovectomy is a stable elbow. Although synovectomy may be considered in select patients with stage 3a disease, it is contraindicated in patients with instability (stage 3b) and arthrofibrosis (stage 4).

The treatment of choice for more advanced stages of rheumatoid arthritis is total elbow arthroplasty (Clinical Table). The surgeon has a choice between two basic designs: resurfacing or semiconstrained. Resurfacing, or unconstrained, designs have the theoretical advantage of less stress transfer to the bone cement interface (28–30). Successful arthroplasty with an unconstrained implant, however, depends on sufficient bone stock and ligamentous integrity (28–30). Therefore, resurfacing arthroplasty may be limited to patients with less advanced disease, stage 2 or 3a.

Semiconstrained implants, on the other hand, have a more universal application that depends less on bone stock and is independent of ligamentous integrity (31–33). Most designs allow for 5° to 10° of both varus-valgus and axial rotation (31–33). Biomechanical studies have shown that for the most part these implants function within the limits of normal elbow kinematics (34). Certainly, the clinical results with semiconstrained implants have been much better than those with the earlier constrained hinge designs (31,35).

Clinical Table: Elbow Arthritis: Surgical Treatment

Procedure	Indications	Technique	Anatomy	Pitfalls
Total elbow arthroplasty	• Rheumatoid arthritis any age • Osteoarthritis, >60 years old • Posttraumatic arthritis, >60 years old	• Triceps sparing approach • Ulnar nerve transposition • Semiconstrained device • Cemented fixation • Antibiotic PMMA	• Triceps • Ulnar nerve • Humeral and ulnar anatomic center of rotation • Collateral ligaments • Radial head	• Intraoperative fracture • Failure to restore COR • Triceps rupture • Nerve injury • Infection
Débridement arthroplasty	• Osteoarthritis, <60 years old	• Medial approach • Ulnar nerve exposure • Anterior and posterior capsular excision • Coronoid and olecranon tip excision • Decompression olecranon and coronoid fossa	• Flexor pronator muscle mass • Ulnar nerve • Medial collateral ligament	• Inadequate decompression • Neurovascular injury • Recurrent impingement • Heterotopic ossification
Distraction arthroplasty with or without fascial interposition	• Posttraumatic arthritis, <60 years old	• Medial or lateral approach • Ulnar nerve transposition • Anterior and posterior capsulectomy • Release intra-articular adhesions • Coronoid and olecranon tip excision • Fascial interposition if articular damage	• Median, ulnar, radial nerves • LUCL • MCL • Distal humerus • COR	• Wound healing • Pin tract infection • Neurovascular injury • Instability • Ulnar and humeral bone loss

PMMA, polymethylmethacrylate; COR, center of rotation.

The primary indications for total elbow arthroplasty in rheumatoid arthritis are pain; limited range of motion; and in some cases, instability. Given that the primary function of the elbow is to position the hand in space, reconstruction of the elbow should be considered only in a patient with a functional hand. In general, elbow reconstruction takes precedence over shoulder reconstruction in cases of equal ipsilateral involvement (36). However, an ankylosed shoulder may result in increased stress transfer at the elbow. Therefore, if inadequate shoulder rotation is present, consideration is given to proceeding with total shoulder arthroplasty first (37).

Absolute contraindications to total elbow replacement include recent or active infection. Relative contraindications include posttraumatic or degenerative arthritis in a young patient and presence of a neurotrophic joint. Ankylosis is not viewed as a contraindication, although the gains in motion are more modest (38).

Fascial interposition arthroplasty has been effectively used to treat patients with rheumatoid arthritis of the elbow and has provided reasonable pain relief (39,40). In terms of stability, range of motion, and pain relief, however, the results from this procedure have been considerably less predictable than those from total elbow replacement (40).

OSTEOARTHRITIS

The primary indication for treatment of osteoarthritis of the elbow is pain, particularly pain at extremes of motion. Loss of range of motion is a secondary indication for surgery (20). Nonoperative measures involve use of nonsteroidal anti-inflammatory drugs (NSAIDs) and activity modification. Surgical options include arthroscopic débridement and three débridement arthroplasty techniques (41–46).

Arthroscopy provides an effective and useful means of removing loose bodies and small osteophytes on the olecranon and coronoid. Experience with the application of arthroscopy to more extensive débridement is limited (41,42). Currently, the primary indication for arthroscopic débridement is for removal of loose bodies or for limited débridement in a patient with near-normal elbow range of motion (greater than −45° to 110°) (41,44). For patients with more limited motion and extensive osteophytes of the coronoid, olecranon, and coronoid fossa, an open method of débridement is preferred (44).

The common goal of débridement arthroplasty procedures is the removal of loose bodies and osteophytes from the coronoid, olecranon, and coronoid fossa. The Outerbridge Kashiwagi arthroplasty, or ulnohumeral arthroplasty, is an effective way to accomplish this surgical goal; the procedure involves a posterior approach and the creation of a fenestration through the coronoid fossa (20,43). In patients with more severe contracture (flexion contracture is greater than 55° to 60°; flexion is less than 110°), it is preferable to use a procedure that allows equal access to the soft tissues anteriorly (44).

Two approaches have been described from the lateral side (44,45): the lateral débridement described by Tsuge and Mizuseki (45) and the lateral column procedure described by Morrey (44). Tsuge and Mizuseki's exposure involves taking down the lateral ligament complex, but Morrey's approach preserves the lateral ulnar collateral ligament while allowing exposure to excise both the anterior and posterior capsule.

Hotchkiss and Kasparyan (46) outlined another approach in which the elbow is approached from the medial side. The advantages are that the surgeon can address the soft tissue contracture both anteriorly and posteriorly, remove osteophytes, and protect or transpose the ulnar nerve. The anterior bundle of the medial collateral ligament is preserved, so that repair and prolonged protection are not necessary. The radiohumeral joint is not exposed; however, as noted, the radiohumeral joint is usually not the source of significant disease in osteoarthritis of the elbow.

For patients older than 60 or 65 years, total elbow arthroplasty may be a reasonable option for symptomatic degenerative arthritis of the elbow.

POSTTRAUMATIC ARTHRITIS

The choice of treatment for posttraumatic conditions of the elbow depends to a large extent on the presence or absence of intra-articular involvement. Posttraumatic ankylosis that results from extra-articular factors, heterotopic ossification, or soft tissue contracture can be managed with excision of bone and/or soft tissue release. Sometimes the release and reconstruction of ligaments is necessary, in which case application of a distraction device (hinge external fixator) allows for immediate stability and early motion while the ligamentous reconstruction heals (3,22,47,48). In patients in whom the joint is involved, distraction arthroplasty with or without fascial interposition may be required. In general, presence of pain and loss of more than 50% of the articular surface are reasons to consider fascial arthroplasty (22).

Distraction arthroplasty with or without fascial interposition is a technically demanding procedure with many potential complications. Both the surgeon and the patient should have a clear understanding of the goals and objectives of surgery preoperatively. The primary goal is range of motion, but not without the risk of instability and almost always some loss of strength (22). Therefore, patients who are manual laborers with a painless, stiff elbow may not be ideal candidates. While increasing the range of motion would certainly improve the overall function of the upper extremity, a loss of strength and potential instability would preclude heavy manual activity. Patients should also understand that the goals are for a functional arc of motion, approximating 30° to 130° of flexion. Patients with flexion contractures less than 45° and flexion to 115° or more are also probably not candidates (44).

Alternative procedures include allograft arthroplasty, which must be considered a salvage procedure for young patients with marked bone loss; resection arthroplasty, reserved almost exclusively for infection; arthrodesis, which is rarely considered because of its functional limitations; and total elbow arthroplasty for older patients.

Operative Treatment

ELBOW ARTHROPLASTY TECHNIQUES

Total Elbow Arthroplasty: Semiconstrained

The surgical approach most commonly used for semiconstrained implants is the posteromedial approach described by Bryan and Morrey (49). The patient is positioned supine in a slight beach chair position with the arm across the chest and a sterile tourniquet high on the humerus. The limb is exsanguinated, and a straight proximal incision over the medial third of the triceps is made and extended distally over the lateral border of the cubital tunnel. The incision then gently curves laterally over the proximal third of the ulna. The ulnar nerve is identified proximally along the medial border of the triceps and dissected along its course from proximal to distal. The nerve is released from the cubital tunnel and dissected along its course between the two heads of the flexor carpi ulnaris, allowing for anterior transposition. A Penrose drain or ves-

sel loop is placed around the nerve to help maintain identification of the nerve (Fig. 24.2A).

An incision is made along the medial border of the proximal ulna; and using sharp dissection, the flexor carpi ulnaris is dissected from the medial border of the ulna. The insertion of the medial collateral ligament is released from the sublime tubercle, taking care to avoid the ulnar nerve. The triceps insertion in continuity with the forearm fascia is sharply elevated from the proximal ulna and reflected laterally. This results in a continuous extensor soft tissue sleeve. A beaver blade is often useful in this portion of the dissection.

The anconeus and lateral collateral ligaments are released from the lateral ulna and, together with the triceps, are retracted laterally to expose the radial head. The radial head is resected with an oscillating saw, proximal to the annular ligament. After release of both medial and lateral collateral ligaments, the shoulder is externally rotated, and the elbow can be dislocated, providing excellent exposure of the proximal ulna. In cases of severe flexion contracture or ankylosis, anterior capsulectomy may be required.

Once the anatomic center of the ulna is determined, a guide is used to mark the proximal ulna, and an oscillating saw is used to make the appropriate bone cuts (Fig.

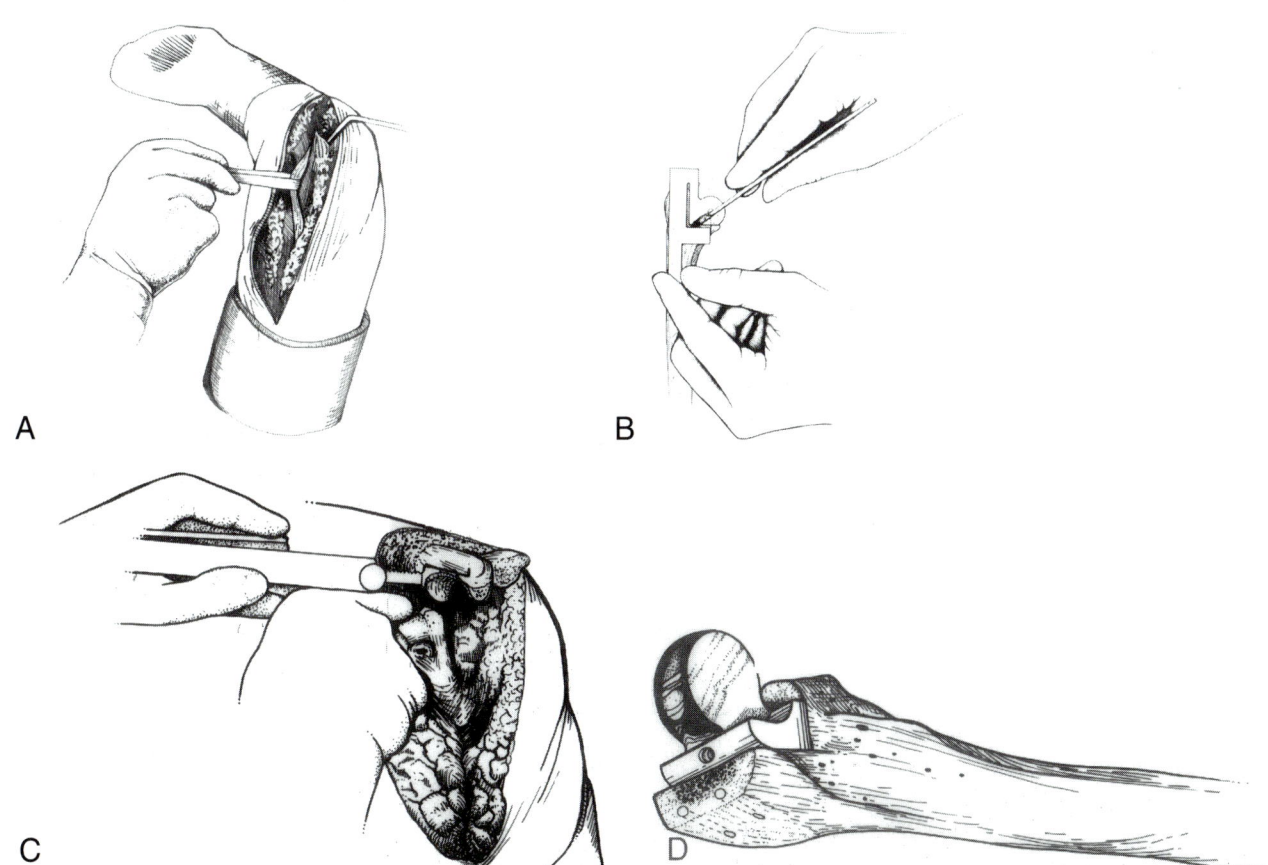

Figure 24.2. A. In the Bryan–Morrey approach to total elbow arthroplasty, the ulnar nerve is released and protected with a Penrose drain. **B.** An ulnar template is used to mark the proximal ulnar os- teotomy, and care is taken to restore the anatomic center of rotation. **C.** The proximal ulnar osteotomy is performed with a microsagittal saw. **D.** The trial ulnar component is then seated.

24.1B,C). The medullary canal of the ulna is then identified with a small awl, and the proximal ulna is prepared with the appropriate size rasps. Adequate preparation can be confirmed with a trial ulnar component (Fig. 24.1D).

Preparation of the distal humerus begins with resection of the central portion of the articular surface and identification of the humeral medullary canal with an awl (Fig. 24.3A). Cutting jigs, which are based on an intramedullary alignment guide, are then used to make the distal humerus bone cuts (Fig. 24.3B,C). An important consideration in planning the distal humerus cuts is restoration of the anatomic center of rotation. Furthermore, care must be taken not to violate the supracondylar ridges. Notching or excessive force used when broaching the distal humerus can result in fracture. Once the bone cuts have been made, the distal humerus is rasped to the appropriate size (Fig. 24.3D).

At this point, the trial components are seated, and the elbow is reduced and taken through a range of motion. The elbow should flex beyond 130° and extend beyond 20°. Pronation and supination are also checked, but they may be limited by the extent of wrist involvement. Any bony impingement or soft tissue restriction should be released. The radial neck should be evaluated to ensure that it does not impinge against the implant. In addition, the coronoid

process should be checked to ensure that it does not limit flexion. The tip of the coronoid can be excised to relieve impingement.

Once satisfactory motion is established, the trial components are removed, and the intramedullary canals of both the humerus and ulna are prepared by removing loose debris with pulse lavage irrigation. The intramedullary canals are then packed to ensure a dry, cancellous bone bed for cementing. Although methods of uncemented fixation are being explored, the ulnar and humeral components are generally cemented. The cement is introduced into the medullary canal using a syringe. The implants are then seated; the surgeon must take care to restore the anatomic center of rotation of both ulnar and humeral components (Fig. 24.4A). Excess cement is removed, the tourniquet is deflated, and hemostasis is obtained.

The elbow is articulated, and the central axle is locked into place. The extensor mechanism is repaired with two nonabsorbable sutures placed through drill holes in the ulna (Fig. 24.4B). A drain is placed in the deep wound. The ulnar nerve may be transposed or returned to its anatomic position, depending on the surgeon's preference.

The wound is closed in layers. A compressive dressing is applied, and the elbow is splinted at the discretion of

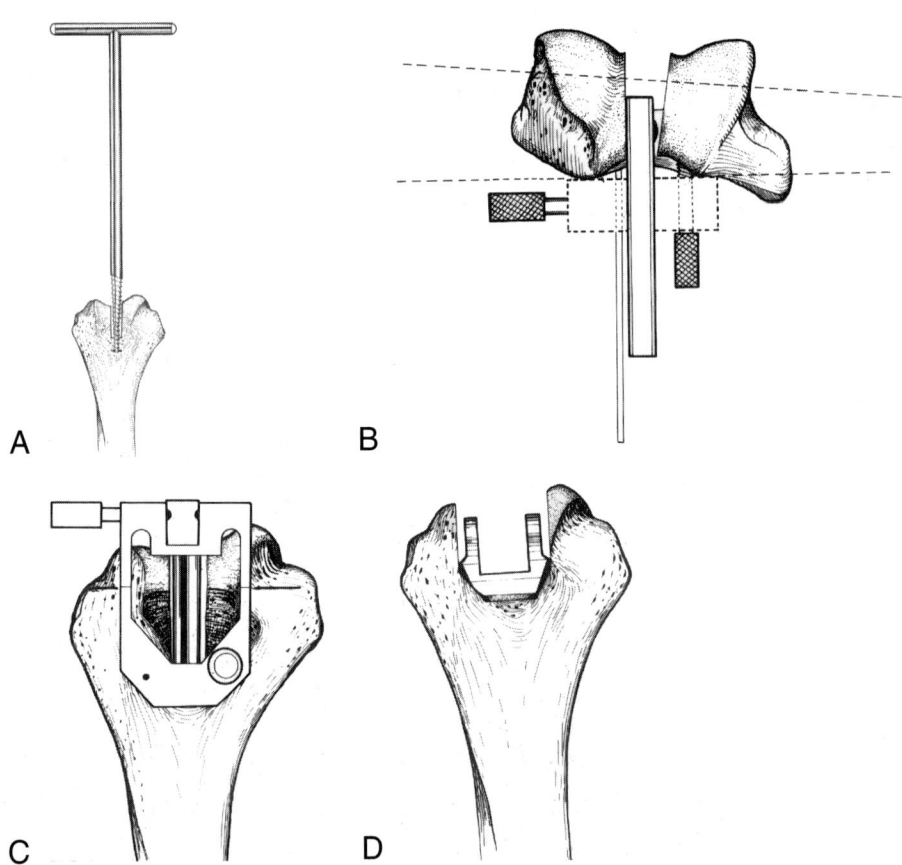

A   B   C   D

Figure 24.3. **A.** After resection of the central portion of the articular surface of the distal humerus, an awl is placed in the intramedullary canal. **B.** The distal humerus cutting guide relies on intramedullary alignment to establish the proper orientation in the coronal and sagittal planes. The guide must be slightly internally rotated in the coronal plane to match the center of rotation axis of the distal humerus. **C.** The distal humerus cutting guide is adjusted proximally and distally to restore the center of rotation. **D.** The humeral canal is rasped, and the trial humeral component is seated.

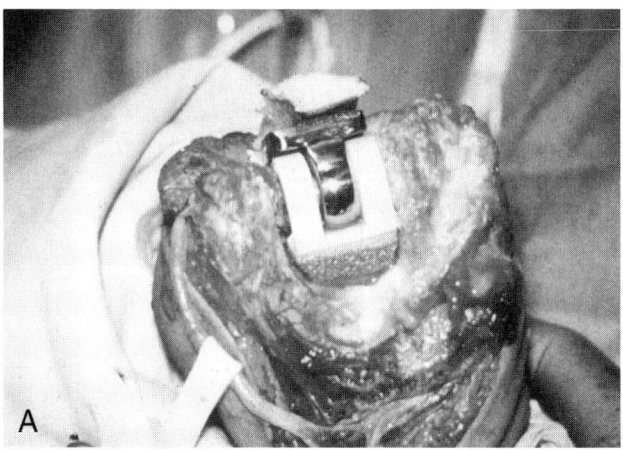
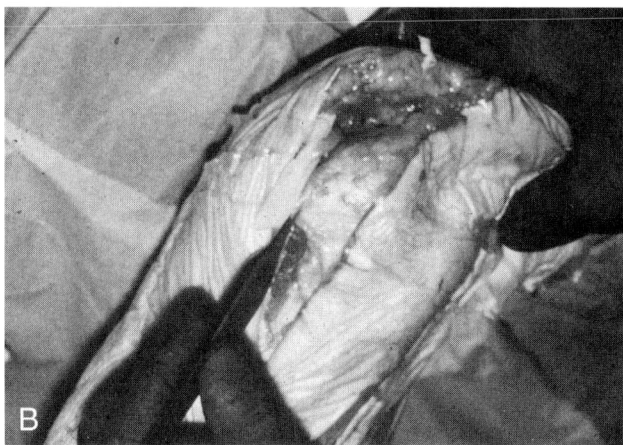

Figure 24.4. A. The ulnar and humeral components have been cemented, the components have been articulated, and the axle has been placed. **B.** The triceps is reduced and repaired with two non-absorbable sutures placed through the olecranon.

the surgeon. Some surgeons prefer to begin early passive range of motion (PROM) exercises with a continuous passive motion (CPM) machine. If a plaster splint is applied, the arm is placed in 30° of flexion, and the splint is removed after 24 to 48 h.

Débridement Arthroplasty

This section discusses débridement arthroplasty from the medial approach (46). The patient is positioned supine with the arm on an arm board. An extensive medial incision is made (Fig. 24.5A). The ulnar nerve is exposed and mobilized from the cubital tunnel, and the intermuscular septum is excised. The proximal portion of the flexor pronator mass is elevated, exposing the anterior humerus and anterior capsule (Fig. 24.5B).

The flexor carpi ulnaris is left attached to the medial epicondyle; the origin of the medial collateral ligament lies underneath. A right angle retractor placed underneath the brachialis protects the neurovascular structures (median nerve and brachial artery). The anterior capsule is then excised (Fig. 24.5C). The tip of the coronoid and hypertrophic osteophytes characteristic of degenerative arthritis are removed with an osteotome. A burr is used to deepen and restore the coronoid fossa on the anterior humerus.

At this point, the triceps is mobilized from the posterior humerus and the posterior capsule is exposed and excised. The triceps insertion may be partially mobilized, as in the Morrey–Bryan approach (49), to facilitate exposure. An osteotome is used to remove the tip of the olecranon (Fig. 24.5D). A burr can be used to deepen the olecranon fossa on the posterior surface of the distal humerus. Then the elbow is taken through its range of motion to ensure absence of bony impingement, complete loose body removal, and adequate soft tissue excision.

The triceps, if partially mobilized, is repaired with nonabsorbable sutures through the olecranon. The pronator flexor origin is repaired, and the ulnar nerve is transposed subcutaneously.

Distraction Arthroplasty with or without Fascial Interposition

The use of a hinged distraction device allows the surgeon to gain immediate stability, obtain early range of motion, and distract the joint while soft tissues and joint surfaces heal (3,22,47,48). Application of such devices is not limited to use in reconstructive procedures for chronic conditions, a distraction device may also be used for acute injury (1). Currently, three types of distraction devices are available: the Brigham Hospital device (3), the device designed by Morrey (22), and the one designed by Hotchkiss et al. (48). Although the specific technique for each of these devices is unique, there are numerous similarities.

The rationale for the use of a distraction device is based on the fact that the elbow's center of rotation is essentially a fixed point at the center of the trochlea and capitellum. The fixed center of rotation allows for distraction of the ulna and maintenance of distraction through a full arc of motion. The Brigham Hospital and Morrey devices include pins that are placed through the center of rotation. Hotchkiss et al.'s device uses a pin to establish the center of rotation, about which the frame is applied; after application, the pin is removed. Humeral fixation is obtained with half pins in the proximal humerus that are placed in stronger cortical bone away from the reconstructive site. Similarly, ulnar fixation is obtained more distal in the ulna with half pins.

With any distraction arthroplasty procedure, joint exposure can be obtained through a variety of approaches. The decision to use a particular surgical approach may be influenced by the degree of ligamentous integrity, previous incisions, and the nature of additional procedures being performed. If the medial collateral ligament has already been compromised, then a posteromedial approach with reconstruction of the ligament would be appropriate. If the medial collateral ligament is intact, then a lateral exposure may be employed, preserving the integrity of the medial collateral ligament.

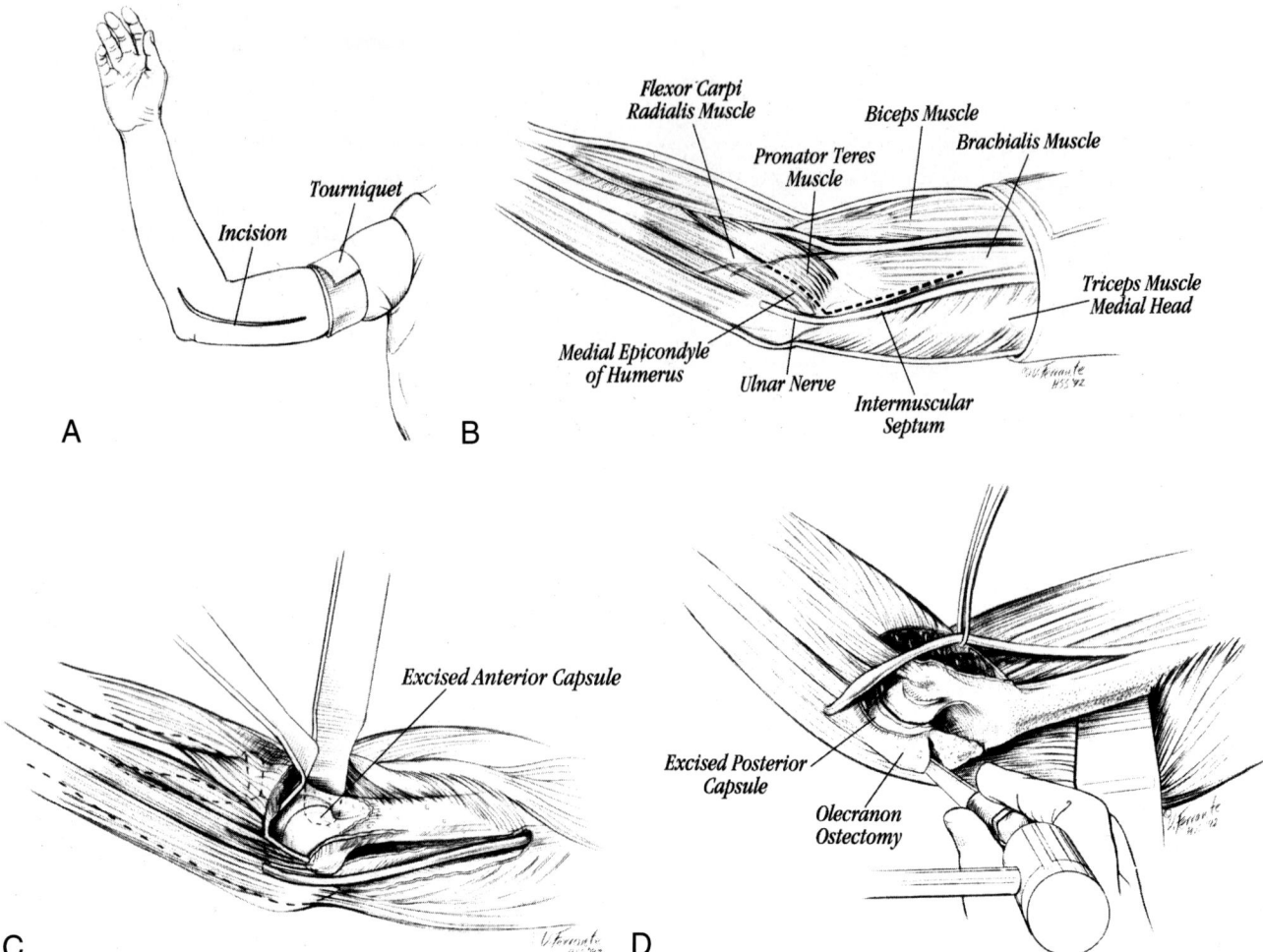

Figure 24.5. A. The medial approach for débridement arthroplasty. **B.** The ulnar nerve is released from the cubital tunnel. The elbow is exposed anteriorly by sharply elevating the origin of the pronator teres together with the brachialis proximally. **C.** A retractor is placed beneath the brachialis, protecting the neurovascular bun-dle; and the anterior capsule is excised. **D.** After partial elevation of the triceps and excision of the posterior capsule, the tip of the olecranon is removed with an osteotome. Courtesy of Robert N. Hotchkiss.

The patient is positioned supine. The arm may be placed on an arm board or across the chest, depending on the surgeon's preference. For the lateral approach, an extensile lateral (Kocher) incision is made. The brachioradialis and extensor carpi radialis longus (ECRL) are elevated from the lateral humerus. Care is taken to preserve the lateral ulnar collateral ligament. The anterior capsule is exposed by elevating the brachialis with a periosteal elevator. At this point, the anterior capsule can be excised. For posterior contracture, the triceps is elevated from the posterolateral humerus; the posterior capsule is excised; the triceps insertion can be sharply elevated from the olecranon; and the tip of the olecranon is removed, because it can serve as a source of impingement. Care must be taken to prevent injury to the ulnar nerve.

If insufficient motion is obtained, the origin of the lateral ulnar collateral ligament is released, allowing extensive intra-articular exposure (22) and more extensive release of soft tissues and intra-articular adhesions. If the joint surfaces are affected by a malunion or loss of articular cartilage, then a fascial interposition can be performed. If the collateral ligament has been released, then a distraction device is applied to protect the ligament reconstruction and allow early range of motion.

The decision to proceed with fascial interposition is based on the loss of articular cartilage (more than 50%) or incongruity secondary to malunion (22). The possible need for fascial interposition may be suggested by preoperative radiographs or clinically by the presence of pain in addition to stiffness (22).

Autogenous fascia lata is commonly used for graft material, although numerous other possibilities exist, including the use of skin (39). Cadaveric Achilles tendon provides a thick graft and avoids the complication of harvesting an autogenous fascia lata graft. As described above, the exposure may be medial or lateral. Once the joint is exposed, the surfaces are prepared to accept the fascial graft. A burr is used to contour the surfaces, with care taken not to remove too much subchondral bone. Too much bone resection may predispose to resorption later, which has been a problem, particularly on the humeral side (22).

When fascia lata is used, it is usually harvested from the contralateral thigh and folded for greater thickness. The graft can be secured to the humeral and ulnar surfaces with Mitek anchors or sutures placed through bone (Fig. 24.6). The elbow is then reduced, and a distraction device is applied.

When a distraction device is applied, the ulnar nerve must be exposed and mobilized so that it will be protected when the pin is placed through the center of rotation (Fig. 24.7). If significant intra-articular adhesions were released or a fascial interposition was performed, then the joint is distracted, usually 2 to 3 mm. The ligament origin is repaired anatomically, and nonabsorbable sutures are placed through the two bone holes. If the triceps insertion was mobilized, it is repaired with nonabsorbable sutures placed through the holes in the olecranon. The ulnar nerve is transposed anteriorly, and the remainder of the wound is closed in a routine manner (Fig. 24.8).

Pitfalls and Common Mistakes

TOTAL ELBOW ARTHROPLASTY

Total elbow arthroplasty requires a familiarity with modern arthroplasty principles and the surgical anatomy of the elbow. It is hoped that the surgeon armed with this understanding can avoid the following common pitfalls and complications.

Fractures

Fractures that occur in total elbow arthroplasty, as in other types of arthroplasty, can be divided into those that occur intraoperatively and those that occur postoperatively. The most common intraoperative fracture occurs at either the medial or the lateral supracondylar ridge of the distal humerus (31,32). Some of these fractures can be pre-

vented by attention to proper sizing of the humeral component, taking care not to notch the distal humeral resection, and proper humeral component alignment. If a fracture occurs, it can be stabilized in a variety of ways and protected postoperatively. Another option is to consider excision of the epicondylar fragment (31).

Another source of intraoperative fracture results from inadvertent perforation of either the ulnar or the humeral medullary canal. These fractures are more common in the revision total elbow and can largely be prevented in the primary elbow by taking care during reaming and broaching.

Fractures that occur in the postoperative period may occur at the supracondylar ridges of the distal humerus, the humeral shaft, or the ulna (31,32). Patients with ipsilateral total elbow and total shoulder replacements may be predisposed to fractures involving the humeral diaphysis, because of a stress riser occurring between the humeral components. The use of shorter-stem humeral components should theoretically decrease the risk of such fractures.

In general, if the implant is stable, many of these fractures may be amenable to splinting. On the other hand, if the implant is loose, revision to a longer-stem component will likely be necessary (31,32).

Infection

Total elbow replacement is associated with a high infection rate (50,51), which is attributed to a number of factors, including the subcutaneous location of the elbow joint. Furthermore, the majority of patients have some type of inflammatory arthritis, and many are on immune-suppressing drugs. Besides careful surgical technique and postoperative wound management, routine use of antibiotics in the cement is believed to be beneficial.

Triceps Insufficiency

Triceps insufficiency can largely be avoided with a triceps-sparing approach (49). Care must be taken not to compromise the soft tissue sleeve while mobilizing the ex-

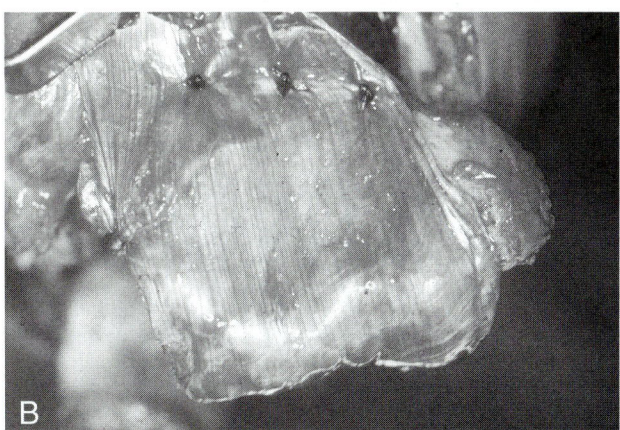

Figure 24.6.   A. An intraoperative view, showing significant articular cartilage damage in a patient with posttraumatic arthritis of the elbow. **B.** An intraoperative view, showing the resurfacing of the distal humerus with a fascia lata graft. Courtesy of Robert N. Hotchkiss.

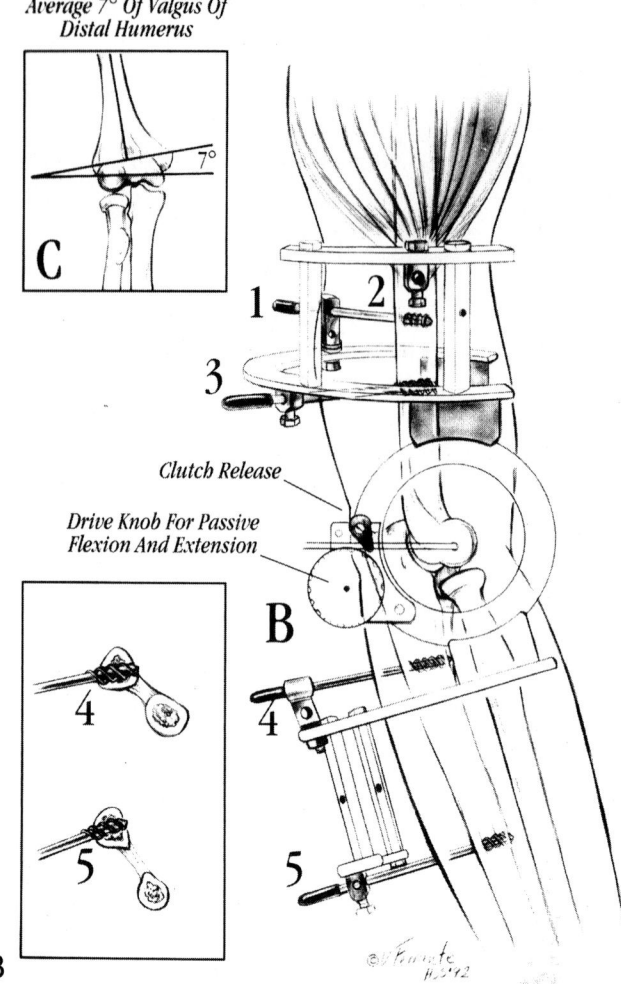

Average 7° Of Valgus Of Distal Humerus

Differential Block Height Compensates For Average 7° Of Valgus Of Distal Humerus

Axis Of Rotation

Clutch Release

Drive Knob For Passive Flexion And Extension

Figure 24.7. A. The application of the Compass elbow hinge and placement of the humeral pins. The hinge is applied after a 3.1-mm Steinmann pin is placed through the axis of rotation of the distal humerus. The Steinmann pin is removed after the hinge is applied. **B.** Lateral view of the Compass elbow hinge and placement of the ulnar pins. **C.** Average valgus angle of distal humerus. Courtesy of Robert N. Hotchkiss.

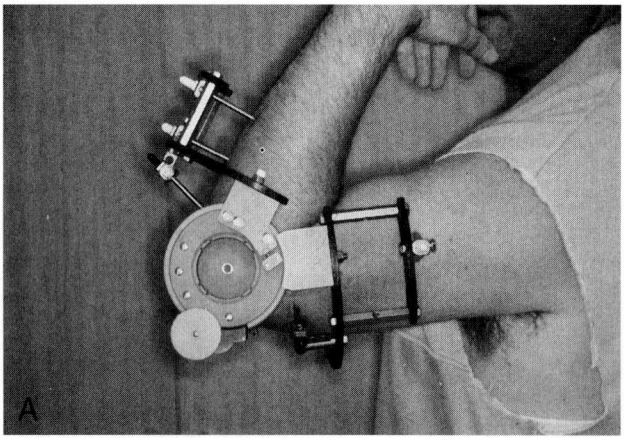
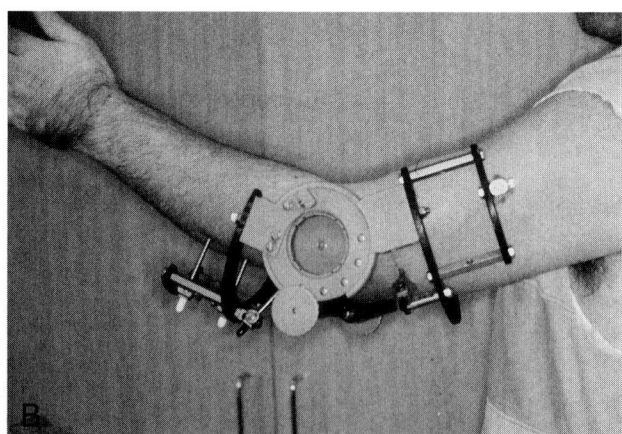

Figure 24.8. Active flexion (**A**) and extension (**B**) with the Compass elbow hinge. Courtesy of Robert N. Hotchkiss.

tensor mechanism and releasing Sharpey's fibers. The tendon is repaired with nonabsorbable sutures at the completion of surgery.

Neural Injury

The ulnar nerve is the most common site of neural injury, especially when the nerve is not identified and protected (31,32). Reasons for injury include trauma from surgical exposure and transposition, inadvertent pressure or injury during the procedure, postoperative hematoma formation, and pressure from the postsurgical dressing. Fortunately, most cases of ulnar neuritis resolve.

DÉBRIDEMENT ARTHROPLASTY

Inadequate Soft Tissue Release and Bony Decompression

Although the literature does not comment specifically on inadequate débridement, the surgeon must be sure to adequately address the sources of painful limitation in extension and flexion. For extension, it is important to resect the hypertrophic olecranon tip and release or resect the fibrotic anterior capsule. Loss of flexion must be addressed by resection of the hypertrophic coronoid process, reconstitution of the coronoid fossa, and resection of the posterior capsule.

Ectopic Ossification

Fortunately, heterotopic ossification after débridement arthroplasty is infrequent (45). Attention should be given to thorough irrigation of the wound and careful removal of all bone debris. In addition, use of an NSAID, such as Indocin, can be used to decrease the incidence of heterotopic ossification.

Neural Injury

Neural injury is infrequent and usually involves the ulnar nerve. Exposure of the nerve from the medial approach or careful retraction from the other approaches should prevent this complication.

Recurrent Impingement

Recurrent radiographic changes and, in some cases, recurrent symptoms have been reported (20,43,45). Unfortunately, there may be little that can be done to prevent recurrence of osteophytes responsible for the impingement. Successful repeat débridement has been reported (45).

DISTRACTION ARTHROPLASTY WITH OR WITHOUT FASCIAL INTERPOSITION

There are many complications associated with distraction arthroplasty, because of the complexity of the procedure, the extent of soft tissue dissection, and other factors related to the injury itself or subsequent treatment.

Wound Healing

The presence of previous incisions, the extensive surgical dissection often required, and postoperative swelling increase the likelihood of wound-healing problems. The risk of deep infection is also increased, particularly in the patient who has had previous surgeries. While some of the wound healing problems may be unavoidable given the extensive releases sometimes required, an awareness of the potential for wound healing problems and early recognition should lead to appropriate treatment when they do occur.

Pin Tract Infection

As with any external fixator, pin loosening and pin tract infection may occur. The devices that require maintenance of a pin at the humeral center of rotation must be followed closely, and device removal is recommended at 3 or 4 weeks (22). One advantage of the Compass hinge designed by Hotchkiss et al. (48) is that it allows the humeral pins to be placed more proximally away from the surgical wound and in better quality bone. If pin tract drainage develops, the pins should be immediately removed, and the patient treated with appropriate antibiotics.

Neural Injury

The nerves most susceptible to injury are the ulnar and posterior interosseous nerves. Ulnar nerve exposure and protection are essential to avoid injury during placement of the pin through the humeral center of rotation. The ulnar nerve is frequently transposed. The posterior interosseous nerve is also at risk, particularly with the extensile Kocher incision. Most of these injuries are caused by excessive traction and generally will recover. Injuries to the median nerve are possible during extensive soft tissue release, particularly with a large flexion contracture (44). Injury to the radial nerve can occur when the proximal lateral humeral pin of the Compass hinge is placed.

Triceps Insufficiency

Triceps weakness is common; however, avulsion of the triceps is less common. Postoperative protection of the extensor mechanism can prevent most of these injuries. Triceps avulsion requires surgical reattachment.

Bone Resorption

Bone resorption has been reported after fascial interposition (22). Bone resorption of both the ulna and humerus can be quite impressive and is believed to be possibly caused by the denervation that results from the extensive surgical exposure. Violation of the subchondral bone may also be a contributing factor. Therefore, resection of subchondral bone should be kept to a minimum.

Postoperative Rehabilitation

TOTAL ELBOW ARTHROPLASTY

The Bryan–Morrey approach (49) to total elbow arthroplasty allows the patient to begin early range of motion, usually on the 2nd postoperative day, if the wound is dry and the drain and splint have been removed. Cryotherapy is continued and the use of a CPM is initiated. The therapist guides the patient through early rehabilitation, but the patient is encouraged to use the arm as much as possible for activities of daily living. Patients are told before surgery that a flexion contracture of 30° or less can be expected. Pronation and supination exercises are also emphasized, but motion may ultimately be limited by preexisting wrist disease. Gentle strengthening exercises may begin after 6 weeks. However, patients are advised against lifting objects heavier than 4.5 kg (10 lb).

DÉBRIDEMENT ARTHROPLASTY

Postoperative rehabilitation from débridement arthroplasty begins immediately, with the institution of CPM in the recovery room. Cryotherapy and a compressive dressing help control swelling. The patient is encouraged to use the arm in daily activities. A physical therapist instructs the patient in active-assisted range of motion exercises. NSAIDs are continued for several weeks after surgery to decrease inflammation and reduce the incidence of heterotopic ossification. Once the wound has healed and the staples have been removed, flexion and extension splints are initiated to obtain final range of motion.

DISTRACTION ARTHROPLASTY

Regardless of the indication for the distraction device, early motion is often prescribed. A CPM machine started in the recovery room. This is often facilitated through the use of a continuous brachial plexus block to reduce pain. Cryotherapy is used to reduce swelling, which can be extensive. Patients are started on a active and/or passive range of motion exercise program. The length of time the distraction device is left in place depends on the type of fixator used. We use the Hotchkiss et al. device and often leave the fixator in place for 6 to 10 weeks, depending on the nature of the procedure. Splinting is often employed after the distraction device is removed to assist in gaining motion.

SUMMARY

The understanding of the pathogenesis and surgical treatment of elbow arthritis continues to evolve. However, advances over the last 15 years have led to more appropriate treatment options and improved clinical results. Increased survivorship with current designs of total elbow replacement has greatly facilitated the treatment of patients with rheumatoid elbows and older patients with noninflammatory or posttraumatic conditions of the elbow. Total elbow replacement in patients with rheumatoid arthritis has resulted in predictable pain relief (more than 90%), improved function through a functional arc of motion, and greater than 90% 5-year survivorship (31,32,35).

Degenerative arthritis has been increasingly recognized as a cause of elbow arthritis. As our knowledge of this entity has increased, more successful surgical treatments have evolved, especially débridement arthro-

plasty. Although motion gains of 10° to 15° in flexion and extension can generally be obtained, the primary goal is relief of pain at the extremes of motion, which can predictably be obtained in 90% of patients (20,43,45). The results have been observed to deteriorate with time (19,43).

Posttraumatic conditions of the elbow continue to present the most difficult reconstructive challenges. The results of total elbow replacement in posttraumatic arthritis have been disappointing (52,53). The surgical treatment of these conditions has improved with application of distraction devices and interpositional arthroplasty. Overall, the results of distraction arthroplasty with or without fascial interposition have been satisfactory in the majority of patients, but not without a high complication rate (22).

REFERENCES

1. Morrey BF. The elbow and its disorders. 2nd ed. Philadelphia: Saunders, 1993.
2. London JT. Kinematics of the elbow. J Bone Joint Surg 1981; 63A:529.
3. Deland JT, Garg A, Walker PS. Biomechanical basis for elbow hinge-distractor design. Clin Orthop 1987;215:305.
4. Morrey BF, Chao EY. Passive motion of the elbow joint. J Bone Joint Surg 1976;58A:501–508.
5. Morrey BF, Askew LJ, An KN, Chao EY. A biomechanical study of normal functional elbow motion. J Bone Joint Surg 1981; 63A:87–89.
6. Morrey BF, An KN. Articular MD ligamentous contributions to the stability of the elbow joint. Am J Sports Med 1983;11:315.
7. Regan WD, Korinek SL, Morrey BF, An KN. Biomechanical study of ligaments around the elbow joint. Clin Orthop 1991;271:170.
8. Morrey BF, An KN. Functional anatomy of the ligaments of the elbow. Clin Orthop 1985;201:84.
9. O'Driscoll SW, Horii E., Morrey BF, Carmichael S. Anatomy of the ulnar part of the lateral collateral ligament of the elbow. Clin Anat 1992;5:296.
10. Schwab GH, Bennett JB, Woods GW, Jullos HS. Biomechanics of elbow instability: the role of the medical collateral ligament. Clin Orthop 1980;146:42–52.
11. O'Driscoll SW, Bell DF, Morrey BF. Postero-lateral rotatory instability of the elbow. J Bone Joint Surg 1991;73A:440.
12. Wolfe AM. The epidemiology of rheumatoid arthritis: a review. Bull Rheum Dis 1968;19:518.
13. DeSeze S, Debetre N, Jan D, Etal A. The elbow joint [Int Congress Ser no. 61]. Amsterdam: Excerpta Medica, 1963.
14. Porter BB, Park N, Richardson C, et al. Rheumatoid arthritis of the elbow. The results of synovectomy. J Bone Joint Surg 1974; 56B:427.
15. Amis AA, Hughes SJ, Wright V. A functional study of the rheumatoid elbow. Rheumatoid Rehabil 1982;21:151.
16. Doherty M, Preston B. Primary osteoarthritis of the elbow. Ann Rheum Dis 1989;48:743.
17. Doherty M, Watt I, Dieppe PA. Influence of primary generalized osteoarthritis on development of secondary osteoarthritis. Lancet 1983;2:8.
18. Kash, Uagi D. Intra-articular changes of the osteoarthritic elbow, especially about the fossa olecrani. Jpn Orthop Assoc 1978; 52:1367.
19. Minami NM. Roentgenological studies of osteoarthritis of the elbow joint. Jpn Orthop Assoc 1977;51:1223.
20. Morrey BF. Primary arthritis of the elbow treated by ulnohumeral arthroplasty. J Bone Joint Surg 1992;74B:409.
21. Husband JB, Hastings H. The lateral approach for operative release of post-traumatic contracture of the elbow. J Bone Joint Surg 1990;72A:1353.

22. Morrey BF. Post-traumatic contracture of the elbow. J Bone Joint Surg 1990;72A:601.

23. Morrey BF. The elbow and its disorders. 1st ed. Philadelphia: Saunders, 1985.

24. Steinbrocker O, Traeger CH, Batterman RC. Therapeutic criteria in rheumatoid arthritis. JAMA 1949;140:659–665.

25. Ferlic DC, Patchett CE, Clayton ML, Freeman AC. Elbow synovectomy in rheumatoid arthritis. Clin Orthop 1987;220:119.

26. Inglis AE, Ranawatt CS, Straub LR. Synovectomy and debridement of the elbow in rheumatoid arthritis. J Bone Joint Surg 1971; 53A: 652.

27. Tulp NJA, Winia WPCA. Synovectomy of the elbow in rheumatoid arthritis: long term results. J Bone Joint Surg 1989;71B:664.

28. Ewald FC, Scheinberg RD, Poss R, et al. Capitellocondylar total elbow arthroplasty: two- to five-year follow-up in rheumatoid arthritis. J Bone Joint Surg 1980;62A:1259.

29. Ewald FC, Simmons ED, Sullivan JA, et al. Capitellocondylar total elbow replacement in rheumatoid arthritis. J Bone Joint Surg 1993; 75A:498.

30. Kudo H, Iwano K, Wajanabe S. Total replacement of the rheumatoid elbow with a hingeless prosthesis. J Bone Joint Surg 1980; 62A:277.

31. Morrey BF, Adams RA. Semiconstrained arthroplasty for the treatment of rheumatoid arthritis of the elbow. J Bone Joint Surg 1992;74A:479.

32. Figgie MP, Inglis AE, Figgie HE III, Mow CS. Semiconstrained total elbow replacement in rheumatoid arthritis. Orthop Trans 1990; 14:104.

33. Gschwend N, Loehr J, Ivosevir-Radovanovic D, et al. Semiconstrained elbow prostheses with special reference to the GSB III prosthesis. Clin Orthop 1988;232:104–111.

34. O'Driscoll SW, An KN, Korinek S, Morrey BF. Kinematics of semiconstrained total elbow arthroplasty. J Bone Joint Surg 1992; 74B:297.

35. Kraay MJ, Figgie MP, Inglis AE, et al. Primary semiconstrained total elbow arthroplasty. Survival analysis of 113 consecutive cases. J Bone Joint Surg 1994;76B:636–640.

36. Friedman RJ, Ewald FC. Arthroplasty of the ipsilateral shoulder and elbow in patients who have rheumatoid arthritis. J Bone Joint Surg 1987;69A:661–667.

37. Goldberg VM, Figgie HE, Inglis AE, Figgie MP. Current concepts review: total elbows arthroplasty. J Bone Joint Surg 1988; 70A:778–783.

38. Figgie MP, Inglis AE, Mow CS, Figgie HE III. Total elbow arthroplasty for complete ankylosis of the elbow. J Bone Joint Surg 1989; 71A:513.

39. Froimson AI, Silva JE, Richey DG. Cutis arthroplasty of the elbow joint. J Bone Joint Surg 1976;58A:863.

40. Hurri L, Pulkki T, Vainiok. Arthroplasty of the elbow in rheumatoid arthritis. Acta Chir Scand 1964;127:459.

41. O'Driscoll S. Morrey BF. Elbow arthroscopy: a critical assessment. J Bone Joint Surg 1992;74A:84.

42. Redden JF, Stanley D. Arthroscopic fenestration of the olecranon fossa in the treatment of osteoarthritis of the elbow. Arthroscopy 1993;9:14.

43. Kashiwagi D. Outerbridge Kashiwagi arthroplasty for osteoarthritis of the elbow joint. In: Kashiwagi D, ed., Proceedings of the International Congress, Kobi Japan. Amsterdam: Excerpta Medica, 1986.

44. Morrey BF. Reconstructive surgery of the joints. 2nd ed. New York: Churchill Livingstone, 1996.

45. Tsuge K, Mizuseki T. Debridement arthroplasty for advanced primary osteoarthritis of the elbow: results of a new technique used for 29 elbows. J Bone Joint Surg 1994;76B:641–646.

46. Hotchkiss RN, Kasparyan G. Medial over-the-top exposure of the elbow: a useful exposure for contracture release and ulnohumeral arthroplasty. Unpublished manuscript.

47. Volkov MV, Oganesian OV. Restoration of function in the knee and elbow with a hinge-distractor apparatus. J Bone Joint Surg 1975;57A:591–600.

48. Hotchkiss RN, An KN, Weiland AJ, O'Brien G. Treatment of severe elbow contracture using the concepts of Ilizarov. Paper presented at the 61st Annual Meeting of the American Academy of Orthopaedic Surgeons, New Orleans, February 28, 1994.

49. Bryan RS, Morrey BF. Extensive posterior exposure of the elbow. Clin Orthop 1982;166:188–192.

50. Morrey BF, Bryan RS. Infection after total elbow arthroplasty. J Bone Joint Surg 1983;65A:330.

51. Wolfe SL, Figgie MP, Inglis AE, Bohn WW, Ranawat CS. Management of infection about total elbow prostheses. J Bone Joint Surg 1990;72A:198–212.

52. Figgie MP, Inglis AE, Figgie HE, Mow CS. Total elbow arthroplasty in traumatic arthritis. Acad Orthop Trans 1990;14:628.

53. Morrey BF, Adams RA, Bryan RS. Total replacement for post-traumatic arthritis of the elbow. J Bone Joint Surg 1991;73B:607.

chapter 25

Marc R. Safran

Elbow Tendinopathy: Surgical Repair of the Epicondylitides

The majority of injuries to the elbow are chronic overuse injuries. These injuries are the result of repetitive intrinsic and/or extrinsic overload, which causes microrupture of the soft tissue. Intrinsic overload is the force from muscular contraction, concentric or eccentric, and can lead to tendinitis or muscular injury. Extrinsic overload is a tensile overload caused by excessive joint torque forces, which stress the soft tissue, resulting in stretching and eventual disruption. Extrinsic overload may also be the result of compression of the tendon, which leads to abrasion or impingement.

Muscles that span more than one joint, such as wrist extensors and flexors, are more susceptible to inflammation and injury because of the additional intrinsic and extrinsic overload. These muscles are exposed to extrinsic forces from stretching as they cross the two joints and intrinsic forces from muscular contraction. The resultant microrupture of the soft tissue is often coupled with an imperfect healing process, leading to chronic tendinitis. As juvenile apophyses undergo ossification, they are susceptible to stress injuries, resulting in local inflammation, disordered or irregular ossification patterns, overgrowth, and pain. Thus skeletally immature patients rarely develop tendinopathies.

RELEVANT ANATOMY AND PATHOGENESIS

The extensor carpi radialis longus (ECRL) arises from the distal one-third of the lateral humeral supracondylar ridge and from the lateral intermuscular septum. Its origin is between the origins of the brachialis and of the ECRB (1–3). The ECRB is located under the ECRL and arises from the common extensor tendon at the inferolateral aspect of the lateral epicondyle of the humerus, the lateral ligament of the elbow, the intermuscular septum, and the overlying fascia. The ECRB origin can be visualized only after the

ECRL tendon has been retracted. The ECRB is the most lateral of the extensor group. The EDC originates from the common extensor tendon and is just medial or ulnar to the ECRB. In the proximal forearm, the muscle fibers of the ECRL and EDC are almost indistinguishable from those of the ECRB. The ECU arises from two heads, one above and one below the elbow joint. The humeral origin is the most medial of the common extensor group originating from the lateral epicondyle of the humerus. The ulnar attachment is along the aponeurosis of the anconeus and at the superior border of this muscle. The lateral ligamentous complex of the elbow originates on the lateral epicondyle of the humerus, deep to the origin of the extensor tendons.

The flexor-pronator muscles arise from the medial aspect of the elbow. The pronator teres is the most proximal of this group and usually has two heads of origin: the larger arises from the anterosuperior aspect of the medial epicondyle, and the smaller one from the coronoid process of the ulna. The FCR originates from the medial epicondyle just inferior to the pronator teres. This interface is the most common site of disorders in medial epicondylitis; but pathologic tissue can also be seen at the FCU origin, the palmaris longus origin, and the undersurface of the flexor digitorum superficialis (FDS) (4,5). The FCU originates more posteriorly than the other muscles from the medial epicondyle and also arises from the medial border of the coronoid and the medial aspect of the proximal ulna.

The ulnar nerve enters the forearm between the two muscular origins of the FCU, the first innervating the FCU. The palmaris longus arises from the septa of the FCR and FCU and from the medial epicondyle. The FDS had a deep origin and arises medially from the common flexor tendon and proximal ulna; its smaller lateral head originates more distally from the proximal radius. The ulnar collateral ligament (UCL) complex originates from the broad anteroinferior surface of the medial epicondyle. The ulnar nerve rests in the posterior aspect of the medial epicondyle but is not intimately related to the fibers of the anterior bundle of the UCL. The anterior portion of the UCL inserts along the medial aspect of the coronoid process.

Tennis elbow is probably the most common elbow injury evaluated by the orthopaedic surgeon. *Tennis elbow* is a broad popular term used to describe an overuse-type injury to the tendon origin of the muscle group of the lateral aspect of the elbow; it has also been applied to the tendon origin of the medial elbow muscle group. Although the injury has also been referred to as tendinitis and epicondylitis, histologic studies of surgical specimens have confirmed that the disorder consists of vascular infiltration and degeneration of the tendon origin, not an inflammatory process (6–8). Intrinsic overload leads to a microtear of the tendon, which heals through fibrosis and granulation tissue production. As this process continues, mucinoid degeneration of the tendinous origin results; and with continued use, this eventually leads to partial failure of the tendon.

Lateral epicondylitis (the condition most often referred to as tennis elbow) is arguably the most common source of elbow pain in the general population. It occurs 7 to 20 times more frequently than does medial epicondylitis (9,10). It was first described more than 100 years ago in a tennis player (11,12) but has since been described in association with many other athletic and nonathletic endeavors.

Lateral epicondylitis is a chronic degeneration and vascular infiltration of the wrist extensor muscles, primarily the extensor carpi radialis brevis (ECRB), owing to overuse in terms of intensity and duration. Surgical studies confirm that the ECRB is the source of pathologic change and pain; however, the anterior extensor digitorum communis (EDC), the underside of the extensor digitorum radialis longus (EDRL), and (rarely) the origin of the extensor carpi ulnaris (ECU) may be involved as well (13,14).

Medial epicondylitis, often referred to as golfer's elbow and medial tennis elbow, is a pathologic change of the tendon of the flexor-pronator muscle group. Because this entity is not well studied, many of the ideas about and approaches to this problem are based on what is known about lateral epicondylitis. Medial epicondylitis primarily involves the pronator teres and flexor carpi radialis (FCR) muscles and, occasionally, the flexor carpi ulnaris (FCU) (14). Valgus stress, from throwing or axial compression, increases distraction or tensile forces to the medial elbow. The primary dynamic stabilizer to this stress is the flexor-pronator muscle mass. With repetitive throwing, the muscle mass may fatigue, injuring the musculotendinous structure and imparting the stress to the ulnar collateral ligament.

Imperfect healing after the microtrauma results in tendinitis of the flexor-pronator mass and attenuation of the ligament. The result is increased forearm valgus caused by ligamentous incompetency and an elbow flexion contracture owing to attempts at repair and stabilization (15). With repetitive valgus stress, patients may develop myotendinous injury to the flexor-pronator muscle group, chondromalacia of the radiocapitellar joint, loose bodies in the posterior or lateral compartments, injury to the ulnar collateral ligament, osteochondritis dissecans, or ulnar neuritis.

The biceps and triceps are two major muscles that cross the elbow anteriorly and posteriorly. These musculotendinous structures do not commonly develop clinically symptomatic tendinitis and thus will not be discussed here.

INITIAL FINDINGS, PHYSICAL EXAMINATION, AND DIAGNOSIS

History

Lateral epicondylitis presents as lateral elbow pain that has an insidious onset, beginning gradually after vigorous activity and progressing to pain with activity. It has been shown that 50% of club tennis players over the age of 30 have experienced symptoms characteristic of tennis elbow (16). Half of these players noted minor symptoms with duration of less than 6 months, whereas the other half had major symptoms that lasted an average 2.5 years. Lateral epicondylitis tends to occur in recreational tennis players who are 35 to 50 years old (average 41 years), play three to four times per week, are inadequately conditioned, and often use poor technique. Several factors are believed to help precipitate this problem: heavier, stiffer, and more tightly strung rackets; incorrect grip size; metal rackets; inexperience; and bad backhand technique (16–19). Advanced tennis players who warm up, use good technique, and are well conditioned rarely suffer from this malady. This problem is also seen with increased incidence in throwing athletes, swimmers, fencers, carpenters, plumbers, meat cutters, and textile workers.

Lateral muscular disruption caused by athletic endeavors is uncommon in patients who have not had a previous cortisone injection (9). These patients complain of severe acute pain, often associated with a pop or snap.

Athletes with medial epicondylitis are often aggressive, advanced players, in contrast to the middle-aged, recreational athlete who is susceptible to lateral tennis elbow (20). Throwers, golfers (trailing arm), swimmers, tennis players, bowlers, carpenters, and others who perform repetitive forceful wrist palmar flexion and pronation are at risk. Patients with medial epicondylitis occasionally note swelling of the medial elbow. The most consistent complaint is medial elbow pain that is worse with wrist flexion, such as with throwing, serving or hitting a forehand in tennis (especially with a lot of topspin on the forehand), and pain when using a screwdriver. Care should be taken to look for symptoms of ulnar neuritis and ulnar collateral ligament injury or laxity. Disruption of the flexor-pronator muscle group is more common than of the extensor muscle group, even though epicondylitis is more common on the lateral side.

Medial epicondylitis occurs during forceful extension of the elbow and pronation of the forearm, although it may also occur with forceful valgus stress. Norwood et al. (21) found a ruptured flexor-pronator muscle group in all four of their patients with acute ulnar collateral ligament tears. Conway et al. (22) found a 13% incidence of flexor-pronator muscle rupture near its origin on the medial epicondyle. The history usually reveals sudden onset of pain along the medial epicondyle, although pain may be insidious with partial ruptures.

Physical Examination

The examination of a patient with lateral epicondylitis reveals tenderness 1 to 2 cm distal to the lateral epicondyle. The patient complains of pain with passive wrist flexion and with resisted wrist extension. This is worsened with elbow extension. Grasping or pinching with the wrist extended (the coffee cup test) usually reproduces pain precisely at the point of tenderness. Lateral muscular disruption is evident by the weakness of wrist extension and forearm supination. Occasionally, a defect—a bulge in the proximal forearm and ecchymosis—is palpated slightly distal to the lateral epicondyle, if the condition is identified in the first few days following disruption.

Patients with medial epicondylitis occasionally note swelling of the medial elbow. These patients are tender over the medial epicondylar origin of the flexor-pronator muscles. Pain occurs when testing the muscles with resisted wrist flexion, resisted pronation, and/or passive wrist extension. The pain is worsened by elbow extension as the flexor-pronator group crosses the elbow and wrist joints. Complete disruption of the flexor-pronator muscle group is associated with weakness of wrist flexion. A palpable gap in the tendon may be felt, and a bulge may be felt or seen in the proximal forearm.

In both instances, the range of motion of both the elbow and the wrist should be full, and there should be no sensory deficits.

Differential Diagnosis

Radial nerve entrapment at the elbow, also known as resistant tennis elbow, can occur by itself or in conjunction with lateral epicondylitis in approximately 5% of cases (23,24). This syndrome occurs when the motor branch of the radial nerve, the posterior interosseous nerve (PIN), becomes entrapped within the radial tunnel (25). These patients complain of symptoms similar to lateral epicondylitis, often with an ache that frequently radiates down the forearm. Because the PIN is a motor nerve, there are no sensory deficits (25). The use of counterforce bracing for presumed lateral epicondylitis may aggravate symptoms if the true cause is radial nerve entrapment. There is tenderness 4 cm distal to the lateral epicondyle over the radial nerve as it passes through the supinator; though occasionally, the pain will be at the junction of the

middle and proximal thirds of the forearm where the nerve exits the supinator. Pain is aggravated by active supination and passive pronation and by resisted extension of the long finger while the elbow is extended, depending on the site of entrapment.

Electromyography is helpful only if positive, which may occur if compression has been present for 7 to 9 months. Concomitant ulnar nerve compression may occur in up to 40% of cases (15,20,26). The symptoms of ulnar neuropathy are generally mild and usually occur after prolonged activity. The repetitive valgus stress seen in throwing athletes may produce concomitant injury and/or laxity of the UCL or injury to only the ligament, masking as medial epicondylitis. Tenderness associated with ulnar collateral ligament injury is usually 2 cm distal to the medial epicondyle.

Intra-articular disorders may mimic symptoms associated with tendinopathy. Radiocapitellar degeneration may give rise to symptoms similar to lateral epicondylitis, whereas intra-articular medial disorders may result in symptoms resembling medial epicondylitis.

RADIOLOGIC STUDIES

Plain radiographs are frequently normal in lateral epicondylitis, although 22% of patients will have evidence of a spur or exostosis at the lateral epicondyle or calcification of the common extensor tendon (8). Radiocapitellar degenerative change may simulate symptoms of lateral epicondylitis; and radiographs reveal any significant radial head or distal humeral osteophytes. For medial epicondylitis or flexor-pronator disruption, plain radiographs (including stress radiographs) are normal, although some calcific deposits may be identified in the tendon. If concomitant ulnar nerve symptoms are present, cubital tunnel views should be obtained to rule out spurs that are compressing the nerve. Plain radiographs should also be assessed for calcification within the ulnar collateral ligament.

Some authors suggest that MRI may help confirm the diagnosis, staging, and the local extent of pathologic tissue; however, I have not used this technique to evaluate or stage tendinopathy. Bone scans have been advocated for ruling out bony pathologies as a cause of medial or lateral elbow pain. Currently, MRI and CT scans have no proven benefit in the evaluation of elbow tendinopathies.

TREATMENT

Nonoperative Alternatives

OVERUSE INJURIES

Treatment of overuse injuries should always start with prevention, which saves time, effort, money, and other resources. Prevention should include education; an increase in overall flexibility, strength, and endurance; a proper warm-up and stretch, and avoidance of fatigue (27–30). Proper equipment, mechanics, and technique are other important factors in preventing tennis elbow (16,19,31). Many physicians advocate icing then stretching after throwing or offending activity as an important technique in prevention of injury (28).

Once a patient develops an overuse injury, an aggressive nonoperative program is begun, using the acronym PRICEMM. First, *p*rotect the elbow from further injury. *R*est the elbow from the offending event, but allow the individual to continue maintaining cardiovascular fitness. The elbow is *i*ced, *c*ompressed with an elastic bandage, and *e*levated. Prescribe *m*edications; nonsteroidal anti-inflammatory drugs (NSAIDs) are quite successful at relieving the pain and inflammation. Several *m*odalities, such as high-voltage galvanic electrical stimulation and iontophoresis, are also helpful (8).

After the acute symptoms have resolved, a rehabilitation protocol should be instituted, with a gradual return to activity. Changes in technique are often required, especially in recurrent cases. When patients have failed a quality rehabilitation program and experience constant pain without activity, pain that affects activity, persistent weakness or atrophy, and/or dysfunction, then surgery may be indicated.

My general approach to rehabilitation of elbow tendinopathy is stretching and strengthening. Passive wrist hyperextension and hyperflexion while the elbow is extended maximally stretch the flexor-pronator and extensor-supinator groups, respectively. Strengthening is performed while resisting low weights (0.5 kg; 1 lb) for wrist extension, flexion, radial deviation, and ulnar deviation. Grip strengthening is achieved via a squeeze ball or Silly Putty, and pronation-supination exercises are also encouraged.

LATERAL EPICONDYLITIS

Initial treatment is conservative (using PRICEMM) and is often quite successful. Tennis players should also strive for proper technique, reduce the tension on their racket strings, use a cushioned synthetic grip, improve their physical conditioning, and use a counterforce brace. Counterforce bracing is quite useful for tennis elbow (32,33). Many theories have been proposed to explain how the counterforce brace works; essentially the brace causes a change in the sequence and direction of muscle pull, which short circuits the force of muscle contraction by shortening the effective length of the muscle.

If the PRICEMM protocol is not effective after 1 to 2 weeks, injection with Xylocaine and corticosteroids just below the ECRB is indicated. If conservative treatment fails to return the athlete to usual activities after 3 to 6 months, which occurs in approximately 10% of cases, many authors recommend surgical intervention (8). Some authors recommend surgery for recurrence following successful resolution by conservative means (34), although most would recommend another trial of conservative treatment first.

MEDIAL EPICONDYLITIS

The mainstay of treatment for medial epicondylitis is a conservative approach using PRICEMM. If after 1 to 2 weeks the symptoms are no better, a local injection with steroid may be of benefit. Care must be taken to not inject into the tendon or ulnar nerve, owing the risk of tendon rupture or nerve damage. If symptoms persist after 3 to 6 months with the PRICEMM protocol, surgical treatment may be necessary.

MUSCULAR RUPTURE

If weakness persists after the pain subsides from a lateral muscular rupture and if all or a major part of the extensor tendon origin is ruptured, then primary surgical repair of the tendon to bone is indicated. Surgical reattachment is mandatory for medial musculotendinous origin rupture, because the common flexor origin is an important stabilizer for the medial elbow. However, repair is difficult and rarely restores competitive function.

Operative Treatment

Many surgical techniques for the different chronic tendinopathies have been described; however, the common salient features include identification and excision of the pathologic tissue and use of the adjacent normal tissue to close the defect, frequently after abrading underlying bone to allow fresh scar to heal in (Clinical Table). This allows the body's healing response to close the defect with healthy scar tissue that can withstand the repetitive stress that the weakened, abnormal tendon could not

Clinical Table: Elbow Tendinopathy: Surgical Repair of the Epicondylitides

Procedures	Indications	Technique	Anatomy	Pitfalls
Lateral epicondylar repair	• Refractory lateral epicondylitis	• Excise • Abrade • Repair • Protect	• ECRB • LUCL • Posterior interosseous nerve	• Deep dissection LUCL injury • PIN syndrome • Aggressive rehabilitation
Medial epicondylar repair	• Refractory medial epicondylitis	• Excise • Abrade • Repair • Protect	• FCR • Pronator teres • Ulnar nerve • UCL	• UCL injury • Leave associated pathologies • MABC nerve injury

MABC, medial antebrachial cutaneous.

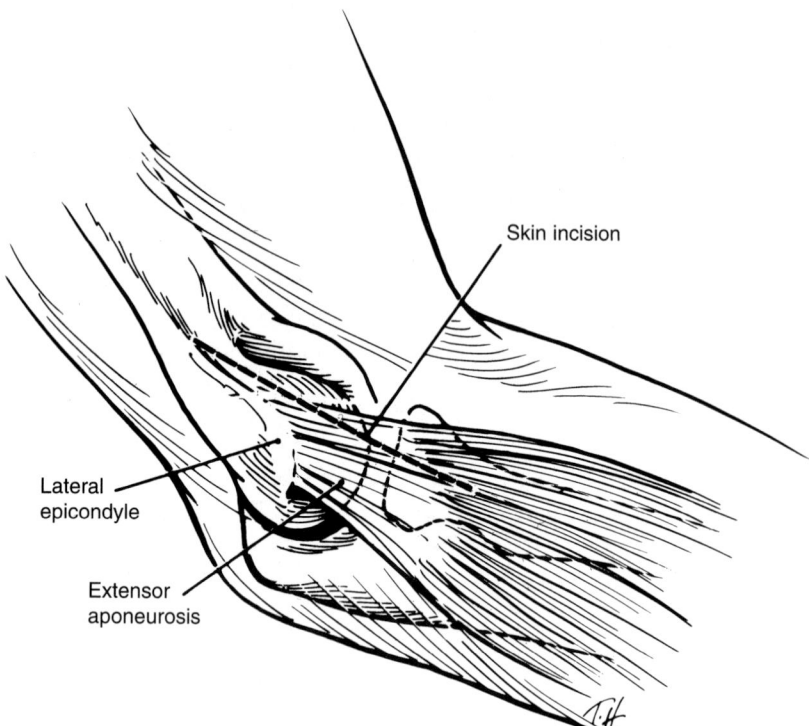

Figure 25.1. The skin incision for lateral epicondylitis extends from 2 to 3 cm proximal to the anterior aspect of the lateral epicondyle to 1 cm distal to the epicondyle (the level of the radiocapitellar joint).

withstand. After the surgery, the tissue is protected, and graded postoperative rehabilitation is performed before the patient can return to sports; this allows the scar tissue to develop and mature to resemble normal tendinous tissue architecture. Other procedures involve releasing the extensor tendons from either the elbow or the wrist and releasing the annular ligament.

APPROACH

As noted above, the general indications for surgical treatment of tendinopathy about the elbow is failure after 3 to 6 months of conservative treatment. Furthermore, some authors recommend surgery for recurrence following successful resolution by conservative means, though most would recommend conservative treatment first.

If weakness persists after the pain subsides and if all or a major part of the extensor tendon origin is ruptured, then primary surgical repair of the tendon to bone is indicated. Surgical reattachment of medial musculotendinous origin rupture is mandatory, since the common flexor origin is an important stabilizer for the medial elbow.

PROCEDURE

Lateral Epicondylitis

The lateral epicondylitis patient is placed supine on the operating table, and anesthesia (general or arm block) is administered. The arm is draped free with a nonsterile tourniquet and placed on an arm board. The incision extends from 2 to 3 cm proximal and just anteromedial to the lateral epicondyle down to the level of the radiocapitellar joint (i.e., 1 cm distal to the epicondyle) (Fig. 25.1). The subcutaneous tissue and superficial fascia are incised and

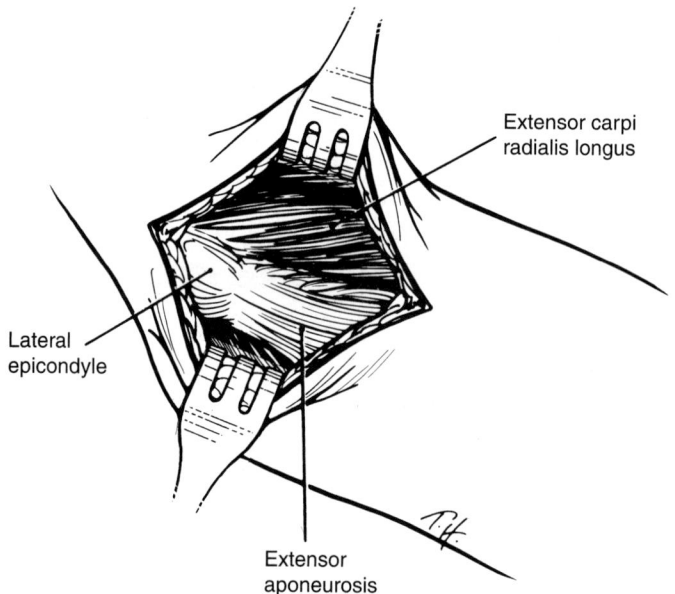

Figure 25.2. Identification of the interval between the ECRL tendon and extensor aponeurosis. The pathologic ECRB is not seen because it lies beneath the ECRL.

retracted, and the interval between the ECRL muscle and the firm anterior edge of the extensor aponeurosis is located. A palpable groove is identified between the thin fascia over the ECRL and the thick, firm anterior edge of the aponeurosis (Fig. 25.2). A 2- to 3-mm-deep incision is made between the ECRL and extensor aponeurosis, starting 2 to 3 cm proximal to the lateral epicondyle and extending distally to the level of the joint line. The ECRL is released by sharp dissection and is retracted anteromedi-

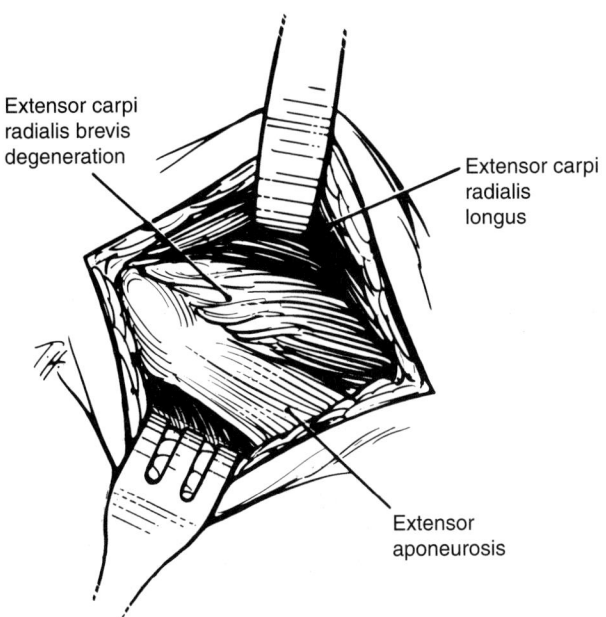

Figure 25.3. An incision in the ECRL–extensor aponeurosis interval allows the ECRL to be retracted and the pathologic ECRB tendon to be exposed. It is important to note that the ECRB is not very deep to the ECRL and interval; thus dissection must not be made more than 2 to 3 mm vertically.

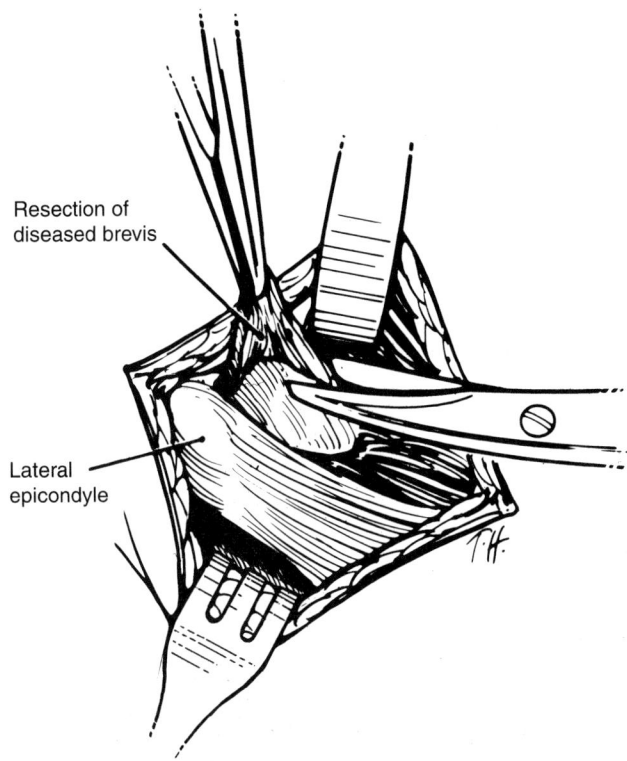

Figure 25.4. The pathologic tissue is completely resected. Take care not to release the extensor aponeurosis completely from the lateral epicondyle.

ally 2 to 3 cm. This brings the ECRB into direct view (Fig. 25.3).

With appropriate exposure, the entire origin of the ECRB is easily identified. Normal tendinous tissue is shiny and firm and has a slightly yellowish white hue. The gross appearance of the pathologic musculotendinous tissue is edematous and friable, with a dull grayish appearance; it may also be ruptured. The pathologic tissue often incorporates the entire ECRB origin; and in Nirschl's (26) series, the anterior 10% edge of the extensor aponeurosis was abnormal in approximately 35% of cases.

Excision of all pathologic tissue in the ECRB origin is performed en bloc. This tissue is somewhat triangular, and the base is distal. The typical size of this triangle is 1 × 2 cm. The ECRB origin is released from the lateral epicondyle and anterior edge of the extensor aponeurosis. If the anterior aponeurosis shows pathologic changes, the pathologic tissue is also removed. Care is taken to not remove or excise normal tendon.

Pathologic tissue is easily identified by its appearance. The Nirschl scratch test (26) is performed by scratching the superficial layers with the scalpel: The friable pathologic tissue easily peels off the normal tissue. When healthy tissue is reached, tissue no longer peels off with the scratching motion. Nirschl has found that this technique is especially helpful when removing the pathologic changes in the anterior edge of the aponeurosis, which is addressed at this time.

In the 20% of cases that present with an exostosis or prominence of the lateral epicondyle, the proximal edge of the aponeurosis is peeled off the epicondyle, allowing

the surgeon then to excise the exostosis with a rongeur and smooth it with a rasp.

Following the resection of the pathologic tissue, a defect is present in the ECRB (Fig. 25.4). The more distal aspect of the ECRB is still attached to the orbicular ligament, distal anterior aponeurosis, and the underside of the ECRL. The ECRB, therefore, does not retract distally, thereby maintaining an essentially normal resting length of its entire musculotendinous unit (i.e., from the elbow origin to the wrist insertion). Care must be taken to ensure a firm, watertight repair of the aponeurosis. Remember that the goal of the operation is resection of all pathologic tissue, not tendon release.

A small arthrotomy may be made at this time to inspect the anterolateral compartment of the joint. I usually find this to be unnecessary, unless the patient presented with clear preoperative intra-articular signs and symptoms.

Two to three small drill holes or punctures with an awl are made into the lateral epicondylar cortical bony bed (at the area of the resected tissue defect) to cancellous bone to enhance the vascular supply (Fig. 25.5). This will theoretically encourage rapid healing of the defect with healthy fibrotendinous tissue.

The interface between the posterior edge of the ECRL and the remaining anterior edge of the extensor aponeurosis is now closed tightly. I use simple interrupted stitches of number 1 Vicryl (Fig. 25.6). It is unnecessary to repair the distal ECRB, since its attachments are maintained to the orbicular ligament, distal aponeurosis, and

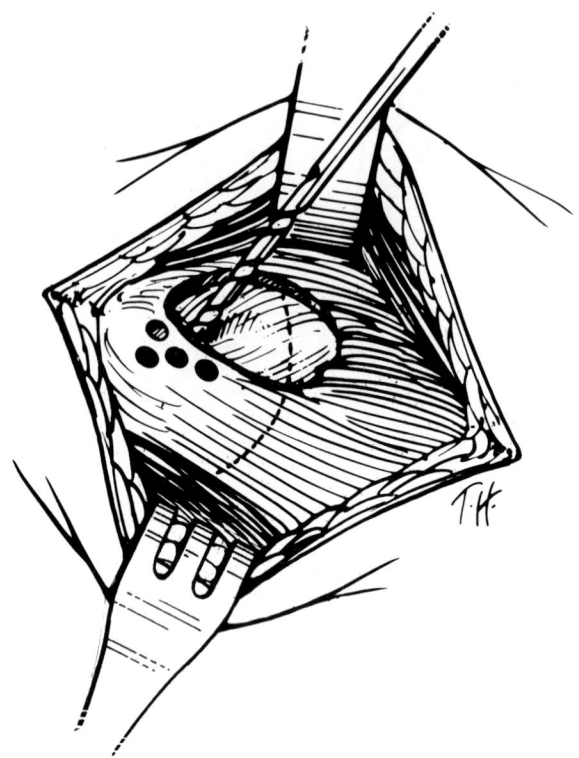

Figure 25.5. Using a small bit, drill from the cortex of the lateral epicondyle into cancellous bone to enhance revascularization. Alternatively, a pick or awl may be used to reduce the risk of thermal injury to the bone.

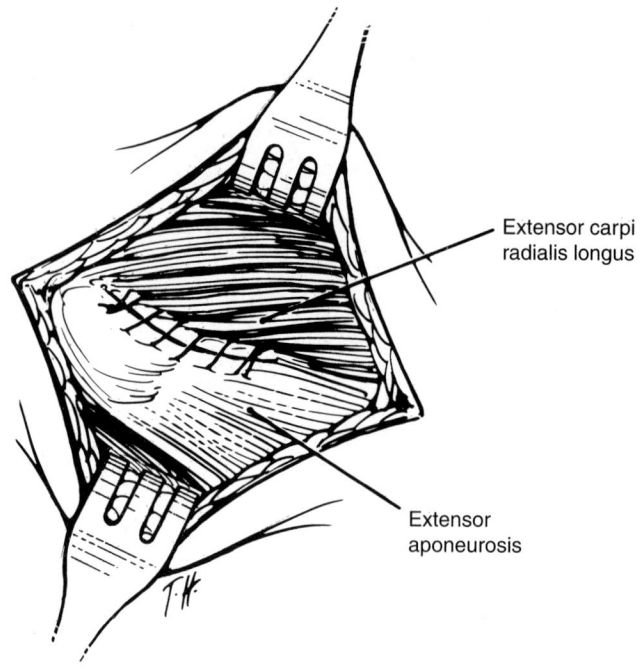

Extensor carpi radialis longus

Extensor aponeurosis

Figure 25.6. The ECRL–extensor aponeurosis is repaired with number 1 Vicryl, affording a watertight closure.

underside of the ECRL distally. The extensor aponeurosis is firmly repaired anteriorly, and its proximal attachment is largely undisturbed; thus rapid postoperative mobilization is possible and encouraged. The skin is closed with subcuticular undyed 4–0 Dexon, benzoin, and Steri-Strips.

Medial Epicondylitis

The medial epicondylitis patient is placed supine on the operating table, and anesthesia (general or arm block) is administered. The arm is draped free with a nonsterile tourniquet and placed on an arm board. A longitudinal incision, approximately 7.5 cm long, is made parallel to the medial epicondylar groove just posterior to the medial epicondyle (Fig. 25.7). The incision extends 2.5 cm proximal to 5 cm distal to the medial epicondyle. This incision avoids injury to the medial antebrachial cutaneous nerve, which tends to run on the anterolateral side of the medial epicondyle.

Dissection is carried through the subcutaneous tissue (which may be substantial) to the deep fascia covering the ulnar head of the FCU. The dissection then progresses anterolaterally over the medial epicondyle. This exposes the common flexor origin. Pathologic changes generally are not observed at this level, but occasionally degeneration is identified at the superficial layer of fibers.

The most common areas of pathologic change are at the pronator teres–flexor carpi radialis interface, extending

distally from the tip of the medial epicondyle for 2 to 5 cm. A thin muscle layer or a layer of normal tendon may cover and hide the deeper pathologic tissue. It is important to know exactly where the patient's primary area of palpable tenderness is before the anesthesia is delivered. The clinical tenderness pinpoints the area of pathologic change.

A longitudinal incision is made in the tendon origins at the area of maximal tenderness, extending from the medial epicondyle distally for approximately 5 cm. The incision is spread, and the pathologic tissue comes into view (Fig. 25.8). The incision is enlarged as needed to clearly identify the full extent of pathologic change.

All of the pathologic tissue is excised longitudinally and elliptically (Fig. 25.8). The resection may continue down to the anteromedial joint as needed (rare). All normal tissue, including tendon insertions, are left intact on the medial epicondyle, because the common flexor origin is an important medial elbow stabilizer (Fig. 25.9). Indiscriminate release of the normal common flexor tendon may result in valgus instability owing to ulnar collateral ligament sectioning.

In cases with concomitant ulnar nerve neuropraxia secondary to compression in the medial epicondylar groove (approximately 40%), decompression is undertaken. Flexion and extension of the elbow should be undertaken to rule out instability of the ulnar nerve. If ulnar nerve subluxation or dislocation is present, a subcutaneous anterior transfer of the nerve is accomplished by generous release between the two origins of the FCU from the level of the medial epicondyle for approximately 7.5 cm distally.

To enhance the vascular supply to the resection area (for healing), two to three small drill holes or punctures

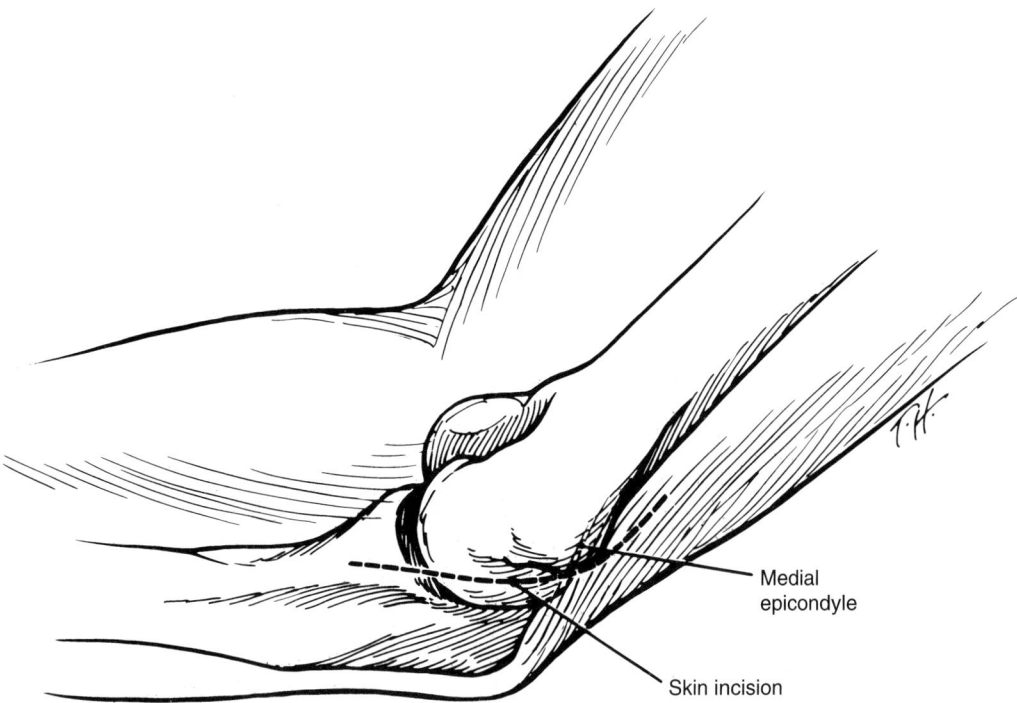

Figure 25.7. The skin incision for medial epicondylitis extends from 2 to 3 cm proximal and posterior to the medial epicondyle to 5 cm distal. This incision allows the surgeon to expose the ulnar nerve and common flexor-pronator origin and to avoid the medial antebrachial cutaneous nerve.

Figure 25.8. The pathologic tissue is completely resected elliptically from the pronator teres and FCR. If necessary, the ulnar nerve is also released. Care is taken not to release the whole common flexor-pronator origin from the medial epicondyle.

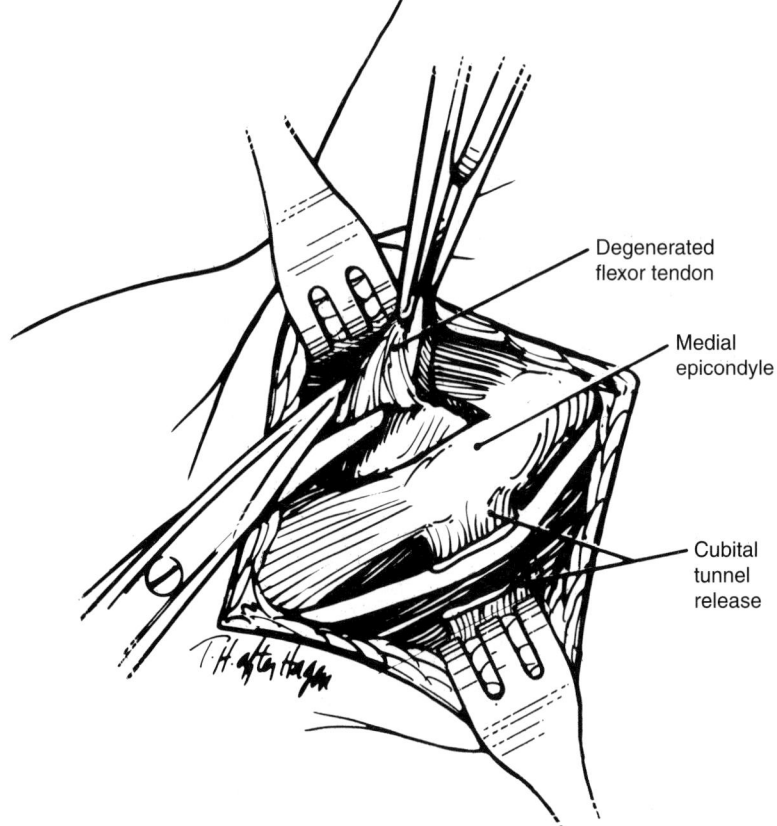

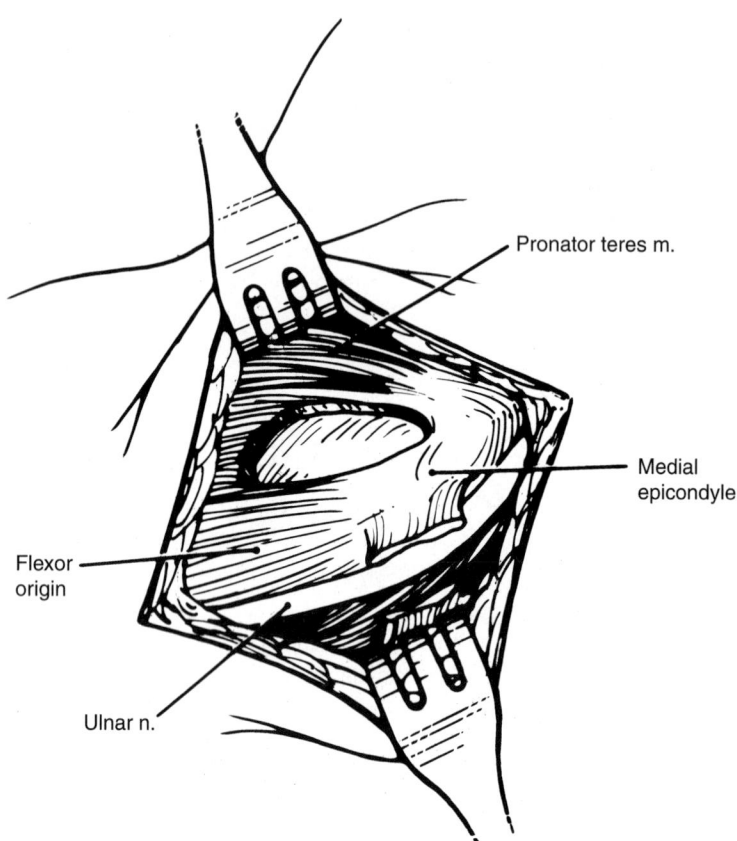

Figure 25.9. After the complete excision of the pathologic tendon and ulnar nerve release, the normal tendon is still attached to the medial epicondyle.

Pronator teres m.

Medial epicondyle

Flexor origin

Ulnar n.

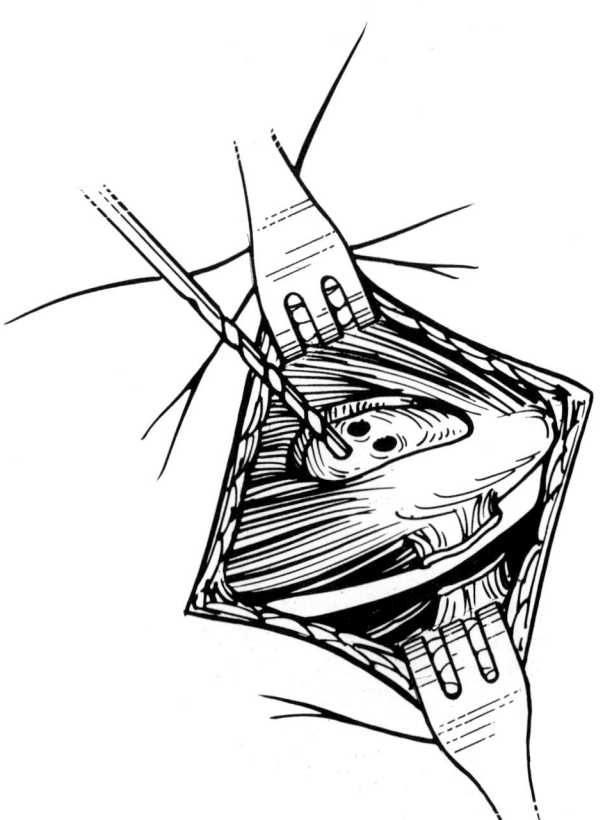

Figure 25.10. Using a small bit, drilling from the cortex of the medial epicondyle into cancellous bone to enhance revascularization. Alternatively, a pick or awl may be used to reduce the risk of thermal injury to the bone.

with an awl are made through cortical bone in the medial epicondyle into cancellous bone (Fig. 25.10).

The elliptical defect from the excised tissue is then closed with simple interrupted number 1 Vicryl sutures (Fig. 25.11). In cases with concomitant ulnar nerve decompression, the closure of the operative tendon defect is easier and tends to help with the decompression, although release of the cubital tunnel is also important.

In the unusual circumstance of subluxating or dislocating ulnar nerve, the nerve is transferred at this time. My preferred technique is a subcutaneous anterior transfer with a fascial sling to prevent further instability. The submuscular transfer substantially increases surgical and functional morbidity and is of unproved advantage.

Subcutaneous tissue is then closed with subcuticular 4–0 Dexon suture, benzoin, and Steri-Strips.

PITFALLS AND MOST COMMON CLINICAL MISTAKES

The most common cause of failure of surgery for lateral epicondylitis is beginning with the incorrect diagnosis. Posterior interosseous nerve syndrome is also known as resistant tennis elbow, because the symptoms persist despite adequate treatment for tennis elbow (34).

A common surgical error for lateral epicondylitis is to dissect too deeply (vertically) beyond the ECRL, as discussed earlier (26). It is also important not to dissect too deeply when developing the plane between the ECRL and the anterior aponeurosis; it should be only 2 to 3 mm deep; otherwise, iatrogenic distortion occurs, and the sur-

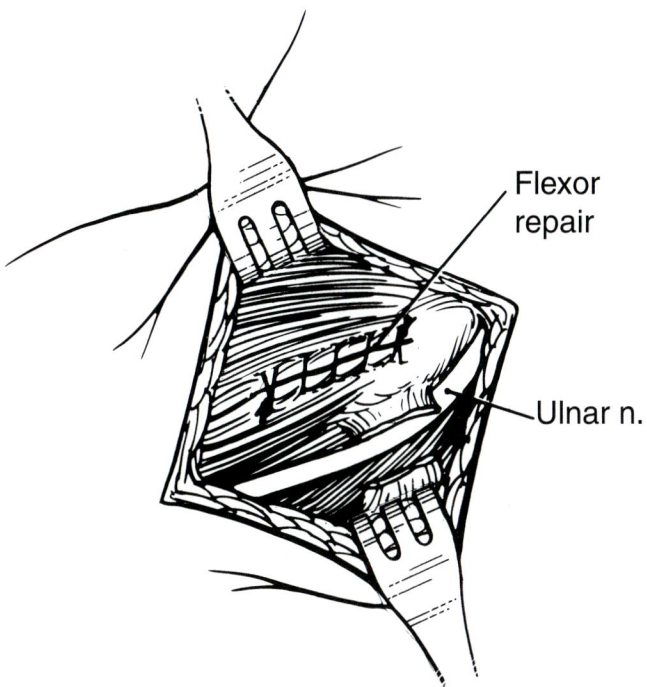

Figure 25.11. The defect left from the excision is repaired with number 1 Vicryl, which affords a watertight closure of the remaining normal tendon. Note that closure of the dead space tends to increase the gap after an ulnar nerve release, enhancing a decompression.

geon may bypass the pathologic tissue of the ECRB. Posterolateral rotatory instability following surgery for lateral epicondylitis has been described, as the lateral ulnar collateral ligament origin is adjacent to the common extensor origin (35). Another pitfall is an aggressive postoperative rehabilitation program that does not allow the wound to heal completely.

One potential problem when treating medial epicondylitis is to fail to address concomitant pathologic conditions, such as ulnar collateral ligament injury and ulnar neuritis, as described above. If these problems are not dealt with, persistent laxity or persistent ulnar nerve symptoms will exist. Furthermore, the UCL is at risk for injury owing to its origination from the medial epicondyle. Care must be taken when calcifications are identified during surgery; removal of calcification of the UCL may result in elbow instability. If the whole flexor-pronator origin is released, medial elbow stability and strength may be compromised. When making the skin incision, the surgeon must be careful to prevent injury to the medial antebrachial cutaneous (MABC) nerve.

Postoperative Management and Rehabilitation

After surgery, the arm is immobilized in a splint with the elbow at 90° flexion and the forearm in neutral. The wrist and hand may be left free. Complete immobilization is used for 2 days. Active elbow motion exercises are usually started within 48 h after surgery (tendon and/or tendon with nerve surgery). Intermittent immobilizer protection is usually maintained for 6 to 7 days, at which time normal activities of daily living are resumed. Counterforce support that provides protection is used until full forearm strength returns (usually 3 to 6 months). The brace is used at times of rehabilitative exercise and more vigorous forearm activities, such as heavy household activities. A gradual return to sports is often initiated at 8 to 10 weeks with brace protection.

SUMMARY

Many surgical procedures for the treatment of lateral epicondylitis have been described (19,36–40). Approximately 85% of patients who undergo surgical treatment return to full activities without pain, 12% improve but still have some pain with vigorous activities, and 3% show no improvement (1,3,4). The results of surgical treatment of medial epicondylitis reveal that 86% of patients have no limitation in elbow use at an average follow-up of 7 years (20).

REFERENCES

1. Anderson JE. Grant's atlas of anatomy. 8th ed. Baltimore: Williams & Wilkins, 1983:6-50–6-70.
2. Hoppenfeld S, deBoer P. Surgical exposures in orthopaedics. The anatomic approach. Philadelphia: Lippincott, 1984:77–108.
3. Morrey BF. Anatomy of the elbow joint. In: Morrey BF, ed. The elbow and its disorders. 2nd ed. Philadelphia: Saunders, 1993:16–52.
4. Nirschl RP. Prevention and treatment of elbow and shoulder injuries in the tennis player. Clin Sports Med 1988;7:289.
5. Nirschl RP. Sports and overuse injuries to the elbow. In: Morrey BF, ed. The elbow and its disorders. 2nd ed. Philadelphia: Saunders, 1993:537–552.
6. Nirschl RP, Pettrone F. Tennis elbow. The surgical treatment of lateral epicondylitis. J Bone Joint Surg 1979;61A:832.
7. Regan W, Wold LE, Coonrad R, et al. Microscopic histopathology of chronic refractory lateral epicondylitis. Am J Sports Med 1992; 20:746–749.
8. Coonrad RW, Hooper WR. Tennis elbow. Its course, natural history, conservative and surgical management. J Bone Joint Surg 1973;55A:1177.
9. Kvitne RS. Epicondylitis. Paper presented at the Shoulder and Elbow in Sports AAOS Meeting, Beverly Hills, CA, October 1992.
10. Coonrad RW. Tendinopathies at the elbow. Instr Course Lect 1991;40:1–87.
11. Major HP. Lawn-tennis elbow. Br Med J 1883;2:557.
12. Runge F. Zur genese und behandlung des schreibekrampfes. Berl Klin Wochenschr 1873;10:245.
13. Nirschl RP. Muscle and tendon trauma: tennis elbow. In: Morrey BF, ed. The elbow and its disorders. Philadelphia: Saunders, 1985:481–496.
14. Leach RE, Miller JK. Lateral and medial epicondylitis of the elbow. Clin Sports Med 1987;6:259–272.
15. King JW, Brelsford HJ, Tullos HS. Analysis of the pitching arm of the professional baseball pitcher. Clin Orthop 1969;67:116.
16. Nirschl RP. Tennis elbow. Orthop Clin North Am 1973;4:787.
17. Gerberich SG, Priest JD. Treatment for lateral epicondylitis: variables related to recovery. Br J Sports Med 1985;19:224–227.
18. Hang YS, Peng SM. An epidemiologic study of upper extremity in-

jury in tennis players with a particular reference to tennis elbow. Taiwan I Hsueh Hui Tsa Chih 1984;83:307–316.

19. Nirschl RP, Sobel J. Conservative treatment of tennis elbow. Phys Sports Med 1981;9:42.

20. Vangsness CT Jr, Jobe FW. Surgical treatment of medial epicondylitis. Results in 35 elbows. J Bone Joint Surg 1991; 73B:409–411.

21. Norwood LA, Shook JA, Andrews JR. Acute medial elbow ruptures. Am J Sports Med 1981;9:16.

22. Conway JE, Jobe FW, Glousman RE, et al. Medial instability of the elbow in throwing athletes: treatment by repair or reconstruction of the ulnar collateral ligament. J Bone Joint Surg 1992; 74A:67–83.

23. Comtet JJ, Lalain JJ, Moyen B, et al. Epicondylalgia with compression of the posterior branch of the radial nerve. Rev Chir Orthop 1985;71(Suppl 2):89–93.

24. Werner KO. Lateral elbow pain and posterior interosseous nerve entrapment. Acta Orthop Scand Suppl 1979;174:1.

25. Roles NC, Maudsley RH. Radial tunnel syndrome. J Bone Joint Surg 1972;54B:499.

26. Nirschl RP. Lateral and medial epicondylitis. In: Morrey BF, ed. Masters techniques in orthopaedic surgery, the elbow. New York: Raven Press, 1994:129–148.

27. Garrett WE Jr, Safran, MR, Seaber AV, et al. Biomechanical comparison of stimulated and nonstimulated muscle pulled to failure. Am J Sports Med 1987;15:448–454.

28. Hotchkiss RN. Common disorders of the elbow in athletes and musicians. Hand Clin 1990;6:507–515.

29. Safran MR, Garrett WE Jr, Seaber AV, et al. The role of warm up in muscular injury prevention. Am J Sports Med 1988;16:123–129.

30. Safran, MR, Seaber AV, Garrett WE Jr. Warm up and muscular injury prevention: an update. Sport Med 1989;8:239–249.

31. Nirschl RP. Arm care. Arlington, VA: Med Sports, 1983.

32. Froimson AI. Treatment of tennis elbow with forearm support band. J Bone Joint Surg 1971;53A:183.

33. Ilfeld FW, Field SM. Treatment of tennis elbow: Use of a special brace. JAMA 1966;195:67.

34. Dobyns JH. Musculotendinous problems at the elbow. In: Evarts CM, ed. Surgery of the musculoskeletal system. 2nd ed. New York: Churchill-Livingstone, 1990:1661–1681.

35. O'Driscoll SW, Bell DF, Morrey BF. Posterolateral rotatory instability of the elbow. J Bone Joint Surg 1991;73A:440–446.

36. Bosworth DH. The role of the orbicular ligament in tennis elbow. J Bone Joint Surg 1955;37A:527.

37. Cyriax JH. The pathology and treatment of tennis elbow. J Bone Joint Surg 1936;18B:921.

38. Garden RS. Tennis elbow. J Bone Joint Surg 1961;43B:100.

39. Goldie I. Epicondylitis lateralis humeri (epicondylalgia or tennis elbow). A pathogenetical study. Acta Chir Scand Suppl 1964;339:1–45.

40. Kaplan EB. Treatment of tennis elbow (epicondylitis) by denervation. J Bone Joint Surg 1959;41A:147.

chapter 26

Entrapment Neuropathy: Neurolysis and Transposition

Robert N. Hotchkiss

Compression of the ulnar nerve at the elbow is the second most common nerve entrapment syndrome in the upper extremity. Despite the frequency of this problem, there is little information available on conservation treatment and little agreement on the optimal surgical treatment.

RELEVANT ANATOMY AND PATHOGENESIS

The ulnar nerve originates from the nerve roots of C8 and T1 and receives contributions from the medial cord of the brachial plexus. The ulnar nerve pierces the medial intermuscular septum in the proximal arm and proceeds distally posterior to the septum (Fig. 26.1). The cubital tunnel begins at the level of the medial epicondyle. At this level, the nerve lies within the groove of the medial epicondyle and is deep to Osborne's fascia. The nerve continues distally between the two heads of the flexor carpi ulnaris (FCU), giving off its first motor branches. The nerve continues through the flexor-pronator mass into the forearm.

Potential sites of nerve entrapment that have been described are cervical disc disease at C6–7 and C7–T1, thoracic outlet syndrome, arcade of Struthers, the intermuscular septum, aponeurosis of the flexor-pronator mass (Osborne's fascia), an anomalous anconeus epitrochlea, articular disease (ganglia, synovial cysts, rheumatoid arthritis), flexor digitorum superficialis fascia, and cubitus valgus deformity. Gabel and Amadio (1) described five levels of potential compression of the ulnar nerve about the elbow. In addition, the nerve is susceptible to direct trauma, chronic subluxation of the nerve, and prolonged flexion from intraoperative positioning. Finally, throwing athletes may have symptoms secondary to repetitive valgus stress.

The cause of cubital tunnel syndrome is poorly understood. Factors contributing to symptoms involve both mechanical and biologic mechanisms. Elbow flexion decreases the cross-sectional area of the cubital tunnel by 55%. Intraneural pressures are also increased by elongation of the nerve. The ulnar nerve has an excursion of 4.7 mm over a full arc of motion. These mechanical factors lead to transient ischemia, which can lead to edema and subsequent demyelination. The topography of the ulnar nerve at the elbow reveals that sensory fibers are located more peripherally than are motor fibers. In addition, motor fibers to the hand are more peripheral than are motor fibers of the forearm. Thus external compression of the nerve leads to sensory changes early, followed by motor involvement of the intrinsics with time.

INITIAL FINDINGS, PHYSICAL EXAMINATION, AND DIAGNOSIS

The clinical presentation of cubital tunnel syndrome correlates with the sensory and motor distribution of the ulnar nerve. While pain and vague discomfort over the medial elbow may be present, numbness of the ulnar two digits is the most common presenting complaint. Numbness over the dorsum of these two digits essentially eliminates wrist and hand sources of entrapment as the dorsal branch of the ulnar nerve branches in the distal forearm. Two-point discrimination should be documented in all patients. Motor weakness, if present, typically develops later than sensory changes. Weakness of the intrinsics may be demonstrated by wasting of the first dorsal interosseous muscle and a positive Froment sign. Weakness of the small finger abductor is associated with ulnar nerve denervation. Motor weakness of the flexor digitorum profundus to the fourth and fifth digits may also be demonstrable. Clawing is a sign of prolonged denervation of the interossei with preservation of the flexor digitorum profundus (FDP) to the ulnar digits.

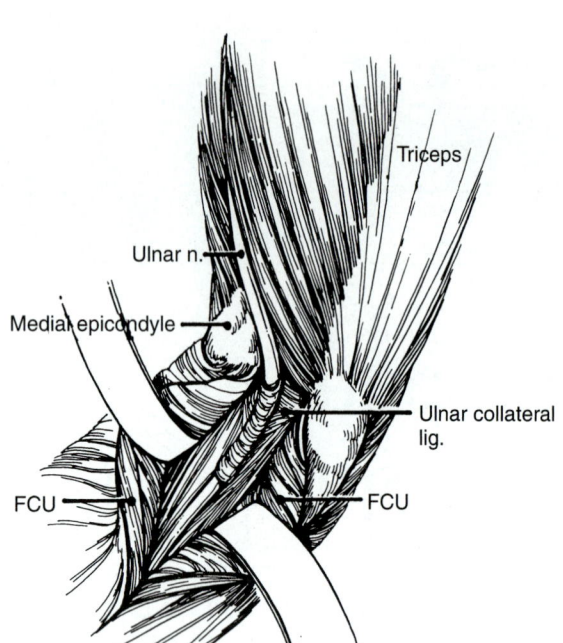

Figure 26.1. The ulnar nerve lies posterior to the medial epicondyle before entering the forearm, where it lies between the two heads of the flexor carpi ulnaris (*FCU*). Reprinted with permission from Eversmann WW Jr. Entrapment and compression neuropathies. In: Green D, ed. Operative hand surgery. 3rd ed. Vol. 2. New York: Churchill Livingstone, 1993:1357.

Provocative testing of cubital tunnel syndrome includes the elbow flexion test and the Tinel sign over the ulnar nerve. Although a positive Tinel sign may help localize the area of entrapment, the test has poor sensitivity. Likewise, reproduction of symptoms with prolonged elbow flexion is helpful when positive, but a negative test does not exclude the diagnosis of cubital tunnel syndrome.

The diagnosis can usually be made on the basis of a careful history and physical examination. Alternate locations of compression, such as thoracic outlet or cervical radiculopathy, should be considered. Electromyogram and nerve conduction velocities (EMG/NCV) help establish the diagnosis. Slowing of the NCV to less than 50 m/s is believed to be the most specific diagnostic factor. EMG changes of denervation suggest a more significant degree of involvement. These two tests also help to rule out other potential sources of nerve entrapment.

TREATMENT

Little has been written about conservative treatment of cubital tunnel syndrome, but conservative measures may be of help in early cases. The majority of authors recom-

mend surgical treatment, either as initial treatment or following failure of conservation measures.

Operative Treatment

Controversy exists regarding the different available surgical options for cubital tunnel syndrome. The five most frequently described procedures are discussed here. Each procedure has proponents and detractors, despite there being little evidence of the superiority or inferiority of any of these procedures (Clinical Table).

TECHNICAL CONSIDERATIONS FOR ANY PROCEDURE

The importance of identifying and protecting the medial antebrachial cutaneous nerve cannot be overstated. The nerve lies anterior to the intermuscular septum and is usually seen in the subcutaneous tissue of the anterior flap. Distally, the nerve and its branches cross the flexor-pronator mass from anterior to posterior. Failure to protect this nerve may result in a painful neuroma.

A transient decrease in blood supply to the ulnar nerve may occur with anterior transposition. Thus one should preserve as much blood supply as possible when conducting this procedure.

The exposure is the same for all the techniques. A longitudinal incision is centered between the medial epicondyle and the olecranon. The medial antebrachial nerve is identified and protected. Flaps are raised directly off the fascia to expose the posterior margin of the biceps and the anterior margin of the triceps. Distally, the anterior and posterior boundaries of the flexor-pronator mass should be defined. This exposure should be visualized prior to proceeding with the planned method of decompression.

To facilitate nerve mobilization, ulnar nerve branches to the flexor-pronator mass can be traced distally. This frees the nerve from its posterior location but preserves the innervation to the muscle.

IN SITU DECOMPRESSION

In situ decompression is believed to prevent constriction of the nerve as the elbow is brought into flexion, similar to the release of the transverse carpal ligament in carpal tunnel syndrome. This procedure, as proposed, is indicated for patients who have well-localized symptoms of a short duration in the absence of subluxation. The theoretical advantages of this procedure are the ease of dissection and preservation of the vascularity to the nerve. Although there are reports of favorable results with in situ decompression, these results were usually achieved in patients with mild symptoms. Unfortunately, the mechanical affect of the medial epicondyle is not addressed by this procedure, and not all potential sites of compression are treated. The nerve remains susceptible to compression with elbow flexion, thereby limiting the use of this procedure.

Clinical Table: Entrapment Neuropathy: Neurolysis and Transposition

Procedure	Indications	Technique	Anatomy	Pitfalls
In situ decompression	• Limited indications • Short duration of symptoms	• Release Osborne's fascia	• Osborne's fascia • Medial antebrachial cutaneous nerve	• Nerve remains susceptible to compression
Medial epicondylectomy	• Cubital tunnel syndrome • Tardy ulnar nerve palsy	• Excise epicondyle along ulnar border of trochlea	• Flexor-pronator mass • Medial epicondyle • Medial antebrachial cutaneous nerve	• Medial collateral ligament injury • Incomplete osteotomy • Heterotropic ossification
Subcutaneous transposition	• Cubital tunnel syndrome • Tardy ulnar nerve palsy	• Fasciodermal or fascial sling	• Flexor-pronator mass • Medial antebrachial cutaneous nerve	• Compression from the sling • Nerve damage • Subcutaneous tissue injury
Intramuscular transposition	• Cubital tunnel syndrome	• Intramuscular bed	• Flexor-pronator mass • Medial antebrachial cutaneous nerve	• Compression from the muscle tissues
Submuscular transposition	• Cubital tunnel syndrome • Tardy ulnar nerve palsy	• Detach flexor-pronator mass	• Flexor-pronator mass • Brachialis fascia • Medial antebrachial cutaneous nerve	• Flexor-pronator weakness

MEDIAL EPICONDYLECTOMY

One advantage of the medial epicondylectomy is the elimination of the fulcrum over which the ulnar nerve is stretched in flexion. The ulnar nerve elongates approximately 47 mm around the medial epicondyle with flexion. Furthermore, the nerve undergoes relatively little dissection, and its local blood supply may be maintained. Some potential disadvantages include weakening of the flexor-pronator mass, injury to the medial collateral ligament, heterotopic ossification, inadequate resection, and elbow flexion contracture.

Once the exposure has been obtained, the intermuscular septum is excised and Osborne's fascia is divided. The ulnar nerve is gently retracted posteriorly. A longitudinal incision is made over the epicondyle in line with the fibers of the flexor-pronator mass. The attachment is elevated subperiosteally with a knife to expose the metaphyseal-diaphyseal junction of the epicondyle. At this junction, the epicondyle along the medial margin of the trochlea is removed with an osteotome. The flexor-pronator fascia is repaired with the elbow in extension. A posterior splint is used for 2 weeks, at which time the sutures are removed and movement is initiated.

SUBCUTANEOUS TRANSPOSITION

Multiple variations of the subcutaneous transposition procedure exist. Anterior transposition with appropriate mobilization releases areas of potential entrapment and removes tension on the nerve throughout the elbow's arc of motion (Fig. 26.2). In addition, loss of the anterior position may be prevented by a variety of methods, including wrapping subcutaneous fat around the nerve, suturing the nerve to the anterior fascia, applying fascial slings, and using the fasciodermal technique (Fig. 26.3). Many of these procedures are similar, and the superiority of any one technique has not been established. No procedure, however, should create a new region of potential compression. The indications for anterior subcutaneous transposition include all potential causes of cubital tunnel syndrome. Some authors argue that anterior transposition places the nerve too superficial and, therefore, should not be used in younger patients or in throwing athletes.

After the exposure is made, the intermuscular septum is excised and Osborne's fascia is divided. The nerve is mobilized to allow for anterior transposition without tension. The fascia over the flexor-pronator mass must usually be released immediately deep to the nerve to avoid kinking. I prefer a patulous fascial sling to prevent posterior subluxation. Aftercare includes a soft dressing and early unprotected movement of the upper extremity.

INTRAMUSCULAR TRANSPOSITION

For intramuscular transposition, originally described by Adson in 1918, the ulnar nerve is transposed anteriorly

Figure 26.2. Mobilization of the nerve for transposition includes the release of the arcade of Struthers and the fascia overlying the two heads of the flexor carpi ulnaris. Reprinted with permission from Eversmann WW Jr. Entrapment and compression neuropathies. In: Green D, ed. Operative hand surgery. 3rd ed. Vol. 2. New York: Churchill Livingstone, 1993:1360.

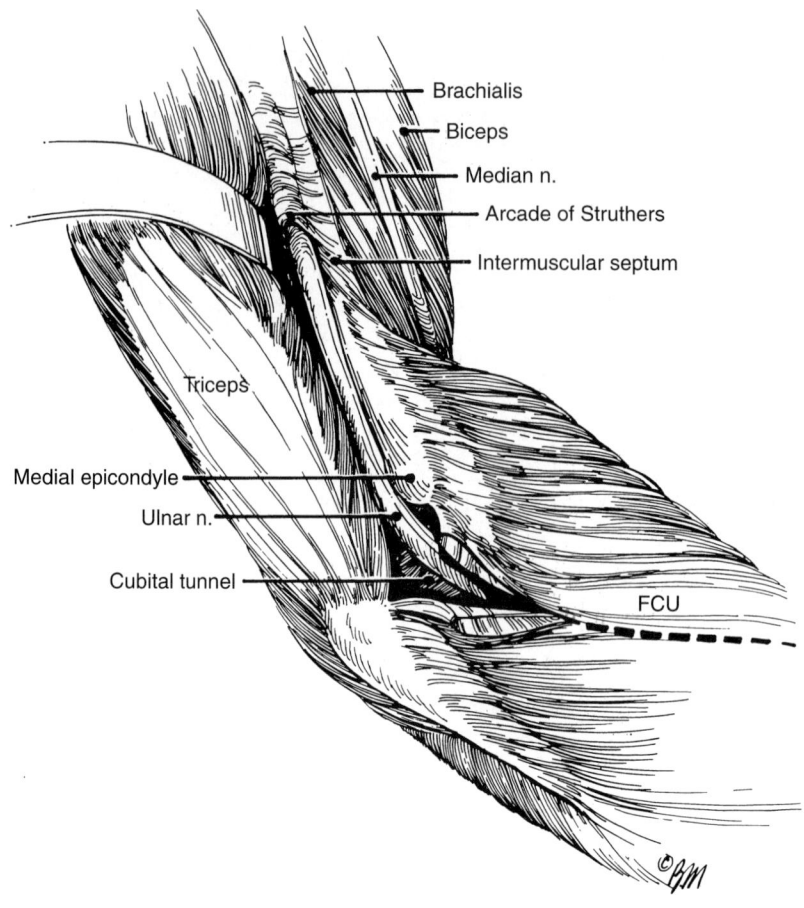

Figure 26.3. After anterior subcutaneous transposition, the nerve rests on the forearm fascia. The cubital tunnel may be closed to prevent the nerve from returning to its original position behind the medial epicondyle. Reprinted with permission from Eversmann WW Jr. Entrapment and compression neuropathies. In: Green D, ed. Operative hand surgery. 3rd ed. Vol. 2. New York: Churchill Livingstone, 1993:1359.

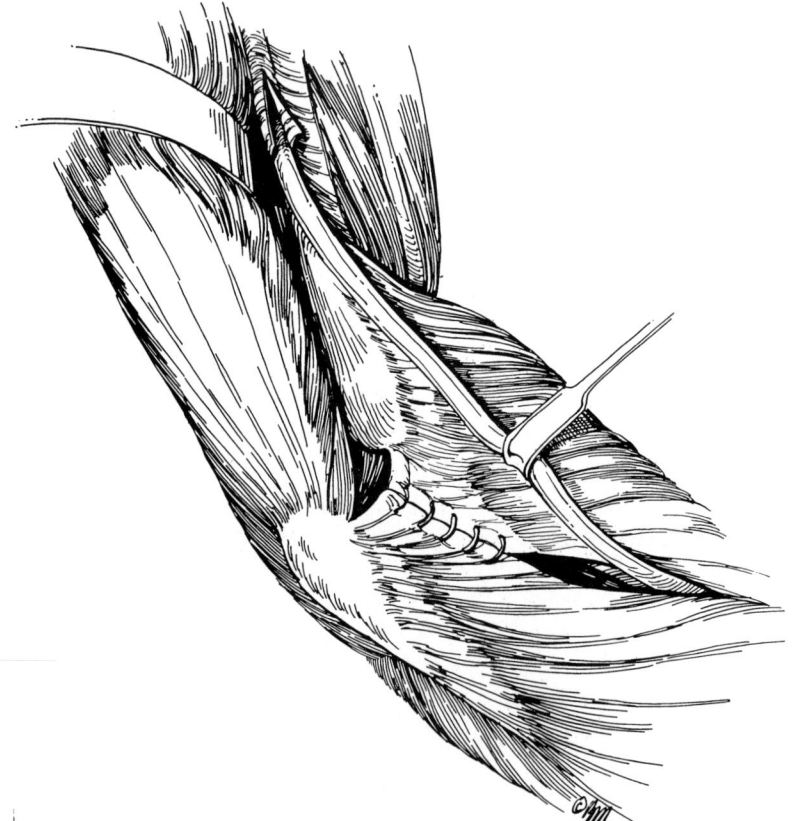

and placed within the substance of the flexor-pronator muscle mass. Advocates of this procedure claim that the nerve is more protected than when it is placed subcutaneously and that it is in a well-vascularized bed. Critics state that the intramuscular position is likely to be subjected to traction forces and that scar formation in the muscle bed may occur.

Once the exposure has been obtained, the intermuscular septum is excised and Osborne's fascia is divided. The nerve is fully mobilized and then draped over the flexor-pronator mass to outline the ideal placement, which is marked. The nerve is then gently retracted posteriorly, and the fascia is incised along the marked line. The muscle fibers and septa are then divided sharply in the same line as the fascia. The nerve is placed in this groove, and the fascia is closed over the nerve. The tourniquet should be released before closure to allow for adequate hemostasis. A posterior splint is used for 2 weeks, at which time the sutures are removed and movement is initiated.

SUBMUSCULAR TRANSPOSITION

Anterior submuscular transposition entails the complete detachment of the flexor-pronator mass. With this exposure, the nerve will lie on the brachialis fascia, adjacent to the median nerve (Fig. 26.4). The reported advantages of this procedure include placement of the nerve in a favorable bed and complete release of tension and potential entrapment. Potential problems include prolonged healing secondary to the degree of dissection, the weakening of the flexor-pronator mass, and the need for postoperative immobilization. Submuscular transposition has been advocated for throwing athletes in whom a concomitant medial collateral ligament reconstruction will be done. It has perhaps its broadest support as revision for a failed primary procedure.

Once the exposure has been obtained, the intermuscular septum is excised and Osborne's fascia is divided. The anterior and posterior margins of the flexor-pronator mass are identified, and the median nerve may also be identified. The origin of the flexor-pronator mass is elevated from the medial epicondyle and is retracted distally (Fig. 26.5). The well-mobilized ulnar nerve is then brought anterior and placed adjacent to the median nerve over the brachialis fascia. The flexor-pronator mass is reattached to its origin with heavy nonabsorbable suture (number 5 Ethibond) through drill holes in the epicondyle. Care is taken to avoid impingement of the nerve distally. An al-

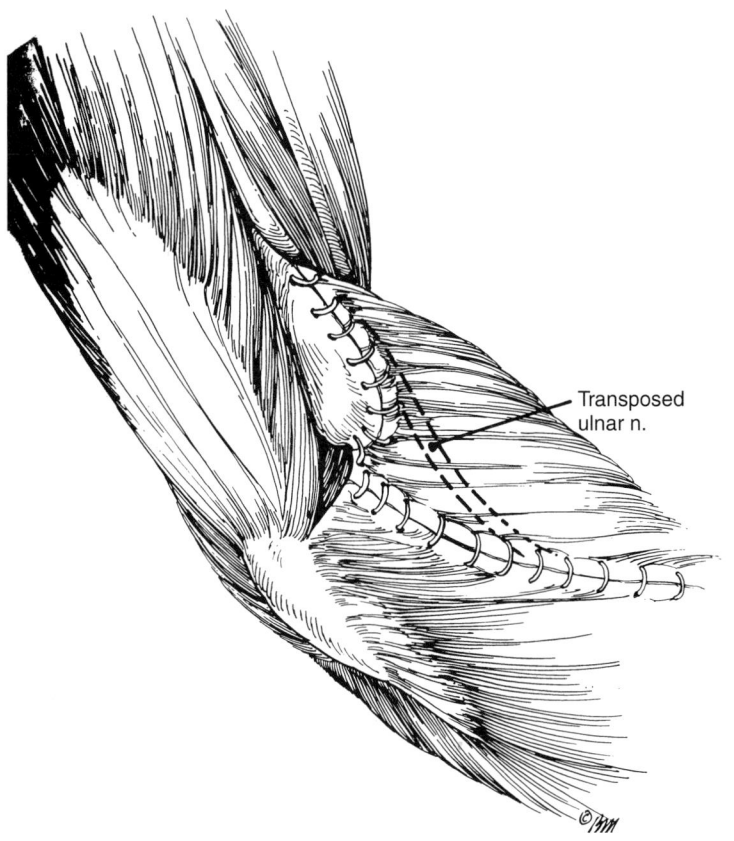

Figure 26.4. For the submuscular transposition, the nerve is transposed anteriorly and is placed deep to the flexor-pronator muscle. Reprinted with permission from Eversmann WW Jr. Entrapment and compression neuropathies. In: Green D, ed. Operative hand surgery. 3rd ed. Vol. 2. New York: Churchill Livingstone, 1993:1361.

Transposed ulnar n.

Figure 26.5. The common flexor-pronator origin is elevated from the medial epicondyle, and the anterior part of the ulnar collateral ligament is cut. The osteotomy follows the plane of the medial border of the trochlea. Reprinted with permission from Eversmann WW Jr. Entrapment and compression neuropathies. In: Green D, ed. Operative hand surgery. 3rd ed. Vol. 2. New York: Churchill Livingstone, 1993:1363.

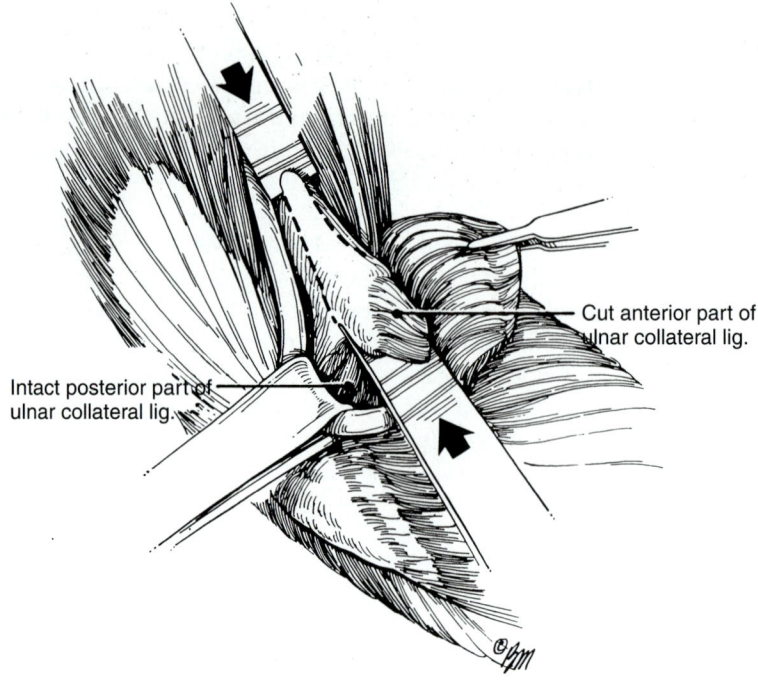

Cut anterior part of ulnar collateral lig.

Intact posterior part of ulnar collateral lig.

ternative to this procedure is to step-cut the origin of the flexor-pronator mass and repair the fascia in a slightly lengthened position. Aftercare consists of splinting the elbow in 90° of flexion with slight pronation and slight wrist flexion for 2 weeks.

Rehabilitation

For in situ decompression and subcutaneous transposition, motion of the elbow and forearm may begin immediately following surgery. After a medial epicondylectomy, intramuscular transposition, or submuscular transposition, 2 weeks of immobilization is recommended. The elbow is flexed to 90°, and the forearm and wrist are placed in slight pronation and flexion. Sutures are removed at 2 weeks after surgery, and motion is begun at that time. Supervised therapy is rarely indicated.

REFERENCE

1. Gabel GT, Amadio PC. Reoperation for failed decompression of the ulnar nerve in the region of the elbow. J Bone Joint Surg 1990; 72A:213–219.

Suggested Readings

Brougy AS, Leffert RD, Smith RJ. Technical problems with ulnar nerve transposition at the elbow: findings and results of reoperation. J Hand Surg 1978;3A:85–89.

Craven PR, Green DP. Cubital tunnel syndrome. Treatment by medial epicondylectomy. J Bone Joint Surg 1980;62A:986–989.

Del Pizzo W, Jobe FW, Norwood L. Ulnar nerve entrapment syndrome in baseball players. Am J Sports Med 1977;5:182.

Froimson AI, Zahrawi F. Treatment of compression neuropathy of the ulnar nerve at the elbow by epicondylectomy and neurolysis. J Hand Surg 1980;5A:391–395.

Leffert RD. Anterior submuscular transposition of the ulnar nerve by Learmouth technique. J Hand Surg 1982;7A:147.

Richards RL. Traumatic ulnar neuritis. The results of anterior transposition of the ulnar nerve. Edinburgh Med J 1945;52:14–21.

chapter 27

Jonathan D. Lewin and Kevin D. Plancher

Tendon Transfers for Scapular Winging

Scapular winging is one of the most common abnormalities of the scapulothoracic articulation. The winging can be classified as primary, secondary, or voluntary (Table 27.1). The primary disorders directly affect the scapulothoracic anatomy and articulation. Patients with scapular winging have irreparable lesions of the scapulothoracic muscles with minimal deficits of the muscles that control the glenohumeral joint. The most common type of scapular winging is secondary to spinal accessory and long thoracic nerve palsies (Table 27.2).

RELEVANT ANATOMY AND PATHOGENESIS

Spinal accessory nerve palsy leads to paralysis of the trapezius muscle. The trapezius originates from the medial third of superior nuchal line, ligamentum nuchae, and the spinous processes of C7 to T12 and inserts on the lateral third of the clavicle, acromion, and scapular spine. It elevates, retracts, and rotates the scapula.

Long thoracic nerve palsy leads to scapular winging from a paralysis of the serratus anterior muscle. This sawtoothed muscle originates as fleshy digitations from the external surfaces of the lateral portions of the ribs and inserts on the anterior surface of the medial scapular border. It protracts the scapula and holds it against the thoracic wall.

Secondary disorders are a result of glenohumeral irregularities, which, if treated successfully, resolve the scapular winging. Voluntary winging often represents a psychological disorder. If this rare type of winging is addressed surgically, disastrous complications can arise (1).

INITIAL FINDINGS, PHYSICAL EXAMINATION, AND DIAGNOSIS

A thorough history and physical examination will guide the clinician to diagnose scapular winging as the source of pain in the shoulder. A directed physical examination must be performed in an area of the body often overlooked by many clinicians. Bigliani et al. (2) treated 10 patients surgically, 9 of whom had a missed diagnosis of a trapezius paralysis despite prior screening with orthopaedists, neurologists, and neurosurgeons. The purpose of this chapter is to familiarize the reader with the subtleties of scapular winging as a source of shoulder pain.

The history should include a birth history. Any existing neurologic condition should be discussed with the physician. The patient will often volunteer information about clicking, grinding, or popping that is noted with movement of the shoulder girdle.

The directed physical examination begins with observation of the shoulder girdle from the front, side, and rear. Patients should be evaluated for muscle atrophy (which may indicate fascioscapulohumeral muscular dystrophy) and/or the presence of static winging. The scapulothoracic articulation is placed through a range of motion after all structures about the shoulder have been carefully palpated.

It is helpful to test the winging against resistance (dynamic deformity), as some patients will demonstrate symptoms only when faced with a moderate resisted force. The dynamic deformity can be demonstrated by asking the patient to push against a wall with her or his hands while resisting forward elevation and/or to perform shoulder shrugs at various degrees of abduction. Alternatively, dynamic instability can be tested by asking the patient to stand erect and place his or her arms in 30° of forward flexion. The examiner stands behind the patient and resists further flexion (Fig. 27.1).

Observation of the scapula from behind the patient is simple and may reveal subtle dynamic winging. The physical examination is completed by recording any scapulothoracic crepitus and abnormal scapulothoracic rhythm.

291

table	27.1	Classification of Scapular Winging

Primary
    Birth palsy
    Neurologic origin (brachial plexus injury)
        Spinal accessory nerve (trapezius palsy)
        Long thoracic nerve (serratus anterior palsy)
        Dorsal scapular nerve (rhomboideus palsy)
        Suprascapular nerve (supraspinatus palsy)
        Axillary nerve (deltoid palsy)
        Subscapularis nerve (subscapularis palsy)
    Poliomyelitis
    Osseous origin
        Osteochondromas
        Fracture malunions
    Soft tissue origin
        Contractural winging
        Muscle avulsion or agenesis
        Scapulothoracic bursitis
Secondary
Voluntary

table	27.2	Scapular Winging: Quick Reference Chart

Common causes	Long thoracic nerve palsy; spinal accessory nerve palsy
Diagnosis	Primarily clinical with EMG confirmation
	a. Long thoracic nerve palsy: superior elevation, medial translation of scapula
	b. Spinal accessory nerve palsy: depression and lateral translation of scapula
Treatment	Nonoperative for 12 months: AROM and PROM to avoid stiffness; periscapular strengthening; brace
	Dynamic transfer is the treatment of choice
	a. Marmor–Bechtol: pectoralis major transfer for long thoracic nerve palsy
	b. Eden–Lange: levator scapulae/rhomboid transfer for spinal accessory nerve palsy
	Static procedures: scapulothoracic fusion for failed dynamic procedure or muscular dystrophy
Rehabilitation	Active exercises at 6 weeks (Marmor–Bechtol) or 8 weeks (Eden–Lange)
Results	Nonoperative treatment has variable results (long thoracic nerve palsy has better results than does spinal accessory nerve palsy); surgical treatment has a success rate of >80%

EMG, electromyogram; *AROM*, active range of motion; *PROM*, passive range of motion.

Figure 27.1. The examiner resists forward flexion from behind to test for scapular winging.

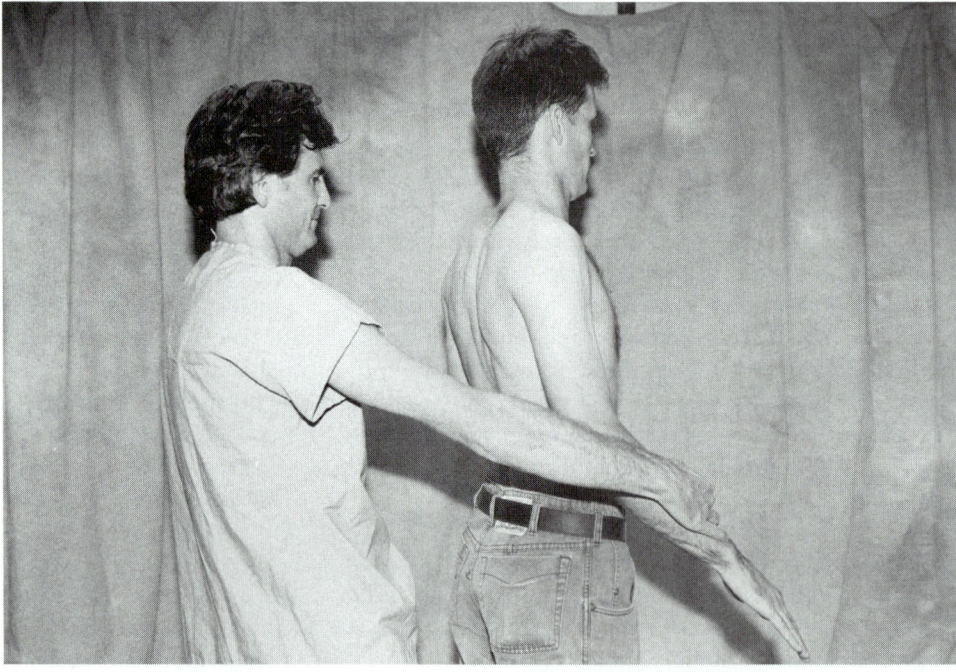

Two of the principal neurologic causes of winging—serratus anterior paralysis and trapezius paralysis—can be easily discerned by a careful physical examination. In trapezius winging secondary to spinal accessory nerve dysfunction, the patient assumes a position with the shoulder depressed and the scapula translated laterally with its inferior angle rotated laterally (Fig. 27.2). Patients attempt to compensate for this deformity by using their rhomboids and levator scapulae. This leads to overuse of these muscles and pain in the scapulothoracic articulation.

In contrast, winging from a serratus anterior paralysis leads to superior elevation of the scapula, medial translation, and medial rotation of the inferior pole (Fig. 27.3).

The presence of a bony prominence, such as an osteochondroma, on the inferior wall of the scapula may cause winging. Similarly, muscular avulsions may leave palpable gaps on the anterior or posterior thorax and may cause the winged scapula. In these cases an electromyogram (EMG) should be performed if the physical examination does not determine the cause of the winged scapula.

We believe that all patients with winging of the scapula in whom surgical repair is being considered should have a baseline EMG study. Lacerations or traumatic nerve disruptions require a different treatment regime if discovered early. When EMG studies are abnormal or show minimal nerve function, nerve grafting and/or neurolysis rather than tendon transfers should be performed. The results of nerve grafting or neurolysis are best done within 6 months of injury (2).

Primary Scapular Winging

The spinal accessory nerve is the only innervation to the trapezius muscle. Its subcutaneous location on the floor of the posterior cervical triangle makes it susceptible to injury from blunt or penetrating trauma. Lymph node dissections and radical neck dissection are common iatro-

genic causes of this nerve injury (3–5). Patients complain of disabling pain and spasm from the change in biomechanics of the scapulothoracic articulation. Many patients will have pain from the secondary effects of winging, which include adhesive capsulitis, subacromial impingement, radiculitis from a brachial plexus traction, and acromioclavicular joint pain. Trapezius wasting with an inability to shrug the shoulders and difficulty with forward elevation of the humerus will also be apparent on physical examination. The physical findings of the depressed shoulder and laterally translated scapula are often obvious.

The serratus anterior receives its innervation from the long thoracic nerve. This nerve originates from the ventral rami of C5–7 and travels beneath the brachial plexus and clavicle over the first rib and then inferiorly superficially along the lateral chest wall (Fig. 27.4). This nerve is susceptible to blunt and penetrating trauma. Athletes who participate in contact sports are especially prone to injury of this nerve (6). Surgical positioning, viral illness (7), inoculation (8), and brachial neuritis have all been implicated as causes for long thoracic nerve palsy. Other reported causes have been bed rest with the arm abducted while propping up to read a book (9). There have also been reports of patients with a C7 radiculopathy who may have symptoms of serratus anterior weakness and winging (10).

Physical examination with a serratus anterior palsy reveals a scapula that is superiorly elevated and is medially

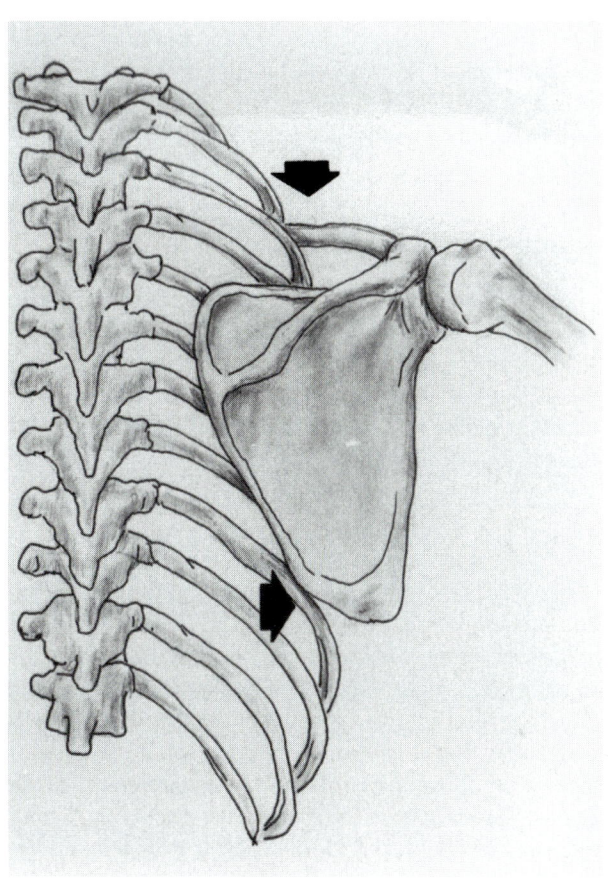

Figure 27.2. Winging of the scapula caused by trapezius palsy.

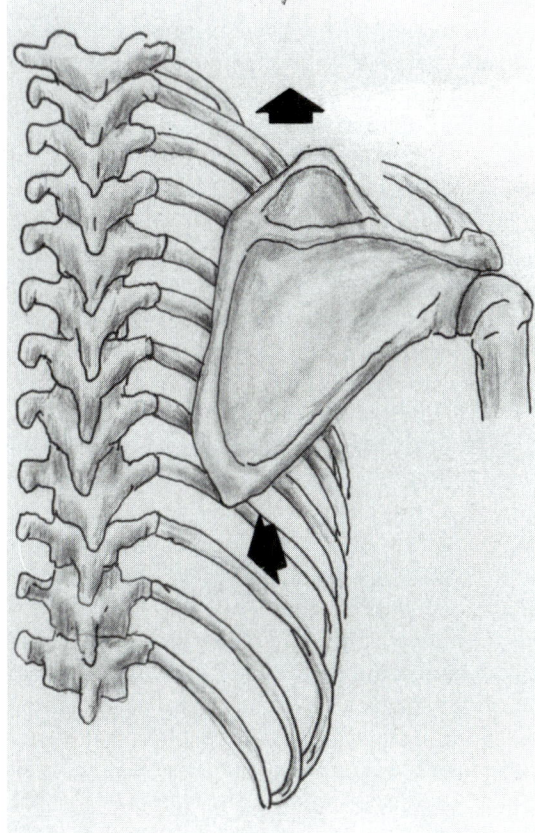

Figure 27.3. Winging of the scapula caused by serratus anterior palsy.

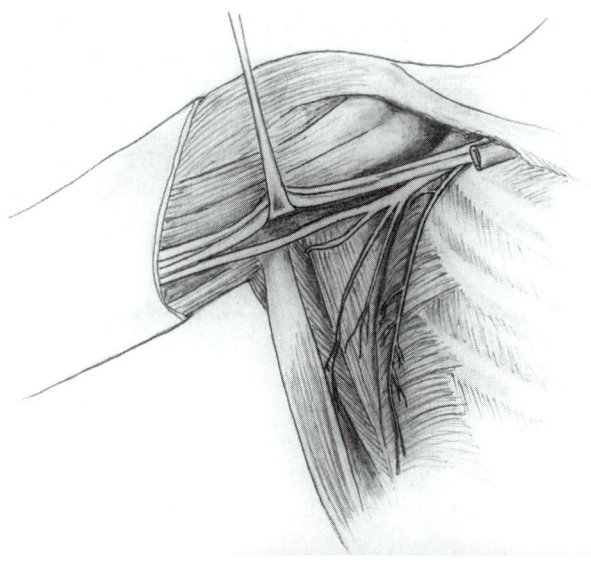

Figure 27.4. Anatomy of the long thoracic nerve.

translated with some rotation (Fig. 27.3). Pain is often present as muscles about the shoulder compensate for the change in the biomechanics of the shoulder girdle. Abduction above 120° accentuates winging and pain, as does tilting the head to the contralateral shoulder.

Rhomboid major or minor weakness is a rare cause of primary scapular winging. Any process that injures the dorsal scapular nerve (which originates from the nerve root of C5 and passes deep to or through the levator scapula) may theoretically cause winging. The patient's history usually reveals pain localized to the medial scapular border. Winging at rest is minimal on examination; there is a slight depression and lateral translation of the scapula similar to the winging caused by a palsy of the trapezius. Atrophy along the medial scapular border may be present, with accentuation of winging when the arm is slowly lowered from the forward elevated position (11). Treatment for this type of winging is trapezius strengthening.

Scapular osteochondromas, the most common scapular tumor, may lead to structural pseudo-winging of the scapula (12). The diagnosis is made on physical examination with audible crepitus on movement of the scapula. Confirmation with tangential x-rays or a CT scan of the scapula is helpful. EMG studies show no abnormalities. When the patient is symptomatic, resection of the tumor leads to arrest of the winging.

The remaining causes of primary scapular winging include malunion of the body of the scapula. This rare cause of pseudo-winging occurs from a structural imbalance (13). Congenital absence of the serratus anterior (14), trapezius, and rhomboid major or minor (15) has been reported as another cause of winging with minimal symptoms. Muscular avulsion of the serratus anterior (16), transection of a scapular muscle from a surgical approach to the back

(12), and trauma in this area can also result in scapular winging. In these latter cases, the amount of tissue damage can be assessed by MRI. Early reattachment is recommended, if the diagnosis is confirmed by imaging.

Primary winging of the scapula may also be secondary to inflamed bursae between the scapula and thorax. Physical examination will reveal scapular crepitus and pain. This type of winging is associated with subscapular bursitis and resolves with management of the bursitis.

Secondary Scapular Winging

Secondary scapular winging is caused by disorders of the glenohumeral joint or subacromial space, such as rotator cuff tears, shoulder instability, and adhesive capsulitis. In throwing athletes with occult instability and secondary impingement, subtle scapula winging may be observed. Unlike primary scapular winging, EMG denervation of the serratus anterior, trapezius, and rhomboids does not occur with secondary winging. Contracture of the glenohumeral joint in patients with congenital fibrosis of the deltoid or obstetrical shoulder trauma can lead to this type of winging of the scapula (17).

Patients with painful shoulders often limit their glenohumeral motion. Limited glenohumeral motion leads to periscapular muscle overuse with a resultant increase of abnormal scapulothoracic motion. The periscapular muscles fatigue, and the secondary scapular winging is found on physical examination. Secondary winging subsides once the primary glenohumeral disorder has been addressed. A scapular rehabilitation program should be initiated to facilitate recovery.

Voluntary Scapular Winging

Voluntary scapular winging is a rare cause of winging and is associated with attention-seeking personalities. The appropriate personnel should be consulted to determine the underlying psychosocial issues. Reassurance and muscle retraining are the mainstays of treatment (12,18).

RADIOLOGIC STUDIES

The diagnosis of scapular winging is performed by a clinical examination. EMG studies should be obtained in all patients being considered for surgical management of their winging. X-rays and other diagnostic modalities play a limited role in the diagnosis of scapular winging. Occasionally x-rays centered on the scapula may demonstrate medial or superolateral displacement of the scapula, depending on the cause of the winging. X-ray or CT studies can be useful for the diagnosis of winging from osteochondromas or fracture malunions.

TREATMENT

Nonoperative Alternatives and Indications for Surgery

The mainstay of treatment for symptomatic scapular winging is physical therapy. The emphasis is on shoulder range of motion to avoid stiffness. In the majority of cases, neurapraxia will resolve in 1 to 2 years. Gregg et al. (6) reported on a series of 10 patients with an isolated serratus anterior paralysis as a result of a traction injury to the long thoracic nerve. Of these, 9 patients had a full recovery, with an average healing time of 9 months. The presence of EMG nerve activity of the long thoracic nerve as it courses along the chest wall portends an early return of function. Overpeck and Ghormley (19) reported equally encouraging results. Despite the decrease in pain and good functional result, patients should be reminded that mild scapular winging might persist, especially in response to stress testing (1).

The results of conservative management for winging secondary to trapezius dysfunction may not be as encouraging. The pain from trapezius dysfunction is more intense than that from winging secondary to long thoracic nerve palsy (20). The pain is caused by traction on the brachial plexus, which occurs in addition to the drooping of the shoulder from a trapezius palsy (2). Bigliani et al. (2) noted that of eight patients treated conservatively for a spinal accessory palsy, only one had a successful outcome. Physical therapy and muscle strengthening were insufficient to relieve the pain from spasm and radiculitis, but they helped alleviate discomfort from a concomitant frozen shoulder. All patients in their series had persistent winging. Other workers have commented on similarly poor results of conservative treatment for trapezius paralysis (21).

No study has proven that early surgical intervention improves outcome. Most patients have at least a 12-month trial of physical therapy. A brace can be used to prevent overstretching of the long thoracic nerve in patients awaiting surgery. The decision to proceed with surgery should be based on the presence of pain and disability rather than the cosmetic appearance of winging. Earlier surgical intervention can be considered for winging from nonneurapraxic causes (e.g., tumor, nerve avulsion directly off the brachial plexus, documented lacerations of the long thoracic or spinal accessory nerves, and the muscular dystrophies).

Operative Treatment

Surgical management for scapular winging can be divided into static and dynamic procedures. The static procedures attempt to immobilize the scapula either by a scapulothoracic fusion or by tethering the scapula to the spine. Dynamic procedures involve a muscle transfer to compensate for the lost function of the serratus anterior or the trapezius (1) (Clinical Table). Scapulothoracic fusions have been discouraged in the past because of the enormity of the surgery and potential for complications, such as pneumothorax, hemothorax, rib fracture, and loss of vital capacity.

Clinical Table: Tendon Transfers for Scapular Winging

Procedure	Indications	Technique	Anatomy	Pitfalls
Scapulothoracic fusion	• Fascioscapulohumeral dystrophy • Failed dynamic procedures for serratus anterior winging	• Luque wires (23)—19-gauge wire with dynamic compression plate	• T4–7 ribs	• Pneumothorax
Fascial sling	• Scapular winging	• Fascia lata graft to 2nd and 3rd dorsal vertebrae and spine of scapula	• Levator scapulae • Dorsal spine	• Pain • Instability • Late recurrence
Eden–Lange (31)	• Trapezius palsy	• Transfers levator scapulae and rhomboid major and minor laterally	• Spine of scapula • Levator scapulae	• Rhomboid major and minor damaged • Avoid dorsal scapular nerve and transverse cervical artery medially • Pneumothorax • Suprascapular nerve palsy
Chaves (27)	• Serratus anterior palsy	• Pectoralis minor and fascial extension graft	• Coracoid inferior border of scapula	• Avoid proximal dissection so as not to injure medial and lateral pectoral nerves
Marmor–Bechtol operation	• Serratus anterior palsy	• Pectoralis major	• Inferior tip of scapula • Shaft of humerus	

STATIC PROCEDURES

Scapulothoracic Fusion

Letournel et al. (22) reported on 16 scapulothoracic fusions in which 9 patients had a diagnosis of fascioscapulohumeral dystrophy. Fascioscapulohumeral dystrophy is an autosomal dominant disease that appears in the second and third decades of life with a selective myopathy of the face, trunk, and limbs. The serratus anterior, trapezius, rhomboids, and teres muscles are affected, but the deltoid and rotator cuff are often spared. The disease can lead to a painful, disfiguring winging of the scapula. Fusion of the scapula to the spine helps increase the mechanical advantage of the functioning deltoid in shoulder abduction and flexion. Three of the ribs from T4–7 are fused to the spine. (Fig. 27.5) The average operating room time for Letournel et al. was 1 h 20 min. They reported three pneumothoraces and one postoperative pleural effusion. With an average follow-up of 24 months, none of the patients had scapular winging, and all said that they could perform most of their activities of daily living. Preoperative shoulder abduction improved from 77° to 102°; and flexion, from 75° to 108°.

Jakab and Gladhill (23) described a simplified technique for a scapulothoracic fusion with the use of Luque wires. Their three patients (all with fascioscapulohumeral dystrophy) had a gain in abduction and flexion of approximately 30°. There were no reported complications, and no postoperative immobilization was used in this series.

Hawkins et al. (24) treated nine patients with ten scapulothoracic fusions. Of these, eight patients (average age = 28 years) were available for follow-up. At an average follow-up of 28 months, five patients had fascioscapulohumeral muscular dystrophy, two patients had a serratus anterior palsy, and one suffered from cleidocranial dysostosis. The technique involves a medial parascapular incision. The infraspinatus and subscapularis muscles are dissected 2 cm off the medial scapular border, and ribs 3, 4, and 5 are denuded of cortical bone. A 19-gauge wire is passed beneath each drill hole and then through the medial scapular border and dynamic compression plate. The scapula is externally rotated on the chest wall 15°. An autogenous bone graft is taken and interposed between the scapula and the ribs before the wires are tightened. On postoperative day 2, a shoulder spica cast is placed on the patient.

Eight of nine patients of Hawkins et al. (24) had less pain after fusion. (Pain was the primary indicator for surgery in all cases.) Forward elevation improved in all patients except the patient with cleidocranial dysostosis. The greatest gains in forward elevation were found in the two patients with isolated serratus anterior palsy. Complications included one patient who had a pneumothorax that required a chest tube. Four of the nine patients had pseudarthrosis, which caused clunking when the shoulder was moved but was not disabling. The authors believed long-term pain management was, by far, superior to a scapulothoracic fusion; and range of motion could increase in the long term only in patients with an isolated serratus anterior palsy, not those with muscular dystrophy.

Post (25) reported on two patients with a scapulothoracic fusion. Both patients had a serratus anterior paralysis; after surgery, both had a decrease in pain and gains in shoulder (glenohumeral) motion.

We believe that a scapulothoracic fusion has its greatest role in the management of failed dynamic procedures, in laborers with disabling serratus anterior winging, and in cases in which more than one muscle group contributes to decreased motion and winging (e.g., the muscular dystrophies).

Fascial Sling Operation

The fascial sling operation is another type of static procedure for treating scapular winging. The goal is to tether the scapula to the surrounding spinal musculature or vertebrae. Fascial grafts from the fascia lata, or elsewhere, are often used. The scapula is left fixed in position to avoid its contracture toward the spine (Fig. 27.6).

Combination fascial sling and dynamic procedures have been used for the winging associated with a trapezius paralysis (5). The fascia lata graft is anchored to the spines of the second and third dorsal vertebrae and spine of scapula. The levator scapulae is then transferred laterally to the lateral spine. The levator now rotates around a fixed point in an attempt to mimic the forces of the paralyzed trapezius (Fig. 27.7).

Fascial slings have lost popularity recently because of reports of loss of strength (26) and late failure secondary to stretching of the sling. Bigliani et al. (2) reported on two patients who initially experienced good results from a combination procedure; but at 6 months, the patients noted pain, instability, and a late recurrence of scapular

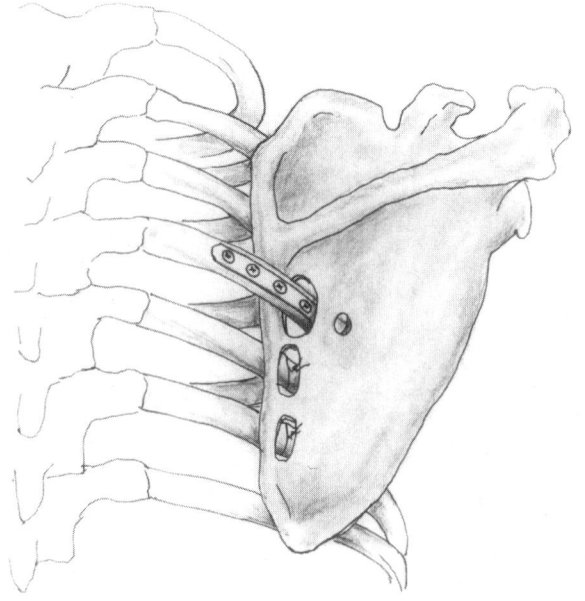

Figure 27.5. Scapulothoracic fusion technique of Letournel et al. (22).

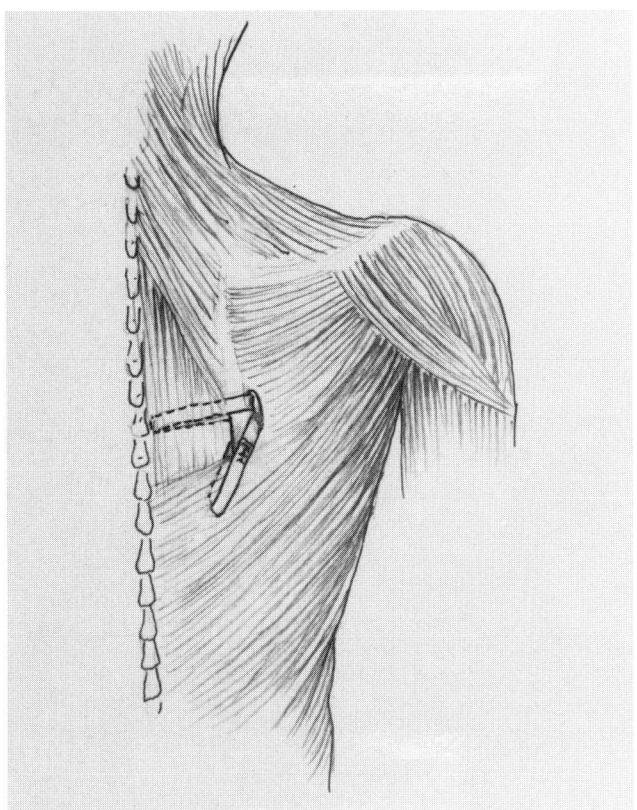

Figure 27.6. In the fascial sling operation, the scapula is tethered to thoracic vertebrae and paraspinal musculature.

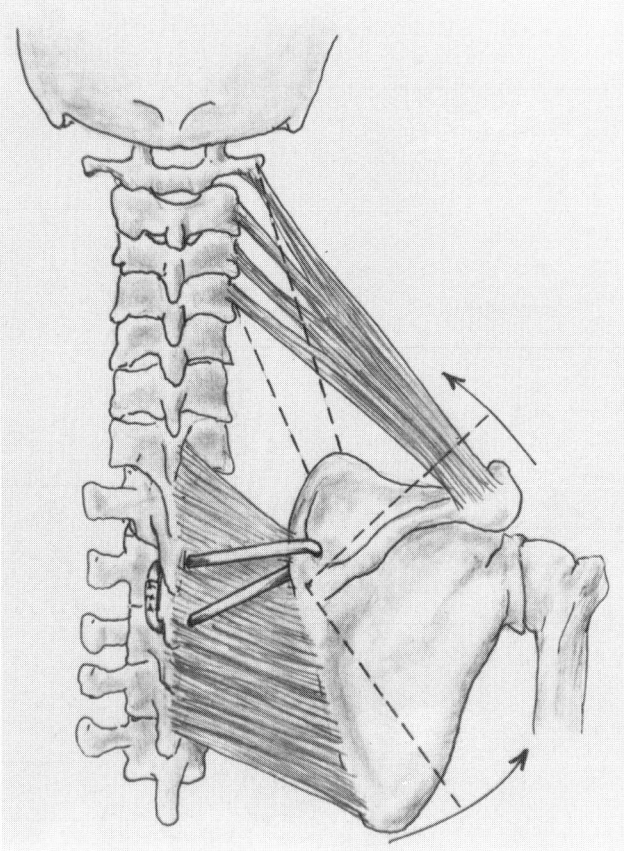

Figure 27.7. Fascial sling operation combined with a levator scapular transfer.

winging. In our hands, the sling procedure has a limited role in the treatment of symptomatic scapular winging.

DYNAMIC PROCEDURES: MUSCLE TRANSFERS FOR PRIMARY SCAPULAR WINGING

The cornerstone of surgical management of scapular winging has become the dynamic tendon or muscle transfer procedures. The dynamic procedures transfer a muscle or tendon unit that compensates for the lost function of the paralyzed muscle. This transfer attempts to alleviate the pain and winging, without the loss of motion that often occurs with static procedures. The choice of the dynamic procedure depends on the affected muscle.

Transfers for Serratus Anterior Palsy

There are several muscle transfers that have been described for treating scapular winging caused by serratus anterior nerve palsy. The pectoralis minor muscle transfer with the use of a fascial extension graft has been described by several authors (27,28). This transfer uses a two-incision technique, and the pectoralis minor is released from the coracoid and subcutaneously tunneled to the inferior border of the scapula.

Transfer of the pectoralis major, known as the Marmor–Bechtol operation (20), is the most widely used procedure for serratus anterior weakness. In this tech-

nique, the patient lies supine on the operating room table with the arm widely abducted and a sandbag placed underneath the scapula. An incision is made across the axilla from the inferior tip of the scapula to the pectoralis major tendon as it inserts onto the shaft of the humerus (Fig. 27.8).

The subcutaneous tissue and fascia is divided, and the pectoralis major tendon is exposed. A plane is developed between the clavicular and sternocostal heads of the pectoralis major muscle. The sternocostal head is resected off of the humerus and freed up proximally (Fig. 27.9). The areolar tissue in the axilla is dissected away to facilitate exposure of the serratus anterior and latissimus dorsi musculature. The tip of the inferior scapula is exposed, and any tissue is cleared away. The ipsilateral thigh is prepared, and a 17.8- × 5-cm (7- × 2-in) fascia lata graft is obtained and tubulized (Fig. 27.10). The graft is sutured with permanent suture into the distal portion of the pectoralis tendon and passed through a foramen made by a drill hole in the inferior tip of the scapula. The graft is sutured onto itself, with maximum tension being applied (Fig. 27.11).

Post (25) described a similar procedure for serratus anterior winging using the pectoralis major that incorporates several modifications of the original Marmor–Bechtol operation. Post found that the operation was easier to per-

Figure 27.8. Incision for the pectoralis major transfer. Modified from Marmor L, Bechtol CO. Paralysis of the serratus anterior due to electric shock relieved by transplantation of the pectoralis major muscles: a case report. J Bone Joint Surg 1963;45A:156–160.

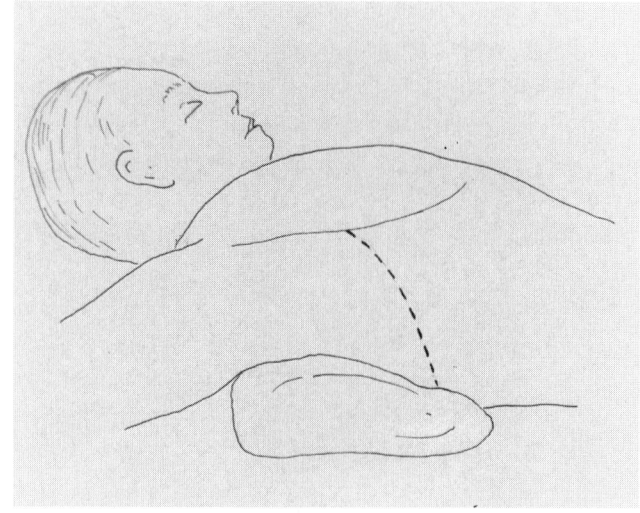

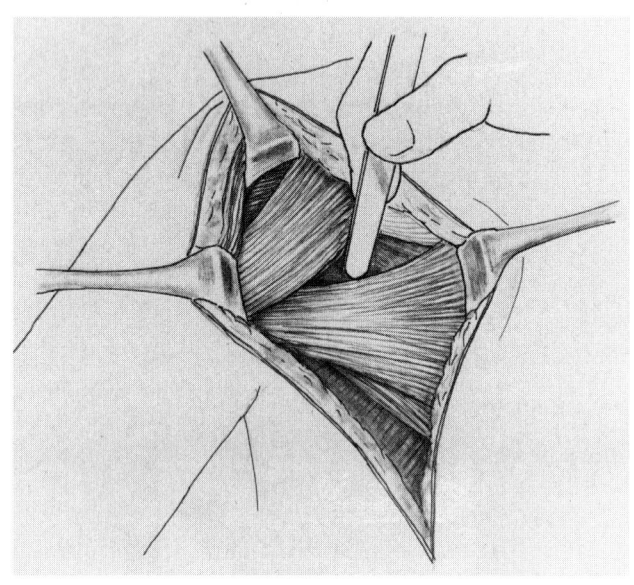

A

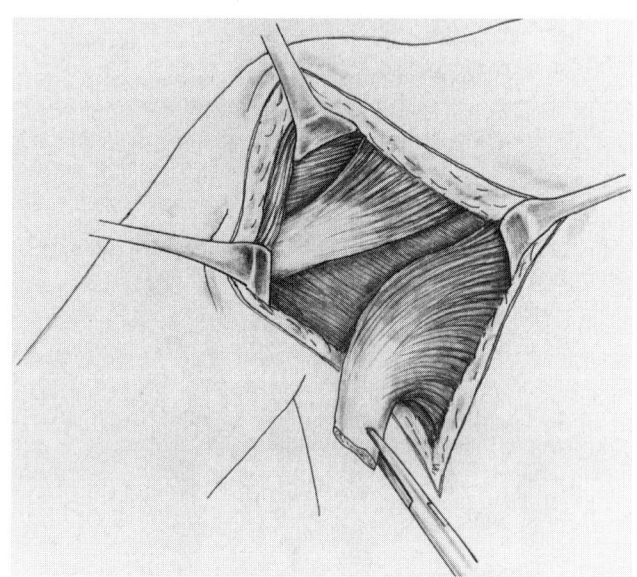

B

Figure 27.9. A. An interval is developed between the sternocostal and clavicular heads of the pectoralis major. **B.** The sternocostal head of the pectoralis major is transected and freed from the proximal humerus.

Figure 27.10. An ipsilateral fascia lata graft is harvested and tubulized.

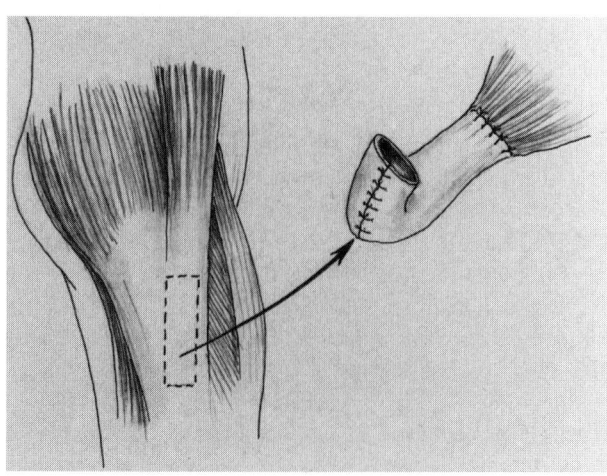

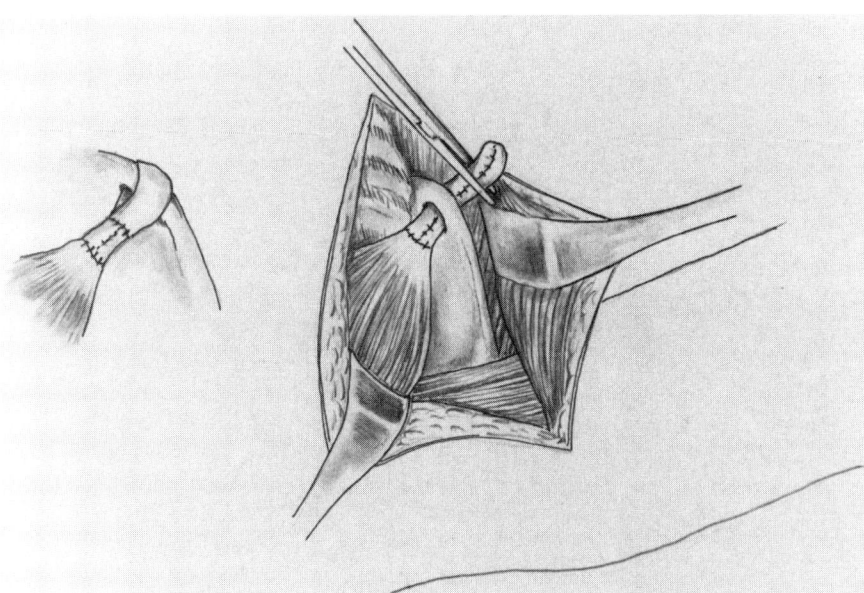

Figure 27.11. The graft is sutured onto itself through a drill hole in the inferior tip of the scapula.

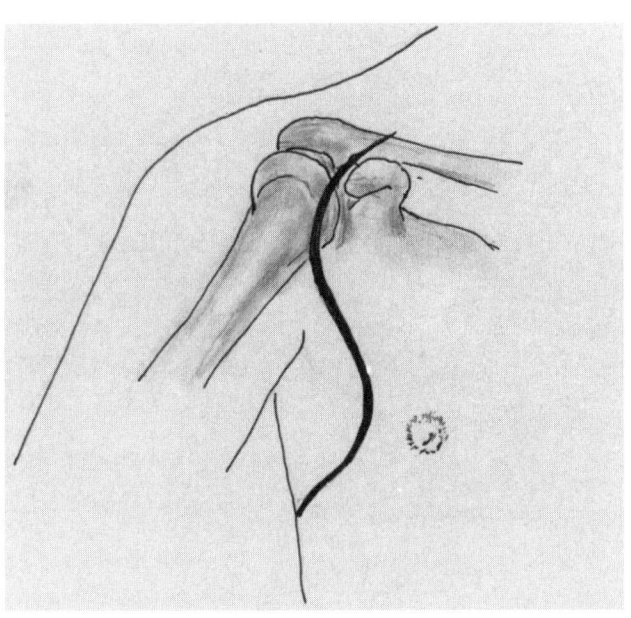

Figure 27.12. Skin incision for correcting serratus anterior winging. Modified from Post M. Pectoralis major transplant for paralysis of the serratus anterior. J Shoulder Elbow Surg 1995;4:1–9.

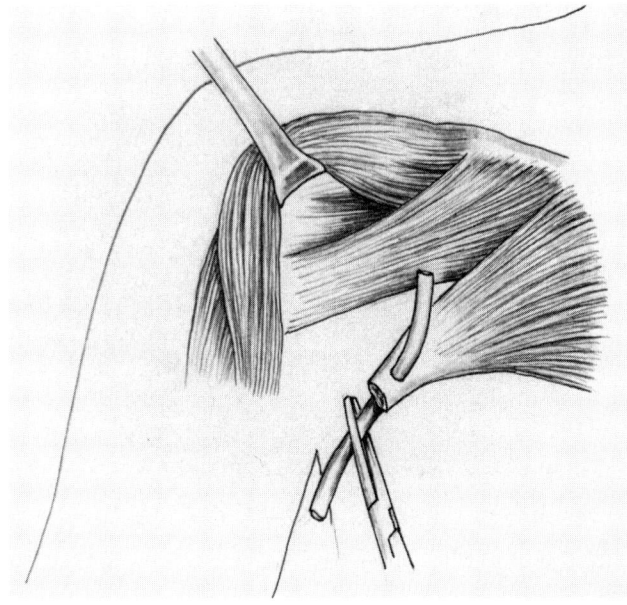

Figure 27.13. The fascia lata is threaded through the myotendinous junction.

form if he placed the patient in the lateral decubitus position (instead of supine), with the torso tilted backward by 35°. The graft is harvested from the posterior fascia lata close to the intermuscular septum; thus the graft is obtained from the thickest region of the fascia lata. The graft is then tubulized by the use of two clamps (one on each end) and then woven with number 5 nonabsorbable suture. Post also modified the axilla skin incision and described it as being curvilinear, beginning below the coracoid and lateral to the nipple and then curving dorsally to the inferior angle of the scapula (Fig. 27.12). The sternal head is transected 1 to 2 mm off of the humerus, and a stab

wound is placed in the myotendinous junction (Fig. 27.13). The fascia lata graft is threaded through this wound and sutured onto itself and the pectoralis tendon with nonabsorbable suture (Fig. 27.14).

The inferior angle of the scapula is mobilized; and the serratus anterior, subscapularis, rhomboid major, and infraspinatus muscles are all elevated off the scapula. An 8- to 10-mm hole is drilled through the membranous portion of the scapula 2.5 cm proximal to the inferior angle and medial to the thickened cortical edge of bone. The graft is placed through this drill hole and tightened appropriately (Fig. 27.15).

Figure 27.14. In Post's technique (25), the fascia lata is sutured onto itself and the pectoralis tendon.

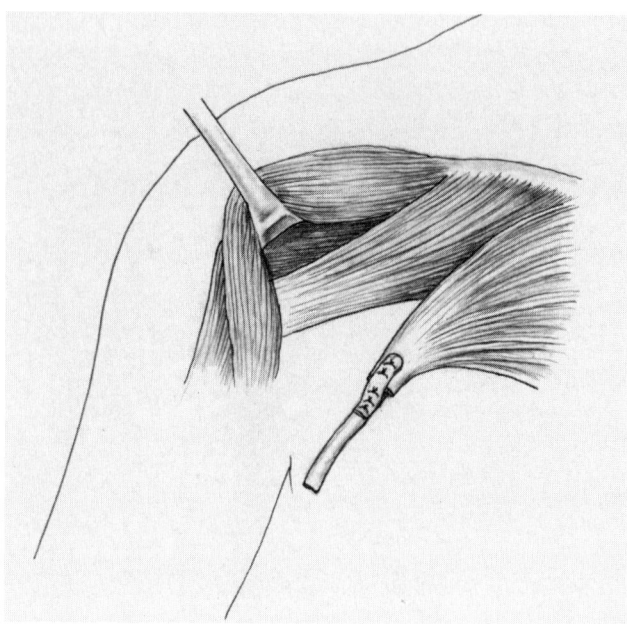

Figure 27.15. Final position of the fascia lata graft in the membranous portion of the scapula.

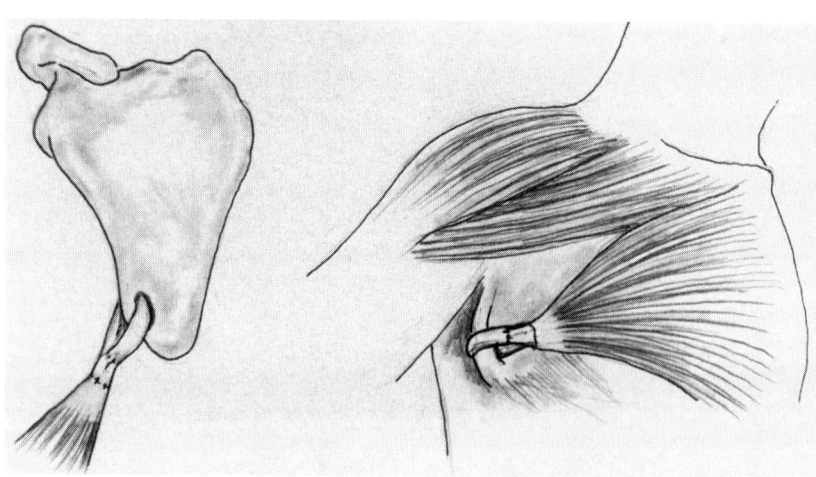

Another approach to the pectoralis major tendon transfer for serratus anterior palsy uses separate anterior and posterior incisions (29) (Fig. 27.16).

Pitfalls and most common technical mistakes. There are certain precautions that surgeons should be aware of before performing the pectoralis major tendon transfer. It is important that the surgeon avoid a proximal dissection when mobilizing the pectoralis major muscle. The proximal dissection puts the medial and lateral pectoral nerves at risk, as they pierce the undersurface of the muscle. We have also found that the inferior angle of the scapula has a large vascular anastomosis that must be avoided. Meticulous dissection and hemostasis should be performed to avoid any blood loss or serious complication. When drilling through the scapula, the surgeon must avoid the cortical edge of the scapula, so the bone is not allowed to fragment.

Rehabilitation. After surgery, the patient is placed in a sling. Passive range of motion is begun at 4 weeks, and ac-

tive motion is started at 6 weeks. Active strengthening begins at 12 weeks. Post (25) encourages the use of a Velpeau cast or orthosis in the noncompliant patient.

Transfers for Trapezius Palsy

The dynamic procedure most often employed in the treatment of trapezius paralysis is the transfer of the levator scapulae and rhomboid major and minor laterally on the scapula. The technique described by Eden (30) and Lange (31) attempts to mimic the vector pull of the upper-middle and lower trapezius muscle masses (Fig. 27.17). Lagenskiold and Ryoppy (32) place the patient in a lateral decubitus position; their incision extends from the dorsal aspect of the acromion to the medial inferior border of the scapula. We prefer a two-incision technique, which was described by Bigliani et al. (2) (Fig. 27.18).

The first incision is made midway between the spinous process and the medial scapular border just above the superior edge of the scapula. This incision courses the length

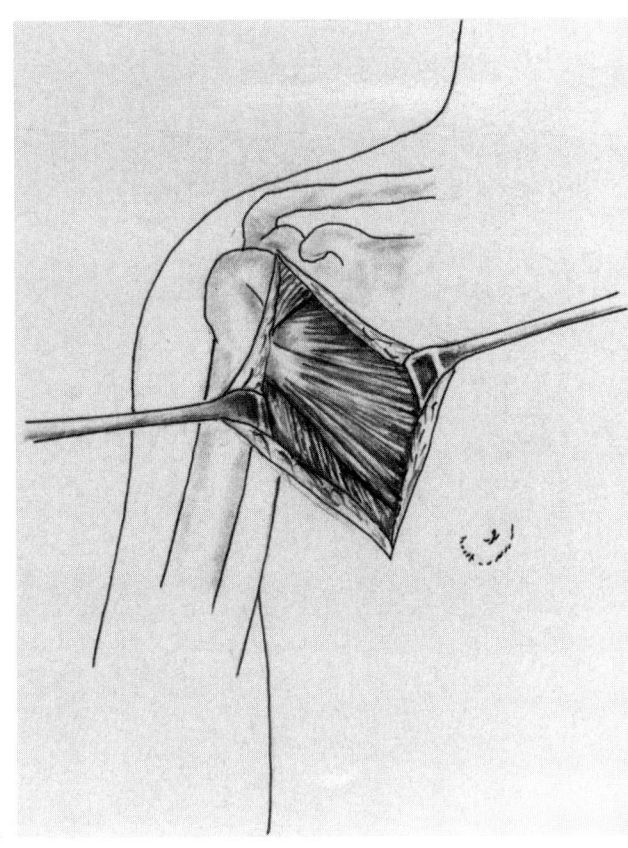
A

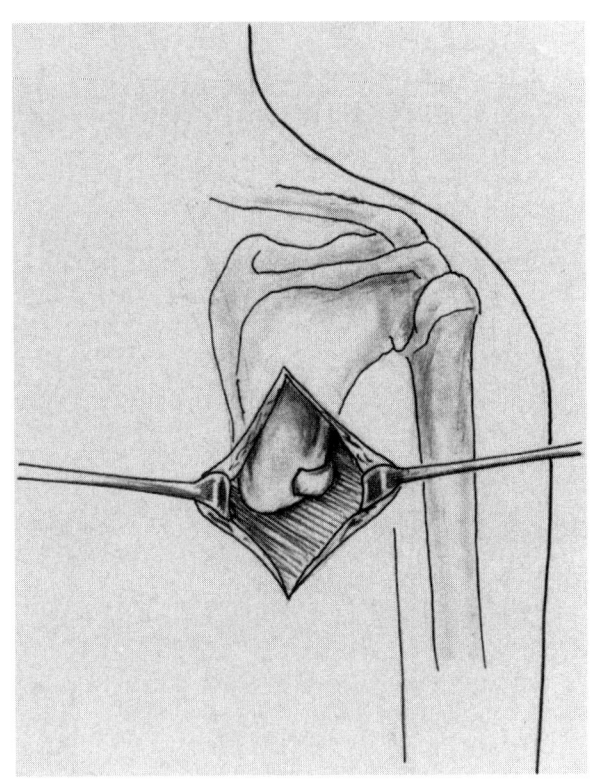
B

Figure 27.16. A. Anterior incision and dissection to harvest the pectoralis major. **B.** Posterior incision showing the pectoralis major and fascia lata graft fixed to the scapula.

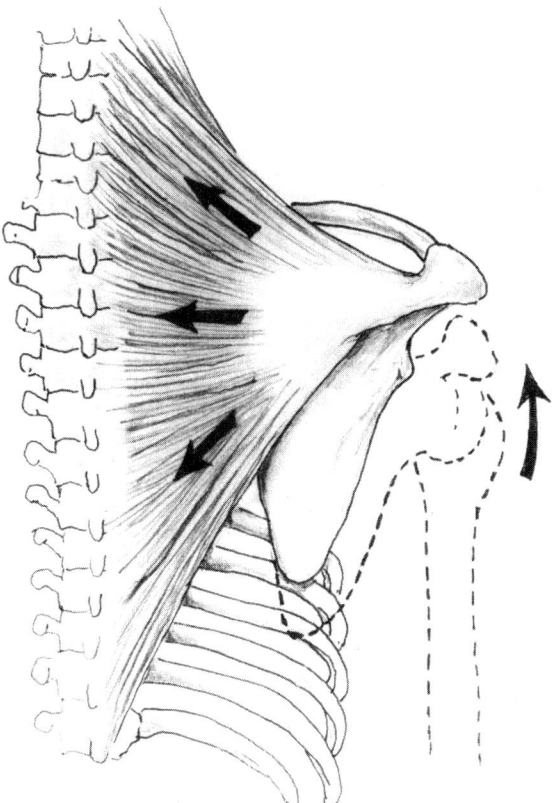

Figure 27.17. Vector pull of the trapezius muscle.

of the scapula. The atrophic trapezius is cut close to the scapular border. The planes between the levator scapula and rhomboid major and minor are identified (Fig. 27.19). These three muscular attachments are released with a small piece of bone from the medial scapula, and the muscles are separated from one another. The levator scapulae must be mobilized to reach the lateral aspect of the scapular spine.

The infraspinatus is elevated from the infraspinatus fossa, and six holes are drilled 1.5 to 2.0 cm apart, beginning 5 cm lateral to the medial border of the scapula. Heavy nylon suture is passed through these holes. The top two holes are used to suture the rhomboid minor and the superior aspect of the rhomboid major. The remaining holes are used for attachment sites for the rhomboid major. All sutures are tied with the scapula held reduced and the arm abducted 90° (Fig. 27.20). The infraspinatus is reattached with suture anchors or drill holes.

The last incision is made over the spine of the scapula and begins 3 cm medial to the posterior tip of the acromion. The trapezius, deltoid, and supraspinatus are elevated, and three drill holes are made through the spine of the scapula. A tunnel is made in line with the medial and lateral incisions and with the fibers of the trapezius. The levator is tunneled through this passageway and sutured to the spine of the scapula (Fig. 27.20).

Figure 27.18. Two-incision technique for the Eden–Lange procedure. Modified from Bigliani LU, Perez-Sanz JR, Wolfe IN. Treatment of trapezius paralysis. J Bone Joint Surg 1985;67A: 871–877.

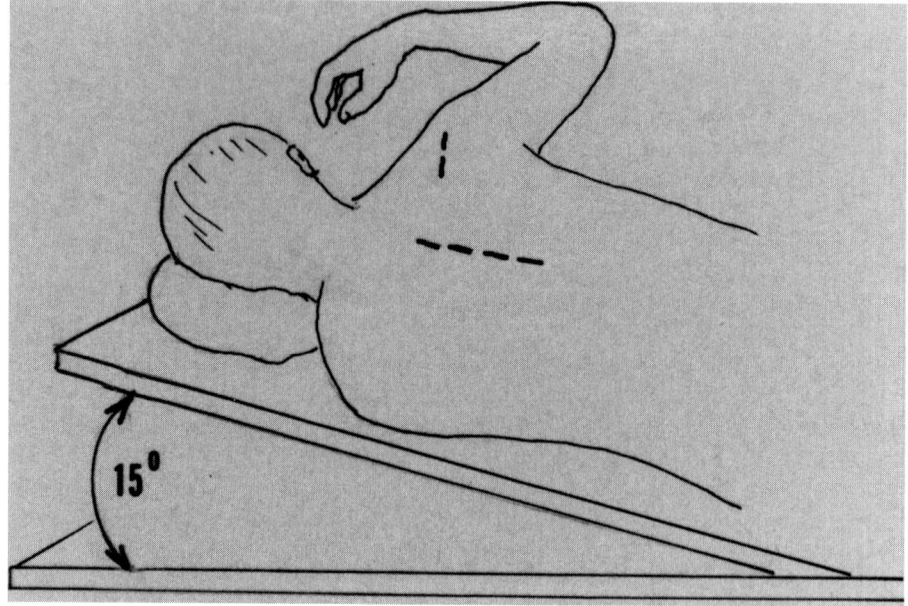

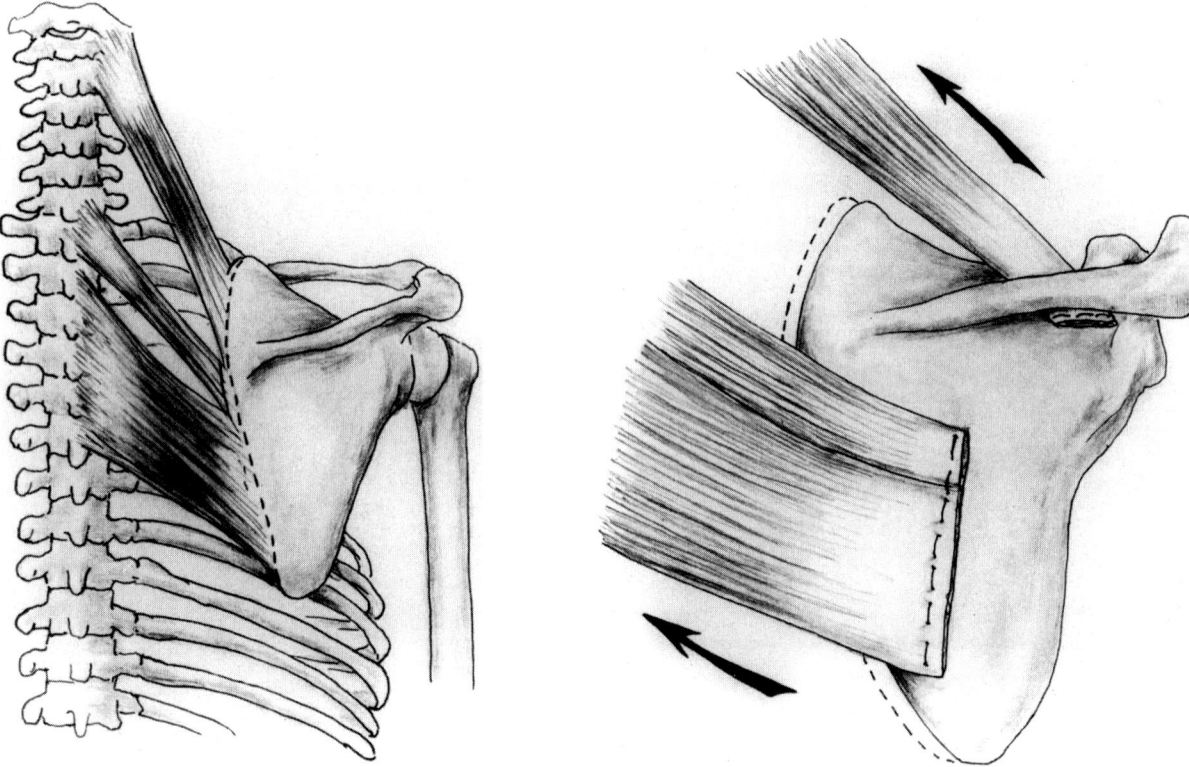

Figure 27.19. With the trapezius removed, the planes of the levator scapula and rhomboid major and minor are identified. *Dashed line* indicates the first incision of the Eden–Lange procedure.

Figure 27.20. When the Eden–Lange procedure is complete, the rhomboid major and minor are tied to the scapula, and the levator scapula is tunneled and sutured to the spine of the scapula.

Pitfalls and most common technical mistakes. To avoid pitfalls and common technical mistakes, the surgeon must keep the following in mind:

- When removing the trapezius off of the scapular border, the surgeon must stay away from the spinous processes, or the rhomboid major and minor will be damaged.

- When attempting to separate the levator scapulae and rhomboids from each other, the surgeon must avoid the dorsal scapular nerve and transverse cervical arteries, which traverse medially.
- When drilling, the surgeon must make sure all drill holes are in bone to avoid a pneumothorax.
- When mobilizing the supraspinatus off the scapular

spine, the surgeon must avoid damaging the suprascapular nerve.

Rehabilitation. Passive range of motion exercises are begun at 6 weeks after surgery. A sling or abduction brace may be used early in the postoperative period. Active range of motion exercises are begun at 8 to 12 weeks after surgery.

Results of Treatment

The results of tendon transfers for the treatment of scapular winging have been encouraging. Post (25) has reported the results of the Marmor–Bechtol procedure for serratus anterior winging. He followed eight patients for an average of 27.1 months and was able to alleviate pain in seven of those patients. He also was able to maintain a full range of motion. All patients returned to work, but five patients were restricted from heavy lifting. He reported one complication in a patient who had a large thigh seroma from the graft site, which required multiple aspirations to resolve. He commented that spiraling the graft was paramount to avoiding graft failure.

Iceton and Harris (33) reported on 16 patients; excellent results were obtained in 9 of the patients. These patients had no pain or winging and good shoulder motion. They noted failures in 4 patients, of which 2 had postoperative fascioscapular humeral dystrophy. The remaining 2 patients had associated preoperative brachial plexus injury. We have learned from our own results that therapy in the immediate postoperative period should not stress the shoulder joint.

The pectoralis minor muscle transfer, while less popular, has also been successful. Vastamaki (28) reported on six patients with a pectoralis minor muscle transfer; four patients had no postoperative pain or winging. One patient, however, had a failure because of a weak pectoralis minor muscle. Iceton and Harris (33) agree with other authors that the pectoralis minor is a weak muscle with a short arc of contracture; they advise against its use for correction of scapular winging.

Leffert (26) reported 2 failed transfers in a series of 10 patients treated with pectoralis major transfer, giving him an 80% success rate. We use the Marmor–Bechtol procedure as the technique of choice for treating isolated serratus anterior palsy; we believe that other muscle transfers do not have the same mechanical advantage or predictable results. Postoperative seroma of the thigh, late failure, and persistence of winging despite relief of pain must be discussed with the patient when obtaining a surgical consent.

The Eden–Lange transfer has been the most widely used and reported procedure for isolated trapezius winging. Bigliani et al. (2) discussed seven patients treated with the Eden–Lange procedure. Five of these patients had excellent results, described as full shoulder use, normal appearance, and no pain. One had intermittent pain and weakness, and the last patient had persistent pain and weakness and was considered the only unsatisfactory result. Leffert (26) reported that all eight patients in his series experienced good to excellent results, with improvement over time. He recommended the Eden–Lange transfer for treatment of isolated trapezius winging.

SUMMARY

Scapular winging is often a missed source of pain in the shoulder. The winging can be primary, secondary, or voluntary. A well-directed physical examination will avoid a missed diagnosis and help many patients who have already seen numerous other physicians. Conservative treatment can resolve many muscle imbalances; but when it is unsuccessful, operative intervention can yield excellent results.

REFERENCES

1. Kuhn JE, Plancher KD, Hawkins RJ. Scapular winging. J Am Acad Orthop Surg 1995;3:319–325.
2. Bigliani LU, Perez-Sanz JR, Wolfe IN. Treatment of trapezius paralysis. J Bone Joint Surg 1985;67A:871–877.
3. Dunn AW. Trapezius paralysis after minor surgical procedures in the posterior cervical triangle. South Med J 1974;67:312–315.
4. Wright YA. Accessory spinal nerve injury. Clin Orthop 1975;108:15–18.
5. Dewar FP, Harris RI. Restoration of function of the shoulder following paralysis of the trapezius by fascial sling fixation and transplantation of the levator scapulae. Ann Surg 1950;132:1111–1115.
6. Gregg JR, Labosky D, Harty M, et al. Serratus anterior paralysis in the young athlete. J Bone Surg 1979;61A:825–832.
7. Radin EL. Peripheral neuritis as a complication of infectious mononucleosis: report of a case. J Bone Joint Surg 1967;49A:535–538.
8. Ball CR. Paralysis following injection of antitetanic serum: case report with serratus magnus involved. US Naval Med Bull 1939;37:305–330.
9. Leffert RD. Nerve injuries about the shoulder. In: Rowe CR, ed. The shoulder. New York: Churchill Livingstone, 1988;435–454.
10. Makin GJ, Brown WF, Ebers GC. C7 radiculopathy: importance of scapular winging in clinical diagnosis. J Neurol Neurosurg Psychiatry 1986;49:640–644.
11. Saeed MA, Gatens PF Jr, Singh S. Winging of the scapula. Am Fam Phys 1981;24:139–143.
12. Fiddian NJ, King RJ. The winged scapula. Clin Orthop 1984;185:228–236.
13. Mendoza FX, Main K. Peripheral nerve injuries of the shoulder in the athlete. Clin Sports Med 1990;9:331–342.
14. Levin SE, Trummer MJ. Agenesis of the serratus anterior muscle: a cause of winged scapula. JAMA 1973;225:748.
15. Wood VE, Marchinski L. Congenital anomalies of the shoulder. In: Rockwood CA, Matsen FA, eds. The shoulder. Philadelphia: Saunders, 1990:98–148.
16. Weeks LE. Scapular winging due to serratus anterior avulsion fracture. Orthop Trans 1993;17:184.
17. Minami M, Yamazaki J, Minami A, Ishii S. A postoperative long-term study of the deltoid contracture in children. J Pediatr Orthop 1984;4:609–613.
18. Rowe CR. Unusual shoulder conditions. In: Rowe CR, ed. The shoulder. New York: Churchill Livingstone, 1988:639–654.
19. Overpeck DO, Ghormley RK. Paralysis of the serratus magnus muscle caused by lesions of the long thoracic nerve. JAMA 1940;114:1994–1996.
20. Marmor L, Bechtol CO. Paralysis of the serratus anterior due to electric shock relieved by transplantation of the pectoralis major muscles: a case report. J Bone Joint Surg 1963;45A:156–160.

21. Olarte M, Adams D: Accessory nerve palsy. J Neurol Neurosurg Psychiatry 1977;40:1113–1116.
22. Letournel E, Fardeau M, Lytle JO, et al. Scapulothoracic arthrodesis for patients who have fascioscapulohumeral muscular dystrophy. J Bone Joint Surg 1990;72A:78–84.
23. Jakab E, Gladhill RB. Simplified technique for scapulocostal fusion in fascioscapulohumeral dystrophy. J Pediatr Orthop 1993;13:748–751.
24. Hawkins RJ, Willis RB, Litchfield RB. Scapulothoracic arthrodesis for scapular winging. In: Post M, Morrey BF, Hawkins RJ, eds. Surgery of the shoulder. St. Louis: Mosby, 1990:356–359.
25. Post M. Pectoralis major transplant for paralysis of the serratus anterior. J Shoulder Elbow Surg 1995;4:1–9.
26. Leffert RD. Pectoralis major transfer for serratus anterior paralysis. Orthop Trans 1992–1993;16:761.
27. Chaves JP. Pectoralis minor transplant for paralysis of the serratus anterior. J Bone Joint Surg 1951;33B:228–230.
28. Vastamaki M. Pectoralis minor transfer in serratus anterior paralysis. Acta Orthop Scand 1984;55:293–295.
29. Durman D. An operation for paralysis of the serratus anterior. J Bone Joint Surg 1945;27:380–382.
30. Eden R. Zur behandlung der trapeziuslahmungmittels-l muskelplastik. Dtsch Z Chir 1924;184:387–389.
31. Lange M. Die operative behandlung der irrepairablem trapeziuslahmung. Tip Fakult Mecmausi 1959;22:137–141.
32. Langenskiold A, Ryoppy S. Treatment of paralysis of the trapezius muscle by the Eden–Lange operation. Acta Orthop Scand 1973;44:383–388.
33. Iceton J, Harris WR. Treatment of winged scapula by pectoralis major transfer. J Bone Joint Surg 1987;69B:108–110.

SPINE

Cervical Spine Trauma: Upper and Lower Cervical Spine Injury

Cervical spine injury with or without neurologic deficit has a major effect not only on the patient but on families, trauma units, and society in general. In particular, the initial evaluation and treatment of the multiply-injured patient raise complex issues that can be addressed only through a systematic approach to acute care. The primary goals of management for cervical injury are to reduce the neurologic deficit and to prevent any additional loss of neurologic function. In the acutely injured patient with a suspected neck injury, the spine must be immobilized to prevent further neural injury. Thereafter, the anatomy of the injury can be further delineated to plan treatment while avoiding the risk of additional injury.

Neurologic injury occurs in 39 to 50% of bony cervical spine injuries. Such damage may occur, particularly in children, without radiographic evidence of fracture (spinal cord injury without radiographic abnormality; SCIWORA). SCIWORA is also found in adults with cervical spinal stenosis. Because it is easy to overrely on static imaging techniques in the acute setting, it is important to remember to assess the clinical condition of subacute instability. Subacute instability is defined as the development of radiographic instability within 3 weeks of cervical spine injury, in association with a normal initial radiographic evaluation and neurologic examination. At follow-up, there may be a neurologic deficit in association with radiographic evidence of instability, as a result of ligamentous and disc injury.

The most common causes of missed cervical spine injury are multiple trauma, altered consciousness, and noncontiguous fractures. Heightened awareness of the possibility of a significant neck injury, with or without bony injury, is thus of paramount importance in the early diagnosis and subsequent management of this potentially devastating condition.

RELEVANT ANATOMY AND PATHOGENESIS

Injury to the cervical spine most commonly occurs in the young adult male, and the peak incidence is in the third decade of life. The causes of injury vary regionally throughout the world. The most frequent mechanisms of injury are motor vehicle accidents (40 to 50%), falls and firearms (30 to 40%), and water sports (10%). Some trauma centers have noted that the rate of motorcycle-related injuries has recently risen significantly. Patients under 30 years of age tend to sustain the trauma from motor vehicle accidents or water-sports activities, whereas older patients are prone to neck trauma from falls and firearms.

The most common anatomic sites of injury are C1, C5, C6, and C7. Approximately 40% of patients present with complete spinal cord injuries, 40% present with incomplete lesions, and 20% are neurologically intact. The overall mortality in the United States for multiply-injured patients with cervical spine injury is 40%; a much lower rate is reported from specialized regional trauma centers. The highest in-hospital mortality from cervical cord injury relates to C4–5-level injuries. Mechanisms of injury and the direction of force required to cause significant neck trauma are discussed below for each type of injury. Many vital structures lie in close proximity within a small area in the cervical spine. Complete familiarity with the three-dimensional anatomy of the bony, ligamentous, muscular, neural, and vascular elements of the cervical spine complex is important for understanding normal function and provides insights into the pathomechanics of cervical injury.

The cervical spine has three primary functions: housing and protecting the spinal cord and nerve roots, allowing for active triplanar motion of the head, and acting as a shock absorber for the head and brain. The cervical spine consists of the first seven vertebrae of the spinal column. With the exception of the atlas, each vertebra consists of a body, upper and lower articular surface, vertebral canal, and vertebral arch. The vertebrae below the axis have a pedicle and a lamina of the vertebral arch. Laterally, the intervertebral foramina serve as portals of entry and exit for blood vessels and nerves.

The lower five cervical vertebrae have many common features. Typically, they increase in size from C3 to C7 to accommodate increasing loads and are essentially oval, short cylinders. The normal cervical lordosis is produced by wedge-shaped intervertebral discs, not by the vertebral bodies. The lateral margins of the superior surface of the vertebral bodies display prominent hook-like projections, called uncinate processes, that hold the lateral surfaces of the vertebra just above between them on both sides and are responsible for the stability and mobility of the cervical spine. When using an anterior approach to surgery of the cervical spine, the surgeon should preserve as much of the uncinate processes as possible to maintain stability of the spine.

The spinous processes of C3–5 and usually C6 are bifid, whereas C7 is longer and tapered at the ends. Because of the length of its spinous process, C7 is also referred to as the vertebra prominens and can be a useful anatomic landmark; however, it is the most prominent process at the cervicothoracic junction in only 79% of women and 59% of men. The spinous process of C6 is the prominent vertebra in 13% of women and 6% of men, and T1 is most prominent in 6% of women and 9% of men. The transverse foramina of C3–6 transmit the vertebral artery and vein and the sympathetic plexus.

For anterior operative approaches to the cervical spine, it is important to appreciate the surface anatomic landmarks that indicate spinal levels. The first cervical vertebra is behind the angle of the mandible, and the transverse process of the atlas is usually palpable between the angle of the mandible and the mastoid process. The hyoid bone lies anterior to C3, whereas the thyroid cartilage is anterior to C4. The cricoid cartilage is opposite C6 and is thus an important landmark for the two common sites of cervical disc disease (e.g., C5–6 and C6–7). The skin incision for an anterior approach to the C7–T1 level is usually just above the clavicle. The preoperative lateral radiograph usually aids in relating palpable landmarks to the spine levels of an individual patient.

The atlas has a unique ring-like structure composed of paired lateral masses that are joined together by a short, thick anterior arch and a long, thinner, more highly curved posterior arch.

The axis is the thickest and strongest of the cervical vertebrae. Its unique feature is that the body of C1 is fused to the axis body at the odontoid process, around which the atlas rotates.

The pedicle or pars interarticularis area of the axis is subject to high shearing forces, which, if large enough, may result in a hangman's fracture. Dorsally, the axis tapers into a short, thick, and usually bifid spinous process. Its transverse foramen is oriented to allow lateral inclination of the vertebral artery to the corresponding foramen of the atlas. The dens protrudes superiorly from the body of the axis, is 14 to 16 mm high, and forms a $-20°$ to $42°$ angle with respect to the body of the atlas in the sagittal plane. It is important to remember the variability of this angle when considering odontoid screw fixation. The neck of the axis is slightly constricted, to 10 mm, which may occasionally limit odontoid fixation of a fracture to a single screw. On the anterior aspect of the dens is a larger oval facet that articulates with the posterior aspect of the anterior arch of the atlas by way of a synovial joint. The superior aspect of the dens is pointed for attachment of the apical ligament, and roughened surfaces on the lateral aspect are for attachment of the alar ligaments.

The anterior and posterior longitudinal ligaments extend over the entire length of the spine and are major stabilizers of the intervertebral joints. The stronger anterior longitudinal ligament is a ribbon-like structure that attaches to the anterior aspect of the axis and extends upward, merging into the anterior arch of the atlas and the anterior atlanto-occipital membrane. Its superficial fibers extend over many vertebrae, whereas its deep fibers are shorter and connect adjacent vertebrae. The posterior longitudinal ligament is widest in the upper cervical spine and narrows caudally. The superficial portion is easily separated from the deep portion at the level of the vertebral body. The deep portion forms a narrow ligament at the middle of the vertebral body and broadens over the disc to become strongly attached to the annulus fibrosus.

Idiopathic ossification of this ligament is now recognized as an important cause of chronic compression of the spinal cord, particularly in men of Asian countries. It occurs in 3 to 5% of Japanese men over the age of 40, and the incidence shows a linear progression with advancing age. The estimated prevalence among U.S. Caucasians is much less, at 0.12%. Idiopathic ossification is frequently associated with ossification of other spinal ligaments and has a predilection for the cervical spine. Its presence makes the traumatized cervical spine particularly prone to cord injury.

The ligamentum flavum attaches to the anterior surface of the inferior half of the upper vertebral lamina and to the superior margin of the lower vertebral lamina. Each ligamentum flavum is separated from its counterpart at the same level by a small fissure. Laterally, they merge with the capsule of the facet joint. The ligamentum flavum is important as a stabilizer of the neck in flexion and has a high elastic fiber content, giving it a characteristic yellow color. In a hyperextension injury, it can buckle into the spinal canal and traumatize the spinal cord.

The interspinal ligaments in the cervical spine that connect adjacent spinous processes are thin, membranous, and poorly developed. The supraspinal ligaments that extend between the tips of the spinous processes are expanded into a midline fibrous sheet that reaches from the external occipital protuberance and median nuchal line to the spinous process of C7. This fibrous sheet is known as the ligamentum nuchae.

The transverse ligament of the axis is a strong transversely oriented ligament that is attached on either side to tubercles on the medial aspect of the lateral masses of the axis. It widens as it passes posterior to the dens, where two relatively narrow vertically running fasciculi are attached to it. The superior longitudinal fasciculus extends from the upper border of the ligament's midportion to the anterior margin of the foramen magnum. The inferior longitudinal fasciculus extends inferiorly to the posterior aspect of the axis body. This arrangement of the transverse ligament and longitudinal fasciculi is called the cruciform ligament.

A narrow apical ligament courses from the apex of the dens to the anterior margin of the foramen magnum. It has no functional significance, but it localizes the site of a type of avulsion dens fracture that may be associated with atlanto-occipital dislocation. The major part of the paired alar ligaments extends from the lateral aspect of the dens to the medial aspect of the occipital condyles. They lie anterior to the cruciform ligament, and the direction of the ligament's fibers depends on the height of the dens relative to the occipital condyles.

The tectorial membrane lines the inner aspect of the anterior wall of the upper aspect of the spinal canal. It is the cranial extension of the posterior longitudinal ligament of the spine. It is fixed to the posterior surface of the body of the axis and extends upward to gain attachment to the anterior and lateral margins of the foramen magnum, where it merges with the spinal dura. The tectorial membrane helps stabilize the atlanto-occipital and atlantoaxial joints.

The spinal cord occupies the middle third of the sagittal plane at the level of the atlas. The anterior third is occupied by the dens, and the posterior third has meninges, epidural fat, veins, and cerebrospinal fluid. This posterior third acts as a safe zone, because narrowing of the spinal canal by up to one-third at this level does not compromise cord function. This relationship was first described by Steele and is known as Steele's rule of thirds. Throughout the cervical spine region, much potential space exists for the spinal cord, which decreases the potential for spinal cord injury. The subaxial cervical spine, however, has less mobility and a smaller cord:canal diameter ratio than does the spine at C1–2, thus contributing to the greater frequency of neurologic injuries in the lower cervical spine. Indeed, the cervical cord enlarges at C3 and reaches its maximal circumference at C6 before tapering down to T3. This enlargement accommodates the nerve supply to the upper limbs.

Surrounding the spinal cord is the cerebrospinal fluid, which cushions the cord during accelerations and decelerations of the neck. Within the meninges, the cord is stabilized by the denticulate ligaments. These ligaments arise as part of the pia, from either side of the whole cord in 19 to 23 pairs that attach to the dura in the intervals between the emerging spinal nerve rootlets. In the upper cervical spine, the cord segments are located at approximately the same level as their corresponding vertebrae. The nerve roots, therefore, exit by passing transversely to the intervertebral foramina. In the lower cervical spine, however, the spinal cord segments are one level higher than the corresponding vertebrae. Consequently, the nerve roots descend obliquely to reach their intervertebral foramina.

Clinically important structures that require protection from avoidable trauma during cervical spine surgery include the vertebral artery, the carotid artery, the recurrent laryngeal nerve, the sympathetic chain, the thoracic duct, and the esophagus. The vertebral artery is the major source for the arteries supplying the cervical cord and cervical spine. The arteries usually enter the transverse foramina of C6 (90%) but may also (rarely) enter at C5, C4, C7, or even C3. The arteries, surrounded by a venous network, ascend in the transverse foramina to the atlas. There, they wind posteriorly around the lateral masses of the atlas and pass over the posterior arch of C1, just behind its lateral mass. This atlas portion of the artery allows for elongation during rotation of the atlas and head. Both arteries then pass through the posterior atlanto-occipital membrane and through the foramen magnum, where they unite to become the basilar artery.

The vertebral artery may be injured during anterior cervical decompressive surgical procedures, with an incidence of less than 1%. If ligated, vertebrobasilar ischemic signs and symptoms may develop postoperatively. This is not a universal occurrence, however, and in many clinical situations occlusion of one vertebral artery may be well tolerated, because of the anatomy of the artery. The left artery is hypoplastic in 5.7% and absent entirely in 1.8% of cases. On the right side, the artery is hypoplastic in 8.8% and absent in 3.1% of cases. Despite the low incidence of neurologic sequelae, the recommended approach is to attempt repair of the artery.

To avoid injury to the carotid artery, internal jugular vein, or vagus nerve, the surgeon must be careful not to enter the carotid sheath laterally. The surgical dissection should not enter the plane between the trachea and esophagus, because the recurrent laryngeal nerve is at risk. Vocal cord paresis may occur as a result of injury to this nerve. Hoarseness occurs in 5% of anterior cervical fusions and is usually temporary. The nerve is less prone to injury on the left side of the neck because of its longer course and more protected position in the tracheoesophageal groove. The use of a sharp self-retaining retractor should be avoided to prevent perforation of the esophagus. This is a rare but serious complication of anterior cervical fusion that occurs in 1 in 500 cases. The use of a nasogastric tube may help identify the esophagus during surgery.

Injury to the cervical sympathetic chain may result from dissection lateral to the longus colli muscles. Such an injury may result in Horner syndrome, which is usually not permanent. The superior thyroid artery is encountered above C4, and the inferior thyroid artery is below C6. The surgeon should be aware of the thoracic duct below C7 when approaching the spine from the left side. This important structure enters the neck on the left side between the spinal column and the esophagus. It passes from medial to lateral behind the carotid artery to enter the left subclavian vein. If it is divided, it should be ligated proximally and distally to prevent a chylothorax.

INITIAL FINDINGS, PHYSICAL EXAMINATION, AND DIAGNOSIS

The first step in management consists of early recognition or suspicion of the condition. Initial treatment should be in line with advanced trauma life support (ATLS) guidelines and begins in the field with emergency personnel using proper patient extrication and spinal immobilization procedures. Field treatment includes establishing an airway, ensuring adequate ventilation, and maintaining circulation. Cardiorespiratory resuscitation takes precedence over consideration of the possible presence of a spinal injury.

To minimize the potential for further injury, however, all patients with a suspected spine injury should be supported on a hard backboard; the cervical spine should be secured in an appropriate rigid cervical orthosis, sandbags should be placed on both sides of the neck, and the head should be taped to the backboard. Particular care should be taken with children; because of their relatively large head in relation to torso size, children's cervical spines are actually flexed when they lie flat on a hard board. Thus support must be placed posteriorly between the scapulae to maintain the cervical spine in the neutral position. There is never an urgency to remove the immobilization apparatus until the spine has been fully assessed.

To obtain an adequate airway, intubation may be performed before a thorough assessment is made of the cervical spine. This scenario may require awake nasal intubation or oral tracheal intubation while maintaining the neutral position of the neck. If the expertise is available, fiberoptic nasal tracheal intubation is generally satisfactory; emergency cricothyroidotomy or tracheostomy is rarely necessary.

The quadriparetic patient may present with a low blood pressure. The clinician must determine the cause before proper treatment can be initiated. Neurogenic, hypovolemic, and cardiogenic shock must be distinguished. Neurogenic shock is characterized by hypotension with a normal pulse or bradycardia, warm extremities, adequate urine output, and a clear neurologic sensorium. The condition results from a loss of sympathetic tone as a result of the neurologic injury. Treatment includes avoiding overhydration; placing the patient in the Trendelenburg position; and in more severe cases, using a pneumatic compression suit, atropine, and/or phenylephrine.

Hemorrhagic shock is characterized by hypotension tachycardia, cold extremities, and diminished urine output, which result from massive extravascular blood loss. Treatment includes control of hemorrhage and rapid infusion of crystalloid and blood products. Cardiogenic shock is characterized by hypotension, tachycardia, low cardiac output, elevated central venous pressure and pulmonary wedge pressure, and pulmonary edema. It may arise from chest trauma, such as tension pneumothorax, pericardial tamponade, cardiac contusion, and with ischemic or valvular heart disease. Treatment is focused on correcting the underlying cause and increasing cardiac output with the use of inotropics or vasodilators.

Once the multiply-injured patient's general condition has been stabilized, the clinician should focus on identifying specific sites of injury. Remember that up to 50% of patients with cervical cord injuries also have significant skeletal or visceral injuries, which are often overlooked. The examination should include the spine, with an emphasis on determining the level and severity of injury. Evidence of trauma to the head suggests the possibility of an associated cervical spine injury. Occipital lacerations indicate a flexion injury mechanism, and frontal or facial injury raises the possibility of an extension injury. Superior injuries involving the vertex of the skull suggest a cervical spine axial loading injury. The spine should be palpated along its entire length for evidence of tenderness, stepoffs, widening of the spinous processes, or open injuries. This is performed by controlled log rolling, using experienced personnel.

A full neurologic examination is performed in the cooperative patient and should include a complete cranial nerve examination; a complete motor and sensory examination; testing of all reflexes, including the bulbocavernosus reflex; and a rectal examination to assess rectal tone. Neurologic examination of the unconscious, intoxicated, or combative patient should include testing for gross pain sensation and motor function by observing withdrawal to noxious stimuli. The patient should also be observed for spontaneous movement of each extremity to assess gross motor function. The Frankel spinal cord injury classification system is simple and widely used. The five grades are listed in Table 28.1.

Incomplete lesions may present as clinical syndromes, such as Brown-Sequard, anterior cord, or central cord syndrome. The presence or absence of distal motor function cannot be precisely determined until the reversal of spinal shock, which is heralded by the return of the bulbocavernosus reflex (contraction of the anal sphincter in response to pinching of the penile shaft), usually between 24 and 48 h after injury. To limit the secondary insult that occurs to the cord, high-dose intravenous steroids are used as a potent inhibitor of free oxygen radicals. A prospective randomized trial showed that this pharmacologic approach might improve motor and sensory function in both complete and incomplete cervical and thoracic spinal cord injury (1). The drug must be given within 8 h of the injury. The loading dose is 30 mg/kg over 1 h followed by 5.4 mg/kg/h for 23 h.

table	28.1	The Frankel Classification System

Frankel Grade	Lesion
A	Complete neurologic injury
B	Sensory preservation only below the level of injury
C	Sensory preservation with useless motor function below the level of injury
D	Sensory preservation with useful motor function below the level of injury
E	Normal function

Patients with a neurologic deficit should be placed in skull traction consisting of either Gardner-Wells tongs or a halo ring to assist in decompression of the cord by realigning fractures and dislocations. Most modern halo rings are made of carbon and have the advantage of being MRI compatible. Halo traction can also be subsequently incorporated into a halo vest and used for the definitive treatment of a significant number of cervical spine injuries.

Traction is applied only after obtaining adequate cervical spine radiographs to assess the type of injury involved. The weight is applied to the skull in a sequential fashion starting at 2 to 4.5 kg (5 to 10 lb) and adding weight in 2-kg (5-lb) increments. Application of a weight or increasing the weight should be preceded by neurologic examination and a lateral plain radiograph to avoid overdistraction of the cervical spine, which could result in neurologic injury. Such an occurrence can be quite catastrophic, for example, when an unrecognized atlantoaxial dissociation undergoes fatal cord distraction. Before changing the weight, enough time should pass to permit ligamentotaxis. Although the use of up to 63 kg (140 lb) has been described, the clinician should avoid using more than 23 kg (50 lb).

Particular care should be taken with cases of facet joint dislocations, because clinically significant anterior disc herniations may coexist. Management of this situation remains controversial and will be discussed later in this chapter. The clinician must be careful when treating patients with ankylosing spondylitis who present with a cervical spine fracture. The initial management should ensure realignment of the neck to the *position of spinal deformity preceding the fracture*, rather than the application of skeletal traction in the neutral position. This usually involves the immediate use of a halo vest or bivector traction.

If adequate closed reduction of the fracture or dislocation is achieved and the patient is neurologically stable, definitive management can generally be delayed until coexisting medical or surgical conditions have been addressed. Urgent decompression is warranted for neurologic deterioration secondary to mechanical cord compression in an otherwise stable patient.

Adjunctive treatment consisting of the following measures should be considered. An indwelling urinary catheter to monitor urine output and to avoid bladder overdistension should be used. Prophylaxis against gastroduodenal ulceration and hemorrhage with intravenous H_2-receptor blockers is recommended. Patients with spinal cord injury should receive prophylaxis against thromboembolic disease via pneumatic compression boots and subcutaneous low-dose heparin (5000 units every 12 h).

Halo Ring and Vest Application

The patient should be in the supine position. Determine the ring size by holding the ring over the head. Allow a clearance of 1 to 2 cm. If a vest is to be used, determine the size by measuring the chest circumference.

Place the sterile ring below the skull equator, and temporarily hold it in place with plastic positioning cups. Locate the pin sites; 4 pins are usually used in an adult. Classically, the anterior pins are positioned 1 cm above the orbital rim at the level of the outer third of the eyebrow. The posterior pins are place roughly diagonal to the anterior pins. Shave the hair at the posterior pin sites, and prepare all sites with a 1% povidone-iodine solution. Anesthetize the pin sites with 1% lidocaine hydrochloride. Advance sterile pins to level of the skin. Tell the patient to close his or her eyes, and then tighten the pins with the manufacturer's torque wrench at 2-in/lb increments in a diagonal fashion. The pins should be tightened to 8 in/lb in an adult. For infants younger than 3 years, a multiple-pin, low-torque technique is used. Generally, 6 to 8 pins are placed with an application torque of 2 to 5 in/lb; 10 to 12 pins may be used.

Apply the lock nuts to the pins. If immediately applying the vest, raise the patient's trunk to 30° while maintaining traction. Apply the posterior portion of the vest before the anterior portion; connect the two portions. Fix the ring to the vest using the upright posts supplied by the manufacturer. Tape the vest-removing tools to the vest, in case of emergency. Custom-made halo vest components may be required for children.

Obtain cervical spine radiographs while the patient is in the halo ring. At 48 h after the halo was applied, retighten the pins once to 8 in/lb.

RADIOLOGIC STUDIES

Significant cervical spine injuries may be missed because of lack of suspicion or a reliance on inadequate imaging studies. For multiply-injured patients a lateral cervical spine radiograph is obtained as part of the initial assessment along with chest, abdomen, and pelvis radiographs. Later, a full cervical spine series is performed to detect any injuries. Five views of the cervical spine should be obtained. The lateral radiograph alone allows the diagnosis of only 70 to 85% of injuries. The addition of AP and open-mouth radiographs (a three-view series) or obliques (a five-view series) increases the sensitivity to 80 to 95%.

When a CT scan is also obtained, the sensitivity is close to 100%. It is important to look for other fractures at adjacent levels, which occur in up to 50% of upper cervical injuries. Noncontiguous cervical spine injuries occur in 16% of cases, and noncontiguous thoracic and/or lumbar injuries occur in about 9% of cases. An assessment of the complete spine is, therefore, of paramount importance.

Plain Radiographs

The lateral radiograph should clearly outline the bony anatomy of the cervical spine from the occiput to T1 (Fig. 28.1). It may be difficult to visualize the lower cervical spine in the unconscious, uncooperative, or muscular patient (Fig. 28.2). If this is the case, the radiograph should be repeated while downward traction is applied to the arms or a swimmer's view should be taken. If visualization remains inadequate, a CT scan of the cervicothoracic region should be obtained.

The following points should be noted on the lateral radiograph.

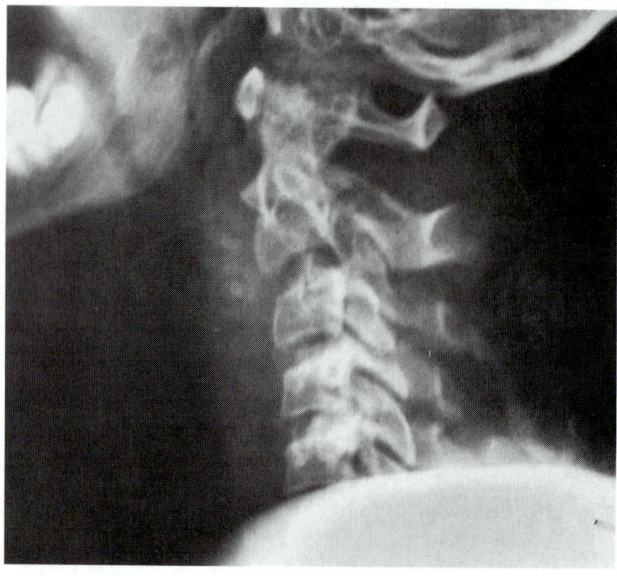

Figure 28.2. Lateral view in which the entire cervical spine is not visualized. Although C2 fractures are seen, associated injuries to the lower cervical spine may be overlooked.

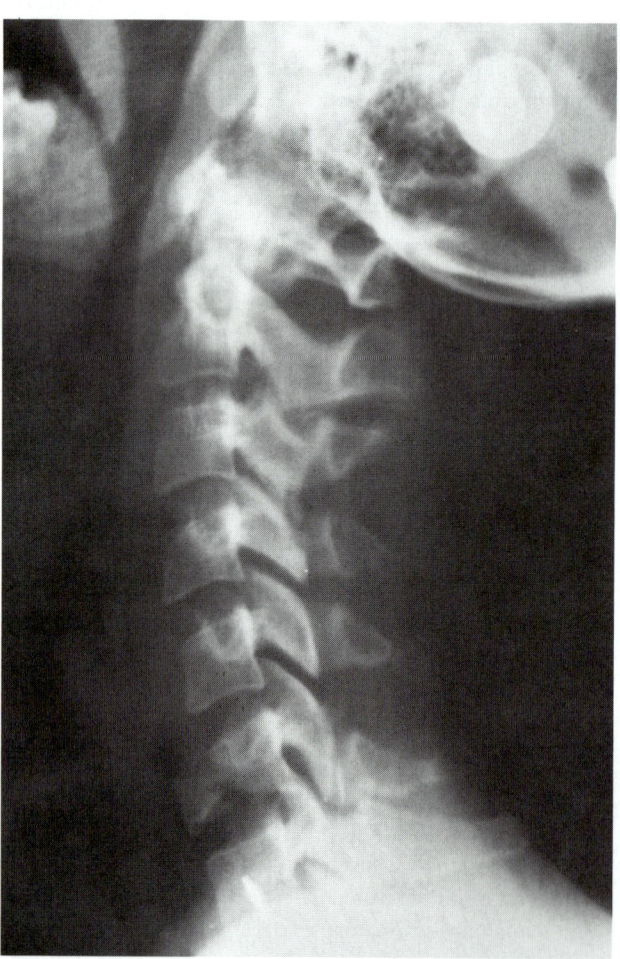

Figure 28.1. The lateral view should clearly outline the bony anatomy of the cervical spine from the occiput to T1.

1. The four smooth lordotic lines, consisting of the anterior spinal line, posterior spinal line, spinolaminar line, and a line along the tips of the spinous processes, should be seen.
2. The basilar line of Wackenheim, drawn along the posterior aspect of the clivus, should be tangent to the posterior cortex of the tip of the odontoid process.
3. Any loss of height, rotational malalignment, or alteration of the normal oblique parallelism of the facets should be recorded for each vertebra.
4. The posterior structures should be examined for spinous process fracture or a relative increase in the space between the spinous processes (suggests posterior ligament disruption from a flexion-type injury).
5. The width of the prevertebral soft tissues should be measured and should not exceed 10 mm at C1, 5 mm at C2, 7 mm at C3–4, and 20 mm at C5–7 (disregard dimensions if endotracheal or nasogastric tube was used, the child was crying, or a penetrating neck injury occurred).
6. The atlantodens interval (ADI) should be assessed; the upper limit of normal is 3 mm in an adult and 5 mm in a child.

Evaluation of the anteroposterior radiograph (Fig. 28.3) should include an examination of the spinous process to rule out asymmetry, which indicates a rotational subluxation (e.g., with a unilateral facet joint dislocation). The interspinous distance should be measured. A vertical widening that is 1.5 times greater than that at adjacent levels indicates a flexion injury. Inspect the lateral masses and facet joints, which should be symmetrical and give the appearance of a single column. Alteration of this appearance suggests a fracture or facet joint disruption.

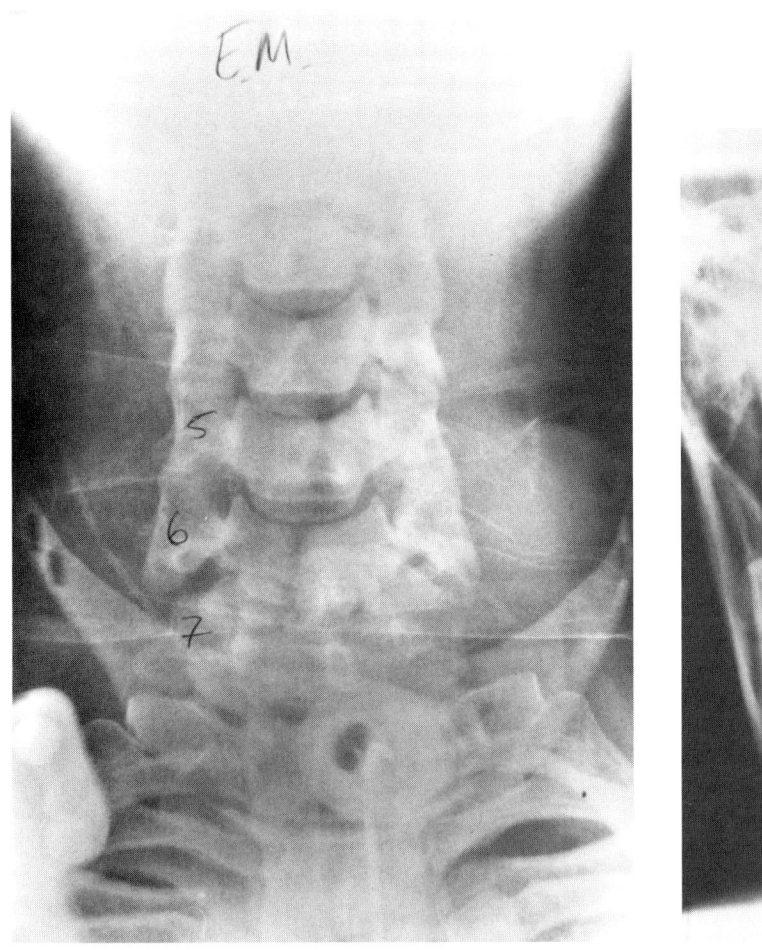

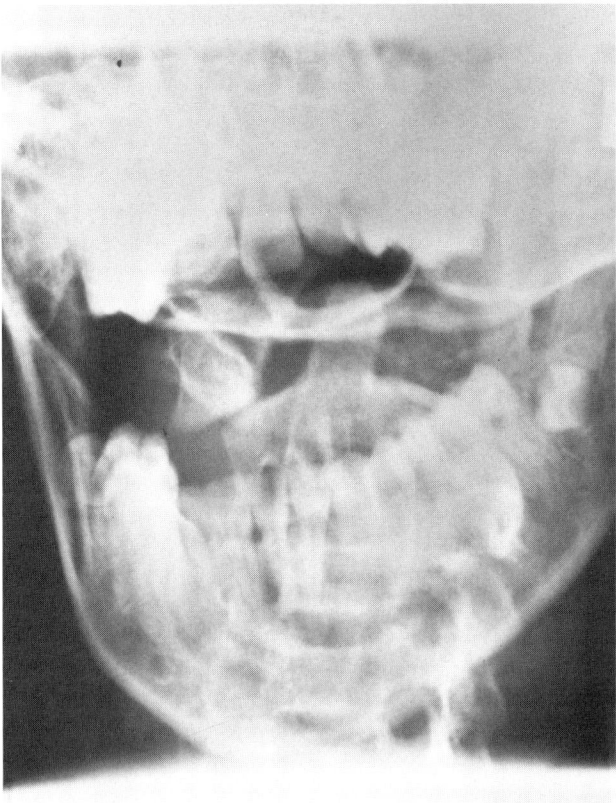

Figure 28.3. AP view showing a C6 fracture.

Figure 28.4. Open-mouth view.

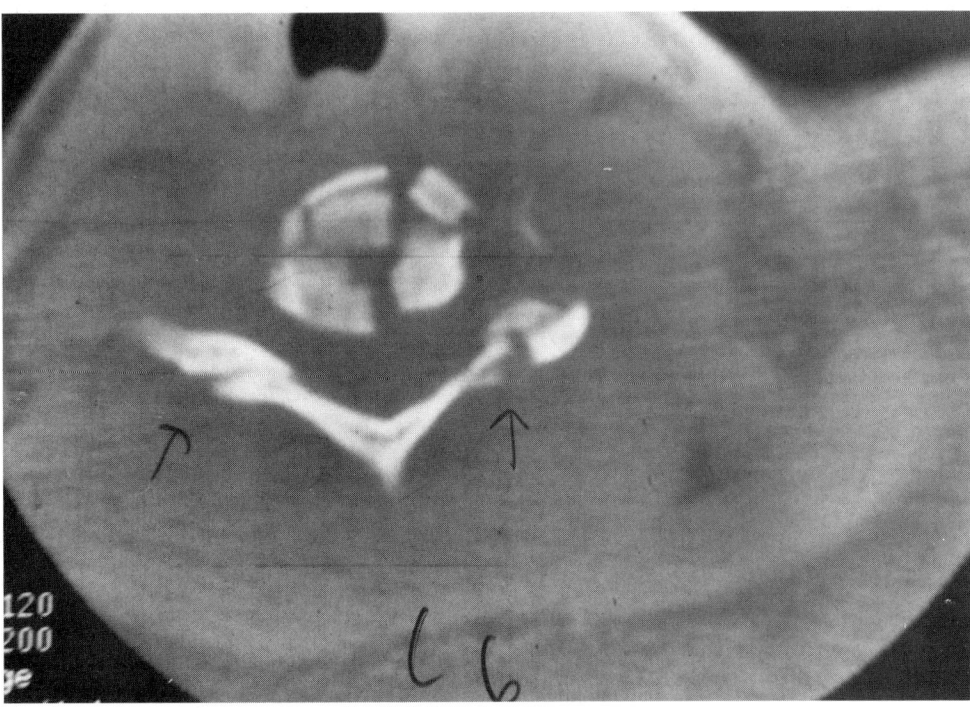

Figure 28.5. Axial view CT study showing a vertebral body fracture.

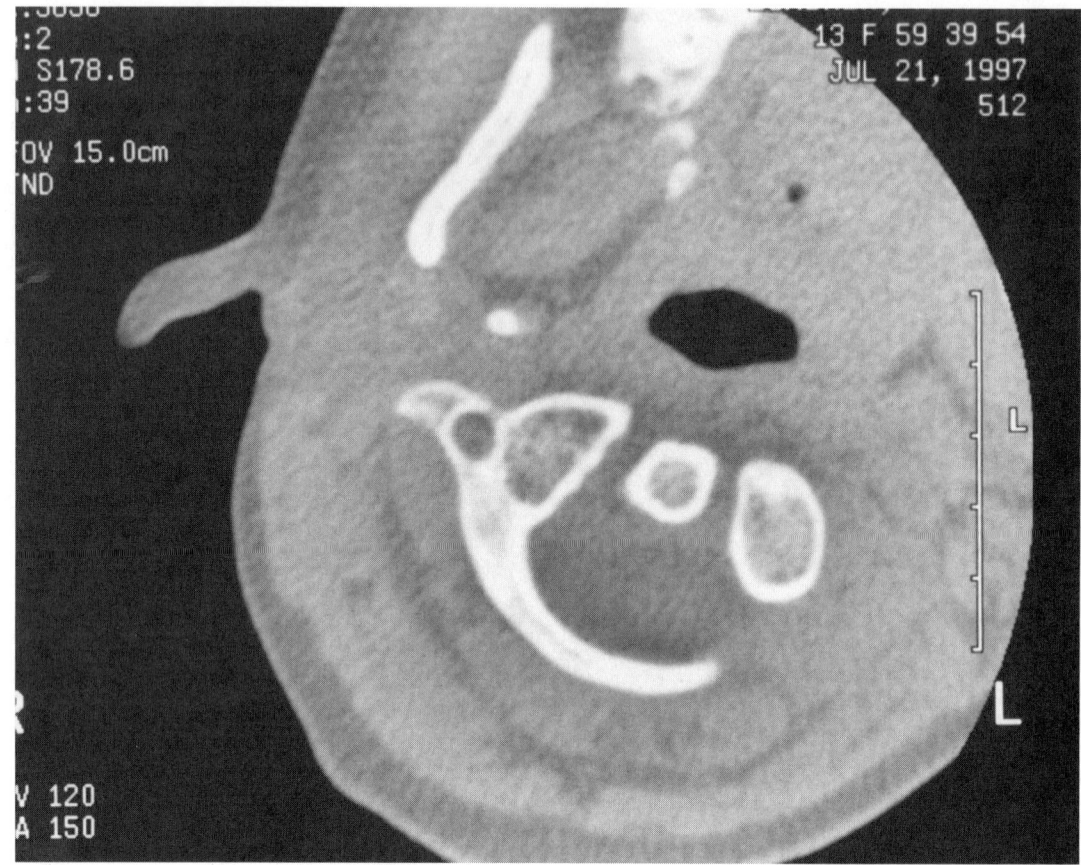

Figure 28.6. Axial view CT study showing a rotatory subluxation.

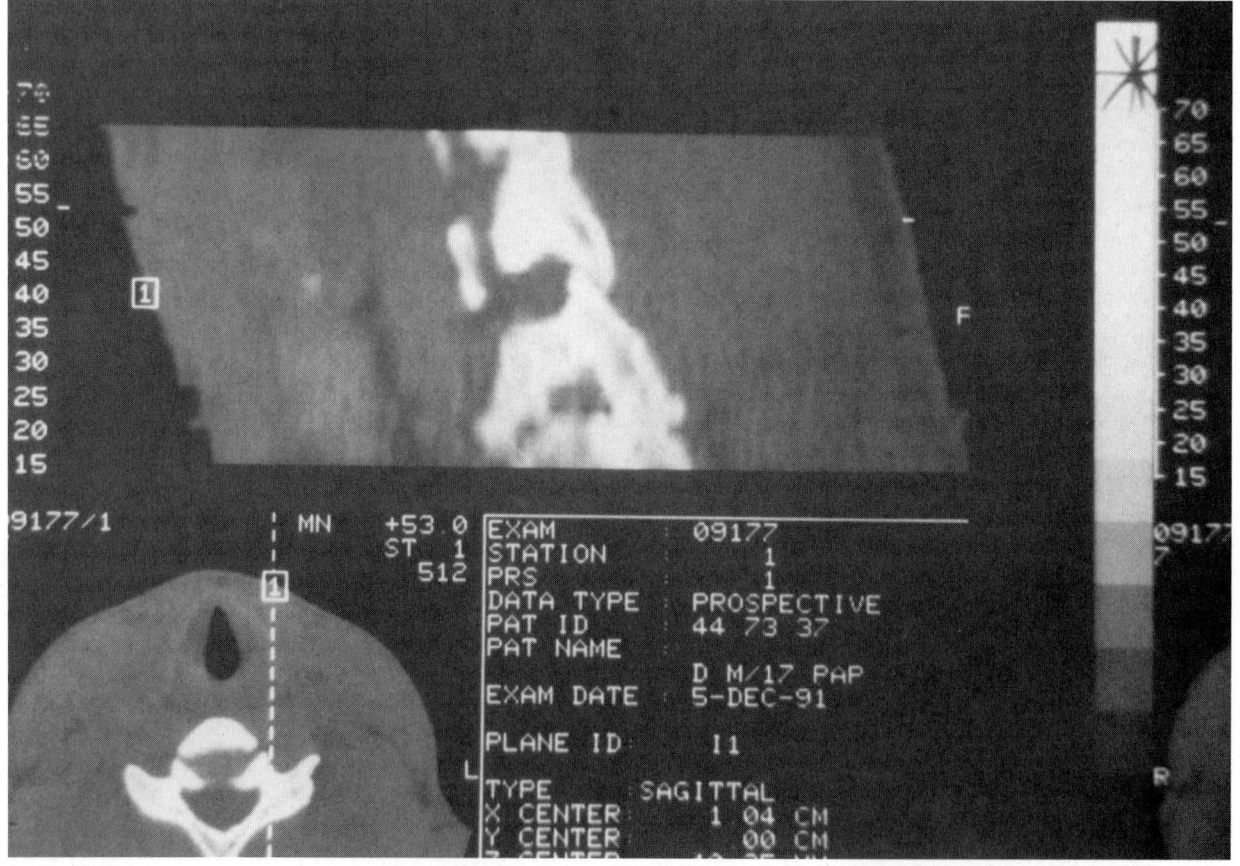

Figure 28.7. Sagittal view CT study showing a subluxation of the facets.

The open-mouth view is essential for the full evaluation of the upper cervical spine (Fig. 28.4). The space between the dens and the medial edge of the lateral masses on either side should be equal; no overhang of the lateral edge of the C1 articular masses on the lateral edge of C2 should be detected. Suspect a fracture of C1 (Jefferson fracture) if the sum of the lateral mass displacement from the dens for both sides is 7 mm or greater.

The odontoid process should be inspected for evidence of fracture. The atlanto-occipital joints may also be inspected. Oblique radiographs are particularly useful for assessing the facet joints. The typical symmetrical overlapping of the lamina should be appreciated. Any alteration of this appearance may suggest a lamina fracture or facet joint disruption. The neural foramina should be assessed for evidence of narrowing from a fracture or facet joint subluxation.

CT Studies

CT studies are useful in the evaluation of suspicious lesions seen on plain radiographs (Figs. 28.5–28.7). A CT scan should also be used to assess the cervicothoracic junction if it cannot be seen on the plain radiographs. The level above and below the area of interest should be included in the scan. The 3-mm cuts should overlap by 1 mm so definition in the reformatting is not lost, which can hide an underlying bony injury. Fractures in the same plane as the tomogram, which includes most odontoid fractures, may be missed by the CT studies. Conventional tomography can help detail the anatomy of injuries in planes other than the sagittal or coronal and thus is particularly useful with facet joint injuries and odontoid fractures.

MRI Studies

MRI is the best imaging modality for assessing of cervical soft tissue, including the intervertebral disc, the anterior and posterior longitudinal ligament, and the spinal cord. It is particularly useful in demonstrating injury to the posterior ligamentous complex, which is seen as increased signal intensity on a T_2-weighted image as a result of the associated edema (Fig. 28.8). It is the best method for assessing the presence of a disc prolapse in association with a subluxation or dislocation of the facet. MRI is indicated when a neurologic deficit is present, because it outlines the degree and cause of spinal cord compression and the extent of cord injury (Fig. 28.9). It is less efficacious than CT at detailing the anatomy of bony injury.

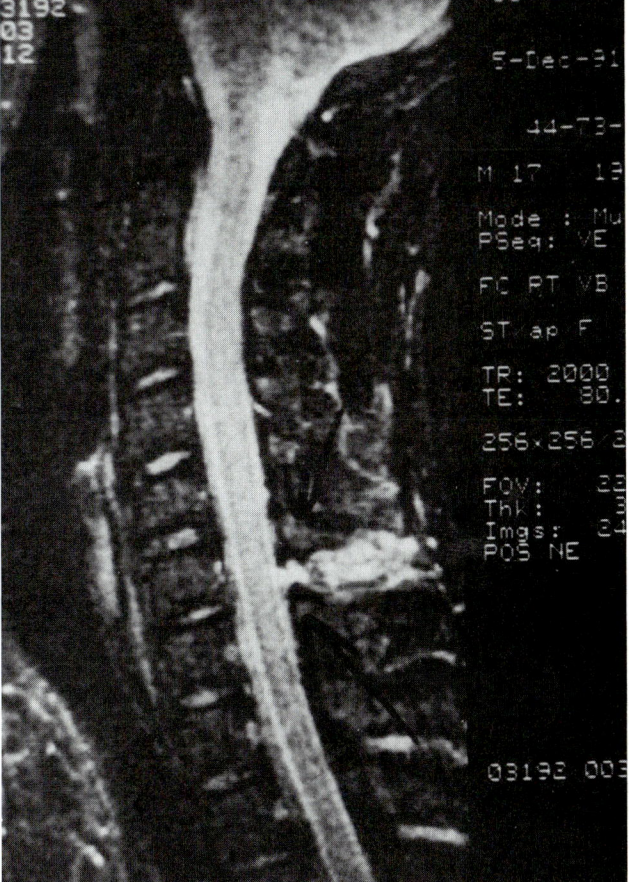

Figure 28.8. MRI study showing signal changes within the supraspinous and infraspinous ligaments.

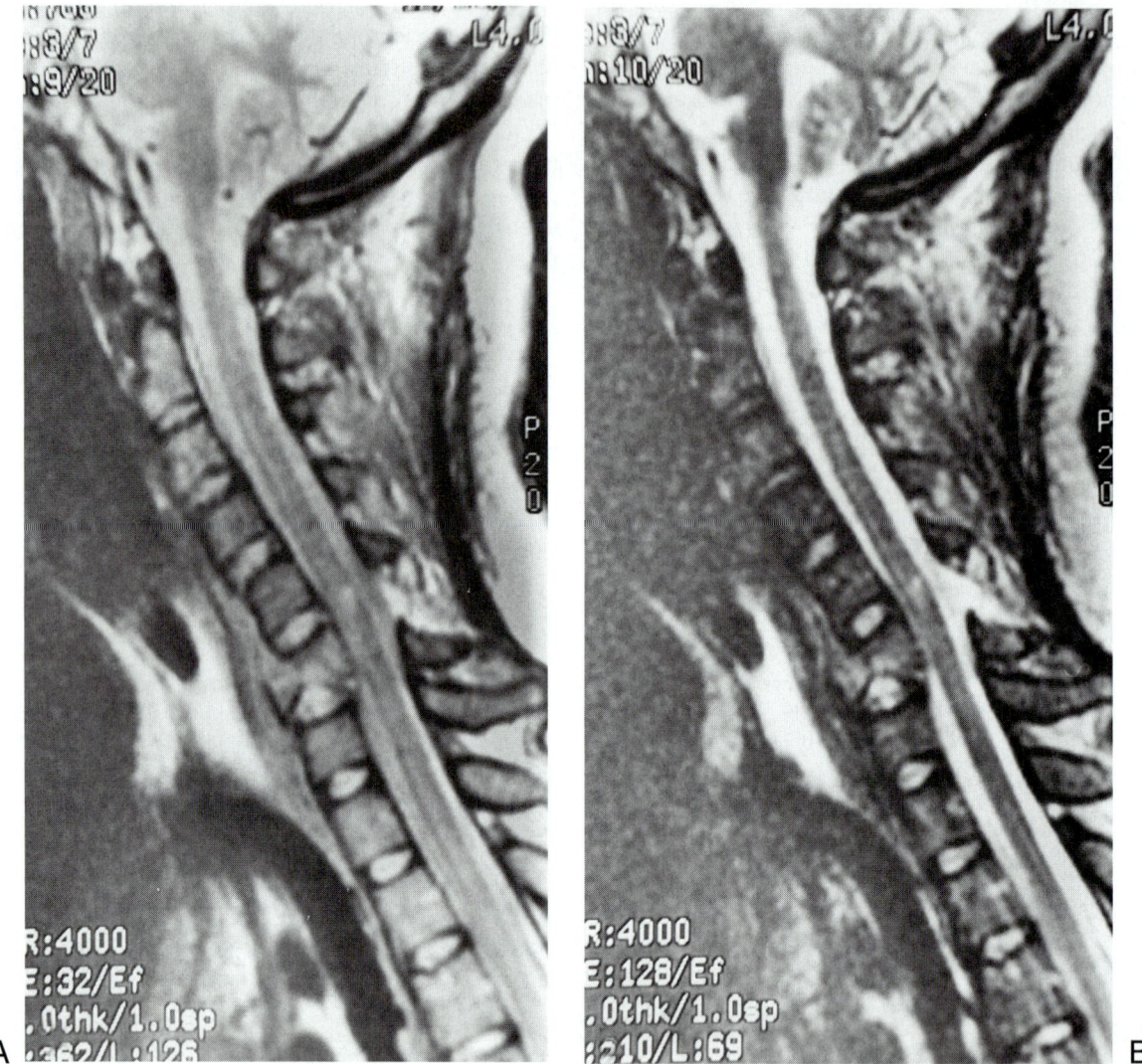

Figure 28.9. T_1- (**A**) and T_2-weighted (**B**) images showing cord compression and signal changes at the level of C6.

TREATMENT

General Principles

The choice between operative and nonoperative treatment of cervical spine injuries depends on the specific injury sustained, the presence of other injuries, and the neurologic state (Frankel grade) of the patient at presentation. In general, operative intervention is required for neural decompression, instability, and residual malalignment. It may also be used in the multiply-injured patient for pulmonary toilet and early rehabilitation (Clinical Table).

Severe ligamentous injury is unlikely to heal without a bone grafting procedure. Use of autogenous graft is preferred to allograft because of the higher rate of fusion. The number of motion segments fused should be limited to preserve function and minimize the rate of pseudarthrosis. The upper cervical spine supplies the largest degree of motion of the cervical spine; thus arthrodesis should be

particularly avoided at this level, if possible, to preserve long-term function. Halo vest treatment may be preferable if there is no definite indication for operative intervention. Acrylic bone cement may assist in providing immediate stability but does not provide long-term stability at adjacent motion segments. Its use should be avoided.

Intraoperative electrophysiologic monitoring is recommended. A meticulous approach to the decortication of bony structures to be incorporated in the fusion is essential to provide the greatest chance of fusion. Internal fixation increases the chance of bony fusion while allowing early mobilization. Modern titanium and polypropylene implants, because of their MRI compatibility, allow postoperative visualization of the neural structures. Cable systems are currently preferred to monofilament wire but are considerably more expensive.

Fixation options for the various levels in the cervical spine include the following. For the occiput, wires, cables,

Clinical Table: Cervical Spine Trauma: Upper and Lower Cervical Spine Injury

Procedure	Indications	Technique	Anatomy	Pitfalls
Halo vest	• Primary treatment of cervical fracture • Supplement to fusion techniques	• Secure halo to skull • Use four pins in an adult, more in an infant • Attach halo to vest	• Place ring below skull equator • Supraorbital nerve • Temporal artery	• Loose vest • Retighten pins at 48 h • Pin site infection
Occipitocervical fusion	• Atlanto-occipital instability	• Posterior approach • Contoured metal loop or plate	• Sagittal sinus • Dura • Cord • Nerve roots	• CSF leak from dural penetration at occiput
Upper cervical decompression	• Cord or medulla compression not relieved by traction	• Transoral resection of odontoid • Or posterior C1 laminectomy	• Use midline avascular plane posteriorly	• High rate of infection with transoral route • Technically demanding
C1-2 fusion	• C1-2 instability • Odontoid fracture nonunion	• Gallie fusion • Brooks fusion • Magerl fusion	• Magerl fusion used if posterior arch of C1 fractured or absent	• Vertebral artery injury
Anterior odontoid screw fixation	• Acute type II odontoid fracture	• Anterior approach • Use two screws	• Use image intensification	• Avoid with anteriorly displaced odontoid • Short neck • Established nonunion
Subaxial cervical fusion	• Subaxial instability	• Anterior interbody fusion • Posterior wiring • Posterior lateral mass plating	• Lateral mass plating preferred if spinous processes absent	• Vertebral artery injury • Operating on wrong level
Subaxial cervical decompression	• Neurologic compression	• Anterior or posterior approach • With multilevel trauma, usually posterior	• Esophagus • Carotid sheath • Laryngeal nerves	• Inadequate decompression • Operating on wrong level

or plates with unicortical or bicortical purchase are used. For the posterior approach to the C1 (the atlas), use sublaminar wire or cable or lateral mass screw purchase with a transarticular C1–2 screw fixation (Fig. 28.10). For the posterior approach to C2 (the axis), wires or cables can be passed through or under the large spinous process or in a sublaminar fashion. Screw fixation through the lateral mass or pedicle is also feasible as part of a plate construct. Anterior C2 vertebral body screw fixation is rarely performed as part of a plate system.

For the posterior approach to C3 through T1, the spinous process is the well-established and technically easiest fixation site using wire or cable constructs. Sublaminar fixation may be used, but the potential for cord damage by the wire exists. Fixation through the pedicle has been described, but this method has inherent risks and is technically demanding. Lateral mass screw fixation with a plate system is technically easy and reasonably safe. Anteriorly, vertebral body screw fixation with bicortical or, more commonly, unicortical purchase is used for attachment to a plate (Fig. 28.11).

Cervical Spine Instability

Clinical instability has been defined by White and Panjabi (2) as "the loss of the ability of the spine under physiologic loads to maintain its pattern of displacement so that there is no initial or additional neurological deficit, no major deformity and no incapacitating pain." Although qualitative, this definition is broadly accepted as a reasonable attempt to define a term that remains confusing to many clinicians and researchers in spine pathology. The ability to measure stability in the acute injury setting is compounded by the fact that the clinician is often relying on static imaging studies, which do not demonstrate the dynamic quality of the injury (Fig. 28.12). Most injuries are part of a spectrum from stable to grossly unstable; however, parameters based on the static and dynamic components of the injury depicted by imaging studies have been determined.

UPPER CERVICAL SPINE

At the atlanto-occipital junction, the upper limit of motion is 1 mm of sagittal plane translation of C0 in relation to

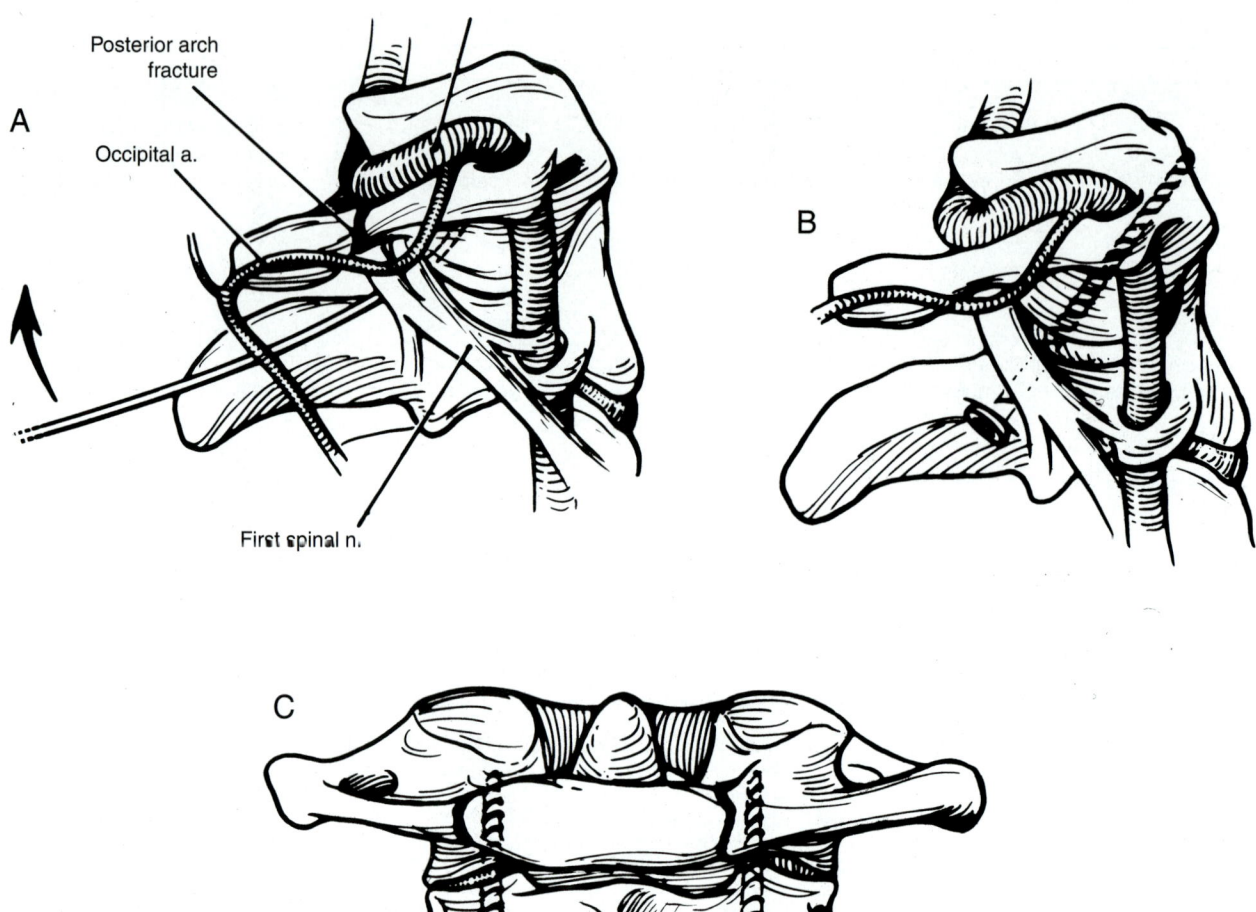

A

Posterior arch
fracture

Occipital a.

First spinal n.

B

C

Figure 28.10. Transarticular screw fixation at C1–2.

C1. At the C1–2 level, bilateral overhang of C1 on C2, as in a Jefferson-type fracture of C1, should not exceed 7 mm. At the C1–2 level, the atlantodental interval should not exceed 3 mm. Acceptable criteria for upper cervical instability are categorized as shown in Table 28.2.

table	28.2	Criteria for Upper Cervical Instability
C0–1		**C1–2**
>8° axial rotation to one side		>7 mm combined overhang of C1 on C2
>1 mm translation		>45° axial rotation to one side
		>4 mm sagittal translation
		<12 mm space available for the cord
		Avulsed transverse ligament

LOWER CERVICAL SPINE

White and Panjabi (2) outlined the biomechanical conditions for subaxial cervical spine instability: (*a*) either all of the anterior or all of the posterior elements are disrupted or unable to function, (*b*) more than 3.5 mm of horizontal displacement of one vertebra on another, and (*c*) more than 11° of rotational difference to that of either adjacent vertebra level. White and Panjabi also suggested criteria for the evaluation of the cervical spine that take into account a number of factors; each is given a numerical value (Table 28.3). According to this evaluation system, a value of five or more implies spinal instability.

Detailed consideration of treatment is best reviewed according to the specific fracture or dislocation sustained. Injuries of the cervical spine can generally be divided into those affecting the upper portion (atlas and axis) and those affecting the lower portion (C3–7). This is because

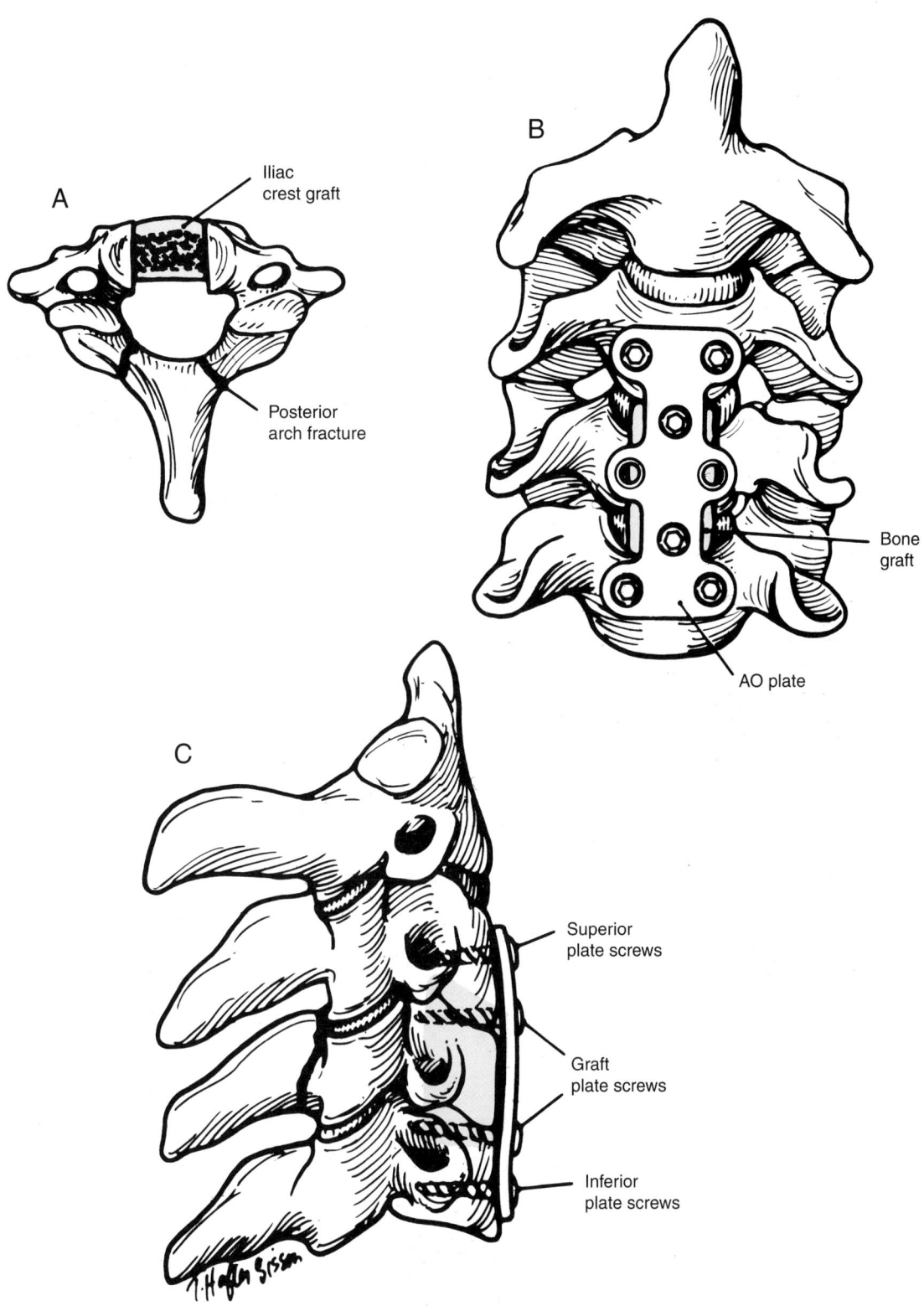

Figure 28.11. Anterior cervical plate fixation.

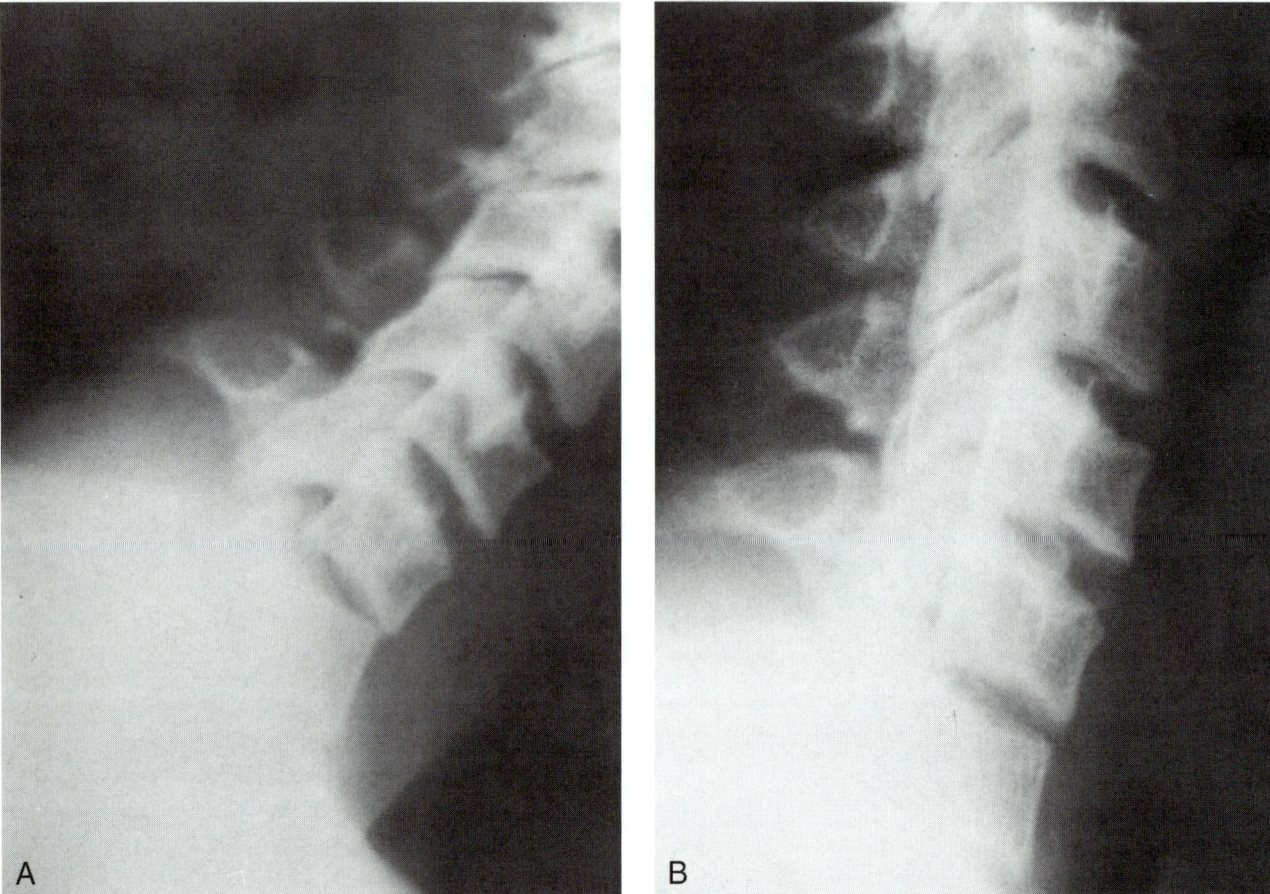

A   B

Figure 28.12. Lateral flexion (**A**) and extension (**B**) views of the cervical spine showing intersegmental instability at C6 and C7.

table	28.3	Diagnosis of Subaxial Clinical Instability

Element	Value[a]
Anterior elements destroyed or unable to function	2
Posterior elements destroyed or unable to function	2
Positive stretch test	2
Radiographic criteria (A *or* B)	
A. Flexion/extension x-rays	
1. Sagittal plane translation > 3.5 mm or 20%	2
2. Sagittal plane rotation > 20°	2
B. Resting x-rays	
1. Sagittal plane displacement > 3.5 mm or 20%	2
2. Relative sagittal plane angulation > 11°	2
Abnormal disc narrowing	1
Developmentally narrow spinal canal (A *or* B)	
A. Sagittal diameter < 13 mm	1
B. Pavlov's ratio < 0.8	1
Spinal cord damage	2
Nerve root damage	1
Dangerous loading anticipated	1

[a]A total of ≥5 implies spinal instability.

the C3–7 vertebrae are more uniform and are structurally and functionally different from both the C1 and C2 vertebrae.

Upper Cervical Spine Injuries

ATLANTO-OCCIPITAL DISLOCATION

Until recently, injuries at the atlanto-occipital level were rarely seen in the live trauma victim because of the accompanying severe neurologic deficit with respiratory arrest. As a result of improvements in emergency medical services, many of these patients are now surviving to arrive at the emergency room. Atlanto-occipital dislocation is caused by high-energy trauma, resulting in severe ligamentous disruption of the alar ligaments, tectorial membrane, and the atlanto-occipital joint capsules.

Cervical traction should be avoided in these patients, because even 2 kg (5 lb) may produce a significant overdistraction of tissues, including the cord. The presence of an avulsion fracture of the tip of the odontoid process suggests this injury. The initial management of atlanto-occipital dislocations is halo vest immobilization followed by posterior occiput to C1 and C2 fusion, as it is a purely ligamentous injury that is unlikely to adequately stabilize with nonoperative treatment. The fusion can be achieved with standard wiring and bone grafting techniques or it can be augmented with occipitocervical plates and screws. Two screws should be placed through the plate into the occiput on either side. Wires should be passed around the posterior arch of C1 and around the plates at this level. Transarticular (Magerl) screw fixation or pedicle screw fixation is performed for purchase through the plate to the C2 vertebra. Because of the severe instability of these injuries, postoperative immobilization in a halo vest should be maintained until union has occurred.

OCCIPITAL CONDYLE FRACTURE

Occipital condyle fracture is an uncommon injury that has been classified into three types by Anderson and Montesano (3). Type I is an impacted condyle fracture, usually occurring on only one side of the skull. This is a stable injury that can be treated in a rigid cervical collar. Type II occipital condyle fractures are associated with a fractured base of the skull. This is less stable and can usually be satisfactorily treated with 12 weeks of immobilization in a halo vest. In the type III injury, occipital condyle fractures are associated with atlanto-occipital instability. Plain film radiographs, CT scans, or tomograms reveal a small fragment of bone that represents an avulsion injury of the insertion of the alar ligament on the medial aspect of the occipital condyle. Overdistraction, as with any atlanto-occipital injury, should be avoided. An occiput to C2 fusion is the definitive treatment.

FRACTURES OF THE ATLAS

Four major types of atlas fracture are recognized: anterior arch fracture or avulsion, posterior arch fracture, lateral mass fracture, and Jefferson fracture. These injuries usually occur as a result of an axial compressive load that drives the occipital condyles into the lateral masses of the atlas. Depending on the extent and direction of the force applied, the C1 ring may break, resulting in a two-, three-, or four-part fracture. Fractures of the atlas are rarely associated with neurologic injury because of the decompressive nature of the applied force. If there are associated neurologic deficits, the clinician should conduct a thorough search for the contiguous or noncontiguous spinal injuries responsible for the deficit.

Atlas fractures are often best appreciated on the open-mouth view radiograph; the sum of the overhang of C1 on C2 bilaterally may exceed 7 mm, which usually indicates a disruption of the transverse ligament. The best imaging modality for classifying these injuries is the axial CT scan. The classic Jefferson fracture is a four-part fracture with bilateral fractures of the anterior and posterior regions of the C1 ring (Fig. 28.13). A rupture of the transverse ligament may be seen on the axial MRI views. Posterior arch fractures have a second fracture in 50% of cases; the most common is a posteriorly displaced odontoid fracture or trau-

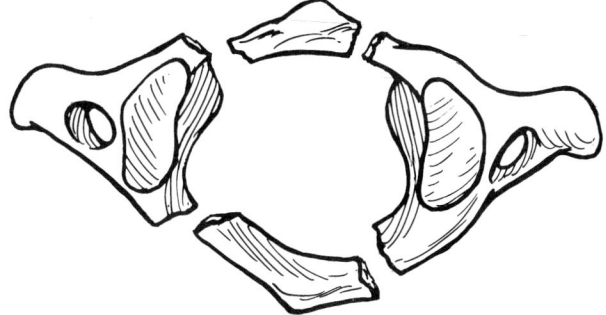

Figure 28.13. Jefferson fracture of the atlas.

matic spondylolisthesis of C2. Fractures of the anterior arch of C1 generally result from avulsion of the longus colli muscles.

Isolated anterior or posterior arch fractures are stable injuries; and after evaluation with flexion and extension x-rays to rule out C1–2 instability, they can be treated in a rigid cervical orthosis for comfort. Once the pain has subsided, the collar may be discarded. Unilateral fractures of the lateral mass of the atlas are, as the name implies, usually limited to one side of the neural arch. An additional fracture on the contralateral side of the posterior arch has been reported in the literature. The asymmetric displacement of the affected lateral mass is usually appreciated on the open-mouth view radiograph.

The Jefferson or burst fracture of the atlas is best managed by initial traction followed by immobilization in a halo vest for 3 months. A clinical evaluation of these fractures revealed that an associated transverse ligament disruption is not associated with the development of late instability as reported by Levine and Edwards (4). The need for reduction of lateral mass displacement remains uncertain. There is no evidence that patients have greater problems from C1–2 facet arthrosis, causing residual pain, when the lateral mass is left in an unreduced position than when it is not. Skeletal traction may be used to achieve reduction in patients with significant lateral mass displacement (more than 7 mm). Prolonged axial traction (a minimum of 6 weeks) is necessary to maintain the reduction, because a halo vest does not provide sufficient distraction for this. The patient then undergoes 6 weeks of halo vest immobilization. Many spinal injury units place the patient directly into a halo vest as soon as medically possible, regardless of the amount of displacement present. With either approach, flexion and extension x-rays should be taken at the end of the treatment period to detect persistent C1–2 instability.

ATLANTOAXIAL INSTABILITY WITHOUT FRACTURE

The atlantoaxial ligamentous complex may rupture, resulting in instability without fracture. This condition may occur following severe flexion loads to the spine or with less force in the presence of preexisting rheumatoid arthritis or other connective tissue diseases. This instability may lead to cervical cord injury, because the odontoid process is free to compress the cord against the posterior arch of the atlas. Cord damage is rare, however, because of the copious residual potential space available (Steele's rule of thirds). The ADI is increased to more than 3 mm in adults in such cases. This is best appreciated on flexion and extension radiographs, and the ligament disruption can be seen on MRI. In the presence of significant pain, this dynamic change may be missed because of the presence of muscle spasm. An ADI greater than 5 mm implies complete disruption of the ligamentous complex. The space between the posterior aspect of the odontoid and the anterior aspect of the posterior C1 arch should also be measured. This represents the space available for the cord (SAC). A space less than 16 mm is abnormal, less than 13 mm implies significant risk for spinal cord injury, and less than 10 mm is critical. Because atlantoaxial instability is purely a ligamentous injury, surgical stabilization is required to prevent chronic instability. This is achieved by a posterior C1–2 fusion, usually with a wire construct.

ATLANTOAXIAL ROTATORY SUBLUXATION

Atlantoaxial rotatory subluxation is a relatively uncommon, subtle injury that primarily affects children, but it may also occur in adults. It has been described as occurring spontaneously, particularly following upper respiratory infection, or it may occur with trauma. Combined distraction and axial rotation results in subluxation of the C1–2 articulation. It generally presents with painful torticollis and extreme apprehension on attempted neck movement. In chronic cases, the subluxation becomes fixed, causing persistent abnormal positioning of the head.

Atlantoaxial rotatory subluxation may be missed on initial radiographic examination. The open-mouth view demonstrates asymmetry of the distance between the lateral masses of the atlas and the odontoid process (Fig. 28.14). The distance between the medial edge of the articular mass and the outer edge of the dens is less on one side. This is known as a wink sign. Dynamic CT with the patient's head turned to the left and right may demonstrate subluxation of the facet with fixed rotation of the atlas (Fig. 28.6).

Acute injuries in children usually respond to a period of cervical traction followed by collar immobilization. Acute injuries in adults usually require skeletal traction for reduction, followed by halo vest immobilization for 3 months (Figs. 28.15 and 28.16). Failure of attempted closed reduction necessitates surgical reduction and posterior C1–2 fusion. Alternatively, direct anterior transoral reduction with anterior C1–2 plate fixation may be used. Closed reduction is rarely successful in injuries greater than 3 months' duration, and fusion is generally required for pain relief.

ODONTOID FRACTURES

Odontoid fractures are categorized by anatomic location as type I, II, or III injuries, according to the classifica-

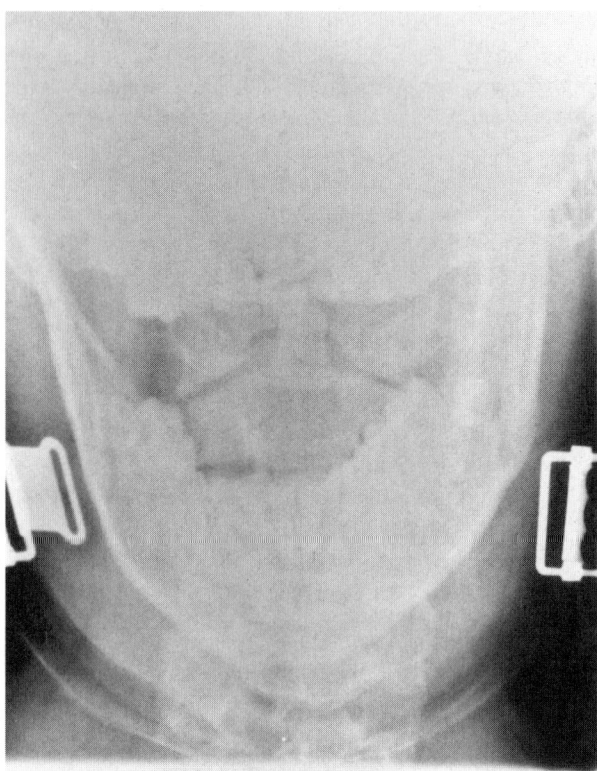

Figure 28.14. Open-mouth view showing rotatory displacement of C1 on C2.

tion system of Anderson and D'Alonzo (5) (Fig. 28.17). Type I fractures are characterized by an avulsion of the tip of the odontoid process at the site of attachment of the alar ligament. These are thought to be stable, insignificant injuries; however, they may be associated with an atlanto-occipital dislocation.

Type II odontoid fractures occur through the neck of the dens in the axial plane. They are the most common odontoid fractures and present management problems because of their instability and high nonunion rate when treated nonoperatively. The significant nonunion rate has been attributed to the poor blood supply of the dens, its small cross-sectional surface area at the fracture site, and the predominance of cortical over cancellous bone. Type II fractures rarely present with neurologic deficit, although they are associated with high-velocity trauma, e.g., motor vehicle accidents or considerable falls.

Halo vest treatment is associated with a nonunion rate of 35%. Factors predisposing to high nonunion rates include age greater than 40 years, displacement more than 4 mm at the fracture site, and posterior displacement of the odontoid in relation to its base. Alternatives for treatment are halo vest immobilization and surgical stabilization. Serious consideration should be given to performing early surgical stabilization in cases with a high risk of nonunion. Both treatment options, along with their risks and benefits, may be outlined to patients with type II fractures. Patients who wish to be treated nonoperatively can be

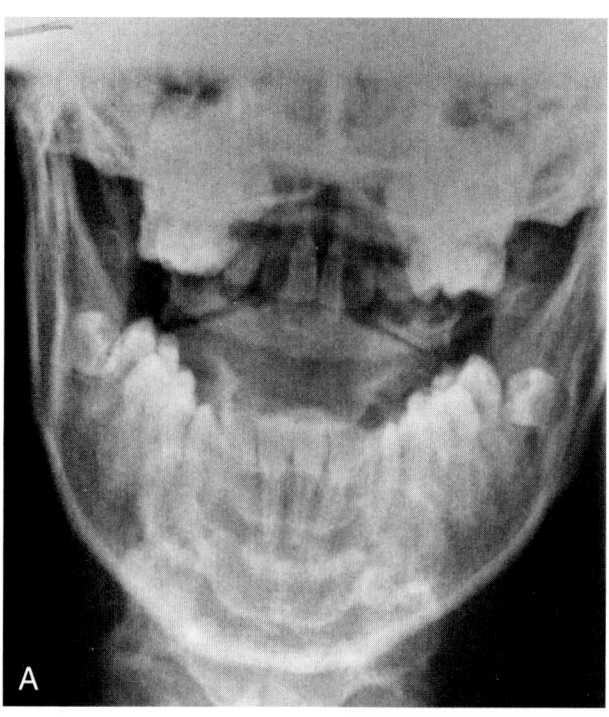

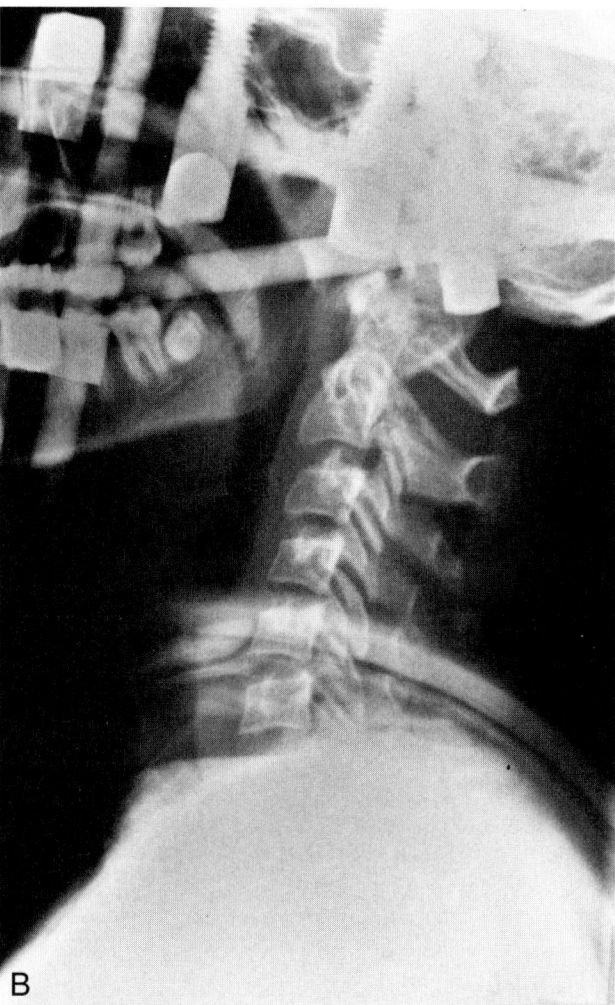

Figure 28.15. **A.** Posttraction open-mouth view showing reduction of the rotatory subluxation.
B. Lateral view showing reduction of C1–2 after halo vest immobilization.

placed in a halo vest for 3 months and then evaluated for fracture healing. If nonunion occurs, a posterior C1–2 fusion is then performed. In the acute stage, patients can be treated operatively, typically with a posterior C1–2 fusion and more recently with anterior odontoid screw fixation. The transoral reduction and anterior plate fixation procedure to preserve C1–2 axial rotation has been described, predominantly from European centers.

Type III odontoid fractures extend down into the base of the odontoid process. These fractures, because of greater cross-sectional fracture surface area, better blood supply, and the presence of abundant cancellous bone compared with type II odontoid fractures, commonly unite. They are usually managed by halo vest immobilization for 12 weeks. Alternatively, impacted nondisplaced fractures can be treated in a rigid cervical orthosis. The rare case of a displaced angulated type III fracture may require internal fixation.

Posterior C1–2 arthrodesis may be achieved by the Gallie, Brooks, or Magerl techniques. The Gallie fusion uses a single wire or cable looped around the posterior

arch of C1 and continued under the spinous process of C2. This wire incorporates an autogenous iliac crest H-shaped graft between C1 and C2. The Brooks fusion involves the use of two sublaminar cables or wires looped under the laminae of C1 and C2 and incorporates a corticocancellous bone graft. The Brooks fusion does not tend to pull the ring of C1 posteriorly toward the lamina of C2 as does the Gallie fusion. Consequently, a Brooks fusion is a more appropriate and stable technique for posteriorly displaced odontoid fractures. These techniques have a reported fusion rate of 90 to 96%.

The Magerl technique of transarticular C1–2 screw fixation has a nonunion rate of less than 1%. When possible, the transarticular fixation should be combined with a Brooks or Gallie wiring and bone grafting technique. It is a technically demanding procedure that has a particular role in the 15% of odontoid fractures that have an associated C1 posterior arch fracture that prevents the use of sublaminar fixation. Other alternatives in this situation include extension of the fusion to the occiput, which should be avoided because of its increased morbidity and higher nonunion

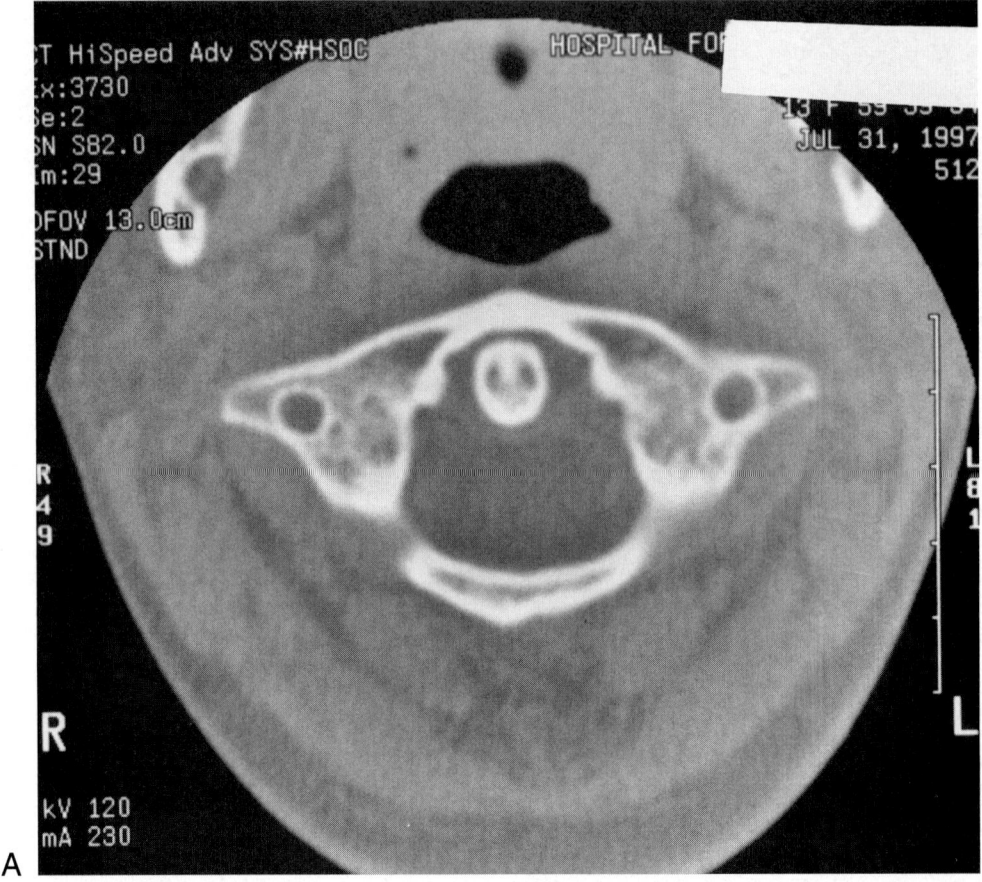

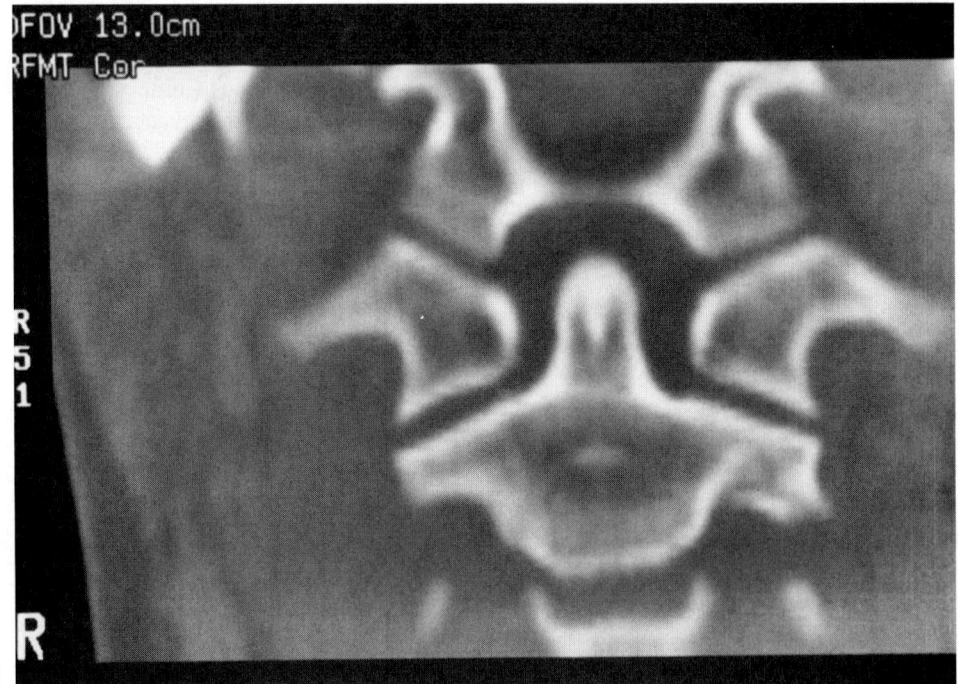

Figure 28.16. Axial view (**A**) and reformatted (**B**) CT studies showing reduction of rotatory subluxation in the patient shown in Figure 28.6.

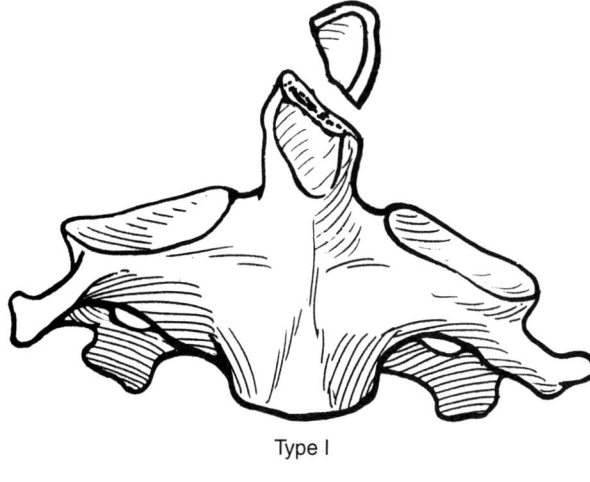

Type I

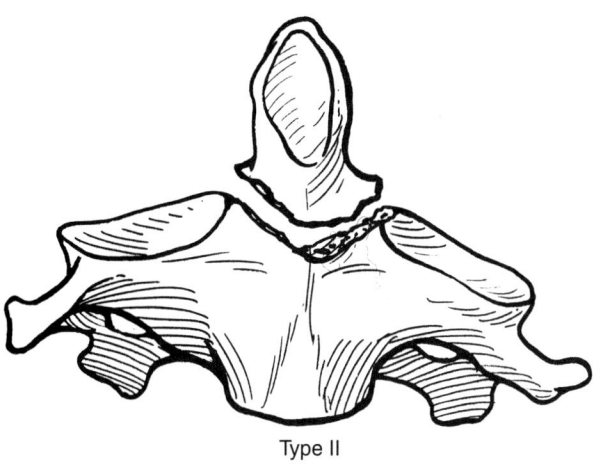

Type II

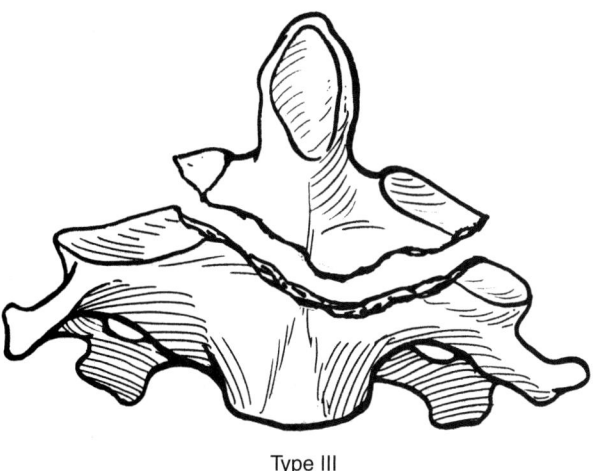

Type III

Figure 28.17. Anderson and D'Alonzo's classification of odontoid fractures.

rate. A more appropriate alternative may be to allow the C1 fracture to heal while immobilized and then to perform a delayed C1–2 arthrodesis.

Another surgical technique is anterior odontoid screw fixation, in which the screw enters at the anteroinferior base of the axis and proceeds up to the tip of the dens. If the cross-sectional area of the odontoid allows, two screws rather than one should be used for rotational stability. This technique should not be used in an anteriorly displaced odontoid fracture that cannot be reduced, in the presence of a significant osteopenia, or for an established nonunion. Only one-third of nonunion cases go on to solid union via this technique. The union rate in acute fractures is greater than 90%. The proposed advantage of anterior screw fixation compared to posterior C1–2 arthrodesis is the preservation of C1–2 motion. A reduced range of motion has been demonstrated in 8 of 13 patients evaluated by CT scan to assess rotation.

HANGMAN'S FRACTURE OF C2

The hangman's fracture of C2, also known as a traumatic spondylolisthesis of the axis, is a fracture through the pedicles of C2, with or without an associated injury of the C2–3 disc and anterior ligaments. Various classification systems have been proposed, and Levine and Edwards' (4) system is the most commonly used.

Type I fractures are through the neural arch at the base of the pedicle, displacement of C2 on C3 is less than 3 mm displacement, and there is no angulation (Fig. 28.2). These type I injuries are the result of hyperextension and axial loading on the cervical spine that is sufficient to fracture the neural arch without significantly injuring the disc or longitudinal ligaments. Flexion and extension view radiographs differentiate this injury from the type II fracture. Type I fractures are intrinsically stable and can be satisfactorily managed with immobilization in a rigid orthosis for 8 to 12 weeks.

There are two classes of type II hangman's fractures. These fractures are characterized by translation greater than 3 mm, angulation of the fracture, and compression of the anterior superior corner of the C3 vertebral body. The initial hyperextension and axial loading leading to fracture are followed by a secondary flexion force that disrupts the C2–3 disc, partially tears the posterior longitudinal ligament, and may strip the anterior longitudinal ligament off the body of C3. The anterior longitudinal ligament, however, remains intact.

Treatment consists of initial fracture reduction by halo traction with the neck in a slightly extended position. Patients with moderate initial displacement (3 to 6 mm) can then be placed in a halo vest for 8 to 12 weeks. Patients with more severe initial displacement (>6 mm) may require more prolonged traction of 4 to 6 weeks to allow early fracture healing in the reduced position, this followed by halo vest immobilization for a total treatment period of 12 weeks. Early mobilization in a halo vest for patients with severely displaced fractures leads to a significant loss of reduction and higher nonunion rates.

An alternative is anterior or posterior C2–3 arthrodesis, which may be indicated in multiply-injured patients for improved pulmonary care and early rehabilitation. The anterior procedure involves an anterior retropharyngeal approach, protection of the hypoglossal nerve, and application of a C2–3 plate. A transoral approach may also be used, but it carries the risk of contamination. The posterior approach consists of a C1–3 wiring technique, bypassing the fragment but including another level in the fusion; or the fracture can be crossed with pedicle screws, and lateral mass screws in C3 span the C2–3 injury with a plate. This limits the fusion to one level by a posterior approach.

Type IIA fractures are characterized by significant angulation with minimal translation and are considered a variant of the type II fracture. This injury is the result of severe flexion and distraction. The fracture line of type IIA fractures is more oblique and posterior than the type II line and lies directly anterior to the facet joints. It is an extremely unstable injury pattern, which may be significantly worsened by traction. Identification before instigating treatment is, therefore, critical. This injury is usually treated by immediate halo vest immobilization for 12 weeks. Satisfactory healing usually ensues, with the formation of an anterior bridge between the C2 and C3 vertebral bodies that spans the disc space.

Type III hangman's fractures are the result of flexion and compression and are characterized by severe angulation, translation, and additional unilateral or bilateral C2–3 facet dislocation, with or without a facet fracture. These cases usually require surgical reduction and fusion by a posterior approach. The surgical options for stabilization are the same as those described for a type II fracture.

Lower Cervical Spine Injuries

Although a comprehensive classification system of lower cervical spine injuries, based on the mechanism of injury, was outlined by Allen et al. (6), we will consider the types of injury according to widely used terminology. The mechanism of injury for each fracture type will be related to the injury.

WEDGE COMPRESSION FRACTURE

Wedge compression fractures occur as a result of a flexion and compression force and are characterized by a loss of anterior vertebral body height. The C4–5 and C5–6 levels are most commonly involved. The posterior aspect of the vertebral body usually remains intact, although the posterior longitudinal ligament may rupture in more severe cases. Imaging studies should include flexion and extension views; CT scan; and an MRI study, particularly for assessing possible cord or posterior longitudinal ligament injury.

The criteria of White and Panjabi (2) may be used as a guideline for instability in these cases. Wedge fractures with less than 25% of anterior height loss and preservation of the posterior vertebral wall are regarded as stable. Treatment in a rigid orthosis for 8 to 12 weeks is usually satisfactory. When there is more than 50% anterior height loss, significant damage to the posterior ligamentous complex has probably occurred. Such cases are treated by operative stabilization and fusion, which is best achieved by spinous process wiring. If the wedge compression fracture

is associated with a posterior element fracture, incorporation of a normal adjacent motion segment by spinous process wiring is required. Although oblique wiring techniques may be used in this setting, the better alternative is lateral mass plating, which restricts the fusion to the involved level only. Posttraumatic kyphotic deformity is a late complication that can be avoided by anterior column reconstruction in cases of severe wedging.

FACET JOINT INJURY

Injury to the facets includes subluxation, dislocation, fracture, and combination injuries. Such injuries can occur unilaterally or bilaterally and may be associated with neurologic deficit. These injuries most often affect the C5–6 and C6–7 levels and are often (40%) initially missed because of inadequate radiographs, presence of associated injuries, or initial lack of symptoms. In cases of frank dislocation, the inferior articular process of the cephalad vertebra comes to rest anterior to the superior articular process of the caudad vertebra. Common causes of facet joint injury are motor vehicle accidents, falls, assaults, and contact sports.

Unilateral facet dislocation is a flexion distraction injury with rotation. The injury is purely ligamentous; the supraspinous ligament, interspinous ligament, ligamentum flavum, and facet capsule are disrupted. On the side of the dislocated facet, the neural foramen is narrowed, giving rise to a high incidence of radiculopathy. Lateral radiographs demonstrate about 25% anterior vertebral displacement and the typical "bow tie" appearance of the laminae. Oblique radiographs demonstrate the dislocation; in cases of subluxation, a perched facet and narrowing of the foramen are seen. Deviation of the spinous process toward the side of dislocation is seen on the AP radiograph. A CT scan assists in defining the anatomy and detecting associated fractures. An empty or naked superior facet of the lower vertebra is seen.

Bilateral facet dislocation involves disruption of ligaments, facet capsules, and often the disc, as a result of the flexion distraction injury. The lateral radiograph will reveal approximately 50% vertebral body subluxation. As a result of spinal canal narrowing, there is a high incidence of spinal cord injury.

The traditional initial treatment for all facet joint dislocations has been early closed reduction by skull traction. Recently, several reports have alluded to possible neurologic deterioration following closed reduction, thought to be the result of an associated herniated disc seen on the postreduction studies (7). Some clinicians now argue for routine CT myelography or MRI studies before attempting reduction in all cases. The safety of closed reduction in an awake cooperative patient is, however, well documented by several large series. Therefore, another approach is to reserve MRI examination before attempted reduction for the unconscious or uncooperative patient. All patients should undergo careful radiographic and neurologic monitoring. Any patient who shows neurologic deterioration during attempted reduction or who is scheduled for operative intervention should be evaluated by MRI examination. Patients presenting with complete neurologic involvement are probably best served by urgent reduction, and MRI studies should be reserved for preoperative planning.

If there is no evidence of disc protrusion, posterior stabilization and fusion are recommended because of the ligamentous nature of the injury. The stabilization is usually achieved with a posterior spinous wiring technique or lateral mass plating. When there is evidence of a significant concomitant disc herniation, anterior cervical discectomy and fusion should be performed before the posterior stabilization. Some centers have resorted to purely anterior decompression, interbody grafting, and anterior plating for this situation; however, the use of anterior plating without a posterior procedure for this posterior injury pattern remains controversial.

Facet fractures are usually seen in association with facet dislocation, but they can occur as isolated injuries. Associated neurologic deficits range from root injuries to spinal cord syndromes. Unilateral cases can usually be reduced by closed means; however, the residual rotational instability often necessitates posterior stabilization and fusion. Patients with facet fractures and root deficits require a cervical foraminotomy as part of the surgical treatment. The severity of instability after bilateral cases depends on the actual site of the superior or inferior facet fracture. Generally, operative stabilization is required for these injuries as well.

VERTEBRAL BODY BURST FRACTURE

Vertebral body burst fractures occur with axial loading, usually in association with a flexion component. The result is a comminuted fracture involving the posterior aspect of the vertebral body with a variable degree of bony retropulsion into the spinal canal. Posterior element involvement, either as ligamentous disruption or fracture, is common and may result in significant kyphosis. Spinal cord injury of variable severity is common in these patients because of the canal encroachment and spinal deformity.

The plain lateral radiograph usually demonstrates the fracture, except for the less common sagittal plane fractures. These fractures are best seen on an AP radiograph or axial CT scan. The CT scan outlines the bony anatomy and details the extent of spinal canal compromise (Fig. 28.5).

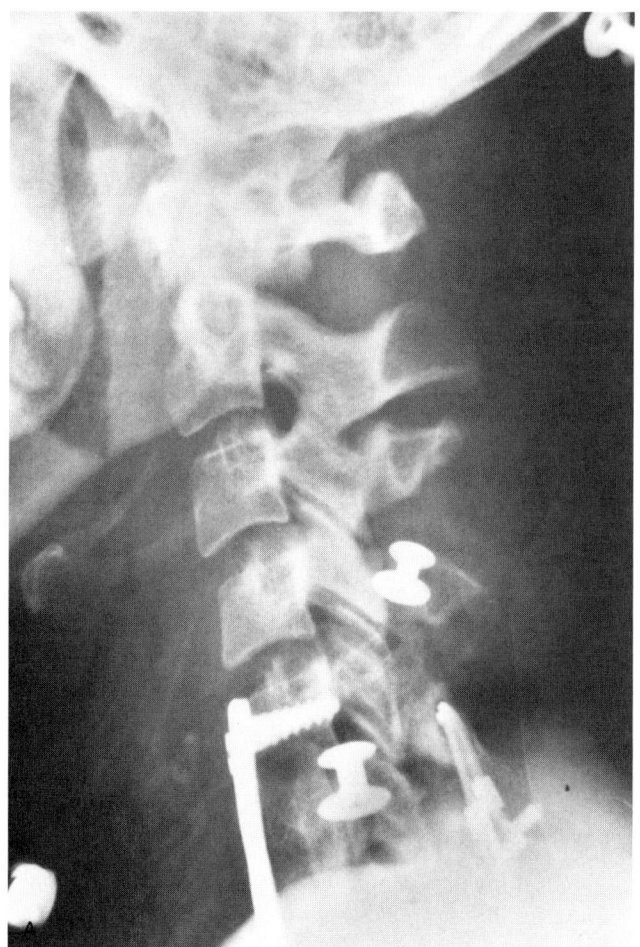
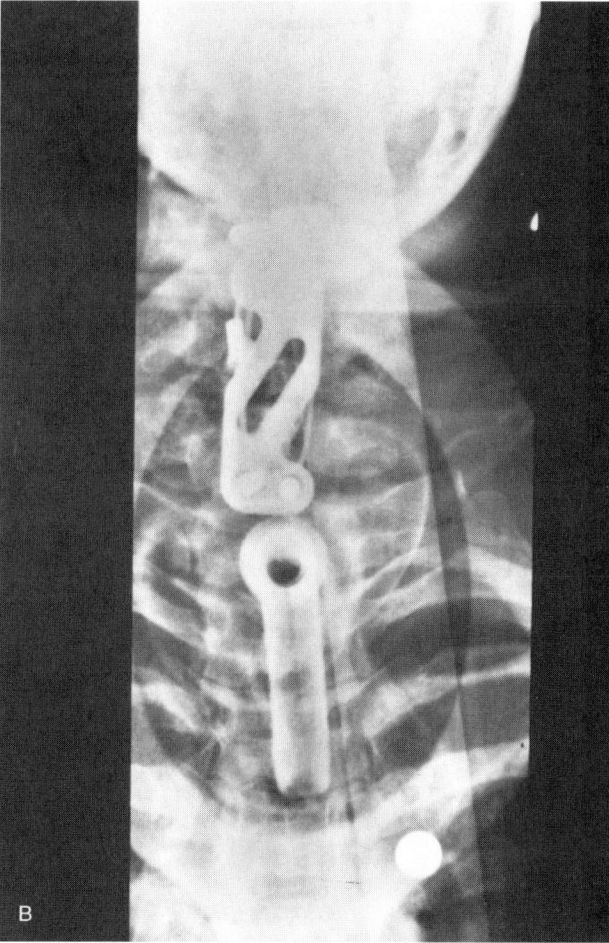

Figure 28.18. AP (**A**) and lateral (**B**) views showing vertebrectomy with decompression of the spinal canal.

MRI aids in assessing the degree of mechanical cord compression and parenchymal cord injury and reveals the integrity of the posterior ligamentous complex (Fig. 28.9).

Initial skeletal traction realigns the spine and assists in indirect reduction of the retropulsed bony fragments by ligamentotaxis. An MRI study is then used to evaluate the degree of canal compromise. Neurologically intact patients who have no canal compromise can be maintained in traction or halo vest immobilization until operative intervention with internal fixation can be scheduled. Urgent anterior surgical decompression is warranted for patients with an incomplete neurologic deficit and residual canal compromise. Surgical intervention for these injuries consists of an anterior corpectomy as part of the decompression procedure and reconstructive anterior load sharing by means of a tricortical iliac crest or fibular strut graft (Fig. 28.18). Stabilizing these major injuries with anterior plating alone remains controversial, particularly if the posterior ligamentous complex is disrupted (Fig. 28.11). In such cases, an additional posterior stabilization procedure by spinous process wiring or lateral mass plating significantly improves the stability of the construct and is, therefore, the preferred approach (Fig. 28.19).

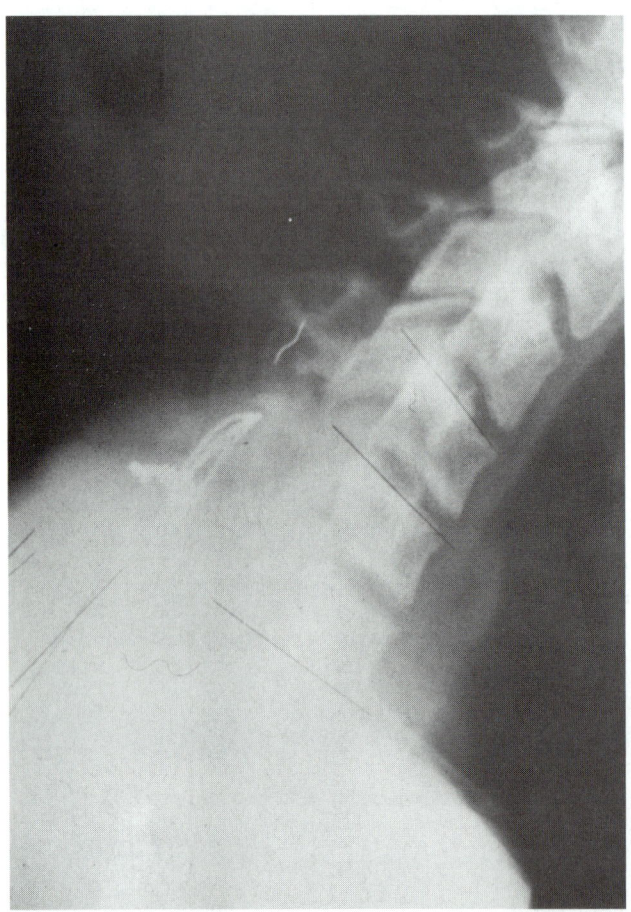

Figure 28.19. Lateral view showing posterior fixation with wiring for a C6–7 segmental instability.

TEARDROP FRACTURE DISLOCATION

Teardrop fracture dislocation is a grossly unstable flexion compression injury that usually occurs at the C5–6; it often has a relatively innocuous appearance on plain radiographs. This injury is characterized by the presence of a displaced fracture of the anteroinferior corner of the superior vertebral body, segmental disc disruption, and posterior ligamentous injury or fracture (Figs. 28.1 and 28.3). Posterior subluxation and angulation of the affected vertebra occurs with widening of the interspinous space. The result is spinal canal narrowing; there is a relatively high incidence of neurologic injury, which ranges from root injury to complete cord injury. The initial evaluation and treatment principles are similar to vertebral body burst fractures.

LAMINA FRACTURE

Isolated fracture of the lamina is rare and is the result of extension and axial loading. This fracture usually occurs in combination with other more major cervical spine injuries. Concomitant pathology should always be suspected, and a comprehensive radiographic evaluation should be performed. Isolated fractures are treated in a rigid orthosis for a minimum of 6 weeks.

LATERAL MASS FRACTURE

Lateral mass fracture involves a complete separation of the lateral mass from the rest of the vertebra because of fracture of the pedicle and ipsilateral lamina and disruption of the facet joints superior and inferior to the involved lateral mass. It is usually associated with other cervical spine injuries but occasionally occurs as an isolated injury. Nondisplaced fractures may be treated nonoperatively. Displaced fractures are unstable and may be associated with nerve injury or (rarely) vertebral artery injury. Surgical reduction, stabilization, and fusion should be performed. Lateral mass plate fixation is currently the preferred stabilization procedure for the isolated case.

SPINOUS PROCESS AVULSION

Spinous process avulsion is also known as a clay-shoveler fracture. It commonly occurs in the lower cervical spine, particularly at the C7 vertebra. The injury consists of an oblique avulsion of the spinous process and is considered to be stable; however, other more significant cervical injuries should be excluded. Pseudarthrosis is common with the isolated injury. A cervical collar is used for symptomatic patients.

SUMMARY

Cervical spine trauma may have devastating consequences for the patient. An aggressive diagnostic approach and an acute awareness of the pitfalls in management maximize the chances of recovery while preventing further deterioration and minimizing complications. A thorough understanding of cervical anatomy and patterns of injury allows the clinician to determine the best treatment plan. Judicious selection of surgical candidates and improved fixation techniques allow early return of function and improve outcome. The newer surgical techniques are technically demanding and require considerable experience. In the multiply-injured patient, a combined general surgical, orthopaedic, neurosurgical, and neuroanesthetic approach optimizes outcome.

REFERENCES

1. Bracken MB, Shepard MJ, Collins WF, et al. A randomized, controlled trial of methylprednisolone or naloxone in the treatment of acute spinal cord injury: results of the second national acute spinal cord injury study. N Engl J Med 1991;324:1829–1838.
2. White AA, Panjabi MM. Clinical biomechanics of the spine. 2nd ed. Philadelphia: Lippincott, 1990.
3. Anderson PA, Montesano PX. Morphology and treatment of the occipital condyle fractures. Spine 1988;13:731–736.
4. Levine AM, Edwards CC. The management of traumatic spondylolisthesis of the axis. J Bone Joint Surg 1985;67A:217–226.
5. Anderson LD, D'Alonzo RT. Fractures of the odontoid process of the axis. J Bone Joint Surg 1974;56A:1663–1674.
6. Allen BL, Fergusen RL, Lehmann R, et al. Mechanistic classification of closed indirect fractures and dislocations of the cervical spine. Spine 1982;7:1–27.
7. Eismont FJ, Arena MJ, Green BA. Extrusion of an intervertebral disc associated with traumatic subluxation or dislocation of the cervical facets. J Bone Joint Surg 1991;73A:1555–1560.

Degenerative Disorders of the Cervical Spine

Degenerative afflictions of the cervical spine are expected to affect all of us, in various degrees, at some point in our lives. The spectrum of presentations and disease entities is wide. This chapter reviews chronic neck pain caused by cervical spondylosis (degenerative disc and joint disease), cervical radiculopathy caused by disc herniation or lateral recess stenosis, and cervical myelopathy or mixed myeloradiculopathy (spinal cord dysfunction) caused by central canal stenosis.

For many patients with pain and/or radiculopathy, these conditions are merely facts of life, manifestations of aging and wear and tear, rather than disease states. Such patients accept the initial presenting symptoms and also deal well with their chronic nature. Other individuals are troubled by either the initial severity or the chronicity of the symptoms. A significant percent of the population will experience disabling neck pain at some point, fewer people will be afflicted by cervical nerve root entrapment, and only a minority of patients will ever be afflicted with disabling myelopathy. The clinician must be familiar with the natural history of the conditions that cause these presentations.

Many syndromes of axial neck pain are self-limited. DePalma et al. (1) reported that 78% of axial cervical pain problems resolve or improve within 3 months. Gore et al. (2) noted that at the 15-year follow-up 21% of patients were unchanged or worse and 33% of the patients who did not have surgery had persistent moderate to severe pain. At the 5-year follow-up of patients with cervical degenerative disc disease, Rothman and Rashbaum (3) found that 23% of patients remained partially or totally disabled secondary to their condition.

Other studies have documented the natural history of spondylotic neck pain (4,5) and of cervical radiculopathy and myelopathy. Many patients with cervical radiculopathy recover without intervention. When myelopathic in-

volvement is long-standing and severe, especially when accompanied with cord atrophy, the prognosis for recovery is poor. Better prognosis with surgical intervention is achieved in younger patients who have experienced symptoms for less than 1 year, especially when unilateral motor loss is a presenting finding (6,7). Thus the general approach to axial neck pain must first be to reassure and educate the patient and to emphasize the use of low-cost and effective treatment modalities. For patients with significant radiculopathy refractory to nonsurgical treatment and for patients with myelopathy, surgery is the treatment of choice.

RELEVANT ANATOMY AND PATHOGENESIS

The subaxial cervical spine anatomy is remarkably similar from one segment to the next. Each motion segment is defined by the interplay of two vertebral bodies separated by disc and paired uncovertebral joints (joint of Luschka) anteriorly and paired facet joints posteriorly. These joint pairs are true synovial joints with typical articular cartilage. Constrained motion is allowed by these structures by virtue of their unique geometry and viscoelastic properties and because of the limiting effect of associated soft tissue structures, including the paravertebral and neck musculature, the interspinous and interlaminar ligaments, capsular tissue, and anterior and posterior longitudinal ligaments. Most of the soft tissue structures have a generous vascular supply and pain receptors. The center of the disc (nucleus pulposus) is an exception; it receives its nutrition through passive diffusion from small vessels in the subchondral vertebral end plate capillary plexus, and it has no neurologic elements.

Each bony element rests on the one below, forming a gentle harmonious curve with its apex anterior (lordosis). The spinal canal itself is wider toward the caudal and cranial extent of the cervical spine but has less space available in its midsection. The cervical cord also expands in this area because of the large number of neural elements in the cord dedicated to upper extremity and hand function. Each respective nerve root exits through a foramen, or window, and is bounded on the front by the posterolateral aspect of the disc, uncovertebral joint, and vertebral end plate and on the back by the facet joint and its capsule. This region is referred to as the lateral recess. Around each nerve root is a capillary and epidural venous plexus. The spinal cord receives its circulation through paired posterior spinal arteries and a single anterior spinal artery. The vertebral artery passes through a foramen in the transverse process.

With aging, trauma, vascular impairment, and repetitive or occult injury, damage can occur to any of these soft tissue structures, resulting in local pain, referred sclerotomal pain, or radicular pain. Central cord compression may lead to painless neurologic dysfunction. Impingement on the vertebral artery by osteophytic proliferation laterally may cause vertebrobasilar circulatory abnormalities.

Many axial pain syndromes are attributed to a subtle injury of the ligament, facet capsule, and disc annulus. Neurogenic pain syndromes are often the result of posterolateral disc herniations that cause nerve root and, in some cases, cord compression. Pain syndromes related to nerve root entrapment by the degenerative enlargement of the uncovertebral joint, the facet joint, or the vertebral end plate (lateral recess stenosis) are also common. Painless neurologic dysfunction can be seen with central cord compression as a result of stenosis of the canal caused by advanced spondylosis; central disc herniation; ossification of the posterior longitudinal ligament (OPLL), particularly common in those of Asian descent; and malalignment or deformity of the cervical spine.

Congenital stenosis may predispose some individuals to problems when combined with lesser degrees of the degenerative conditions mentioned above. For many patients, pain as a result of injury to or deterioration and degeneration of a motion segment may improve with time. Unfortunately, prolonged or neglected nerve root and spinal cord compression may lead to irreversible functional loss.

INITIAL FINDINGS, PHYSICAL EXAMINATION, AND DIAGNOSIS

Increasingly, more patients with early axial neck pain and/or radicular arm pain may be seen by the primary care physician. The responsibility for initial assessment and early conservative management thus may fall in different hands. It is appropriate, however, to follow these basic guidelines.

The diagnosis can usually be made by taking a complete history and physical examination. The examiner must carefully consider the differential diagnosis. Plain radiographs often supplement the diagnostic suspicion and usually show age-appropriate changes. Special imaging is rarely necessary early on. An emphasis should be placed on conservative measures and education about the natural history of recovery and self-healing.

The history should document the timing of the onset of symptoms and the localization and severity of symptoms. Provocative and ameliorating factors should be described. The pattern of referred pain and associated symptoms of numbness, weakness, or incoordination may help localize nerve root involvement. Lower extremity symptoms, gait abnormalities, spasticity, and bowel or bladder dysfunction may suggest spinal cord compression.

The physical examination should detail the patient's areas of tenderness, abnormalities in range of motion, and sensitivities to position or applied load. Specifically, the examiner should observe for radicular pain with axial rotation and extension (Spurling's test), pain referred down the spine with rapid neck flexion (Lhermitte's maneuver), and pain with axial compression. Relief of pain with shoulder abduction suggests cervical root entrapment.

A careful neurologic exam includes a complete evaluation of upper and lower extremity sensation, motor strength and reflex function. Signs of spinal cord (long tract) involvement should be sought by looking for spasticity, atrophy, and hyperreflexia with or without clonus. The extensor withdrawal of the great toe and flaring of the little toes with plantar stimulation (Babinski response) and reflex contraction of the thumb and finger interphalangeal joints with flicking of the distal interphalangeal (DIP) joint of the long finger in extension (Hoffmann's sign) are also helpful signs of cord involvement. A biceps or brachioradialis reflex that is suppressed but generalizes to the finger flexors (inverted radial reflex) may suggest a proximal myelopathy at C5 (8). Gait disturbances should be documented.

To avoid confusion when considering the differential diagnosis for radiculopathy, the clinician should look for signs of shoulder joint dysfunction, vascular disturbances of the upper extremity, thoracic outlet syndrome, peripheral nerve entrapment syndromes, and underlying chest or visceral disease. With each of these entities, patients often complain of arm or proximal shoulder girdle symptoms, and differentiating between the conditions can be challenging. Check for shoulder impingement, point tenderness, limitation of motion, and instability or apprehension to exclude the shoulder as the primary site of symptom origin. Check the radial pulse and observe its disappearance with Adson's maneuver and the military brace maneuver to exclude vascular disturbance and thoracic outlet syndrome in other patients. Check for peripheral sites of nerve entrapment at the elbow, forearm, and wrist in the usual manner to distinguish carpal and cubital tunnel syndrome. Occasionally, multiple sites of symptom origin are found.

RADIOLOGIC AND DIAGNOSTIC STUDIES

To some extent, imaging and further diagnostic studies are confirmatory, supporting the clinician's diagnosis based on the history and physical examination. A rather high percentage of asymptomatic individuals will have abnormal findings on plain film, MRI and CT or myelography. Therefore, an abnormal imaging study must relate to the presenting clinical syndrome. Approximately 75% of plain x-rays reveal spondylosis after the seventh decade (9,10). A prospective study of 63 asymptomatic patients showed disc space abnormalities in 25% of subjects under 40 and in 60% of patients over 40 (11). Cervical myelograms were significantly abnormal in a similar group of asymptomatic individuals in 21% of cases (12).

Patients may be sensitive to being told that their x-ray or MRI is abnormal and may assume that these findings are relevant and not age related. Patient reaction is particularly important when dealing with questions of causality and aggravation, such as when a patient is injured at the work place or in a motor vehicle accident.

Conventional Radiographs

Patients with long-standing neck pain, radiculopathy, and/or myelopathy should have a set of diagnostic radiographs (Fig. 29.1). Patients with a history of trauma, malignancy, or a suspicion of malignancy or infection must also have diagnostic radiographs (Fig. 29.2). AP, lateral, and

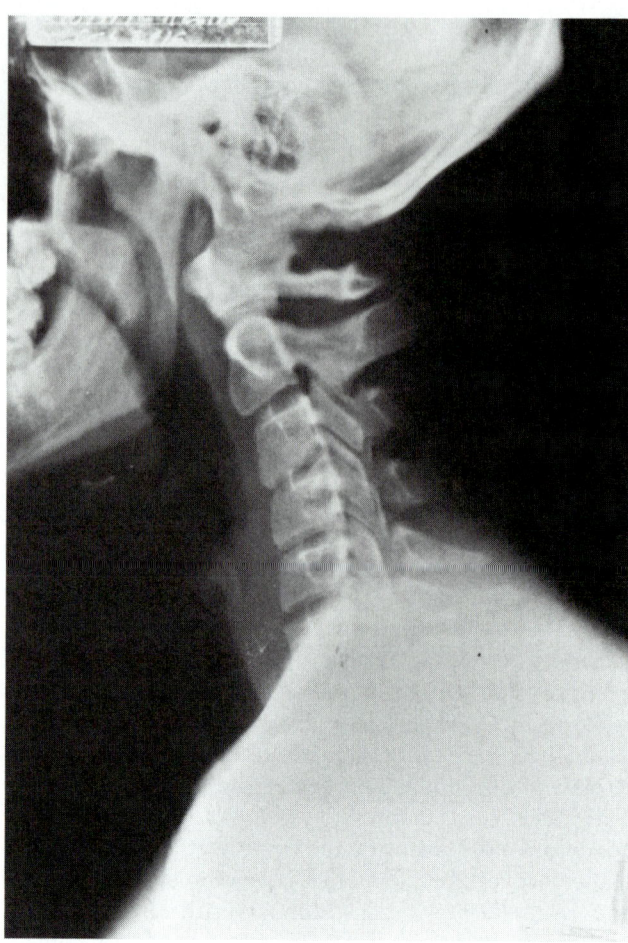

Figure 29.2. Lateral view of a 29-year-old male following an injury while playing football. Loss of cervical lordosis and degenerative disc disease at C3–4 and C4–5 are seen. The neurologic examination was abnormal.

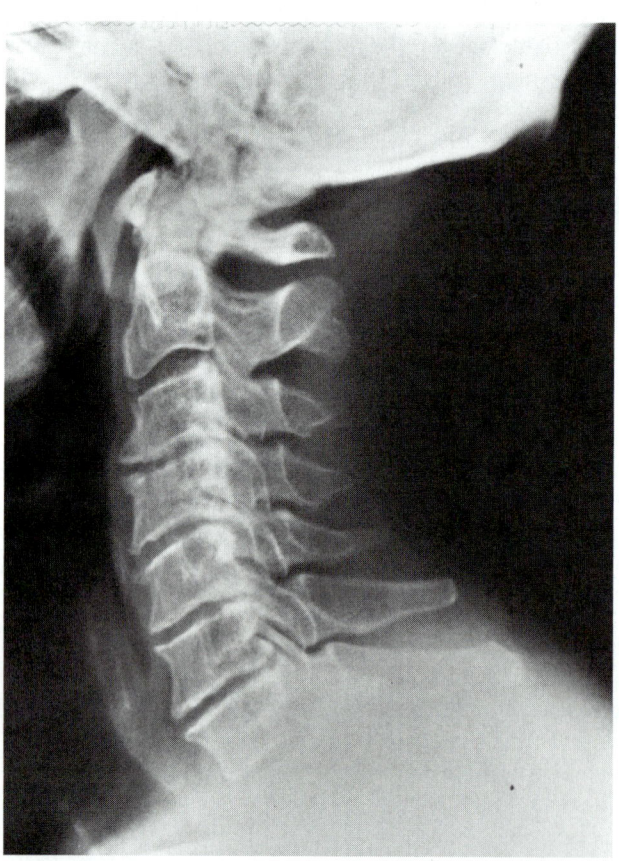

Figure 29.1. Lateral view of a 50-year-old male with several months of left arm pain and an abnormal neurologic examination. Significant cervical spondylosis is seen, with degenerative spondylolisthesis of C7 on T1. Cervical lordosis is maintained.

swimmer's views assist the clinician in detecting unsuspected lesions, disc space narrowing, osteophytic spurs, and degenerative subluxations that may be seen with disc degeneration. Oblique views help define facet arthrosis and bony foraminal stenosis. Dynamic studies are of additional benefit when evaluating traumatic and inflammatory causes or obvious subluxations.

Nuclear Medicine

In a patient in whom malignancy or infection is a consideration, a bone scan may be of benefit. It is not routinely indicated for the evaluation of neck or arm pain, however.

MRI

MRI is the imaging study of choice for evaluating the cervical spine. It provides excellent images of the spinal cord, discs, and ligaments (Fig. 29.3). A change in signal within the spinal cord may represent hematoma or edema. In the ligaments, such signal abnormality may represent rupture. In the disc, signal change may represent the de-

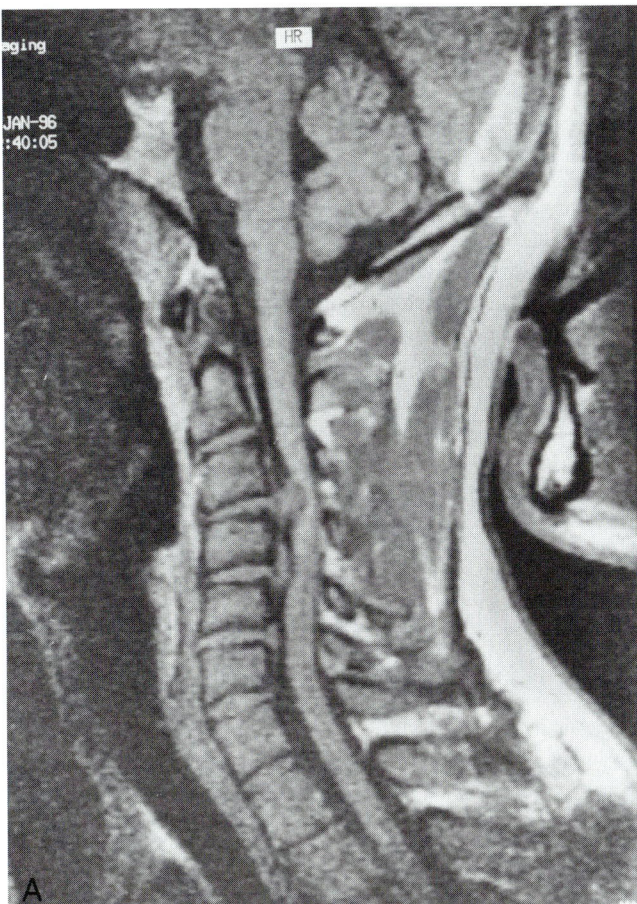 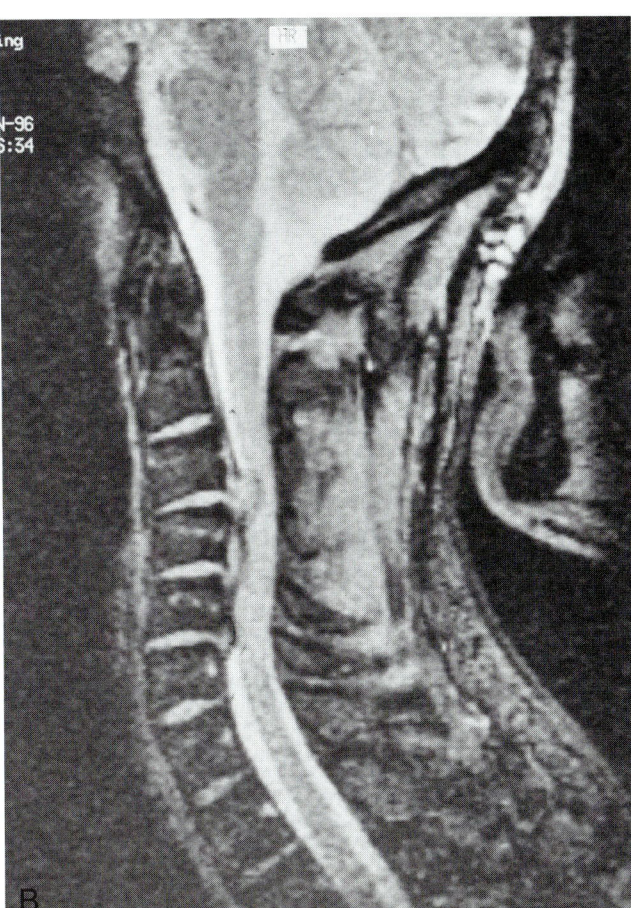

Figure 29.3. MRI studies of the patient shown in Figure 29.2. Note the large herniated nucleus pulposus at C3–4 and C4–5 and the significant spinal cord compression.

gree of desiccation, indicating degeneration. The change in signal arising from the bone may represent reactive degenerative change or a lesion, such as infection or malignancy (Fig. 29.4). It may, however, be difficult to differentiate soft disc from osteophyte in the spondylotic cervical spine via an MRI scan. This can be improved by obtaining a plain CT scan to assess bony abnormalities. The resolution of the MRI is not always optimal; however, with advances in hardware and software technologies it continues to improve.

CT with Intrathecal Contrast

The CT with intrathecal contrast (CT myelogram) has traditionally been the gold standard for imaging of the cervical spine. Its resolution and ability to discriminate between hard and soft tissue abnormalities set it apart from MRI. It is less prone to unusual artifacts and may give a more accurate sense of the degree of stenosis. Unfortunately, it is invasive and carries greater risk to the patient than does MRI. It may be helpful when confronting a diagnostic dilemma and as a supplement to MRI when necessary. Both CT myelography and MRI have been shown to reveal lesions in the cervical spine that are surgically confirmed to be relevant in 80 to 90% of patients (13).

Discography and Facet Blocks

Discography and diagnostic facet blocks may have a role in evaluating chronic neck pain. These modalities are invasive, however. Discography is used as a provocative test for axial neck pain. If positive, surgical fusion may be warranted. Discography of the cervical spine has obvious risks, given the anatomical structures traversing the neck (esophagus, carotid vessels). Facet blocks can be used therapeutically and diagnostically. Most clinicians limit its use to the evaluation of the patient with a cervical acceleration-deceleration injury (whiplash). Therapeutically, it helps relieve facet pain; diagnostically, it helps determine the symptomatic facet. Again, cervical fusion may be warranted in such a patient.

Neurodiagnostic Studies

Neurophysiologic studies of nerve root and spinal cord function may assist the clinician in evaluating radiculopathy and myelopathy. Each helps confirm the impression formed from the history, physical findings, and imaging studies. Neurodiagnostic studies may establish the exact location of dysfunction, when it remains in question; may confirm multiple sites of neurologic dysfunction; may es-

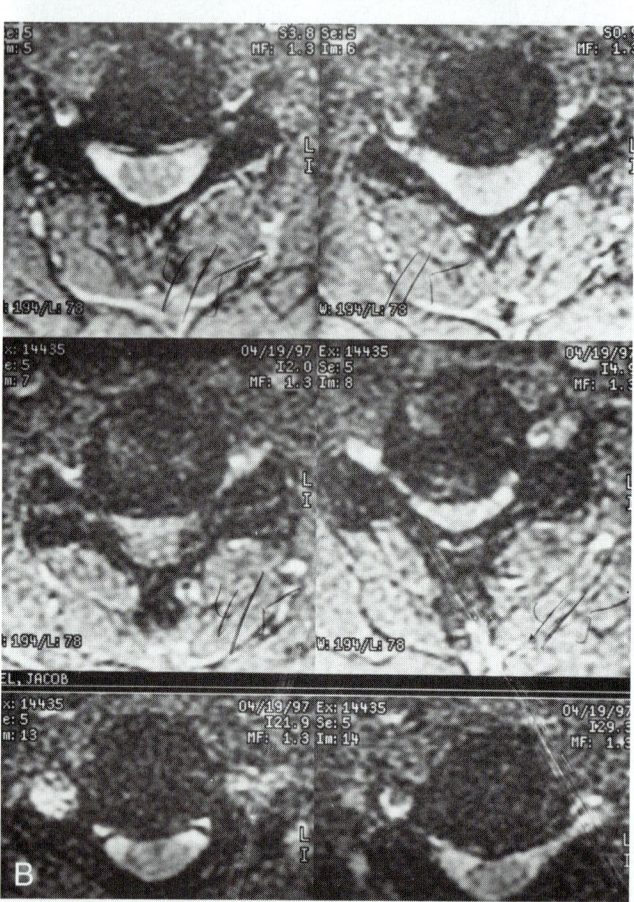

column transmission and are indicative of spinal cord function, which helps in the evaluation of the patient with myelopathy.

Laboratory Studies

Laboratory studies may be helpful for the occasional patient with suspected infection, tumor, or inflammatory or metabolic condition. Complete blood count with differential; erythrocyte sedimentation rate (ESR); blood cultures; metabolic studies; serum protein electrophoresis (SPEP); thyroid function test (TFT); prostate-specific antigen (PSA); and when appropriate, rheumatologic studies (HLA-B27, antibody to nuclear antigens [ANA], rheumatoid factor) may be helpful. Selection of laboratory studies depends on the presenting clinical picture, and specific details are beyond the scope of this chapter.

TREATMENT

Nonoperative Treatment

Several nonoperative measures are available for treating the patient with neck and/or arm pain (14). Myelopathic conditions as a result of cervical stenosis should be treated definitively, however, without using temporizing measures in most patients. For patients with myelopathy, the literature supports a more favorable improvement rate in those who are decompressed within the first year of onset of symptoms than in those who are not.

Reassurance, education, and the development of a professional relationship committed to close observation of symptoms and physical findings help patients better understand the origin and natural history of their condition. Given the natural history of recovery, early emphasis should be on education and simple symptomatic treatment, such as the use of nonsteroidal anti-inflammatory drugs (NSAIDs) and activity modification.

For persistent or more severe neck or radicular arm pain, other measures may be required. Patients should avoid provocative activities, which may require modification of the work and home environments. Treatment consists of outpatient physiotherapy that emphasizes education; isometric exercises; aerobic conditioning as tolerated; in-line manual traction; postural training; and modalities, such as warm moist heat, ultrasound, and transcutaneous stimulation. Home cervical traction units may help patients who have benefited from manual in-line traction. Chiropractic techniques may improve some patients who have acute neck pain; but we recommend against manipulative treatment in the presence of radiculopathy, especially when accompanied by myelopathic findings. A trial of NSAIDs is usually indicated for those tolerant of these medications. Patients should be cautioned about and evaluated for the development of renal insufficiency, hypertension, dyspepsia, and bleeding disorders. The short-term use of a muscle relaxant may reduce spasm-type symptoms. Do not to use these in the presence of heart disease.

Figure 29.4. A. The sagittal view MRI of a 50-year-old patient shows signal changes within the spinal cord at the level of C4–5, which is secondary to the severe spinal cord compression. **B.** The axial view MRI shows significant cord compression at C4–5.

tablish the presence of underlying systemic neuropathies; and may establish a presurgery baseline. Nerve conduction velocity and electromyography (EMG) are useful in the differential diagnosis of radicular arm pain. Somatosensory evoked potentials (SSEP) monitor dorsal

If these measures fail, a short trial of low-dose rapidly tapered oral steroids (such as the 6-day Medrol Dosepak) may help some patients overcome or temporize their symptoms. Occasionally, adverse reactions can be seen even with low doses. Opioids should be avoided.

Minimally invasive therapeutic techniques may benefit many patients. An epidural steroid may reduce radicular arm symptoms, cervical facet blocks may reduce pain from well-localized areas of spondylotic disease, and trigger-point injection may help reduce muscular pain. These techniques carry some risk of neural injury and infection and are relatively expensive.

Some patients may ask about the safety and efficacy of acupressure, acupuncture, and massage. Though not well documented in the literature, these techniques may help some patients.

In all, 6 and perhaps up to 12 weeks of conservative measures should be employed for radicular arm symptoms, depending on the symptom severity. It is usually recommended that 6 to 12 months of conservative treatment be tried for chronic neck pain. Early surgical intervention is necessary for the patient with myelopathy.

Operative Treatment

The absolute indications for surgical intervention are severe and/or progressive neurologic deficit and loss of bowel or bladder control. Operative techniques should be considered for any patient with myelopathy resulting from cervical stenosis and for patients with more than 6 weeks of upper extremity radiculopathy or 6 to 12 months of axial neck pain caused by spondylosis, if a reasonable trial of conservative measures has failed.

The choice of technique depends on the disease entity itself and the region(s) of neural compression; surgeon and patient preferences and host factors are also important considerations (Clinical Table). There are few studies in the literature that compare anterior to posterior procedures for herniated disc with radiculopathy. The prospective study of Herkowitz et al. (15) suggests that anterior procedures may have a slight edge in terms of favorable outcome. Advanced age, smoking history, steroid exposure, and diabetes are relative contraindications for some surgeons to consider an arthrodesis. The inconvenience of bracing for those considering an arthrodesis also may influence their choice of treatment. Basic guidelines for selecting each technique are discussed below.

It is suitable to start with some general comments about the preparations for cervical surgery, the intraoperative setup, and the postoperative care. Conventional intubation is appropriate, except for patients with significant myelopathy, instability, and/or intolerance of extension posturing of the neck. In these instances, an awake nasotracheal fiberoptic intubation is usually employed. In an-

Clinical Table: Degenerative Disorders of the Cervical Spine

Procedure	Indications	Technique	Anatomy	Pitfalls
ACDF, 1 level	• Radiculopathy • Myelopathy	• Anterior approach • Decompression of cord and/or nerve roots • Tricortical autogenous iliac graft	• Recurrent laryngeal nerve • Esophagus • Thoracic duct • Carotid sheath	• Inadequate decompression • Loss of lordosis • Pseudarthrosis • Displacement of graft
ACDF, 2 or more levels		• Use of anterior plate • Allograft • Fibula		• Failure of instrumentation • Possible need for posterior instrumentation
Laminotomy	• Posterolateral disc herniation • Foraminal disc herniation	• Foraminotomy • Disc excision	• Epidural plexus • Nerve root • Spinal cord	• Missed fragment • Cord injury • Late instability
Laminectomy	• Cervical stenosis	• Remove the laminae • Partial facetectomy	• Spinal cord • Nerve root	• Late instability or kyphosis • Loss of lordosis • Postdecompression radiculopathy
Laminaplasty	• Multilevel OPLL	• Expand the canal by opening the lamina	• Spinal cord • Nerve root	• Late instability or kyphosis • Loss of lordosis • Postdecompression radiculopathy
Posterior fusion	• Salvage for anterior pseudarthrosis • Instability	• Fusion with autogenous graft • Interspinous wiring • Lateral mass plate	• Spinal cord • Nerve root • Absence of posterior element	• Failure of instrumentation • Nerve root injury • Vertebral artery injury

ACDF, anterior cervical discectomy and fusion.

terior procedures, endotracheal tube and cuff pressures should be rechecked after self-retaining retractors are placed to avoid additive compression on the airway and the recurrent laryngeal nerve. For surgeries done in the sitting position, a central venous catheter is important, as this position has an increased risk of air embolism.

For supine positioning in anterior cases, a Mayfield horseshoe headrest may be used with a small roll positioned horizontally below the shoulders. Significant hyperextension of the neck should be avoided. The shoulders are taped to the side using 10-cm (4-in) tape secured to the shoulder laterally with adhesive spray. The elbows should be padded. A horizontal incision in a flexion skin crease can usually be selected for a one- or two-level discectomy and fusion or for a one-level corpectomy. An oblique incision along the medial aspect of the sternocleidomastoid muscle is preferable when greater degrees of exposure are required. The anterior ilium should be prepped out when an autograft is needed. Intraoperative confirmation of the level selected should be obtained with a short needle placed in a disc space above the radiographic shadow of the shoulders.

For prone positioning in posterior cases, a three-point positioning frame or Gardner-Wells tongs with a Mayfield headrest is used to prevent pressure on the orbits. These are sterile, but the hair is not shaved. The neck is placed in slight flexion, and the chin must clear the upper edge of the table. The shoulders are carefully tucked and taped at the patient's side. The knees and legs rest on pillows. Reverse Trendelenburg positioning is used. When a posterior fusion is not contemplated, the sitting position can be considered. The sitting position has the advantage of decreasing intraoperative blood loss, which is sometimes considerable in the prone position. When a fusion is needed and autografting is planned, the posterior ilium should be prepped out as well. An x-ray for confirmation of level is used, when necessary. Exposure should be limited to the region requiring visualization but should not compromise technique. The dissection should stay in the midline and in a subperiosteal plane to avoid excessive muscular bleeding.

ANTERIOR CERVICAL DISCECTOMY AND FUSION

The anterior cervical discectomy and fusion (ACDF), a time-tested technique, is ideal for treating larger central or posterolateral disc herniations with cord or root compression and for treating limited regions of cervical spondylosis in patients with long-standing complaints of axial neck pain. It is also a reasonable alternative to a posterior keyhole foraminotomy for a foraminal disc herniation. In the past, discectomy was sometimes performed without bone grafting. Most contemporary surgeons perform interbody grafting with a tricortical autogenous iliac crest graft using a horseshoe configuration (Smith-Robinson technique) (16,17), whereas others prefer a cylindrical graft with careful preparation and grafting of the uncovertebral joints (Cloward technique) (18). Each procedure allows for a thor-

ough decompression of the neurologic elements. The posterior longitudinal ligament can be taken down to visualize the dura.

Many surgeons believe that the posterior osteophytes will slowly resorb with a successful arthrodesis. Thus, when the osteophytes are not directly implicated in neural compression, they may be left; however, an osteophyte that causes direct neural compression should be removed.

Success rates are high in terms of relieving neurogenic arm symptoms, easing axial spinal discomfort, and achieving an arthrodesis. Many patients experience little neck discomfort with the surgical incision, do not complain of postoperative limitation of motion, and note an excellent cosmetic incision. These results have made ACDF a popular technique.

A transverse skin incision is made, generally on the left side. The dissection requires splitting the platysma longitudinally and developing the interval between the sternocleidomastoid muscle and the strap muscles. The pretracheal fascia is incised, and the interval between the carotid sheath and the trachea and esophagus is identified. The prevertebral fascia is opened, allowing the surgeon to visualize the vertebral bodies and disc spaces. Retraction is maintained by atraumatic retractors placed under the elevated margins of the longus colli muscles. Interbody retraction pins, 14 to 16 mm long, help achieve segmental distraction and restore lordosis. The dissection is facilitated by operative loupes and a headlight or an operating microscope. A thorough removal of the disc and cartilaginous end plate is essential to achieving a good arthrodesis. An adequate decompression of the neural elements requires careful attention to detail and often gentle distraction of the vertebral bodies using ligamentotaxis. Most surgeons prefer a 7-mm or larger graft. Spinal instrumentation is generally not required for a one-level arthrodesis.

Procedure-specific risks include postoperative hematoma; postoperative wound infection involving the donor site; and esophageal injury leading to possible mediastinitis, which can be devastating. Low right-sided exposures can lead to recurrent laryngeal nerve injury, causing permanent hoarseness, whereas low left-sided exposures can lead to injury to the thoracic duct. Generally, a left-sided exposure is used, because the path of the recurrent laryngeal nerve is less variable. More proximal exposures may require takedown of the superior thyroid artery and may jeopardize the superior laryngeal and hypoglossal nerve, among other structures. A sore throat, mild hoarseness, and some difficulty swallowing can be expected in most patients. There is a low rate of nerve root and spinal cord injury with this procedure.

Common technical mistakes include inadequate attention to hemostasis or to structures at risk with the surgical approach. Inadequate decompression can lead to ongoing radicular pain; and inadequate preparation of the interspace can lead to pseudarthrosis, resulting in axial neck pain.

Patients wear a rigid collar for 2 months following surgery. Individuals should expect to lose a small amount of normal motion, perhaps as much as 10% per subaxial level fused. Most surgeons eventually allow their patients to return to unrestricted activity and do not mandate a period of postoperative physical therapy.

MULTILEVEL ACDF OR CORPECTOMY WITH AN INTRACERVICAL BONE GRAFT

Multilevel adjacent segment degeneration as a result of either soft disc disease or spondylosis may require attention to two or move levels (19). Both central and lateral recess stenoses can be addressed in this manner. When significant central stenosis and myelopathy are concerns, corpectomy affords greater ease in taking down the posterior longitudinal ligament and directly visualizing the anterior cord to assess the adequacy of the decompression. In addition, a corpectomy may be required when a stenosis exists behind the midbody as a result of OPLL or of caudal or cranial migration of a disc fragment. Fusion rates may be slightly higher when a corpectomy is performed; but the length of the structural graft is longer, which may lead to greater morbidity associated with harvesting. With either technique, it is reasonable to use adjuvant instrumentation to stabilize the grafts against dislodgement and to promote a higher likelihood of arthrodesis. Most patients who undergo these procedures enjoy a good result; however, the pseudarthrosis rate rises arithmetically with each additional motion segment fused (20).

The surgical exposure is identical to that used for single-level disease, but an oblique longitudinal skin incision along the medial border of the sternocleidomastoid muscle may be necessary for three or more levels. If the surgeon elects a multilevel ACDF to treat multilevel disease, attention must be paid to adequacy of decompression of the joints of Luschka. A high-speed burr, fine cervical curettes, 2-mm-thick cervical footplate, and Kerrison rongeurs are necessary. Furthermore, if anterior instrumentation is used, the surgeon must be familiar with its application. Intermediate screw capture of the intervening host bone is recommended, and care must be taken not to place a screw into the bone graft, graft–host bone interface, disc, or end plate. Plates should be applied flush with the vertebral bodies (Fig. 29.5).

When performing a corpectomy, it is preferable first to initiate the adjacent discectomies and then advance into the intervening bone. A complete corpectomy can be done in conjunction with take down of the posterior longitudinal ligament. A tricortical intracervical bone graft (ICBG) strut can be used for a one- or two-level corpectomy, and instrumentation is suggested. In some patients, there may be a need for intermediate screw capture of the structural graft.

A pitfall of the multilevel ACDF is inadequate decompression of the neural elements resulting from inadequate visualization, limited working space, and concern for preserving a bridge of host bone for arthrodesis. Ideal screw

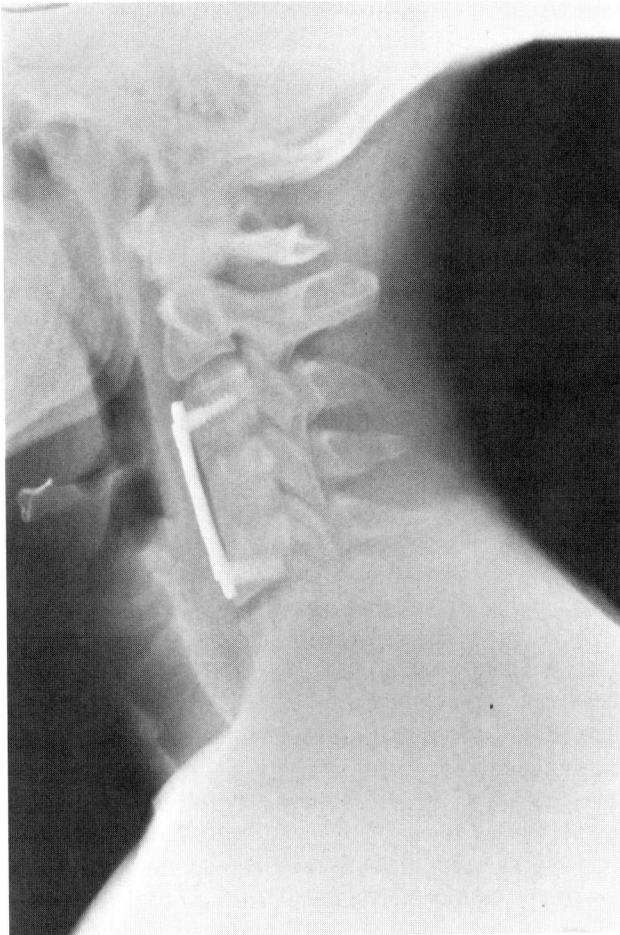

Figure 29.5. This patient underwent decompression and fusion of C3–5 with an anterior plate.

placement may also be problematic, given the large number of host–graft bone interfaces to avoid. When performing a corpectomy, it is essential to avoid straying far lateral into the vertebral body, as this may jeopardize the vertebral artery in some patients. Careful attention to the joints of Luschka and thorough removal of soft tissue from the lateral margins of the graft will aid in obtaining a lateral arthrodesis. The lateral aspect of the graft may be fenestrated with a 2-mm pencil-point burr to further promote lateral arthrodesis.

In the event of pseudarthrosis, salvage can commonly be obtained by considering a posterior interspinous wiring with an autogenous ICBG. Because of loosening or fatigue, the plate may eventually need to be removed; patients should be informed of this and followed carefully for any clinical or radiographic signs of this occurrence.

The aftercare and rehabilitation of patients undergoing a multilevel procedure are similar to those for single-level procedures. Greater degrees of motion are lost with multilevel procedures than with single-level ones, and patients may need to modify their lifestyles and work habits and limit their arc of motion to promote longevity of the adjacent motion segments.

MULTILEVEL CORPECTOMY WITH FIBULAR STRUT GRAFT

Patients with severe stenosis and myelopathy resulting from anterior disease involving three or more levels are best treated with a laminectomy, laminaplasty, or multilevel corpectomy with anterior reconstruction. Because the disease process is anterior, many surgeons prefer the anterior approach. Reconstruction can be facilitated by the use of structural autograft, alloplastic materials filled with morcellized autograft, allograft, or autograft fibular struts. It is essential to decompress all levels contributing to cord compression. If initiated early, some patients will see neurologic recovery, but the goal of treatment for most patients is to prevent progression of neurologic loss. Patients with myelopathic findings for 1 year or longer are less likely to see significant neurologic improvement with surgery.

The technique is similar to that described for a corpectomy. An extensile exposure should always be used. Techniques for harvesting and insetting the fibular strut graft have been described (21,22). Autograft fibulae have significantly higher union rates than do allograft fibulae (23). Some surgeons now recommend the use of anterior instrumentation to provide additional internal stability, which can be an attractive alternative to cumbersome orthotics or a halo vest.

The risks and pitfalls of the procedure are similar to those of the corpectomy. Careful insetting and good security of the fibular graft are essential for preventing catastrophic dislodgement. Complete preparation of the end plate is critical to obtaining an adequate arthrodesis.

Aftercare typically requires the use of a structural brace or a halo vest, depending on internal stability. Patients should be prepared to accommodate to the inherent loss of motion and the restriction in activity that accompany this procedure.

LAMINOTOMY AND KEYHOLE FORAMINOTOMY

A posterolateral keyhole foraminotomy is an excellent operative procedure for patients with lateral recess stenosis and radiculopathy resulting from foraminal disc herniation or spondylosis (24–26). The goal of the procedure is to make more space available for the involved roots by dorsally unroofing them. Free disc fragments can be retrieved. Approximately 90% of patients experience significant relief of their radicular arm pain after a well-performed foraminotomy. No loss of motion is expected and instabilities generally are not seen. Spine surgeons managing degenerative cervical disorders should become facile with this technique.

As noted, either a sitting or a prone position is used. A midline incision with dissection unilateral to the involved facet(s) is adequate. A skeleton keyhole opening is fashioned over the involved root after radiographic confirmation of level. A small burr—first cutting, then diamond—and a 2-mm cervical Kerrison rongeur facilitate the creation of the foraminotomy. The long arm of the opening is roughly 1 cm in length. An unnamed membrane is encountered and this should be taken down with small tenotomy scissors. Deep to this is a venous epidural plexus over the root, which can bleed vigorously. Bipolar electrocautery with nonstick tips is essential to control this. If a disc fragment is present, it can often be retrieved under the axillae of the root.

Perhaps the most common technical mistake with this procedure is to inadequately decompress the root either because of inadequate resection of the facet or failure to remove an associated disc fragment. Bleeding can be vigorous. Hemostasis and a head-up position can help minimize this problem. The surgeon must not mistake the more dorsally situated motor rootlet for a disc fragment and must not stray medially toward the cord when manipulating the root. In addition, the unnamed membrane should not be mistaken for an inflamed root.

Most patients require a 2-day hospital stay and benefit from the short-term use of a soft collar on an as-needed basis. Most individuals can return to their normal activities without restriction in 2 to 6 weeks.

MULTILEVEL CERVICAL LAMINECTOMY AND LAMINAPLASTY

Multilevel cervical laminectomy and laminaplasty are alternatives for the patient with multilevel stenosis and myelopathy who does not require an anterior arthrodesis (Fig. 29.6). These techniques should also be considered for patients who are at significant risk for not healing an arthrodesis. Most patients will have at least three-level disease. Generally, laminectomy is used in older patients with concentric stenosis who have maintained lordosis. Open door laminaplasty has become a mainstay for managing patients with OPLL; the operative technique has been discussed in the literature (27–29).

The operative setup and exposure for laminectomy are much like those for the laminotomy and foraminotomy discussed above, but a bilateral exposure is made of the dorsal elements. For the laminectomy, bilateral resection of the laminar arch and appropriate foraminotomies are done. Some favor prophylactic foraminotomies in the mid-cervical region of lordosis, because the cord will commonly displace posteriorly and place tension over the dorsal aspect of the roots if not unroofed, resulting in a postoperative radiculopathy. This most commonly affects the C5 nerve root (30). A similar root injury is treated in Japan with open door laminaplasty when the cord displaces and rotates into the new space available for it dorsally. Care must be taken to do appropriate foraminotomies in this instance as well.

There are risks of paralysis and root dysfunction, and some patients will develop instabilities and postlaminectomy or postlaminaplasty kyphosis and sagittal imbalance. Recurrent stenosis resulting from a postlaminectomy membrane and residual stenosis as a result of untreated anterior disc affect some patients.

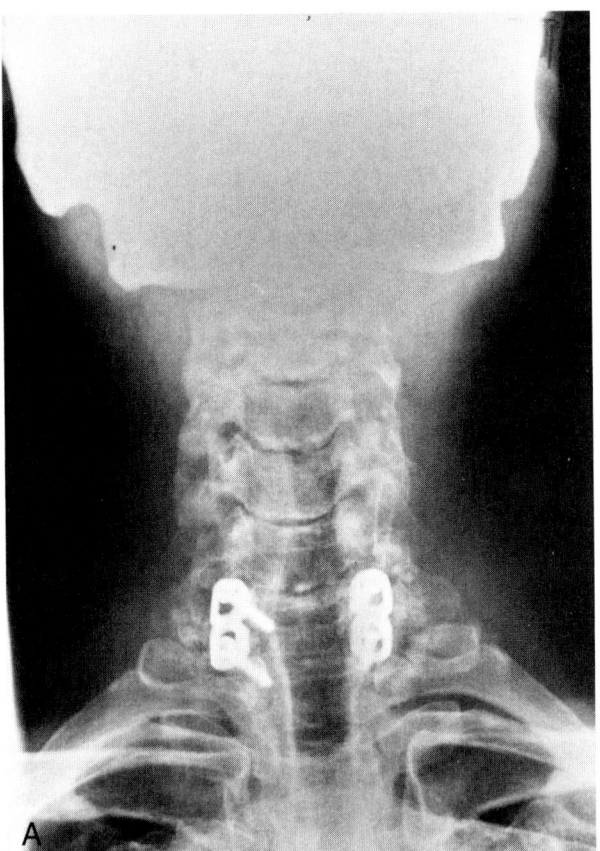

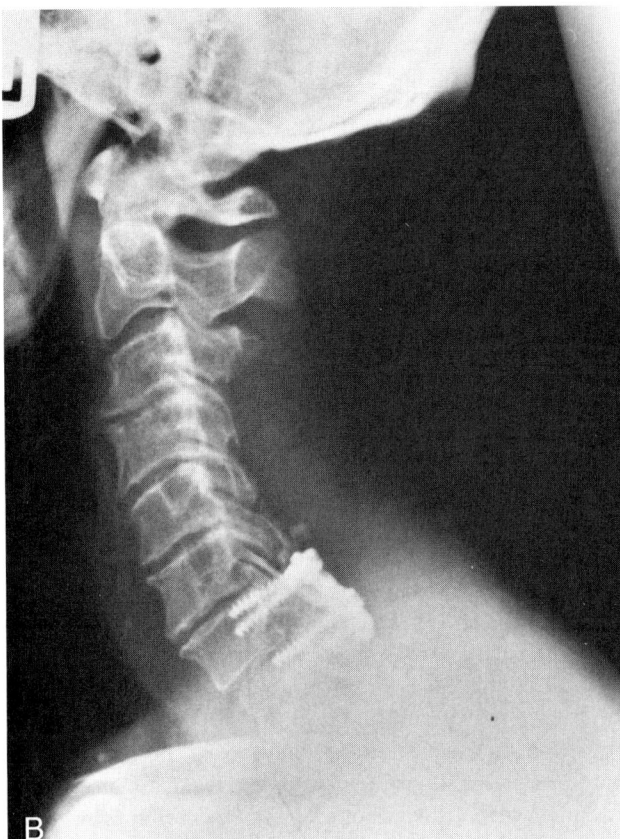

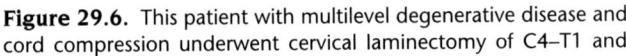

Figure 29.6. This patient with multilevel degenerative disease and cord compression underwent cervical laminectomy of C4–T1 and posterior fusion with pedicle fixation to stabilize a C7 on T1 degenerative spondylolisthesis.

In general, the aftercare of a patient undergoing laminectomy is similar to that described for foraminotomy. After laminaplasty, more rigid postoperative stabilization is necessary to allow the bone used in maintaining canal expansion to heal. This may require a halo vest or rigid cervical collar.

POSTERIOR FUSION: ISOLATED OR IN CONJUNCTION WITH ANTERIOR FUSION

Posterior spinal fusion can be considered when there is need for arthrodesis for spondylosis, but this is not a common indication. More frequently, this technique is used to treat pseudarthrosis after an anterior procedure (31), to address instabilities when a posterior approach is favored for decompression, and to serve as an adjuvant to anterior procedures when there is severe three-column disease or when poor host factors exist for a three-level arthrodesis and anterior instrumentation is not an option.

Techniques for posterior spinal fusions are varied in the subaxial cervical spine. Onlay autogenous ICBG is usually used in conjunction with interspinous wiring. Various techniques for wiring have been described, all with the goal of restoring a tension band and/or containing the graft. Traditionally, hospital-grade (16- to 20-gauge) wire has been used; but recently, braided wires of stainless steel, titanium, or polyethylene strand have become popular.

The latter has excellent ultimate and fatigue strength and does not create any significant artifact on postoperative imaging. Care should be taken to carefully decorticate and graft the facet joint but to avoid displacing graft into any foraminotomy site.

Lateral mass plates popularized by Roy-Camille et al. (32), Magerl, and Anderson are available in an array of styles and sizes. These devices do not presently have FDA approval for spine applications. Rigid fixation is possible with lateral mass plates, however; and they are invaluable in sparing a fusion level in the presence of deficient posterior elements. When a laminectomy has been done and lateral mass plates are used, the surface area for biologic arthrodesis is less and great care must be taken to get fusion within the facet joints.

Risks with posterior interspinous wiring for arthrodesis are few, and this is a time-tested and generally safe technique. Lateral mass plating carries with it the concern for inadvertent injury to the root in the foramen if the screws are directed too horizontally and for injury to the vertebral artery if the screws are long and directed too medially. A careful preoperative review of the MRI and/or CT studies is essential, as are careful placement of the screws and selection of screw length. In the future, computerized stereotactic image guidance systems used intraoperatively will help minimize risk. For patients undergoing circumferential arthrodesis, extra care must be paid to maintaining an airway, given the global swelling in the neck that accompanies these procedures. Some surgeons favor intubation overnight.

The aftercare for patients undergoing posterior spinal fusions or circumferential cervical arthrodesis will be much like that of the anterior procedures, although more surgical neck pain resulting from the dissection and retraction of muscles can be expected.

SUMMARY

Cervical degenerative disorders lead to a wide spectrum of presentations. Often a subtle mix of axial neck pain, radicular upper extremity dysfunction, and even myelopathic states exist. The natural history of recovery should always be considered, particularly when recommending early diagnostic and treatment options. Safe and effective conservative measures should always be employed and exhausted for painful afflictions of the neck and for cervical radiculopathy. Major motor weakness and myelopathy are indications for early evaluation and definitive surgical treatment. Surgical options are varied, and the guidelines for selecting an approach or combination of approaches were reviewed. Extreme caution and attention to detail in technique will often yield an excellent result in well-selected patients.

REFERENCES

1. DePalma AF, Rothman RH, Lewinnek GE, et al. Anterior interbody fusion for severe cervical disc degeneration. Surg Gynecol Obstet 1972;134:755–758.
2. Gore D, Sepic S, Gardner G, et al. Neck pain: a long term follow up of 205 patients. Spine 1987;12:1–5.
3. Rothman RH, Rashbaum RF. Pathogenesis of signs and symptoms of cervical disc degeneration. Instr Course Lect 1978;27:203–215.
4. Lees F, Aldren-Turner JW. Natural history and prognosis of cervical spondylosis. Br Med J 1963;5373:1607–1610.
5. Lestini WF, Wiesel SW. The pathogenesis of cervical spondylosis. Clin Orthop 1989;239:69–93.
6. Nurick S. The pathogenesis of the spinal cord disorder associated with cervical spondylosis. Brain 1972;95:78–100.
7. Signorini GL, Beltramello A, Pinna G, et al. The significance of preoperative neurologic disorders in predicting outcome in cervical spondylitic myelopathy after surgery. J Neurosurg Sci 1984; 28:89–92.
8. Connell MD, Wiesel SW. Natural history and pathogenesis of cervical disk disease. Orthop Clin North Am 1992;23:369–380.
9. Fenlin JM Jr. Pathology of degenerative disease of the cervical spine. Orthop Clin North Am 1971;2:371–387.
10. Friedenberg ZB, Miller WT. Degenerative disc disease of the cervical spine. J Bone Joint Surg 1963;45A:1171–1178.
11. Boden SD, McCowin PR, Davis DO, et al. Abnormal magnetic-resonance scans of the cervical spine in asymptomatic subjects. J Bone Joint Surg 1990;72A:1178–1184.
12. Hitselberger WE, Witten R. Abnormal myelograms in asymptomatic individuals. J Neurosurg 28:204–206, 1968
13. Modic MT, Masaryk TJ, Mulopulos GP, et al. Cervical radiculopathy: prospective evaluation with surface coil MR imaging, CT with metrizamide and metrizamide myelography. Radiology 1986; 161:753–759.
14. Garfin SR, Herkowitz HH, eds. The degenerative neck. Orthop Clin North Am 1992;23:369–515.
15. Herkowitz HN, Kurz LT, Overholt DP. Surgical management of cervical soft disc herniation: a comparison between the anterior and posterior approach. Spine 1990;15:1026–1030.
16. Smith GW, Robinson RA. The treatment of certain cervical spine disorders by anterior removal of the intervertebral disc and interbody fusion. J Bone Joint Surg 1958;40A:607.
17. Robinson RA, Walker E, Ferlic DC, et al. The results of anterior interbody fusion of the cervical spine. J Bone Joint Surg 1962; 44A:1569.
18. Cloward RB. The anterior approach for ruptured cervical disc. J Neurosurg 1958;15:602.
19. Bohlman HH. Cervical spondylosis with moderate to severe myelopathy. Spine 1977;2:151–162.
20. Bohlman HH, Emery SE, Goodfellow DB, et al. Robinson anterior cervical discectomy and arthrodesis for cervical radiculopathy. J Bone Joint Surg 1993;75A:1298–1307.
21. Zdeblick TA, Bohlman HH. Myelopathy, cervical kyphosis and treatment by anterior corpectomy and strut grafting. J Bone Joint Surg 1989;71A:170–182.
22. Whitecloud TS, LaRocca H. Fibular strut graft in reconstructive surgery of the cervical spine. Spine 1976;1:33–43.
23. Fernyhough JC, White JI, LaRocca H. Fusion rates in multilevel cervical spondylosis comparing allograft fibulae with autograft fibulae in 126 patients. Spine 1991;16(Suppl):561–564.
24. Henderson CM, Hennessy RG, Shuey HM Jr, et al. Posterior-lateral foraminotomy as an exclusive operative technique for cervical radiculopathy: a review of 846 consecutively operated cases. Neurosurgery 1983;13:504–512.
25. Dillin W, Simeone FA. Treatment of cervical disc disease, selection of operative approaches. Contemp Neurosurg 1986;8:1–6.
26. Brodsky AE. Management of radiculopathy secondary to acute cervical disc degeneration and spondylosis by the posterior approach. In: The cervical spine (CSRS). Philadelphia: Lippincott-Raven, 1983:395–402.
27. Hirabayashi K, Watanabe K, Wakano K, et al. Expansive open-door laminaplasty for cervical spinal stenotic myelopathy. Spine 1983;8:693–699.
28. Herkowitz HN. Surgical management of cervical disc disease: open-door laminaplasty. Semin Spine Surg 1989;1:245–253.
29. Epstein NE. The surgical management of ossification of the posterior longitudinal ligament in 43 North Americans. Spine 1994; 19:664–672.
30. Epstein JA. The surgical management of cervical spinal stenosis, spondylosis and myeloradiculopathy by means of the posterior approach. Spine 1988;13:864–869.
31. Farey ID, McAfee PC, Davis RF, et al. Pseudarthrosis of the cervical spine after anterior arthrodesis. Treatment by posterior nerve-root decompression, stabilization and arthrodesis. J Bone Joint Surg 1990;72A:1171–1177.
32. Roy-Camille R, Mazel CH, Sullant G. Treatment of cervical spine injuries by a posterior osteosynthesis with plates and screws. In: Kehr P, Weidner A, eds. Cervical spine. Vol. 1. New York: Springer-Verlag, 1987:163–174.

30

Bernard A. Rawlins and Oheneba Boachie-Adjei

Thoracolumbar Fractures

Approximately 50,000 spine fractures occur each year. Of these, 80% are within the thoracic or lumbar spine. There are 10,000 survivors of new spinal cord injuries each year, with a male:female ratio of 4:1, and a mean age in the middle 20s. The causes of spinal cord injury are motor vehicle accidents (45%), falls (20%), sports-related injuries (15%), violence (15%) and miscellaneous injuries (5%).

RELEVANT ANATOMY AND PATHOGENESIS

The spine protects the neural elements within the spinal canal and is divided into the thoracic segments (T1–11), the thoracolumbar segments (T12–L1), and the lumbar segments (L2–5). The thoracic section is the most stable because of the ribs and its relatively shorter discs and because it is essentially kyphotic in the sagittal plane. The thoracolumbar region is relatively straight; and the lumbar region is relatively mobile, has taller discs, and is lordotic. The thoracolumbar region is vulnerable because it lies at the junction between the stable thoracic area and mobile lumbar region.

The cord extends from the base of the brain down to its caudal extent at L2, called the conus terminalis. The position of the conus terminalis may vary along the spinal canal. Distal to the conus terminalis is the subarachnoid space, containing the anterior and posterior roots, which form the cauda equina. Injuries to the thoracic or thoracolumbar spine have the potential to produce cord symptoms, whereas injuries at the level of the cauda equina have the potential to produce root-related symptoms. Fractures of the thoracic spine have a high likelihood of association with chest-related injuries, fractures of the thoracolumbar junction have a high incidence of abdominal injuries, and fractures of the lumbar spine may have associated pelvic injuries.

INITIAL FINDINGS, PHYSICAL EXAMINATION, AND DIAGNOSIS

The initial standard trauma evaluation of the airway, breathing, and circulation (ABCs) should be initiated; and

the patient's immediate life-threatening injuries should be stabilized. The history and mechanism of injury should be obtained, which may help assess the degree of risk for significant spine trauma and instability. The entire length of the spine should be examined. The clinician should palpate the spinous processes for areas of focal tenderness, interspinous widening, or obvious kyphotic deformity.

A detailed neurologic evaluation should assess the presence of a sensory level, levels of muscle weakness, the existence of peripheral reflexes, Babinski reflex, and the bulbocavernosus reflex. In males, the bulbocavernosus reflex is elicited by pulling on the Foley catheter or squeezing the glans penis while performing a rectal exam. Increased tone in the rectum with this maneuver is a positive response. In females, tapping the clitoris should initiate the same response.

Spinal shock refers to a physiologic disruption of spinal cord function, which occurs below the level of the anatomic lesion. Resolution of spinal shock occurs within 24 to 48 h in 99% of cases and is marked by the return of the bulbocavernosus reflex. Therefore, an adequate assessment of a patient's complete lesion cannot be made until spinal shock has resolved. The return of the bulbocavernosus reflex in the face of complete absence of distal motor function suggests that significant neurologic function is unlikely to return.

An evaluation of the patient's ability to voluntarily void, or the existence of bladder control, is an important preoperative assessment. In the trauma patient, a catheter may already be in place, and a genitourinary evaluation may be necessary for complete assessment.

The existence of any motor or sensory function below the level of injury suggests an incomplete lesion. Incomplete lesions can be divided into four classic syndromes based on the neural damage within the spinal cord. Central cord syndrome is the most common and presents clinically with greater proximal muscle weakness than distal muscle weakness. Functional recovery is expected in 75% of the cases with this lesion. In anterior cord syndrome, the anterior cord is damaged, while the posterior cord is spared. There is a resulting complete loss of motor function, deep pain, and temperature sensation. This relatively common injury has a functional recovery in about 10% of cases. Posterior cord syndrome is rare and is associated with damage to the posterior cord but preservation of the anterior spinothalamic tracts. Brown-Sequard syndrome is an uncommon injury, characterized by loss of ipsilateral motor function, light touch proprioception and vibratory sense, and contralateral loss of deep pain and temperature sense. Functional recovery, however, is seen in more than 90% of patients.

Neurogenic shock is a common cause of hypertension in patients with thoracolumbar spine injuries and is characterized by bradycardia and hypertension. The hypertension is the result of increased circulatory capacity resulting from loss of sympathetic tone and unopposed vagal parasympathetic vasodilation. Neurogenic shock is also characterized by hypovolemia, hypotension, and tachycardia; and evidence for hypovolemia, such as local hemorrhage, should always be investigated, given the potential risk of other injuries.

Steroids should be administered to all patients with spinal cord injuries, with full awareness of the potential complications of gastric ulcers and infection. The protocol was established by Bracken et al. (1), using a 30-mg methylprednisolone bolus per kilogram of body weight, followed by 5.4 mg/kg/h of continuous infusion over a total period of 23 h. The recommended time to administer steroids is within 6 h of the acute injury. Despite criticism of the Bracken et al. study, this approach to early steroid treatment is considered the standard of care.

Grading Schemes

Various grading schemes provide a means to monitor the extent of neurologic injury and its progression and to assess the efficacy of different treatment methods. The Frankel grading scheme (Table 30.1) has the advantage of being well known, widely used, and simple to apply. Its disadvantages are that it does not assess rectal or bladder function and is not sensitive to the neurologic improvement within grade D. Furthermore, it does not take into account the level of injury and degree of dysfunction. For example, a quadriplegic would be assigned the same grade as a paraplegic.

A more comprehensive classification scheme was proposed by Lucas and Ducker, who used a standard motor examination that incorporated 14 muscle groups. The American Spinal Injury Association (ASIA) modified Lucas and Ducker's motor index and created a 100-point grading system based on motor tests of 20 specific muscles (Table 30.2). Each muscle group is assigned a number from 0 through 5, using the standard technique for muscle testing. The drawback of this system is that it does not assess bowel or bladder function.

Classification of Spine Fractures

A classification system should be simple, be complete, reflect the mechanism of injury as it relates to the anatomic abnormality, assist in treatment, and reflect prognosis. Broadly speaking, fractures are either stable or unstable. A stable spine is defined as a spine able to withstand stress without progressive deformity, neurologic change, or pain under physiologic loads. It is difficult to predict a significant mechanism of injury based solely on the final position of a spine on radiographs. Therefore, some consideration should be given to a history of neurologic change at the time of trauma. This implies significant motion within the spine to have allowed transient neurologic symptoms at the time of injury.

The three-column concept of the spine was developed by Denis (2,3) in an effort to assess and quantify stability in the fractured spine. This is the most popular system to date (Fig. 30.1). The anterior column consists of the anterior longitudinal ligament, the anterior annulus, and the anterior portion of the vertebral body. The middle column consists of the posterior longitudinal ligament, the posterior annulus, and the posterior aspect of the vertebral body. The posterior column consists of the osseous neural arch, the interspinous ligament, the superior spinous ligament, and the ligamentum flavum. Failure of two or more columns results in spine instability.

table	30.1	Frankel Classification

Grade	Characteristics
A	Motor and sensory function absent below a given level
B	Sensation present, complete motor paralysis
C	Sensation present, motor function not useful (grade 2–3/5)
D	Sensation present, motor function weak but useful (grade 4/5)
E	Neurologically intact

table	30.2	Motor Index Score Adapted by the ASIA[a]

Grade on the Right	Muscle	Grade on the Left
0–5	C5	0–5
0–5	C6	0–5
0–5	C7	0–5
0–5	C8	0–5
0–5	T1	0–5
0–5	L2	0–5
0–5	L3	0–5
0–5	L4	0–5
0–5	L5	0–5
0–5	S1	0–5

[a]Highest possible score per side = 50; highest possible total score = 100.

Denis identified four major fracture patterns: compression fractures, burst fractures, seat belt-type injuries, and fracture-dislocations (Fig. 30.2). The four major fracture patterns are identified by the mode of failure of the three columns. The compression fracture is a failure of one column and is inherently stable.

The burst fracture is a failure under axial load that affects both the anterior and middle columns; the burst fracture can be divided into five subtypes (Fig. 30.3). Type A is a burst fracture that affects both end plates, type B is a fracture of the superior end plate, type C is a fracture of the inferior end plate, type D is a burst fracture with rotation, and type E is a burst fracture with lateral flexion. These subtypes are believed to have inherent instability, increasing from A to E.

The seat belt-type injury is a failure of the posterior and middle columns under tension. These injuries may be entirely through bone, as is a Chance fracture, or may have bony and ligamentous components.

The fracture-dislocation is a failure of three columns under compression, tension, rotation, or shear and represents the most unstable fracture type. There are three types of fracture-dislocations: flexion-rotation, shear-type, and flexion-distraction fracture dislocations.

McAfee et al. (4) developed a classification system that is based on the three forces that act on the middle column: axial compression, axial distraction, and translation within the transverse plane. They identified six principal injuries based on this concept: wedge compression fracture, stable burst fracture, unstable burst fracture, Chance fracture, flexion-distraction injury, and translational injuries. The wedge compression fracture occurs with isolated failure of the anterior column, only; the middle column is intact. In the stable burst fracture, the anterior and middle columns fail in compressive loads, with no posterior column loss of integrity. The posterior column is disrupted in the unstable burst fracture. In the Chance fracture, the middle column fails in distraction. With a flexion-distraction injury, the middle column fails in tension with the posterior column, and the anterior column fails in compression. With translational injuries, all three columns fail in shear.

Magerl et al. (5) proposed a comprehensive classification of spine fractures based on the three basic forces of compression, distraction, and rotation. These forces produce the main injury types A, B, and C, which represent compression, distraction, and rotation, respectively. Each type is divided into subcategories 1 through 3, based on severity. For example, type A fractures are divided into body impaction (A1), splitting (A2), and burst (A3). Type A1-1 is an end plate impaction fracture, whereas type A1-3 is a compression lesion with complete body collapse. This

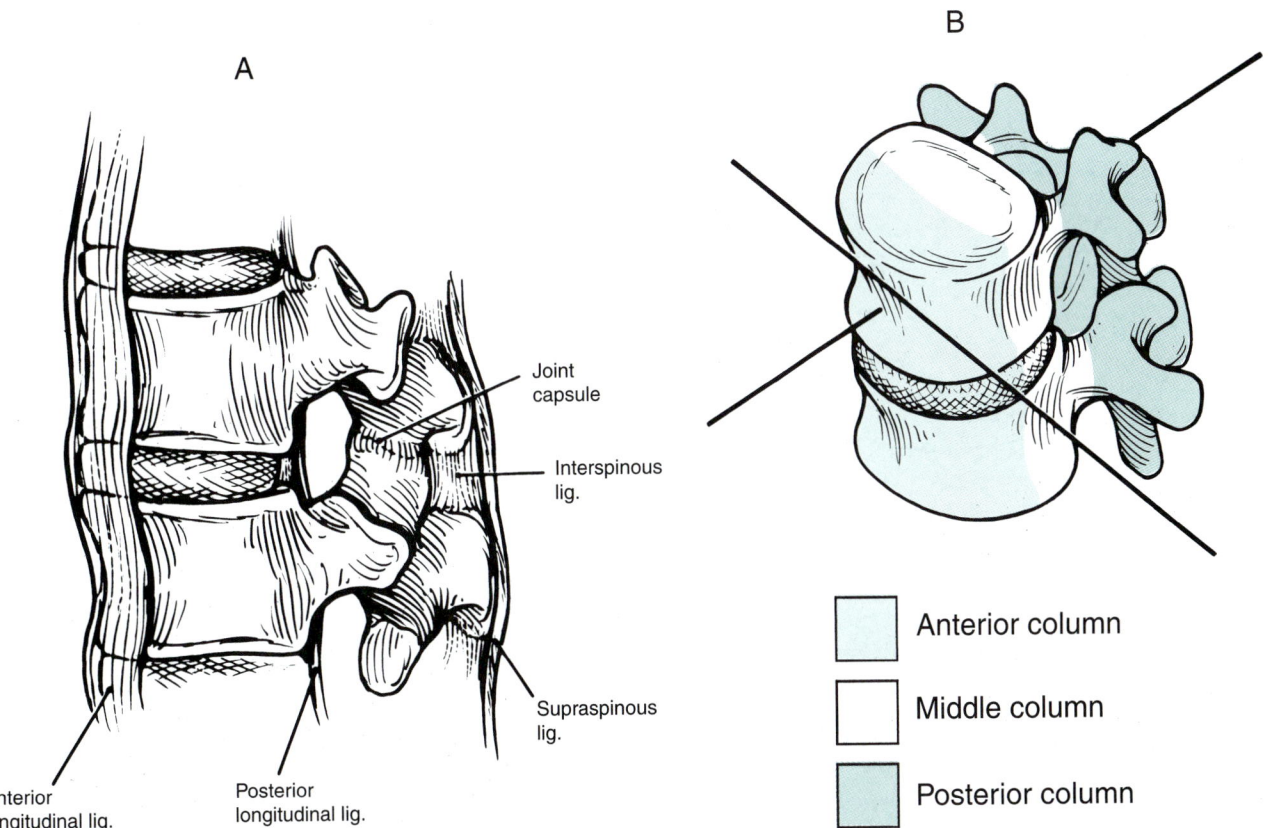

Figure 30.1. Three-column spine.

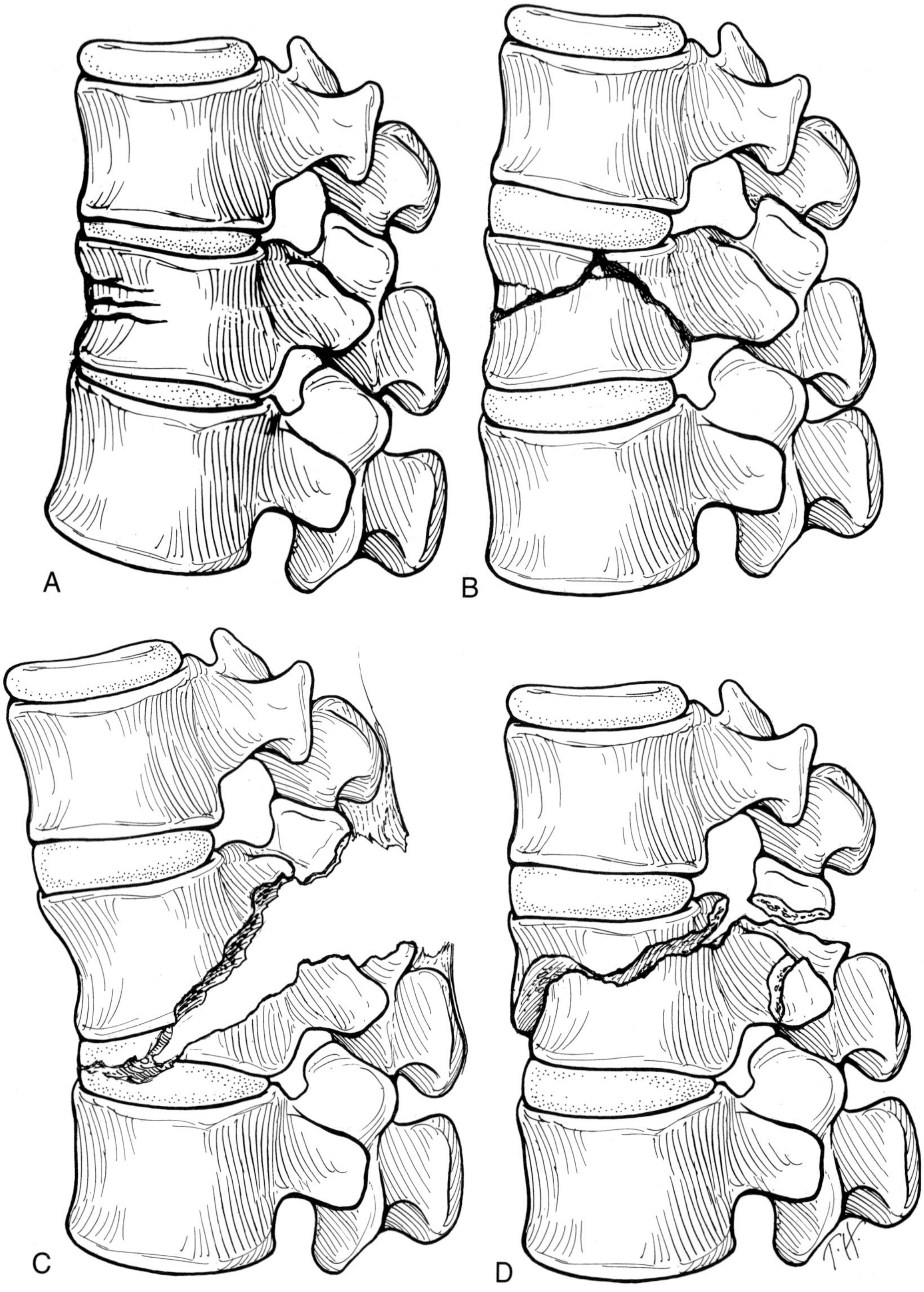

Figure 30.2. Four major fracture patterns identified by Denis: compression fracture (**A**), burst fracture (**B**), seat belt-type injury (**C**), and fracture-dislocation (**D**).

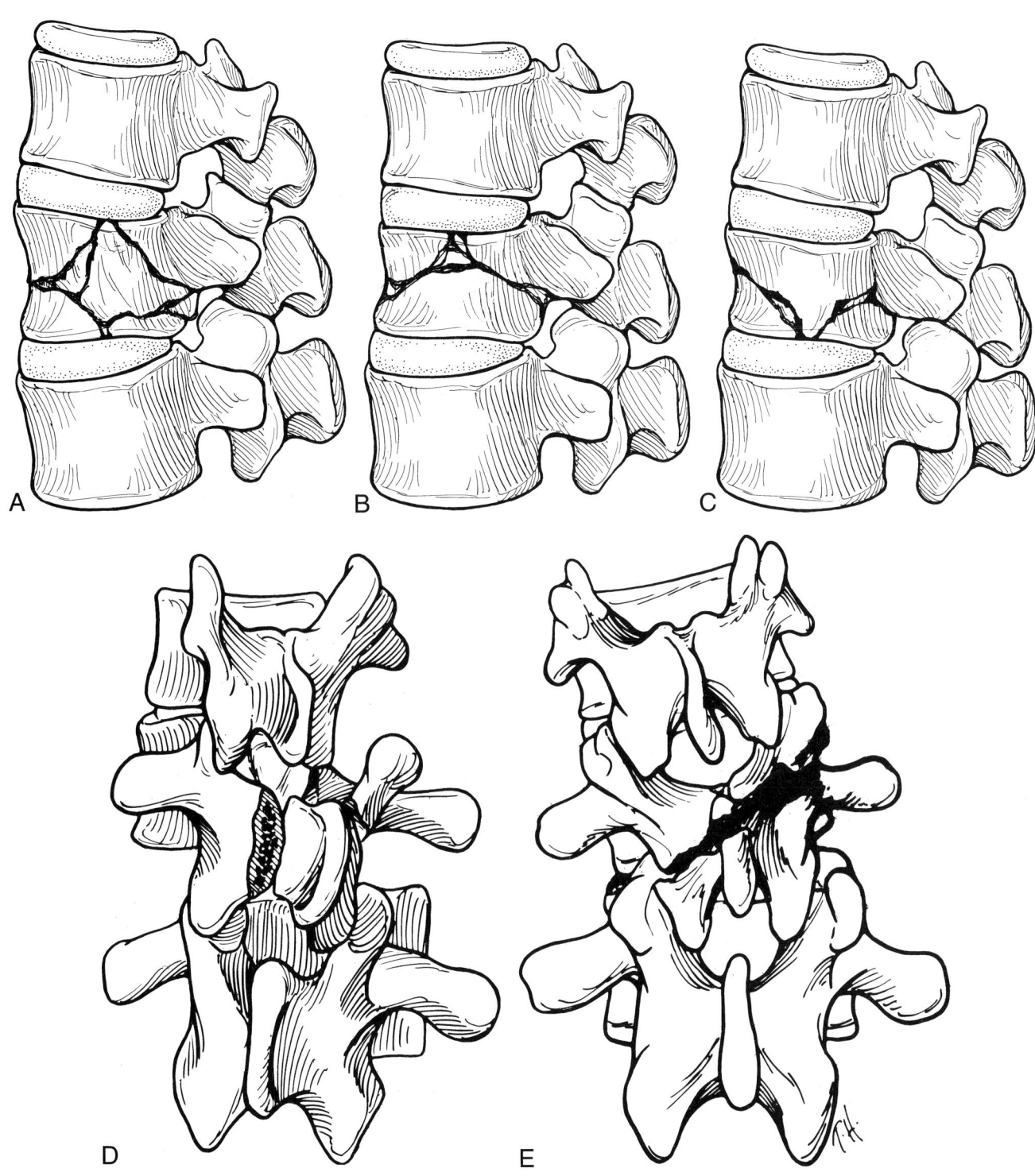

Figure 30.3. Five subtypes of the burst fracture.

classification system is comprehensive, but may be difficult to use. It presently is under evaluation.

In addition to column disruption, geometric considerations of the spine fracture are a means of identifying potential instability. A fracture is considered stable if there is less than 50% loss of vertebral body height or if the angle of deformity is less than 20°. Gertzbein (6) reported on a multicenter study of more than 1000 patients who had spinal fractures. He found that patients with more than 30° of kyphosis had an increased incidence of significant back pain. For contiguous deformities, the percentage of compression and degree of angulation should be summed.

RADIOLOGIC STUDIES

Initial radiographs consist of AP and lateral views of the spine. Given the high association of thoracolumbar fractures with other spine injuries, consideration should be given to a survey of the entire spinal canal. In 70 to 90% of cases, a single cross-table lateral x-ray shows significant spine injury (Fig. 30.4). The AP radiograph identifies sig-

nificant pedicle widening or evidence of posterior element involvement by widening of the spinous processes (Fig. 30.5). Vertical laminar fractures and transverse laminar fractures also can be identified on the AP radiograph. If there is pedicle widening, the clinician should suspect middle column involvement. Significant interspinous widening is an indication of posterior column involvement.

In the pediatric population, a high index of suspicion of spinal cord injury should be entertained, because it can exist without evidence of significant osseous injury. This phenomenon has been described as spinal cord injury without radiographic abnormality (SCIWORA). Therefore, for a comprehensive evaluation of a child, CT or MRI studies should be considered.

The clinician should have a high index of suspicion of spinal cord injury in patients with ankylosing spondylitis and diffuse idiopathic skeletal hyperostosis (DISH). Patients with these underlying diseases can have significant fractures with relatively minor trauma, but the fractures can be difficult to visualize with routine radiographs.

Figure 30.4. Lateral view of a 45-year-old woman who was hit by a car. Note the L2 burst fracture.

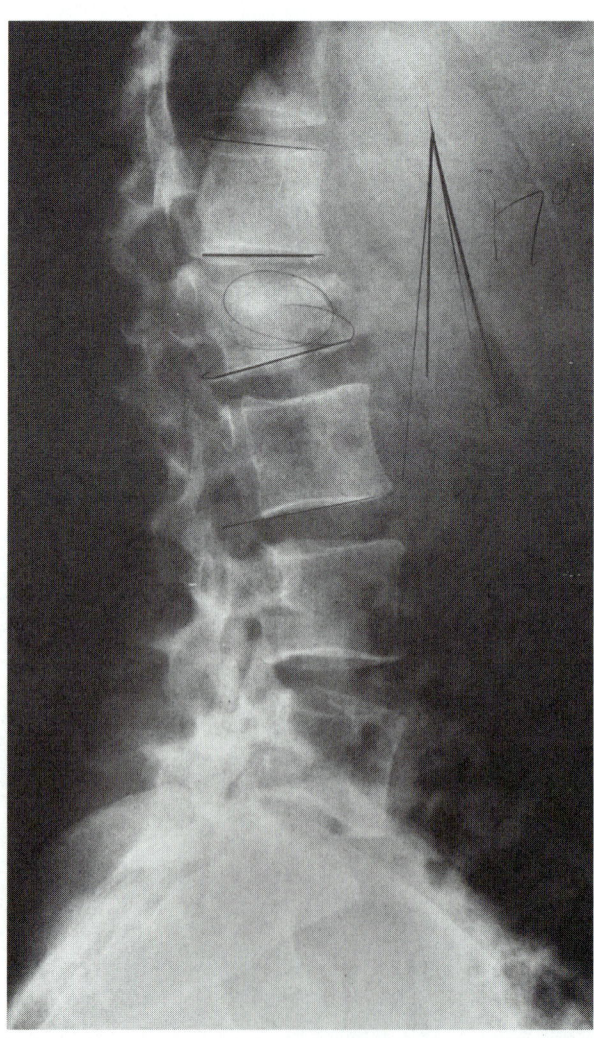

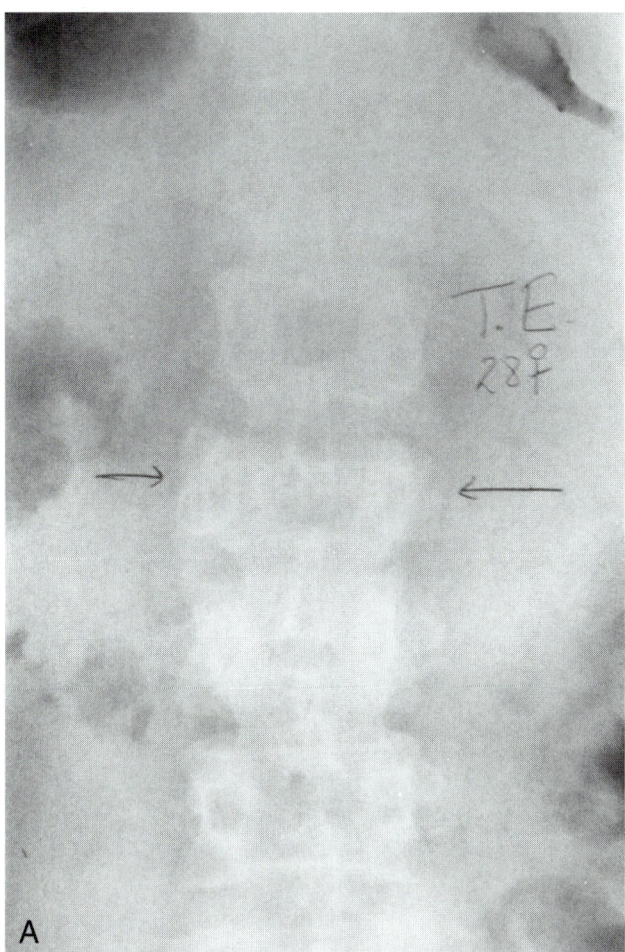

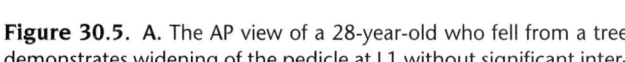

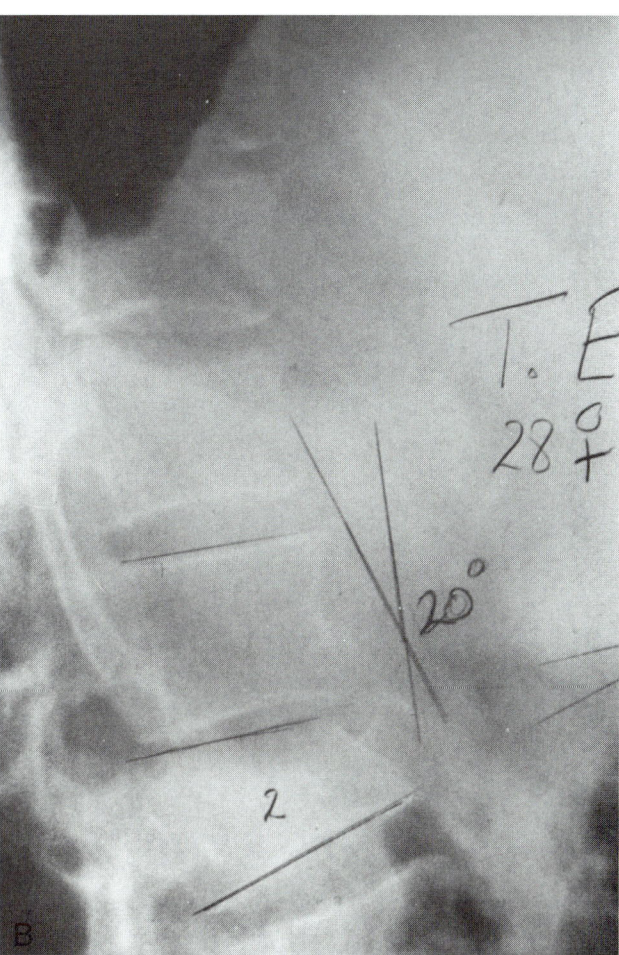

Figure 30.5. **A.** The AP view of a 28-year-old who fell from a tree demonstrates widening of the pedicle at L1 without significant inter- spinous involvement. **B.** The lateral view shows loss of vertebral body height and 20° of angulation.

In particular, the patient with ankylosing spondylitis and significant back pain related to trauma should be treated as if he or she had a fracture.

CT Scan

A CT scan should be performed on all patients who have evidence of fracture. This mode of evaluation gives excellent information on bony detail and degree of canal compromise. Attention should be given to the relative facet joint relationships, which will provide information on the degree of displacement. The integrity of the lamina and pedicles can be easily evaluated. Coronal and sagittal reconstructions, although not always essential, can give additional information about the structure of the fracture, which may help the surgical decompression.

MRI

MRI serves as a useful complement to CT studies but should not be used in lieu of a CT scan. A CT scan gives ex- cellent detail on the bony anatomy; and the MRI provides excellent demonstration of the status of intervertebral discs, potential ligamentous injury, epidural hematoma, and significant impingement on the cord (Fig. 30.6). Cord hemorrhage can be identified as a hypointense region on T_1-weighted images; cord edema can be identified as a hy- perintense region on T_2-weighted images. We conduct MRI studies on all patients with neurologic symptoms and all significant fractures in the area of the cord and conus ter- minalis, with or without symptoms of cord injury, to evalu- ate the degree of cord and conus compression (Fig. 30.7). These studies cover fractures between the upper thoracic segments down to the expected level of the conus termi- nalis.

Myelogram

With the advent of MRI, a myelogram is rarely in- dicated. In instances in which an MRI is not obtainable (particularly with the presence of cardiac pacemakers, ferromagnetic implants, claustrophobia) or when the eval-

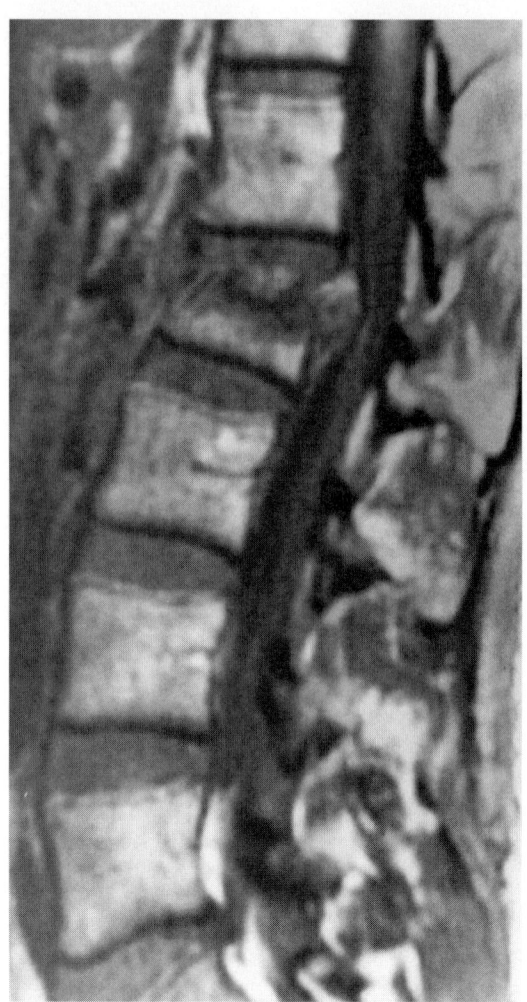

Figure 30.6. Sagittal view MRI study showing canal compromise from a retropulsed fragment resulting from an L2 burst fracture.

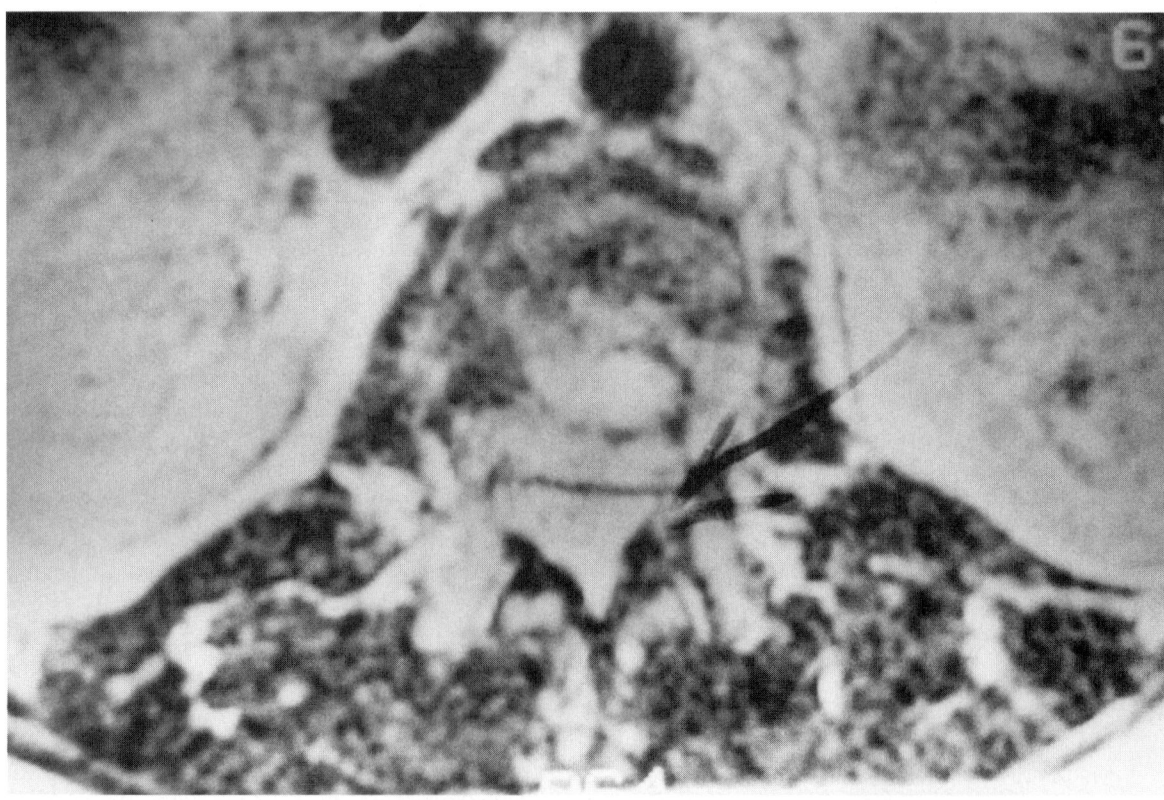

Figure 30.7. MRI study showing a compromised cord and a displaced conus terminalis.

uating physician finds the MRI quality to be suboptimal, a myelogram should be performed. The myelogram may be particularly useful in identifying dural tears.

TREATMENT

The goals of treatment should be to establish a painless, balanced, stable spinal column; to obtain optimal neurologic function while immobilizing the least number of spine segments; and to provide enhanced rehabilitation. These goals can be met through a nonoperative or an operative approach.

Nonoperative treatment of spine fractures frequently requires a brace, which is a thoracolumbosacral orthosis for the thoracolumbar regions. Nonoperative treatment is used for fractures that are considered stable; this approach has been supported in the literature. It is believed that in some cases, bone within the spinal canal resorbs over a long period of time (7). An unstable fracture is generally treated surgically. Surgical treatment of spine fractures may be provided by a posterior approach, an anterior approach, or a combined anterior and posterior procedure (Clinical Table).

Nonoperative Treatment

Nonoperative treatment should be considered for stable fractures, i.e., fractures that involve one column and have no evidence of significant local kyphosis. The stable burst fracture may also be treated nonoperatively. Injuries at the level of T8 and proximal should be considered for a cervicothoracolumbar orthosis. Patients with fractures distal to T8 should be considered for a thoracolumbosacral orthosis. The preferred orthosis is custom molded, with a posterior opening, using standard Velcro straps. The orthosis is worn for 3 to 6 months. Healing is gauged by improvement in pain. The fracture is monitored radiographically for evidence of instability throughout the bracing treatment to identify any evidence of kyphosis.

Operative Treatment

Surgical treatment is indicated in the unstable spine. Controversy exists regarding the treatment of the unstable spine without evidence of neurologic deficit. Denis et al. (8) reviewed patients with thoracolumbar fractures without neurologic deficit and reported that all patients treated operatively were able to return to work, whereas 25% of the patients treated nonoperatively were unable to return to work. In addition, 17% of the patients in the nonsurgical group developed late neurologic problems. It is difficult to predict which patient will develop a potential kyphosis; and although 20° of angulation has been considered the arbitrary limit of potential instability, other issues must be considered, including the potential size of the patient, which will provide a larger kyphosing moment.

We prefer an anterior approach for decompression of all patients with neurologic injury resulting from retropulsed bony fragments. This has been shown to give improved anterior decompression and offers the potential for neurologic recovery (Fig. 30.8) (9,10). Decompression is performed at the level of the vertebral body injury, and a strut graft is used to span the adjacent disc space and vertebral body to the adjacent vertebral levels (Fig. 30.9). Our preferred technique is anterior instrumentation with use of the Kaneda device. A good tricortical autograft is placed posteriorly on the vertebral body and spans the coronal

Clinical Table: Thoracolumbar Fractures

Procedure	Indications	Technique	Anatomy	Pitfalls
Anterior decompression and fusion with instrumentation	• Unstable fracture with retropulsed fragment	• Thoracolumbar or retroperitoneal approach	• Aorta and vena cava • Ureter • Diaphragm • Posterior longitudinal ligament	• Poor structural graft placement • Unicortical screw purchase • Unrecognized laminar fracture • Unrecognized posterior spine injury
Posterior fusion with instrumentation	• Laminar fracture • Unstable fracture without neurologic injury • Unstable fracture with complete injury	• Posterior approach	• Facet joints • Transverse process • Lamina	• No anterior load sharing • Fusion too short for very unstable fractures
Anterior and posterior decompression and fusion with posterior instrumentation	• Unstable fracture with retropulsed fragment and posterior element disruption	• Thoracoabdominal or retroperitoneal approach	• Aorta and vena cava • Diaphragm • Ureter • Facets • Transverse processes	• Inadequate anterior load sharing • Fusion too short for severely unstable fractures

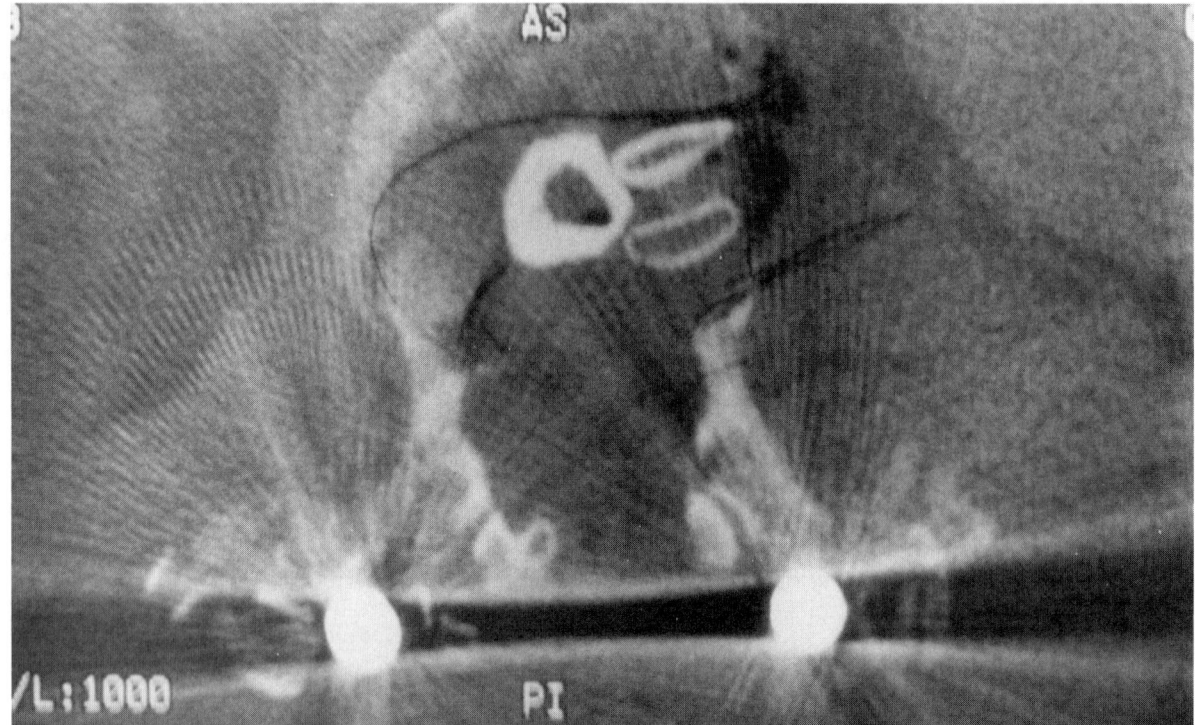

Figure 30.8. Postoperative CT scan of the patient shown in Figure 30.7. Note the excellent canal decompression.

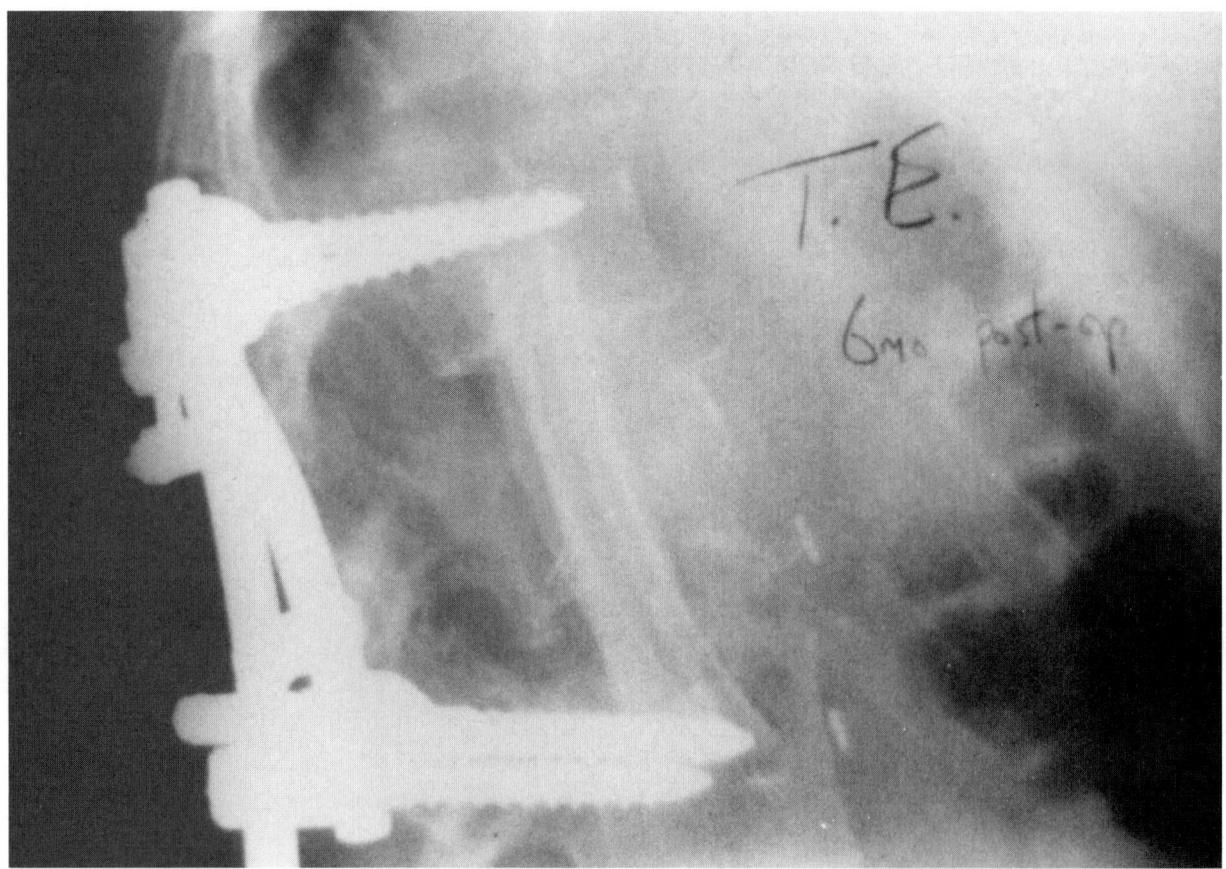

Figure 30.9. Postoperative lateral view radiograph of the patient shown in Figure 30.5. This patient underwent an anterior decompression, fibula and rib strut graft, and a posterior instrumental fusion. The alignment has been maintained since the surgery.

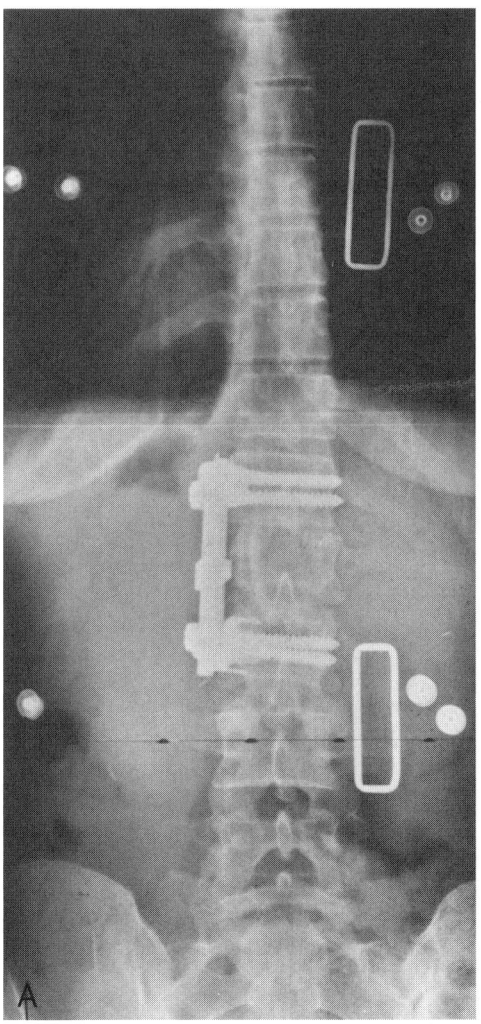

Slice of bone

Chips of bone

Figure 30.10. Anterior bone grafting with a tricortical strut graft and anterior Kaneda instrumentation.

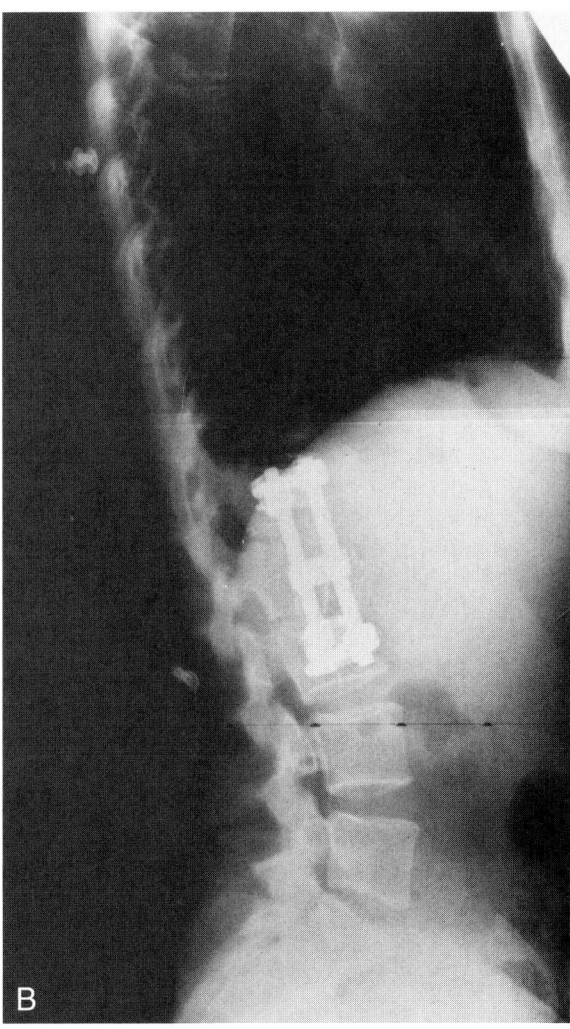

Figure 30.11. Postoperative standing AP (**A**) and lateral (**B**) views of a patient with an L2 burst fracture with retropulsed fragments. The patient underwent an anterior decompression and autologous iliac strut graft with Kaneda instrumentation. Note the good postoperative alignment.

depth of the vertebral body. Careful protection of the neural elements posteriorly is accomplished with use of Gelfoam. Anterior bony chips from the vertebral body or a rib, if one is resected for the approach, are used anterior to the strut graft. The Kaneda device provides excellent fixation and avoids a posterior procedure (Figs. 30.10 and 30.11).

Kaneda et al. (11) reviewed their results with the use of this approach on 150 consecutive patients who had burst fractures associated with neurologic deficits of the thoracolumbar spine. A total of 10 patients developed pseudarthrosis, which was successfully treated with posterior spine instrumentation and fusion. The Kaneda device broke in 9 patients, which was attributed to poor strut graft technique. Solid fusion was obtained by a posterior instrumented fusion. Approximately 95% of patients improved a minimum of one Frankel grade, 72% of patients with bladder dysfunction recovered completely, and 96% of patients who were employed before the surgery were able to return to work. These data are extremely good (mean follow-up = 8 years; range = 5 to 12 years).

The anterior approach is particularly suited to unstable burst fractures, translational injuries, and fracture-dislocation injuries with failure of all three columns. In these cases, the anterior approach increases the fusion and is complemented by a posterior instrumented fusion, as well.

The posterior approach must be considered first in all burst fractures with associated laminar fractures when there is neurologic involvement. Cammisa et al. (12) studied 60 patients who had burst fractures of a thoracolumbar vertebral body and who were treated with posterior instrumentation and arthrodesis. There were 30 laminar fractures, 11 of which had dural lacerations and 4 had an entrapped neural element. Their study has heightened our awareness of potential neural entrapment in patients with laminar fractures and associated burst fractures. The surgical approach to the decompression is from the contralateral side of the laminar fracture; removal of the contralateral lamina hinges at the site of the laminar fracture, preventing further injury to the neural elements when the laminar fracture is decompressed (13).

The posterior instrumented fusion may be performed in a patient with complete neurologic deficit resulting from an upper thoracic injury and burst fracture with a laminar fracture or segmental deformity at the thoracolumbar junction without neurologic deficit. Indirect decompression from the posterior approach may be obtained through the pedicle or through a wide laminectomy performed posteriorly. This procedure, however, is indirect, may be particularly difficult around the cord, and may be less hazardous distal to the conus terminalis. Pedicle screw instrumentation provides for limited fusion posteriorly; one level below the indicated fracture provides more free segments in the lumbar spine. Early reports of instrumentation failure with a short segment fusion (14), however, have advocated the need for anterior fusion as well, to help with load sharing anteriorly.

REFERENCES

1. Bracken MB, Shepard MJ, Collings WF, et al. A randomized controlled trial of methylprednisolone or naloxone in the treatment of acute spinal cord injury: results of the second national acute spinal cord injury study. N Engl J Med 1990;322:1405–1411.
2. Denis F. The three column spine and its significance in the classification of acute thoracolumbar spinal injuries. Spine 1983; 8:817–831.
3. Denis F. Spinal instability as defined by the three-column spine concept in acute spinal trauma. Clin Orthop 1984;189:65–76.
4. McAfee PC, Yuan HA, Fredrickson BE, Lubicky JP. The value of computed tomography in thoracolumbar fractures. J Bone Joint Surg 1983;65A:461–473.
5. Magerl F, Harms J Gertzbein S, Aebi M. Classification of spinal fractures. Paper presented at the Annual American Association of Orthopaedic Surgeons Meeting, Vail, CO, 1989.
6. Gertzbein SD. Scoliosis Research Society. Multicenter spine fracture study. Spine 1992;17:528–540.
7. Weinstein JN, Collalto P, Lehmann TR. Thoracolumbar "burst" fractures treated conservatively: a long-term follow-up. Spine 1988;13:33–38.
8. Denis F, Armstrong GW, Searls K, Matta L. Acute thoracolumbar burst fractures in the absence of neurologic deficit: a comparison between operative and nonoperative treatment. Clin Orthop 1984;189:142–149.
9. Bradford DS, McBride G. Surgical management of thoracolumbar spine fractures with incomplete neurologic deficits. Clin Orthop 1987;218:201–216.
10. McAfee PC, Bohlman HH, Yuan HA. Anterior decompression of traumatic thoracolumbar fractures with incomplete neurological deficit using a retroperitoneal approach. J Bone Joint Surg 1985; 67A:89–104.
11. Kaneda K, Taneichi H, Abumi K, et al. Anterior decompression and stabilization with the Kaneda device for thoracolumbar burst fractures associated with neurological deficits. J Bone Joint Surg 1997;79A:69–83.
12. Cammisa FP, Eismont FT, Green BA. Dural lacerations occurring with burst fracture and associated lamina fractures. J Bone Joint Surg 1989;71A:1044–1052.
13. Denis F, Burkus K. Diagnosis and treatment of cauda equina entrapment in the vertebral lamina fracture of lumbar burst fractures. Spine 1991;16:S433.
14. McLain RF, Sparling E, Benson DR. Early failure of short-segment pedicle instrumentation for thoracolumbar fractures: a preliminary report. J Bone Joint Surg 1993;754A:162–167.

chapter 31

Federico P. Girardi and Oheneba Boachie-Adjei

Pediatric Deformities of the Spine

I Pediatric Spinal Deformity

Deformities of the spine are common and vary in intensity from mild to severe. It is important to remember that scoliosis is only a physical finding, not a disease in itself. The clinician must determine the diagnosis, the deformity's severity and rigidity or flexibility, the effect of the deformity on the child's ability to function, and the child's exact state of growth and maturity (Table 31.1). The terminology used in the study, diagnosis, and treatment of spinal deformities is reviewed below.

Curvatures are measured by the Cobb-Lippman system. The vertebrae at the upper and lower ends of the curve (i.e., the vertebrae that are maximally tilted from the horizontal apical vertebrae) are identified. The angle formed by the intersection of lines drawn perpendicular to the end vertebral lines (at the end plates or pedicle level) is measured for each curve.

Structural scolioses are lateral curvatures of the spine that persist in the supine position. Bending radiographs reveal a segment of the spine that lacks normal flexibility. In contrast, nonstructural scolioses are lateral curvatures of the spine that disappear in the supine position and have normal flexibility, especially when the irritative lesion has been eliminated. The characteristics of structural curves can be remembered via the mnemonic DWARF: displacement of the apex away from the midline, wedging of the vertebral body or disc space, angulation, rotation, and (lack of) flexibility.

Scoliosis is a three-dimensional deformity consisting of a combination of angulation, rotation, and translation that occurs along the axes of all three planes. Nevertheless, it is common practice to assess scoliosis with a single AP radiograph for purposes of observation. Scoliosis is described by the direction of the convexity of the curve as a right or left curve. The primary or major curve is the more structural, has the least flexibility, usually came first, and has the greatest clinical deformity.

Although there are numerous causes of spinal deformity in the pediatric population, idiopathic scoliosis, postural "round back," and Scheuermann's disease account for most of these conditions. By definition, adolescent idiopathic scoliosis (AIS) is a structural lateral curvature of the spine that occurs at or near the onset of puberty and for which no cause is established (1). It is the most common of all spinal deformities in children.

RELEVANT ANATOMY AND PATHOGENESIS

Although there are many studies and theories regarding the cause of AIS (genetic, growth disturbances, disc changes, collagen disease, muscle or CNS equilibrium dysfunction, etc.), it remains unknown. Enneking and Harrington (2) concluded that the deformity is produced by an extraosseous cause and that change in bone and cartilage are secondary adaptations.

Scoliosis in the adolescent patient is rarely associated with pain; thus it is the discovery of back asymmetry that prompts evaluation by a family physician or pediatrician. The most common means of early detection of spinal deformity is by school screening programs; more than 3 million children are screened annually (3). Such screening has revealed a prevalence of 1.4% in the general population (4); 0.2 to 0.3% of patients require bracing or surgery. Scoliosis occurs almost equally in males and females, but it progresses to the point of treatment more often in females than in males. Epidemiologic and natural history studies indicate that less than 1% of the screened populations and fewer than 10% of positively screened patients (those with a curve greater than 10°) will require active treatment.

table	31.1	The Scoliosis Research Society's Classification of Pediatric Deformities

Scoliosis
  Nonstructural
    Postural
    Secondary to leg length discrepancy
    Secondary to irritative lesion
      Disc herniation
      Spondylolisthesis
      Tumor
    Hysterical
  Structural
    Idiopathic
      Infantile (0–3 years)
      Juvenile (3–10 years)
      Adolescent (10+ years)
    Congenital
    Defects of formation
      Defects of segmentation
      Mixed
    Neuromuscular
      Neuropathic
      Myopathic
    Neurofibromatosis
    Mesenchymal defects
      Marfan's syndrome
      Ehlers-Danlos syndrome
    Osteochondrodystrophies
      Achondroplasia
      Spondyloepiphyseal dysplasia
      Dystrophic dwarfism
      Other
    Postradiation
    Secondary to multiple rib resection
    Other
Kyphosis
  Postural
  Scheuermann's disease
  Congenital
  Postlaminectomy
  Postradiation
  Osteochondrodystrophies
    Achondroplasia
    Mucopolysaccharidosis
    Dystrophic dwarfism
  Tuberculosis
  Other
Lordosis
  Postural
  Secondary to hip flexion contracture
  Congenital
  Neuromuscular
  Secondary to ventriculoperitoneal shunting
  Other

Data are from Winter RB. Spinal deformity. In: Pang D, ed. Disorders of the pediatric spine. New York: Raven, 1995:309–348.

INITIAL FINDINGS, PHYSICAL EXAMINATION, AND DIAGNOSIS

The objective of the evaluation is to exclude unusual causes of spinal deformity. To diagnose abnormalities of spinal alignment the clinician must know the normal range of spinal curvature and alignment. In the coronal, or frontal, plane (represented by an AP radiograph) no deviation from the midline should be present. There is a wider range of normal curvature in the sagittal plane (represented by a lateral radiograph) of the spine. The normal range of thoracic kyphosis is 25° to 50°. The apex of thoracic kyphosis normally lies at the T6–8 level, and the apex of lumbar lordosis generally falls at the L3–4 level. There should be minimal or no rotation of the spine, which is assessed by viewing the location of the pedicles on an AP radiograph of the spine.

The history should include accurate information about when the deformity was first noted, whether it has been progressive, and whether it has caused problems for the patient (such as cosmetic, pain, dyspnea, or neurologic compromise). The presence of pain may be an ominous symptom. The patient should be asked if the onset of deformity was sudden and/or related to an acute traumatic event.

It is also important to know the patient's general medical condition. A detailed review of systems, including birth history, developmental history, and history of childhood illnesses, must be obtained. Family history may suggest inheritance of conditions such as Marfan's syndrome. Finally, the clinician must know the precise status of the child's growth: Has growth been completed? Has a female patient begun menstruating?

The first step in the physical examination is to evaluate the curve. Determine the area involved and the direction of the curve. Note any signs of tenderness and associated dysraphism or other disorder (e.g., hair patches, dimples, café-au-lait spots, hemangiomas). Measure the height of the rotational prominence. Determine the relative flexibility by bending the patient from side to side. Assess the posture by noting shoulder or pelvic asymmetry or abnormal flank creases, drop a plumb line to measure torso decompensation, and conduct the Adams forward bend test (have the patient bend forward with the knees extended). Rotational prominence is then measured with a scoliometer (normal = less than 5° to 7°) or by using a linear measurement of the prominence (Fig. 31.1).

A thorough neurologic examination should be performed. Gait and reflexes are assessed, noting any pathologies such as ankle clonus and Babinski sign. A subtle finding of an asymmetric abdominal reflex may indicate intraspinal abnormalities. Leg length should be assessed. Leg length inequality causes pelvic obliquity and secondary scoliosis that may be corrected with a shoe lift. Determine the standing and sitting height spans to evaluate patients who may have Marfan's syndrome.

The next step is to evaluate the whole child. Note any eye or ear deformities. Determine whether the child's hairline is low set. Record any anomalies of the extremities, especially a cavus foot, and any signs of limb atrophy. Finally, assess the physiologic state of the child, including the Tanner stage.

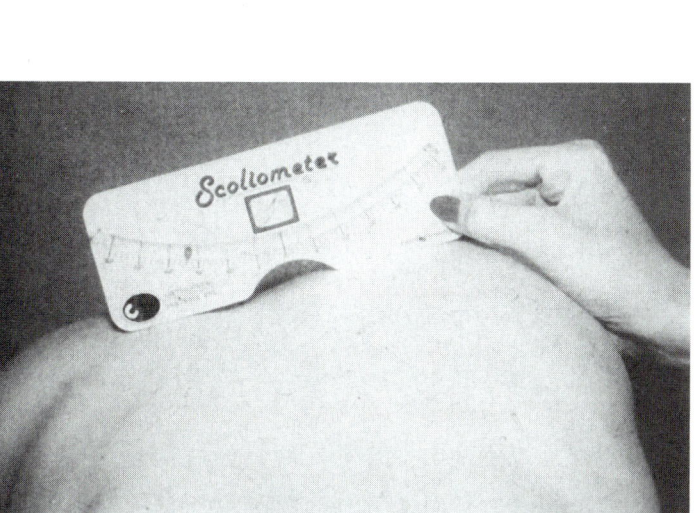
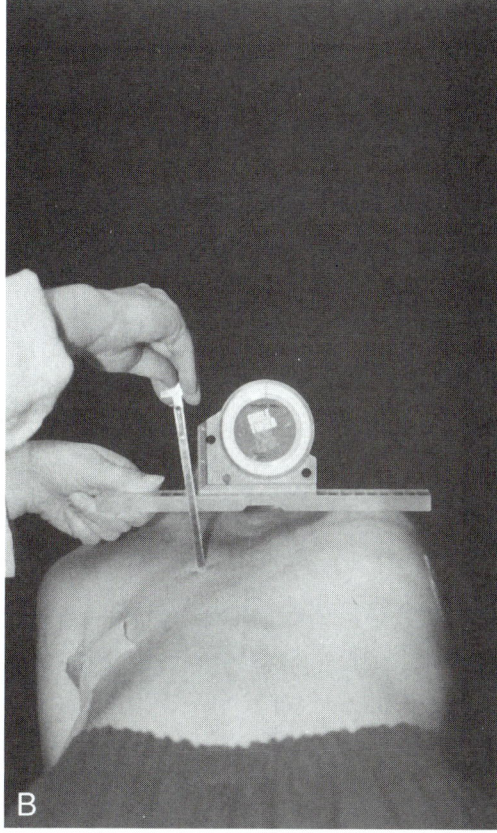

Figure 31.1. A. Using a scoliometer to measure the angle of rotational prominence.
B. Determining the linear measurement of the prominence.

RADIOLOGIC STUDIES

Radiologic examination of a child with spine deformity is done to determine the cause and the severity of the problem. The basic film is a standing AP radiograph (with shield) of the spine from occiput to the sacrum. AP radiographs should include the iliac crest, the triradiate cartilage, and the growth plate of the acetabulum. The most common finding in idiopathic scoliosis is a right thoracic and left lumbar curve. A left thoracic curve is unusual and may be neuromuscular in origin, necessitating additional tests. Vertebral and rib anatomy is evaluated to exclude congenital abnormalities, and the pedicles and interpedicle distances are also studied. Skeletal maturity is best determined by bone age at the wrist using the Greulich and Pyle atlas, the ossification of the iliac apophysis is noted and graded using the Risser scale, and the vertebral ring apophysis is rated on an AP spine film (Fig. 31.2).

Additional radiographic tests may include additional views or special imaging tests. A lateral view should be done when evaluating associated kyphosis or lordosis; a Stagnara view should be done to evaluate a rotational deformity. Radiographs taken with blocks under a short limb or with the patient seated may show a correction of the scoliosis. Supine right and left lateral bending films show

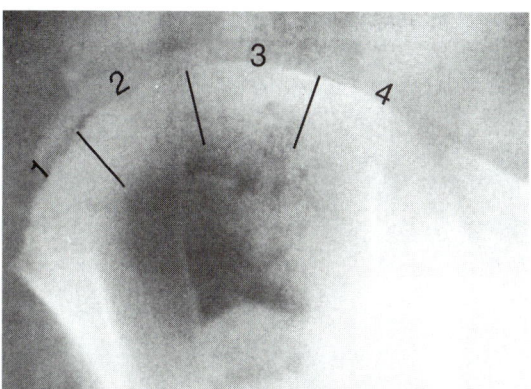

Figure 31.2. Grading the iliac apophysis using the Risser scale.

curve flexibility and are important if brace or surgical treatment is planned.

MRI or CT myelography is used to rule out intraspinal abnormalities in an individual with neurologic abnormalities. A bone scan is ordered when there is pain with scoliosis and a bone tumor or infection is suspected.

The spinal deformity is described by the location of the apex (e.g., thoracic or thoracolumbar) or by a description

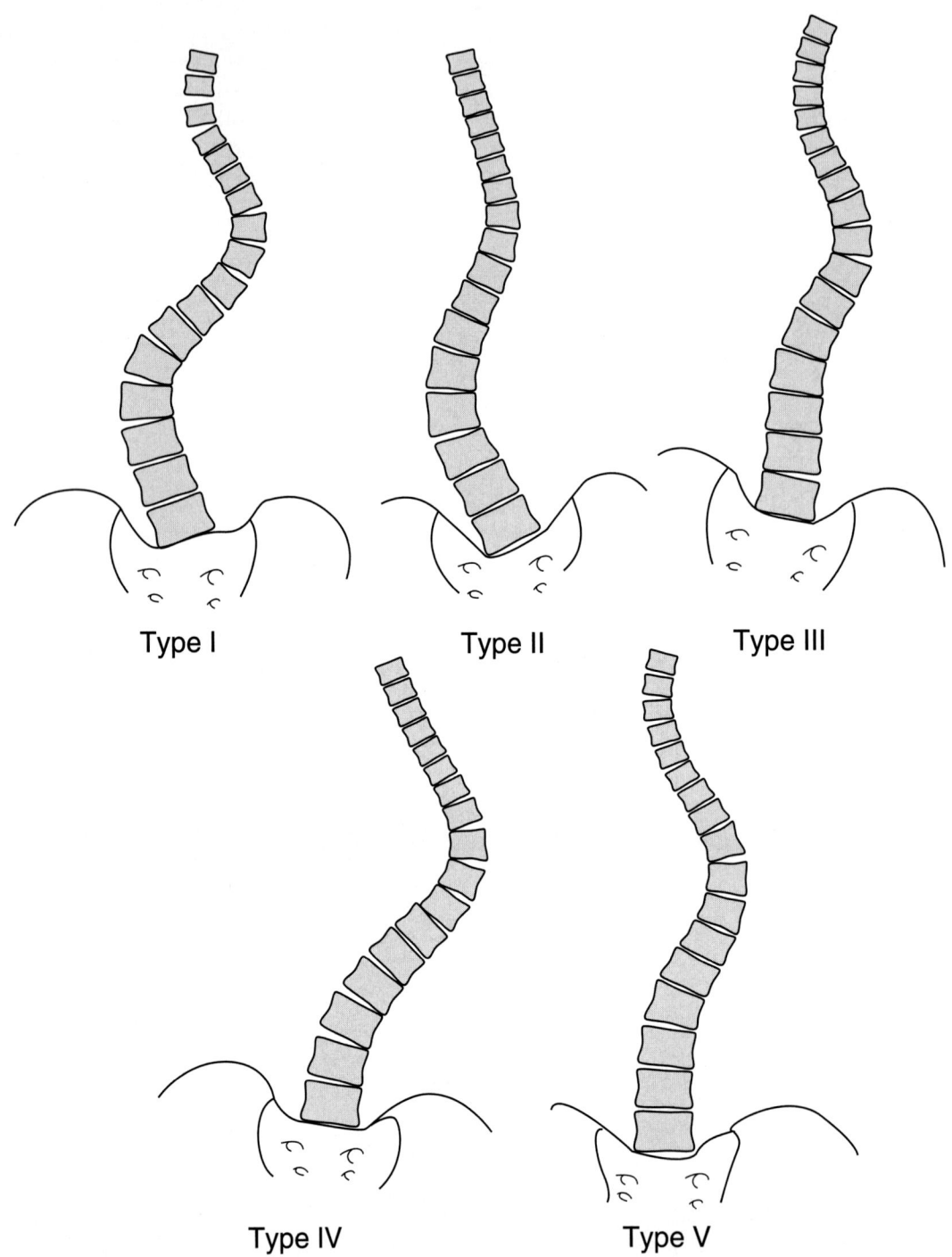

Type I   Type II   Type III

Type IV   Type V

Figure 31.3. King-Moe classification of spinal curves. *Type I curve:* The lumbar curve is larger than the thoracic curve, or the thoracic curve is more flexible than the lumbar curve. *Type II curve:* The thoracic curve is larger than the lumbar curve. The lumbar curve crosses the midline and is more flexible than the thoracic curve on side bending. *Type III curve:* The thoracic curve is larger than the lumbar curve. The lumbar curve does not cross the midline and is much more flexible than the thoracic curve. *Type IV curve:* The thoracic curve is a long curve initiating off a tilted L4. *Type V curve:* A double thoracic curve in which T1 is tilted into the concavity of the upper curve. The lumbar curve may have a type II or III appearance.

of the curve pattern. The King-Moe classification of AIS is universally acknowledged and has been used for determining the levels of fusion in patients requiring surgery (Fig. 31.3) (3).

NATURAL HISTORY

It is imperative that physicians treating patients with scoliosis have a thorough knowledge of the natural course of this condition so that they can offer treatment options that alter the natural history of the disorder in a positive way.

Skeletally Immature Patients

The progression of deformity in a child depends on the amount of growth remaining at the time of diagnosis. A number of parameters have been used to assess growth potential. Essentially, the younger the patient, the lower the Risser stage, and the later the onset of menarche, the greater the risk of progression in the skeletally immature patient. In addition, certain curve factors are associated with progression, including magnitude and location. Thus double-curve patterns, large curves, and thoracic spine curves have a greater tendency to progress.

Skeletally Mature Patients

There are five considerations in the natural history of untreated AIS: back pain (lumbar curvature less than 60°), pulmonary function (thoracic curvature less than 100° or thoracic lordosis), psychologic effects, mortality (more than 100°), and curve progression (1).

Curve Progression

Duriez (5) demonstrated that curves may continue to progress throughout life. The most marked progression was noted in curves of more than 50° at skeletal maturity. In the thoracic curve pattern, the Cobb angle, Mehta angle (less than 20°), and apical vertebral rotation (more than 30%) are important factors in curve progression after maturity. Lumbar curves of more than 30° at maturity generally lead to progression. Right lumbar curves tend to progress twice as often as do left lumbar curves (6).

Scoliosis has not been shown to have a significant effect on pregnancy in terms of delivery and well-being of the fetus. Pregnancy does not cause progression of curvature in patients with spinal deformity (7).

TREATMENT

The aims of treatment are the control of the curve, prevention of progression, avoidance of surgery, and improvement of cosmesis. After AIS is diagnosed, a treatment decision is made (Table 31.2). The three choices of treatment are observation, orthotic treatment, and surgi-

cal treatment. The two most important factors in the treatment decision are the magnitude of the curve and the growth potential of the child. Growth potential is assessed by determining where the child's growth is in relation to the adolescent growth spurt. In general, the onset of the growth spurt coincides with the appearance of secondary sex characteristics: pubic hair development in both sexes and breast budding in girls. Menarche in girls and the appearance of axillary hair in boys occur in the decreased-growth phase. At this time, approximately 18 months of growth remain. The key to successful treatment is early detection.

table	31.2	Treatment Guidelines Based on Curve Pattern and Severity
Curve Magnitude	Active Growth	No Active Growth
0–19°	Observation	Observation, discharge
20–29°	Observation or bracing	Observation
30–39°	Bracing	Observation
>40°	Surgery	Observation or surgery

Data are from King HA, Lonstein JE. Adolescent idiopathic scoliosis: natural history, nonoperative and operative treatment. Paper given at the 62nd Annual Meeting of the American Academy of Orthopaedic Surgeons, Orlando, FL, February 18, 1995.

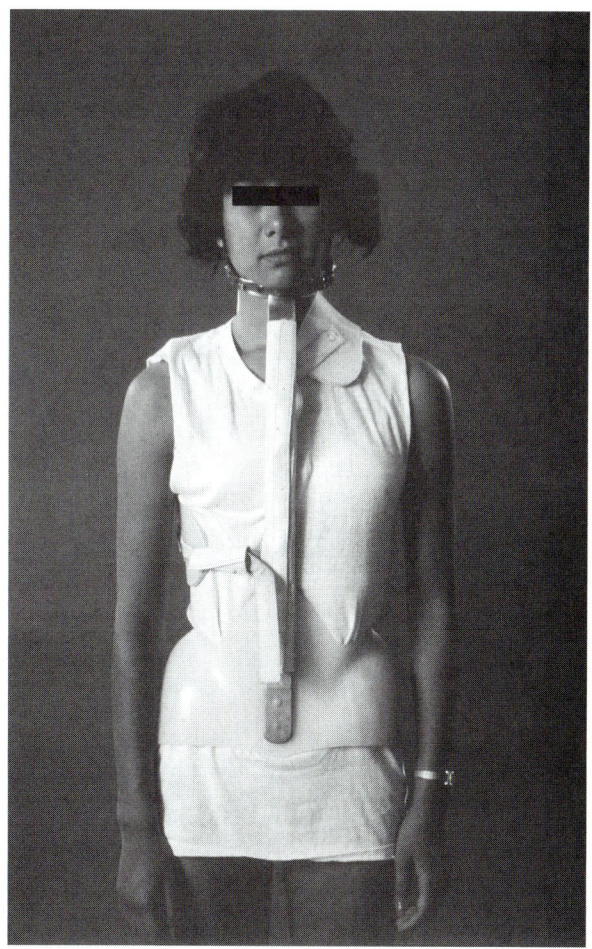

Figure 31.4. Patient in a Milwaukee brace.

Nonoperative Treatment

When observation is the treatment of choice, two questions arise, what constitutes progression? and how often should the curve be evaluated? A minimum change of 6° is significant. A baseline for treatment or follow-up is established with adequate initial assessment of a child and confirmation of the diagnosis of AIS.

BRACING

The efficacy of bracing for AIS was found to be 40% more effective than treatment with observation alone or with electric stimulation (8). In the standard procedure for bracing, the patient wears the brace for 23 h/day until skeletal maturity, at which time the patient is gradually weaned from the brace over a period of several months. The curves generally reach their pretreatment magnitude when the brace treatment has been terminated.

The Milwaukee brace is limited primarily to the treatment of major thoracic curves that have an apex above the level of T7 and of high thoracic and cervicothoracic curve patterns (9) (Figs. 31.4 and 31.5).

Thoracolumbar spinal orthoses (TLSOs) or underarm orthoses were developed during the 1960s and 1970s. The basic concept of these braces is similar; and biomechanically, these braces are completely passive. TLSOs are most effective in patients with thoracic curves that have an apex below the level of T7 and in those with thoracolumbar and lumbar curves (Fig. 31.6). These patients make up the majority of candidates for brace treatment (10).

The problems related to brace treatment are diminished pulmonary function, skin problems, altered renal function, chest cage constriction, and psychologic disturbance. To ameliorate these limitations, part-time bracing regimens have been developed: good results were achieved when patients wore the brace 16 h/day (11).

Operative Treatment

The surgery itself is a spine fusion, the welding together of separate vertebrae into a solid mass of bone. This is done by excision of the facet joints, decortication of the laminae and transverse processes, and the addition of a bone graft. Correction is achieved with some type of internal fixation. After the decision to operate has been made, the surgeon must determine the levels of the spine to be fused and the type of spinal instrumentation to be used (Clinical Table).

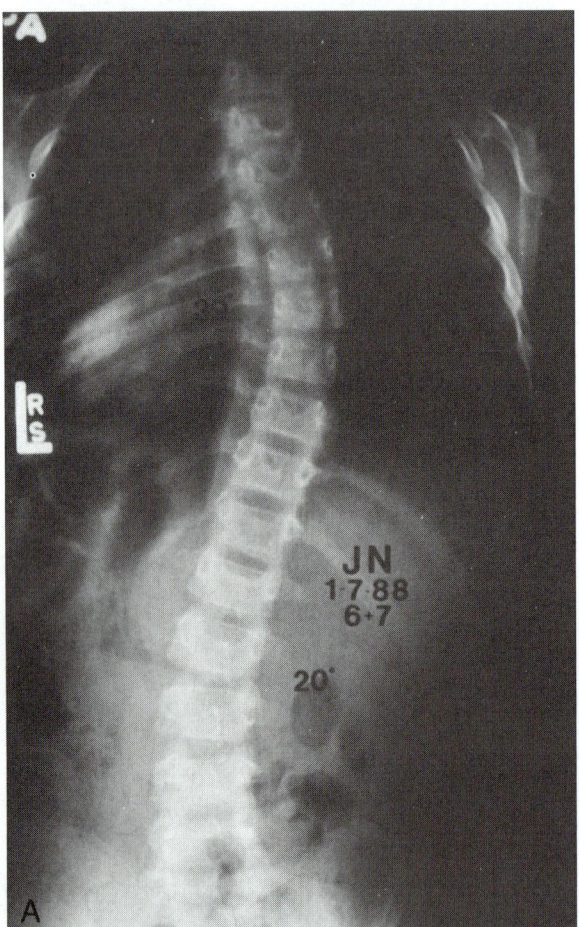
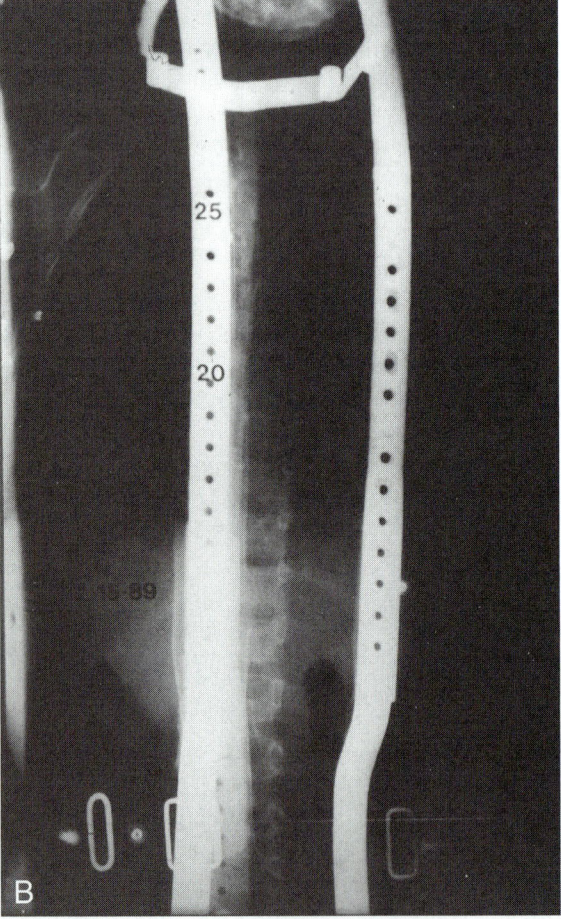

Figure 31.5. Patient with light thoracic scoliosis before (**A**) and after (**B**) correction with a Milwaukee brace.

Clinical Table: Pediatric Deformities of the Spine

Procedure	Indications	Technique	Anatomy	Pitfalls
Posterior subfascial/submuscular rodding without fusion	• Infantile idiopathic scoliosis • Flexible infant or juvenile idiopathic scoliosis or congenital scoliosis	• End vertebral fusion • Subfascial rod placement • Two-rod technique preferred • Lengthening procedure performed every 6 months as needed • Rod exchange every year or when lengthening exceeds rod length	• Spinal muscle dissection • Transverse processes, lamina, and pediatric facet joints	• End vertebral fusion very important; avoid exposure of midvertebral segments • Utilize downsized low-profile hooks for proximal and distal fixation • If supralamina hooks are used, avoid excessive canal intrusion
Posterior spinal fusion in situ without instrumentation	• Stable balanced congenital scoliosis of the cervicothoracic and thoracic spine • Suitable for congenital kyphosis in the very young patient (<5 years old) with <50° kyphosis on hyperextension	• Index curve arthrodesis for scoliosis • Bilteral facet fusion with autologous bone graft • Hyperextension casting may be required for kyphosis patient	• Congenital hemivertebra • Unsegmented bar	• Avoid apex fusion only • Beware of spina bifida and inadvertent canal penetration by instrument
Posterior spinal fusion with instrumentation	• Juvenile and adolescent idiopathic scoliosis • Congenital scoliosis and kyphosis in the adolescent or patient with adequate bone size to receive instrumentation	• Spinal exposure, facet fusion; segmental instrumentation preferred • Dual-rod technique with distal lumbar pedicle screw fixation preferred; rod rotation for double major curves. • Translational correction for severe curves • Thoracoplasty for rib prominence reduction	• Transverse process, lamina, and ligamentum flavum • Epidural space • Spinal pedicles • Costovertebral and costotransverse ligament • Spinal nerve root • Spinal cord	• Identify levels with radiographs • Utilize low-profile instrumentation system (internal and external) to avoid excessive metal in the spinal canal • Take care with sublaminal wire placement to avoid injury to the spinal cord and dura
Anterior spinal fusion with or without instrumentation	• Adolescent thoracolumbar and lumbar scoliosis	• Exposure of intervertebral disc spaces • Segmental vessel ligation • Identify the psoas margin for thoracolumbar and lumbar deformity • Complete discectomy and annular excision • Screw placement in the midvertebral body posterior aspect • Bicorticar screw fixation at each chosen level • Structural grafts to maintain lordosis • Rod rotation to restore lumbar lordosis • Rod rotation before compression	• Intervertebral disc • Segmental vessels • Psoas muscle • Great vessels: aorta and vena cava for lumbar deformity • Spinal canal and neural elements • Anterior longitudinal ligament	• Discectomy must be complete • Spinal canal exposure not necessary • Complete discectomy and end plate decortication • Bicortical screw fixation necessary • Rigid rods preferred: single $\frac{1}{4}$-in or double $\frac{3}{16}$-in rod

continued

Clinical Table: Pediatric Deformities of the Spine (continued)

Procedure	Indications	Technique	Anatomy	Pitfalls
Anterior and posterior spinal fusion with or without instrumentation	• Large curves in immature patients with a potential to crankshaft • Severe curves in the adolescent and juvenile patient	• One-stage anterior and posterior spinal fusion preferred • Lateral decubitus position with convex side up • Total discectomy in the area of the index curve • Autologous bone graft if instrumentation is to be used posteriorly • For posterior procedure, one incision and selection of fusion levels as utilized for adolescent idiopathic scoliosis • Facet fusion, decortication, segmental instrumentation	• Same as for anterior spinal fusion with or without instrumentation	• Same as for anterior spinal fusion with or without instrumentation
Convex anterior and posterior hemiepiphyseodesis and hemiarthrodesis	• Congenital scoliosis • Fully segmental thoracolumbar or lumbar hemivertebra in a young patient < 5 years of age • Curve 60° with no kyphosis	• Anterior approach with convex side up • Convex half of the apex, intervertebral disc, and the index curve • Posterior convex fusion only	• Intervertebral discs • Segmental vessels • Vertebral body • Lamina • Transverse processes	• Do not approach concave side anteriorly or posteriorly • Do not utilize procedure for patient with associated kyphosis
Hemivertebral excision and wedge resection	• Rigid decompensated congenital scoliosis • Fully segmented lumbar and lumbosacral hemivertebra	• Hemivertebral, vertebral bodies, intervertebral discs, segmental vessels, great vessels of the lumbar and lumbosacral spine	• Anterior and posterior hemivertebral excision with the convex side approach for the anterior and posterior procedures • Instrumentation optional for larger patients • Early excision preferred	• Preferred procedure for lumbosacral and lumbar fully segmented hemivertebra • Complete vertebral body resection to avoid inadvertent entry of retropulsed fragments into spine

Subfascial or subcutaneous rods can occasionally be used without fusion in the very young child; however, all instrumentation methods are accompanied by fusion of all instrumented levels. Like other mechanical devices, spinal instrumentation will fatigue and break or eventually become displaced in the absence of spinal fusion (Fig. 31.7). The goal of spinal instrumentation and fusion is safe and lasting curve correction with restitution or maintenance of trunk balance.

Preoperative considerations include medications, pulmonary evaluation, and blood transfusion (autologous blood, intraoperative cell saver). It is best to avoid inhalation agents such as halothane and isoflurane if the surgery will include spinal cord monitoring using the technique of evoked potentials. Hypotensive anesthesia has been used to reduce blood loss. There is also a technique for reduction of red cell mass, called the acute normovolemic hemodilution method (12).

Perhaps the most common method of spinal cord monitoring involves the so-called Stagnara wake-up test. The anesthesia is decreased after correcting the spinal deformity to bring the patient to a conscious level. The patient is asked to move both lower extremities before the surgical procedure is completed. Once movement is noted, anesthesia is returned to appropriate levels, and the surgical procedure continues. The somatosensory evoked potential monitoring system can alert the surgeon to evolving spinal cord injury.

SURGICAL APPROACH

There are three approaches for spinal surgery. The anterior approach is used when correcting thoracolumbar

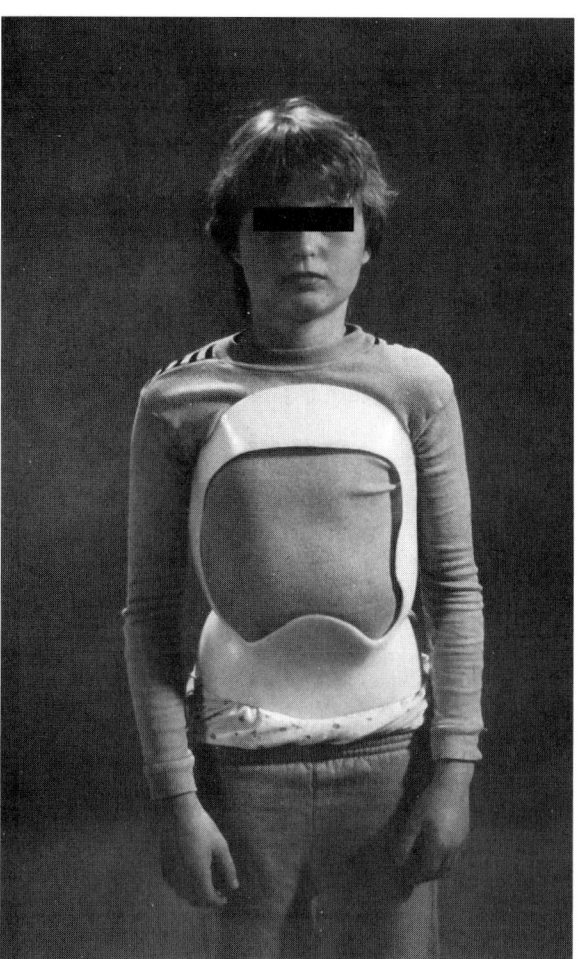

Figure 31.6. Patient in a TLSO used to treat a right thoracic scoliosis.

and lumbar curves, and the posterior approach can be used for all curves. The combined anterior and posterior approach is used for severe curves (more than 80°), curves with a kyphosis component greater than 50°, and curves that need an anterior release. The combined approach is also used when there is concern about pseudarthrosis and crankshaft phenomenon (in younger patients with a Risser scale score less than 1) (13). A posterior fusion in the presence of an intact anterior growth obligates the spine to a progressive lordoscoliosis with rotation in the direction of the original rotatory deformity (14).

Posterior Approach

For the posterior approach, the prone position is used, with no pressure on the abdomen and bony prominences. The hip should be extended to allow a physiologic lordotic posture in the lumbar spine. The posterior approach is done in the usual fashion by making a straight incision in the midline. Thorough subperiosteal dissection is performed to expose the segments being fused. The facet joints are excised, the laminae and transverse processes are decorticated, and graft is added. An autologous bone

graft is the best option, but there are many bone substitutes (allograft, ceramic, bovine, etc.). The method of application depends on the type of instrumentation being employed.

Anterior Approach

The incision for the anterior approach to the spine is generally on the convex side of the scoliosis. In the chest area, the incision should be along the rib leading to the superior vertebra to be fused. If the vertebrae to be fused are at the T10 level or above, a posterolateral thoracotomy is sufficient; but if the vertebral fusion level extends to T11–L1, the thoracotomy should be combined with a retroperitoneal approach and diaphragmatic detachment. The L1–5 levels are reached readily by a retroperitoneal approach.

When the spine is exposed, the next step is complete disc removal to the posterior annulus. The cartilaginous end plate should be removed, and attention should be directed to the posterior lateral corner of the disc and the annulus. This area should be released to facilitate derotation and lordization of the spine. The vertebral body screws are then placed, beginning with the apical vertebra and progressing to each end of the curve; the screws are directed in a posteroanterior direction. The apical screw should be placed as far as possible, and the starting point at each successive screw is moved slightly anterior to the previous one. Bone graft should be placed between the vertebral bodies. Beginning with the apical screw, the vertebral screws are then compressed until the end plates are parallel. Because of the potential risk of injury to the common iliac vessels by the instrumentation, it is recommended that anterior instrumentation not be used distal to L4.

SELECTION OF FUSION LEVELS

The selection of levels to be fused is different for the anterior and posterior procedures. The choice of specific fusion levels is based on the identification of the curves to be fused. Other factors, such as presence of shoulder or trunk imbalance, also are considered. The decision is based on standing AP films, side bending films, and (sometimes) traction films.

King-Moe Classification

The King-Moe type I curve is the only curve that necessitates a fusion to L3 or L4 (Figure 31.3). The remaining curves generally can be fused at the thoracic curve only. The lower level of fusion is selected by creating a line perpendicular to the iliac crest that bisects the midline of the sacrum. This line is called the center sacral line or center gravity line. The lower extension of fusion should include all measured segments of the curve to the vertebra most closely bisected by the center sacral line (stable vertebra). The surgeon must be careful not to correct the thoracic curve beyond the flexibility of the lumbar curve.

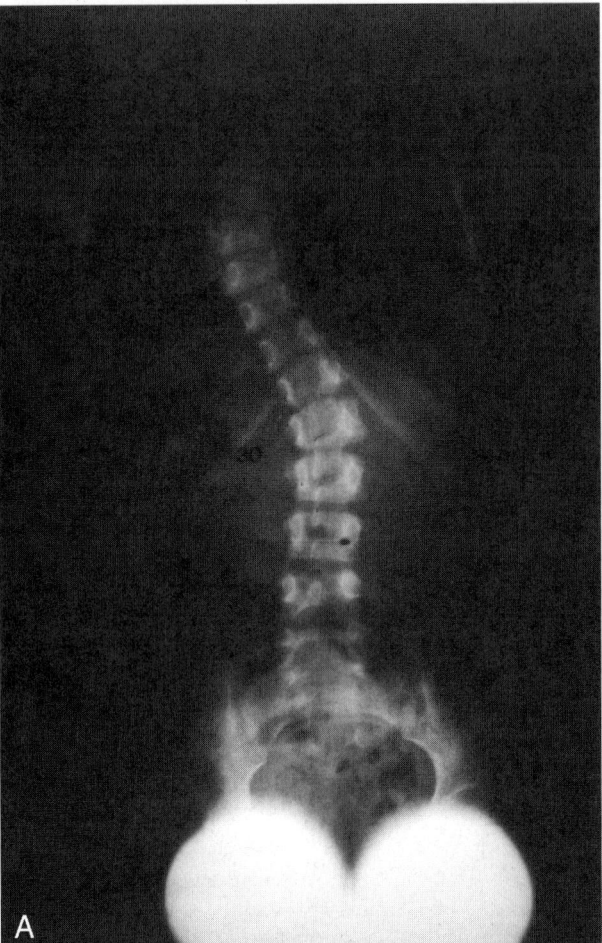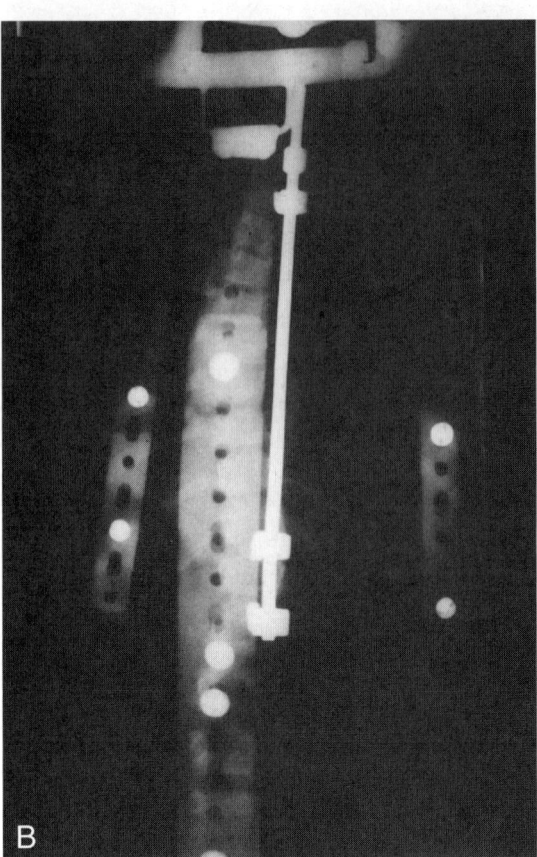

Figure 31.7. **A.** Four-year-old with idiopathic scoliosis. **B.** Postoperative view showing the placement of a subcutaneous rod and brace application.

A decompensated spine may be the result of overcorrecting the thoracic curve. Trunk decompensation in type II curves has been a problem seen by many authors. Ibrahim and Benson (15) established subtypes A and B for the type II pattern. Type IIA is characterized by a lumbar curve of less than 35° that corrects more than 70% on side bending. The apical lumbar vertebral body touches the center sacral line, and the lumbosacral fractional curve measures 12° or less. The type IIB curve has a lumbar curve of more than 35°; the flexibility of this curve is less than 70%. The apical lumbar vertebra extends beyond the sacral center line, and the lumbosacral curve measures more than 12°. Type IIB tends to be unbalanced, unless the inferior end is extended to the horizontal lumbar disc. These large, less flexible curves may not be able to adapt to the amount of thoracic correction obtained at surgery (16).

For the double thoracic, or type V, curve the patient must have a balanced correction. The term *positive* T1 *tilt* indicates a full (not fractional) high left curve. Both curves must always be fused. If the left shoulder is elevated on presentation or if a left trapezial prominence is observed, then the high left curve must be included in the fusion (17).

Thoracolumbar and Lumbar Scoliosis

Thoracolumbar and lumbar curves are not included in the King-Moe classification, and surgical treatment is dictated by the pattern and flexibility of the primary curve, compensatory curves, or both. Anterior instrumentation for AIS is limited to the treatment of thoracolumbar (T12–L1 apex) and lumbar curves because of anatomic constraints. In general, the fusion levels for curves treated anteriorly consist only of those vertebrae that are structural components of the curve. This method assumes that the compensatory curve above and the fractional curve below are flexible.

The authors' preferred method of selecting fusion levels includes thoracolumbar and lumbar curves of less than 60° in adolescents or young adults. For the apex vertebra, fusion includes one level above and one below the apex. If the apex falls at the disc space, fusion includes two levels above and two levels below the apex. Emphasis is placed on overcorrection.

The structural vertebrae of these curves are identified using supine side bending radiographs to determine which vertebrae continue to define the curve. Contraindications include associated kyphosis (18).

INSTRUMENTATION

Posterior Instrumentation

Posterior instrumentation includes three types:

- First generation: Harrington and modified versions
- Second generation: Luque and modified versions
- Third generation: Cotrel-Dubousset and modified versions

Cotrel-Dubousset instrumentation. The Cotrel-Dubousset (CD) rod system, introduced in 1985, emphasizes the three-dimensional correction of scoliosis. The CD system uses two identical rods, multiple open or closed hooks (laminar or pedicle) on each rod, pedicle screws for the lumbar spine, and two or more cross-linking devices. The scoliosis is corrected by a combination of initial longitudinally applied forces with a subsequent rod/vertebral rotation, which converts the scoliosis to either thoracic kyphosis or lumbar lordosis.

The side with concavity in the thoracic region and convexity in the lumbar region is the first side to be instrumented. As the contoured rod is rotated from a lateral curvature position to a contour in the sagittal plane, the scoliosis is corrected. The rod should appear straight when seen from posterior to anterior. The second rod is contoured in the sagittal plane and inserted, with little further scoliosis correction needed in most cases.

The principal advantages of this system are versatility, ability to preserve sagittal alignment, and slightly improved rotational correction (19). For curves of more than 75°, however, the residual spine curve may be of such magnitude that it is difficult to contour a single rod into the desired sagittal curve position. In such instances, multiple rods on the concavity with transverse connectors are used. Size and cost must also be considered. The reported incidence of neurologic complication with the CD system was 3 times that reported by those using other posterior systems (20). Overcorrection of the thoracic curve in type II curves tended to transmit rotational forces into the lumbar curve and aggravate the lumbar deformity, resulting in coronal plane decompensation. No postoperative brace is necessary.

Isola instrumentation. Isola instrumentation allows for correction of deformity in the coronal, sagittal, and axial planes (Fig. 31.8). The Isola concept emphasizes torsional correction of major scoliotic (torsional) deformities; the system employs segmental instrumentation via the use of hooks, wires, and distal lumbar pedicle screw placement to a prebent, anatomically contoured rod. Because of multiple fixation points, no cast or brace is required after surgery. The Isola instrumentation can correct deformities that are greater than 60%. These instrumentation sequences involve three-dimensional analysis of biplanar radiographs (Fig. 31.9).

End instrumented vertebral selection. The upper instrumented vertebra should be midway between the sides of the rib cage and have a normal sagittal and transverse plane angular position. It is usually one or two vertebrae above the upper end vertebra for major thoracic curves but is the upper end vertebra for double thoracic and compensatory thoracic curves. For single and double thoracic curves, the lower instrumented vertebra is usually one below the lower end vertebra but may be the end (double thoracic) or two below (single thoracic). It should not have transverse plane angulation (less than 10°) and should be the stable vertebra following the instrumentation. In the sagittal plane, the upper end vertebra is the first vertebra above a normal intersegmental alignment.

Anterior Instrumentation

The principal advantage of anterior instrumentation is the possibility of fusing fewer segments than is necessary with a posterior approach. Anterior spinal instrumentation and fusion for scoliosis treatment is used for flexible thoracolumbar and upper lumbar curves (T12, L1, and L2 apex) and as the initial stage of a two-stage anterior and posterior procedure. The contraindications are kyphosis above the planned upper instrumentation level and a compensatory curve that does not correct to 20° on supine lateral bending films.

Anterior instrumentation functions as a compression device that is applied to the convexity of the curve. The instrumentation should include all levels that have a wider disc space on the curve convexity as seen on preoperative bending radiographs. If the regional apex (the most laterally displaced portion of the Cobb curve) is a vertebra, then the apex vertebra and one vertebra above and below are instrumented. If the regional apex is a disc, instrumentation is applied to two vertebrae above and below the apex. There are many anterior instrumentation systems, including Dwyer, Zielke, TSRH, and Isola (Fig. 31.10).

Zielke instrumentation. The implants in the Zielke system include screws that are used to attach half-staples or washers to the vertebral body and a solid rod, fitted with hexagonal nuts, that passes through the screw heads to obtain and hold correction. Correction has been excellent, with 60 to 80% curve correction and 40 to 50% rotational correction. The primary potential problem, despite the use of anterior bone blocks, is localized kyphosis at the site of fusion. Rod breakage has been reported in obese individuals.

THORACOPLASTY

In patients who have significant rib prominence (rib hump greater than 3 cm and scoliometer measurement greater than 15°), thoracoplasty, or rib resection, can be performed to reduce it and provide bone graft (21). The midline incision can be used by elevating a skin flap by subcutaneous dissection. The ribs are exposed subperiosteally in a circumferential fashion. Every attempt is made not to violate the periosteum on the anterior surface of the rib, so that the pleural space is not entered. The wound is checked for hemostasis and for any violation of the pleura. If a pleural leak occurs, the defect is identified and closed with sutures. A chest drain connected to an underwater seal is inserted.

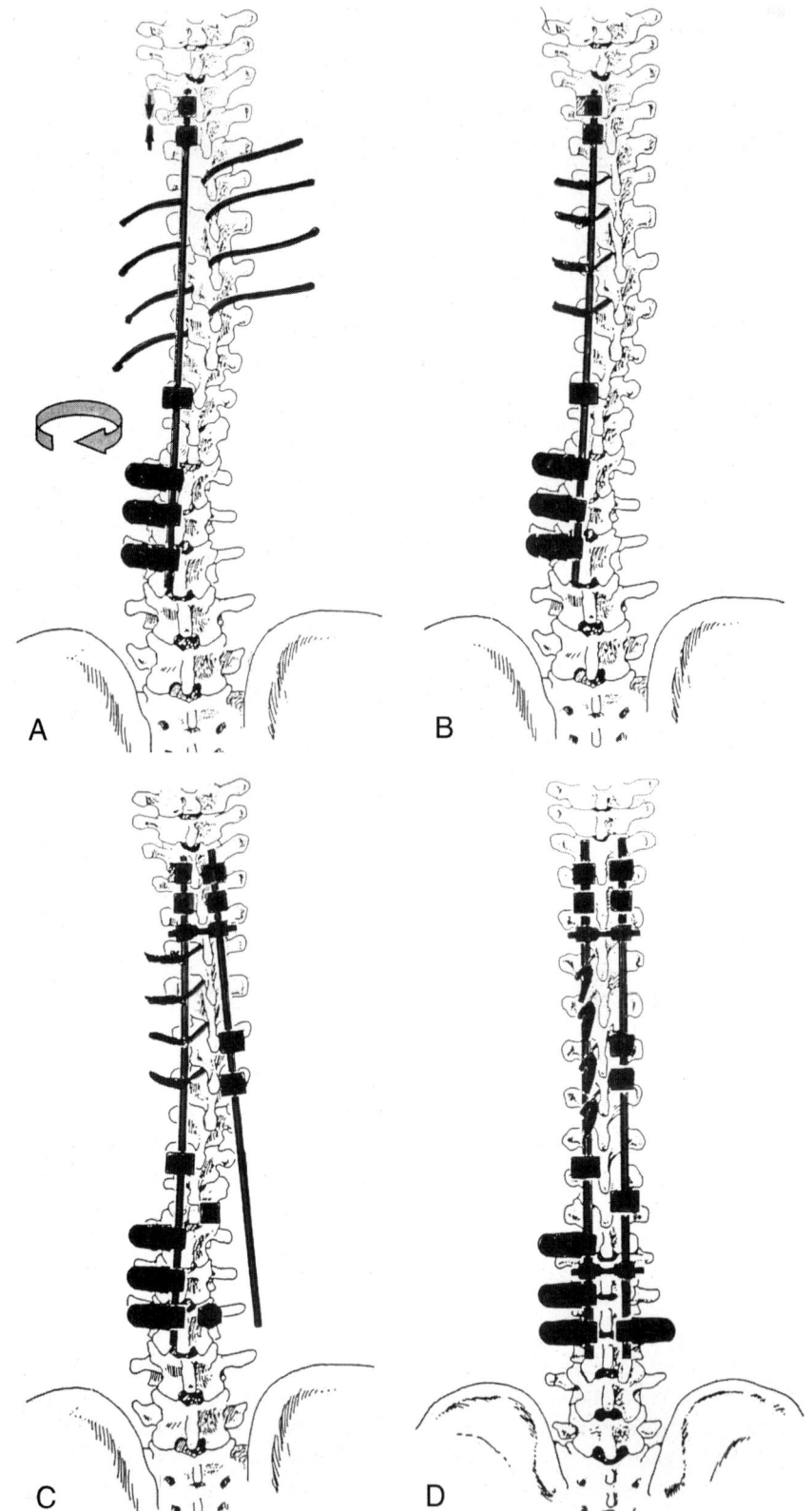

A

B

C

D

Figure 31.8. **A.** In the Isola instrumentation sequence, the left rod is placed and rotated (*arrow*) to correct the lumbar rotational deformity. Sublaminar wires are then introduced. **B.** The right thoracic concave wire is tightened for posteromedial translation and correction of the thoracic deformity. Note the anatomically contoured rod is placed without regard to the coronal plane deformity. **C.** The right rod is placed, and the transverse connector is set to obtain the proximal foundation. **D.** The distal end of the right rod is set. Finally, left convex compression and distal right lumbar distraction are performed to force the last instrumented vertebra into the horizontal plane.

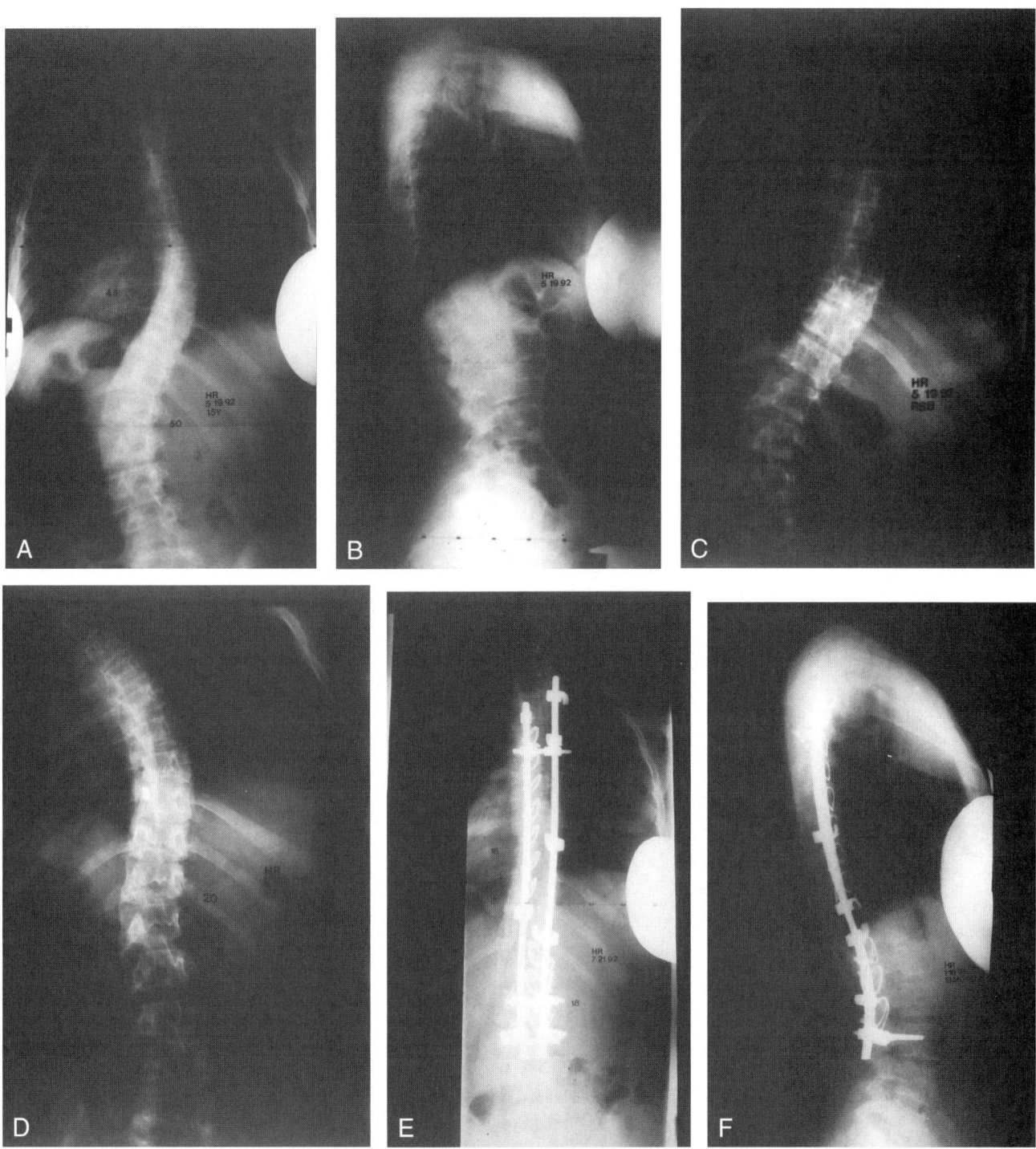

Figure 31.9. Preoperative AP (**A**) and lateral (**B**) views of a patient with a double thoracic lumbar scoliosis. The right side bending view (**C**) shows flexibility of the right thoracic curve; the left side bending view (**D**) shows flexibility of the lumbar curve. Postoperative AP (**E**) and lateral (**F**) views showing sagittal plane alignment.

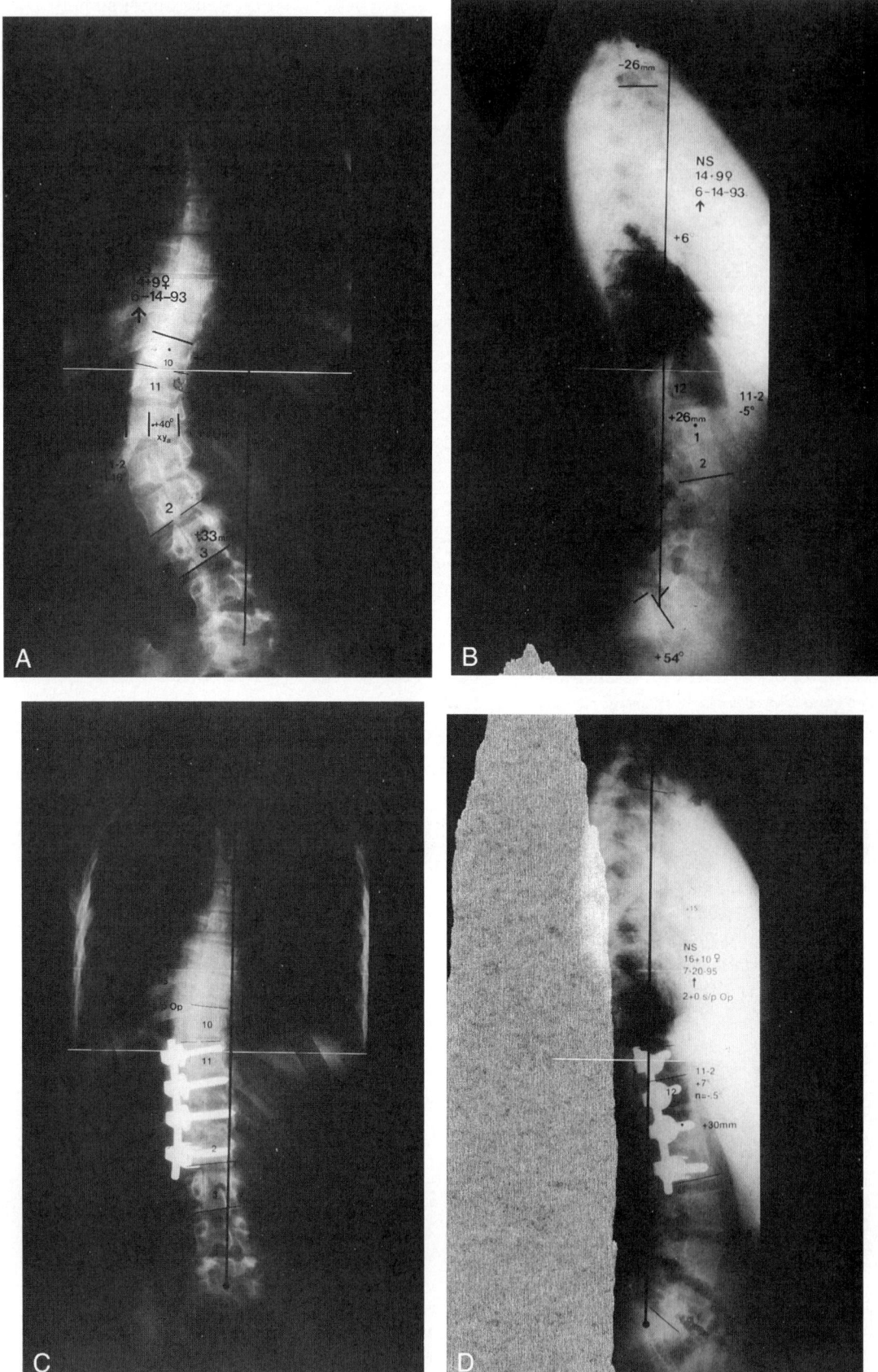

Figure 31.10. Preoperative AP (**A**) and lateral (**B**) views of a patient with a single left thoracolumbar scoliosis. Postoperative AP (**C**) and lateral (**D**) views showing the anterior instrumentation for the screw construct at T11–L2 and the maintenance of the lumbar lordosis. Figure courtesy of Marc Asher.

Complications and Pitfalls

EARLY COMPLICATIONS

Neurologic injury during surgery occurs in less than 1% (probably less than 0.5%) of patients undergoing instrumentation (20). Injury may occur by inadvertent entry of surgical instruments into the spinal canal, but neurologic injury is most likely to occur during the time of instrument correction of the scoliosis. Because rates of recovery from iatrogenic neurologic injury are better if the implants are removed within 2 to 3 h of the onset of neurologic problems, spinal cord monitoring should lead to earlier detection of neurologic injury and an increased chance of reversibility.

The rate of postoperative wound infection is less than 1%. If a wound infection is diagnosed, the wound is opened widely and thorough irrigation and débridement are performed. The implants and the majority of the bone graft are left in, and the wound is closed over subfascial and subcutaneous suction drains.

Patients who require two-stage corrective procedures may become malnourished as a result of the limited oral caloric intake associated with closely spaced major surgical procedures. Some surgeons have advocated use of parenteral hyperalimentation immediately after the first procedure. The combined anterior-posterior procedure performed during the same anesthesia session has been shown to decrease the problem of malnutrition and associated complications, especially wound healing (22).

At the time of subperiosteal posterior spine exposure, the pleura may be opened inadvertently, especially between the thoracic spine transverse processes on the concave side of the scoliosis. The pleura also may be opened during the thoracoplasty. Observation is appropriate if the pneumothorax is less than 10 to 20%, but chest tube insertion is needed for a larger pneumothorax.

A dural tear may occur at the time of ligamentum flavum removal or at the time of hook or wire insertion. Repair of all dural tears should be attempted using 5–0 or 6–0 Prolene suture. If the tear is large, freeze-dried dura, muscle augmentation, or cryoprecipitate can be used to facilitate repair.

Some instrumentations produce torsional changes in the instrumented and uninstrumented spine that could result in spinal imbalance. King-Moe type II curves have a greater risk of imbalance. Spinal imbalance after this type of instrumentation can be reduced by avoiding overcorrection and by including mobile transition segments.

The surgeon must be careful to choose the correct levels for fusion. There are three methods for identifying the correct vertebral levels: (a) identification of the lowest rib by palpation, (b) identification of the sacrum by visual inspection, and (c) identification of the vertebrae by radiographic examination.

The syndrome of inappropriate secretion of antidiuretic hormone (SIADH) is characterized by a decline in urinary output on the evening after surgery. If serum and urine osmolality are both elevated, the patient is likely to be hypovolemic, but if the serum osmolality is diminished and the urine osmolality is elevated, SIADH should be diagnosed and fluid overload avoided (14).

LATE COMPLICATIONS

The pseudarthrosis rate is approximately 1%. The fusion should be solid by 6 months after surgery. If there is continued loss of correction after this time or if pain is present in the fusion area, nonunion should be suspected. A fusion tomography may be useful in the diagnosis.

Two major factors appear to lead to back pain: fusion below the level of L4 and elimination of lumbar lordosis at the time of instrumentation and fusion. If instrumentation and fusion eliminate the physiologic lumbar lordosis, disability and unsightly posture result. Prevention of this malalignment is most important; if present, the only treatment is extension osteotomy of the fusion mass, usually at the second or third lumbar level.

Two other late complications are rod or wire breakage and kyphosis above the instrumentation. With the modern systems, the creation of a kyphosis postoperatively stopping the fusion at the T12 level is not a problem as long as there was no true kyphosis preoperatively (14).

SUMMARY

Scoliosis is a physical finding. The diagnosis must be determined; and the clinician must record the severity and flexibility of the deformity and the state of growth and maturation of the child. Scoliosis is a three-dimensional abnormality, and the clinician must be familiar with the normal three-dimensional range of spinal curvature and alignment when analyzing biplanar radiographs.

It is imperative that the physician treating patients with scoliosis have a complete knowledge of the natural course of the disease so they can offer treatment options that alter the natural history of the disorder in a positive way. The younger the patient, the lower the Risser stage, and the later the onset of the menarche, the greater risk of progression in the skeletally immature patient. In addition, certain curve factors are associated with progression, including magnitude and location.

The aims of treatment are to control the curve, prevent progression, avoid surgery, and improve cosmesis. The three choices of treatment are observation, nonsurgical treatment (orthosis), and surgical treatment. The two most important factors in treatment decisions are the magnitude of the curve and the growth potential of the child.

The spinal approach for the surgical treatment may be anterior, posterior, or a combined anterior and posterior approach. Thoracoplasty reduces significant rib prominence and provides bone graft for the spine fusion.

II Congenital Spinal Deformity

Congenital deformities are those caused by specific anomalies of vertebral development. The three major patterns of congenital spinal deformity are lordosis, kyphosis, and scoliosis. These anomalies are present at birth, and the curve may be present then or develop later. Females tend to progress more than males, thoracic curves tend to progress more than lumbar curves (23).

RELEVANT ANATOMY AND PATHOGENESIS

Congenital scoliosis or congenital kyphosis results from vertebral malformation and is classified as being caused by failure of formation, failure of segmentation, or mixed anomalies.

Congenital spinal anomalies are divided into two basic groups: defects of formation and defects of segmentation (Fig. 31.11). A classic example of a defect of formation is a hemivertebra that has a mobile disc both caudal and cephalad to it (a so-called free hemivertebra). A classic example of a defect of segmentation is a unilateral unsegmented bar in which one side of the spine has failed to segment over the length of several vertebrae while the other side has segmented normally (23). Although congenital scoliosis can be caused by a defect of formation or by a defect of segmentation, combined defects are by far the most common.

Generally, 25% of the curves do not progress, 25% progress slowly, and 50% progress severely. The propensity for progression is related especially to the type of anomaly but also to the rate of growth of the patient (24). The most progressive of all lesions is the unilateral unsegmented bar on the concavity with a hemivertebra on the convexity (Table 31.3). This type of curve can progress at a rate of 10° to 12° a year. Next in severity is the unilateral bar, followed by double-convex hemivertebrae. A single hemivertebra may or may not cause a progressive curvature, depending on whether there is balanced or unbalanced growth potential. Curves progress because of growth imbalance, and they progress more rapidly during rapid growth (ages 0 to 3 and during the pubertal growth spurt). The most important step in the evaluation of these patients is to estimate whether the spine is balanced and will remain balanced during growth; the greater the potential growth discrepancy between the two sides, the greater the likelihood that the deformity will progress (24). It is very important to know whether a curve is progressing. This determination depends on accurate and precise monitoring, both clinically and radiographically. The clinician should examine the child every 6 months, checking that the shoulders are level, the pelvis is balanced, the curve is unchanged, and there is no sign of decompensation.

Embryologically, these anomalies must develop between the 5th and 8th weeks of gestation. A positive family history of congenital spinal deformity is rare; however, hereditary congenital scoliosis has been described by several investigators (25).

INITIAL FINDINGS, PHYSICAL EXAMINATION, AND DIAGNOSIS

There is a frequent association of congenital deformities with other anomalies. These may be either inside or outside the spine. The most common associated lesion is spinal dysraphism, a group of conditions currently considered to include any congenital anomaly of the neural axis. Diastematomyelia, in which the midline structures have fused but a spike of bone projects anteriorly from a fused vertebral arch, is an example of spinal dysraphism. Other spinal abnormalities include Arnold-Chiari malformation,

| table | 31.3 | Rate of Deterioration Without Treatment for Congenital Scoliosis[a] |

	Type of Congenital Anomaly					
			Hemivertebra			
Site of Curvature	Block Vertebrae	Wedged Vertebrae	Single	Double	Unilateral Unsegmented Bar	Unilateral Unsegmented Bar and Contralateral Hemivertebrae
Upper thoracic	<1°–1°	*–2°	1°–2°	2°–2.5°	2°–4°	5°–6°
Lower thoracic	<1°–1°	2°–2°	2°–2.5°	2°–3°	5°–6.5°	6°–7°
Thoracolumbar	<1°–1°	1.5°–2°	2°–3.5°	5°–*	6°–9°	>10°–*
Lumbar	<1°–*	<1°–*	<1°–1°	*	>5°–*	*
Lumbosacral	*	*	<1°–1.5°	*	*	*

Reprinted with permission from McMaster MJ, Ohtsuka K. The natural history of congenital scoliosis: a study of 251 patients. J Bone Joint Surg 1982;64A:1144.
Open outline, no treatment required; *shaded,* may require spinal fusion; *solid outline,* requires spinal fusion;*, too few or no curves.
[a]Median yearly rate of deterioration (in degrees) without treatment for each type of single congenital scoliosis in each region of the spine (all patients). The numbers on the left in each column refer to patients who were seen before the age of 10 years; the numbers on the right refer to patients who were seen at or after the age of 10 years.

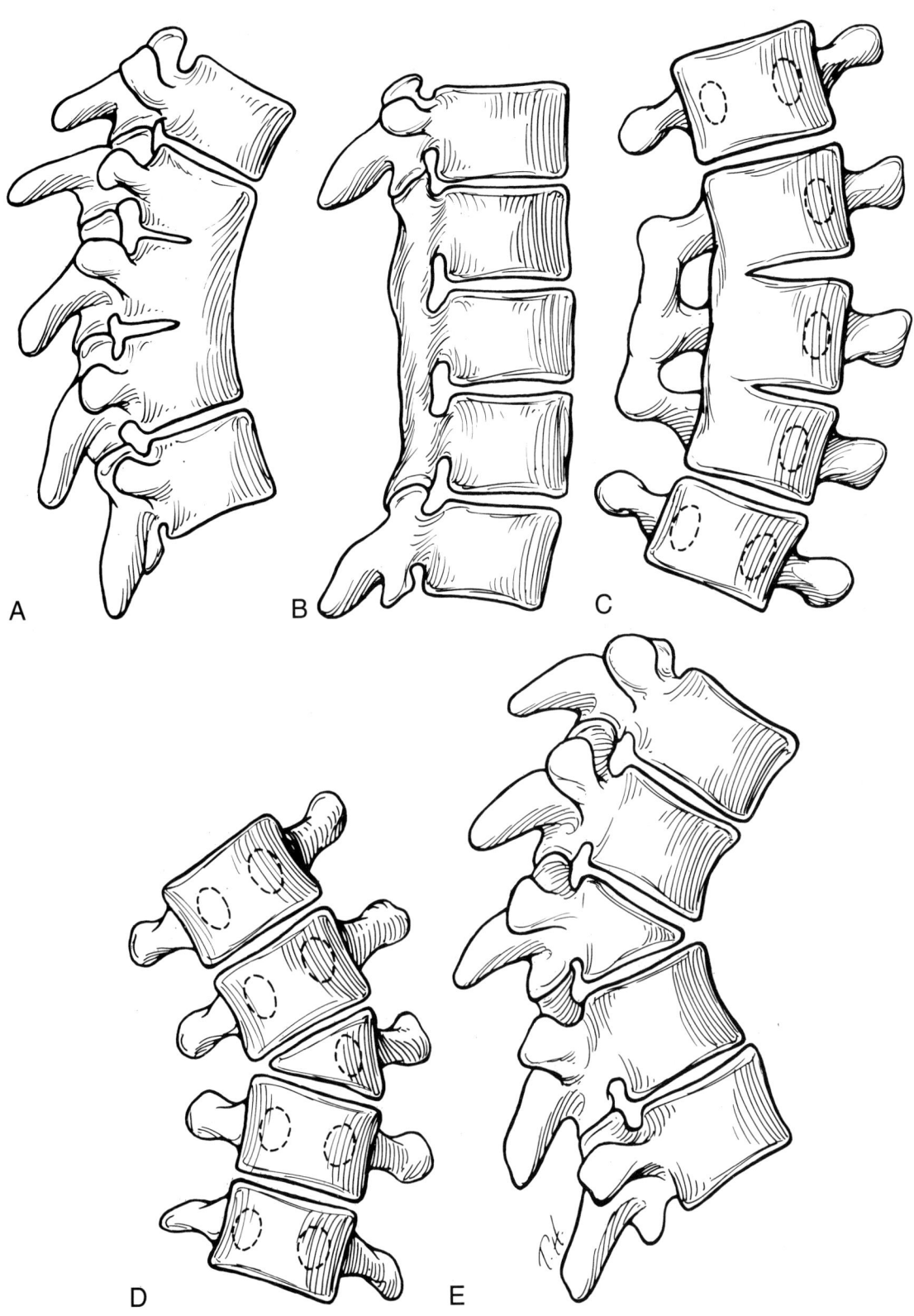

Figure 31.11. **A.** Anterior failure of segmentation leads to kyphosis. **B.** Posterior failure of segmentation leads to lordosis. **C.** Lateral failure of segmentation leads to scoliosis. **D.** Lateral failure of formation leads to scoliosis. **E.** Anterior failure of formation leads to kyphosis.

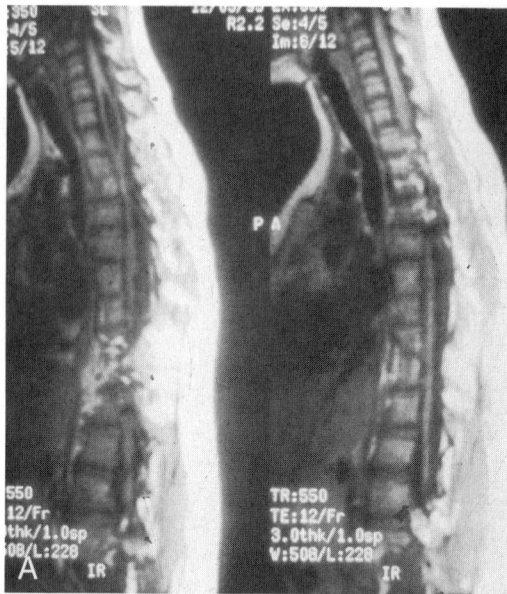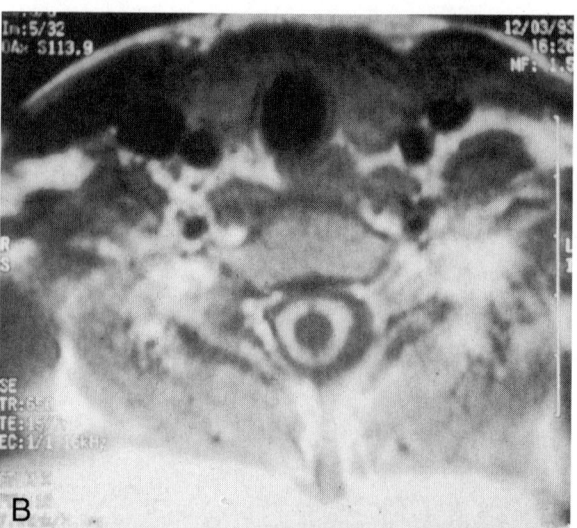

Figure 31.12. Preoperative MRI study of a patient with thoracic scoliosis showing a cervical syringomyelia.

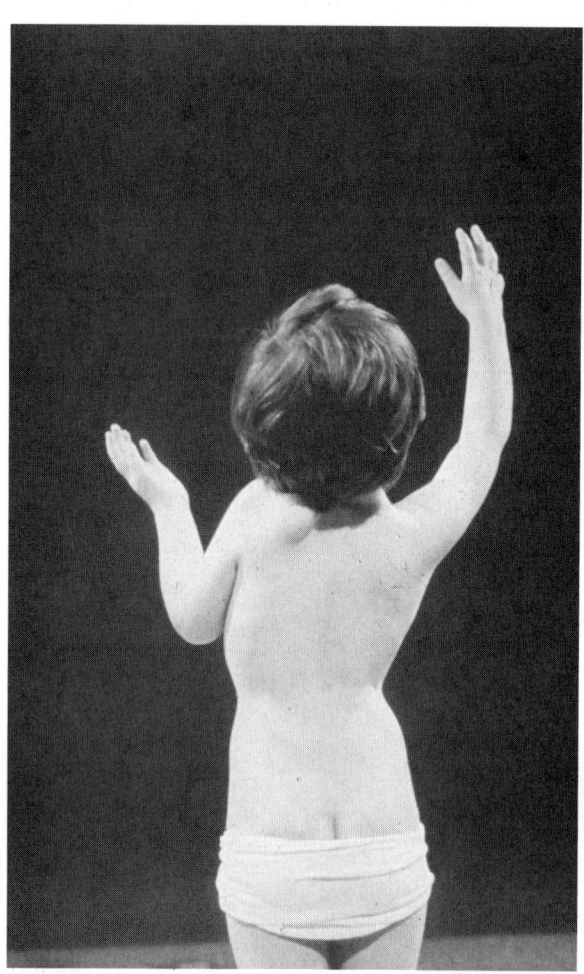

Figure 31.13. Patient with cervicothoracic congenital scoliosis associated with frank Sprengel's deformity. Note the inability to elevate the left upper extremity. Figure courtesy of Robert B. Winter.

syringomyelia, diplomyelia, and intraspinal tumors. These lesions may be associated with a cutaneous hairy patch, a nevus, or a detectable neurologic deficit (Fig. 31.12).

Anomalies of the genitourinary system occur in 20 to 30% of congenital scoliosis patients. Cardiac anomalies are less frequent but must be detected (24). Extremity anomalies include amelia, absent digits, radial club hand, and congenital elevation of the shoulder (Sprengel's deformity). A child with one foot smaller than the other has a dysraphic neural axis until proven otherwise (Fig. 31.13).

Congenital lordosis is the least common of the three major patterns of congenital spinal deformity and is caused by a defect of segmentation posteriorly in the presence of active growth anteriorly. The deformity associated with congenital lordosis is usually progressive. When the deformity occurs in the thoracic spine, it inevitably produces respiratory compromise, and early death can result (26). When the deformity occurs in the lumbar spine, it results in hyperlordosis, with the spine approaching the anterior abdominal wall.

Congenital kyphosis is the result of posterior growth continuing in the absence of anterior growth. The more severe the anterior defect, the more progressive the deformity. A defect of segmentation tends to produce a round kyphosis rather than a sharp angular gibbus; thus paraplegia is rarely a problem (27). The main clinical symptom, apart from the visible deformity, is low back pain caused by the necessary compensatory hyperlordosis. The deformity tends to progress slowly.

Congenital kyphosis with a defect of formation has a much worse prognosis. Paraplegia resulting from the natural progression of the lesion is a very real possibility (28,29). In North America, congenital kyphosis is the most common cause of paraplegia arising from spinal deformity. Paralysis can occur at any age but is most common during the pubertal growth spurt, when the deformity progresses suddenly.

RADIOLOGIC STUDIES

Congenital scoliosis is more difficult to measure than either idiopathic or neuromuscular scoliosis, since the radiographs often do not show the vertebral end plates clearly (Fig. 31.14). At every visit, the current radiograph should be compared with both the previous and the original radiograph. Tomography is useful in defining bony anatomy. Congenital scoliosis patients should also be examined via renal sonography or intravenous pyelography, ECG, and echocardiography to rule out any abnormalities.

TREATMENT

The treatment of congenital lordosis is purely operative. Bracing cannot halt the progression of this deformity. There are two types of operations: one for stabilization and the other for correction. The stabilizing operation can be done when the surgeon has the opportunity to see the patient before major deformity (and loss of pulmonary function) has developed. An arthrodesis of the entire involved area and one or two vertebrae cephalad and caudal to the lesion must be done (Clinical Table).

The corrective operation is done when the patient has a major deformity and, usually, a substantial loss of pulmonary function (30). The goal is to improve not only spinal alignment but also pulmonary function. The entire area of deformity must be approached both anteriorly and posteriorly. Through the anterior approach, the discs should be completely excised, as should the wedges of bone cephalad and caudal to them. The posterior portion of the operation consists of multiple osteotomies of the laminar synostosis, performed at the same levels from which the discs were excised anteriorly. Sublaminar wires are then passed and twisted over a kyphotically contoured, stiff rod, and are tightened gradually, to correct the lordosis.

Congenital kyphosis must be treated operatively. Defects of segmentation can be treated with a prompt posterior arthrodesis, which should include the entire kyphosis and one vertebra cephalad and caudal to the lesion. This procedure can prevent further progression, but it cannot correct an existing deformity. If correction is the goal, an anterior approach is needed, with multiple osteotomies of the anterior bar of bone followed by the posterior arthrodesis. For larger patients, posterior compression instrumentation is desirable. If the patient is too

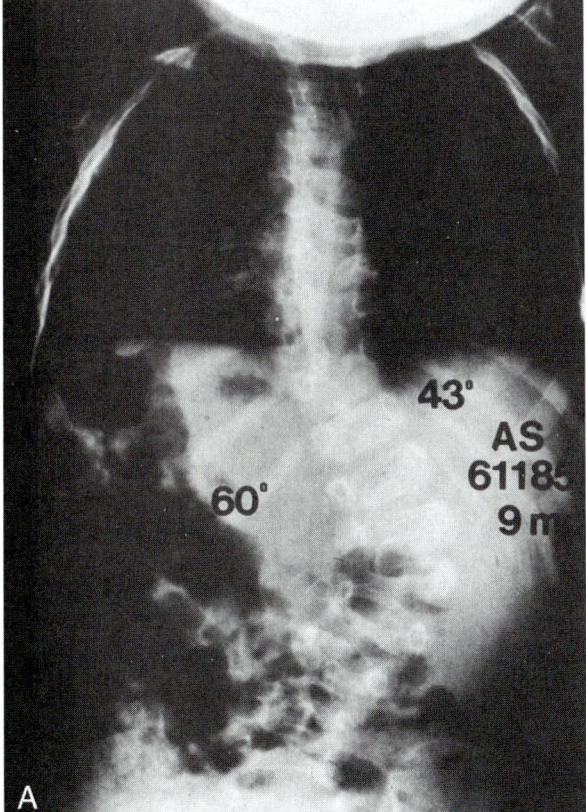
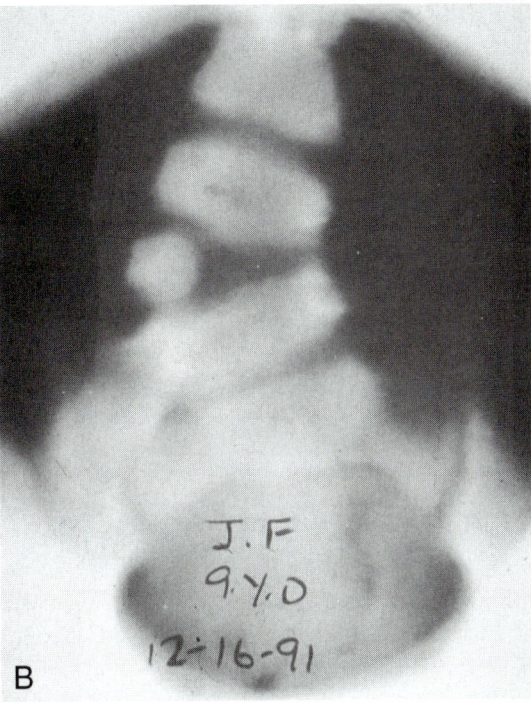

Figure 31.14. A. AP view of 9-month-old showing severe lumbar scoliosis due to hemivertebra at L2. **B.** AP view tomography showing a fully segmental hemivertebra.

small for instrumentation, hyperextension casting is needed to maintain the correction until the area of the arthrodesis has fused. For defects of formation, the main goal is the prevention of paraplegia.

If the defect is detected early (less than 5 years) and there is less than 50° of kyphosis on a supine radiograph, posterior fusion alone will produce the desired outcome. The child must wear a hyperextension cast (not a brace) for 6 months. When fusion is achieved, the remaining anterior growth produces a gradual correction of the deformity.

When the deformity is large or the patient is an older child or an adult, a combined anterior and posterior arthrodesis is mandatory (31). The anterior arthrodesis is done first, with radical excision of the shortened anterior longitudinal ligament, the discs, and the related ligaments. Then a posterior arthrodesis with compression instrumentation or a hyperextension cast is done. If the patient presents with severe neurologic deficit (loss of motor, bowel, or bladder function), the anterior and posterior arthrodeses must be combined with an anterior decompression of the spinal cord.

The treatment of congenital scoliosis falls into one of three categories: periodic observation, orthotics, or surgery. Periodic observation is only indicated for children with minimal deformity and no evidence of progression. Orthotic treatment plays a limited role. Bracing has been found to be effective for controlling long, flexible curves, until the time of pubertal growth spurt. All short, sharp curves; all rigid curves; and all kyphotic or lordotic curves are contraindications to brace. Since a high percentage of congenital scolioses progress and since few of them can be treated by orthoses, a large number of cases require surgical treatment.

The four basic operations for treatment of these anomalies are posterior arthrodesis, combined posterior and anterior arthrodesis, convex growth arrest (epiphysiodesis), and hemivertebra excision (23). Correction of the curve can be achieved with internal instrumentation or with a cast or brace. Instrumentation should never be used without a preoperative evaluation of the spinal canal. An intraoperative evaluation with a wake-up test should be done whenever spinal instrumentation is used.

Posterior spinal arthrodesis is the standard of care. Many congenital scolioses can be managed with this procedure. The entire curve should be fused. Critics of isolated posterior arthrodesis have implied that a combined anterior and posterior arthrodesis is needed to prevent bending of the fusion mass over time (the crankshaft effect). Convex growth arrest is appropriate only for patients with some growth potential remaining in the concave side. It must be done early (less than 5 years old) and before the curve has progressed beyond 50° to 60°. After surgery, the child wears a corrective cast for 6 months. The presence of any degree of kyphosis is a contraindication for this procedure. Hemivertebra excision is indicated for patients with a fixed decompensation in whom adequate alignment cannot be achieved with other procedures (e.g., hemivertebra at L5) (Fig. 31.15). This procedure has higher risks than the other procedures, including greater blood loss and increased risk of neurologic injury.

There is an increased incidence of neurologic complications in surgery for patients with congenital scoliosis because of intraspinal anomalies. It is important to remember that a patient who has congenital scoliosis typically has no growth potential on the concave part of the curve. There is growth potential only on the convex side, and this growth is not productive of vertical height, only of deformity. The child will be taller if arthrodesis is done earlier, since increasing deformity results in shortening of the trunk. We believe it is better to be short and relatively straight than to be shorter and more crooked.

SUMMARY

Patients with congenital spinal deformities have a high frequency of associated anomalies, both within and outside the spine; thus a thorough evaluation is essential. The natural history ranges from no progression to extremely severe deformity, pulmonary compromise, paraplegia, and early death.

Appropriate management involves careful evaluation of the patient, careful and precise monitoring for progression of the deformity clinically and radiographically, and prompt action when progression is observed. Bracing is useless for the treatment of congenital kyphosis, congenital lordosis, and congenital scoliosis with a short and stiff curve pattern. Bracing can be useful for scoliosis with a long and flexible curve pattern. Spinal arthrodesis is the mainstay of treatment.

III Juvenile Kyphosis

After the advent of x-rays, Scheuermann, in 1920, first outlined the radiographic manifestations of juvenile kyphosis (Fig. 31.16). In 1964, Sorenson (31a) further described the disease process and suggested that Scheuermann's disease is characterized by three central adjacent vertebrae with wedging of at least 5°. Scheuermann's disease is second only to idiopathic scoliosis in prevalence. It occurs in 0.5 and 8% of the population, depending on whether the diagnosis is based on radiographic or clinical criteria (32). There is an increased prevalence in the male population (33). The age of onset of the disease is difficult to establish because radio-

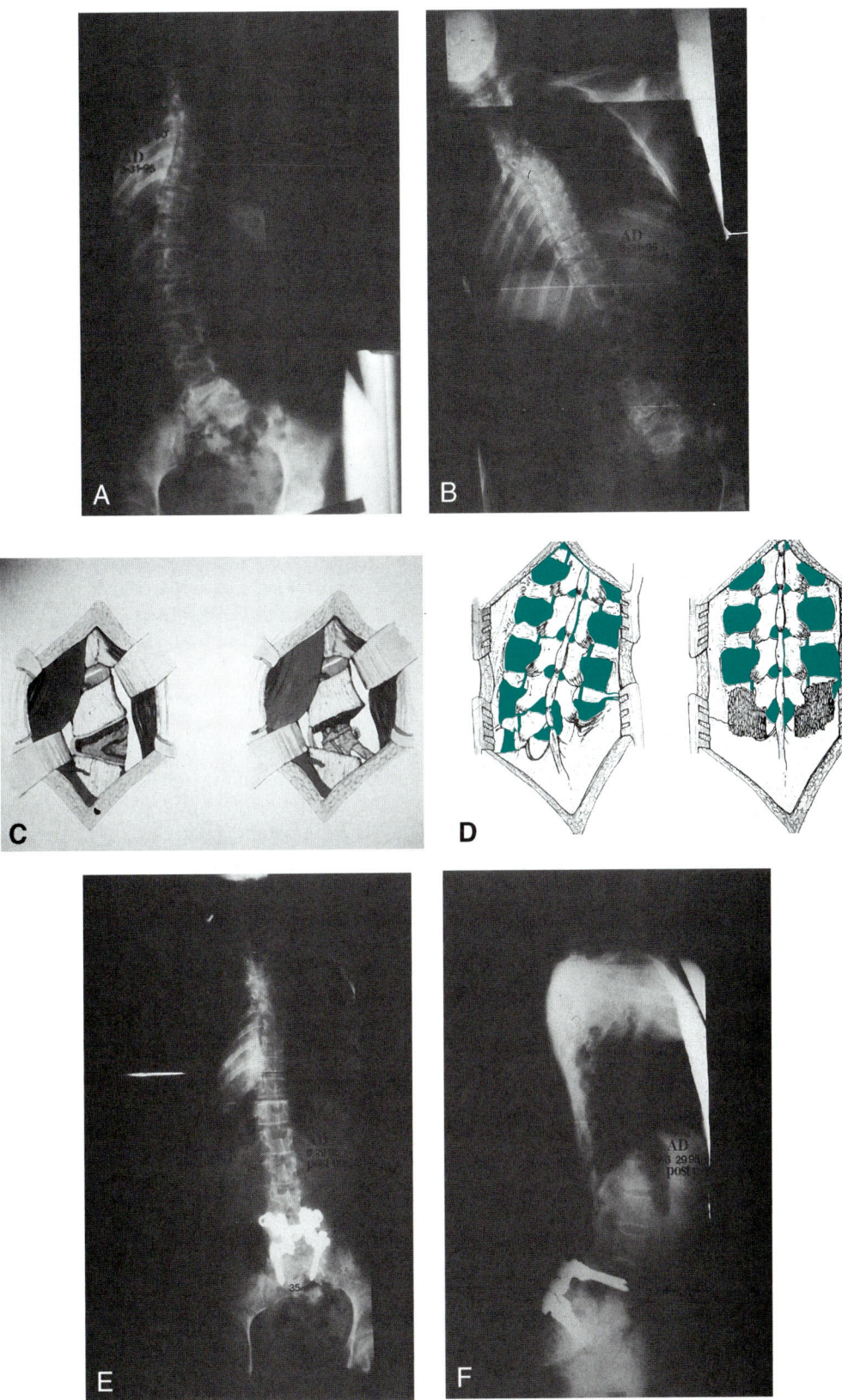

Figure 31.15. A. AP view of a patient with congenital lumbosacral hemivertebra showing the oblique takeoff in a lumbar scoliosis. **B.** Bending view showing the flexibility of the lumbar curve. **C.** Surgical approach for an anterior hemivertebra excision through a retroperi- toneal approach. **D.** Posterior view of a posterior hemivertebra arch resection and correction. Postoperative views showing the correction of the lumbar curve (**E**) and sagittal plane alignment (**F**) following re- section of the lumbosacral hemivertebra.

graphic changes typical of Scheuermann's disease are rarely demonstrable before age 10 or 11. By the time the child is 12 to 13 years old, however, typical vertebral changes along with wedging and kyphosis are usually present.

Based on radiographic features, Scheuermann's disease is characterized by an increased kyphosis that exceeds 45° and is associated with 5° or more wedging of at least three adjacent vertebrae at the apex of the kyphosis. Curves greater than 65° to 70° may increase even after skeletal maturation is complete. Small degrees of kyphosis in the lumbar and thoracolumbar spine may be more clinically apparent than thoracic deformities, as a greater distortion of sagittal contour at this level is more obvious. The incidence of thoracic pain in the untreated adult ranges from 10 to 42% of patients in reported series (34). After the completion of growth, low back pain in Scheuermann's disease seems to be common. Cord compression may develop secondary to the angular deformity alone or in association with a herniated thoracic intervertebral disc. It is exceedingly rare.

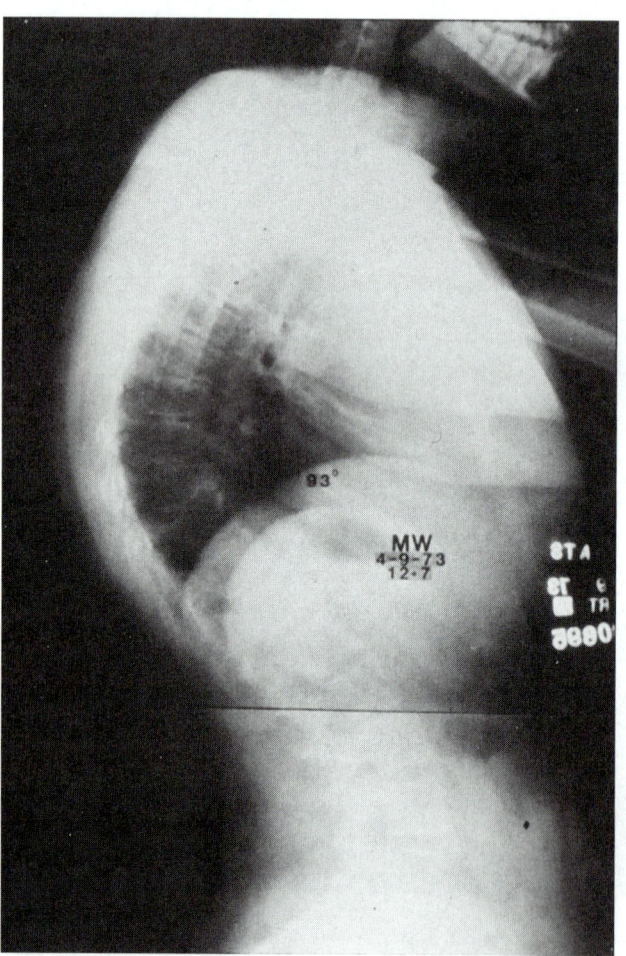

Figure 31.16. Lateral view of a patient with Scheuermann's disease (thoracic kyphosis). Note the wedging of the apical vertebra.

RELEVANT ANATOMY AND PATHOGENESIS

A thoracic kyphosis ranging from 20° to 50° (or 45°) in a growing child is normal; one greater than 45° to 50° should be considered excessive. The cause of Scheuermann's disease remains unknown. Many theories, hypotheses, and speculations have been presented to describe isolated findings (pathologic, structural, biochemical, biomechanical, endocrine, and metabolic findings). Abnormalities have been identified histologically; whether they are primary or secondary to altered mechanics or secondary to repeated stress or trauma is unknown.

INITIAL FINDINGS, PHYSICAL EXAMINATION, AND DIAGNOSIS

Initial complaints relate to the deformity and its location. Approximately 20% of patients have pain. The incidence is much higher in patients with a kyphosis involving L1 or L2 (32,35). In adults, increased compensatory lumbar and cervical lordosis may also contribute to discomfort. As the patient moves beyond middle age, particularly females, physiologic osteoporosis of the spine, degeneration of discs, and arthritic collapse of the apophyseal joints will greatly increase or accelerate the process of kyphosis.

Scheuermann's disease may predispose the patient to spondylolysis, and this problem should be ruled out in symptomatic patients. Increased lumbar lordosis places increased stress on the pars interarticularis (36).

Deformities greater than 65° to 70° are noticeable on physical examination, and the child presents with a round back appearance. The thoracic hump may be increased with forward-bending as seen in the lateral view (Fig. 31.17). Thoracolumbar or lumbar kyphosis is not easily visible. Muscle tightness, particularly of the hamstrings and anterior shoulder girdle, is common. In the adolescent with postural kyphosis, mostly due to poor posture, the kyphotic posture is easy to correct either on command or by manipulation. Patients should undergo careful neurologic examination to rule out a spastic paraparesis, manifested by ataxia and hyperreflexia, which may present on rare occasions secondary to spinal cord compression (37).

Scheuermann's disease should be distinguished from postural round back deformity. Children with postural deformity have only a slight increase in thoracic kyphosis (40° to 60°). Clinically, the kyphosis is mobile, easily and voluntarily correctable, and unassociated with muscle contractures. Radiographs show normal vertebral wedging without end plate changes. Because radiographic changes of Scheuermann's disease may not be present until the age of 10 to 12, it is possible that early Scheuermann's disease could be incorrectly diagnosed as a postural round back deformity.

There is an atypical form of Scheuermann's disease that may present in one of two types: (*a*) vertebral body changes without wedging or increased kyphosis or (*b*) in-

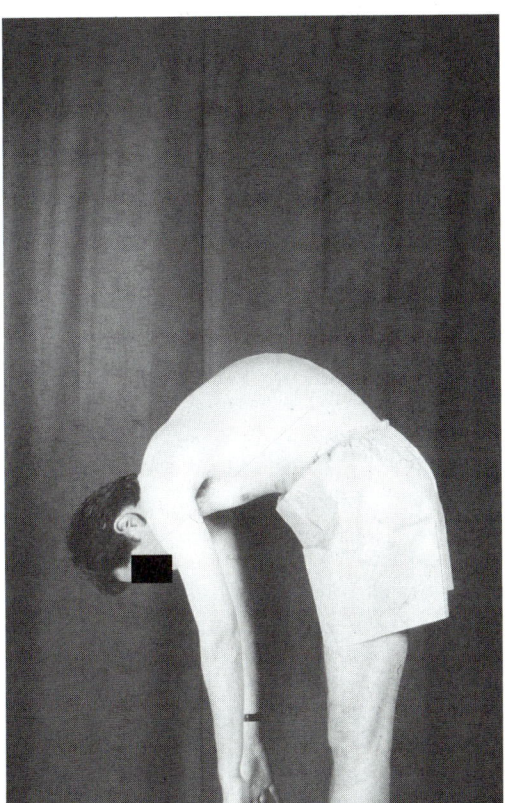

Figure 31.17. Teenaged male with thoracolumbar Scheuermann's disease showing the increased kyphosis with forward bending.

creased kyphosis without vertebral body changes. In the first type, patients often have back pain and spasm, radiographic changes showing end plate irregularity, disc space narrowing, and Schmorl nodules.

Scheuermann's disease must be differentiated from other types of kyphosis, including infectious spondylitis, traumatic injuries, osteochondrodystrophies (e.g., Morquio's disease), tumors, neuromuscular conditions, postlaminectomy kyphosis, and congenital kyphosis. Lumbosacral anomalies should be ruled out. Spondylolisthesis at L5–S1 can produce a severe lumbar lordosis with, consequently, a compensatory thoracic kyphosis.

RADIOLOGIC STUDIES

Radiographs show the classic findings of disc space narrowing, end plate irregularity, apical vertebral wedging of 5° or more, and sometimes a hyperkyphosis. A standing lateral view (with the arms straight forward and resting on a ladder) evaluates the magnitude and cause of the problem. To evaluate flexibility, a supine lateral cross-table film is done with the patient hyperextended over a firm bolster at the apex of the kyphosis. Skeletal maturation should be assessed. Note that a mild scoliosis (10° to 20°) is seen in 20 to 30% of patients.

TREATMENT

Nonoperative Treatment

In the growing child, a painful or progressive deformity should be treated; and the treatment of choice is orthotics. All nonoperative methods, which must be done during the rapid growth period of the child, should produce a mechanical correction of the spinal deformity and maintain the correction until full skeletal maturity is reached.

When the deformity is relatively mild (less than 50°), treatment centers around observation, serial lateral radiographs, postural exercises, and extension exercises. In a skeletally immature patient in whom progression is noted or who presents with a high magnitude of deformity, bracing should be considered. A hyperextension cast applied in one or two stages has proved effective as a method of treatment.

If the disease is in the midthoracic spine, its usual area of presentation, a Milwaukee brace should be used. The lumbar hyperlordosis common to this condition must be controlled by the pelvic girdle. A pad is fixed to each of the posterior uprights just below the apex of the kyphosis to permit active extension against the pressure exerted by the kyphosis (34,38).

If the apex of the deformity is caudal to T8, bracing with an underarm TLSO can be attempted. The TLSO can be modified for treatment of kyphosis by using the principle of pelvic control and maintaining the anterior portion high on the chest with the posterior portion trimmed just below the apex of the deformity. Unlike bracing for AIS, bracing in patients with juvenile kyphosis often results in a permanent correction of the deformity after the treatment is discontinued (39). Bracing may also help control pain. The majority of the patients should wear the brace longer than 18 months to obtain an optimal result. To avoid loss of correction, the brace should be worn until vertebral wedging is 5° or less (38).

Surgical correction is still possible in the older patient, even though the iliac apophysis may be closed. As long as the ring apophyses of the vertebral bodies are open, some skeletal remodeling potential is still possible. A severe degree of kyphosis (more than 75°), skeletal maturity, and vertebral wedging that averages more than 10° are factors limiting the degree of correction.

Operative Treatment

On rare occasions, a progressive curve will not respond to an orthosis, and surgery will be needed. Surgery is reserved for patients with large deformities (70° or more), for those who exhibit progression despite bracing, or for those who develop significant back pain.

If the deformity is flexible, posterior fusion only is adequate. Anterior and posterior fusion with posterior instrumentation is recommended for patients with kyphosis of more than 70° or with a deformity that does not correct to less than 50° on a hyperextension lateral radiograph (22). It is extremely important to restore the normal sagittal alignment, thoracic kyphosis apex (T7–T8), and lumbar lordosis apex (L3).

POSTERIOR APPROACH

For the posterior approach, we position the patient prone on a suspension frame. A subperiosteal dissection is done to expose the spinous processes, laminas, apophyseal joints, and the transverse process. We find the Isola segmental instrumentation ideal for this surgery (Fig. 31.18). We use three claws proximal and three claws distal, which are mounted on longitudinal bilateral rods that are connected with two or three transverse connector devices. The sagittal rods should be contoured to the degree of desired correction. All facets and transverse processes are prepared for fusion by decortication. Autogenous bone grafts are preferred.

After closure of the wound, a chest x-ray for possible pneumothorax should be taken. Luque rods with sublaminar wires should be avoided. Junctional kyphosis is common in this type of fixation. Instrumentation of the total extent of the curvature is necessary to restore sagittal plane balance and prevent subsequent "adding on" with junctional kyphosis (40, 41).

Some authors (42) have reported satisfactory results with surgical correction by single-stage anterior instrumentation and fusion. We do not favor this approach because of the extension of the kyphosis over multiple segments and because a single anterior implant may not be sufficient to stabilize and produce a normal sagittal alignment.

ANTERIOR APPROACH

Anterior surgery is done through a left-side thoracotomy if the segments to be fused are between T4 and T10. For adequate access, the sixth, seventh, or eighth rib is removed, depending on the highest level of fixation. If a lower level of exposure is needed (T11 to upper lumbar), a combined left thoracoabdominal transdiaphragmatic retroperitoneal approach is used, and the eighth or ninth rib is removed. After exposing the spine, anterior releases, discectomies, osteotomies of vertebral end plates, and wedge grafting are performed, and the intervertebral disc spaces are filled with chipped rib bone graft. The pleura is closed over the spine, the diaphragm is repaired,

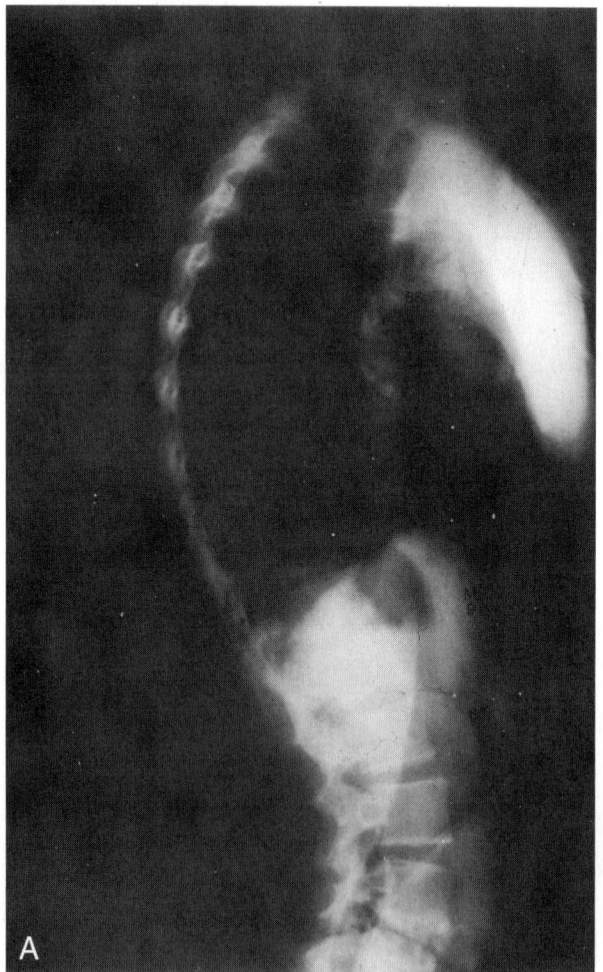 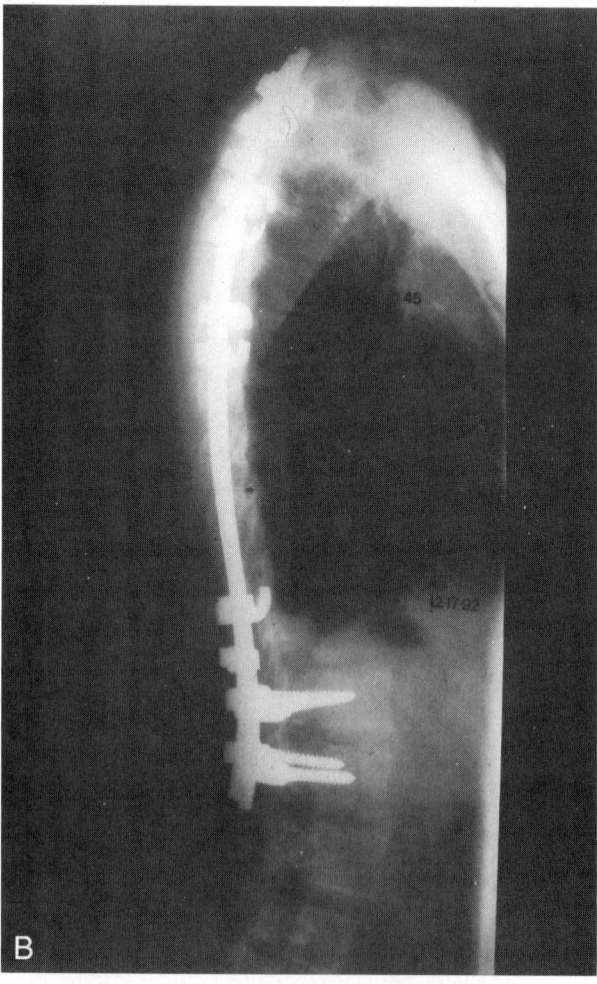

Figure 31.18. Preoperative (**A**) and postoperative (**B**) views of a patient who underwent posterior spinal fusion with Isola instrumentation for thoracic Scheuermann's disease.

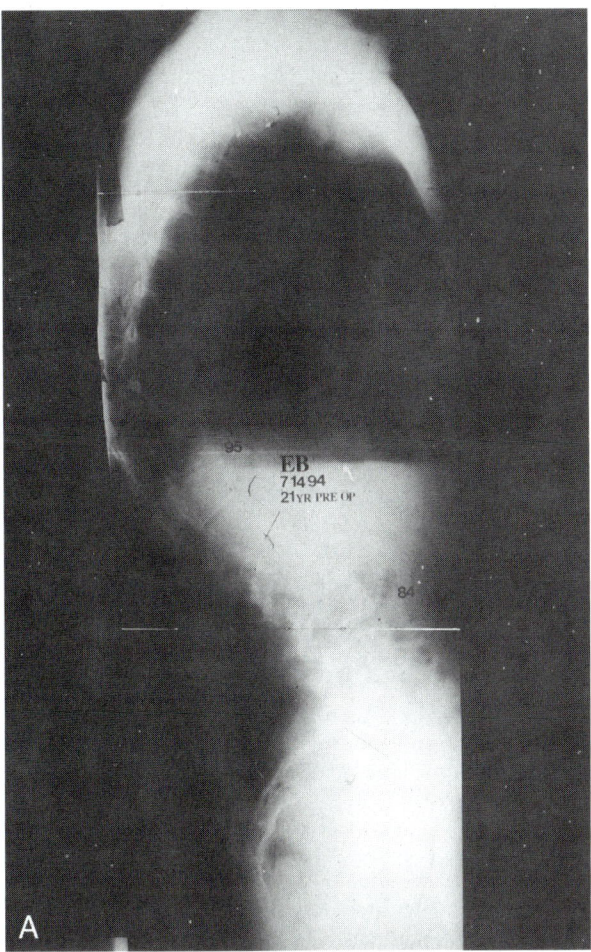
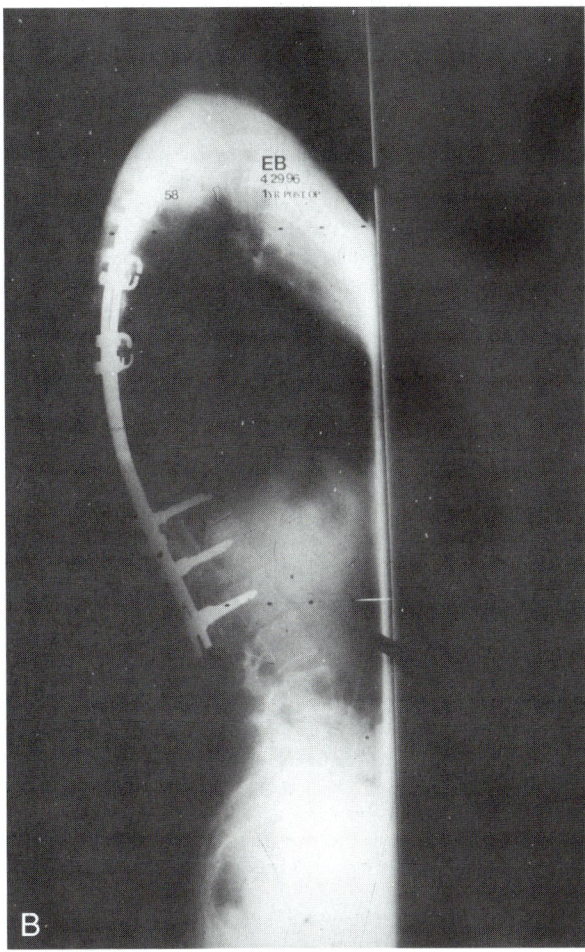

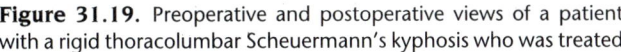

Figure 31.19. Preoperative and postoperative views of a patient with a rigid thoracolumbar Scheuermann's kyphosis who was treated with anterior multilevel discectomy and posterior spinal fusion with segmental Isola instrumentation.

chest tubes are placed in the pleural cavity, and the wound is closed.

ONE-STAGE ANTERIOR AND POSTERIOR SURGERY

The advantages of a one-stage anterior and posterior procedure are a relatively shorter recuperative time and avoidance of in-between anterior and posterior stage morbidity problems that can result in delays of the second surgery (Fig. 31.19).

SUMMARY

It is important to detect juvenile kyphosis as early as possible during the rapid growth period in the child. Treat it first with therapeutic exercises; if there is no improvement or at the first sign of progression, promptly brace. If bracing is used, continue the treatment until skeletal maturity is reached. If surgery is indicated, prepare the correction by anterior spine soft tissue releases, discectomies, and fusion (if the kyphosis is beyond 70° and not flexible), followed by posterior fusion and strong segmental fixation.

REFERENCES

1. Weinstein SL. Adolescent idiopathic scoliosis: prevalence and natural history. Instr Course Lect 1989;38:115–128.
2. Enneking WF, Harrington P. Pathological changes in scoliosis. J Bone Joint Surg 1969;51A:165–184.
3. Lonstein JE. Adolescent idiopathic scoliosis: screening and diagnosis. Instr Course Lect 1989;38:105–113.
4. Lonstein JE, Bjorklund S, Wanninger MH. Voluntary school screening for scoliosis in Minnesota. J Bone Joint Surg 1982; 64A:481–488.
5. Duriez J. Evolution de la scoliose idiopathique chez l'adulte. Acta Orthop Belg 1967;33:547–550.
6. Weinstein SL, Ponseti IV. Curve progression in idiopathic scoliosis. J Bone Joint Surg 1983;65A:447–455.
7. Betz RR, Bunnel WP, Lamrecht-Mulier E, MacEwen GD. Scoliosis and pregnancy. J Bone Joint Surg 1987;69A:90–96.
8. Nachemsom AL, Peterson LE. Effectiveness of treatment with a brace in girls who have idiopathic scoliosis. J Bone Joint Surg 1995; 77A:815–822.
9. King HA, Moe JH, Bradford DS, Winter RB. The selection of fusion levels in thoracic idiopathic scoiosis. J Bone Surg 1983;65A: 1302–1313.
10. Keller RB. Nonoperative treatment of adolescent idiopathic scoliosis. Instr Course Lect 1989;38:129–135.

11. Green NE. Part-time bracing of adolescent idiopathic scoliosis. J Bone Joint Surg 1986;68A:738–742.

12. Engler GL. Preoperative and intraoperative considerations in adolescent idiopathic scoliosis. Instr Course Lect 1989; 38:137–141.

13. Dubousset J, Herring JA, Shufflebarger H. The crankshaft phenomenon. J Pediatr Orthop 1989;9:541–550.

14. Tolo VT. Surgical treatment of adolescent idiopathic scoliosis. Instr Course Lect 1989;38:143–156.

15. Ibrahim K, Benson L. Cotrel-Dubousset instrumentation for double major right thoracic left lumbar scoliosis; the relation between frontal balance, hook configuration and fusion levels. Orthop Trans 1991;15:114.

16. Thompson JP, Transfeld EE, Bradford DS, et al. Decompensation after Cotrel-Dubousset instrumentation of idiopathic scoliosis. Spine 1990;15:927–931.

17. Winter RB, Denis F. The King V curve pattern. Its analysis and surgical treatment. Orthop Clin North Am 1994;25:353–362.

18. Puno R, Mehta S, Abbott Byrd J. Surgical treatment of idiopathic thoracolumbar and lumbar scoliosis in adolescent patients. Orthop Clin North Am 1994;25:275–286.

19. Denis F. Cotrel-Dubousset instrumentation in the treatment of idiopathic scoliosis. Orthop Clin North Am 1988;19:291–311.

20. Scoliosis Research Society. Morbidity and Mortality Committee report. Vancouver: Scoliosis Research Society, 1987.

21. Krajbich JL. Thoracoplasty. In: Weinstein SL, ed. The pediatric spine: principles and practice. New York: Raven, 1994:1459–1465.

22. Herndon WA, Emans JB, Micheli LG, et al. Combined anterior and posterior fusion for Scheuermann's juvenile kyphosis. Spine 1981;6:125–130.

23. Winter RB, Lonstein JE, Boachie-Adjei O. Congenital spinal deformity. J Bone Joint Surg 1996;78A:300–311.

24. Boachie-Adjei O, Lonner B. Spinal deformity. Pediatr Clin North Am 1996;43:885–897.

25. Roberts AP, Conner AN, Tolmie JL, Connor JM. Spondylothoracic and spondylocostal dysostosis. Hereditary forms of spinal deformity. J Bone Joint Surg 1988;70B:123–126.

26. Winter RB, Moe JH, Bradford DS. Congenital thoracic lordosis. J Bone Joint Surg 1978;60A:806–810.

27. Mayfield JK, Winter RB, Bradford DS, Moe JH. Congenital kyphosis due to defects of anterior segmentation. J Bone Joint Surg 1980;62A:1291–1302.

28. Cotrel Y, Dobousset J. Nouvelle technique d' osteosynthèse rachidienne segmentaire par voie postérieure. Rev Chir Orthop 1984;70:489–495.

29. Montgomery SP, Hall JE. Congenital kyphosis. Spine 1982; 7:360–364.

30. Rawlins BA, Winter RB, Lonstein JE, et al. Reconstructive spine surgery in pediatric patients with major loss in vital capacity. Orthop Trans 1994;18:95–96.

31. Winter RB, Moe JH, Lonstein JE. The surgical treatment of congenital kyphosis. A review of 94 patients age 5 years or older, with 2 years or more follow-up in 77 patients. Spine 1985;10:224–231.

31a. Sorenson KH. Scheuermann's juvenile kyphosis. Copenhagen: Munksgaard, 1964.

32. Bradford DS. Juvenile kyphosis. In: Lonstein JE, Bradford DS, Winter RB, eds. Moe's textbook of scoliosis. 3rd ed. Philadelphia: Saunders, 1995:349–367.

33. Murray PM, Weinstein SL, Spratt KF. The natural history and long term follow-up of Scheuermann's kyphosis. J Bone Joint Surg 1993;75A:236–248.

34. Bradford DS, Moe JH, Montalvo FJ, Winter RB. Scheuermann's kyphosis and roundback deformity. Results of Milwaukee brace treatment. J Bone Joint Surg 1974;56A:740–758.

35. Marrero GH. Juvenile kyphosis. Spine 1990;4:173–185.

36. Ogilvie JW, Sherman J. Spondylosis in Scheuermann's disease. Spine 1987;12:251–253.

37. Yablon JS, Kasdon DL, Levine H. Thoracic cord compression in Scheuermann's disease. Spine 1988;13:896–898.

38. Montgomery SP, Erwin WE. Scheuermann's kyphosis. Long term results of Milwaukee brace treatment. Spine 1978;6:5.

39. Bradford DS, Brown DM, Moe JH. Scheuermann's kyphosis, a form of juvenile osteoporosis? Clin Orthop 1976;118:10.

40. Coscia MF, Bradford DS, Ogilvie JW. Scheuermann's kyphosis-results in 19 cases treated by spinal arthrodesis and L-rod instrumentation. Orthop Trans 1988;12:255.

41. Lowe TG. Double L-rod instrumentation in the treatment for severe kyphosis secondary to Scheuermann' s disease. Spine 1987; 12:336–341.

42. Kostuik JP. Anterior Kostuik-Harrington distraction systems for the treatment of kyphotic deformities. Spine 1990;15:169–180.

chapter 32

Baron S. Lonner and Oheneba Boachie-Adjei

Adult Scoliosis

Spinal deformity occurring in the adult patient shares some features with that presenting in skeletally immature individuals. Nevertheless, the pathogenesis, natural history, clinical presentation, and operative indications for spinal deformity in the adult are generally distinct from those in the younger patient.

RELEVANT ANATOMY AND PATHOGENESIS

Spinal deformity may occur in the coronal plane, sagittal plane, or both. In fact, deformity occurs in three dimensions along three axes. In the coronal or frontal plane, the spine should be straight. A deviation of 10° or more (Cobb method) is abnormal. A plumb line dropped from C2 or T1 should fall within 1 cm of the S1 spinous process. In the sagittal plane, alignment is more complex, consisting of a series of lordotic and kyphotic curves in sequence from the cervical to the sacrococcygeal regions, which allows the head and torso to be balanced over the pelvis. On the lateral radiograph, a vertical line extending from the midportion of the body of the first thoracic vertebra should project just anterior to the second sacral vertebra. The normal range of thoracic kyphosis is 20° to 45°, and the range for lumbar lordosis is 30° to 60°. The thoracolumbar junction represents a transitional zone in which the normal curvature ranges from 0° to 5° of kyphosis. The apex of kyphosis is found at the T6–7 level, and the apex of lordosis lies at the L3–4 level.

Adult spinal deformity may be classified by the plane in which it occurs, i.e., scoliosis in the coronal plane and kyphosis or lordosis in the sagittal plane. Deformity is also classified by its pathogenesis.

Scoliosis in the adult may be idiopathic with its onset during adolescence or earlier. There is a propensity toward progression of curvature in patients with curves greater than 50° at a mean rate of 1°/year (1). Less common causes of scoliosis with onset in childhood, such as congenital scoliosis, rarely present for first-time treatment in adulthood.

The most common cause of scoliosis that presents de novo in the adult is degenerative scoliosis of the lumbar spine, caused by asymmetric wear of the disc space and facet joints, leading to wedging of the disc and, secondarily, the vertebrae themselves (2). This is most progressive in individuals with osteoporosis. Degenerative curves are generally not highly progressive and are usually no larger than 30° to 40°.

Kyphosis in the adult may have its onset in childhood in the form of Scheuermann's disease. Patients may present in adulthood because of progressive pain or deformity. Kyphosis is commonly seen secondary to osteoporosis and multiple compression fractures in the elderly and in women with premature onset of menopause. Kyphosis may also develop in young adults following high-energy blunt trauma in which a burst fracture or compression-type fracture is treated nonoperatively.

Iatrogenic causes of deformity include postlaminectomy kyphosis, flat back deformity, and junctional deformities following prior spinal arthrodesis. The former more commonly occurs in children after laminectomy but may occur in the adult after wide laminectomy, compromising the facet articulations. This most commonly leads to spondylolisthesis in the lumbar spine following decompression for stenosis. Postlaminectomy kyphosis may also occur in the adult if anterior and middle-column supports are inadequate, such as occurs in the face of malignancy, infection, or osteoporosis. Rarely, a swan-neck deformity may occur in the cervical spine after decompression for cervical spondylotic myelopathy if the facet joints are compromised.

Flat back syndrome (3) occurs as a result of inadequate preservation of lumbar lordosis with scoliosis fusions to L4 or L5. This has been one of the major disadvantages of distraction instrumentation using the Harrington system, which is effective in correcting coronal plane deformity but does not adequately preserve sagittal plane alignment. In these patients, the remaining unfused caudal motion segments initially compensate for the relative lumbar kyphosis with segmental hyperlordosis. In time, however, the motion segments degenerate and collapse, leading to lumbar kyphosis. Flat back syndrome is characterized by an inability to maintain an upright posture; easy fatigability; low back pain; and in some patients, neurogenic claudication caused by spinal stenosis. Junctional deformities may occur when a previous fusion and instrumentation were poorly planned. Fusions of inadequate length that do not extend to the stable and neutral vertebrae may result in curve progression distal or proximal to the fusion. In addition, fusions ending at or near the apex of the thoracic kyphosis may be complicated by a junctional kyphosis.

Other causes of deformity include pyogenic or granulomatous infection, neoplastic disease leading to loss of the structural integrity of the vertebral column, ankylosing spondylitis, and paralysis caused by spinal cord injury.

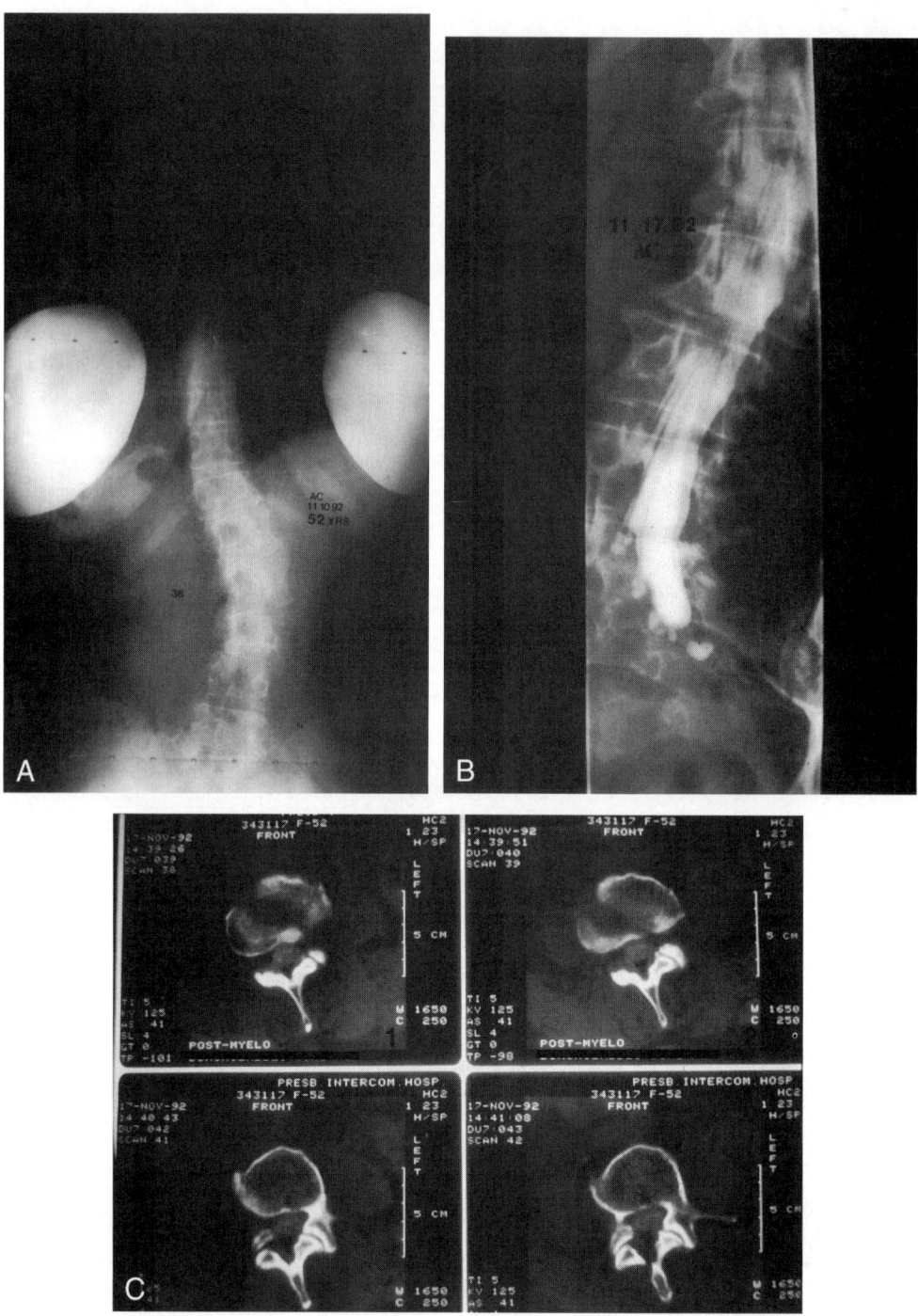

Figure 32.1. A. AP view of a patient with degenerative lumbar scoliosis and neurogenic claudication. **B.** AP view myelogram showing a segmental extradural defect in the midlumbar spine. **C.** Postmyelographic discography showing central and foraminal stenoses.

INITIAL FINDINGS, PHYSICAL EXAMINATION, AND DIAGNOSIS

Unlike children and adolescents with scoliosis, adults with spinal deformity commonly present with pain. Other reasons for seeking medical care include progressive deformity, neurologic deficits, and respiratory difficulties caused by thoracic volume changes.

Pain in adult spinal deformity has a number of different origins and presentations. For treatment to be effective, it must be directed at the pain generators. While taking the history, the clinician should ask about the pain's location, radiation into the lower extremities, intensity, interference with activities of daily living, and quality (e.g., paresthesia, dysesthesia, aching); the patient's medication requirements should also be determined. Pain is often related to muscle strain and is commonly found on the convexity of the curve. Pain may be concentrated in the concavity of the curve and related to facet arthrosis and disc degeneration. Intercostal neuralgias may occur on the concave aspect of the thorax; they are related to the impingement of intercostal nerves by abutting ribs or foraminal encroachment, causing radicular pain. Another source of pain is rib tip impingement of the 11th or 12th rib on the posterior iliac crest in severe collapsing deformity. Low back pain may be related to disc and facet degeneration below an idiopathic deformity or within a primary degenerative scoliosis. Discography may play a role in identifying symptomatic levels in the lumbar spine below a spinal deformity, although this remains controversial (4). Radiculopathy may also occur secondary to disc herniation and/or lateral recess stenosis below an idiopathic deformity or within a degenerative curve.

In some patients, spinal deformity may be progressive. As discussed previously, idiopathic deformity has a tendency to progress with curvatures of 50° or greater. Curvatures of 30° or less are unlikely to progress in the adult (1). Progression of kyphosis is common, particularly in postmenopausal women with osteoporosis. Progressive torso decompensation, diminishing height, and changes in the waistline are all indicative of worsening deformity.

Neurologic involvement may occur, particularly in patients with degenerative scoliosis. These patients often have symptoms of neurogenic claudication, with back, buttocks, groin, and thigh pain or a sense of heaviness in the extremities occurring with ambulation. Radicular patterns of pain below the knee may also occur, commonly in the young adult; and may result from foraminal narrowing on the concavity of a curve, lateral disc herniation, or a tension neurapraxia on the convexity of a lumbar or thoracolumbar curvature (5) (Fig. 32.1). Ability to ambulate distances is severely limited. There is often a paucity of neurologic findings on physical examination. Patients with severe stenosis may have resting neurologic deficits, including bladder and/or bowel dysfunction.

Pulmonary function is affected, and restrictive disease occurs in thoracic curves of 60° or greater (6). Clinically significant changes in pulmonary function occur with curvatures greater than 90° to 100°. Significant pulmonary deficits also occur with smaller magnitudes of curvature in the presence of thoracic lordosis or marked hypokyphosis (7,8).

Physical examination of the adult with spinal deformity should focus on assessment of deformity, localization of pain, and evaluation of neurologic status. Abnormal spinal curvature, shoulder and pelvic obliquity, rib prominence, and plumb line deviation from the midline are noted. The spine is palpated for areas of tenderness. The patient's gait is assessed; for example, an antalgic gait may be associated with radiculopathy or hip abnormality. A forward-stooped gait is consistent with spinal stenosis or ankylosing spondylitis. Finally, a thorough neurologic examination is performed. The information gathered from a complete history and physical examination, combined with data gathered from imaging studies, provides the basis for formulating a treatment plan.

RADIOLOGIC STUDIES

Standard radiographic studies of the spine for deformity are the standing (sitting in nonambulators) full-length AP and lateral view x-rays of the spine. These radiographs provide the basis for a three-dimensional analysis of the spine. Coronal and sagittal curvature is measured using the Cobb method. Shoulder and pelvic obliquity are quantified on the AP radiograph. The neutral and stable vertebrae are determined. The neutral vertebra is the first nonrotated vertebra at the caudal extent of a curvature. The stable vertebra is the one most closely bisected by the center sacral line, a line drawn vertically from the spinous process of the first sacral vertebra. In addition, plumb line deviation (from T1) from the first sacral vertebra on the coronal and sagittal views is determined. Finally, the apical vertebra, the vertebra with the greatest translation from the midline in each curvature, is noted. The magnitude of deviation from the midline and the amount of rotation of each apical vertebra are recorded.

These data are used to compare radiographs taken at 1-year intervals to determine if there has been progression of deformity. The data are also important for preoperative planning. Supine right and left bending x-rays or a traction AP radiograph provides information on the flexibility of the deformity, which is also useful for operative planning. Flexibility of a kyphotic deformity is assessed from a hyperextension cross-table lateral radiograph, which is taken with a wedge placed at the apex of the kyphosis.

Additional detail is obtained with coned-down views of specified areas of the spine. Further definition of the bony anatomy in congenital deformity, for example, is achieved with CT or conventional tomography. MRI or CT combined with myelography is used to assess neural element compression in patients with neurologic deficits and neurogenic claudication. Although the combined study provides excellent bony detail, it should be reserved, because of its invasive nature, for patients who are indicated for surgery. Because up to 40% of patients with congenital spinal deformities have intraspinal anomalies, these patients are also candidates for MRI or CT plus myelography (9).

As noted, discography may play a role in delineating painful segments within a curvature or in the region below a deformity. Facet injections, selective nerve root blocks, and electromyography may also be useful in this regard. These tests must be interpreted carefully and used in conjunction with data collected from the history, physical examination, and other diagnostic studies (8).

TREATMENT

Nonoperative Alternatives

Nonoperative management is aimed at controlling pain and improving function. Regardless of whether symptoms are related directly to the deformity or are typical of low back pain seen in patients without spinal deformity, initial treatment is the same. Nonsteroidal anti-inflammatory drugs (NSAIDs) to control pain and muscle relaxants to control muscle spasms are the mainstay of medical management. Care should be taken when prescribing NSAIDs, particularly in patients with a history of peptic ulcer disease and kidney disease. Narcotics should be avoided because of their addictive potential and tendency to affect bowel function, especially in elderly patients.

Counseling on activity modification and body mechanics is an important aspect of treatment. Aerobic and muscular conditioning may also prove beneficial in limiting disability and improving function. Modalities that have not been shown to improve outcome include traction, transcutaneous electrical nerve stimulation (TENS), ultrasound, trigger-point injections, facet injections, lumbar corsets, and acupuncture (10). Brief periods of bed rest—not to exceed 2 to 4 days—may help control acute severe symptoms. Epidural steroid injections may be beneficial for patients with neurogenic claudication who are unresponsive to the above measures. Finally, in elderly patients who are poor candidates for surgery and who have not responded well to the above modalities, orthoses, such as the Knight-Taylor brace or a custom-molded thoracolumbar sacral orthosis, may be useful (Fig. 32.2). In these patients, muscular conditioning must be encouraged to avoid the deconditioning effects of bracing on truncal musculature. Bracing will generally not halt a progressive deformity.

Evaluation of patients for osteoporosis is also essential. Laboratory tests should be performed; and bone mineral density should be assessed with dual-energy x-ray absorptiometry, if available, in patients with evidence of osteoporosis. Appropriate therapy should be instituted in patients with or without osteoporosis, ranging from exercise and calcium supplementation to estrogen, calcitonin, and/or biphosphonate treatment.

Operative Approaches

Indications for surgical treatment of patients with adult spinal deformity include

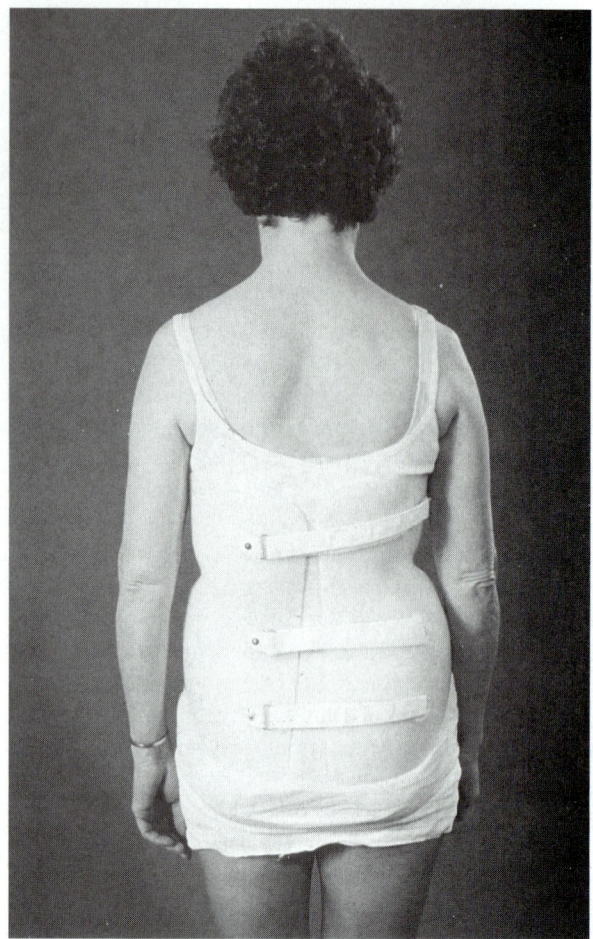

Figure 32.2. Posterior view of a patient with degenerative scoliosis treated with a thoracolumbosacral orthosis.

1. Progressive spinal deformity
2. Painful thoracic and/or lumbar curvature unresponsive to nonoperative treatment (generally, thoracic curvature is not associated with disabling pain until the deformity reaches approximately 50°; lumbar deformity may be painful at lesser magnitudes)
3. Neurologic symptoms, including patients with degenerative scoliosis associated with stenosis and neurogenic claudication and/or radicular symptoms (may occur below a deformity in patients with idiopathic disease)
4. Restrictive pulmonary disease in patients with severe thoracic deformity or with deteriorating pulmonary function caused by progressive deformity
5. Cosmesis (patient's self-image is rarely the primary indication for surgery, but it is often an important consideration, especially in the young adult)

The goals of surgical treatment of adult spinal deformity are to correct and stabilize a progressive deformity, creating a balanced, fused spine (balance must be achieved in the coronal and sagittal planes); to offer pain relief to all painful spinal segments, including painful degenerative

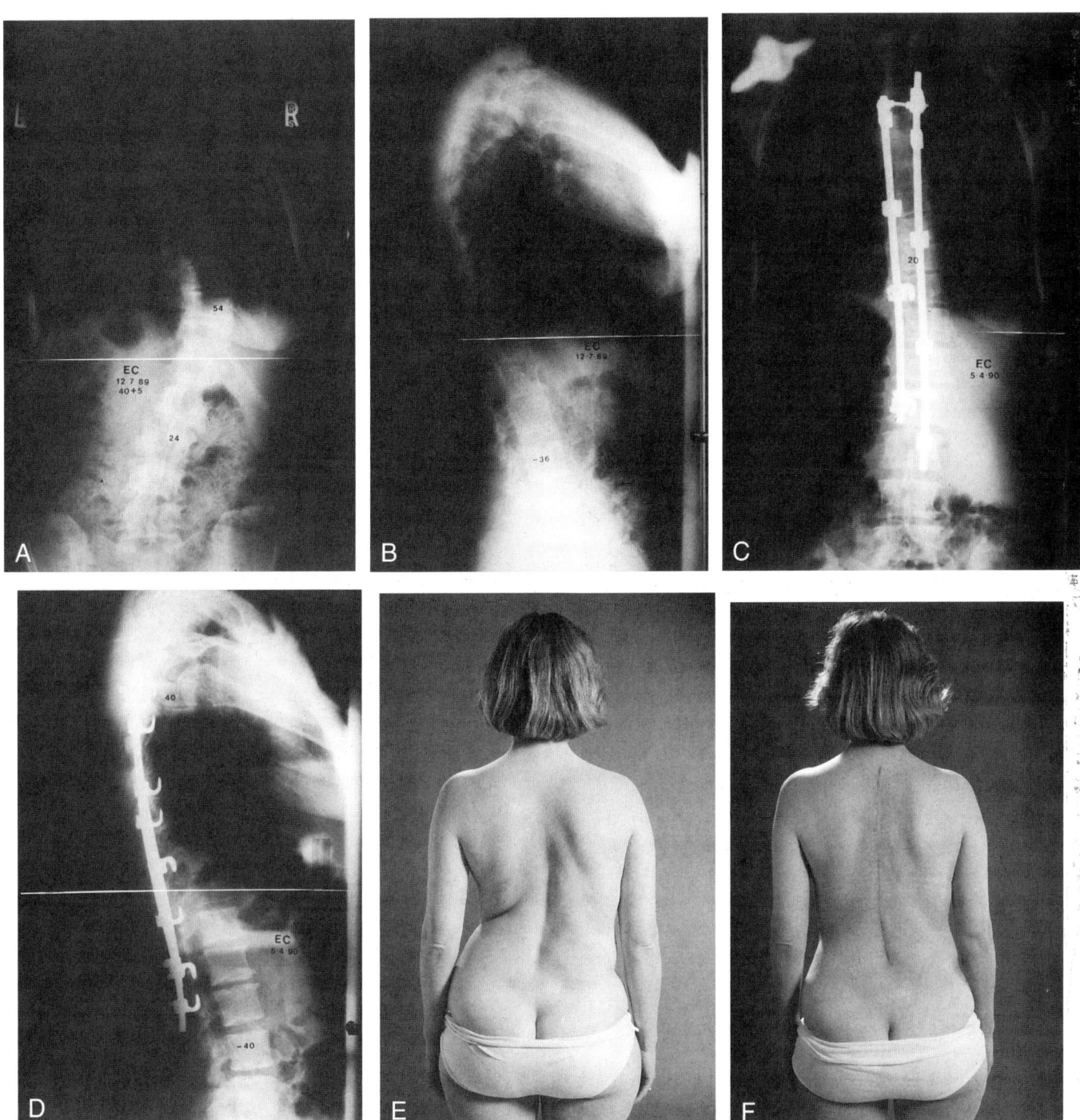

Figure 32.3. A. AP view of a patient with right thoracic scoliosis. **B.** Lateral view showing normal sagittal alignment and disc degeneration with narrowing of the lumbar disc spaces. **C.** Postoperative AP view of the patient showing balanced correction. **D.** Lateral view showing restoration of sagittal alignment. **E.** Before surgery, the pa-tient had a right thoracic curve, scapular protrusion, and left flank crease. **F.** After a single-stage posterior spinal fusion and segmental instrumentation, the patient has a balanced correction with level shoulders and pelvis.

levels below a deformity; and to decompress stenotic levels and include decompressed levels in the arthrodesis.

POSTERIOR FUSION WITH INSTRUMENTATION

The majority of patients with symptomatic adult spinal deformity refractory to nonoperative modalities are effectively managed with a posterior spinal arthrodesis with instrumentation (Fig. 32.3). Curvature of less than 70° in the thoracic spine and less than 60° in the lumbar spine that is flexible on bending films is amenable to this approach. Balanced correction and stabilization can be achieved with current segmental instrumentation systems (Clinical Table).

The arthrodesis must extend to the stable and neutral vertebrae caudally. It may be necessary to extend the

Clinical Table: Adult Scoliosis

Procedure	Indications	Technique	Anatomy	Pitfalls
Posterior spinal fusion with instrumentation	• Adult thoracic, thoracolumbar curves of <60°	• Selective thoracic fusion for thoracic curves to stable vertebra; include levels that show instability or translational deformity or degenerative changes presenting with back pain • Facet fusion; intertransverse fusion and segmental fixation dual rods with distal lumbar pedicle screws • Rod rotation for lumbar curves • Translational correction with sublamina wires for rigid thoracic and thoracolumbar deformities	• Spinal and interspinal ligaments, spinous process, ligamentum flavum, epidural space, lumbar pedicles, costovertebral and costotransverse ligaments • Spinal nerve roots and spinal cord	• Proper selection of fusion levels • Include all degenerative segments in the distal fusion levels selected • Care with sublamina wire placement to avoid injury to spinal cord and nerve roots
Anterior spinal fusion with instrumentation	• Flexible thoracolumbar and lumbar curves with mild to moderate thoracic deformity	• Approach thoracoabdominal transdiaphragmatic for T10 to distal lumbar fusion T11 or T12 retropleural for retroperitoneal T12 to distal lumbar fusion levels • Intervertebral disc exposure • Segmental vessel ligation; complete discectomy; screw placement midvertebral body and posterior aspect • Bicortical fixation • End vertebral staple placement and intervening vertebral screw washer or staple • Rod rotation to correct deformity and restore lumbar lordosis; structural grafts to maintain lordosis	• Intervertebral discs, segmental vessels, diaphragm, psoas muscle • Great vessels: aorta and vena cava • Spinal canal and neural elements • Anterior longitudinal ligament • Sympathetic chain	• Complete exposure of the posterior aspect of the vertebral body to place screws posteriorly; screws to be directed anterior and bicortical • Complete decortication of end plate; rigid rods for patients with good bone, $\frac{1}{4}$-in or double $\frac{3}{16}$-in rods; spinal canal exposure not necessary

Clinical Table: Adult Scoliosis *(continued)*

Procedure	Indications	Technique	Anatomy	Pitfalls
Combined anterior and posterior spinal fusion with posterior instrumentation	• Rigid thoracic deformity of <75° • Decompensated large rigid thoracolumbar, lumbar scoliosis	• First-stage anterior convex side up transthoracic for thoracic deformity • Thoracoabdominal for thoracolumbar deformity • Retropleural retroperitoneal for lower thoracic T11 to distal lumbar spine • Retroperitoneal dissection for L1–4 • Complete discectomy and procedure as for anterior approach above • Posterior second stage under the same anesthetic; patient placed prone in full extension to restore lordosis • Complete facetectomy and facet decortication • Distal lumbar pedicle screws; no rod rotation for thoracic curves • Sublamina wire for translational correction; rod rotation for lumbar curves or double major curves • Facet fusion and intertransverse fusion; sublamina wire placement just prior to curve manipulation; iliac crest bone graft or thoracoplasty through same approach	• Same as for posterior and anterior procedures	• One-stage procedure preferred but use staged procedure if medically unstable or if blood loss exceeds more than half the patient's blood volume on the first stage; the total operating time should not exceed 12 h; otherwise, it should be staged • Thoracoplasty—avoid injury to pleura; test for air leak
Arthrodesis to the sacrum	• Patients with deformity and significant low back pain • Stenosis and/or disc herniation of the lumbosacral region; L4–L5 end vertebra with spondylolisthesis or lateral listhesis below this level • Oblique takeoff of L5; low bone mineral density for end selected fusion level	• Same as for one-stage combined anterior and posterior fusion to the lower lumbar spine • Anterior procedure L4–5, L5–S1 down through the anterior approach • Structural grafts with femoral ring allograft tricortical iliac crest, or metal cages and baskets for L4–5, L5–S1 • Bifurcation of the iliac vessels should be dissected for L5–S1 approach • Medial sacral vessels ligation and division • Preservation of sympathetic chain	• Same as for single-stage or combined anterior and posterior spinal fusion • Aortic and vena cava bifurcation	• Same as for single-stage anterior and posterior spinal fusion and combined procedures • Beware of vascular injury; if unfamiliar with anatomy and dissection, utilize general or vascular surgeon's assistance

arthrodesis more caudally to include painful degenerated segments (11). Fusion to L5 can be performed to preserve the lowest motion segment, if a number of criteria are met: The L5–S1 disc should have normal height without foraminal narrowing; there should be no stenosis or posterior column deficiency, such as spondylolysis; and the spine should be able to be balanced without extending the fusion to the sacrum (12). Generally, this requires less than 15° of coronal tilt of the end vertebrae. The L5 vertebral body should have normal bone mineral density to prevent postsurgical collapse.

Painful thoracic hyperkyphosis may also be managed by this approach. Kyphosis of 75° or less that corrects to 50° on a hyperextension lateral radiograph can be treated with a posterior approach (13). In these patients, correction is maximized by performing thorough facetectomies and partial lamina resection at each level to be fused, thereby shortening and compressing the posterior column of the spine.

In some patients with de novo degenerative scoliosis, arthrodesis may be avoided. In patients with nonprogressive scoliosis and foraminal stenosis, a laminotomy and foraminotomy alone (with or without discectomy) may be performed as long as there is no existing central stenosis. This approach has the advantage of decreasing operative morbidity related to arthrodesis while achieving the desired decompression and not affecting spinal stability. Most patients with degenerative scoliosis and stenosis who are surgical candidates require complete laminectomy and foraminotomies combined with an instrumented fusion. In addition to a direct decompression, an indirect decompression is achieved by distraction on the concavity of the curvature, increasing foraminal height (5).

ANTERIOR SPINE FUSION WITH INSTRUMENTATION

Anterior spinal arthrodesis with instrumentation often allows the surgeon to save a distal level in thoracolumbar or lumbar curves in the adolescent patient in whom a relatively flexible deformity exists (14) (Fig. 32.4). In adults, spinal deformity tends to be more rigid because of facet arthrosis, disc degeneration, and stabilizing osteophytes.

Anterior surgery without posterior release is of limited value for stiff curves. However, relatively young patients with flexible lumbar or thoracolumbar curves may benefit from this operation, which characteristically has a lower blood loss associated with it than do the posterior procedures.

COMBINED ANTERIOR AND POSTERIOR SPINE FUSIONS WITH POSTERIOR INSTRUMENTATION

In patients with rigid, severe thoracic deformities (greater than 75°) anterior release with excision of the anterior longitudinal ligament, the intervertebral disc, and vertebral end plate improves correction and arthrodesis rates. This is particularly helpful for patients in whom a long arthrodesis and a large correction are required. Anterior column support is most useful at the L3–4, L4–5,

and L5–S1 levels. A structural femoral ring allograft packed with cancellous autograft or anterior metallic cages with autograft may be used to provide anterior column support, protecting the posterior construct until fusion occurs (Fig. 32.5). Care must be taken in using anterior structural support in elderly osteoporotic patients, because collapse of the bony end plate and subsidence of the graft may occur, leading to loss of correction and potential failure of the posterior instrumentation.

ARTHRODESIS TO THE SACRUM

Arthrodesis to the sacrum is indicated in patients with scoliosis in the following instances:

1. Significant low back pain below a deformity along with degenerative disc disease and/or facet arthrosis that is unlikely to improve with balancing of the spine; MRI and/or discography may help guide the decision to fuse to the sacrum.
2. Stenosis and/or disc herniation in the lumbosacral region when the stenotic segment is contiguous with or within the spinal deformity.
3. When L4 or L5 is the end vertebra of a planned arthrodesis for a posterior column deficiency (i.e., spondylolysis, spondylolisthesis, or lateral listhesis).
4. When there is an oblique takeoff of L5.

An arthrodesis may be terminated at L5 if the L5–S1 disc height is well maintained, there is no stenosis at this segment, and there is no pain related to lumbosacral degenerative disease. Patients fused to L5 must be warned of the need to extend to the sacrum at a later time.

Successful arthrodesis to the sacrum in long fusions from the thoracic spine requires a greater fixation than is used in short fusions to the sacrum. When pedicle screws into the sacrum are used as the only form of fixation for long fusions, there is a high rate of failure because of the long lever arm and excessive forces concentrated on the lumbosacral junction. Pedicle screw fixation alone suffices for three- or four-level fusions performed for degenerative curves.

A number of techniques have been advocated for improving the arthrodesis rate and diminishing the incidence of instrumentation failure at the lumbosacral junction. Anterior arthrodesis with a structural allograft at L4–5 and L5–S1 is often the primary procedure, followed by posterior arthrodesis and instrumentation either under the same anesthesia or in a staged fashion. We prefer sacral pedicle fixation combined with Galveston fixation with either iliac screws (Isola system) or rod contouring placed into iliac drill holes (Fig. 32.6) (15,16). Alternative forms of fixation include transsacral rod fixation into the sacral ala (Jackson technique), iliosacral screw fixation, first and second sacral pedicle fixation, and simultaneous first sacral pedicle and alar screw fixation (Chopin block).

Osteotomies are useful for restoring spinal alignment and balance for patients in whom previous arthrodesis or congenital bars have resulted in sagittal and/or coronal

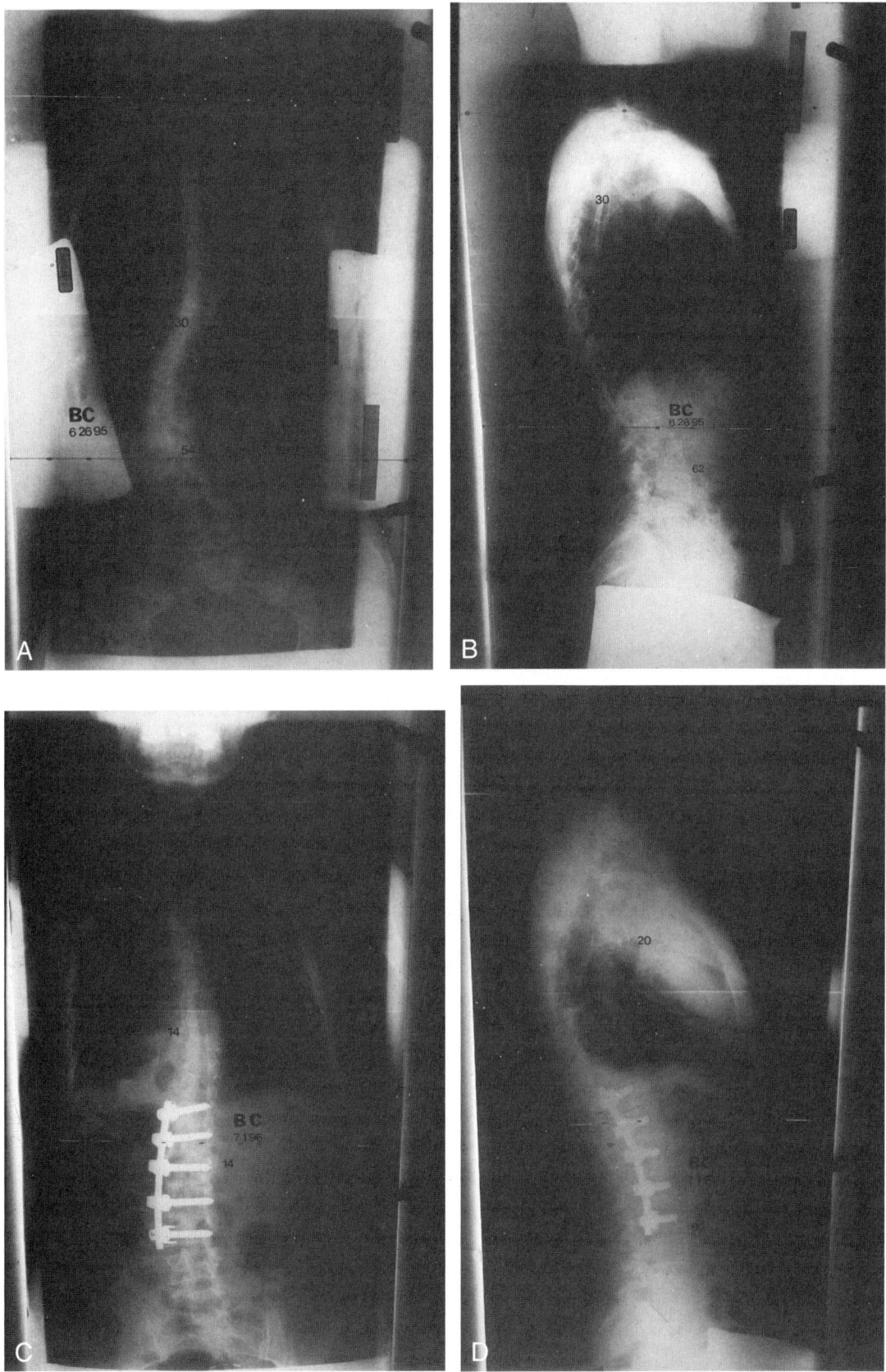

Figure 32.4. **A.** AP view of a patient with a major left thoracolumbar scoliosis, showing the left thoracolumbar curve. **B.** Lateral view showing normalization of the sagittal alignment after a single-stage anterior spinal fusion with instrumentation. **C.** AP view showing balanced correction after correction of the major deformity to 10°. **D.** Postoperative lateral view showing restoration of sagittal alignment.

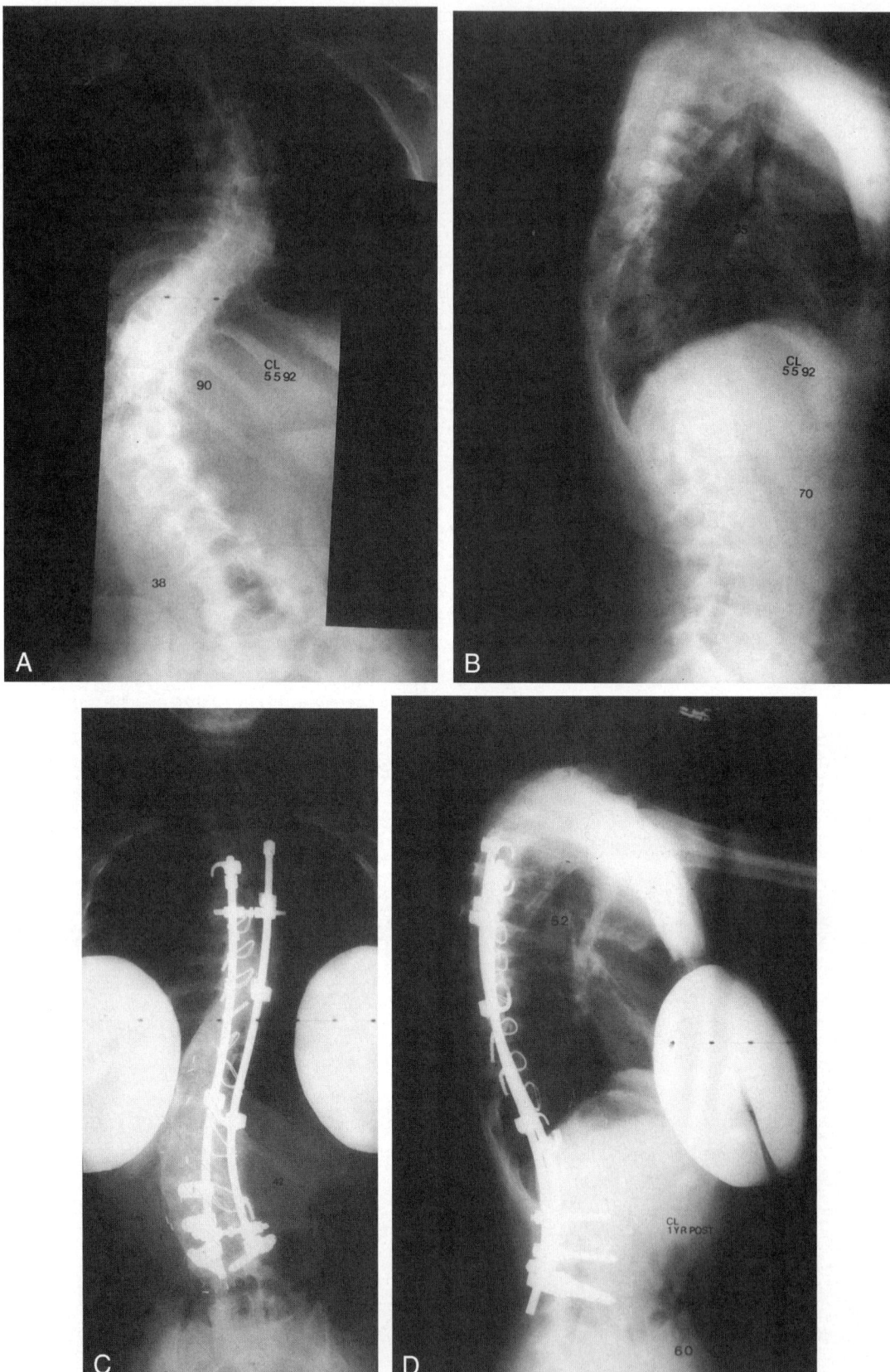

Figure 32.5. A. AP view of a patient with a major right thoracic and left thoracolumbar curve of 90°. Note the 28° fractional curve. **B.** Sagittal alignment showing thoracolumbar kyphosis. **C.** Postoperative AP view 1 year after an anterior and posterior single-stage reconstruction. Note the solid arthrodesis and segmental Isola instrumentation of the thoracic and lumbar curves to L4. **D.** Postoperative lateral view showing the restoration of sagittal alignment.

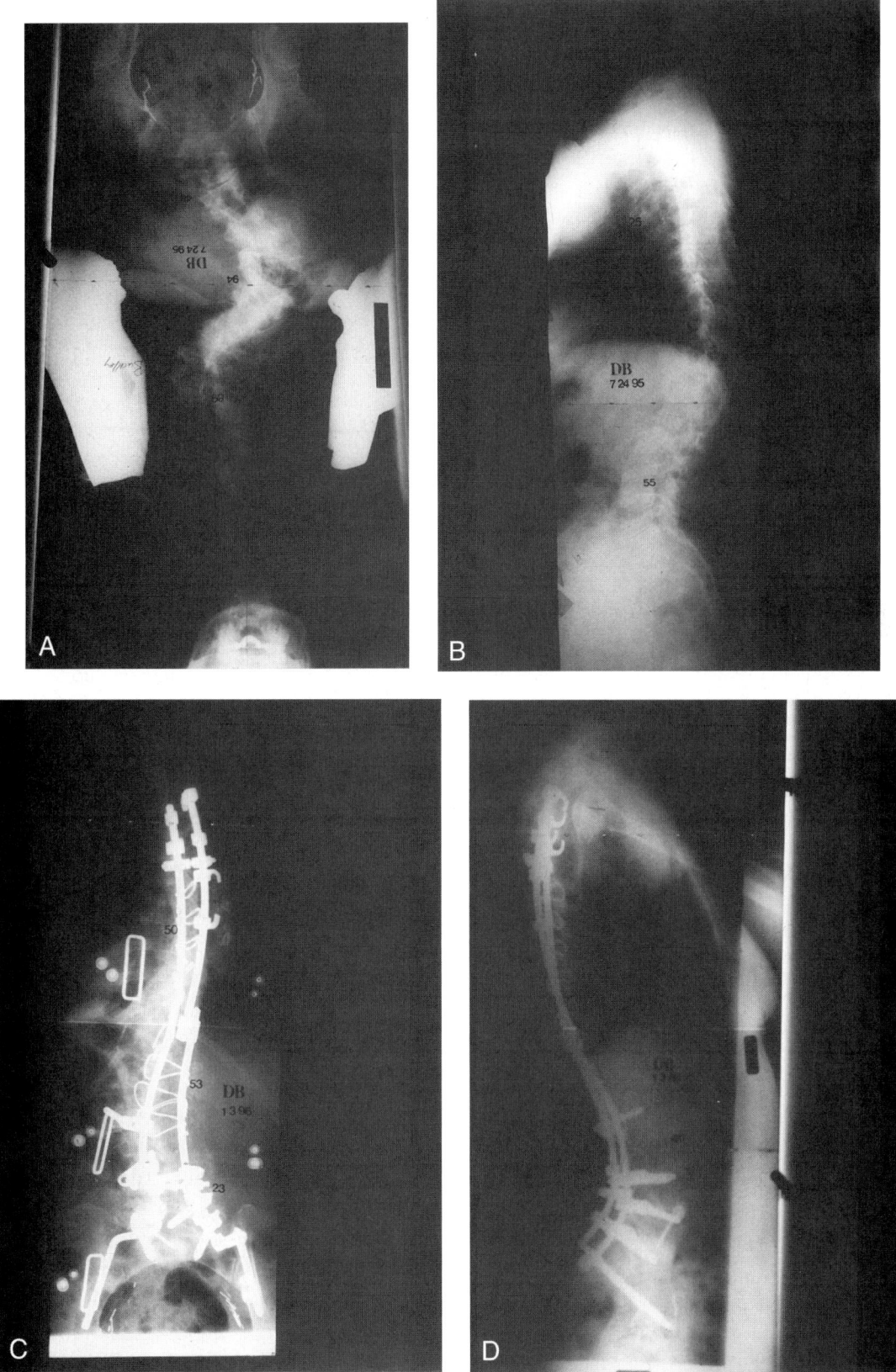

Figure 32.6. A. Preoperative AP view of a patient with a double major curve and lumbosacral degeneration. **B.** Preoperative lateral view showing associated thoracolumbar kyphosis. **C.** Postoperative AP view showing the long posterior fusion to the sacropelvis with Galveston fixation and balanced correction. **D.** Postoperative lateral view showing the restoration of the sagittal alignment.

plane imbalance. Osteotomies through the fusion mass at multiple segments can be expected to achieve up to 50° of correction. A high-speed drill is used to approach the inner cortex of the fusion mass and to enter the spinal canal in a small area. The exposed tips of the transverse processes are used as a landmark above which osteotomies are performed. Once this is achieved, a Kerrison rongeur is used to complete the osteotomy. The edges of the osteotomy are undercut in the midline and laterally in the foraminal region to prevent nerve root and dural entrapment with closure of the osteotomy. Closure is performed by extending the hips and performing segmental compression instrumentation. Anterior osteotomies or partial vertebral resection may be required in the face of previous anterior arthrodesis.

Instrumentation of a fused spine can be performed by placing hooks in the fusion mass or by using segmental pedicle fixation. Biplanar correction can be achieved by multiple posterior osteotomies done in a trapezoidal configuration to correct coronal and sagittal malalignment. Alternatively, anterior vertebral column resections or wedge osteotomies at the appropriate level can be performed in addition to posterior osteotomies (17,18). To minimize the number of levels that must achieve arthrodesis and decrease the potential for pseudarthrosis, the surgeon should limit the number of osteotomies performed.

Pitfalls and Complications

NEUROLOGIC COMPLICATIONS

Direct injury of neural elements from instrumentation components (e.g., hooks, wires, and screws) or indirect injury caused by ischemic insult or neurapraxia related to distractive forces occurs in less than 5% of all cases. Intraoperative spinal cord monitoring and the use of the Stagnara wake-up test are useful in limiting these potential complications (19).

SPINAL DECOMPENSATION

In performing corrective instrumentation for spinal deformity, the surgeon must be attentive to achieving balance in both coronal and sagittal planes. Spinal decompensation is most commonly related to improper selection of levels of fusion. If instrumentation is terminated proximal to the neutral and/or stable vertebra or if significant tilt of the end vertebra remains, progressive decompensation and deformity caudal to the arthrodesis may occur. Thus the distal fused motion segment must be coronally and sagittally balanced. Another potential mistake is to terminate instrumentation at or just below the sagittal apex, most commonly in the thoracic spine. This may result in a progressive junctional kyphosis, requiring a later reconstructive procedure. Iatrogenic flat back deformity from distraction in the lumbar spine is rarely a problem with current segmental spinal instrumentation systems but serves as an important reminder of the need

for appropriate sagittal rod contouring and fixation at multiple points.

Overcorrection in selective thoracic fusions using derotation maneuvers for King type II curves may result in progressive coronal plane imbalance from progression of the lumbar curve (20,21). Failure to fuse all structural curves may also cause decompensation. For example, a selective thoracic fusion for a double structural thoracic and lumbar curve (thoracic curve larger and stiffer than the lumbar curve; lumbar curve exceeds 45°) that is significantly rotated and laterally displaced from the midsacral line (King type IIb) may result in coronal imbalance (Isola sequence). Selective thoracic fusions are effective when curves are repaired within the correctability of the lumbar curve on side-bending films. Finally, failure to fuse the upper thoracic curve of a double thoracic curve (King type V) will result in coronal decompensation with elevation of the left shoulder. The King type V pattern is characterized by a proximal left thoracic curve in which the first thoracic vertebra is tilted into the concavity. Fusion of both thoracic curves will prevent decompensation. The upper instrumented vertebra usually is T1 or T2.

POSTERIOR ELEMENT FAILURE

Adult deformity is often rigid and associated with osteoporosis. This combination may lead to fracture of the lamina or transverse process fixation point during corrective instrumentation. To minimize this problem, a large number of fixation points should be used with a combination of hooks, wires, and screw anchors. In addition, for large, rigid curves, anterior discectomies and osteotomies combined with posterior osteotomies as needed provide for a more supple, correctable deformity, and less corrective force is required at each fixation point. When possible, the lamina rather than the transverse or spinous process should be used for hook placement. Pedicle screws at the caudal end of an arthrodesis provide a strong foundation for a long construct.

ANTERIOR SPINAL FUSION WITH INSTRUMENTATION

Sagittal Plane Imbalance

Anterior instrumentation may lead to thoracolumbar kyphosis or loss of lumbar lordosis. This may be avoided by placing the screws posteriorly in the vertebrae and, if necessary, placing structural autograft in the disc spaces to maintain lordosis.

Coronal Plane Imbalance

Coronal plane imbalance may occur if there is a relatively large fractional lumbosacral curve or proximal compensatory curve when the primary curve is overcorrected.

COMBINED ANTERIOR AND POSTERIOR FUSION WITH POSTERIOR INSTRUMENTATION

The long arthrodesis to the sacrum is characterized by a large-lever arm on the lowest level of fixation, i.e., the sacrum. There is a significant rate of failure of lumbosacral fixation and pseudarthrosis as a result of the forces acting at this level (22). We favor the use of Galveston-type fixation with either a contoured rod or iliac screws in combination with anterior structural support in the form of femoral ring allograft packed with cancellous autograft.

OSTEOTOMIES AND DECANCELLATION

Undercorrection

In performing reconstructive osteotomies the surgeon must achieve the desired sagittal alignment. We have been able to perform 40° of correction with a single-level osteotomy and decancellation procedure. Beyond this, multiple levels must be used.

Coronal Decompensation

In biplanar deformities, posterior osteotomies alone may result in worsening of coronal deformity. It is difficult to obtain a balanced biplanar correction with a posterior approach alone. This may require a trapezoidal osteotomy that is challenging to accurately execute. We favor a combined anterior and posterior osteotomy for deformity occurring in both coronal and sagittal planes.

Neural Element Entrapment

Nerve root or dural entrapment may result if the edges of the osteotomy and the foramina are not carefully undercut to allow for adequate space for these elements on completion of the correction. Evoked potential monitoring in addition to the Stagnara wake-up tests should routinely be employed during these procedures.

Postoperative Rehabilitation

By 48 h after surgery, patients are assisted from bed to chair. Ambulation is gradually increased within the patient's tolerance limits. Custom thoracolumbar sacral orthoses are often given to the patient to be worn when the patient is out of bed. In patients who have good bone quality and in whom satisfactory fixation has been achieved, a brace may not be required. Bending and lifting is prohibited until solid arthrodesis has been achieved, generally at 6 to 12 months. Ambulation is encouraged, and aerobic exercise on a stationary bicycle may be instituted as fusion mass consolidation is noted. Gradual resumption of full activities is permitted by 6 to 9 months. Contact sports are generally prohibited for 1 or 2 years.

SUMMARY

The pathogenesis, natural history, clinical presentation, and operative indications for adult scoliosis are generally distinct from adolescent idiopathic scoliosis. The most common clinical presentation is pain. Clinical evaluation using diagnostic imaging studies is more complex and will include a CT scan, myelogram, MRI scan, discography, and bone scans when needed. Adults who have failed conservative treatment should be considered for surgical treatment, and indications include progressive deformity, painful deformity of the thoracic and lumbar curvature, restrictive pulmonary disease, neurologic symptoms, and cosmesis. Most adults with flexible thoracic and thoracolumbar balanced curves do well with posterior spinal fusion alone. Anterior and posterior spinal fusion with posterior instrumentation is recommended for adults with rigid thoracic curves over 75° that do not bend to less than 30 to 40%. Adults with decompensated thoracolumbar, lumbar, rigid, and large curves require one-stage anterior discectomy and fusion and posterior spinal fusion with instrumentation. Single-stage anterior release and fusion with instrumentation can be performed for the adult with mild to moderate thoracolumbar, lumbar curve.

Arthrodesis to the sacrum is indicated in patients with significant low back pain, stenosis, and/or disc herniation of the lumbosacral region and in patients with a curve extending to the L4–5 level. This also includes patients with significant bone mineral density loss that may produce postoperative distal junctional fracture and collapse. Combined anterior and posterior spinal reconstruction is best performed in one stage to reduce morbidity, problems associated with wound healing, and nutritional decompensation in staged procedures. For staged procedures, interval hyperalimentation or enteral support is recommended.

Complex deformities with either spontaneous ankylosis or revision require adjunctive procedures such as osteotomy and decancellation.

REFERENCES

1. Weinstein SL, Ponsetti IV. Curve progression in idiopathic scoliosis. J Bone Joint Surg 1983;65A:447–455.
2. Grubb SA, Lipscomb HJ, Coonrad RW. Degenerative adult onset scoliosis. Spine 1988;13:241–245.
3. Lagrone MO, Bradford DS, Moe JH, et al. Treatment of symptomatic flatback after spine fusion. J Bone Joint Surg 1988; 70A:569–580.
4. Kostuik JP. Decision making in adult scoliosis. Spine 1979; 4:521–525.
5. Simmons EH, Jackson RP. The management of nerve root entrapment syndromes associated with the collapsing scoliosis of idiopathic lumbar and thoracolumbar curves. Spine 1979;4:533–541.
6. Weinstein SL, Zavala DC, Ponsetti IV. Idiopathic scoliosis: long-term follow-up and prognosis in untreated patients. J Bone Joint Surg 1981;63A:702–712.
7. Winter RB, Lovell WW, Moe JH. Excessive thoracic lordosis and loss of pulmonary function in patients with idiopathic scoliosis. J Bone Joint Surg 1975;57A:972–977.
8. Jackson RP, Simmons EH, Stripinis D. Coronal and sagittal plane spinal deformities correlation with back pain and pulmonary function in adult idiopathic scoliosis. Spine 1989;14:1391–1397.
9. Bradford DS, Heithoff KB, Cohen M. Intraspinal abnormalities and congenital spine deformities: a radiographic and MRI study. J Pediatr Orthop 1991;11:3641.
10. Deyo RA. Fads in the treatment of low-back pain. N Engl J Med 1991;325:1039–1040.
11. Grubb SA, Lipscomb HJ. Diagnostic findings in painful adult scoliosis. Spine 1992;17:518–527.

12. Bridwell KH, DeWald RL, Ogilvie JW. Posterior surgery for adult spinal deformity. Paper presented at the 62nd Annual Meeting of the American Academy of Orthopaedic Surgeons, Orlando, FL, February 18, 1995.

13. Lowe TG. Current concepts review. Scheuermann's disease. J Bone Joint Surg 1990;72A:940–945.

14. Moe JH, Purcell GA, Bradford DS. Zielke instrumentation (VDS) for the correction of spinal curvature. Analysis of results in 66 patients. Clin Orthop 1983;180:133–153.

15. Allen BL, Ferguson RL. The Galveston technique for L-rod instrumentation of the scoliotic spine. Spine 1982;7:276–284.

16. Saer EH, Winter RB, Lonstein JE. Long scoliosis fusion to the sacrum in adults with nonparalytic scoliosis. Spine 1990; 15:650–653.

17. Boachie-Adjei O, Bradford DS. Vertebral column resection and arthrodesis for complex spinal deformities. J Spinal Dis 1991; 4:193–202.

18. Leatherman KD, Dickson RA. Two stage corrective surgery for congenital deformities of the spine. J Bone Joint Surg 1979; 61B:324–328.

19. Vauzelle C, Stagnara P, Jouvinroux P. Functional monitoring of spinal cord activity during spinal surgery. Clin Orthop 1973; 93:173–178.

20. Thompson JP, Transfeldt EE, Bradford DS, et al. Decompensation after Cotrel-Dubousset instrumentation of idiopathic scoliosis. Spine 1990;15:927–931.

21. Bridwell KH, McAllister JW, Betz RR, et al. Coronal decompensation produced by Cotrel-Dubousset "derotation" maneuver for idiopathic right thoracic scoliosis. Spine 1991;16: 769–777.

22. Kostuik JP. Treatment of scoliosis in the adult thoracolumbar spine with special reference to fusion to the sacrum. Orthop Clin North Am 1988;19:371–381.

*Kenneth K. Hansraj, Frank P. Cammisa, Jr., Federico P. Girardi,
and Patrick F. O'Leary*

Herniated Nucleus Pulposus in the Lumbar Spine

Low back pain (LBP) is a common symptom, affecting 60 to 80% of individuals at some point in their lives. It is the most frequent and most costly musculoskeletal impairment. It ranks third behind arthritis/rheumatism and heart disease as a cause of disability in people in their working years. While LBP is common from the second decade on, herniated lumbar disc is most prominent in otherwise healthy people in the third and fourth decades of life. Most patients relate their back and leg pain to a traumatic injury. However, further questioning may show a history of back pain for months and even years preceding their acute episode.

RELEVANT ANATOMY AND PATHOGENESIS

The motion segment is the basic anatomic unit of the spine. It is composed of two adjacent vertebrae, the intervertebral disc, and their intervening soft tissues. The disc forms the primary articulation between the vertebral bodies and is the major constraint to motion; it is made up of two parts. The annulus fibrosus (the outer part of the disc) consists of approximately 90 bonded type I collagen sheets. The fibers of the collagen sheets are oriented vertically at the periphery, but they become progressively more oblique with each underlying layer. These layers derive strength from the lamination. The nucleus pulposus (inner part of the disc) is made up of type II collagen, although in young adults it is generally 90% water. The remaining structure consists of collagen and proteoglycans, which bind water.

A lumbar herniated nucleus pulposus (HNP) may be classified as bulging, extruded, or sequestrated. A bulging disc is protruding, but the annulus is still intact. An extruded disc has herniated through the annulus but is contained by the posterior longitudinal ligament. A sequestrated disc is free in the canal.

The intervertebral lumbar disc is injured predominantly through rotation and shear, which produce circumferential and radial tears. The inner layer weakens and becomes torn, which adds stress on the outer layers, leading to a radial tear. When the outer layers are torn, the inner layers of the annulus and segments of the nucleus may be forced through the weak areas.

The outer areas of the annulus are richly innervated, thus the severe LBP experienced by the patient. The herniated nuclear substance may cause a chemical neuritis with inflammation. Spasm and pain are mediated through the sinuvertebral nerve, which branches from the posterior primary ramus. Substance P, vasoactive intestinal peptide (VIP), and calcitonin gene-related peptide (CGRP) have been identified in the outer annulus and the supraspinous and interspinous ligaments. The dorsal root ganglion may serve as a storage area. Over time, the herniated nucleus pulposus extrudes, causing mechanical compression of the nerve, resulting in sciatica and/or radiculopathy.

INITIAL FINDINGS, PHYSICAL EXAMINATION, AND DIAGNOSIS

The patient is generally a healthy 20- to 40-year-old. There may be a history of rotational and torsional activities in sports. Most patients cite a specific traumatic incident; however, after being questioned further, many will relate that they have had LBP for months or years secondary to annulus degeneration. The pain is typically brought on by heavy exertion, repetitive bending, twisting, heavy lifting, and sometimes reaching.

Severe back pain precedes leg pain. Back pain generally lessens as the leg pain begins to predominate. Symptoms increase with activity, especially sitting. Symptoms are exacerbated with a flexion episode and may be relieved by rest.

Numbness and weakness in both legs with rectal pain, sensory changes in the perineum, paralysis of the sphincters, and/or sudden loss of bladder or bowel control should alert the physician to cauda equina syndrome, which is a surgical emergency.

Acutely, the patient may experience paraspinal spasm, sciatica, scoliosis or list, loss of normal lordosis, or tenderness of the involved spinous process. Weakness and paresthesia may or may not be present in a dermatomal distribution.

Straight leg raising (SLR) is a delicate and accurate test. The lower extremity is flexed at the hip with the knee held in full extension. When the limit of straight leg raising has been reached, further tension is caused by dorsiflexion of the ankle (Lasègue's test), which puts further stress on the sciatic nerve. During SLR the first 15° to 30° of elevation causes little or no movement of the nerve root at the foraminal level. At 30° there is traction on the sciatic nerve. The greatest disturbance of root movement occurs when the SLR has brought the leg to an angle of 60° to 80°. The greatest degree of movement occurs in the L5 nerve root. There is slight movement at L4 and essentially no movement at L3 and L2. A positive SLR is of great value in helping locate disc herniation at the L5–S1 and L4–5 levels, but its absence does not argue against a disc herniation existing at a higher level.

The contralateral straight leg raise is equally objective and informative. Reproduction of symptoms in the involved extremity by elevation of the noninvolved leg is a positive test. On rare occasions, the contralateral SLR is elicited with a negative ipsilateral SLR test.

The posterior tibial nerve test (bowstring sign) is even more accurate in evaluating the L5 or S1 root. The SLR is performed as usual. At the limit of the SLR, the knee is flexed, reducing the tension on the sciatic root and hamstrings. The hips are further flexed, and the knee is again extended until pain is produced. At this point, the posterior tibial nerve is stretched like a bowstring across the popliteal fossa. Firm pressure is applied with the ball of the thumb over the nerve in the popliteal fossa. The patient is asked to describe the pain. A positive test provokes pain in a dermatomal distribution either retrograde or antegrade. Pain or discomfort locally in the popliteal fossa is not significant.

The femoral nerve roots are not well evaluated with the above tests. The femoral nerve passes into the thigh in front of the pubic ramus, and SLR will relieve any tension on these roots. The femoral nerve stretch test is performed with the patient placed prone or lying on the side. The femoral nerve is stressed by extending the hip with a flexed knee.

L4 root compression is generally indicative of a posterolateral L3–4 disc herniation or extraforaminal far lateral L4–5 herniation (Table 33.1). Motor deficit includes the tibialis anterior and, to various degrees, the quadriceps and the adductor musculature. Sensory deficit is along the posterolateral thigh, anterior knee, and medial leg. Reflex changes may be found in the patellar tendon.

L5 root compression is generally indicative of a posterolateral L4–5 disc or a far lateral L5–S1 herniation. Motor deficit includes the extensor hallucis longus, gluteus medius, medial hamstrings, and extensor digitorum longus and brevis. Sensory deficit is along the anterolateral leg, the dorsum of the foot, and the great toe. Reflex changes are not usually found. Tibialis posterior reflexes are difficult to elicit.

S1 root compression is generally indicative of L5–S1 disc herniation. Motor deficit includes the peroneus longus and brevis, the gastrocnemius–soleus complex, and the gluteus maximus (hip extensors). Sensory deficit is along the lateral malleolus, lateral foot, heel, and web of the fourth and fifth toe. Reflex changes may be found in the Achilles tendon.

Differential Diagnosis

The differential diagnosis of lumbar HNP may be divided into sources extrinsic and intrinsic to the spine. Sources extrinsic to the spine include the urogenital, gastrointestinal, vascular, endocrine, extraspinal nervous, and extrinsic musculoskeletal systems. Sources intrinsic to the spine include infections, tumors, metabolic disturbances, congenital abnormalities, associated diseases of aging, the local hematopoietic system, the spinal musculoskeletal system, the local neurologic system, trauma, and immune diseases. A thorough spinal evaluation includes consideration for ankylosing spondylitis, multiple myeloma, vascular insufficiency, arthritis of the hip, osteoporosis with stress fractures, extradural tumors, peripheral neuropathy, and herpes zoster. Sources causing sciatica not related to lumbar herniated nucleus pulposus include synovial cysts, rupture of the medial head of the gastrocnemius,

| table | 33.1 | Clinical Manifestations of Compressed Lumbar Nerve Roots |

Nerve Root	Posterolateral Herniation	Far Lateral Herniation	Motor Deficit	Sensory Deficit	Reflex
L4	L3–4	L4–5	Tibialis anterior; quadriceps; adductors	Posterolateral thigh; anterior knee; medial leg	Patellar tendon
L5	L4–5	L5–S1	Extensor hallucis longus; gluteus medius; extensor digitorum longus and brevis	Anterolateral leg; dorsum or foot	Usually none; posterior tibialis
S1	L5–S1		Peroneus longus and brevis; gastrocnemius-soleus complex	Lateral malleolus; lateral foot, heel, and web of 4th and 5th toes	Achilles tendon

sacroiliac joint dysfunction, sacral lesions, pelvic lesions, and ischial tuberosity fractures.

RADIOLOGIC STUDIES

X-rays should include a lumbar spine series: AP, lateral, and oblique views and, when clinically indicated, flexion and extension views. The following radiographic parameters have no association with LBP: disc space narrowing,

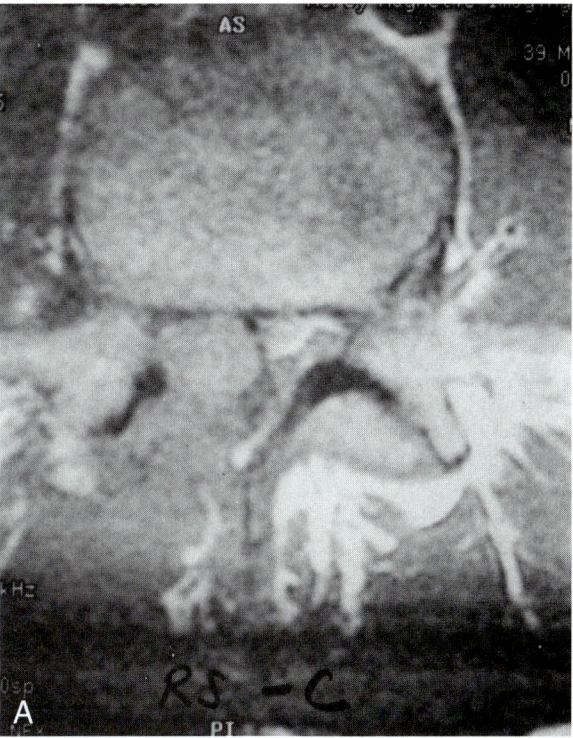

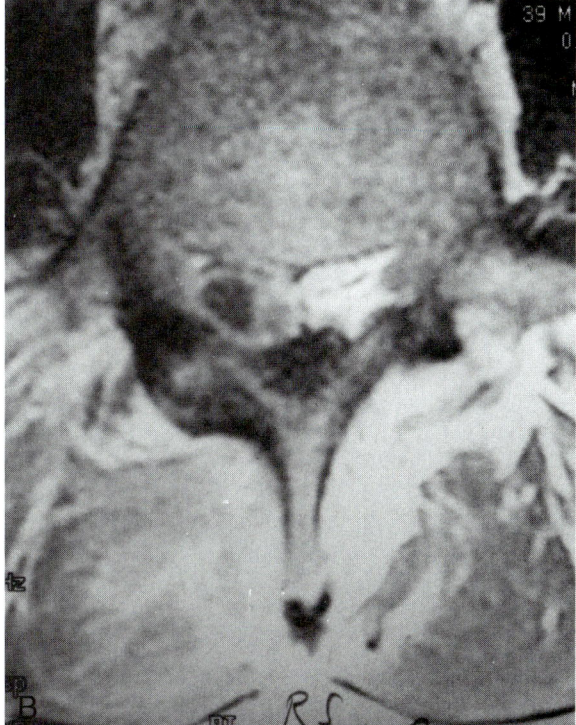

Figure 33.2. A. MRI scan without gadolinium showing recurrent L4–5 right herniated nucleus pulposus. **B.** MRI scan with gadolinium reveals the recurrent fragment surrounded by fibrosis.

transitional vertebrae, Schmorl's nodes, lumbar lordosis, disc vacuum sign, claw spur, scoliosis, level of pelvic inter-cristal line, disc space wedging, length of the transverse processes of L3 and L4, and spina bifida occulta.

Myelography followed by a CT scan may be used in the evaluation of herniated nucleus pulposus. It is an invasive study but has an accuracy of 67 to 100%. It is no longer the

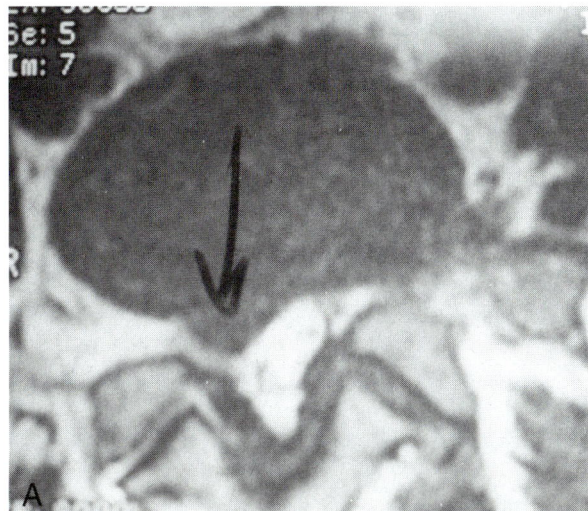

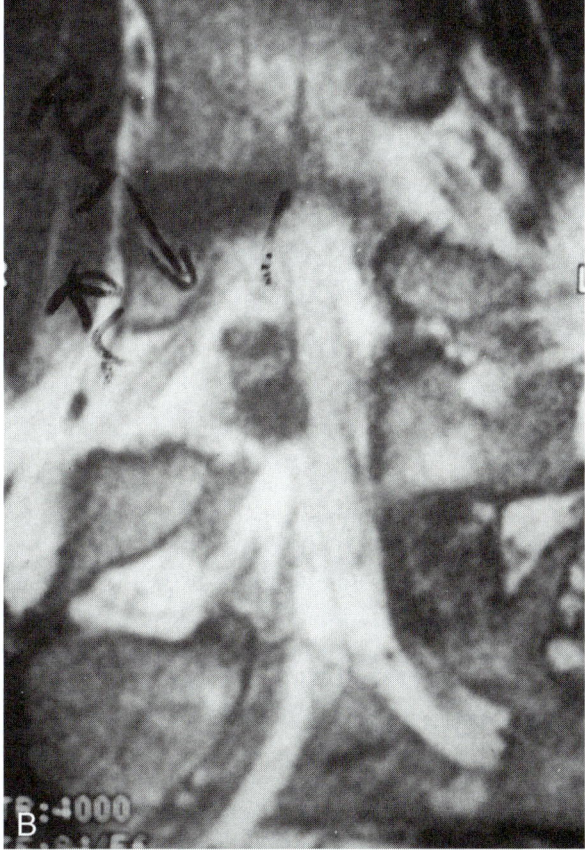

Figure 33.1. A. Axial view MRI showing a right L4–5 disc herniation that is compressing the dural sac and right L5 nerve root. **B.** Coronal view showing a disc herniation that has migrated cephalad and is compressing the right L4 nerve root.

imaging technique of choice, although it is useful when disc herniations may be associated with deformity, instability, or previous surgery.

CT alone requires a lower radiation dose than when used with myelography. It may be a sufficient diagnostic study for a simple disc herniation and lateral or foraminal herniated discs.

MRI is now the imaging modality of choice. It provides cross-sectional and orthogonal images similar to CT, and it is superior in terms of soft tissue differentiation (Fig. 33.1). MRI helps differentiate the annulus fibrosus from the nucleus pulposus, identify degenerative changes within the spine, and document changes within the disc itself. It also can rule out unusual pathologies such as conus lesions, bone lesions, and infection. Myelograms can produce false-negative indications of lateral disc herniation (1). MRI scans can identify the lateral disc as intraforaminal (located in the foramen anterior to the superior facet of the inferior vertebra), extraforaminal (located beyond the facet), or mixed.

Myelography is not a reliable method of distinguishing between recurrent disc herniation and fibrotic scar in the postoperative patient; the differentiation may also be difficult with CT. Gadopentetate dimeglumine can be used to enhance the appearance of tissue with adequate vascular supply on the MRI (Fig. 33.2). Because postoperative scar is vascular, it is enhanced on the MRI; but the recurrent disc is not.

Discography with CT may be used to study HNP. The morphology of the disc is demonstrated on contrast-enhanced radiographs (Fig. 33.3). The ideal study reproduces the patient's pain. In one study, abnormal results were found in 37% of asymptomatic patients. The physician cannot be sure of the precise source of pain in these patients. Discography with CT may also be used to study recurrent HNP and/or far lateral disc herniations.

Electromyelogram (EMG) helps assess the physiologic integrity of the nerve root, determine peripheral neuropathy (e.g., diabetes), and distinguish peroneal neuropathy from L5 radiculopathy. EMG may be used to determine the presence of generalized myopathy and assess peripheral polyneuropathy.

TREATMENT

Nonoperative Treatment

When a patient presents with acute low back and leg pain, the most conservative treatment recommendation is for 2 days of bed rest. Most of the pressure on the disc and affected nerve root will be relieved if the patient lies in a semi-Fowler position or on the side with the hips and knees flexed and a pillow between the legs. Prolonged bed rest should be avoided. Extended bed rest can cause muscle atrophy, generalized deconditioning, and osteopenia. Patients may get up for bathroom functions and for meals. Sitting, especially in low or soft chairs, should be avoided.

Aspirin provides pain relief with an anti-inflammatory effect. Time-limited use of oral muscle relaxants, analgesics, and tricyclic antidepressants may provide symptomatic relief. Passive modalities (heat or ice, massage,

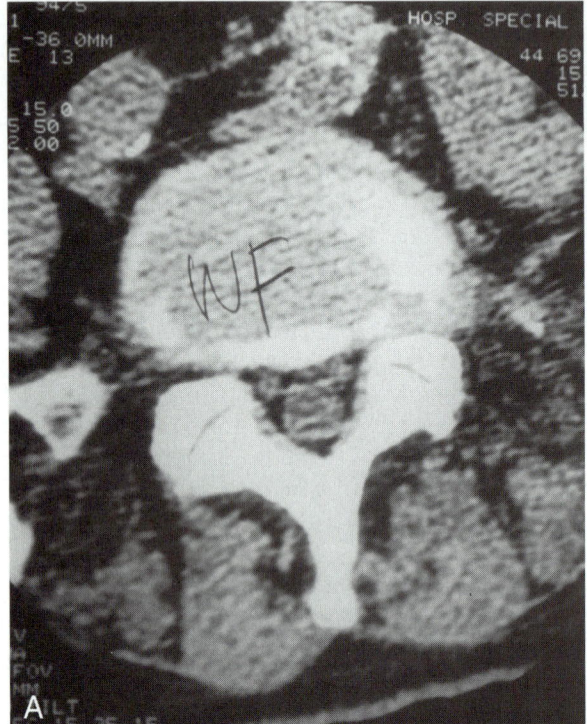
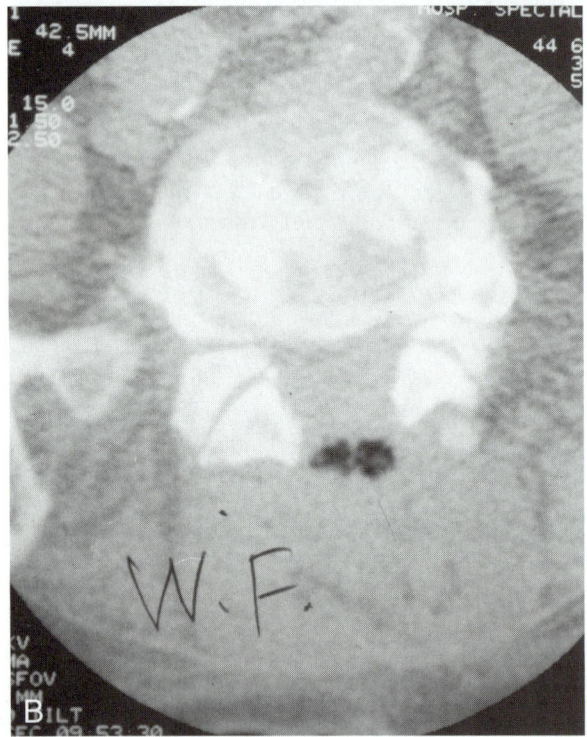

Figure 33.3. A. Preoperative CT scan showing left L5–S1 far lateral disc herniation with compression of the left L5 nerve root. This was not recognized at the time of surgery, which involved a laminectomy for lumbar spinal stenosis. The patient had persistent postoperative left L5 radiculopathy. **B.** Postdiscography CT scan showing a far lateral disc herniation that is compressing the left L5 nerve root.

acupuncture, transcutaneous electrical nerve stimulation, ultrasound) may be recommended for short periods. The efficacy of the following frequently prescribed modalities has not been proven scientifically: strong narcotics, muscle relaxants, oral steroids, antidepressants, transcutaneous electrical nerve stimulation (TENS), traction, back braces, corsets, ultrasound therapy, and diathermy.

Physical therapy should be used judiciously. The exercises should be fitted to the symptoms and not regimented to the patient. An individualized program requires careful consideration of the clinical situation. Generally, range of motion or stretching exercises precede muscle-strengthening techniques; low-impact aerobic exercises, if tolerated by the patient, can then be done. The McKenzie extension regimen can help centralize the pain pattern and diminish extremity radiation of herniated lumbar nucleus pulposus with radiculopathy. The Williams flexion exercises are useful in mechanical LBP syndromes without a major radicular component. Modern-day back care emphasizes patient education, especially in the areas of prevention, fitness and strength, lifestyle habits, and stress management.

Long-acting steroids with anesthetics may be administered in the epidural space. Studies show a 60 to 85% short-term success rate and a 30 to 40% long-term (6 months) rate. The best results are in chronic leg pain without previous surgery. Epidural steroid injections are contraindicated in infection, neurologic disease, bleeding diathesis, cauda equina syndrome, and rapidly progressive neural deficit. Complications of epidural steroid injections include failure to place the needle into the epidural space, intrathecal injection, transient hypotension, difficulty in voiding, severe paresthesias, cardiac angina, headache, transient hypercorticoidism, and bacterial meningitis.

Operative Treatment

OPEN TECHNIQUES FOR DISCECTOMY

Absolute indications for surgery include cauda equina syndrome and progressive neurologic deficit. Relative indications for surgery are pain and static neurologic deficit (Clinical Table).

The traditional open technique uses general or epidural anesthesia (2). The abdomen is allowed to hang free on a four-poster table. Alternatively, the knee–chest position can be used. The surgeon may use loupes with magnification and a headlamp to better visualize the local anatomy. Bipolar cautery leads to less thermal trauma to the tissues and secures hemostasis.

The surgeon must identify the affected level carefully, usually using an x-ray. A limited skin incision is followed through the fascia and then through a subperiosteal dissection to the lamina. With the lamina and ligamentum flavum exposed, a curette is used to remove ligamentum flavum from the inferior surface of the lamina. A Kerrison rongeur is used to remove bone. The ligamentum flavum is elevated and dissected back to expose the dura and epidural fat below. The dura and nerve root are retracted to expose the disc, which is removed using tissue forceps and graspers. It is important to inspect above and below the posterior longitudinal ligament and in the root axilla for fragments. Menostasis is an important consideration throughout the procedure.

A microsurgical lumbar discectomy is performed in a similar fashion. However, visualization of the local anatomy is through the operating microscope with a 400- or 200-mm lens. Special microretractors and microinstrumentation, including a micropituitary rongeur, are used. Some surgeons recommend using a combination suction nerve root retractor. The skin incision is made precisely above the involved level. The epidural space is entered by penetration of ligamentum flavum. A micro-45 Kerrison rongeur may be used to remove the ligamentum flavum. The annular defect is dilated with a Penfield number 4 dissector, and the herniated lumbar nucleus pulposus is decompressed with discectomy forceps.

The traditional open discectomy has a reported good/excellent rate of 80 to 97% (2); and microdiscectomy has a good/excellent rate of 80 to 88% (3). Complications of either open technique are uncommon, but include wound infection, discitis, cerebral spinal fluid leak, and nerve root injury (4–6). Cauda equina syndrome, retroperitoneal vascular injury, thrombophlebitis, pulmonary embolism, and other systemic complications have also been reported.

CHEMONUCLEOLYSIS

Chemonucleolysis is currently in disfavor in the United States. It has, however, been in use for 30 years, first investigationally and then for general use in 1982 after Food and Drug Administration (FDA) approval. Presently, the technique is used much more frequently in Europe than in the United States. The indication for chemonucleolysis is a symptomatic contained lumbar disc that is refractive to conservative measures. Contraindications include sensitivity to papaya and its derivatives, severe spondylolisthesis, progressive neurologic deficit, paralysis, spinal cord tumor, cauda equina syndrome, and previous use of the enzyme (7, 8).

Reported good/excellent results for chemonucleolysis are between 76 and 90%. Case reports of transverse myelitis, cerebral hemorrhage, and deaths have dampened the enthusiasm to use this enzyme.

PERCUTANEOUS LUMBAR DISCECTOMY

In 1975, Hijikata (9) performed the first percutaneous nucleotomy, using modified pituitary forceps. In 1985, Davis et al. (10) introduced an automated cutting/suction device for disc removal. Various innovators have modified the percutaneous lumbar discectomy technique to include microendoscopic instrumentation and lasers (11). In 1986, Choy et al. (12) was credited with being the first to use the Nd:YAG laser for decompression of the lumbar disc. In 1996, Chiu pioneered the combined use of mechanical decompression with microinstrumentation, the reciprocating cutting/suction device, and holmium laser at low-level energy to tighten and shrink the disc.

Clinical Table: Herniated Nucleus Pulposus in the Lumbar Spine

Procedure	Indications	Technique	Anatomy	Pitfalls
Open disc excision	• Absolute — Cauda equina syndrome — Progressive neurologic deficit • Relative — Pain — Static neurologic deficit	• Posterior midline approach • Subperiosteal dissection • Flavectomy • Discectomy • Laminotomy • Hemilaminectomy	• Each nerve root must be identified and protected	• Incomplete decompression of the disc • Dural tear • Venous plexus bleed • Nerve root damage • Missed fragment
Microlumbar disc excision	• Absolute — Cauda equina syndrome — Progressive neurologic deficit • Relative — Pain — Static neurologic deficit	• Posterior midline approach • Subperiosteal dissection • Flavectomy • Discectomy • Microinstruments	• Appropriate nerve root • Microscopic identification	• Incomplete or incorrect identification of appropriate nerve root • Dural tear • Venous plexus bleed • Nerve root damage • Missed fragment
Chemonucleolysis	• Symptomatic contained lumbar disc	• Lateral decubitus position • Hips and knees flexed • Fluoroscopic guidance	• Abdominal contents at risk with poor technique	• Transverse myelitis • Inject outside of the disc space
Automated percutaneous lumbar discectomy (APLD)	• Symptomatic contained lumbar disc	• Lateral decubitus position • Hips and knees flexed • Fluoroscopic guidance • Nucleotome	• Abdominal contents at risk with poor technique	• L5–S1 is a difficult entry because of high-riding iliac crests • Discitis • Rapid degeneration of the disc
Percutaneous lumbar laser discectomy	• Symptomatic contained lumbar disc	• Lateral decubitus position • Hips and knees flexed • Fluoroscopic guidance • Laser	• Abdominal contents at risk with poor technique	• L5–S1 is a difficult entry because of high-riding iliac crests • Discitis • Rapid degeneration of the disc
Endoscopic-assisted APLD	• Symptomatic contained lumbar disc	• Lateral decubitus position • Hips and knees flexed • Fluoroscopic guidance • Microinstruments • Discectomy • Laser • Endoscope	• Abdominal contents at risk with poor technique	• L5–S1 is a difficult entry because of high-riding iliac crests • Discitis • Rapid degeneration of the disc

The indication for percutaneous lumbar discectomy is intractable pain with radicular symptoms (numbness, weakness, and reflex changes) and a positive MRI or CT scan for a contained disc in a consistent dermatome that has failed conservative management. Contraindications for percutaneous lumbar discectomy include evidence of acute or progressive degenerative spinal cord diseases, neurologic or vascular processes mimicking a disc, presence of bone spurs blocking entry into the disc space, evidence of central canal or lateral recess stenosis, and presence of an extruded disc.

The surgical technique for percutaneous lumbar discectomy is as follows. The patient is placed in the lateral decubitus position, and a towel roll is placed under the flank. Both hips and knees are flexed at 90°, and a pillow is placed between the legs. The patient is prepared, draped, and injected with 2% Xylocaine at the entry point. Entry is at the respective level, 8 to 12 cm away from the midline. An 18-gauge trocar is introduced approximately 50° laterally from the midline. The trocar tip is checked on the fluoroscope in both the AP and lateral planes. Using a guidewire, the surgeon places a cannula within the disc. With the use of a fluoroscope, the surgeon uses microinstruments, a reciprocating cutting/suction device, or a laser probe to decompress the disc. As noted, the Nd:YAG laser was once the predominant laser; recently, however, the holmium laser has been used to decompress and tighten the disc (*thermodiscoplasty*). The endoscope permits visualization of the decompression and may be used to assess residual disc and debris.

The good/excellent results of percutaneous lumbar discectomy range from 44 to 100% (13). These results reflect the lack of consistent inclusion criteria, the lack of a consistent rating system, the lack of consistent factors that are evaluated, and the wide variation in follow-up. The technique and modalities of treatment vary greatly by surgeon. Reported complications of this technique include neurologic injury, vascular injury, disc space infection, abdominal injuries, and retroperitoneal hematoma (14,15).

SUMMARY

Herniated nucleus pulposus in the lumbar spine is particularly disabling because it is most prominent in otherwise healthy people in the third and fourth decades of life. A number of nonoperative treatments can be effective, although cauda equina syndrome and progressive neurologic deficit remain absolute indications for surgical treatment. In those patients with continued pain with nonoperative treatment and a static neurologic deficit, surgery also is frequently considered.

Newer surgical methods including percutaneous lumbar discectomy provide encouraging results, though evaluation of the success of these methods needs to be more consistent among clinicians.

REFERENCES

1. Postacchini F, Montanaro A. Extreme lateral herniations of lumbar disks. Clin Orthop 1979;138:222–227.
2. Spangfort EV. The lumbar disc herniation. A computer-aided analysis of 2,504 operations. Acta Orthop Scand Suppl 1972;142:1–95.
3. Spengler DM, Ouellette E, Battie M, et al. Elective discectomy for herniation of a lumbar disc. J Bone Joint Surg 1990;72A:230–237.
4. Garrido E, Rosenwasser RH. Painless footdrop secondary to lumbar disk herniation: report of two cases. Neurosurgery 1981;8:484–486.
5. Hodge CJ, Binet EF, Kieffer SA. Intradural herniation of lumbar intervertebral discs. Spine 1978;3:346–350.
6. Harbison SP. Major vascular complications of intervertebral disc surgery. Ann Surg 1954;140:342.
7. Crenshaw C, Frazer AM, Merriam WF, et al. A comparison of surgery and chemonucleolysis in the treatment of sciatica: a prospective randomized trial. Spine 1984;9:195.
8. Hall BB, McCulloch JA. Anaphylactic reactions following the intradiscal injection of chymopapain under local anesthesia. J Bone Joint Surg 1983;65A:1215–1219.
9. Hijikata, S. Percutaneous nucleotome new concept technique and 12 years experience. Clin Orthop 1989;289:9–23.
10. Davis GW, Onik G, Helms, O. Automated percutaneous discectomy. Spine 1991;16:359–363.
11. Sherk HH. Lasers in orthopaedics. Philadelphia: Lippincott, 1990.
12. Choy DS, Case RB, Fielding W, et al. Percutaneous laser nucleolysis of lumbar disks. N Engl J Med 1987;317:771–772.
13. Bernhardt M, Gurganious LR, Bloom DL, White AA III. Magnetic resonance imaging analysis of percutaneous discectomy. A preliminary report. Spine 1993;18:211–217.
14. Gill K. New-onset sciatica after automated percutaneous discectomy. Spine 1994;19:466–467.
15. Gill K. Retroperitoneal bleeding after automated percutaneous discectomy. A case report. Spine 1990;15:1376–1377.

Lumbar Spinal Stenosis

The syndrome of lumbar spinal stenosis was not widely diagnosed until 1954, when Verbiest (1) described findings of middle-aged and older adults with back and lower extremity pain precipitated by standing and walking and aggravated by hyperextension. He determined that congenital narrowing of the spinal canal was a contributing factor in many patients and noted that the secondary development of degenerative changes further narrowed the lumbar canal and precipitated symptoms.

RELEVANT ANATOMY AND PATHOGENESIS

Lumbar spinal stenosis has been defined as a condition involving any type of narrowing of the central spinal canal, lateral recesses, or intervertebral foramina (2,3). It may be caused by bone or soft tissue. Spinal stenosis may also be found in the cervical and thoracic spine. Stenosis of the lumbar spine is classified by the site of pathologic change: central stenosis (stenosis of the central canal), lateral recess stenosis, foraminal stenosis (compression of the nerve root between the pedicles), and extraforaminal stenosis (compression of the nerve beyond the pedicles).

There may be associated pathologies with lumbar spinal stenosis. Congenital stenosis occurs when the canal is inherently small and is usually associated with widened pedicles (e.g., as is found in achondroplastic dwarfs). The congenital type of spondylolisthesis, scoliosis, and kyphosis may be associated causes. Idiopathic lumbar spinal stenosis occurs when there is no apparent associated cause. Degenerative and inflammatory types of stenosis occur when osteoarthritis, inflammatory arthritis, diffuse idiopathic skeletal hyperostosis (DISH), scoliosis, kyphosis, and degenerative forms of spondylolisthesis are involved. Metabolic causes for stenosis include Paget's disease and fluorosis.

Spinal stenosis may be classified by time of onset and by its pathomechanics (4). Congenital stenosis is based on development, e.g., in achondroplastic dwarfs. Stenosis can

be acquired through time, e.g., with degenerative stenosis, which includes central, lateral recess, or foraminal stenosis or a combination thereof. Spondylolisthesis or a spondylolytic defect may include a lateral recess, foraminal or extraforaminal stenosis. There are iatrogenic causes of lumbar spinal stenosis, including postlaminectomy defects and postfusion (anterior or posterior) and late posttraumatic changes.

Patients with congenital stenosis present in their early 30s, patients with degenerative stenosis present from their late 50s into their 80s, and patients with stenosis resulting from degenerative spondylolisthesis present in their 50s. Males tend to be affected more frequently than are females; however, more females than males present with degenerative spondylolisthesis. According to Eisenstein (5), the average canal size is smaller in blacks than in Caucasians; however, clinically significant stenosis is rare in blacks.

The anterior boundaries of the canal consist of the disc, the posterior longitudinal ligament, and the vertebral body. The posterior boundaries consist of the ligamentum flavum and the lamina. The lateral boundaries are the pedicles. The anterior boundaries of the neuroforamina consist of the disc and the vertebral body, and the posterior boundaries are the facet joints. The superior and inferior boundaries of the neuroforamina are the pedicles.

Disc degeneration often initiates the degenerative process. With aging there is a decrease in the water and proteoglycan content of the nucleus pulposus and an increase in the keratin sulfate:chondroitin sulfate ratio. Fibrocartilaginous metaplasia occurs within the nucleus; the proportion of type I collagen increases, type III collagen is formed, and irreducible cross-links are formed. The most commonly involved sites are L5–S1, L4–5, and L3–4. There may be loss of disc height with subsequent bulging and frank herniation with or without the presence of osteophytes (6).

The facet is the posterior support in the three-joint spine motion segment unit. With aging, the facet hypertrophies, joint space is lost, and osteophytes are formed. Nerve root compression may occur between the superior articular facet and the pedicle. The ligamentum flavum may hypertrophy, compressing the canal posteriorly; it becomes broader and wider with increasing lordosis. The pedicles become larger and have broad inferior surfaces in the lower lumbar spine. It is hypothesized that with spinal stenosis there is an increased capillary permeability, leading to intraneural edema, which increases pressure and results in a mini-compartment syndrome.

MORPHOLOGIC OBSERVATIONS

The spinal canal at the lower lumbar and lumbosacral levels widens and flattens and has a more variable shape. Canal morphology was described by Eisenstein (5) in a cadaver study. The capacity of the lumbar canal was noted to be significantly greater in flexion.

Nerve root tunnels are shown to have both an inner and an outer diameter. Eisenstein (5) noted that the AP diameter of the nerve root tunnel is reduced in stenotic vertebrae. Generally, a nerve root tunnel diameter of 15 mm is considered the limit of normal; most authors recognize a diameter of 12 mm as pathologic. Verbiest (7) classified stenoses on the basis of the nerve root diameter: (a) a pure absolute stenosis has a midsagittal diameter of 10 mm or less, (b) a pure relative stenosis has a midsagittal diameter between 10 and 12 mm, and (c) a mixed stenosis has an interpedicular distance that does not contribute to the stenosis.

Bolender et al. (8) obtained CT scans of the dural sac. They found that a cross-sectional area of the dural sac of less than 100 mm^2 is consistent with stenosis and a cross-sectional area between 100 and 130 mm^2 indicates early stenosis. In the control population, the canal measured 180 ± 50 mm^2.

Physical Findings

Wiltse et al. (9) described the classic physical findings of lumbar spinal stenosis, which are presented in Table 34.1.

table	34.1	Classic Physical Findings of Lumbar Spinal Stenosis (9)

Pain in the back
Sciatic-type pain in the legs
Pain on standing, which is relieved by lying or sitting down
Cramping and pain in the calves after walking short distances
Paresthesia and numbness in one or both legs after walking relatively long distances
Walking uphill is easier than walking downhill
Bike riding, even over long distances, is easy
Hyperextension of the back produces pain
Circulation is normal
Patient's age is older than 50
Males and females equally affected

The office findings may be vague. It is important to evaluate distal pulses to rule out vascular claudication. Evaluate the range of motion of the hips to assess for osteoarthritis. Straight leg raising, sciatic tension tests, and neurologic examination are all commonly normal; however, the neurologic evaluation may be abnormal if the patient is allowed to walk to the limit of pain. Gait and posture after walking may reveal a positive stoop test: the patient walks in a stooped posture or sits bent forward in a chair to ease his or her symptoms. If the stoop test is negative (i.e., there is no resolution of symptoms), there may be a coexistent problem, such as vascular claudication, degenerative disc disease, primary osteoarthritis of the hip, or meralgia paresthetica.

The differential diagnosis for lumbar spinal stenosis includes atherosclerotic peripheral vascular disease; retroperitoneal disease, including tumors and renal abnormalities; hip or pelvic disease; peptic ulcer disease; aortic aneurysm; and depression.

RADIOLOGIC STUDIES

Myelogram followed by CT scan was historically considered the gold standard for assessing the central canal, lateral recess, and foramina (Fig. 34.1). Unfortunately, it is invasive and carries limited risks. MRI is noninvasive and may be used to assess neuroelement compression and unusual pathologies, such as tumor and infection. A combination of MRI and noncontrast CT scan is usually sufficient to define the pathologic anatomy (Fig. 34.2). In cases of associated deformity, myelopathy, and scoliosis, however, CT is best.

The use of a lumbar root block with or without contrast may indicate the symptomatic root if all pain is relieved with one block. Psychologic testing may help predict outcome. Electromyelogram (EMG) may be used to rule out polyneuropathy or neuromuscular diseases that are not common in the elderly.

TREATMENT

Nonoperative Treatment

Rest, nonsteroidal anti-inflammatory drugs (NSAIDs), and decreased activity may be all that is necessary to make the patient asymptomatic. Epidural steroid injections may be beneficial. It is important to teach the patients how best to deal with their back problems. Braces that hug the patient in a mildly forward flexed position may also be helpful.

Operative Treatment

INDICATIONS FOR AND PRINCIPLES OF SPINAL STENOSIS SURGERY

Indications for surgery are (a) increasing pain resistant to conservative measures, (b) progressively limited walk-

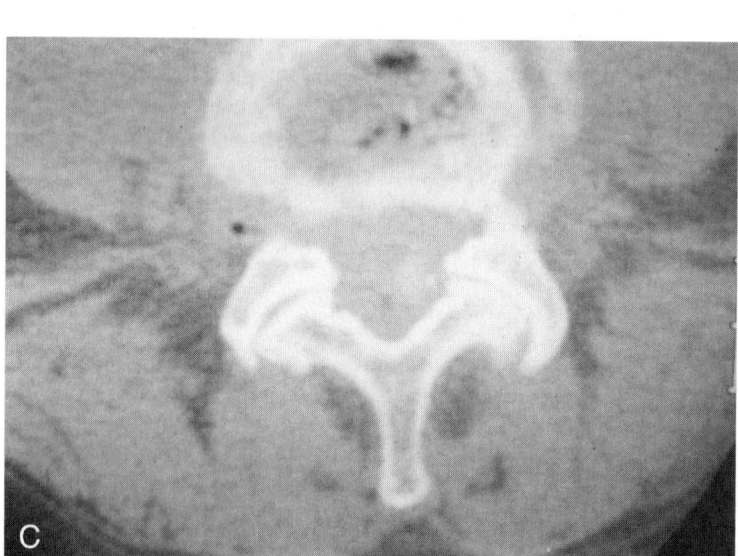

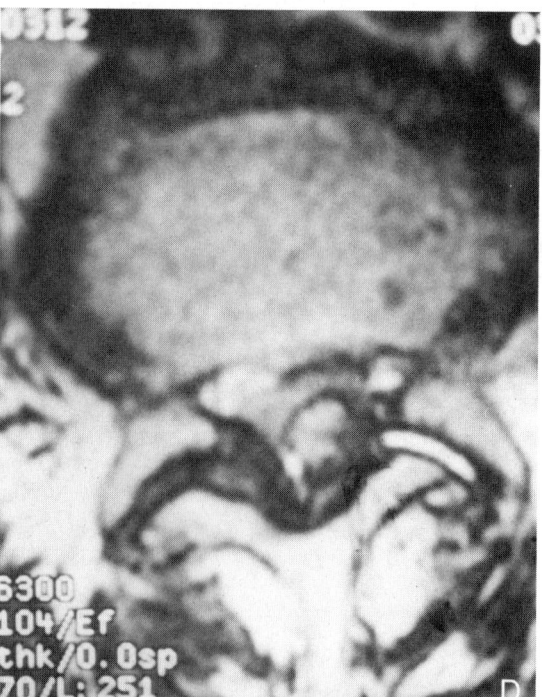

Figure 34.1. AP view (**A**) and lateral view (**B**) myelograms showing cauda equina compression at the L4–5 level. **C.** CT scan taken after the myelograms, showing calcification near the left L4–5 facet joint. **D.** MRI study showing a synovial cyst in contact with the left L4–5 facet.

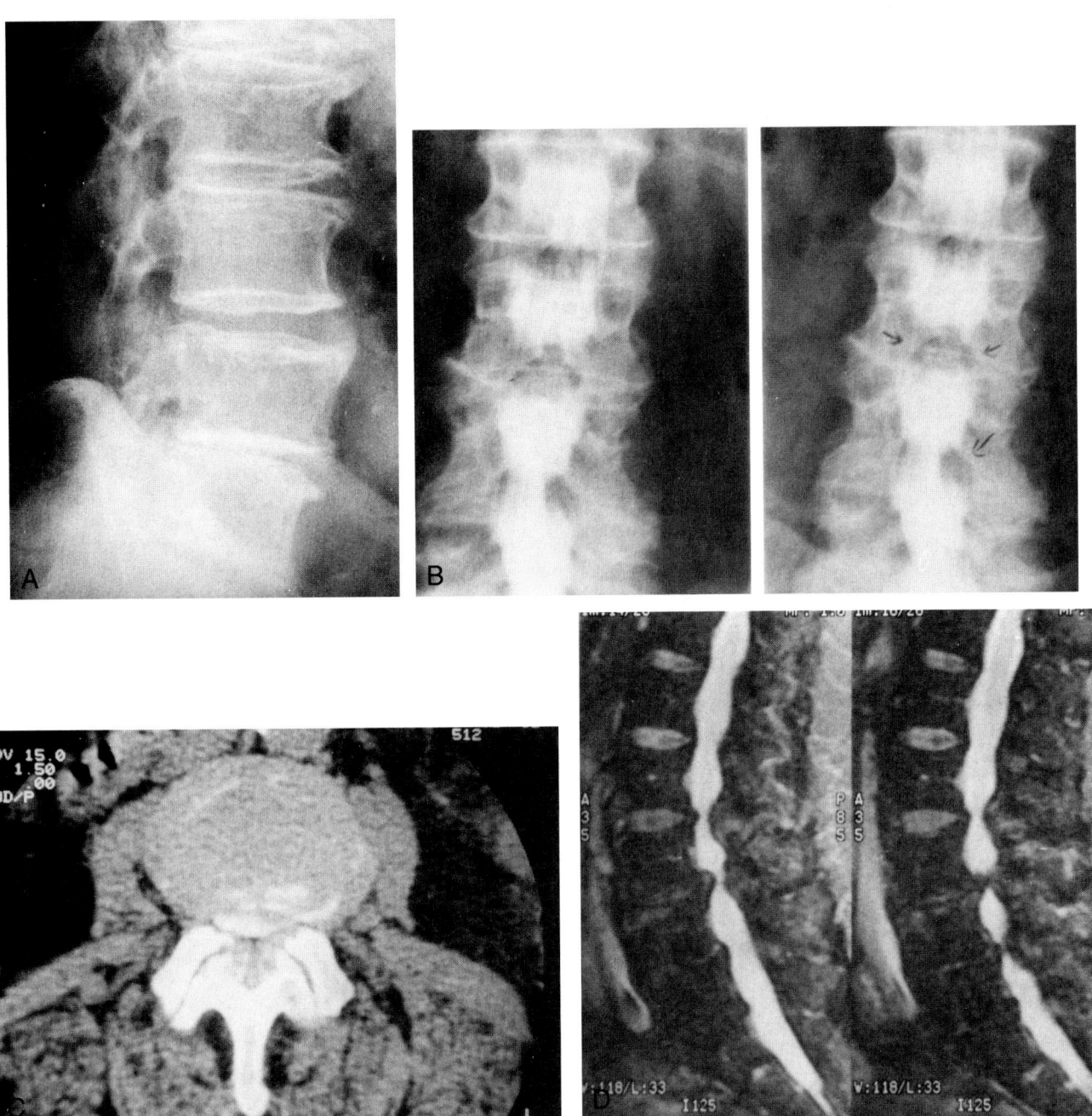

Figure 34.2. A. Lateral view radiograph showing degenerative spondylotic changes at multiple levels. **B.** AP view myelogram showing compression at multiple levels. **C.** CT scan taken after the myelograms, showing central and lateral recess stenosis. **D.** Sagittal view MRI showing multiple degenerative disc disease and compression of the dural sac.

ing distances or standing endurance, (c) major neurologic deficits, (d) progressive neurologic compromise, and (e) bowel or bladder dysfunction (Clinical Table).

The goal of spinal stenosis surgery is to decompress the neural elements but maintain stability and prevent the future occurrence of deformity. The classical procedure is laminectomy with partial medial facetectomy and partial foraminotomy (Fig. 34.3).

It is important to remove a sufficient amount of the cephalad lamina to expose the disc and nerve root.

Removing relatively more of the superior edge of the caudal lamina (angled anteriorly) permits visualization of the nerve root at the level of the pedicle. Sometimes it is necessary to remove the medial and inferior portion of the pedicle as a part of the decompression. It is imperative to maintain the pars interarticularis for stability.

It is generally recognized that removal of more than one whole facet, either by complete ablation unilaterally or by 50% ablation bilaterally, risks late instability. It is important to precisely localize the origin of pain anatomically.

Clinical Table: Lumbar Spinal Stenosis

Procedure	Indications	Technique	Anatomy	Pitfalls
Decompression	• Symptomatic spinal stenosis with failure of conservative management	• Posterior midline approach • Laminectomy • Decompression of inferior and superior facets • Foraminal decompression	• Cauda lamina • Pedicle • Facet • Nerve root	• Inadequate decompression • Dural tear • Venous plexus bleed • Segmental arterial bleed • Nerve root damage
Decompression and fusion	• Associated spondylolisthesis	• Posterior midline approach • Intertransverse fusion	• Superior cluneal nerves with harvesting of iliac crest bone graft	• Pseudarthrosis
Decompression, fusion, and instrumentation	• Instability • Associated spondylolisthesis • Associated scoliosis • Mechanical destabilization (removal of pars, radical discectomy)	• Posterior midline approach • Laminectomy • Decompression of inferior and superior facets • Foraminal decompression • Pedicle screws instrumentation • Intertransverse fusion	• Pedicle • Facet • Lamina • Nerve root • Transverse process	• Infection • Increased blood loss • Nerve root damage with placement of pedicle screws
Anterior fusion	• Associated spondylolisthesis • Associated scoliosis • Radical discectomies • Vertebral body fracture • Previous infection	• Anterior approach —Transthoracic —Transperitoneal —Retroperitoneal	• Aorta • Inferior vena cava • Ureter • Sympathetics	• Retrograde ejaculation • Extrusion of graft

Fusion, with or without instrumentation, may be necessary in cases of documented instability, iatrogenic instability (when too much bone is removed at surgery), associated spondylolisthesis, associated scoliosis, or revision surgery. The use of instrumentation depends on the individual characteristics of the patient and surgeon.

Surgeons that promote concomitant fusion for lumbar spinal stenosis with associated spondylolisthesis believe that the pain is related to osteoarthritic changes at the intervertebral joints, that decompressed segments become unstable later on, that continuous motion may produce osteophytes, that progressive instability may occur, and that progressive compression of nerve roots may occur. Surgeons that do not promote concomitant fusion point out that the stability of the decompressed spine can be maintained with meticulous dissection and preservation of the pars and a majority of the facet and that degenerative changes (including osteophytes) decrease disc height, and calcified ligaments increase the stability of the spine.

Decompression should be considered as the only mode of treatment for lumbar spinal stenosis associated with scoliosis, a rigid curve, a lack of curve progression, no predominant radiculopathy within the concavity of the curve, maintained lumbar lordosis, no evidence of lateral spondylolisthesis, and mild curves. Conversely, decompression with arthrodesis and instrumentation should be considered with curve flexibility, evidence of curve progression, predominant radiculopathy within a curve, loss of lumbar lordosis, the presence of lateral spondylolisthesis, and severe curve magnitude (Fig. 34.4).

Some cases require an anterior approach and fusion. Indications for anterior procedures include lumbar spinal stenosis with associated spondylolisthesis, scoliosis, and destabilization of the anterior column (e.g., radical discectomies, fracture of the vertebral body, and previous infection). It is important to note, however, that each case must be approached individually. The major concepts of neuroelement compression, stability, and alignment/defor-

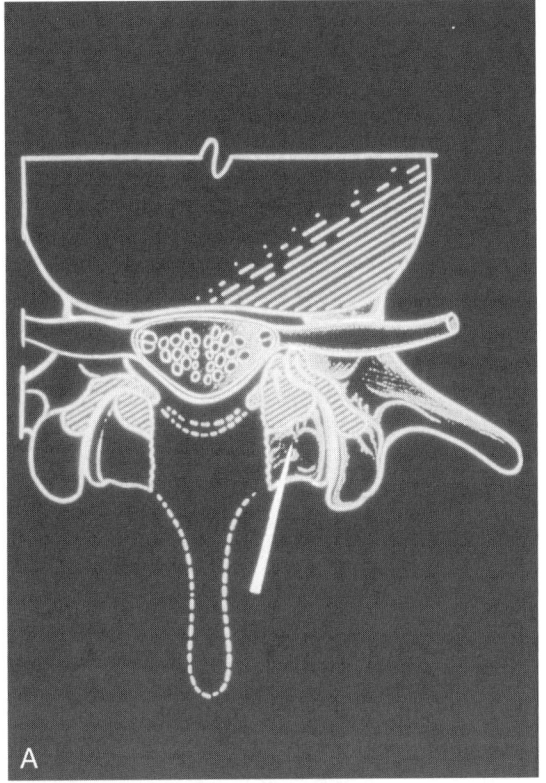

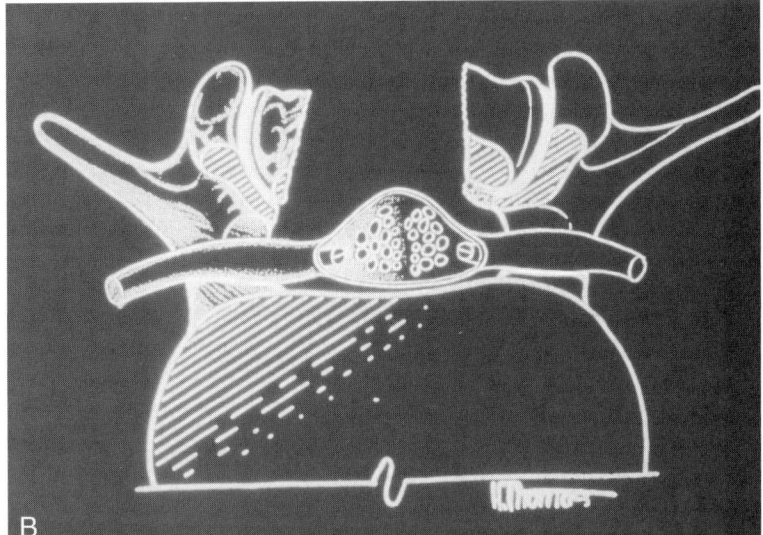

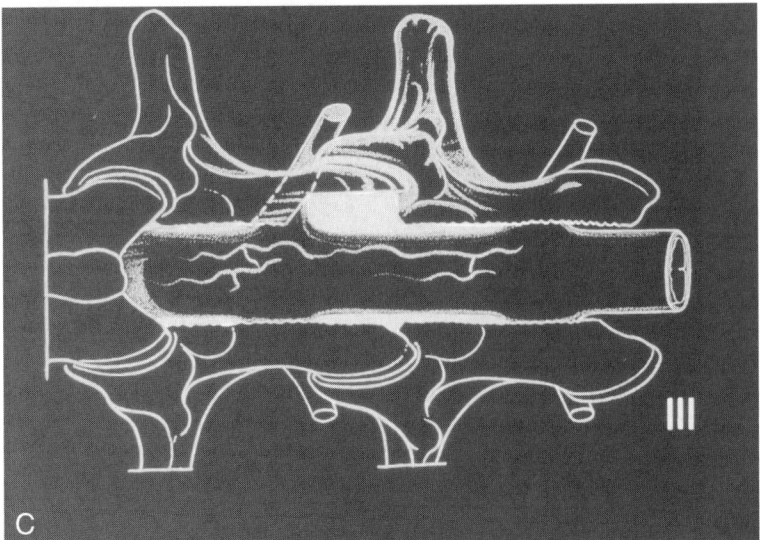

Figure 34.3. A. After central decompression (removal of the spinous process and lamina), attention is directed to the facets *(arrow)*. The medial third of the facetectomy is done with an osteotome. **B.** Bilateral medial facetectomy results in a satisfactory lateral recess decompression. **C.** Decompression that preserves the pars interarticularis and the majority of the facet.

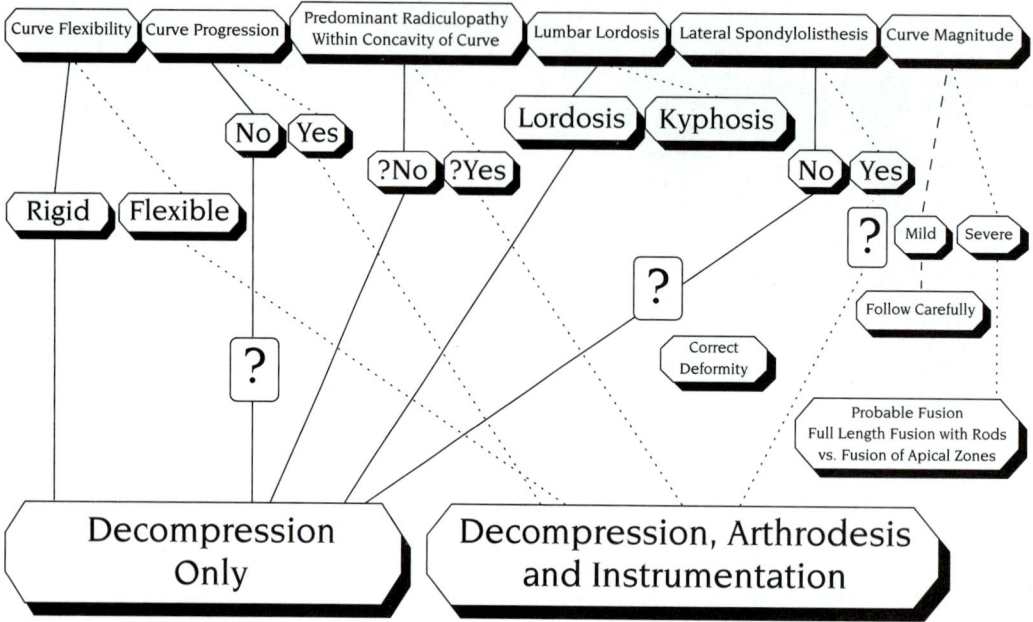

Figure 34.4. Factors involved in the management of lumbar spinal stenosis with associated scoliosis.

mity must be addressed when planning any spinal surgical procedure.

SUMMARY

Lumbar spinal stenosis remains a serious, significant, and often incapacitating cause of lower back pain in middle-aged and older adults. It is not infrequently confused with a variety of other lower back and lower extremity pain syndromes, including claudication, hip, and knee diseases. Its treatment, because it frequently occurs in the older age population, is difficult because both nonoperative and operative treatment methods may be particularly burdensome in the older age group.

In this age group as in other age groups with chronic back and leg pain that fails to respond to nonoperative treatment, the goal of spinal stenosis surgery is not only to decompress the neural elements but also to maintain stability and prevent a future occurrence of deformity.

Although technically challenging, the results of clearly identified and clearly documented spinal stenosis surgery remain good. Careful clinical and radiographic evaluation is key to diagnosis of symptomatic lumbar spinal stenosis.

REFERENCES

1. Verbiest H. A radicular syndrome from developmental narrowing of the lumbar vertebral canal. J Bone Joint Surg 36B:230–237.
2. Kirkaldy-Willis WH, Paine KW, Cauchoix J. Lumbar spinal stenosis. Clin Orthop 1974;99:30–50.
3. Kirkaldy-Willis WH, Wedge JH, Yong-Hing K, Reilly J. Pathology and pathogenesis of lumbar spondylosis and stenosis. Spine 1978; 4:319.
4. Arnoldi CC, Brodsky AE, Cauchoix J. Lumbar spinal stenosis and nerve root entrapment syndromes: definition and classification. Clin Orthop 1976;115:4–5.
5. Eisenstein S. Lumbar vertebral canal morphology for computerised tomography in spinal stenosis. Spine 1983;8:187–191.
6. Spengler DM. Current concepts review: Degenerative stenosis of the lumbar spine. J Bone Joint Surg 1979;61A:479.
7. Verbiest H. Pathomorphologic aspects of developmental lumbar stenosis. Orthop Clin North Am 1975;6:177–196.
8. Bolender NF, Schonstrom NS, Spengler DM. Role of computer tomography and myelography in the diagnosis of central spinal stenosis. J Bone Joint Surg 1985;67A:240–246.
9. Wiltse LL, Kirkaldy-Willis WH, McIvor GW. The treatment of spinal stenosis. Clin Orthop 1976;115:83–91.

chapter 35

Dwight Tyndall, Luis Alvarez, and Oheneba Boachie-Adjei

Spondylolysis and Spondylolisthesis of the Lumbar Spine

Spondylolisthesis is the forward slippage of a superior vertebral body on an inferior vertebral body. The word is derived from the Greek words *spondylos* ("vertebra") and *olisthesis* ("to slide or a slide"). Spondylolysis describes a defect located in the pars interarticularis. The suffix *lysis* means "losing, coming apart, or dissolving." Spondyloptosis is a more severe slip in which the superior vertebral body rests anterior to the inferior body.

The process was first described in 1854 by Kilian (1), who believed that the entire vertebral body slipped forward with its posterior element intact. There is no identifiable inheritance pattern for spondylolisthesis, although Wynne-Davies and Scott (2) found that relatives of patients with dysplastic spondylolisthesis had a 1 in 3 risk of developing spondylolisthesis and a 1 in 7 chance for developing isthmic spondylolisthesis.

CLASSIFICATION OF SPONDYLOLISTHESES

Several classification systems have been presented for spondylolisthesis (Fig. 35.1). The most commonly used classification is based on Wiltse and Hutchinson (3) and Wiltse et al. (4).

Type I: Dysplastic or congenital spondylolisthesis
Type II: Isthmic spondylolisthesis
Type III: Degenerative spondylolisthesis
Type IV: Traumatic spondylolisthesis
Type V: Pathologic spondylolisthesis
Type VI: Postsurgical spondylolisthesis

Type I: Dysplastic or Congenital Spondylolisthesis

Dysplastic or congenital spondylolisthesis is characterized by dysplasia of the sacrum and facet joints. Wiltse and Hutchinson (3) and Wiltse et al. (4) believe sacral dysplasia causes an instability and subsequent slippage as a result of incompetent facets. Because the facets are oriented in the pure sagittal or the axial plane, they seem to be unable to fully resist the translation forces placed on the L5–S1 articulation. A subset of type I spondylolisthesis develops a pars defect, but unlike type II (isthmic) spondylolisthesis, the pars defect is the result of the slip and subsequent stresses rather than the cause of the spondylolisthesis.

Dysplastic spondylolisthesis is typically seen in the first decade (ages 5 to 9). There are two subtypes, based on the orientation of the facets of the L5–S1 articulation. In type IA, the facets are axially oriented and are often accompanied by spina bifida, which can result in an early high-grade slip. In a series of 12 patients with congenital spondylolisthesis, Wynne-Davies and Scott (2) found that 11 had spina occulta. If the pars elongates as part of the disease, it can be difficult to distinguish this type IA from type IIB spondylolisthesis. In type IB, the facets are sagittally oriented. The neural arch remains intact, thus a high-grade slip is unlikely.

Type II: Isthmic Spondylolisthesis

The essential causative abnormality in isthmic spondylolisthesis is a spondylolytic defect in the pars. This is unlike type I, which is located within the facets. It is thought

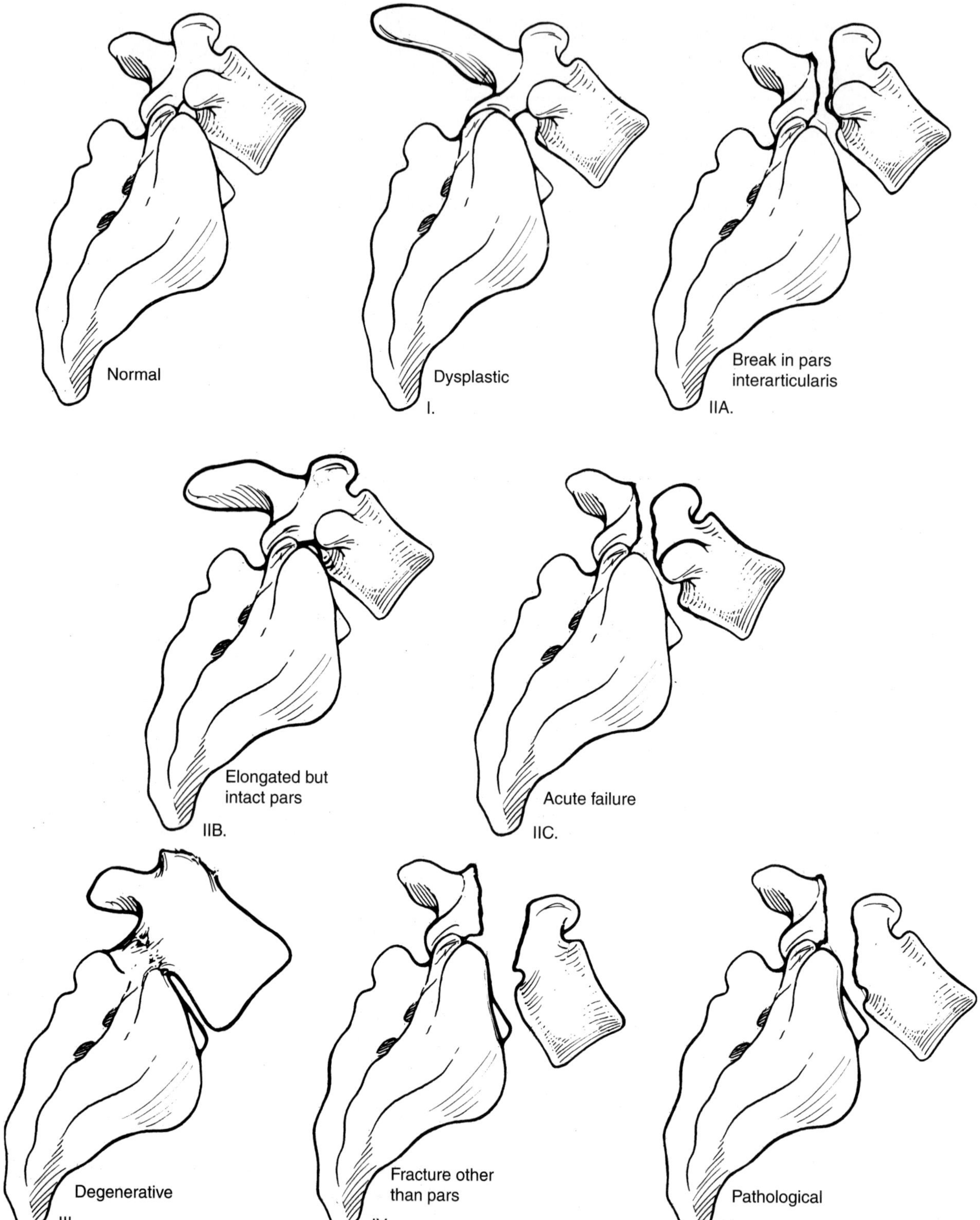

Figure 35.1. Classification of spondylolistheses.

that nonambulators do not have this spondylitic defect because the pars does not experience the forces created by the normal biped gait. Rosenberg et al. (5) studied 143 nonambulatory patients aged 11 to 93 and found no evidence of spondylolysis or spondylolisthesis in this population. There were various underlying diagnoses for these patients, but the predominant one was cerebral palsy.

The presence of spondylolisthesis in other disease processes has been reported. Ogilvie and Sherman (6) found an increased incidence of asymptomatic spondylolysis in 18 patients with Scheuermann's disease and recommended that such patients be evaluated for spondylolysis. Fisk et al. (7) found that of 500 patients with idiopathic scoliosis, 6.2% had spondylolysis; this incidence is slightly higher than that of the general population (5%). Fisk et al. recommended that both pathologies be treated as indicated. Goldstein et al. (7a) cautioned that when treating scoliosis that involves the lumbar spine, care must be taken to ensure that the lumbosacral junction is not fused in an "uncorrected" position with too much lumbosacral kyphosis. He did not address the issue of reduction in such cases.

Isthmic spondylolisthesis occurs in the lumbar spine at the L5–S1 level in 82.1%, at L4–5 in 11.3%, at L3–4 in 0.5%, and at L2–3 in 5.8% of cases. There appears to be a racial and gender difference in the occurrence of isthmic spondylolisthesis. Hensinger (8) found the lowest prevalence in black women and the highest in Caucasian males. Athletes who engage in sports that require lumbar extension and twisting seem to be at higher risk for developing spondylolisthesis. Weight lifters have the highest prevalence. Gymnasts, football linemen, and judoists are also at risk.

Isthmic spondylolisthesis is also divided into two subtypes. Type IIA is characterized by a lytic pars interarticularis defect, possibly the result of a stress fracture (3,4). It is uncertain if the defect arises from a congenitally weakened pars or simply from continued stress of the biped gait or strenuous athletic activities. O'Neil and Micheli (9) believe that type IIA spondylolisthesis is the result of fatigue stresses, since the pars defect heals with immobilization. The typical age of presentation is 11 to 16 years, which is older than that of congenital spondylolisthesis. Risk factors for progression include young age at presentation, female, high degree of slip, high lumbosacral kyphosis, and loss of sacral inclination.

Type IIB is characterized by an elongated pars resulting from repetitive stress fractures and healing. The demographics and age of presentation are similar to type IIA; however, since the posterior arch remains intact, there is an increased likelihood of neurologic symptoms with high-grade slips. The L5 nerve root is usually affected, since it is trapped by the posterior elements of L5.

Type III: Degenerative Spondylolisthesis

This type III spondylolisthesis is characterized by long-standing spondylosis with facet and disc degeneration. With loss of disc height, there is a rotational and transla-tion force placed on the L4–5 articulation, which might be already weakened with age. Unlike types I and II, this type of spondylolisthesis is often seen at the L4–5 level; the next most frequently affected site is the L3–4 level.

Degenerative spondylolisthesis can be seen with segmental instability, which has implications regarding treatment. Rosenberg (10) found an increased incidence in women over 40 years of age. Other risk factors include sacralization of L5 and increased sagittal alignment of the L4–5 facet, which then does not serve as an adequate buttress. There is an increased sagittal alignment of facets in patients with degenerative spondylolisthesis when compared with the normal population. It is believed the sacralization of L5 passes additional stresses onto the L4–5 level, leading to degenerative changes and spondylolisthesis.

With age-related changes in the L4–5 disc, the axis of rotation shifts posteriorly, placing more stress on the facets. Unlike the L5–S1 facets, which are in a more coronal plane, the L4–5 facets are more sagittally oriented and are, therefore, less able to resist rotatory and translatory forces. As the spondylolisthesis develops, neural symptoms can occur as the posterior elements compress the exiting nerve roots. Slips rarely exceed 25 to 30%; only 30% of patients have slips exceeding 30%. Type III spondylolisthesis can occur in conjunction with spinal stenosis, or it may be a form of dynamic stenosis.

Type IV: Traumatic Spondylolisthesis

The type IV lesion is a pars defect that occurs acutely for traumatic reasons. Traumatic spondylolisthesis is extremely rare; only isolated cases are reported in the literature. Cope (11) reported on a 34-year-old male who fell 12 feet, sustaining a severe compression fracture of L1 and fractures of the L4 and L5 vertebral bodies. In addition, the patient sustained a fracture of the pars of L5 with a type I spondylolisthesis. Treatment included bed rest followed by gradual mobilization with a brace. There was subsequent healing of the pars defect in 14 weeks, and no adverse sequelae were reported. Klinghoffer and Murdock (12) reported a similar case.

Type V: Pathologic Spondylolisthesis

Type V spondylolisthesis is the result of an isolated or generalized pathologic process involving the pars or posterior elements that leads to slip and/or instability. Type VA spondylolisthesis involves a generalized skeletal process—such as Albers-Schönberg disease, arthrogryposis, Recklinghausen's disease, Marfan's syndrome, and Larsen's disease—that leads to a pars defect. In type VB, a local bony destruction, such as a metastasis or a posterior element tumor, causes a pars defect.

Type VI: Postsurgical Spondylolisthesis

Type VI spondylolisthesis is characterized by instability resulting from the loss of supportive posterior elements caused by extensive surgical decompression. This type is not well reported in the literature.

CLINICAL FINDINGS

In isthmic and dysplastic spondylolistheses, pain is the most common symptom. Most patients with a spondylitic defect do not, however, complain of pain. The pain is musculoskeletal and is described as a dull ache localized to the lower back or as radicular (8). The exact cause of the pain is unclear. Radicular pain is unusual but is associated with a high-grade slip and L5 radiculopathy.

Other physical findings in nondegenerative spondylolisthesis include hamstring tightness, palpable defect in the lumbar spine, increased lumbar lordosis, flattening of the sacral inclination, and a waddling gait. Hamstring tightness may stem from the body's attempt to place itself in a more vertical position or to rotate the pelvis to a more horizontal position. Hamstring tightness usually resolves 7 to 8 months after surgery, when the fusion is solid.

As the slip increases, the patient undergoes physical changes to compensate for the increased lumbosacral kyphosis, including a more horizontal alignment of the pelvis, which gives the impression of a flattened and wide buttock known as the "sweetheart pelvis." Increased translation caused by the slip creates truncal shortening and protrusion of the ribs anteriorly as they come to rest on the anterior pelvis as the patient tries to maintain an upright posture. The patient must flex the knees and extend the hips. Wiltse noted that the degree of physical changes correlated with the degree of slip and that changes can be seen with a slip of only 50%.

The clinical picture for degenerative spondylolisthesis depends on the presence of spinal stenosis associated with the slip. Patients with only spondylolisthesis often present with complaints of back pain alone. Those with spinal stenosis often have back pain along with leg pain, which can be unilateral or bilateral. Leg symptoms are usually brought on by walking and are relieved by sitting or flexing the spine. The symptoms are usually activity related; therefore, patients with significant pain at rest should be evaluated for other causes. The L5 nerve root is often involved with an L4–5 slip, but the L4 nerve root may also be affected.

Physical examination may reveal mild weakness in the extremities in 15 to 20% of patients. Reflex loss is nonspe-

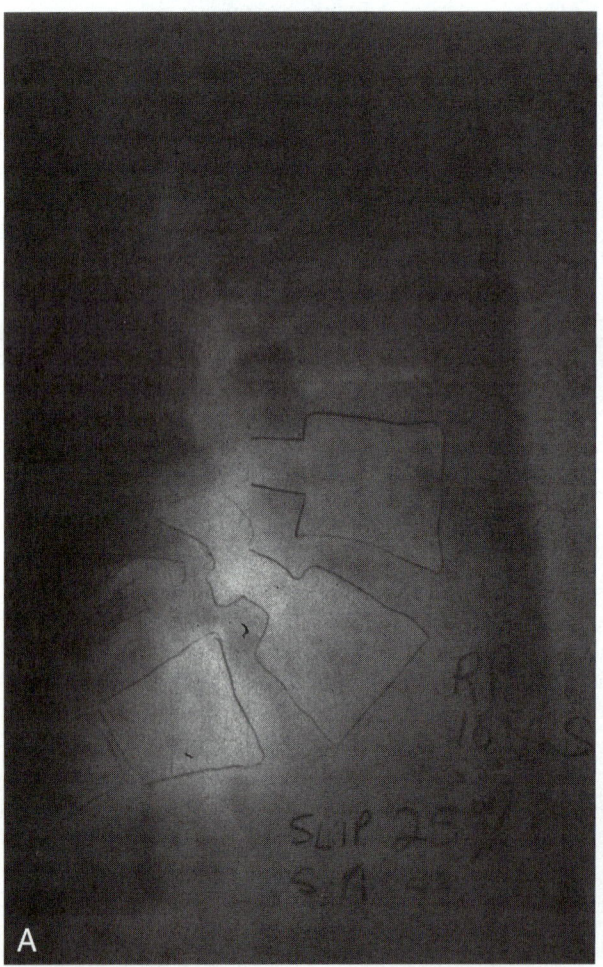
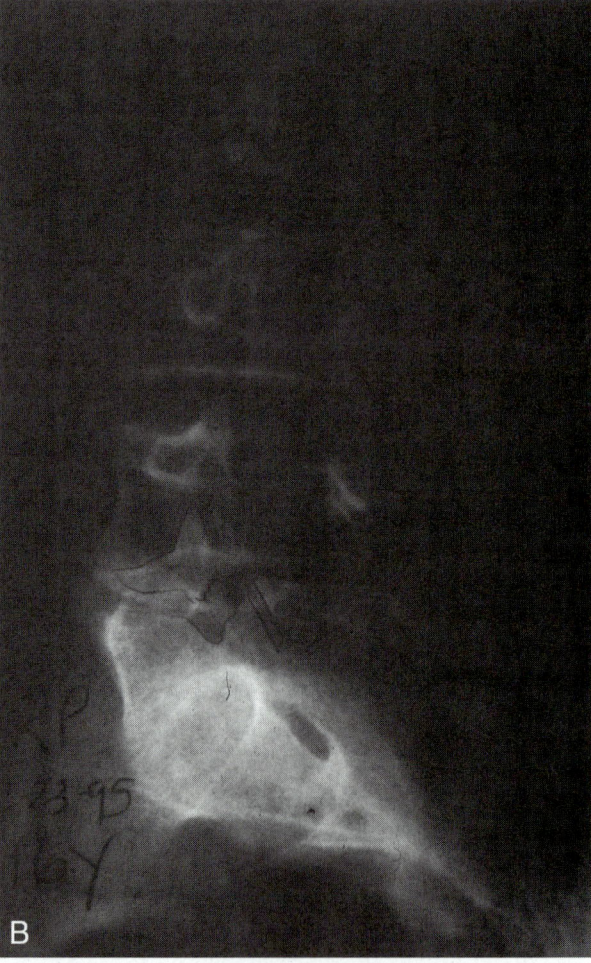

Figure 35.2. A. Lateral view of a patient with an isthmic spondylolisthesis, showing a defect in the pars interarticularis (the slip is 25%). **B.** Oblique view showing the pars interarticularis lesion, represented by the collar of the Scottie dog.

cific, since ankle and patellar reflexes are often lost with aging. Straight leg raising is rarely positive in this population, unless there is an advanced slip with a disc protrusion. Bladder problems, such as poor control and dribbling, are common in this age group and usually are not caused by the underlying stenosis. Another source of leg pain in this population is vascular claudication, which the examination should address.

RADIOLOGIC STUDIES

In dysplastic and isthmic spondylolisthesis, initial radiographic studies should include standing lateral, AP, and oblique views (Fig. 35.2). Oblique views help delineate the pars defect noted in isthmic spondylolisthesis: the so-called collar seen around the neck of the Scottie dog. Since 20% of pars defects are unilateral (6,9), oblique radiographs are especially helpful in the evaluation.

Other defects, such as spina bifida, can be noted on the radiographs. Ferguson views, helpful in detecting anomalies if regular radiographs are nondiagnostic, are obtained with a 20° cranial tilt of the x-ray beam and can be obtained for anterior, lateral, and oblique views.

Various radiographic measurement methods are used to evaluate the severity of a slip (Fig. 35.3). Each of these methods has proponents, and all seem applicable; it is important to be consistent, using the same method each time the patient is examined. Perhaps the most universal method is that of Meyerding (13). The inferior vertebral body is subdivided into four equal parts, and the translation of the superior vertebral body is measured as a percentage of the inferior vertebral body. With a severe slip spondyloptosis, the AP view reveals an upside down Napoleon hat in front of the body of S1 (Fig. 35.4).

The slip angle describes the rotational relationship between L5 and S1. The angle is measured from a line drawn along the superior or inferior end plates of the fifth vertebral body to a line drawn perpendicular to a line along the

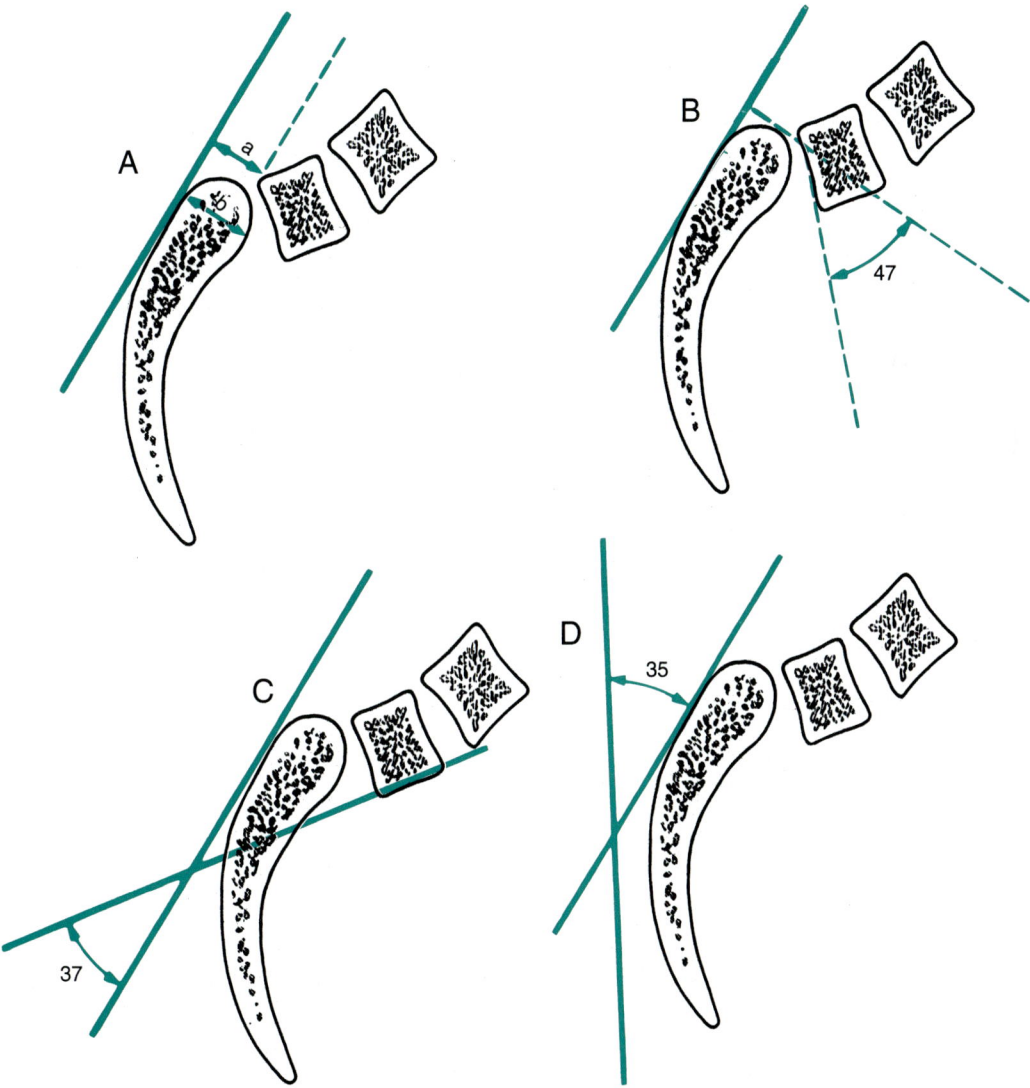

Figure 35.3. A. The percent of slippage of a spondylolisthesis equals $a \times b \times 100$. Here it is 72%. The slip angle (**B**), sagittal rotation (**C**), and sacral inclination (**D**) are also measured.

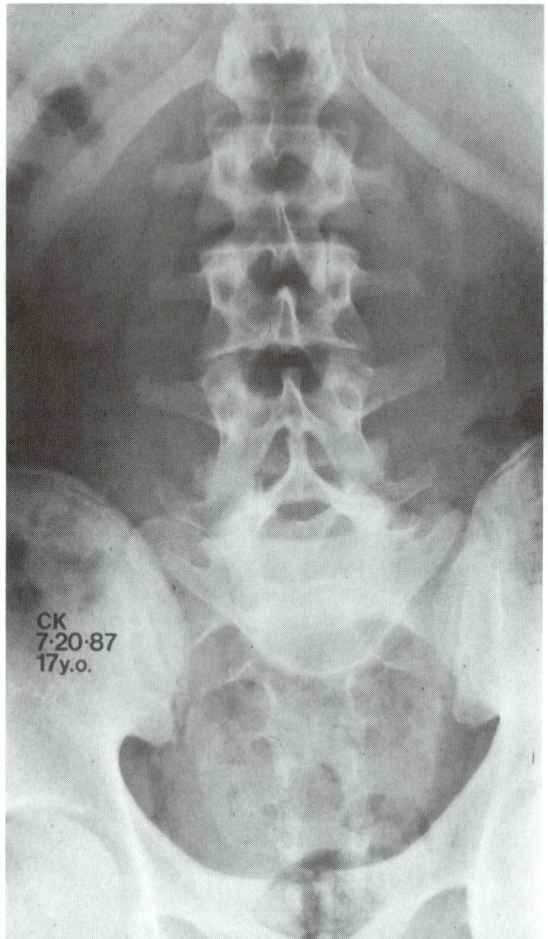

Figure 35.4. AP view of a patient with a severe spondylolisthesis. Note the upside-down Napoleon hat deformity at the L5–S1 level.

posterior margin of the sacrum (Fig. 35.3). This angle increases as the degree of slip increases. The sacral inclination and sacrohorizontal angles are used to assess the position of the sacrum to the vertical and horizontal, respectively (14) (Fig. 35.3). These angles are complementary; as one increases, the other decreases. The lumbar lordosis measurement, which increases with the severity of the slip, is another useful guide for gauging the degree of slip.

Bone scans are helpful for evaluating acute spondylolisthesis but are less so for chronic slip (15). Bone scans are especially useful for athletes and help the clinician evaluate the success of healing of the pars defect and judge the patients' ability to return to competition. CT studies of the pars defect may be useful if bone scans are nondiagnostic. CT can also help evaluate a fibrocartilaginous pars mass, which is often implicated as the cause of the pain associated with spondylolisthesis.

In degenerative spondylolisthesis, the radiologic evaluation is similar to that of isthmic and dysplastic spondylolisthesis, except for use of the bone scan. Plain radiographs should include standing lateral and AP views along with flexion and extension views for evaluating gross instability. Instability is defined as translation motion of at least 4 mm of increased forward movement on flexion with excessive angular motion of more than 10°.

Additional studies should include an MRI scan and CT with myelography. The MRI scan, useful for all types of spondylolistheses, examines the involved disc and surrounding discs to help the surgeon determine fusion levels. In degenerative spondylolisthesis, MRI can help determine whether a herniated L4–5 disc is responsible for stenotic symptoms. CT myelography is used to evaluate other areas of stenosis, which occurs in 15 to 20% of cases (16).

TREATMENT

Nonoperative Treatment

The goals of nonsurgical management are to improve the patient's quality of life by reducing pain, improving exercise, and tolerating activities of daily living (ADL). Most patients with spondylolysis can be treated conservatively. Bed rest for 2 to 3 days with anti-inflammatory medication may be helpful. If symptoms persist, physical therapy with modalities, including ultrasound, heat, and/or massage, is the next step. A lumbosacral corset used daily for 3 to 6 weeks may help control lower back symptoms. A brace also can be used for up to 3 months to decrease symptoms and (perhaps) to heal the spondylitic defect.

Once the patient's symptoms are controlled, physical therapy may begin. The physical therapy program should include general aerobic conditioning, abdominal flexion exercises, weight loss as needed, and general back strengthening exercises.

Younger patients who present with acute pain and positive bone scans indicating acute lesions may benefit from forgoing active sports and wearing a lumbosacral brace for 3 to 4 months, even though healing may not be expected. Symptomatic improvement may be expected in the majority of these patients (8).

For patients with a degenerative slip, epidural steroids may help alleviate symptoms, although the effect of these drugs is unpredictable.

Operative Treatment

Initial treatment for spondylolisthesis, except for a high-grade slip, is usually conservative. Surgical management is indicated if nonsurgical management fails. Other indications for surgical treatment are the presence of (a) progressive neurologic loss, (b) progressive slip, (c) persistent back and leg pain that is resistant to nonsurgical management, and (d) significant decrease in quality of life. Surgical options include Gill's operation (17), pars interarticularis repair, and in situ fusion with either posterolateral fusion or posterior interbody fusion (Clinical Table).

Surgical management historically has included decompressive laminectomy (Fig. 35.5), including Gill's operation (18). Osterman et al. (17) reviewed 130 patients

Clinical Table: Spondylolysis and Spondylolisthesis of the Lumbar Spine

Procedure	Indications	Technique	Anatomy	Pitfalls

Posterior spinal fusion in situ	• Low-grade (less than 50%) spondylolisthesis in an adolescent or young adult patient
	• Spondylolysis without spondylolisthesis with significant back pain
	• Single level of fusion L4–5 or L5–S1
		• Bilateral lateral fusion, intertransverse fusion
		  —Midline excision, dissection through fascia on either side, paraspinous muscles split, exposure of transverse processes
		  —Decortication of transverse processes and iliac crest bone graft.
		• Midline exposure, facet exposure, intertransverse exposure
		  —Transverse fusion and facet fusion
		  —L4–S1 for high-grade slip of >50%
			• Spinous process
			• Facet joint
			• Transverse process
			• Pars interarticularis
			• Spinal nerve root
				• Identification of proper levels by radiograph
				• Avoid exposure of facet capsule

Decompression fusion and instrumentation	• Patients with radiculopathy and spinal stenosis • Most common nerve root L5 for the L5–S1 lesion	• Prone position in full extension; intraoperative x-ray to mark levels • Midline exposure; exposure of loose posterior element of L5; transverse processes L4–sacrum; removal of loose arch • Decompression of foramina L5–S1 and removal of scar tissue in the pars interarticularis • Visualization of L5 nerve root bilaterally • Temporally, distraction to visualize nerve root; disc L5–S1 not needed to be removed • Posterolateral fusion at L4–sacrum; iliac crest bone graft utilized; pedicle screw fixation L4 and S1 • Reduction not necessary for patients with mild slip angles; L5 pedicle screw if slip angle minimal and can be reached; S1 to L5 fibular graft for patient with large slip angles not requiring reduction	• Posterior spinal elements • Spinous process, loose posterior arch L5 • Pars interarticularis • Ligamentum flavum • Intervertebral disc L5–S1 • Spinal nerve roots L5 and S1 • Transverse processes • Spinal pedicle • Epidural vessels	• Proper selection of fusion • Proper identification of L5 nerve root; nerve conduction dermatome, SSEP, or EMGs to help visualize and identify L5 nerve root; proper screw placement in pedicles L4, L5, S1

EMGs, electromyograms; *SSEP,* somatosensory evoked potential.

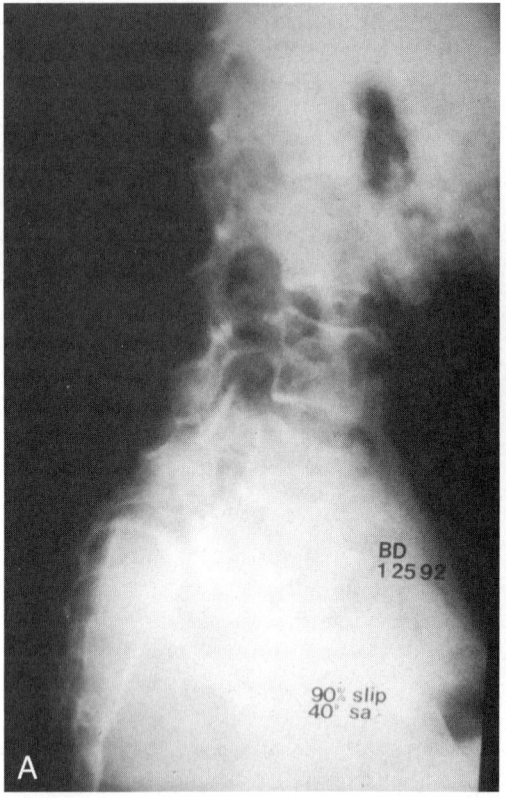

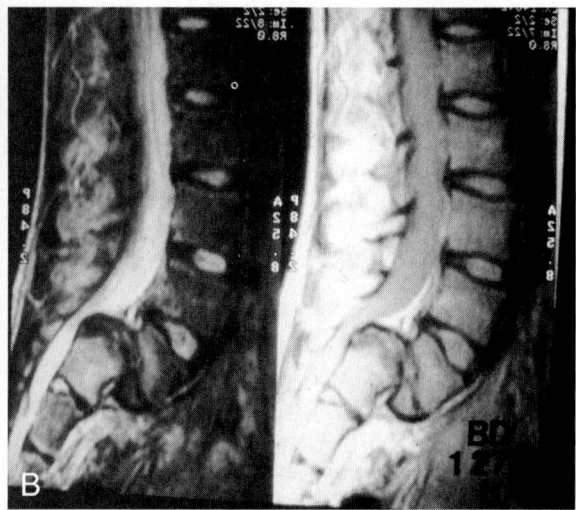

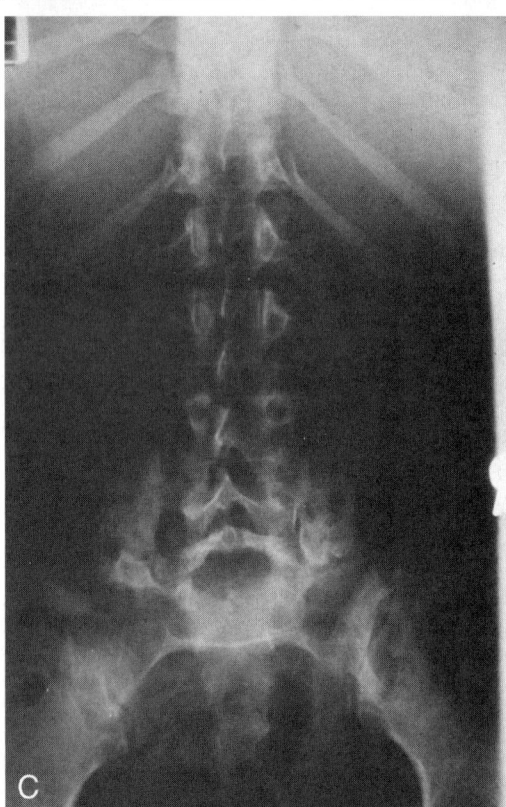

Figure 35.5. A. Lateral view radiograph of a patient with severe spondylolisthesis. Note the high-grade slip. **B.** MRI study showing the deformity of the lumbosacral angle and a severe slip angle of 40°. **C.** Postoperative radiograph showing the posterolateral fusion mass incorporation following posterior decompression and fusion at L4–S1 without reduction.

treated for spondylolisthesis with the Gill procedure and reported good to excellent results in 85% of patients at the 1-year follow-up; this dropped to 75% at 5 years. They attributed the worsening of the patients' complaints to additional degeneration of the disc. Progression of spondy-

lolisthesis was observed in 27% of patients. Osterman et al. concluded that Gill's operation is contraindicated in adolescents, except in cases involving cauda equina, and recommended the operation only for patients over 40 with painful spondylolisthesis and nerve root symptoms. This procedure has fallen out of favor recently because some authors have reported increased slippage and lumbosacral kyphosis after this treatment.

Pars reduction is often advocated for a low-grade slip and a competent disc. In the face of an incompetent disc that might produce pain, the wisdom of a pars fusion can be questioned. Various techniques have been described in which fixation is obtained at the pars with a loop of wire passed around the posterior elements. The pars defect is roughened, and bone graft is placed at the defect site (19–22).

The treatment for patients with spinal stenosis and degenerative spondylolisthesis is simple decompression. Lombardi and Wiltse (23) reviewed 47 patients who had undergone surgical treatment for this condition and noted that those with complete decompression (including the facets) had poor outcomes compared to patients who had a more limited decompression. The best outcome was noted in patients who had decompression and posterolateral fusion. Recent studies have echoed these conclusions (16,20,24–26). Herkowitz and Kutz (25) published the results of a prospective study of 50 patients with spinal stenosis and degenerative spondylolisthesis. The patients who underwent fusion had better outcomes and less slippage after surgery than those who did not. The role of instrumentation in this patient population was also addressed by the recent studies.

Bridwell and Sedgewick (26) reviewed 44 patients treated for spinal stenosis and degenerative spondylolisthesis and examined three treatment options: no fusion, fusion with instrumentation, and fusion without instrumentation. They noted that the group with decompression and pedicle screw fixation had a higher fusion rate than did the noninstrumented group (87% versus 30%). The instrumented group had a better outcome in terms of symptoms and a higher fusion rate (Fig. 35.6).

However, not all patients who have spinal stenosis and degenerative spondylolisthesis will need fusion and instrumentation after decompression. Decompression alone may be adequate for patients with a stiff and significant osteoarthritic spine, minimum slippage, and no movement on flexion and extension lateral radiographs and who require less extensive decompression that spares the facets (20).

Despite the appearance of solid fusion, additional slippage can occur; routine follow-up is warranted, especially in younger patients (27,28). Slip progression has been associated with Gill's laminectomy, lack of postoperative immobilization, and high initial slip angle (17).

Other treatment options for a high-grade slip include reduction with anterior and/or posterior fusion. The advantages of reduction are restoration of lumbar lordosis, reduction of lumbosacral kyphosis, and establishment of normal sagittal alignment. For a severe slip, anterior fusion with posterior fusion and reduction to reestablish sagittal alignment may be indicated. The reduction maneuver can be accomplished by the anterior procedure, Gaines' pro-

cedure (vertebrectomy) (29), or posterior procedure with interbody graft and fusion.

The primary danger of reduction is neurologic injury: cauda equina syndrome and nerve root injury. For an L5–S1 high-grade spondylolisthesis, the L5 nerve root is at particular risk during reduction. Precautions include posterior decompression and (perhaps) stopping short of a complete reduction. In a cadaver study, Petraco and Spivak (30) noted that during the reduction of high-grade slips, the greatest stretch on the L5 nerve occurs during the second half of the reduction. They found that the amount of stretch on the nerve could be reduced by correcting the lumbosacral kyphosis.

Although preoperative extension and flexion radiographs help predict the amount of reduction, a lateral radiograph obtained on the operating table is a better predictor. Montgomery and Fischgrund (31) studied 24 patients with degenerative and isthmic slips. They noted a slip reduction of 6 to 24% on the operating room table with patients under anesthesia. They concluded that translation motion of the spondylolisthesis is greater than predicted on preoperative flexion and extension radiographs.

Bradford and Boachie-Adjei (32) reported on 22 patients who had gradual reduction and then anterior fusion after posterior decompression and fusion. The slip angle was improved from 71° to 28° on follow-up. Posterior decompression and fusion were performed to decrease the chance of injury to the cauda equina. A total of 4 patients had pseudarthrosis, which resolved with additional surgery. There was 1 case of cauda equina syndrome, which occurred after the first stage and which resolved with additional decompression. Bradford and Hu (33) examined 16 patients with high-grade slips; they reported three incidences of postoperative neurologic loss, one of which eventually resolved. O'Brien et al. (34) reported similar results in 22 patients with high-grade slips (at least grade 3). A total of 2 patients had a loss of reduction, one from noncompliance and the other from pseudarthrosis. The pseudarthrosis was repaired by additional anterior surgery. Minor neurologic damage occurred in 2 patients.

Gaines and Nichols (29) reported on a two-stage L5 vertebrectomy and reduction of L4 onto S1 with posterior fusion in two patients. The initial procedure consisted of an anterior L5 vertebrectomy with the L4–5 and the L5–S1 discs. The second procedure was accomplished after 2 weeks of bed rest. The posterior elements were then removed, and the L4 posterior elements were compressed onto the posterior elements of S1 with Harrington compressive instrumentation. Bed rest was continued for another week before the patients were allowed to ambulate in a brace with a leg extension. Both patients obtained solid fusion with no complication after reexploration and additional grafting at an average of 4.5 months. Total bed rest averaged 5 months. They recommended this procedure for only spondyloptosis.

In another approach to slip reduction, Fabris and

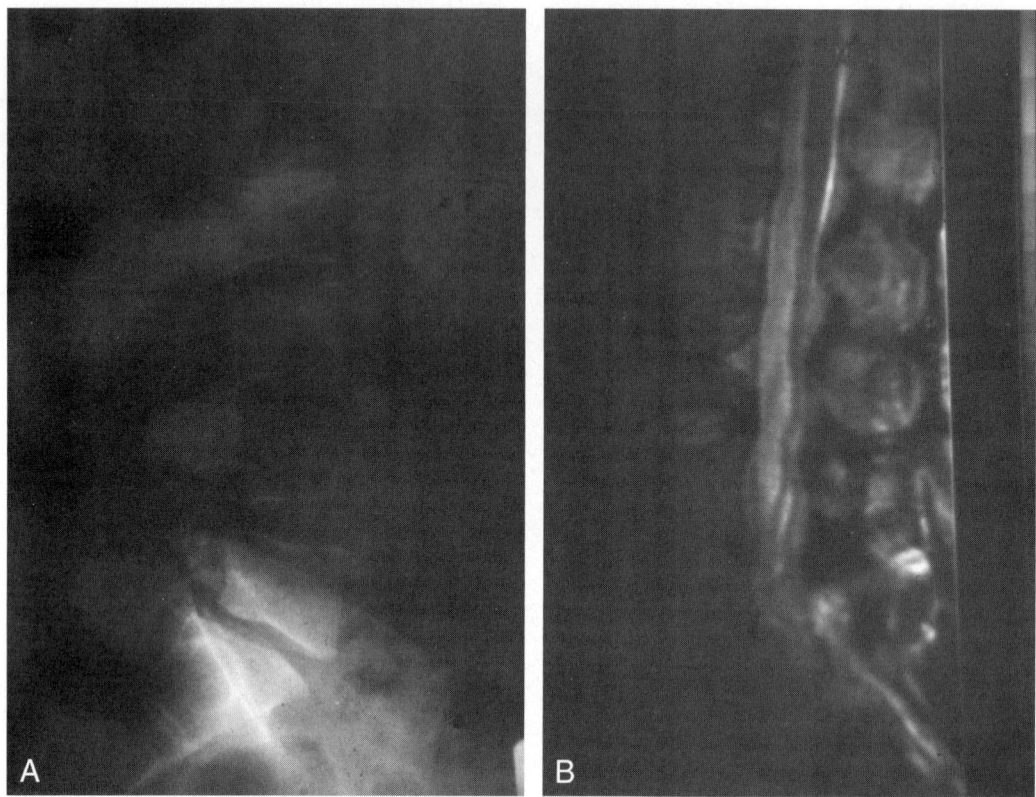

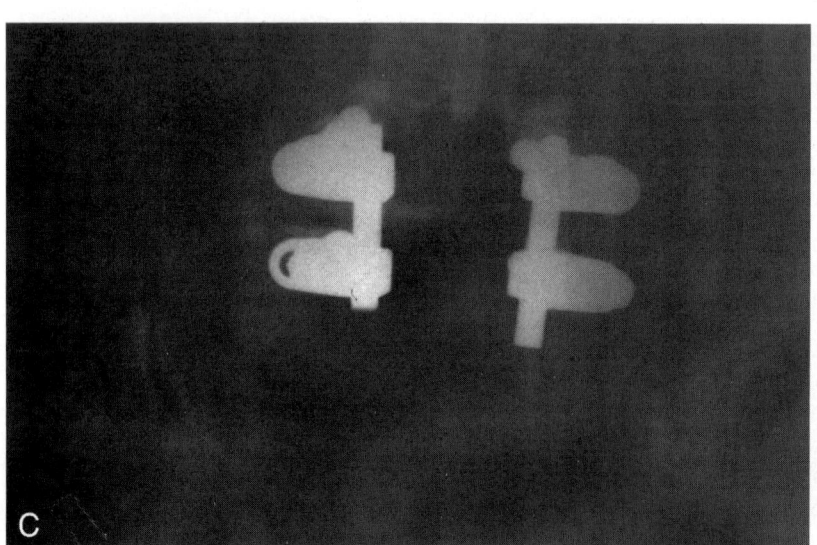

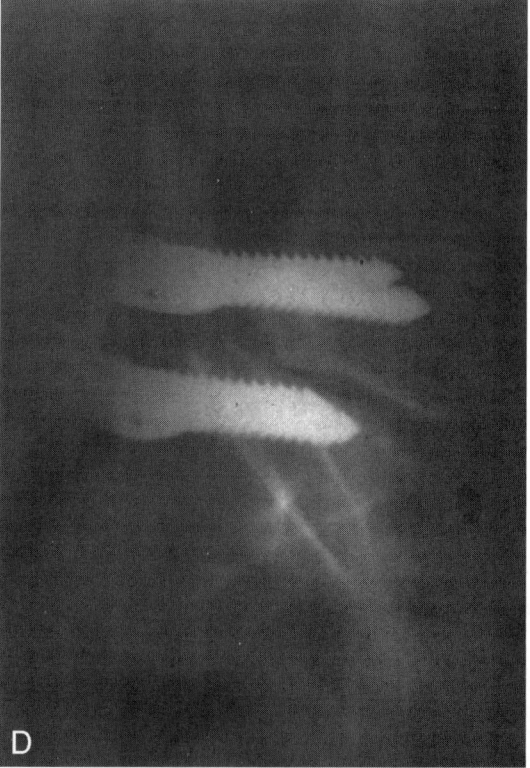

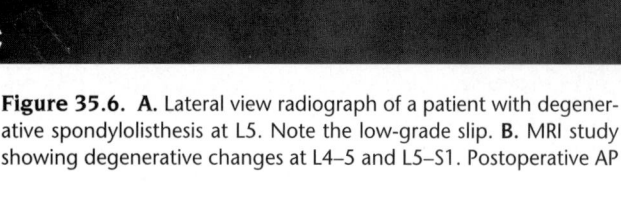

Figure 35.6. A. Lateral view radiograph of a patient with degenerative spondylolisthesis at L5. Note the low-grade slip. **B.** MRI study showing degenerative changes at L4–5 and L5–S1. Postoperative AP (**C**) and lateral (**D**) view radiographs showing the posterolateral fusion with segmental fixation at L5–S1.

Costantini (35) studied 12 patients with high-grade slips (59 to 85%) who had arch decompression, complete posterior L5–S1 discectomy, and reduction with a distractive device placed between L1 and S1. The patients then underwent posterior interbody strut grafting and posterolateral fusion with pedicle screw fixation. There were no intraoperative or postoperative neurologic complications, and all patients had solid fusion at follow-up. Mean correction of the initial slip was 79%.

Abdu and Wilber (36) reported on pedicular transvertebral fixation for high-grade spondylolisthesis slips in three patients. No attempts at reduction were made. The authors noted that this technique offers immediate three-column fixation and is safer than methods of fixation that rely on some sort of anterior fixation, by either posterior or anterior methods.

Traumatic spondylolisthesis, which has not been extensively reported in the literature, should be considered potentially unstable; the instability is comparable to a fracture dislocation and thus has a great propensity to progress (11,27). Hilibrand and Urquhart (27) reported on five patients with traumatic spondylolisthesis following major trauma. The three patients with grade 1 slips and the one patient with a grade 3 slip progressed. All patients were treated with posterolateral fusion. Two of grade 1 patients were initially treated nonsurgically with a body cast.

SUMMARY

Isthmic spondylolysis presents as the most common pathologic abnormality resulting in spondylolisthesis in adolescents and young adults. The most common presentations are back pain and deformity. Nonoperative treatment including activity modification and brace immobilization results in symptomatic improvement in a majority of patients despite lack of healing of the spondylitic defect. Posterior spinal fusion in situ has excellent results in the majority of patients with low-grade slips. Adolescents and young adult patients with high-grade slip and lumbosacral kyphosis benefit best from a posterior spinal fusion. Combined anterior and posterior spinal fusion is reserved for patients with high-grade slips. Reduction of the slip angle is most critical in restoring sagittal alignment. Reduction of translational slip is not necessary for optimal results.

Degenerative spondylolisthesis is most common at the L4–5 level in patients over 40 years of age. Symptoms related to neurogenic claudication, spinal stenosis, and back pain from mechanical instability are the most common presentations. Conservative treatment including anti-inflammatory medication, physical therapy, and epidural steroid injections helps the majority of patients treated nonoperatively. For patients who have failed conservative treatment, surgical decompression with or without fusion and instrumentation is the procedure of choice. Pedicle screw fixation for segmental instrumentation provides the best results for stabilization procedures.

REFERENCES

1. Kilian JF. Schilderungen neur backenformen und ihrer verhalten im leben. Mannhein: Bassermann & Mathy, 1854.
2. Wynne-Davies R, Scott JH. Inheritance and spondylolisthesis. J Bone Joint Surg 1979;61B:301–305.
3. Wiltse LL, Hutchinson RH. Surgical treatment of spondylolisthesis. Clin Orthop 1964;35:116–135.
4. Wiltse LL, Newman PH, Macnab I. Classification of spondylolysis and spondylolisthesis. Clin Orthop 1976;117:23–29.
5. Rosenberg NJ, Bargar WL, Friedman B. The incidence of spondylolisthesis and spondylolysis in nonambulatory patients. Spine 1981;6:35–38.
6. Ogilvie JW, Sherman J. Spondylolysis in Scheuermann's diseases. Spine 1987;12:251–253.
7. Fisk JR, Moe JH, Winter RB. Scoliosis, spondylolysis and spondylolisthesis. Their relationship as reviewed in 539 patients. Spine 1978;3:234–245.
7a. Goldstein LA, Haake PW, DeVanny JR, Chou PK. Guidelines for the management of lumbosacral spondylolisthesis associated with scoliosis. Clin Orthop 1976;117:135.
8. Hensinger RN. Spondylolysis and spondylolisthesis in children. Instr Course Lect 1983;32:132–151.
9. O'Neil DB, Micheli LJ. Post-operative radiographic evidence for fatigue fracture as the etiology in spondylolysis. Spine 1989;14:1342–1355.
10. Rosenberg NJ. Degenerative spondylolisthesis: predisposing factors J Bone Joint Surg 1975;57A:112–120.
11. Cope R. Acute traumatic spondylolysis. Report of a case and review of the literature. Clin Orthop 1988;230:162–165.
12. Klinghoffer L, Murdock MG. Spondylosis following trauma. A case report and review of the literature. Clin Orthop 1982;166:72–74.
13. Meyerding HW. Spondylolisthesis. Surg Gynecol Obstet 1932;54:371–377.
14. Speck GR, McCall IW, O'Brien JP. Spondylolisthesis: the angle of kyphosis. Spine 1984;9:659–660.
15. Lowe J, Schachner E, Hirschberg E, et al. Significance of bone scintigraphy in symptomatic spondylolysis. Spine 1984;9:653–655.
16. Herkowitz HN. Spinal stenosis: clinical evaluation. Instr Course Lect 1992;41:183–185.
17. Osterman K, Lindholm TS, Laurent LE. Late results of removal of the loose posterior elements (Gill's operation) in the treatment of lytic lumbar spondylolisthesis. Clin Orthop 1976;117:121–128.
18. Gill GG, Manning JG, White HL. Surgical treatment of spondylolisthesis without spine fusion. J Bone Joint Surg 1955;37A:492.
19. Buck J. Further thoughts on direct repair of the defect in spondylolysis. J Bone Joint Surg 1979;61B:123.
20. Pederson A, Hagen R. Spondylolysis and spondylolisthesis treatment by internal fixation and bone grafting of the defect. J Bone Joint Surg 1988;70A:15–24.
21. Roche MB. Healing of bilateral fracture of the pars interarticularis of a lumbar neural arch. J Bone Joint Surg 1950;32A:428–429.
22. Rombold C. Treatment of spondylolisthesis by posterolateral fusion, resection of the par interarticularis and prompt mobilization of the patient. J Bone Joint Surg 1966;48A:1282–1300.
23. Lombardi J, Wiltse L. Treatment of degenerative spondylolisthesis. Spine 1985;10:821–827.
24. Johnsson KE, Willner S, Johnsson K. Postoperative instability after decompression for lumbar spinal stenosis. Spine 1986;11:107–110.
25. Herkowitz HN, Kutz LT. Degenerative lumbar spondylolisthesis with spinal stenosis. A prospective study comparing decompression with decompression and intertransverse progressive arthrodesis. J Bone Joint Surg 1991;73A:802–808.
26. Bridwell K, Sedgewick T. The role of fusion and instrumentation in the treatment of degenerative spondylolisthesis with spinal stenosis. J Spinal Disorders 1993;6:467–472.

27. Hilibrand AS, Urquhart AG. Acute spondylotic spondylolisthesis. Risk of progression and neurologic complications. J Bone Joint Surg 1995;77A:190–196.

28. Riley PM, Gillespie R, Koreska J. Severe spondylolisthesis and spondyloptosis: results of posterolateral fusion in children and adolescents J Bone Joint Surg 1986;68B:856.

29. Gaines RW, Nichols WK. Treatment of spondyloptosis by two stage L5 vertebrectomy and reduction of L4 onto S1. Spine 1985;10:680–685.

30. Petraco DM, Spivak JM. An anatomic evaluation of L5 nerve stretch in spondylolisthesis reduction. Spine 1996;21:1133–1138.

31. Montgomery DM, Fischgrund JS. Passive reduction of spondylolisthesis on the operating room table: a prospective study. J Spinal Disord 1994;7:167–172.

32. Bradford D, Boachie-Adjei O. Treatment of severe spondylolisthesis by anterior and posterior reduction and stabilization. J Bone Joint Surg 1990;72A:1060–1065.

33. Hu SS, Bradford DS. Reduction of high-grade spondylolisthesis using Edwards instrumentation. Spine 1996;21:367–371.

34. O'Brien JP, Mehdian H, Jaffray D. Reduction of severe lumbosacral spondylolisthesis. Clin Orthop 1994;300:64–69.

35. Fabris DA, Costantini S. Surgical treatment of severe spondylolisthesis in children and adolescents. Results of intraoperative reduction, posterior interbody fusion and segmental fixation. Spine 1996;21:728–733.

36. Abdu WA, Wilber RG. Pedicular transvertebral screw fixation of the lumbosacral spine in spondylolisthesis. A new technique for stabilization. Spine 1994;19:710–715.

chapter 36

Spinal Infections

Andrew V. Slucky

Before the era of antibiotic treatment, spinal infections were diseases of high morbidity and mortality. The advent of antibiotic chemotherapy, coupled with improved surgical and anesthetic techniques, has dramatically improved the disease prognosis. Despite current progress, the insidious nature of the disease and the crippling sequelae of inadequate treatment require a heightened vigilance and close coordination of the orthopaedic and infectious disease specialties.

CLASSIFICATION

Spinal infections can be classified by host immune response, anatomic location, or infectious route. Bacterial pathogens typically cause a pyogenic host immune response, whereas *Mycobacterium*, fungi, and syphilis will induce a granulomatous reaction. Infection can involve the vertebral bodies, intervertebral discs, epidural space, or adjacent soft tissues. The route of infection can be hematogenous, contiguous, or postoperative. Histologic response provides the most basic classification of spinal infections.

EPIDEMIOLOGY

Pyogenic Infections

Pyogenic spinal osteomyelitis represents 2 to 8% of all cases of osteomyelitis, third in frequency only to involvement of the femur and tibia (1–3). Although osteomyelitis affects all age groups, Sapico and Montgomerie (4) reported that 52% of presenting patients were older than 50. Intravenous drug abusers account for an increasingly younger patient population. There is also a predilection for men, at a ratio of 2:1; elderly men are particularly susceptible to the disease.

Granulomatous Infections

Mycobacterium sp. is the most common causative organism, and M. *tuberculosis* is the most common pathogen, of granulomatous infections. Extrapulmonary tuberculosis involves the skeletal system in 1% of patients in Western countries and 10% of patients in endemic regions. Up to 50% of affected patients will have tuberculosis of the spine. Tuberculosis of the spine is most common in underdeveloped regions that have problems of malnutrition and overcrowding; it affects all age groups, including infants and children (5,6). In these areas, 10 to 40% of patients will develop a neurologic deficit (6). In the United States, tuberculosis of the spine affects primarily elderly adults and chronic abusers of alcohol or other substances.

Fungal infections and other nontuberculous spinal granulomatous infections are uncommon. These infections typically occur in immunocompromised people. Diagnosis is often delayed because of an indolent infectious course.

PATHOGENESIS

Pyogenic Infections

In the majority of cases, the primary route of pyogenic infection appears to be hematogenous spread secondary to bacteremia. The most common sources of identifiable infection include the genitourinary tract (29%), soft tissue (13%), upper respiratory tract (11%), and intravenous drug abuse (1 to 2%), typically in younger age groups (4,6). Less frequent causes include salmonellosis, infective endocarditis, ostitis media, dental manipulations, and hemodialysis. The source of infection is unidentified in 37% of cases reported in the literature (4).

Although genitourinary infections are more common in females than in males, the increased incidence of pyogenic spondylitis in males may possibly be related to the longer male urethra, which is surrounded by heavily vascularized tissue that makes the development of metastatic infection more likely after urologic manipulation.

Immunocompromised individuals appear to be at increased risk of spinal infection (4). Diabetic patients, in general, show an increased frequency of osteomyelitis compared to the general population. This increase is presumed secondary to diabetic-related vascular disease and peripheral neuropathy, resulting in soft tissue ulceration and urinary stasis, both of which can produce systemic bacteremia. An increased incidence of pyogenic osteomyelitis has not been noted in patients with AIDS, although increased involvement with atypical *Mycobacterium* granulomatous infections has been reported.

Gram-positive organisms predominate as the primary infectious agent. *Staphylococcus aureus* accounts for greater than 50% of reported vertebral osteomyelitis cases (4). Gram-negative organisms, including *Escherichia coli*, *Pseudomonas*, and *Proteus* sp., are the most frequently associated genitourinary pathogens. *Pseudomonas* is typically associated with intravenous drug abuse. *Salmonella* osteomyelitis is rare and typically occurs following an acute intestinal infection; a propensity for infection in areas of preexisting osseous disease has been noted. Anaerobic infections are unusual and are generally associated with penetrating trauma, foreign bodies, or diabetes mellitus. Hematogenous infection by multiple organisms is rare.

Hematogenous spinal infection typically begins in the vertebral metaphysis. Wiley and Trueta (7) demonstrated a rich arterial anastomosis of end arterioles within the metaphyseal region of the vertebral body that could allow for the spread of infection. Batson (8) described the paraspinous venous plexus as a route for the metastasis of infection through the spine. Using injection studies, Batson noted that dye flowed retrograde into the valveless venous plexus when pressure was applied to the lower abdominal wall. It is most likely that both mechanisms are responsible for spread of infection within the vertebral metaphysis.

Metaphyseal infection may spread through the intervertebral disc periphery or rupture through the end plate, resulting in enzymatic destruction of the intervertebral disc. This is in contrast to tuberculous infections in which the adjacent end plates are destroyed but the disc is preserved because of a lack of proteolytic enzymes. Untreated pyogenic infection can spread through adjacent soft tissue planes to form a paraspinal or epidural abscess. Infections of the lumbar spine can produce a psoas abscess that may be large and contain in excess of 1 L purulent fluid.

Destruction of the vertebral body and intervertebral disc can lead to structural instability with kyphosis and collapse. Spinal cord or nerve damage can result from direct compression by bony elements or abscess mass or by ischemic damage from septic thrombosis or inflammatory infiltration of the dura.

Tuberculous Infections

The primary route of tuberculous infection appears to be hematogenous spread from extraspinal foci, most frequently from pulmonary or genitourinary sources (9). Direct inoculation can occur from adjacent visceral lesions.

Vertebral involvement typically presents in one of three forms: peridiscal, central, or anterior. Dobson (10) reported peridiscal involvement in 33%, central involvement in 12%, and anterior involvement in 2% of cases; in his series, 53% of cases demonstrated disease too extensive to determine the foci of origin. Primary posterior involvement is unknown because of typical association with extensive disease, but it is estimated to occur in up to 10% of cases.

In cases of peridiscal origin, infection begins in the anterior portion of the vertebral metaphysis with subsequent destruction of the adjacent end plate. Spread to adjacent vertebrae occurs by extension beneath the anterior longitudinal ligament. Central infections tend to remain isolated within one vertebral body. Vertebral weakening results in central collapse and significant deformity. The lesions are frequently mistaken for tumor. Cases of anterior involvement begin underneath the anterior longitudinal ligament and demonstrate an anterior vertebral scalloping, typically over several contiguous levels.

In contrast to pyogenic infections, tuberculous infections typically spare the intervertebral disc because of a lack of enzymatic degradation (9). At time of operation, the disc can be often found intact within an area of necrotic bone. The pathologic changes tend to occur over a prolonged period, resulting in greater deformity; large paraspinal abscesses are more common in tuberculous than in pyogenic infections.

Neurologic compromise can occur from direct compression by displaced bone or disc, epidural granuloma formation, or the development of kyphotic deformity.

Other Granulomatous Infections

Nontuberculous spinal granulomatous lesions are rare (6). Spinal infection typically occurs through hematogenous routes, although spread to bone can occur from direct invasion to the lungs in cases of *Aspergillosis*, *Blastomycosis*, *Cryptococcus*, and *Coccidioidomycosis*. Abscess formation with lytic destruction of osseous elements is common with these organisms.

CLINICAL PRESENTATION

The clinical course of spinal infections is variable and depends on the virulence of the infective organism and the host's resistance. The presentation may be acute, subacute, or insidiously chronic with few signs of general illness. In a large review of patients, Sapico and Montgomerie (4) documented symptom duration of less than 3 weeks in 20% of patients, 3 weeks to 3 months in 30%, and symptoms of greater than 3 months duration in 50% before presentation. In general, pyogenic infections demonstrate a more acute presentation than do granulomatous infections.

In acute presentations, patients may demonstrate focal spine pain, fever, and muscle spasm. Lumbar spine involvement can produce a positive Lasègue sign, pain with weight bearing, or hip flexion contracture secondary to psoas involvement. Torticollis, dysphagia, and fever may be the only presenting signs with cervical involvement. The patient with tuberculous spondylitis classically presents with complaints of spine pain and systemic findings of weight loss, malaise, and intermittent fevers.

In subacute or chronic presentations, the history may be vague and the symptoms less clear. Up to 15% of patients may present with atypical symptoms, such as chronic chest, abdominal, or hip pain secondary to root irritation (4). A fever higher than 37.7°C (100°F) is documented in only 52% of patients at presentation. Delay in diagnosis is common because associated symptoms overshadow the underlying complaint of neck and back pain.

In pyogenic infections, 48% of patients present with lumbar spine involvement, followed by the thoracic spine in 35%, cervical spine in 6.5%, thoracolumbar in 5%, and lumbosacral junctions in 5% of cases (11). Conversely, tuberculous disease most frequently occurs in the thoracic spine, followed closely by the lumbar spine and thoracolumbar junction; it is rarely found in the cervical or sacral regions (10).

Neurologic deficit has been reported in 4 to 17% of pyogenic infections (6). Eismont et al. (12) identified several factors that predisposed patients to paralysis: diabetes, rheumatoid arthritis, systemic steroid use, age over 50 years, a more cephalad infectious involvement, and infection with S. *aureus*. Neurologic compromise is most often secondary to direct compression of neural elements or kyphosis of the spine but may also result from inflammatory infiltration or septic thrombosis of the spinal cord.

Because of delays in diagnosis, neurologic deficits develop in up to 40% of patients with granulomatous disease (6,13). The incidence is higher when the disease affects the thoracic spine. Paraplegia as the first sign of tuberculous spondylitis is more common in adults than in children, for whom kyphosis is typically the first sign.

DIAGNOSIS

The diagnosis of spinal infections relies primarily on appropriate imaging studies and definitive identification of the infectious pathogen. An algorithm for the evaluation of patients with spinal infection is shown in Figure 36.1.

Routine laboratory studies are required in the general management of patients with suspected spinal infections, although the erythrocyte sedimentation rate (ESR) is the only study, other than Gram stain and culture, that is consistently valuable for the diagnosis of pyogenic spinal infection (4). The leukocyte count is a less sensitive indicator; only 42% of patients demonstrate a leukocyte count

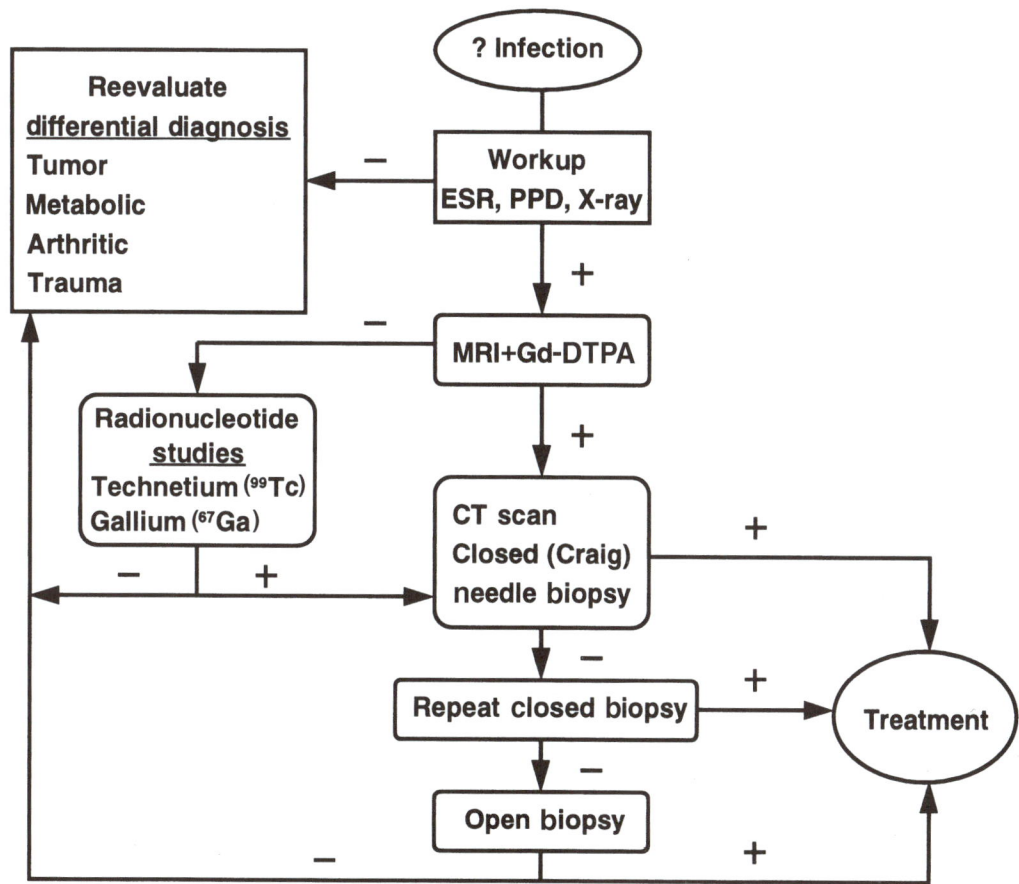

Figure 36.1. Diagnostic evaluation of spine infections. *ESR,* erythrocyte sedimentation rate; *PPD,* purified protein derivative; *Gd-DPTA,* gadolinium-diethylenetriamine pentaacetic acid.

greater than 10,000/mm^3 (10) on admission. Conversely, the ESR may be normal in occult infections with a low-virulence organism.

The sedimentation rate is most useful in assessing response to treatment. Sapico and Montgomerie (4) reported that the ESR decreased to two-thirds the original value after successful antibiotic treatment in all patients and decreased by half the original value in the majority of patients at the end of treatment.

In cases of tuberculous disease, the Mantoux test—the tuberculin purified protein derivative (PPD) skin test—is usually positive and indicates exposure to M. *tuberculosis* and other less common, atypical mycobacterial infections (6). False-negative reactions are seen with anergy that is typically associated with immunologic compromise, malnutrition, overwhelming tuberculosis, or advanced age. With tuberculous spondylitis, the ESR is generally elevated, although not as high as it is with pyogenic disease. Paus (11) noted that an ESR greater than 50 mm/h contradicted a diagnosis of spinal tuberculosis unless there were complications of concomitant pyogenic disease.

Radiographic studies are helpful in assessing spinal involvement at later stages of infection. In both pyogenic and granulomatous disease, there are no radiographic changes early in the disease process. Characteristic changes do not become evident for at least 2 to 4 weeks and will typically lag 2 to 3 months behind the clinical response.

In pyogenic infections, narrowing of the disc space is the earliest and most characteristic finding and is noted in 74% of patients at presentation (4). Later findings include localized osteopenia with decreasing end plate density followed by lytic destruction, typically in the anterior aspect of the vertebral body adjacent to the end plate.

Similarly, tuberculous infections will also initially show findings of disc space narrowing and adjacent bony destruction; however, initial radiographs often show far advanced bony changes with vertebral destruction because of the insidious nature of the disease. Central body involvement results in rarefaction and bony collapse, often resembling a tumor. With anterior multilevel involvement, scalloped erosions occur at the anterior aspect of several adjacent vertebral bodies. With peridiscal involvement, the disc space is narrowed, although typically preserved, and is followed by adjacent vertebral destruction similar to that seen in pyogenic infections.

Radionucleotide studies are useful in the early diagnosis of pyogenic infections. Conversely, in the majority of granulomatous cases, radionucleotide studies are not needed to make the diagnosis because the vertebral changes are obvious at the time of clinical presentation (6).

The technetium-99m (^{99m}Tc) bone scan is a sensitive test that can detect vertebral pyogenic infections in the early stages before radiographic changes are evident. Modic et al. (14) found that ^{99m}Tc scans have a sensitivity of 90%, a specificity of 78%, and an accuracy of 86% in the

diagnosis of pyogenic spondylitis. The likelihood of a positive bone scan increases to near absolute with the duration of symptoms. False-negative scans have been reported in young children and the elderly and are attributed to regional ischemia of the affected area.

Gallium-67 (^{67}Ga) scans have also been useful in the early detection of pyogenic disease; the method has a reported sensitivity of 89%, a specificity of 85%, and an accuracy of 86% in diagnosis of disc space infection (6). ^{99m}Tc scans show a diffusely increased uptake in an infectious region and remain positive for a significant period after infection resolution. In contrast, ^{67}Ga scans show increased uptake in a characteristic butterfly pattern about the infected spine and become normal during healing. Thus the ^{67}Ga scan may be useful in assessing treatment response. False-positive ^{67}Ga scans have been reported in leukopenic patients.

Indium-111–labeled leukocyte imaging has been found to have poor sensitivity in spinal infection; it has a reported sensitivity of 17%, a specificity of 100%, and an accuracy of only 31% (6). False-negative results have been correlated with previous antibiotic therapy, radiation therapy, and metastatic disease and to the reduced leukocytic inflammatory response in chronic spinal infections.

MRI is emerging as the diagnostic modality of choice because of its demonstration of both soft tissue and bony involvement in pyogenic and granulomatous spinal infections (14). The addition of gadolinium-diethylenetriamine pentaacetic acid (Gd-DPTA)—a vascular-based enhancement of MRI—has improved the anatomic resolution of standard MRI, allowing the clinician to differentiate neural structures, assess paravertebral and intravertebral involvement, and determine the presence of epidural abscess. Modic et al. (14) reported that MRI has a sensitivity of 96%, a specificity of 93%, and an accuracy of 94% in the diagnosis of spinal infections.

MRI reveals changes that are characteristic of pyogenic spinal infection, including a confluent decreased signal intensity of the vertebral bodies and adjacent disc on T_1-weighted sequences and increased signal intensity within the affected vertebral bodies and disc on T_2-weighted sequences. Gd-DPTA enhancement results in increased signal intensity on T_1- and T_2-weighted sequences; striking enhancement of epidural abscesses are seen on T_1-weighted sequences.

MRI findings characteristic of tuberculous spinal infections include demonstration of the normal intervertebral disc signal and single body vertebral involvement in cases of central infection (disc and adjacent vertebral body erosion is characteristic of pyogenic spinal infections).

Regardless of the imaging modality, definitive diagnosis rests with vertebral biopsy and bacteriologic or microscopic evaluation of the specimen. False-negative results have been reported with all imaging modalities, particularly in occult infections involving organisms of low virulence. The only situation in which the diagnosis can be made without direct biopsy is in cases with positive blood culture at two separate settings and obvious signs of spondylitis. However, blood cultures are positive in less than 25% of pyogenic cases on presentation (4). Urine cultures are even less reliable, and septic patients often exhibit a coincidental urinary tract infection with a different organism (12).

Fluoroscopic or CT-guided closed-needle biopsy is the preferred technique. A Craig biopsy needle is recommended because it can collect a larger sample size and it has bone-boring capability. All areas of the spine are accessible, although open biopsy may be preferred under certain circumstances in the cervical or thoracic regions. Further indications for an open biopsy include a failed, unsafe, or nondiagnostic closed-needle biopsy. Failure of diagnosis by biopsy often is related to previous treatment with antibiotics.

TREATMENT

Nonoperative Treatment

The goals of treatment of spinal infections are to establish a definitive diagnosis, eradicate the infection, prevent or reverse any neurologic deficit, and ensure spinal stability. The advent of modern antibiotics has led to a substantial decrease in morbidity and mortality; however, attention to medical care is of vital importance to the overall success of treatment.

Treatment begins with identification of the inciting organism. Biopsy, either open or closed, is mandatory in all cases, with the possible exception of patients with positive blood cultures and a strong clinical evidence of spinal infection. If possible, antibiotic treatment should be withheld until positive identification of the organism is made. In cases of severe sepsis or patients with clinical evidence of spinal infection but negative cultures from open biopsy, a full course of broad-spectrum antibiotics is recommended after the biopsy is completed.

In cases of pyogenic infection, selection of antibiotics of maximal specificity and least toxicity depends on the culture and the sensitivity of the test results. Current recommendations regarding route and duration of antibiotic therapy are for maximal dose parenteral antibiotic administration for a period of 6 weeks. Parenteral therapy for less than 4 weeks results in a 25% rate of infectious recurrence (4,6). Antibiotic serum concentration levels should be routinely checked to maximize bactericidal effects and minimize systemic toxicity.

The effectiveness of therapy can be monitored by serial evaluation of the ESR. In most patients, the ESR will decrease to two-thirds the original value after successful antibiotic treatment. If the sedimentation rate does not improve through the course of therapy, the possibility of repeat biopsy should be considered; imaging studies, preferably ^{67}Ga scans, may need to be repeated (6).

The treatment of choice for tuberculous infection is short-course chemotherapy for 6 months (6,15). The recommended regimen for newly diagnosed patients is 2 months of oral isoniazid, rifampin, and pyrazinamide daily, followed by 4 months of isoniazid and rifampin given daily. Patients of recent immigration from tuberculous-endemic regions or areas of increased drug resistance should receive the standard regimen plus oral ethambutol for the first 2 months. In cases of suspected multiple-drug resistance, a parenteral drug (e.g., amikacin, capreomycin) and a fluoroquinolone should be added.

Fungal lesions are typically treated with intravenous amphotericin B and require close monitoring by an infectious disease specialist. In such cases, surgery is frequently required because of significant spinal element destruction and to reduce fungi concentration, maximizing parenteral treatment.

In both pyogenic and granulomatous presentations, immobilization and brace therapy should be implemented for pain control and prevention of deformity and neurologic deterioration. Most authors recommend at least a 3- to 4-month course of bracing. Cervical and cervicothoracic lesions are best immobilized in a halo brace. Upper thoracic lesions can be managed in a Yale brace or a modified thoracolumbosacral orthosis (TLSO) with a chin piece. Lower thoracic or lumbar lesions can be effectively braced with a molded TLSO.

Operative Treatment

The indications for surgery in cases of spinal infection are limited and concise: (a) when closed biopsy is negative or deemed unsafe, to obtain an infectious agent; (b) when the patient is refractory to prolonged nonoperative treatment and shows no clinical improvement; (c) when a clinically significant abscess is present (spiking temperatures and septic course); (d) when spinal cord compression causes neurologic deficit; and (e) when significant deformity or vertebral body destruction is present, particularly in the cervical spine (6) (Clinical Table).

An anterior approach to the spine is recommended in the majority of cases because it allows for direct access to infected tissues for débridement, allows for stabilization of the spine by bone grafting, promotes rapid healing without collapse, and facilitates rehabilitation (13,16) (Fig. 36.2). In regions of the spinal cord, laminectomy is contraindicated because of numerous reports of neurologic deterioration and increased postoperative instability. Exceptions are lesions below the level of the conus, where adequate decompression can be carried out posteriorly, provided there is no associated psoas abscess that would require drainage or severe destruction of the anterior vertebral bodies that would necessitate débridement and grafting.

For lesions of the thoracic spine, a transthoracic approach is recommended. In certain cases, a limited costotransversectomy can be used for biopsy or when minimal decompression with limited grafting is necessary or with cases of grossly purulent abscesses requiring drainage. If a

Clinical Table: Spondylolysis and Spondylolisthesis of the Lumbar Spine

Procedure	Indications	Technique	Anatomy	Pitfalls
Diagnostics				
White cell count (WBC)	• Suspected spinal infection (fevers, axial pain)	• Phlebotomy		• Elevated in less than 50% of patients on admission
Erythrocyte sedimentation rate (ESR)	• Suspected spinal infection (fevers, axial pain)	• Phlebotomy		• Sensitive; not specific • May be normal in occult infections
Purified protein derivative (PPD)	• Suspected tuberculous infection (fever, axial pain, exposure history)	• Skin test		• False-negative with anergy conditions (immunologic compromise, malnutrition, advanced age)
Radiographs	• Suspected spinal infection (fevers, axial pain)	• Radiography	• Vertebral body/disc space	• Pathologic findings lag clinical symptoms or response by 2 to 8 weeks
MRI + gadolinium-DPTA (MRI–Gd-DPTA)	• Suspected spinal infection (elevated ESR, (+) PPD)	• MRI with Gd-DPTA contrast enhancement	• Prevertebral fascia • Vertebral body/disc space • Epidural space	• High accuracy • Recommended diagnostic
Technetium (^{99m}Tc) bone scan	• Suspected spinal infection (elevated ESR, (+) PPD), MRI-Gd unavailable	• Radionucleotide injection study	• Dependent on osseous vasculature	• False-negative scans in children and elderly due to regional ischemia
Gallium (^{67}Ga) scan	• Suspected spinal infections • Assessment of treatment response	• Radionucleotide injection study	• Dependent on labeled neutrophil migration	• False-negative scans in neutropenic patients
Indium (^{111}I) scan	• Not indicated • Poor accuracy in axial infections	• Radionucleotide injection study	• Dependent on labeled leukocyte migration	• False-negative scans in chronic spinal infections or previous antibiotic or radiation treatment
Surgical Treatments				
Anterior approach Cervical	• Abscess instability, neurologic compromise, refractory treatment, unknown pathogen	• Anterior discectomy or vertebrectomy with bone graft reconstruction	• Trachea • Esophagus • Carotid arteries	• Esophageal perforation • Vascular injury
Thoracic	• Abscess instability, neurologic compromise, refractory treatment, unknown pathogen	• Transthoracic (as above)	• Aorta • Vena cava • Pleura/lungs	• Vascular injury
Lumbar	• Abscess instability, neurologic compromise, refractory treatment, unknown pathogen	• Retroperitoneal approach (as above)	• Aorta • Vena cava • Ureters	• Vascular injury
Posterior approach Cervical	• Dorsal epidural abscess	• Laminectomy	• Lamina • Thecal sac-spinal cord	• Postlaminectomy instability
Thoracic	• Dorsal epidural abscess	• Laminectomy	• Lamina • Thecal sac-spinal cord	• Postlaminectomy instability • Indirect drainage of retropleural abscess
Lumbar	• Isolated discitis • Epidural abscess	• Laminectomy	• Lamina • Thecal sac-cauda equina	• Postlaminectomy instability • Indirect drainage of psoas abscess

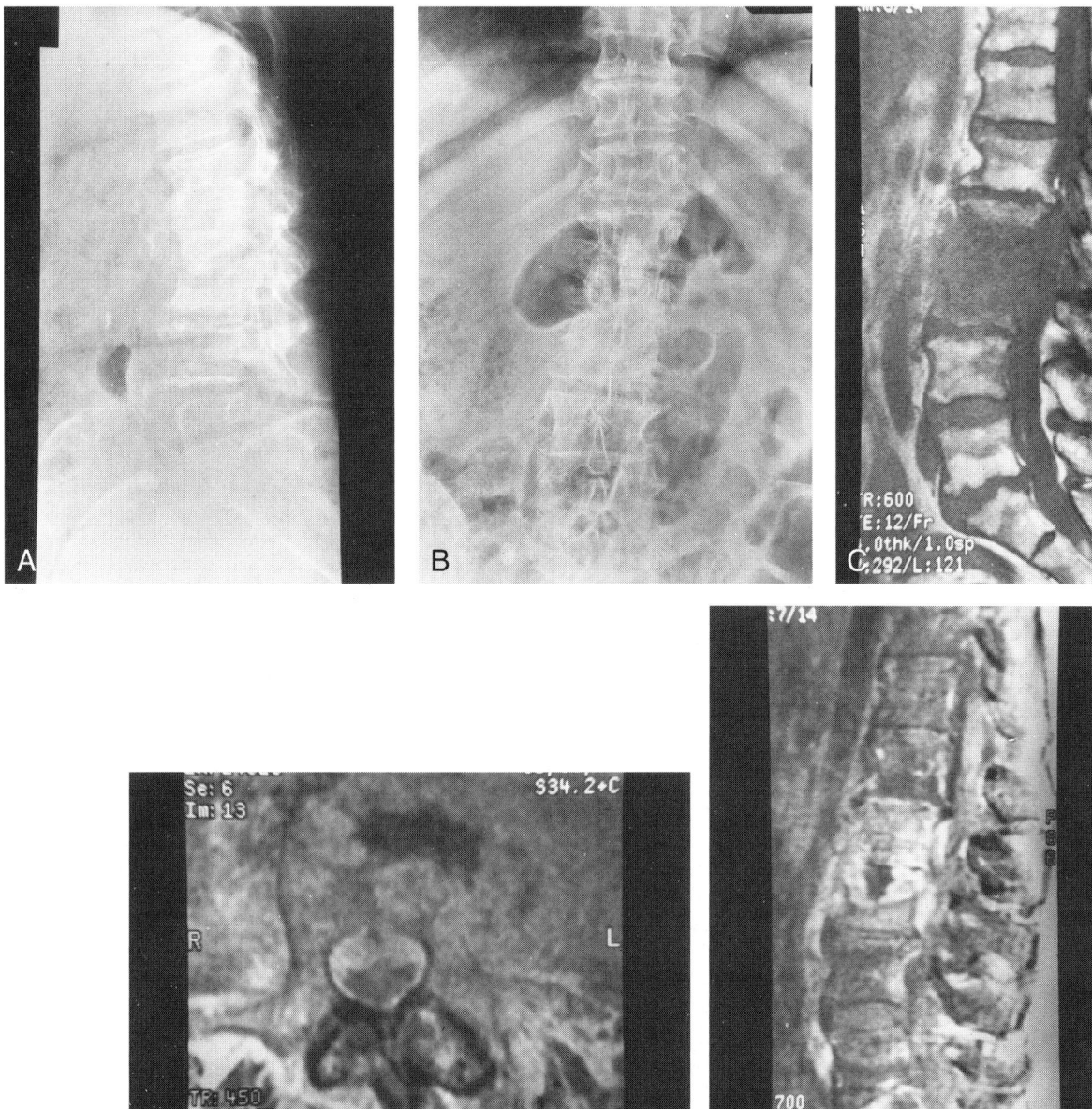

Figure 36.2. Lateral (**A**) and AP (**B**) views of a 63-year-old female with a history of diabetes mellitus who presented with acute-onset low back pain and difficulty urinating. Urine and blood cultures were positive for methicillin-resistant *S. aureus,* and the patient was treated with a 5-day course of intravenous antibiotics. Three weeks later, she demonstrated continued febrile episodes and developed a neurogenic bowel and bladder. Note the disc space collapse and erosion of the L2 and L3 vertebral bodies and the left lateral listhesis. **C.** Sagittal view T$_1$-weighted MRI study (*TR* = 600; *TE* = 12) showing a confluent decreased signal intensity of the L2 and L3 vertebral bodies with loss of the disc space. **D.** Sagittal view Gd-DPTA-enhanced T$_1$-weighted MRI study (*TR* = 700; *TE* = 12) showing an increased signal intensity in the L2 and L3 vertebral bodies, anterior paravertebral tissues, and the ventral L2–3 epidural space. **E.** Axial view Gd-DPTA-enhanced T$_1$-weighted MRI study (*TR* = 450; *TE* = 12) showing significant left paraspinal mass and ventral spinal canal compromise. The patient was treated with an immediate anterior retroperitoneal decompression and fusion followed by a 6-week course of antibiotics. Tissue cultures grew methicillin-resistant *S. aureus.* She had resolution of her infection but no change in her bowel or bladder function.

laminectomy is performed for lesions of the lumbar spine, extreme care should be taken to preserve the facets, and a discectomy débridement should be performed. In addition, an autogenous lateral transverse process fusion is recommended to prevent spondylolisthesis and foraminal narrowing secondary to progressive disc collapse (6).

Cases with significant bony destruction and kyphotic deformity should be approached as staged procedures (6). Anterior reconstruction with autogenous bone grafting after extensive débridement should be the first stage; subsequent posterior instrumentation and fusion should be performed in cases with severe kyphosis or facet compromise, provided the patient can tolerate the stress of an additional procedure. Reconstruction using autogenous iliac crest graft is recommended following débridement of the infected focus. In certain cases, a good-quality rib graft, harvested during the transthoracic approach, can be used for short segment stabilization in cases without kyphosis.

SUMMARY

Advances in diagnostic capabilities and antibiotic treatments have reduced patient mortality to less than 5% (6). Patients at increased risk are the elderly and those with underlying systemic disease (e.g., rheumatoid arthritis, diabetes).

The majority of cases can be treated nonoperatively with early detection, treatment, and bracing (to prevent kyphotic deformity). For patients who require anterior surgical débridement, primary bone grafting, and parenteral antibiotics, the prognosis is good. Most modern series report a high rate of recovery with solid fusion and minimal deformity. The mortality of operative procedures is proportional to the severity of the presenting neurologic deficit.

REFERENCES

1. Waldvogel FA, Medoff G, Swartz MN. Osteomyelitis: a review of clinical features, therapeutic considerations and unusual aspects. N Engl J Med 1970;282:198–206.
2. Waldvogel FA, Medoff G, Swartz MN. Osteomyelitis: a review of clinical features, therapeutic considerations and unusual aspects (second of three parts). N Engl J Med 1970;282:260–266.
3. Waldvogel FA, Medoff G, Swartz MN. Osteomyelitis: a review of clinical features, therapeutic considerations and unusual aspects.
3. Osteomyelitis associated with vascular insufficiency. N Engl J Med 1970;282:316–322.
4. Sapico FL, Montgomerie JZ. Vertebral osteomyelitis. Infect Dis Clin North Am 1990;4:539–550.
5. Martin NS. Tuberculosis of the spine: a study of the results of treatment during the last twenty-five years. J Bone Joint Surg 1970;52B:613–628.
6. Slucky AV, Eismont FJ. Spinal infections. In: Bridwell KH, de Wald RL, eds. The textbook of spinal surgery. 2nd ed. Philadelphia: Lippincott-Raven, 1996:1500–1543.
7. Wiley AM, Trueta J. The vascular anatomy of the spine and its relationship to pyogenic vertebral osteomyelitis. J Bone Joint Surg 1959;41B:796–809.
8. Batson OV. The function of the vertebral veins and their role in the spread of metastasis. Ann Surg 1940;112:138–149.
9. Compere EL, Garrison M. Correlation of pathologic and roentgenologic findings in tuberculosis and pyogenic infections of the vertebrae: the fate of the intervertebral disk. Ann Surg 1936;104:1038–1067.
10. Dobson J. Tuberculosis of the spine. An analysis of the results of conservative treatment and of the factors influencing the prognosis. J Bone Joint Surg 1951;33B:517–531.
11. Paus B. Tumour, tuberculosis and osteomyelitis of the spine: differential diagnostic aspects. Acta Orthop Scand 1973;44:372–383.
12. Eismont FJ, Bohlman HH, Soni PL, et al. Pyogenic and fungal vertebral osteomyelitis with paralysis. J Bone Joint Surg 1983;65A:19–29.
13. Hodgson AR, Stock FE, Fang HSY, Ong GB. Anterior spinal fusion: the operative approach and pathologic findings in 412 patients with Pott's disease of the spine. Br J Surg 1960;48:172–178.
14. Modic MT, Feiglin DH, Piraino DW, et al. Vertebral osteomyelitis: assessment using MR. Radiology 1985;157:157–166.
15. Medical Research Council Working Party on Tuberculosis of the Spine. A controlled trial of six-month and nine-month regimens of chemotherapy in patients undergoing radical surgery for tuberculosis of the spine in Hong Kong. Tubercle 1986;67:243–259.
16. Emery SE, Chan DP, Woodward HR. Treatment of hematogenous pyogenic vertebral osteomyelitis with anterior debridement and primary bone grafting. Spine 1989;14:284–291.

Rheumatoid Arthritis of the Spine

Rheumatoid arthritis is the most common form of inflammatory arthritis, affecting 1% of the population worldwide, with an age-related increase in frequency from the third decade onward. Approximately 5% of the population over the age of 70 years are affected. Although the limb joints—hand, wrist, knee, and foot—are commonly afflicted, the spine is frequently involved. In the spine, the lumbar and thoracic regions are rarely affected; the cervical spine is the most commonly affected site (1).

Clinical involvement of the cervical spine was first described by Garrod (2) in 1890, and subluxations of the motion segments were reported shortly thereafter. Fatal medullary compression with atlantoaxial involvement, however, was first described in 1951 by Davis and Markley (3). On the basis of clinical examination, Garrod diagnosed cervical spine involvement in 36% of 500 patients. The reported prevalence of cervical spine involvement has since ranged from 20 to 90% of all patients, depending on the series reviewed. The wide range of reported occurrence is due to differences in patient populations studied (in terms of severity and longevity of disease) and differences in the clinical or radiographic criteria used for diagnosis.

RELEVANT ANATOMY AND PATHOGENESIS

The hallmark of rheumatoid arthritis is synovitis; and the spinal anatomic abnormalities that occur are the result of destruction of joints, ligaments, and bone by this inflammatory process. Although the cause remains unknown, it is probably multifactorial; genetically predisposed individuals are exposed to an environmental factor that initiates the synovitis, and altered immune reactivity aids disease progression.

In the affected joints of the cervical spine, articular cartilage is destroyed, and the rheumatoid inflammatory tissue (pannus) enlarges to involve adjacent structures. Ligaments undergo distention, attenuation, and rupture. Erosion of bone with osteoporosis and cyst formation occurs. The pannus can involve the disc itself, resulting in a spondylodiscitis. This destruction of the anatomic integrity of the spine leads to an alteration in vertebral alignment in both the upper and the subaxial cervical spine. Vertebral malalignment in conjunction with direct invasion by the pannus causes a narrowing of the spinal canal, which in some cases results in spinal cord compression. Three basic patterns are recognized: atlantoaxial subluxation (AAS), atlantoaxial impaction (AAI), and subaxial subluxation (SAS). Frequently, these patterns occur in combination.

The natural history of the condition remains somewhat unclear because of variability in reported series. Neck pain is reported in 40 to 88% of patients with rheumatoid arthritis. If involvement of the cervical spine is to occur, it seems to commence early in the disease; and its progression appears to correlate with that of erosive destruction in peripheral joints (1,4). Cervical spine subluxations are observed in 43 to 86% of patients and are commoner in males, despite the much greater tendency for rheumatoid arthritis to occur in females.

In a prospective study of 106 patients with rheumatoid arthritis, the incidence of radiographic cervical spine involvement increased from 43 to 70%, and 36% had progressive neural involvement over a 5-year period. Approximately 13% of patients required arthrodesis for pain and instability associated with neural dysfunction. A 20-year follow-up of 73 patients with rheumatoid involvement of the cervical spine demonstrated neural dysfunction in 42 patients (58%), of which 35 (48%) had an arthrodesis (5). From a postmortem study of 104 rheumatoid patients, Nekulowiski et al. (6) estimated that 10% of patients may die from previously unrecognized medullary compression. Once cervical myelopathy occurs, a high probability of mortality ensues. Nonoperative treatment is associated with a 100% mortality, usually as a result of the cord compression or comorbid factors.

Atlantoaxial Subluxation

AAS is the most common manifestation of rheumatoid disease in the cervical spine, representing 65% of all subluxations and occurring in as many as 70% of patients with advanced disease (7). It is caused by erosive synovitis of the atlantoaxial, atlanto-odontoid, and atlanto-occipital joints and of the synovium-lined bursa between the odontoid and transverse ligament. The majority of AAS patients have anterior subluxation, although lateral subluxation (greater than 2 mm) occurs in 20%, and posterior subluxation occurs in less than 10%. The anterior subluxation beyond the normal limit of 3.5 mm (atlantodental interval; ADI) occurs as a result of destruction by the direct inflammatory infiltration of the ligamentous complex, which holds the odontoid process to the anterior arch of the atlas. This includes the transverse, apical, and alar ligaments. The adjacent synovitis also causes bony erosion of the odontoid, which in the most severe cases results in its complete absence. This is the main mechanism for posterior subluxation. Anterior subluxation beyond 9 to 10 mm leads to encroachment on the spinal cord.

Atlantoaxial Impaction

AAI is also termed cranial settling, pseudo-basilar invagination, and vertical migration of the odontoid. AAI has been found in 5 to 32% of rheumatoid patients surveyed. It accounts for approximately 20% of all rheumatoid subluxations, occurring either alone or in combination with AAS. In patients undergoing surgery for rheumatoid cervical disease, 37% of patients are affected (8). AAI is caused by progressive destruction of the atlanto-occipital, atlanto-odontoid, and atlantoaxial joints, leading to vertical translation of the odontoid and settling of the occiput. Progression eventually results in compression of the spinal cord as it enters the foramen magnum or the medulla oblongata. Cause of death is cord compression; vertebral artery obstruction; or occlusion of the flow of cerebrospinal fluid, which produces increased intracranial pressure and hydrocephalus.

Subaxial Subluxation

SAS results from widespread involvement of structures important for the integrity of the subaxial cervical spine. It occurs in 10 to 20% of all patients with rheumatoid arthritis. SAS involves destruction of facet joints, interspinous ligaments, and intervertebral discs (spondylodiscitis). Therefore, all major components involved in providing stability to the cervical spine motion segment are affected.

Subaxial subluxation often occurs at multiple levels, most commonly at the C2–4 levels, giving a stepladder appearance. In the subaxial region, there is much less risk of spinal cord subluxation than in the atlantoaxial region, because of the relatively narrow dimensions of the canal in relation to the cord at this level. Although myelopathy may occur purely from the subluxation, compression may occur anteriorly from the spondylodiscitis or posteriorly from extensive pannus at the facet joints (9).

INITIAL FINDINGS, PHYSICAL EXAMINATION, AND DIAGNOSIS

Rheumatoid involvement of the cervical spine may be completely asymptotic, or the patient may present with pain or neurologic deficit. The rheumatoid patient is also prone to sudden death, as some 10% of patients may die from previously unrecognized medullary compression (6). The severely afflicted patient with polyarticular involvement who is receiving corticosteroids or immunosuppressive medication is most commonly affected by clinical rheumatoid disease.

Neck pain is reported in 40 to 88% of rheumatoid arthritis patients. Other local symptoms are common, including occipital headache, craniocervical junction pain, shoulder pain, interscapular pain, neck stiffness, and creatinase. The occipital pain is the result of upper cervical instability, direct irritation of the greater occipital nerve, or referred pain from the posterior ramus of the C1 nerve root. Patients with cervical myelopathy may have multiple neurologic symptoms, which can be quite vague. A subtle loss of upper or lower limb function with weakness or a loss of endurance—often signaled by deterioration in writing quality—may occur. The patient may describe paresthesias in the hands or an electric shock sensation throughout the body with neck movement (Lhermitte's sign). Urinary incontinence or retention may be the first indication of myelopathy in these patients. The presentation may be that of vertebrobasilar insufficiency with vertigo, tinnitus, dysphagia, diplopia, visual disturbance, and loss of equilibrium.

Physical examination demonstrates loss of neck movement, particularly rotation. Neurologic evaluation of the patient for evidence of myelopathy is particularly difficult because of concomitant severe peripheral joint disease. Objective weakness and upper motor neuron signs may be present in advanced cases. A high index of suspicion with a careful search for subtle signs of cord compression, such as hyperreflexia or a positive Babinski sign, is warranted in all cases. The degree of cervical myelopathy may be classified according to the Japanese Orthopedic Association scale for myelopathy; however, this classification requires an evaluation of the use of chopsticks, making it difficult to apply in the Western world. Thus the Ranawat grading system is often employed in the United States (10) (Table 37.1).

table	37.1	Ranawat Grading Scale

Class	Characteristics
I	Normal
II	Weakness, hyperreflexia, dysesthesia
IIIA	Paresis and long tract findings but can ambulate
IIIB	Quadriparesis and inability to ambulate

RADIOLOGIC STUDIES

Plain Radiographs

Plain radiographs—AP, open-mouth, lateral, oblique, and flexion and extension lateral views—are part of the evaluation of the rheumatoid patient even if he or she has no neck symptoms (Fig. 37.1). These studies form a baseline for future comparison and may assist in the diagnosis of instability at an early stage. Furthermore, all patients requiring an operative procedure that may involve general anesthesia with endotracheal intubation should have a preoperative radiographic evaluation to detect instability.

The specific measurements that should be assessed include the anterior atlantodental interval (AADI) on the lat-

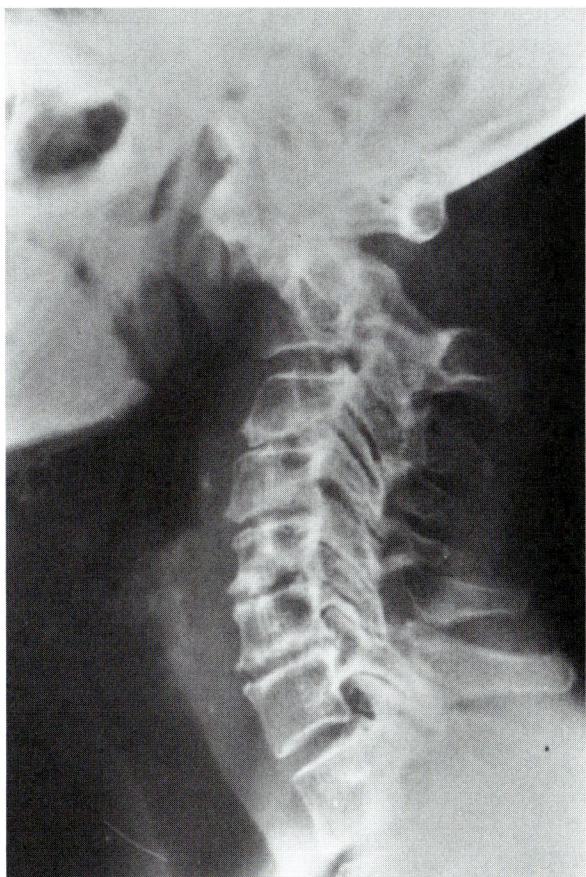

Figure 37.2. Lateral view of the cervical spine showing pronounced C1–2 subluxation and mild C2–3 subluxation.

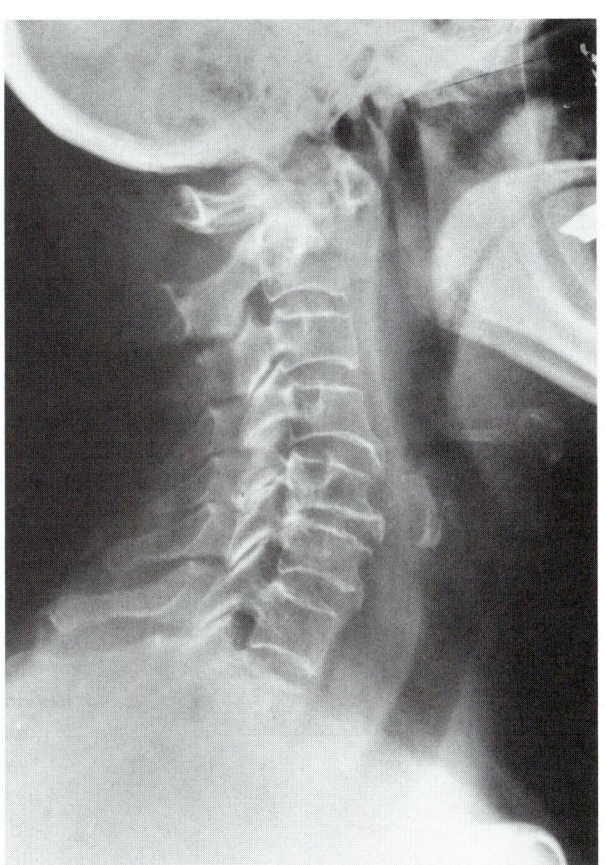

Figure 37.1. Lateral extension and flexion view showing the AAS of C1 on C2, which worsened on the flexion film. Note the degenerative changes at C4–5, C5–6, and C6–7 and the erosion of the odontoid.

eral view. This should not exceed 3.5 mm on either the neutral, flexion, or extension lateral radiograph. An absolute subluxation of 8 to 10 mm is regarded as significant (Fig. 37.2); however, the difficulty in using this measurement to predict risk of neurologic compression has recently been highlighted (5). An alternative measurement is the posterior atlantodental interval (PADI), measured from the posterior wall cortex of the dens to the anterior aspect of the C2 lamina. If this is greater than 14 mm, there is a 94% chance (negative predictive value) that the patient will not have paralysis. The 14-mm cutoff yields a sensitivity of 97% and a specificity of 52%. Boden et al. (5) concluded that the PADI is a better predictor of paralysis than the AADI.

AAI may be measured in a variety of ways on plain radiographs. McGregor's line measures the distance on a lateral view from the superior tip of the odontoid to a line drawn from the base of the hard palate to the base of the occiput. The odontoid should not project more than 4.5 mm above this line. The odontoid on a lateral view should lie below McRae's line, which connects the anterior and posterior margins of the foramen magnum (basion to opisthion). Chamberlain's line joins the posterior margin of the hard palate to the posterior margin of the foramen magnum. The odontoid should not project more than 3 mm above this line, and 6 mm is definitely abnormal. The Redlund-Johnell line passes from McGregor's line to the caudal end plate of the axis; this distance should be greater than 34 mm in men and 29 mm in women. On the open mouth view, the Fischgold and Metzger measurement may be used. The digastric line is drawn from the base of the mastoid where it joins the base of skull. The tip of the odontoid should lie 1 cm or more below this line.

Because it is difficult to delineate the necessary anatomic structures for the diagnostic measurements on plain films, the Ranawat index was devised (10). This index is based on landmarks that are readily identified on a lateral plain radiograph and avoids the use of the odontoid or hard palate. A line is drawn connecting the midpoints of the anterior and posterior arches of the atlas. The center point of the pedicles of the axis is selected and a line is drawn perpendicular from this point to the midaxis line. A distance of less than 15 mm for men and 13 mm for women is regarded as significant for impaction. The Ranawat index is also specific for documenting the severity of AAI caused by atlantoaxial disease rather than atlanto-occipital disease. The use of these measurement techniques has been somewhat superseded by direct visualization of the cord and medullary compression on MRI.

CT Studies

CT is excellent at detailing the bony anatomy in the cervical spine and helps in the evaluation of rotatory subluxation (Fig. 37.3). Conventional tomography may also be

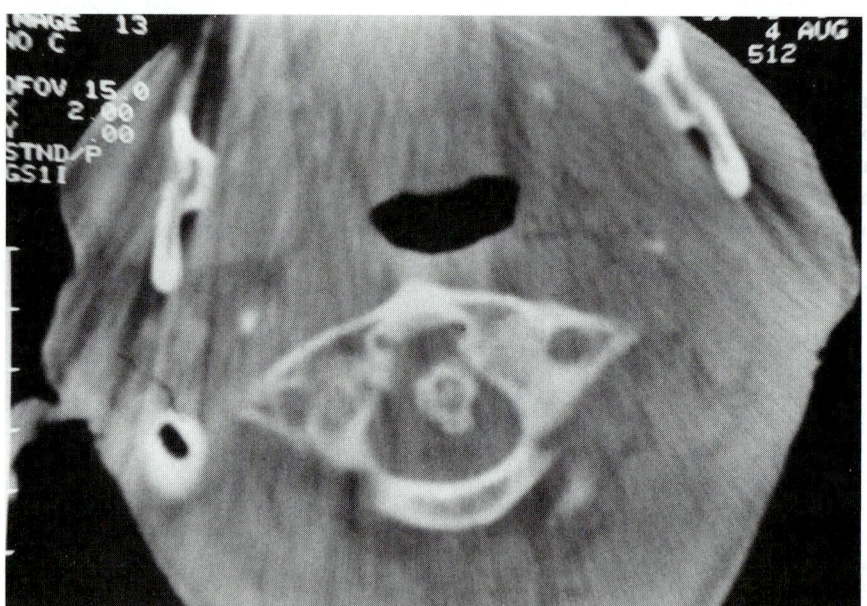

Figure 37.3. Axial view CT study of the cervical spine showing incompetence of the transverse ligament.

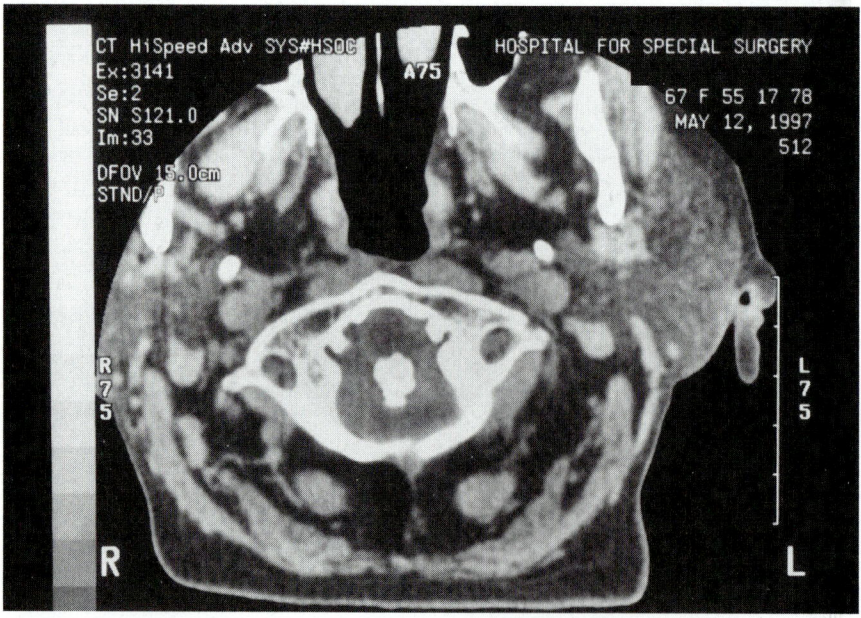

Figure 37.4. CT study showing the remnant of the odontoid and the anterior subluxation of C1 on C2.

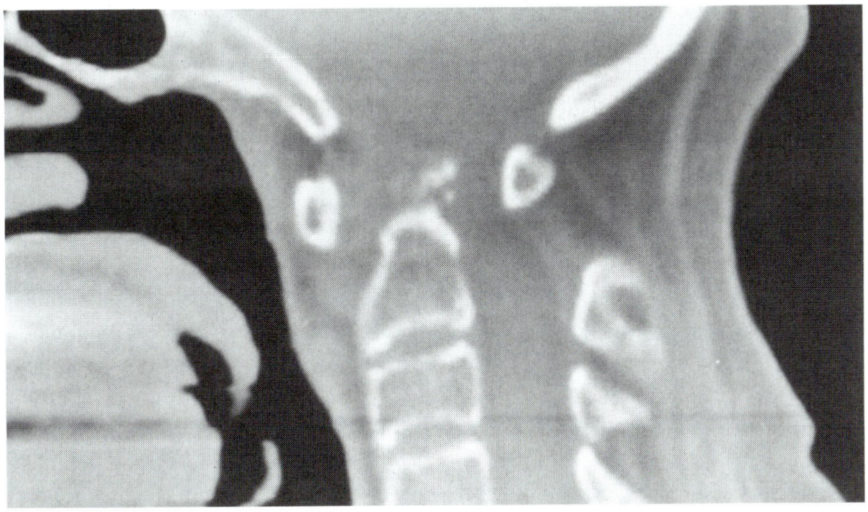

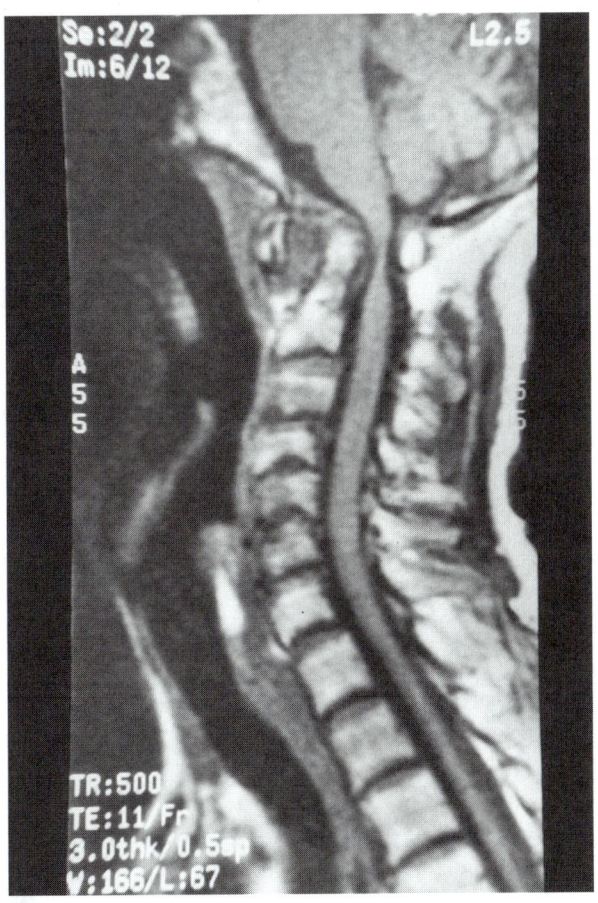

Figure 37.5. Reformatted CT study showing the erosion of the odontoid and an increased ADI. Note that the space available for the cord has narrowed.

used for this purpose and may avoid the loss of detail that occurs with improper reformatting to produce sagittal images using CT (Figs. 37.4 and 37.5). If combined with myelography, CT can be used to determine the extent and site of cord compression in the cervical spine.

MRI Studies

MRI, including dynamic imaging, has now become the imaging modality of choice for the evaluation of the soft tissue component of the disease and for detailing any possible neurologic compression in both the upper and the lower cervical spine (Fig. 37.6). In particular, it is useful in detecting cord compression caused by an extensive pannus rather than vertebral malalignment. A pannus of 3 mm or more seen on MRI at the level of the dens has been shown to contribute to neural compression (Fig. 37.7) (11). Flexion-extension MRI can demonstrate dynamic com-

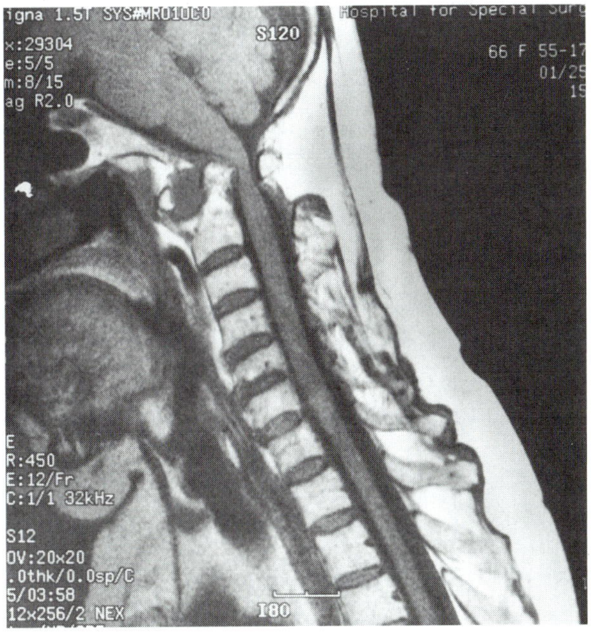

Figure 37.6. Sagittal view MRI showing cord compression secondary to an enlarged atlantodens interval and a reduced space available for the cord.

Figure 37.7. MRI study showing evidence of spinal cord compression secondary to atlantoaxial subluxation. A pannus is evident between the arch of C1 and the dens.

pression of the cord by the pannus behind the dens. This pannus has been shown on MRI to regress after fusion. MRI is also a useful technique in identifying the significant levels of compression in multilevel disease.

TREATMENT

Nonoperative Treatment

The best method of treatment for rheumatoid arthritis of the spine still lies in the area of prevention, as with most diseases. Since spinal involvement is associated with severe peripheral joint disease, an aggressive attempt at halting progression early by medical intervention should be successful. Continued monitoring of the spine by radiographic and neurologic examination throughout the disease process is an important aspect of the nonoperative management. Specific nonoperative therapy for cervical symptoms is supportive. Cervical collars may help relieve local discomfort, but they have not been shown to prevent progression of the disease process to cervical malalignment and cord compression. Other local modalities, such as massage, heat therapy, gentle exercises, and transcutaneous electrical nerve stimulation, may be tried, but none has a proven benefit. Anti-inflammatory medication, muscle relaxants, and trigger point injection may provide pain relief.

Operative Treatment

A small subset of patients with rheumatoid involvement of the cervical spine eventually require operative intervention. In one study, 13 of 46 patients with documented cervical involvement required surgical stabilization by the end of the 5-year follow-up (12). The indications for surgery include neurologic abnormality with instability, intractable pain, clinical findings of vertebral artery compromise, and impending neurologic deficit (Clinical Table). Surgical intervention to prevent the onset of neurologic compromise by arthrodesis has been advocated for some time and has more recently received further support (5,10,13,14).

Guidelines for surgical intervention have been developed from attempts at defining patients at risk for neurologic compromise. An AADI greater than 9 mm indicates a significant risk, requiring stabilization and fusion. Boden et al. (5) suggested that a PADI of 14 mm or less indicates a cord at risk at the atlantoaxial level. These parameters should be used in conjunction with an MRI evaluation (11,15). If the MRI study demonstrates a cervicomedullary angle of less than 135°, a cord diameter in flexion of less than 6 mm, or a space available for the cord (SAC) of less than 13 mm, stabilization is recommended (16). Patients with AAI of more than 5 mm and AAS are also at risk. MRI, particularly in flexion, usually demonstrates cord or

Clinical Table: Rheumatoid Arthritis of the Spine

Procedure	Indications	Technique	Anatomy	Pitfalls
Halo vest	• Supplement to fusion techniques	• Secure halo to skull with four pins in an adult	• Place ring below skull equator • Avoid supraorbital nerve • Temporal artery	• Loose vest • Retighten pins at 48 h
Occipitocervical fusion	• Atlantoaxial impaction with subluxation	• Posterior approach • Contoured metal loop or plate	• Sagittal sinus • Dura • Cord • Nerve roots	• CSF leak from dural penetration at occiput
Upper cervical decompression	• Cord or medulla compression not relieved by traction	• Transoral resection of odontoid • Or posterior C1 laminectomy	• Use midline avascular plane posteriorly	• High rate of infection with transoral route • Technically demanding
C1–2 fusion	• C1–2 instability	• Gallie's fusion • Brooks' fusion • Magerl's technique	• Magerl's fusion used if posterior arch of C1 is absent	• Vertebral artery injury
Subaxial cervical fusion	• Subaxial instability	• Posterior wiring • Lateral mass plating	• Lateral mass plating preferred if spinous processes are absent	• Vertebral artery injury • Operating on wrong level
Subaxial cervical decompression	• Neurologic compression	• Anterior or posterior approach • With multilevel disease, usually posterior	• Esophagus • Carotid sheath • Laryngeal nerves	• Inadequate decompression • Operating on wrong level

CSF, cerebrospinal fluid.

medullary compression in patients warranting stabilization. In the subaxial cervical spine, patients with SAS greater than 3.5 mm, or 20%, and a sagittal diameter of the spinal canal of 14 mm or less should be further evaluated by MRI. If the true SAC on flexion and extension MRI is less than 13 mm or if there is hypermobility, arthrodesis should be considered (16).

Having established the indication for surgical intervention, the clinician must now consider the general health status of the patient. Patients tend to be significantly debilitated with extensive peripheral polyarticular disease accompanied by advanced systemic manifestations. They may be nonambulatory as a result of polyarticular disease or myelopathy. Wound healing is often compromised, osteoporotic bone makes fixation problematic, and rates of nonunion and infection are generally high. Anesthetic risks are high as a result of difficulties in airway management, coexistent interstitial lung disease, and compromised respiratory function in a debilitated or paretic patient.

Awake nasotracheal intubation using a fiberoptic laryngoscope is the least traumatic means of establishing an airway before surgery. The patient is then positioned, and neurologic function is checked before induction of anesthesia. Preoperative halo traction may assist in the gradual reduction of subluxations or impaction and can be achieved in a wheelchair or in bed to allow mobility while preventing the problems of prolonged recumbency.

The operative procedure to be performed depends on the preoperative evaluation of the level or levels of instability or neurologic compression. In cases of isolated C1–2 instability (AAS), a posterior C1–2 arthrodesis is performed. Significant AAS associated with AAI requires occiput to C2 fusion. A decompressive procedure is included if there is significant compression on the cord or medulla not relieved by preoperative skeletal traction. This can be performed anteriorly by resection of the odontoid via a transoral approach or posteriorly by C1 laminectomy. In patients with SAS, a posterior subaxial arthrodesis to include the involved levels is performed. A posterior decompression is included in cases of cord compression. For patients with significant upper and lower cervical involvement, the fusion should incorporate all the unstable segments.

C1–2 FUSION

C1–2 fusion may be performed by a variety of techniques using a posterior approach to the upper cervical spine. The patient is intubated while awake and turned prone before general anesthesia is administered, to allow confirmation of motor function. Skeletal traction is maintained with the cervical spine in the neutral position. A lateral radiograph to evaluate the alignment on image intensifier is useful before draping. Spinal cord monitoring may also be used.

A posterior midline skin incision is made from the external occipital protuberance downward to allow adequate exposure as far as the C3 level. The dissection is kept midline and subperiosteally to expose the spinous processes and laminae of C2 and C3 as far lateral as the facet joints.

Exposure of the posterior arch of the atlas is performed with care. It often still lies somewhat anteriorly, and lateral exposure should be limited bilaterally to 1.5 cm to avoid vertebral artery injury. The occiput is exposed if it is to be included in the fusion, and hemostasis is achieved by electrocautery. Three basic techniques of stabilization are described below: Gallie's fusion, Brooks' fusion, and Magerl's transarticular screw fixation.

Gallie's Fusion

Gallie's fusion involves the passage of a loop of 18-gauge wire in the midline under the posterior arch of the atlas, from inferior to superior. An H-shaped autogenous corticocancellous bone graft is then placed on the superior aspect of the C2 spinous process resting against the posterior arch of C1. This is locked in position by passing the wire loop over the bone graft and around the spinous process of the axis. The two ends of the wire are then tied down over the graft. A modification of this technique is to place the two free ends of the wire through holes in the graft before tying.

Brooks' Fusion

For Brooks' fusion, a double-wire technique is used (Fig. 37.8). Each double wire is passed under the laminae of

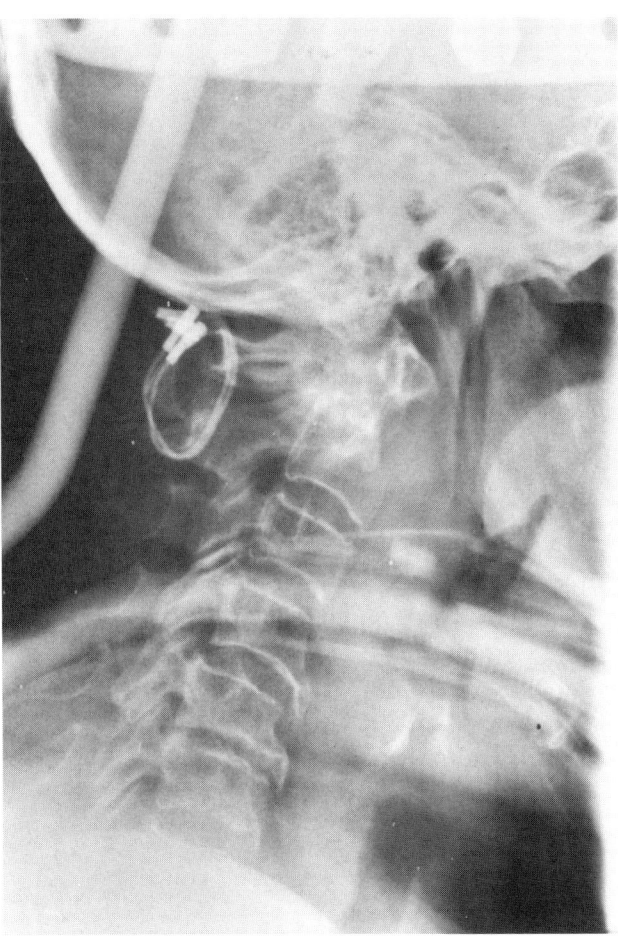

Figure 37.8. Postoperative lateral view of a patient who underwent sublaminar C1–2 wiring (Brooks' fusion) with a corticocancellous bone graft.

both C1 and C2 bilaterally on either side of the midline. An autogenous corticocancellous bone graft is then placed between the laminae of C1 and C2 bilaterally. The double wire is then tightened over the bone graft on both sides. The advantage of this technique is its enhanced stability, but it requires extra dissection in the sublaminar area of C2.

Magerl's Transarticular Screw Fixation

Magerl's transarticular screw fixation in conjunction with Gallie's technique is the most stable construct for C1–2 fixation. It is particularly useful without Gallie's fusion in cases of posterior element C1 or C2 deficiency. For Magerl's fixation, 3.5-mm screws are passed bilaterally across the C1–2 joints, using a posterior approach. The procedure is technically demanding. The bony anatomy and relative position of the vertebral artery should be assessed in the preoperative imaging studies.

Fluoroscopic guidance is used to confirm the reduction of C1 on C2 and to assist in the safe anatomic placement of the screws. Using a 2.5-mm drill, the starting hole is made 2 mm superior and lateral to the midpoint of the medial border of the inferior articular process. The drill is then advanced in the sagittal plane, directed toward the middle or superior aspect of the anterior arch of C1, and confirmed on image intensification. The drill bit is left in place to maintain the reduction, and the hole for the second screw

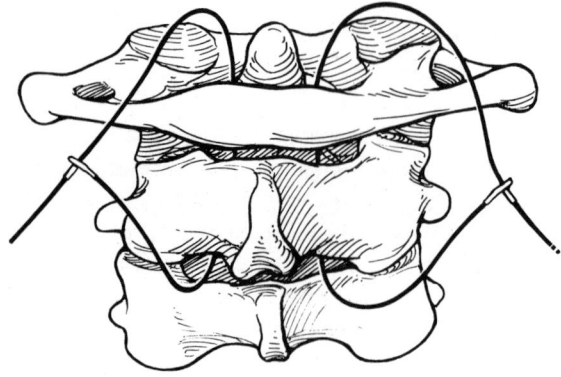

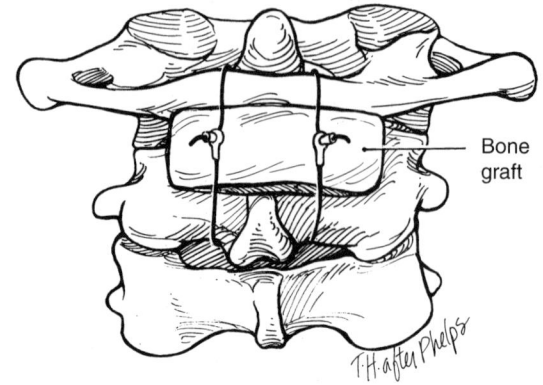

Bone graft

Figure 37.10. Brooks' procedure for C1–2 wiring and fixation. Note the bone graft is placed under the wires between C1 and C2 to prevent excessive compression and obtain anatomic alignment.

on the contralateral side is drilled. The distance is measured and the appropriate length screw is used. If there is posterior element deficiency, Gallie's fusion cannot be conducted, and the atlantoaxial joints should be decorticated and grafted to allow a fusion to occur. Stainless-steel cables have been designed for use in the spine; they are stronger than monofilament wire. Titanium wires, or cables, and screws may be used to allow better visualization of the region on postoperative NM.

A rigid orthosis is usually used for a minimum of 6 to 12 weeks. In rheumatoid patients, the surgeon may prefer supplementation of internal fixation with a halo brace, because of poor bone quality and risk of nonunion.

OCCIPITOCERVICAL FUSION

A variety of techniques have been described for fusing the cervical spine to the occiput since Newman's original graft onlay technique. These include the use of sublaminar and suboccipital wired bone graft procedures, wires and methylmethacrylate mesh that is wired in place (with or without cement), contoured metal loops that are wired to the occiput and laminae, and reconstruction plates that are contoured to the occiput and lateral masses and screw fixation. The latter two techniques provide good stability and have largely superseded previous techniques (17–19). These procedures can be used in conjunction with transoral anterior decompression or posterior C1 arch excision

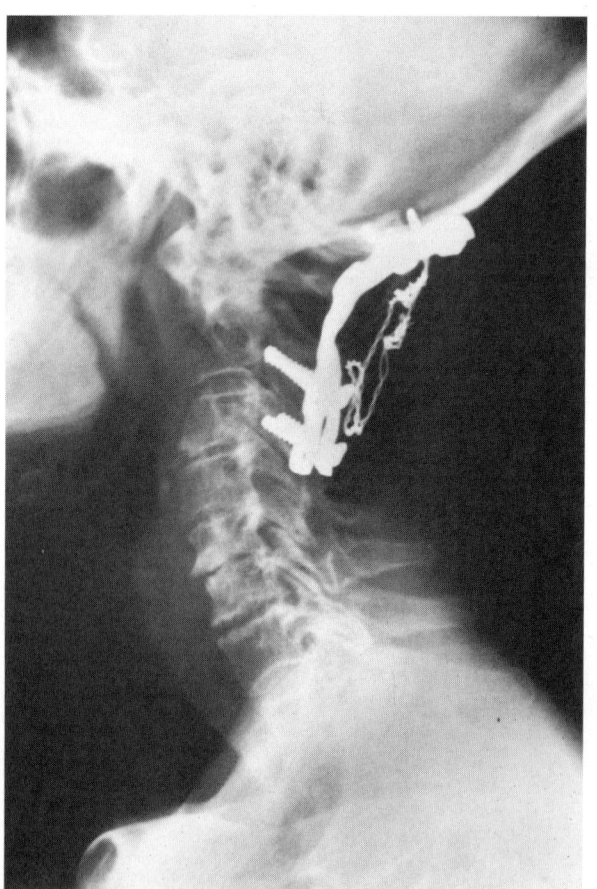

Figure 37.9. Postoperative lateral view of the cervical spine showing satisfactory reduction and fixation.

and posterior widening of the foramen magnum, if there is significant cord compression. Methylmethacrylate should be avoided if possible, as it may obstruct the potential for bony fusion.

With the contoured reconstruction plate technique, 6- to 8-mm-deep fixation or, preferably, bicortical purchase is used in the occiput. Two or, preferably, three screws are used in the occiput bilaterally. Overpenetration into the dura may give rise to a cerebrospinal fluid leak. Bone wax is placed in the hole, and the screw inserted as normal. Lateral mass screws are placed in C2 through the contoured plate; they have unicortical purchase and require drilling under fluoroscopic control. Additional fixation may be obtained by passing wire underneath the arch of C1 and through the adjacent holes of the reconstruction plate.

Both the contoured rod and plating techniques can be extended into the subaxial spine, if required (Fig. 37.9).

The postoperative management using such methods is simply the use of a cervical collar rather than a halo brace in most cases.

SUBAXIAL FUSION

Subaxial fusion is accomplished by a variety of wiring techniques or by lateral mass plate fixation (20–23). Lateral mass plating has been shown biomechanically to provide the most rigid construct. It is particularly useful in situations of deficient posterior elements or if a laminectomy is performed to achieve posterior decompression (Figs. 37.10 and 37.11). Wiring techniques, however, are simple, inexpensive, and effective in most patients. If the spinous

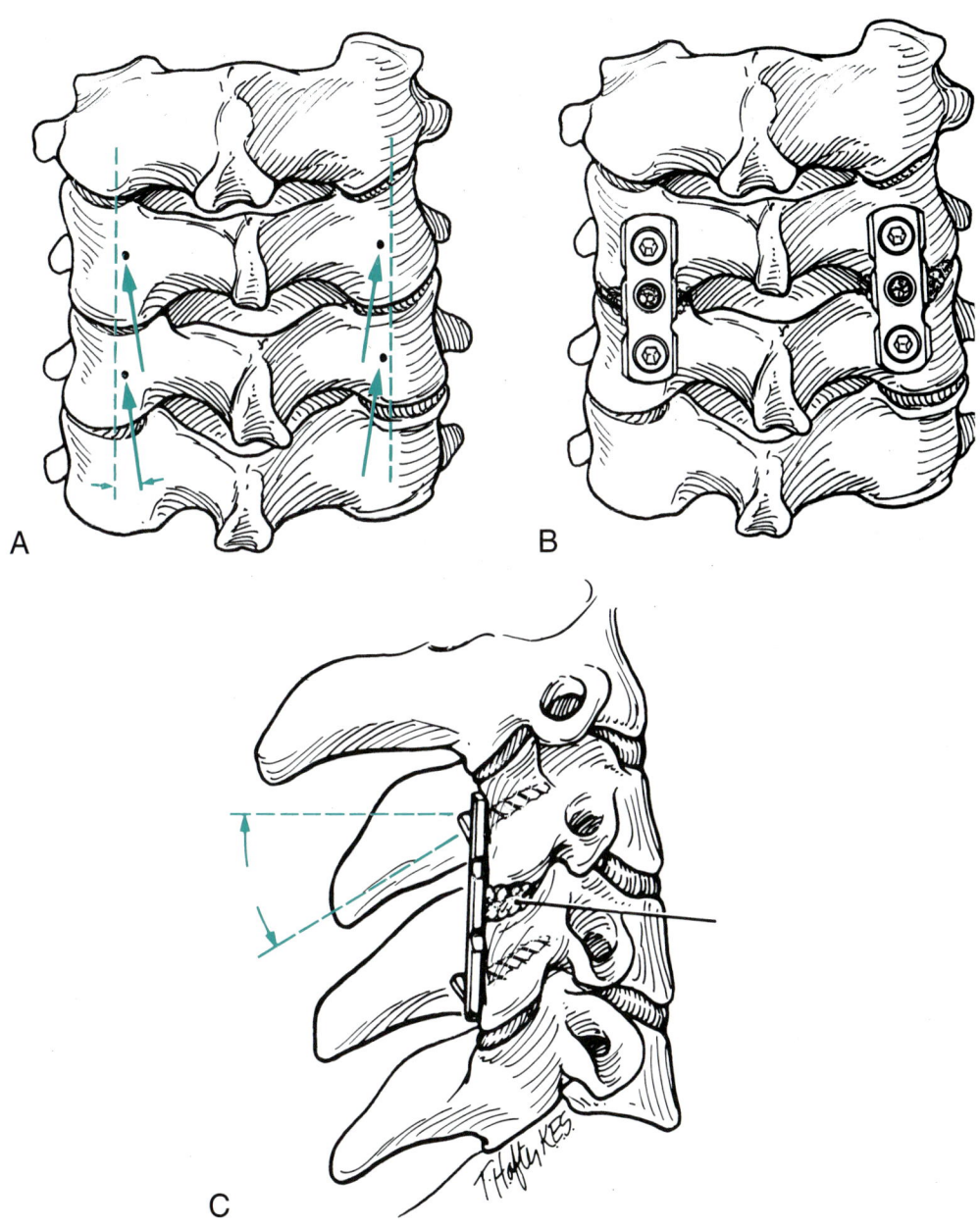

Figure 37.11. A. For posterior subaxial lateral mass plating, the screw holes are started past medial to the midline of each lateral mass. **B.** Each screw is placed parallel to the lateral mass on the sagittal view. **C.** On the normal view, the screw is laterally directed. This up-and-out direction prevents damage to the nerve root and vertebral entry.

processes are intact, the Bohlman triple-wire technique is preferred by most authors (22). Facet wiring techniques, as described by Robinson and Southwick (23), may be used in patients with compromised posterior elements. As with all fusion procedures, it is essential to perform adequate decortication and bone grafting to achieve union.

The outcome for surgical management in cervical rheumatoid disease has improved in recent reported series; the mortality rate has declined from 30 to 10%. Pain relief is usually excellent in 80 to 100% of patients. Neurologic improvement has been reported in 42 to 100% of patients; it is related to the severity of the preoperative neurologic deficit (5,10).

Nonunion rates in the occipitocervical region with wire techniques vary from 0 to 50%. Gallie's and Brooks' techniques have an overall nonunion rate of 5 to 15% in more recent series. High fusion rates approaching 100% in occipitocervical fusion and in the subaxial cervical spine have been reported with plating techniques.

SUMMARY

The cervical spine is commonly involved in rheumatoid arthritis and is potentially the most disabling and life threatening of the skeletal manifestations of the disease. The primary goal in management is the prevention of the onset of neurologic deficit. Early and serial evaluation of the neck with neurologic evaluation and imaging studies will identify the patients at risk for neural compression. The goal of surgery is to relieve pain, reduce deformity and prevent progression. Early surgical intervention in these patients is advocated to preserve function with less perioperative complications than if surgery is delayed. Pain relief is good when a solid arthrodesis is achieved. Newer fixation techniques provide rigid fixation, no longer mandating the use of a cumbersome halo vest or cast in an otherwise debilitated patient.

REFERENCES

1. Benhamou CL, Roux C, Viala JF, Gervais T. Thoracic and lower cervical spine involvement in a case of rheumatoid arthritis. Rheumatol Int 1989;9:39.
2. Garrod AE. A treatise on rheumatism and rheumatoid arthritis. London: Griffin, 1890.
3. Davis FW, Markley NH. Rheumatoid arthritis with death from medullary compression. Ann Intern Med 1951;35:341–345.
4. Winfield J, Cooke D, Brook AS, Corbett M. A prospective study of the radiologic changes in early rheumatoid disease. Ann Rheum Dis 1981;40:109–114.
5. Boden SD, Dodge LD, Rechtine GR, Bohlman HH. Rheumatoid arthritis of the cervical spine. A twenty-year analysis with predictors of paralysis and recovery. J Bone Joint Surg 1993;75A:1282–1297.
6. Nekulowiski P, Wolheim FA, Rotmil P, Olsen I. Sudden death in rheumatoid arthritis with atlantoaxial dislocation. Acta Med Scand 1975;198:445–451.
7. Conlon PN, Isdale IC, Rose BS. Rheumatoid arthritis of the cervical spine. Ann Rheum Dis 1966;25:120–128.
8. Clark CR, Keggi KJ, Panjabi MM. Methylmethacrylate stabilization of the cervical spine. J Bone Joint Surg 1984;66A:40–46.
9. Kudo H, Iwano K. Surgical treatment of subaxial cervical myelopathy in rheumatoid arthritis. J Bone Joint Surg 1991;73B:474–480.
10. Ranawat CS, O'Leary P, Tsairis P, et al. Cervical spine fusion in rheumatoid arthritis. J Bone Joint Surg 1979;61A;1003–1010.
11. Dvorak J, Grob D, Baumgartner H, et al. Functional evaluation of the spinal cord by magnetic resonance imaging in patients with rheumatoid arthritis and instability of the upper cervical spine. Spine 1989;14:1057–1064.
12. Pellici PK, Ranawat CS, Tsairis P, Bryan WJ. A prospective study of the progression of rheumatoid arthritis of the cervical spine. J Bone Joint Surg 1981;63A:342–350.
13. Ferlic DC, Clayton ML, Liedholt JD, et al. Surgical treatment of the symptomatic unstable cervical spine in rheumatoid arthritis. J Bone Joint Surg 1975;57A:349–354.
14. Clark CR, Goetz DD, Menzes AH. Arthrodesis of the cervical spine in rheumatoid arthritis. J Bone Joint Surg 1989;71A:381–392.
15. Kawaida H, Sakou T, Morijono Y, et al. Magnetic resonance imaging of upper cervical disorders in rheumatoid arthritis. Spine 1989;14:1144–1148.
16. Boden SD. Rheumatoid arthritis of the cervical spine. Surgical decision making based on predictors of paralysis and recovery. Spine 1994;19:2275–2280.
17. Ransford AO, Crockard HA, Pozo JL, et al. Craniocervical instability treated by a contoured loop fixation. J Bone Joint Surg 1986;68B:173–177.
18. Smith MD, Anderson P, Grady S. Occipitocervical arthrodesis using contoured plate fixation. Spine 1993;14;1984–1990.
19. Sasso RC, Jeanneret B, Fischer Y, Magerl F. Occipitocervical fusion with posterior plate and screw instrumentation. Spine 1994;19:2364–2368.
20. Grady MS, Anderson PA. Lateral mass plate stabilization of the cervical spine. Tech Orthop 1994;9:75–79.
21. Rogers WA. Fractures and dislocations of the cervical spine: an end result study. J Bone Joint Surg 1957;39A:341–376.
22. McMee PC, Bohlman HH, Wilson WL. The triple wire fixation technique for stabilization of acute fracture-dislocations: a biomechanical analysis. Trans Orthop 1985;9:142.
23. Robinson RA, Southwick WO. Indications and technics for early stabilization of the neck in some fracture dislocations of the cervical spine. South Med J 1960;53:565–579.

Suggested Readings

Brooks AL, Jenkins EB. Atlanto-axial arthrodesis by the wedge compression method. J Bone Joint Surg 1978;60A:297.
Gallie WE. Fractures and dislocations of the cervical spine. Am J Surg 1939;46:494–499.
Smith K, Anderson PA. Occipitocervical fusion. Tech Orthop 1994;9:37–42.
Winfield J, Young A, Williams P, Corbett M. Prospective study of the radiological changes in hands, feet, and cervical spine in adult rheumatoid disease. Ann Rheum Dis 1983;42:613–618.

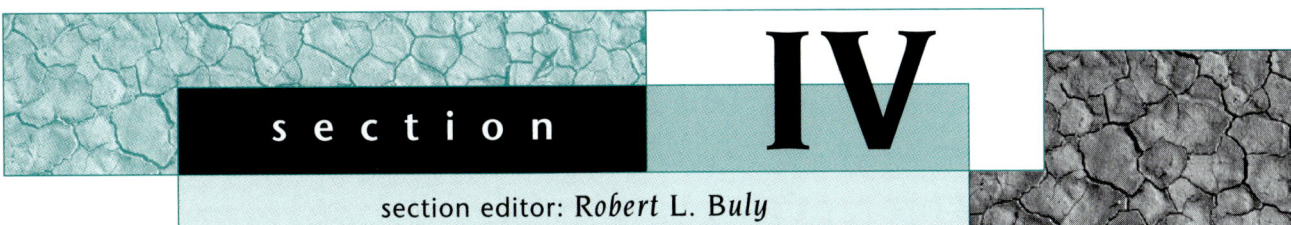

HIP

chapter 38

Craig S. Bartlett III, Robert L. Buly, and David L. Helfet

Intertrochanteric and Subtrochanteric Fractures of the Proximal Femur

Extracapsular fractures of the proximal femur include those of the intertrochanteric and subtrochanteric regions. Each type must be approached differently, based on its pattern. Successful management—maximizing the likelihood of healing and restoration of function with minimal complications—requires the consideration of biomechanical, biologic, and social factors. It is also important to remember that the responsibility for fracture reduction is the surgeon's, not the implant's. Thus, regardless of the treatment method selected, poor technique will guarantee poor results.

Intertrochanteric fractures most commonly occur in patients aged 75 to 80 years (1–11) and carry higher rates of morbidity and mortality than do fractures of the femoral neck (12–17). The term *hip fracture* is appropriate when referring to cervical and intertrochanteric fractures but should not be applied to fractures in the subtrochanteric region. Subtrochanteric fractures, which make up 7 to 15% of fractures of the proximal femur (18–22), are essentially a subgroup of shaft fractures and present unique mechanical and biologic problems (18,21–27).

Distinctions among fractures are often blurred. Subtrochanteric extension is present in one-fourth of intertrochanteric fractures, and proximal fracture extension is not uncommon with subtrochanteric fractures (28,29). Subtrochanteric fractures commonly occur in two age groups, with equal frequency: younger adults in their 40s who suffer high-energy trauma and elderly patients in their 80s who incur low-energy injuries (18,27,30–32).

Because hip fractures account for more than 70% of all fracture surgery in patients over the age of 70 and fractures of the femoral shaft make up another 16% (33), it is obvious that these injuries represent a significant problem for the elderly and their orthopaedic surgeons. Alarmingly, the risk for hip fracture doubles with each decade of life after the age of 50; and by 90 years, 32% of women and 17% of men will have sustained one (34). Hip fractures occur in 250,000 to 300,000 Americans each year and are the fourth largest cause of death in the elderly (18,35–39). In part because of the increasing average age of the population, the prevalence of hip fractures has doubled since the 1960s and is expected to double again within the next 50 years (18,37,38,40–44). In addition to the human costs, fractures of the proximal femur consume a major portion of national health care resources, ranging from $5.5 to $8.7 billion annually, which is more than for all other fractures combined (1,18,35,38,39,45,46).

DEMOGRAPHICS

In young adults, transverse or short oblique fractures of the proximal femur (particularly in the subtrochanteric region) typically result from high-energy trauma from a lofty fall, motor vehicle accident, or (less commonly) gunshot wound (18,23,27,47). Other, often interrelated, risk factors that are associated with fractures of the proximal femur include falls, female gender, advanced age, decreased bone mass (osteoporosis), osteomalacia, low body weight, muscle weakness, impaired vision, neurologic impairment (poor balance, altered reflexes), physical inactivity, malnutrition, race (Caucasian), smoking, alcohol consumption, and geography (18,34,39,40,43,48–57).

Falls are responsible for the increased incidence of fractures, particularly in females, over the age of 50 and the dramatic rise after the age of 65 (14,55). As a result, nearly 90% of hip fractures in the elderly are the result of a fall (12,38). Long oblique fractures with minimal comminution are commonly seen in elderly patients who sustain such low-energy injuries. Significant comminution, while variable in presentation, tends to occur more commonly in elderly patients who suffer violent injuries, particularly a direct blow to the greater trochanter (27).

Owing to their lower peak bone mass, rapid postmenopausal bone loss, and greater risk of falls, women are two to eight times more likely to sustain a hip fracture than are men (1,9,10,14,17,54,58). Although menopause itself does not appear to be a risk factor, both estrogen supplementation and a high daily intake of calcium (1000 mg premenopausal; 1500 mg postmenopausal) have protective effects (55,57,59).

Progressive loss of trabecular bone, diaphyseal cortical thinning, and intramedullary canal widening occur with increasing age or with metabolic bone disease (23). In addition, arthritic conditions have varied effects on the risk for fracture and the outcome of its treatment. Osteoarthritis may actually provide protection against hip fracture, as a result of the presence of thickened sclerotic bone (60). In contrast, rheumatoid patients with intertrochanteric fractures reportedly have higher rates of avascular necrosis (AVN) (10%), nonunion (7%), and secondary displacement (24%) than would be expected in the nonrheumatoid general population (61). Although osteoporosis has been demonstrated in 80% of hip fracture patients aged 80 years or more, other reports have failed to associate its presence with an increased risk of fracture (52,62).

Fractures in the geriatric population and in 30-year-olds appear to unite over a similar period of time (33,63,64); therefore, management should not differ greatly in response to the age of the patient. The primary goals remain good fracture alignment and enough stabilization to allow early mobilization and functional rehabilitation. Significant medical comorbidities, advanced physiologic age, and poor quality of available bone stock are, however, major risk factors that must be incorporated into the treatment algorithm.

RELEVANT ANATOMY AND PATHOGENESIS

The anatomy of the proximal femur dictates the optimal positioning of implants. The decussation of medial compression and lateral tension trabeculae in the compact cancellous bone of the center of the femoral head create an area of maximal bone density, approximately 25 mm from the subchondral cortex (25,65). In contrast, the femoral neck is composed of weaker cancellous bone that is more dense peripherally and a central area (Ward's triangle) that progressively thins with advancing age (23) (Fig. 38.1). An appreciation of trabecular patterns helps gauge the likelihood of success of internal fixation. To this end, the Singh index attempts to estimate the degree of osteoporosis by the roentgenographic grading of trabecular patterns using a scale of 1 (severe osteoporosis) to 6 (normal bone) (5,65,66). The index's subjective nature, however, limits its prognostic reliability (67–70).

Neck geometry must also be appreciated when directing implants into the femoral head or intramedullary canal. The normal human femoral neck–shaft angle decreases from 150° in newborns to an average of 135° in adults to as low as 120° in elderly patients (71,72). In adults, anteversion averages 7° to 16°. Proximal to the lesser trochanter, the sagittal plane anterior bow of the shaft reverses to a convex bow posteriorly (23). This aligns the intramedullary canal with the piriformis fossa; thus most intramedullary implants must be inserted through this region or through the posterior prominence of the greater trochanter. Because the greater trochanter is a posterior structure, care must be taken to direct the implants more anteriorly. If they are carelessly placed through the center of the trochanter or more posteriorly, they may exit through the posterior portion of the neck and damage the blood supply to the femoral head.

The intertrochanteric region is composed of highly vascularized, compact cancellous bone and is bounded by the greater and lesser trochanters, which serve as musculotendinous insertion sites for the gluteal (medius and minimus) and iliopsoas muscles, respectively. Distally, the thin metaphyseal cortical shell gradually tapers into thicker diaphyseal bone (72). Since no anatomic features mark the border of this transition, the subtrochanteric region has arbitrarily been defined as a zone extending from either the top or bottom of the lesser trochanter to a point as close as 5 cm distal or as far as the isthmus of the shaft (22,23,25,73–75).

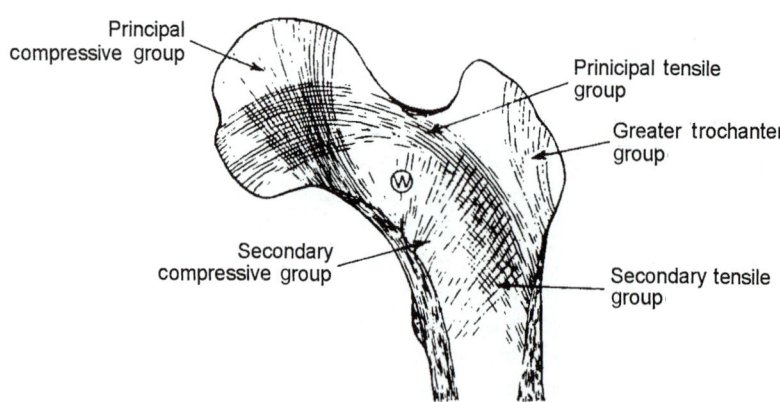

Figure 38.1. The five groups of normal trabecular bone that course through the proximal femur. *W,* Ward's triangle. Reprinted with permission from Singh M, Nagrath AR, Maini PS. Changes in trabecular pattern of the upper end of the femur as an index of osteoporosis. J Bone Joint Surg 1970; 52A:457–467.

Principal compressive group

Prinicipal tensile group

Greater trochanter group

Secondary compressive group

Secondary tensile group

The calcar femorale is a condensed vertical bony thickening that extends from the posterior neck, through the posteromedial portion of the intertrochanteric region just anterior to the lesser trochanter, to the posteromedial cortex of the subtrochanteric area (23,71). Many authors have emphasized the tremendous compressive and tensile stresses that are transmitted through this region during weight bearing (25,76–79).

Biomechanics

The magnitude and direction of applied forces and the degree of osteoporosis contribute to the variable fracture patterns seen in the proximal femur and hip joint. Direct forces include blows to the greater trochanter and impingement of the acetabular rim on the femoral neck. Indirect forces usually consist of axial stresses along the femur and the pull of the abductors on the greater trochanter (40). The lesser trochanter is commonly involved when an individual falls with the hip in an extended position (80). A fall from a standing position produces energy that actually exceeds by many times the amount required to create a fracture. Some of this potential energy is dissipated when the individual uses the upper extremities to brace the fall and by the elastic properties of soft tissues and other components of the skeleton. Unfortunately, the contraction of older, slower, and weaker muscles often cannot dissipate enough energy to prevent a fracture (40).

The proximal femur is a cantilevered arch that supports the trunk. Pauwels (81) calculated a single limb, stance phase, joint reaction force of 3 times the body weight, applied at a 159° angle to the vertical plane. While confirming these data, other authors noted that this force can range from 1.5 to 3 times the body weight during supine straight leg raising, from 2.5 to 4 times the body weight while getting on and off a bedpan, from 4 to 5 times the body weight during running, and to 7 times the body weight during stair climbing (3,22,23,72,82–84). These are important factors to consider when choosing an implant and planning rehabilitation.

The most extreme stresses occur in the subtrochanteric region (Fig. 38.2A). In 1917, Koch (76) calculated a maximal compressive force greater than $8,274 \times 10^3$ Pa (1,200 psi) at 2.5 to 7.5 cm distal to the lesser trochanter. More proximally, he noted peak lateral cortex tensile stresses of $6,895 \times 10^3$ Pa (1,000 psi). More recently, Rybicki et al. (77) calculated a maximal stress of $11,583 \times 10^3$ Pa (1,680 psi). Moreover, the inclusion of hip abductor muscle tension in these calculations leads to a fourfold increase in stress, which approaches the tensile strength of the femur (Fig 38.2B) (22,77). During normal walking, this increase can be offset by approximately 90 kg (200 lb) of tensor fasciae latae tension, which reduces stress on the femur by a factor of 3 and strain energy by a factor of 10 (77).

Bony defects along the medial femoral cortex resulting from comminution or displacement of large fragments will reduce fracture stability and increase the bending moment on bone–implant composites, thereby shortening their fatigue life (25,82). To prevent this, the reconstitution of the proximal medial femoral cortex is a crucial goal. Although it is not known how large a defect is required to significantly affect the stability of intertrochanteric and subtrochanteric fractures, Apel et al. (85) have shown that fixation of the entire medial cortex and a majority of the posterior cortex increases the load to failure by 57%. In contrast, stabilization of a small lesser trochanter fragment produces only a 17% increase in the load to failure. Other factors, including the type of fixation, biomechanical state of the fracture, geometry of the reduction, bone quality, and rate of healing, may play more important roles in achieving stability than do size, shape, or location of the medial fragment(s) (23).

Poor-quality bone predisposes the patient to fracture, makes fixation more tenuous, diminishes the potential of a stable interference fit by intramedullary devices, and increases the risk of implant failure or subsequent fracture just distal to the implant. In contrast, the typically excellent bone quality of younger patients provides greater fixation stability and improved surgical outcomes. Varus reductions produce a longer moment arm and, hence, increased deforming force on both implants and the healing fracture than do valgus reductions, which result in less stress (23,65,86,87). Bending loads on an implant can also be reduced by translating the implant closer to the center of the weight-bearing axis. Intramedullary fixation, for example, will support between three and four times the body weight, in contrast to plate constructs, which fail at loads from one to two times the body weight (82).

INITIAL FINDINGS, PHYSICAL EXAMINATION, AND DIAGNOSIS

All patients with traumatic injuries require a rapid and concise evaluation. Approximately 50% of patients sustaining a high-energy subtrochanteric fracture will have associated major injuries, including viscus ruptures and other fractures of the extremities, pelvic ring, and spine (18,26,30,32). Hemodynamic instability can result from blood loss, which averages 580 to 1500 mL for fractures in the subtrochanteric and diaphyseal regions (32,47,88). Neurovascular injury is rare (40). The absence of high-energy trauma does not diminish the importance of a thorough examination, because elderly patients living alone may lie undiscovered for hours or even days after a fall, delaying medical treatment and leading to dehydration and confusion. Neurologic conditions such as Parkinson's disease, stroke, and dementia require special surgical considerations but are not contraindications for either internal fixation or prosthetic replacement (40,89).

Although clinical deformity may be lacking in a nondisplaced intertrochanteric fracture, physical findings usually include pain, an inability to stand or walk, shortening, and external rotation of the extremity. Acutely, there may be swelling in the hip region; later, there may be ecchymosis over the greater trochanter. In the subtrochanteric pattern,

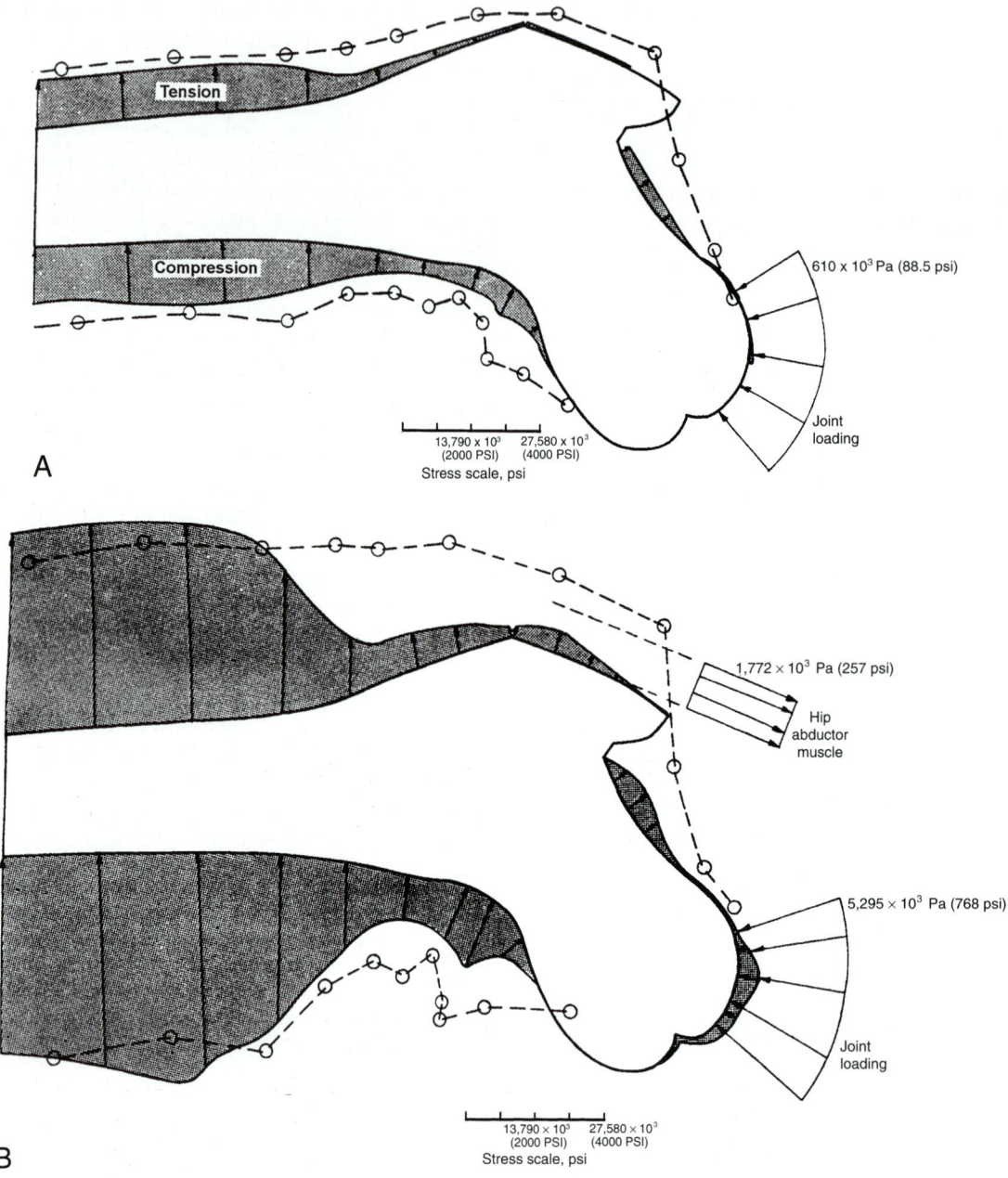

Figure 38.2. A. Calculated stress distribution as a result of joint loading for the proximal third of the femur (muscle forces excluded). **B.** Calculated stress distribution as a result of joint loading and hip abductor muscle force for the proximal third of the femur. *Solid line,* finite element analysis; *broken line with open circles,* beam analysis. Reprinted with permission from Rybicki EF, Simonen FA, Weiss EB. On the mathematical analysis of stress in the human femur. J Biomech 1972;5:203.

powerful muscle spasm abducts (gluteal), flexes (iliopsoas), and externally rotates (short external rotators) the proximal fragment while displacing the distal fragment medially (adductors). This leads to marked shortening and external rotation of the extremity, with a bulge at the thigh (18,23,80,90,91).

RADIOLOGIC STUDIES

Three roentgenographic views are mandatory to evaluate the proximal femur (Fig. 38.3): an AP view of the pelvis to allow comparison with the contralateral side and provide general information regarding the acetabula and pelvic ring; an AP view of the hip to demonstrate fractures in the intertrochanteric region and to delineate the neck anatomy (if taken in internal rotation); and a lateral view to detect a missed subcapital fracture and identify any posterior comminution, displacement, or extension into the greater trochanter or piriformis fossa (a cross-table lateral is better tolerated) (18,75,91). Additional oblique views may be required to better evaluate fracture comminution or a suspected nonunion (91). For subtrochanteric fractures, the entire femur should be imaged, including the knee joint.

Continued complaints by an elderly individual who had

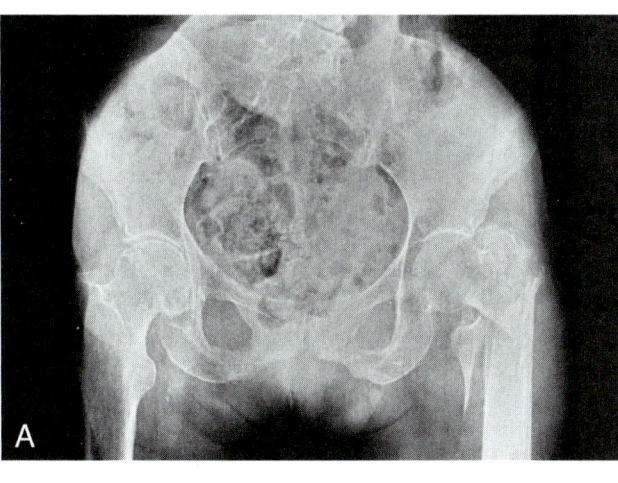

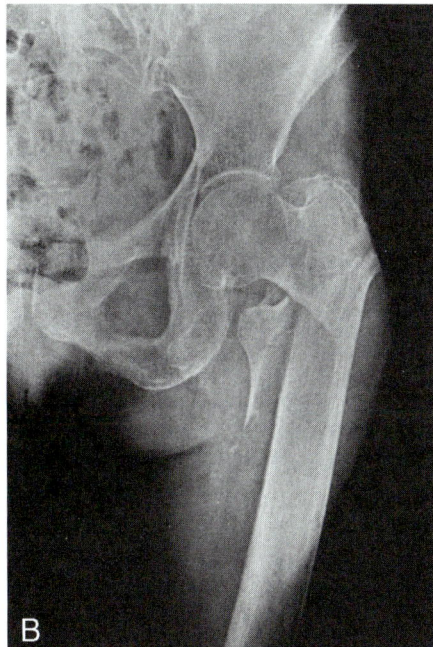

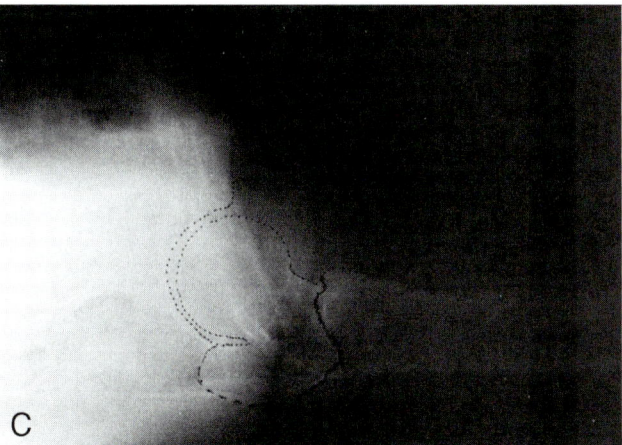

Figure 38.3. AP view of the pelvis (**A**), AP view of the left hip (**B**), and lateral view of the left hip (**C**) of a patient who sustained a fall.

normal roentgenograms should prompt the clinician to suspect an occult fracture. Such fractures often present with a vague history of minimal trauma, hip pain, variable discomfort on motion, and an inability to bear weight (92). Only 2.5% of patients with such complaints, however, will develop a displaced hip fracture (93); and many atraumatic diagnoses, including neoplasm, arthritis, trochanteric bursitis, avascular necrosis, and spinal conditions can have similar presentations. Therefore, if suspicion is low or the patient is not a candidate for further imaging studies, non-weight bearing should be instituted and new roentgenograms obtained in 1 week. If suspicion is high, then technetium-99m (^{99m}Tc) bone scanning should be conducted; it has a reported 100% sensitivity and specificity and has been the traditional diagnostic procedure of choice (92,94). It may be necessary to postpone the bone scan for several days to improve sensitivity, which increases costs and delays treatment (Fig. 38.4) (3,95). The

use of MRI has gained popularity because of its rapid procurement, excellent specificity, and ability to delineate fracture lines (96). Furthermore, because no contrast material is needed, MRI studies can be obtained in patients with renal or urinary tract problems.

TREATMENT

Initial Treatment and Timing of Surgery

After an intertrochanteric fracture, light skin traction (2.2 kg; 5 lb) can provide some immobilization and maintenance of extremity length; however, care must be exercised in the patient with peripheral vascular or sensory changes. Because of the significant deforming forces present, fractures involving the subtrochanteric region often require tibial or distal femoral pin traction, especially if treatment is to be delayed for several days.

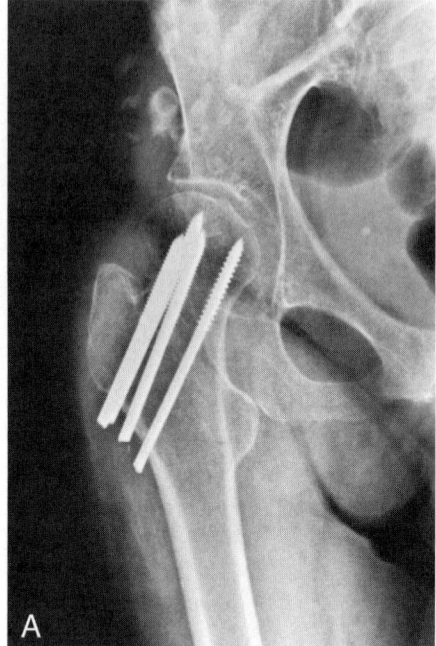

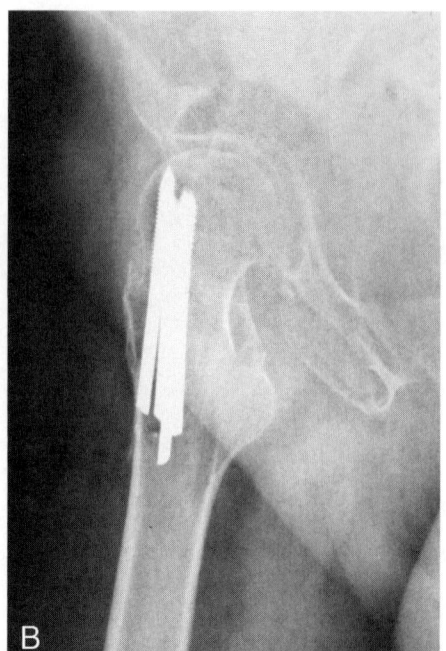

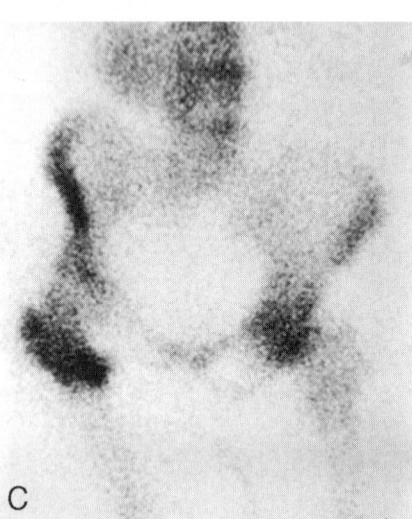

Figure 38.4. **A.** AP view of the right hip of an elderly woman who sustained a fall. Note the small but suspicious lucent area. This patient suffered a previous right femoral neck fracture that was treated with internal fixation. **B.** Lateral view showing no obvious fracture. **C.** Bone scan taken 1 week later, revealing a marked area of uptake in the right intertrochanteric region that is consistent with an intertrochanteric fracture.

Most authors have noted that early operative treatment reduces both mortality and morbidity (2,18,37,97–103). Early stabilization of the femur fracture in polytrauma patients is particularly desirable because it lowers the incidence of pulmonary complications and promotes rapid mobilization and recovery (99–102). Elderly individuals with isolated injuries, however, may benefit from a proper medical evaluation and optimization of associated medical problems over a period of time not exceeding 48 h (6,14,37,97).

Sexson and Lehner (37) noted that early surgery decreases the mortality rate of healthy patients from 15 to 3% but increases the rate from 22 to 33% in patients with three or more comorbidities. Zuckerman et al. (97) reported that a delay of 2 days or more was associated with 50% reduction of 1-year mortality for patients with three or more comorbidities, but they noted a threefold increase in mortality for patients with fewer comorbidities. In contrast, Kenzora et al. (6) noted a high (28%) 1-year mortality rate for relatively healthy patients who were taken to surgery within 24 h compared with those undergoing surgery in 2 to 5 days (4%).

Open fractures should be treated by standard open fracture protocols with emergent surgical débridement and stabilization. The patient must be returned to the operating room repeatedly until the wounds are clean, and antibiotics should be given until closure or coverage has been achieved.

There are several techniques available for the surgical stabilization of a proximal femur fracture (Clinical Table). For each individual case, the selection of the optimal technique is affected by the location of the fracture (intertrochanteric versus subtrochanteric), fracture pattern, bone quality, soft tissue involvement, presence of associated injuries, preexisting comorbidities, personality of the patient, and experience of the surgeon.

Clinical Table: Intertrochanteric and Subtrochanteric Fractures of the Proximal Femur

Procedure	Indications	Technique	Anatomy	Pitfalls
ORIF hip screw	• Intertrochanteric fracture • Stable subtrochanteric fracture	• Formal open reduction • Indirect reduction • Bone graft (subtrochanteric)	• Straight lateral approach	• Lag screw penetration • Malalignment • Overimpaction
ORIF DCS	• Reverse oblique intertrochanteric fracture • Subtrochanteric fracture with piriformis fossa involvement	• Formal open reduction • Indirect reduction • Bone graft	• Straight lateral approach • Detach portion of the vastus lateralis	• Lag screw penetration • Malalignment
ORIF blade plate	• Reverse oblique intertrochanteric fracture • Subtrochanteric fracture with piriformis fossa involvement	• Formal open reduction • Indirect reduction • Bone graft	• Straight lateral approach • Detach portion of the vastus lateralis	• Implant penetration • Malalignment, especially between the implant and femoral shaft
Intermedullary nailing (first generation)	• Low subtrochanteric fracture with comminution of fossa • Piriformis fossa intact	• Closed nailing (with or without reaming) • Limited open reduction	• Split the gluteus maximus • Entry point through the piriformis fossa or posterior cortex	• Rotational malalignment
Intermedullary nailing (second generation)	• High subtrochanteric fracture with comminution of fossa • Piriformis fossa intact	• Closed nailing (with or without reaming) • Limited open reduction	• Split the gluteus maximus • Entry point through the piriformis fossa or posterior cortex	• Implant penetration • Rotational malalignment
Intermedullary hip screw	• Unstable intertrochanteric fracture • Subtrochanteric fracture with piriformis fossa involvement	• Closed nailing (with or without reaming) • Limited open reduction	• Split the gluteus maximus • Entry point through the tip of the greater trochanter	• Comminution of the greater trochanter • Lag screw penetration • Rotational malalignment

Intertrochanteric Fractures

Introduced in the 1930s, fixed-angle devices, such as the Thornton (104), Jewett (105), and strong Holt (13) nails, were among the first implants to successfully treat intertrochanteric femur fractures (Fig. 38.5). These devices consisted of a single-piece triflanged nail, like the Smith-Peterson nail, fixed to a side plate at angles ranging from 130° to 150°. The McLaughlin nail (106) allowed the plate to be adapted to the femoral shaft after the nail had been driven into the femoral head. Although these devices were effective for stable patterns, settling and impaction occurred in unstable fractures, leading to failure rates as high as 44 to 53% (107–109). Problems included hip joint penetration, cutout through the superior portion of the head, breakage of the implant, and separation of the plate and screws from the shaft (54,107–115).

In an effort to improve fracture reduction and stability, a variety of surgical techniques and implant modifications were introduced during the 1950s and 1960s. Successful techniques included the Dimon-Hughston medial displacement (107,108,116), the Sarmiento valgus (117), and the Wayne County lateral displacement (118) osteotomies. The introduction of sliding nail plate devices allowed controlled and stable impaction to occur at the fracture site, leading to medial displacement of the shaft and a shortened lever arm with less extremity shortening than with a formal displacement osteotomy (80,119). Schumpelick and Jantzen (120) and Clawson (113) substituted a blunt-tipped screw with a large outer thread diameter for the proximal nail-like portion of the earlier sliding devices. This screw better resists cutout of the femoral head and penetration into the hip joint (121). Additional rotational stability has been obtained by "keying" the screw into the

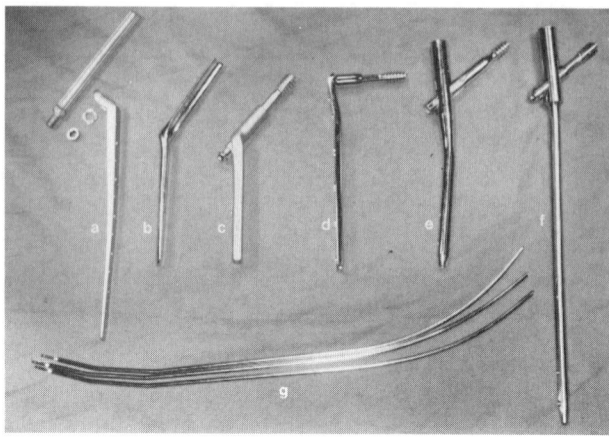

Figure 38.5. Devices for stabilizing intertrochanteric femur fractures: *a,* McLaughlin adjustable nail plate; *b,* Jewett nail plate; *c,* compression hip screw; *d,* Dynamic condylar screw (DCS); *e,* Gamma nail; *f,* intramedullary hip screw (Smith Nephew Richards; Memphis, TN); and *g,* Ender nails.

barrel of the plate (82). A recent variant of the sliding hip screw has the additional capacity for axial compression along the femoral shaft (122,123). These and other refinements have resulted in the modern sliding hip screw devices, which tolerate stress better, lead to fewer complications, and result in more superior outcomes than most static implants (3,54,109,110,112,114,118,124–130).

Some authors believe that the inherent stability of the reduction remains a more important determinant of healing at the fracture site (68,108,131,132). Although modern sliding hip screw devices have reported failure rates of 5% or less for stable fractures, their use in unstable intertrochanteric and subtrochanteric variants has lead to failure in 4 to 21% of cases (11,19,70,109,110,112, 116,122,126,129,133). The majority of technical failures are related to an improperly placed lag screw cutting out of the femoral head or complete telescoping of the implant, effectively making it a fixed nail plate device (69,110,116,134–137). Secondary overimpaction causes telescoping in up to 60% of unstable fractures (109). Even without implant failure, this results in 1 to 2 cm of extremity shortening and a shortened hip abductor lever arm, which can lead to pain and a poor functional result (70,98,113,129,138–140). Bendo et al. (139) noted some degree of collapse in 32% of patients who underwent sliding screw fixation of unstable intertrochanteric fractures compared with a 0% incidence in those with stable fracture patterns. Although patients with minimal collapse remained asymptomatic, 93% of patients with moderate to severe collapse had poor functional results.

The combination of a medial displacement osteotomy with a sliding screw plate device decreased the incidence of implant failure to 1.7 and 5.5% in two studies (98,141). Other authors, however, have presented biomechanical and clinical data that fail to reveal any significant advantage of medial displacement or valgus osteotomy over anatomic reduction (65,118,128,142–144). Chang et al.

(128) demonstrated that medial displacement osteotomy results in decreased compression across the calcar region and twice the plate strain associated with anatomic reduction. Even when the posteromedial (calcar) fragment was discarded in the latter group, strain was 50% less. Osteotomy also increases blood loss and anesthesia time (142).

Introduced in 1970, Ender nails have been promoted as an alternative for stabilization of intertrochanteric fractures; they offer a shortened operative time, decreased blood loss, and low rates of nonunion, infection, and mortality (54,145–151). Presently, this technique is not recommended for fractures of the proximal femur, except perhaps for some pediatric cases or (rarely) elderly debilitated patients with a stable fracture who can tolerate only a minimally invasive procedure (18,54,133). The technique is demanding and has a reported complication rate of 16 to 76% (8,19,54,103,109,127,130,133,147,148,152). Complications are likely in the presence of unstable fracture patterns and include blood loss, shortening, varus and external rotation deformities, irritation and loss of motion at the knee, pin migration, cortical penetration, and supracondylar femoral fractures. Even after pin removal, scar excision, and steroid injections, some patients have continued to experience pain at their medial femoral condyle insertion sites (153). Early reoperation ranges from 5 to 20% of cases but can be as high as 35% for intertrochanteric fractures and 68% for subtrochanteric fractures (8,19,54,109,133,147,152). If used, Ender nails should be prebent into anteversion and driven deeply into the femoral head to avoid an external rotational deformity (54). A titanium condylocephalic implant, promoted by Harris (154) for both intertrochanteric and subtrochanteric femur fractures has not been successful in other hands (127).

The Gamma nail (Howmedica; Rutherford NJ), introduced in the 1980s, combines the features of a sliding hip screw with those of a rigidly locked intramedullary nail (125,155–157). Its theoretical technical and biomechanical advantages include ease of insertion, limited fracture exposure, minimal blood loss, short operating time, and low bending moment (short lever arm) acting on the implant. Serious complications have included difficulties with distal locking, intraoperative comminution of the greater trochanter, cortical penetration at the time of insertion, cutting out of the screw through the femoral head, and femoral fracture at the lower end of the implant (11,75,125,155–162). The incidence of femoral fracture has ranged from 2 to 17% (11,155,156,159,161–163). In addition, recent biomechanical and clinical studies have failed to demonstrate any advantage of these implants over the sliding hip screw system for the treatment of intertrochanteric fractures (162–166). Shaw and Wilson (164) determined that both the Gamma nail and sliding screw device exhibited sufficient structural integrity to carry loads up to 273 kg (600 lb); however, the nail prevented fracture compression and permitted greater motion at the fracture site. Rosenblum et al. (165) found that with decreasing fracture stability the rigid nail transmitted decreasing loads to the calcar but increasing stress distally, near its tip.

In defense of intramedullary hip screw systems, some authors suggest that intraoperative difficulties and postoperative complications may be related to improper surgical technique and not to inherent defects in implant design (11,75,125,156,157,159). Technical errors have included erroneously placed drill holes for distal locking screws, insufficient reaming, and the introduction of a double-curved nail with the forceful blows of a hammer. In the largest series reported (628 cases), Boriani (157) noted that the 1% incidence of intraoperative shaft fracture was associated with 1 mm of overreaming. No intraoperative fractures occurred with 2 mm of overreaming, and four of the five postoperative fractures were related to acute trauma. Recent clinical and biomechanical studies regarding newer and longer intramedullary hip screw devices suggest that the problems associated with the original Gamma nail may have been related to its short length (29,156,161,167).

CLASSIFICATION

Many classification systems for intertrochanteric fractures exist, but Evans' (168) system is perhaps the easiest to understand and use in clinical practice (Fig. 38.6). Evans, recognizing the importance of the posteromedial

cortical buttress, designated fractures as either stable (type 1) or unstable (type 2). In type 1 fractures, this area remains intact or is minimally comminuted. Therefore, collapse of the fracture is minimal; and regardless of the fixation method, stability is obtained by restoration of medial cortical contact. Type 2 fractures include those with comminution of the posteromedial cortex, subtrochanteric extension, and the reverse oblique pattern (an oblique fracture line extending from the proximal-medial cortex to the distal-lateral cortex) (54). In these fractures, implants with advanced designs are required. Although Evans' classification system provides insight into the definition of a stable reduction, it has been documented to have poor reproducibility (54).

Boyd and Griffin's (28) classification system, modified by Kyle (110), is useful because it subdivides stable fractures (Fig. 38.7) (169). Type I fractures are nondisplaced, stable, and lack comminution. Type II fractures are stable, minimally comminuted, and displaced (reduction leads to a stable construct). Type III fractures are unstable and have significant posteromedial comminution. The relatively rare unstable type IV fracture involves subtrochanteric extension and is the most difficult to stabilize because of the great forces in the area (110,151).

Muller et al.'s comprehensive classification system identifies fractures with a multipart label (Fig. 38.8). For example, an intertrochanteric fracture is labeled 31-A: the 3 refers to the femur, the 1 to the proximal area, and the A

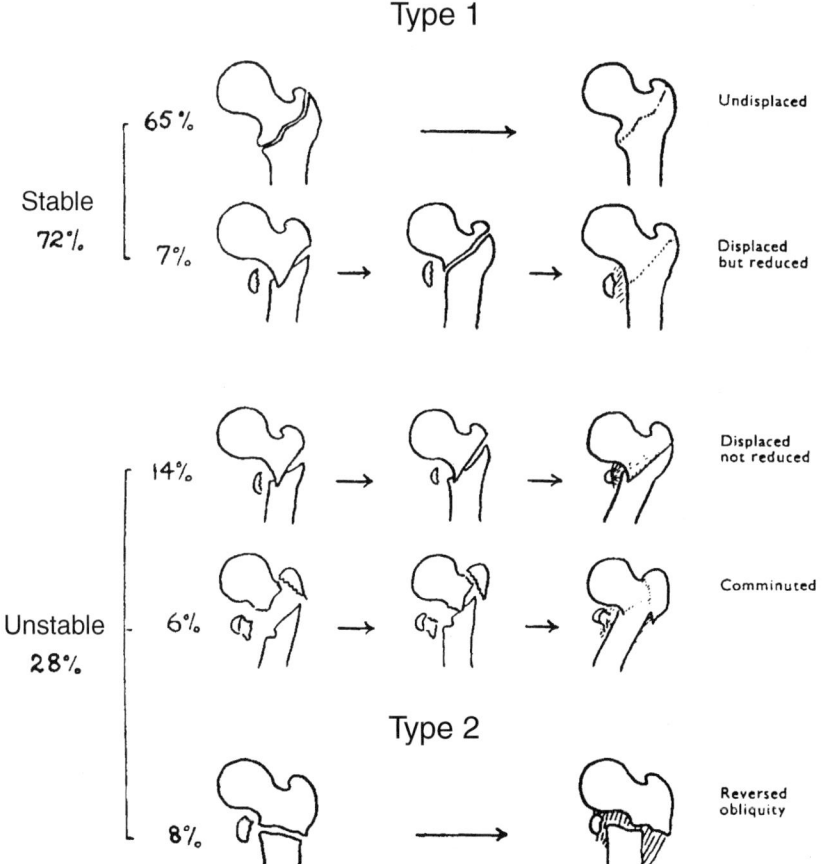

Type 1

Stable
72%

65%

7%

Unstable
28%

14%

6%

Type 2

8%

Undisplaced

Displaced
but reduced

Displaced
not reduced

Comminuted

Reversed
obliquity

Figure 38.6. Evans' classification of intertrochanteric fractures. Reprinted with permission from Evans EM. The treatment of trochanteric fractures of the femur. J Bone Joint Surg 1949;31B:190–203.

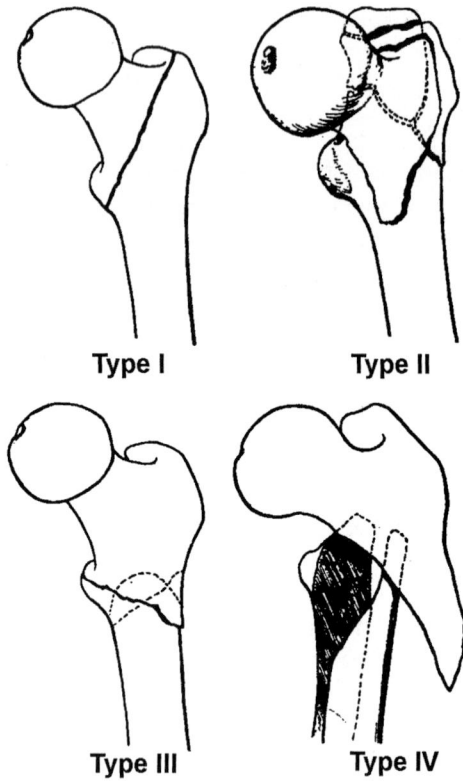

Figure 38.7. Boyd and Griffin's classification of intertrochanteric fractures. Reprinted with permission from Boyd HD, Griffin LL. Classification and treatment of trochanteric fractures. Arch Surg 1949;58:853–866.

tient has a fracture united in a shortened malaligned position. Thus surgical stabilization of the fracture is preferable in the majority of cases. Intertrochanteric fractures require 2 to 4 months of healing, depending on the stability of the fracture and the integrity of its fixation (70,98,108,123,129, 149,171). These factors are in turn related to the fracture pattern and the quality of the bone.

Nonoperative treatment is associated with significant morbidity and mortality and is suitable for only a small proportion of patients (172–176). Hornby et al. (173) noted no significant differences in fatality, leg pain, or unhealed decubiti among patients with intertrochanteric fractures treated either conservatively or with surgical stabilization. The latter group, however, required 26 fewer days of hos-

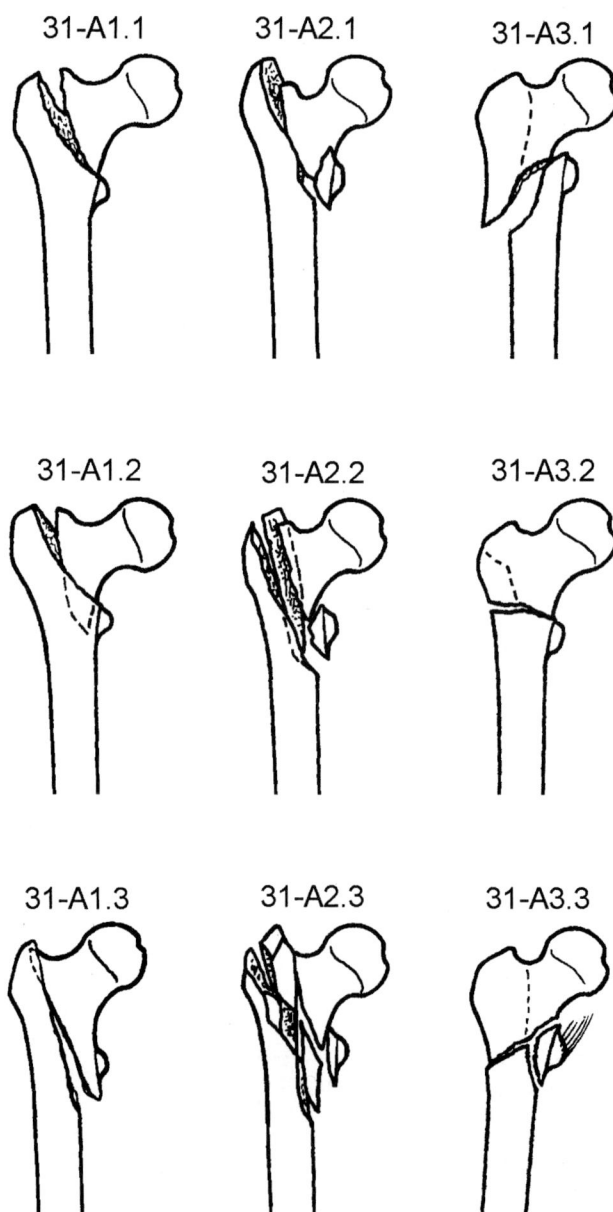

Figure 38.8. AO comprehensive classification as adapted by Muller et al. (170).

to the trochanteric region. Fractures are more specifically described by a two-part number that follows the letter; trochanteric area fractures are classified as follows:

31-A1.1: a pertrochanteric simple fracture along the intertrochanteric line
31-A1.2: a pertrochanteric simple fracture through the greater trochanter
31-A1.3: a pertrochanteric simple fracture below the lesser trochanter (subtrochanteric extension)
31-A2.1: a pertrochanteric multifragmentary fracture with one intermediate fragment
31-A2.2: a pertrochanteric multifragmentary fracture with several intermediate fragments
31-A2.3: a pertrochanteric multifragmentary fracture that extends more than 1 cm below the lesser trochanter (subtrochanteric extension)
31-A3.1: a simple oblique intertrochanteric fracture
31-A3.2: a simple transverse intertrochanteric fracture
31-A3.3: a multifragmentary intertrochanteric fracture

NONOPERATIVE TREATMENT AND INDICATIONS FOR SURGERY

The goals of treatment are to provide early mobilization and a good functional outcome. These are difficult to achieve when the patient is in pain, confined to a bed, and at risk for serious medical complications and when the pa-

pitalization, incurred lower financial and social costs, and was only half as likely to have lost independence. Patients with conservatively treated unstable fractures had the worst results. Although early mobilization and meticulous nursing care can reduce the risks of decubiti, urinary tract infections, deep venous thrombosis, and pulmonary complications, such a regimen is demanding and difficult to maintain (45). In addition, limited or non–weight-bearing ambulation is difficult for frail, elderly patients.

SELECTION OF IMPLANT AND TECHNIQUE

Successful treatment of an intertrochanteric fracture depends on a stable osteosynthesis, which can be achieved by open reduction and internal fixation (ORIF) or an intramedullary device. External fixation has little place in the treatment of intertrochanteric hip fractures (171). Because complex unstable fractures and poor bone quality can predispose the implant to failure, osteotomies, bone cement, and hemiarthroplasty are occasionally required (33,54,107,117,140,177,178).

Although ORIF is associated with relatively low mortality, it does not eliminate complications; nor does it always allow immediate full weight bearing, a desirable condition for frail elderly patients. Therefore, primary hip arthroplasty has been used in a limited number of elderly patients who have comminuted unstable intertrochanteric fractures (18,54,140,179). Haentjens et al. (179) performed 91 bipolar hemiarthroplasties and nine total hip arthroplasties in this population and obtained good to excellent functional results in 78% of cases. The dislocation rate after total hip arthroplasty was 45%, compared with 3% in the hemiarthroplasty group. In patients without dislocations, rehabilitation was easier and more rapid and the incidences of decubitus ulcers, pulmonary infection, and atelectasis were significantly lower than in historical controls. At present, the indications for arthroplasty for the treatment of acute intertrochanteric fracture remain undefined.

The preferred method of surgical stabilization remains the sliding compression hip screw device, which easily achieves a valgus reduction and medial shaft displacement (Figs. 38.9 and 38.10) (18,113,128,141,180). This technique shortens the lever arm of the force acting at the center of the weight-bearing axis, minimizing the bending moment applied to the proximal femur and reducing the risk of varus collapse and fixation failure (86,87). The sliding compression hip screw device also permits the lateral cortex to take on some of the compressive load normally borne by the medial calcar. Although this device usually provides satisfactory fixation of the proximal fragment, its success depends on many other factors, including the fracture configuration, reduction, quality of the cancellous bone present, operative technique, and postoperative care.

Currently, most sliding hip screw systems provide plates in 5° increments from 130° to 150° (181). The 150° implants have been popular because of their small varus mo-

ment and their alignment with the vertically oriented forces across the hip joint, which theoretically improve telescoping through the barrel and the implant's resistance to failure (81,115,182,183). The increased angle of these devices, however, moves the lag screw's insertion site more distally into diaphyseal bone and accentuates the technical difficulty of proper screw placement into the center of the femoral head. Moreover, clinical studies have failed to demonstrate any advantages of the 150° plate (116,184), and a biomechanical study by Meislin et al. (181) found that its high angle produced neither optimal compressive medial femoral loading nor decreased plate tensile loading. The 150° implant has a significant tendency to cut out of the femoral head; therefore, most authors prefer the 135° and 140° plates (54,114,116,181,184). With these devices, placement of the screw into the femoral head is easy, and its insertion site lies in metaphyseal bone, where any stress-riser effects are minimized (54). When the piriformis fossa is not intact, a hip screw with a long side plate, limited interfragmentary fixation, and supplementary bone grafting can be used (18).

Although reverse oblique fractures are frequently treated with sliding hip screws, they are probably better stabilized with the devices used for subtrochanteric fractures: intramedullary nails; intramedullary hip screws; blade plates, such as the 95° condylar plate (Synthes; Paoli, PA); and the Dynamic condylar screw (DCS; Synthes; Paoli, PA). The latter two implants provide improved fixation of the proximal fragment and avoid insertion directly through the fracture site, whereas intramedullary stabilization has superior load-bearing capacity and prevents medialization of the shaft fragment (18,166,185).

Intramedullary hip screws have not been proven superior to sliding hip screw devices for the treatment of intertrochanteric hip fractures, but they may have select indications. These include reverse oblique patterns and fractures with subtrochanteric extension, which would require a long side plate. Relative contraindications for intramedullary implants are the presence of severe intertrochanteric comminution, a widely displaced coronal fracture of the proximal femur, and extension into the piriformis fossa (18,23,47,54,91). Newer intramedullary devices that allow insertion through the tip of the greater trochanter may overcome these obstacles.

SURGICAL APPROACH, PROCEDURES, AND PITFALLS

The patient is placed supine on a fracture table with the affected extremity in traction. The ipsilateral groin is placed against a padded perineal post, with care taken to avoid injuring the labia or scrotum. The contralateral leg is abducted, flexed at the hip and knee, and allowed to rest on a support to facilitate positioning of the image intensifier. A closed reduction under fluoroscopic guidance is performed first. After gentle longitudinal traction is applied with the leg externally rotated to disengage the fracture fragments, internal rotation completes the reduction. AP and lateral views will either confirm the reduction or

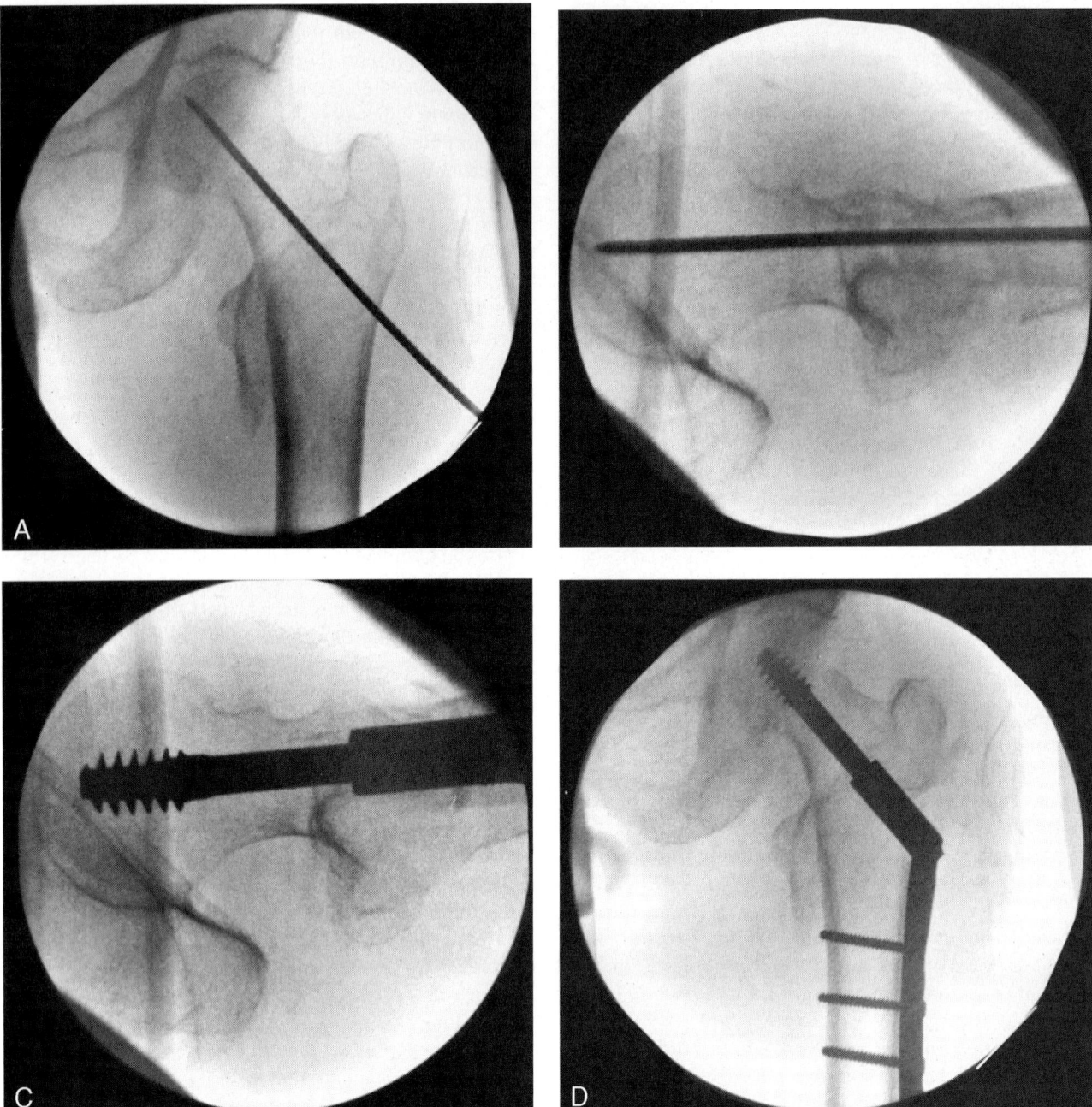

Figure 38.9. Intraoperative fluoroscopic images of the patient shown in Figure 38.3. **A.** AP view showing the guidewire in the appropriate position within the femoral head and neck. **B.** Lateral view confirming the proper placement of the guidewire. **C.** Lateral view showing the lag screw in place. **D.** Postoperative AP view showing the fixation device.

identify problems, such as varus angulation, posterior sag, and malrotation. Varus can be corrected by repeating the reduction maneuver with additional traction. An inadequate reduction after several repeated gentle attempts is an indication for a limited exposure of the fracture site during surgery to permit proper positioning of the fracture fragments.

The surgical approach entails a lateral skin incision, incision of the fascia lata, and exposure of the shaft by dissection of the vastus lateralis from its lateral aspect with a periosteal elevator. The midsubstance of the vastus lateralis can be split in the direction of its fibers, or the muscle can be detached posteriorly from its insertion into the linea aspera. The advantage of the latter technique is that implants are easily covered by unmolested muscle. Greater care must be exercised, however, to identify and ligate the large perforating vessels entering the muscle from its posterior aspect. Upon exposure of the fracture, any remaining posterior sag of the fracture can be corrected by upward pressure applied to the buttocks or fe-

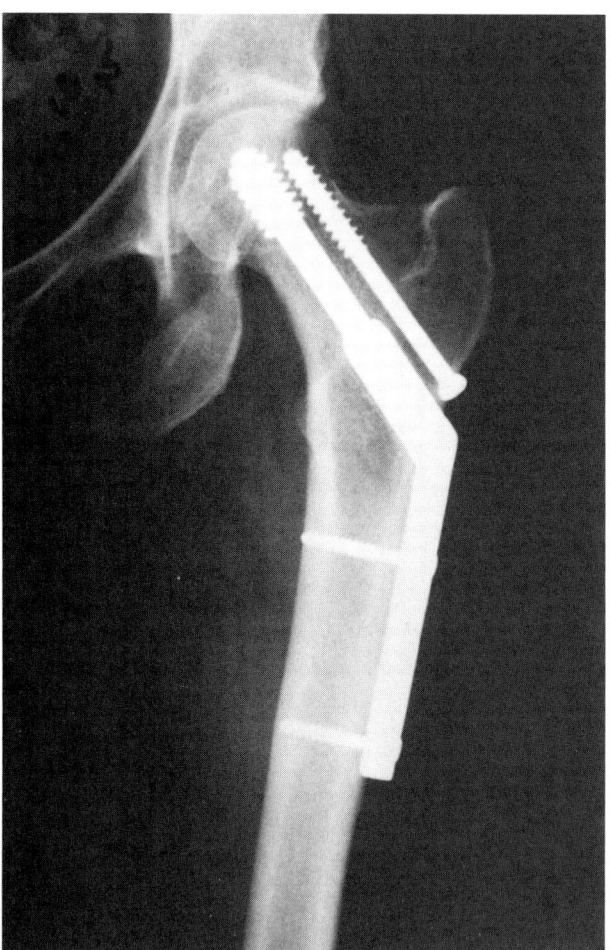

Figure 38.10. AP view showing augmented fixation with an antirotation screw for a basicervical fracture of the proximal femur.

mur. Failing this, a periosteal elevator or bone hook should be inserted at the fracture site and used to manually correct the deformity.

Reverse oblique fractures make up 8% of intertrochanteric fractures and are distinguished from the other types by the location and direction of the major fracture line, which prevents the normal impaction achieved with a sliding screw device (168). The pull of the adductor and psoas muscles results in medial displacement of the shaft; and the hip abductors cause abduction, flexion, and lateral displacement of the proximal fragment (18,54). In these fractures, excessive traction can actually cause additional displacement. Therefore, to obtain a reduction, the surgeon may have to release the traction and rotate the fracture fragments slightly before reducing them manually to the side plate (18).

The most critical and technically demanding aspect of the procedure is proper and secure placement of the sliding screw into the femoral head (18,54,65,68,69,111,183). Using a preselected angled guide, the surgeon drills a guidepin from a point approximately 1 cm below the vastus ridge up into the femoral neck and head. A small drill bit can be used initially to create a hole in the lateral cortex, which allows rapid repositioning of the guidepin. During advancement, the proper orientation of this pin should be confirmed with AP and lateral views under image intensification (Fig. 38.9A,B). The shaft of the guidepin should lie in the central third of the femoral neck, with its tip in a central position 5 to 12 mm from the subchondral bone of the femoral head (5,18,54,68,69,116,141,144,184.) If this is not possible, then a posteroinferior position is acceptable. Anterosuperior positioning, especially within 8 mm of the subchondral line places the screw in the weakest area of the femoral head and must be avoided to prevent superior screw cutout (5,54,136,186,187). A guidewire or screw that has been positioned outside of the central two-thirds of the femoral head is at risk for penetrating into the joint.

Although the sliding hip screw device permits postoperative fracture impaction, it is essential to obtain a stable impacted reduction at the time of surgery. This can be obtained by releasing traction and manually impacting the distal fragment into the proximal fragment with the screw and side plate in place but before fixing the plate to the shaft. If excessive postoperative impaction allows the threads of the screw to come into contact with the barrel of the plate, the maximal capacity for telescoping of the implant has been reached and it becomes the biomechanical equivalent of a rigid nail plate. In fact, a sliding capacity of less than 10 mm has been associated with a sixfold increase in fixation failure (136). Because the average screw shortening in unstable intertrochanteric fractures has ranged from 7 to 16 mm, the screw should be long enough to allow at least 20 mm of impaction (108,111,114, 136–139,188). Thus 86 mm is the shortest length screw that can be used safely; it is calculated by adding 20 mm to the length of the standard Dynamic hip screw (DHS; Synthes; Paoli, PA) barrel (38 mm) and the minimum length of the threaded part of the screw that protrudes at the maximal slide (27.5 mm). If a shorter screw length is desired, then the short barrel side plate (25 mm) should be used (136).

After the sliding screw is inserted, a side plate corresponding to the guidewire angle should be secured to the lateral aspect of the shaft with a Verbrugge clamp (Fig. 38.9C). The length of the plate is based on the fracture pattern and the security of the fixation. Although a recent study demonstrated that a three-hole plate with three bicortical screws (six cortices) distal to the fracture is often sufficient (189), most authors prefer a four-hole plate with four bicortical screws (eight cortices) to obtain an adequate margin of safety (23,31,54,190). In osteoporotic bone, five or six screws should be used (18,31). Once coronal, sagittal, and rotational alignments have been verified visually and with the image intensifier, the plate is fixed to the shaft (Fig. 38.9D).

Because the proximal and distal fragments may move independently in unstable fractures and because malrotation usually results from internal rotation of the distal fragment at the time of internal fixation, the distal fragment should be fixed in neutral to slight external rotation (54). If there is a large posteromedial fragment, then traction should be released and an attempt made to capture it with lag screw fixation, but without additional dissection or periosteal stripping (Fig. 38.11). An anatomic reduction of this fragment is not required if it can be brought back to the area of the posteromedial defect to provide a buttress against varus displacement. Although cerclage wiring may also achieve this end, it is less desirable because of potential devascularization of bone fragments. External rotation of the extremity and release of the iliopsoas tendon have rarely been required for exposure and reduction of this fragment; and fixation may be difficult, particularly if comminution is present.

In fractures with extension into the cervical region (basicervical type), gross instability may allow rotation of the proximal fragment during reaming, sliding screw insertion, and postoperative rehabilitation. Because this rotation can lead to malreduction or devascularization of the fragment, the addition of a second wire in a more superior position, known as an antirotation wire, should be considered before insertion of the sliding screw over the inferior wire (116). Afterward, a large cannulated screw (6.5 or 7.3 mm) can be placed over the antirotation wire, if desired (Fig. 38.10).

Fractures with comminution and displacement of the greater trochanter require additional fixation to maintain optimal abductor function. This can be accomplished by a figure-eight tension band; a cerclage wire is passed under the abductor tendon and around the barrel of the plate and then tightened after the plate has been fixed to the shaft (54). Special cables and grips, such as the Dall-Miles system (Howmedica; Rutherford, NJ), can be quite useful in these situations.

Methyl methacrylate has been advocated as an adjunct in the internal fixation of unstable comminuted intertrochanteric fractures in osteoporotic patients over the age of 70 (178,191,192). Although Bartucci et al. (191) demonstrated its effectiveness, they noted that the cement tended to inhibit telescoping of sliding hip screws in their barrels and was associated with poorer functional outcome at follow-up. Therefore, methyl methacrylate use with sliding hip screw fixation for nonpathologic fractures is not routinely recommended (54). Autologous bone grafting of defects secondary to medial comminution is rarely required for intertrochanteric fractures but may promote early healing (18).

Subtrochanteric Fractures

In 1891, Allis (193) described the difficulties and poor results after conservative treatment of subtrochanteric fractures. Lambotte (194) later recommended the use of internal fixation. Because of the inferior design and mistrust of early implants, however, traction in a position of flexion, abduction, and external rotation to match the alignment of the proximal fragment, as advocated by Hibbs (195), remained the preferred method of management. Thus patients continued to suffer from shortening, nonunion, varus malunion, and the complications of recumbency. In the 1940s, the successful treatment of in-

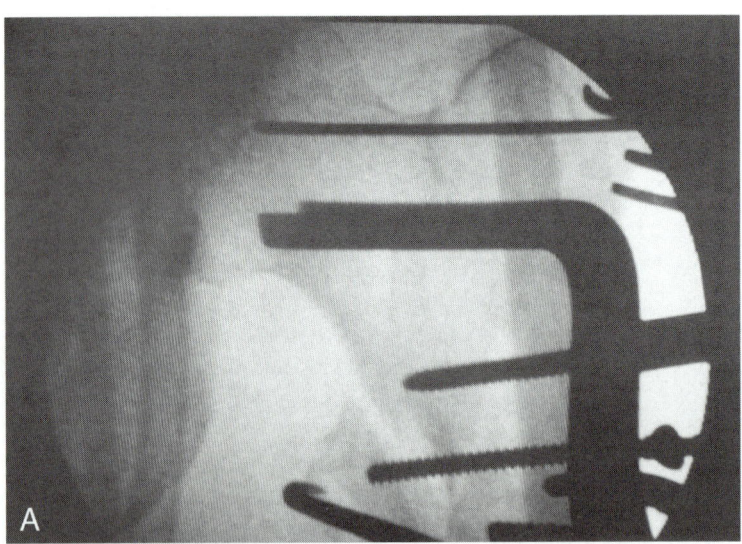
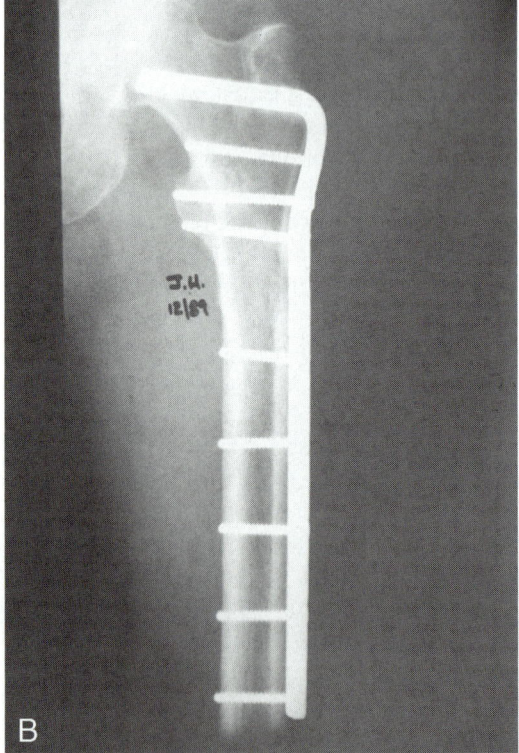

Figure 38.11. Restoration of the medial buttress. **A.** Capturing the lesser trochanter. **B.** Stabilization with lag screws.

tertrochanteric fractures with fixed-angle plates rekindled an interest in internal fixation of fractures in the subtrochanteric region (Fig. 38.12). Because the majority of fixation methods at that time were still grossly inadequate for stabilization of subtrochanteric fractures, nonunion rates ranged from 26 to 57%, malalignment rates were 70%, and implant failure rates ranged from 17 to 50% (21–23,28,64,78,90,196–199).

The transition to sliding screw devices, improved designs, and modern metallurgy lead to improved outcomes, particularly for low-energy injuries (18,23,25,27,86,87,200). High-angled devices, however, remained a poor choice for most fractures (27,166,201). The screw holes in these devices start several centimeters below the lesser trochanter, limiting fixation of the proximal segment and increasing stresses on the neck of the implant. This deficiency stimulated the development of the condylar (blade) plate and the DCS. These implants permit the insertion of two or three additional screws into the proximal fragment and are biomechanically more rigid and clinically more effective than their higher-angled counterparts (20,25,31,73,74, 91,166,202,203). Sanders and Regazzoni (31) treated 32 consecutive subtrochanteric femur fractures with DCSs, achieving union in 77% of cases with good to excellent functional outcome in 68% of cases.

Although technical failures and unsatisfactory results have been reported after the use of both the blade plate and the DCS (27,31,199,204), most problems can be attributed to inadequate indications or failure to restore the medial buttress. The latter is required to allow these devices to function as tension-band plates. Senter et al. (73) noted that 31 of 36 subtrochanteric fractures treated with either the angled-blade plate or the sliding hip screw achieved equally satisfactory results if reconstitution of the medial cortex was achieved by either an anatomic reduction and stabilization or a liberal bone grafting. The indirect reduction techniques of Kinast et al. (74) and Blatter and Janssen (203) are also associated with low failure rates. Kinast et al. (74) obtained a 100% rate of union and a 0% rate of infection by using indirect reduction techniques, tensioning the condylar plate properly, and avoiding medial dissection. Classical formal ORIF by these authors had previously lead to a 17% rate of delayed union or nonunion and a 21% rate of infection. Contoured plates have produced good results in the hands of some authors and may be an alternative method of treatment (205,206); however, we do not advocate their routine use.

An alternative to ORIF for subtrochanteric femur fractures is closed intramedullary nailing, developed by Küntscher (207) in the 1930s. Although applicable to proximal shaft fractures extending into the subtrochanteric region, neither the classic Küntscher nail nor its modification (the double or Y nail) could adequately control extremity length or rotational alignment (23,69,158,208–210). The Zickel nail, with its proximal locking capabilities and good purchase, produced excellent rates of union and satisfactory results (21,23,32,197,208,211,212). Unfortunately, technical problems have plagued inexperienced users, e.g., the need for open reduction, fractures of the greater trochanter during insertion, improper seating of the triflanged locking bolt into the head of the femur, and iatrogenic fractures during extraction (18,23,25,27,91,197,208, 211,213–215). Because the nail was not designed for distal locking screws, length and rotation have been difficult to control without supplementary fixation, required in up to 35% of cases (Fig. 38.13) (18,27,30,32,91,208,216).

The reamed first-generation locking nails in the 1980s, including the Grosse-Kempf nail, addressed these deficiencies and resulted in consistent maintenance of alignment, low rates of infection, rare implant failure, and high rates of union for both shaft and subtrochanteric fractures (18,47,63,75,82,217–224). Brien et al. (47) achieved a 97% union rate for subtrochanteric fractures using closed locked intramedullary nailing. This method results in less blood loss and fewer complications than either the Zickel nail or the condylar plate. Further design changes have included increased thickness, especially at the proximal section of the nail, and enlarged tunnels for larger, stronger locking screws (18,75). Modern second-generation designs often allow for proximal interlocking into the femoral head with either a blade, screws, or a sliding screw.

As discussed earlier, intramedullary hip screws, such as the Gamma nail, have had mixed results. Although the Gamma nail is significantly stronger and more rigid than the extramedullary devices used for the subtrochanteric fracture fixation, the limited length of the device may create an undesirable stress riser and increase the risk of femur fracture (166,185). In this regard, newer, longer intramedullary hip screw implants hold promise (29,156,161,167). Cole and Ansel (29) treated 50 predominantly unstable intertrochanteric and subtrochanteric femur fractures with long-stem intra-

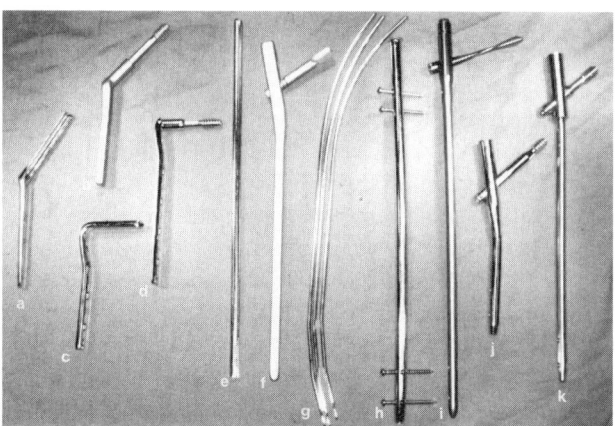

Figure 38.12. Devices for stabilizing subtrochanteric fractures. *a,* Jewett nail plate; *b,* compression hip screw; *c,* condylar plate; *d,* Dynamic condylar screw; *e,* Küntscher nail; *f,* Zickel nail; *g,* Ender nails; *h,* Grosse-Kempf nail; *i,* unreamed femoral nail with spiral blade (Synthes; Paoli PA); *j,* Gamma nail; *k,* intramedullary hip screw (Smith Nephew Richards; Memphis, TN).

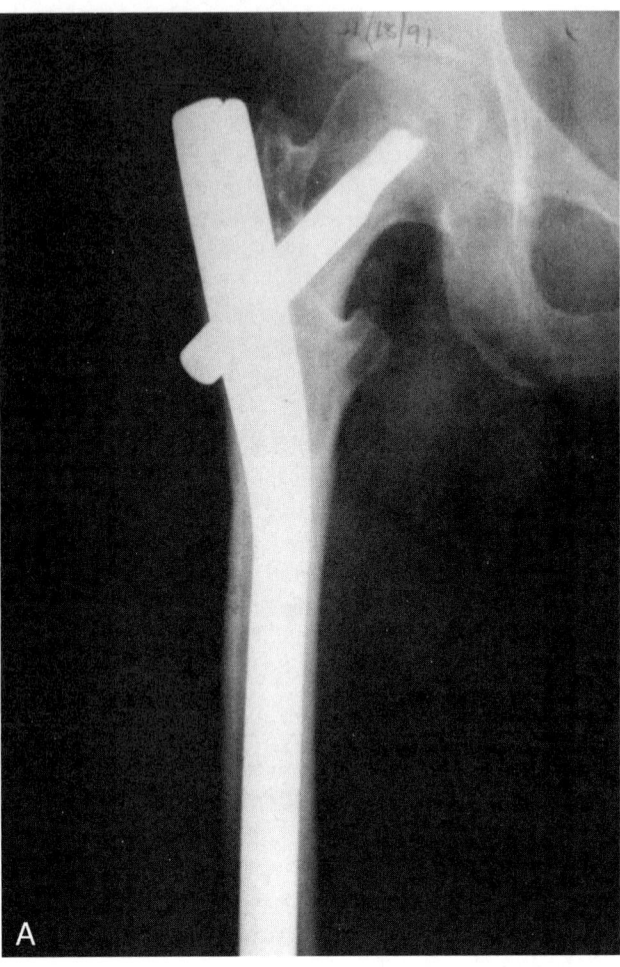 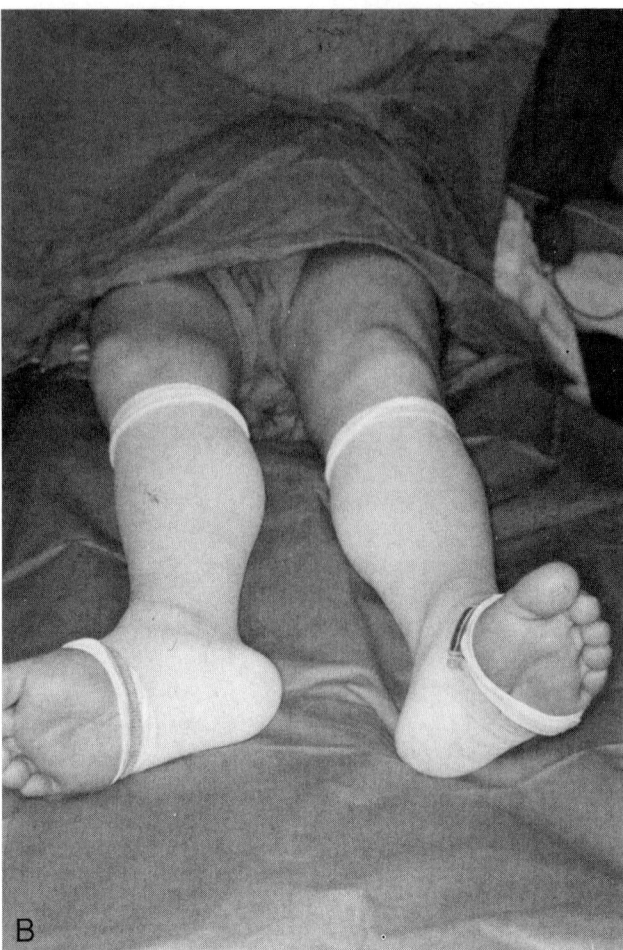

Figure 38.13. A. AP view of the right hip and femur after fixation with a Zickel nail device for a subtrochanteric fracture. **B.** Note the rotational malalignment of the right femur.

medullary hip screws; they reported no cases of femur fracture and only one implant failure. Similarly, Stapert et al. (161) treated 92 patients with subtrochanteric or intertrochanteric–subtrochanteric femur fractures. A total of 32 patients developed complications, 25 of which were related to complicated revision cases after failure of initial treatment. By the end of the study, 96% of patients were able to walk.

Ender nails have been successfully used to treat subtrochanteric femur fractures (147,148,150,198,225–227). The frequent problems encountered during their use for intertrochanteric patterns are more likely to occur in the case of complex unstable subtrochanteric fractures: Pain at the insertion site, the need for adjunctive fixation, early loss of fixation, and reoperation rates have been high (19,23,147,148,150,152,225,226). Whitelaw et al. (19) reported 0% intraoperative and 16% postoperative complication rates with the compression screw but 20% and 32%, respectively, with Ender nails. Of the patients treated with the compression screw, 98% achieved satisfactory fracture reduction and 86% realized acceptable device position compared with 64% and 16%, respectively, of patients treated with Ender nails. Postoperative time to ambula-

tion, knee pain, and reoperation rates were significantly higher in the Ender nail group.

CLASSIFICATION

Subtrochanteric fractures can essentially be divided into intertrochanteric–subtrochanteric and distal (shaft) types. In response to the varied fracture patterns seen in this region, many anatomic classification systems have been proposed, although few contribute to understanding or selection of proper treatment (23,27,64,170,208). The first classification system was proposed in 1949 by Boyd and Griffin (28) (Fig. 38.8). Unfortunately, this system is too simple, classifying subtrochanteric fractures as a subset of trochanteric fractures (types III and IV).

Seinsheimer (199), recognizing various instability patterns, introduced the first classification system dedicated to the subtrochanteric fracture (Fig. 38.14). In this system, outcomes are based more on the fracture configuration and the method of fixation rather than on location. Seinsheimer's system is complicated, ignores limb length, and does not address the medial calcar or piriformis fossa. Type I fractures are nondisplaced (<2 mm of displacement). Type II fractures are two-part fractures; this group is further subdi-

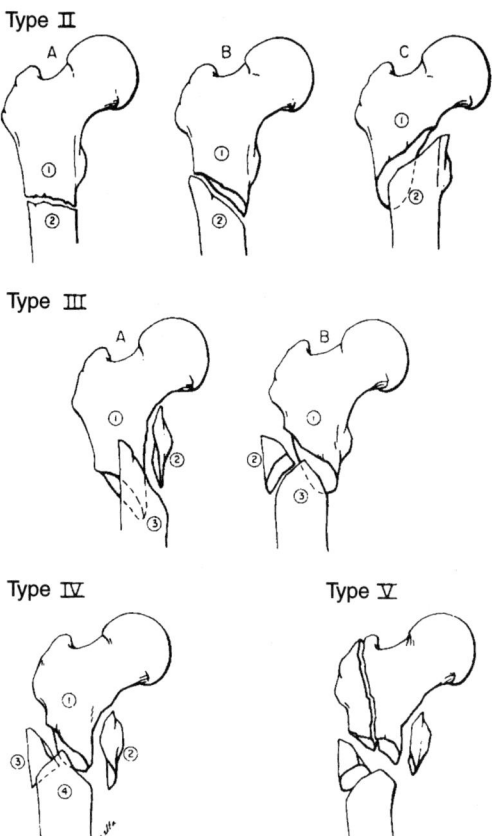

Figure 38.14. Seinsheimer's classification of subtrochanteric femur fractures. Reprinted with permission from Seinsheimer F. Subtrochanteric fractures of the femur. J Bone Joint Surg 1978;60A: 300–305.

vided into type IIA, transverse fractures; type IIB, spiral fractures with the lesser trochanter attached to the proximal fragment; and type IIC, spiral fractures with the lesser trochanter attached to the distal fragment. Type III fractures have an additional butterfly-shaped fragment (three-part fracture) and are further subdivided into type IIIA, spiral fractures with the lesser trochanter attached to the butterfly fragment (an inferior cortical spike is often present), and type IIIB, spiral fractures with the lesser trochanter attached to the proximal fragment. Type IV fractures are comminuted with four or more fragments, and type V are subtrochanteric fractures with intertrochanteric extension.

Muller et al.'s (170) comprehensive classification for pure subtrochanteric fractures is 32: 3 refers to the femur, and 2 refers to the diaphyseal area (Fig. 38.15). The limitation of this system is its complexity, particularly when it incorporates femoral shaft fractures. It does, however, provide a precise and detailed anatomic description, which is useful for data collection and the analysis of results. Fractures are more specifically described by a letter and a two-part number; subtrochanteric fractures are classified as follows:

32-A1.1: a simple subtrochanteric spiral fracture
32-A2.1: a simple subtrochanteric oblique fracture of 30° or more

32-A1.3: a simple subtrochanteric transverse fracture of less than 30°
32-B1.1: a subtrochanteric spiral wedge fracture
32-B2.1: a subtrochanteric bending wedge fracture
32-B3.1: a subtrochanteric fragmented wedge fracture
32-C1.1: a complex spiral diaphyseal fracture with two intermediate fragments
32-C1.2: a complex spiral diaphyseal fracture with three intermediate fragments
32-C1.3: a complex spiral diaphyseal fracture with more than three intermediate fragments
32-C2.1: a complex segmental diaphyseal fracture with two intermediate fragments
32-C2.2: a complex segmental diaphyseal fracture with three intermediate fragments
32-C2.3: a complex segmental diaphyseal fracture with more than three intermediate fragments
32-C3.1: an irregular complex diaphyseal fracture with two or three intermediate fragments
32-C3.2: an irregular complex diaphyseal fracture with limited shattering (less than 5 cm)
32-C3.3: an irregular complex diaphyseal fracture with extensive shattering (5 cm or more)

Simple classification systems for implant and technique include those proposed by Russell and Taylor (228)

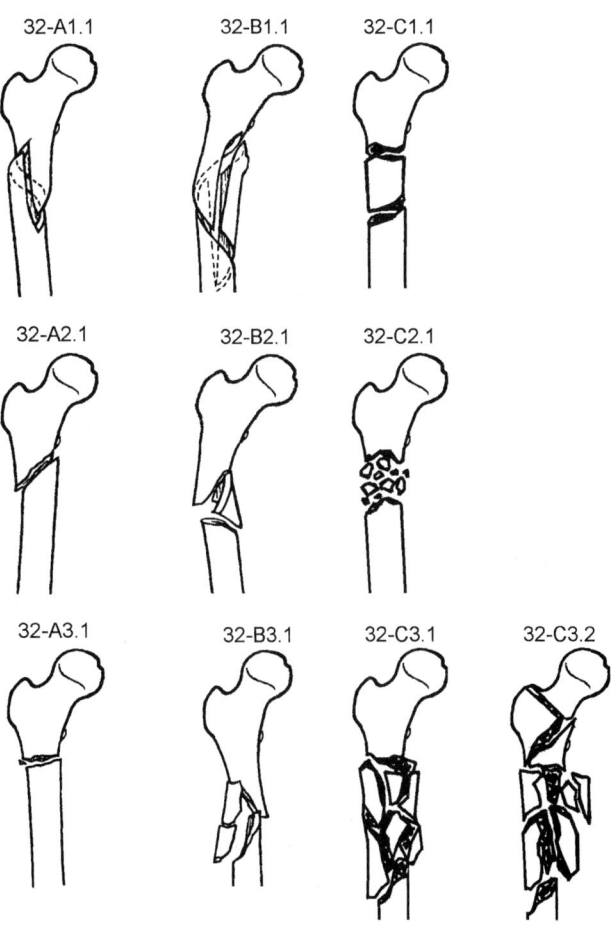

Figure 38.15. AO comprehensive classification for subtrochanteric femur fractures as adapted by Muller (170).

and Kyle et al. (18,110) (Figs. 38.16 and 38.17). These systems address the integrity of the medial calcar and the presence of a coronal plane fracture that extends into the piriformis fossa, which can complicate intramedullary fixation. Russell and Taylor group I fractures have an intact piriformis fossa, and group II fractures extend into this area. Both groups are further subdivided, based on whether the medial wall and lesser trochanter are intact (groups IA and IIA), or not intact (groups IB and IIB). In addition, both groups may include either simple or comminuted fractures, with extension into the shaft. Kyle et al. type I fractures are high subtrochanteric fractures that extend into the lesser trochanter; the type II fractures are low subtrochanteric fractures with an intact lesser trochanter. The integrity of the piriformis fossa affects the implant of choice for each of these types.

NONOPERATIVE TREATMENT AND INDICATIONS FOR SURGERY

As with fractures in the intertrochanteric region, the goals of treatment are to provide early mobilization and good functional outcome. Fractures in the subtrochanteric region usually take 15 to 17 weeks to achieve union (74, 87,203,205,225). Stable low-energy injuries that are treated with bone grafts may take only 8 weeks to heal, but high-energy injuries may take as long as 26 weeks (25,47,75,86,229). No more than 1 to 1.5 cm of shortening, 5° to 7° of malalign-

ment in the frontal plain, or 7° to 10° of malalignment in the sagittal plain should be accepted (230).

Although subtrochanteric fractures have been successfully treated with traction and bracing as well as with pins and plaster, the application of these regimens in the adult population has been problematic; unsatisfactory results are reported in up to 50% of cases (26,27,229,231). Mortality (ranging from 20 to 40%) and morbidity (e.g., deep venous thrombosis, decubiti, and other complications of recumbency) are significant problems (22,23,26,27, 87). Furthermore, subsequent displacement while in traction, varus and rotational malunion, early refracture, and nonunion are not uncommon, even under the most experienced of hands (23,27,230). Typically, bed rest and traction (14 to 18 kg) are required for 4 to 12 weeks (91,230,231). Even after this long risk-filled period, progress is slow, and a spica cast or bracing may be required for several more months to assist ambulation.

In light of the criteria for an acceptable reduction, the pitfalls of conservative care, the refinement of techniques and implants since the 1960s, and the good results reported after surgical stabilization, there is little place today for the nonoperative treatment of a subtrochanteric fracture in an adult patient (22,25,75,91,225). For patients under 8 to 10 years old, traction followed by spica casting or bracing at 4 to 6 weeks can be effective (75,230). Some authors are concerned about the control of the proximal

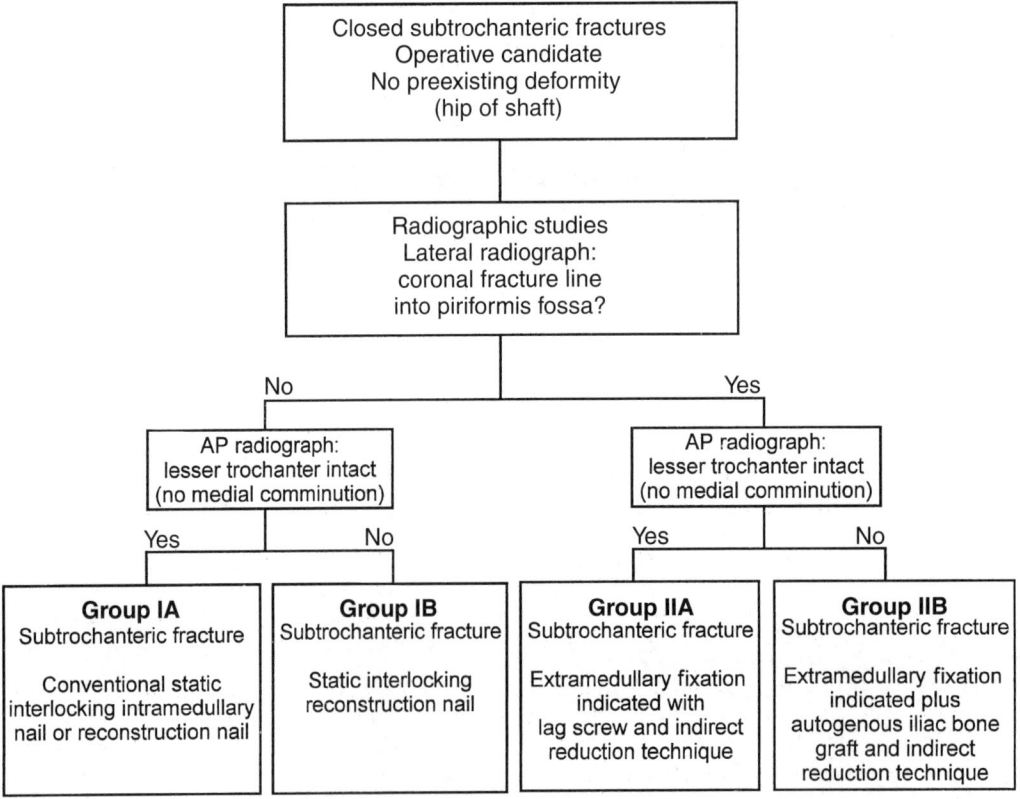

Figure 38.16. Russell and Taylor's (228) classification of subtrochanteric fractures.

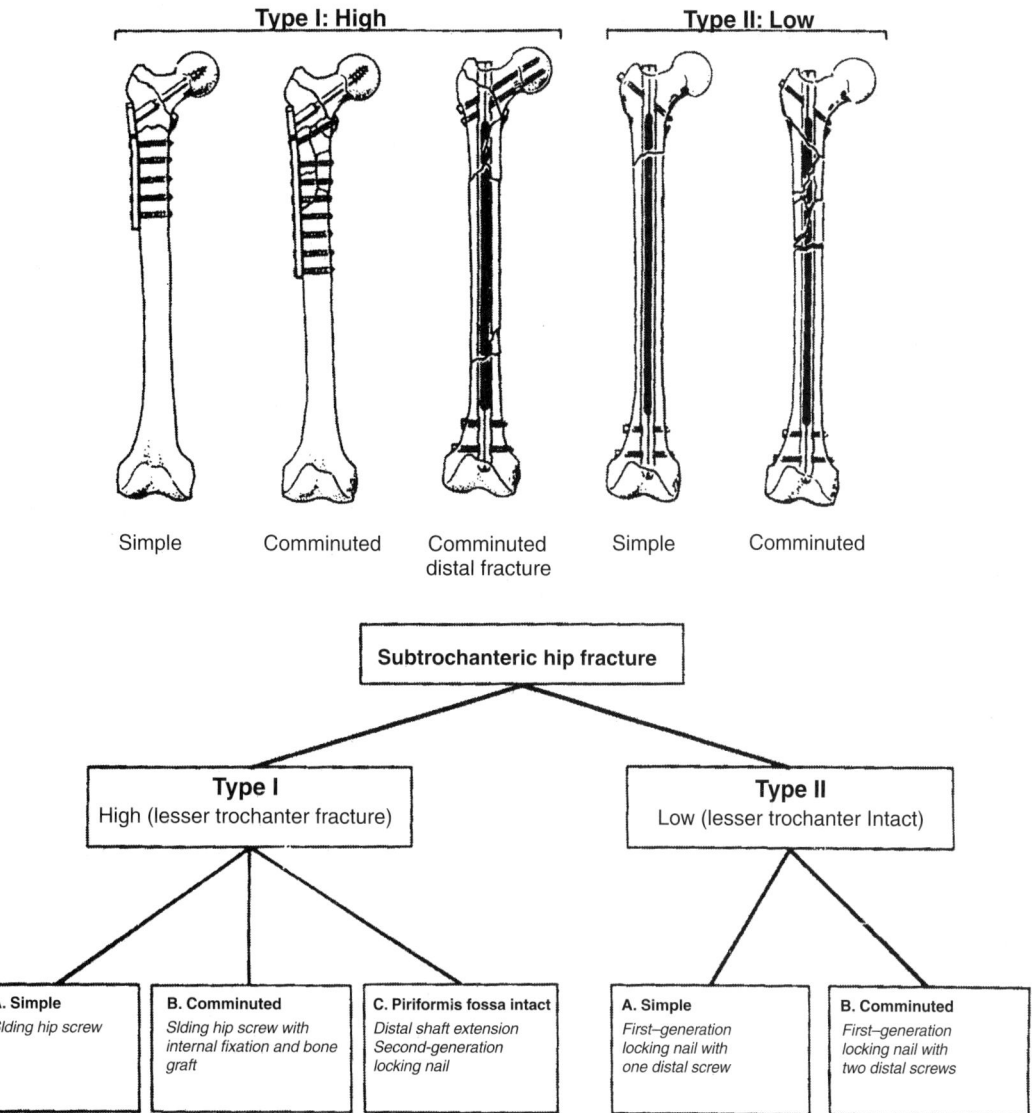

Figure 38.17. Classification of subtrochanteric fractures of Kyle et al. Reprinted with permission from Gustilo RB, Kyle RF, Templeman DC. Fractures and dislocations. Vol. 2. St. Louis: Mosby, 1993:819.

fragment and recommend plate fixation, even in the young population (206).

SELECTION OF IMPLANT AND TECHNIQUE

The selection of the proper surgical technique for subtrochanteric fractures is based largely on the presence of additional injuries (polytrauma) and the fracture pattern, especially any extension into the piriformis fossa, femoral neck, or lesser trochanteric (medial calcar) region. Treatment options include ORIF with fixed-angle plates or compression hip screws and intramedullary stabilization (Fig. 38.18). Primary hip arthroplasty may be indicated in a limited number of patients with subtrochanteric fractures; however, its role remains undefined (179).

Although implant construction is important, it appears that the stability of the fracture is the most significant determinant to a good outcome. Senter et al. (73) found that

regardless of the fixation device, healing was similar in all cases if the medial cortex was restored. Even the strongest of implants are likely to fail if there is loss of the medial calcar. This was clearly demonstrated by Seinsheimer (199), who documented the highest rates of implant failure (44%) for his type IIIA fractures (loss of medial buttress), usually resulting from bending or breakage of the plate near the fracture site. Failure was especially common in the presence of a spiral component measuring more than 8 cm in length. Other authors have confirmed that Seinsheimer types IIIA, IV, and V fractures are associated with the greatest fracture instability and complication rates (30,31,86).

The favorable biologic, biomechanical, and structural characteristics of modern intramedullary devices make closed locked intramedullary nailing the technique of choice for most nonpathologic subtrochanteric femur frac-

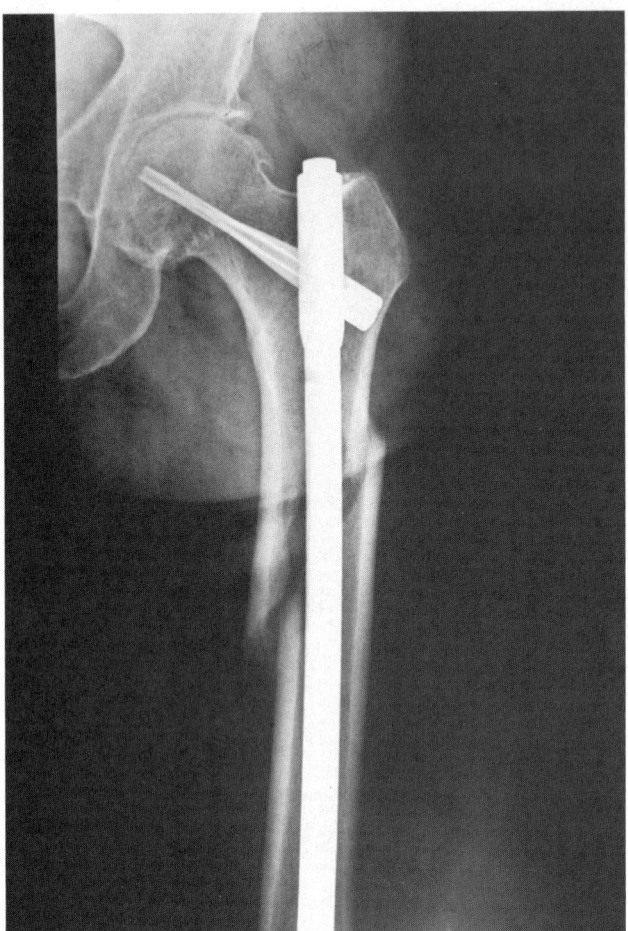

Figure 38.18. Intramedullary stabilization of a subtrochanteric fracture with an unreamed femoral nail which is locked proximally with a spiral blade (Synthes; Paoli, PA).

tures, regardless of fracture pattern or the degree of comminution (21,47,75,82). This technique is particularly useful for many pathologic fractures and fractures with extensive medial comminution. Closed locked intramedullary nailing will benefit elderly patients who are unable to tolerate a more extensive procedure or cooperate with protected weight bearing (23). Rapid healing can be attributed to the preservation of peripheral soft tissue attachments and intramedullary stabilization, which greatly reduces the lever arm and allows load sharing of the deforming forces between bone and implant. Furthermore, modern nails are stronger, have larger diameters, and are more fatigue resistant than their predecessors.

The technique of intramedullary nailing with reaming provides the benefit of autogenous reamer bone graft to the fracture site and allows the insertion of a stronger and larger-diameter nail. The disadvantages of reaming include a longer procedure time; damage to the osseous blood supply; blood loss; potential infection in grossly contaminated open fractures; and possible deterioration of pulmonary function, particularly when thoracic trauma is present (232,233). Several recent large clinical series have

not demonstrated increased vascular or pulmonary problems (234,235). Therefore, although still controversial, reaming is probably best used for isolated closed fractures; and unreamed nailing techniques should be used for severe open fractures and polytrauma, particularly in patients with thoracic injuries.

Ender's technique may rarely be a viable alternative for the pediatric population (91). Anterograde placement is preferred for pure subtrochanteric fractures; and retrograde placement, above the epiphysis of the distal femur, is preferred for fractures that extend upward into the intertrochanteric area (91). Small-diameter reconstruction nails are also viable alternatives, but they should be reserved for older children of at least 12 years (91). External fixation can also be considered in the pediatric population.

A relative contraindication for the use of intramedullary implants is the presence of intertrochanteric comminution or extension into the piriformis fossa (Fig. 38.19) (18,23,47,54,91). A fracture through the piriformis fossa is susceptible to extension or displacement when an entry hole is created or an intramedullary device is inserted in this area. A comminuted and widely displaced coronal fracture that extends into the piriformis fossa may also allow the implant to fall out the back of the proximal femur. Modern nails with anterograde locking into the femoral head and newer intramedullary hip screw designs allow insertion through the tip of the greater trochanter and may overcome the obstacle of piriformis fossa fracture involvement. As with extramedullary fixation, intramedullary nailing can be complicated by varus deformity and implant cutout (230).

Patients who complain of hip pain after an intramedullary nailing should not be ignored, as an associated occult femoral neck fracture may be present (236). In such cases, depending on the proximal locking fixation, cannulated screw fixation of the neck may be performed. If the combination of a cervical and subtrochanteric fracture is diagnosed before surgery, then alternatives include cannulated screw fixation in conjunction with a standard nail, an anterograde locking implant, and ORIF of the two fractures.

Because the torsional rigidity of even statically locked nails is only one-tenth that of extramedullary devices, plate fixation may be more suitable for stable subtrochanteric fractures and nonunions where bone-to-bone contact allows load transfer and compression across the fracture surfaces (82). The condylar plate and DCS devices allow two additional screws (6.5 mm cancellous or 4.5 mm cortical) to be placed through their proximal holes into the proximal fragment. Designed to function as tension-band plates, these implants depend on the existence of an intact medial buttress or the capacity for its rapid restoration by anatomic reduction and rigid stabilization. The alternative of bypassing the segment using the biobuttress technique depends on rapid bony healing before failure of the implant. If none of these scenarios is possible, then liberal autologous cancellous bone grafting should be performed.

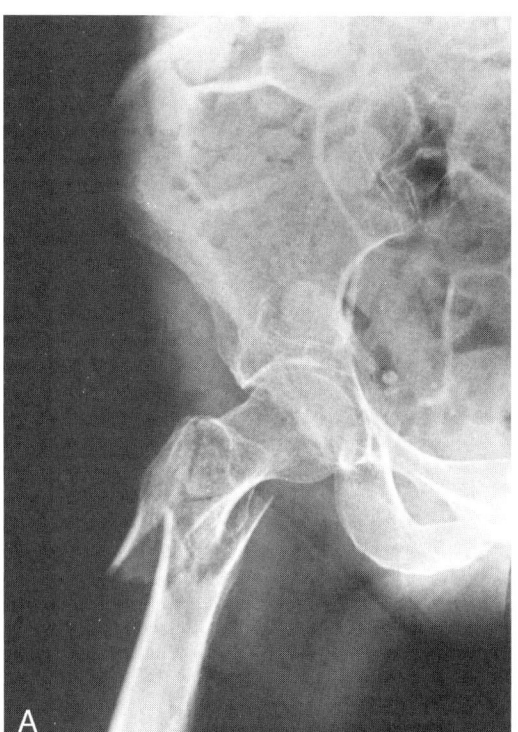

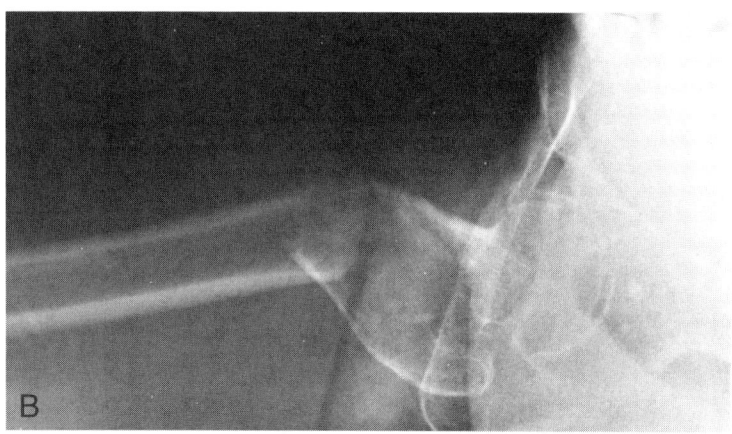

Figure 38.19. A. Preoperative AP view of a right hip showing a subtrochanteric fracture with extension into piriformis fossa. **B.** Preoperative AP view showing the flexion-abduction-external rotation deformity. Interoperative AP (**C**) and lateral (**D**) views showing the placement of the summation wire. **E.** Postoperative AP view showing reduction and internal fixation with a DCS.

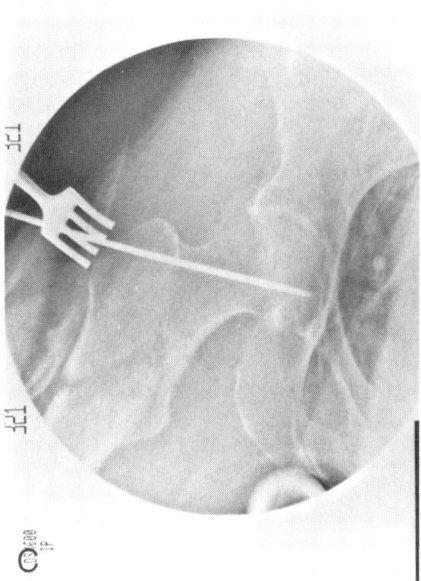

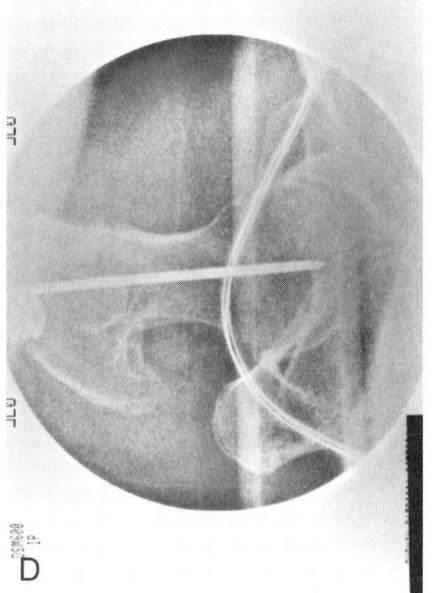

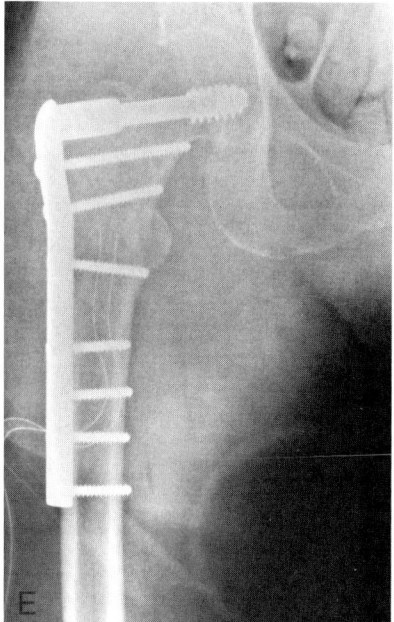

The restoration of the medial buttress is technically easier to achieve in less complex fractures (e.g., transverse, short, or long oblique patterns with or without lesser trochanteric avulsion) where lag screw fixation can be used to provide additional stability (Fig. 38.11) (31). The blade plate and DCS are also well suited for low or distal subtrochanteric fractures and those with intertrochanteric extension or comminution (73,74,82). Still, extramedullary devices are generally required only when the less invasive techniques of intramedullary nailing cannot be used. Sanders and Regazzoni (31) suggested that

extensive bony comminution is a contraindication for the use of the DCS, because of its association with technical failure in their series of patients. Because the configuration of the subtrochanteric fracture does not allow for impaction by the angled DHS, this implant should be considered only in intertrochanteric–subtrochanteric fractures for which a degree of settling is desired, and in those with extension into the piriformis fossa (87,200,230).

Internal techniques can vary from formal open approaches to indirect reductions. Each has its benefits and limitations. Traditional open approaches have achieved

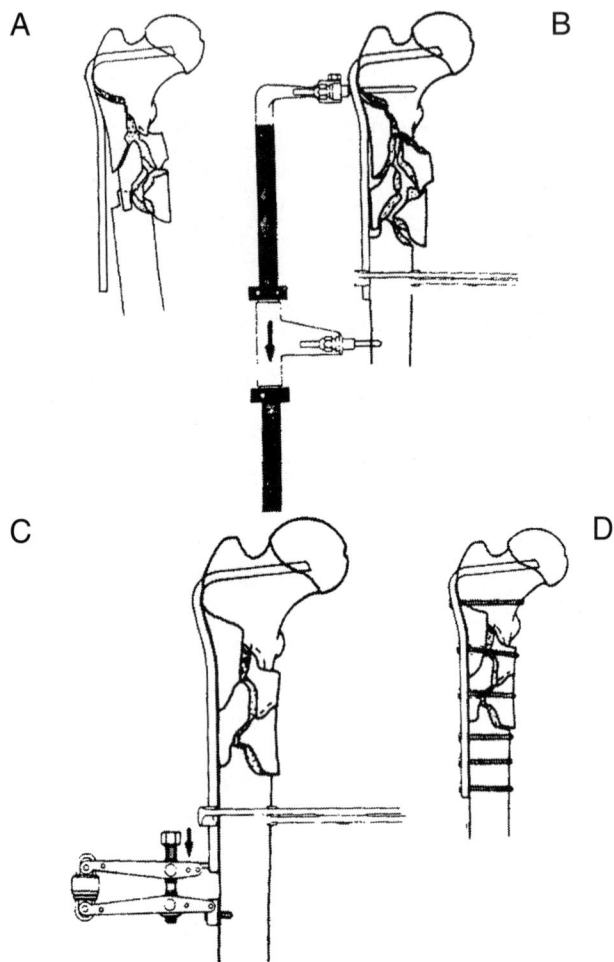

Figure 38.20. A. Indirect reduction techniques include placing the implant into the proximal fragment with minimal stripping of soft tissues. **B.** The femoral distractor can be used as an indirect reduction tool. Once the fracture has been distracted to its proper length, the fragments are pulled into position by soft tissue tension. Additional gentle mobilization of any incompletely reduced fragments completes the reduction. The plate is affixed to the distal fragment with a clamp. **C.** A tensioning device can be used to compress a reduced and stable fracture. **D.** Final fixation is achieved with lag screws into the calcar.

95% union rates and satisfactory results in 50 to 85% of cases (27,73,78,237,238). This involves exposure of the fracture site, anatomic reduction of bone fragments, and interfragmentary compression, which decreases the stresses on the plate by directing load transfer from fragment to fragment (25). Oblique and spiral fractures are first reduced and fixed with lag screws before the selected side plate is inserted (25). Overzealous periosteal stripping devascularizes the fracture fragments, leading to delayed healing and offsetting any initial gains in fracture stability. For this reason, the osteosynthesis techniques of Kinast et al. (74) and Blatter and Janssen (203), which promote the biologic principles of limited dissection of fracture fragments and indirect reduction, have revolutionized surgical treatment (Fig. 38.20). For indirect reduction, tension is applied to the soft tissue attachments of the bony frag-

ments, which contributes to progressive fracture stability as the fragments are pulled into their anatomic positions.

Although intramedullary stabilization is the treatment of choice in most cases, it is up to the surgeon to evaluate each case separately when making preoperative decisions. To this end, the Russell and Taylor and Kyle et al. classification systems provide simple guidelines. For Russell and Taylor group IA fractures (Kyle et al. type II fractures), the intact piriformis fossa and medial cortex permit treatment with less expensive, conventional first-generation interlocking nails (the proximal locking screw is placed retrograde from the greater to the lesser trochanter). Russell and Taylor group IB fractures (Kyle et al. type I fractures with an intact piriformis fossa) are better addressed with second-generation nails that proximally lock into the femoral head.

Russell and Taylor group IIA fractures (Kyle et al. type II fractures with fossa extension) carry a high risk for comminution and failure of intramedullary fixation because of piriformis fossa involvement. Therefore, internal fixation should be initially considered (18,23,47,54). An alternative treatment method is the intramedullary hip screw, which can be inserted through the tip of the greater trochanter (Fig. 38.21). Russell and Taylor group IIB fractures (Kyle et al. type I fractures with fossa extension) are stabilized in a similar fashion; but if they are addressed with plate fixation, the medial buttress must be restored. This can be achieved by indirect reduction techniques or, if medial dissection is required, autologous bone grafting.

SURGICAL APPROACH, PROCEDURES, AND PITFALLS

Intramedullary Nailing

For closed intramedullary nailing, the patient is typically placed in the supine position on a fracture table with the affected leg externally rotated and under traction. For obese patients, the lateral position may be better, but this position increases the risk of malunion (particularly valgus and external rotation) and restricts the ability to obtain a lateral image (18,91). Polytrauma patients should always be treated in the supine position to allow ease of access to the airway and to facilitate treatment of the other injuries (18).

A 6- to 8-cm incision is made, beginning at the tip of the greater trochanter and extending proximally and slightly posteriorly. The fascia of the gluteus maximus are split in line with the muscle's fibers. The subfascia is dissected and the surgeon identifies the tip of the greater trochanter and piriformis fossa by palpating with a finger. An entry portal will be created at one of these two sites, depending on the implant used (Fig. 38.22) (239). If the entry portal is to be placed in the piriformis fossa, a large blunt clamp can help clear tissue from the fossa to enable accurate placement of an awl or drill bit. This point should be in line with the medullary canal on the AP radiograph and lie just anterior to the piriformis fossa on the lateral radiograph (18).

During the surgical exposure, entry portal placement, and reaming, the surgeon must remain cognizant of the

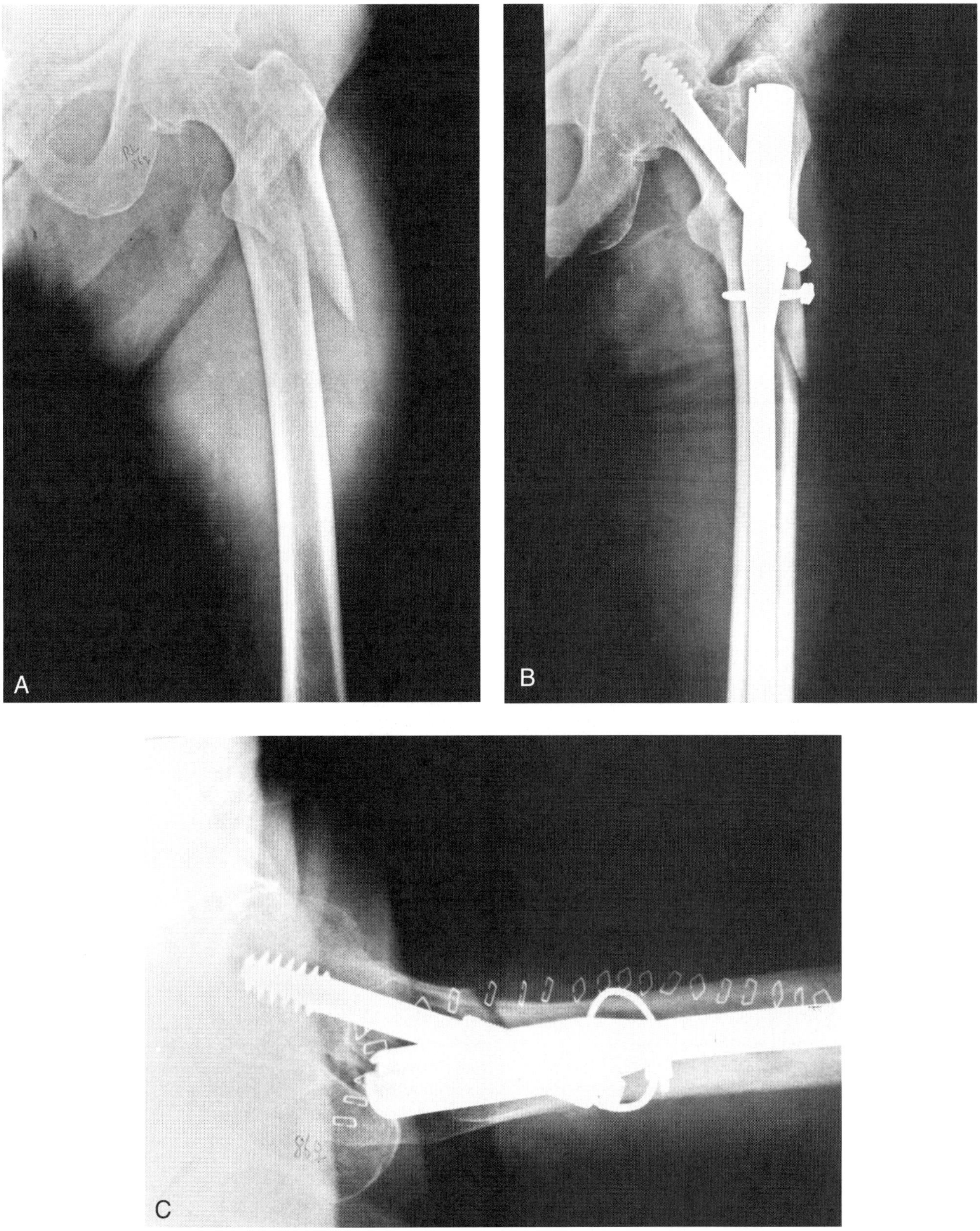

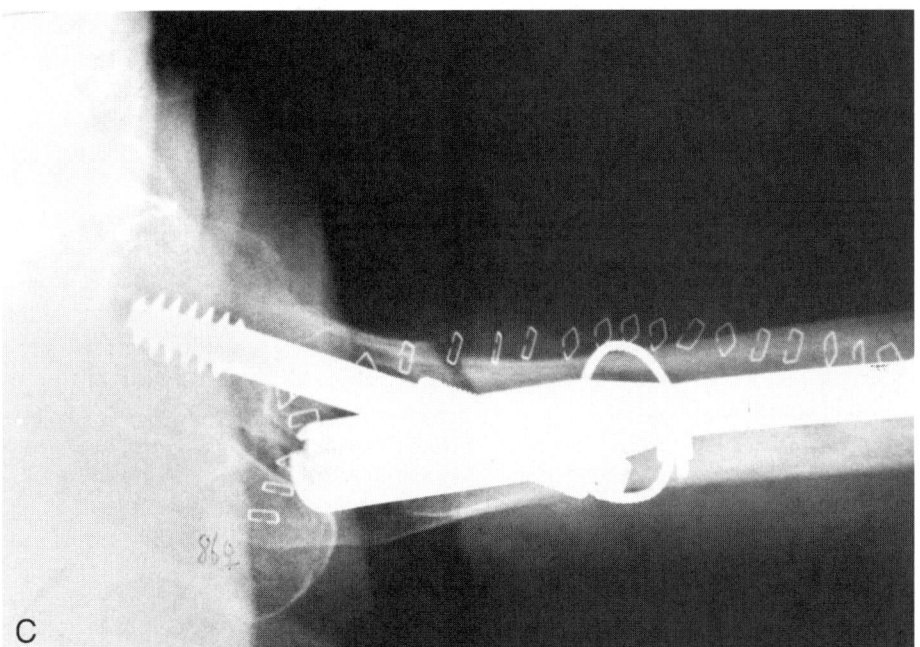

Figure 38.21. **A.** AP view of a left hip showing a subtrochanteric fracture with proximal extension. **B.** AP view showing intramedullary stabilization with an intramedullary hip screw (Smith Nephew Richards; Memphis, TN). **C.** Postoperative lateral view showing proper placement of the lag screw.

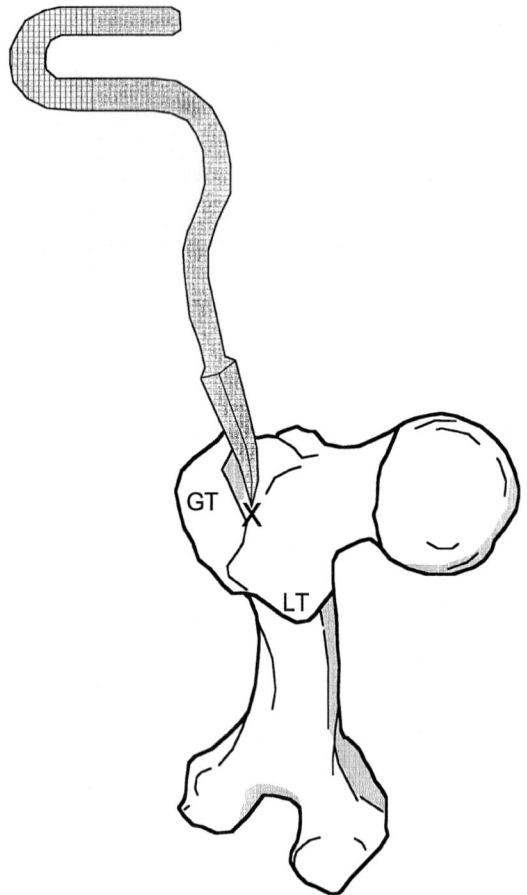

Figure 38.22. Proper location of the portal in the piriformis fossa. *GT,* greater trochanter; *LT,* lesser trochanter.

flexion-abduction-external rotation deformity associated with this fracture (Fig. 38.9B). The flexed and abducted greater trochanter can lie against the ilium, making access difficult, particularly in obese patients (18). If this is the case, then the torso should be tilted away from the affected extremity, which is also further adducted. All efforts should be made to place the entry portal in the correct location. A portal placed too anteriorly without consideration of the flexed proximal segment will direct the screw posteriorly out the back of the femur, leading to further fracture comminution. Anterior translation of the insertion site can also lead to increased hoop stress and decreased load to failure in the femoral neck region (239).

If the surgeon initially uses a T-handled reamer, the insertion of the curved bead-tipped guidewire will be easier. If passing the wire across the fracture site proves difficult, the surgeon should apply pressure on the anterior aspect of the proximal fragment with either the hand or an instrument (e.g., a small-diameter nail) to aid in the reduction (18). If this fails or difficulty exists in maintaining the reduction, then the fracture site can be opened with a limited incision, and an elevator placed anteriorly to push down the distal end of the proximal fragment while the guidewire is placed. Unlike isthmic shaft fractures, proximal fractures do not simply reduce when an intramedullary device is inserted. It is thus essential to maintain the reduction and

proper alignment during reaming because reaming across an unreduced fracture can lead to malposition of the implant. Reaming should proceed in 1-mm increments until cortical contact is obtained; it is then advanced in 0.5-mm increments until cortical chatter is significant. To ease insertion, improve rotational alignment, and decrease stress, the canal should be overreamed 1.5 to 2 mm greater than the diameter of the nail to be inserted (18,157).

Using a plastic exchange tube, the surgeon exchanges the beaded wire for the nonbeaded driving wire and the proper-length intramedullary nail. Nail length is determined by using a guidewire of known length and measuring the amount that protrudes from the femur. Preoperative radiographs of the contralateral intact femur also provide an estimation of the proper nail length, particularly for comminuted fractures. The nail is inserted over the driving wire.

For unreamed nailing, the entry portal must be enlarged to prevent too tight a fit of the widened proximal section of the implant. The advantage of these strong, solid implants is that they often make excellent reduction tools during placement. After the proximal nail is inserted to the level of the fracture site, it can be used to lever the flexed abducted proximal fragment into its proper alignment with the shaft portion of the fracture. Once this has been accomplished, the tip of the implant is advanced across the fracture site into the distal fragment.

Because second-generation locking nails are thicker and more rigid than earlier implants, care must be taken to not fracture the femur during nail insertion (18). It is also essential to confirm the proper rotational alignment of the extremity before locking the nail. As with diaphyseal fractures, static locking is required when using an intramedullary device for acute fractures in the subtrochanteric region (75,91). This is critical in the presence of comminution, because locking screws prevent rotation, shortening, and collapse at the fracture site. Although callus formation occurs more slowly in fractures treated with the newer-generation nails, most statically locked constructs allow enough motion at the fracture site to create a favorable milieu for healing (91).

Proximal locking should be performed per the requirements of the individual implant. If anterograde locking into the femoral head is desired, then special attention must be paid to the version of the neck, and superior placement in the head should be avoided. Proximity to the subchondral bone allows for improved fixation, but nontelescoping devices are associated with an increased rate of cutout when placed within 10 mm of the joint surface (65,69). Distal locking is performed by whichever technique the surgeon finds comfortable. The preferred method at our institution involves a freehand technique with a radiolucent drill after first obtaining round holes on the lateral fluoroscopic view (18,230).

Open Reduction and Internal Fixation

Generally, the surgical exposure for ORIF is similar to that for the intertrochanteric fracture, except that the origin of the vastus lateralis may have to be detached to some degree when using 95° implants. Although traction on the fracture table has been advocated as an indirect reduction tool, it may fail to control the subtrochanteric fracture because of the external rotation-flexion-abduction deformity of the proximal fragment and the sagging of the unsupported distal segment (Fig. 38.19B) (25,203). In fact, as with reverse oblique intertrochanteric fracture variants, traction can actually interfere with manipulation of the limb and tighten the tissue envelope. This makes the exposure and reduction of spiral and torsional butterfly fragments particularly difficult (25). A more effective indirect reduction is obtained by using the femoral distractor with the patient's leg prepped and draped free on a radiolucent table (Fig. 38.20B) (74). Additional distraction can be provided by the reversed tension device, which is affixed to the distal portion of the plate after the proximal portion has undergone fixation.

To guide insertion of the condylar plate or DCS, a Kirschner wire (K wire) should be inserted along the anterior surface of the neck (anteversion wire), and a second wire should be inserted at a 95° angle to the shaft (coronal plane alignment). The orientation of these wires dictates the placement of a summation wire. For the condylar plate, the third wire or a drill bit is inserted approximately 1 cm below the tip of the greater trochanter and advanced into the inferior quadrant of the femoral neck and head. Using the blade plate drill guide, starter holes are made to guide the seating chisel. The seating chisel and blade plate must be inserted along the anterior border of the posteriorly aligned greater trochanter so they do not exit through the posterior portion of the neck, damaging the blood supply to the femoral head.

For the DCS, the summation wire is introduced just anterior to the midpoint of the greater trochanter and parallel to the middle of the femoral shaft in the sagittal plane. Using a 95° guide, the wire is directed up into the subchondral bone of the femoral head. After proper placement has been verified on AP and lateral fluoroscopic views, reaming is performed to within 10 mm of the subchondral bone, and the DCS lag screw is inserted (Fig. 38.19C,D). For osteoporotic patients, Sanders and Regazzoni (31) suggested advancing the screw to within 5 mm of subchondral bone, if necessary. This may improve fixation, but an increased rate of cutout has been reported for nontelescoping devices placed within 10 mm of the joint surface (65,69). Although the DCS telescopes to some degree, motion is limited because of its 95° angle.

It is important to avoid fixation of the fracture in a distracted position. In the absence of comminution and following reduction of the fracture with correction of the length and rotation, the tension device can be used in a compression mode (Fig. 38.20C), which increases stability and provides greater compression of the fracture than is afforded by the eccentric placement of cortical screws through the plate. This crucial step prestresses the plate, providing additional dynamic axial compression (25). Once optimal compression (if possible) has been obtained, then distal fixation is performed.

As discussed earlier, the length of the plate used should usually allow for 8 to 10 cortices (four to five bicortical screws) transfixed in the shaft component. In younger patients, however, as few as 6 cortices may be adequate (23,31,190). If there is a large posteromedial fragment, then traction should be released and an attempt made to capture it with lag screw fixation, without extensive dissection or periosteal stripping. Similarly, although supplemental fixation with wires or cables (e.g., with a Dall-Miles system) has been advocated by many authors for more unstable fractures, this technique involves additional stripping and devascularization of bone; thus it should be minimized or avoided altogether (Fig. 38.23) (47,91,159).

Most authors perform routine bone grafting, especially for comminuted and unstable fractures treated with ORIF (25–27,30,31,73,74,91,203,206,219,240,241). A cancellous graft, while failing to provide initial support, soon becomes an osteoid bridge, linking the proximal and distal fragments, contributing to load bearing, and decreasing cyclical loading of the plate (25). Unfortunately, additional soft tissue stripping is required to place the graft medially where it is most needed. This somewhat counteracts the benefits of grafting. A solution to this dilemma was suggested by Wiss et al. (91), who insert the bone graft directly through the fracture site, placing it up against the comminuted area.

Pathologic Fractures

Pathologic fracture of the femur is not rare, accounting for 30% of all metastatic osseous disease (24). The most common primary tumor associated with impending or pathologic fracture of the proximal femur is malignancy of the female breast (45%), followed by myeloma (20%) and bronchial tumors (11%) (242). Because prognosis is directly related to the primary tumor—with an average survival of 3.6 months for lung and 22.6 months for breast carcinoma (3)—a biopsy should be considered. Care must be taken to sample only the area of the lesion and not the fracture callus, which can be confused with sarcomatous changes (243).

Because 50 to 75% of patients presenting with metastatic long-bone fractures will be alive 1 year later, aggressive management should be undertaken for these and any impending fractures (3,24,244). The goals of surgical stabilization are to decrease pain, improve function, permit early mobilization, and reduce the time of hospitalization. Although the treatment principles remain similar to those for nonneoplastic fractures, there is no role for plating techniques in the presence of metastatic shaft lesions, and both hemiarthroplasty and supplemental methacrylate assume more prominent roles because of poor bone quality (3,21,24,27,75,206,243). Intramedullary stabilization is often the preferred technique for destructive disease that involves the subtrochanteric region; however, it does not necessarily permit ambulation for debilitated patients (245). When treating suspected metastatic renal cell or thyroid carcinomas, the surgeon should respect the exten-

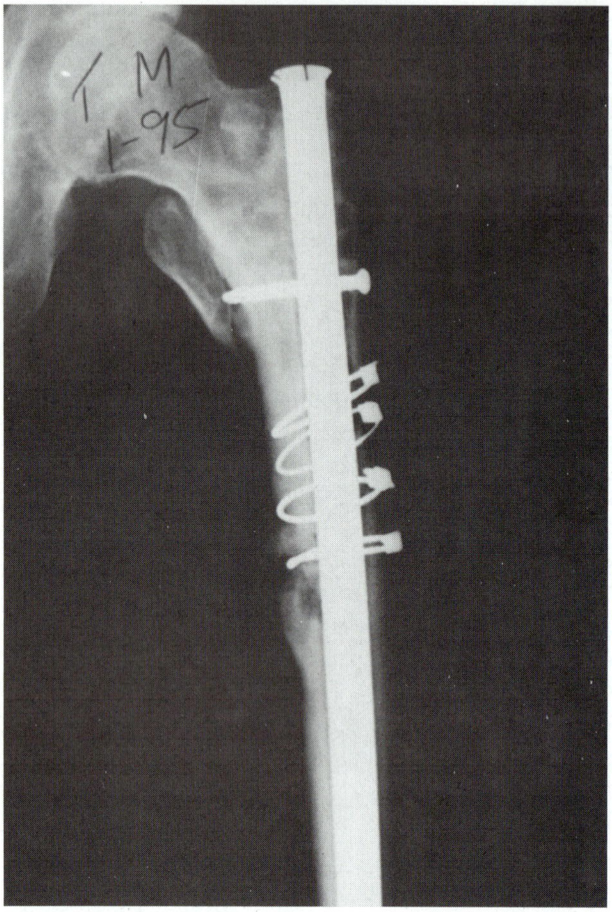

Figure 38.23. AP view of the left hip and femur showing open intramedullary stabilization with a Grosse-Kempf nail and overzealous use of cerclage wires. Note the devascularization of the fracture site and diaphyseal nonunion.

sive vascular supplies of these tumors (243). Before surgery, a skeletal survey is recommended to identify other lesions, which may affect the treatment plan.

Patients with osteitis deformans (Paget's disease) who sustain an intertrochanteric fracture can be treated via standard techniques. In contrast, pagetic fractures in the subtrochanteric region are particularly difficult to manage (246,247). Improved results can be achieved with preoperative medical treatment and bone scanning to assess the fracture, followed by second-generation intramedullary anterograde nailing (246,247).

Postoperative Care and Rehabilitation

A first-generation cephalosporin should be given just before the incision is made, and it should be continued for at least the first 24 h after surgery. Suction drains should be placed before closure to prevent hematoma formation, which can serve as a culture medium for infection. In the postoperative period, some form of antithrombotic prophylaxis is essential.

Regardless of weight-bearing status, postoperative care must be directed toward early mobilization to avoid

the complications of recumbency. Up to one-third of hip fracture patients develop a decubitus ulcer within 2 weeks of admission, often on the day of surgery; half of these patients develop multiple sores (248). As manifestations of local skin and subcutaneous tissue ischemia, decubiti occur most commonly at the sacrum, heels, and buttocks. These sores are difficult to manage, prolong hospitalization, and are associated with a mortality rate of 27% (248). Fortunately, they are easily prevented by surveillance and by turning the patient every 2 h.

If pain permits, the patient should be allowed to sit on the day after surgery. Strengthening and range of motion exercises are instituted immediately. Ambulation should begin early; the patient can use parallel bars on the 2nd or 3rd day postsurgery. The specific postoperative weight-bearing status remains a controversial topic for patients with intertrochanteric fractures. To prevent shortening and overimpaction of the fracture, some authors recommend restricted weight bearing until evidence of healing, but the majority of authors note that unrestricted weight bearing has no deleterious effects (5,40,54,98,108,116,129,144,157, 177,184). In light of the present knowledge of hip joint forces, the latter view seems the more prudent. Thus immediate weight bearing as tolerated is advocated for patients with stable reductions of intertrochanteric fractures. Patients who have undergone fixation of unstable fractures and those with severely osteoporotic bone have an impaired weight-bearing ability, even when implants are used properly. In these cases, protected weight bearing must be strongly considered until a callus is evident on follow-up radiographs (18,177).

In contrast to the aggressive regimen followed by patients recovering from intertrochanteric fractures, a period of protected weight bearing is recommended for patients recovering from subtrochanteric fractures with significant shaft or intertrochanteric extension and those treated with intramedullary or fixed-angled extramedullary devices. Unstable fractures are under significant stress, are often comminuted, and are stabilized with implants that are not designed to allow stabilizing fracture impaction and medial shaft translation. Therefore, patients with these fractures should be mobilized immediately but restricted to protected partial weight bearing for 3 to 6 weeks (27,91,166,208,230). This is particularly important for younger, active, and obese patients, who are more likely to subject their fracture fixation to excessive stress. Other authors have suggested toe-touch weight bearing for up to 12 weeks for patients with unstable fracture patterns that required static locking nails (230). In the elderly, who are intolerant of restricted ambulation, immediate full weight bearing is an acceptable compromise (23).

Patients who have undergone dynamically locked nailing of a stable fracture configuration may begin weight bearing almost immediately. Rapidly progressing to 50% weight bearing, these patients usually achieve full weight bearing by 4 to 6 weeks (91,161,230). Some implants, e.g., the Gamma nail, are designed to allow immediate full weight bearing (155,157,161,166), although this goal is not always achieved, partly due to unwillingness of both the patient and the surgeon.

Patients who have undergone hemiarthroplasty by a posterior surgical approach require dislocation precautions, including high chairs and toilets and an abduction pillow to prevent flexion and adduction (the position of least stability). For added security in noncompliant or demented patients, the use of a knee immobilizer will limit flexion of the hip.

Of occasional concern during the postoperative period is a tendency for the leg to lie in an externally rotated position. Rarely a sign of malalignment, this finding disappears once the patient begins to walk and bear weight (150). Whatever technique is chosen for stabilization, it must be remembered that no device is a panacea and that complications, such as nonunion and fixation failure, are not uncommon. Because these may not be evident for 6 to 12 months, patients must be carefully monitored until healing has been achieved. Radiographs should be obtained at 1 and 2 weeks to ensure that proper impaction of the fragments is occurring without fixation problems. Additional follow-up at 4 and 6 weeks, then monthly for the first 6 months after the fracture, is recommended. Patients should also undergo extended rehabilitation for at least 3 months, as they will continue to demonstrate gains in terms of pain, range of motion, and strength after this time (249). After complete healing, implants may be removed at 15 to 18 months in young, active, or symptomatic patients (18).

Complications

It is often difficult to compare reports of outcomes and complications of the treatment of fractures of the proximal femur because of the many different implants used, modern medical management, and the evolution of surgical techniques since the 1950s. Many series that have reported high mortality rates were published before the initiation of routine prophylactic antibiotic and deep venous thrombosis (DVT) treatment protocols for surgical patients. Different lengths of reported follow-up and the lack of classification of fractures into different anatomic locations prevent specific comparisons.

THROMBOEMBOLISM

Deep venous thrombosis (DVT) is the most common major postoperative complication following a fracture of the hip and a significant diagnostic problem. As many as 50% of patients will display no clinical signs or symptoms (250). Although its clinical incidence has generally ranged from 2 to 44%, rates have been as high as 60 to 70% in some studies (173,250–254). The latter figures are more in line with the 58% rate (18% proximal) that was determined via contrast venography by Geerts et al. (255) in a trauma population. DVT is also a danger for the preoperative hip fracture patient, with documented rates of 9% (venographic)

and 12% (ultrasonographic) (250,254). Intertrochanteric fractures have been reported to have a lower risk (4%) than those in the cervical area (17%) (250).

The variability of these reports is a result of the different prophylactic regimens (nothing, aspirin, warfarin, low-dose or low-molecular-weight heparin, dextran, intermittent external pneumatic compression, and inferior vena caval filters) and diagnostic modalities (physical examination, duplex ultrasonography, MRI, venography) used by the medical community. Although the complications related to prophylactic anticoagulation may outweigh its benefits in select cases, the majority of patients with a fracture of the proximal femur should receive some form of prophylaxis (37,256). Although no one strategy has proven clearly superior in this population, warfarin is perhaps the most effective, having reduced the rate of fatal pulmonary embolism from 8 to 1% (252). Unfortunately, warfarin is contraindicated in patients with gastrointestinal dysfunction, has a delayed onset of action, requires laboratory monitoring, is difficult to reverse if additional surgery is required, and leads to an increased risk of postoperative bleeding if the prothrombin time is not kept within the range of 1.2 to 1.5 times control (18,252,255,257–259).

Other successful pharmacologic antithrombotic regimens include low-dose aspirin (less than 1000 mg/day) and low-molecular-weight heparin (98,251,252,255,257,258, 260); however, some studies have questioned the efficacy of these agents, and both have been associated with wound problems, including hematoma formation (251,253,255,261,262). Aspirin, while inexpensive, presents a significant risk for gastrointestinal hemorrhage (251). Dextran is effective in preventing DVT in hip fracture surgery, but it is costly, can cause volume overload or anaphylaxis, and has not demonstrated superiority to aspirin or heparin (251,252,260). Low-dose heparin is relatively ineffective in the prevention of thromboembolic disease in trauma and hip fracture patients (255,257).

Nonpharmacologic agents include inferior vena caval filters and external compression devices. The former reduce mortality but are expensive ($5000), have uncertain long-term safety, and have been evaluated only in uncontrolled studies (255). Compression devices are effective because of their ability to reduce venous stasis and enhance blood fibrinolytic activity (263–265). Combining a compression device with low-dose heparin, Demers et al. (265) noted a reduction from 46 to 20% of DVT in hip fracture patients, including fewer proximal thrombi (from 30 to 6%). Unfortunately, these devices are costly, uncomfortable, and often improperly applied (266,267).

With a reported incidence of 1 to 8%, fatal pulmonary embolism is the most feared sequela of DVT (14,98,252). This rate compares unfavorably to a 2% rate after total hip arthroplasty and approximates the 2 to 22% rate observed in the trauma population (252,255). Proximal thrombi are the most dangerous, presenting a much greater risk for pulmonary emboli than distal thrombi (268). Pulmonary emboli are probably more prevalent than present data suggest. In a postmortem study of patients dying from multiple causes, Fitts et al. (269) found that 38% of patients had actually died of a pulmonary embolism—nearly 20 times the expected rate. Therefore, once there is a clinical suggestion of DVT, evaluation and treatment must be aggressive. The diagnosis should be confirmed with duplex ultrasonography or venography, and a ventilation-perfusion scan should be performed if there is suspicion for a pulmonary embolism. Intravenous heparin should be instituted as soon as possible, followed by subsequent conversion to warfarin. On discharge, oral anticoagulation is recommended for an additional 3 months.

MORBIDITY AND MORTALITY

Before the introduction of modern surgical principles of internal fixation, in-hospital mortality rates following conservative treatment of intertrochanteric and subtrochanteric fractures typically ranged on the higher end of 10 to 44% (4,17,22,28,86,87,168,175,270). By the 1950s and 1960s, the introduction of operative treatment had reduced mortality to a still unacceptable 10 to 26% (4,7,14,15,17,80,113,115,168). Today, advancements in surgical, medical, and nursing management have further reduced in-hospital mortality to 3 to 10% (3,10,14,30,70, 133,271,272). Overall mortality rates (10 to 50%) are still greater than age- and sex-matched controls for the 6 to 12 months after injury, and the majority of deaths occur within the first 4 months (4,6–9,12,14–16,27,28,32,37, 54,64,70,78,86,87,116,122,129,130,154,173,175,204,269, 271–277).

Although subtrochanteric fractures appear to have a higher mortality rate than do intertrochanteric fractures, comparisons are difficult because patients presenting with intertrochanteric fractures tend to be young and thus have a good prognosis for recovery. Other important variables adversely affecting morbidity and mortality include psychiatric or other central nervous system disorders; multiple preexisting or poorly controlled medical conditions, including cardiac disease, diabetes, chronic obstructive pulmonary disease, and rheumatoid arthritis; low weight; environment; immobilization; and poor previous level of function (6,7,9,10,12,14,37,39,45,103,172,176,178, 272,273, 278–282). Wood (282) noted that the most alarming of these factors were dementia, postoperative chest or wound infection, neoplasia, and advanced age. Within 6 months of fracture, 74% of demented patients over the age of 85 were dead. Miller (273) found that patients with chronic organic brain syndrome, cerebrovascular disease, or psychosis had a 1-year mortality rate of 47% compared with 18% for those with intact cognition. Magaziner et al. (272) countered that it is not patients with dementia but normally cognitive patients who suffer delirium on admission who have three times the risk of dying.

Physical condition and level of function are also critical factors affecting survival (6,7,10,16,37). Kenzora et al. (6) reported a 1-year mortality of 11% for patients with less than four medical comorbidities compared with 25% for those with four or more. White et al. (7) noted a high degree of correlation with the grading system used by the American Society of Anesthesiologists. Patients classified as grade I or II (healthy or mild systemic disease) had a 1-year mortality of 8%, whereas those classified as grade III or IV (severe or incapacitating systemic disease) had a mortality rate of 49%. The 1-year mortality rates for dependent patients approach 60 to 70%, compared with 7 to 13% for those previously independent (16,37). As discussed earlier, prompt surgical intervention can reduce mortality; however, if the patient has significant comorbidities, a period of medical optimization may be more beneficial.

Postoperative complications have been consistently associated with increased morbidity and mortality (6,10,14,37,40). Sexson and Lehner (37) noted a 38% mortality rate in patients with postoperative complications compared with an 11% rate for those without complications. Beals (14) reported that in a series of hip fracture patients pneumonia was the most common cause of death (42%), followed by wound infection (37%) and myocardial infarction or heart failure (12%). Urinary tract infection, which occurs in as many as 30% of patients, has been associated with a 24% mortality rate (279). Malnutrition, decubiti, and postoperative confusion have also been associated with increased mortality after surgery (45).

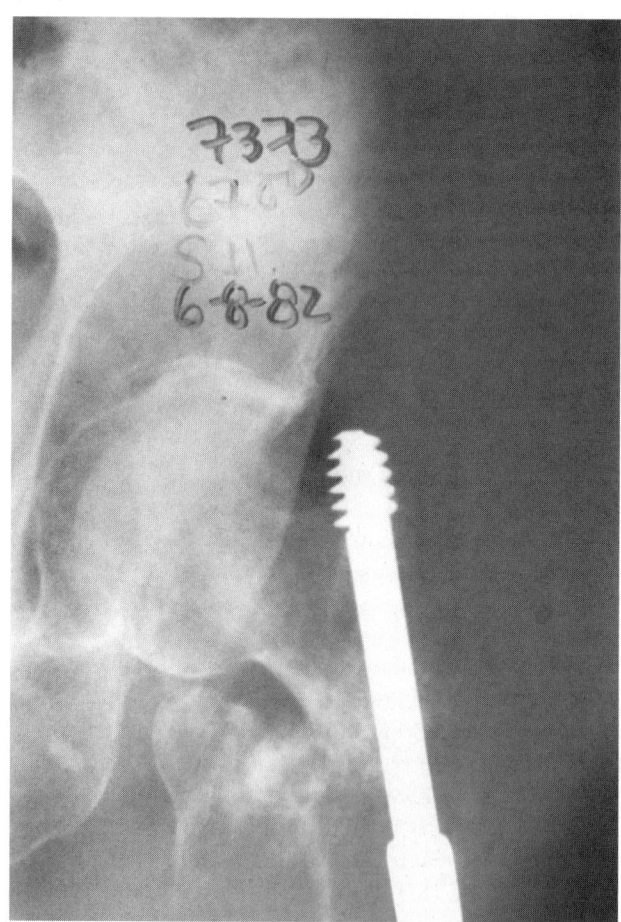

Figure 38.24. AP view of the left hip showing that the lag screw has cut out of the femoral head.

Other factors may be linked to mortality but are controversial. Being 75 to 85 years of age or older has been associated with increased mortality after a fracture in the trochanteric region (6,9,10,12,16,37,45,272–274,280,281). There is some evidence that a proper coordination of orthopaedic and geriatric health care services may reduce mortality and improve outcomes (2,45,271,283–285). Paradoxically, some authors have noted that younger patients were actually more likely to die (7,272). Although there are reports that male mortality rates are two to three times that of female rates, when other risk factors are controlled (e.g., the greater number of comorbidities in men), mortality rates seem to be more similar (6–10,12,14, 16,37,45,272,273,280,281).

The time under anesthesia and the type of anesthesia used have not been consistently associated with mortality rates (7,45,286–288). One study noted that early deaths were less likely to occur with regional anesthesia (proba- bly as a result of reduced thromboembolism); but by 8 weeks, mortality rates did not differ (288).

FAILURE OF FIXATION, NONUNION, AND MALUNION

The development of modern high-strength stainless-steel and titanium alloys and the introduction of computer-assisted design have reduced stress risers and eliminated weak areas in fixation devices, reducing the frequency of implant breakage to less than 1% (18). However, the most common mode of failure remains the cutting out of an implant through an osteoporotic femoral head, leading to varus collapse and a variable amount of rotation (Fig. 38.24) (18,54,69,128,156,211). Another mode of failure is caused by a varus moment acting on the screws and side plate, which fractures the implant or pulls the screws out of the bone (Figs. 38.25 and 38.26) (116,137,289). Most of these failures are associated with delayed fracture healing and various technical factors

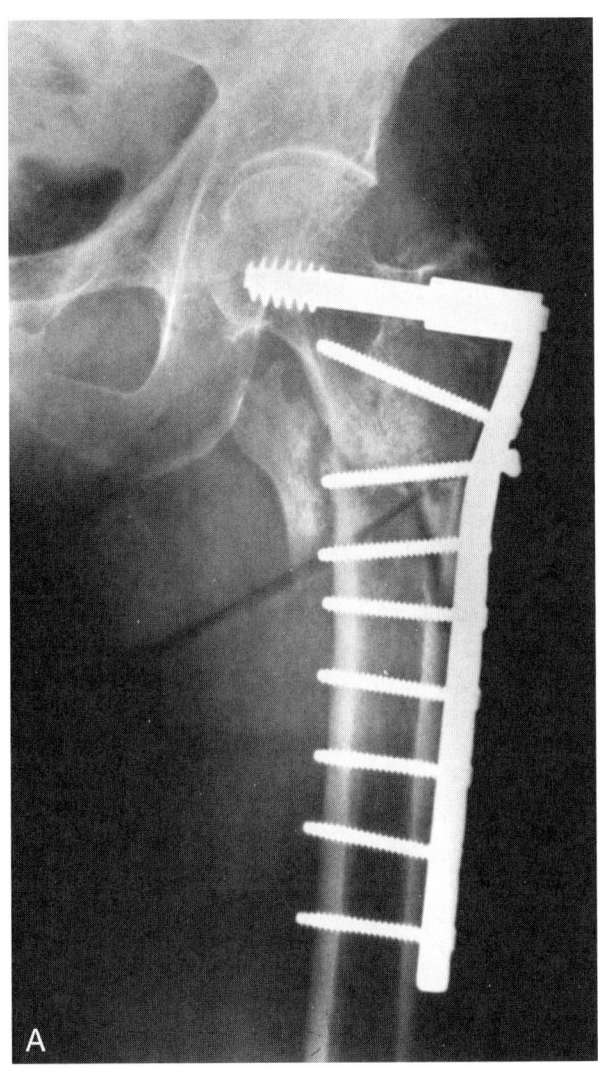
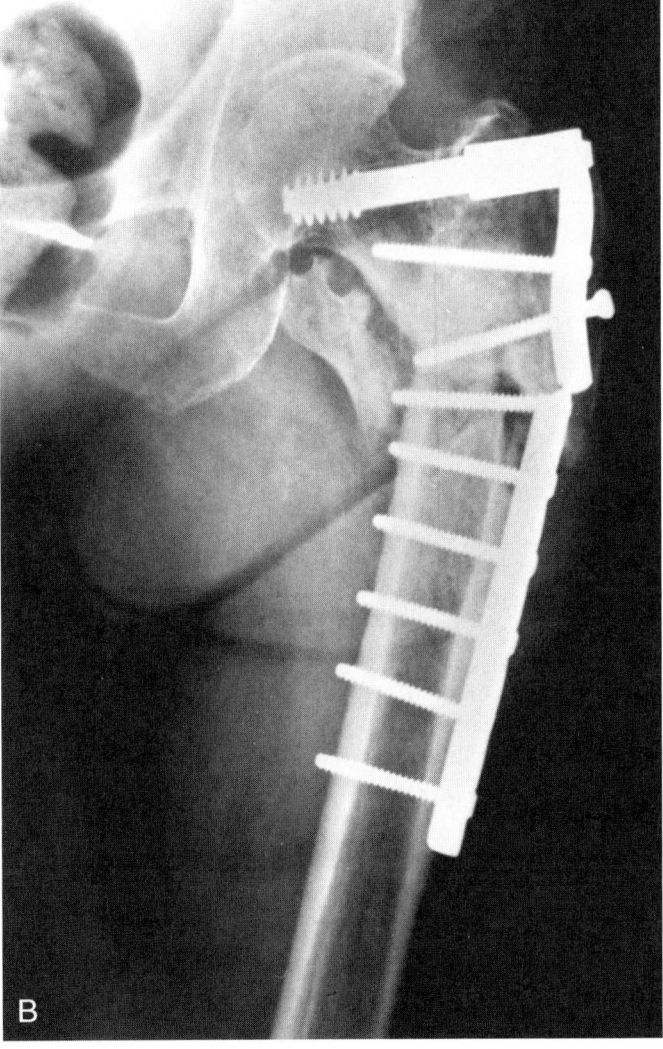

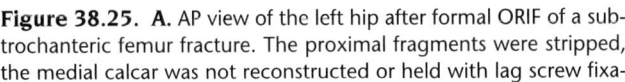

Figure 38.25. A. AP view of the left hip after formal ORIF of a subtrochanteric femur fracture. The proximal fragments were stripped, the medial calcar was not reconstructed or held with lag screw fixa- tion, and no bone grafting was performed. **B.** AP view taken 4 months later, showing nonunion of the fracture and fatigue failure of the implant.

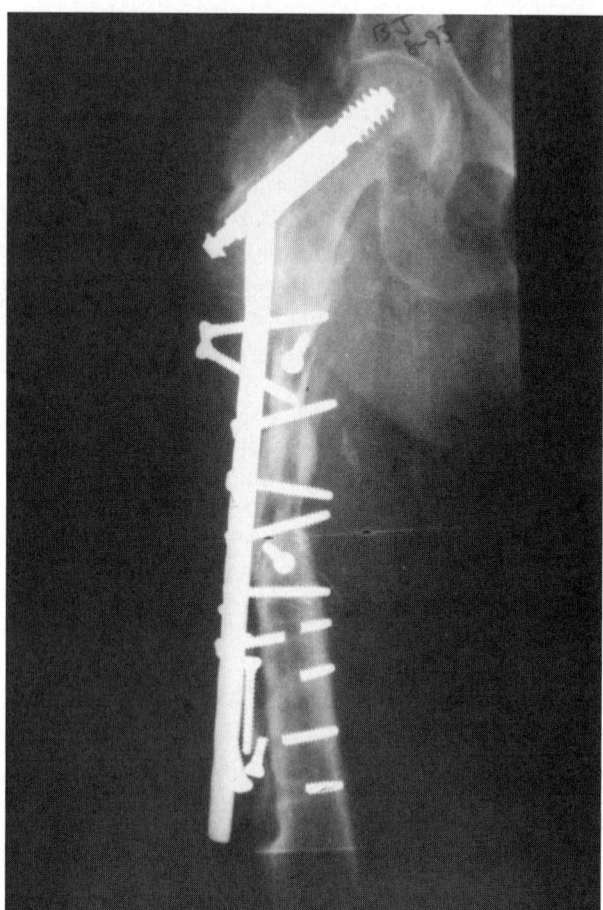

Figure 38.26. AP view of the right hip and femur showing an infected nonunion of a subtrochanteric femur fracture that has been complicated by implant failure.

(290). Technical problems include improper placement of an implant into the femoral head, which increases the risk of failure by three; poor reaming technique; an inability to obtain a stable reduction because of a lack of posteromedial support; severe osteoporosis; excessive fracture collapse that exceeds the sliding capacity of the implant; and inhibited sliding caused by inadequate screw–barrel engagement (18,65,69,116,136,137,289).

Because of the extracapsular nature of intertrochanteric and intertrochanteric–subtrochanteric fractures and their occurrence through well-perfused cancellous bone, healing is rarely a problem, and reported nonunion rates range from 0 to 10% (8,13,18,19,54,70,98,110,129,130,141,156, 157,290). In contrast, the less copious blood supply, more cortical nature, and greater stresses in the subtrochanteric region have contributed to higher rates of nonunion and implant failure (22,79,86,291); however, diaphyseal nonunion after intramedullary stabilization is rare (218). Thus the high failure rates of subtrochanteric fractures reported in earlier studies may have been related more to the treatment regimens than to the fractures themselves. With the evolution of implant design and operative technique, rates of nonunion and failure of fixation after surgi-

cal stabilization in this region now range from 0 to 13% (19,21,27,30,32,47,75,86,87,156,203,208,225,241). Malunion and rotational deformity occur in only 3 to 8% of cases, although subtrochanteric fractures are more problematic (13,47,87,129,156,157).

Management options for implant failure, nonunion, and malunion include conservative treatment and acceptance of the deformity, a second attempt at surgical reduction and stabilization, and conversion to arthroplasty. The former treatment should be considered only in nonambulatory patients who are poor surgical risks (54). In the absence of infection, the majority of patients with a nonunion in the intertrochanteric region can be successfully treated by revision of the fixation, including a more valgus position of the proximal fragment and bone grafting (18,290,292). A blade plate is often optimal in the case of poor remaining bone stock, because it presents a broader surface for support. Using this approach, Mariani and Rand (290) achieved an 82% union rate at 6 months and functional results that were better than those for patients treated with arthroplasty. A symptomatic varus malunion can similarly be managed with an intertrochanteric valgus osteotomy (Fig. 38.27).

Delayed unions after intramedullary nailing of the subtrochanteric region can be successfully treated with dynamization of the nail at 6 months, which is required in approximately 25% of cases (75). Nonunions of the proximal shaft and subtrochanteric regions are best treated with a thick, reamed, locked nail. For a symptomatic rotational deformity, an open or closed derotational osteotomy with a locked intramedullary rod should be considered. In these cases, preoperative CT anteversion studies can help assess any limb length discrepancy and/or rotational malalignment.

Although the patient may have avoided complications associated with fracture healing, there is a theoretically increased risk for new fractures adjacent to the implant (Fig. 38.28). The difference between the moduli of elasticity of the implant and of the bone creates a stress riser, which, combined with a variable amount of trauma and quality of bone stock, may result in fracture. Although technically challenging, these fractures can often be addressed with standard methods of fixation.

When revision surgery is undesirable or impossible after failed internal fixation of proximal femur fractures, salvage hip arthroplasty is a successful alternative, usually done with a calcar-replacement prosthesis (Fig. 38.29) (54,161,293,294). Haentjens et al. (276) reported that patients who underwent hemiarthroplasty rehabilitated more easily and faster—with a reduced incidence of decubiti, pulmonary infections, and atelectasis—than did a historical group of patients who underwent internal fixation. At one year, 82% of the hemiarthroplasty patients had a good or better functional rating, according to d'Aubigne's scale, compared with 60% for the internal fixation group. The former group did, however, have a 9% rate of dislocation.

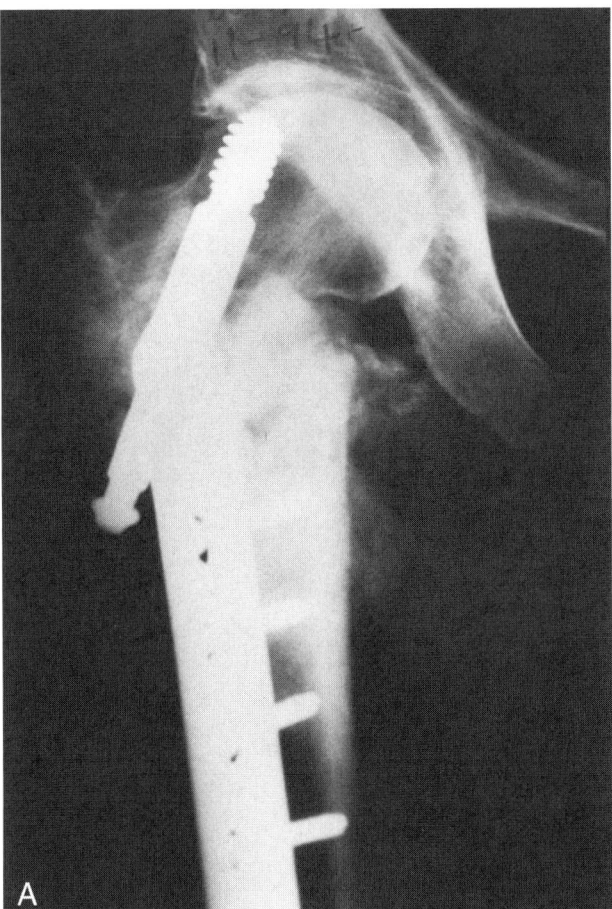 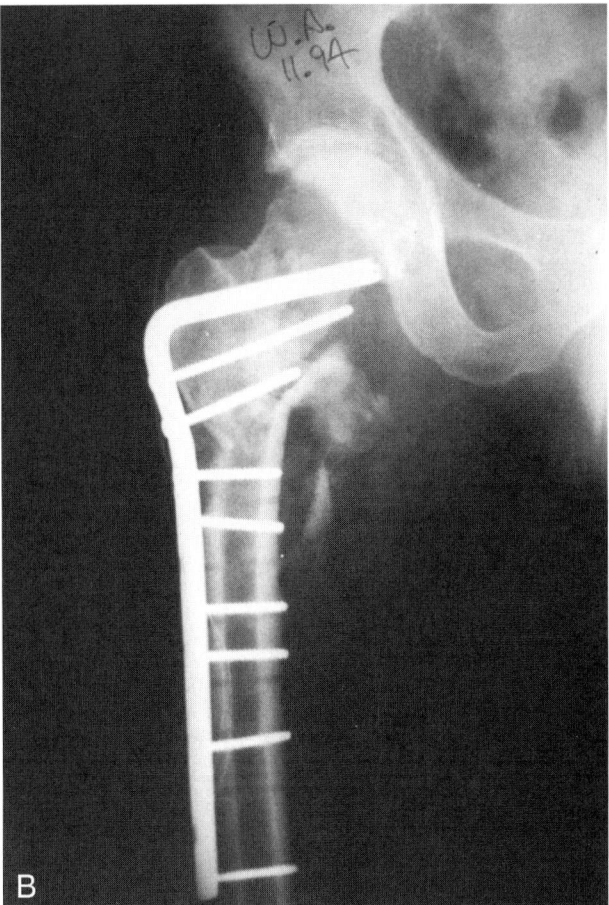

Figure 38.27. A. AP view of the right hip showing varus collapse after fracture fixation. **B.** AP view showing revision with valgus intertrochanteric osteotomy.

The surgeon must use insight and good judgment when returning to the operating room with frail elderly patients, who may have only limited demands. Even after fixation failure, up to 61% of these patients may still be easily mobilized because of lack of pain (65), and postoperative shortening can be partially overcome with a shoe lift. Surgery should be considered in this population only if the implant cuts out or causes severe pain.

AVASCULAR NECROSIS

Osteonecrosis, or avascular necrosis (AVN), of the femoral head following intertrochanteric and subtrochanteric femur fractures is quite rare, with an incidence of less than 1% (18,54,80,98,108,110,203,276,295–297). In a group of 1600 patients with intertrochanteric fractures, Mann (296) observed only 5 cases of AVN, all presenting between 2 and 4 years after the original fracture surgery. Although no association has yet been found between the fracture pattern or the location of the fracture fixation in the proximal fragment and the development of AVN, significant fracture displacement may play a role (54,295).

The relatively high rate of AVN (10%) in rheumatoid patients is probably related to associated corticosteroid treatment (61,298).

INFECTION

Prophylactic antibiotics for the patients undergoing hip fracture surgery have reduced major postoperative wound and urinary tract infections to the lower end of 0 to 7% (8,13,14,32,47,98,129,130,133,141,157,161,201,203,208,299). The somewhat higher rate of infection associated with subtrochanteric fractures may reflect the greater technical difficulties and longer operative times required to treat this injury (14,74). This theory was substantiated by Kinast et al. (74), who were able to reduce infection rates from 21 to 0% by using indirect reduction techniques and avoiding medial dissection.

A deep infection early in the perioperative period requires aggressive irrigation and débridement followed by intravenous antibiotics for approximately 6 weeks, depending on the organism. Should the infection become chronic, then further débridement, removal of the implants, and placement of antibiotic beads are recom-

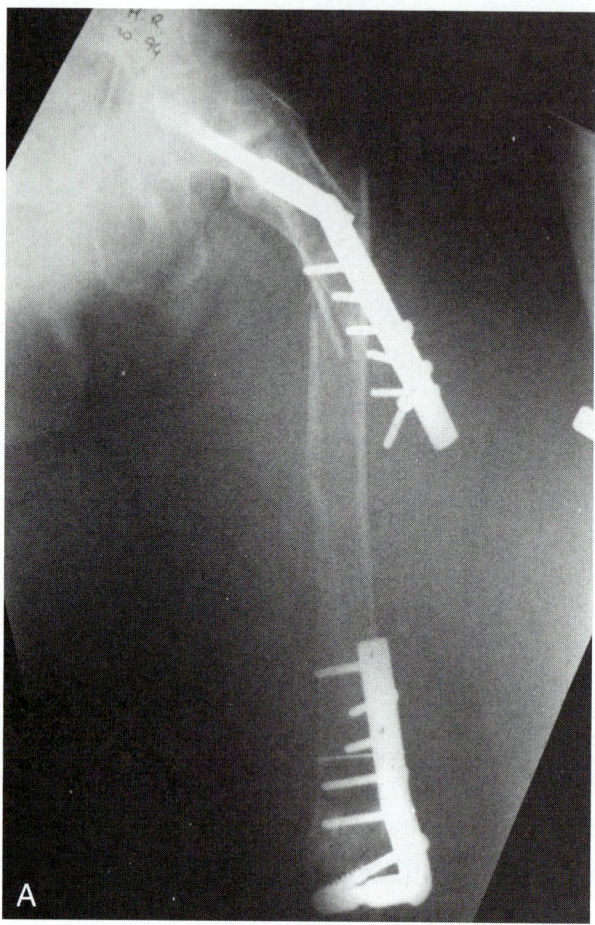

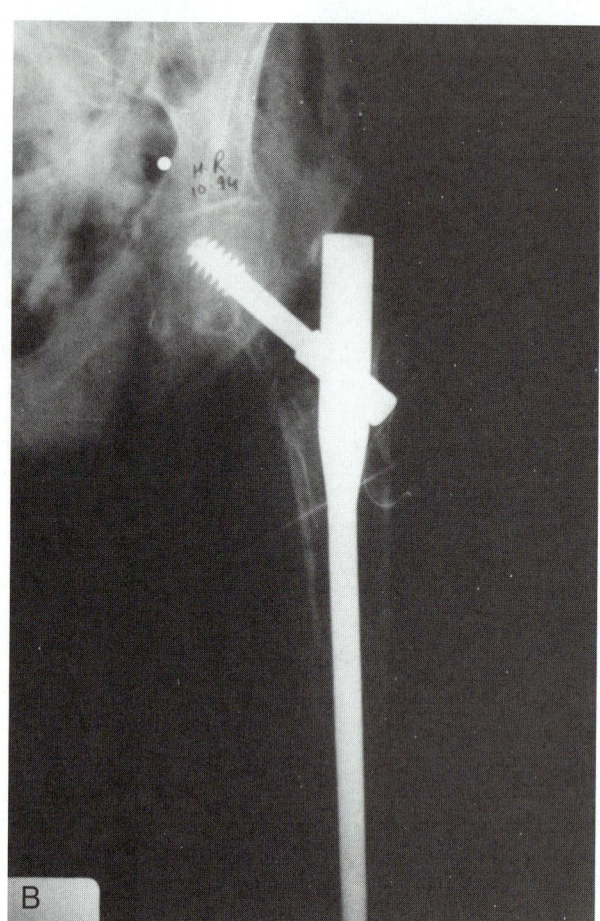

Figure 38.28. A. AP view of an elderly individual who suffered a fall, showing a subtrochanteric femur fracture below a compression hip screw that was used to stabilize an intertrochanteric fracture sev- eral years earlier. **B.** AP view showing stabilization of the new fracture with an intramedullary hip screw.

mended (Fig. 38.30). Generally, the antibiotic beads are retained for 6 weeks. After a course of antibiotic therapy, revision fixation can be considered.

LOSS OF FUNCTION

From 25 to 50% of patients lose their ability to ambulate unassisted after a fracture of the proximal femur (4,32,45,98,116,209,273,300). Many also fail to regain their preinjury ability to perform either basic (feeding, bathing, dressing, toileting) or instrumental (shopping, cooking, housework, using public transportation) activities of daily living (ADLs) (2,14,274,300,301). As a result, 24 to 60% of patients require a prolonged period of institutionalized care (1,8,301,302). Risk factors predictive of such a need include age greater than 60 to 80 years, female sex, poor general condition, cognitive deficits, limb contractures, abductor muscle weakness, inability to ambulate 2 weeks postsurgery, the need for assistance with ADLs, rehospi- talization, limited social contacts or living alone, and de- pendency before fracture (1,2,10,14,45,273,274,278, 301–306).

An interdisciplinary hospital program developed by Zuckerman et al. (285) has lead to fewer postoperative complications, fewer intensive care unit transfers (10% versus 20%), significantly improved ambulatory capacity at discharge (56% independent with assistive devices versus 18%), and proportionally fewer discharges to nursing homes (8% versus 19%).

Bergman et al. (32) noted that 25% of patients with sub- trochanteric fractures could not ambulate at discharge, but only 4% remained nonambulatory at follow-up; failure to ambulate was primarily the result of medical problems. Sanders and Regazzoni (31) reported similar results: 72% of subtrochanteric fracture patients treated with ORIF re- turned to work. These findings reflect the fact that younger patients are more likely to recover their preinjury level of function than are older patients.

SUMMARY

A wide spectrum of fracture patterns are produced in the intertrochanteric and subtrochanteric regions of the proximal femur. It is important to appreciate the greater forces involved with the latter as well as its association with other injuries. Because of the different biomechanical nature of these two fracture types, different implants are

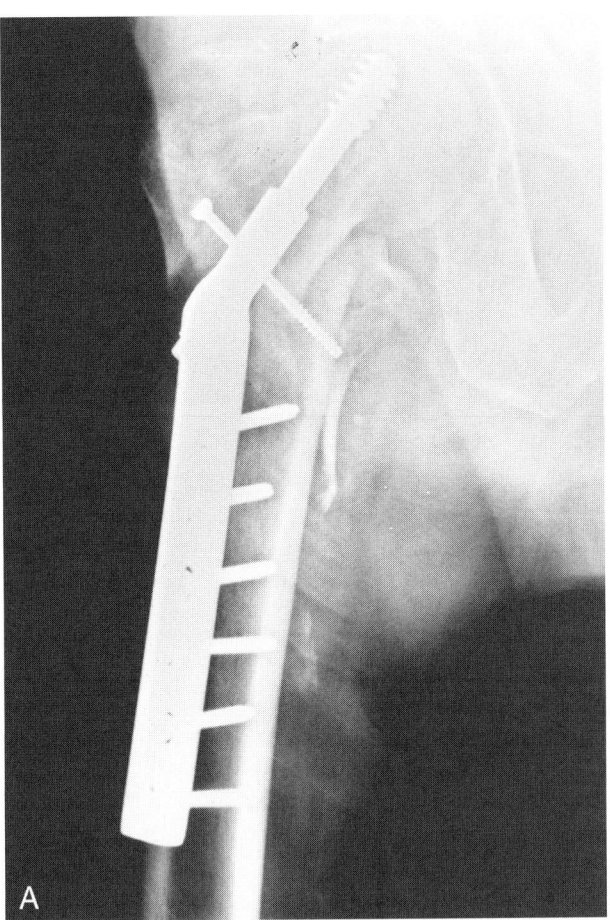

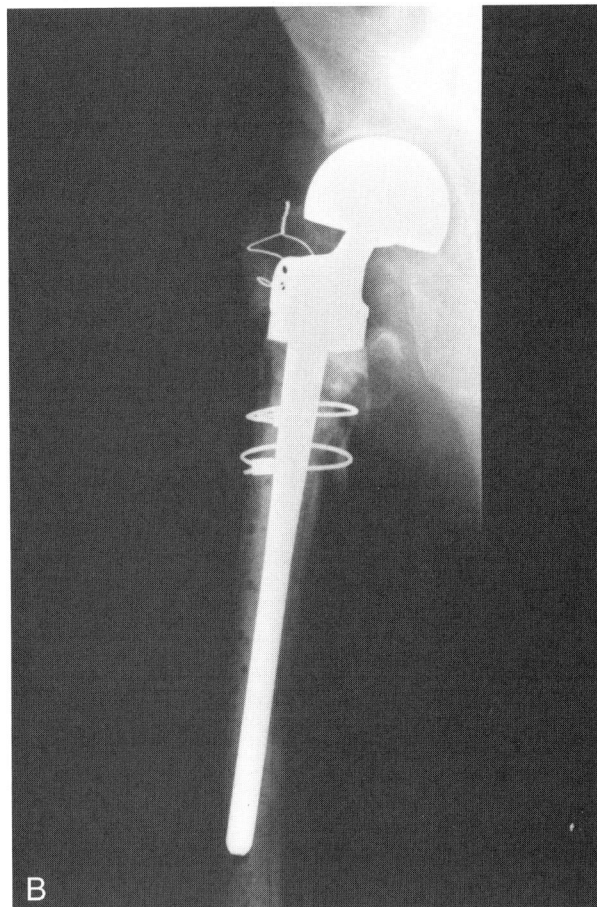

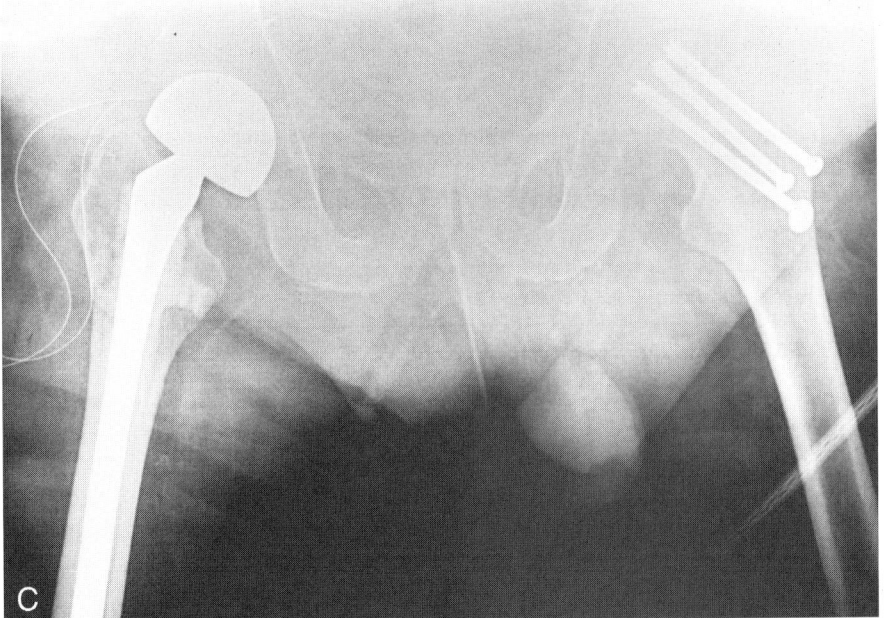

Figure 38.29. **A.** AP view of the right hip of an 87-year-old-male, showing failure of fixation 2 weeks after ORIF of a highly unstable four-part intertrochanteric fracture. Note the comminution of the greater trochanter. **B.** Postoperative AP view showing the cemented calcar replacement hemiarthroplasty. **C.** Postoperative AP view of a patient who underwent hemiarthroplasty for an intertrochanteric–subtrochanteric fracture below the cannulated screws that were used to treat a previous femoral neck fracture. Note that the proximal calcar fragment has been preserved and incorporated as a "napkin-ring" segment.

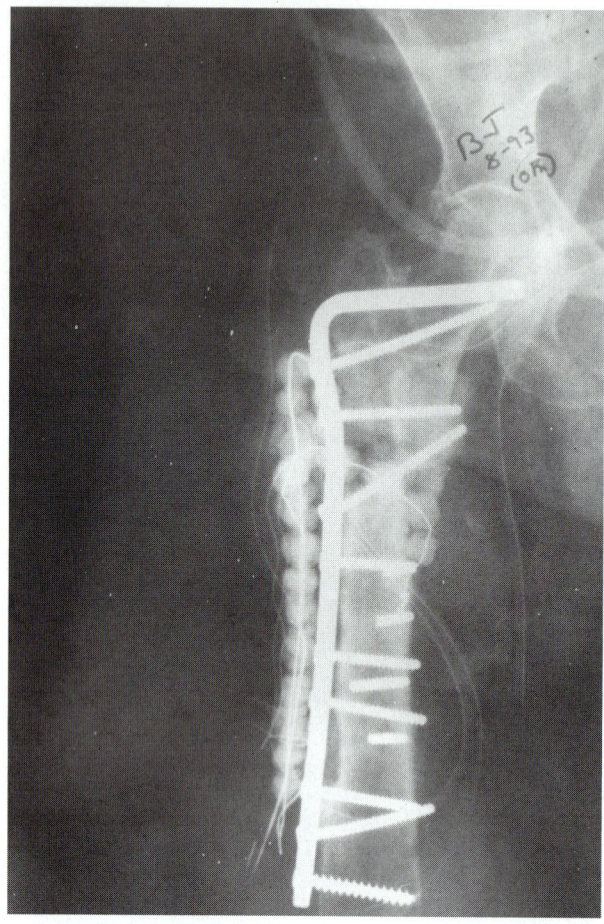

Figure 38.30. Postoperative AP view of the patient shown in Figure 38.26. The infected nonunion has been débrided and stabilized with a condylar plate and lag screws.

required for their stabilization. Although sliding screw-plate devices are generally preferred for intertrochanteric fractures and intramedullary devices are generally preferred for subtrochanteric fractures, each patient must be individually assessed. The great variability of fracture patterns and the common existence of extension from one area to the other prevent the consistent use of one implant for all fracture types.

REFERENCES

1. Borgquist L, Lindelow, Thorngren KG. Costs of hip fracture. Acta Orthop Scand 1991;62:39–48.
2. Ceder L, Thorngren KG, Wallden B. Prognostic indicators and early home rehabilitation in elderly patients with hip fractures. Clin Orthop 1980;152:173–184.
3. Lyden JP. Fracture management of the elderly patient. In: Sculco TP, ed. Orthopaedic care of the geriatric patient. St. Louis: Mosby, 1985:269–287.
4. Niemann KMW, Mankin HJ. Fractures about the hip in an institutionalized patient population. II. Survival and ability to walk again. J Bone Joint Surg 1968;50A:1327–1340.
5. Larsson S, Friberg S, Hansson LI. Trochanteric fractures. Influence of reduction and implant position on impaction and complications. Clin Orthop 1990;259:130–139.
6. Kenzora JE, McCarthy RE, Lowell JD, et al. Hip fracture mortality. Clin Orthop 1984;186:45–56.
7. White BL, Fisher WD, Laurin CA. Rate of mortality for elderly patients after fracture of the hip in the 1980's. J Bone Joint Surg 1987;69A:1335–1345.
8. Sernbo I, Johnell O, Gentz F, Nilsson JA. Unstable intertrochanteric fractures of the hip: treatment with Ender pins compared with a compression hip-screw. J Bone Joint Surg 1988;70A:1297–1303.
9. Dahl E. Mortality and life expectancy after hip fracture. Acta Orthop Scand 1980;51:163–170.
10. Jensen JS. Determining factors for the mortality following hip fractures. Injury 1984;15:411.
11. Aune AK, Ekeland A, Odegaard B, et al. Gamma nail versus compression screw for trochanteric femoral fractures. Acta Orthop Scand 1994;65:127–130.
12. Alffram PA. An epidemiologic study of cervical and trochanteric fractures of the femur in an urban population. Analysis of 1,664 cases with special references to etiologic factors. Acta Orthop Scand 1964;(Suppl 65):1–109.
13. Holt EP. Hip fractures in the trochanteric region: treatment with a strong nail and early weight-bearing. J Bone Joint Surg 1963;45A:687–705.
14. Beals RK. Survival following hip fracture. Long follow-up of 607 patients. J Chronic Dis 1972;25:235–244.
15. Fitts WT, Lehr HB, Schor S, Roberts B. Life expectancy after fracture of the hip. Surg Gynecol Obstet 1959;108:7–12.
16. Gordon PC. The probability of death following a fracture of the hip. Can Med Assoc J 1971;105:47–51.
17. McGoey PF, Evans J. Fractures of the hip: immediate versus delayed treatment. Can Med Assoc J 1960;83:260–263.
18. Kyle RF, Cabanela ME, Russell TA, et al. Fractures of the proximal part of the femur. J Bone Joint Surg 1994;76A:924–950.
19. Whitelaw GP, Segal D, Sanzone CF, et al. Unstable intertrochanteric/subtrochanteric fractures of the femur. Clin Orthop 1990:238–245.
20. Nungu KS, Olerud C, Rehnberg L. Treatment of subtrochanteric fractures with the AO Dynamic condylar screw. Injury 1993;24:90–92.
21. Zickel RE. Subtrochanteric femoral fractures. Orthop Clin North Am 1980;11:555–568.
22. Fielding JW. Subtrochanteric fractures. Clin Orthop 1973;92:86–99.
23. Trafton PG. Subtrochanteric-intertrochanteric femoral fractures. Orthop Clin North Am 1987;18:59–71.
24. Haberman EJ, Sachs R, Stern RE, et al. The pathology and treatment of metastatic disease of the femur. Clin Orthop 1982;169:70–82.
25. Schatzker J, Waddell JP. Subtrochanteric fractures of the femur. Orthop Clin North Am 1980;11:539–554.
26. Velasco R, Comfort TH. Analysis of treatment problems in subtrochanteric fractures of the femur. J Trauma 1978;18:513–523.
27. Waddell JP. Subtrochanteric fractures of the femur: a review of 130 patients. J Trauma 1979;19:582–591.
28. Boyd HD, Griffin LL. Classification and treatment of trochanteric fractures. Arch Surg 1949;58:853–866.
29. Cole JD, Ansel LJ. Intramedullary nail and lag-screw fixation of proximal femur fractures. Operative technique and preliminary results. Orthop Rev 1994;Suppl:35–44.
30. Lechner JD, Rao JP, Stashak G, Adibe SO. Subtrochanteric fractures: A retrospective analysis. Clin Orthop 1980:140–145.
31. Sanders R, Regazzoni P. Treatment of subtrochanteric femur fractures using the Dynamic condylar screw. J Orthop Trauma 1989;3:206–213.
32. Bergman GD, Winquist RA, Mayo KA, Hansen ST Jr. Subtrochanteric fracture of the femur. Fixation using the Zickel nail J Bone Joint Surg 1987;69A:1032–1040.
33. Pennig D. Principles of fracture management in elderly patients. In: Newman RJ, ed. Orthogeriatrics: comprehensive orthopaedic care for the elderly patient. Oxford: Butterworth-Heinemann, 1992:420–435.

34. Gallagher JC, Melton RJ, Riggs BL, Bergstrath E. Epidemiology of fractures of the proximal femur in Rochester, Minnesota. Clin Orthop 1980;150:163–171.

35. Praemer A, Furner S, Rice DP. Musculoskeletal conditions in the United States. Chicago: American Academy of Orthopaedic Surgeons, 1992.

36. Anonymous. Statistics NHCfH. Advance data from Vitaland health statistics: 1985 summary: nutritional hospital discharge summary. Hyattsville, MD: Public Health Service, 1986.

37. Sexson SB, Lehner JT. Factors affecting hip fracture mortality. J Orthop Trauma 1987;1:298–305.

38. Cummings SR, Rubin SM, Black D. The future of hip fractures in the United States. Numbers, costs, and potential effects of postmenopausal estrogen. Clin Orthop 1990;252:163–166.

39. Cummings SR, Kelsey JL, Nevitt MC, O'Dowd KJ. Epidemiology of osteoporosis and osteoporotic fractures. Epidemiol Rev 1985;7:178–208.

40. Koval KJ, Zuckerman JD. Hip fractures. I. Overview and evaluation and treatment of femoral neck fractures. J Am Acad Orthop Surg 1994;2:141–149.

41. Ogilvie-Harris, Botsford DJ, Hawker RW. Elderly patients with hip fractures: improved outcomes with the use of care maps with high-quality medical and nursing protocols. J Orthop Trauma 1993;7:428–437.

42. Anonymous. Office CS. Social trends no. 17. London: Her Majesty's Stationery Office, 1987.

43. Obrant KJ, Bengner U, Johnell O, et al. Increasing age-adjusted risks of fragility fractures: a sign of increasing osteoporosis in successive generations? Calcif Tissue Int 1989;44:157–167.

44. Wallace WA. The scale and financial implications of osteoporosis. Int Med 1987;12 (Suppl):3–4.

45. Koval KJ, Zuckerman JD. Functional recovery after fracture of the hip. J Bone Joint Surg 1994;76A:751–758.

46. Fitzgerald JF, Moore PS, Dittus RS. The care of elderly patients with hip fracture. Changes since implementation of the prospective payment system. N Engl J Med 1988;319:1392–1397.

47. Brien WW, Wiss DA, Becker V Jr., Lehman T. Subtrochanteric femur fractures: a comparison of the Zickel nail, 95 degrees blade plate, and interlocking nail. J Orthop Trauma 1991;5:458–464.

48. Aaron JE, Gallagher JC, Anderson J, et al. Frequency of osteomalacia and osteoporosis in fractures of the proximal femur. Lancet 1974;1:229–233.

49. Boyce WJ, Vessey MP. Habitual physical inertia and other factors in relation to risk of fracture of the proximal femur. Age Ageing 1988;17:319–327.

50. Cooper C, Barker DJP, Morris J, Briggs RSJ. Osteoporosis, falls and age in fracture of the proximal femur. Br Med J 1987;295:13–15.

51. Davidson BJ, Ross RK, Paganini-Hill A, et al. Total and free estrogens and androgens in postmenopausal women with hip fractures. J Clin Endocrinol Metab 1982;54:115–120.

52. Demarest GB, Osler TM, Clevenger FW. Injuries in the elderly: evaluation and initial response. Geriatrics 1990;45:36–42.

53. Evans JG. Falls and fractures. Age Ageing 1988;17:361–364.

54. Koval KJ, Zuckerman JD. Hip fractures. II. Evaluation and treatment of intertrochanteric fractures. J Am Acad Orthop Surg 1994;2:150–156.

55. Michel BA, Bloch DA, Fries JF. Physical activity and fractures over the age of fifty years. Int Orthop 1992;16:87–91.

56. Riggs BL, Melton LJ. Involutional osteoporosis. N Engl J Med 1986;314:1676–1686.

57. Hedlund R, Lindgren U, Ahlbom A. Age- and sex-specific incidence of femoral neck and trochanteric fractures. An analysis based on 20,538 fractures in Stockholm County, Sweden, 1972–1981. Clin Orthop 1987;222:132–139.

58. Greenspan SL, Myers ER, Maitland LA, et al. Fall severity and bone mineral density as risk factors for hip fracture in ambulatory elderly patients. JAMA 1994;271:128–133.

59. Heaney RP, Gallagher JC, Johnston CC, et al. Calcium nutrition and bone health in the elderly. Am J Clin Nutr 1982;36:986–1013.

60. Biyani A, Simison AJ, Klenerman L. Intertrochanteric fractures of the femur and osteoarthritis of the ipsilateral hip. Acta Orthop Belg 1995;61:83–91.

61. Bogoch ER, Ouellette G, Hastings DE. Intertrochanteric fractures of the femur in rheumatoid arthritis patients. Clin Orthop 1993;294:181–186.

62. Firooznia H, Rafii M, Golimbu C, et al. Trabecular mineral content of the spine in women with hip fracture: CT measurement. Radiology 1986;159:737–740.

63. Moran CG, Gibson MJ, Cross AT. Intramedullary locking nails for femoral shaft fractures in elderly patients. J Bone Joint Surg 1990;72B:19–22.

64. Fielding JW, Magliato HJ. Subtrochanteric fractures. Surg Gynecol Obstet 1966;122:555–560.

65. Laros GS, Moore JF. Complications of fixation in intertrochanteric fractures. Clin Orthop 1974;101:110–119.

66. Singh M, Nagrath AR, Maini PS. Changes in trabecular pattern of the upper end of the femur as an index of osteoporosis. J Bone Joint Surg 1970;52A:457–467.

67. Lane JM, Vigorita VJ. Current concepts review: osteoporosis. J Bone Joint Surg 1983;65A:274–278.

68. Walsh ME, Wilkinson R, Stother IG. Biomechanical stability of four-part intertrochanteric fractures in cadaveric femurs fixed with a sliding screw-plate. Injury 1990;21:89–92.

69. Davis TR, Sher JL, Horsman A, et al. Intertrochanteric femoral fractures: mechanical failure after internal fixation. J Bone Joint Surg 1990;72B:26–31.

70. Rao JP, Banzon MT, Weiss AB, Rayhack J. Treatment of unstable intertrochanteric fractures with anatomic reduction and compression screw fixation. Clin Orthop 1983;175:65–71.

71. Hoaglund FT, Low WD. Anatomy of the femoral head and neck, with comparative data from Caucasians and Hong Kong Chinese. Clin Orthop 1980;152:10–16.

72. Rydell N. Biomechanics of the hip joint. Clin Orthop 1973;92:6.

73. Senter B, Kendig R, Savoie FH. Operative stabilization of subtrochanteric fractures of the femur. J Orthop Trauma 1990;4:399–405.

74. Kinast C, Bolhofner BR, Mast JW, Ganz R. Subtrochanteric fractures of the femur. Results of treatment with the 95 degrees condylar blade-plate. Clin Orthop 1989:122–130.

75. Wiss DA, Brien WW. Subtrochanteric fractures of the femur. Results of treatment by interlocking nailing. Clin Orthop 1992;283:231–236.

76. Koch JC. The laws of bone architecture. Am J Anat 1917;21:177–298.

77. Rybicki EF, Simonen FA, Weiss EB. On the mathematical analysis of stress in the human femur. J Biomech 1972;5:203.

78. Watson HK, Cambell RD, Wade PA. Classification, treatment and complications of the adult subtrochanteric fracture. J Trauma 1964;4:457.

79. Frankel VH, Burstein AH. Orthopaedic biomechanics: the application of engineering to the musculoskeletal system. Philadelphia: Lea & Febiger, 1970.

80. Massie WK. Extracapsular fractures of the hip treated by impaction using a sliding nail-plate fixation. Clin Orthop 1962;22:180–202.

81. Pauwels F. Der schenkenholsbruck em mechanisches probem. Grundlagen des heilungsvorganges prognose und kausale therapie. Stuttgart: Ferdinand Enke, 1935.

82. Tencer AF, Johnson KD, Johnston DW, Gill K. A biomechanical comparison of various methods of stabilization of subtrochanteric fractures of the femur. J Orthop Res 1984;2:297–305.

83. Nordin M, Frankel VH. Biomechanics of the hip. In: Frankel VH, Nordin M, eds. Basic biomechanics of the skeletal system. Philadelphia: Lea & Febiger, 1989:135–151.

84. Rydell NW. Forces acting on the femoral head-prosthesis. Acta Orthop Scand Suppl 1966;88:1–132.

85. Apel DM, Patwardhan A, Pinzur MS, Dobozi WR. Axial loading studies of unstable intertrochanteric fractures of the femur. Clin Orthop 1989;246:156–64.

86. Ruff ME, Lubbers LW. Treatment of subtrochanteric fractures with a sliding screw plate device. J Trauma 1986;26:75–80.

87. Wile PB, Panjabi MM, Southwick WO. Treatment of subtrochanteric fractures with a high-angle compression hip screw. Clin Orthop 1983;175:72–78.

88. Lieurance R, Benjamin JB, Rappaport WD. Blood loss and transfusion in patients with isolated femur fractures. J Orthop Trauma 1992;6:175–179.

89. Coughlin L, Templeton J. Hip fractures in patients with Parkinson's disease. Clin Orthop 1980;148:192–195.

90. Froimson AI. Treatment of comminuted subtrochanteric fractures of the femur. Surg Gynecol Obstet 1970;131:465–472.

91. Wiss DA, Browner BD, Heppenstall RB, Whitelaw GP. Symposium: subtrochanteric femoral fractures: current concepts in treatment. Contemp Orthop 1994;29:213–232.

92. Rizzo PF, Lyden JP, Schneider RN. Occult hip fractures: diagnosis and treatment. Contemp Orthop 1993;27:339–345.

93. O'Dwyer FG, Harper WM, Finlay DB. Do elderly patients with hip pain following trauma require hospital admission? Injury 1992;23:295–296.

94. Fairclough J, Colhoun E, Johnston D, Williams LA. Bone scanning for suspected hip fractures: a prospective study in elderly patients. J Bone Joint Surg 1987;69B:251–253.

95. Geslien GE, Thrall JH, Espinosa JL, Older RA. Early detection of stress fractures using 99mTc polyphosphate. Radiology 1976;1121:683–687.

96. Yao L, Lee JK. Occult intraosseous fracture: detection with magnetic resonance imaging. Radiology 1988;167:749–751.

97. Zuckerman JD, Skovron ML, Fessel K, et al. The role of surgical delay in the long-term outcome of hip fractures in geriatric patients. Orthop Trans 1992;16:750.

98. Laskin RS, Gruber MA, Zimmerman AJ. Intertrochanteric fractures of the hip in the elderly. Clin Orthop 1979;141:188–195.

99. Charash WE, Fabian TC, Croce MA. Delayed surgical fixation of femur fractures is a risk factor for pulmonary failure independent of thoracic trauma. J Trauma 1994;37:667–672.

100. Pape HC, Auf'm'Kolk M, Paffrath T, et al. Primary intramedullary femur fixation in multiple trauma patients with associated lung contusion—a cause of posttraumatic ARDS? J Trauma 1993;34:540–548.

101. Bone LB. Early versus delayed stabilization of femoral fractures. J Bone Joint Surg 1989;71A:336–340.

102. Seibel R, LaDuca J, Hassett JM, et al. Blunt multile trauma (ISS 36), femur traction, and the pulmonary failure septic state. Ann Surg 1985;202:283–295.

103. Sherk HH, Snape WJ, Loprete FL. Internal fixation versus nontreatment of hip fractures in senile patients. Clin Orthop 1979;141:196–198.

104. Thornton L. The treatment of trochanteric fractures of the femur. Piedmont Hosp Bull 1937;10:21–28.

105. Jewett EL. One-piece angle nail for trochanteric fractures. J Bone Joint Surg 1941;23A:803–810.

106. McLaughlin HL. An adjustable fixation element for the hip. Am J Surg 1947;73:150–161.

107. Dimon JH, Hughston JC. Unstable intertrochanteric fractures of the hip. J Bone Joint Surg 1967;49A:440–450.

108. Harrington KD, Johnston JO. The management of comminuted unstable intertrochanteric fractures. J Bone Joint Surg 1973;55A:1367.

109. Jensen JS, Sonne-Holm S, Tondevold E. Unstable trochanteric fractures. A comparative analysis of four methods of internal fixation. Acta Orthop Scand 1980;51:949–962.

110. Kyle RF, Gustilo RB, Premer RF. Analysis of six hundred and twenty two intertrochanteric fractures. A retrospective and prospective study. J Bone Joint Surg 1979;61A:219–221.

111. Steinberg GG, Desai SS, Kornwitz NA, et al. The intertrochanteric hip fracture: a retrospective analysis. Orthopedics 1988;11:265–273.

112. Jensen JS, Tondevold E, Sonne-Holm S. Stable trochanteric fractures. A comparative analysis of four methods of internal fixation. Acta Orthop Scand 1980;51:811–816.

113. Clawson DK. Trochanteric fractures treated by the sliding screw plate fixation method. J Trauma 1964;4:737–752.

114. Jacobs RR, McClain O, Armstrong HJ. Internal fixation of intertrochanteric hip fractures. Clin Orthop 1980;146:62–70.

115. Sarmiento A. Intertrochanteric fractures of the femur. J Bone Joint Surg 1963;45A:706–722.

116. Wolfgang GL, Bryant MH, O'Neill JP. Treatment of intertrochanteric fracture of the femur using sliding screw plate fixation. Clin Orthop 1982;163:148–158.

117. Sarmiento A, Williams EM. The unstable intertrochanteric fracture. Treatment with a valgus osteotomy and I beam nailplate. J Bone Joint Surg 1970;52A:1309–1310.

118. Kaufer M, Matteus LS, Sonstegard D. Stable fixation of intertrochanteric fractures. A biomechanical evaluation. J Bone Joint Surg 1974;56A:899–907.

119. Pugh WL. A self-adjusting nail-plate for fractures about the hip joint. J Bone Joint Surg 1955;37A:1085–1093.

120. Schumpelick W, Jantzen PM. A new principle in the operative treatment of trochanteric fractures of the femur. J Bone Joint Surg 1955;37A:693–698.

121. Malerich MM, Laros GS, Wade T, Yamada R. Four fragment intertrochanteric hip fractures—a biomechanical study. Trans Orthop Res Soc 1977;2:242.

122. Lunsjo K, Ceder L, Stigsson L, Hauggaard A. One-way compression along the femoral shaft with the Medoff sliding plate. The first European experience of 104 intertrochanteric fractures with a 1-year follow-up. Acta Orthop Scand 1995;66:343–346.

123. Medoff RJ, Maes K. A new device for the fixation of unstable pertrochanteric fractures of the hip. J Bone Joint Surg 1991;73A:1192–1199.

124. Bonamo JJ, Accettola AB. Treatment of intertrochanteric fractures with a sliding nail-plate. J Trauma 1982;22:205–215.

125. Goldhagen PR, O'Connor DR, Schwarze D, Schwartz E. A prospective comparative study of the compression hip screw and the Gamma nail. J Orthop Trauma 1994;8:367–372.

126. Heyse-Moore GH, MacEachern AG, Evans DC. Treatment of intertrochanteric fractures of the femur. A comparison of the Richards screw-plate with the Jewett nail-plate. J Bone Joint Surg 1983;65B:262–267.

127. Sherk HH, Foster MD. Hip fractures: condylocephalic rod versus compression screw. Clin Orthop 1985:255–259.

128. Chang WS, Zuckerman JD, Kummer FJ, Frankel VH. Biomechanical evaluation of anatomic reduction versus medial displacement osteotomy in unstable intertrochanteric fractures. Clin Orthop 1987;225:141–146.

129. Ecker ML, Joyce JJ, Kohl EJ. The treatment of trochanteric hip fractures using a compression screw. J Bone Joint Surg 1975;57A:23–27.

130. Nungu S, Olerud C, Rehnberg L. Treatment of intertrochanteric fractures: comparison of Ender nails and sliding screw plates. J Orthop Trauma 1991;5:452–457.

131. Pitsaer E, Samuel AW. Functional outcome after intertrochanteric fractures of the femur: does the implant matter? A prospective study of 100 consecutive cases. Injury 1993;24:35–36.

132. Barrios C, Walheim G, Brostrom L, et al. Walking ability after internal fixation of trochanteric fractures with Ender nails or sliding hip screw. Clin Orthop 1992;294:187–192.

133. Cobelli NJ, Sadler AH. Ender rod versus compression screw fixation of hip fractures. Clin Orthop 1985;201:123–129.

134. Doherty JH, Lyden JP. Intertrochanteric fractures of the hip treated with the hip compression screw. Clin Orthop 1979;141:184–187.

135. Manoli A. Malassembly of the sliding screw-plate device. J Trauma 1986;26:916–922.

136. Gundle R, Gargan MF, Simpson AH. How to minimize failures of fixation of unstable intertrochanteric fractures. Injury 1995; 26:611–614.

137. Simpson AH, Varty K, Dodd CA. Sliding hip screws: modes of failure. Injury 1989;20:227–231.

138. Flores LA. The stability of intertrochanteric fractures treated with a sliding-screw plate. J Bone Joint Surg 1990;72B:34–40.

139. Bendo JA, Weiner LS, Strauss E, Yang E. Collapse of intertrochanteric hip fractures fixed with sliding screws. Orthop Rev 1994;(Suppl):30–37.

140. Broos PL, Rommens PM, Deleyn PRJ, et al. Pertrochanteric fractures in the elderly: Are there indications for primary prosthetic replacement? J Orthop Trauma 1991;5:446–451.

141. Harper MC. The treatment of unstable intertrochanteric fractures using a sliding screw-medial displacement technique. J Trauma 1982;22:792–796.

142. Desjardins AL, Roy A, Paiement G, et al. Unstable intertrochanteric fracture of the femur. A prospective randomised study comparing anatomical reduction and medial displacement osteotomy. J Bone Joint Surg 1993;75B:445–447.

143. Hopkins CT, Nugent JT, Dimon JH. Medial displacement osteotomy for unstable intertrochanteric fractures: Twenty years later. Clin Orthop 1989;245:169–172.

144. Clark DW. Treatment of unstable intertrochanteric fractures of the femur: a prospective trial comparing anatomical reduction and valgus osteotomy. Injury 1990;21:84–88.

145. Ender J, Simon-Weidner R. Die fixierung der trochanterer bruche mit runden elastischen kondylennageln. Acta Chir Aust 1970; 1:40.

146. Moehring HD. Flexible intramedullary fixation of femoral fractures. Clin Orthop 1988;227:190–200.

147. Harper MC, Walsh T. Ender nailing for peritrochanteric fractures of the femur. An analysis of indications, factors related to mechanical failure, and postoperative results. J Bone Joint Surg 1985;67A:79–88.

148. Pankovich AM, Tarabishy IE. Ender nailing of intertrochanteric and subtrochanteric fractures of the femur. J Bone Joint Surg 1980;62A:635–645.

149. Russin LA, Sonni A. Treatment of intertrochanteric and subtrochanteric fractures with Ender's intramedullary rods. Clin Orthop 1980;148:203–212.

150. Waddell JP. Remote nailing of intertrochanteric and subtrochanteric fractures of the femur. Instr Course Lect 1983; 32:303–316.

151. Waddell JP. Ender nailing in intertrochanteric fractures of the femur. Instr Course Lect 1984;33:218–221.

152. Levy RN, Siegel M, Sedlin ED, Siffert RS. Complications of Ender-pin fixation in basicervical, intertrochanteric, and subtrochanteric fractures of the hip. J Bone Joint Surg 1983;65A: 66–69.

153. Levy RN, Sherry HS, Siffert RS. Surgical management of metastatic disease of bone at the hip. Clin Orthop 1982:62–69.

154. Harris LJ. Closed retrograde intramedullary nailing of peritrochanteric fractures of the femur with a new nail. J Bone Joint Surg 1980;62A:1185–1193.

155. Lueng KS, So WS, Hui PW. Gamma nails and Dynamic hip screws for peritrochanteric fractures. J Bone Joint Surg 1992;74B: 345–351.

156. Halder SC. The Gamma nail for peritrochanteric fractures. J Bone Joint Surg 1992;74B:340–344.

157. Boriani S. Results of the multicentric Italian experience on the Gamma nail: a report of 648 cases. Orthopedics 1991; 14:1307–1314.

158. Sukhbir S, Deep SK, Chander SR. Modified Kuntscher nail: treatment alternative for adult subtrochanteric fractures. Contemp Orthop 1996;32:298–302.

159. Lyddon DW. The prevention of complications with the Gamma locking nail. Am J Orthop 1996;25:357–363.

160. Williams WW, Parker BC. Complications associated with the use of the Gamma nail. Injury 1992;23:291–292.

161. Stapert JW, Geesing CL, Jacobs PB, et al. First experience and complications with the long Gamma nail. J Trauma 1993; 34:394–400.

162. Mahomed N, Harrington I, Kellam J, et al. Biomechanical analysis of the Gamma nail and sliding hip screw. Clin Orthop 1994; 304:280–288.

163. Bridle SH, Patel AD, Bircher M, Calvert PT. Fixation of intertrochanteric fractures of the femur. A randomised prospective comparison of the Gamma nail and the Dynamic hip screw. J Bone Joint Surg 1991;73B:330–334.

164. Shaw JA, Wilson S. Internal fixation of proximal femur fractures: a biomechanical comparison of the Gamma locking nail and the Omega compression hip screw. Orthop Rev 1993;22:61–68.

165. Rosenblum SF, Zuckerman JD, Koval FJ, Tam BS. A biomechanical evaluation of the Gamma nail. J Bone Joint Surg 1992; 74A:352–357.

166. Curtis MJ, Jinnah RH, Wilson V, Cunningham BW. Proximal femoral fractures: a biomechanical study to compare intramedullary and extramedullary fixation. Injury 1994;25:99–104.

167. Bostrom MP, Lyden JP, Ernberg JJ, et al. A biomechanical evaluation of the long stem intramedullary hip screw. J Orthop Trauma 1995;9:45–52.

168. Evans EM. The treatment of trochanteric fractures of the femur. J Bone Joint Surg 1949;31B:190–203.

169. Boyd HB, Anderson LD. Management of unstable trochanteric fractures. Surg Gynecol Obstet 1961;112:633–638.

170. Muller ME, Allgower M, Schneider R, Willenegger H. Manual of internal fixation. Berlin: Springer-Verlag, 1991.

171. Dhal A, Varghese M, Bhasin VB. External fixation of intertrochanteric fractures of the femur. J Bone Joint Surg 1991; 73B:955–958.

172. Frew JFM. Conservative treatment of intertrochanteric fractures. J Bone Joint Surg 1972;54B:748–749.

173. Hornby R, Evans JG, Vardon V. Operative or conservative treatment for trochanteric fractures of the femur. J Bone Joint Surg 1989;71B:619–623.

174. Winter WG. Nonoperative treatment of proximal femora fractures in the demented nonambulatory patient. Clin Orthop 1987;218:97–103.

175. Murray RC, Frew JFM. Trochanteric fractures of the femur: a plea for conservative treatment. J Bone Joint Surg 1949;31B:204–219.

176. Lyon LJ, Nevins MA. Management of hip fractures in nursing home patients: to treat or not to treat? J Am Geriatr Soc 1984; 32:391–395.

177. Chow SP, Tang SC, Pun WK, et al. Treatment of unstable trochanteric fractures with Dimon-Hughston osteotomy displacement fixation and acrylic cement. Injury 1987;18:123–127.

178. Muhr G, Tscherne H, Thomas R. Comminuted trochanteric femoral fractures in geriatric patients. The results of 321 cases treated with internal fixation and acrylic cement. Clin Orthop 1979;138:41–44.

179. Haentjens P, Casteleyn PP, Opdecam P. Primary bipolar arthroplasty or total hip arthroplasty for the treatment of unstable intertrochanteric and subtrochanteric fractures in elderly patients. Acta Orthop Belg 1994;1:124–128.

180. Greider JL Jr, Horowitz M. Clinical evaluation of the sliding compression screw in 121 hip fractures. South Med J 1980; 73:1343–1348.

181. Meislin RJ, Zuckerman JD, Kummer FJ, Frankel VH. A biomechanical analysis of the sliding hip screw: the question of plate angle. J Orthop Trauma 1990;4:130–136.

182. Kyle RF, Wright TM, Burstein AH. Biomechanical analysis of the sliding characteristics of compression hip screws. J Bone Joint Surg 1980;62A:1308–1314.

183. Den Hartog BD, Bartal E, Cooke F. Treatment of the unstable intertrochanteric fracture: effect of placement of the screw, its an-

gle of insertion, and osteotomy. J Bone Joint Surg 1991;73A: 726–733.

184. Mulholland RC, Gunn DR. Sliding screw plate fixation of intertrochanteric femoral fractures. J Trauma 1972;12:581–591.

185. Friedl W. Relevance of osteotomy and implant characteristics in inter- and subtrochanteric osteotomies. Experimental examination under alternating and static load after stabilisation with different devices including Gamma nail osteosynthesis. Arch Orthop Trauma Surg 1993;113:5–11.

186. Thomas AP. Dynamic hip screws that fail. Injury 1991;22:45–46.

187. Mainds CC, Newman RJ. Implant failures in patients with proximal fractures of the femur treated with a sliding screw device. Injury 1989;20:98–100.

188. Jacobs RR, Armstrong HJ, Whittaker JH, Pazell J. Treatment of intertrochanteric hip fractures with a compression hip screw and a nail plate. J Trauma 1976;16:599–603.

189. Reich SM, Jaffe WL, Kummer FJ. Biomechanical determination of the optimal quantity of plate fixation screws for the sliding hip screw device. Poster presented at the 61st Annual Meeting of the American Academy of Orthopaedic Surgeons, New Orleans, February 28, 1994.

190. Seinsheimer F. Concerning the proper length of femoral side plates. J Trauma 1981;21:42–45.

191. Bartucci EJ, Gonzalez MH, Cooperman DR, et al. The effect of adjunctive methylmethacrylate on failures of fixation and function in patients with intertrochanteric fractures and osteoporosis. J Bone Joint Surg 1985;67A:1094–1107.

192. Harrington KD. The use of methylmethacrylate as an adjunct in the internal fixation of unstable comminuted intertrochanteric fractures in osteoporotic patients. J Bone Joint Surg 1975; 57A:744–750.

193. Allis OH. Fractures in the upper third of the femur, exclusive of the neck. Med News 1891;59:585–590.

194. Lambotte A. L'intervention operatoire dans les fractures recentes et anciennes; envisagee pariculierement au point de vue de l'osteosynthese avec la description de plussieurs techniques nouvelles. Brussels: Lamertain, 1907.

195. Hibbs RA. The management of the tendency of the upper fragment to tilt forward in fractures of the upper third of the femur. N Y State J Med 1902;75:177–179.

196. Teitge RA. Subtrochanteric fractures of the femur. J Bone Joint Surg 1976;58A:282.

197. Thomas WG, Villar RN. Subtrochanteric fractures: Zickel nail or nail-plate? J Bone Joint Surg 1986;68B:255–259.

198. Waddell JP. Surgical treatment of subtrochanteric fractures of the femur. Paper presented at the 53rd Annual Meeting of the American Academy of Orthopaedic Surgeons, New Orleans, February 1986.

199. Seinsheimer F. Subtrochanteric fractures of the femur. J Bone Joint Surg 1978;60A:300–305.

200. Mullaji AB, Thomas TL. Low-energy subtrochanteric fractures in elderly patients: results of fixation with the sliding screw plate. J Trauma 1993;34:56–61.

201. Ganz R, Thomas RJ, Hammerle CP. Trochanteric fractures of the femur. Clin Orthop 1979;138:30–40.

202. Schatzker J, Mahomed N, Schiffman K, Kellam J. Dynamic condylar screw: a new device. A preliminary report. J Orthop Trauma 1989;3:124–132.

203. Blatter G, Janssen M. Treatment of subtrochanteric fractures of the femur: reduction on the traction table and fixation with Dynamic condylar screw. Arch Orthop Trauma Surg 1994; 113:138–141.

204. Warwick DJ, Crichlow TP, Langkamer VG, Jackson M. The Dynamic condylar screw in the management of subtrochanteric fractures of the femur. Injury 1995;26:241–244.

205. Rowe SM, Chung JY, Moon ES, Song EK. Bent plate fixation in combined intertrochanteric and subtrochanteric fractures of the femur. Orthopedics 1991;14:1123–1128.

206. Cech O, Sosna A. Principles of the surgical treatment of subtrochanteric fractures. Orthop Clin North Am 1974;5:651–662.

207. Küntscher G. Dauerbruch und umbauzone. Bruns Beitr Klin Chir 1939;169:557–572.

208. Zickel RE. An intramedullary fixation device for the proximal part of the femur. J Bone Joint Surg 1976;58A:866–872.

209. Davis TR, Sher JL, Checketts RG, Porter BB. Intertrochanteric fractures of the femur: a prospective study comparing the use of the Kuntscher-Y nail and a sliding hip screw. Injury 1988; 19:421–426.

210. Cuthbert H, Howat TW. The use of the Kuntscher Y nail in the treatment of intertrochanteric and subtrochanteric fractures of the femur. Injury 1976;8:135.

211. Templeton T, Saunders EA. A review of fractures in the proximal femur treated with the Zickel nail. Clin Orthop 1979;141:213–216.

212. Zickel RE. A new fixation device for subtrochanteric fractures of the femur: preliminary report. Clin Orthop 1967;54:115–123.

213. Davis AD, Meyer RD, Miller ME, Killian JT. Closed Zickel nailing. Clin Orthop 1985;201:138–146.

214. Yelton C, Low W. Iatrogenic subtrochanteric fracture: a compression of Zickel nails. J Bone Joint Surg 1986;68A:1237–1240.

215. Ovadia DN, Chess JL. Intraoperative and postoperative subtrochanteric fracture of the femur associated with removal of the Zickel nail. J Bone Joint Surg 1988A;70:239–243.

216. Reynders PA, Stuyck J, Rogers RK, Broos PL. Subtrochanteric fractures of the femur treated with the Zickel nail. Injury 1993; 24:93–96.

217. Kempf I, Grosse A, Beck G. Closed locked intramedullary nailing. J Bone Joint Surg 1985;67A:709–720.

218. Winquist RA, Hansen ST, Clawson DK. Closed intramedullary nailing of femoral fractures. J Bone Joint Surg 1984;66A:529–539.

219. Johnson KD, Johnson DWC, Parker B. Comminuted femoral shaft fractures: treatment by roller traction, cerclage wires, and an intramedullary nail, or an interlocking intermedullary nail. J Bone Joint Surg 1984;66A:1222–1235.

220. Thoreson BO, Alho A, Ekeland A, et al. Interlocking intramedullary nailing in femoral shaft fractures. A report of forty-eight cases. J Bone Joint Surg 1985;67A:1313–1320.

221. Brumback RJ, Uwagie-Ero S, Lakatos RP, et al. Intramedullary nailing of femoral shaft fractures. Part II. Fracture healing with static interlocking fixation. J Bone Joint Surg 1988;70A:1453–1462.

222. Wiss DA, Brien WW. Interlocked nailing for the treatment of femoral fractures due to gunshot wounds. J Bone Joint Surg 1991; 73A:598–606.

223. Wiss DA, Brien WW. Interlocked nailing for treatment of segmental fractures of the femur. J Bone Joint Surg 1990; 72A:724–728.

224. Wiss DA, Fleming CH, Matta JM, Clark D. Comminuted and rotationally unstable fractures of the femur treated with an interlocking nail. Clin Orthop 1986;212:35–47.

225. Dobozi WR, Larson BJ, Zindrick M, et al. Flexible intramedullary nailing of subtrochanteric fractures of the femur. A multicenter analysis. Clin Orthop 1986;212:68–78.

226. Zain EBS, Olerud S, Karlstrom G. Subtrochanteric fractures: classification and results of Ender nailing. Arch Orthop Trauma Surg 1984;103:241–250.

227. Slater JD, Taylor JC, Russell TA, et al. Complex subtrochanteric fractures of the femur. Paper presented at the 58th Annual Meeting of the American Academy of Orthopaedic Surgeons, Anaheim, CA, March 1991.

228. Russell TA, Taylor JC. Subtrochanteric fractures of the femur. In: Browner BD, Jupiter JB, Levine AM, Trafton PG, eds. Skeletal trauma. Vol. 2. Philadelphia: Saunders, 1992:1485–1524.

229. Garland DE, Chick R, Taylor J, Salisbury RB. Treatment of proximal-third femur fractures with pins and thigh plaster. Clin Orthop 1981;160:86–93.

230. Wiss D. Subtrochanteric fractures of the femur. In: Chapman MW, ed. Operative orthopaedics. Philadelphia: Lippincott, 1993: 605–620.

231. De Lee JC, Clanton TO, Rockwood CA Jr. Closed treatment of subtrochanteric fractures of the femur in a modified cast-brace. J Bone Joint Surg 1981;63A:773–779.

232. Pape HC, Dwenger A, Regel G, et al. Pulmonary damage after intramedullary femoral nailing in traumatized sheep—is there an effect from different nailing methods? J Trauma 1992;33:574–581.

233. Pape HC, Regel G, Dwenger A, et al. Influences of different methods of intramedullary femoral nailing on lung function in patients with multiple trauma. J Trauma 1993;35:709–716.

234. Bone LB, Babikian G, Stegemann PM. Femoral canal reaming in the polytrauma patient with chest injury. A clinical perspective. Clin Orthop 1995;318:91–94.

235. Bosse MJ, MacKenzie E, Riemer BL, et al. Comparison of ARDS, pneumonia and mortality in MIP with pulmonary injury and femur fractures acutely treated with either reamed IM nails or plates. Paper presented at the 11th Annual Meeting of the Orthopaedic Trauma Association, Tampa, FL, Sept 29, 1995.

236. Swiontkowski MF. Ipsilateral femoral shaft and hip fractures. Orthop Clin North Am 1987;18:73–84.

237. Asher MA, Tippet JW, Rockwood CA, Zilber S. Compression fixation of subtrochanteric fractures. Clin Orthop 1976;117:202–208.

238. Whatley JR, Garland DE, Whitecloud TS III, Wickstrom J. Subtrochanteric fractures of the femur: treatment with ASIF blade plate fixation. South Med J 1978;71:1372–1375.

239. Miller SD, Burkart B, Damson E, et al. The effect of the entry hole for an intramedullary nail on the strength of the proximal femur. J Bone Joint Surg 1993;75B:202–206.

240. Malkawi H. Bone grafting in subtrochanteric fractures. Clin Orthop 1992;168:69–72.

241. Hanson GW, Tullos HS. Subtrochanteric fractures of the femur treated with nail-plate devices: a retrospective study. Clin Orthop 1978;131:191–194.

242. Behr JT, Dobozi WR, Badrinath K. The treatment of pathologic and impending pathologic fractures of the proximal femur in the elderly. Clin Orthop 1985;198:173–178.

243. Wilkins RM, Sim FH, Springfield DS. Metastatic disease of the femur. Orthopaedics 1992;15:621–630.

244. Harrington KD. Orthopaedic management of metastatic bone disease. St. Louis: Mosby, 1988.

245. Fasano FJ Jr, Olysav DJ, Stauffer ES. Intramedullary stabilization of neoplastic destructive disease involving the subtrochanteric region of the femur. Orthopedics 1988;11:1699–1704.

246. Barlow IW, Thomas NP. Reconstruction nailing for subtrochanteric fractures in the pagetic femur. Injury 1994;25:426–428.

247. Bidner S, Finnegan M. Femoral fractures in Paget's disease. J Orthop Trauma 1989;3:317–322.

248. Verluysen M. Pressure sores in elderly patients. The epidemiology related to hip operations. J Bone Joint Surg 1985;67B:10–13.

249. Walheim G, Barrios C, Stark A, et al. Postoperative improvement of walking capacity in patients with trochanteric hip fracture: a prospective analysis 3 and 6 months after surgery. J Orthop Trauma 1990;4:137–143.

250. Roberts TS, Nelson CL, Barnes CL, et al. The preoperative prevalence and postoperative incidence of thromboembolism in patients treated with dextran prophylaxis. Clin Orthop 1990;255:198–203.

251. Feldman DS, Zuckerman JD, Walters I, Sakales SR. Clinical efficacy of aspirin and dextran for thromboprophylaxis in geriatric hip fracture patients. J Orthop Trauma 1993;7:1–5.

252. Haake DA, Berkman SA. Venous thromboembolic disease after hip surgery. Risk factors, prophylaxis, and diagnosis. Clin Orthop 1989;242:212–231.

253. Monreal M, Lafoz E, Navarro A, et al. A prospective double-blind trial of a low molecular weight heparin once daily compared with conventional low-dose heparin three times daily to prevent pulmonary embolism and venous thrombosis in patients with hip fracture. J Trauma 1989;29:873–875.

254. Girasole GJ, Coumo F, Denton JR, et al. Diagnosis of deep vein thrombosis in elderly hip fracture patients using duplex scanning technique. Orthop Rev 1994;23:411–416.

255. Geerts WH, Jay RM, Code KI, et al. Low-dose heparin versus low-molecular-weight heparin to prevent venous thromboembolism. N Engl J Med 1996;335:701–707.

256. Lotke PA, Day L. Prophylaxis against deep-vein thrombosis [Letter]. JAMA 1988;259:687–688.

257. Alho A, Stangeland L, Rottingen J, Wiig JN. Prophylaxis of venous thromboembolism by aspirin, warfarin, and heparin in patients with hip fracture. A prospective clinical study with cost-benefit analysis. Ann Chir Gynaecol 1984;73:225–228.

258. Gerhart TN, Yett HS, Robertson LK, et al. Low-molecular-weight heparinoid compared with warfarin for prophylaxis of deep-vein thrombosis in patients who are operated on for fracture of the hip: a prospective, randomized trial. J Bone Joint Surg 1991;73A:494–502.

259. Hamilton HW, Crawford JS, Gardiner JH, Wiley AM. Venous thrombosis in patients with fracture of the upper end of the femur. A phlebographic study of the effect of prophylactic anticoagulation. J Bone Joint Surg 1970;52A:268–289.

260. Bergqvist D, Kettunen K, Fredin H, et al. Thromboprophylaxis in patients with hip fractures: a prospective, randomized, comparative study between Org 10172 and dextran 70. Surg 1991;109:617–622.

261. Channon GM, Wiley AM. Aspirin prophylaxis of venous thrombolic disease following fracture of the upper femur. Can J Surg 1979;22:468–472.

262. Morris GK, Mitchell JRA. Preventing venous thromboembolism in elderly patients with hip fractures: studies of low-dose heparin, dipyridamole, aspirin, and flurbiprofen. Br Med J 1977;1:535.

263. Knight MTN, Dawson R. Effect of intermittent compression of the arms on deep venous thrombosis in the legs. Lancet 1976;2:1265–1268.

264. Hull RD, Raskob GE, Gent M, et al. Effectiveness of intermittent pneumatic compression for preventing deep vein thrombosis after total hip replacement. JAMA 1990;263:2313–2317.

265. Demers C, Ginsburg JS, Brill-Edwards P, et al. Heparin and graduated compression stockings in patients undergoing fractured hip surgery. J Orthop Trauma 1991;5:387–391.

266. Comerota AJ, Katz ML, White JV. Why does prophylaxis with external pneumatic compression fail for deep vein thrombosis? Am J Surg 1992;164:265–268.

267. Gersin K, Grindlinger GA, Lee V, et al. The efficacy of sequential compression devices in multiple trauma patients. J Trauma 1994;37:205–208.

268. Moser KM, LeMoine JR. Is embolic risk conditioned by location of deep vein thrombosis. Ann Int Med 1981;94:439.

269. Fitts WT, Lehr HB, Bitner RL, Spelman JW. An analysis of 950 fatal injuries. Surgery 1964;56:663–668.

270. Taylor GM, Neufeld AJ, Janzen J. Internal fixation for intertrochanteric fractures. J Bone Joint Surg 1944;26:707–712.

271. Gilchrist WJ, Newman RJ, Hamblen DL, Williams BO. Prospective randomized study of an orthopaedic geriatric inpatient service. Br Med J 1988;297:1116–1118.

272. Magaziner J, Simonsick EM, Kashner TM, et al. Survival experience of aged hip fracture patients. Am J Pub Health 1989;79:274–278.

273. Miller CW. Survival and ambulation following hip fracture. J Bone Joint Surg 1978;60A:930–934.

274. Jensen JS, Bagger J. Long-term social prognosis after hip fractures. Acta Orthop Scand 1982;53:97–101.

275. Elmerson S, Zetterburg C, Andersson BJ. Ten-year survival after fractures of the proximal end of the femur. Gerontology 1988;34:186–191.

276. Haentjens P, Casteleyn PP, De Boeck H, et al. Treatment of unstable intertrochanteric and subtrochanteric fractures in elderly

patients. Primary bipolar arthroplasty compared with internal fixation. J Bone Joint Surg 1989;71A:1214–1225.

277. Johnson LL, Lottes JO, Arnot JP. The utilization of the Holt nail for proximal femoral fractures. J Bone Joint Surg 1968;50A:67–78.

278. Barnes B, Donovan K. Functional outcomes after hip fracture. Phys Ther 1987;67:1675–1679.

279. Craxford AD, Stevens J. Proximal femoral fractures in psychiatric patients. Injury 1979;11:19–22.

280. El Banna S, Raynal L, Gerebtzof A. Fractures of the hip in the elderly: therapeutic and medico-social considerations. Arch Gerontol Geriatr 1984;3:311–319.

281. Evans JG, Prudham D, Wandless I. A prospective study of fractured proximal femur: Factors predisposing to survival. Age Ageing 1979;8:246–250.

282. Wood DJ. Fractures in the elderly. Masters thesis, University of London, United Medical and Dental, 1990.

283. Harrington MR, Brennant M, Hodkinson HM. The first year of a geriatric-orthopaedic liaison service: An alternative to "orthogeriatric" units? Age Ageing 1988;17:129–133.

284. Reid J, Kennie DC. Geriatric rehabilitation care after fractures of the proximal femur: one year follow up of a randomized clinical trial. Br Med J 1989;299:25–26.

285. Zuckerman JD, Sakales SR, Fabian DR, Frankel VH. Hip fractures in geriatric patients. Results of an interdisciplinary hospital care program. Clin Orthop 1992;274:213–225.

286. Davis FM, Woolner DF, Frampton C, et al. Prospective multicentre trial of mortality following general or spinal anesthesia for hip fracture surgery in the elderly. Br J Anaesth 1987;59:1080–1088.

287. Valentin N, Lomholt B, Jensen JS, et al. Spinal or general anesthesia for surgery of the fractured hip? A prospective study of mortality in 578 patients. Br J Anaesth 1986;58:284–291.

288. McKenzie PJ, Wishart HY, Smith G. Long-term outcome after repair of fractured neck of the femur. Comparison of subarachnoid and general anaesthesia. Br J Anaesth 1984;56:581–584.

289. Amis AA, Bomage JD, Larvin M. Fatigue fracture of a femoral sliding compression screw-plate device. Biomaterials 1987; 8:153–157.

290. Mariani EM, Rand JA. Nonunion of intertrochanteric fractures of the femur following open reduction and internal fixation. Clin Orthop 1987;218:81–89.

291. Shelton ML. Subtrochanteric fractures of the femur. Arch Surg 1975;110:41.

292. Boyd HB, Lipinski SW. Nonunion of intertrochanteric and subtrochanteric fractures. Surg Gynecol Obstet 1957;104:463–470.

293. Haentjens P, Casteleyn PP, Opdecam P. Hip arthroplasty for failed internal fixation of intertrochanteric and subtrochanteric fractures in the elderly patient. Arch Orthop Trauma Surg 1994; 113:222–227.

294. Stoffelen D, Haentjens P, Reynders P, et al. Hip arthroplasty for failed internal fixation of intertrochanteric and subtrochanteric fractures in the elderly patient. Acta Orthop Belg 1994;1: 135–139.

295. Shih LY, Chen TH, Lo WH. Avascular necrosis of the femoral head—an unusual complication of an intertrochanteric fracture. J Orthop Trauma 1992;6:382–385.

296. Mann RJ. Avascular necrosis of the femoral head following intertrochanteric fractures. Clin Orthop 1973;92:108–115.

297. Taylor GM, Neufeld AJ, Nickel VL. Complications and failures in the operative treatment of intertrochanteric fractures of the femur. J Bone Joint Surg 1955;37A:306–316.

298. Haddon WA, Abernathy PJ, Haw C. Hip fractures in rheumatoid arthritis. Clin Orthop 1982;170:252–259.

299. Burnett JW, Gustilo RB, Williams DN, Kind AC. Prophylactic antibiotics in hip fractures: a double-blind, prospective study. J Bone Joint Surg 1980;62A:457–462.

300. Jette AM, Harris BA, Cleary PD, Campion EW. Functional recovery after hip fracture. Arch Phys Med Rehabil 1987;68:735–740.

301. Magaziner J, Simonsick EM, Kashner TM, et al. Predictors of functional recovery one year following hospital discharge for hip fracture: a prospective study. J Gerontol 1990;45:101–107.

302. Thorngren KG, Ceder L, Svensson K. Predicting results of rehabilitation after hip fracture. Clin Orthop 1993;287:76–81.

303. Bonar SK, Tinetti ME, Speechley M, Cooney LM. Factors associated with short-versus long-term skilled nursing facility placement among community-living hip fracture patients. J Am Geriatr Soc 1990;38:1139–1144.

304. Broos PL, Stappaerts KH, Luiten EJ, Gruwez JA. Home-going: prognostic factors concerning the major goal in treatment of elderly hip fracture-patients. Int Surg 1988;73:148–150.

305. Cummings SR, Phillips SL, Wheat ME, et al. Recovery of function after hip fracture. The role of social supports. J Am Geriatr Soc 1988;36:801–806.

306. Mullen JO, Mullen NL. Hip fracture mortality: a prospective, multifactorial study to predict and minimize death risk. Clin Orthop 1992;280:214–222.

chapter 39

Charles N. Cornell

Intracapsular Fractures of the Femoral Neck

Intracapsular fractures of the femoral neck, as a subset of hip fractures, are common and often devastating injuries. Intracapsular fractures are epidemic in the elderly population, occurring with a frequency as high as 63.3 per 100,000 U.S. women (1). In the geriatric population, these fractures result in significant morbidity and mortality and have a profound impact on the economics of health care in the United States. It is estimated that $10 billion is spent each year to manage the 300,000 hip fractures that occur in the United States. The incidence of these fractures is expected to double by the year 2050. In young patients, femoral neck fractures occur from significant violence and carry a high incidence of disabling complications, such as osteonecrosis of the femoral head. Because intracapsular fractures are common and have the potential for extremely poor patient recovery, it is imperative that all orthopaedic surgeons become facile and competent in the management of this injury (1).

RELEVANT ANATOMY AND PATHOGENESIS

The adult anatomy of the femoral neck is established after closure of the capital femoral epiphysis. The femoral neck shaft angle is relatively constant at $130° \pm 7°$. The femoral neck is anteverted with respect to the shaft; the average anteversion is $10° \pm 7°$.

The osseous anatomy of the femoral head and neck dictate the ideal position for placement of internal fixation devices. The center of the femoral head represents the area of maximal bone density, as it is the region of confluence of the bony trabeculae. The calcar femorale is a dense plate of bone that projects vertically along the posteromedial portion of the femoral neck. This region of the femoral neck plays an important role in the biomechanics of femoral neck fracture and is the keystone for reduction and stable internal fixation of intracapsular fractures.

The vascular anatomy of the femoral head is a crucial element affecting the outcome following a femoral neck fracture (2) (Fig. 39.1). Most of the vascular flow to the femoral head is supplied by the posterior branch of the medial femoral circumflex, a branch of the profunda femoris artery. The medial and lateral femoral circumflex arteries form a ring around the base of the femoral neck. Ascending cervical branches arise from this network and enter the capsule at its insertion. These small, delicate vessels run along the superior neck and perforate the femoral head near its base. Thus femoral neck fractures often result in disruption of the femoral head blood supply (3). Claffey (4), however, demonstrated that fractures of the femoral neck might occur with only kinking of these vessels, leaving the potential for revascularization of femoral head blood flow following prompt reduction of the fracture.

The capsule of the hip joint inserts along the intertrochanteric line. The intact capsule is able to tamponade bleeding; therefore, little bleeding is associated with intracapsular fractures. The unyielding capsule can cause the development of high intracapsular pressure following fractures, which may contribute to the reduction of blood flow to the femoral head. Some authors argue that capsulotomy may be an important step in the reduction and fixation of intracapsular fractures (5).

In the elderly, decreased bone mineral density and a tendency to fall are the predominate risk factors for the development of hip fractures. Fractures of the hip are occurring with increasing frequency as the longevity of the senior population has increased. White women have the highest risk of sustaining hip fractures, and this risk can be directly correlated to the bone mineral density of the femoral neck. Women who have supplemented their diets with calcium and vitamin D and those that have maintained physically active lifestyles have lower risk (6,7). Black women and men characteristically have a low risk for

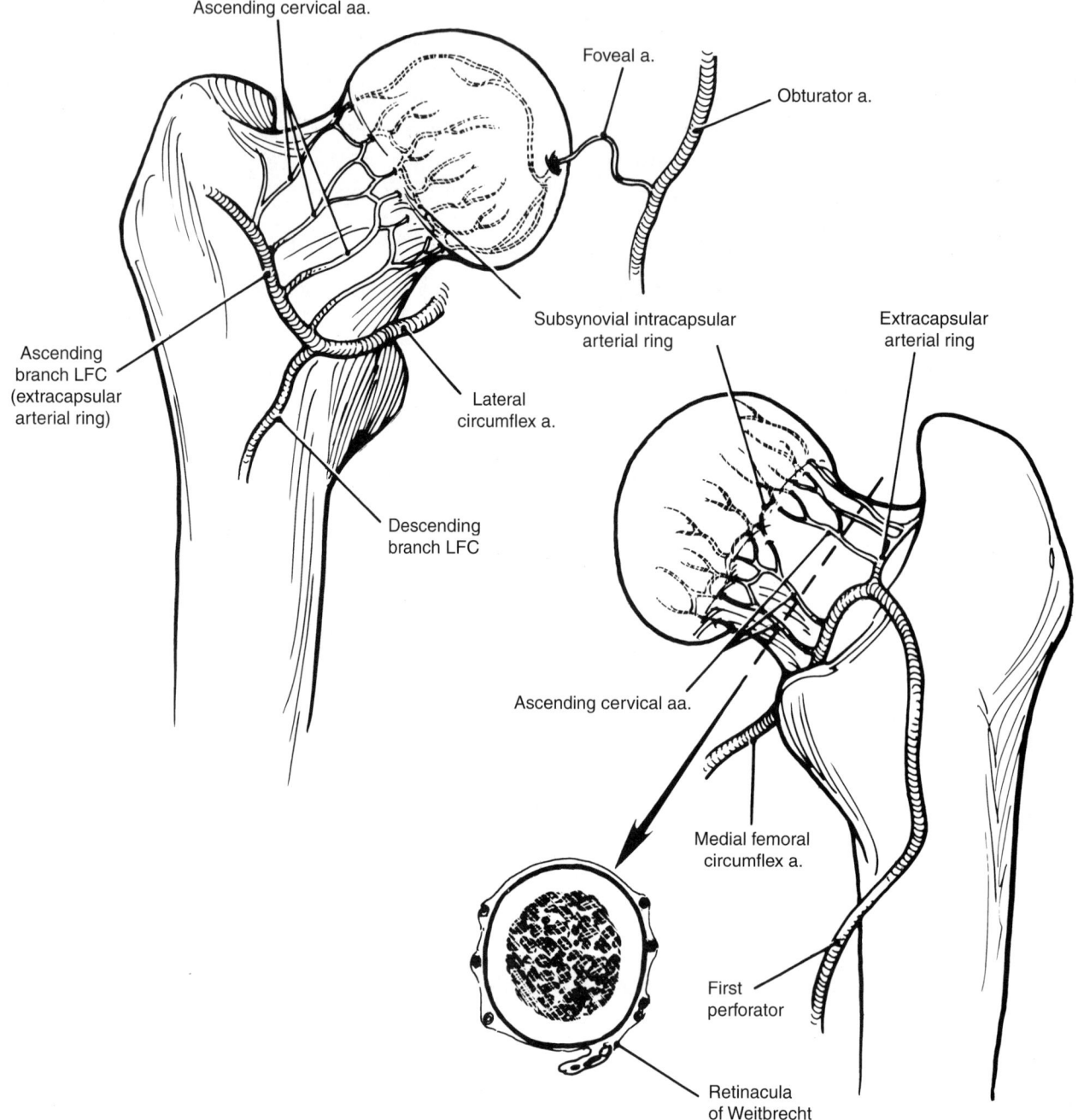

Ascending cervical aa.

Foveal a.

Obturator a.

Subsynovial intracapsular arterial ring

Extracapsular arterial ring

Ascending branch LFC (extracapsular arterial ring)

Lateral circumflex a.

Descending branch LFC

Ascending cervical aa.

Medial femoral circumflex a.

First perforator

Retinacula of Weitbrecht

Figure 39.1. The vascular anatomy of the femoral head. Modified from DeLee JC. Fractures and dislocations of the hip. In: Rockwood CA, et al., eds. Rockwood and Green's fractures in adults. 3rd ed. Philadelphia: Lippincott, 1991:1483.

developing osteoporosis and have the lowest risk of hip fracture.

Despite the importance of bone density as causative factor of femoral neck fractures, few such fractures result from fatigue or occur spontaneously. The majority of fractures occur as the result of a fall from a standing position. Courtney et al. (8) suggest that falls onto the side that cause an impact on the greater trochanter result in proximal femoral fractures. This helps account for the fact that the elderly with chronic medical and neuromuscular dis-

ease and those with a history of sedentary lifestyles are at the highest risk. The risk of a second hip fracture is twice that of the first as the result of an increased likelihood of falling.

Prevention of hip fractures must, therefore, be approached from two perspectives. Prevention of osteoporosis with early screening, education, and adoption of healthy diet and activity levels must become a national health priority. Second, research directed at prevention of falls is needed. If the home environment can be made safer and appropriate physical conditioning methods can be developed for the elderly, then the risk of falls both in and out of the home can be reduced. Furthermore, a greater awareness by the entire medical profession of the iatrogenic causes of falls and the importance of physical rehabilitation after any major medical illness will go a long way to improving the safety of the geriatric population.

Femoral neck fractures in younger individuals are relatively uncommon. They usually result from severe violence with vertical loading of the femur with the hip abducted. In this setting, femoral neck fractures occur despite normal bone density. In such cases, severe associated injuries are common and must be sought in the trauma evaluation. Stress fractures of the femoral neck do occur in individuals who suddenly increase their physical activity, for example, in military recruits or in those with severe metabolic bone disorders, such as osteomalacia or chronic renal failure. It is believed that the fractures occur in the first group as a result of the weakening caused by the initial phases of remodeling that is stimulated by the increased skeletal loads that result from training (9). In the second group, poor bone quality results in a skeletal structure that is unable to withstand normal loading conditions. Stress fractures in either group must be aggressively diagnosed and treated to prevent displacement and avoidable morbidity.

INITIAL FINDINGS, PHYSICAL EXAMINATION, AND DIAGNOSIS

Virtually all patients who sustain intracapsular fractures present with the complaint of having severe groin pain and an inability to walk following a fall. For many elderly who live alone it may take hours or days before they receive appropriate medical intervention and thus can present with severe dehydration, confusion, and decompensation of chronic medical conditions that need to be corrected before surgery (10).

The range of clinical deformity of the affected extremity varies with the severity of the fracture. Classically, the patient with a displaced femoral neck fracture presents with a shortened and externally rotated leg. Stable, impacted, or nondisplaced fractures may present with little deformity. A bruise over the greater trochanter is further evidence that a fracture of the hip should be sought.

RADIOLOGIC EXAMINATION

The standard radiographic examination includes an AP view of the hip and pelvis and a cross-table lateral view. To fully evaluate the femoral neck, the injured leg should be internally rotated at least to neutral, which better aligns the femoral neck for visualization (Fig. 39.2). This is espe-

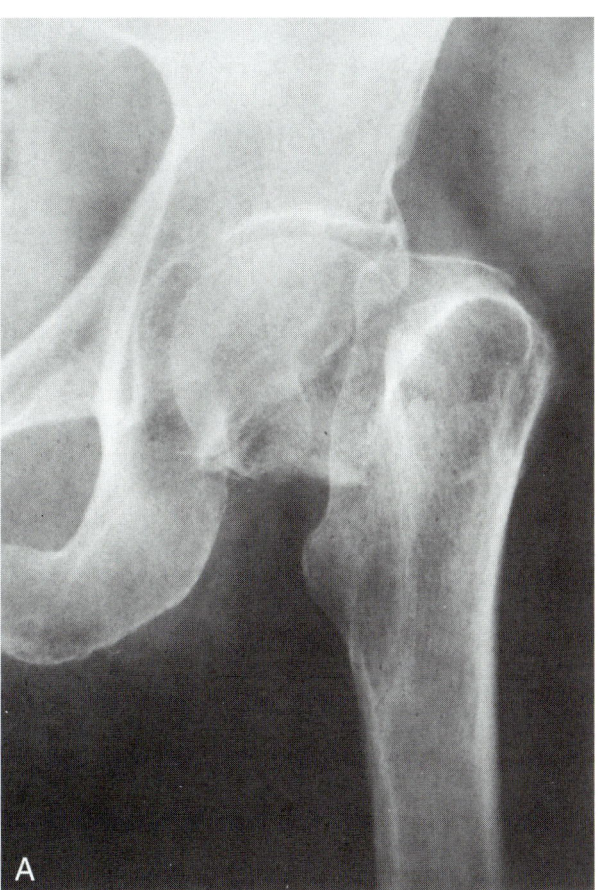
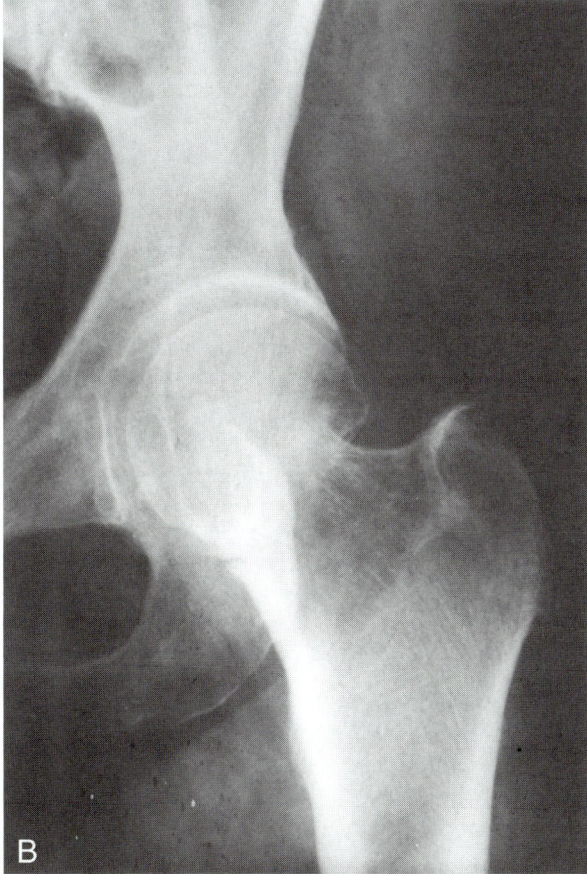

Figure 39.2. External (**A**) and internal (**B**) rotation views of the leg.

Figure 39.3. MRI study showing a femoral neck fracture.

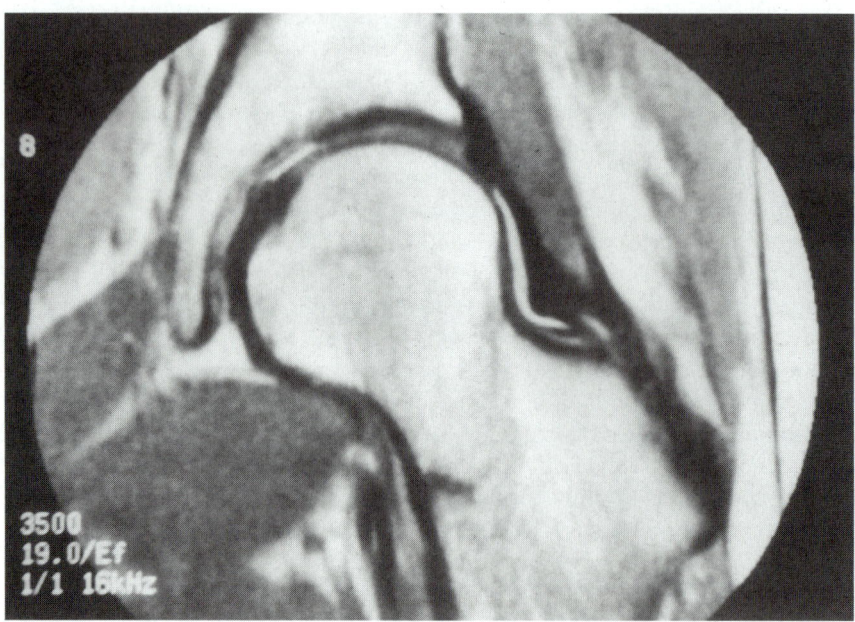

cially important in evaluating minimally displaced or occult fractures. If a femoral neck fracture is suspected on clinical grounds (e.g., an elderly women has fallen and presents with groin pain) but a fracture is not apparent on plain films, then technetium bone scanning or MRI are required. The bone scan is highly sensitive to occult femoral neck fractures, but are sometimes unreliable earlier than 48 h postfracture. MRI, although more costly, is highly accurate within the first 24 h postinjury (Fig. 39.3).

The classification of femoral neck fractures quoted most often in the literature is the Garden classification (11) (Fig. 39.4). In this system, femoral neck fractures are divided into four grades on the basis of the degree of displacement of the fracture fragments. Grade I fractures are incomplete or valgus-impacted fractures. Grade II fractures are complete but are not displaced. Grade III fractures are displaced but some contact between the femoral head and neck is maintained. Grade IV fractures are completely displaced. In practice it is often difficult to reliably distinguish these four types. In addition, most treatment decisions are based on the degree of fracture displacement. Therefore, it is currently believed to be more clinically relevant to distinguish only two types of fractures: displaced (Garden grades III and IV) and nondisplaced (Garden grades I and II).

TREATMENT

When one considers that the goal of treatment of intracapsular fractures is maximal return of function and avoidance of the complications of bed rest in the elderly, it becomes obvious that nearly all femoral neck fractures should be treated operatively (Clinical Table). In rare instances when a patient is too infirm to tolerate surgery or is unlikely to functionally benefit (e.g., a paraplegic) then nonoperative management is tenable.

Nondisplaced Fractures

There is general agreement that Garden grade I and II fractures should be treated by stabilization in situ with multiple cannulated screws. Some authors argue that impacted fractures are stable and can be managed without fixation, but Bentley (12) reported a late displacement rate of 8 to 15%. Furthermore, nonoperative management requires a prolonged period of non-weight bearing, which is poorly tolerated in these patients. There is no consensus on the optimal number of screws that are required for adequate fixation of nondisplaced fractures. Since cannulated screws tend to have large diameters and achieve good initial compression, two or three screws are sufficient.

TECHNIQUE

Cannulated screw fixation of the femoral neck is best performed on a fracture table with the injured leg in traction. The uninjured leg is positioned to allow safe and easy access of the image intensifier (Fig. 39.5). Although the leg is placed in the traction apparatus, no traction is applied, so that the fracture is not disimpacted. Internal rotation of 20° to 30° improves visualization of the femoral head and neck and makes exposure easier.

Although cannulated screws can be inserted percutaneously, it is easier and more nearly accurate to place them through a small incision that exposes the flair of the greater trochanter. A 3- to 4-cm incision centered over the flair of the greater trochanter and placed in the midlateral line is usually sufficient (Fig. 39.6). Once the exposure is complete, the guidewires are placed into the femoral head. A 4.5-mm drill bit can be used to create pilot holes in the lateral femoral cortex, which makes accurate and deliberate positioning of the guidewires possible. The guidewires should be placed parallel with as much spread

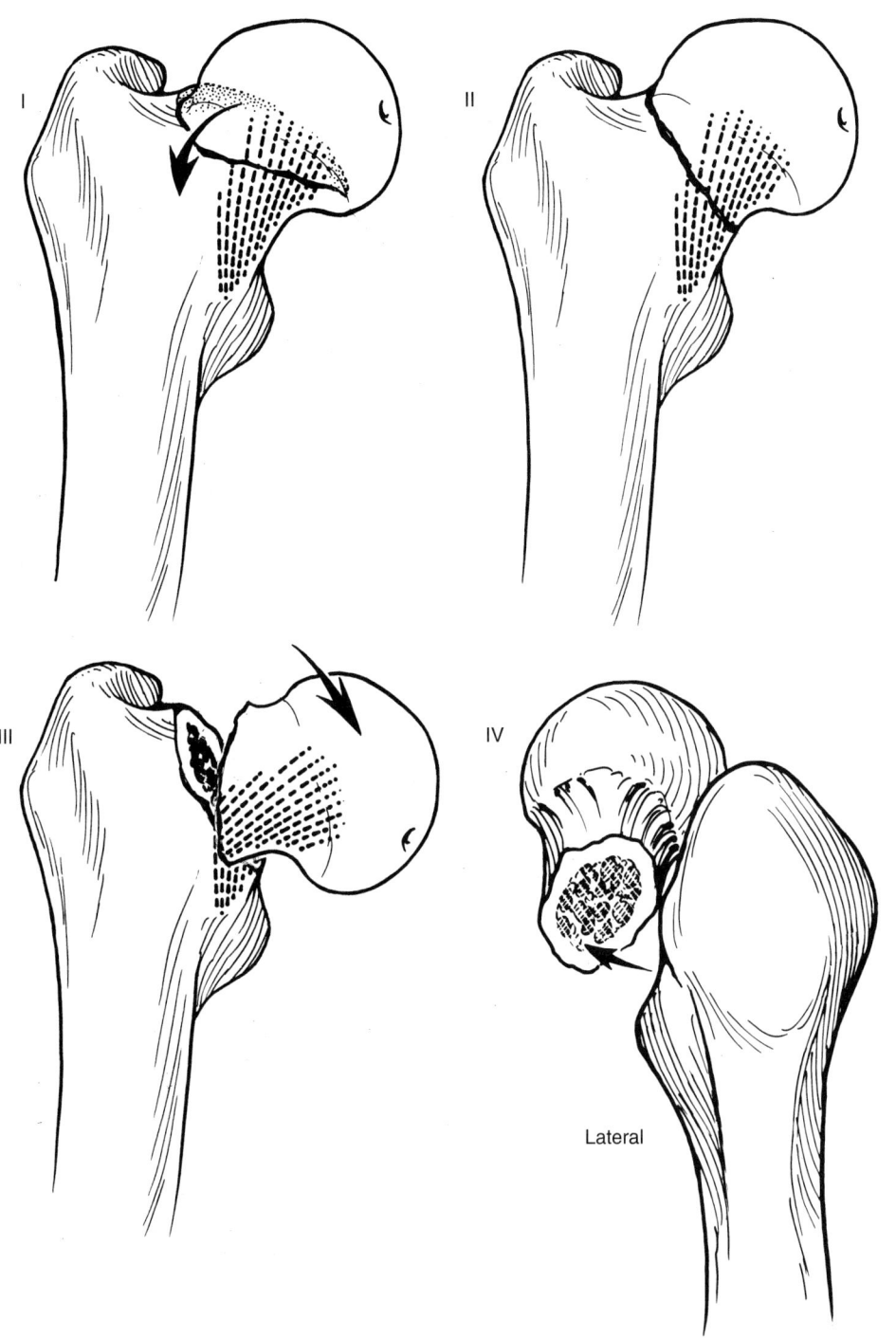

Figure 39.4. The Garden classification of femoral neck fractures. Modified from Browner B, Jupiter JB, Levine A, et al., eds. Skeletal trauma. Philadelphia: Saunders, 1992.

Clinical Table: Intracapsular Fractures of the Femoral Neck

Procedure	Indications	Technique	Anatomy	Pitfalls
Internal fixation	• Undisplaced fractures in patients > 65 years • All fractures in patients < 65 years	• Watson-Jones approach • Reduce fracture through traction • Use image intensifier • Place cannulated pins	• Anterior capsule • Femoral neck • Medial femoral circumflex vessels	• Poor reduction • Malpositioned pins • Femoral head perforation
Hemiarthroplasty	• Displaced fractures in patients > 65 years with low activity levels	• Preoperative planning • Posterior or lateral approach • Remove femoral head • Neck resection • Size the acetabulum • Cement the prosthesis (bipolar or monopolar)	• Hip capsule • Acetabular fossa • Sciatic nerve • Superior gluteal vessels	• Leg length inequality • Hip instability • Neurovascular injury • Damage to the acetabulum
Total hip arthroplasty	• Displaced fractures in patients > 65 years with high activity levels • Fractures with preexisting arthritis • Fractures with preexisting femoral head necrosis	• Preoperative planning • Posterior or lateral approach • Remove femoral head • Neck resection • Size the acetabulum • Cemented or porous socket • Cemented femoral stem	• Hip capsule • Acetabular fossa • Sciatic nerve • Superior gluteal vessels	• Leg length inequality • Hip instability • Malpositioned components • Neurovascular injury

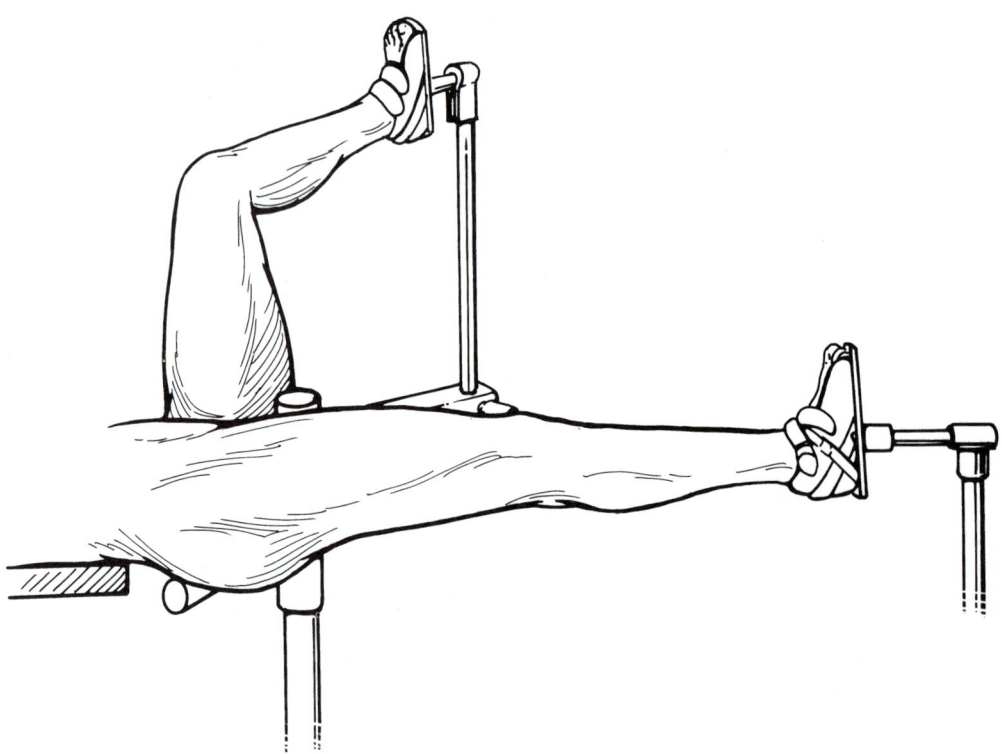

Figure 39.5. Patient positioned on the fracture table.

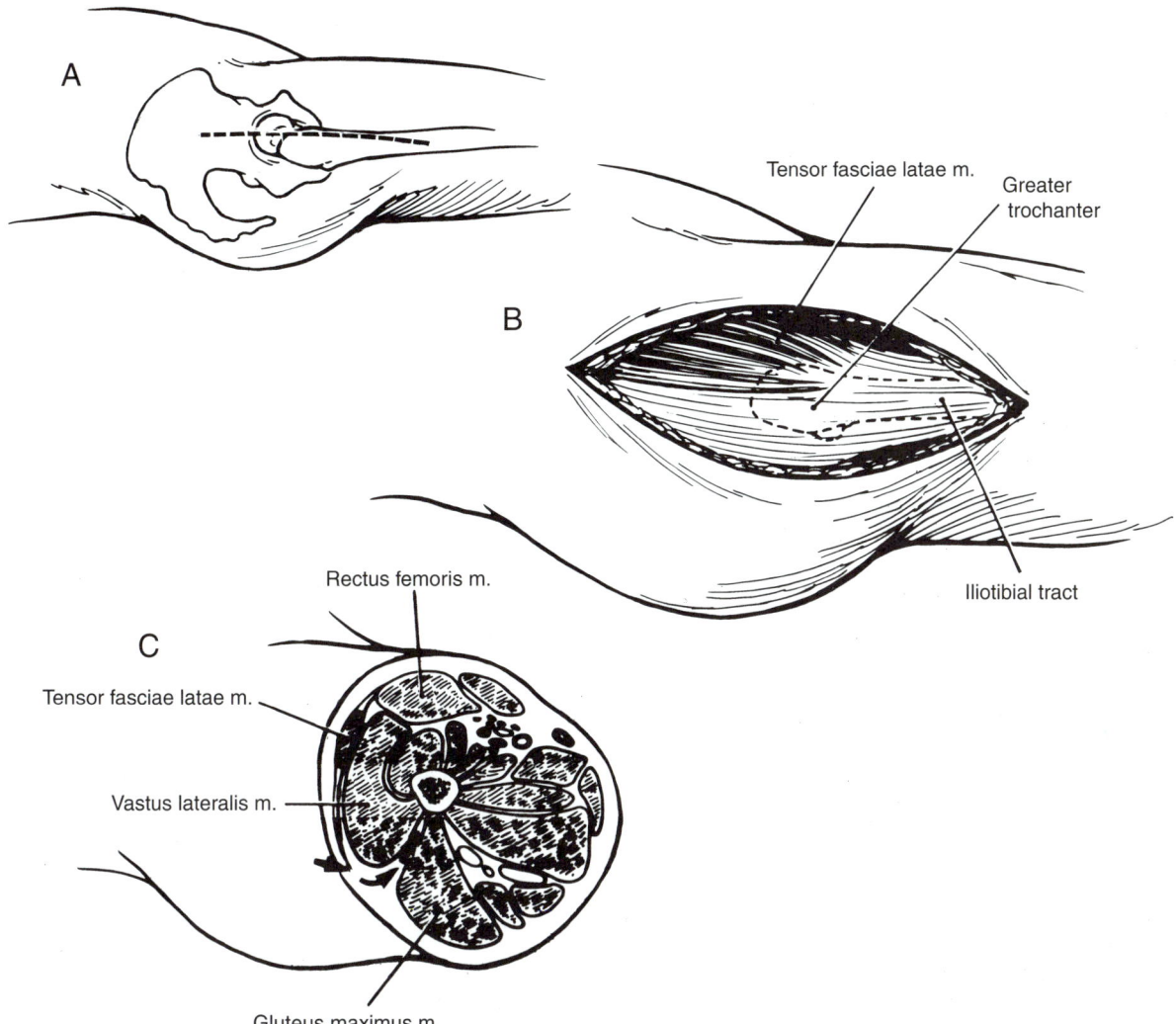

A

B

Tensor fasciae latae m.

Greater trochanter

Iliotibial tract

C

Rectus femoris m.

Tensor fasciae latae m.

Vastus lateralis m.

Gluteus maximus m.

Figure 39.6. Exposure of the greater trochanter.

as practicable, and the surgeon should try to achieve as much cortical contact within the femoral neck as possible. When three screws are used, they should be placed in an inverted triangular pattern.

With the advent of large-diameter cannulated screws, the incidence of iatrogenic subtrochanteric fractures has increased (Fig. 39.7). These fractures probably result from stress failure of the lateral subtrochanteric cortex, which is weakened by the introduction of the screws. I have observed that most of these stress fractures occur when the screws are placed at the level just below the lesser trochanter and when an upright triangle screw pattern is used. The bone just below the lesser trochanter is purely cortical and narrows rapidly to a small diameter; thus screw holes in this area may lead to significant stress concentration. Therefore, be sure to place all screws at or above the midpoint of the lesser trochanter, using a low insertion angle and an inverted triangular pattern, which places two screws more proximal (Fig. 39.8). In small pa-

tients, use just two parallel screws placed in the midlateral plane. Four screws are rarely, if ever, indicated.

Displaced Fractures

Treatment of displaced intracapsular fractures of the femoral neck (Garden grades III and IV) remains one of the ongoing controversies in modern-day fracture care. The controversy revolves around the benefits of closed versus open reduction and internal fixation versus prosthetic replacement of the femoral head.

Reduction by open or closed means with internal fixation using pins or screws is time honored and preserves the patient's own hip joint. This procedure has significant advantages for younger patients, for whom prosthetic replacement is undesirable. The downside of reduction and internal fixation is the high incidence of nonunion and avascular necrosis and the frequent need for reoperation. Lu-Yao et al. (13) authored a meta-analysis of 106 pub-

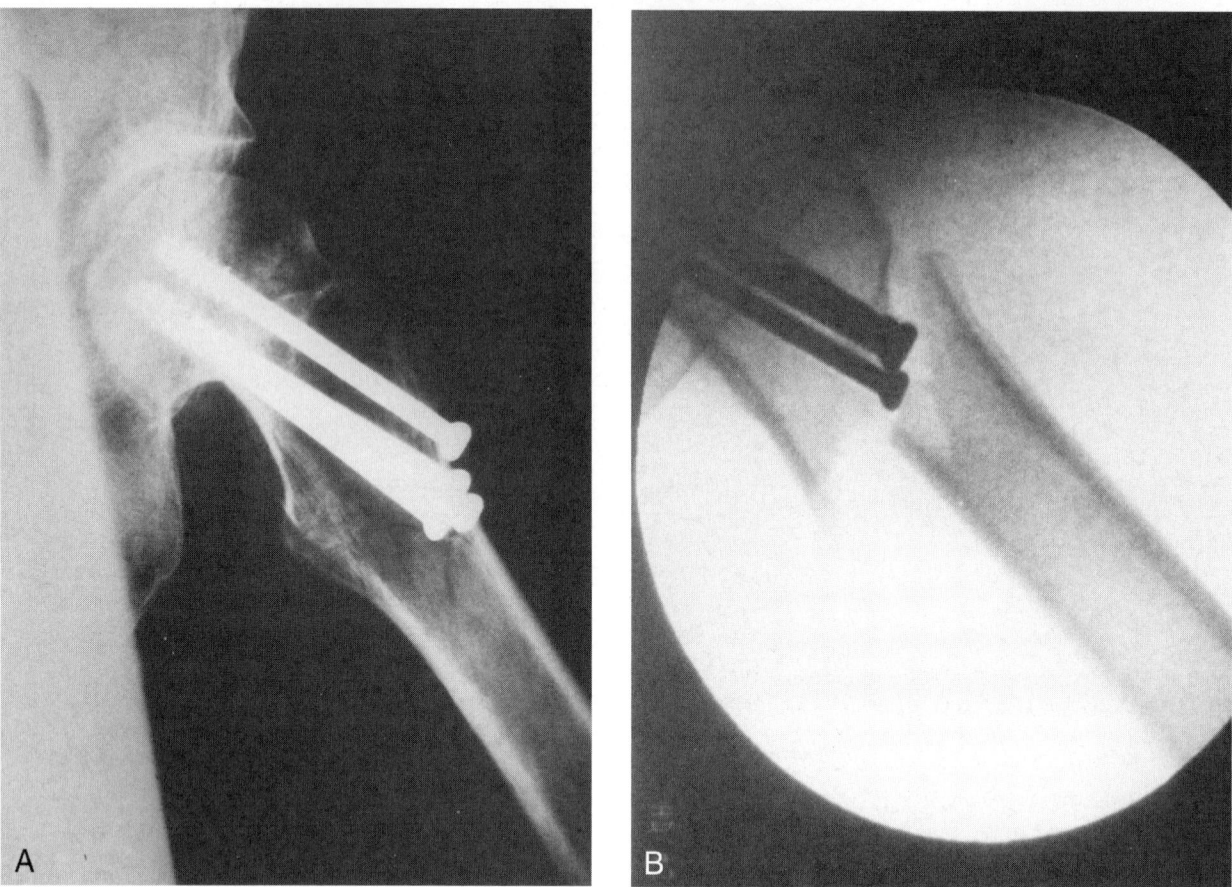

Figure 39.7. Subtrochanteric fracture caused by the cannulated screws.

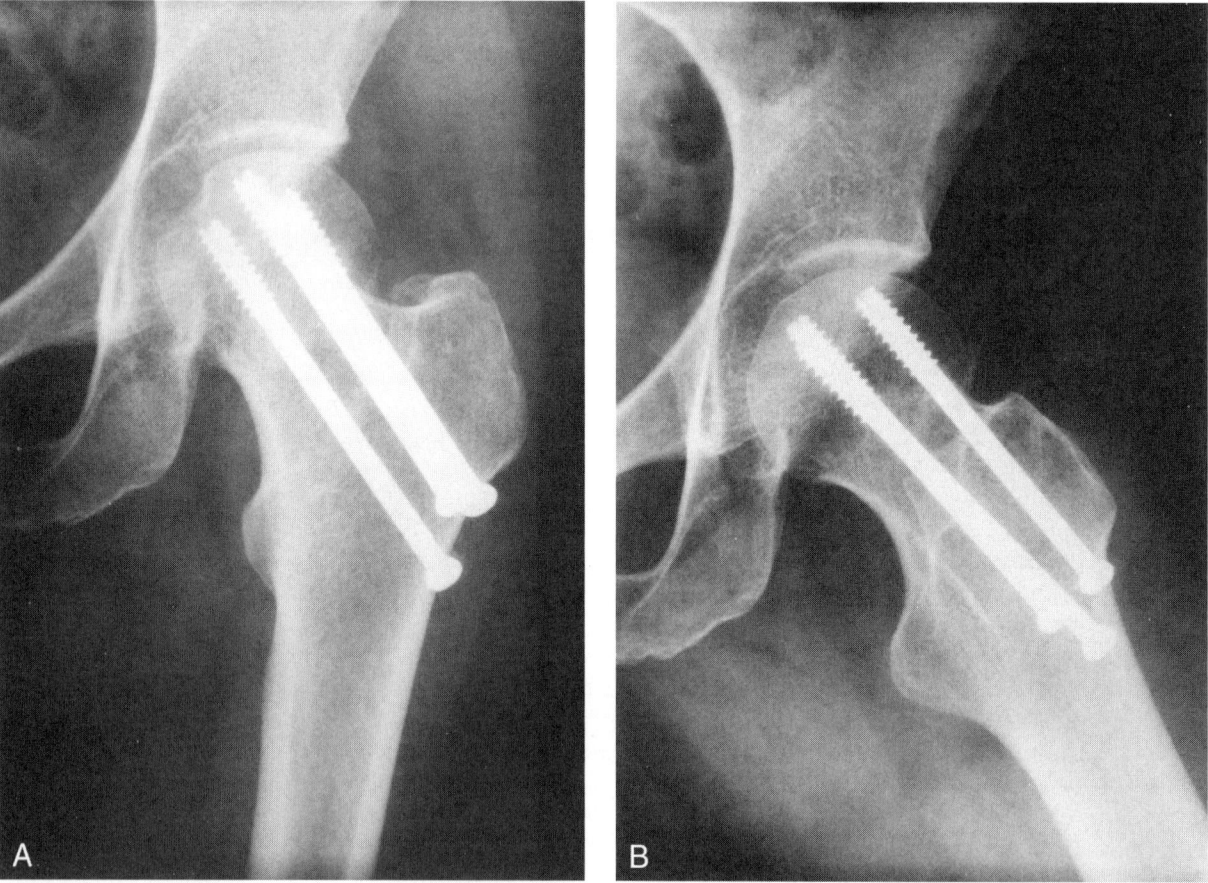

Figure 39.8. Proper placement of the cannulated screws.

lished reports of the outcome of treatment of displaced femoral neck fractures. When internal fixation was compared to prosthetic replacement, there was no statistically significant difference in the 30-day mortality rate. At 6 months, 16% of patients treated by reduction and pinning had failure of fixation, whereas only 2 to 3% of patients treated by arthroplasty suffered dislocations. At the 2-year follow-up, 32% of patients treated with internal fixation had nonunion and 16% had avascular necrosis. No advantage was gained by using larger internal fixation devices, such as sliding hip screws; and in fact, significant disadvantages were noted due to disruption of bone stock. Approximately 11% of bipolar hemiarthroplasty patients had erosion of the acetabular cartilage or loosening of the stem. The need for reoperation in the prosthetic replacement group was substantially lower than in the fixation group at the 2-year follow-up.

Arnold (14) found that only 75% of displaced femoral neck fractures could be adequately reduced in an elderly population; furthermore, in those patients adequately reduced and treated with Knowles pins, 50% required reoperation for nonunion or avascular necrosis within 2 years. On the other hand, long-term experience using bipolar hemiarthroplasty has been excellent, with a 3% dislocation rate, no need for revision secondary to acetabular erosion or loosening of the prosthetic stem, and excellent pain relief and function in all patients who survived to the 5-year follow-up (15).

These data strongly support the use of prosthetic replacement for patients who are acceptable candidates for hip arthroplasty. There are a variety of prosthetic designs available for use, ranging from uncemented, Press-Fit, monopolar stems (such as the Austin Moore) to cemented bipolar designs that use a typical total hip replacement stem. It is clear from the literature that a well-cemented bipolar prosthetic provides better function and pain relief and is associated with lower rates of acetabular erosion and stem loosening (13,16). To date, however, the superiority of bipolar designs has not been conclusively demonstrated, and new designs of monopolar heads that attach to modular cemented stems may be comparable. In general, patients 70 years of age and older or younger patients with a sedentary lifestyle are better served by a cemented bipolar hemiarthroplasty than by reduction and internal fixation. Monopolar prostheses inserted with or without cement should be reserved for elderly or debilitated patients who have low functional demands. Younger, more active patients who elect prosthetic replacement over internal fixation may be best treated by total hip replacement (5).

Special mention should be made of management of femoral neck fractures in young patients injured by high-energy mechanisms. In these cases, all efforts to preserve the femoral head must be made. Considerable evidence suggests that the more rapidly the intracapsular fracture is reduced in this patient population, the greater the likelihood of avoiding femoral head necrosis. Therefore, these fractures should be treated as emergently as possible us-

ing closed or open reduction and internal fixation. Several authors also argue the benefits of open capsulotomy to decompress the hematoma and increased pressure within the hip joint (5).

TECHNIQUE

The technique of reduction and internal fixation of displaced intracapsular fractures is similar to that used for nondisplaced fractures, except that the step of internal fixation is preceded by the reduction maneuver, which is usually performed (16); open reduction is occasionally necessary. As with all hip surgery, regional anesthesia using spinal or epidural block is preferred.

The patient is positioned on the fracture table with the affected limb in traction. The majority of hip fractures can be reduced by simply applying longitudinal traction at a pull equivalent to 7 to 9 kg (15 to 20 lb) and then maximally internally rotating the distal limb. The reduction is checked using the image intensifier and analyzing AP and lateral views. An acceptable reduction is one in which the femoral head is reduced into a valgus position with respect to the neck and the medial cortex of the distal fragment is fully supported on the femoral neck (Fig. 39.9). In the lateral view, the ideal reduction restores the anteversion of the neck, but up to 10° of posterior angulation is acceptable. Any varus angulation on the AP view or lack of support of the proximal fragment is unacceptable.

If the initial reduction maneuver is not successful, the leg is released from traction and the hip is gently flexed and externally rotated to disimpact the fragments; then the hip is extended, traction is applied, and the limb is internally rotated. Repeated attempts at reduction are not advised, as this only contributes further injury to the blood supply to the femoral head. Fractures that cannot be reduced should be treated by open reduction or prosthetic replacement.

Open reduction is best performed by extending the lateral incision proximally and more anteriorly. For the Watson-Jones approach to the hip, a natural extension of the lateral approach, the interval between the gluteus medius and the tensor fascia lata muscles is developed. After the incision is made, the deep fascia is opened and the interval between these muscles is bluntly split. The muscle bellies are retracted to expose the anterior capsule of the hip, which lies directly beneath this interval. The capsule is opened to provide direct inspection and reduction of the femoral neck. A bone hook, or other instrument, is placed into the fracture site, allowing disimpaction of the fracture fragments and direct reduction. The fracture is held reduced while preliminary fixation is accomplished using cannulated screw guidepins. Three pins should be placed, using an inverted triangular pattern. Cannulated screw fixation is then performed.

Prosthetic replacement is ideally performed using regional anesthesia. The most commonly used approach is the posterior approach to the hip, with the patient in the lateral decubitus position. A hypobaric spinal anesthesia or epidural block is helpful, because the patient can be

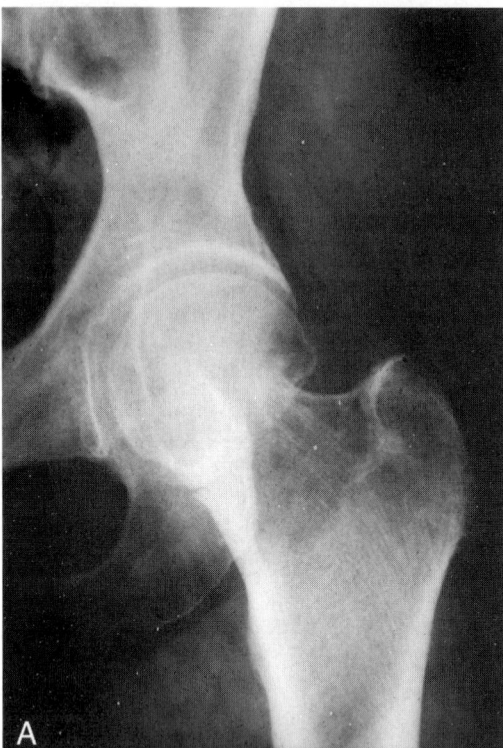

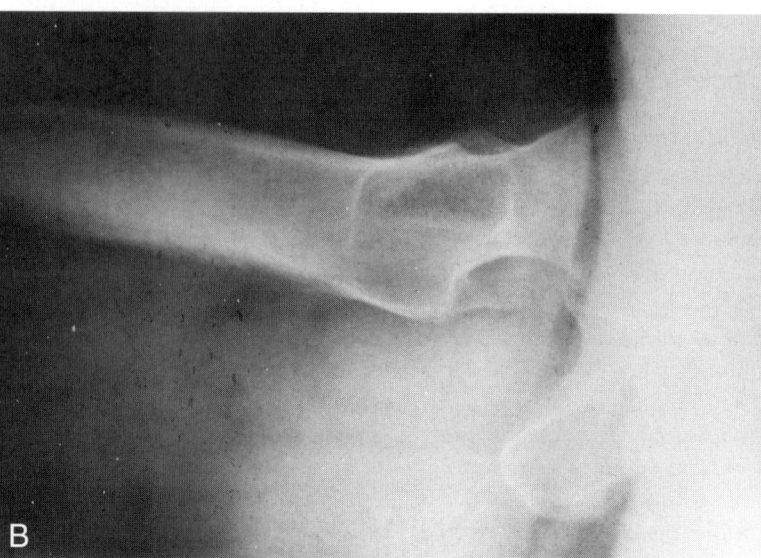

Figure 39.9. Acceptable reduction of the femoral neck.

positioned for surgery as the block sets without having to reposition the patient. Before prepping the patient, careful preoperative planning is performed, using the AP pelvis radiograph to properly size the desired implant and plan the level of the femoral neck resection (Fig. 39.10). This step is needed to ensure proper leg length and offset, which improves ambulatory function and lowers the risk of postoperative dislocation.

The posterior approach to the hip is made. The short external rotators and posterior capsule should be incised with a careful repair in mind. I prefer to detach the tendons from bone at the piriformis fossa and create a posteriorly based flap of capsule; the structures are tagged with heavy nonabsorbable suture for later repair. The femoral neck fracture is then exposed by maximally internally rotating and flexing the leg. The femoral neck resection is performed according to the preoperative plan. The femoral head is then extracted from the acetabulum and its outer diameter is measured so the surgeon can choose the appropriately sized prosthetic head. Soft tissues in the acetabulum, such as the ligamentum teres, should not be resected; and the labrum and acetabular cartilage should not be disturbed. Trial heads are inserted into the acetabulum and tested. The trial head must fit completely into the acetabulum and not load equatorially. It should have relatively free movement but at the same time should create a good suction seal and be difficult to extract. I tend to use the smaller size if the actual fit seems to be between two trial sizes. The acetabulum is then packed with a moist sponge and the femoral component is inserted, using

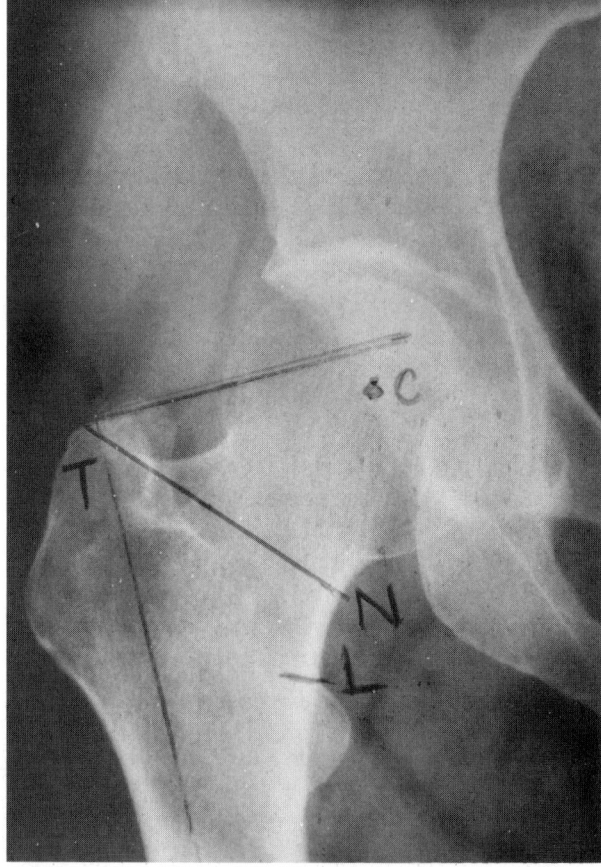

Figure 39.10. Preoperative planning for internal fixation and bipolar hemiarthroplasty.

standard techniques to optimize cement pressurization. After assembly of the modular head, the hip is reduced into the acetabulum, after the surgeon is sure that no debris has been left behind.

The hip range of motion and stability should be checked. Then the surgeon performs a careful repair of the short external rotators and capsule through drill holes to the greater trochanter.

Postoperative Care and Rehabilitation

Prophylactic antibiotics are given within 2 h of the start of surgery and should be continued for 24 h postsurgery. Prophylaxis against deep venous thrombosis and pulmonary embolism is recommended. Low-molecular-weight heparin or low-dose Coumadin combined with external pneumatic compression boots is an ideal protocol. Anticoagulation should probably be discontinued on discharge, unless a specific indication for its continued use is identified.

Physical therapy should begin immediately and should consist of exercises that help the patient regain strength, range of motion, and voluntary control of the limb. Most elderly patients comply poorly with partial– or non–weight-bearing exercise; therefore, these patients should be allowed to bear weight to tolerance. Arnold (14) has shown conclusively that the postoperative weight-bearing status makes little difference in the outcome and that no negative effect of weight bearing on reduced and fixed femoral neck fractures can be found.

All patients should receive information about how to prevent falls and should be evaluated for treatment of osteoporosis. Patients should be evaluated nutritionally and receive supplements as needed. Medical and psychiatric consultants should round out the medical team to manage common medical decompensation, delirium, and depression as they arise. Social work assistance in discharge planning should begin immediately to carefully plan for postacute care and long-term rehabilitation. An assessment of the home environment is needed to be sure the patient's home and social supports are safe and adequate. After the acute healing period, all patients should be encouraged to enroll in a vigorous, supervised physical therapy program to strengthen the lower extremities and improve gait and balance.

MANAGEMENT OF COMPLICATIONS

The risk of avascular necrosis and nonunion associated with intracapsular fractures was discussed above. In the elderly, nonunion and avascular necrosis are best treated by total hip replacement. In younger patients, nonunion can be managed by performing a valgus, intertrochanteric osteotomy that encourages union by increasing compression loads along the nonunion.

Nonunion and osteonecrosis can often coexist, and osteonecrosis usually does not become apparent until the

nonunion heals. Posttraumatic osteonecrosis of the hip does not respond to core decompression and carries a poor prognosis for future collapse and debilitating arthrosis. Salvage procedures in the face of osteonecrosis are probably not justified; total hip replacement is the more successful option. MRI scanning should be performed to help clarify the viability of the femoral head before proceeding with intertrochanteric osteotomy.

SUMMARY

All femoral neck fractures are optimally treated surgically. Nondisplaced fractures (Garden grades I and II) require screw fixation in situ to prevent disimpaction and complete displacement. Results of fixation in situ are excellent, but osteonecrosis occurs in 10% of cases. The treatment of displaced femoral neck fractures must be individualized, but protocols can be employed. Active elderly patients, the majority of cases, are best treated with a cemented bipolar or newer monopolar prosthesis using standard techniques for fixation of the femoral component. Patients that are physiologically younger than 65 years should be considered for reduction and internal fixation. If arthroplasty is selected based on clinical findings or the patient's wishes, a total hip replacement will probably provide better painless function and better long-term results than will hemiarthroplasty. Very elderly and debilitated patients are well served with less expensive Press-Fit prostheses, such as the Austin Moore.

REFERENCES

1. Praemer A, Furner S, Rice DP, eds. Musculoskeletal condition in the United States. Park Ridge, IL: American Academy of Orthopaedic Surgeons, 1992.
2. Trueta J, Harrison MHM. The normal vascular anatomy in the femoral head of adult man. J Bone Joint Surg 1953;35B:442–461.
3. Sevitt S. Avascular necrosis and revascularization of the femoral head after intracapsular fracture: a combined arteriographic and histologic necropsy study. J Bone Surg 1964;46B:270–296.
4. Claffey TJ. Avascular necrosis of the femoral head:an anatomical study. J Bone Joint Surg 1960;42B:802–809.
5. Swiontkowski MF. Current concepts review: intracapsular fracture of the hip. J Bone Joint Surg 1994;76A:129–138.
6. Chapey MC, Arlot ME, Duboeuf F, et. al. Vitamin D$_3$ and calcium to prevent hip fracture in elderly women. N Engl J Med 1992; 327:1637–1642.
7. Michel BA, Block DA, Fries JF. Physical activity and fractures over the age of fifty years. Int Orthop 1992;16:87–91.
8. Courtney AC, Wachtel EF, Myers ER, Hayes WC. Age-related reductions in the strength of the femur tested in a fall-loading configuration. J Bone Joint Surg 1995;77A:387–395.
9. Ross J. A review of lower limb overuse injuries during basic military training. Part 1: types of overuse injuries. Mil Med 1993; 158:410–415.
10. Kenzora JE, McCarthy RE, Lowell JD, et al. Hip fracture mortality: relation to age, treatment, preoperative illness, time of surgery and complication. Clin Orthop 1984;186:45–56.
11. Garden RS. Reduction and fixation of subcapital fractures of the femur. Orthop Clin North Am 1974;5:683–712.
12. Bentley G. Treatment of nondisplaced fractures of the femoral neck. Clin Orthop 1980;152:93–101.

13. Lu-Yao GL, Keller RB, Littenberg B, Wennberg JE. Outcomes after displaced fractures of the femoral neck: a meta-analysis of one hundred and six published reports. J Bone Joint Surg 1994; 76A:15–25.

14. Arnold WD. The effect of early weight-bearing on the stability of femoral neck fractures treated with Knowles pins. J Bone Joint Surg 1984;66A:847–852.

15. Goldhill VB, Lyden JP, Cornell CN, Bochner RM. Bipolar hemi-arthroplasty for fracture of the femoral neck. J Orthop Trauma 1991;5:318–324.

16. Arnold WD, Lyden JP, Minkoff J. Treatment of intracapsular fractures of the femoral neck: with special references to percutaneous Knowles pinning. J Bone Joint Surg 1974;56A:254–262.

chapter 40

Craig S. Bartlett III, Paul K. Kosmatka, and David L. Helfet

Acetabular Fractures

The treatment of acetabular fractures has evolved rapidly since the late 1960s, consistently leading to decreased morbidity and improved outcomes (1–5). To a great extent, this is the result of the revolutionary techniques introduced by Judet and Letournel (1,3,6,7), who stimulated interest in the surgical reduction and stabilization of a fracture rarely operated on in earlier years. Clearly, however, the surgical outcome depends on many factors, especially the ability of the surgeon to make an accurate diagnosis, choose the appropriate approach, and employ the proper techniques. Thus, although some acetabular fracture patterns are amenable to treatment by the general orthopaedic surgeon via familiar approaches, the majority of these fractures, especially the more complex ones, are best treated by an experienced orthopaedic traumatologist. Therefore, to better discriminate between simple fractures and those that are best referred to orthopaedic traumatologists, all orthopaedic surgeons should be familiar with the classification and general treatment of these injuries.

RELEVANT ANATOMY AND PATHOGENESIS

Anatomically, the pelvis is formed from three primary centers of ossification: the ischium, the pubis, and the il-

ium. These come together at the triradiate cartilage, where fusion takes place at 16 to 18 years of age (8). Conceptually, the acetabulum can be thought of as being composed of two pillars, or columns, of bone: one anterior and one posterior (Fig. 40.1). These columns resemble an inverted Y, joined together superiorly in the ilium and inferiorly by a strut called the ischiopubic ramus. These columns can be disrupted alone or in combination. The iliac wing is inclined 45° in the sagittal plane with respect to the long axis of the body, and the major axis of each iliac wing is oriented at a right angle to its respective obturator ring.

Numerous perforators on both the inner and outer tables provide the blood supply to the pelvis; major contributions come from the superior gluteal and iliolumbar arteries. The acetabulum is surrounded by an extensive soft tissue envelope: the gluteal muscles on its external surface, the iliacus on its internal surface, and the short external rotators posteroinferiorly. The close proximity of several important neurovascular structures leads to their frequent injury. The sciatic nerve exits through the greater sciatic notch, along with the superior and inferior gluteal vessels and nerves. The pudendal nerve exits the greater sciatic notch and then courses around the ischial spine, to reenter the pelvis through the lesser sciatic notch.

Figure 40.1. Inner (**A**) and outer (**B**) views of the pelvis showing the anterior and posterior columns of the acetabulum.

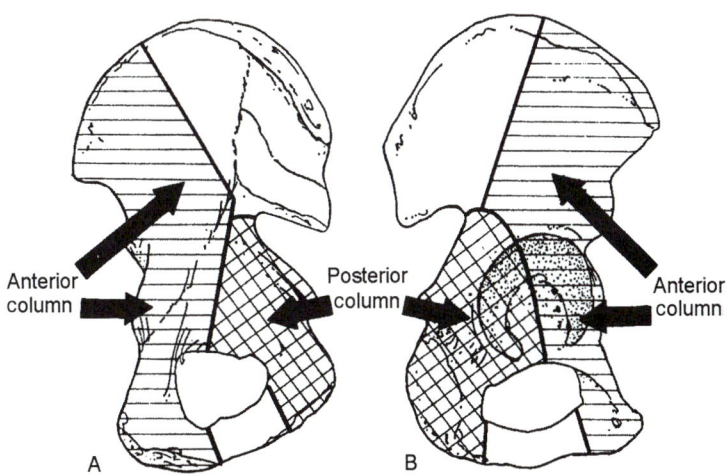

Anterior column

Posterior column

Anterior column

A

B

Judet et al. (6) proposed a widely accepted classification system for acetabular fractures that is based on the identification of fractured anatomic landmarks visualized on an AP view of the pelvis and oblique views of the acetabulum. The fracture patterns are divided into five elemental and five associated (complex) types (Fig. 40.2). The associated fractures are so named because they include at least two of the elementary forms. The five elemental types are fractures of the posterior wall, posterior column, anterior wall, and anterior column and transverse fractures. The associated fracture patterns are T-shaped fractures, posterior wall and column fractures, transverse plus

Figure 40.2. A. The five elemental acetabular fractures: *1,* posterior wall fracture; *2,* posterior column fracture; *3,* anterior wall fracture; *4,* anterior column fracture; *5,* transverse fracture. **B.** The five associated acetabular fractures: *1,* fracture of the posterior column and posterior wall; *2,* transverse and posterior wall fracture; *3,* T-type fracture; *4,* anterior column and posterior hemitransverse fracture; *5,* both-column fracture.

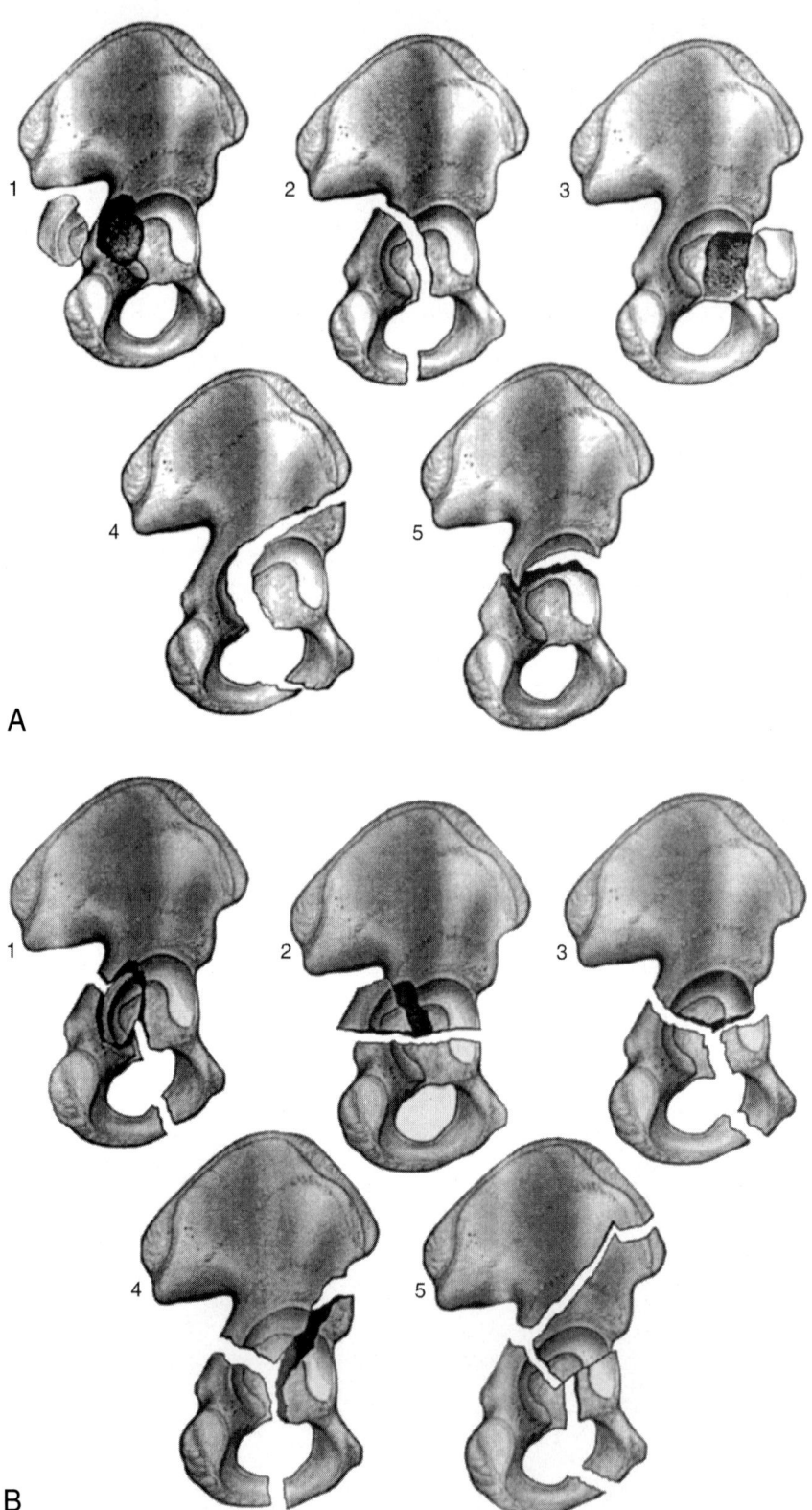

posterior wall fractures, anterior (column or wall) fractures with a posterior hemitransverse, and associated both-column fractures.

For simplicity, three fracture patterns are grouped with others: The posterior column and anterior hemitransverse fracture is grouped with the T-shaped fractures. The anterior wall fracture and anterior column fractures are grouped together. The anterior wall and posterior hemitransverse fracture and anterior column and posterior hemitransverse fractures are grouped together and collectively referred to as anterior fractures with a posterior hemitransverse fracture.

The Letournel-Judet system has now been incorporated into the AO alphanumeric classification scheme for computerized documentation and evaluation of these injuries (9) (Fig. 40.3). The three broad categories are one-column and/or wall partial articular fractures (type A), transverse-oriented partial articular fractures (type B), and complete articular (associated both-column) fractures (type C).

INITIAL FINDINGS, PHYSICAL EXAMINATION, AND DIAGNOSIS

Although the patient with an acetabular fracture may have no outward signs of trauma to the region, a careful history will often reveal clues that suggest its presence. Most acetabular fractures occur as a result of high-energy trauma sustained by motor vehicle trauma as a pedestrian, bicyclist, or car occupant or as the result of a fall from a height (3). Unrestrained car occupants whose knees have struck the dashboard are at particularly great risk. The mechanism of injury is usually from indirect trauma, transmitted to the acetabulum via the femur. Direct blows to the greater trochanter, the flexed knee, or the foot with the knee extended can all result in a fracture of the acetabu-

lum. The exact position of the femoral head in relation to the acetabulum at the time of impact determines the pattern of fracture. Increasing hip external rotation causes anterior fractures, whereas internal rotation produces posterior fractures. A neutral position tends to produce a transverse fracture (3) (Fig. 40.4).

Because of high-energy involvement, there is a significant incidence of associated injuries, including pelvic ring and long bone fractures, spinal and head trauma, and abdominopelvic visceral injuries (3). As the majority of these injuries can be fatal in and of themselves, the initial management of a patient with an acetabular or pelvic fracture requires prompt evaluation and resuscitation by a trained multidisciplinary trauma team, followed by stabilization of any life-threatening injuries. Once the patient has been stabilized, definitive evaluation and treatment of the acetabular fracture should be undertaken by an experienced orthopaedic traumatologist.

Palpation of bony fragments on rectal or vaginal exam is an indication of significant bony pelvic disruption. The presence of an open fracture heralds a poor prognosis. Hematuria is frequently seen in the trauma patient, even without pelvic fracture, and should be carefully assessed. The position of the lower extremities can suggest the fracture pattern. Windswept legs, i.e., one externally rotated and one internally rotated, can occur with a pelvic fracture with a transverse acetabular fracture pattern. A shortened, internally rotated limb is common with posterior dislocation.

All patients complaining of hip or pelvic pain must undergo a thorough examination. Pain with gentle logrolling of the hip or tenderness to palpation about the hip should increase the clinician's suspicion. Patients may have signs of direct trauma to the pelvis, including contusions or abrasions. Contusions and abrasions directly over the greater trochanter or iliac crest herald the presence of the Morel-

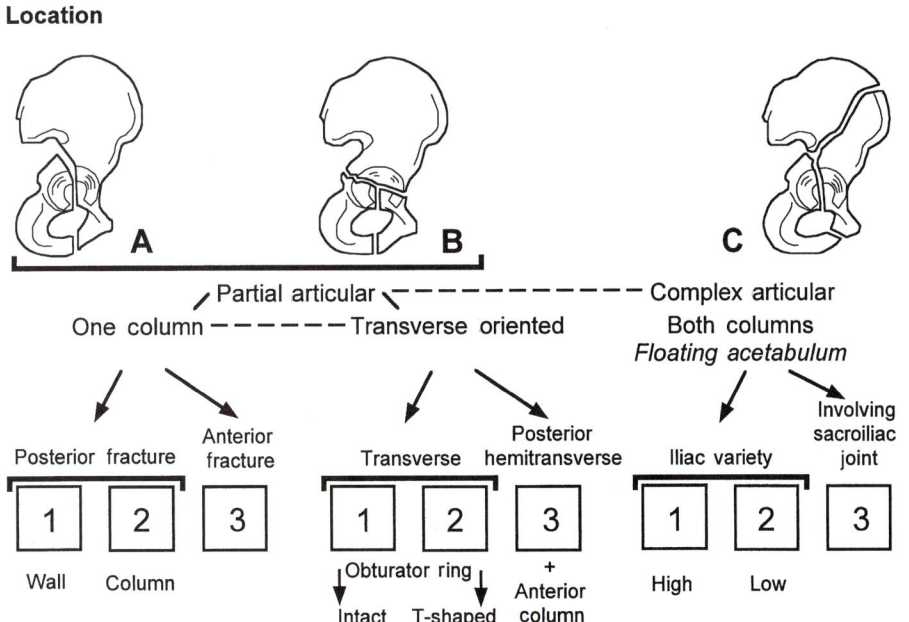

Figure 40.3. AO alphanumeric classification of acetabular fractures. Adapted from Tile M, Helfet DL, Kellam JF. Comprehensive classification of fractures in the pelvis and acetabulum. Berne, Switzerland: Muller Foundation, 1995.

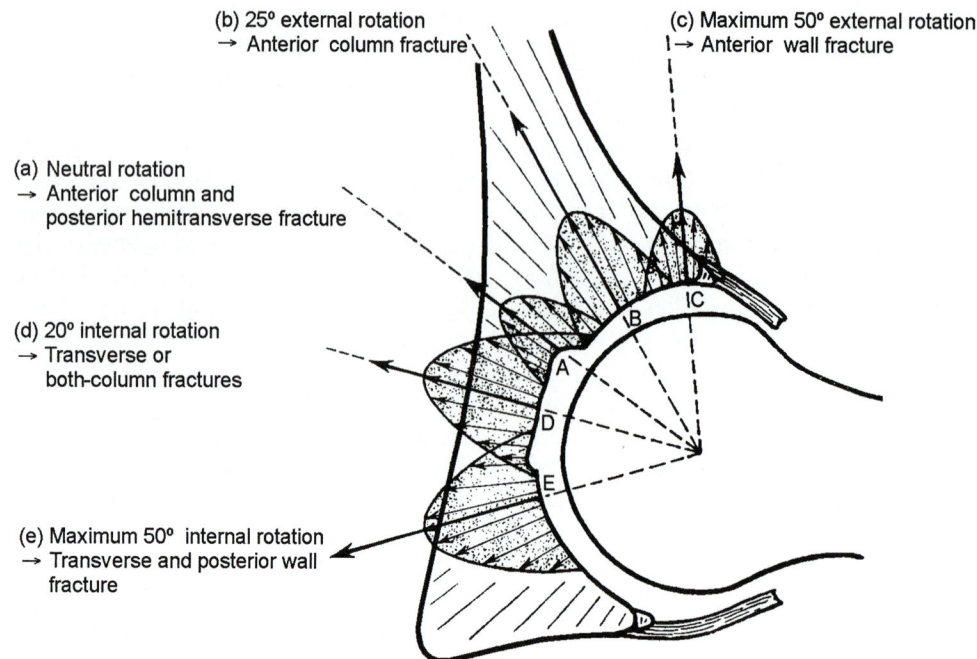

(b) 25° external rotation
→ Anterior column fracture

(c) Maximum 50° external rotation
→ Anterior wall fracture

(a) Neutral rotation
→ Anterior column and
   posterior hemitransverse fracture

(d) 20° internal rotation
→ Transverse or
   both-column fractures

(e) Maximum 50° internal rotation
→ Transverse and posterior wall
   fracture

Figure 40.4. The fracture pattern is related to the position of the femoral head relative to the acetabulum. Reprinted with permission from Letournel E, Judet R. Fractures of the acetabulum. 2nd ed. Berlin: Springer-Verlag, 1993.

Lavele lesion, an area of fluctuance secondary to a large hematoma and fat necrosis developing under the degloved skin and subcutaneous tissues. These lesions have a surprising rate of secondary bacterial contamination, despite their closed nature; and most authors recommend surgical decompression, débridement, and drainage before definitive care of the fracture (10).

An associated anterior or posterior hip dislocation occurs in 48% of acetabular fractures (3). This is considered an orthopaedic emergency and must be reduced as soon after injury as possible to decrease the risk of avascular necrosis. Reduction should be performed before proceeding to further diagnostic testing, such as CT, unless there are immediate life-threatening reasons for delaying reduction. After reduction, stability should be assessed. If there is any tendency toward redislocation, skeletal traction is indicated. A distal femoral traction pin is safest, particularly if the ligamentous status of the knee is unknown. The amount of traction weight should be no greater than one-sixth the body weight.

Patients should be carefully evaluated for neurologic and vascular deficits. An accurate neurologic examination is mandatory, as the incidence of preoperative, posttraumatic sciatic nerve compromise following acetabular fractures can range from 12 to 38% (3,4,11–18). The peroneal division of the sciatic nerve is most often involved. A thorough examination by a neurologist to document the initial neurologic status is important, particularly if there is later deterioration.

Injuries to the superior gluteal artery occur in association with acetabular fractures either as a result of the fracture pattern or as an iatrogenic insult during surgery (19,20). Letournel and Judet (3) reported an incidence of 3.5% in their series. This potentially lethal injury is most likely to occur in acetabular fractures with severe displacement of the greater sciatic notch (e.g., high transverse fractures with marked medial rotation) (5,19). Patients with unexplained hemodynamic instability or a significant drop in hematocrit should undergo pelvic angiography to evaluate for such a vascular injury. Certainly, hemodynamic instability in the presence of a documented arterial injury must be addressed, usually with arteriographic embolization of the superior gluteal artery. Once stabilized, however, concerns exist about the viability of the gluteal muscle flap.

Orthopaedic trauma patients are at high risk for developing a deep vein thrombosis (DVT) (21,22). Those with acetabular or pelvic fractures are at greatest risk, especially for proximal thrombosis with reported rates of 30 to 40% with adequate screening. Therefore, all of these patients should receive prophylaxis, especially if a delay in surgery is anticipated. Our preferred method of screening is magnetic resonance venography, which has proved to be extremely sensitive and reliable (23). Patients presenting with an increased risk of DVT and those with documented preoperative DVT are managed with an inferior vena cava filter and intravenous heparin before surgery.

RADIOLOGIC STUDIES

A thorough understanding of the complex pathoanatomy involved in the acetabular fracture is extremely important before operative fixation. An accurate diagnosis of the basic fracture pattern can be accomplished with three basic roentgenograms described by Judet et al. (6): an AP view of the pelvis, an iliac oblique view of the acetabulum, and an obturator oblique view of the acetabulum (the latter two are the so-called Judet views). These three roentgenographic views are based on the geometry of the pelvis and provide information that allows the surgeon to map the fracture pattern on a pelvic model as part of the preoperative plan. When there are associated pelvic ring disruptions, inlet and outlet views should also be obtained.

The iliac oblique view is obtained by rolling the patient 45° toward the injured side. This provides an en face view of the iliac wing and a profile of the obturator ring. The obturator oblique view, obtained by rolling the patient 45° toward the uninjured side, provides an en face view of the obturator ring, and a profile of the iliac wing. Whenever possible, the patient should be rolled and supported with foam wedges during exposure of Judet views. Tilting the X-ray beam, rather than rolling the patient, results in distorted images, making interpretation difficult.

There are six radiographic lines that must be identified and evaluated when interpreting acetabular fracture radiographs (Fig. 40.5). The two lines representing the anterior and posterior lips (walls) of the acetabulum can be differentiated by the smooth contour of the latter. The iliopectineal line represents the anterior column line and is the radiographic marker of the pelvic brim. The ilioischial line represents the posterior column and delineates the bone tangential to the quadrilateral surface, extending to the ischium. The line tangential to the superior margin of the acetabular dome, known as the roof or sourcil, represents only a 2- to 3-mm strip of bone and, therefore, does not give any indications of the overall integrity of the anatomical roof, which encompasses an arc of 50° to 60° (3). Finally, the teardrop is formed by a U-shaped continuous surface of bone, the outer part of which is the cotyloid fossa. Its inner part is the area of bone where the outer wall

of the obturator canal merges with the quadrilateral surface of the ischium. Disruption of any of these lines represents a fracture involving the corresponding bony structure.

All six lines can be identified on the AP pelvic radiograph, though incompletely. For better delineation, the iliac oblique projection demonstrates the ilioischial line and anterior lip, and the obturator oblique view demonstrates the iliopectineal line and posterior lip. It is often helpful to transfer the fracture lines from these radiographic studies to a model pelvis. Such a three-dimensional perspective can assist the surgeon in the selection of the optimal surgical approach, reduction technique(s), and method(s) of fixation for the major fracture fragments. By systematically studying these radiographic features and understanding the classification system, the surgeon can classify the fractures into one of the 10 patterns described by Letournel and Judet. The level of the fracture on all three views can be quantified with roof arc measurements. The roof arc angle is determined by extending 2 lines from the geometric center of the acetabulum, one toward the center of the roof and the other toward the intra-articular portion of the fracture.

In addition to these six lines, the surgeon must pay attention to the remainder of the bony structures seen on the plain films to avoid missing associated injuries that need concomitant stabilization or that affect the choice of surgical exposure. The obturator ring, well seen on the obturator oblique view, should be examined for fracture lines extending to the ischium, indicative of a T-type fracture. The remainder of the pelvic ring should be evaluated to assess the integrity of the sacrum, the sacroiliac joints, and the symphysis. The femoral head and neck should be scrutinized for fractures as well.

Conventional CT scans with axial cuts allow the clinician to assess the extent of injury to the acetabulum and iden-

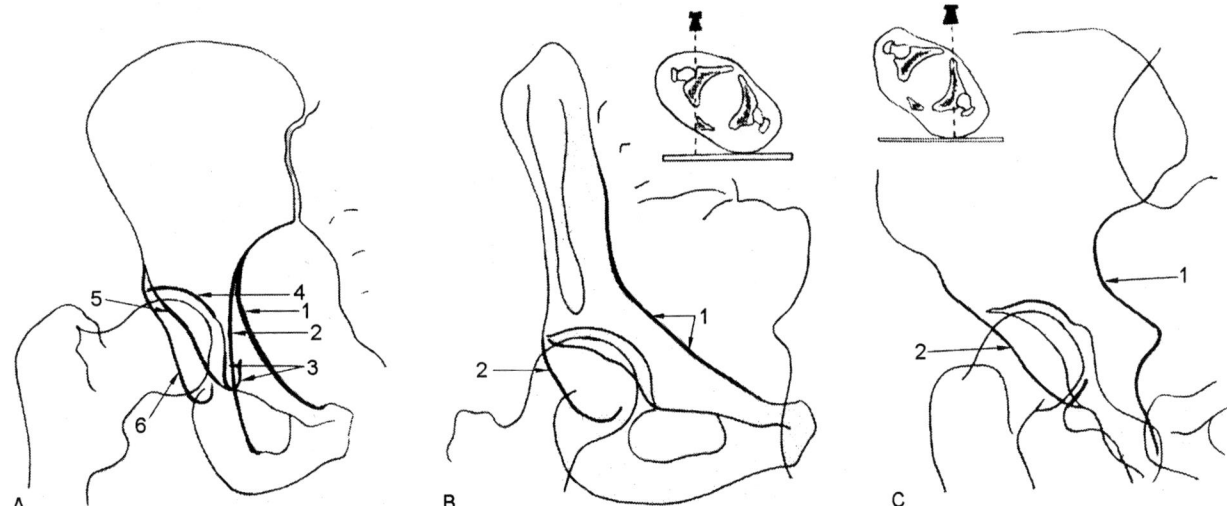

Figure 40.5. A. AP view showing the six radiographic lines. *1,* Iliopectineal line; *2,* ilioischial line; *3,* teardrop; *4,* roof; *5,* anterior wall; and *6,* posterior wall. **B.** Obturator oblique view showing the iliopectineal line (anterior column) (*1*) and the posterior wall (*2*). **C.** Iliac oblique view showing the ilioischial line (posterior column) (*1*) and the anterior wall (*2*). Reprinted with permission from Muller ME, Allgower M, et al. Manual of internal fixation: techniques recommended by the AO-ASIF group. Berlin: Springer-Verlag, 1991.

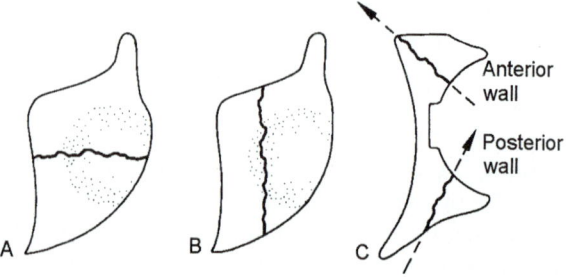

Figure 40.6. A. On a CT scan, a horizontal fracture line implies a fracture of one or both columns. **B.** A vertical fracture line is seen with transverse fractures. **C.** An oblique fracture line suggests a fracture of the wall. Reprinted with permission from Letournel E, Judet R. Fractures of the acetabulum. 2nd ed. Berlin: Springer-Verlag, 1993.

tify the size and number of posterior wall fragments, marginal impaction injuries, rotation of the columns, intra-articular fragments, and femoral head fractures (Fig. 40.6). Axial CT scans can also demonstrate associated injuries to the posterior aspect of the pelvis, such as a sacroiliac joint disruption or sacral fracture. The orientation of fracture lines on the CT study gives a clue to the type of fracture, although CT should not be a substitute for careful scrutiny of the plain films (Fig. 40.6). Fractures of one or both columns will tend to orient in the coronal plane, whereas transverse fractures are directed more in the sagittal plane. Fractures of the walls will usually be directed obliquely. Preoperative evaluation of plain films and CT scans is important for assessing the obliquity of the fracture lines (especially transverse fractures) and to best plan the proper placement of lag screws.

Advances in imaging software technology have led to the development of the three-dimensional CT, which facilitates a better understanding of the spatial relationship of the fracture pattern relative to the pelvis as a whole. Although its role is not fully defined, three-dimensional CT can be useful when viewed at real-time on a monitor that allows visualization of the fracture from various projections. Three-dimensional CT scans can be used in conjunction with plain roentgenograms, including Judet views and axial CT scans, for teaching and for facilitating preoperative planning, especially for acetabular nonunions and malunions.

TREATMENT

When selecting the proper management of an acetabular fracture, the surgeon must assess the risks and benefits of surgical intervention as opposed to nonoperative treatment. Because acetabular fractures should be treated with the same principles governing other intra-articular fractures, the primary goal in their management is to perform an accurate reduction of the articular surface to obtain a congruent hip joint, thus restoring normal joint mechanics. Malreduction or subluxation of the hip joint can lead to abnormal loading of the articular cartilage and subsequent joint arthrosis.

Judet and Letournel were among the first to recommend operative fixation of all displaced acetabular fractures to anatomically restore the weight-bearing articular surface of the acetabulum and obtain a concentric reduction of the hip. Today, most authors agree that these steps are essential to lessen the likelihood of posttraumatic arthritis and obtain long-term satisfactory results (1,3,4,6,15–17,24–38). The explanation for this shift in thinking over the past 30 years is directly related to the advances made in surgical technique. In the hands of a skilled acetabular surgeon, the risk–benefit analysis usually shifts in favor of open reduction and internal fixation (ORIF). Therefore, nonoperative treatment is rarely indicated, particularly for displaced fractures of the acetabulum. No matter what the fracture pattern or personality of the injury, however, poor surgical planning and technique will guarantee poor results.

When determining the optimal management of an acetabular fracture, certain findings unquestionably mitigate in favor of operative stabilization: displacement of the articular surface, incongruence of the joint, unacceptable roof arc measurements of less than 45° (15), incarceration of an intra-articular fragment within the joint, and any subluxation of the femoral head. It must be remembered, however, that the requirement for a successful outcome is a stable hip joint with a concentric reduction, regardless of the presence of a plate and screws. Nondisplaced fractures that satisfy these criteria will heal readily and can often be treated nonoperatively.

Conservative management may also be considered for displaced fractures that do not extend into the weight-bearing dome. Among this group are low anterior column fractures, which involve only the inferior portion of the anterior acetabulum, and small posterior wall fractures, which involve less than 25% of the posterior wall measured by CT. Low transverse fractures with roof arc angles greater than 45° on all three x-ray views are considered appropriate for nonoperative treatment. Associated both-column fractures with excellent secondary congruence are occasionally considered for conservative treatment, particularly in low-demand individuals.

Patient-based factors must also be considered when determining a treatment plan. Severe preexisting medical comorbidities may increase the risks of prolonged anesthesia or blood loss and thus favor conservative management; however, subsequent reconstructive surgery (ORIF or arthroplasty) of an acetabular malunion or nonunion is quite difficult. Therefore, medical conditions should be aggressively managed perioperatively to permit surgical intervention, when indicated. Nonoperative treatment typically enforces a period of prolonged bed rest, with its own inherent risks. Severe osteoporosis limits the ability to achieve rigid and secure fixation and is a relative contraindication to internal fixation. Preexisting osteoarthrosis may also affect the treatment plan. Early degenerative changes do not necessarily preclude ORIF. If significant osteoarthritis or associated femoral head damage is present, then primary total hip arthroplasty should be given consideration (Fig. 40.7).

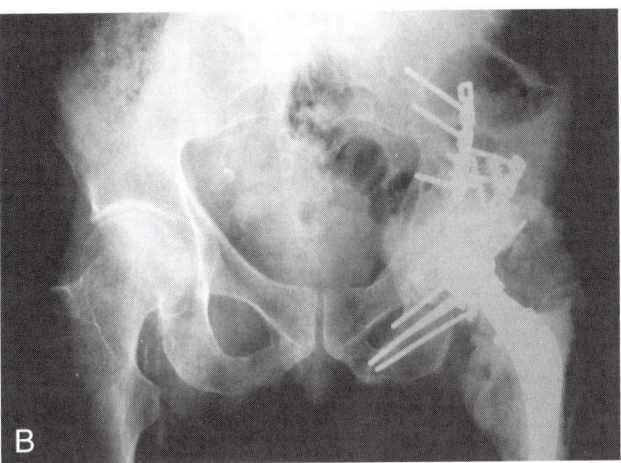

Figure 40.7. A. CT study of an 85-year-old patient showing an acetabular fracture and impaction injury to the femoral head. **B.** Postoperative view showing extensive heterotopic ossification around the acetabulum.

Operative Treatment

TIMING AND CHOICE OF SURGICAL APPROACH

The timing of surgery depends on several factors, including the availability of an experienced surgeon; stabilization of associated visceral, skeletal, and soft tissue injuries; and completion of all imaging studies necessary for preoperative planning. A femoral head dislocation or an incarcerated intra-articular fragment following closed reduction needs to be addressed promptly to minimize the incidence of femoral head avascular necrosis and post-traumatic arthritis.

The goal of the surgeon is to restore joint congruency with the least morbidity. To this end, the approach used is often dictated by the experience of the operating surgeon but should provide the greatest chance of anatomic reduction and stabilization of the joint surface. Mayo (5) noted five major factors that affect this selection: the fracture pattern, the local soft tissue conditions, the presence of associated major systemic injuries, the age and projected functional status of the patient, and the delay to surgery. When open treatment is indicated, the majority of acetabular fractures can be managed through a single surgical approach after an appropriate preoperative evaluation of the fracture pattern (29,39,40). Helfet and Schmeling (40) treated 93 acetabular fractures involving two columns. Using the technique of indirect reduction, they found that 84 cases required only a single ilioinguinal, or Kocher-Langenbeck, approach. A satisfactory reduction was achieved in 91% of cases, the deep infection rate was 0%, and the incidence of significant heterotopic ossification was 2%.

For more complex fracture patterns involving both acetabular columns, most authors have recommended the use of an extensile or combined anterior and posterior approaches for greater visualization and reduction (1,3,17, 24,25,32,34,36–38). Compared to dual approaches, extensile exposures appear to involve greater patient morbidity, including increased operative time, blood loss, infection, postoperative nerve injury, abductor weakness, joint stiffness and heterotopic ossification (17,24,26, 32,34,37,38,41). Both extensile and dual approaches have their own indications, and one does not replace the other.

The three most frequently used approaches for acetabular fracture surgery remain the Kocher-Langenbeck, the ilioinguinal, and the extended iliofemoral (Clinical Table). The Kocher-Langenbeck approach gives access to the retroacetabular surface of the innominate bone from the ischium to the greater sciatic notch (Fig. 40.8A). Access to the quadrilateral surface is possible by palpation through the greater and lesser sciatic notches, which allows assessment after the reduction of fractures involving the quadrilateral plate and anterior column. The greater sciatic notch provides a window for placing clamps to manipulate and reduce these fractures. The superior gluteal neurovascular bundle limits access to the superior iliac wing in this approach.

Nonoperative Treatment

Nonoperative treatment consists of bed rest, with or without traction, depending on the stability of the hip joint. An optional abduction pillow helps position the hip and reduces the likelihood of dislocation. Active motion should be encouraged for hip joints with stable reductions. Patients with small posterior wall fractures can be mobilized rapidly; but hip flexion beyond 60° to 80° and weight bearing greater than 9 kg (20 lb) should be avoided until adequate healing is present. Similarly, patients with low transverse fractures can be mobilized as comfort allows, with toe-touch weight bearing. To lessen the risk of redislocation, patients with unstable hip joints require 6 to 8 weeks of bed rest, with or without traction, before mobilization. While recumbent, an aggressive regimen of pulmonary toilet must be maintained. Immobilized and bedridden patients are also at extremely high risk for DVT, and prophylaxis with warfarin or a vena cava filter is mandatory.

Clinical Table: Acetabular Fractures

Procedure	Indications	Technique	Anatomy	Pitfalls
Kocher-Langenbeck approach	• Posterior wall • Posterior column • Transverse • Transverse with posterior wall • Some T-types	• Leave capsule intact	• Sciatic nerve • External rotators • Posterior column and wall of acetabulum	• Indirect reduction of anterior component of transverse fracture
Ilioinguinal approach	• Anterior column • Associated both-column • Anterior column with posterior hemitransverse	• Leave fascia intact over femoral vessels • Penrose around inguinal canal, femoral vessels, iliopsoas, and femoral nerve • Detach iliopectineal fascia	• Femoral vessels and nerve • Lateral femoral cutaneous nerve • Internal surface of ilium and pubic ramus	• Indirect reduction of posterior column
Extended iliofemoral approach	• Late associated both-column • Complex transverse • T-type	• Detach abductors from greater trochanter • Repair with nonabsorbable suture • Capsulotomy at rim	• Abductors of hip • Sciatic nerve • Combines posterior approach with Smith-Peterson approach	• Heterotopic ossification • Risk of abductor flap necrosis

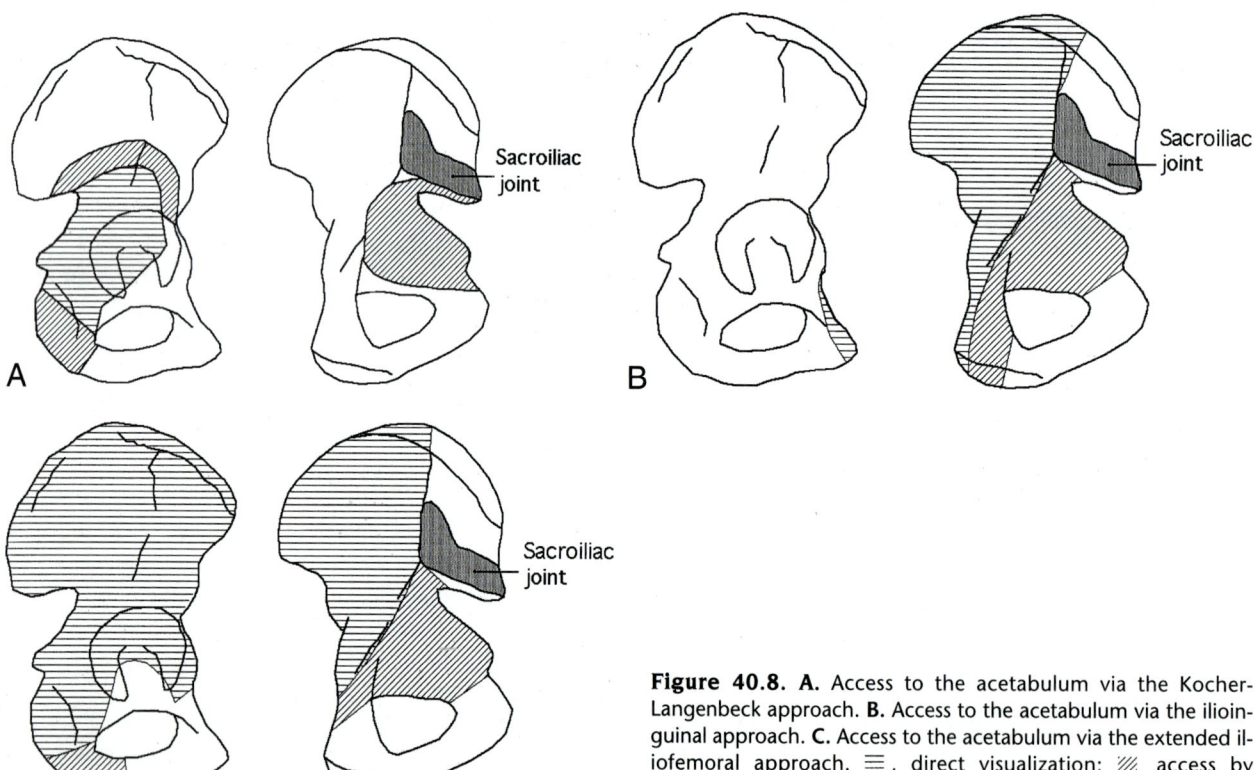

Figure 40.8. A. Access to the acetabulum via the Kocher-Langenbeck approach. **B.** Access to the acetabulum via the ilioinguinal approach. **C.** Access to the acetabulum via the extended iliofemoral approach. ≡, direct visualization; ▨, access by palpation.

The ilioinguinal approach, introduced by Letournel and Judet (1–3), offers direct visualization of the iliac wing, anterior sacroiliac joint, the entire anterior column, and the pubic symphysis (Fig. 40.8B). The extended iliofemoral approach, also introduced by Letournel, is an anatomic approach that follows an internervous plane, reflecting the muscles innervated by the femoral nerve anteriorly and the muscles innervated by the superior and inferior gluteal nerves posteriorly (Fig. 40.8C). The posterior flap is mobilized as a unit, without damaging its neurovascular bundles (3).

Posterior wall, posterior column, and comminuted posterior variants are fracture patterns that can be consistently reduced through a standard Kocher-Langenbeck approach. For transverse and T-type fractures, the proper approach depends on the obliquity of the transverse fracture, the direction of rotation, and the column with the major displacement. If the major displacement is posterior, particularly in an infratectal or juxtatectal fracture, and there is an associated posterior wall fracture, then the Kocher-Langenbeck approach should be used. If the major displacement or rotation is primarily anterior, then the ilioinguinal approach should be employed. T-type or high transtectal transverse patterns (among the most difficult patterns to treat) that involve the weight-bearing dome often require an extensile approach to gain adequate access to the roof of the acetabulum.

Anterior column and/or wall fractures are directly visualized through the ilioinguinal approach. Both-column acetabular fractures are also ideally approached and stabilized through the ilioinguinal approach. This requires an indirect reduction of the posterior column and hence cannot be performed if the fracture is more than 2 to 3 weeks old. In addition, significant involvement of the posterior wall, comminuted fractures of the posterior column, involvement of the sacroiliac joint, and the presence of lateral dome involvement preclude this approach and require an extensile exposure

Because they have the greatest morbidity of any surgical approach to the acetabulum, extensile approaches are not the first choice for most fractures (3–5,42,43); however, they are preferred for the difficult fracture patterns already discussed and in other situations. Infection rates with the ilioinguinal approach are high in the presence of nearby suprapubic catheters and colostomies (34). Surgical treatment of acetabular fractures after a delay of 2 to 3 weeks is difficult without significant exposure, and the ability to obtain an anatomic reduction drops from 75 to 62% of cases, because of the difficult task of meticulously taking down increasing amounts of callus (3,44). The major technical limitation of the extended iliofemoral exposure is access to the low anterior column (5). Dissection becomes more difficult and dangerous as the surgeon dissects medial to the iliopectineal eminence, where the psoas muscle and iliopectineal fascia block progress.

Alternatives to the extensile approach are a simultaneous approach and a sequential anterior and posterior approach. Using the latter, Routt and Swiontkowski (36) were able to obtain an anatomic reduction in 96% of 108 complex acetabular fractures. Complications included iatrogenic nerve injury in 5%, deep infection in 3%, pulmonary embolism in 3%, and functionally significant heterotopic ossification in 5% of cases. The theoretical advantage of separate anterior and posterior approaches is the avoidance of complete detachment of the gluteal flap from the iliac wing. While performing the extended iliofemoral approach, the detachment retains only one major blood supply to the flap: the superior gluteal artery. This has lead to concern that damage to this structure, either at the time of injury or at the time of the extensile approach, will lead to complete ischemic necrosis of the flap (5,45).

In fact, the incidence of complete ischemic necrosis of the abductor flap is relatively low (3,46). Letournel, Matta, Mast, and Martimbeau reported no such cases in more than 400 acetabular fractures addressed with an extended iliofemoral approach (3). Furthermore, a recent canine study by Tabor et al. (47) confirmed that, although some ischemic necrosis of the gluteal muscle does occur after the extended iliofemoral approach, following a complete ligation of the gluteal vessels complete necrosis is rare. Thus the case for abductor necrosis may be overstated. This is important, because a combined surgical approach in the floppy lateral position provides suboptimal visualization of the fracture pattern from either approach. Extensile approaches still remain a viable strategy, especially for high transtectal T-type fractures and fractures treated more than 2 weeks postinjury.

In cases when the surgeon is uncertain regarding his or her ability to reduce a complex acetabular fracture through a single approach (e.g., with a both-column or T-type fracture), the patient should be prepared and draped in the floppy lateral position. This will permit the use of a combined anterior and posterior approach, if necessary. The initial approach should be directed at the column with the greater displacement, and the initial attempt should be to obtain an indirect reduction of the less-involved column through the single nonextensile incision. If necessary, the patient can be turned and the beanbag adjusted, to allow ORIF through a second approach. A second option is to close the wounds of the first approach, and then reprepare and drape the patient.

Blunt trauma to the gluteal muscle mass and peritrochanteric region is perhaps the most troubling finding when planning a posterior or extensile approach, because a Morel-Lavele (closed degloving injury) lesion may be present. A last and relative contraindication for an extensile approach is the presence of a closed-head injury that has the potential in and of itself to lead to massive heterotopic ossification (48).

OPERATING ROOM PREPARATION

The patient is placed on a radiolucent operating table that allows intraoperative traction and fluoroscopy. All cases should be performed under general anesthesia with hypotension, if possible, to decrease blood loss. Epidural catheterization is beneficial because less inhaled anesthetic is required, blood loss is reduced, and postoperative pain relief is improved (5). A Foley catheter should be placed in the patient's bladder. Vascular access with two large-bore intravenous catheters is required, as there is a capacity for significant blood loss during these lengthy procedures. Patients with advanced age or significant medical conditions may require arterial or central line placement. An intraoperative cell saver permits recycling of about 20 to 30% of the effective blood loss (49) and minimizes the patient's exposure to banked blood.

Both somatosensory evoked potentials (SSEPs) and electromyography (EMG) have been shown to afford a degree of protective surveillance (11,13,14). These techniques are especially important for patients at risk for developing an iatrogenic sciatic nerve injury, i.e., those already demonstrating preoperative nerve compromise and those with a fracture pattern that includes a posterior column or wall fracture. The entire extremity is prepared free, and sterile subdermal electrodes are inserted. For intraoperative EMG, motor electrodes are placed within the tibialis anterior, peroneus longus, flexor hallucis brevis, and abductor hallucis muscles. Sciatic nerve compromise can be detected through intraoperative monitoring of real-time EMG activity or by significant unilateral changes in amplitude and latency of the SSEPs. When such compromise is detected, a prompt response is required. Traction should be released, and retractors that have been placed against the nerve should be removed until the EMG activity ceases or the potentials return to baseline.

SURGICAL ANATOMY

Many neurovascular structures are encountered during ORIF of an acetabular fracture. The relative risk of damage to each structure depends on the approach used, but those generally at greatest risk and that require the most vigilance and care during dissection are discussed below.

Sciatic Nerve

The sciatic nerve is at risk during exposure of the posterior column and needs to be identified along the belly of the quadratus femoris muscle and then protected behind the conjoined tendons of the obturator internus and gemelli (Fig. 40.9). Traction along the nerve should be avoided by maintaining the hip extended and the knee flexed at all times. This structure is at particular risk during the Kocher-Langenbeck and extended iliofemoral approaches.

Lateral Femoral Cutaneous Nerve

The lateral femoral cutaneous nerve is at risk when dissecting along the anterior superior iliac spine. It can also sustain a traction injury during mobilization of the soft tissues. Releasing some of its fibrous attachments to the abdominal musculature can often reduce tension on this structure. Patients should be warned preoperatively to expect the complication of lateral thigh paresthesia. This

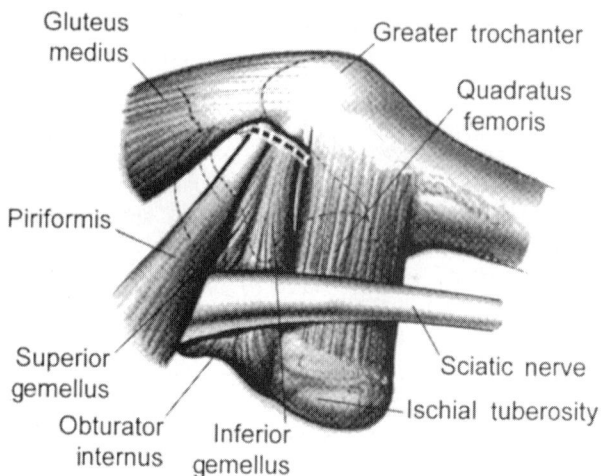

Figure 40.9. The sciatic nerve crosses underneath the piriformis but above the obturator internus and gemelli. Reprinted with permission from Hoppenfeld S, deBoer P. Surgical approaches in orthopaedics: the anatomic approach. Philadelphia: Lippincott, 1984:341.

structure is at particular risk with the ilioinguinal and extended iliofemoral approaches.

Superior Gluteal Neurovascular Bundle

Superior gluteal neurovascular bundle injury can result from severe displacement of the sciatic notch caused by a high transverse fracture with marked medial rotation or from an iatrogenic insult during surgery (5,19,20). Letournel and Judet (3) reported an incidence of 3.5% in their series. The neurovascular bundle is at greatest risk during exposure of the greater sciatic notch, irrespective of the approach, and must be protected from undue traction or damage by retractors.

Femoral Neurovascular Structures

The femoral nerve is at risk during mobilization and excessive retraction of the iliopsoas muscle during the ilioinguinal approach. Hip flexion provides some relaxation of the iliopsoas muscle and minimizes the need for any undue retraction. The femoral vessels are especially at risk during mobilization of the vascular compartment off the iliopectineal fascia. They must be isolated with a broad Penrose drain and protected throughout the procedure. Leaving the conjoined tendon intact over their surface protects them from undue dissection and retraction. The femoral neurovascular structures are also at great risk when dissecting past the medial extent of the extended iliofemoral approach (iliopsoas muscle and iliopectineal eminence) without an additional ilioinguinal incision.

Pudendal Nerve

The pudendal nerve is at risk as it exits the pelvis through the greater sciatic notch, wraps around the ischial spine, and travels back into the pelvis through the lesser sciatic notch. It is at particular risk during the Kocher-Langenbeck and extended iliofemoral approaches.

Inguinal Canal

An inadequate closure of the floor of the inguinal canal can lead to a direct hernia. A sound closure of the insertion of the transversalis abdominis muscle and the internal oblique muscle to the inguinal ligament is necessary. The contents of the spermatic cord are at risk during exposure of the external inguinal ring and should be carefully isolated and retracted with a Penrose drain.

Medial Femoral Circumflex Artery

The medial femoral circumflex artery is at risk during exposure of the posterior column. Its branches lie deep in the belly of the quadratus femoris muscle and can be injured if the muscle is released at its insertion on the femur.

Corona Mortis

During the ilioinguinal approach, it is important to search for the corona mortis, a variable retropubic anastomosis that should be ligated if identified.

Obturator Artery and Nerve

The obturator artery and nerve are also at risk during exposure of the quadrilateral surface and must be protected with carefully placed retractors.

KOCHER-LANGENBECK APPROACH

For the Kocher-Langenbeck approach, the patient is positioned in either the lateral decubitus or prone position, depending on the fracture pattern. We typically position patients with an isolated posterior wall fracture laterally, which has the advantage of easier intraoperative management, especially anesthetic concerns. For transverse fractures, the weight of the leg will often interfere with reductions from the lateral decubitus position. In these cases, a prone position is often preferred. During the Kocher-Langenbeck approach, the sciatic nerve is in danger and constant vigilance and protection of the nerve is mandatory. The maintenance of knee flexion and hip extension throughout the procedure lessens tension on the sciatic nerve, affording a degree of protection.

The incision is centered over the posterior half of the greater trochanter and is extended distally along the shaft of the femur for approximately 8 cm. Proximally, the incision is curved posteriorly toward the posterior superior iliac spine for another 8 cm (Fig. 40.10). The fascia lata is then split in line with the skin incision distally, and the gluteus maximus and its fascia are split in line with the muscle fibers proximally by blunt dissection. Distally, the gluteus maximus tendinous insertion onto the femur is sharply released. The sciatic nerve can be consistently identified and isolated along the medial aspect of the quadratus femoris fascia.

The short external rotators, particularly the piriformis and the conjoined tendons of the gemelli and obturator

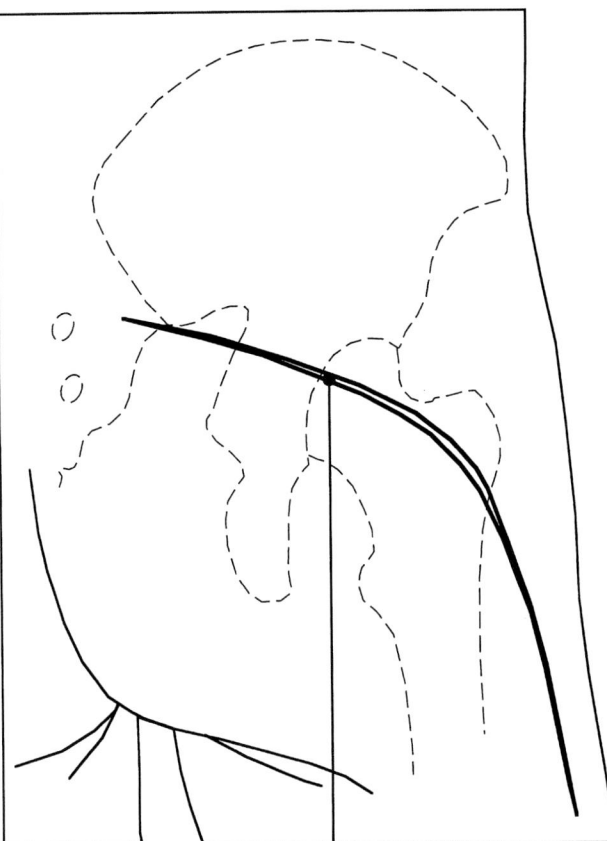

Figure 40.10. Skin incision for the Kocher-Langenbeck approach.

internus are visualized, placed on stretch by internal rotation of the hip, tagged, and reflected from their femoral insertions. The obturator internus muscle can be traced back to its origin from the lesser sciatic notch. Retraction of this tendon, provides both access to the lesser sciatic notch and protection to the sciatic nerve, which passes superficial to the tendon. Retraction of the piriformis tendon provides access to the greater sciatic notch but fails to protect the sciatic nerve, which exits the notch deep to the tendon (Fig. 40.11).

Two blunt Hohmann retractors are carefully placed in the greater and lesser sciatic notches to provide visualization of the entire retroacetabular surface. It is critical to maintain the latter consistently with the tendon of the obturator internus to provide a protective layer of soft tissue between the retractor and the sciatic nerve. If necessary, the distal portion of the posterior column can be visualized to the ischial tuberosity by sharply releasing some of the origin of the hamstring muscles.

In the region of the ischial spine, take care to protect the pudendal nerve as it passes over the external surface of the spine. Caution should also be taken in identifying and protecting the superior gluteal neurovascular bundle as it exits the greater sciatic notch in the region of the sciatic buttress. Excess traction on the bundle may tear the artery or stretch the nerve, leading to disastrous conse-

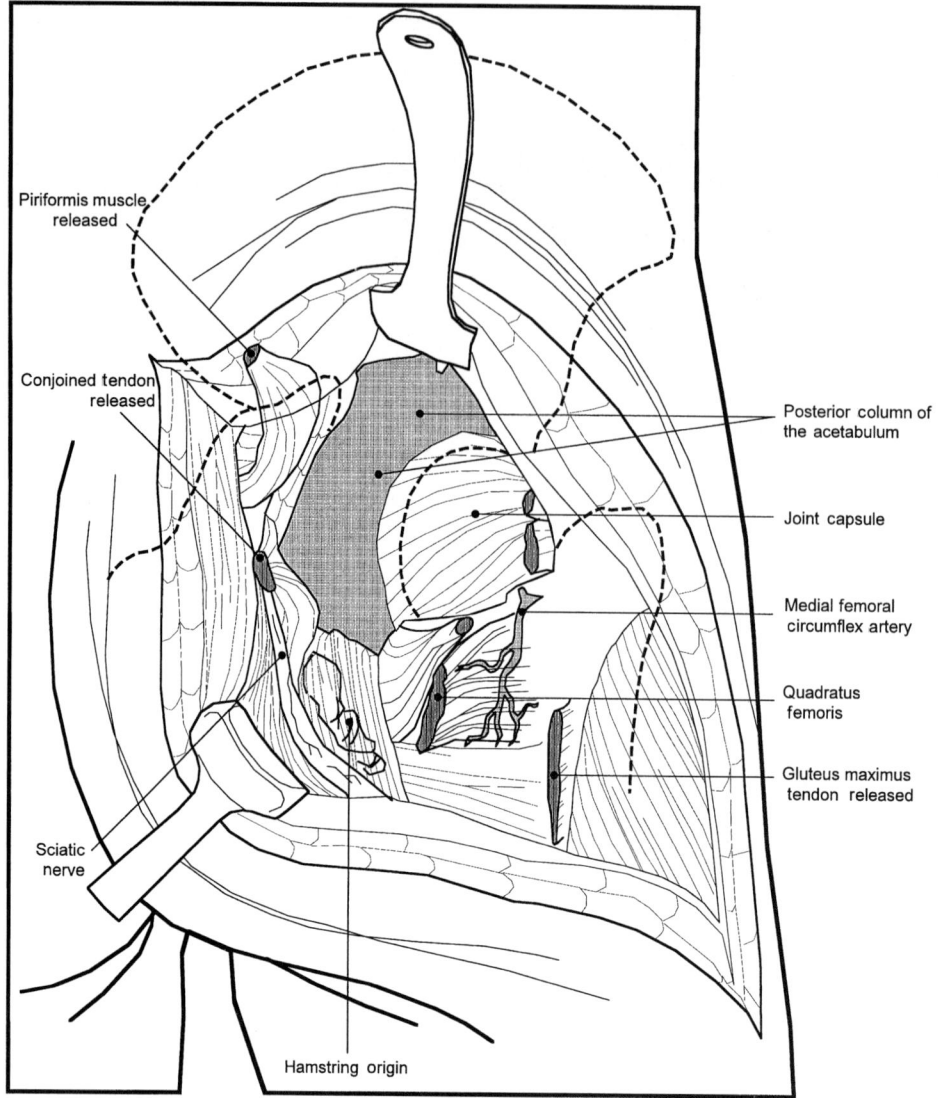

Figure 40.11. Deep exposure for the Kocher-Langenbeck approach.

quences. Once the retractors have been placed and the exposure completed, vigilance must be maintained.

Uncommonly, such as in high transtectal transverse or T-type fractures, an osteotomy of the greater trochanter is required to gain access to the superior weight-bearing surface of the acetabulum. The advantages of this technique are improved exposure of the superior aspect of the acetabulum to the anterior inferior iliac spine and decreased tension on the superior gluteal neurovascular bundle (24); however, the greater trochanter is at risk for nonunion. Furthermore, the increased gluteal muscle stripping associated with this technique results in a significantly greater risk for heterotopic ossification (41).

Reduction Techniques

Intraoperative traction is crucial because it leads to an indirect reduction of fragments that have retained their capsular or soft tissue attachments. Distal traction can also be used to subluxate the femoral head inferiorly from within the acetabulum, allowing visualization of the joint, removal of loose fragments, and reduction of the fracture, especially with margin impaction injuries. Traction can be applied by several means. The classic method is the use of the Judet table, which permits lateral and longitudinal traction, in concert with the image intensifier (3,32); however, fractures of the contralateral superior and inferior pubic rami preclude the use of the fracture table, since the perineal post tends to increase the pelvic deformity.

The preferred alternative is to position the patient on a radiolucent table and drape the leg free, allowing manipulation of the hip joint throughout the procedure. Once the fracture is exposed, the AO universal large distractor (Synthes; Paoli, PA) is applied with two 5-mm Schanz pins, one into the sciatic buttress proximally and the other into the femur at the level of the lesser trochanter (Fig. 40.12). Other supplemental forms of traction include direct

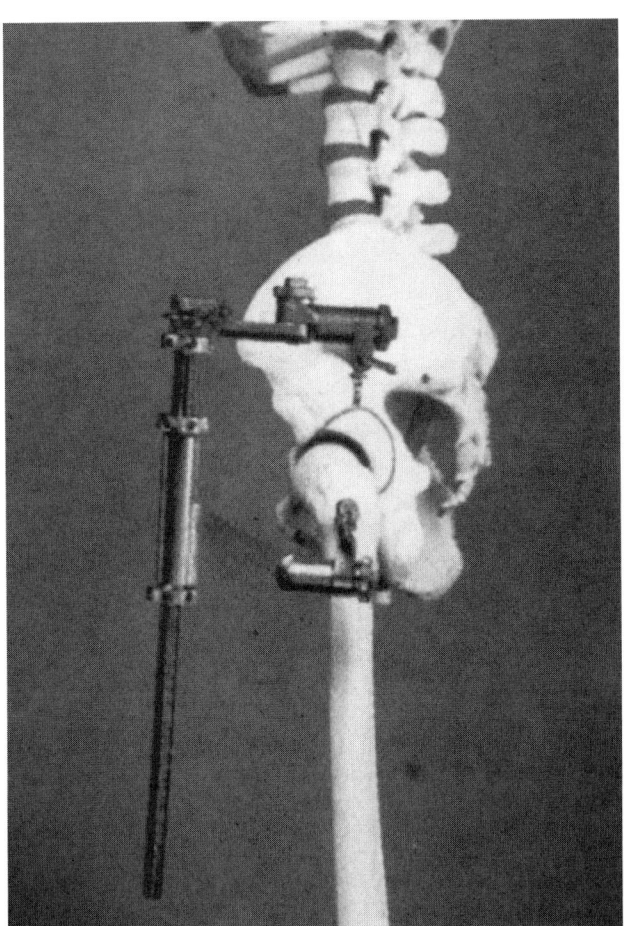

Figure 40.12. An AO universal large distractor is placed to allow distraction of the hip joint for inspection and débridement. The Schanz pin in the ilium is placed to avoid interference with the fixation plate.

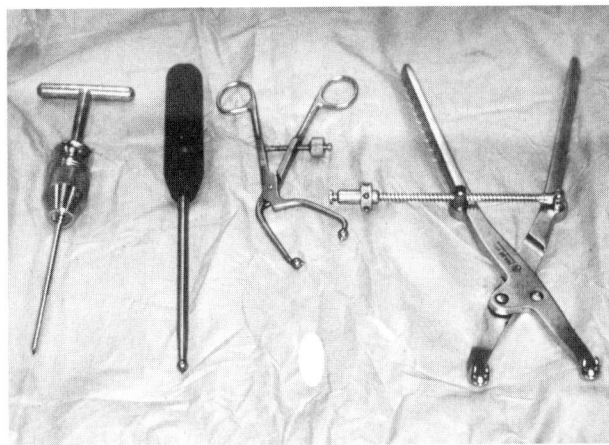

Figure 40.13. Reduction tools. *Left to right:* Schanz pin on T-handle chuck, ball-spiked pusher, angled-jaw reduction forceps, and screw-holding reduction clamp.

manual traction through the thigh using a Schanz pin attached to the AO universal T-handle chuck (Synthes; Paoli, PA) placed laterally into the femoral head.

A wide variety of reduction tools are available for use at different sites along the bony pelvis (Figs. 40.13 and 40.14). Typically, more than one reduction forceps is required to correct each of the displacement vectors. Modifications of pointed reduction forceps, including king-tong and queen-tong clamps, permit application from the outer and inner pelvic surfaces or from the greater sciatic notch to the anterior inferior iliac spine. These are particularly useful for manipulating the quadrilateral surface in transverse or T-type fracture patterns. The Lambotte-Farabeuf clamp and the large screw-holding AO pelvic reduction clamp (Synthes; Paoli, PA) are designed to anchor to screw heads on each side of a major fracture line. These clamps provide substantial leverage and rotational control of fracture fragments and can be used to obtain initial distraction of the fracture, followed by a controlled reduction and then compression of the fracture.

Posterior wall fractures. Single large fragments are often easily reduced and stabilized, which might lead the sur-

geon to the conclusion that isolated posterior wall fractures are simple fractures to treat. Unfortunately, this belief is incorrect. Posterior wall fractures are frequently complicated by comminution and marginal impaction, which significantly increases their level of surgical difficulty; thus these fractures have some of the poorest outcomes of the acetabulum fractures, especially when associated with a posterior column or transverse fracture pattern (3,4,50).

Marginal impaction of the articular surface occurs in 16 to 23% of cases and is usually associated with a posterior hip dislocation (3,50). As the femoral head dislocates, it not only fractures the posterior wall but implodes the articular surface. The CT scan should be scrutinized to assess the status of the posterior wall and to determine any evidence of comminution or marginal impaction (Fig. 40.15). If the latter diagnosis is missed or not addressed, a poor result is almost guaranteed.

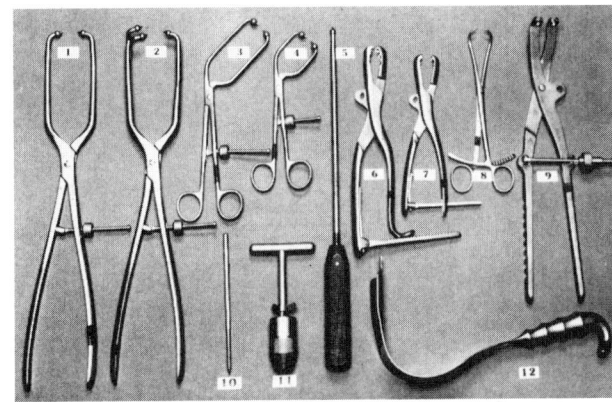

Figure 40.14. Reduction clamps. *1,* King-tong clamp; *2,* queentong clamp; *3,* large angled-jaw reduction clamp; *6* and *7,* Lambotte-Farabeuf reduction clamp; *8,* Weber clamp. Reprinted with permission from Muller ME, Allgower M, et al. Manual of internal fixation: techniques recommended by the AO-ASIF group. Berlin: Springer-Verlag, 1991.

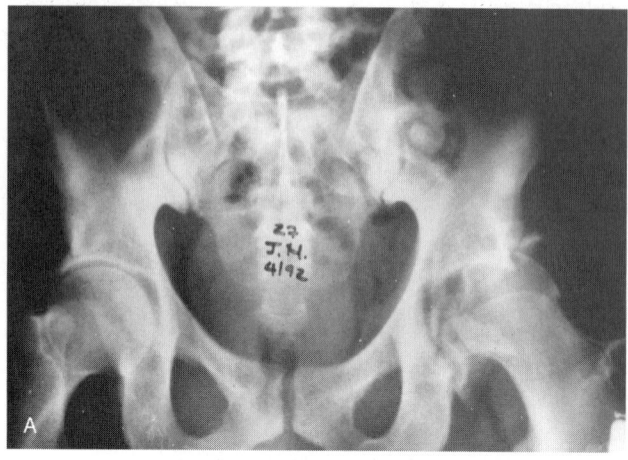

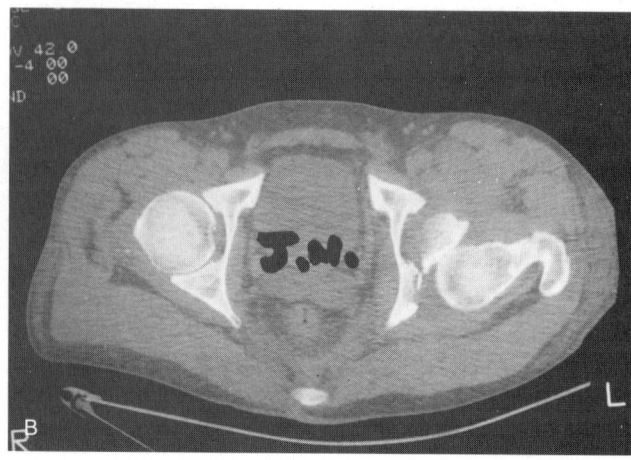

Marginal impaction of the dome

Posterior

Hip joint

Anterior

Femoral head

Figure 40.15. **A.** AP view showing comminuted posterior wall fracture with posterior dislocation. **B.** CT scan showing a large intra-articular fragment that renders the hip irreducible. Note the marginal impaction of posterior wall. **C.** Intraoperative view showing marginal impaction of the acetabular joint surface. **D.** Postoperative AP view.

Subluxation of the femoral head from the joint permits inspection of the articular surface and débridement of loose bodies or redundant ligamentum teres, which will prevent a concentric reduction. Once an adequate débridement is completed, the femoral head is anatomically reduced and used as a template for the articular reduction. Any impacted fragments are gently elevated into a position congruent with the femoral head. Most often, when a marginally impacted piece of articular surface is elevated, there is a metaphyseal defect underlying the articular fragment. Autologous cancellous bone, obtained through a small window in the greater trochanter, is used to buttress these fragments. Next, reduction of the cortical wall fragments is easily performed using the straight ball

spike pusher (Synthes; Paoli, PA), followed by provisional fixation with Kirschner (K) wires.

In the course of dissection, the medial aspect of each wall fragment should be cleared of enough soft tissue to permit visualization of its reduction, but the surgeon should retain as much capsular attachment as possible to preserve the blood supply. The surgeon must be aware of the orientation and geometry of the wall fragments to avoid placing the screws in the intra-articular space. Thus each wall fragment should be inspected before its final reduction and provisionally fixed with a K wire. Provisional reduction and immobilization of small fragments can also be achieved by using the straight ball spike pusher. The assistant should not exert excessive pressure with this instrument, since these fragile pieces are easily comminuted.

A 3.5-mm reconstruction plate is then applied in the buttress mode over the reduced posterior wall and anchored to the ilium proximally and the ischium distally. An underbent plate, in relation to the posterior wall, will help reduce the construct and compress the fracture. To best prevent fracture displacement, one or more lag screws should be placed through the plate and posterior wall into the posterior column.

When the posterior wall is significantly comminuted, it is not possible to restore all the small articular fragments with individual lag screws. In this situation, the surgeon can use spring-hook plates. These are two-, three-, or four-hole one-third tubular plates that have had an end cut off through a hole; the prongs thus created are bent downward to create hooks that are placed into the small fragments on the cortical surface (15,51) (Fig. 40.16). When overcontoured, they further reduce the small fragments to the femoral head.

Posterior column fractures. A posterior column fracture rarely occurs as an isolated injury; it is more frequently associated with a posterior wall fracture. The posterior col-

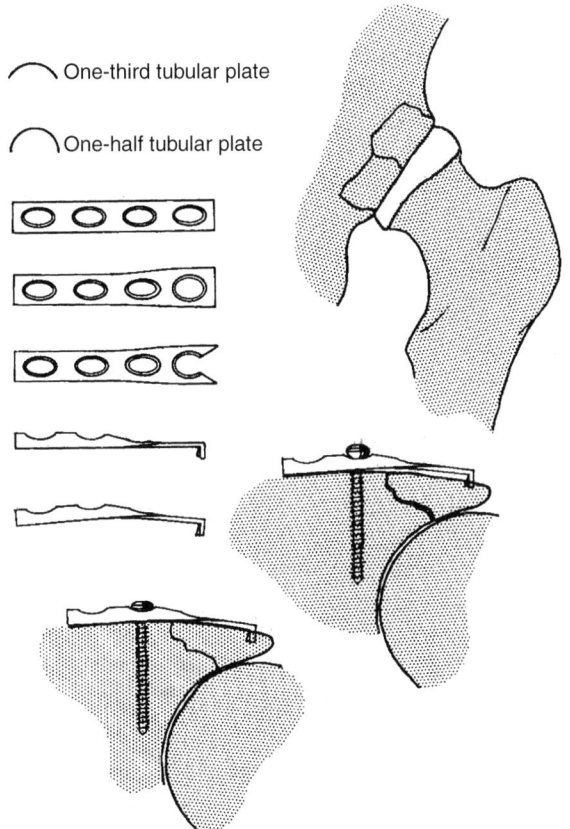

One-third tubular plate

One-half tubular plate

Figure 40.16. The one-third tubular plate is used as a spring plate to fix small fragments of the posterrior wall. Reprinted with permission frm Mast JW, Ganz R, Jakob RP. Planning and reduction technique in fracture surgery. New York: Springer-Verlag. 1989:244

umn is typically displaced posteriorly and medially, and internally rotated.

Dissection should be performed to allow the surgeon to place a finger through the greater sciatic notch to palpate the proximal fracture line along the quadrilateral surface. Reduction of the displaced posterior column fragments is usually accomplished with the spiked AO pelvic reduction forceps (Synthes; Paoli, PA). This clamp is applied to each of the main column fragments, away from the eventual location of the plate. Derotation of the inferior portion of the posterior column fragment can be facilitated by placing a 5-mm Schanz pin, attached to an AO universal T-handle chuck, into the ischium. Direct visual inspection of the posterior fracture line best assesses displacement of the column. Rotation is best judged by digital palpation along the quadrilateral surface, which should be smooth after a proper reduction.

The surgeon must be aware of the location of the gluteal neurovascular bundle throughout the reduction, because displacement of the bundle into the fracture site or a stretch injury is possible. Once reduction has been accomplished, a K wire is used to provisionally fix the fracture fragments and to allow the application of a 3.5-mm reconstruction plate from the sciatic buttress to the ischium, spanning the posterior column. A lag screw across the fracture and into the anterior column is necessary to prevent redisplacement. In the case of an associated posterior wall fracture, the wall fragment should be treated as previously described, with separate buttress plates for both the wall and the column fractures.

Transverse fractures. Reduction and stabilization of transverse fractures employ techniques similar to those used for posterior column fractures. The reduction, however, is more difficult because the anterior column is also involved. Displacement can be controlled by using an AO pelvic reduction clamp and 4.5-mm screws placed on opposite sides of the fracture (Fig. 40.17). Rotation can be controlled with either a Schanz pin placed in the medial portion of the ischial tuberosity or a pelvic reduction forceps with pointed ball tips placed in the sciatic notch. An elegant technique is to use a plate secured into one of the fracture fragments, which is then manipulated and drawn to facilitate reduction of the other fragment. Once reduced, these fragments are provisionally fixed with K wires, unless a plate has been used, in which case it is fixed with screws. The reduction is assessed by inspecting the retroacetabular surface and by palpation along the quadrilateral surface. Once provisional fixation of the transverse component with a K wire has been performed, the fracture is stabilized with a plate and lag screw(s).

When applying the 3.5-mm reconstruction plate to the retroacetabular surface, the plate must be overcontoured, because compression of the anterior column will occur as the plate is tightened down to the posterior column. Care must be taken not to undercontour the plate (a desirable configuration for a posterior wall fracture), as this will lead to distraction of the anterior column. A posterior-to-anterior

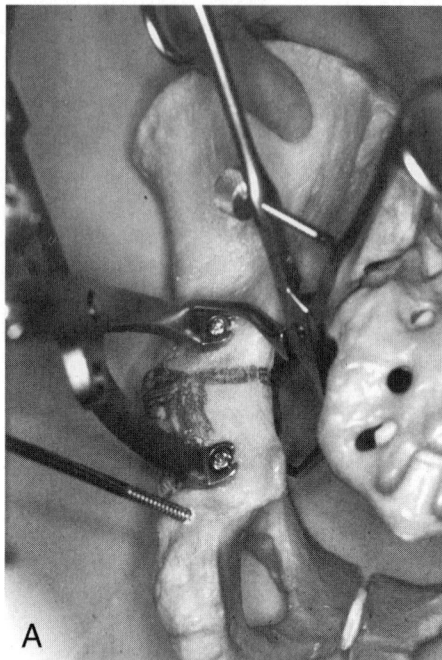

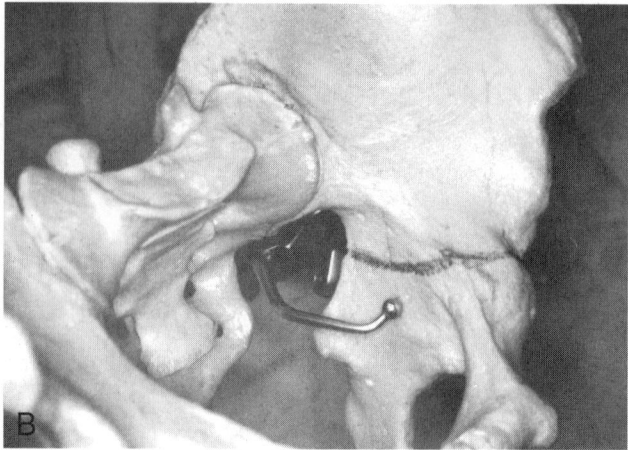

Figure 40.17. A. Posterior approach showing a pelvic reduction clamp used to reduce a transverse acetabular fracture. Note one screw is placed on each side of transverse fracture and a Schanz pin is placed in the ischium to help control rotation. The large angled-jaw reduction clamp is placed with one tong above and one below the fracture site. **B.** Position of the angled-jaw clamp on the quadrilateral surface below the fracture.

column lag screw is required for all transverse fracture types to prevent displacement of the anterior column. This screw can usually be placed through the posterior buttress plate; and in low transverse fractures, it must be oriented parallel to the quadrilateral surface to avoid joint penetration.

T-type fractures. The T-type fracture pattern is probably the most difficult of all acetabular fracture types to manage. It is a complex variant of the transverse fracture pattern, which presents significant additional problems in regard to reduction. In the transverse fracture pattern, the inferior fracture fragment is composed of a single ischiopubic segment. In the T-type pattern, however, the inferior segment is separated by a vertical stem component into two distinct pieces: one anterior and one posterior. Therefore, reduction of one column does not guarantee reduction of the opposite column.

To a great extent, the success of fixation of this fracture through the posterior approach depends on the surgeon's ability to palpate the anterior column and stem component through the greater sciatic notch. Pointed reduction clamps placed into the sciatic notch can be used to manipulate the anterior column fragment after the posterior column has been provisionally stabilized. In addition, a small bone hook or pusher gently introduced along the quadrilateral plate can be used to derotate and pull posteriorly the displaced portion of the anterior column into the acute angle between the intact proximal anterior column and the reconstructed posterior column.

Care must be taken that provisional or definitive fixation of one column does not cross into the opposite column, hindering or preventing its reduction (37). Once an acceptable reduction has been accomplished, stabilization is achieved by the application of a posterior buttress plate and posterior-to-anterior lag screws, as in transverse fractures.

Closure

Closure is rarely problematic. The external rotators are sutured to the cuff of tissue on the posterior aspect of the greater trochanter or are reattached through drill holes. The gluteus maximus tendon insertion into the femur is repaired. Deep and superficial drains should be placed. The fascia lata and fascia over the gluteus maximus are repaired, followed by subcutaneous and skin closures.

ILIOINGUINAL APPROACH

For the ilioinguinal approach, the patient is positioned supine on a fluoroscopic table and protected at all bony prominences. The incision begins at the midpoint of the iliac crest, curves toward the anterior superior iliac spine, and continues parallel to the inguinal ligament, ending 2 cm superior to the pubic symphysis (Fig. 40.18). The proximal aspect of the approach is performed first by identifying the avascular fascial periosteal layer at the iliac crest and dividing it sharply between the attachments of the external oblique and abductor muscles, to minimize bleeding. Next, the abdominal and iliacus musculature is elevated in continuity by subperiosteal dissection off the internal iliac fossa. With this dissection, a nutrient artery of the ilium is often encountered, which requires hemostasis by electrocautery or bone wax. Once the internal iliac fossa has been exposed, it is packed with a sponge, and attention is directed to the inguinal dissection.

Using sharp dissection, the subcutaneous tissue is incised down to the level of the external oblique aponeurosis. This is the most superficial layer of the deep dissection. Proceeding medially, the surgeon must be sure to identify the termination of the inguinal canal, or the external inguinal ring. This structure transmits the spermatic cord in the male and the round ligament in the female. The

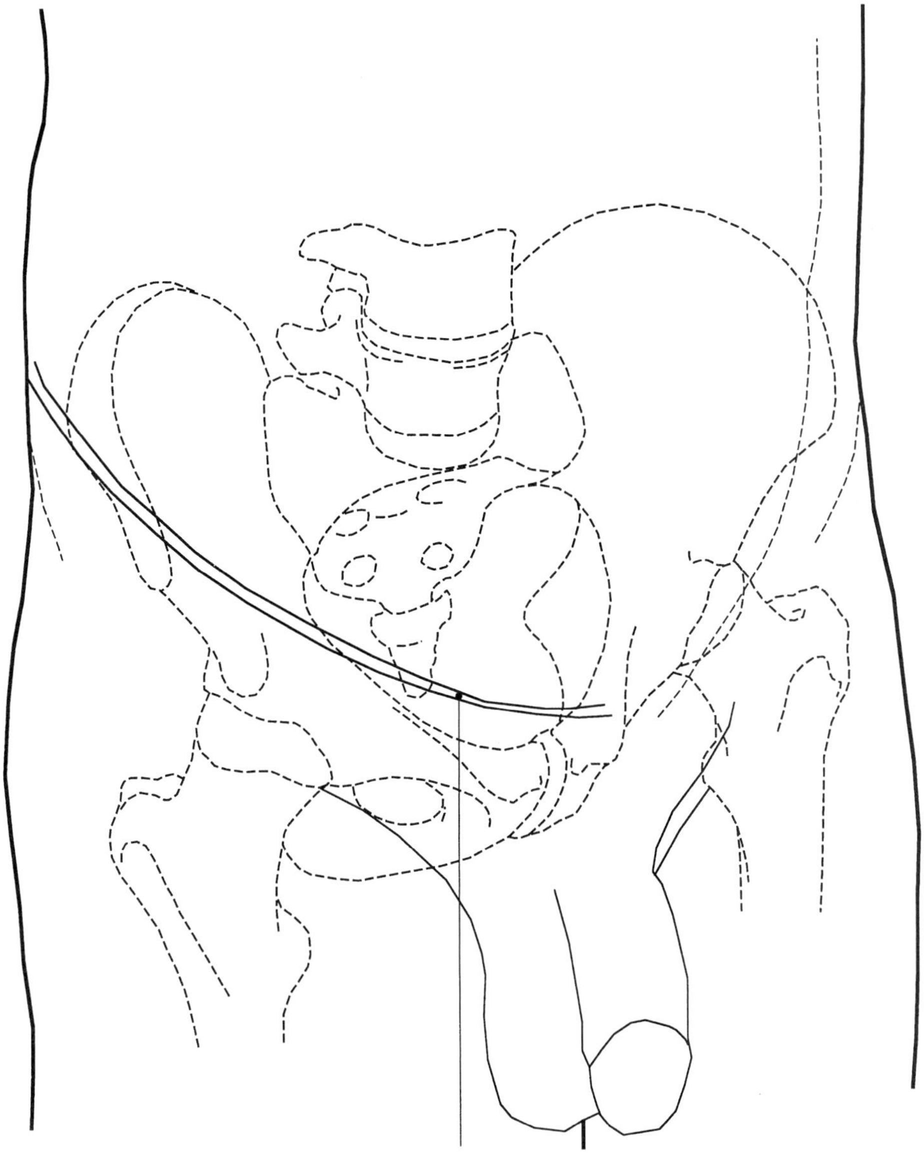

Figure 40.18. Skin incision for the ilioinguinal approach.

ilioinguinal nerve should also be identified. Once mobilized, these structures should be isolated with a Penrose drain. Next, the external oblique aponeurosis is incised 5 mm from its insertion on the inguinal ligament, from the anterior superior iliac spine to the external inguinal ring. This exposes the conjoined tendon of the internal oblique and transversalis abdominis muscles.

Laterally, this conjoined tendon is incised from the inguinal ligament with a 2-mm cuff. The lateral femoral cutaneous nerve is at risk immediately underneath the lateral extent of the conjoined tendon just medial to the anterior superior iliac spine. As the incision proceeds medially, the reflected fascia from the iliopectineal fascia will be encountered. This nearly vertical fascia reflects off of the iliopsoas muscle to merge into the undersurface of the conjoined tendon (Fig. 40.19). The iliopectineal fascia separates the true and false pelvis, and its excision allows access to the quadrilateral surface. At this point of the dissection, extreme care must be exercised, because the femoral vascu-

lar bundle lies just medial to the iliopectineal fascia. For this reason, we prefer to leave the conjoined tendon intact where it covers the femoral artery, vein, and lymphatics. This avoids unnecessary dissection and protects these neurovascular structures from undue retraction.

Medial to the vessels, the conjoined tendon can be incised, if required, and the ipsilateral rectus abdominis muscle can be released from the pubic tubercle to the pubic symphysis, allowing access to the space of Retzius. With anterior pelvic ring injuries, the rectus abdominis muscle is often already avulsed from the pubic tubercle and ramus, in which case, the bladder is at increased risk of iatrogenic injury during the exposure. Keeping the bladder decompressed with a Foley catheter decreases this risk. Associated anterior pelvic ring injuries may require fixation across the pubic symphysis, necessitating a partial release of the contralateral rectus abdominis muscle.

The last portion of the deep exposure is also the most critical and the most hazardous. Laterally, the iliopsoas

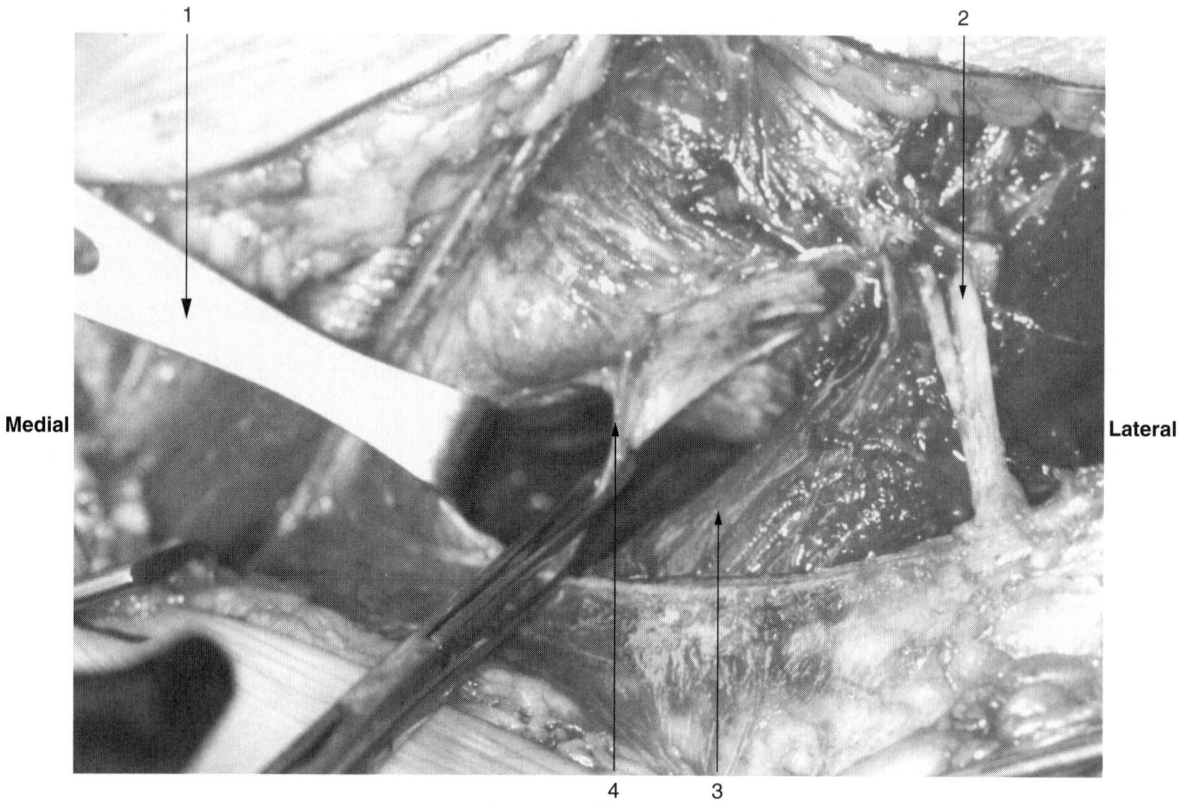

Figure 40.19. Intraoperative view showing the retractor around the femoral vessels (*1*), the lateral femoral cutaneous nerve (*2*), the iliopsoas (*3*), and the iliopectineal fascia (*4*).

muscle and the femoral nerve are bluntly separated off the iliopectineal fascia and mobilized with a broad (2.5-cm) Penrose drain. The femoral vasculature and lymphatics are next carefully dissected off the pectineal fascia medially, maintaining these structures as a unit with the overlying conjoined tendon. Once the iliopectineal fascia has been isolated, it is excised along the pelvic brim from the pectineal eminence to just anterior to the sacroiliac joint. This effectively connects the lacuna musculorum with the lacuna vasorum.

Using gentle dissection with a periosteal elevator and blunt dissection with a fingertip, the femoral vessels are mobilized from the underlying ramus. Before performing this mobilization, the area along the superior ramus should be palpated and a visual inspection performed. A dangerous retropubic communication between the external iliac artery and the obturator or deep epigastric arteries—called the corona mortis—can be encountered and should be ligated if identified. Finally, a broad Penrose drain is passed around the femoral vessels, lymphatics, and the overlying conjoined tendon. Access to the acetabulum through the ilioinguinal approach is now complete.

Medial retraction of the iliopsoas muscle and femoral nerve allows access to the internal iliac fossa and anterior sacroiliac joint, the first window of the ilioinguinal approach (Fig. 40.20). The second window is visualized by lateral retraction of the iliopsoas muscle and the femoral nerve and medial retraction of the femoral vasculature, allowing access to the pelvic brim, the quadrilateral surface, and the posterior column. Gentle retraction will prevent injury and thrombosis of the vessels. The third window is exposed through lateral retraction of the femoral vasculature and lymphatics, allowing access to the superior ramus and pubic symphysis. The obturator neurovascular structures are visualized through either the second or third window and require protection during exposure and reduction of the fracture.

Reduction Techniques

Reduction can be aided by hip flexion, which relaxes the structures crossing anterior to the hip joint. A Schanz screw inserted through the lateral aspect of the femur into the femoral head followed by distal traction can be extremely helpful, because it facilitates fracture reduction through ligamentotaxis. This is especially useful in cases in which the femoral head has protruded through the quadrilateral surface.

An accurate reduction of all the fracture fragments is imperative, since the articular surface is not directly visualized through the ilioinguinal approach. Before attempted reduction, all the fracture lines are carefully irrigated and débrided to remove fracture hematoma and any small comminuted fragments. The hip joint is also irrigated, and loose fragments are removed through the displaced portion of the articular fracture.

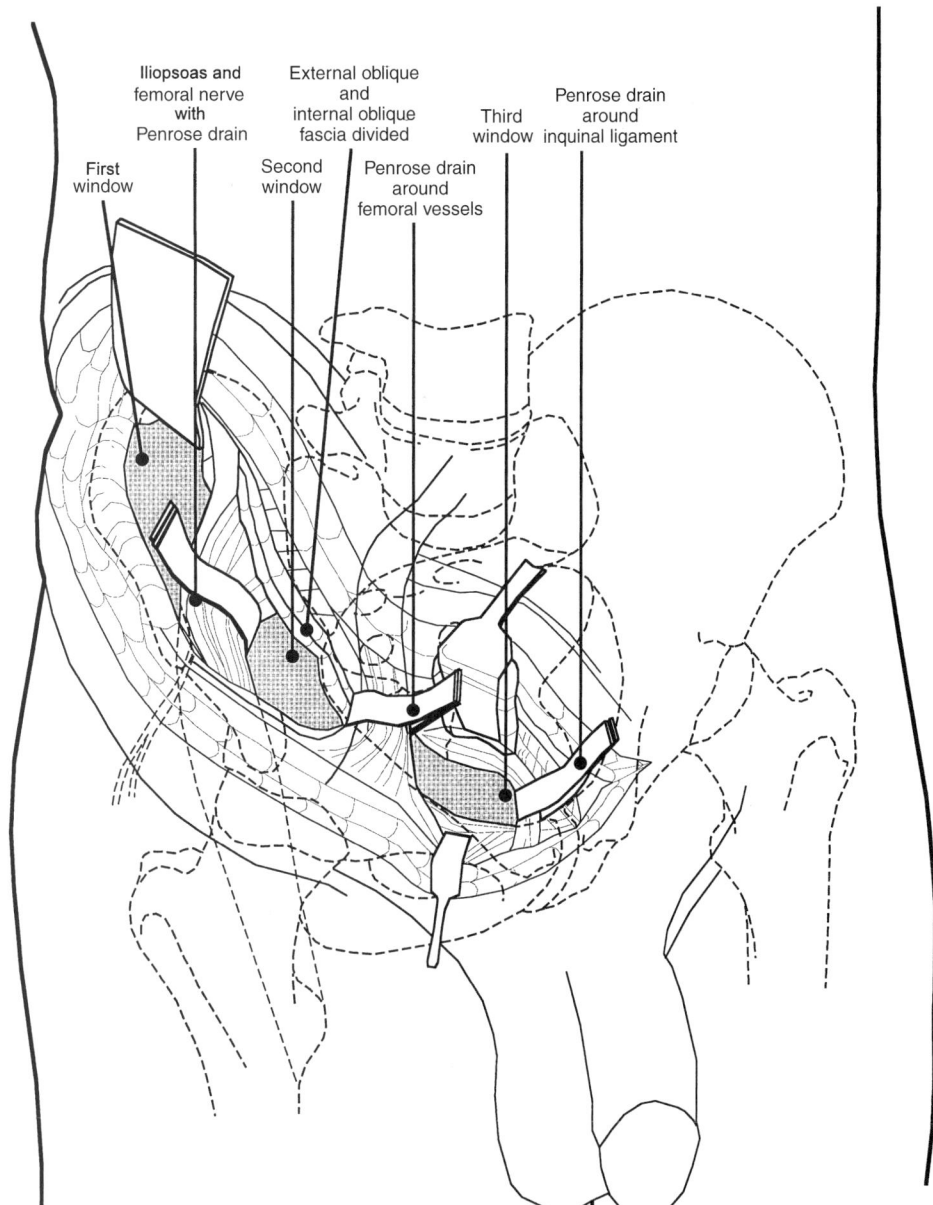

Figure 40.20. Deep exposure afforded by ilioinguinal approach.

Anterior wall and column fractures. In dealing with an isolated anterior wall or anterior column fracture, sequential reduction is achieved starting at the outer portions of the iliac crest. These fragments can be reduced with pointed reduction clamps or with the specially designed pelvic reduction clamps. Gliding holes for lag screw fixation can be created before fracture reduction to ensure optimal lag screw position within the thin cortical cap of the iliac crest. The crest is then stabilized by any combination of lag screws and 3.5-mm reconstruction plates. Next, the anterior column is reduced to the intact iliac wing and temporarily stabilized with a K wire (and/or a 3.5-mm lag screw) into the sciatic buttress through the first window of the ilioinguinal approach. Then through the second win-

dow, any anterior wall fracture is reduced. Finally, any superior pubic rami and displaced pubic column fractures are reduced through the third window.

A 3.5-mm reconstruction plate can then be molded along the iliac fossa, across the iliopectineal eminence to the pubic tubercle and pubic column. This should not cross the symphysis pubis, unless there are associated fractures in the pubic ramus or there is an associated pelvic ring injury with involvement of the symphysis pubis. It is essential that this plate is perfectly molded, otherwise fixation of the plate to the pelvis can lead to a malreduction of the acetabular fracture. The plate is stabilized to the internal iliac fossa, superior to the acetabulum, with 3.5-mm cortical screws and medially to the pubic tu-

Figure 40.21. Fracture fixation of an anterior column fracture with a 3.5-mm reconstruction plate and lag screws across the posterior hemitransverse component.

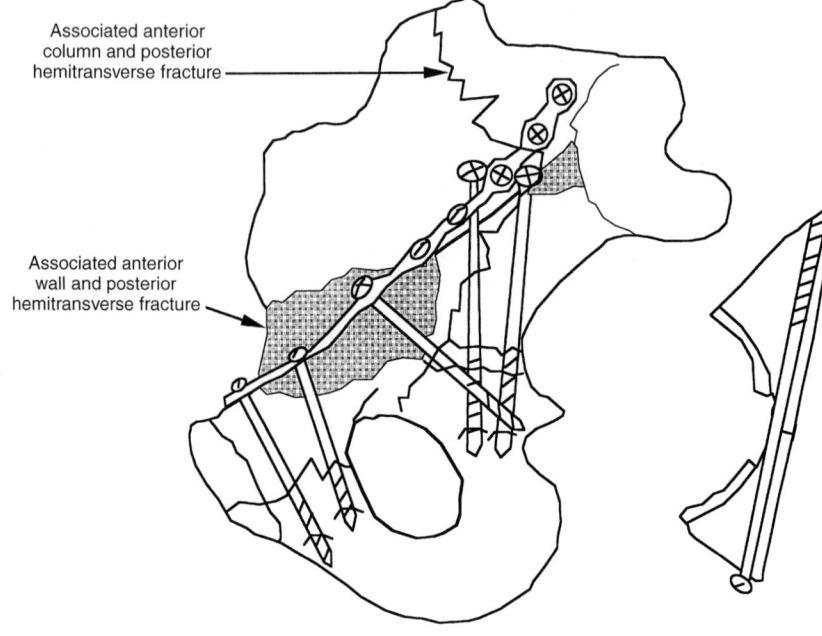

Associated anterior column and posterior hemitransverse fracture

Associated anterior wall and posterior hemitransverse fracture

Figure 40.22. Screws that are parallel to the quadrilateral surface and pass partially through the cotyloid fossa will not interfere with the femoral head.

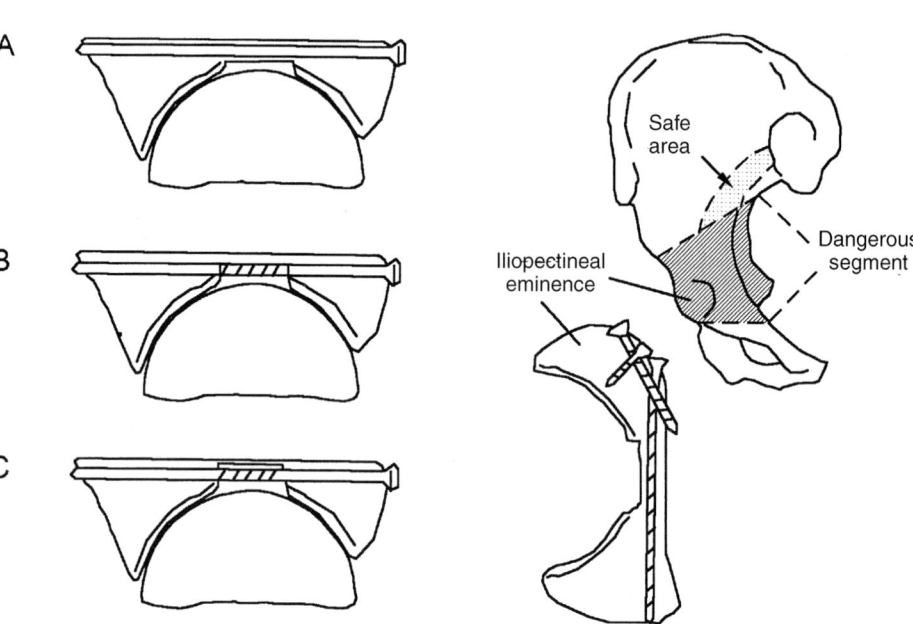

A

B

C

Safe area

Iliopectineal eminence

Dangerous segment

bercle and ramus (Fig. 40.21). In the central area of the iliac fossa lies a region of thin bone that provides minimal purchase of screws. This area should be avoided. In contrast, the area of the sciatic buttress and quadrilateral plate, proximal to the acetabulum, provides excellent purchase for stabilization of the anterior column to the iliac wing and posterior column. These screws must parallel the quadrilateral plate to avoid joint penetration (Fig. 40.22). Fracture reduction is assessed by finger palpation of the quadrilateral plate. Fluoroscopic Judet views are necessary to assess the adequacy of the reduction and to confirm the extra-articular position of the hardware.

Associated both-column fractures. Upon initial exposure of the associated both-column fracture, translational displacement is readily apparent, while rotational displace-

ment is much more difficult to visualize. It is important to appreciate this, as understanding the three-dimensional deformity is paramount to its correction by indirect techniques through this approach. Fracture reduction should begin in a sequential manner, beginning with reduction of the individual peripheral fracture fragments to portions of the intact pelvis. Working from the periphery toward the articular surface, the surgeon sequentially and patiently reduces and provisionally stabilizes the fragments. At every step, the quality of reduction is critical to the outcome of the procedure. What may initially appear to be a small extra-articular error in fracture reduction will magnify as the reconstruction proceeds toward the joint.

The anterior column is reduced first then stabilized with a 3.5-mm reconstruction plate, as previously de-

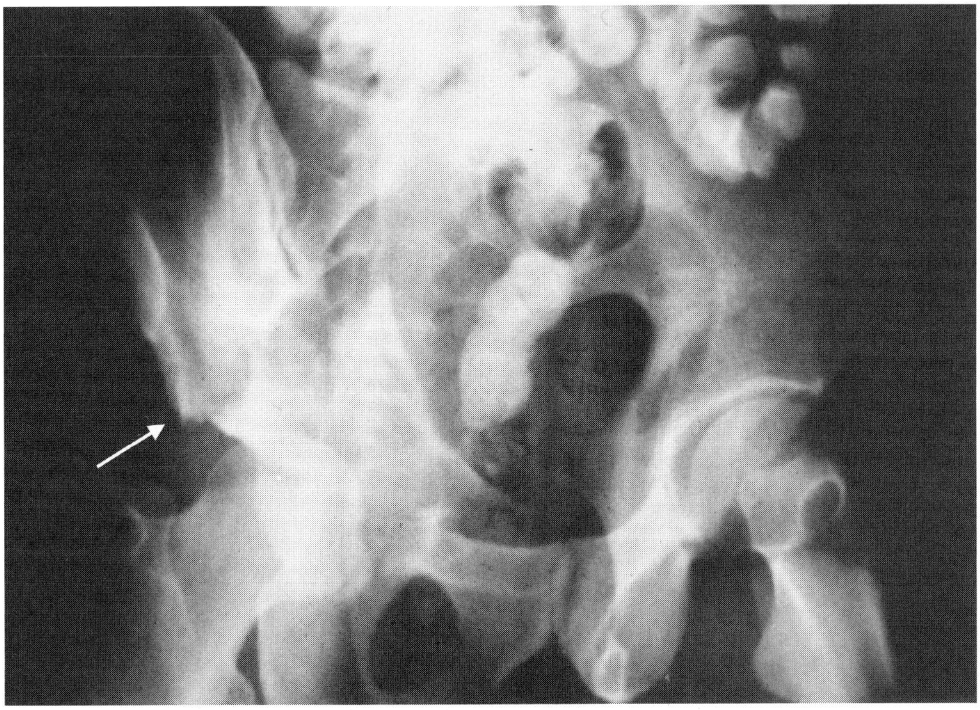

Figure 40.23. Obturator oblique view of an associated both-column acetabular fracture showing the spur sign *(arrow),* which represents the intact ilium that has no portion of the articular surface of the acetabulum attached to it.

scribed for anterior fractures. This must be performed perfectly from the iliac crest to the symphysis pubis, to provide an anatomic template for subsequent reduction of the posterior column to the reduced anterior column. If the anterior column fracture is incomplete, it may have to be completed to accomplish this reduction adequately. The anterior column segment of a both-column fracture is typically shortened and externally rotated. To properly reduce this segment to the intact iliac wing, known as the spur sign (Fig. 40.23), a significant amount of longitudinal traction is required. An assistant can provide the traction by pulling on an AO universal T-handle chuck that is attached to a Schanz pin anchored in the femoral head.

After anatomic reduction and stabilization of the anterior column are achieved, the rotated and medially displaced posterior column can be reduced to the restored anterior column. This often requires lateral and anterior traction of the hip, via the Schanz screw in the femoral head, and specially designed pelvic reduction clamps. One tine of the clamp is placed on the outer surface of the ilium through a small limited exposure and the other tine is placed on the quadrilateral plate and/or posterior column through the first or second window of the ilioinguinal exposure (Fig. 40.24). In addition, it is often helpful to place a small bone hook down the quadrilateral plate, hooking it around the ischial spine to pull the posterior column up to the anterior column. Following this reduction, 3.5-mm lag screws are inserted through the pelvic brim superior to the acetabulum into the posterior column. These screws should parallel the quadrilateral surface and be aimed at the ischial spine (Fig. 40.25). With a

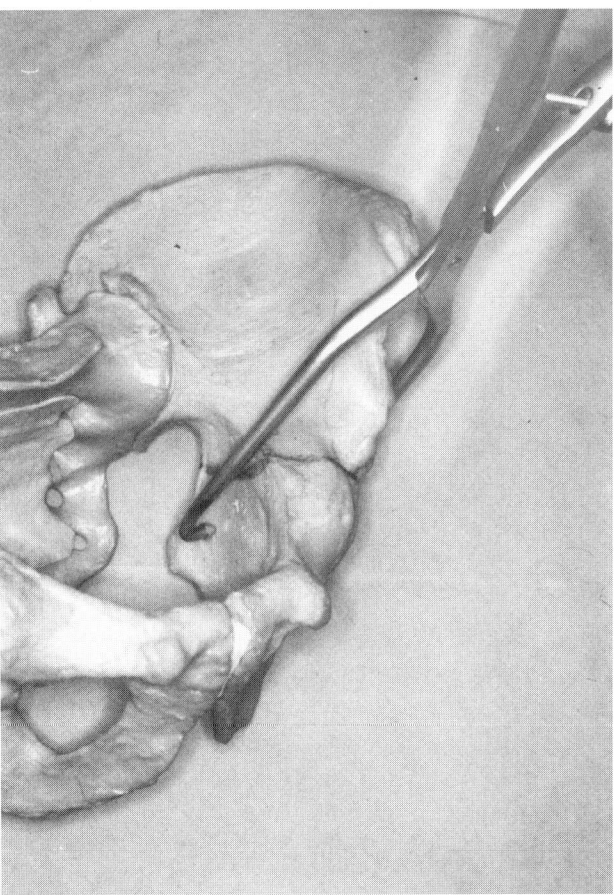

Figure 40.24. Placement of the king-tong clamp for reduction of the posterior column portion of an associated both-column acetabular fracture, as visualized from the ilioinguinal exposure.

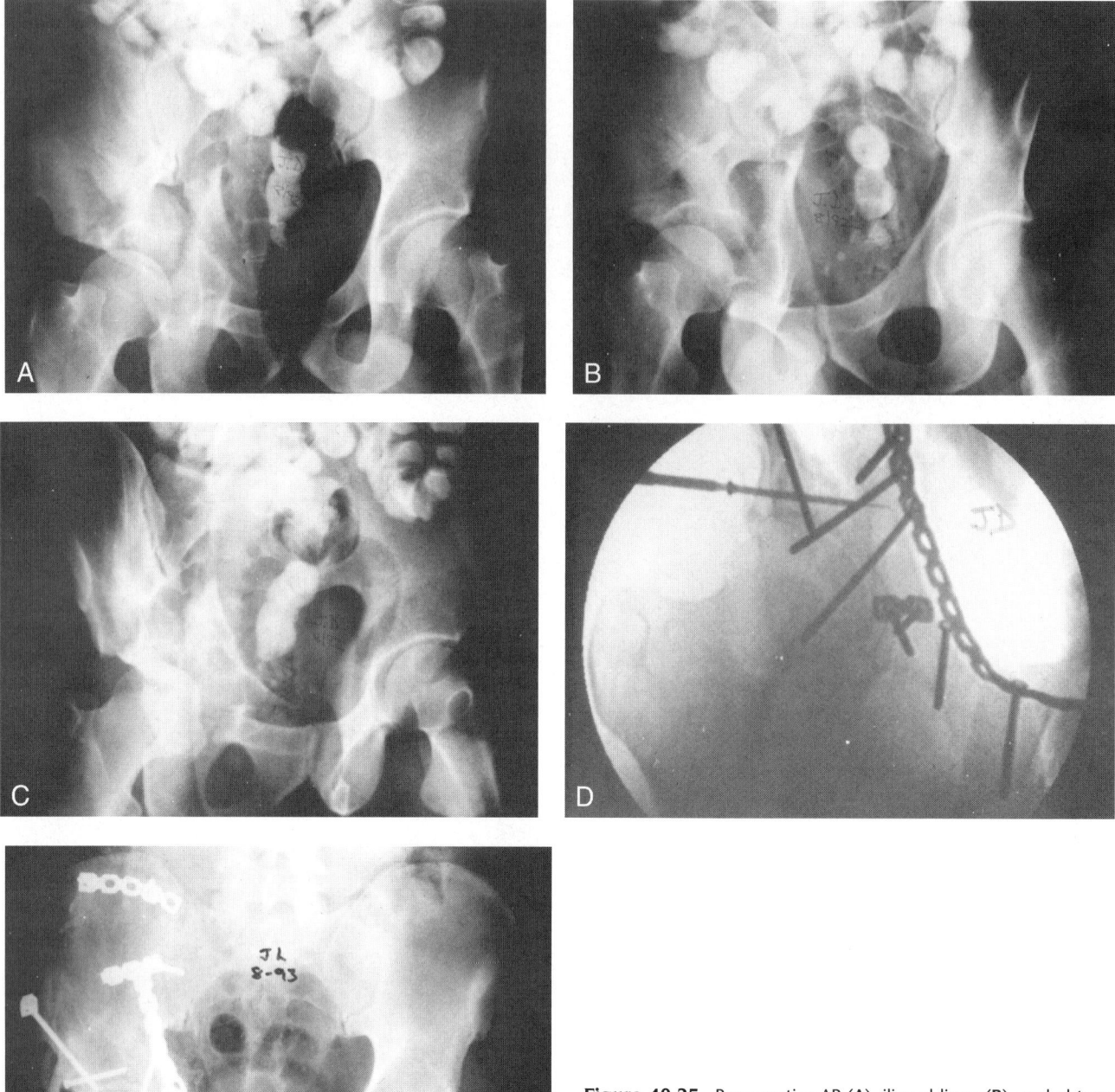

Figure 40.25. Preoperative AP (**A**), iliac oblique (**B**), and obturator oblique (**C**) views showing an associated both-column acetabular fracture extending into iliac wing. **D.** Intraoperative image intensifier view showing the reduced and stabilized fracture. Note the lag screws from the anterior column to the posterior column. **E.** Postoperative AP view taken at the 1-year follow-up, showing maintenance of the reduction and preservation of the joint space.

more proximal starting point in the iliac fossa, the surgeon can aim for the ischial tuberosity, often obtaining fixation with long screws. The direction of screw placement is dictated by the position of the articular surface and, therefore, requires a careful appreciation of the location of the acetabulum relative to the fixed pelvic landmarks.

Closure

Once the fracture is reduced and stabilized, drains are inserted from the internal iliac fossa to the space of Retzius. If the rectus abdominis muscle has been detached, it is reattached to the pubis by suturing it to the cuff of tissue remaining on the anterior aspect of the pubis. If this repair is tenuous, suture anchors can be helpful. The floor of the inguinal canal is repaired by suturing the conjoined tendon to the inguinal ligament with nonabsorbable sutures. The roof of the inguinal canal is restored by repair of the external oblique aponeurosis and external inguinal ring. This portion of the repair continues laterally, as the external oblique muscle is reattached to the inguinal ligament and the iliac crest with nonabsorbable sutures. The skin is then closed over a superficial suction drain.

EXTENDED ILIOFEMORAL APPROACH

For the extended iliofemoral approach, the patient is supported on a beanbag and placed in the lateral decubitus position on a radiolucent operating table or fracture table, depending on the surgeon's preference. There are three main stages to the dissection, which provides simultaneous extensile exposure of both columns: elevation of all the gluteal muscles and the tensor fascia lata, division of the external rotators of the hip, and an extended capsulotomy along the lip of the acetabulum (3). The extended iliofemoral approach exposes the outer aspect of the ilium and the whole posterior column inferiorly to the upper part of the ischial tuberosity (Fig. 40.8C).

The incision is in the form of an inverted J, beginning at the posterior-superior iliac spine and extending along the iliac crest toward the anterior-superior iliac spine (ASIS) (Fig. 40.26). From here, the distal arm of the incision proceeds along the anterolateral aspect of the thigh for 15 to 20 cm, toward a point 2 cm lateral to the superolateral pole of the patella (3,5). The avascular fascial-periosteal layer at the iliac crest is identified and divided sharply between the attachments of the external oblique and abductor muscles to minimize bleeding. Using an elevator, the musculature along the external surface of the iliac wing is released up to the superior border of the greater sciatic notch and anterosuperior aspect of the hip joint capsule. Care must be taken to identify the superior gluteal neurovascular bundle, which is at risk as it exits from the notch.

Attention then turns to the anterior portion of the approach. The distal limb of the incision is carried through the fascial sheath covering the tensor fascia lata muscle, which is entered 10 to 15 cm below the ASIS. From this point, the dissection progresses superiorly toward the spine and distally as necessary. It is important to stay within the bounds of this sheath to remain lateral to the lateral femoral cutaneous nerve and the majority of its branches. Next the muscle belly is reflected off its posterior fascia and retracted laterally and upward to expose the floor of the sheath and fascia overlying the rectus femoris muscle. Small vessels from the superficial circumflex artery are divided and coagulated close to the bone between the superior and inferior spines (3). Distally, the incision must be long enough to expose the inferior aspect of the muscle belly. This facilitates further release of the gluteal muscles from the crest.

The fascia overlying the rectus muscle is divided longitudinally and horizontally, and its reflected head and direct heads are retracted downward and medially to expose the aponeurosis over the vastus lateralis muscle. When the rectus is retracted, a constant small vascular pedicle along the lateral border of the muscle will often require coagulation (3). The aponeurosis can be divided longitudinally to expose the ascending branches of the lateral

circumflex vessels, which must be isolated and ligated. Next, the thin sheath of the iliopsoas muscle is exposed and longitudinally incised. This allows the use of an elevator to strip the fibers of the psoas from the anterior and inferior aspects of the hip capsule. The exposure of the iliac wing is complete when the reflected head of the rectus femoris is sharply released from its insertion.

Attention is then directed to the gluteus minimus tendon, where it inserts into the anterior edge of the greater trochanter. This tendon is tagged and transected, leaving a 3- to 5-mm cuff for repair (3). Release of the extensive attachments of the gluteus minimus muscle to the superior aspect of the hip capsule may also be required. Posteriorly and superiorly, the 15- to 20-mm long gluteus medius tendon is isolated, tagged, and transected, leaving a 3- to 5-mm cuff. The tensor fascia lata and gluteal muscles are held in continuity as a flap and reflected posteriorly to expose the external rotators and sciatic nerve. From this point, the dissection is similar to the Kocher-Langenbeck approach: The tendons of the piriformis, obturator internus, and the inferior and superior gemelli are tagged and transected; the tendinous femoral insertion of the gluteus maximus is identified, tagged, and released with a cuff for repair; the quadratus femoris is preserved; and retractors are placed into the two sciatic notches. The dissection is now complete (Fig. 40.27).

Although medial exposure of the anterior column is limited by the iliopsoas muscle and the iliopectineal fascia, further access to the internal iliac fossa and acetabulum is possible. This is obtained by subperiosteal dissection of the sartorius and direct head of the rectus or by osteotomizing the superior and inferior iliac spines. The iliacus muscle and the insertion of the external oblique muscle onto the crest can be subperiosteally released to reveal the inner table of the pelvis. Although devascularization of the iliac wing is rare, Matta and Merritt (34) noted its occurrence in associated both-column fractures. To avoid this problem, they suggested leaving the direct head of the rectus femoris and anterior hip capsule attached to the anterior column.

Extensive acetabular fractures often present with tears in the hip joint capsule. If capsular disruption is not present, then exposure of the acetabular articular surface can be obtained with a marginal capsulotomy, leaving a cuff of tissue for repair. Once the hip joint is exposed, distraction with either a Schanz screw placed into the femoral head or a femoral distractor will facilitate visualization. As with other approaches, this visualization is necessary to evaluate the articular reduction, identify intra-articular hardware, and remove any incarcerated osteochondral fragments.

Because this approach creates significant soft tissue flaps, it is important to keep them moist with wet sponges and periodic irrigation throughout the procedure. During reduction and stabilization, the surgeon has several columns of bone at his or her disposal for placing the screws, ranging from 50 to 120 mm. These columns include

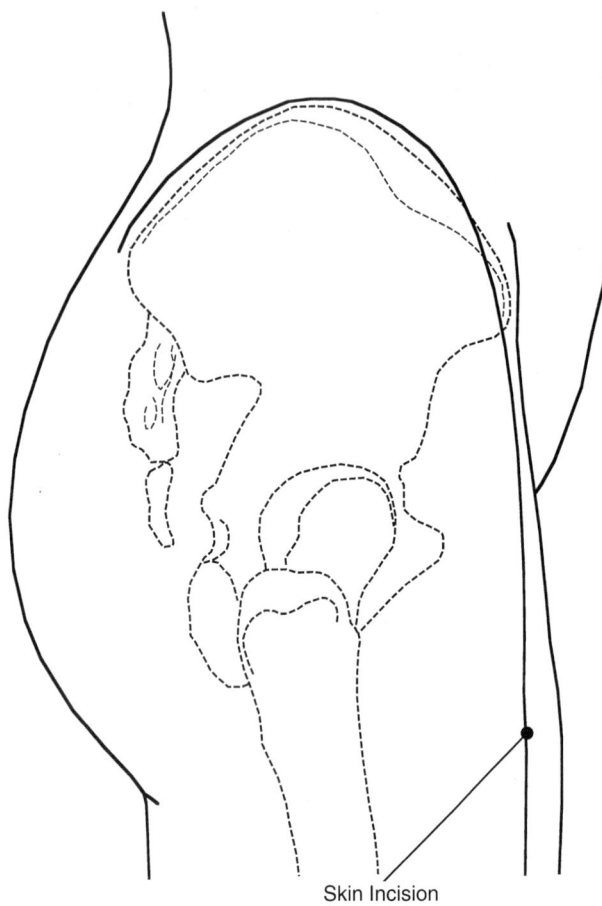

Skin Incision

Figure 40.26. Skin incision for the extended iliofemoral approach.

the iliac crest, the gluteal ridge, the sciatic buttress, the anterior column, and the posterior column (49).

Reduction Techniques

Transverse and T-*type fractures.* In a transverse fracture, there is rotational malalignment of the displaced inferior portion of the acetabulum. The T-type fracture pattern is more complex, because the anterior and posterior fragments are separate and both columns become displaced and malrotated (Fig. 40.28). The anterior segment is usually medially displaced, increasing the radius of curvature of the acetabulum over that of the femoral head (45). For the reduction of the T-type and more comminuted variants, the anterior column may be reduced first with respect to the residual acetabular roof portion of the ilium (45).

Several reduction maneuvers for these fractures are similar to those described for the Kocher-Langenbeck approach. The pelvic reduction clamp with 4.5-mm screws—one proximal and one distal to the posterior column fracture—can be used to provide distraction, allowing débridement of the fracture surfaces and then reduction. A laminar spreader in the fracture site can also facilitate exposure of the joint (Fig. 40.29). Additional rotational control of the fracture fragments and their subsequent re-

duction can be facilitated by a Schanz screw in the ischium and by a pelvic clamp in the greater sciatic notch.

The adequacy of reduction of the posterior column can be visualized by direct assessment of the articular surface and with digital palpation through the greater and lesser sciatic notches. Before definitive reduction, a gliding hole can be inserted into the proximal aspect of the posterior column from superior to inferior, ensuring the position of the gliding hole in the middle of the posterior column. Following reduction, it is then possible to insert a 4.5- or 3.5-mm cortical lag screw down the posterior column. Additional stabilization is accomplished with a 3.5-mm reconstruction plate molded to the posterior column.

A lag screw can also be inserted from the lateral aspect of the iliac wing into the anterior column, distal and medial to the articular surface. Generally, this requires the placement of a gliding hole three fingerbreadths proximal to the superior aspect of the articular surface and one fingerbreadth posterior to the gluteal ridge. The lag screw is then angled from posterosuperior to anteroinferior directly down the superior pubic ramus to secure the anterior column of the acetabulum. This can be accomplished with a 4.5-mm cortical screw in large individuals, but a 3.5-mm cortical screw is preferred in females and small individuals. This is a challenging screw to place safely, and intraoperative fluoroscopy too guide the insertion is mandatory. Care must be taken to ensure that the screw remains extra-articular and does not penetrate the anterior aspect of the superior ramus, in the area of the iliopectineal eminence where the femoral vasculature is closely adherent.

Associated both-column fractures. As in the ilioinguinal approach, when reducing both-column acetabulum fractures through the extended iliofemoral approach, the surgeon should work from the periphery toward the acetabulum, reducing each fracture fragment sequentially. Once the iliac wing is stabilized with lag screws and/or by 3.5-mm reconstruction plates, the posterior column is reduced to the iliac wing with direct visualization of the acetabular articular surface.

Fixation is accomplished in the same manner as for transverse and T-type fractures, using a posterior column lag screw and a 3.5-mm reconstruction plate. The anterior column is then attached to the posterior column, using 4.5-mm lag screws inserted from the anterior-superior spine into the sciatic buttress and/or anterior column lag screws from the lateral aspect of the iliac wing, as described previously. The adequacy of the reduction is then assessed by direct visualization of the acetabulum and by finger palpation of the greater and lesser sciatic notches and quadrilateral plate and, if necessary, the internal iliac fossa. The use of fluoroscopy is essential to confirm the adequacy of reduction and the position of the fixation.

Closure

After completion of the operative reconstruction, suction drains are placed along the external surface of the il-

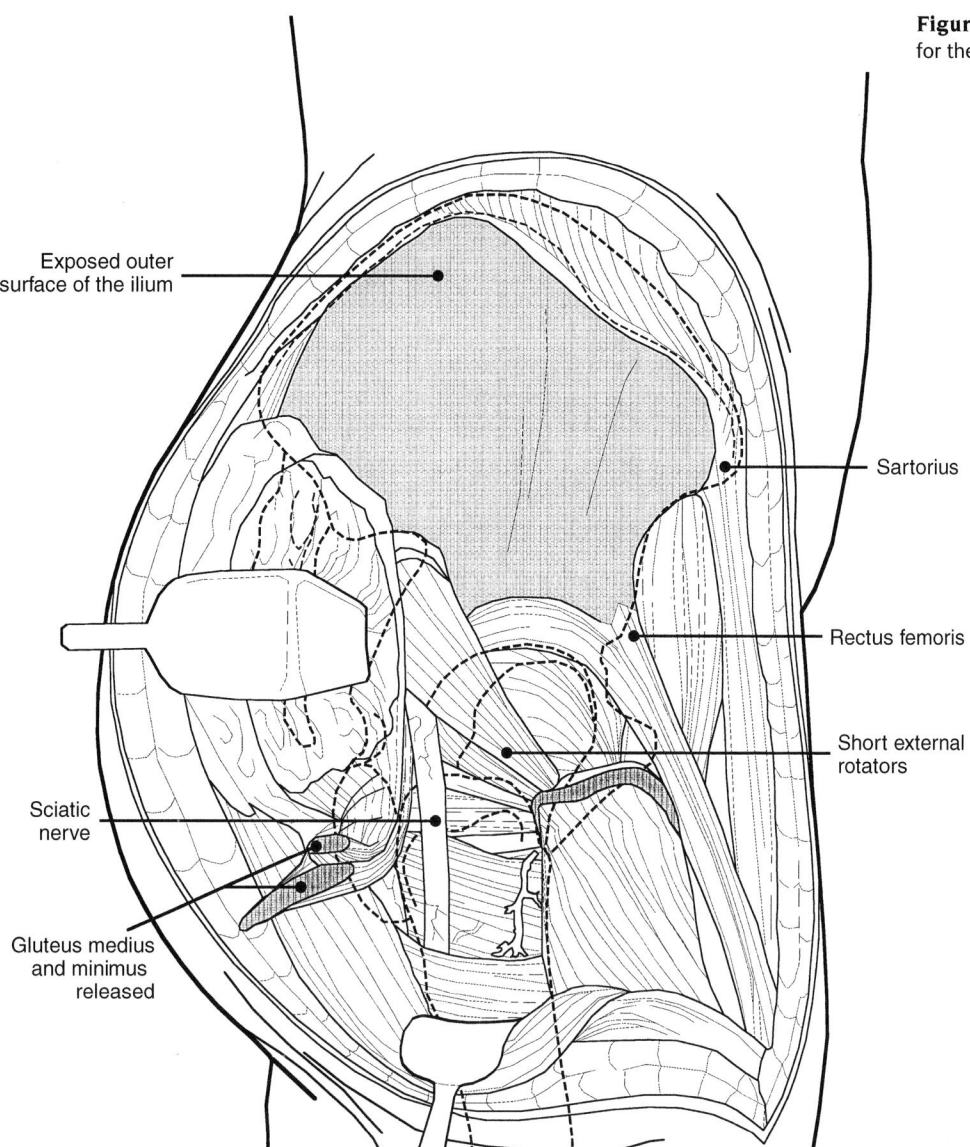

Figure 40.27. Completed dissection for the extended iliofemoral approach.

Exposed outer surface of the ilium

Sartorius

Rectus femoris

Short external rotators

Sciatic nerve

Gluteus medius and minimus released

iac wing, in the vicinity of the posterior column and vastus lateralis muscle. If the internal iliac fossa has been exposed, a third drain is placed there. All drains should exit anteriorly.

The hip capsule is repaired first, followed by reattachment of the tendinous insertions of the short external rotators to the greater trochanter and the reattachment of the femoral insertion of the gluteus maximus. Next, the trochanteric insertions of the gluteus medius and minimus muscles are repaired, using five or six sutures for each tendon, as recommended by Letournel and Judet (3). Finally, the tensor fascia lata and gluteal muscles are reattached to their origins on the iliac crest.

If a medial exposure has been performed, then the origins of the sartorius and direct head of the rectus femoris muscles are reattached through drill holes (or lag screws, if osteotomies have been performed). Finally, the fascia overlying the proximal thigh is repaired, followed by placement of a subcutaneous suction drain and skin closure.

INTRAOPERATIVE ASSESSMENT OF REDUCTION

Before closure, all acetabular fracture reductions should be assessed with intraoperative radiographs to confirm that a satisfactory reduction has been achieved and to ensure that hardware has not been inadvertently placed in the intra-articular area. Intraoperative fluoroscopic images are useful for this purpose, especially the AP and Judet views (Fig. 40.30). A fluoroscopic view should be obtained for any anterior column lag screws that appear close to the joint. The beam should be parallel to the quadrilateral surface, aiming down the lag screw.

With a finger on the quadrilateral surface, the surgeon should place the hip through a range of motion of the hip to detect the presence of any crepitation in the joint, indicative of residual bony fragments or intra-articular hardware. The adequacy of the reduction of the posterior column to the anterior column can be determined by palpation along the quadrilateral surface.

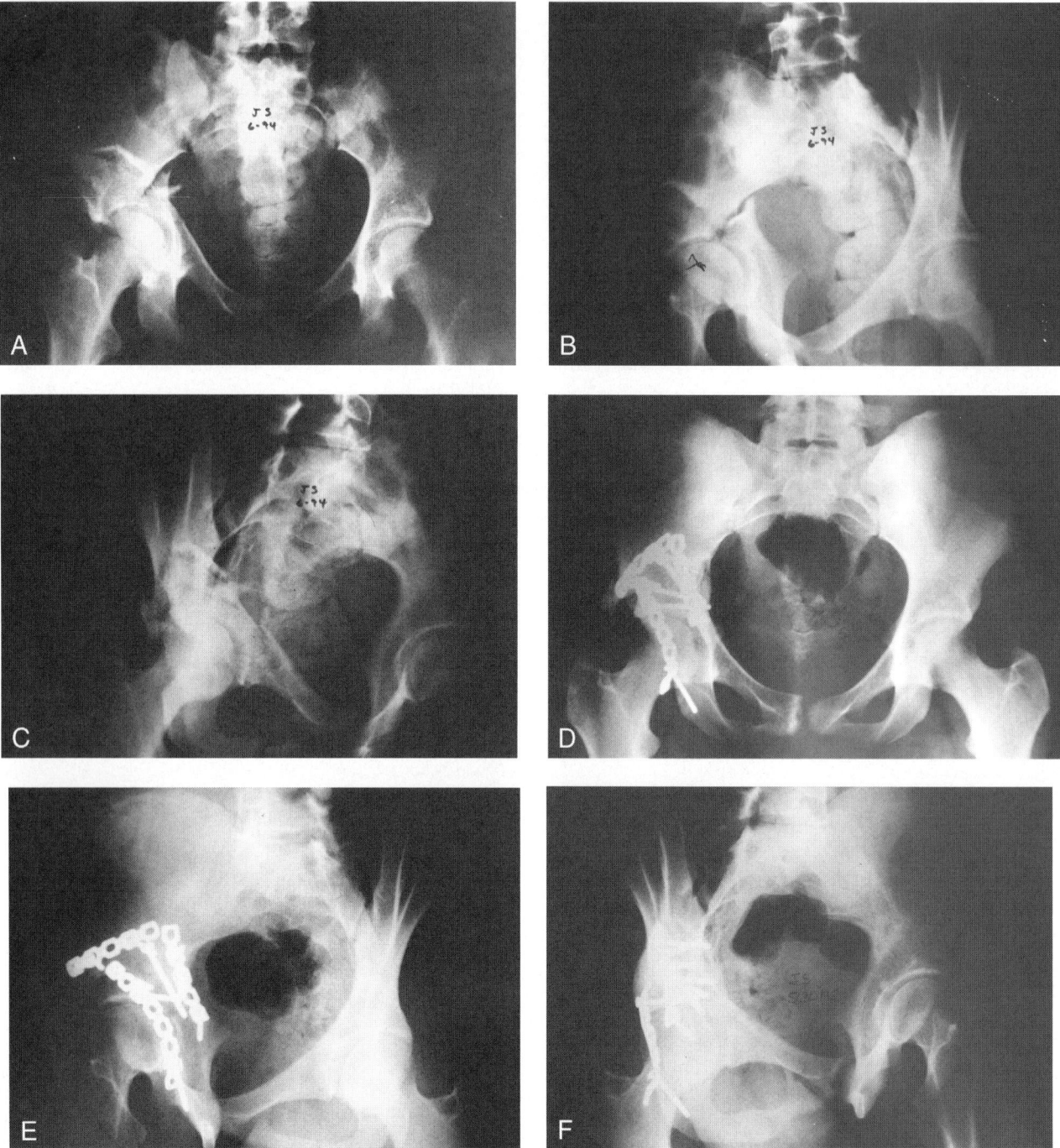

Figure 40.28. Preoperative AP (**A**), iliac oblique (**B**), and obturator oblique (**C**) views of a transtectal T-type fracture with dome comminution in a 34-year-old male. This was approached through an ex- tended iliofemoral approach. Postoperative AP (**D**), iliac oblique (**E**), and obturator oblique (**F**) views.

POSTOPERATIVE CARE

Postoperatively, patients are maintained on intravenous cefazolin for 48 to 72 h. Our anticoagulation regimen includes compression boots while the patient is hospitalized and 6 weeks of warfarin. Heterotopic ossification

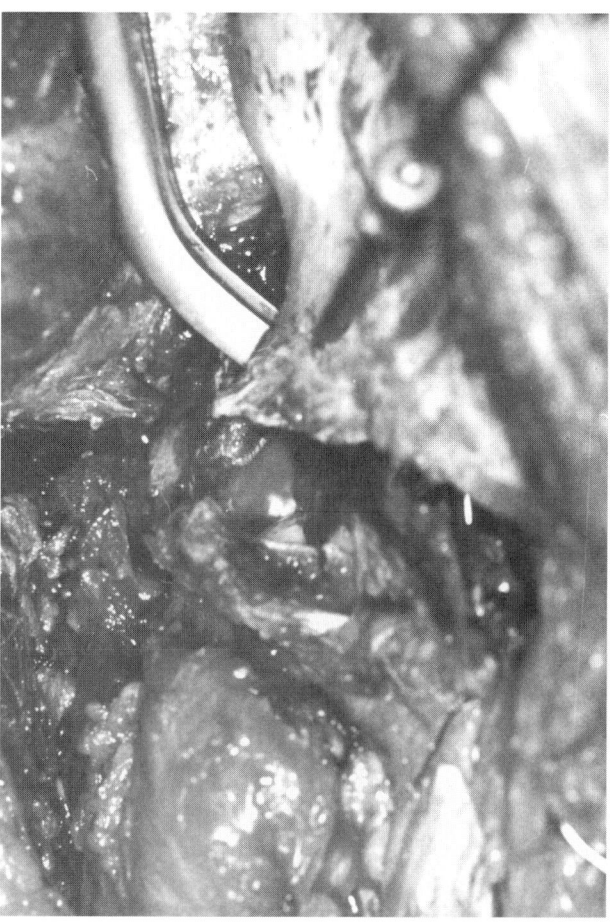

Figure 40.29. A lamina spreader is used to distract the fracture line, allowing visualization of the hip joint from the extended iliofemoral approach.

prophylaxis is mandatory after the Kocher-Langenbeck and extended iliofemoral approaches; it is necessary after ilioinguinal approaches when the external surface of the iliac wing required stripping. We prefer indomethacin (75 mg po sustained-release once daily) for 6 weeks.

Early mobilization should be stressed, and patients are encouraged to dangle their legs and sit in a chair within the first 24 to 48 h following surgery. We do not use continuous passive motion (CPM), because we have not had difficulty regaining hip motion in our patient population.

After the drains are removed, usually by 48 to 72 h, patients are allowed toe-touch weight bearing to (9 kg) (20 lb), using crutches. Strengthening exercises along with gait training are initiated by the physical therapist. Weight bearing is not advanced for the first 6 to 8 weeks after surgery. When an extended iliofemoral approach or a trochanteric osteotomy has been performed, active abduction is avoided for 6 to 8 weeks. During the 3rd month postsurgery, depending on roentgenographic evidence of healing, the patient is allowed to progress to full weight bearing as tolerated.

Intraoperative radiographs displaying an adequate fracture reduction and a congruent hip joint can sometimes be misleading. Thus we routinely obtain postoperative roentgenograms (AP pelvis and Judet views) and a CT scan to critically assess the fracture reduction and hardware position and to identify any residual loose fragments.

RESULTS

After acetabular fractures, functional outcome depends on several factors, some controllable, but others injury related and inevitable. The most important surgical factors are obtaining an anatomic reduction of the articular surface and avoiding both acute and late complications. Factors out of the surgeon's control are the degree of cartilage damage at the time of injury, the loss of vascularity sustained by the femoral head, and the associated soft tissue injuries.

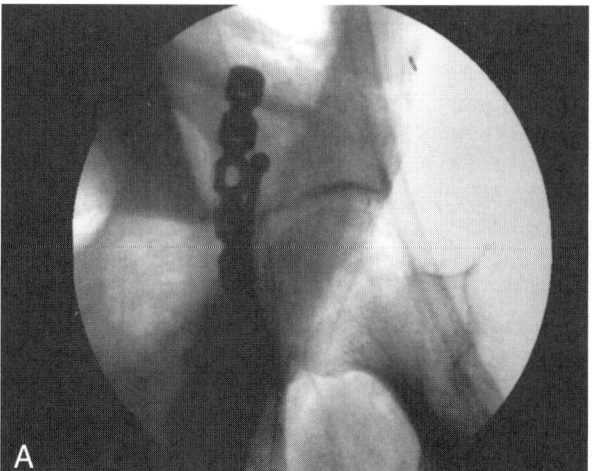

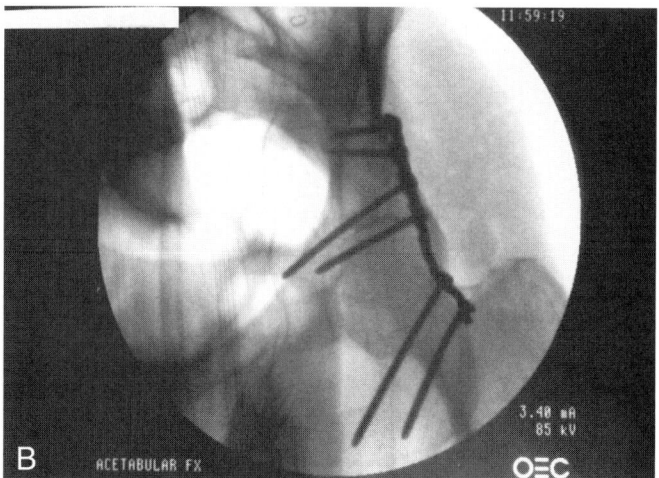

Figure 40.30. Intraoperative AP (**A**) and obturator oblique (**B**) views confirming the extra-articular placement of the hardware.

Long-term clinical outcome correlates closely with the quality of reduction achieved during surgery. Rowe and Lowell (52) reviewed 93 acetabular fractures treated non-operatively and noted poor results for all 10 patients in whom the weight-bearing dome was not anatomically reduced. The results of Letournel and Judet (3) and others (4,15,29,46,53) further support this finding. In a review of 569 acetabular fractures treated within 3 weeks of injury, Letournel and Judet (3) achieved an anatomic reduction (a maximum of 1 mm of displacement on any of three views) in 74% of cases, and 82% of these patients had very good clinical outcomes at a follow-up of as much as 33 years. On the other hand, for patients with an imperfectly reduced fracture, very good results were obtained in 54% of cases when the femoral head was centered under the dome but in only 23% of cases when there was residual subluxation of the femoral head.

The amount of incongruity that is acceptable is still open to debate, but most authors would agree that more than 1 to 2 mm of incongruity is unsatisfactory. In early retrospective studies, Matta et al. (15) and Kebaish et al. (53) noted good long-term results after restoration of the articular surface to within 3 and 4 mm, respectively. Matta's (4) prospective study, however, demonstrated that these criteria are not acceptable. Matta achieved an anatomic reduction in 71% of 262 acetabular fractures, and 83% of patients had good to excellent results at an average follow-up of 6 years. Of the 29% of patients with an imperfectly reduced acetabulum, good to excellent results were obtained in 68% of cases when the defect measured 2 to 3 mm but only 50% when the defect was greater than 3 mm. The most predictive factor initially for a poor result was damage to the femoral head at the time of injury. These results are in agreement with Helfet and Schmeling (29), who noted that an articular stepoff of greater than 2 mm or a gap of more than 3 mm was associated with a fourfold increase in joint-space narrowing at early follow-up (46). Finally, cadaver models further support the idea that 2 mm or less is the appropriate definition of an acceptable reduction (27,31).

COMPLICATIONS

Complications following operative treatment of acetabular fractures are best divided into three groups: intraoperative, early, and late. Intraoperative complications include neurovascular injury, malreduction, articular penetration of hardware, and death. Early postoperative complications include DVT, pulmonary embolism (PE), skin necrosis, infection, loss of reduction, arthritis, and death. The late group includes heterotopic ossification (HO), chondrolysis, avascular necrosis, and posttraumatic arthrosis.

HO is the most common complication following the operative fixation of acetabular fractures, with an incidence ranging from 18 to 90% (Fig. 40.31) (3,4,41,42,54,55); however, it has been reported to cause functional limitation in only 5 to 10% of cases (34,37,46,49). The greatest risk for heterotopic bone formation is in patients who require an extended iliofemoral approach and elevation of the whole external surface of the iliac wing (3,4,42,46,54,55). Both indomethacin and low-dose radiation therapy (single or multiple fractions) have displayed prophylactic efficacy when given early (3,42,48,54,56).

Iatrogenic sciatic nerve injury or worsening of a preexisting deficit is a significant problem. Patients at increased risk include those with preoperative sciatic nerve compromise and those with fracture patterns that involve the posterior wall or column (14). The experience of the surgical team appears to be the most significant factor in reducing the incidence of iatrogenic sciatic nerve injury. Letournel and Judet (3) and Matta et al. (15) have reported a significant decrease in the incidence of iatrogenic nerve injuries with greater experience. Letournel and Judet initially noted an 18.4% incidence of postoperative iatrogenic sciatic nerve injury using the Kocher-Langenbeck approach, which was subsequently reduced to 3.3%. None of their 114 patients treated with an extensile approach developed this complication. Matta et al. initially reported a 9% incidence of iatrogenic nerve palsy which was reduced to 3.5% with further experience. Furthermore, only two of nine neurologic injuries involved the sciatic nerve. The use of intraoperative sciatic nerve monitoring using somatosensory-evoked potentials has reduced the incidence of iatrogenic sciatic nerve injury to 2% (13,14). This risk is further lessened by the addition of intraoperative monitoring of motor pathways (57).

Letournel and Judet (3) reported a 2.3% incidence of in-hospital death following operative fixation of acetabular fractures; the majority of the deaths occurred in patients over the age of 60 years. Though the exact incidence of DVT is unknown, it plays a major role in postoperative morbidity and mortality. Letournel and Judet (3) reported a 3% incidence of clinically evident DVT, with 4 fatal and 8 minor pulmonary emboli in a series of 569 patients, although the majority of patients received anticoagulant prophylaxis. Using a preoperative and postoperative

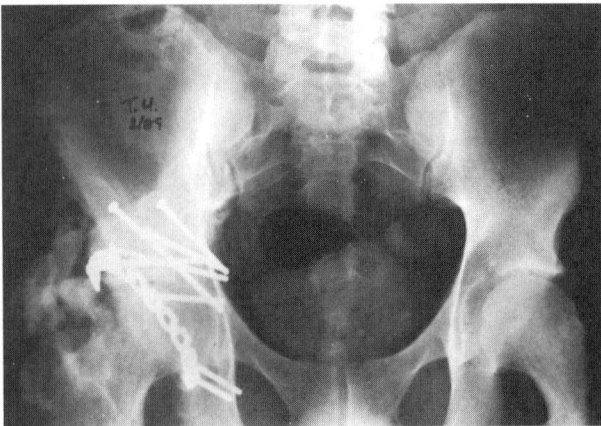

Figure 40.31. HO in a 56-year-old male who underwent ORIF of a posterior column with posterior wall fracture dislocation 5 months earlier. Note the avascular necrosis with femoral head collapse.

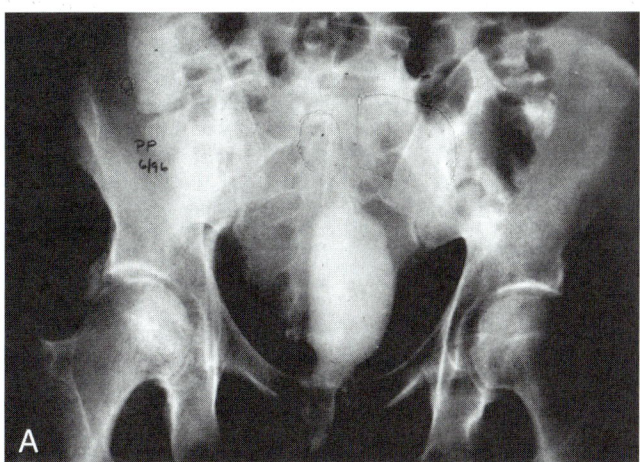

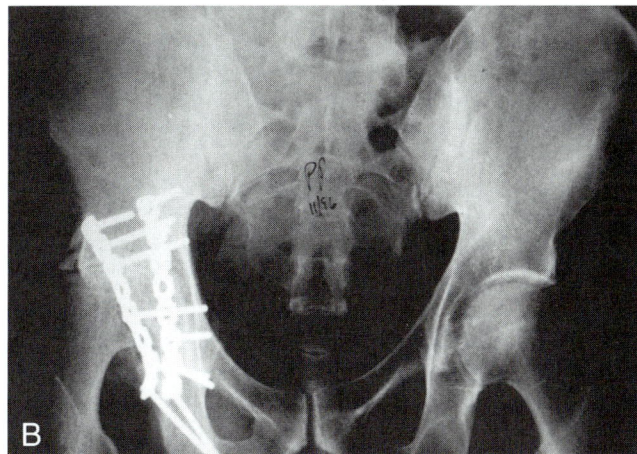

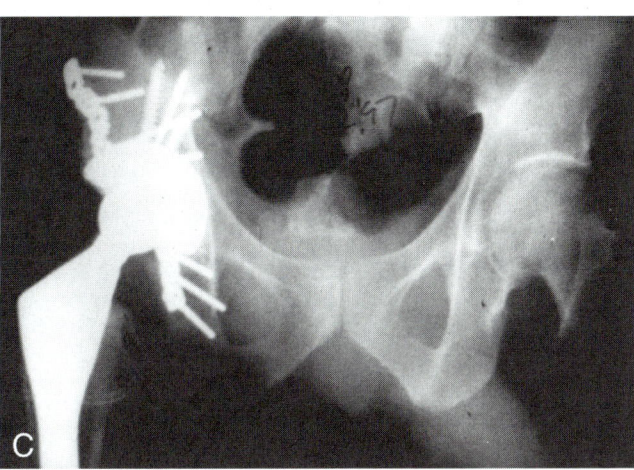

Figure 40.32. A. Preoperative AP view. **B.** AP view at the 5-month follow-up showing decreased joint space and collapse of the femoral head. **C.** After conversion to a total hip arthroplasty.

treatment protocol, Stickney and Helfet (22) significantly decreased the incidence of DVT. Improved detection of venous thromboembolism by using magnetic resonance venography has also lead to more aggressive treatment and, therefore, a lower incidence of pulmonary embolism (23).

The incidence of infection lies between 4 and 5%, but has been reported to be as high as 9% (3,4,34,40,46,52). Skin necrosis was noted in 1.8% (10.2% of extended iliofemoral approaches) and hematomas in 6.7% of Letournel and Judet's cases. To minimize wound problems, they advocated the use of prophylactic antibiotics, the use of multiple suction drains in all recesses to prevent hematoma formation, surgical evacuation of hematomas, and débridement of any existing Morel-Lavele lesions.

The incidence of avascular necrosis of the femoral head following operative treatment of acetabular fractures has generally ranged from 3 to 9%; the majority of cases are identified between 3 and 18 months following surgery (3,4,15). Delay in treatment may be a risk factor, because Letournel and Judet (3) have noted an increased incidence of avascular necrosis in cases presenting after 3 weeks. They also noted an increased risk in injuries associated with a posterior fracture/dislocation, suggesting that the fate of the femoral head is determined at the time of the initial injury (Fig. 40.32).

SUMMARY

Fractures of the acetabulum are among the most difficult of fractures encountered by the orthopaedic traumatologist. Of paramount importance to both understanding and treatment is determining the pattern of the fracture. The system of Letournel group fracture types as either elemental (anterior or posterior wall, anterior or posterior column, and transverse) or associated (anterior wall and column, posterior wall and column, anterior with a posterior hemitransverse, T-type, and both-column). This improves preoperative planning, including the selection of the optimal surgical approach (generally a Kocher-Langenbeck, ilioinguinal, extended iliofemoral, or combined approach) and the contemplation of the required intraoperative reduction maneuvers. As the patient's outcome is directly related to the adequacy of reduction and complications can be disastrous, these challenging fractures should be managed only by experienced surgeons.

REFERENCES

1. Letournel E. Acetabulum fractures: classification and management. Clin Orthop 1980;151:81–106.
2. Letournel E. Surgical treatment of acetabular fractures. Paper presented at the 15th Open Scientific Meeting of the Hip Society, San Francisco, CA, 1987.

3. Letournel E, Judet R. Fractures of the acetabulum. Berlin: Springer-Verlag, 1981, 1993.
4. Matta JM. Fractures of the acetabulum: accuracy of reduction and clinical results. J Bone Joint Surg 1996;78A:632–645.
5. Mayo KA. Surgical approaches to the acetabulum. Tech Orthop 1990;4:24–35.
6. Judet R, Judet J, Letournel E. Fractures of the acetabulum: classification and surgical approaches for open reduction. Preliminary report. J Bone Joint Surg 1964;46A:1615–1646.
7. Judet R, Lagrange J. La voie postero externe de ceibson. Presse Med 1958;63(3):263–264.
8. Smith RW, Staple TW. Computerized tomography (CT) scanning: technique for the hindfoot. Clin Orthop 1983;177:34–38.
9. Orthopaedic Trauma Association Committee for Coding and Classification. Fracture and dislocation compendium. J Orthop Trauma 1996;10:71–75.
10. Hak DJ, Olson SA, Matta JM. Management of the Morel-Lavele lesion. Paper presented at the 3rd Annual International Consensus on Surgery of the Pelvis and Acetabulum. Pittsburgh, October 5–11, 1996.
11. Helfet DL, Anand N, Malkani AL, et al. Intraoperative monitoring of motor pathways during operative fixation of acute acetabular fractures. J Orthop Trauma 1977;11:2–6.
12. Helfet DL, Borrelli JD Jr, DiPasquale TG, Sanders RW. Stabilization of acetabular fractures in elderly patients. J Bone Joint Surg 1992;74A:753–765.
13. Helfet DL, Hissa EA, Sergay S, Mast JW. Somatosensory evoked potential monitoring in the surgical management of acute acetabular fractures. J Orthop Trauma 1991;5:161–166.
14. Helfet DL, Schmeling GJ. Somatosensory evoked potential monitoring in the surgical treatment of acute, displaced acetabular fractures: results of a prospective study. J Orthop Trauma 1992;6:484.
15. Matta JM, Anderson LM, Epstein HC, Hendricks P. Fractures of the acetabulum: a retrospective analysis. Clin Orthop 1986;205:241–250.
16. Matta JM, Mehne DK, Roffi R. Fractures of the acetabulum: early results of a prospective study. Clin Orthop 1986;205:241–250.
17. Pennal GF, Davidson J, Garside H, Plewes J. Results of treatment of acetabular fractures. Clin Orthop 1980;151:115–123.
18. Vrahas M, Gordon RG, Mears DC, et al. Intraoperative somatosensory evoked potential monitoring of pelvic and acetabular fractures. J Orthop Trauma 1992;6:50–58.
19. Bosse MJ, Poka A, Reinert CM, et al. Preoperative angiographic assessment of the superior gluteal artery in acetabular fractures requiring extensile surgical exposures. J Orthop Trauma 1989;2:303–307.
20. Johnson EE, Eckhardt JJ, Letournel E. Extrinsic femoral artery occlusion following internal fixation of an acetabular fracture. A case report. Clin Orthop 1987;217:209–213.
21. Geerts WH, Code KI, Jay RM, et al. A prospective study of venous thromboembolism after major trauma. N Engl J Med 1995;332:1448–1449.
22. Stickney JL, Helfet DL. Deep vein thrombosis prevention in orthopaedic trauma patients [Abstract]. J Orthop Trauma 1991;5:227.
23. Montgomery KD, Potter HG, Helfet DL. Magnetic resonance venography to evaluate the deep venous system of the pelvis in patients who have an acetabular fracture. J Bone Joint Surg 1995;77A:1639–1649.
24. Bray TJ, Esser M, Fulkerson L. Osteotomy of the trochanter in open reduction and internal fixation of acetabular fractures. J Bone Joint Surg 1987;69A:711–717.
25. D'Aubigne RM. Management of acetabular fractures in multiple trauma. J Trauma 1968;8:333–349.
26. Goulet JA, Bray TJ. Complex acetabular fractures. Clin Orthop 1989;240:9–20.
27. Hak DJ, Olson SA, Hamel AJ, et al. Consequences of transverse acetabular fracture malreduction on load transmission across the hip joint. Paper presented at the 12th Annual Meeting of the Orthopaedic Trauma Association, Boston, Sept 27–29, 1996.
28. Heeg M, Ostvogel H, Klasen H. Conservative treatment of acetabular fractures: the role of the weightbearing dome and anatomic reduction in the ultimate results. J Trauma 1987;27:555–559.
29. Helfet DL, Schmeling GJ. Management of complex acetabular fractures through single nonextensile exposures. Clin Orthop 1994;305:58–68.
30. Hofmann AA, Dahl CP, Wyatt RW. Experience with acetabular fractures. J Trauma 1984;24:750–752.
31. Malkani AL, Voor MJ, Rennirt G, et al. Increased peak contact pressure following incongruent reduction of transverse acetabular fractures: a cadaveric model. Paper presented at the 12th Annual Meeting of the Orthopaedic Trauma Association, Boston, Sept 27–29, 1996.
32. Matta JM. Operative indications and choice of surgical approach for fractures of the acetabulum. Tech Orthop 1986;1:13–22.
33. Matta JM, Letournel E, Browner BD. Surgical management of acetabular fractures. Instr Course Lect 1986;35:382–397.
34. Matta JM, Merritt PO. Displaced acetabular fractures. Clin Orthop 1988;230:83–97.
35. Mayo KA. Fractures of the acetabulum. Orthop Clin North Am 1987;18:43–57.
36. Routt MLC, Jr., Swiontkowski MF. Operative treatment of complex acetabular fractures: combined anterior and posterior exposures during the same procedure. J Bone Joint Surg 1990;72A:897–904.
37. Tile M. Fractures of the acetabulum. Orthop Clin North Am 1980;11:481–506.
38. Tile M, Burgess A, Helfet DL, Kellam JP. Fractures of the pelvis and acetabulum. Baltimore: Williams & Wilkins, 1995.
39. Helfet DL, Bartlett CS, Lorich D. The use of a single limited posterior approach and reduction techniques for specific patterns of acetabular fractures. Oper Tech Orthop 1997;7:196–205.
40. Helfet DL, Schmeling GJ. The management of acute, displaced complex acetabular fractures using indirect reduction techniques and limited surgical approaches. Orthop Trans 1991;15:833–834.
41. Kaempffe FA, Bone L, Border JR. Open reduction and internal fixation of acetabular fractures: heterotopic ossification and other complications of treatment. J Orthop Trauma 1991;5:439–445.
42. Bosse MJ, Poka A, Reinert CM, et al. Heterotopic ossification as a complication of acetabular fracture: prophylaxis with low-dose irradiation. J Bone Joint Surg 1988;70A:1231–1237.
43. Leenen LP, van der Werken C, Schoots F, Goris RJ. Internal fixation of open unstable pelvic fractures. J Trauma 1993;35:220–225.
44. Johnson EE, Matta JM, Mast JW, Letournel E. Delayed reconstruction of acetabular fractures 21–120 days following injury. Clin Orthop 1994;305:20–30.
45. Mears DC, Rubash HE. Extensile exposure of the pelvis. Contemp Orthop 1983;6:21–31.
46. Alonso JE, Davila R, Bradley E. Extended iliofemoral versus triradiate approaches in management of associated acetabular fractures. Clin Orthop 1994;305:81–87.
47. Tabor OB, Bosse MJ, Greene KG, et al. The effects of the abductor muscles of surgical approaches for acetabular fractures associated with gluteal vascular injury. Paper presented at the 12th Annual Meeting of the Orthopaedic Trauma Association, Boston, MA, September 27–29, 1996.
48. Skura DS, Buchsbaum S. Prophylactic low-dose postoperative irradiation for the prevention of heterotopic ossification in acetabular fractures [Abstract]. Orthop Trans 1992;16:221.

49. Mears DC, Gordon RG. Internal fixation of acetabular fractures. Tech Orthop 1990;4:36–51.

50. Brumback RJ, Holt ES, McBride MS, et al. Acetabular depression fracture accompanying posterior fracture dislocation of the hip. J Orthop Trauma 1990;4:42–48.

51. Mast JW, Ganz R, Jakob RP. Planning and reduction technique in fracture surgery. New York: Springer-Verlag, 1989.

52. Rowe CR, Lowell JD. Prognosis of fractures of the acetabulum. J Bone Joint Surg 1961;43A:30–59.

53. Kebaish AS, Roy A, Rennie W. Displaced acetabular fractures: long-term follow-up. J Trauma 1991;31:1539–1542.

54. Moed BR, Maxey JW. The effect of indomethacin on heterotopic ossification following acetabular fracture surgery. J Orthop Trauma 1993;7:33–38.

55. Tile M, Kellam JF, Joyce M. Fractures of the acetabulum: classification, management protocol and results of treatment. J Bone Joint Surg 1985;67B:173.

56. McLaren AC. Prophylaxis with indomethacin for heterotopic bone. J Bone Joint Surg 1990;72A:245–247.

57. Goodman SB, Adler SJ, Fyhrie DP, Schurman DJ. The acetabular teardrop and its relevance in acetabular migration. Clin Orthop 1988;236:199–204.

41

Michael H. Huo and Barry J. Waldman

Cemented Total Hip Replacement

Total hip replacement (THR) is an excellent treatment option for patients with end-stage degenerative hip disease. In the 35 years since Sir John Charnley first reported his experience, THR has become one of the most commonly performed reconstructive procedures in orthopaedic surgery. Excellent results are obtained in the majority of patients, but long-term fixation of the components to bone continues to be the outstanding challenge. Moreover, wear of the articulating surfaces and the resulting osteolysis have emerged as the major mechanisms of failure. In this chapter, we discuss some general issues related to hip anatomy, indications of hip replacement, surgical techniques, implant design, cement preparation, and clinical results of THRs done with cement.

RELEVANT ANATOMY AND PATHOGENESIS

The hip is a constrained joint that is further reinforced by a fibrocartilaginous labrum and a strong joint capsule. The capsular ligaments originate on the ilium and ischium and insert onto the intertrochanteric ridge of the femur. The capsule is composed of the iliofemoral ligament anteriorly (Y ligament of Bigelow) and the ischiofemoral ligament posteriorly. The acetabulum is at the confluence of the ischium, ilium, and pubis. It is formed from ossification of the triradiate cartilage during development. It is lined with articular cartilage, except inferiorly. The transverse acetabular ligament connects the posterior and anterior labrum, crossing the inferior margin of the acetabular fossa.

The hip is surrounded by several muscles that provide dynamic stability to the joint and stabilize the trunk during gait. The gluteus maximus originates from the posterior iliac crest and inserts on the fascia lata and posterior proximal femur. The gluteus medius and minimus are broad, fan-shaped muscles that originate from the lateral iliac wing and insert onto the greater trochanter. Together, these three muscles abduct the hip and prevent lateral sway of the trunk during gait. The tensor fascia lata also arises from the iliac crest and inserts on the iliotibial band distally. The vastus lateralis arises from the intertrochanteric ridge and the linea aspera along the lateral femur. It becomes a part of the quadriceps complex and helps extend the knee. The rectus femoris arises from the anterior inferior iliac spine and hip capsule. It inserts on the quadriceps tendon and acts to flex the hip and extend the knee. The iliacus arises from the medial iliac wing and joins in a common tendon with the psoas, which takes its origin off the transverse processes, vertebral bodies, and disks of T12–L4. The common iliopsoas tendon inserts onto the lesser trochanter and acts to flex the hip.

The piriformis originates from the greater sciatic notch and inserts on the posterior greater trochanter in the piriformis fossa. It is the most proximal external rotator of the hip. The other external rotators are the obturator internus, the inferior and superior gemelli, and the quadratus femoris. The obturator externus and gemelli originate from the posterior ischium. The quadratus femoris originates from the posterior aspect of the pubis. All four of the short external rotators insert posteriorly along the intertrochanteric crest.

The femoral vein, artery, and nerve can be found medial to the rectus femoris and iliopsoas after they pass under the inguinal ligament. The lateral and medial femoral circumflex vessels surround the femoral neck and provide blood supply to the proximal femur. The femoral nerve provides innervation to the quadriceps muscles. The superior gluteal vessels exit the pelvis from the greater sciatic notch superior to the piriformis. The superior gluteal nerve supplies the gluteus medius, minimus, and tensor fascia lata. The inferior gluteal nerve exits inferior to the piriformis and supplies the gluteus maximus. Finally, the sciatic nerve exits the greater sciatic notch and runs down the femur posterior to the short external rotators. It supplies the lower leg through its tibial and peroneal divisions. The external rotators receive their innervation from individual nerves that arise from the lumbosacral plexus.

Causes of Hip Degeneration

The most common causes of end-stage degeneration of the hip joint are osteoarthritis, rheumatoid arthritis, osteonecrosis of the femoral head, posttraumatic arthritis, infection, and neoplasia. Less common conditions include arthritis associated with Paget's disease, hemophilia, sickle-cell anemia, and ankylosing spondylitis. Congenital conditions, such as developmental dysplasia of the hip and Legg-Calvé-Perthes disease, may result in severe arthritis in adulthood. The incidence of severe joint degeneration secondary to developmental problems may be much higher than can be documented at the time of adult presentation. The severity of joint destruction in end-stage disease often obscures any distinguishing radiographic signs of developmental dysplasia. Many of these patients may carry a diagnosis of osteoarthritis or idiopathic degenerative joint disease.

INITIAL FINDINGS AND PHYSICAL EXAMINATION

The common clinical presentations of the disease entities associated with hip degeneration are pain, decreased motion, gait abnormalities, and loss of function. Leg length discrepancy occurs as a result of decreased cartilage thickness, deformity of the femoral head, and development of flexion and adduction contractures. The patient's gait should be assessed for Trendelenburg's sign (abductor lurch) and motion of the hip, knee, and ankle. The lumbar spine and knee should be carefully examined. These areas are common sources of pain that may radiate to the hip.

RADIOLOGIC STUDIES

Radiographs should be obtained in all patients under consideration for surgical treatment. An AP view of the pelvis and a lateral view of the hip are recommended. The lateral radiograph is commonly taken in the frog-leg position (with the hip abducted and flexed). Some patients may not be able to abduct sufficiently for this view to be taken. As an alternative, a Lauenstein or pass-through lateral may be substituted. CT, though not routinely obtained, may be useful for patients who have severe deformity and for those who may require a custom-designed prosthesis. MRI is useful in the diagnosis of osteonecrosis but is of limited use for presurgical planning.

Radiographic features may differ depending on the cause of degenerative arthritis; however, end-stage degeneration often has a characteristic appearance. The majority of radiographs will display narrowing of the joint space, indicating degeneration of the articular cartilage. Bony abnormalities are commonly seen. Osteophytes may be present along the acetabular rim, especially superiorly. Subchondral cysts and sclerosis can be seen in both the acetabulum and the femoral head, usually in weight-bearing areas. With advanced degrees of arthritis, the femoral head may become flattened and deformed. Developmental dysplasia, which may leave the patient with a shallow acetabulum, resulting in subluxation or dislocation of the femoral head, often articulates with a false acetabulum.

TREATMENT

Nonoperative Treatment

Patients with hip arthritis may have long-term relief of pain and improvement in function with nonoperative therapy. A number of modalities are available. Nonsteroidal anti-inflammatory drugs (NSAIDs) can relieve pain and decrease inflammation. Patients should undergo a trial for at least 3 to 4 weeks for the clinician to evaluate the efficacy of any new anti-inflammatory. Many patients will respond well to one medication but not to others. Walking aids, such as a cane or walker, are excellent for relieving pain by unloading the affected hip. Physical therapy, muscle conditioning, weight reduction, and modification of activities can all result in clinical improvement.

Other surgical alternatives should be considered, especially for younger patients. Arthrodesis of the hip results in a pain-free joint that can support weight-bearing loads indefinitely (1,2). However, the loss of motion may be unacceptable to some patients. Moreover, altered biomechanical alignment and stresses often result in degeneration of the ipsilateral knee joint, the opposite hip, and the lumbosacral spine. Realignment osteotomy of the proximal femur can reduce pain by unloading the most degenerated areas of cartilage and medializing the femur (3). Biomechanically, additional varus of the proximal femur increases the abductor lever arm, resulting in reduced joint reaction force. Young patients with an underdeveloped acetabulum secondary to congenital hip dysplasia may benefit from a pelvic osteotomy, with or without concomitant femoral osteotomy.

Indications for THR Surgery

Patients are considered surgical candidates after failure of nonoperative therapy and stabilization of any chronic medical conditions. Relief of pain and improvement in function are the goals of any THR surgery. Indications for surgery should include moderate to severe pain or disability and radiographic evidence of joint degeneration. Preoperative education is crucial to the success of THR. Patients with unrealistic expectations may not be satisfied with what the surgeon believes to be an excellent reconstruction.

Contraindications to THR are few. Active systemic or local infection and unstable medical conditions present absolute contraindications. Obesity has been considered a relative contraindication because of the increased mechanical loads placed on the prostheses. Age is also an important consideration. Higher loosening and revision rates are reported with patients younger than 50 years old. Every effort should be made to treat these patients with other modalities before considering THR.

Operative Treatment

DESIGN AND CEMENTING TECHNIQUES

Many changes have evolved in the design of prostheses inserted with cement since Charnley's original work. Not all changes have been improvements; however, some design changes have resulted in improved clinical performance and durability of cemented THRs. This section will focus primarily on the discussion of femoral stem design and cementing techniques.

Cement acts as a grout between the prosthesis and the bone, transferring stress between the two. Cement must be inherently strong and the mantle sufficiently thick to resist the stresses to which it is exposed. Changes in the preparation and delivery of cement have been introduced since the late 1970s, along with changes in prosthetic design and biomaterials. It is important to understand the terminology that is currently used in the discussion of cemented THR. Each cementing technique has its own clinical success rate.

It is necessary to be familiar with the concept of generations in cementing techniques (4). First-generation techniques involved manual mixing and hand packing the cement into the femoral canal and acetabulum. No distal plug or pressurization devices were used. Later studies showed that the uniformity and thickness of the cement mantle were among the most important factors in the durability of fixation (5).

A number of techniques have since been developed to improve the biomechanical properties and delivery of the cement. Second-generation cementing techniques include the use of an intramedullary plug, pulsatile lavage of the bony bed to remove debris, introduction of cement with a gun in a retrograde fashion, and pressurization of the cement. The distal plug, which can be made of polyethylene, cement, or bone, allows the cement to be pressurized without filling the entire intramedullary canal of the femur.

Third-generation techniques were developed to further the goals of providing stronger cement and a uniform cement mantle. In addition to the second-generation techniques, new procedures include porosity reduction of the cement and surface modification of the prosthesis. Porosity reduction of the cement can be accomplished with centrifugation or vacuum-mixing devices (6,7). Surface modifications of the stem may include changes in texture, precoating with methylmethacrylate, and the use of a distal centralizer or proximal spacers. These modifications allow for a stronger interface between the prosthesis

and the cement, central placement of the stem, and increased pressurization of the cement (5).

Stem

The mechanical properties of any material used to fabricate prostheses for THR must be strong enough to tolerate cyclic loading with a force that may be many times the patient's weight. Moreover, the biologic response to stress transfer by the material to the host bone and to any debris generated by wear and corrosion must be carefully considered. The most commonly used biomaterials in fabricating femoral stems for insertion with cement are cobalt-based (Co-based) super alloys that include chromium (Cr) as the other major chemical component. Titanium-based (Ti-based) alloys are less preferable for either the stem or the articulating surface because of its wear characteristics, especially if the prosthesis has loosened (8–10). Because of its lower modulus of elasticity, Ti-alloy stems generate greater stresses in the cement mantle than do Co-Cr-alloy stems. The increased stress can theoretically lead to cracks within the cement, resulting in loss of fixation.

Biomechanical analyses have demonstrated that the ideal stem design for use with cement has a broad medial surface, rounded shoulders laterally, and a tapered wedge shape. A broad cross-sectional geometry of the stem proximally has been shown to decrease the stress in the cement mantle, theoretically providing longer durability of fixation (11). The surface of the stem should offer a texture that facilitates cement bonding. The surface may be precoated with a layer of cement, molded with grooves or ridges, or produced with a sand-blasted-type finish. These surface treatments can enhance stress transfer to the cement mantle and surrounding bone, but they can also represent stress concentration points that encourage crack initiation and propagation within the cement mantle itself, especially if debonding occurs.

The use of a collar remains controversial. Biomechanical analyses have demonstrated increased loading of the proximal medial calcar when there is collar-calcar contact in cemented stems. This may in turn reduce the stress-shielding effects of the stem on the femoral bone. The clinical significance of this design feature remains to be fully documented (12).

Currently, many stem designs offer spacers and centralizers both distally and proximally to ensure a desirable thickness of cement and to guide the stem down the center of the mantle during insertion (5). Biomechanical studies of the cement mantle around the femoral stem have demonstrated a minimum thickness of 2 to 3 mm to be necessary. Furthermore, the mantle should be at least 3 to 4 mm in the proximal medial zone (Gruen zone 7) and nearly 1 cm in the distal area (Gruen zone 4).

Cup

The acetabular cup can be made with a metal backing or entirely from ultrahigh-molecular-weight polyethylene

(UHMWPE). Metal backing of the cup was at one time popular due to the theoretical advantage of decreasing stress transfer from the articulating surface to the underlying cement (13). The clinical performance of metal-backed cups inserted with cement, however, has been reported to be inferior to non–metal-backed cups (14). Metal backing has the expense of decreased polyethylene thickness, which can result in accelerated wear and debris generation, leading to significant osteolysis and loosening of fixation. In contrast, some authors have recently reported no increased loosening or wear rates in metal-backed cups inserted with cement (15) (Fig. 41.1). Regardless of the controversy, the majority of surgeons currently would use an all-polyethylene cup if cement fixation is selected.

Reduction of wear at the articulating surface can also be accomplished by improving the femoral head component. Surface treatment of metal, such as nitrogen ion implantation, may offer improved wear characteristics of the femoral head. Ceramics, such as aluminum oxide or zirconium oxide, also serve as excellent biomaterials for the articulating surface. They offer greater wear resistance and less friction than do metal-on-polyethylene couplings (16). Ceramics, however, are more prone to fractures (17,18). This potential catastrophic failure mode is related to the grain size and crystallinity of the ceramic-manufacturing process and, in particular, the design of the Morse taper junction.

SURGICAL TECHNIQUE

Preoperative surgical planning is crucial for the successful performance of any cemented THR. Routine AP views of the pelvis should be available along with a lateral projection of the affected hip for templating. Templating is performed to plan for the size and position of the components. The leg length and femoral offset must be reconstructed to match the contralateral hip whenever possible.

Surgical Approaches

Various surgical approaches may be used to expose the hip joint for a THR. All have advantages and disadvantages. The surgeon should understand the limitations and use the surgical exposure that meets the specific anatomy and reconstructive goals of each patient. Charnley originally used the transtrochanteric approach. It is currently used less often for primary surgery than for revision situations. This section focuses on the two most commonly used surgical exposures for performing primary THR: lateral and posterior.

Lateral approach. The lateral, or Hardinge, approach has the advantage of exposing the acetabulum in a directly lateral orientation, allowing for easy and proper placement of the cup (19). It does not disrupt the posterior capsule, thus minimizing postoperative dislocations. This exposure, however, is at the expense of releasing part of the abductor muscle, which can result in a persistent limp after surgery.

The patient is placed in the lateral decubitus or supine position using a pelvic positioner or a sandbag. A straight lateral incision is made over the greater trochanter. The fascia lata is exposed and split along the line of the skin incision, centered on the greater trochanter and extended distally. The proximal exposure is made in the interval between the tensor fascia lata and the gluteus maximus to expose the underlying gluteus medius. This interval can be identified by palpating the undersurface of the fascia lata. Distal dissection of the fascia lata is extended to the level of the tendinous insertion of the gluteus maximus. The underlying trochanteric bursa is excised, exposing the insertion of the gluteus medius and the origin of the vastus lateralis on the greater trochanter.

The gluteus medius is split from the greater trochanter proximally, leaving the posterior one-third of the muscle attached to the greater trochanter (Fig. 41.2A). This portion

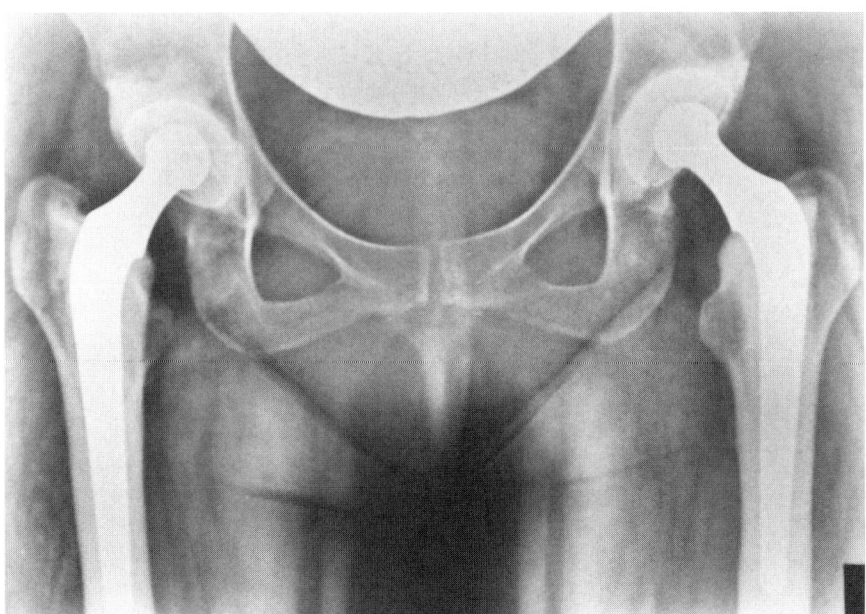

Figure 41.1. AP view showing the 8-year follow-up of a bilateral cemented THR with metal-backed cups and stable fixation.

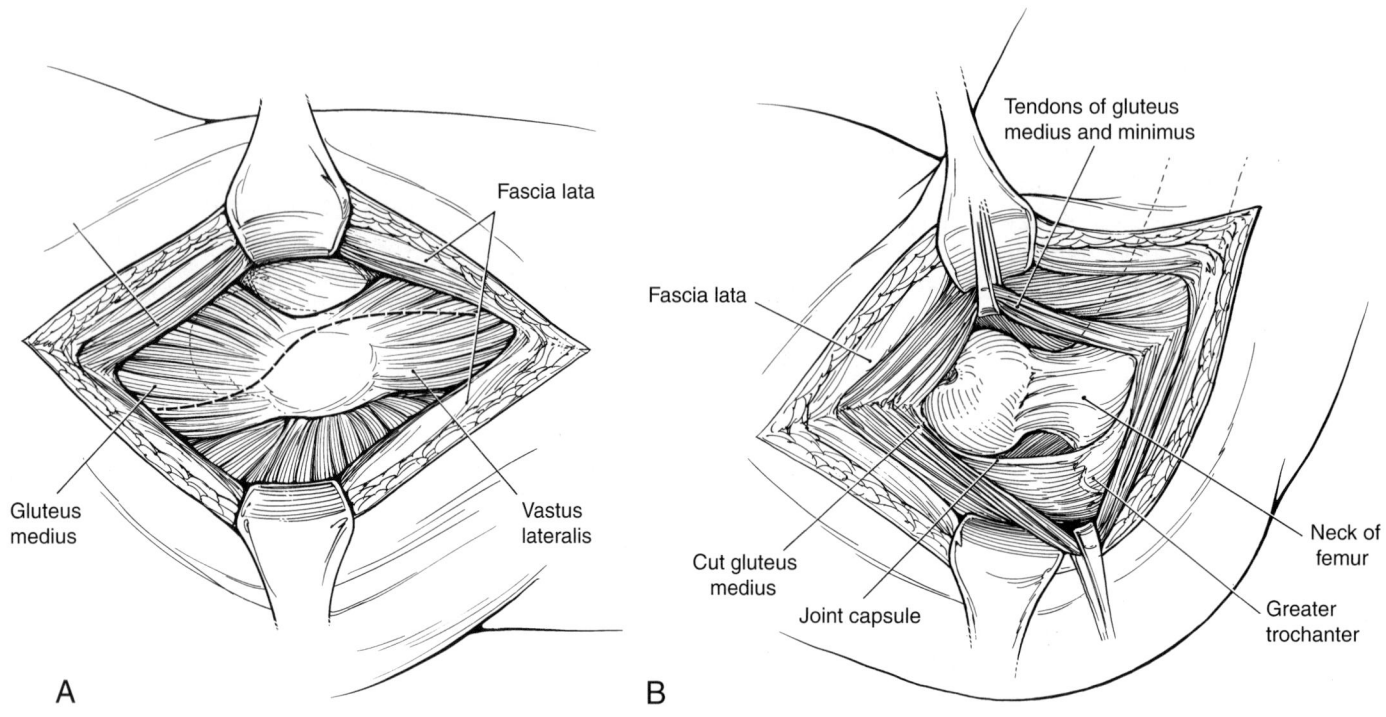

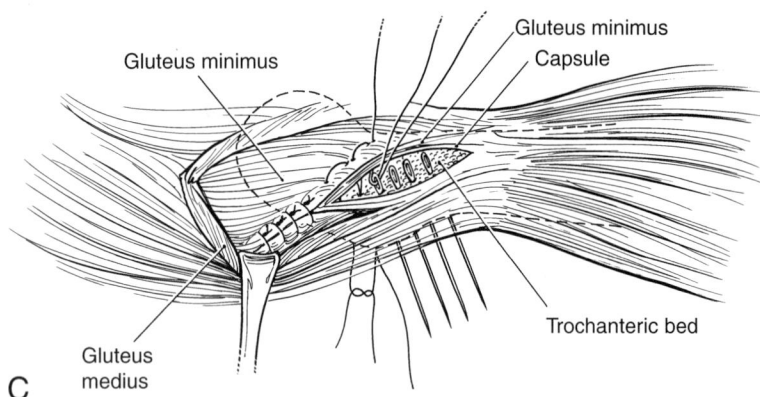

Figure 41.2. A. Dissection of the gluteus medius is done along the anterior two-thirds, leaving the posterior tendon attached to the greater trochanter. A cuff of the vastus lateralis is dissected to create a continuous musculotendinous sleeve. **B.** The anterior hip joint capsule is exposed and released. The femoral head can be dislocated with extension, external rotation, and adduction of the femur. Modified from Hoppenfeld S, deBoer P. Surgical exposures in orthopaedics: the anatomic approach. Philadelphia: Lippincott, 1984:334. **C.** The abductor tendon sleeve is reattached to the greater trochanter.

is more tendinous and can be palpated before the muscle is split. It is critical to limit the separation of the gluteus medius muscle to no more than 4 cm proximal to the superior edge of the acetabulum. Further splitting can injure the superior gluteal nerve and vessels. This dissection is extended distally, splitting the origin of the vastus lateralis 2 to 3 cm distal to the trochanteric ridge. This extension creates a sleeve of tendon anteriorly that can be repaired later. The anterior sleeve is then dissected off the proximal femur anteriorly in the direction of the joint capsule. The gluteus minimus tendon is then released, along with the anterior two-thirds of the gluteus medius, revealing the joint capsule. If the gluteus medius tendon is atrophic or scarred from previous surgeries, a wafer of bone from the trochanter can be mobilized to create a musculoosseous sleeve to allow for more secure reattachment.

The anterior joint capsule is identified, and a capsulectomy is performed to expose the femoral neck (Fig. 41.2B).

Leg length measurements may be taken at this time. The joint is then dislocated by flexing, adducting, and externally rotating the femur. The femoral neck osteotomy can then be done at the appropriate level, according to preoperative planning. Routine acetabular preparation can be easily done by placing retractors over the anterior, inferior, posterior, and superior acetabulum. Femoral preparation is performed by placing the leg across the table into a side pocket, similar to the transtrochanteric approach. It is important to protect the remaining gluteus medius during reaming and broaching.

The gluteus medius muscle is reattached to the greater trochanter after insertion of the components (Fig. 41.2C). This can be achieved with nonabsorbable sutures through drill holes into bone. The sutures should be passed through the gluteus medius and minimus to ensure secure reattachment. Routine closure of the fascia and the superficial layers completes the procedure.

Posterior approach. The posterior approach uses the interval between the gluteus maximus and the gluteus medius. The advantages include ease of dissection, excellent exposure of the acetabulum and the femur, no disruption of the abductor muscles, and fast postoperative rehabilitation. The primary disadvantage is increased risk of dislocations (20). This complication can be minimized by proper orientation of the components, careful repair of the posterior soft tissues, and adherence to dislocation precautions during rehabilitation.

The patient is placed in the lateral decubitus position. The incision is made over the greater trochanter, and the proximal extension is curved toward the sacrum posteriorly in line with the fibers of the gluteus maximus. The incision will appear straight if the hip is flexed to 90°. The fascia lata is incised in line with the skin incision and centered on the greater trochanter. The distal exposure should be made to the level of the gluteus maximus tendon and the proximal portion about 5 cm proximal to the greater trochanter. The gluteus maximus muscle, which is adherent to the fascia lata, is split along its fibers proximally. The gluteus maximus tendon can be partially released from its bony insertion to better mobilize the femur.

The trochanteric bursa can then be excised to reveal the external rotators. The external rotators of the hip—piriformis, gemelli, obturator internus, and quadratus femoris—are exposed by placing retractors over the superior and inferior neck of the femur (Fig. 41.3A). The

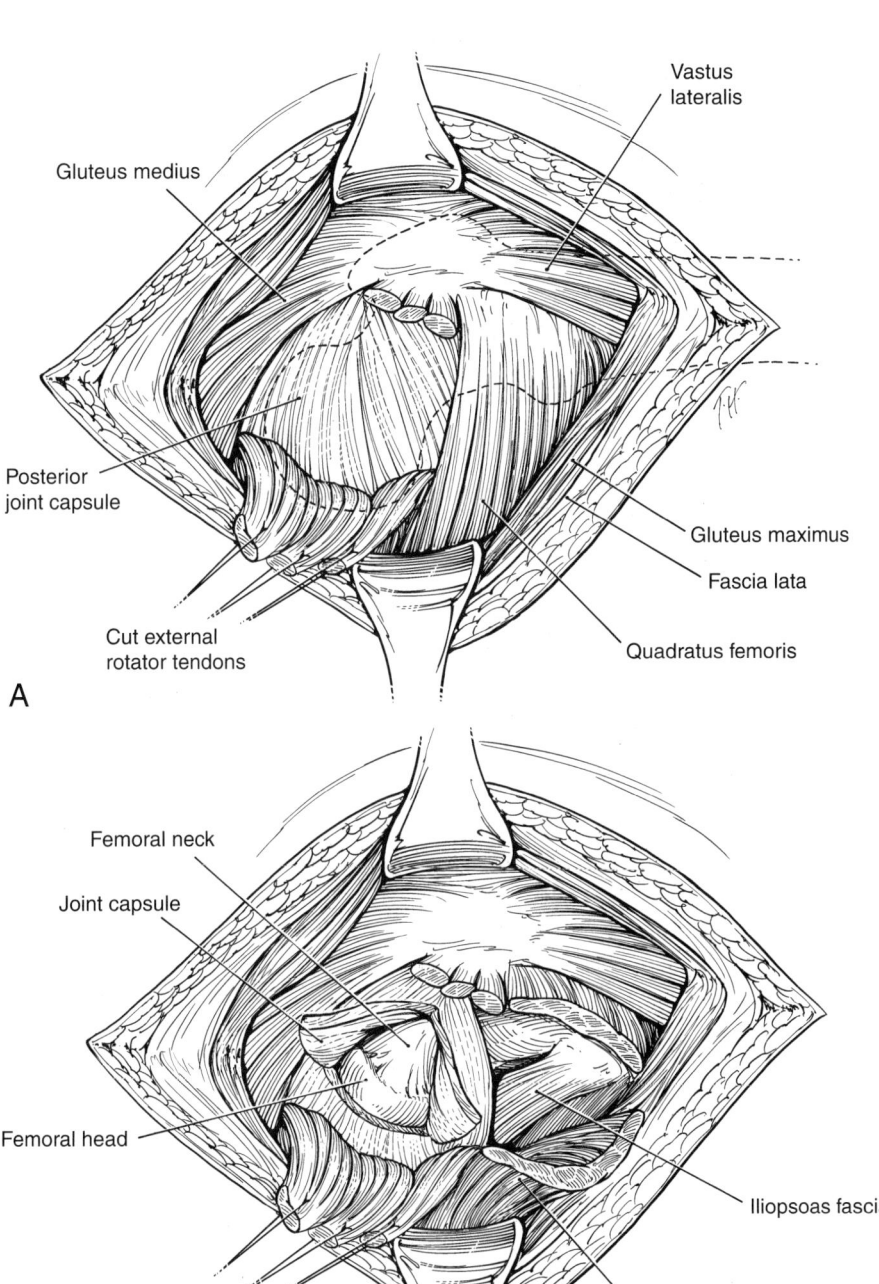

Figure 41.3. A. The short external rotators of the hip are exposed. Note the close relationship of the sciatic nerve to the direction of the surgical dissection. **B.** The posterior hip joint capsule is released; and the femoral head can be dislocated with flexion, internal rotation, and adduction of the femur.

posterior joint capsule is identified after releasing the external rotators from the greater trochanter. A complete capsulectomy or a posterior capsular flap can be performed to expose the joint. Dislocation of the femoral head is performed by internal rotation, flexion, and adduction (Fig. 41.3B). The femoral neck osteotomy is then performed at the appropriate level according to preoperative planning.

The acetabulum is exposed by placing retractors over the anterior rim, inferior transverse acetabulum ligament, posterior wall, and the superior-lateral wall. Routine preparation of the acetabulum can be easily completed. Visualization can be facilitated by banking the operating table toward the surgeon.

The femoral canal is accessed by placing the femur in internal rotation, flexion, and adduction. A retractor is used to elevate the neck of the femur from the posterior soft tissue flap. A retractor is also placed over the piriformis fossa to protect the abductor muscles. Reaming and broaching of the canal can easily be performed in this position. Following insertion of the trial components, the hip is reduced. Stability can then be assessed. After the permanent components are cemented in place, the short external rotators and the posterior capsular flap (if preserved) can be sutured back to the greater trochanter through drill holes. Routine closure of the fascia and the superficial layers completes the procedure.

The major structure at risk during the posterior approach is the sciatic nerve. We have not routinely dissected out the nerve in uncomplicated primary surgeries. Care is taken to avoid excessive traction of the posterior soft tissues with retractors during surgery. Furthermore, overlengthening is avoided by careful selection of the proper neck length.

Insertion of the Acetabular Cup with Cement

The acetabulum is exposed in a similar manner as it is for insertion of a cup without cement. Complete resection of the labrum and capsular tissues is necessary to prevent interposition between the component and the cancellous bone bed. Efforts should be made to preserve the transverse acetabulum ligament inferiorly. This structure is often helpful in preventing cement extrusion inferiorly and assists in containing and pressurizing the cement.

The acetabular fossa is expanded to the lateral cortex of the medial wall using a small-diameter reamer; larger- and larger-diameter reamers are used sequentially until a complete bony bed is exposed and all soft tissues are removed. Care should be taken not to ream more than necessary to expose the subchondral bone. The thickness of the anterior and posterior acetabular walls should be assessed throughout reaming to ensure adequate bone to support the prosthesis. Trial components can be used to select the proper size. It is important to select a cup approximately 2 mm smaller in diameter than the final reamer to ensure an adequate cement mantle around the prosthesis.

Three or four cement anchoring holes are routinely placed over the dome of the acetabulum (Fig. 41.4). The holes can be made by using a curved Cobb bone elevator, a medium-diameter drill bit, or a 10-mm bone punch. Larger holes should be made into the pubis, ischium, and the ilium at the dome of the acetabulum. Holes should not be attempted in the medial wall to prevent perforation and cement extrusion. We have routinely used a 10-mm punch, which allows for impaction of the cancellous bone into the end of each hole. This is intended to enhance pressurization of the cement.

Next, the acetabular fossa is irrigated to remove all the loose debris. We have routinely used either thrombin or hydrogen peroxide in sponges to improve hemostasis. The cement is mixed using contemporary techniques, such as centrifugation or vacuum-mixing devices. The cement is delivered by hand, and initial digital pressurization is performed. Several commercially available cement-pressurization devices are available and can be used for further pressurization. We have used the back side of a simple bulb suction syringe to achieve pressurization.

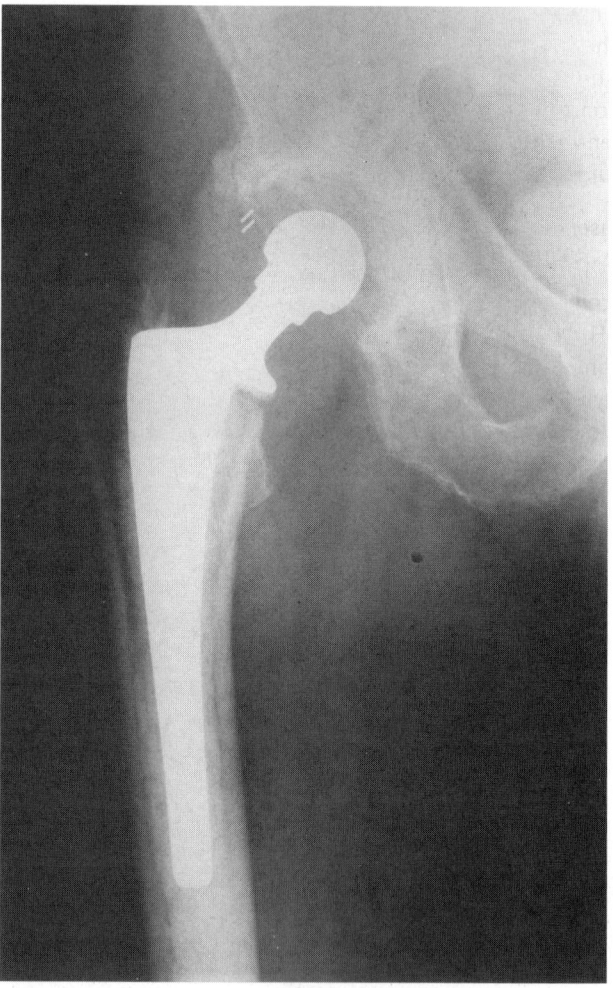

Figure 41.4. AP view showing a cemented THR using an all-polyethylene cup and multiple cement anchoring holes in the superior-medial segment of the acetabulum.

The acetabular cup is then inserted in the proper orientation (Clinical Table). It is important to ensure medial placement of the component as much as possible while leaving approximately 2 mm of medial cement. The surgeon can often use the edges of the cup and acetabulum as a guide. Lateralization of the cup carries far more deleterious effects on long-term fixation stability than does superior placement. The ideal position of the cup is similar to insertion of a cup without cement. We have routinely attempted to achieve 40° to 45° of abduction, along with 25° to 30° of anteversion. Excess and extruded cement should be removed after polymerization and secure fixation of the cup. If not removed, the cement can act as a source of impingement on the neck of the prosthesis and limit range of motion or lead to dislocation.

It is critical to remember that the position of the cup becomes permanent, since fixation is with cement. The surgeon should be especially attentive to the positioning of the cup as the cement dries. Many of the current designs offer an extended polyethylene lip, which may become a source of impingement in cases of excessive malpositioning. Impingement may lead to dislocation in the anterior direction. If this occurs during trial reduction, adding neck lengths on the femoral side will not correct the problem. The surgeon is left with two options: removing the malpositioned cup and inserting another cup in the correct position or using a high-speed burr to remove part of the extended lip of the cup. If this measure is insufficient, the surgeon must then revise the cup.

Insertion of the Femoral Stem with Cement

Preparation of the femoral canal for insertion of the stem with cement is similar to performing cementless THR. The intramedullary canal is located by using the canal finder. Excess bone in the femoral neck is removed by using an osteotome and bone rongeur (Clinical Table). Most current prostheses systems offer straight reamers (rigid or flexible) for preparation of the diaphysis distally. The largest reamer indicates the distal diameter of the distal stem that will be used. Tapered cylindrical reamers are then used to prepare the proximal portion of the femur. Sequential broaching is performed to complete the preparation of the femoral canal. The largest possible stem

should be selected to ensure proper placement and pressurization of the cement during insertion. It is crucial to achieve a cement mantle of at least 2 mm around the prosthesis. A trial reduction is then performed with various neck lengths. The final neck length is selected to maximize stability and re-create the proper soft-tissue tension and leg length.

The cement is mixed using porosity-reduction techniques, such as centrifugation or vacuum. The femoral canal is cleaned using a brush and pulsatile lavage to remove all the loose cancellous bone, blood clots, and other debris. It is especially important to remove all the cancellous bone over the calcar region to allow for direct contact of the cement mantle with the endocortex, maximizing rotational stability. A cement plug is placed at the appropriate level in the canal. Further hemostasis can be accomplished by using hypotensive anesthesia, packing dry sponges into the canal, or using hydrogen peroxide or thrombin-soaked sponges. When the cement reaches a doughy state it is injected, using a gun in a retrograde fashion. Pressurization of the cement is done by using a rubber pressurizer that plugs the femoral canal proximally. The stem is then inserted into the canal. We have generally inserted the stem in about 10° to 15° of anteversion. Unless there was a preoperative deformity of the proximal femur, this position mirrors the natural anteversion of the femoral neck, which can be used as a guide. Excess cement is then removed. After polymerization of the cement, the head component is then impacted onto the neck taper (Fig. 41.5).

PITFALLS AND MOST COMMON TECHNICAL MISTAKES

There are many potential complications in performing a cemented THR. Some of these are related to surgical dissection, and others are related to bone preparation and positioning of the components. The risks of injury to the abductors with the lateral approach and to the sciatic nerve with the posterior approach were mentioned earlier.

Pitfalls in bone preparation include insufficient reaming of the acetabulum to expose the cancellous bed for ideal cement interdigitation, insufficient number of anchoring holes for the cup, eccentric reaming that compromises the posterior wall and column of the acetabulum,

Clinical Table: Cemented Total Hip Replacement

Procedure	Indications	Technique	Anatomy	Pitfalls
Cemented cup	• Selective for >70 years old	• Reaming to cancellous bones • Large anchoring holes • Proper position	• Sciatic nerve (posterior approach) • Abductors (lateral approach)	• Insufficient medialization • Excessive anteversion
Cemented stem	• Any age	• Sequential broaching • Third generation cementing techniques • Adequate thickness of cement mantle	• Sciatic nerve (posterior approach) • Abductors (lateral approach)	• Fracture of the femur • Insufficient cement mantle • Varus position of stem

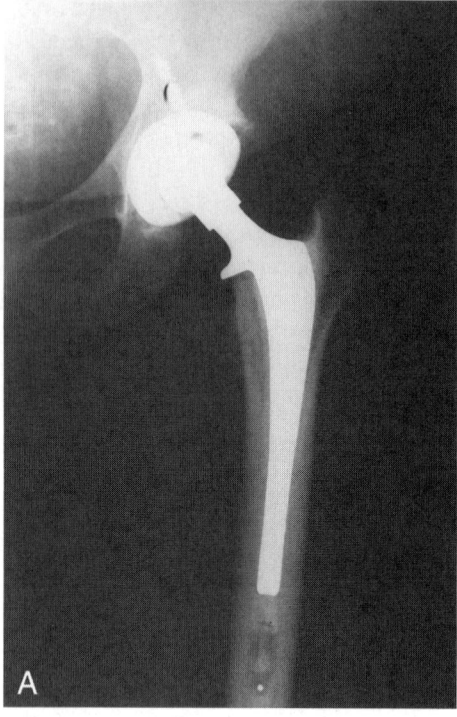
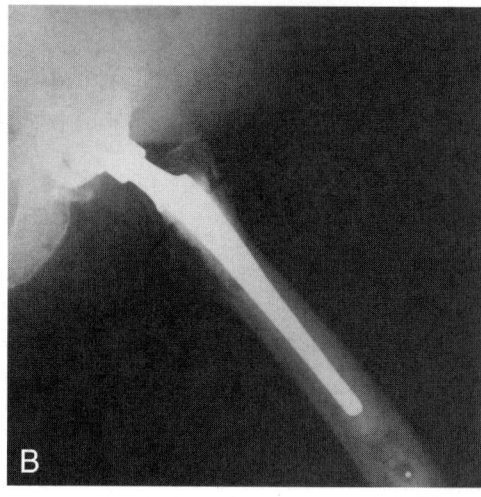
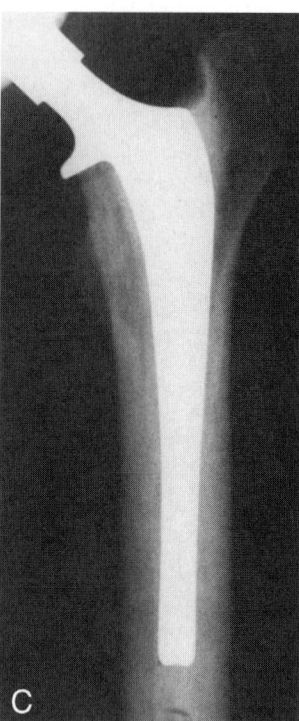

Figure 41.5. AP (**A**) and lateral (**B**) views showing the central placement of the femoral stem with a good cement mantle. **C.** Close-up of the femoral cement mantle showing a complete white-out, which indicates good pressurization technique.

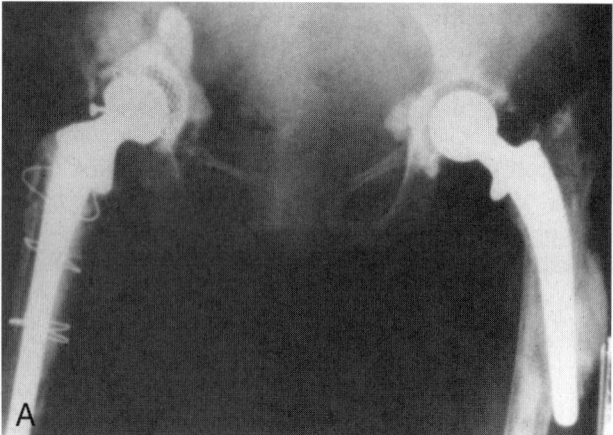
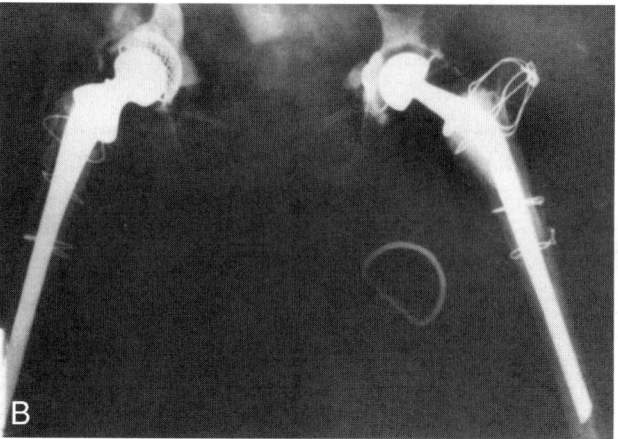

Figure 41.6. A. AP view of the pelvis showing perforation of the left femoral shaft by the stem, which occurred during the insertion with cement. **B.** AP view of the pelvis showing the femoral revision using a long-stemmed femoral component that was inserted with cement. Note the cerclage wires and bone graft around the defect.

and overbroaching the femur that results in fracture of the calcar. Occasionally, perforation of the femoral canal occurs, resulting in suboptimal fixation of the stem (Fig. 41.6).

Technical mistakes in insertion of the acetabular component include insufficient or excessive anteversion and vertical placement, resulting in postoperative dislocation. Problems with the femoral component can occur from selecting too small a stem and inserting it in a varus or valgus position. Inadequate preparation of the cement and canal can result in radiolucencies between the bone and cement and voids within the mantle. Also, selection of an inappropriate neck length can cause instability; leg length discrepancy; and even nerve injury, if excessive lengthening has occurred. All of these can lead to patient dissatisfaction; suboptimal clinical outcome; and most important, decreased durability of the THR.

Rehabilitation

Mechanical stability of the prosthesis is achieved immediately at the time of surgery when inserted with cement. Patients are allowed to begin full-weight-bearing ambulation on the first postoperative day. Patients should initially use a walker or two crutches to assist with balance and to compensate for abductor and extensor muscle weakness from the surgery. They can then be advanced to a cane once muscle strength has become adequate. Partial-weight-bearing ambulation is encouraged for 4 to 6 weeks when the lateral approach is used to protect the repair of the abductor muscles. Patients should be encouraged to perform hip abductor and extensor exercises until strength has become sufficient to prevent limping.

Patients are carefully instructed in dislocation precautions. The operated leg can be placed in a balanced suspension sling in abduction while in bed, or an abduction pillow can be used. In high-risk cases, a small immobilizer can be used over the ipsilateral knee to minimize flexion of the hip. Hip dislocation precautions are followed strictly for at least 3 months. Low-impact athletic activities, such as golf, bicycling, and swimming, are allowed after regaining sufficient control of hip motion and muscle strength. High-impact activities, such as contact sports, skiing, tennis, and running, are generally discouraged.

Patients are seen initially in follow-up at 4 to 6 weeks after surgery and then at 6- and 12-month postsurgery intervals. Annual follow-up thereafter is recommended. Standard AP and frog-leg lateral radiographs should be obtained at each follow-up to evaluate the position of the components, radiolucencies, wear, and osteolysis. Some measure of clinical outcome is necessary. This can be assessed by using standard patient-oriented questionnaires or by using surgeon-oriented hip rating scales, such as the Harris hip scale (13,21).

Follow-up Results of Cemented THR

There have been an enormous number of publications since the 1960s that have reported the clinical and radiographic results of cemented THRs. Several limitations exist in the interpretation of published data. The first relates to the complexity of analyzing and comparing results reported from different institutions. The second limitation relates to the definition of *failure*. Whether revision or radiographic loosening is used as the end point, the incidence of failure is based on each surgeon's or institution's criteria for either recommending revision surgery or identifying looseness. Moreover, clinical performance of the THR measured by various hip scales has generally remained satisfactory, even in the presence of radiographic loosening of the prostheses.

The third limitation relates to the various surgical techniques and prosthetic designs that have evolved over the past three decades. It is important to interpret results based on the type of cementing technique used. The

fourth limitation relates to the methodologies used in reporting the results. Survivorship analysis has been used by many investigators as a means of representing outcome; however, only the most recent reports include confidence intervals, which accurately define the limitations of the data (21).

It is important to differentiate between clinical and radiographic failure. Clinical failures include revision surgery for loosening, infection, recurrent dislocation, or any other cause. They also include patients who have become dissatisfied, as judged by hip scales or by patient-oriented outcome measurement tools. Assessment of radiographic failure is a complex process. Several investigators have each proposed different criteria for the definition of *radiographic failure*. Interpretation is further complicated if good-quality serial radiographs—taken with similar techniques and positions—are not available.

Most surgeons would agree that a cemented femoral stem is definitely loose if one of the following criteria exist: (*a*) subsidence of the stem, (*b*) fracture of the cement mantle, (*c*) new stem–cement radiolucencies, or (*d*) fracture of the stem. Some have further defined stem loosening into probable and possible categories, based on the number and extent of radiolucencies present in the bone–cement interface (22).

Most surgeons would agree that a cemented acetabular cup is definitely loose if there is migration of the cup or if there is a complete circumferential radiolucency between bone and cement around the cup (13). In addition, evidence of polyethylene wear and associated osteolysis should be considered, as they may result in eventual aseptic loosening (Fig. 41.7). It has become customary for investigators to report the results in terms of the mechanical failure rate, which, for any particular prosthetic design or series of patients, is defined by the percent of cases requiring revision surgery plus the percent of cases determined to be radiographically loose. The reported results of cemented THRs are summarized below.

THR WITH FIRST-GENERATION CEMENTING TECHNIQUES

THRs with first-generation cementing techniques were performed in the late 1960s and early 1970s; we reviewed series that had a minimum follow-up of 15 years. Results are reported in Table 41.1. One important common feature in these series is that the surgeries were performed by experienced senior surgeons at centers specializing in THRs. Most patients remained satisfied with their prostheses even after 20 years.

In general, the revision and radiographic failure rates were higher for the cups than for the stems. This difference was especially pronounced in younger patients. Sullivan et al. (26) observed greater revision and radiographic loosening rates for the cups than for the stems in a series of patients who underwent surgery when they were younger than 50 years. Moreover, the cup revision and loosening rates were greater in this series than in a series of older pa-

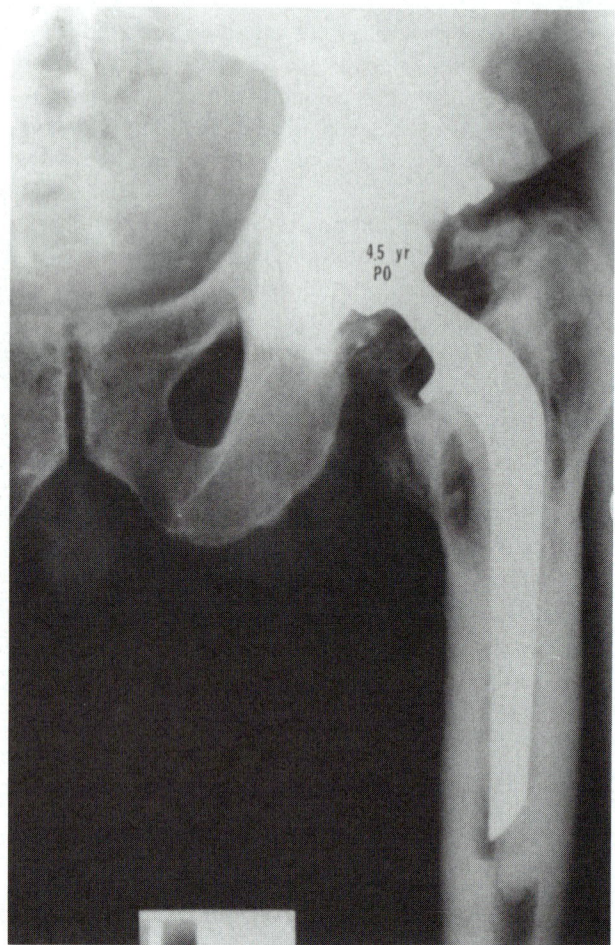

Figure 41.7. AP view showing significant femoral endosteolysis in multiple zones secondary to wear debris.

table	41.1	First-Generation Cementing Techniques

Number of Hips	Mean Follow-up (Years)	Revision Rate (%)	Mechanical Failure Rate (%)[a]	Reference
100	15.3	Stem: 4 Cup: 1	Stem: 7 Cup: 15	23
330	20–22	Stem: 3 Cup: 10	Stem: 8.7 Cup: 19	24
112	20, minimum	Overall: 16	Stem: 32 Cup: 8.7	25
89	18	Stem: 2 Cup: 13	Stem: 8 Cup: 50	26
240	17	Overall: 6	Stem: 29 Cup: 5	27

[a]Revision *rate* plus radiographic loosening rate.

tients operated on by the same surgeon (24). Neumann et al. (27), however, did not confirm this observation; they found similar revision rates in the younger and older age groups. Neumann et al., however, reported a higher loosening rate for the stems than for the cups (29 to 5%); this

was observed equally in the younger and older age groups.

THR WITH IMPROVED CEMENTING TECHNIQUES

THRs with improved cementing techniques were performed from the late 1970s to early 1980s (Table 41.2). All the hips were done with second-generation techniques, including the use of an intramedullary plug, pulsatile lavage, and the injection of cement using a gun in a retrograde fashion. The results at 5 years after surgery were encouraging; mechanical failure rates were less than 2% for both the cups and the stems. The successful results were maintained for the stems up to a mean 15 years of follow-up. Conversely, there was a high rate of mechanical failure for the cups at the longer follow-up interval.

THR WITH HYBRID FIXATION TECHNIQUES

Surgeons have become increasingly impressed with the results obtained when using modern cementing techniques, especially on the femoral side. Meanwhile, ad-

table	41.2	Improved Cementing Techniques

Number of Hips	Mean Follow-up (Years)	Revision Rate (%)	Mechanical Failure Rate (%)[a]	Reference
117	6.2	Stem: 0.8	Stem: 1.7	21
251	5.6	Stem: 0 Cup: 0	Stem: 1.2 Cup: 0.4	28
105	11.2	Stem: 1.9 Cup: 4.9	Stem: 2.9 Cup: 42.7	29
50	12	Stem: 0 Cup: 22	Stem: 2 Cup: 44	30
89	7	Stem: 1.1 Cup: NA	Stem: 1.1 Cup: NA	31
162	15	Stem: 2 Cup: 10	Stem: 6 Cup: 35	32

NA, not available.
[a]Revision rate plus radiographic loosening rate.

table	41.3	Hybrid Techniques

Number of Hips	Mean Follow-up (Years)	Revision Rate (%)	Mechanical Failure Rate (%)[a]	Reference
67	6.5	Stem: 0 Cup: 0	Stem: 0 Cup: 0	33
100	5	Stem: 1 Cup: 2	Stem: 1 Cup: 2	34
38	6	Stem: 0 Cup: 0	Stem: 0 Cup: 0	35
106	8–9	Stem: 6.1 Cup: 0	Stem: 6.1 Cup: 0	36
152	5.6	Stem: 2.2 Cup: 1.4	Stem: 2.2 Cup: 2.1	37
150	8.6	Stem: 0 Cup: 1.4	Stem: 1.4 Cup: 2.1	38
125	6	Stem: 3 Cup: 0	Stem: 5 Cup: 0	39

[a]Revision rate plus radiographic loosening rate.

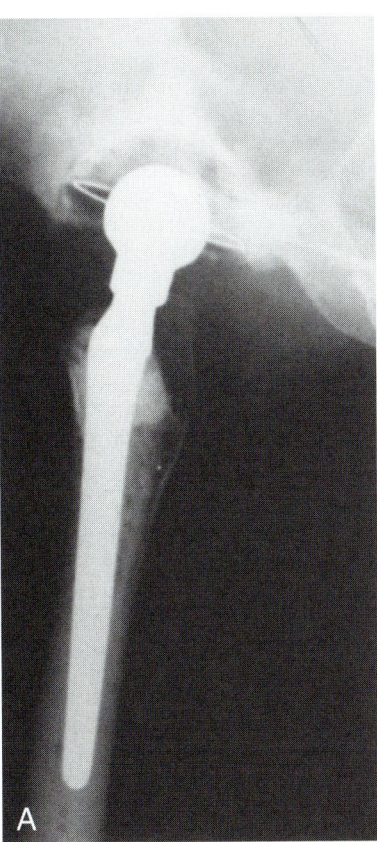
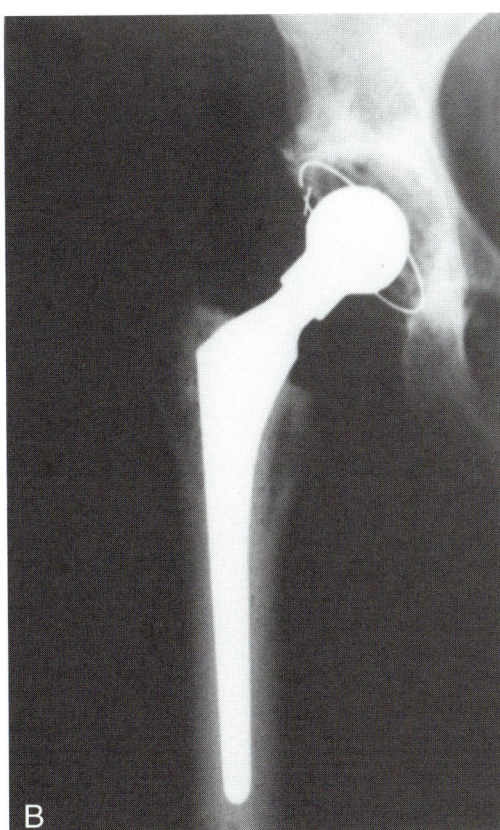

Figure 41.8. Lateral (**A**) and AP (**B**) views showing the 10-year follow-up of a THR that was inserted with cement using second-generation techniques.

vances in cementless fixation continue to be made, especially for the cups. Some surgeons, therefore, have begun performing THR using a combination of the two types of prostheses—a stem inserted with cement using modern techniques and a cup inserted without cement—the so-called hybrid technique.

Many of the hips in the series shown in Table 41.3 were performed with third-generation cementing techniques. The clinical and radiographic results on medium-term follow-up have been excellent. Woolson and Haber (39) reported on the results of 125 hybrid THRs performed by a single surgeon with minimum follow-up of 4.6 years (mean 6 years). The mechanical failure rate for the cups was 0% and for the stems, 5%. Among the 6 hips for which mechanical failure occurred, 2 were caused by stem fracture, 2 required stem revision due to aseptic loosening, and 2 were radiographically loose.

SUMMARY

Cement remains an excellent option for the prostheses in performing a THR. The clinical and radiographic results of cemented THRs performed by experienced surgeons using contemporary techniques have been excellent (Fig. 41.8). On long-term follow-up, the cups do carry a higher risk of failure. Fixation and performance of the femoral stem, however, remain excellent even after 10 years. Based on the literature, the best option for routine primary THRs is perhaps reconstruction using the hybrid

technique. Regardless of fixation choice, osteolysis due to wear debris can occur. Future efforts in improving the performance and durability of cemented THRs should emphasize articulating surface materials, tolerance in the manufacturing of the articulating surfaces, and continued enhancement of the mechanical properties of cement and its bonding to the prostheses.

REFERENCES

1. Callaghan JJ, Brand RA, Petersen DR. Hip arthrodesis. A long-term follow-up. J Bone Joint Surg 1985;67A:1328–1335.
2. Sponseller PD, McBeath AA, Perpich M. Hip arthrodesis in young patients. A long-term follow-up study. J Bone Joint Surg 1984;66A:853–859.
3. Trousdale RT, Ekkernkamp A, Ganz R, Wallrichs S. Periacetabular and intertrochanteric osteotomy for the treatment of osteoarthritis in dysplastic hips. J Bone Joint Surg 1995;77A:73–85.
4. Maloney WJ, Jasty M, Burke DW, et al. Biomechanical and histologic investigation of cemented total hip arthroplasties: a study of autopsy-retrieved femurs after in-vivo cycling. Clin Orthop 1989;249:129–140.
5. Noble PC, Tullos HS, Landon GC. The optimum cement mantle for total hip replacement: theory and practice. Instr Course Lect 1991;40:145–150.
6. Burke DW, Gates EI, Harris WH. Centrifugation as a method of improving tensile and fatigue properties of acrylic cement. J Bone Joint Surg 1984;66A:1265–1273.
7. Wixson RL, Lautenschlager EP, Novak MA. Vacuum mixing of acrylic cement. J Arthroplasty 1987;2:141–149.
8. Agins HJ, Alcock NW, Bansal M, et al. Metallic wear in failed titanium-alloy total hip replacements. A histologic and quantitative analysis. J Bone Joint Surg 1988;70A:347–356.

9. Buly RL, Huo MH, Salvati EA, et al. Titanium wear debris in failed cemented total hip replacement: analysis of 71 cases. J Arthroplasty 1992;7:51–56.

10. Huo MH, Salvati EA, Lieberman JR, et al. Metallic debris in femoral endosteolysis in failed cemented total hip arthroplasties. Clin Orthop 1992;276:157–168.

11. Huiskes R. Failed innovation in total hip replacement. Diagnosis and proposals for a cure. Acta Orthop Scand 1993;64:699–716.

12. Kwong KSC. The biomechanical role of the collar of the femoral component of a hip replacement. J Bone Joint Surg 1990;72B:664–665.

13. Harris WH, White RE Jr. Socket fixation using a metal-backed acetabular component for total hip replacement: a minimum five-year follow-up. J Bone Joint Surg 1982;64A:745–748.

14. Ritter MA, Keating EM, Faris PM, Brugo G. Metal-backed acetabular cups in total hip arthroplasty. J Bone Joint Surg 1990;72A:672–677.

15. Markel DC, Huo MH, Katkin PD, Salvati EA. The use of a cemented all-polyethylene and metal-backed acetabular components in total hip arthroplasty: a comparative study. J Arthroplasty 1995;10:S1–S8.

16. Huo MH, Martin RP, Zatorski LE, Keggi KJ. Total hip replacements using the ceramic Mittelmeier prosthesis. Clin Orthop 1996;332:143–150.

17. Callaway GH, Flynn W, Ranawat CS, Sculco TP. Fracture of the femoral head after ceramic-on-polyethylene total hip arthroplasty. J Arthroplasty 1995;10:855–859.

18. Hummer CD, Rothman RH, Hozack WJ. Catastrophic failure of modular Zirconia-ceramic femoral head components after total hip arthroplasty. J Arthroplasty 1995;10:848–850.

19. Hardinge K. The direct lateral approach to the hip. J Bone Joint Surg 1982;64B:17–19.

20. Vicar AJ, Coleman CR. A comparison of the anterolateral, transtrochanteric, and posterior surgical approaches in primary total hip arthroplasty. Clin Orthop 1984;188:152–159.

21. Dorrey F, Amstutz HC. The validity of survivorship analysis in total joint arthroplasty. J Bone Joint Surg 1989;71A:544–548.

22. Harris WH, McGann WA. Loosening of the femoral component after use of the medullary-plug cementing technique: follow-up note with a minimum five-year follow-up. J Bone Joint Surg 1986;68A:1064–1066.

23. McCoy TH, Salvati EA, Ranawat CS, Wilson PD Jr. The fifteen-year study of one hundred Charnley low-friction arthroplasties. Orthop Clin North Am 1988;19:467–476.

24. Schulte KR, Callaghan JJ, Kelley SS, Johnston RC. The outcome of Charnley total hip arthroplasty with cement after a minimum twenty-year follow-up. The results of one surgeon. J Bone Joint Surg 1993;75A:961–975.

25. Kavanagh BF, Wallrichs S, Dewitz M, et al. Charnley low-friction arthroplasty of the hip. Twenty-year results with cement. J Arthroplasty 1994;9:229–234.

26. Sullivan PM, MacKenzie JR, Callaghan JJ, Johnston RC. Total hip arthroplasty with cement in patients who are less than fifty years old. A sixteen to twenty-two-year follow-up study. J Bone Joint Surg 1994;76A:863–869.

27. Neumann L, Freund KG, Sorensen KH. Total hip arthroplasty with the Charnley Prosthesis in patients fifty-five years old and less. Fifteen to twenty-one-year results. J Bone Joint Surg 1996;78A:73–79.

28. Russotti GM, Coventry MB, Stauffer RN. Cemented total hip arthroplasty with contemporary techniques. Clin Orthop 1988;235:141–147.

29. Mulroy RD Jr, Harris WH. The effect of improved cementing techniques on component loosening in total hip arthroplasty. J Bone Joint Surg 1990;72B:757–760.

30. Barrack RL, Harris WH. Improved cementing techniques and femoral component loosening in total hip arthroplasty. J Bone Joint Surg 1992;74B:385–389.

31. Oishi CS, Walker RH, Colwell CW. The femoral component in total hip arthroplasty. J Bone Joint Surg 1994;76A:1130–1136.

32. Mulroy WF, Estok DM, Harris WH. Total hip arthroplasty with use of so-called second-generation cementing techniques. A fifteen-year-average follow-up study. J Bone Joint Surg 1995;77A:1845–1852.

33. Schmalzried TP, Harris WH. Hybrid total hip replacement. J Bone Joint Surg 1993;75B:608–615.

34. Mohler CG, Kull LR, Martell JM, et al. Total hip replacement with insertion of an acetabular component without cement and a femoral component with cement. J Bone Joint Surg 1995;77A:86–96.

35. Goetz DD, Harris WH. The prevalence of femoral osteolysis associated with components inserted with or without cement in total hip replacements. J Bone Joint Surg 1993;76A:1121–1129.

36. Callaghan JJ, Ghassan ST, Olejniczak JP, et al. Primary hybrid total hip arthroplasty. Clin Orthop 1996;333:118–125.

37. Lewallen DG, Cabanela ME. Hybrid primary total hip arthroplasty. Clin Othop 1996;333:126–133.

38. Berger RA, Kull LR, Rosenberg AG, Galante JO. Hybrid total hip arthroplasty. Clin Orthop 1996;333:134–146.

39. Woolson ST, Haber DF. Primary total hip replacement with insertion of an acetabular component without cement and a femoral component with cement. J Bone Joint Surg 1996;78A:698–705.

Suggested Reading

Hoppenfeld S, deBoer P. Surgical exposures in orthopaedics: the anatomic approach. Philadelphia: Lippincott, 1984.

chapter 42

Bryan J. Nestor and Robert L. Buly

Cementless Total Hip Arthroplasty

The concept of biologic fixation of metal to bone dates back to 1910 when the first patent was issued for a tooth implant (1). Since that time a considerable amount of both clinical and laboratory investigation has confirmed the validity of this concept. Application of biologic fixation to hip implants began in earnest in the United States in 1977. A clinical trial was initiated for a single-size, fully coated femoral prosthesis with a Moore-type femoral stem geometry (2). In 1983, this device (AML; DePuy, Inc., Warsaw, IN) became the first device without cement to be approved by the U.S. Food and Drug Administration for use in humans.

Enthusiasm for cementless total hip arthroplasty (THA) began to grow significantly in the early to mid 1980s, primarily for three reasons: (a) a concern over the durability and long-term viability of first-generation cemented total hip arthroplasty, particularly in the young patient (3,4); (b) encouraging results with early reports of uncemented hip implants (5,6); and (c) a generally held perception that the osteolytic process that led to loosening was entirely due to bone cement, a concept that led to the term *cement disease* (7).

Cementless total hip arthroplasty continues to be a viable reconstructive option for patients with hip disease, particularly in the young patient. Enthusiasm for the use of cementless acetabular components remains high, and there is widespread application. The enthusiasm for cementless femoral components, however, has been tempered by reports of improved results with second-generation cement techniques, including in younger patients (8–11), and by results of 5- to 10-year follow-up reports that reveal an increased incidence of osteolysis and thigh pain and similar rates of revision compared with cemented stems (12–20).

As with cemented total hip arthroplasty, cementless component design and surgical technique continue to evolve. The purpose of this chapter is to review the surgi-cal technique of cementless total hip arthroplasty, including the biology of bone ingrowth; some of the design considerations for cementless total hip components; and the indications, results, and complications of cementless hip arthroplasty.

BIOLOGY OF INGROWTH AND IMPLANT DESIGN

The requirements of successful cementless total hip arthroplasty include (a) obtaining stable immediate (or primary) fixation, so that secondary fixation via bone ingrowth can occur, and (b) using the materials, technique, and mode of biologic fixation that will minimize potential complications and produce a long-lasting clinical result.

Primary Fixation

FEMUR

The first prerequisite for bone ingrowth into or onto an implant surface is limited motion at the bone–prosthesis interface. Although the exact threshold of acceptable micromotion is not known (possibly as small as 30 to 40 μm), the point beyond which bone ingrowth is impossible has been shown to be 150 μm or more (21). This is consistent with data obtained from human autopsy retrieval. In a study that measured micromotion of retrieved femoral components, 13 well-fixed femoral components had less than 40 μm of micromotion in areas of porous coating compared to 150 μm of micromotion in the area of porous coating of one stem with fibrous ingrowth only (22).

Axial micromotion has been shown experimentally to be minimal, not to change significantly with activity, and to be essentially the same for cemented and cementless femoral stems in vitro immediately after implantation (23).

On the other hand, the same in vitro study showed that rotatory micromotion in the transverse plane was significantly greater with stair climbing compared to a single-limb stance and was greater in uncemented stems (mean = 103.1 μm; range = 13.0 to 280.0 μm) than in cemented stems (mean = 26.23 μm; range 2.0 to 76.0 μm) immediately after implantation. The implications of these data are twofold: First, micromotion that is detrimental to successful bone ingrowth occurs with rotation; therefore, rotational stability is an important implant design consideration. Second, activities that result in increased torsional forces, such as unprotected stair climbing, should be avoided as much as possible after surgery to allow time for adequate fixation.

Porous femoral components can be grouped in two design categories based on stem geometry: straight versus curved (Fig. 42.1). Straight stems may be either proximally coated or more extensively coated, depending on the intended mode of fixation (proximal or distal).

Proximally coated straight stems generally have a wedge-shaped proximal geometry that favors metaphyseal "fit and fill" in both the anteroposterior (AP) and the mediolateral planes. The nonporous distal stem may be cylindrical, tapered, fluted, or modular. Although the nonporous distal stem can contribute to initial stability with a proper diaphyseal fit, the effect is lost with time as osseous integration occurs proximally (24). A recent experimental study comparing torsional stability of a number of different distal stem designs found that a solid fluted design was the only design that provided significant torsional stability independent of proximal fixation (25).

Extensively coated straight stems designed for distal fixation rely on diaphyseal fit for both initial and secondary fixation. Those that favor distal fixation argue that the variation in proximal femoral geometry makes proximal fixation difficult and less predictable. The primary concerns with distal fixation are the long-term effects of stress shielding.

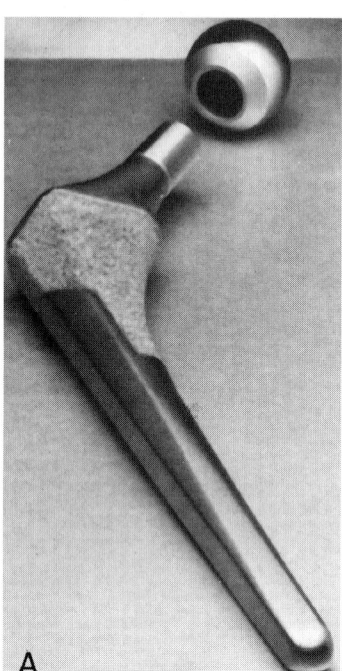
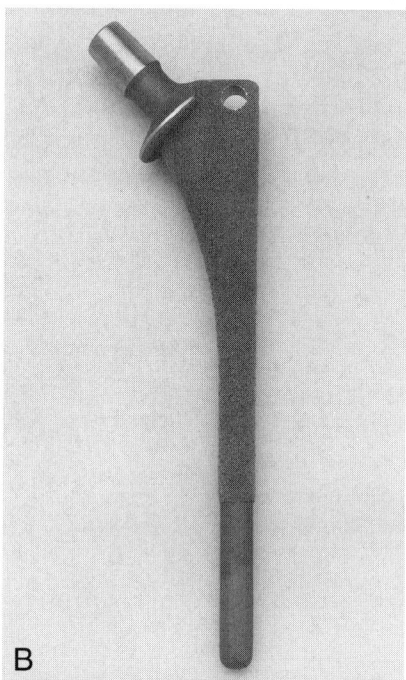

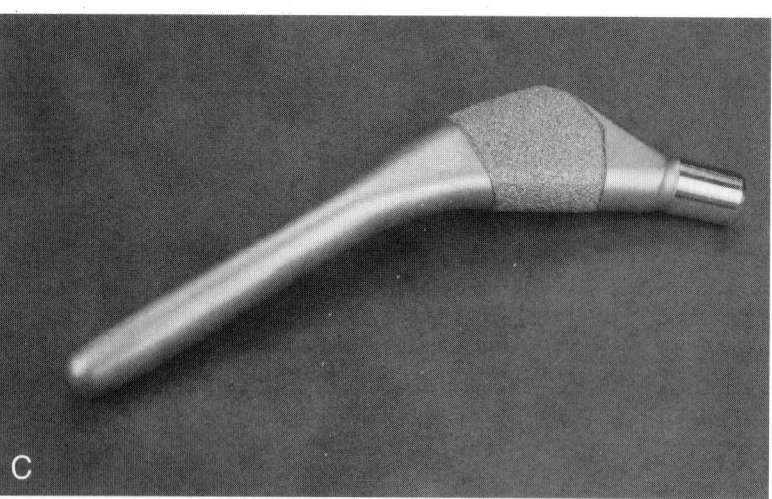

Figure 42.1. A. The Omnifit microstructured stem is a proximally coated, straight-stem model designed for proximal fixation. Reprinted with permission from Osteonics Corporation, Allendale, NJ. **B.** The AML femoral component is an extensively coated, straight-stem model designed for a diaphyseal fit. Reprinted with permission from DePuy, Inc., Warsaw, IN. **C.** The Ranawat-Burstein femoral component is a curved, anatomic stem model designed for proximal fixation. Reprinted with permission from Biomet, Inc., Warsaw, IN.

Curved anatomic stems are proximally coated and have proximal geometries designed for metaphyseal "fit and fill." Experimental evidence suggests that the curved stem geometry contributes to rotational stability (26,27). However, both straight and curved stems have enjoyed similar clinical success.

The type and extent of porous coating has not been shown to significantly contribute to initial femoral implant stability (28). Similarly, use of a collar does not significantly improve rotational stability (29,30). Although the collar may add to axial stability and prevent subsidence (29,30), axial micromotion is probably not significant (23). Furthermore, the collar may prevent complete seating of the component, jeopardizing proximal fixation. Therefore, some authors prefer uncemented stems without a collar.

The ability to obtain immediate stable fixation is influenced by other factors independent of component design, including the surgical technique, the selection of the proper size of implant (discussed below), and the patient's bone quality.

ACETABULUM

Acetabular implants in use today are generally hemispherical. Variations in design include peripheral radial expansion and peripheral geometries that are slightly larger than the radius of curvature of the medial cup, to improve immediate fixation (Fig. 42.2). In addition, adjuvant fixation is available in the form of spikes, peripheral fins, or screws. In one study, three spikes, two pegs, and three screws were shown to provide similar fixation; however, the load to failure was highest with three screws (31). Although screws are effective, there have been concerns about problems related to their application, significantly limiting their use. A number of studies have documented the effectiveness of underreaming in obtaining sufficient initial stability without the use of adjuvant fixation (32–34). One potential disadvantage of underreaming is the creation of gaps between the bone and prosthesis, thereby decreasing the contact surface area available for ingrowth (35,36). Clinically, this has not created a problem, and the significance of such gaps remains to be seen. Without adjuvant fixation, cup geometry becomes increasingly important. True hemispherical cups have been shown to provide better fixation than low-profile cups designed to reduce inferior impingement (34). Experimental data regarding the efficacy of peripheral radial expansion are variable (33,34). The type and extent of surface coating do not seem to contribute significantly to initial acetabular fixation (34).

Most of the acetabular implants available have modu-

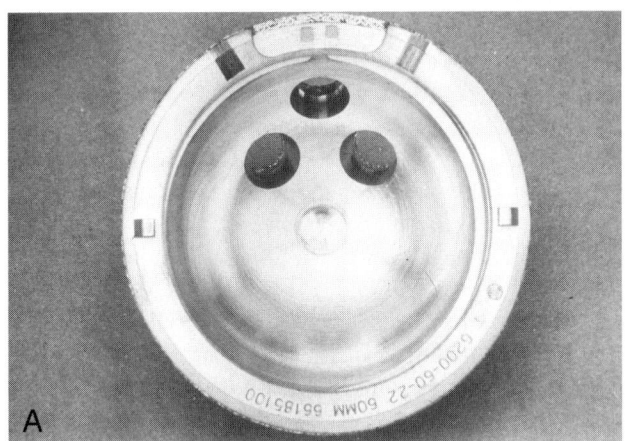

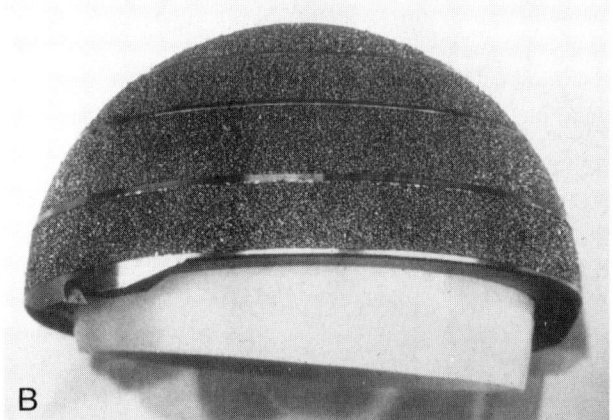

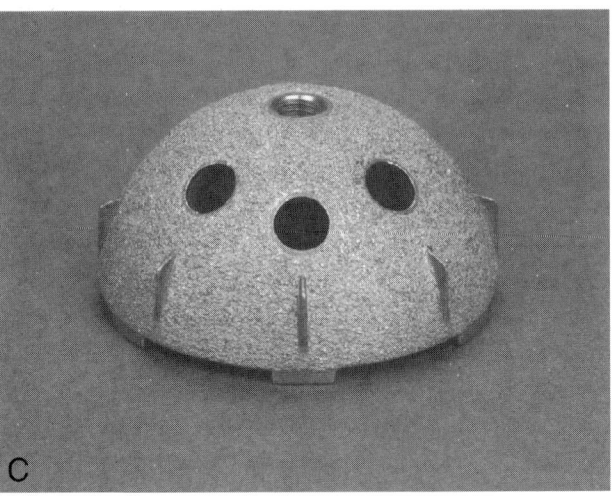

Figure 42.2. A. The Trilogy acetabular component is a modular hemispherical cup with a porous coating. It is available with screw holes, limited screw holes (cluster), or no screw holes. Reprinted with permission from Zimmer, Inc., Warsaw, IN. **B.** The Implex acetabular component is a nonmodular, elliptical cup with a porous coating. It does not have screw holes. Reprinted with permission from Implex Corporation. Allendale, NJ. **C.** The Mallory-Head acetabular component is a spherical cup with a porous coating. It has fins that augment fixation. Reprinted with permission from Biomet, Inc., Warsaw, IN.

lar polyethylene inserts. Concern over increased wear with modular polyethylene, however, has prompted the initiation of clinical trials using nonmodular cementless acetabular components at our institution.

Secondary Fixation

There are two basic types of biologic fixation: macrolock, which requires bone growth onto the surface of a smooth metal substrate, and microlock, which allows for bone ingrowth into a textured surface. While ongrowth of bone, particularly on a titanium substrate, can sufficiently stabilize a femoral component, clinical results have been less predictable with macrolock femoral stems (37). Therefore, the majority of implants used today have a porous surface, allowing for a biologic microlock.

Porous implants available for cementless use are made of either cobalt or titanium alloys. Titanium is often cited as having a greater affinity for bone than cobalt (38); however, both metal substrates are capable of bone ingrowth. Titanium has a modulus of elasticity that allows for more stress transfer to bone than does cobalt, thereby decreasing proximal stress shielding (39,40). Recent clinical data using dual x-ray absorptiometry to measure proximal bone loss found little difference between cobalt and titanium, except along the calcar, suggesting that choice of material may play only a minor role in proximal bone loss to stress shielding (41).

Titanium has better biocompatibility than does cobalt. Cobalt chrome is known to be more cytotoxic and must be considered a potential carcinogen. Recent in vitro studies, however, revealed that titanium alloys result in greater macrophage release of cellular mediators that are implicated in osteolysis than cobalt chrome (42,43). Cobalt has the theoretical advantages of being a harder metal with less tendency for wear and less notch sensitivity to porous surface application than titanium. While there is general agreement that cobalt is the material of choice for cemented stems, there is no clear consensus regarding the best material for uncemented stems.

There are four basic types of surface treatment. The three surface treatments intended to allow bone ingrowth into a porous surface are sintered beads of cobalt or titanium, diffusion bonding of titanium fibers, and plasma spray of titanium powder. Although the optimal surface for ingrowth remains controversial, all three have been associated with clinical success. Plasma spray has the advantage of significantly decreasing the notch sensitivity of titanium (44). Regardless of the surface, it is well accepted that the optimal pore size for ingrowth is in the range of 100 to 400 μm. (45,46). Rough or grit-blasted titanium is the fourth surface treatment and is intended to achieve secondary stabilization by means of bone ongrowth onto the roughened prosthetic surface. Both laboratory (47,48) and clinical (49–51) studies have demonstrated success with rough or grit-blasted titanium surfaces.

Additional surface considerations include circumferential coating (complete or incomplete), the area of coating (proximal or extensive), and the application of ceramic coatings. Because of concerns regarding the intramedullary access of wear particles, most surgeons favor a complete circumferential coating, which also offers greater surface area for bone contact.

While arguably better clinical results have been obtained with more extensive porous coating (2,52), concerns about proximal bone loss secondary to stress shielding have led many surgeons to use only proximally coated femoral stems for primary THA. Both clinical and laboratory studies have documented increased bone loss with more extensive coating (39,52–57).

The use of coatings, such as hydroxyapatite or tricalcium phosphate, to enhance bone osseointegration remains experimental. Both laboratory and early clinical results are encouraging; however, experimental studies in dogs have shown that calcium phosphate coatings will not significantly increase the ultimate amount of bone ingrowth and will not enhance bone growth across gaps at the prosthesis–bone interface (58). Concerns remain regarding the long-term effects of the coating. The coating may generate particulate debris that can act both as a source of third body wear and as a stimulus for osteolysis (59,60).

Studies that analyzed bone ingrowth in retrieved prostheses revealed variable results (61–67). Part of the variability in results is explained by differences in techniques and methods of measurement. In addition, some of the studies were based on specimens retrieved from revision rather than from autopsy, which may not accurately reflect the conditions of well-functioning implants. Interpretation of the available data leads to the following general observations: Bone ingrowth occurs in up to 100% of acetabular and femoral components. The extent of surface with ingrowth is less than 40%, and the percentage of pore volume filled with bone is less than 25% and, in most cases, less than 5 to 10%. Acetabular ingrowth is perhaps less predictable than femoral ingrowth and is most extensive adjacent to areas with adjuvant fixation. Radiographs cannot accurately predict the extent or presence of bone ingrowth. Limited bone ingrowth with extensive fibrous tissue ingrowth is compatible with a successful clinical result.

INDICATIONS FOR CEMENTLESS THA

The indications for cementless versus cemented THA have been the subject of considerable controversy. Although the controversy continues, the following guidelines are generally accepted. The physiologic age of the patient is an important consideration. For patients less than 40 years old, alternatives to hip arthroplasty should be considered. If the patient is a candidate for hip arthroplasty, cementless implants are generally used, unless the patient has a chronic systemic disease (such as rheumatoid arthritis) or requires chronic use of steroids. One exception would be the very young patients with juvenile rheumatoid arthritis (JRA) in whom cementless, sometimes custom implants are also used. Patients are advised to avoid impact-loading activities. The potential for thigh pain, osteolysis, and future revision are emphasized.

The intermediate (10-year) clinical experience of patients between the ages of 40 and 65 with cementless acetabular components continues to support their use. The choice of femoral implant is individualized and depends on physiologic age and bone quality. Patients who are physiologically young, active, and/or heavy may be candidates for cementless femoral components. The quality of bone can be assessed on the preoperative x-ray. A cemented femoral component is recommended when the cortical index is less than 48% (68) or the canal flare index

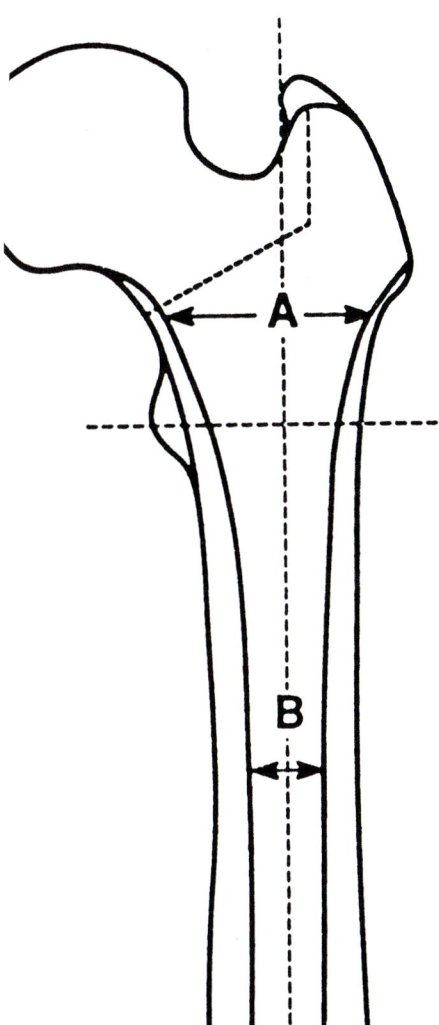

Figure 42.3. The canal flare index is equal to *A/B*. Reprinted with permission from Noble PC, Alexander JW, Lindahl LJ, et al. The anatomic basis of femoral component design. Clin Orthop 1988; 235:148–165.

is less than 3 (69) (Fig. 42.3). Although there is considerable variability in the orthopaedic community and within our institution, the majority of patients between the ages of 50 and 65 are treated with hybrid total hip arthroplasty. For those less than 50, cementless femoral components are more commonly used.

There is general agreement that for patients over 65 years old, the femoral component should be cemented. The use of all polyethylene cemented acetabular components is increasing in this age group. Currently, however, cemented acetabular components are reserved for elderly patients with a life expectancy of less than 10 years.

TREATMENT

Preoperative Planning

Preoperative planning begins with appropriate radiographs, which include an AP view of the pelvis to show both hips, an AP view of the effected hip that extends below the isthmus, and a lateral view. Preoperative templating is helpful in selecting properly sized implants. Templates are available in varying degrees of magnification, usually between 110 and 120%. The acetabulum is templated on the AP pelvis x-ray. The templates are placed so that the subchondral bone is approximated, the anatomic hip center is restored, and the cup is inclined 40° to 45° from horizontal. In cases of severe protrusion, the method described by Ranawat and Zahn (70) can be used to determine the anatomic location of the acetabulum (Fig. 42.4). In the case of significant superolateral deficiencies, plans are made for autogenous bone grafting and restoring the hip center to its anatomic position. The optimally sized acetabular implant is determined intraoperatively and is usually limited by the anteroposterior diameter.

Templating of the femoral component is done on both the AP and lateral hip x-ray. It is essential that the surgeon understand the design rationale of the prosthesis to be used. For proximally coated implants designed for proximal fixation, implant size is based on metaphyseal fit and fill. For components designed for distal fixation, implant size is based more on diaphyseal fit and fill (Clinical Table). After the size of the implant has been selected, the optimal level of neck resection is determined. Although restoration of the femoral offset is important, preference is given to restoration of equal leg lengths.

Surgical Approach

The choice of surgical approach is a matter of surgeon's preference. Regardless of approach, the surgeon should feel comfortable with a more extensive exposure in the case of femoral fracture. At our institution, the posterior approach is used almost exclusively.

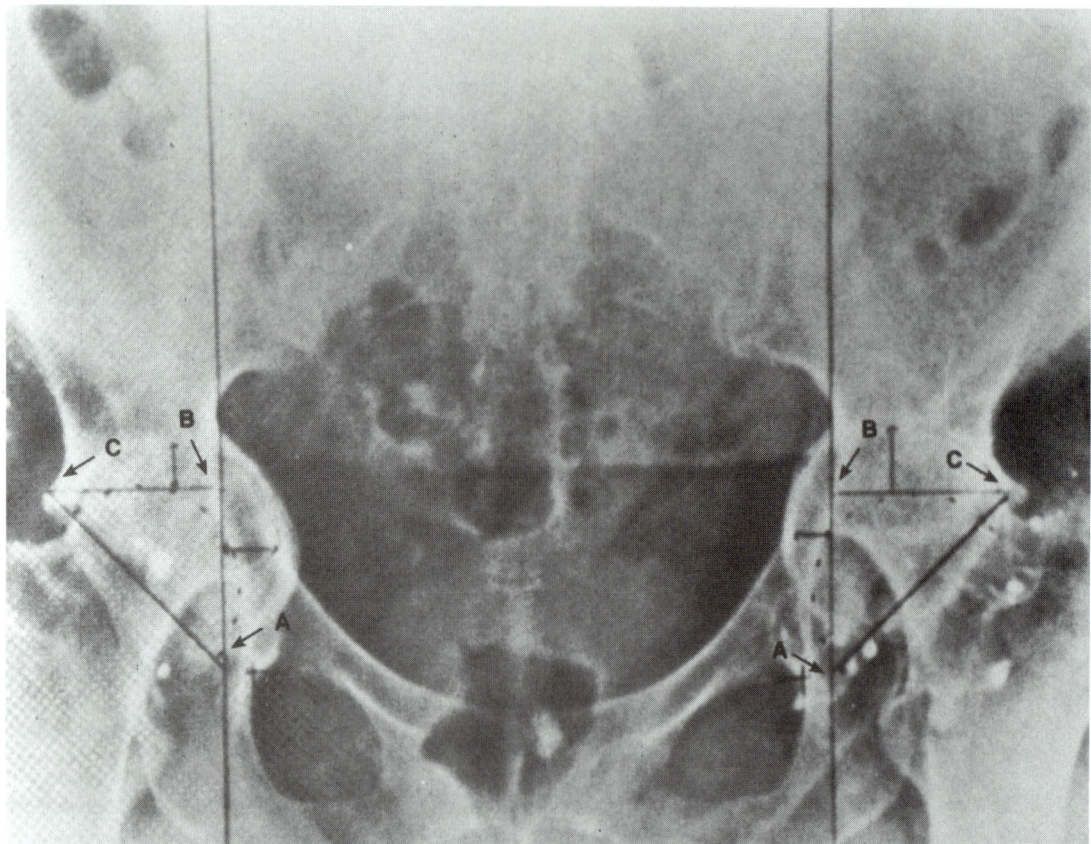

Figure 42.4. Ranawat and Zahn method for determining the acetabular component location. Two parallel horizontal lines are drawn: one tangential to the top of the iliac crests and one tangential to the ischial tuberosities. Point *A* is then established 5 mm lateral to the intersection of Shenton's and Kohler's lines. A line perpendicular to the first two lines is drawn through point *A*. Point *B* is estab-lished on this vertical line by measuring one-fifth the distance between the two horizontal lines. Then line *BC,* perpendicular to and equal in length to *AB,* is drawn. Reprinted with permission from Ranawat CS, Zahn MG. Role of bone grafting in correction of protrusio acetabuli by total hip arthroplasty. J Arthroplasty 1986; 1:131–137.

Clinical Table: Cementless Total Hip Replacement

Procedure	Indications	Technique	Anatomy	Pitfalls
Diaphyseal fitting femoral component	• <40 years old • >40 to <65 years old, selective	• Preoperative template • Diaphyseal reamer determines size • Torsional stability	• Sciatic nerve • External rotators (posterior) • Abductors (anterolateral) • Calcar	• Diaphyseal femoral fracture • Sciatic nerve injury • Undersized stem • Heterotopic ossification
Proximal fit and fill femoral component	• <40 years old • >40 to <65 years old, selective	• Preoperative template • Broach that fills proximal determines size • Torsional stability	• Sciatic nerve • External rotators (posterior) • Abductors (anterolateral) • Calcar	• Proximal femoral fracture • Sciatic nerve injury • Undersized stem • Heterotopic ossification
Hemispherical acetabular component	• Any age	• Preoperative template • Underream • Screw fixation optional (poor bone quality)	• Acetabular fossa • Transverse acetabular ligament • Femoral and sciatic nerves • External and internal iliac arteries and veins • Obturator artery, vein, and nerve	• Acetabular fracture • Intrapelvic neurovascular injury • Femoral, sciatic, or obturator nerve injury • Heterotopic ossification

Acetabular Reconstruction

Acetabular reconstruction begins with removal of peripheral soft tissue, curettage of residual cartilage, and identification of bony landmarks. The ischium and pubis are helpful landmarks that are readily palpable. In primary cases, the transverse acetabular ligament can usually be identified. A retractor is placed below this ligament and behind the inferior aspect of the medial wall (teardrop). The presence of a medial (curtain) osteophyte may obscure the acetabular fossa. The osteophyte is removed along with the pulvinar to allow identification of the medial wall, which is an important landmark for determining the depth of acetabular reaming.

The goal of reaming is to contour the acetabulum into a hemisphere of bleeding subchondral bone, preserving the true acetabular floor and allowing for maximal prosthetic containment. Loss of subchondral bone results in a significant decrease in strength of the bone. Therefore, care is taken to preserve subchondral bone. There are two technical points worthy of consideration. First, in some patients, the subchondral bone is soft and easily violated. Particular care should be taken in patients who have not been weight bearing on the hip for some time; patients with inflammatory arthritis, particularly those on steroids; and patients with significant osteoporosis. Second, in some patients the subchondral bone may be so sclerotic that the reamer is deflected, causing eccentric reaming and, in some cases, violation of the subchondral bone. Therefore, care must be taken in directing the reamer; and

sometimes, the sclerotic bone should be removed with a burr before reaming is continued.

Initial reaming is directed medially and establishes the depth; the surgeon should take care to preserve the inner table (medial wall). Reaming proceeds with sequential increases in size, usually in 2-mm increments. It is helpful to have reamers available in 1-mm increments, allowing the surgeon to use a single set of reamers for many different brands of acetabular components and offering the surgeon more flexibility in selecting the amount of interference fit. The size of the acetabular component is usually limited by the AP diameter of the acetabulum.

Once reaming is completed, an acetabular component is selected that is at least 1 mm, preferably 2 mm, greater in peripheral diameter than the last reamer. In younger patients with hard bone, a 1-mm interference fit is appropriate. When bone quality is poor, an interference fit of 3 mm may be appropriate. Note that underreaming by 4 mm has been shown to be associated with a high incidence of acetabular fracture, requiring an impaction force of 3000 N or greater (71). Positioning guides are available for impaction of the acetabular component; however, their proper use depends on the patient's pelvis being positioned perpendicular to the floor. Therefore, a change in pelvic position that is not accommodated for may lead to component malposition. In most primary cases, excluding perhaps congenital dislocation of the hip (CDH) and severe protrusio, the anatomic acetabular rim can serve as a guide. In general, the ideal component position is 30° to 40° of abduction from horizontal with at least 15° of ante-

Figure 42.5. The ideal acetabular component is impacted in 30° to 40° of abduction from the horizontal plane with 15° to 25° of anteversion.

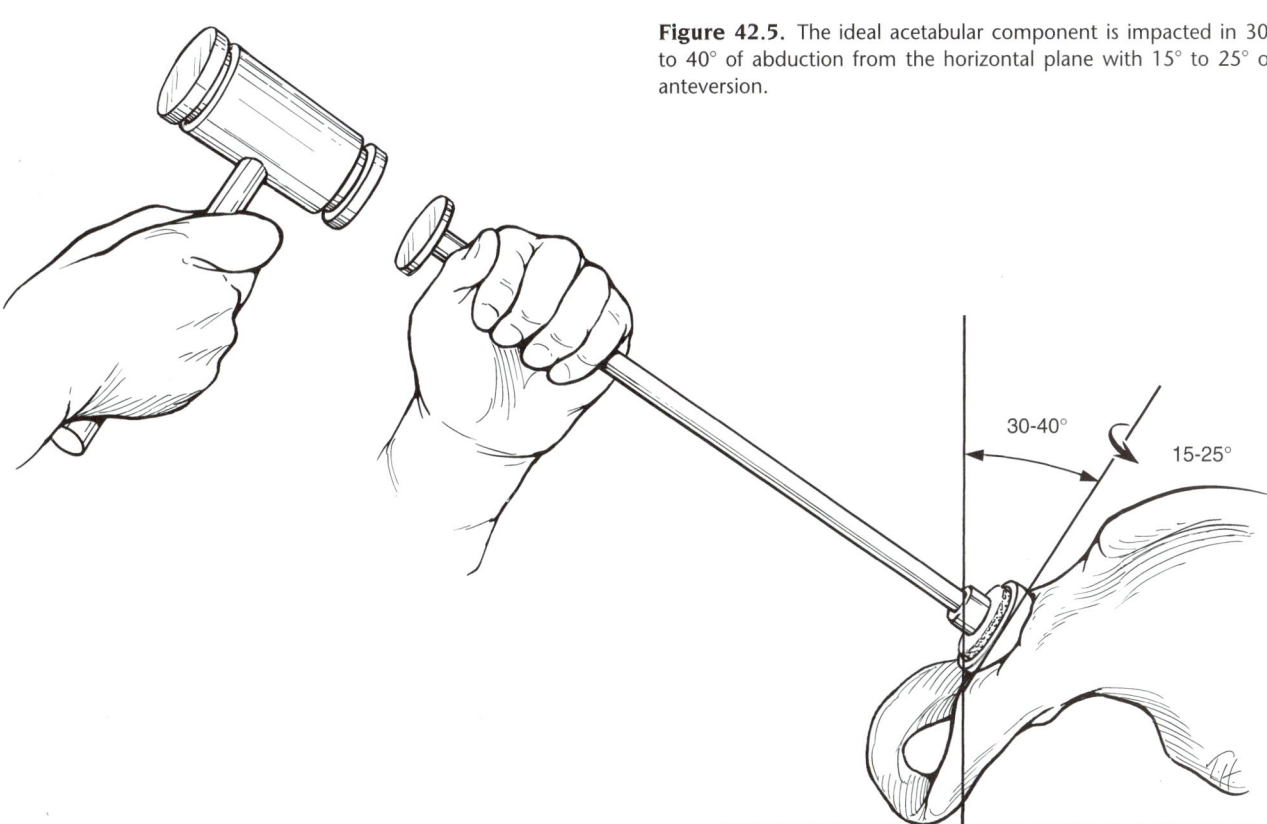

version (Fig. 42.5). Increased anteversion (20° to 25°) may be preferred when the posterior approach is used. Once the component is seated, peripheral osteophytes that may cause impingement are removed.

The use of adjuvant fixation remains controversial. The use of screws can optimize fixation, and retrieval studies have shown that the majority of ingrowth occurs around the screws (31,61,66). Concerns about wear generation and access of particulate debris, however, have led most authors to reserve the use of screws to cases clearly requiring adjuvant fixation. Press-Fit fixation without screws is used in more than 90% of primary cases at our institution. When screws are used, the surgeon must be familiar with both the medial pelvic structures that are at risk and the areas that are safe, posterosuperior and posteroinferior (72,73) (Fig. 42.6). Biomechanical studies have shown that the best screw fixation is obtained in the superior ilium, and bicortical fixation is better than unicortical (74).

When selecting the polyethylene liner, the surgeon should take into consideration issues of wear and the thickness of available polyethylene. In general, a 26- or 28-mm liner is used, which provided a compromise between linear and volumetric wear (75). In smaller acetabular components, however, a 22-mm liner is preferable to provide adequate polyethylene thickness. Many polyethylene liners come with a 10° or 20° buildup, or extension of the rim.

The 10° liner has been shown clinically to result in a decreased dislocation rate at 2 years of follow-up compared to a standard liner (76). Theoretical concerns do remain regarding the possibility of increased polyethylene wear as the result of femoral neck impingement on the elevated acetabular rim. Recent retrieval data at the time of revision confirm significant wear of the elevated rim in 4 of 10 acetabular components with elevated liners (77).

Femoral Reconstruction

The first consideration in cementless femoral reconstruction is the level of neck resection. In general, this can be determined from preoperative templating. Most implant systems have a neck resection guide. A femoral neck osteotomy made too high may lead to undersizing of the femoral component or to a femoral fracture. A femoral neck osteotomy made too low may compromise rotational stability of the implant.

The next step in femoral preparation is reaming the medullary canal. The goal of serial reaming is to shape the bone to fit the prosthesis. The type of reamers used depends on the design of the femoral component. For curved anatomic stems a flexible reamer is often used. For straight stems, a rigid straight reamer is used.

If the straight stem is designed for proximal fixation, then

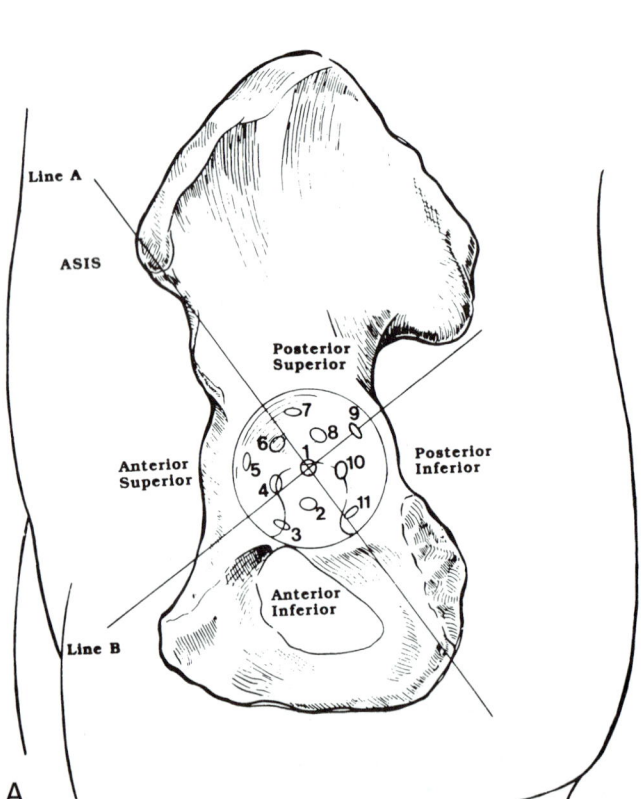

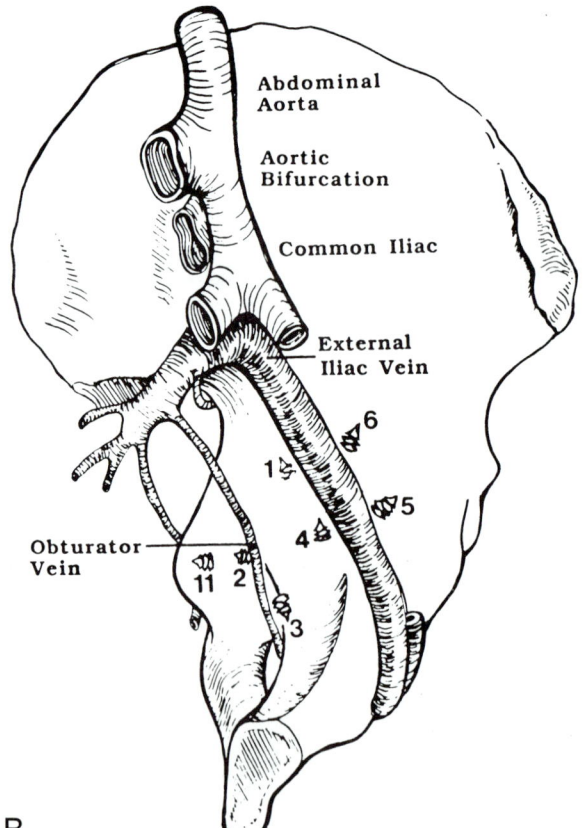

Figure 42.6. A. The quadrant system for determining safe screw placement. The anterior quadrants should be avoided. **B.** Note the proximity of the anterior acetabular screws to vital intrapelvic neurovascular structures. *1–11,* screw positions; *ASIS,* anterior superior iliac spine. Reprinted with permission from Wasielewski RC, Cooperstein LA, Kruger MP, Rubash HE. Acetabular anatomy and the transacetabular fixation of screws in total hip arthroplasty. J Bone Joint Surg 1990;72A:501–508.

either a tapered or cylindrical reamer is used (Fig. 42.7A). In general, for stems designed for proximal fixation, the femur is reamed to allow a line-to-line fit or is slightly over-reamed. However, the size to which the surgeon reams is determined by the size of the stem that provides the best proximal fit. Some of these designs require more cortical bone removal than do stems designed for distal fixation.

A cylindrical reamer is used for straight stems designed for distal or diaphyseal fixation. For stems designed for distal fixation, the femur is usually underreamed by 0.5 to 1 mm. The surgeon determines the size of the reamer by the stem diameter that provides the best diaphyseal fit.

Regardless of femoral stem design and type of reamer, the following principles are noteworthy. From preoperative templating, the surgeon should have a good idea of the size of femoral reamer required. If during serial reaming the surgeon meets significant resistance at a smaller than templated size, it is essential that he or she reevaluate the pilot hole and direction of the reaming. Failure to do so may result in femoral canal perforation and/or fracture. A common tendency is for the reamer to be in varus, particularly when there is excessive trochanteric overhang. This is easily corrected with lateralization of the reamer. Excessive flexion or extension of the reamer relative to the shaft may also lead to eccentric reaming. If resistance per-

sists after readjustment of the reamer, then an intraoperative x-ray may be necessary.

Preparation of the proximal femur is accomplished with serial broaching (Fig. 42.7B). For proximal fixation stem designs, the appropriately sized broach is determined by the size that most intimately fills the proximal femoral metaphysis and provides rotational stability. For distal fixation designs, the broach size is determined by the size of reamer used to obtain the best diaphyseal fit.

Once the broach is fully seated, there should be no evidence of gross motion to torsion. Care must be taken in testing for rotational stability, as injudicious testing may result in femoral fracture. If the appropriately sized broach is difficult to fully seat, the surgeon should check the level of femoral neck resection. An inadvertently low femoral neck resection may give a false impression that the broach is not fully seated. Attempts to further impact the broach in such a case may result in femoral fracture. In addition, if the surgeon has difficulty seating the broach, he or she should check that the last reamer used corresponds to the broach size being used.

At this point, a trial reduction is usually performed to assess hip stability. The hip is flexed and internally rotated to ensure adequate anteversion of both the acetabulum and femoral component. The hip is then extended

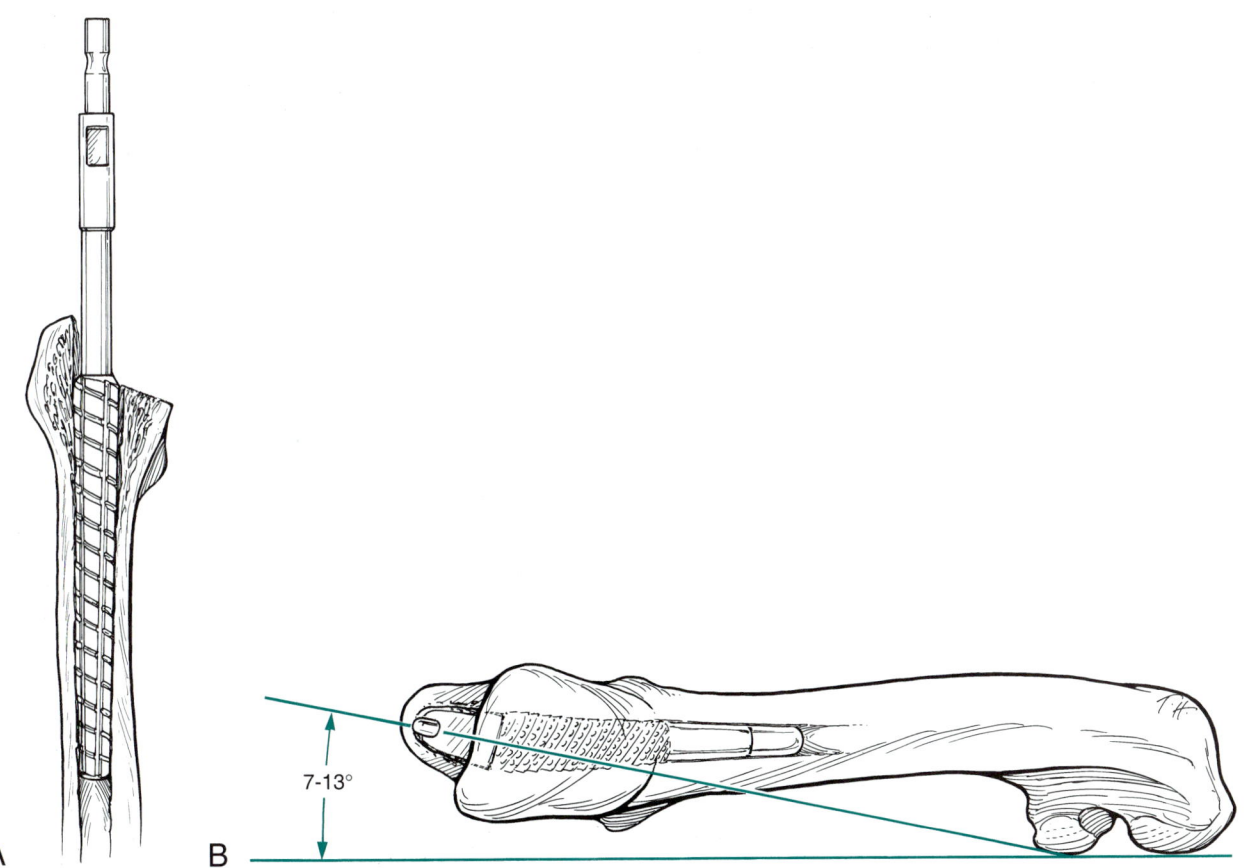

7-13°

A   B

Figure 42.7. A. Tapered reamer. **B.** Femoral broach.

and externally rotated to ensure that one or both components have not been excessively anteverted.

Impaction and final seating of the femoral component is undertaken after removal of the trial components. For stems designed for proximal fixation, there is little resistance to insertion until 1 to 2 cm from final seating. Insertion of stems designed for distal fixation may, conversely, require considerable force to overcome the resistance. Therefore, familiarity with a particular design and methods of insertion are important.

Provided proper fit has been obtained, the femoral component should be stable to torsion. As mentioned above, the surgeon can check for torsional stability with the broach. In addition, he or she can get an impression of stability during impaction. Some implant designs provide a torque wrench to assess torsional stability; but as noted above, care must be taken not to fracture the femur during torque testing.

Pitfalls and Common Mistakes

Intraoperative complications common to both cemented and uncemented components are discussed in Chapter 41. Here we focus on pitfalls and common mistakes unique to uncemented total hip arthroplasty.

INTRAOPERATIVE FEMORAL FRACTURES

Intraoperative femoral fractures in primary THA occur more commonly with cementless than with cemented femoral components (78–80). The reason for the increased incidence of intraoperative fractures with uncemented devices can be explained by the need for rigid initial fixation, which requires intimate bone prosthesis contact, and the narrow range of tolerance between the prosthesis and the femoral canal that can produce large hoop stresses leading to fracture (81). In addition, many authors have acknowledged the presence of a learning curve; the incidence of fractures decreases with the experience of the surgeon (78–80,82).

The pattern of fracture varies with the type of uncemented femoral implant selected. Proximal fixation devices tend to result in fractures of the proximal femur, usually beginning medially or anteromedially and extending distally. These fractures are readily treated with cerclage wiring and have little reported impact on the final result, if the implant has stable fixation (78–80). Distal femur fractures occur more commonly with distal fixation femoral components (78). The same principles apply: If the fracture is complete, it requires some type of internal fixation; and if the implant is stable, there are no long-term sequelae (78).

Factors within the surgeon's control that can help prevent fractures include proper selection of the appropriate implant size and design, being familiar with the use of the chosen implant, maintaining proper alignment during instrumentation of the femur and insertion of the femoral component, and prophylactic wiring in high-risk patients. The use of a 2-mm cable for prophylactic cerclage has

been shown to significantly decrease the microstrain in the proximal femur during instrumentation (83). This is a particularly helpful technique when using an uncemented device after removal of retained hardware with stress risers at the previous screw holes.

INTRAOPERATIVE ACETABULAR FRACTURES

Intraoperative fractures of the acetabulum that result from insertion of oversized acetabular components probably occur more frequently than is commonly appreciated. Experimental data on the rate of fracture in cadaveric specimens reveal that the use of oversized components resulted in fractures of 60% of specimens (71). The fracture rate was 93% for components that were oversized by 4 mm and 27% for components that were oversized by 2 mm (71). The tendency to fracture was independent of the size of the specimen.

The limited evidence for clinical problems resulting from acetabular fractures probably reflects a failure to recognize the fracture and a strong propensity for spontaneous healing. Kim et al. (71) detected only 56% on routine AP and lateral views and could not detect 17% of fractures radiographically.

Patients with persistent postoperative groin pain and normal x-rays may likely have an occult fracture. Depending on the extent of symptoms and radiographic appearance, a period of protected weight bearing may be indicated. Fortunately, available clinical data suggest that the prognosis is good. The majority of these fractures heal spontaneously with no lasting adverse effect.

UNDERSIZING OF THE FEMORAL COMPONENT

Implantation of a too small femoral component results in suboptimal initial fixation and subsequent aseptic failure. Avoidance of this problem begins with careful preoperative templating and a familiarity with the prosthetic design and its mode of fixation. The level of neck resection is also important. A neck resection left long may result in undersizing of the implant, particularly with a design that relies on proximal fixation. Care must be taken while instrumenting the femur to ensure that proper alignment is maintained in all three planes. Judicious torque testing can also help assess torsional stability. Finally, if any question persists, an intraoperative x-ray can be obtained to assess femoral fit.

HETEROTOPIC OSSIFICATION

Heterotopic ossification occurs in both cementless and cemented total hip arthroplasty, and the risk factors are well established. An increased risk of heterotopic ossification has been reported with the use of cementless femoral components, presumably from an increased escape of bone debris and marrow elements normally sealed off by the cement in cemented stems (84). Some authors have failed to show an increased risk of heterotopic ossification with the use of uncemented stems (85,86).

Prevention begins with careful surgical technique. The posterior approach has been shown to have a lower incidence of heterotopic ossification (86). Atraumatic technique, limited muscle retraction, meticulous hemostasis, and lavage are factors under the surgeon's control that may help decrease heterotopic ossification.

The prophylaxis of heterotopic ossification in uncemented devices requires special consideration. Any measures used to inhibit heterotopic ossification will also have an effect on bone ingrowth. Indomethacin, aspirin, and ibuprofen have all been shown to have a significant inhibitory effect on bone ingrowth in an animal model after 4 weeks (87). Clinically, however, short-course indomethacin (10 days) has been effective in preventing heterotopic ossification, with no deleterious effect on clinical outcome (88). Postoperative radiation with Cerrobend (Cerro Metal Products, Bellefonte, PA) shields to protect the ingrowth surfaces has been shown to be another effective means of prophylaxis for heterotopic ossification (89).

INTRAPELVIC NEUROVASCULAR INJURY

While the routine use of adjuvant screw fixation remains controversial, there are occasions even in primary THA when adjuvant fixation may be desired. Therefore, the surgeon must be familiar with the structures at risk with screw placement and, more importantly, how to avoid them. Anatomical studies have clearly outlined the structures at risk: the external iliac artery and vein and the obturator artery, vein, and nerve (72,73). Prevention of intrapelvic neurovascular injury is best accomplished by careful screw placement into regions of the pelvis away from the structures at risk. Fortunately, this is easily accomplished by dividing the pelvis into quadrants (72,73). A line from the anterior superior iliac spine to the ischial tuberosity divides the pelvis into anterior and posterior halves. If the surgeon avoids the anterior half of the pelvis, he or she can avoid most neurovascular injuries (72,73).

Results

In general, a review of the clinical and radiographic results of uncemented THA reveals that successful osseous fixation is possible. Because of the variation in prosthetic design, surgical technique, the surgeon's experience, and patient selection factors, definitive conclusions regarding the efficacy of cementless total hip arthroplasty compared to cemented total hip arthroplasty are not possible. A review of the published clinical and radiographic results of cementless total hip arthroplasty, however, allows the following observations (the results are presented separately for acetabular and femoral components).

ACETABULAR COMPONENTS

As mentioned previously, use of cementless acetabular components has gained widespread acceptance. A review of published intermediate clinical and radiographic results of cementless acetabular components supports their widespread use. Rates of aseptic loosening for hemispherical acetabular components with and without adjuvant screw fixation range from 0 to 1.2%, with no revisions

for aseptic loosening (13,19,90–92). A recent report of 157 patients with hemispherical porous-coated acetabular (PCA) components after a 7- to 10-year follow-up reveals possible loosening in 5%, no revisions for aseptic loosening, radiolucencies in 41%, and osteolysis in 4% (93). Radiolucencies about the acetabular components have been observed in up to 60% of patients, but have seldom been progressive and have not correlated with clinical success (90,92). With longer follow-up on the PCA component, loosening rates from 2.6 to 11% have been reported, pelvic osteolysis have been noted in up to 36% of cases, and acetabular revisions were required in up to 10% of patients (14,15,17). Despite the increasing rates of failure in the PCA components, the results compare favorably with results of cemented acetabular components.

Although the clinical results from intermediate follow-up support the continued use of uncemented acetabular components, long-term follow-up is necessary before any definitive conclusions can be made. Of concern are recent reports of increased wear rates in uncemented hemispherical acetabular components (94,95). Catastrophic failure (96) and liner dissociation (97–99) are additional potential problems with uncemented acetabular components.

FEMORAL COMPONENTS

The intermediate clinical and radiographic results of cementless femoral devices will be considered separately for proximally coated designs and extensively coated designs. The rates of aseptic loosening for proximally coated prostheses with at least 5 years of follow-up range from 2 to 10%; rates of revision range from 2 to 5% (13–15,17,19,49). The incidence of thigh pain ranges from 16 to 50% (13,17), and the incidence of femoral osteolysis ranges from 8 to 31% (13–15,17,19,100).

Intermediate follow-up on extensively coated prostheses reveals slightly better results: Rates of aseptic loosening were less than 2%, and revision rates ranged from 0.5 to 2% (2,12). The incidence of thigh pain was less than 4% (2,12); however, osteolysis was noted in up to 41% of implants in which both the femur and acetabulum were cementless (2). Other concerns with extensively coated implants include stress shielding and difficulty in stem removal.

A follow-up of at least 10 years on the AML femoral prosthesis revealed a femoral aseptic loosening rate of 2.9%, femoral revision rate of 1.7%, activity-limiting thigh pain in 3.9%, and osteolysis in 39% (101).

SUMMARY

The clinical and radiographic results of cementless acetabular components seem to be superior to cemented components with similar follow-up, supporting their widespread use with both cemented and cementless femoral components. Only long-term follow-up will determine whether the intermediate success of cementless acetabular components is enduring. Increased rates of polyethylene wear and osteolysis reported with cementless acetabular components are causes for concern.

The clinical results of cementless femoral stems are comparable to cemented stems using modern cement techniques. The success of cementless stems, particularly in the younger patient (less than 40 years old), supports their continued use.

The increased incidence of thigh pain and increased rates of wear and osteolysis in cementless compared to cemented total hip arthroplasty has tempered the enthusiasm of many surgeons. Concern over issues related to wear and osteolysis and improved results with modern cement techniques have limited the use of cementless femoral components in our practice to younger patients (less than 40 years old) and only selectively in patients older than 40 years.

REFERENCES

1. Spector M. Historical review of porous-coated implants. J Arthroplasty 1987;2:163–177.
2. Engh CA, Hooten J Jr., Zettl-Schaffer KF, et al. Porous-coated total hip replacement. Clin Orthop 1994;298:89–96.
3. Chandler HP, Reineck FT, Wixson RL, McCarthy JC. Total hip replacement in patients younger than thirty years old. A five-year follow-up study. J Bone Joint Surg 1981;63A:1426–1434.
4. Dorr LD, Takei GK, Conaty JP. Total hip arthroplasties in patients less than forty-five years old. J Bone Joint Surg 1983;65A:474–479.
5. Engh CA. Hip arthroplasty with a Moore prosthesis with porous coating. A five-year study. Clin Orthop 1983;176:52–66.
6. Hedley AK, Kabo M, Kim W, et al. Bony ingrowth fixation of newly designed acetabular components in a canine model. Clin Orthop 1983;176:12–23.
7. Jones LC, Hungerford DS. Cement disease. Clin Orthop 1987;225:192–206.
8. Ballard WT, Callaghan JJ, Sullivan PM, Johnston RC. The results of improved cementing techniques for total hip arthroplasty in patients less than fifty years old. A ten-year follow-up study. J Bone Joint Surg 1994;76A:959–964.
9. Schmalzried TP, Harris WH. Hybrid total hip replacement. A 6.5-year follow-up study. J Bone Joint Surg 1993;75B:608–615.
10. Oishi CS, Walker RH, Colwell CW Jr. The femoral component in total hip arthroplasty. Six to eight-year follow-up of one hundred consecutive patients after use of a third-generation cementing technique. J Bone Joint Surg 1994;76A:1130–1136.
11. Barrack RL, Mulroy RD Jr, Harris WH. Improved cementing techniques and femoral component loosening in young patients with hip arthroplasty. A 12-year radiographic review. J Bone Joint Surg 1992;74B:385–389.
12. Pellegrini VD Jr, Hughes SS, Evarts CM. A collarless cobalt-chrome femoral component in uncemented total hip arthroplasty. Five- to eight-year follow-up. J Bone Joint Surg 1992;74B:814–821.
13. Kim YH, Kim VE. Results of the Harris-Galante cementless hip prosthesis. J Bone Joint Surg 1992;74B:83–87.
14. Kim YH, Kim VE. Uncemented porous-coated anatomic total hip replacement. Results at six years in a consecutive series. J Bone Joint Surg 1993;75B:6–13.
15. Owen TD, Moran CG, Smith SR, Pinder IM. Results of uncemented porous-coated anatomic total hip replacement. J Bone Joint Surg 1994;76B:258–262.
16. Havelin LI, Espehaug B, Vollset SE, et al. The Norwegian arthroplasty register. A survey of 17,444 hip replacements 1987–1990. Acta Orthop Scand 1993;4:245–251.
17. Heekin RD, Callaghan JJ, Hopkinson WJ, et al. The porous-coated anatomic total hip prosthesis, inserted without cement. Results after five to seven years in a prospective study. J Bone Joint Surg 1993;75A:77–91.
18. Haddad RJ Jr, Skalley TC, Cook SD, et al. Clinical and roentgenographic evaluation of noncemented porous-coated anatomic medullary locking (AML) and porous-coated anatomic (PCA) total hip arthroplasties. Clin Orthop 1990;258:176–182.
19. Martell JM, Pierson RH III, Jacobs JJ, et al. Primary total hip reconstruction with a titanium fiber-coated prosthesis inserted without cement. J Bone Joint Surg 1993;75A:554–571.
20. Smith SE, Garvin KL, Jardon OM, Kaplan PA. Uncemented total hip arthroplasty. Prospective analysis of the Tri-lock femoral component. Clin Orthop 1991;269:43–50.
21. Pilliar RM, Lee JM, Maniatopoulos C. Observations on the effect of movement on bone ingrowth into porous-surfaced implants. Clin Orthop 1986;208:108–113.
22. Engh CA, O'Connor D, Jasty M, et al. Quantification of implant micromotion, strain shielding, and bone resorption with porous-coated anatomic medullary locking femoral prostheses. Clin Orthop 1992;285:13–29.
23. Burke DW, O'Connor DO, Zalenski EB, et al. Micromotion of cemented and uncemented femoral components. J Bone Joint Surg 1991;73B:33–37.
24. Jasty M, Krushell R, Zalenski E, et al. The contribution of the nonporous distal stem to the stability of proximally porous-coated canine femoral components. J Arthroplasty 1993;8:33–41.
25. Kendrick BJ II, Noble PC, Tullos HS. Distal stem design and the torsional stability of cementless femoral stems. J Arthroplasty 1995;10:463–469.
26. Callaghan JJ, Fulghum, CS, Glisson RR, Stranne SK. The effect of femoral stem geometry on interface motion in uncemented porous-coated total hip prostheses. Comparison of straight-stem and curved-stem designs. J Bone Joint Surg 1992;74A:839–848.
27. Schneider E, Kinast C, Eulenberger J, et al. A comparative study of the initial stability of cementless hip prostheses. Clin Orthop 1989;248:200–209.
28. Biegler FB, Reuben JD, Harrigan, TP, et al. Effect of porous coating and loading conditions on total hip femoral stem stability. J Arthroplasty 1995;10:839–847.
29. Whiteside LA, Easley JC. The effect of collar and distal stem fixation on micromotion of the femoral stem in uncemented total hip arthroplasty. Clin Orthop 1989;239:145–153.
30. Manley PA, Vanderby R, Kohles S, et al. Alterations in femoral strain, micromotion, cortical geometry, cortical porosity, and bony ingrowth in uncemented collared and collarless prostheses in the dog. J Arthroplasty 1995;10:63–73.
31. Lachiewicz PF, Suh PB, Gilbert JA. In vitro initial fixation of porous-coated acetabular total hip components. A biomechanical comparative study. J Arthroplasty 1989;4:201–205.
32. Curtis MJ, Jinnah RH, Wilson VD, Hungerford DS. The initial stability of uncemented acetabular components. J Bone Joint Surg 1992;74B:372–376.
33. Stiehl JB, MacMillan E, Skrade DA. Mechanical stability of porous-coated acetabular components in total hip arthroplasty. J Arthroplasty 1991;6:295–300.
34. Adler E, Stuchin SA, Kummer FJ. Stability of Press-Fit acetabular cups. J Arthroplasty 1992;7:295–301.
35. MacKenzie JR, Callaghan JJ, Pedersen DR, Brown TD. Areas of contact and extent of gaps with implantation of oversized acetabular components in total hip arthroplasty. Clin Orthop 1994;298:127–136.
36. Kim YS, Brown TD, Pedersen DR, Callaghan JJ. Reamed surface topography and component seating in Press-Fit cementless acetabular fixation. J Arthroplasty 1995;10(Suppl):S14–S21.
37. Duparc J, Massin P. Results of 203 total hip replacements using a smooth, cementless femoral component. J Bone Joint Surg 1992;74B:251–256.
38. Kang JD, McKernan DJ, Kruger M, et al. Ingrowth and formation

of bone in defects in an uncemented fiber-metal total hip-replacement model in dogs. J Bone Joint Surg 1991;73A:93–105.

39. Bobyn JD, Glassman AH, Goto H, et al. The effect of stem stiffness on femoral bone resorption after canine porous-coated total hip arthroplasty. Clin Orthop 1990;261:196–213.

40. Sumner DR, Galante JO. Determinants of stress shielding: design versus materials versus interface. Clin Orthop 1992; 274:202–212.

41. Hughes SS, Furia JP, Smith P, Pellegrini VD Jr. Atrophy of the proximal part of the femur after total hip arthroplasty without cement. A quantitative comparison of cobalt-chromium and titanium femoral stems with use of dual x-ray absorptiometry. J Bone Joint Surg 1995;77A:231–239.

42. Haynes DR, Rogers SD, Hay S, et al. The differences in toxicity and release of bone-resorbing mediators induced by titanium and cobalt-chromium-alloy wear particles. J Bone Joint Surg 1993;75A:825–834.

43. Spencer E, Nestor BJ, Crow M, et al. Quantitative analysis of human macrophage response to particulate debris: a comparison of titanium, cobalt, polyethylene, and polymethylmethacrylate [Unpublished manuscript], 1997.

44. Bourne RB, Rorabeck CH, Burkart BC, Kirk PG. Ingrowth surfaces. Plasma spray coating to titanium alloy hip replacements. Clin Orthop 1994;298:37–46.

45. Bobyn JD, Pilliar RM, Cameron HU, Weatherly GC. The optimum pore size for the fixation of porous-surfaced metal implants by the ingrowth of bone. Clin Orthop 1980;150:263–270.

46. Robertson DM, Pierre L, Chahal R. Preliminary observations of bone ingrowth into porous materials. J Biomed Mater Res 1976; 10:335–344.

47. Goldberg VM, Stevenson S, Feighan J, Davy, D. Biology of grit-blasted titanium alloy implants. Clin Orthop 1995;319:122–129.

48. Feighan JE, Goldberg VM, Davy D, et al. The influence of surface-blasting on the incorporation of titanium-alloy implants in a rabbit intramedullary model. J Bone Joint Surg 1995;77A:1380–1395.

49. Robinson RP, Deysine GR, Green TM. Uncemented total hip arthroplasty using the CLS stem: a titanium alloy implant with a corundum blast finish. J Arthroplasty 1996;11:286–292.

50. Blaha JD, Gruen TA, Grappiolo G, et al. Porous coating: do we need it? Orthopedics 1994;17:779–780.

51. Zweymuller KA, Lintner FK, Semlitsch MF. Biologic fixation of a Press-Fit titanium hip joint endoprothesis. Clin Orthop 1988; 235:195–206.

52. Bobyn JD, Mortimer ES, Glassman AH, et al. Producing and avoiding stress shielding. Laboratory and clinical observations of noncemented total hip arthroplasty. Clin Orthop 1992; 274:79–96.

53. Engh CA, Bobyn JD. The influence of stem size and extent of porous coating on femoral bone resorption after primary cementless hip arthroplasty. Clin Orthop 1988;231:7–28.

54. Huiskes R. The various stress patterns of Press-Fit, ingrown, and cemented femoral stems. Clin Orthop 1990;261:27–38.

55. Sumner DR, Turner TM, Urban RM, Galante JO. Remodeling and ingrowth of bone at two years in a canine cementless total hip-arthroplasty model. J Bone Joint Surg 1992;74A:239–250.

56. Engh CA, McGovern TF, Bobyn JD, Harris WH. A quantitative evaluation of periprosthetic bone-remodeling after cementless total hip arthroplasty. J Bone Joint Surg 1992;74A:1009–1020.

57. Kilgus DJ, Shimaoka EE, Tipton JS, Eberle RW. Dual-energy x-ray absorptiometry measurement of bone mineral density around porous-coated cementless femoral implants. Methods and preliminary results. J Bone Joint Surg 1993;75A:279–287.

58. Jasty M, Rubash HE, Paiement GD, et al. Porous-coated uncemented components in experimental total hip arthroplasty in dogs. Effect of plasma-sprayed calcium phosphate coatings on bone ingrowth. Clin Orthop 1992;280:300–309.

59. Howie DW, Haynes DR, Rogers SD, et al. The response to particulate debris. Orthop Clin North Am 1993;24:571–581.

60. Nakashima Y, Shuto T, Hayashi K, et al. The stimulatory effects of ceramic particles on the production of the bone-resorbing mediators in vitro. Paper presented at the 41st Annual Meeting of the Orthopaedic Research Society, Orlando, FL, February 13–16, 1995.

61. Cook SD, Barrack RL, Thomas KA, Haddad RJ Jr. Quantitative analysis of tissue growth into human porous total hip components. J Arthroplasty 1988;3:249–262.

62. Engh CA, Hooten JP Jr, Zettl-Schaffer KF, et al. Evaluation of bone ingrowth in proximally and extensively porous-coated anatomic medullary locking prostheses retrieved at autopsy. J Bone Joint Surg 1995;77A:903–910.

63. Collier JP, Mayor MB, Chae JC, et al. Macroscopic and microscopic evidence of prosthetic fixation with porous-coated materials. Clin Orthop 1988;235:173–180.

64. Collier JP, Bauer TW, Bloebaum RD, et al. Results of implant retrieval from postmortem specimens in patients with well-functioning, long-term total hip replacement. Clin Orthop 1992; 274:97–112.

65. Engh CA, Zettl-Schaffer KF, Kukita Y, et al. Histological and radiographic assessment of well functioning porous-coated acetabular components. A human postmortem retrieval study. J Bone Joint Surg 1993;75A:814–824.

66. Pidhorz LE, Urban RM, Jacobs JJ, et al. A quantitative study of bone and soft tissues in cementless porous-coated acetabular components retrieved at autopsy. J Arthroplasty 1993;8:213–225.

67. Cook SD, Barrack RL, Thomas KA, Haddad RJ Jr. Tissue growth into porous primary and revision femoral stems. J Arthroplasty 1991;6(Suppl):S37–S46.

68. Maynard MJ, Ranawat CS, Flynn WF. The hip. In: Sculco TP, ed. Surgical treatment of rheumatoid arthritis. St. Louis: Mosby, 1992:211–236.

69. Noble PC, Alexander JW, Lindahl LJ, et al. The anatomic basis of femoral component design. Clin Orthop 1988;235:148–165.

70. Ranawat CS, Zahn MG. Role of bone grafting in correction of protrusio acetabuli by total hip arthroplasty. J Arthroplasty 1986; 1:131–137.

71. Kim YS, Callaghan JJ, Ahn PB, Brown TD. Fracture of the acetabulum during insertion of an oversized hemispherical component. J Bone Joint Surg 1995;77A:111–117.

72. Keating EM, Ritter MA, Faris PM. Structures at risk from medially placed acetabular screws. J Bone Joint Surg 1990;72A:509–511.

73. Wasielewski RC, Cooperstein LA, Kruger MP, Rubash HE. Acetabular anatomy and the transacetabular fixation of screws in total hip arthroplasty. J Bone Joint Surg 1990;72A:501–508.

74. Stranne SK, Callaghan JJ, Elder SH, et al. Screw-augmented fixation of acetabular components. A mechanical model to determine optimal screw placement. J Arthroplasty 1991;6:301–305.

75. Livermore J, Ilstrup D, Morrey B. Effect of femoral head size on wear of the polyethylene acetabular component. J Bone Joint Surg 1990;72A:518–528.

76. Cobb TK, Morrey BF, Ilstrup DM. The elevated-rim acetabular liner in total hip arthroplasty: relationship to postoperative dislocation. J Bone Joint Surg 1996;78A:80–86.

77. Murray DW. Impingement and loosening of the long posterior wall acetabular implant. J Bone Joint Surg 1992;74B:377–379.

78. Schwartz JT Jr, Mayer JG, Engh CA. Femoral fracture during noncemented total hip arthroplasty. J Bone Joint Surg 1989; 71A:1135–1142.

79. Fitzgerald RH Jr, Brindley GW, Kavanagh BF. The uncemented total hip arthroplasty. Intraoperative femoral fractures. Clin Orthop 1988;235:61–66.

80. Mont MA, Maar DC, Krackow KA, Hungerford DS. Hoop-stress fractures of the proximal femur during hip arthroplasty. Management and results in 19 cases. J Bone Joint Surg 1992;74B:257–260.

81. Jasty M, Henshaw RM, O'Connor DO, Harris WH. High assembly strains and femoral fractures produced during insertion of uncemented femoral components. A cadaver study. J Arthroplasty 1993;8:479–487.

82. Callaghan JJ, Heekin RD, Savory CG, et al. Evaluation of the learning curve associated with uncemented primary porous-coated anatomic total hip arthroplasty. Clin Orthop 1992; 282:132–144.

83. Herzwurm PJ, Walsh J, Pettine KA, Ebert FR. Prophylactic cerclage: a method of preventing femur fracture in uncemented total hip arthroplasty. Orthopedics 1992;15:143–146.

84. Maloney WJ, Krushell RJ, Jasty M, Harris WH. Incidence of heterotopic ossification after total hip replacement: effect of the type of fixation of the femoral component. J Bone Joint Surg 1991; 73A:191–193.

85. Rockwood PR, Horne JG. Heterotopic ossification following uncemented total hip arthroplasty. J Arthroplasty 1990; 5(Suppl):S43–S46.

86. Bischoff R, Dunlap J, Carpenter L, et al. Heterotopic ossification following uncemented total hip arthroplasty. Effect of the operative approach. J Arthroplasty 1994;9:641–644.

87. Trancik T, Mills W, Vinson N. The effect of indomethacin, aspirin, and ibuprofen on bone ingrowth into a porous-coated implant. Clin Orthop 1989;249:113–121.

88. McMahon JS, Waddell JP, Morton J. Effect of short-course indomethacin on heterotopic bone formation after uncemented total hip arthroplasty. J Arthroplasty 1991;6:259–264.

89. Jasty M, Schutzer S, Tepper J, et al. Radiation-blocking shields to localize periarticular radiation precisely for prevention of heterotopic bone formation around uncemented total hip arthroplasties. Clin Orthop 1990;257:138–145.

90. Schmalzried TP, Harris WH. The Harris-Galante porous-coated acetabular component with screw fixation. Radiographic analysis of eighty-three primary hip replacements at a minimum of five years. J Bone Joint Surg 1992;74A:1130–1139.

91. Schmalzried TP, Wessinger SJ, Hill GE, Harris WH. The Harris-Galante porous acetabular component Press-Fit without screw fixation. five-year radiographic analysis of primary cases. J Arthroplasty 1994;9:235–242.

92. Incavo SJ, Di Fazio FA, Howe JG. Cementless hemispheric acetabular components. 2–4-year results. J Arthroplasty 1993; 8:573–580.

93. Tompkins GS, Jacobs JJ, Kull LR, et al. Primary total hip arthroplasty with a porous-coated acetabular component. J Bone Joint Surg 1997;79A:169–184.

94. Hernandez JR, Keating EM, Faris PM, et al. Polyethylene wear in uncemented acetabular components. J Bone Joint Surg 1994; 76B:263–266.

95. Nashed RS, Becker DA, Gustilo RB. Are cementless acetabular components the cause of excess wear and osteolysis in total hip arthroplasty? Clin Orthop 1995;317:19–28.

96. Berry DJ, Barnes CL, Scott RD, et al. Catastrophic failure of the polyethylene liner of uncemented acetabular components. J Bone Joint Surg 1994;76B: 575–578.

97. Brien WW, Salvati EA, Wright TM, et al. Dissociation of acetabular components after total hip arthroplasty. Report of four cases. J Bone Joint Surg 1990;72A:1548–1550.

98. Kitziger KJ, De Lee JC, Evans JA. Disassembly of a modular acetabular component of a total hip-replacement arthroplasty. a case report. J Bone Joint Surg 1990;72A:621–623.

99. Wilson AJ, Monsees B, Blair VP III. Acetabular cup dislocation: a new complication of total joint arthroplasty. AJR Am J Roentgenol 1988;151:133–134.

100. Goetz DD, Smith EJ, Harris WH. The prevalence of femoral osteolysis associated with components inserted with or without cement in total hip replacements. A retrospective matched-pair series. J Bone Joint Surg 1994;76A:1121–1129.

101. Engh JR, Culpepper WJ, Engh CA. Long-term results of use of the anatomic medullary locking prosthesis in total hip arthroplasty. J Bone Joint Surg 1997;79A:177–184.

Alastair S. E. Younger, Bassam A. Masri, and Clive P. Duncan

Infected Total Hip Replacement

Infection continues to be one of the most devastating complications following total hip arthroplasty, converting the potential of renewed mobility and reduced discomfort to the potential of a sedentary existence with increased pain and poor function. At present, the incidence of deep infection following total hip replacement is less than 1% (1), which is significantly lower than an early report of about 10% (2). This reduction is generally a reflection of the use of prophylactic antibiotics at the time of the initial hip replacement.

Unlike soft tissue infections, a deep prosthetic infection is exceedingly difficult to eradicate without sophisticated surgical treatment (3). The prosthesis is relatively isolated within the bone, creating a barrier to the patient's normal immune system. Furthermore, some prosthetic materials (e.g., cement) have been shown to impair the host's local immune response (4). Finally, the infecting organism can induce the formation of a layer of polysaccharide around the bacterial colonies; known as glycocalyx (5), this layer blocks the penetration of the host's inflammatory cells and antibodies as well as exogenously administered antibiotics. Because the bacteria are relatively immune, infection can progress slowly, leading to chronic infection, steady destruction of bone stock, and failure of the implant. Thus the periprosthetic infections present a challenge.

Because of the devastating nature of these deep infections, every effort should be made to prevent them following total hip arthroplasty. The modern operating room is well equipped with adequate filters and air-exchange cycles to meet the requirements of low airborne organism counts. For total hip and knee arthroplasty, the addition of vertical laminar flow has been shown to reduce the risk of deep infection. These data, however, remain controversial; and not all centers use this modality in the operating room during total joint arthroplasty. Body isolation suits

have been advocated by many surgeons, yet there has been no definitive study demonstrating their definite efficacy in the prevention of infection.

Perioperative prophylactic antibiotics continue to be the most important factor in the prevention of deep infection following total hip arthroplasty. A first- or second-generation cephalosporin, such as cefazolin or cefuroxime, continues to be the most commonly used antibiotic for the prevention of sepsis. The duration of administration of antibiotics varies from 1 day for a primary hip replacement to 5 days for a revision total hip arthroplasty. In the latter situation, antibiotics are continued until negative intraoperative cultures are confirmed.

The addition of antibiotics to the bone cement used to fix the implants has been shown to reduce the risk of postoperative infection (6). The use of prophylactic systemic antibiotics, however, is just as effective. Antibiotic-loaded cement is thus not routinely used for the prevention of infection following primary total hip arthroplasty. On the other hand, it is not uncommon to add antibiotics to the cement for revision procedures with cemented fixation, because of the slight risk of a missed infection on preoperative evaluation and because of the increased risk of infection following secondary procedures.

INITIAL FINDINGS, PHYSICAL EXAMINATION, AND DIAGNOSIS

An infected total hip replacement may present in a variety of ways. It is easy to diagnose a nonprosthetic joint that is infected with bacterial organisms: The area is hot, inflamed, swollen, and painful and has a limited range of motion. These symptoms may be absent in an infected prosthetic joint, and the patient may simply complain of a painful arthroplasty many years after a successful and well-functioning hip replacement. On the other hand, the patient may present with an acutely infected joint that displays systemic symptoms, abscess formation, and draining sinuses.

Deep infection following total hip arthroplasty is best classified based on its pathogenesis and initial presentation (7,8). Occult infection is defined by the appearance of unexpected positive intraoperative cultures at the time of initial total hip arthroplasty. In this case, the patient presents with symptoms, signs, and radiographic features consistent with aseptic loosening of the implants; thus the surgeon proceeds to revise the components. At the time of surgery, routine intraoperative cultures are obtained, which test positive for bacteria.

Early postoperative infection is a deep intraoperative infection that may be related to infection at the time of surgery or to an infected hematoma. Generally, this type of infection occurs within the first 3 to 4 weeks after surgery. The patient often presents with delayed wound healing, persistent wound drainage, increased warmth and erythema around the wound, (possibly) fever, and persistent or worsening pain and dysfunction.

Late hematogenous infection has a similar presentation to early postoperative infection, although it occurs months to years following a successful hip replacement. The patient often presents with an infection of a few days' duration that is related to hematogenous spread of infection elsewhere. Common sources of infections include dental infections, genitourinary infections or manipulations, cutaneous infections, and (rarely) infected indwelling catheters or cannulae.

Chronic infection is a low-grade, often indolent infection. In general, the patient presents with a prolonged history of a painful arthroplasty. On further questioning, the patient often notes that the hip replacement was never pain-free or that the result has been somewhat disappointing from the start. The patient often complains of nocturnal pain, as well as pain at rest. There is often a history of delayed wound healing, a superficial infection, or simply prolonged wound drainage. This history, however, is not always present. Systemic symptoms and signs of infection are often lacking, and physical examination may occasionally reveal evidence of abscess formation and sinus tracts; but more commonly, it is not distinguishable from the examination of a noninfected, failed total hip arthroplasty.

It is important to understand the differences between these types of infections, because the treatment of each is unique.

The diagnosis of an acutely infected total hip arthroplasty (early postoperative infection or late hematogenous infection) with local symptoms and signs and possibly systemic symptoms of infection is not difficult. The appearance of the wound, with purulent drainage or abscess and sinus tract formation, is unmistakable in most cases. One simply must confirm the presence of infection by means of ancillary laboratory investigations: white blood cell count; erythrocyte sedimentation rate (ESR) (9);

and acute-phase reactant serum levels, such as the C-reactive protein (CRP), which are often elevated (10). Definitive identification of the infecting organism is of utmost importance, and every effort should be made to identify it before the administration of any antibiotics. An aspiration of the hip joint, under fluoroscopic guidance and aseptic conditions, is mandatory. Cultures of surface drainage or sinus tracts are unreliable and are best avoided.

The diagnosis of a chronically infected total hip replacement is rather difficult (11). The rule of thumb is to always maintain a high index of suspicion whenever a patient presents with a painful total hip arthroplasty. Plain radiography is the first step in the investigation. If the components are solidly fixed and the patient is experiencing significant pain and disability, the index of suspicion for occult infection should be raised.

Although radiographic signs are never clearly diagnostic of infection, the presence of marked or rapidly progressive endosteal scalloping and/or periosteal reaction around the femur suggests infection (12) (Fig. 43.1). The presence of endosteal erosions in isolation is not pathognomonic of infection, as they can be seen in aseptic loosening as well. When these erosions are extensive or rapidly progressive, the likelihood of infection is increased. In contrast, the presence of lacy periosteal reaction around the femur, particularly medially, is almost always pathognomonic of infection. Unfortunately, this finding is seen in only 1 to 2% of infected total hip replacements. Rapidly progressive osteolysis is also an ominous sign. If the implants are loose, the patient may have either septic or aseptic loosening. If there is nothing in the history or physical examination to suggest infection, screening with laboratory investigation should suffice, provided the results of these screening tests are normal.

The ESR and CRP are the laboratory screening tests of choice for the diagnosis of infected total hip arthroplasty. They should always be obtained in the investigation of the painful or failed total hip arthroplasty. The clinician must clearly exclude inflammatory conditions and associated collagen-vascular diseases when interpreting these tests. The ESR and CRP are unreliable in patients with these inflammatory conditions; in our opinion, routine aspiration of the hip joint should be used as a definitive test for infection in these patients. The sensitivity of the ESR by itself is 82% (13), and the specificity is 85%. CRP is perhaps more sensitive and specific. In our series (excluding patients with inflammatory conditions), the sensitivity of CRP alone is 96%, the specificity is 92%, the predictive value of a positive test is 74%, and the predictive value of a negative test is 99%. The interpretation of these data suggests that when these screening tests are negative, one can be reasonably confident that infection is not present. When the tests are positive, however, the likelihood of infection is much higher, although there is still a 20 to 25% chance that the hip is not infected. Therefore, if the ESR and CRP are elevated and no other reason is found for their eleva-

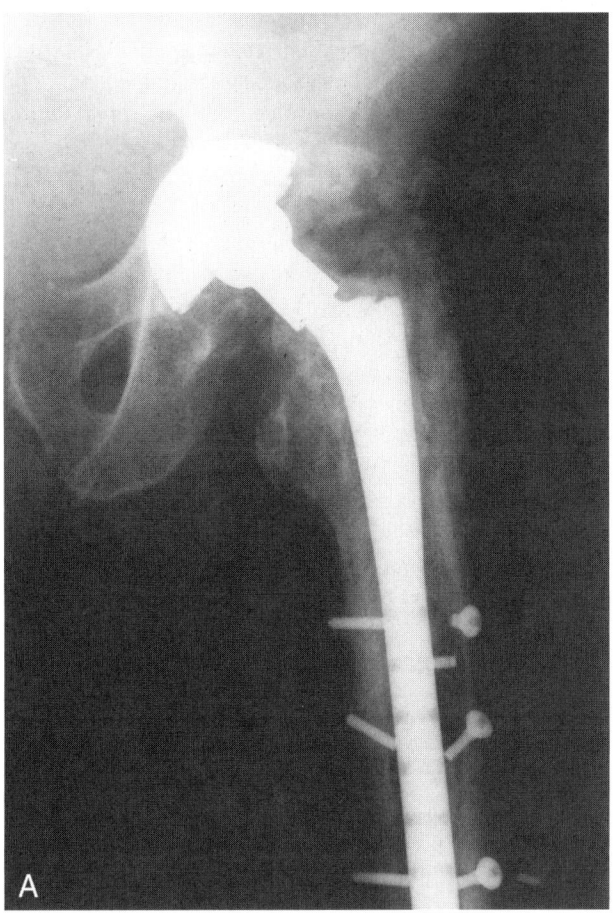

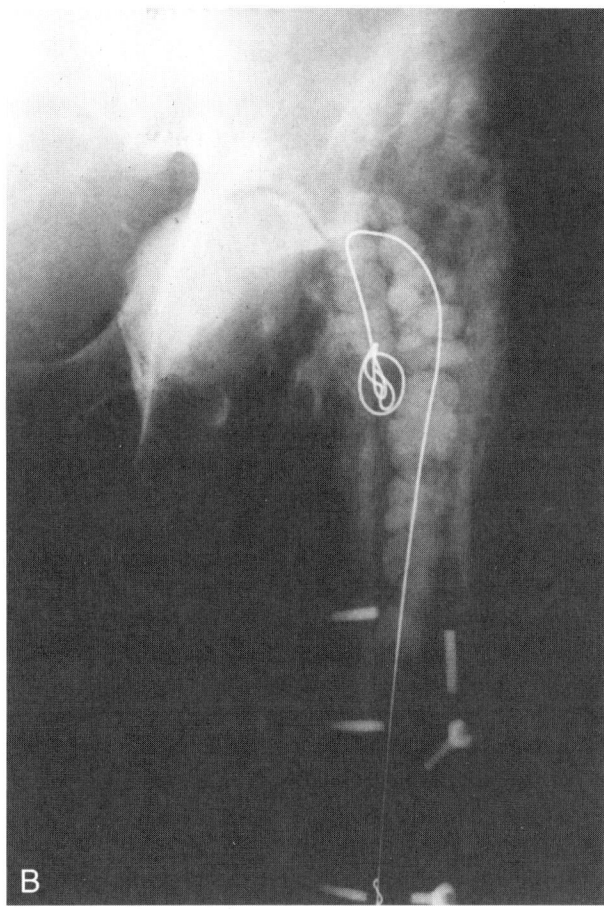

Figure 43.1. A. An 88-year-old patient who presented with a failed and infected Kent prosthesis (Biomet; Warsaw, IN) and broken screws within the medullary canal of the femur. Significant periosteal reaction suggests pan-diaphyseal osteomyelitis. **B.** Because of the patient's age and degree of infection, he was treated with a definitive Girdlestone arthroplasty. Antibiotic-loaded cement was left within the joint cavity and medullary canal of the femur as an antibiotic depot, supplementing intravenous antibiotic therapy.

tion (e.g., no systemic disease or chronic inflammatory condition), the clinician should be concerned about the possibility of infection, and further investigations are essential.

Whenever infection is suspected, either because of abnormal hematologic screening tests or because of suspicious clinical or radiographic features, an aspiration of the hip joint is mandatory. We recommend that these aspirations be performed by experienced personnel, such as a dedicated musculoskeletal radiologist, under strict aseptic techniques and under fluoroscopic guidance. A minimum of three samples should be obtained. If all three samples are negative, infection is unlikely. If all three samples are positive, infection is almost definite. If only one of three samples is positive, the aspiration should be repeated. Before performing an aspiration of the hip joint, the patient should be off all forms of antibiotics for a minimum of 4 weeks. A history of antibiotic use should always be sought before proceeding with an aspiration biopsy. Although routine hip joint aspiration has been recommended in the past, there is clear evidence in the literature that it is not necessary, particularly if the hematologic

screening tests are negative and the history and physical findings do not suggest infection.

Occasionally, the surgeon is faced with a difficult diagnostic challenge in which ancillary diagnostic modalities are necessary, for example, a patient with peritoneal dialysis on chronic antibiotic therapy for the prevention of acute peritonitis who presents with a painful total hip arthroplasty. The ESR and CRP are often elevated, for reasons that are unrelated to the total hip arthroplasty; and the results of the hip joint aspiration, when negative, must be interpreted with caution because of the confounding influence of antibiotic therapy.

Although generally of limited use, scintigraphic imaging may be of value in these and similar circumstances. Neither technetium-99m (^{99m}Tc) bone scanning nor gallium-67 (^{67}Ga) scanning alone is of value for the diagnosis of the infected total hip arthroplasty (14). Although indium-111 (^{111}In)-labeled white blood cell scans are not specific enough for the diagnosis of infection following total hip arthroplasty; sequential scanning, first with ^{99m}Tc and then with ^{111}In-labeled white blood cells, improves the specificity of this test (15). The interpretation of the sequential scanning tests is highly subjective, because a positive test refers to an increased uptake on the ^{111}In scan relative to the ^{99m}Tc scan. Thus the accuracy of the investigation depends on the experience and interest of the radiologist. The reported sensitivity of an ^{111}In-labeled white blood cell scan alone is 100%, whereas the specificity is only 50% and the accuracy is 65%. When combined with ^{99m}Tc scanning, the sensitivity is between 87 and 100%, and the specificity is between 50 and 94%, depending on the series (16,17).

Because of the relative lack of specificity of currently used nuclear imaging modalities, newer techniques, such as ^{111}In-labeled IgG, are being investigated. The ^{111}In-labeled IgG test has been used with encouraging results in the investigation of bone and joint infections, although inflammatory responses caused by wear debris may confound the diagnosis. This test is, therefore, no better at distinguishing between low-grade sepsis and aseptic loosening due to wear debris-induced osteolysis than are other imaging modalities.

Technetium-99m-labeled monoclonal antibody scanning promises to be more specific than the ^{111}In-labeled IgG test, although its validation and cost-effectiveness need to be determined. Until more encouraging results are published, this technique does not have a role in the diagnosis of the infected total hip arthroplasty.

Immunologic and molecular biologic techniques for the diagnosis of infection following total joint replacement surgery are currently under investigation, for example, measuring the levels of various cytokines (interleukin 2 and γ-interferon). Another new technique is to use polymerase chain reaction (PCR) methods to determine the genetic code of the infecting organism within the patients' periprosthetic tissues (3). This test is exquisitely sensitive but, unfortunately, cannot distinguish between live and dead microorganisms following successful treatment of the infection. The utility of both of these tests is at present uncertain, and further laboratory and clinical trials are necessary.

Despite every effort to diagnose infection preoperatively, the surgeon will occasionally be faced with a situation in which the intraoperative appearance of the tissues suggests infection, either because of frank pus or, more commonly, because of the inflamed nature of the joint lining (magenta discoloration and wet edematous tissues). In these cases, additional tests must be performed at the time of surgery to better define the likelihood of infection in that particular patient. Intraoperative cultures should always be taken at the time of revision total hip arthroplasty. The results of these cultures, however, often take between 2 and 5 days, thus more rapid tests are indicated.

In our experience, the Gram stain is universally misleading in the diagnosis of infection. It is often negative, despite obvious evidence of infection. We strongly recommend that a negative intraoperative Gram stain not be used as evidence against possible infection. A biopsy of the most inflamed part of the pseudocapsule and fibrous membrane around the components should be sent to the histopathologic laboratory for a frozen section (17). If more than 5 polymorphonuclear leukocytes per high power field are found in any of the samples, the surgeon should suspect infection (18). Recently, Lonner et al. (19) suggested that the accuracy of the test is improved if the criterion of infection is 10 or more polymorphonuclear leukocytes per high power field. Using 5 or more polymorphonuclear leukocytes per high power field as the criterion of infection, they reported a sensitivity of 84%, a specificity of 96%, a positive predictive value of 70%, and a negative predictive value of 98%. Using 10 or more leukocytes, they reported a sensitivity of 84%, a specificity of 99%, a positive predictive value of 89%, and a negative predictive value of 98%.

TREATMENT

Nonoperative Management

INDICATIONS

Although the majority of infected total hip replacements require surgical treatment, there is a limited role for antibiotic therapy alone in the management of the infected total hip arthroplasty. When a revision total hip arthroplasty has just been performed for presumed aseptic loosening and the intraoperative cultures are positive, a 6-week course of intravenous antibiotics is indicated, if analysis of clinical and laboratory data does not indicate a laboratory contaminant. The frail, elderly, and debilitated patient who cannot withstand surgical treatment or who is reluctant to consent to surgical management should be considered for life-long antibiotic suppression. The choice of antibiotic is often difficult, and combination therapy is commonly indicated. Antibiotic therapy is best supervised by an infectious disease consultant rather than by an orthopaedic surgeon. Antibiotics alone are not indicated for the otherwise healthy patient who presents with an infected total hip arthroplasty.

OUTCOME

A 6-week course of intravenous antibiotics is successful in 90% of patients with positive intraoperative cultures at the time of revision total hip arthroplasty (8). The management is successful in 50% of debilitated patients who are treated with antibiotic suppression alone (20); success is defined as the retention of the prosthesis for at least 3 years after the initial diagnosis. Although the failure rate increases with time, this method of treatment is not used in patients who are expected to survive for a number of years.

Operative Management

In the early days of total hip arthroplasty, excision arthroplasty was recommended for the treatment of the infected total hip arthroplasty. With the introduction of antibiotic-loaded bone cement, it became feasible to revise infected total hip replacements and retain a well-functioning implant rather than subject the patient to the morbidity of excision arthroplasty (21). In addition to excision arthroplasty (22,23), an infected hip replacement may be simply débrided, while retaining the original components, or may be revised in one or two stages. For two-stage revisions, a functional or nonfunctional antibiotic-loaded spacer may be used between stages (Clinical Table). Each of these procedures has its indications, advantages, and disadvantages. Because of the extensive use of antibiotic-loaded cement in the management of the infected total hip arthroplasty, an understanding of the properties and rational use of this composite material is mandatory.

ANTIBIOTIC-LOADED BONE CEMENT

Buchholz et al. (6) introduced the concept of local antibiotic delivery by mixing gentamicin with Palacos R bone cement (Smith, Nephew & Richards; Memphis, TN). Using this material, Buchholz et al. were able not only to reduce the risk of postoperative infection following total hip arthroplasty but also to treat infected total hip prostheses by revising them using antibiotic-loaded bone cement, with a 73% rate of infection eradication. Other antibiotics besides gentamicin have been successfully mixed with bone cement.

It is crucial that the rules be met when antibiotics are mixed with bone cement (24). (a) Because of the increased temperatures at the time of polymerization of bone cement, the antibiotic must be thermostable. This excludes antibiotics such as chloramphenicol and tetracycline. (b) The proposed antibiotic must be available in powder form; it is not recommended that aqueous antibiotic solu-

tions be mixed with bone cement because of their water content. Large amounts of aqueous antibiotics cannot be added to the cement because the volume of liquid makes it impossible for the cement to set. Commonly used antibiotics that are available in powder form include tobramycin, vancomycin, penicillin G, ciprofloxacin, and cephalosporin; although it was the original antibiotic used in bone cement, gentamicin is not available in powder form in North America. (c) The antibiotic cannot have a high allergenic potential. Aminoglycoside allergy is exceedingly uncommon, making these antibiotics ideal for use in bone cement. (d) Elevated systemic levels of antibiotics must not be achieved when the antibiotic is combined with bone cement. Luckily, this is not a problem for most antibiotics. Because antibiotics elute rapidly early on, we recommend that a cell saver not be used following the insertion of antibiotic-loaded cement into the wound, because of the risk of reinfusing the blood with high concentrations of antibiotics, particularly when blood loss is excessive. (e) The chosen antibiotic must be effective against the infecting organism.

The elution properties of a large number of antibiotics have been determined, including aminoglycosides, such as gentamicin, tobramycin, streptomycin, and amikacin; vancomycin; penicillin G; clindamycin; erythromycin; cephalosporins; and colistin. For most patients, the combination of tobramycin and vancomycin should suffice. Tobramycin elution continues to be superior to that of vancomycin; initial elution levels are greater than 200 mg/L. Therapeutic levels of tobramycin are maintained for 2 to 3 months if adequate doses of tobramycin are added to the cement.

Clinical Table: Infected Total Hip Replacement

Procedure	Indications	Technique	Pitfalls
Débridement and irrigation	• Acute early infection • Acute hematogenous infection	• Wide exposure • Avoid devascularization • Exchange modular components	• Components loose • Débridement too late • Inadequate débridement
Girdlestone arthroplasty	• Debilitated patient • Uncooperative patient • Recurrent infection	• Extensile exposure • Femoral osteotomy if necessary • Antibiotic beads • Special techniques for removing solidly fixed components	• Poor function • Worse function if deficient bone stock
One-stage exchange	• Infection with less virulent organism • No draining sinuses • Adequate bone stock for cemented femoral fixation	• Special techniques for removing solidly fixed components • Reconstruct with antibiotic-loaded cement.	• Lower infection control rate • Cannot use cementless femoral fixation • Cannot use bone graft
Two-stage exchange	• Used for most patients • Avoid in unwell or uncooperative patients	• First operation similar to Girdlestone • May use an articulated spacer • Intravenous antibiotics for 6 weeks • Then reimplant	• Long treatment protocol • Expensive

We recommend the use of 2.4 to 3.6 g tobramycin and 1 to 1.5 g vancomycin per package of bone cement, as long as the organism is sensitive and the cement is used as a spacer and not for structural support. The addition of large amounts of antibiotics to bone cement can weaken it, leading to premature failure of the implant. If antibiotic-loaded cement is used for fixation of the implant, we recommend adding no more than 0.6 g tobramycin per package of bone cement.

The antibiotic elution profile depends not only on the type of antibiotic but also on the type of bone cement. The elution profile of antibiotics from Palacos R bone cement is superior to that of Simplex P bone cement (Howmedica; Rutherford, NJ). Palacos R cement has a higher viscosity than Simplex P cement. It is difficult to use Palacos R for the fixation of a cemented implant because of the problems using modern cement techniques with a more viscous cement. On the other hand, when antibiotic-loaded cement is used as a temporary spacer, Palacos R cement is recommended because of its improved antibiotic elution profile.

SURGICAL TREATMENT ALGORITHM

Early Postoperative Infections or Acute Hematogenous Infections

In early florid infections or in similar infections presenting late secondary to hematogenous spread of another infection, débridement and attempted retention of the implant is indicated (Fig. 43.2). This, however, must be performed within 3 weeks of the onset of infection.

Chronic Infection

In the healthy patient, the treatment of choice in North America is two-stage exchange arthroplasty (25), with or without an interim antibiotic-loaded spacer. Occasionally, one-stage exchange arthroplasty (26) may be performed, although the indications for a one-stage exchange arthroplasty are more stringent and much less flexible than are those for a two-stage exchange arthroplasty. Excision arthroplasty is still a viable option for recurrent infections following a previous two-stage exchange arthroplasty in patients who are not thought to be good candidates for

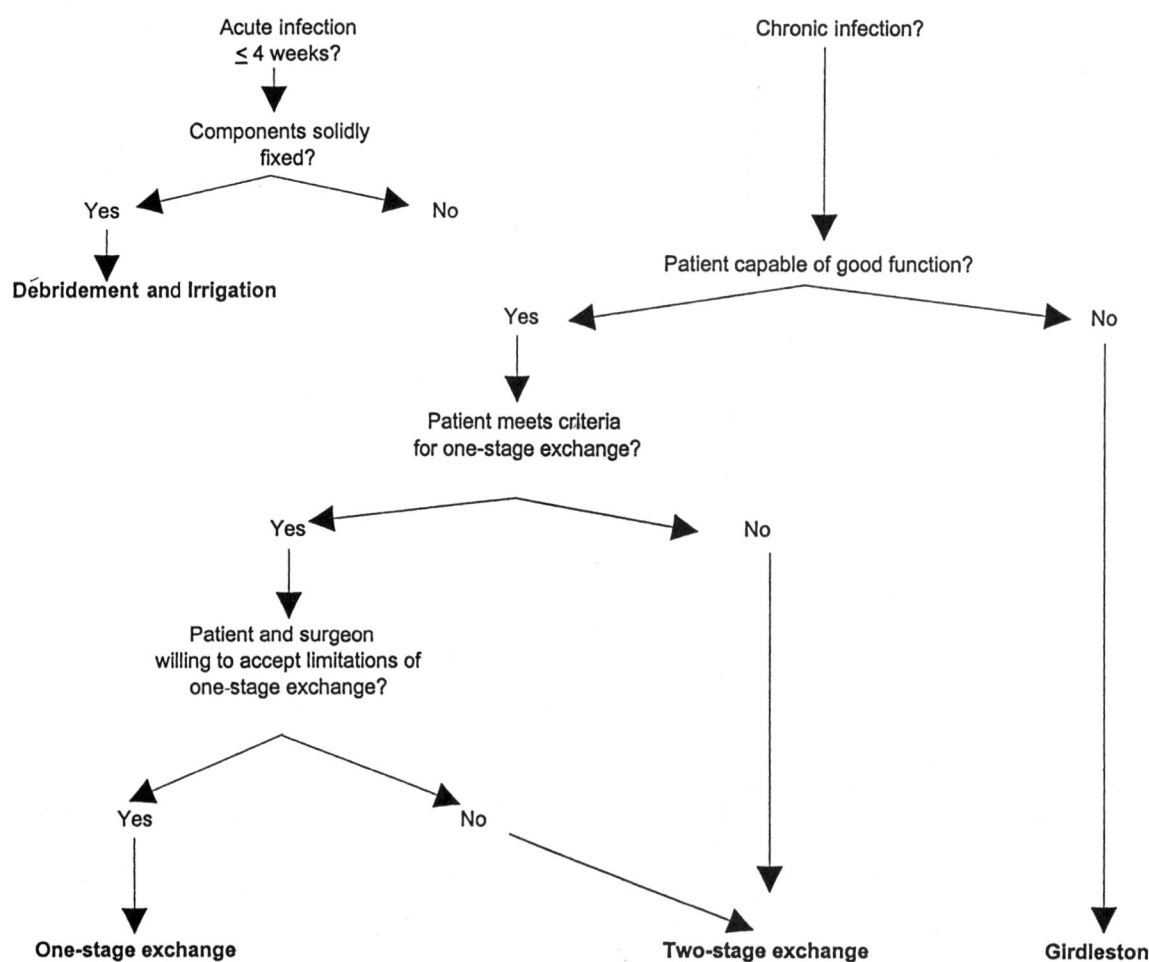

Figure 43.2. Surgical treatment algorithm for infected total hip arthroplasty.

reimplantation of a hip replacement, such as elderly patients who are not capable of independent mobilization; in uncooperative patients, such as intravenous drug abusers; or in patients who are severely immunocompromised.

DÉBRIDEMENT AND RETENTION OF THE COMPONENTS

Indications

Débridement and retention of the components are indicated for early postoperative infection that is diagnosed within 3 to 4 weeks of the onset of infection and for late acute onset hematogenous infection that is diagnosed within 3 to 4 weeks of onset. This procedure is contraindicated for chronic infection (more than 4 weeks) when the components are not solidly fixed.

Technique

For débridement and retention of the components, the patient is positioned in the lateral position. In early postoperative infections, the original surgical approach is used again. In late hematogenous infections, a soft tissue approach, such as the lateral or posterior approach to the hip, is preferred. A trochanteric osteotomy is best avoided in these cases. Adequate tissue cultures are obtained, and intravenous antibiotics are then administered by the anesthesiologist. All devitalized or obviously infected tissues are removed. The hip is dislocated, and the femoral head and acetabular liner are removed, if they are modular. The hip is thoroughly irrigated with a large amount of saline. At the end of the débridement and irrigation, the tissues must have the appearance of noninfected tissue. A new polyethylene liner and a new femoral head are then inserted. The wound is then closed in layers over a suction drain.

After surgery, intravenous antibiotics are continued for 6 weeks under the supervision of an infectious disease consultant.

Outcome

Débridement has the greatest chance of eradicating infection if it is performed immediately after the development of infection; the chances of eradication decrease with time. The infection may be acquired hematogenously from another focus or may present in the early postoperative period. If the débridement is performed within 4 weeks after the development of infection, there is a 71% chance of eradication (8). Earlier débridements may be more successful. One report has raised concern about the possible increased risk of a failed débridement in patients with cementless components, because the cementless surface may harbor bacteria (8). It is much easier to remove cementless components before any bone ingrowth has occurred. For this reason and because of the relatively high rate of failure of débridement and irrigation, we recommend removal of the implants and proceeding with a two-stage exchange arthroplasty—if bone ingrowth is not present at the time of surgery—in early postoperative infections with cementless acetabular and femoral components.

Pitfalls

The technique of débridement and retention of the components is doomed to failure if an adequate débridement is not performed. A superficial débridement without dislocation of the hip and removal of modular components is unlikely to be effective. A complete 6-week course of intravenous antibiotics is also essential. Débridement and irrigation alone in the face of a late hematogenous infection and loose implants are futile and should be avoided.

ONE-STAGE EXCHANGE ARTHROPLASTY

Indications

One-stage exchange arthroplasty—a revision total hip arthroplasty combined with a meticulous débridement and irrigation—is indicated in the chronically infected total hip replacement and following failure of débridement and irrigation in the patient who is medically unfit for two-stage exchange arthroplasty. At our center, only a small minority of patients with infected total hip replacements undergo one-stage treatment. A number of criteria must be met before this procedure can be recommended (Table 43.1).

Technique

The surgical technique of one-stage exchange arthroplasty is similar to that of revision total hip arthroplasty for aseptic loosening, with a few exceptions. Unlike aseptic loosening, a thorough débridement and copious irrigation of the wound are required when infection is present. The surgeon must carefully search for any abscesses or fluid collections, particularly along the iliopsoas tendon and deep to the abductors. Unlike revision surgery, in one-stage exchange arthroplasty for infection, all foreign material must be removed to lower the risk of infection recurrence. This means that any intrapelvic cement must be removed, including cement in the distal femur. Care also must be taken not to devascularize bone with excessive soft tissue stripping. Finally, cementless fixation on both the acetabular and femoral sides is not appropriate, because antibiotic-loaded cement must be used for adequate infection control.

table	43.1	Criteria for One-Stage Exchange Arthroplasty

Infection with less virulent organism (gram-negative organisms and enterococci are contraindications)
No draining sinuses
Adequate bone stock for cemented femoral fixation
Antibiotic-loaded cement must be used
Intravenous antibiotics must be used for 6 weeks postsurgery

The surgical approach should allow adequate exposure of the components and adequate access to the pelvis and distal femur, as necessary to remove cement or foreign material. The choice of surgical approach depends on the complexity of the procedure. The surgical approaches that require excessive soft tissue stripping of the proximal femur, such as the McFarland-Osborne approach and the trochanteric slide, should be avoided. We have found the extended trochanteric osteotomy an ideal approach for revisions of infected total hip arthroplasties (27), particularly in the cases of the solidly fixed, extensively coated, cementless stem and the solidly fixed, cemented stem with a long cement column.

The retroperitoneal approach is occasionally of value when a large bolus of intrapelvic cement or an intrapelvic acetabular component needs to be removed. Alternatively, a defect in the floor of the acetabulum can be widened to remove intrapelvic cement. Following adequate exposure of the hip joint, a thorough débridement (described above) is performed. The components are then removed, and the wound in thoroughly irrigated with copious amounts of saline. Removal of loose components is generally not difficult, provided adequate exposure is achieved. The removal of solidly fixed implants is more challenging and deserves further explanation.

Removal of femoral stems. A solidly fixed proximally coated cementless stem is removed with the aid of flexible osteotomes, which are inserted within the interface between the porous ingrowth surface and the proximal femur. Following debonding of the implant, the stem is extracted from above. In general, a trochanteric osteotomy or an extended trochanteric osteotomy is required for exposure.

A solidly fixed extensively coated cementless stem is more difficult to remove. With proper preoperative planning and the use of adequate extraction equipment, it should be possible to remove these implants without destroying the upper end of the femur. An extended trochanteric osteotomy should be used and should be extended to just below the origin of the uniform cylindrical portion of the femoral stem. The stem is then cut using a metal cutting burr. The proximal portion of the stem is debonded with the use of a Gigli saw through the cut in the stem. The surgeon must be prepared to use a number of these wire saws before breaking the bonds between the stem and the femur. Once the proximal portion of the implant is removed, the distal portion is cored out using a trephine.

A solidly fixed cemented stem is released by removing the stem from within the cement mantle first; then the cement is removed by using a variety of hand tools, high-speed burrs, or ultrasonic devices. Appropriate exposure of the solidly fixed cement mantle is mandatory, which may be accomplished by performing an adequate femoral osteotomy, such as an extended trochanteric osteotomy (Fig. 43.3), or an anterior cortical window, with generous dimensions and rounded corners. The muscle attachment to the cortical window should be maintained so that it is not devascularized. An intraoperative radiograph can help ensure complete removal of the cement mantle. Occasionally, the femoral stem cannot be removed from the cement mantle, particularly when the stem had been precoated with a layer of methyl methacrylate. In this case, we use an extended trochanteric osteotomy for exposure and remove the femoral stem from the cement mantle with the aid of a fine-tipped, high-speed burr. Great care should be taken not to exert an excessive amount of force and to avoid fracturing the femur.

Removal of solidly fixed acetabular components. Solidly fixed cementless acetabular components are removed using sequential curved osteotomes and careful dissection between metal and bone to preserve bone stock. Great care must be taken not to remove an excessive amount of bone.

Solidly fixed cemented cups should be debonded from the cement. Controlled fractures are then made within the cement mantle, and the fragments are removed. Care has to be taken to remove the cement from within the keying holes.

Once the components are removed, a standard revision total hip arthroplasty is performed using a cementless acetabular component and a cemented femoral component. If an extended osteotomy is used, it is repaired with cerclage wires before cementing the femoral component. The component is then inserted as if a standard posterior approach to the hip had been used. An extended osteotomy or a cortical window should be bypassed with a longer cemented stem. By definition, when a one-stage exchange arthroplasty is performed, the bone stock is adequate; and no special effort should be made to reconstruct it.

Outcome

One-stage exchange results in slightly lower rates of infection eradication than does two-stage exchange; infection eradication rates are between 70 and 80% (Table 43.2). In Buchholz et al.'s (21) initial series of one-stage exchange arthroplasties, an infection control rate of 73% was obtained without the use of systemic antibiotics; the rate increased to 77% with the use of systemic antibiotics. It is misleading, however, to compare the results of one-stage exchange arthroplasty to those of two-stage exchange arthroplasty, because more complex revisions are possible with the latter procedure. The revision of a persistently infected total hip arthroplasty, particularly when a long-stem femoral component is used, is indeed difficult, carrying a relatively high morbidity and risk of failure; the surgeon must keep this in mind before recommending one-stage exchange arthroplasty.

Pitfalls

The one-stage exchange has a lower success rate than does the two-stage exchange arthroplasty. It should not be used in young, robust patients who are unwilling to accept the limitations of the procedure. Moreover, the strict crite-

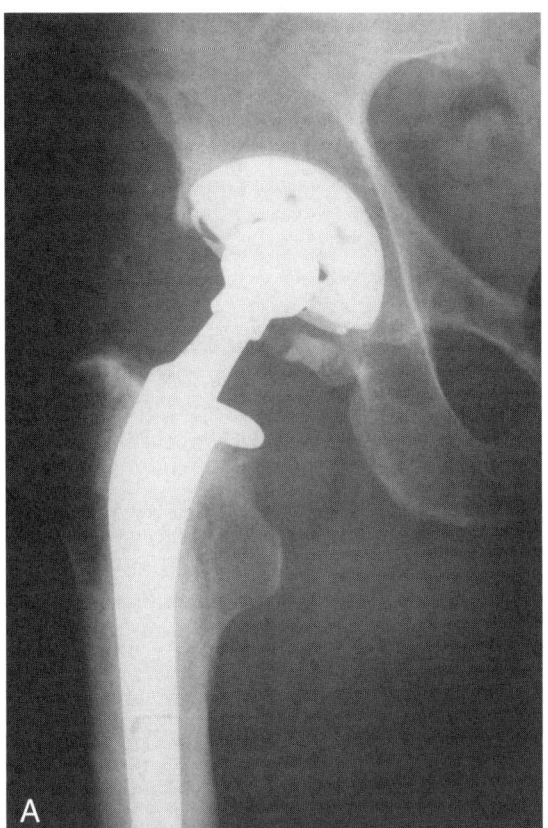

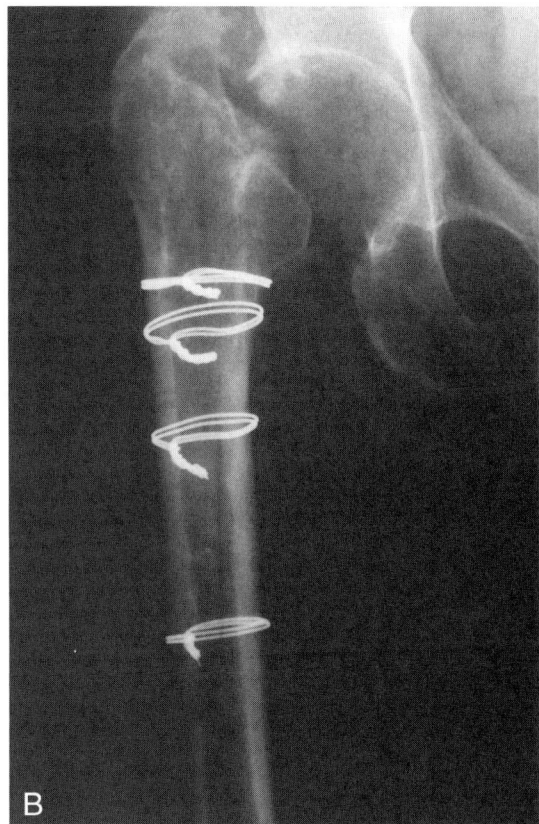

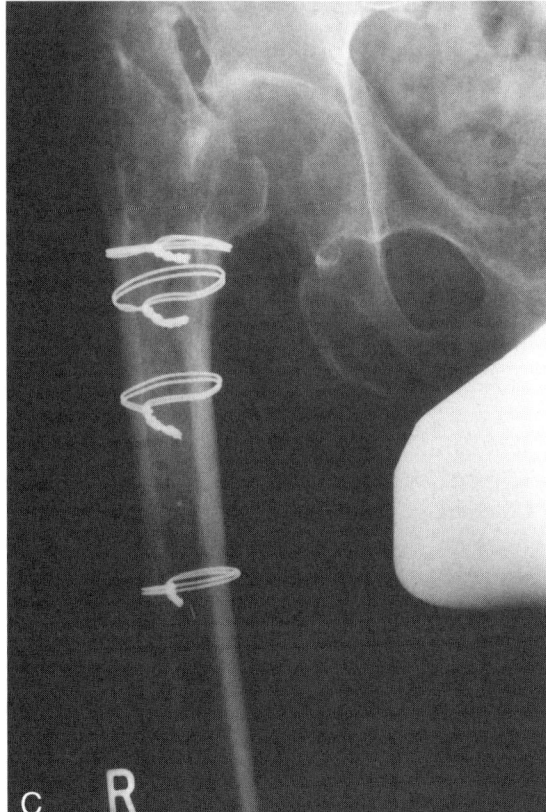

Figure 43.3. **A.** This solidly fixed cemented stem was removed by using an extended trochanteric osteotomy. **B.** Because the patient's history of drug abuse made exchange arthroplasty unwise, a definitive Girdlestone procedure was performed. Note that the osteotomy site can still be seen. **C.** At 3 months following surgery, the osteotomy is well healed, and the patient is pain free.

<table>
<tr><td>t a b l e</td><td>43.2</td><td>Limitations of One-Stage Exchange Arthroplasty</td></tr>
</table>

Criteria in Table 43.1 must be met
Infection control rate is lower than with two-stage exchange arthroplasty
If long-stem cemented femoral components are used, revision may be difficult in the case of recurrent infection
Cementless femoral fixation, which is potentially better for revision total hip replacement, is not possible

ria noted earlier must be met for a predictable outcome. A meticulous débridement is critical, and failure to adequately remove infected, necrotic, or devitalized tissue or failure to remove all foreign material can compromise the outcome of the procedure; yet excessive soft tissue stripping may predispose the patient to treatment failure. Finally, failure to use antibiotic-loaded cement in the reconstruction and failure to carefully administer intravenous antibiotics for a minimum of 6 weeks may contribute to a higher failure rate.

EXCISION (GIRDLESTONE) ARTHROPLASTY

Indications

An excision, or Girdlestone, arthroplasty is indicated in frail, elderly patients who either are unable to tolerate an extensive procedure or are unlikely to become independent ambulators even with revision total hip arthroplasty. The procedure is also indicated in patients at increased risk of reinfection, such as immunocompromised patients and intravenous drug abusers; those with a limited life expectancy; and those with recurrent infection following two-stage exchange arthroplasty.

Technique

Excision arthroplasty is identical to the one-stage exchange arthroplasty, to the point of implant removal. With a Girdlestone arthroplasty, another prosthesis is not inserted (Fig. 43.3). The femoral neck is resected to the level of the lesser trochanter, and the superior rim of the acetabulum is excised if it impinges against the greater trochanter. A stable, pain-free pseudarthrosis is created. Great care must be taken to not detach the iliopsoas tendon to avoid excessive telescoping of the limb.

After a thorough débridement, a bolus of antibiotic-loaded cement is inserted within the acetabular cavity, and a string of antibiotic-loaded cement beads is inserted within the medullary canal of the femur. The surgeon must carefully document the number of beads inserted in case their removal ever becomes necessary. The addition of a small amount of dye, such as chlorophyll (an ingredient in Palacos R cement) or methylene blue (often added to Simplex P cement), makes it easy to identify the beads at the time of their removal.

In the past, a 3-week course of traction was recommended by some authors. We have not found this to be necessary, because an average shortening of 5 cm is the rule, regardless of whether traction is used. Initially, the patient is mobilized with minimal weight bearing for 6 weeks; weight bearing is gradually increased over the following 6 weeks.

Outcome

Most patients obtain some pain relief, but postoperative function is often poor and deteriorates with increased loss of femoral bone stock. Leg length discrepancy can be significant, averaging about 5 cm. Most patients require the permanent use of assistive walking devices, such as a crutch or a walker, in addition to a raise on the ipsilateral shoe. Mobility is more restricted than that following revision total hip arthroplasty, because of the increased energy requirement for ambulation, which is double that of normal walking. Infection control rates following Girdlestone arthroplasty are around 95%.

Pitfalls

The pitfalls of the Girdlestone procedure include inadequate débridement, resulting in increased failure rates; excessive bone loss, making walking difficult; and release of the iliopsoas tendon, creating instability of the limb. Because of its functional limitations, this procedure is best avoided in the active patient.

TWO-STAGE EXCHANGE

Indications

The two-stage exchange is the most common procedure for infected total hip arthroplasty in North America. It is indicted for an infected total hip arthroplasty in healthy patients for whom optimization of infection control and flexibility in reconstruction are desirable and in those for whom retention of a hip arthroplasty is desirable but one-stage exchange is contraindicated.

Technique

The first stage in the two-stage exchange is equivalent to a Girdlestone arthroplasty; the second involves reimplantation of a total hip arthroplasty (Fig. 43.4). Between stages, the patient is treated with at least 6 weeks of intravenous antibiotics. The response to treatment is carefully assessed between stages, and reimplantation is not performed if there is ongoing evidence of sepsis. If necessary, a second débridement may be performed, although this is not often necessary. The ESR and CRP are excellent tests for monitoring the effect of treatment, and a steady decline in both parameters suggests infection eradication. An aspiration biopsy between stages may also help rule out ongoing infection.

The surgical technique for the first stage was described in detail under "Excision (Girdlestone) Arthroplasty." Following removal of the implants, it is usual to implant antibiotic-loaded bone cement to fill the dead space and improve antibiotic delivery to the hip joint. A bolus of antibiotic-loaded cement may be placed within the acetabulum, or a number of beads may be strung on monofilament

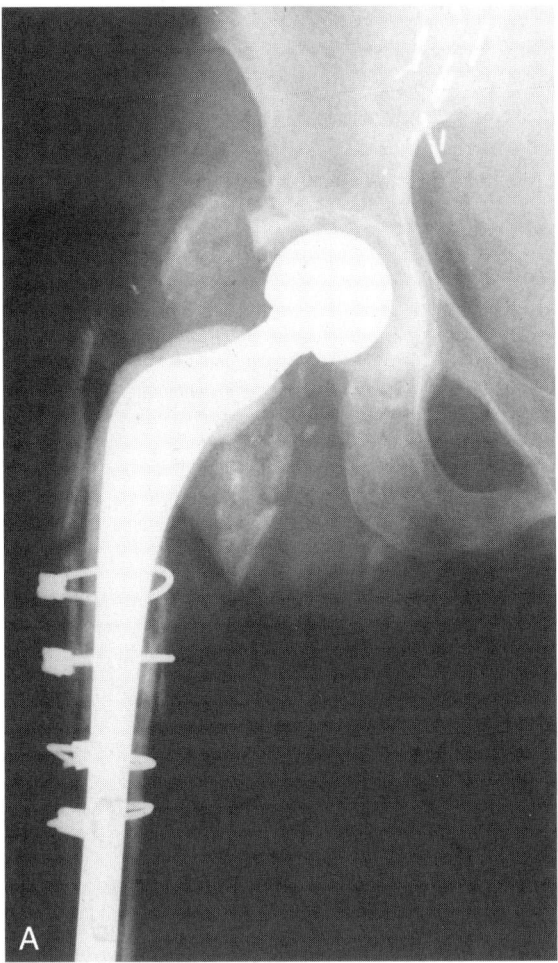 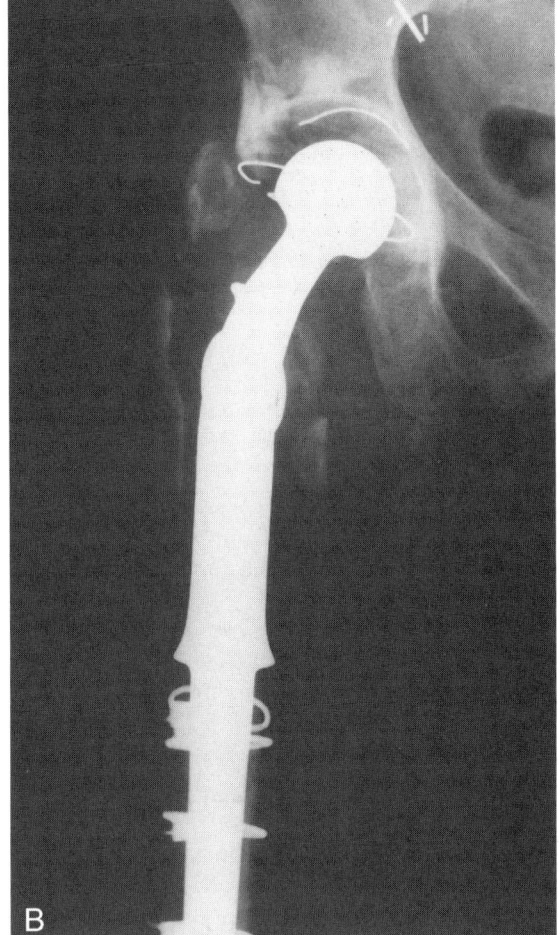

Figure 43.4. A. Because of this patient's extensive bone loss, a one-stage exchange arthroplasty was not possible. Instead, a two-stage exchange arthroplasty was performed. **B.** The final reconstruction used a proximal femoral replacement prosthesis, fixed with antibiotic-loaded bone cement. An allograft was not used because of the low demands of this patient.

wire and inserted within the acetabular fossa. A chain of beads is also inserted into the medullary canal of the femur.

Precautions must be followed when using antibiotic-loaded cement beads. The antibiotic used in the cement must meet the criteria outlined above. The beads should be carefully counted and their number recorded in the operation report, so that all beads may be removed at the time of the second-stage procedure. A dye should be added to the antibiotic-loaded beads so that they become more conspicuous at the time of their removal. Palacos R cement contains chlorophyll dye, and the addition of another dye is not necessary. Simplex P bone cement can be dyed with two drops of methylene blue, which will allow easy detection at the time of removal.

Some authors have recommended traction between stages; however, we have found no advantage to traction and do not currently recommend it. Between the stages, patients experience a loss of function and an associated leg length discrepancy, persistent pain, and relative immobility. Two-stage exchange is more expensive than other procedures, in part because the patient will be in the hospital for a longer period as a result of immobility between stages.

Antibiotic-loaded bone cement may be used as a temporary articulated and functional spacer to hold the joint out to length and allow some hip motion and independent walking. The use of a spacer is particularly important in cases of marked proximal femoral bone loss. Such patients have significant defects after the first stage of the procedure; and without a spacer, traction is almost always mandatory. The articulated temporary spacer that we use is the prosthesis of antibiotic-loaded acrylic cement (PROSTALAC), which consists of a series of femoral molds and a series of metallic endoskeletons. An antibiotic-loaded facsimile of a femoral component is manufactured with antibiotic-loaded bone cement. On the acetabular side, a 45 × 32-mm acetabular component is cemented loosely within the acetabular fossa. Postsugery, the patient is allowed partial weight bearing with crutches until the second stage of the procedure can be performed. Other temporary spacers using old implants may be used, as long as most of the implant is coated with antibiotic-loaded bone cement.

At the time of the second stage of the procedure, any temporary spacers, antibiotic-loaded cement beads, or retained foreign body from the first procedure are removed. Multiple tissue samples are obtained for culture and sensitivity. If there is any doubt about the control of infection, a sample is sent to the laboratory, and a frozen section is examined for acute inflammatory cells.

The subsequent reconstruction is best performed with cemented components, using antibiotic-loaded cement. For sensitive organisms, we use 0.6 g tobramycin per package of bone cement.

Outcome

In a review of 12 reports of two-stage exchange with the use of antibiotic-impregnated cement, Garvin and Hanssen (3) found the overall rate of infection eradication to be 91%. When antibiotic-loaded cement was not used, the cumulative success rate was 82% in 9 studies. These figures are somewhat higher than the cumulative reports of one-stage procedures.

Variables that affect the outcome of two-stage exchange protocols include the duration of postoperative systemic antibiotic therapy, timing of reimplantation, use of allograft bone in the reconstruction, and use of cemented prosthesis. Another factor is the use of antibiotic-loaded cement—as beads or temporary spacer devices—between the first and second stages.

The ideal duration of antibiotic therapy and route of administration have not been determined. Most reported protocols note 4 to 6 weeks of intravenous antibiotic administration. A convenient method of ensuring adequate antibiotic doses is to measure minimal serum bactericidal titers; a minimum titer of 1:8 is recommended for optimal infection control. Titers are measured by obtaining a sample of the patient's serum following administration of antibiotics; after serial twofold dilutions, the bactericidal effect of the serum is checked. The maximum dilution at which the serum remains bactericidal against the actual infecting organism is the minimal bactericidal titer. There is some evidence that parenteral therapy for less than 4 weeks is associated with a higher recurrent infection rate; presently, the consensus is that therapy between stages should be 4 to 6 weeks.

There is no need for a long delay between the stages of the procedure, even though intervals as long as 1 year were once recommended. The most important factor is documented infection control between stages, determined either by a fall in the ESR or by a negative aspirate from the hip joint before reimplantation.

The use of allograft bone at the time of the second stage is often desirable because of the bone loss seen with infection. There is no convincing evidence in the literature that the use of allograft increases the risk of recurrent infection; therefore, a graft may be used in two-stage exchange arthroplasty. Indeed, one of the advantages of the two-stage compared to the one-stage exchange arthroplasty is that the use of allograft at the time of the one-stage exchange surgery may be unwise.

Antibiotic-loaded cement has been recommended for fixation of the stem at the time of the second stage. At present, there is no convincing evidence in the literature for or against cementless fixation of the stem at the second stage. In our initial series of 48 patients using the PROSTALAC articulated spacer, the infection eradication rate was similar to other series of two-stage exchange arthroplasty: 94% of patients were infection free more than 2 years after the reconstruction. The antibiotic-loaded interval spacer allows patient mobility between stages, and there is a significant improvement in the Harris hip score (HHS) after the first stage. Approximately 80% of patients at review had an HHS greater than 80 or an improvement of more than 30 points.

Pitfalls

Pitfalls of the two-stage exchange arthroplasty include inadequate exposure of the joint at the first stage, which may necessitate excessive soft tissue stripping and a potentially increased risk of infection because of devascularization of the femur. Inadequate exposure may also make it difficult to remove all foreign material. Failure to completely débride the joint and remove all foreign material at the first stage may result in failure of treatment. Performance of the second stage of the procedure despite ongoing infection will result in failure of treatment. Failure to use a functional spacer when there is excessive bone loss may result in poor functional outcome between stages and may make reimplantation difficult. Failure to complete a 4- to 6-week course of intravenous antibiotics may decrease the chance for infection eradication.

SUMMARY

The treatment of the infected hip replacement continues to be an area of significant difficulty. For most patients, antibiotics alone are not an acceptable method of treatment, and at least two surgical procedures are necessary. With the increasing cost of delivery of health care, more expedient treatment alternatives may have significant appeal, including the use of articulated spacers in two-stage exchange arthroplasty procedures so patients may be discharged from hospital as soon as possible after the first stage and the use of one-stage exchange arthroplasty when appropriate. Antibiotic therapy in addition to surgery remains important, and the expertise of an infectious disease consultant should be sought when managing patients with infected total hip arthroplasty.

REFERENCES

1. Salvati EA, Robinson RP, Zeno SM, et al. Infection rates after 3175 total hip and total knee replacements performed with and without a horizontal unidirectional filtered air-flow system. J Bone Joint Surg 1982;64A:525–535.
2. Charnley J. Postoperative infection after total hip replacement with special reference to air contamination in the operating room. Clin Orthop 1972;87:167–187.

3. Garvin KL, Hanssen AD. Infection after total hip arthroplasty. J Bone Joint Surg 1995;77A:1576–1588.

4. Gristina AG, Kolkin J. Current concepts review: total joint replacement and sepsis. J Bone Joint Surg 1983;65A:128–134.

5. Gristina AG, Costerton JW. Bacterial adherence and the glycocalyx and their role in musculoskeletal infection. Orthop Clin North Am 1984;15:517–535.

6. Buchholz HW, Elson RA, Heinert K. Antibiotic-loaded acrylic cement: current concepts. Clin Orthop 1984;190:96–108.

7. Fitzgerald RH Jr, Nolan DR, Ilstrup DM, et al. Deep wound sepsis following total hip arthroplasty. J Bone Joint Surg 1977; 59A:847–855.

8. Tsukayama DT, Estrada R, Gustilo RB. Infection after total hip arthroplasty: a study of the treatment of one hundred and six infections. J Bone Joint Surg 1996;78A:512–523.

9. Covey DC, Albright JA. Current concepts review: clinical significance of the erythrocyte sedimentation rate in orthopaedic surgery. J Bone Joint Surg 1987;69A:148–151.

10. Shih L-Y, Wu J-J, Yang D-J. Erythrocyte sedimentation rate and C-reactive protein values in patients with total hip arthroplasty. Clin Orthop 1987;225:238–246.

11. Fitzgerald RH: Infected total hip arthroplasty: diagnosis and treatment. J Am Acad Orthop Surg 1995;3:249–262.

12. Barrack RL, Harris WH. The value of aspiration of the hip joint before revision total hip arthroplasty. J Bone Joint Surg 1993; 75A:66–76.

13. Spangehl M J, Duncan CP, O'Connoll JX, Masri BA. Prospective analysis of preoperative and intraoperative studies for the diagnosis of infection in revision total hip arthroplasties. Paper presented at the Annual Meeting of the American Academy of Orthopaedic Surgeons, San Francisco, CA, February 1997.

14. Reing CM, Richin PF, Kenmore PI. Differential bone-scanning in the evaluation of a painful total joint replacement. J Bone Joint Surg 1979;61A:933–936.

15. Pring DJ, Henderson RG, Rivett AG, et al. Autologous granulocyte scanning of painful prosthetic joints. J Bone Joint Surg 1986; 68B:647–652.

16. Palestro CJ, Kim CK, Swyer AJ, et al. Total-hip arthroplasty: periprosthetic indium-111-labeled leukocyte activity and complementary technetium-99-m-sulfur colloid imaging in suspected infection. J Nucl Med 1990;31:1951–1955.

17. Feldman DS, Lonner JH, Desai P, Zuckerman JD. The role of intraoperative frozen sections in revision total joint arthroplasty. J Bone Joint Surg 1995;77A:1807–1813.

18. Mirra JM, Amstutz HC, Matos M, Gold R. The pathology of the joint tissues and its clinical relevance in prosthesis failure. Clin Orthop 1976;117:540–546.

19. Lonner JH, Desai P, DiCesare PE, et al. The reliability of analysis of intraoperative frozen sections. J Bone Joint Surg 1996;78A: 1553–1558.

20. Goulet JA, Pellicci PM, Brause BD, Salvati EA. Prolonged suppression of infection in total hip arthroplasty. J Arthroplasty 1988; 3:109–116.

21. Buchholz HW, Elson RA, Engelbrecht E, et al. Management of deep infection of total hip arthroplasty. J Bone Joint Surg 1981; 63B:342–353.

22. Charnley JC: Low friction arthroplasty of the hip. Berlin: Springer-Verlag, 1979.

23. Grauer JD, Amstutz HC, O'Carroll PF, Dorey FJ. Resection arthroplasty of the hip. J Bone Joint Surg 1989;71A:669–678.

24. Duncan CP, Masri BA. The role of antibiotic-loaded cement in the treatment of an infection after hip replacement. J Bone Joint Surg 1994;76A:1742–1751.

25. Salvati EA, Chekofsky KM, Brause BD, et al. Reimplantation in infection: a 12-year experience. Clin Orthop 1982;170:62–75.

26. Wroblewski BM. One-stage revision of infected cemented total hip arthroplasty. Clin Orthop 1986;211:103–107.

27. Younger TI, Bradford MS, Magnus RE, Paprosky WG. Extended proximal femoral osteotomy. J Arthroplasty 1995;10:329–338.

Revision Total Hip Replacement

Total hip replacement (THR) is one of the most gratifying procedures in orthopaedic surgery. Long-term success requires stable fixation of the implant to bone, either with cement or by bone ingrowth. The materials must sustain loads of two to three times the body weight during routine activities of daily living and peak loads of possibly six to eight times the body weight at an average of 1 million cycles per year (1,2). The materials must be biologically inert and have acceptable wear rates, to minimize the generation of wear debris. This chapter reviews the causes of THR failure and the options available for revision surgery.

CAUSE OF FAILURE

Material Failure

The concept of low-friction arthroplasty was introduced by Charnley (3) in 1959 as a means to improve the results obtained with metal on metal implants. The initial material selected for the cup was Teflon, which has extremely poor wear characteristics, quickly leading to failure. Vast improvements were seen when manufacturers switched to high molecular weight polyethylene, which is still in widespread use today. Wear resistance is markedly reduced by the combined effects of γ-irradiation, oxidative degradation, aging, and polyethylene fusion defects (4–6). Improved manufacturing techniques to eliminate these problems has increased the durability of polyethylene.

Earlier total hip designs used either stainless steel or cast cobalt chrome for the stems. After years of service, fatigue fractures were not uncommon (7). These fractures have been greatly diminished (but not completely eliminated) by the use of stronger alloys of stainless steel, forged cobalt chrome, or titanium (8).

Loss of Fixation

Cement (polymethyl methacrylate) has been used since the late 1950s to anchor both the acetabular and the femoral components in bone (9). Cement has the benefit of immediate intraoperative stability and the capability for full weight bearing in the postoperative period. Cyclic loading of the cement over the years may lead to fatigue failure and cracking, which starts a vicious circle of increased stress, additional fatigue failure, and implant loosening (10). Failure rates escalate when cementing techniques are poor, when the cement mantle is thin (less than 1 mm), and when the implant imparts high stresses onto portions of the cement mantle (11). Numerous series of primary total hip replacements report failure rates ranging from 5 to 50% for acetabular components and 2 to 32% for femoral stems at 11 to 22 years (12–18). The higher rates for sockets is thought to reflect the difficulty in obtaining a dry bony bed and cement pressurization.

Cementless total hip replacement (bone ingrowth) was introduced to circumvent the high failure rates of cemented THR, especially in young active patients (19–21). Cementless THR is less forgiving than cemented THR, and intraoperative stability is crucial to successful biologic fixation. Poor design, lack of a method for bone attachment (i.e., Press-Fit stems), and undersizing the implants may lead to unsuccessful bone ingrowth, with resultant pain and implant migration. Fractures of either the femur or acetabulum at the time of implantation may also lead to instability and failure. Primary cemented and cementless total hip replacement are discussed in detail in Chapters 41 and 42.

Mechanical Failure

Implants may be made of sound materials but may experience catastrophic failure due to design flaws. Polyethylene may undergo extremely rapid wear or fracture if it is less than 5 mm thick (22,23). Modular stems or cups may disassociate (24). Bone ingrowth surfaces may debond from the substrate. Modularity, which allows considerable intraoperative flexibility, increases the risk of mechanical failure, as well as adding to the cost of the procedure.

Wear Debris

Implants that achieve stable fixation with either cement or bone ingrowth may ultimately fail owing to the generation of wear debris. The debris is generated over time and may consist of polyethylene (25), cement (26), metal (27,28), or ceramic particles (29). Modular components may hasten the generation of debris (30,31). The particles incite an inflammatory reaction that is mediated by macrophages and giant cells, which can cause profound osteolysis and implant failure (32). Wear debris generation remains the weak link in long-term success and is the subject of intensive research that is focused on improving the wear characteristics and minimizing debris generation.

Infection

Acute or chronic deep sepsis of the total hip replacement usually requires removal of the implants and/or revision. Infection occurs in approximately 1% of primary hip replacements over the life of the prosthesis, and revisions have a rate twice as high (33). Management of the infected total hip replacement is discussed in detail in Chapter 46.

Instability of Component

One of the major causes of early revision is component instability. The acetabular component may be excessively anteverted or retroverted or was placed too vertical, leading to recurrent dislocation. Stem malposition, although less frequent, can cause instability, especially if retroverted. Impingement between the implant neck and anterior acetabular osteophytes allows the head to lever out of the socket. A deficient abductor mechanism may cause instability, as can impingement of the greater trochanter and posterior rim in external rotation. Instability may be the result of mismatched components (e.g., a 28-mm head in a 32-mm polyethylene insert). Fracture of the acetabulum or femur during implant insertion (especially with uncemented implants) may cause fixation failure or dislocation.

If the THR causes excessive shortening, the leg length inequality may make the patient feel unbalanced; if it is severe enough, instability may result. If the offset is too short, with a decreased abductor lever arm, the result may be instability and/or abductor muscle weakness. Reoperation for dislocation is most successful when the underlying cause is determined and corrected (34).

INITIAL FINDINGS, PHYSICAL EXAMINATION, AND DIAGNOSIS

Assessment of the patient with a problematic THR must include a thorough history and physical examination. Most patients who require a revision have had years of service with the replacement followed by a gradual and progressive onset of symptoms. Pain is usually the major indication that something has gone awry. Other symptoms include decreased walking endurance; shortening of the leg; diminished range of motion; and increased dependence on ambulatory aids, such as a cane or crutches. The pain associated with loosening is usually worse with weight bearing or during activities that stress the implants (stair climbing or rising from a chair). The pain is usually located in the groin or buttock but may be concentrated in the thigh if the problem is the femoral component.

Pain that has been present since the time of implantation is worrisome, since it may represent either an infection or a failure to achieve initial implant stability. Pain associated with infection may have no relation to weight bearing. Other sources of pain, such as lumbar spinal disorders, bursitis, tumor, abscess, and hernia, must be ruled out.

Gait characteristics may include an antalgic component (diminished stance time on the involved leg, with the torso leaning toward the affected side to minimize joint forces). There may be a Trendelenburg component to the gait that is manifested by a Trendelenburg or abductor lurch during stance (the pelvis dips toward the opposite side during stance on the affected side). A Trendelenburg sign (inability to stand on the involved leg and maintain a level pelvis) may be present. These are caused by abductor muscle weakness and can occur alone or in concert with the antalgic component.

With a catastrophic failure (e.g., fracture of the femur or stem, dislocation) weight bearing may be impossible. Crepitation may be present if there has been implant dissociation or fracture of the polyethylene liner.

Range of motion may be become limited as loosening increases, especially with implant migration or synovitis. Thigh atrophy indicates disuse from pain. The incision must be examined for areas of tenderness, fluctuance, erythema, or sinus tracts.

It is helpful to note leg length. If the involved leg is short, note whether it is a new finding or has been present since the original operation. Progressive shortening usually indicates that the stem is subsiding into the femoral canal or the socket is migrating into the pelvis.

RADIOLOGIC STUDIES

Standard radiographic views include an AP view of the pelvis and the involved hip and some type of lateral view. Most patients with hip pathology cannot perform the typical frog lateral maneuver, in which the involved leg is flexed, abducted, and externally rotated to obtain a true lateral of the upper femur while the patient lies supine. An easier position is the Löwenstein lateral, which is achieved by having the patient roll toward the involved side, placing the lateral side of the knee and thigh against the x-ray plate. The object is to obtain a true lateral of the femoral component. A cross table lateral is helpful to assess the version of the acetabular component and the remaining bone stock in the posterior column. Judet views are also helpful for assessing pelvic bone stock. Fluoroscopic views may be used to determine component version (35).

It is often helpful to compare the current radiographs with postoperative views to assess implant migration. Progressive implant migration is pathognomonic for loosening. Other radiographic signs of loosening of cemented implants include progressive radiolucencies at the bone–cement or implant–cement interfaces and fracture of the cement mantle (36) (Fig. 44.1). Signs of failure with cementless implants include radiolucencies around the ingrowth areas of the component, broken screws, pedestal formation (intramedullary condensation of bone below the tip of the stem), and shedding of the metal ingrowth substrate (37) (Fig. 44.2).

Radiographs must be examined for signs of implant fracture, deformation, or dissociation. The degree of polyethylene wear can be measured by noting the degree of eccentricity of the head within the polyethylene liner (38). Osteolysis may be present, even without implant loosening, as a consequence of polyethylene, cement, or metal debris. In severe cases, the degree of osteolysis may be profound (Fig. 44.3).

CT scans help assess pelvic bone loss and the proximity of the pelvic viscera; they may be combined with intravenous contrast to visualize the major vessels (39). MRI has a limited role at present but may be used to assess the periarticular soft tissues (40). Technetium-99m bone scans show increased uptake in the presence of loosening and/or infection, and enhanced specificity is obtained with an indium-111-labeled white blood cell scan (41). Aspiration arthrograms should be performed if there is any clinical suspicion for infection (42). Injection of lidocaine after the aspiration may help distinguish a failed total hip replacement from other sources of pain.

There are no laboratory studies that reliably confirm implant loosening. The white blood cell count may be nor-

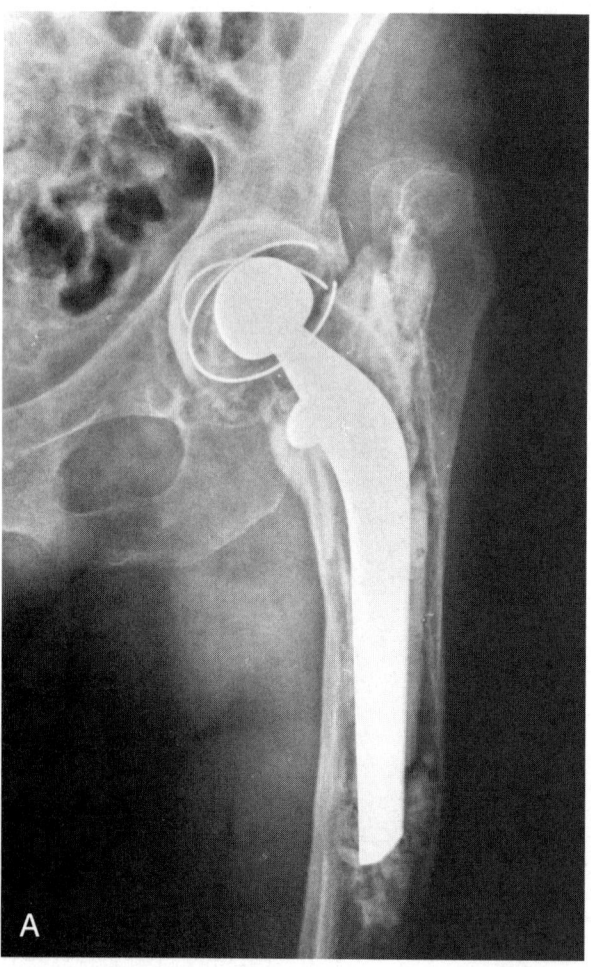
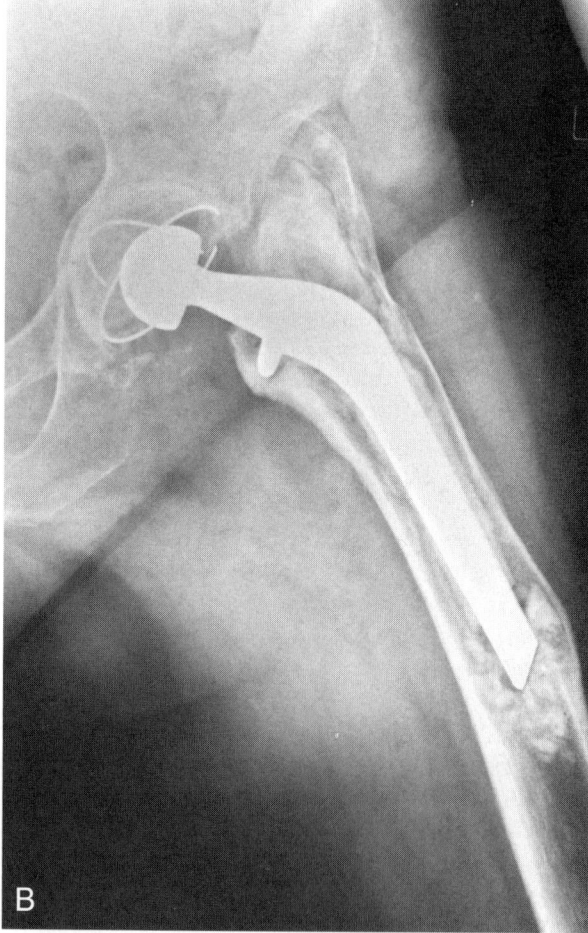

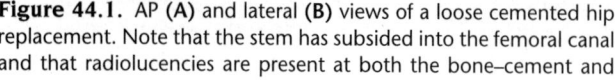

Figure 44.1. AP (**A**) and lateral (**B**) views of a loose cemented hip replacement. Note that the stem has subsided into the femoral canal and that radiolucencies are present at both the bone–cement and implant–cement interfaces. The femoral cement mantle has fractured and extensive osteolysis of the femur has occurred.

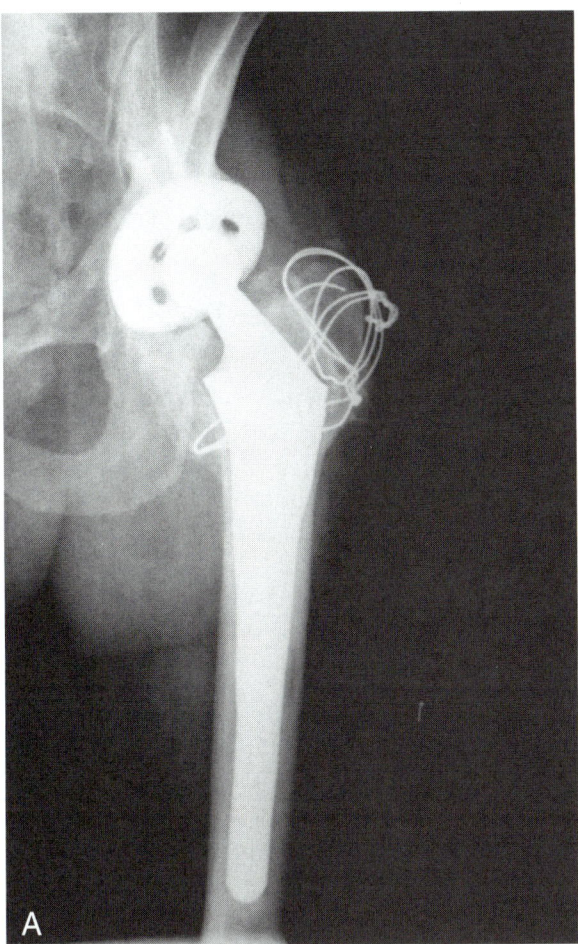

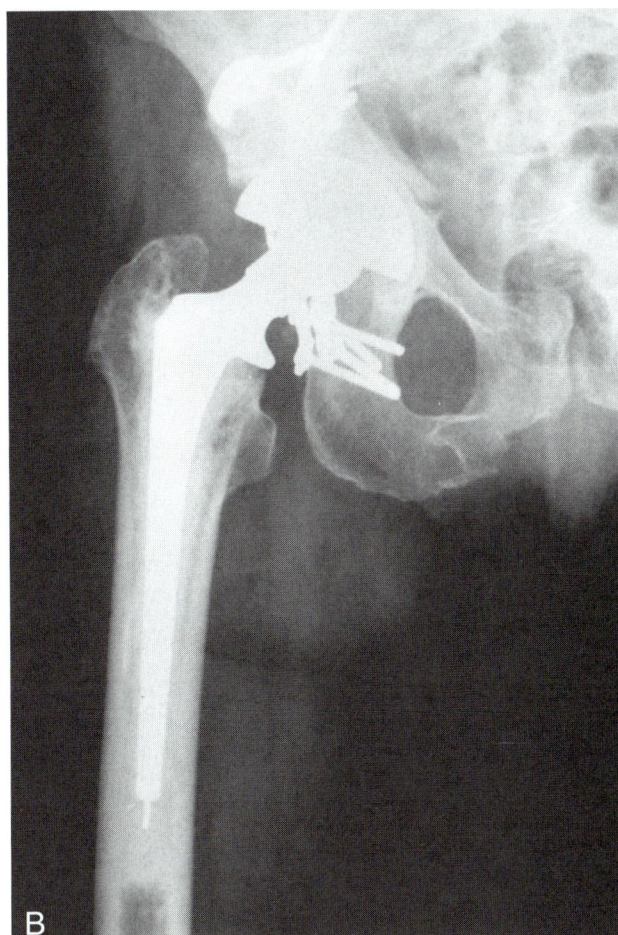

Figure 44.2. A. A loose uncemented femoral component. Note that the stem has subsided 2 cm, a bony pedestal has formed at the tip of implant, and radiolucencies are present between the bone and implant surfaces. **B.** A loose acetabular component. Note that the implant has migrated superiorly 5 mm and has global radiolucency.

mal with a deep-seated infection, although the sedimentation rate and C-reactive protein are usually elevated (43). Once revision surgery is performed, intraoperative frozen sections have been shown to be reliable laboratory indicators of septic loosening (44).

TREATMENT

Nonoperative Treatment

If a THR has become infected or has undergone catastrophic failure, there may be little recourse other than reoperation. If the reason for revision is gradual loosening and diminished function, a nonoperative course may be prudent. Weight loss, activity modification, and the use of ambulatory aids along with anti-inflammatory medications may help temporize the situation. If this course is taken, frequent follow-up care is needed, including radiographic monitoring of osteolysis and implant migration. If bone stock is disappearing rapidly, a revision may be required, even if the symptoms are minimal. Nonoperative management may also be necessary in patients who are too ill to undergo the rigors of revision surgery.

Operative Treatment

PREOPERATIVE PLANNING

One of the most critical steps in revision THR is preoperative planning. Intraoperative surprises may squander resources and time, embarrass the surgeon, and are a disservice to the patient. If the original surgery was done elsewhere, obtain the operative note. If one of the implants is not to be revised, it may be necessary to have a replacement femoral head or polyethylene liner available for the original components. Certain implant systems have equipment that may greatly aid component extraction. The surgeon should know how the locking mechanisms work.

In addition to implants, the surgical team must make sure that all the necessary instruments are available, including cement osteotomes, flexible osteotomes, high-speed pneumatic burrs, stem extractors, cerclage cables, trochanteric attachment hooks, pneumatic or ultrasonic cement chisels, and flexible reamers (Fig. 44.4). A structural and/or morcellized bone graft may be required. Powdered antibiotics (usually tobramycin) may be incorporated into the cement. A cell saver is useful in extensive

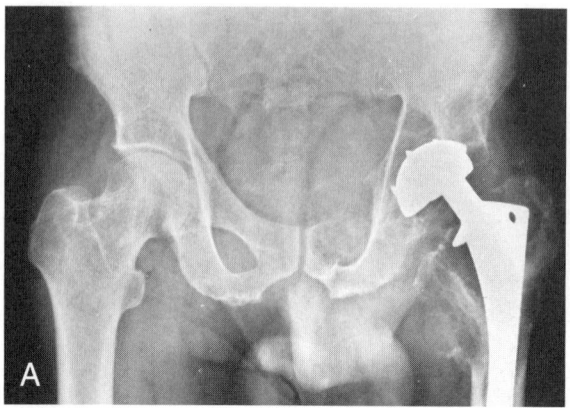

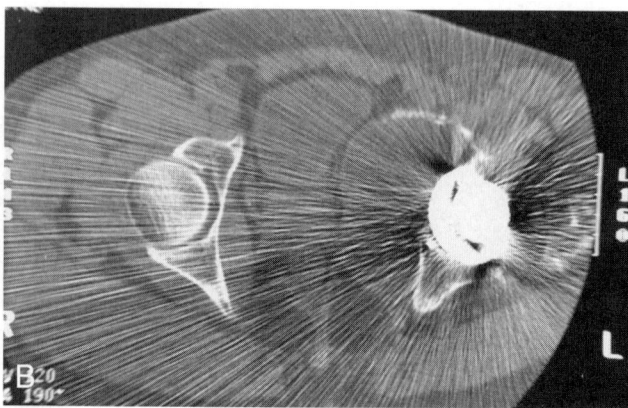

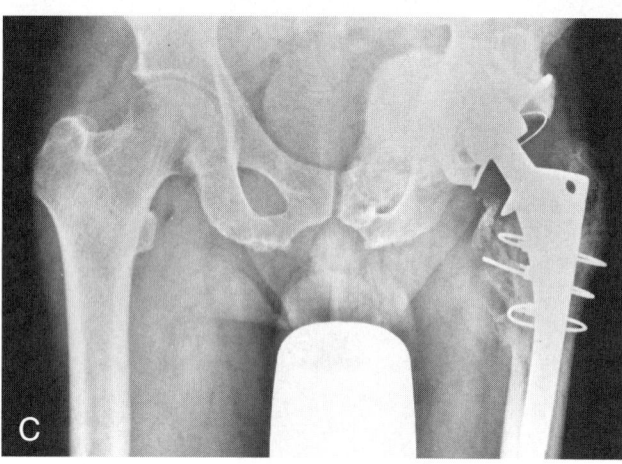

Figure 44.3. A. AP view of 48-year-old-male 8 years after a cementless THR. Note the eccentricity of the head in the socket as a result of polyethylene wear, and the massive osteolysis of the pelvis. **B.** CT scan showing pelvic bone loss and granuloma presenting as a massive tumor. **C.** AP view 1 year after socket revision and bone grafting of the pelvic and femoral defects. Note that the lytic areas have been replaced with new bone.

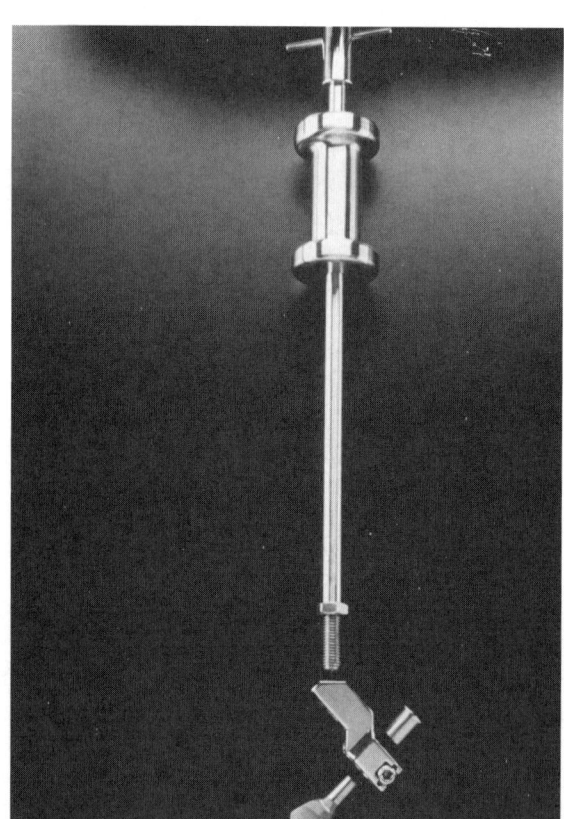

Figure 44.4. Bohn extractor for modular stems.

cases, especially if autologous blood is not available. Fluoroscopy may be required in rare cases to facilitate the complete removal of the femoral cement, especially if reamers, high-speed drills, or ultrasonic tips are used (Fig. 44.5).

Decision Making and Implant Selection

A careful analysis of the radiographs is an important first step for preoperative planning. The surgeon must ascertained whether the revision will involve the stem, cup, or both. Implant loosening can usually be determined before surgery. Well-fixed components should not be revised. Rarely, it may be necessary to remove a well-fixed femoral stem for exposure, especially with nonmodular designs (Clinical Table).

Femur

Another important issue is to determine the type of fixation to be used. Cemented fixation works best in the primary situation when there is plenty of cancellous bone for cement intrusion. Dohmae et al. (45) simulated femoral revisions in cadaver femora. The interface shear strength falls to 20% of that found in the primary cemented stem after one revision and to 6% after the second revision. Cemented revisions perform well if there is some remaining cancellous bone, especially if good cement techniques are used.

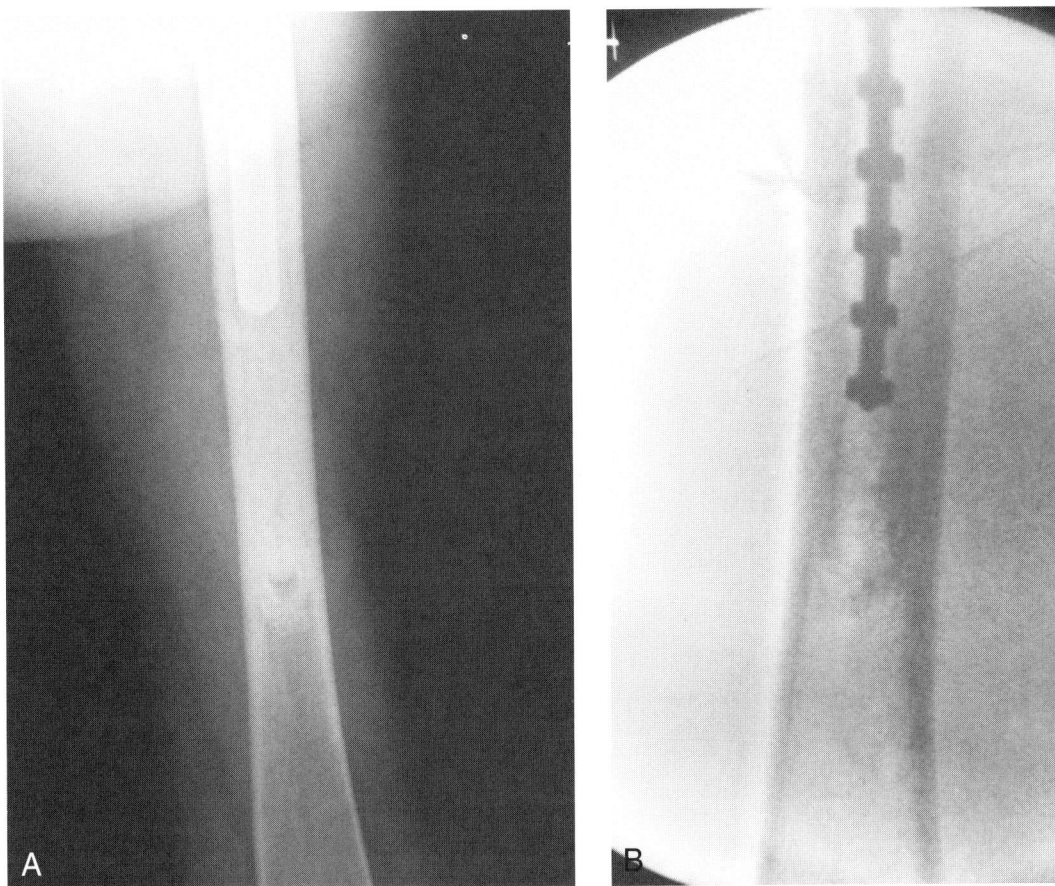

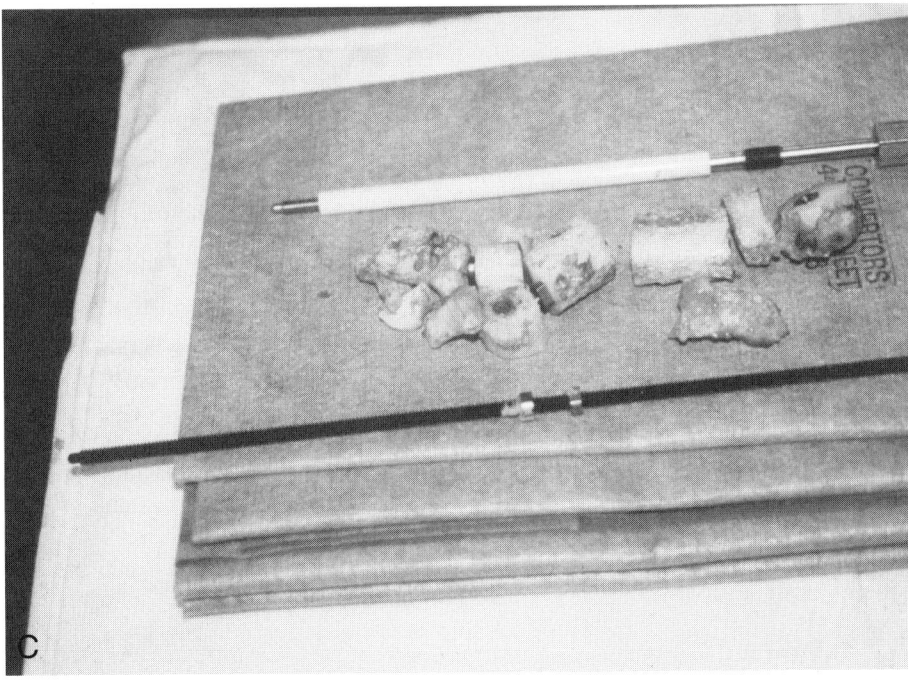

Figure 44.5. **A.** Infected stem with a large, well-fixed cement plug. **B.** Intraoperative fluoroscopy view after ultrasonic coring of the bone and placement of the Segmental Cement Extraction System ("Seg-CES") threaded rod. **C.** Complete removal of the cement plug.

Clinical Table: Revision Total Hip Replacement

Procedure	Indications	Technique	Anatomy	Pitfalls
Cemented cup revision	• Bone insufficient for cementless • Metal reinforcement ring is required	• Cement anchor holes • Good cement mantle • Bone graft defects	• Femoral neurovascular supply • Gluteal neurovascular supply • Sciatic nerve	• Poor technique • Bottom out cup • Malpositioning • Intrapelvic cement
Cementless cup revision	• Sufficient pelvic bone stock to anchor the cup	• Ream and impact cup • Add screws if needed • Bone graft defects	• Femoral neurovascular supply • Gluteal neurovascular supply • Sciatic nerve	• Lack of intraoperative stability • Malpositioning • Neurovascular injury from screws
Cemented femoral revision	• Elderly patient • Good cancellous bone for cement • Unable to attain stability with porous components	• Remove old cement and soft tissue • Good cement techniques • May cement into morcellized graft	• Femoral neurovascular supply • Gluteal neurovascular supply • Sciatic nerve	• Poor technique or interdigitation • Early polymerization with extensive cementing • Fat embolization
Cementless femoral revision	• Cancellous bone gone • Good bone stock	• Proximal coated if bone stock permits • Fully coated if proximally deficient • Obtain intraoperative stability	• Femoral neurovascular supply • Gluteal neurovascular supply • Sciatic nerve	• Femoral fracture • Lack of intraoperative stability • Wrong type of implant for the status of femoral bone

Bone stock classification systems are helpful for preoperative planning and implant selection (46). We have found the Mallory's classification system for femoral defects to be useful (47) (Fig. 44.6). If there is an intact cortex with remaining cancellous bone (type I defect), either cemented or cementless implants should work. In a type II defect, the cortex is intact but most of the cancellous bone is gone. Because there is little chance for cement intrusion, a bone ingrowth implant may work best. If the cortex is gone to the level of the lesser trochanter (type IIIA), it may be necessary to use a calcar replacement stem to provide secure fixation and restore length. In the type IIIB defect, bone may be lost down to the level of the isthmus. If cement is to be used, it may be necessary to use a proximal femoral allograft. Cementless implants may require extensive porous coating to fix the implant distally in the diaphyseal bone. In the type IIIC defect, bone loss extends to the isthmus and beyond. Again, a proximal femoral allograft may be used. It may be difficult to achieve secure fixation distally with an extensively porous-coated stem, since the canal is now diverging below the isthmus. Another approach is to cement the distal portion of the stem into the canal and to reconstruct the upper portion of the femur around a porous-coated stem, with bone graft if necessary, to restore bone stock.

Acetabulum

The classification of acetabular defects described by Paprosky et al. (48) is helpful for implant selection and de-termining the need for bone grafting (Fig. 44.7). Acetabular components may be inserted with or without cement to achieve bone ingrowth. The use of porous ingrowth, hemispherical acetabular components has become popular in both the primary and the revision setting, because it may be difficult to obtain cement intrusion into the wet, sclerotic bone of the acetabulum.

Cementless hemispherical cups can be used only if there is enough bone remaining to anchor the implant. In the type 1 defect, there is little migration and osteolysis. Because the rim is intact, an uncemented hemispherical cup may be used. In the type 2 defect, the superior migration of the socket is less than 2 cm. The type 2A defect is characterized by superomedial migration and an intact rim. Type 2B displays superolateral migration and segmental loss of the superior rim. Type 2C has teardrop lysis, indicating the loss of the medial wall. It is still possible to use uncemented hemispherical sockets, but larger-diameter sizes may be required. The oblong defects created by superior migration of the loose cup (type 2B) may be best managed with an elliptical cup. Morcellized bone graft is usually required for the cavitary bone loss, but structural allografts are not. Segmental defects of the rim or column require structural bone grafts that are secured with internal fixation. If the host rim bone is insufficient, the cup should be cemented, preferably inside a metal acetabular reinforcement ring.

The type 3 defect requires structural allograft to augment the missing acetabular rim or column. The type 3 de-

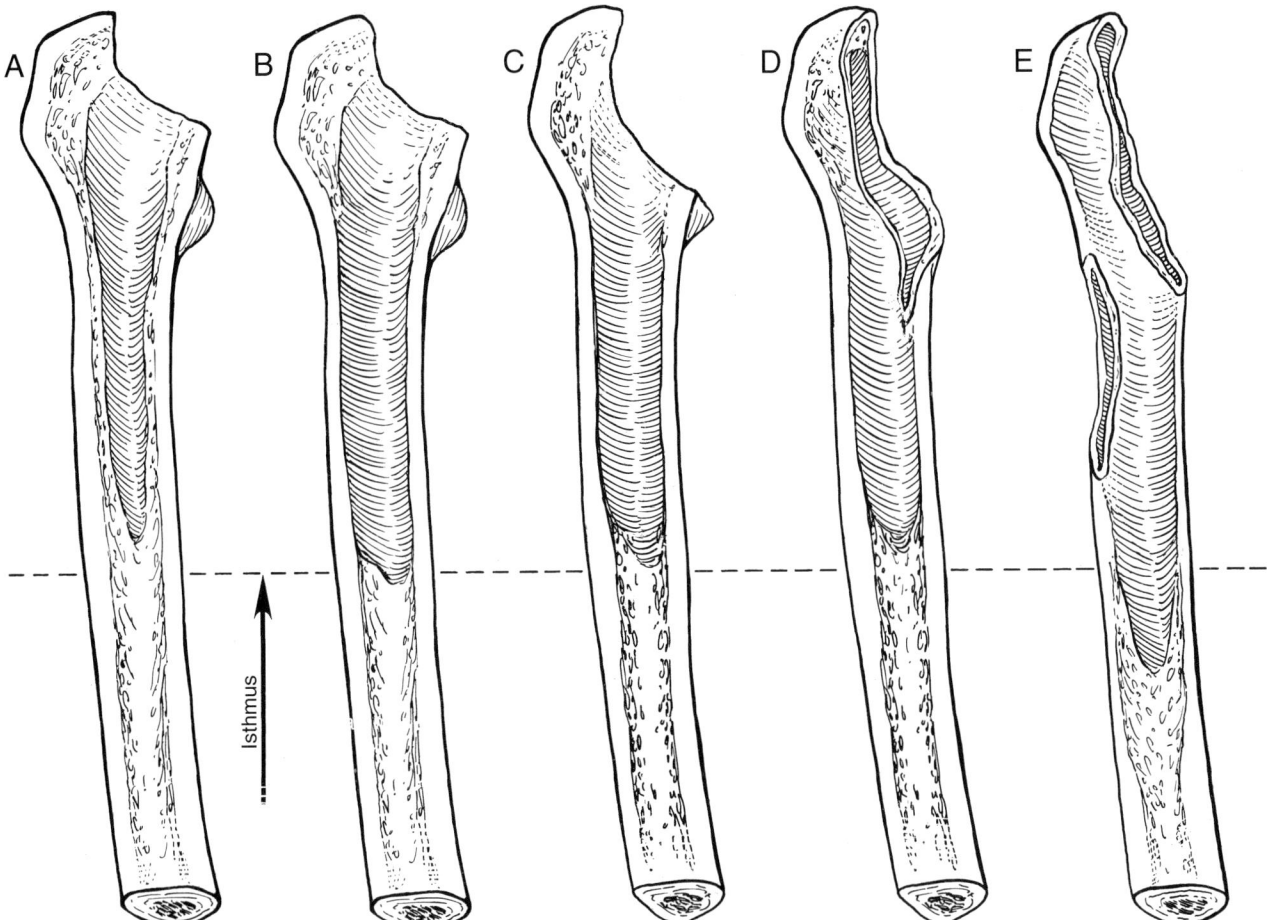

Figure 44.6. Mallory's classification of femoral bone loss in revision THR. **A.** Type I. **B.** Type II. **C.** Type IIIA. **D.** Type IIIB. **E.** Type IIIC.

fect has more than 2 cm of socket migration along with ischial osteolysis. Kohler's line is disrupted in the type 3B defect. If a pelvic discontinuity is present, antiprotrusio cages can be used to span the defect; pelvic reconstruction plates can be used to stabilize the defect and permit bone healing. Entire acetabular allografts may be required in the case of massive bone loss.

SURGICAL APPROACHES

The surgeon should use the approach with which he or she is most comfortable. The old incision should be used whenever possible. The incision is extended down to the deep fascia. Subcutaneous undermining should be minimized to prevent postoperative drainage. After incising the deep fascia, anterior and posterior flaps are mobilized off the vastus lateralis, the greater trochanter, and the abductor muscles. Any hypertrophic bursa tissue is removed. Releasing the insertion of the gluteus maximus into the femur helps mobilize the femur in an anterior direction during exposure of the acetabulum. The joint can be entered either from the back or from the front of the greater trochanter. The sciatic nerve should be dissected out if its position cannot be ascertained.

The anterolateral approaches require peeling off a portion of the abductor muscles from the front of the greater trochanter and proximal splitting of the abductor fibers (49,50). Care must be taken to avoid injuring the superior gluteal nerve. A meticulous repair must be done to minimize postoperative abductor muscle weakness and limp.

In the posterior approach, the external rotators are usually scarred into the posterior capsule, which is peeled off of the greater trochanter. Once the components are exposed, the capsule must be released from the perimeter of the acetabulum and from the femoral neck. The psoas tendon should be left intact, if possible. The femoral head is then dislocated. If the stem is to be revised, it is removed at this time. There should be enough mobility of the femur to expose the socket, even if the femoral component is not revised. It may be necessary to release the anterior capsule if exposure and mobilization of the femur are insufficient.

If the exposure is still inadequate, it may be necessary to perform either a trochanteric osteotomy or a trochanteric slide (51). For a trochanteric osteotomy, a flat or chevron-shaped osteotomy is made just distal to the vastus ridge to the medial side of the greater trochanter. The capsule is re-

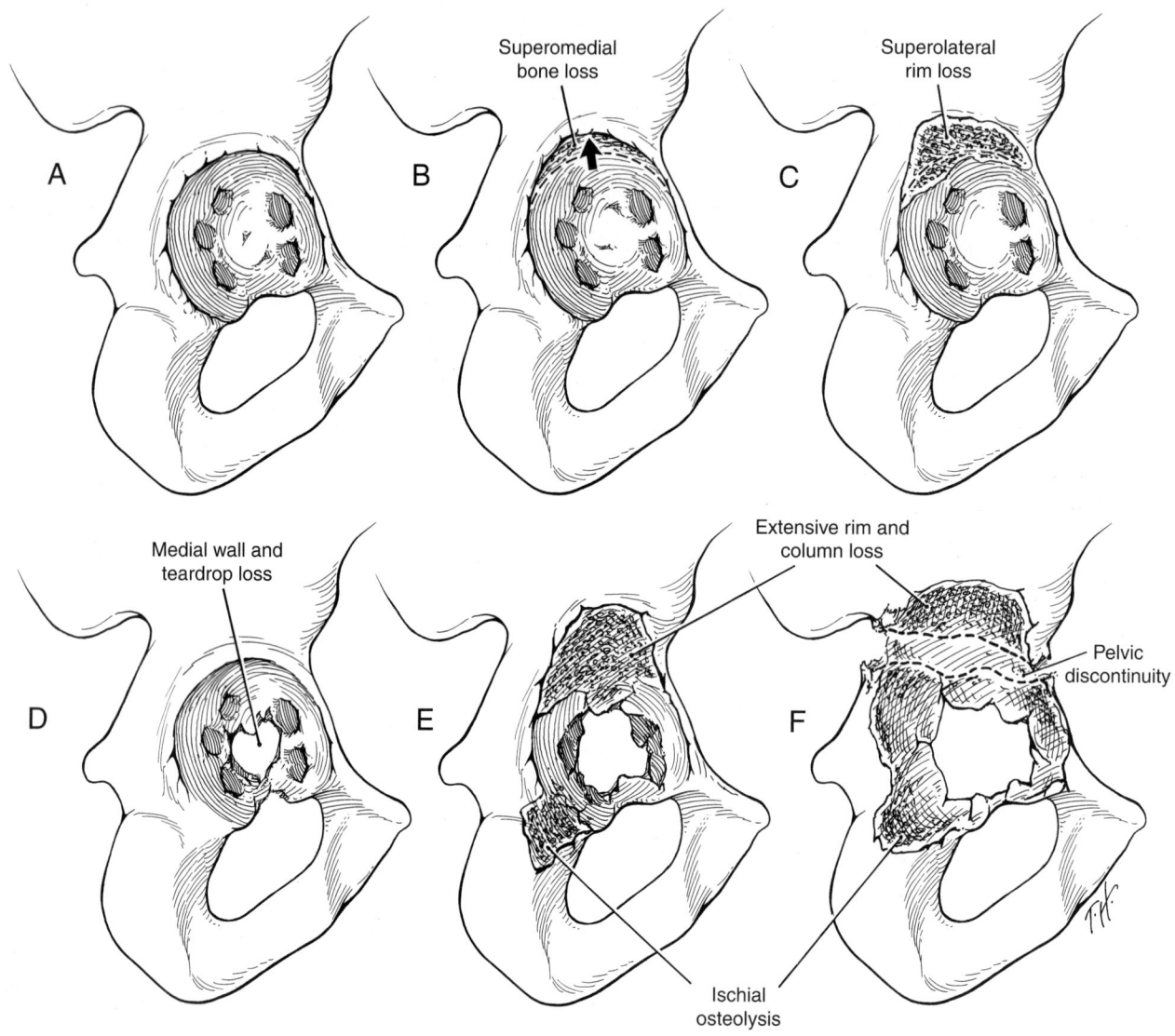

Figure 44.7. Paprosky et al.'s classification of acetabular bone loss in revision THR. **A.** Type 1. **B.** Type 2A. **C.** Type 2B. **D.** Type 2C. **E.** Type 3A. **F.** Type 3B.

leased from both the anterior and posterior sides. The superior capsule is incised, leaving the abductor muscle fibers intact, to allow mobilization of the greater trochanter in a cephalad direction (Fig. 44.8). For the trochanteric slide, a similar cut is made, but the vastus lateralis is left attached to the fragment of the greater trochanter (52) (Fig. 44.9). With either approach, the head can be dislocated in an anterior or posterior direction. Keeping the vastus attached to the greater trochanter maintains more blood supply to the trochanteric fragment and tethers it, helping to prevent nonunion and proximal migration. The anterior osteotomy of the greater trochanter is a variation of the anterolateral approach (53). The intention is to prevent migration of the trochanteric fragment and thus promote healing and preserve abductor strength.

If additional exposure is needed to remove well-fixed cemented or porous-coated stems from the femoral canal, the transfemoral approach is extremely useful (54). This approach is also useful when the upper femur is so deficient that removing the stem and cement from above, in the usual fashion, is futile. For the transfemoral approach, the first osteotomy is longitudinal and splits the greater trochanter in the coronal plane (Fig. 44.10). This split is extended cephalad into the abductor muscle fibers. The osteotomy is then extended distally just posterior to the vastus lateralis and anterior to the linea aspera. The distal extent is determined by preoperative planning and usually extends to the tip of the stem or cement mantle. The transverse component of the osteotomy is marked out by two drill holes at the posterolateral and anterolateral corners. The key is to keep the vastus lateralis attached to the lateral cortex.

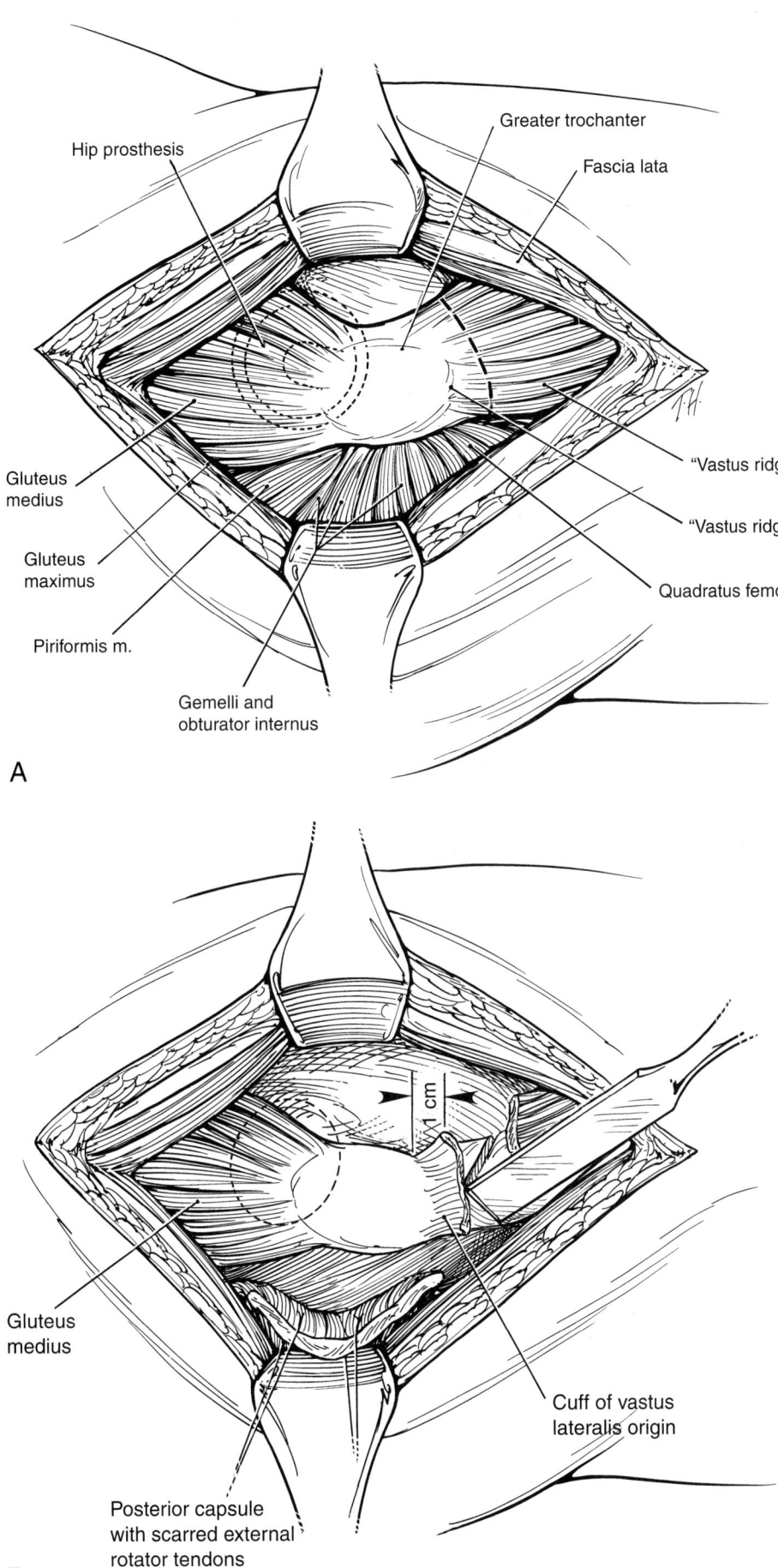

Greater trochanter

Fascia lata

Hip prosthesis

Gluteus
medius

Gluteus
maximus

Piriformis m.

"Vastus ridge"

"Vastus ridge"

Quadratus femoris

Gemelli and
obturator internus

A

Gluteus
medius

Cuff of vastus
lateralis origin

Posterior capsule
with scarred external
rotator tendons

B

Figure 44.8. A. For a trochanteric osteotomy, the vastus lateralis origin is incised 1 cm distal to the vastus ridge **B.** The osteotomy may be flat or chevron shaped; the anterior and posterior capsular attachments are released. *(continued)*

Figure 44.8. *(continued)* **C.** The greater trochanter is reflected proximally with the abductor muscles.

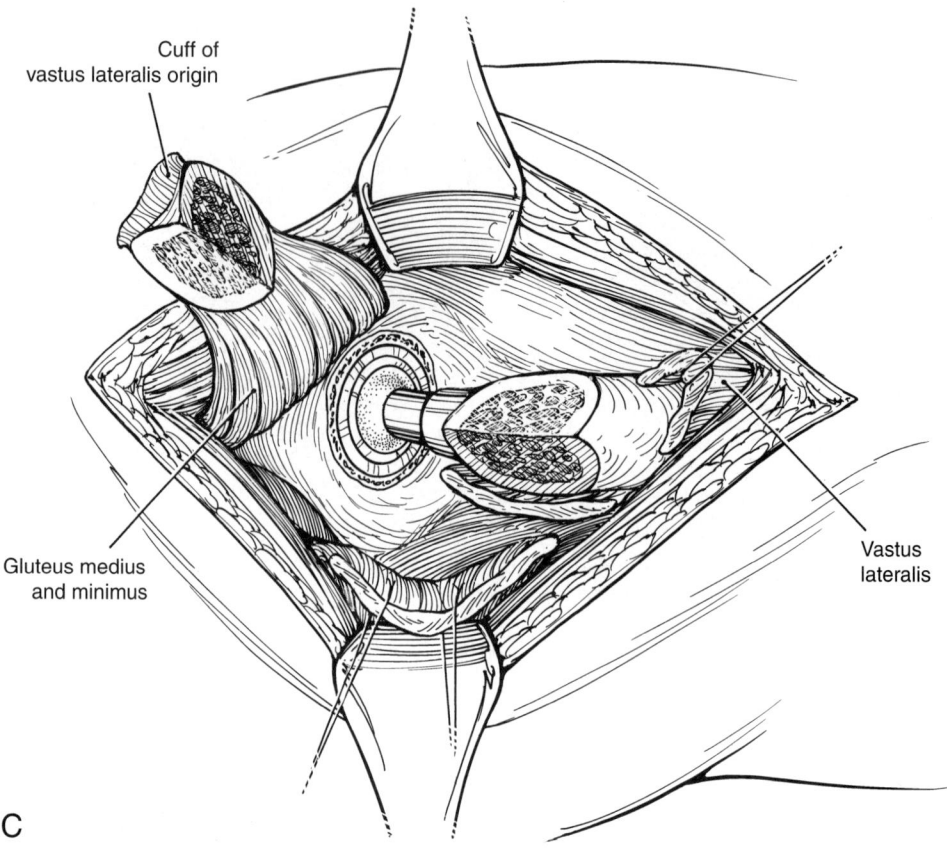

Cuff of vastus lateralis origin

Vastus lateralis

Gluteus medius and minimus

C

Figure 44.9. A. For a trochanteric slide, the osteotomy may be flat or chevron shaped; the vastus lateralis remains attached. *(continued)*

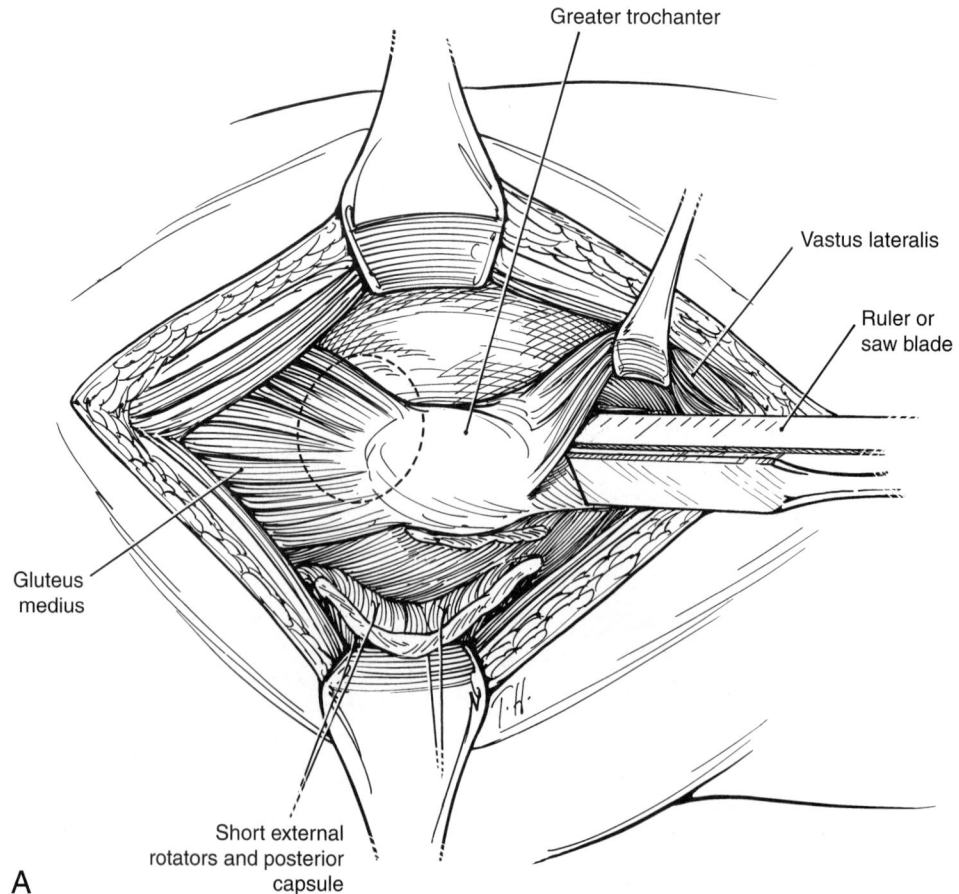

Greater trochanter

Vastus lateralis

Ruler or saw blade

Gluteus medius

Short external rotators and posterior capsule

A

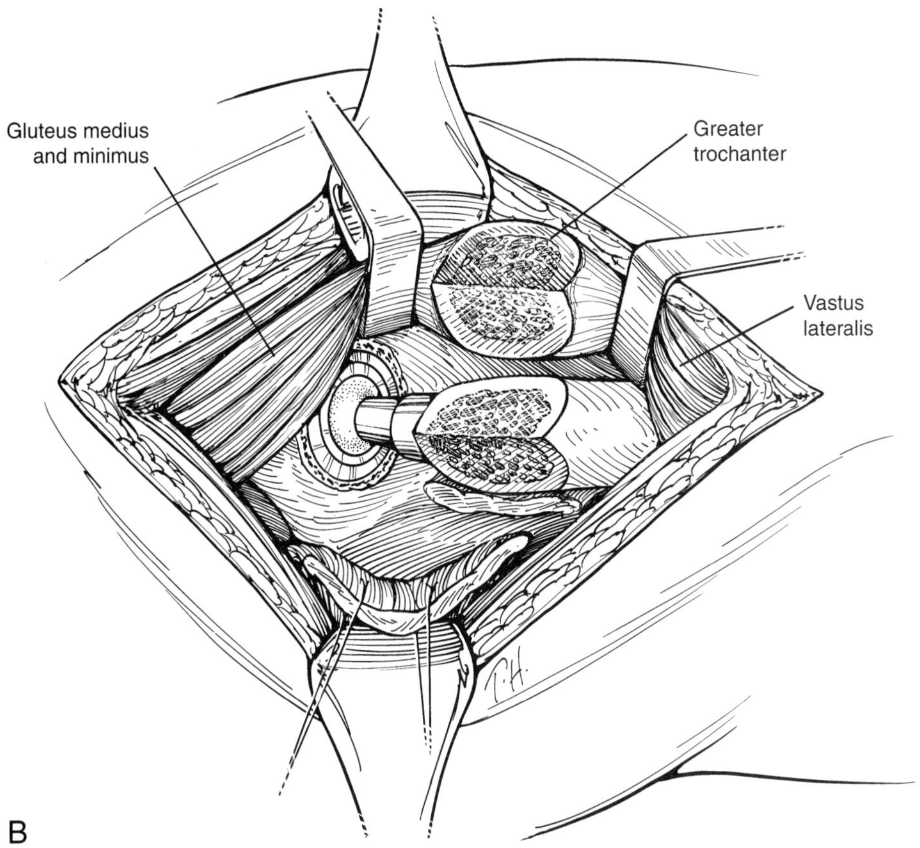

Figure 44.9. *(continued)* **B.** The greater trochanter is reflected anteriorly to expose the hip joint.

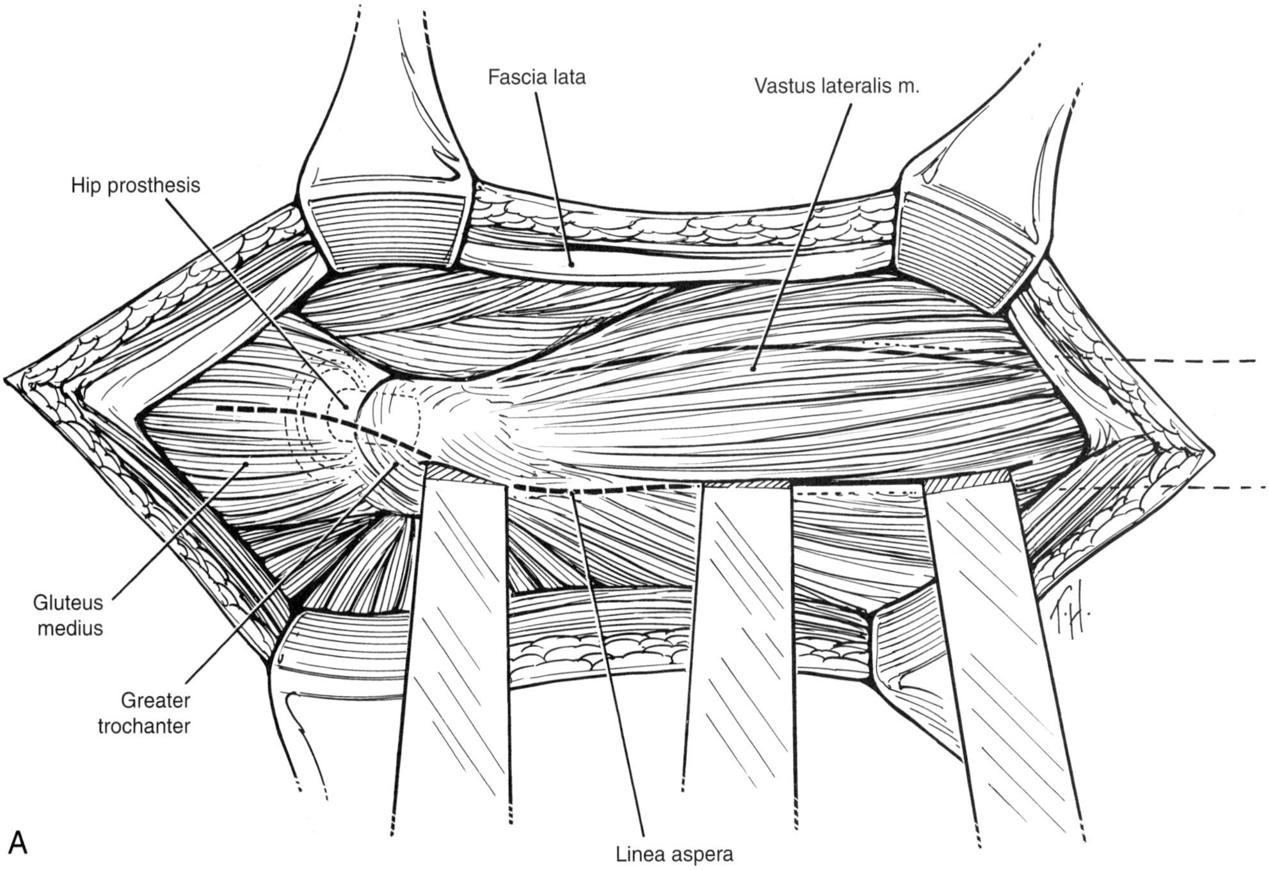

Figure 44.10. A. For the transfemoral approach, the posterior limb is made near the linea aspera and bisects the greater trochanter. *(continued)*

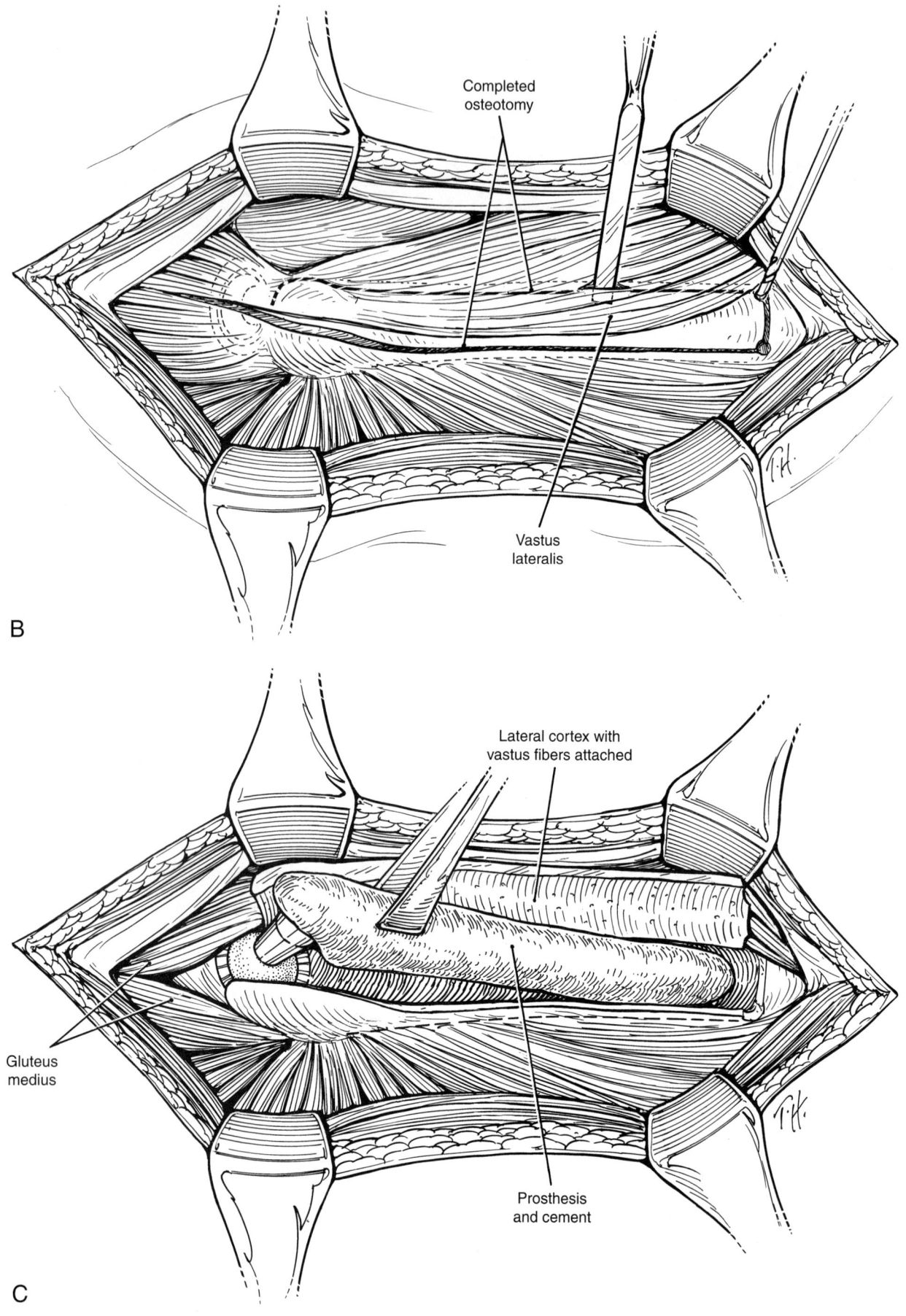

B

Completed
osteotomy

Vastus
lateralis

C

Lateral cortex with
vastus fibers attached

Gluteus
medius

Prosthesis
and cement

Figure 44.10. *(continued)* **B.** The distal extent of the osteotomy is delineated with drill holes, and the anterolateral limb is made with a narrow osteotome through the fibers of the vastus lateralis. The mus-cle fibers must remain on the lateral cortical fragment. **C.** The lateral cortex is flipped open to expose the canal. *(continued)*

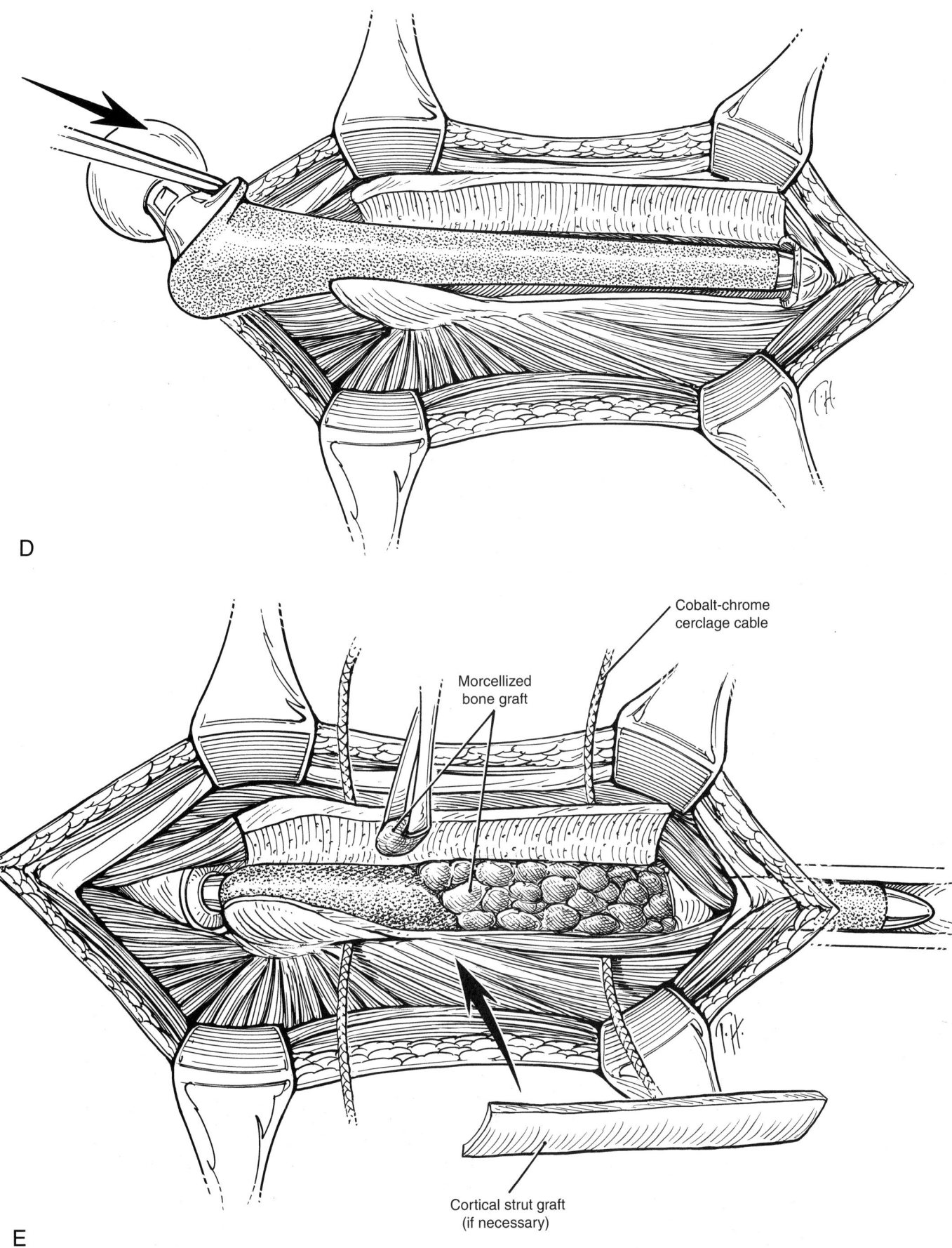

D

E

Figure 44.10. *(continued)* **D.** The stem is inserted (*arrow*). **E.** The osteotomy site is repaired with bone grafts.

From the anterolateral hole, a number of cortical perforations are made through the fibers of the vastus lateralis to delineate the anterior border of the cortical window. These perforations are then taken up to the anterior border of the greater trochanter. With wide osteotomes, the lateral cortex, with the vastus lateralis attached, is hinged open by cracking through the anterolateral perforations. At closure, the lateral cortex is reapproximated with cerclage cables or heavy sutures and supplemented with cortical onlay struts or morcellized bone graft, as needed. If the soft tissues are maintained, the bone healing is quite remarkable. A variation is the extended proximal femoral osteotomy in which the entire trochanter is removed with a lateral cortical extension (55).

IMPLANT REMOVAL

Cemented Implants

Depending on the situation, the components may be easily removed from their beds or may be extremely well-fixed and difficult to remove. Monoblock stems may be removed with slap-hammer extractors with a loop that fits over the head. It is helpful to use chisels to remove any cement that is accessible. Trochanteric bone overgrowth may block the extraction path and must be removed to prevent fracture of the trochanter. If necessary, attempt to break up the bone–cement or stem–cement interface with osteotomes. Stems that were coated with polymethy methacrylate (PMMA) may be extremely difficult to extract from the cement mantle, and in some cases it may be necessary to split the femur to effect removal. Once the stem is out, the cement mantle may be removed with chisels, high-speed drills, reamers, pneumatic chisels, or ultrasonic curettes. An alternative with an intact, well-fixed cement mantle is to add the new cement and a threaded rod with reinforcing nuts into the old cement mantle. Once the new cement has hardened, the rod is removed; the threaded extractors are screwed in; and the mantle is extracted with a slap hammer, 1 cm at a time (56).

The cement plug beyond the tip of the stem is often the most difficult piece to extract. The ultrasonic plug extractor or chisel tips may work. If the plug is long and well-fixed, a high-speed drill may be used; fluoroscopy helps prevent perforation. Once a pilot hole is made, cement hand drills or cannulated reamers may be used. If all else fails, a cortical window can be used to extract the plug under direct vision (57).

If the new stem is to be cemented, it is possible to leave a well-fixed cement mantle (58). This is especially true when the revision is being done to correct malposition or leg length inequality in patient that has no loosening or fracture of the old mantle. If the revision is being done to eradicate infection, it is important to remove all of the old cement.

Acetabular components can usually be broken out of the old cement mantle. The cement is then removed with osteotomes. The surgeon should be sure to look for cement anchoring plugs in the ilium, ischium, and pubis. A well-fixed, all-polyethylene cup can be quartered with the high-speed drill if it is difficult to remove.

Porous Ingrowth Components

Stems may be easy to extract if bone ingrowth is lacking. Stems with proximal porous coating can be removed once the bone–implant interface is disrupted. Flexible osteotomes, both straight and curved, may be used to pass between implant and bone. It may be necessary to remove the collar with a diamond-tipped pneumatic burr to access the medial cortex. A modular head cannot be used for extraction. A threaded extractor is available for some components. A Bohn (Biomet; Warsaw, IN) extractor or similar device that clamps onto the trunnion after removal of the modular head is useful (see Fig. 44.4).

Stems with extensive porous coating may be extremely difficult to remove. If the bone ingrowth is good, it may be necessary to window the femur and cut the stem in half. The distal half may then be removed, after passing a trephine around the distal stem (59). If this is not possible, the entire stem can be exposed with the transfemoral approach.

Porous-coated cups may also be difficult to remove. The interface is disrupted with curved chisels inserted either by hand or under pneumatic power or with ultrasonic devices. An alternate method is to notch the metal shell twice 180° apart and then lock on a pneumatic impaction tool to torque the cup free (60).

PROSTHESIS IMPLANTATION AND BONE GRAFTING

Femur

Implant selection is part of the preoperative plan. Because of the uncertainty of intraoperative findings, it may be necessary to have several different devices on hand. The surgeon must decide whether to use cemented implants or to use cementless implants that provide either proximal or distal fixation.

Before the new implant can be inserted, femoral bone defects must be addressed. Because the cortical tube is intact and some cancellous bone remains in type I defects, bone grafting is not necessary. In type II defects, the cortical shell is intact, albeit thin. The surgeon may fill the canal with cement, but cement intrusion into wet and sclerotic bone surface is poor. It may be necessary to go with a longer stem to achieve adequate cement fixation. This does not restore bone stock, and the next revision will be even more difficult, with cortical ectasia extending beyond the isthmus. Type II defects are amenable to cancellous bone impaction grafting (61). The morcellized bone graft is placed into the canal and impacted firmly. A stem is then cemented into the new bed, and the bone graft eventually consolidates. This technique may also be used with uncemented stems that are fully coated to achieve distal fixation or with modular uncemented stems, such as the S-ROM (Johnson & Johnson; Raynham, MA) (Figs. 44.11 and

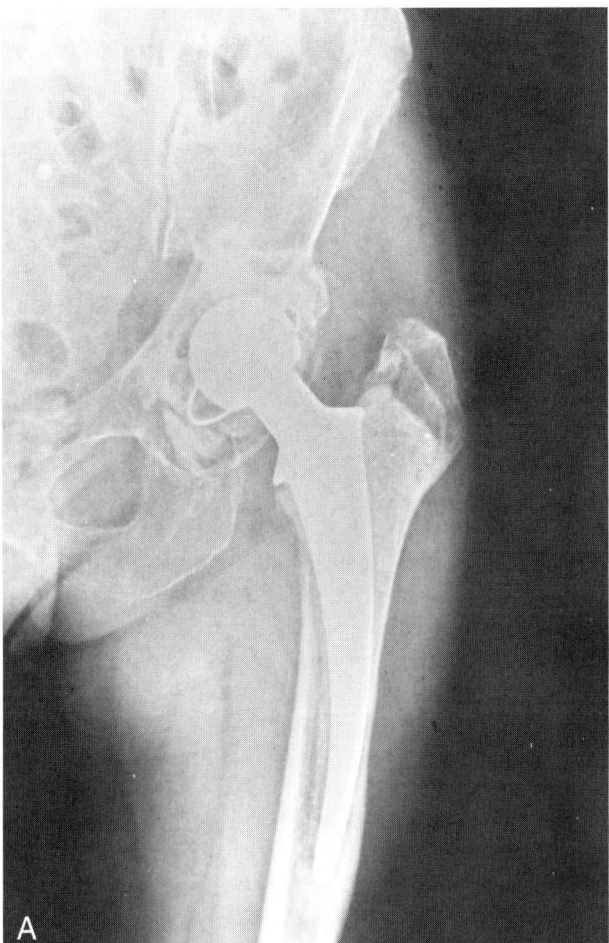

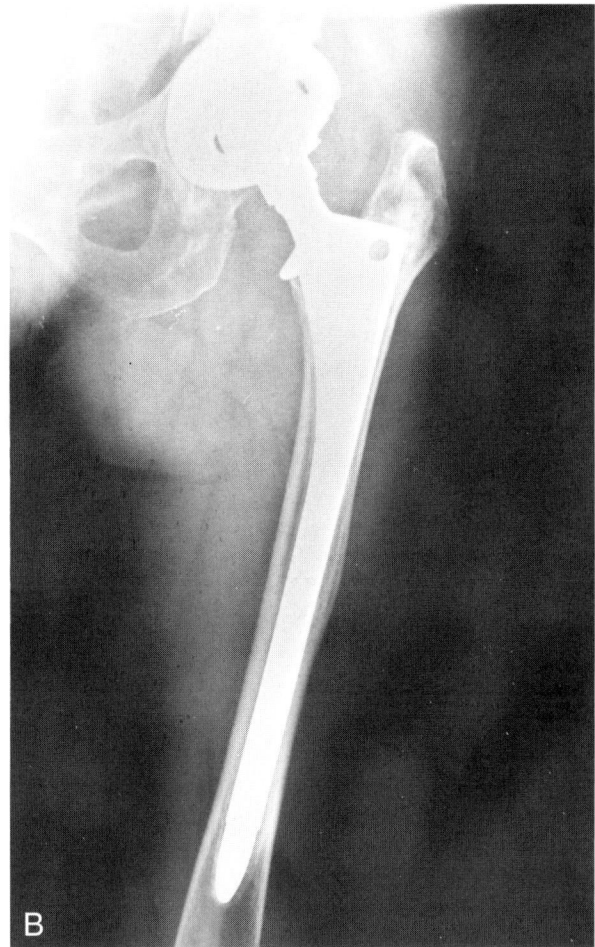

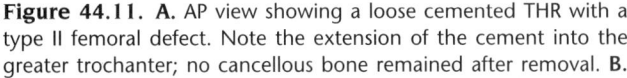

Figure 44.11. A. AP view showing a loose cemented THR with a type II femoral defect. Note the extension of the cement into the greater trochanter; no cancellous bone remained after removal. **B.** AP view 1 year after a cementless revision with a fully coated stem and grafting of the trochanter defect. The type 2C acetabular defect was reconstructed with an uncemented socket.

44.12). The S-ROM stem requires enough proximal cortical bone to obtain solid fixation of the sleeve. The canal is packed with morcellized graft using a trial stem; and then the stem that couples to the sleeve is put in place.

More extensive grafts may be required for type III defects. For a type IIIA defect, napkin-ring-type grafts of the medial calcar have not performed well. The use of a calcar replacement stem, with or without cement, is probably the best choice with fixation in the canal to the level of adequate bone stock. The augmented proximal portion of the component rests on the medial calcar and restores femoral length (Fig. 44.13). Cemented stems have a platform that sits on top of the medial bone column; uncemented stems have an elongated metaphyseal segment (Fig. 44.14). Most stems have a means to allow greater trochanter attachment to anchoring holes in the implant.

With Type IIIB defects, cortical destruction extends from the lesser trochanter to the isthmus of the femur. Uncemented, fully-coated stems may be impacted into the distal femur. These stems must have intraoperative stability and must be able to resist subsidence (axial load), bending moments, and rotation. Uncemented im-

plants that are not stable are doomed to failure. The transfemoral approach is useful because it greatly facilitates removal of the old stem and cement. In this type of defect, the bone is often so deficient proximally that it is not worth saving as an intact tube. The transfemoral approach may even restore proximal bone stock, especially if supplemental grafting is employed (Fig. 44.15).

Another alternative, if cement is to be used, is the use of proximal femoral allograft. While these huge constructs do not revascularize to any appreciable degree, they can heal at the junction with host bone (62). The implant is then cemented into both the allograft and the remaining distal femur, thus spreading interface stresses over a large area. The greater trochanter, if present, may also be reattached to the allograft. With type IIIC defects, the area of bone loss extends beyond the isthmus. A proximal femoral allograft may still be used, but a larger graft and a longer stem are required. It is difficult to use a fully-coated stem without cement in this situation, because the cortical area available for fixation is short and the canal is divergent below the isthmus, making it difficult to jam in an uncemented stem with sufficient stability. It is possible to

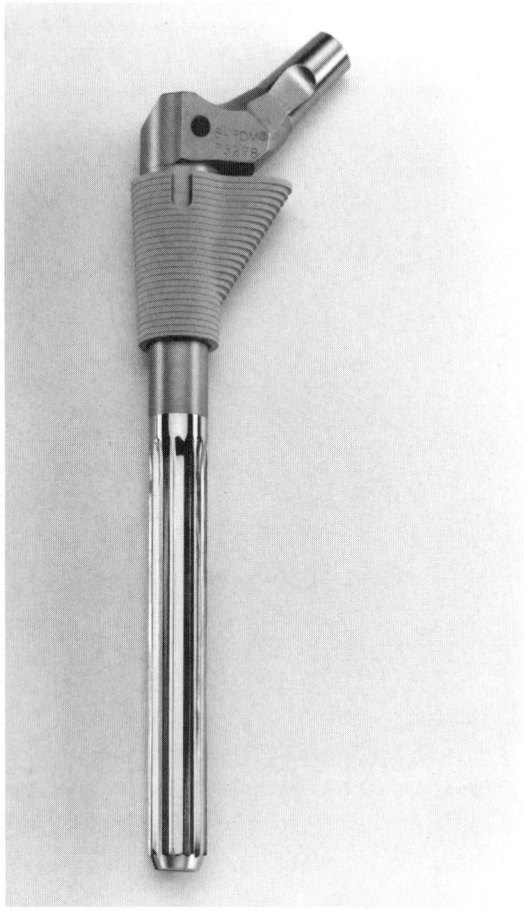

Figure 44.12. The modular design of the S-ROM uncemented femoral stem provides a precise fit both proximally and distally and allows proximal bone ingrowth.

perform a femoral hybrid. A transfemoral approach is performed in the proximal portion of the femur. A long, fully-coated stem is cemented into the distal section. The remnants of the proximal femur are cerclaged around the porous-coated stem with supplemental morcellized and/or cortical onlay graft as needed. This construct attains intraoperative stability, and postoperative healing of the proximal femur augments the bone stock (Fig. 44.16).

When cementing long stems, avoid heating the PMMA powder, which prevents rapid polymerization. The implant is cemented into the proximal femur allograft off the field, the construct is then cemented into the host distal femur. Tobramycin power can be added to the cement (1.2 g/40 g PMMA powder) to lessen the chance of perioperative infection.

Acetabulum

Acetabular components may be inserted with or without cement. As with the femur, bony deficits must be addressed. If there is no bone deficit, a new component may be cemented into place. The bony bed should be as dry as possible. Cement-anchoring holes may be placed in the ilium, ischium, and pubis. The surgeon should avoid bottoming out the cup to allow for a uniform cement mantle around the implant. If a portion of the rim is missing, reinforcement rings, such as a Müller ring, help provide a secure foundation on which to cement the cup (Fig. 44.17). If a medial wall defect is present, bone graft of either morcellized or cancellous wafers can be placed medial to the ring.

If the rim is intact, uncemented sockets may be used. The acetabulum is reamed until a bed of healthy, bleed-

Figure 44.13. The degree of porous coating on the Mallory Head (Biomet; Warsaw, IN) uncemented femoral stem varies, depending on the amount of femoral bone remaining.

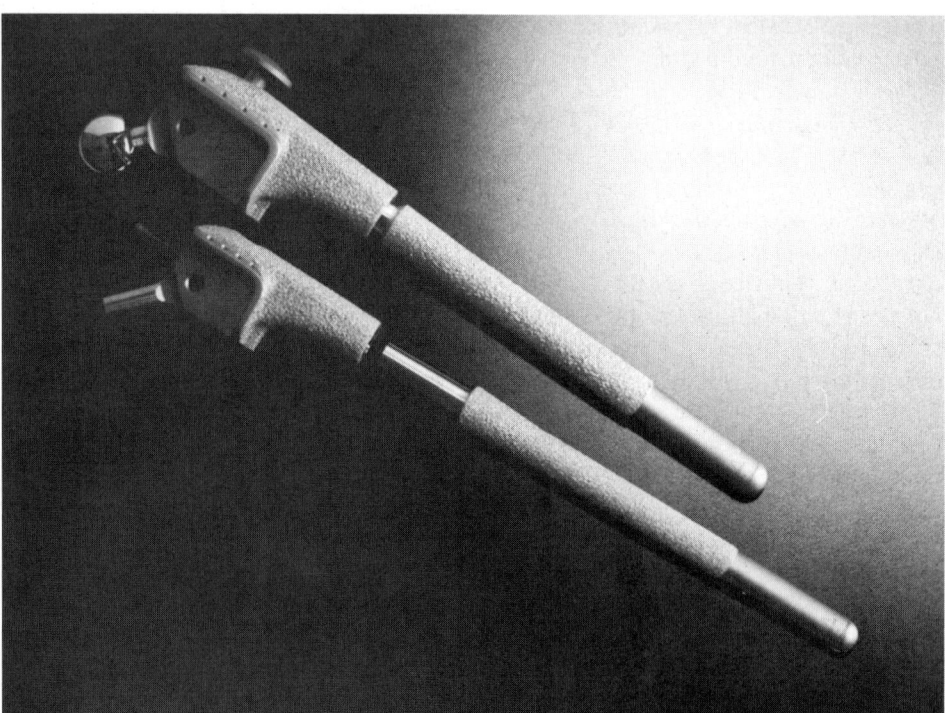

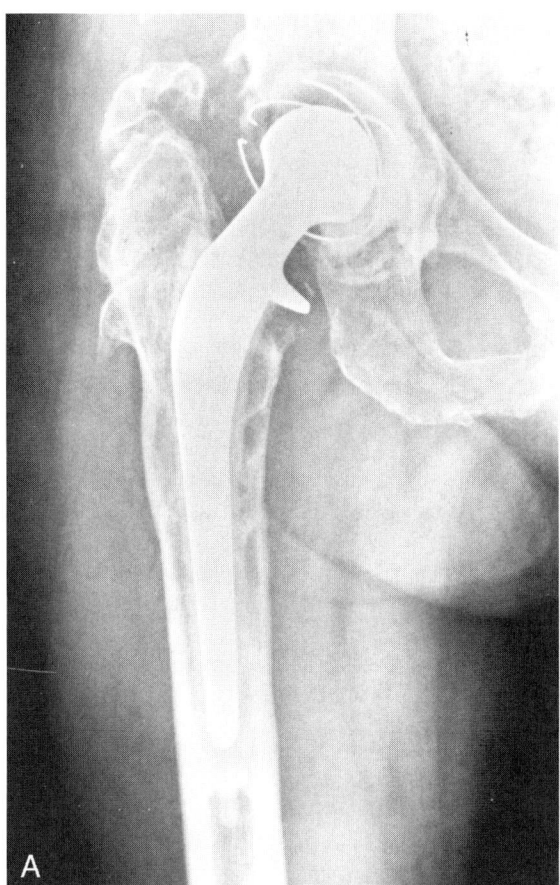

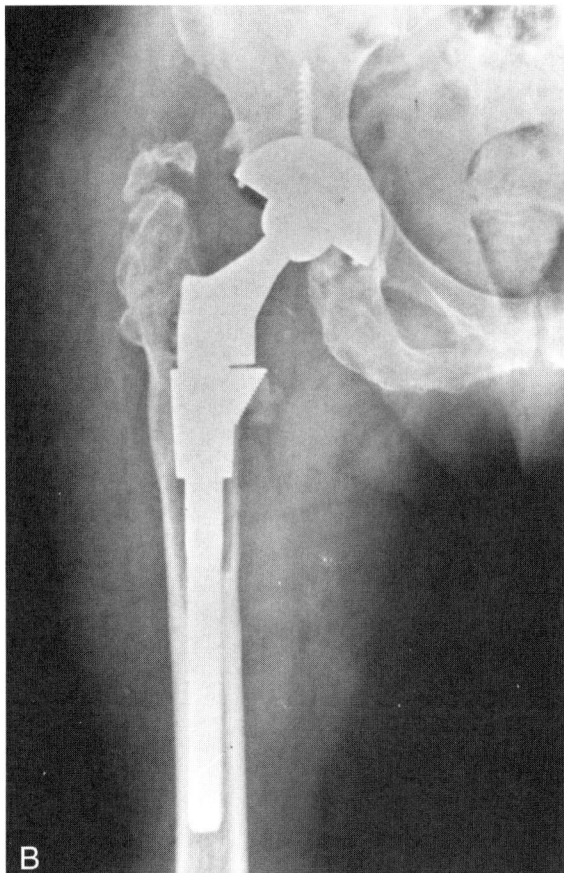

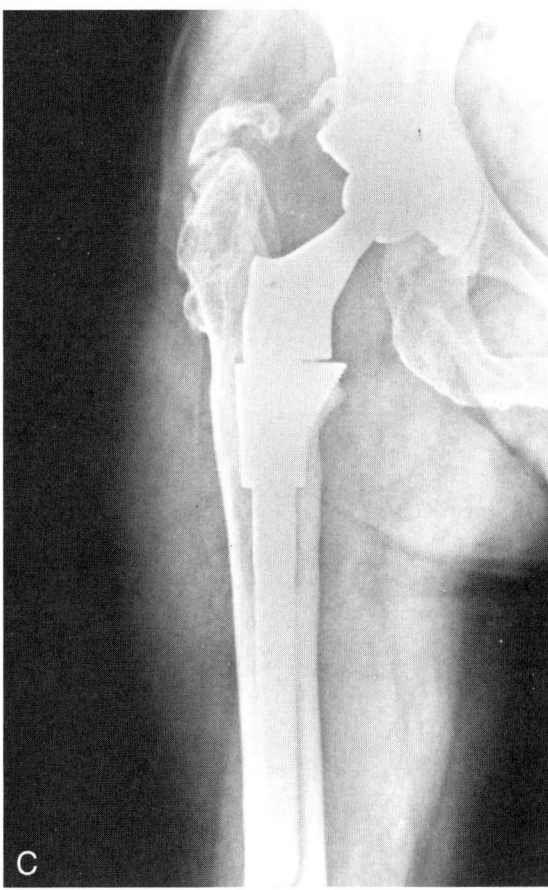

Figure 44.14. A. A loose cemented THR with a type IIIA femoral defect. **B.** An immediate postoperative view showing reconstruction with an uncemented socket and a calcar-type S-ROM stem to restore leg length. **C.** After 9 months, hypertrophy of medial cortex in response to proximal bone ingrowth and stress transfer has occurred.

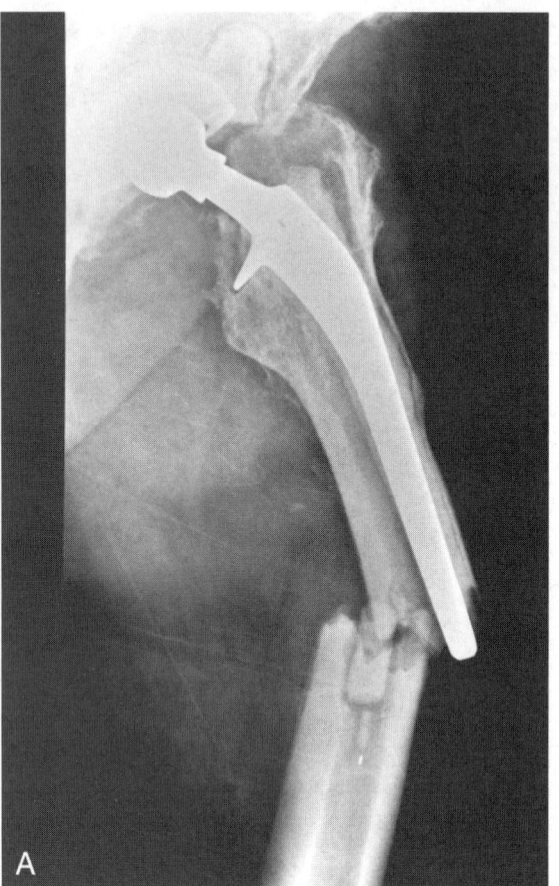

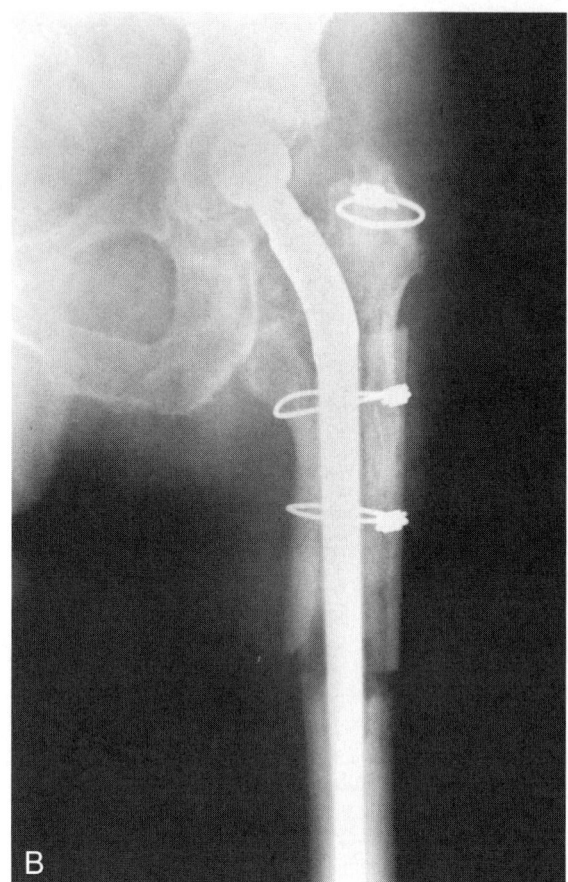

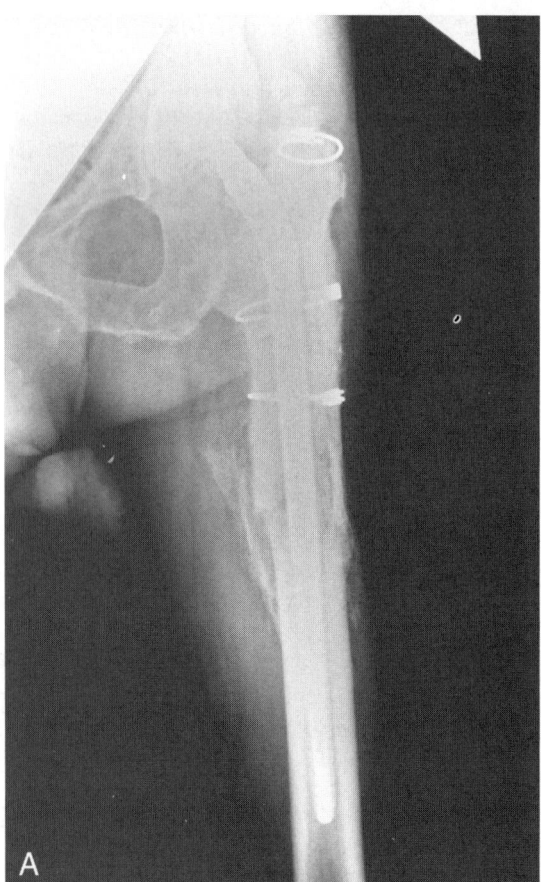

Figure 44.15. A. A periprosthetic fracture of the femur with extensive lateral cortical bone loss (type IIIB) and implant loosening. **B.** Immediate postoperative view showing the transfemoral approach with a distally fixed uncemented stem. **C.** After 2 years the osteotomy has healed and the proximal bone stock has been reconstructed.

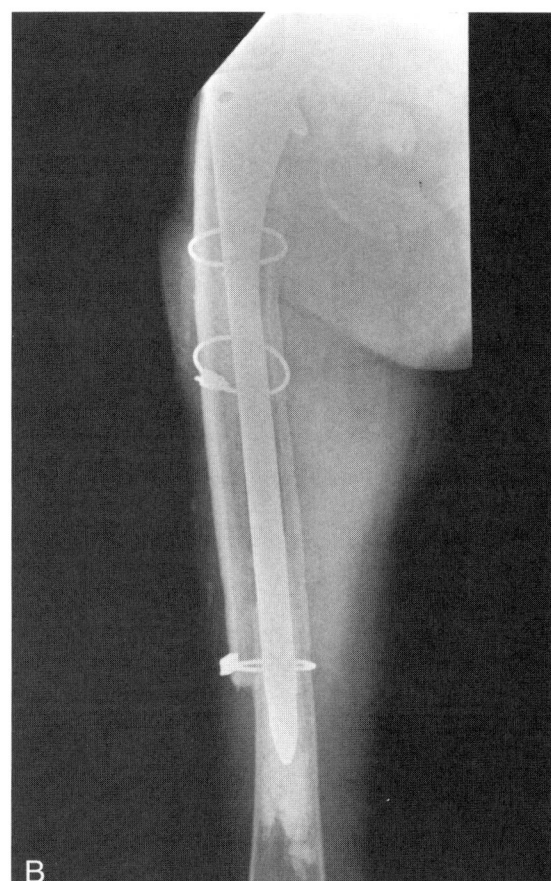

Figure 44.16. A. A type IIIC defect after two previous cemented femoral revisions. **B.** The 1-year follow-up of the femoral hybrid pro-cedure showing the proximal bone reconstruction; only the lower third of stem was cemented to provide postoperative stability.

ing bone is left. The cup selected is usually 2 mm larger than the last reamer used to provide Press-Fit stability. The construct can be made even more secure by the addition of bone screws through the shell, directed into the ilium or ischium. As with any uncemented device, there must be enough intraoperative stability to prevent postoperative migration and failure and enough host bone present to ensure not only stability but postoperative bony attachment (Fig. 44.11).

If large portions of the acetabular walls or columns are deficient, the problem must be addressed. In certain types of defects, such an elliptical defect (type 2B), an unusual implant such as an oblong cup or a hemispherical cup with modular augments may fill the voids and provide stability (Fig. 44.18). It may be possible to place a small uncemented cup into the upper portion of the oblong defect; this does not restore length or the center of rotation to an anatomic position. In addition, the bone stock is usually deficient in this area high up on the iliac wing. In certain situations, however, it may be desirous to add bulk bone allografts. Depending on the amount required, humeral or femoral heads, distal femora, or proximal tibiae may be used. These grafts must be secured to the pelvis with screws and/or plates.

The acetabulum is reamed, and the cup is placed into an anatomic position. The amount of host bone contact required for successful ingrowth is estimated to be approximately 40%, provided that bulk allograft bone is used to provide the additional coverage (63). In a situation in which a massive allograft of the acetabulum is required, cementing in the socket is a better option.

In cases of pelvic discontinuity, the problem of inadequate bone stock is compounded by a disconnection of the pelvic bone proximal and distal to the acetabulum. The ischium may actually fall away from the ilium. Bone grafting is still necessary; but in addition, the periacetabular bone must be secured by internal fixation. An alternative is to use an oversized reinforcement ring, such as the Burch-Schneider ring (Sulzer; Winterthur, Switzerland) (Fig. 44.17), which acts as an oversized plate, bridging the discontinuity defect. The cup is then cemented into the ring. If the defect is massive, it may be necessary to perform an acetabular transplant. After securing the graft to host bone, the cup is cemented to the allograft, preferably inside a metal reinforcement ring (64).

PITFALLS

Thorough preoperative planning is one of the most important aspects of successful surgery. It is difficult to do justice to the task at hand without preoperative planning.

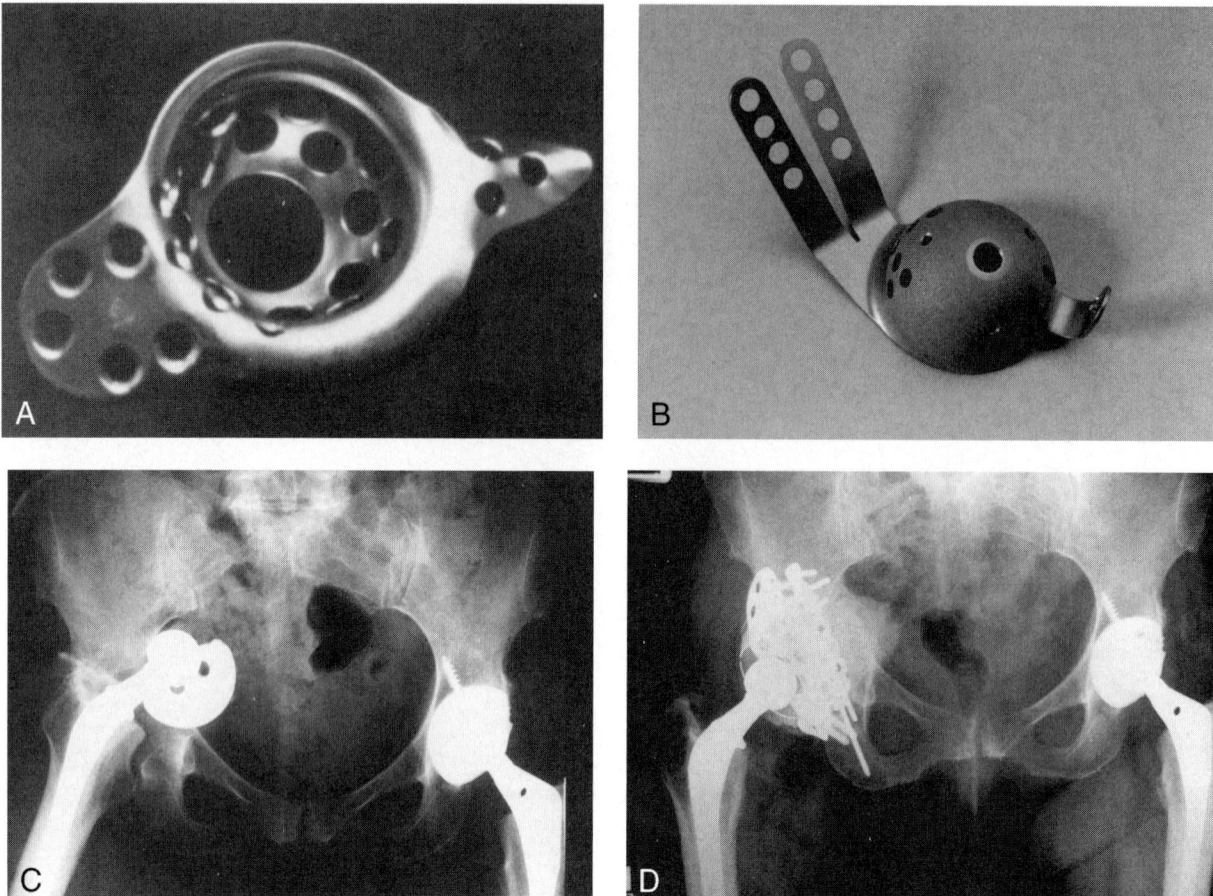

Figure 44.17. A. A Burch-Schneider ring is a type of antiprotrusio cage. **B.** The GAP (Osteonics; Allendale, NJ) cup has a teardrop hook and ilium plates to counteract protrusio **C.** Pelvic discontinuity fol- lowing intraoperative fracture and socket migration. **D.** AP view 2 years after reconstruction with a Burch-Schneider ring and morcel- lized bone graft.

The surgeon should read the old operative note. By run- ning through a checklist of necessary equipment and steps of execution, the surgeon may prevent nasty intraopera- tive surprises. Furthermore, success depends on having the correct implants. The surgeon must determine before- hand all the necessary implants and various types of bone grafts.

Inadequate exposure can lead to intraoperative prob- lems. There are a variety of exposures that can be used to get the job done; but the exposure must be sufficient to expose, remove, and insert the implants. Without suffi- cient release, the femur cannot be mobilized enough to expose the acetabulum, to increase leg length, and/or cor- rect offset. The surgeon must be cognizant of the neu- rovascular structures.

When femoral bone stock is compromised, it is easy to perforate the femur, especially with power instruments. The femur may be fractured simply during the rotation re- quired to dislocate the hip. If it is difficult to guide power tools down the medullary canal, fluoroscopy should be used. Unrecognized perforations can lead to cement ex- trusion into the soft tissues and can be stress risers that promote fractures. The femur may be fractured if long un- cemented stems are inserted without adequate prepara- tion of the canal. Following insertion of these stems, intra- operative radiographs should be obtained to detect any unrecognized femoral fractures.

The surgeon must be aware of the location of the neu- rovascular structures. If extensive bone grafting is required of the posterior column, electromyographic monitoring helps prevent injury to the sciatic nerve (65). With protru- sio defects, preoperative visualization of the great vessels can be done with either contrast-enhanced CT scans or ar- teriograms. The surgeon should avoid placing acetabular screws into the anterior cup quadrants (66). Excessive lengthening may cause a stretch injury of the nerves. The dislocation position should be kept to a minimum to avoid prolonged kinking of the great vessels. If the leg is dislo- cated anteriorly with the leg in a dependent position off the table, set the foot on a stool to avoid excessive stretch on the sciatic nerve.

Leg length inequality is another surgical pitfall. The sur- geon should know the leg length situation before surgery and should determine if the patient notices a leg length in- equality. It is important to know how much of the inequal- ity is due to the leg and how much is due to spine involve- ment with pelvic tilting. Preoperative planning should predict what will happen to the leg length with various

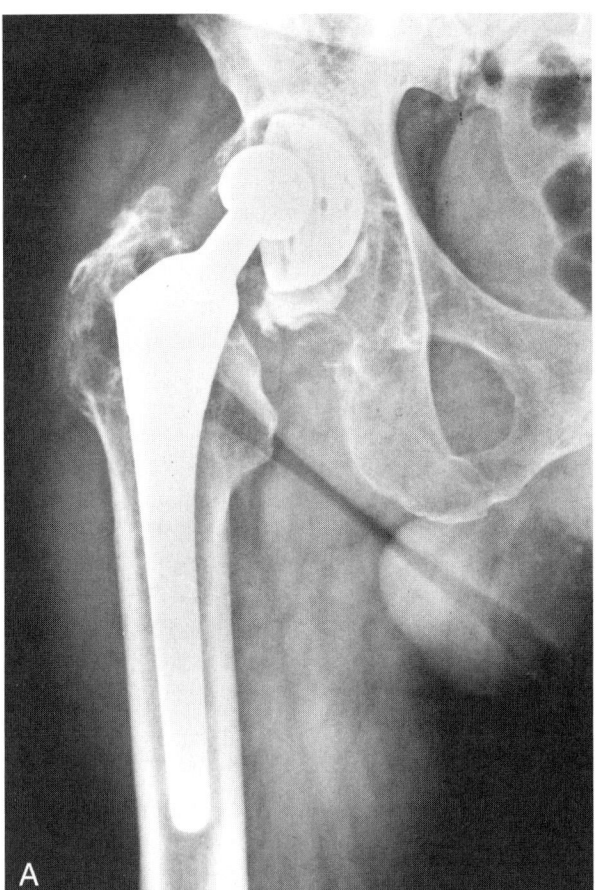

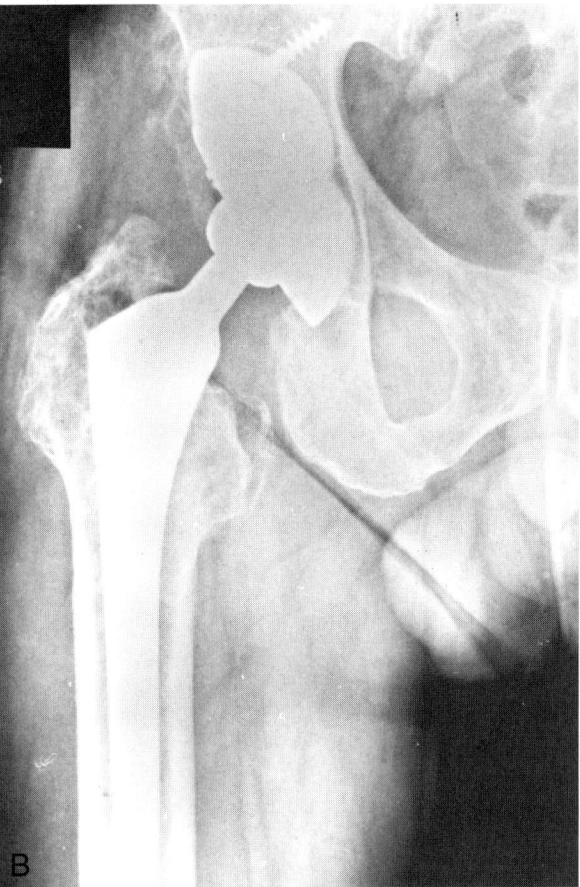

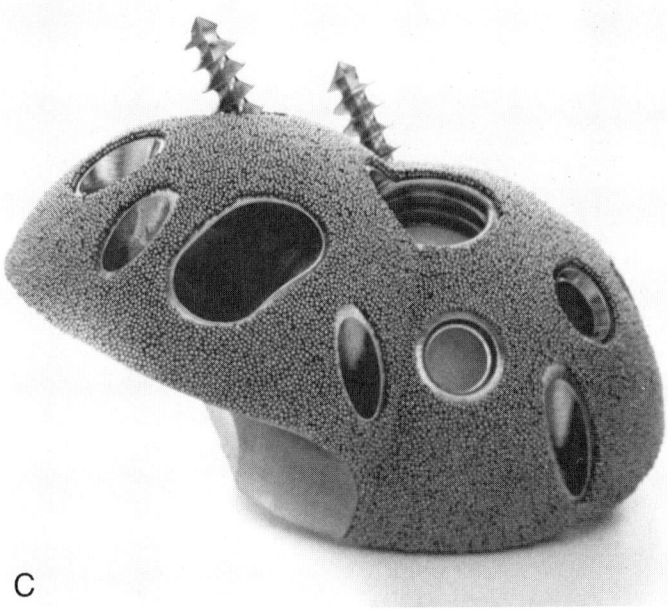

Figure 44.18. A. A type 2B acetabular defect. **B.** Reconstruction with an oblong acetabular component at the 1-year follow-up. **C.** An oblong acetabular component (Johnson & Johnson; Raynham, MA).

components in various positions. Leg length can be monitored during the operation by placing a Steinmann pin in the side of the ilium, and then using a caliper to mark the vastus lateralis fascia at a predetermined distance from the pin (usually 10 cm) before dislocation. This distance can be checked at trial reduction by noting the change in the distance from the pin to the mark on the vastus fascia.

The surgical team should not leave the operating room until it is sure that the hip will be stable in the postoperative environment. A trial reduction should always be performed. The hip should not dislocate anteriorly at full extension and external location. It should be possible to flex the hip beyond 90° without dislocation. At 90° of flexion, it should be possible to internally rotate the hip at least 30° before posterior dislocation occurs. If this not possible, dislocation may occur in the postoperative period. The surgeon should look for impingement of either the greater trochanter in external rotation or the neck of the stem against anterior osteophytes in flexion. Excessive anteversion and any retroversion of the socket should be avoided, and the cup should not be placed too vertically. Leg length and offset are critical for maintaining the proper soft tissue tension.

Poor cement technique can lead to postoperative problems. All of the old cement and soft tissues should be removed from the bony surfaces. The bone surfaces should be freshened, if sufficient bone stock remains, to allow for increased cement intrusion. If possible, the cement should be pressurized.

Cementless implants must be stable at the time of implantation. The components should not be undersized, and the implant should be appropriated for the amount of bone remaining. Screws should be used for cup fixation, unless the Press-Fit stability is exceptionally good. Cement should be used if that is the only way to obtain intraoperative stability.

An un-united trochanter can lead to pain, abductor weakness, and/or hip instability. Trochanteric osteotomy should be avoided, unless it is needed for exposure. The chevron-shaped osteotomy increases the surface area for healing and has more inherent stability than the flat osteotomy. Performing a trochanteric slide, which leaves the vastus lateralis attached, tethers the greater trochanter and helps prevent proximal migration. Fixation must be secured with either monofilament wires, braided cables with a trochanteric hook, or implant bolts that fasten the greater trochanter to the implant.

Patient should be assessed for risk of heterotopic bone formation (i.e., hypertrophic osteoarthritis or ankylosing spondylitis). Trauma to the soft tissues should be minimized, and the hip should be irrigated to remove all fine bone debris. Patients at risk should be treated with either postoperative radiation therapy or anti-inflammatories, such as indomethacin, to prevent bone formation.

REHABILITATION

Patients should be out of bed as soon as possible after surgery to improve pulmonary status, minimize decubitus ulcers, resolve postoperative ileus, and prevent deep venous thrombosis. Patients with a cemented stem can attempt weight bearing as tolerated. Those with an uncemented stem should probably be placed on partial weight bearing until bone ingrowth occurs, at about 6 weeks after surgery. An uncemented cup can usually withstand weight bearing as tolerated if there is excellent bony support. If a structural bone graft was required, weight bearing should be restricted for 6 to 12 weeks.

Patients should use a walker or crutches until muscle weakness resolves, usually between 3 and 12 weeks after surgery. Patients should avoid picking things up off the floor or putting on their socks and shoes without an extender (flexing the hip beyond 90°) until the capsule becomes secure, usually by 3 months after surgery. An elevated toilet seat and sleeping with a pillow between the legs helps for the first 6 weeks after revision surgery. If they are compliant and will walk and perform strengthening exercises, many patients do not need formal physical therapy. With more extensive procedures or with significant preoperative stiffness or weakness, prolonged physical therapy or even transfer to an inpatient rehabilitation center may be necessary. Patients with a trochanteric osteotomy should be managed with partial weight bearing and restricted active hip abduction until trochanteric healing is evident.

RESULTS

Cemented Acetabular Revision

The earliest revision series documented only cases done with cement, since uncemented implants were either unavailable or not in widespread use. In reported series, the definition of *failure* must be ascertained. Certainly, any revision must be viewed as a failure, but the definition must also include the radiographic criteria of loosening (Chapters 41 and 42). In seven studies the rerevision rate was low, ranging from 0 to 5% at 2 to 11 years of follow-up (67–73). The radiographic loosening rate, however, ranged from 17 to 71% in these series. A loose acetabular component seems to have greater forgiveness than does a loose cemented femoral component; patients may continue to function at a reasonable level despite having an acetabular component that is radiographically loose. Berry and Müller (74) reported on the use of an antiprotrusio cage in the face of massive structural defects of the acetabulum. The failure rate was 24% at an average of 5-years follow-up in these very difficult cases. The failures were split evenly between infection and loosening.

Cementless Acetabular Revision

Because of the increased failure rate seen with cemented components, there has been a shift toward uncemented components, especially when bone stock is adequate. Three series reported results with a porous hemispherical cup at 3.5 to 4.5 years of follow-up. The revision rate was low, 0% in two and 0.7% in the third. Unlike the cemented revision series, the radiographic loosening rate was also low, ranging from 0 to 2.9% (75–77).

Cemented Femoral Revision

As noted, it is difficult to achieve cement interdigitation in the femoral revision, which is so important to long-term success. Early studies reported rerevision rates of 9 to 40% at 2 to 10 years of follow-up (67,73,78). The failure rate was even higher if radiographic loosening was included, in one series adding an additional 29% (79).

Better cementing techniques can improve the results. Two studies reported rerevision rates of 9.5 and 10.5%, at 10 and 11 years, respectively (70,80). Radiographic failures were an additional 16 and 11%, which is an improvement over previous studies but still represents 25.5 and 29.5% failure in 10 years or more.

Cemented femoral revisions may be more promising with the Ling technique, by which cement is combined with intramedullary cancellous allografting to address bone loss. Elting et al. (81) reported a 5% fracture rate and a 93% bone incorporation rate at 31 months of follow-up. Gie et al. (61) also reported evidence of bone incorporation at 30 months of follow-up. There was a 3.6% fracture rate, but no stems were revised for loosening.

Cementless Femoral Revision

Because of the difficulty of cemented fixation in the revision situation, interest has increased in cementless femoral revision. Results are poor if the stem used was designed for primary THR and was simply lengthened. One study noted that the Bias (Zimmer; Warsaw, IN) implant had a 0% revision rate but a 32% incidence of subsidence at 4.5 years (82). Another series examined the Osteonics (Allendale, NJ) uncemented stem and noted an 8.7% revision rate and a 57% subsidence rate at 3 years, along with a 46% intraoperative fracture rate (83).

The bony environment is markedly different in revision than in the primary surgery. The upper metaphyseal bone may be atrophic or deficient. An uncemented stem must have intraoperative stability. Proximal-coated designs must fill the metaphysis completely with circumferential porous coating. Alternatively, fully-coated stems may be jammed into the uncompromised bone of the diaphysis below the old prosthetic bed. When these designs are used, the results are much better.

The S-ROM stem is a modular, uncemented device that achieves excellent fit at both the proximal and the distal aspects of the femur. McCarthy et al. (84) reported on a series at an average of 5 years of follow-up and noted a 1.5% revision rate and an additional 4% subsidence rate. Chandler et al. (85) found a 4% revision rate and a 6% subsidence rate at an average of 3 years. Cameron (86) recorded a 6.8% revision rate with the shorter primary length stem but a 16% failure rate in cases requiring a longer revision prosthesis at an average of 3.5 years.

Two series focused on fully-coated stems made by DePuy (Warsaw, IN). Lawrence et al. (87) noted a 5.7% rerevision rate and a 1.1% rate of additional radiographic loosening at an average follow-up of 8.4 years with the AML prosthesis. Paprosky et al. (88) found a 6% rerevision at 5.8

years using the Solution prosthesis. It will be interesting to see if these good results will persevere after a decade of service.

SUMMARY

In summary, the surgeon should be able to execute any of the various surgical approaches that may be necessary to perform the revision procedure. Cemented or cementless implants may not be optimal in all situations. The surgeon must assess the bone quality as part of the preoperative planning and have available the most appropriate implants for the reconstruction. Depending on the complexity of the revision, a large array of revision tools and bone grafting materials may be required. Preoperative planning is mandatory to ensure that intraoperative surprises are kept to a minimum.

REFERENCES

1. Davy DT, Kotzar GM, Brown RH, et al. Telemetric force measurements across the hip after total arthroplasty. J Bone Joint Surg 1988;70A:45–50.
2. Hodge WA, Carlson KL, Fijan RS, et al. Contact pressures from an instrumented hip endoprosthesis. J Bone Joint Surg 1989;71A: 1378–1386.
3. Charnley J. Low friction arthroplasty of the hip: theory and practice. Berlin: Springer-Verlag, 1979.
4. Li S, Chang JD, Barrena EG, et al. Nonconsolidated polyethylene particles and oxidation in Charnley acetabular cups. Clin Orthop 1995;319:54–63.
5. Rimnac CM, Klein RW, Betts F, Wright TM. Post-irradiation aging of ultra-high molecular weight polyethylene. J Bone Joint Surg 1994;76A:1052–1056.
6. Gomez-Barrena E, Chang JD, Li S, et al. The role of polyethylene properties in osteolysis after total hip replacement. Instr Course Lect 1996;45:187–197.
7. Callaghan JJ, Pellicci PM, Salvati EA, et al. Fracture of the femoral component. Analysis of failure and long-term follow-up of revision. Orthop Clin North Am 1988;19:637–647.
8. Cook SD. Materials consideration in total joint replacement. In: Callaghan JJ, Dennis DD, Paprosky WG, Rosenberg AG, eds. Hip and knee reconstruction. Rosemont, IL: American Academy of Orthopaedic Surgeons, 1995:27–34.
9. Charnley J. Anchorage of the femoral head prosthesis to the shaft of the femur. J Bone Joint Surg 1960;42B:28.
10. Jasty M. Why cemented femoral components become loose. Instr Course Lect 1991;40:151–159.
11. Noble PC, Tullos HS, Landon GC. The optimum cement mantle for total hip replacement: theory and practice. Instr Course Lect 1991;40:145–150.
12. McCoy TH, Salvati EA, Ranawat CS, Wilson PD, Jr. A fifteen-year follow-up study of one hundred Charnley low-friction arthroplasties. Orthop Clin North Am 1988;19:467–476.
13. Schulte KR, Callaghan JJ, Kelley SS, Johnston RC. The outcome of Charnley total hip arthroplasty with cement after a minimum twenty-year follow-up. The results of one surgeon. J Bone Joint Surg 1993;75A:961–975.
14. Kavanagh BF, Wallrichs S, Dewitz M, et al. Charnley low-friction arthroplasty of the hip. Twenty-year results with cement. J Arthroplasty 1994;9:229–234.
15. Sullivan PM, MacKenzie JR, Callaghan JJ, Johnston RC. Total hip arthroplasty with cement in patients who are less than fifty years old. A sixteen to twenty-two-year follow-up study. J Bone Joint Surg 1994;76A:863–869.
16. Neumann L, Freund KG, Sorensen KH. Total hip arthroplasty with

the Charnley prosthesis in patients fifty-five years old and less. Fifteen- to twenty-one-year results. J Bone Joint Surg 1996; 78A:73–79.

17. Mulroy WF, Estok DM, Harris WH. Total hip arthroplasty with use of so-called second-generation cementing techniques. A fifteen-year-average follow-up study. J Bone Joint Surg 1995;77A: 1845–1852.

18. Barrack RL, Mulroy RD Jr, Harris WH. Improved cementing techniques and femoral component loosening in young patients with hip arthroplasty. A 12-year radiographic review. J Bone Joint Surg 1992;74B:385–389.

19. Dorr LD, Luckett M, Conaty JP. Total hip arthroplasties in patients younger than 45 years. A nine- to ten-year follow-up study. Clin Orthop 1990;260:215–219.

20. Collis DK. Long-term (twelve to eighteen-year) follow-up of cemented total hip replacements in patients who were less than fifty years old. A follow-up note. J Bone Joint Surg 1991;73A: 593–597.

21. Chandler HP, Reineck FT, Wixson RL, McCarthy JC. Total hip replacement in patients younger than thirty years old. A five-year follow-up study. J Bone Joint Surg 1981;63A:1426–1434.

22. Bartel DL, Bicknell VL, Wright TM. The effect of conformity, thickness, and material on stresses in ultra-high molecular weight components for total joint replacement. J Bone Joint Surg 1986; 68A:1041–1051.

23. Bono JV, Sanford L, Toussaint JT. Severe polyethylene wear in total hip arthroplasty. Observations from retrieved AML PLUS hip implants with an ACS polyethylene liner. J Arthroplasty 1994; 9:119–125.

24. Barrack RL, Burke DW, Cook SD, et al. Complications related to modularity of total hip components. J Bone Joint Surg 1993; 75B:688–692.

25. Schmalzried TP, Jasty M, Harris WH. Periprosthetic bone loss in total hip arthroplasty. Polyethylene wear debris and the concept of the effective joint space. J Bone Joint Surg 1992;74A:849–863.

26. Horowitz SM, Doty SB, Lane JM, Burstein AH. Studies of the mechanism by which the mechanical failure of polymethylmethacrylate leads to bone resorption. J Bone Joint Surg 1993;75A:802–813.

27. Agins HJ, Alcock NW, Bansal M, et al. Metallic wear in failed titanium-alloy total hip replacements. A histological and quantitative analysis. J Bone Joint Surg 1988;70A:347–356.

28. Buly RL, Huo MH, Salvati E, et al. Titanium wear debris in failed cemented total hip arthroplasty. An analysis of 71 cases. J Arthroplasty 1992;7:315–323.

29. Lerouge S, Huk O, Yahia L, et al. Ceramic-ceramic and metal-polyethylene total hip replacements: comparison of pseudomembranes after loosening. J Bone Joint Surg 1997;79B: 135–139.

30. Huk OL, Bansal M, Betts F, et al. Polyethylene and metal debris generated by non-articulating surfaces of modular acetabular components. J Bone Joint Surg 1994;76B:568–574.

31. Salvati EA, Lieberman JR, Huk OL, Evans BG. Complications of femoral and acetabular modularity. Clin Orthop 1995;319:85–93.

32. Jacobs JJ, Sumner DR, Galante JO. Mechanisms of bone loss associated with total hip replacement. Orthop Clin North Am 1993; 24:583–590.

33. Fitzgerald RH, Nasser S. Infection following total hip arthroplasty. In: Callaghan JJ, Dennis DD, Paprosky WG, Rosenberg AG, eds. Hip and knee reconstruction. Rosemont, IL: American Academy of Orthopaedic Surgeons, 1995:157–161.

34. Daly PJ, Morrey BF. Operative correction of an unstable total hip arthroplasty. J Bone Joint Surg 1992;74A:1334–1343.

35. Ghelman B. Three methods for determining anteversion and retroversion of a total hip prosthesis. AJR Am J Roentgenol 1979; 133:1127–1134.

36. Harris WH, McGann WA. Loosening of the femoral component after use of the medullary-plug cementing technique. Follow-up note with a minimum five-year follow-up. J Bone Joint Surg 1986; 68A:1064–1066.

37. Engh CA, Massin P, Suthers KE. Roentgenographic assessment of the biologic fixation of porous-surfaced femoral components. Clin Orthop 1990;257:107–128.

38. Livermore J, Ilstrup D, Morrey B. Effect of femoral head size on wear of the polyethylene acetabular component. J Bone Joint Surg 1990;72A:518–528.

39. Fehring TK, Guilford WB, Baron J. Assessment of intrapelvic cement and screws in revision total hip arthroplasty. J Arthroplasty 1992;7:509–518.

40. Potter HG, Montgomery KD, Padgett DE, et al. Magnetic resonance imaging of the pelvis. New orthopaedic applications. Clin Orthop 1995;319:223–231.

41. Palestro CJ, Kim CK, Swyer AJ, et al. Total-hip arthroplasty: periprosthetic indium-111-labeled leukocyte activity and complementary technetium-99m-sulfur colloid imaging in suspected infection. J Nucl Med 1990;31:1950–1955.

42. Barrack RL, Harris WH. The value of aspiration of the hip joint before revision total hip arthroplasty. J Bone Joint Surg 1993;75A: 66–76.

43. Shih LY, Wu JJ, Yang DJ. Erythrocyte sedimentation rate and C-reactive protein values in patients with total hip arthroplasty. Clin Orthop 1987;225:238–246.

44. Feldman DS, Lonner JH, Desai P, Zuckerman JD. The role of intraoperative frozen sections in revision total joint arthroplasty. J Bone Joint Surg 1995;77A:1807–1813.

45. Dohmae Y, Bechtold JE, Sherman RE, et al. Reduction in cement-bone interface shear strength between primary and revision arthroplasty. Clin Orthop 1988;236:214–220.

46. Masri BA, Duncan CP, Masri BA, et al. Classification of bone loss in total hip arthroplasty. Instr Course Lect 1996;45:199–208.

47. Mallory TH. Preparation of the proximal femur in cementless total hip revision. Clin Orthop 1988;235:47–60.

48. Paprosky WG, Perona PG, Lawrence JM. Acetabular defect classification and surgical reconstruction in revision arthroplasty. A 6-year follow-up evaluation. J Arthroplasty 1994;9:33–44.

49. Hardinge K. The direct lateral approach to the hip. J Bone Joint Surg 1982;64B:17–19.

50. Frndak PA, Mallory TH, Lombardi AV Jr. Translateral surgical approach to the hip. The abductor muscle split. Clin Orthop 1993; 295:135–141.

51. McGrory BJ, Bal BS, Harris WH. Trochanteric osteotomy for total hip arthroplasty: six variations and indications for their use. J Am Acad Orthop Surg 1996;4:258–267.

52. Glassman AH, Engh CA, Bobyn JD. A technique of extensile exposure for total hip arthroplasty. J Arthroplasty 1987;2:11–21.

53. Dall D. Exposure of the hip by anterior osteotomy of the greater trochanter. A modified anterolateral approach. J Bone Joint Surg 1986;68B:382–386.

54. Wagner H. Revision prosthesis for the hip joint in severe bone loss. Orthopäde 1987;16:295–300.

55. Younger TI, Bradford MS, Magnus RE, Paprosky WG. Extended proximal femoral osteotomy. A new technique for femoral revision arthroplasty. J Arthroplasty 1995;10:329–338.

56. Schurman DJ, Maloney WJ. Segmental cement extraction at revision total hip arthroplasty. Clin Orthop 1992;285:158–163.

57. Klein AH, Rubash HE. Femoral windows in revision total hip arthroplasty. Clin Orthop 1993;291:164–170.

58. Lieberman JR, Moeckel BH, Evans BG, et al. Cement-within-cement revision hip arthroplasty. J Bone Joint Surg 1993;75B: 869–871.

59. Glassman AH, Engh CA. The removal of porous-coated femoral hip stems. Clin Orthop 1992;285:164–180.

60. Lachiewicz PF, Anspach WED. Removal of a well fixed acetabular component. A brief technical note of a new method. J Bone Joint Surg 1991;73A:1355–1356.

61. Gie GA, Linder L, Ling RS, et al. Impacted cancellous allografts and cement for revision total hip arthroplasty. J Bone Joint Surg 1993;75B:14–21.

62. Gross AE, Hutchison CR, Alexeeff M, et al. Proximal femoral allo-

grafts for reconstruction of bone stock in revision arthroplasty of the hip. Clin Orthop 1995;319:151–158.

63. Paprosky WG, Magnus RE. Principles of bone grafting in revision total hip arthroplasty. Acetabular technique. Clin Orthop 1994; 298:147–155.

64. Gross AE, Allan DG, Catre M, et al. Bone grafts in hip replacement surgery. The pelvic side. Orthop Clin North Am 1993;24:679–695.

65. Helfet DL, Anand N, Malkani AL, et al. Intraoperative monitoring of motor pathways during operative fixation of acute acetabular fractures. J Orthop Trauma 1997;11:2–6.

66. Wasielewski RC, Cooperstein LA, Kruger MP, Rubash HE. Acetabular anatomy and the transacetabular fixation of screws in total hip arthroplasty. J Bone Joint Surg 1990;72A:501–508.

67. Kavanagh BF, Ilstrup DM, Fitzgerald RH, Jr. Revision total hip arthroplasty. J Bone Joint Surg 1985;67A:517–526.

68. Pellicci PM. Results of revision total hip replacement. Instr Course Lect 1986;35:150–151.

69. Callaghan JJ, Salvati EA, Pellicci PM, et al. Results of revision for mechanical failure after cemented total hip replacement, 1979 to 1982. A two to five-year follow-up. J Bone Joint Surg 1985;67A: 1074–1085.

70. Estok DM II, Harris WH. Long-term results of cemented femoral revision surgery using second-generation techniques. An average 11.7-year follow-up evaluation. Clin Orthop 1994;299:190–202.

71. Marti RK, Schuller HM, Besselaar PP, et al. Results of revision of hip arthroplasty with cement. A five to fourteen-year follow-up study. J Bone Joint Surg 1990;72A:346–354.

72. Engelbrecht DJ, Weber FA, Sweet MB, Jakim I. Long-term results of revision total hip arthroplasty. J Bone Joint Surg 1990;72B: 41–45.

73. Amstutz HC, Ma SM, Jinnah RH, Mai L. Revision of aseptic loose total hip arthroplasties. Clin Orthop 1982;170:21–33.

74. Berry DJ, Müller ME. Revision arthroplasty using an anti-protrusio cage for massive acetabular bone deficiency. J Bone Joint Surg 1992;74B:711–715.

75. Padgett DE, Kull L, Rosenberg A, et al. Revision of the acetabular component without cement after total hip arthroplasty. Three to six-year follow-up. J Bone Joint Surg 1993;75A:663–673.

76. Tanzer M, Drucker D, Jasty M, et al. Revision of the acetabular component with an uncemented Harris-Galante porous-coated prosthesis. J Bone Joint Surg 1992;74A:987–994.

77. Engh CA, Glassman AH, Griffin WL, Mayer JG. Results of cementless revision for failed cemented total hip arthroplasty. Clin Orthop 1988;235:91–110.

78. Pellicci PM, Wilson PD Jr, Sledge CB, et al. Revision total hip arthroplasty. Clin Orthop 1982;170:34–41.

79. Pellicci PM, Wilson PD Jr, Sledge CB, et al. Long-term results of revision total hip replacement. A follow-up report. J Bone Joint Surg 1985;67A:513–516.

80. Katz RP, Callaghan JJ, Sullivan PM, Johnston RC. Results of cemented femoral revision total hip arthroplasty using improved cementing techniques. Clin Orthop 1995;319:178–183.

81. Elting JJ, Mikhail WE, Zicat BA, et al. Preliminary report of impaction grafting for exchange femoral arthroplasty. Clin Orthop 1995;319:159–167.

82. Hussamy O, Lachiewicz PF. Revision total hip arthroplasty with the BIAS (Biologic Ingrowth Anatomic System) femoral component. Three to six-year results. J Bone Joint Surg 1994;76A: 1137–1148.

83. Malkani AL, Lewallen DG, Cabanela ME, Wallrichs SL. Femoral component revision using an uncemented, proximally coated, long-stem prosthesis. J Arthroplasty 1996;11:411–418.

84. McCarthy JC, Mattingly D, Turner RH. Revision of the deficient femur with a modular femoral component. Orthop Trans 1993; 17:965–966.

85. Chandler HP, Ayres DK, Tan RC, et al. Revision total hip replacement using the S-ROM femoral component. Clin Orthop 1995; 319:130–140.

86. Cameron HU. The two- to six-year results with a proximally modular noncemented total hip replacement used in hip revisions. Clin Orthop 1994;298:47–53.

87. Lawrence JM, Engh CA, Macalino GE. Revision total hip arthroplasty. Long-term results without cement. Orthop Clin North Am 1993;24:635–644.

88. Paprosky WG, Jablonsky W, Magnus RE. Cementless femoral revision in the presence of severe proximal bone loss using diaphyseal fixation. Orthop Trans 1993;17:965–966.

Osteotomy and Arthrodesis of the Hip

Most patients with osteoarthritis of the hip develop disabling symptoms in their seventh or eighth decade. When the situation becomes intolerable, total hip arthroplasty will provide predictable pain relief and functional improvement. A certain subset of patients, however, develop disabling symptoms at a much younger age. The majority of these cases are attributable to known disorders, especially developmental dysplasia and slipped capital femoral epiphysis (1–7). The greater the anomaly, the earlier the onset of symptoms. Other less common causes of disabling hip symptoms, such as trauma or avascular necrosis, can occur at any age.

Great strides have been made in the field of total hip arthroplasty. The problems of wear debris generation and osteolysis remain, however, particularly for young patients because of their longevity and increased activity levels, which result in higher failure rates (8–10). Total hip arthroplasty, especially in the younger patient, should be considered the operation of last resort. If the biomechanical situation of the hip can be improved by timely, alternative surgical intervention, it may be possible to postpone total hip arthroplasty for many years. A total hip arthroplasty can still be performed, if needed, when the patient is older and much less active.

It is important not only to recognize which patients are candidates for a nonreplacement surgical procedure but also to determine the timing of intervention. Surgical intervention must take place before hip joint destruction renders any option but total hip arthroplasty untenable. This chapter discusses the various surgical options for the young adult with arthritis of the hip.

INITIAL FINDINGS, PHYSICAL EXAMINATION, AND DIAGNOSIS

Patients who had hip dysplasia as an infant may have had a dislocated hip that required open or closed reduc-

tion, casting, or bracing in childhood. Subsequent hip pain is usually insidious in origin and may be present only with athletic activities. The age of onset of hip pain and degeneration depends on the degree of dysplasia (11). An intoeing gait may be present, if the dysplasia is associated with excessive femoral anteversion.

Patients with an old slipped capital femoral epiphysis may recall a period of hip or knee pain in adolescence and will often have restricted range of motion, especially internal rotation. Patients with avascular necrosis may have sudden onset of hip symptoms.

Symptoms in patients with dysplasia may be related to abnormalities of the acetabular labrum and to articular cartilage loss (12,13). The pathology of the labrum is proportional to the degree of dysplasia. Labral tears or detachments along with osseous or extraosseous ganglia are the rule rather than the exception. When present, symptoms such as clicking, catching, and locking may occur along with pain.

Initially, the range of motion is normal in patients with hip dysplasia. Excessive femoral anteversion will result in limited external rotation. If osteophytes develop, there may be limited range of motion in any axis, depending on the location. Along with decreased range of motion, there may be impingement pain at the extreme limits of motion or night pain with a posterior acetabular osteophyte. Patients with avascular necrosis may develop mechanical symptoms along with increased pain once subchondral collapse occurs. As synovitis and chondrolysis progress, pain may become increasingly severe and motion restricted. At this point, alternatives such as hip osteotomy may no longer provide relief.

RADIOLOGIC STUDIES

All patients should have an AP view of the pelvis along with some type of lateral view, depending on the abnormality. Functional views are taken, if indicated, to simulate the correction possible with various osteotomies.

Dysplasia

Patients with pain in the early stages of dyplasia may have subtle radiographic findings. Radiographs obtained should include an AP view of the pelvis, a frog lateral view and a faux profile (false profile, or lateral) of the involved hip and, if indicated, an abduction film (14). The bone morphology may suggest acetabular insufficiency, indicated on the AP pelvis view by deficient lateral coverage of the femoral head and a center-edge angle of Wiberg of less than 25° (Fig. 45.1) (15,16). Anterior acetabular coverage is usually deficient as well, and there may even be a global loss of femoral head coverage (17). The amount of anterior coverage can be determined by the faux profile view. An anterior center-edge angle of 25° or less indicates dysplasia. Both anterior and lateral center-edge angles should be determined, as the coverage deficiency may not be symmetric at the anterior and lateral locations. A bone cyst seen at the superolateral corner of the acetabulum usually indicates an intraosseous ganglion arising from the abnormal labrum. With more severe degrees of deformity, the head may be subluxed superiorly.

An abduction view should be obtained to determine whether the head reduces into the acetabulum (Fig. 45.2). This view is useful for assessing how the joint should appear if a varus osteotomy of the femur or a derotation osteotomy of the acetabulum were performed. Other functional views may be helpful: An adduction of the leg can be done to simulate a valgus osteotomy, and a flexion view of the hip to simulate an extension osteotomy. Angling the x-ray beam in a caudad direction simulates a flexion osteotomy of the hip (18,19); and a frog lateral radiograph gives a true orthogonal view of the femoral head for assessing its shape (spherical or ovoid) and documenting osteophytes. The joint space must be assessed for narrowing, which indicates articular cartilage loss. The neck-shaft angle should be noted for the presence of either coxa valga or vara, either of which may exist with acetabular dysplasia. Patients treated for dislocation of the hip in infancy may have sustained a growth arrest of the head, which creates a short femoral neck with relative overgrowth of the greater trochanter (20) (Fig. 45.3).

Avascular Necrosis of the Femoral Head

If the vascular insult occurred before skeletal maturity, as in Perthes disease, the femoral head may not be spher-

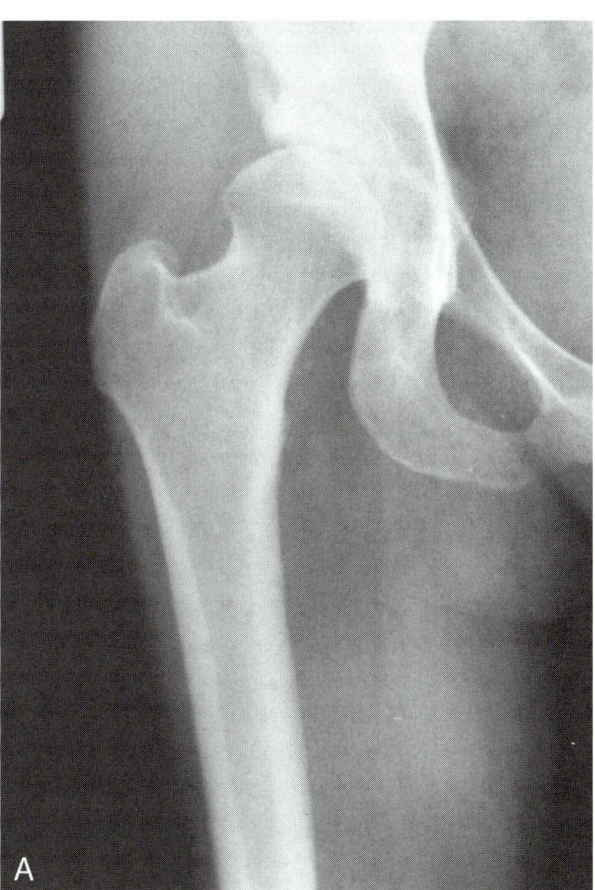
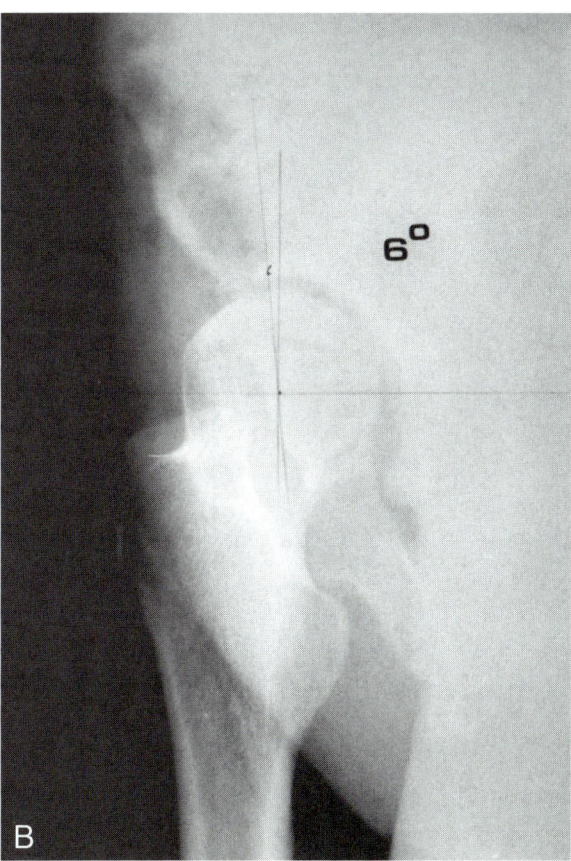

Figure 45.1. AP (**A**) and false profile lateral (**B**) views of a 27-year-old female with a dysplastic left hip. *(continued)*

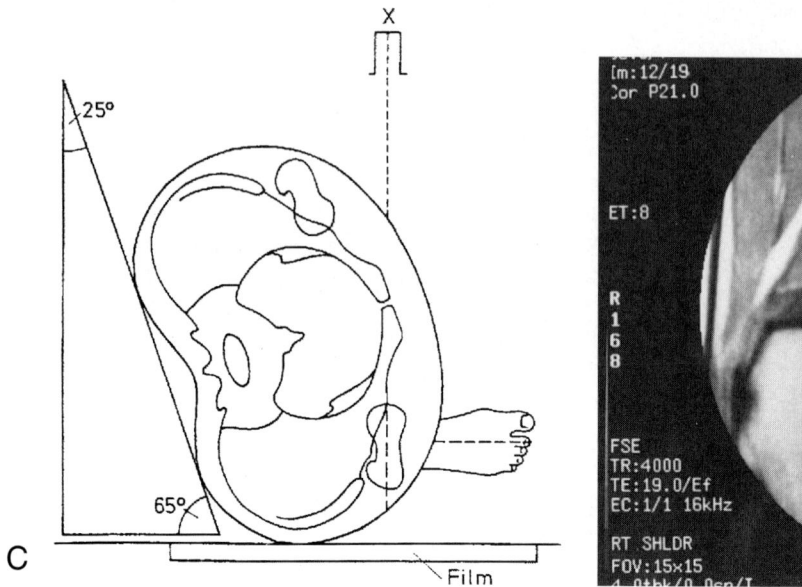

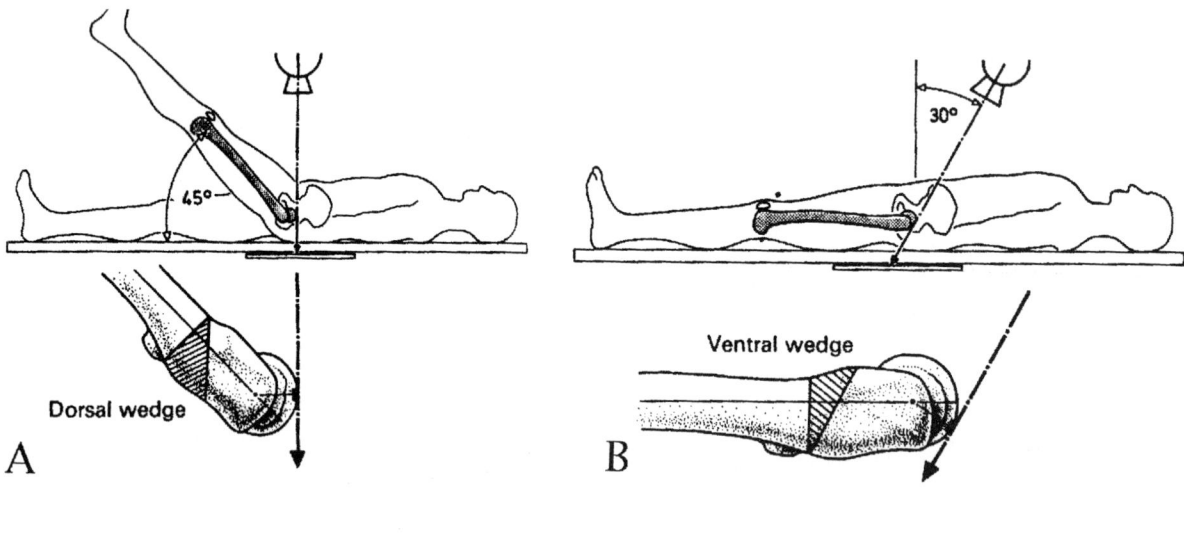

Figure 45.1. *(continued)* **C.** Technique for the obtaining the false profile lateral view. Reprinted with permission from Tonnis D. Congenital dysplasia and dislocation of the hip in children and adults. New York: Springer-Verlag, 1984:102. **D.** MRI study showing the labral pathology and ganglion formation associated with dysplasia.

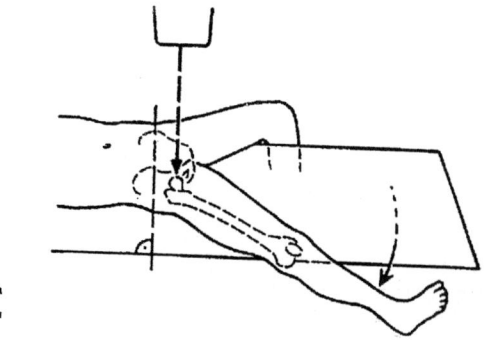

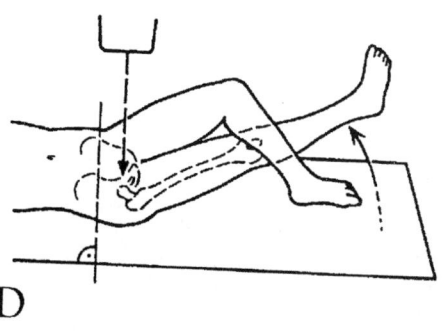

Figure 45.2. A. Flexion of the hip simulates an extension intertrochanteric osteotomy. **B.** Angling the x-ray beam in a caudad direction simulates a flexion osteotomy. Abduction (**C**) and adduction (**D**) views simulate varus and valgus correction in the coronal plane. Reprinted with permission from Schatzker J, ed. The intertrochanteric osteotomy. New York: Springer-Verlag, 1984.

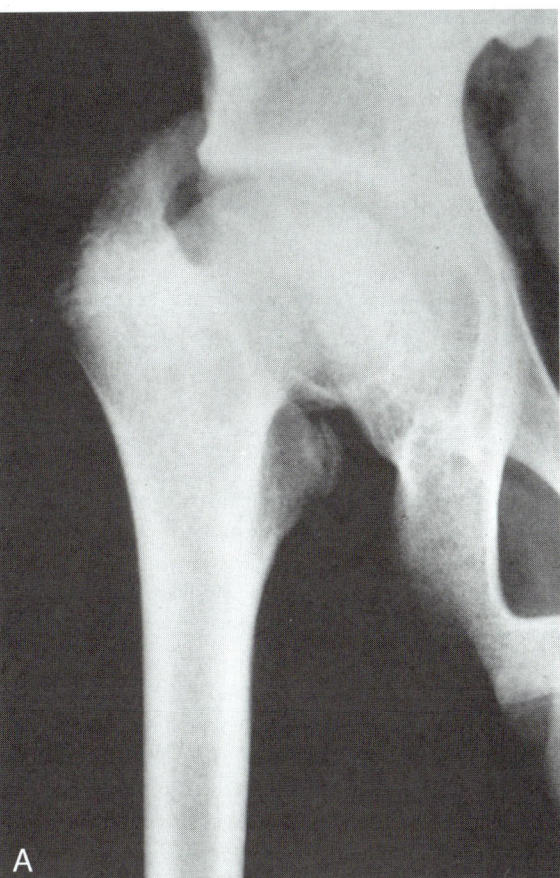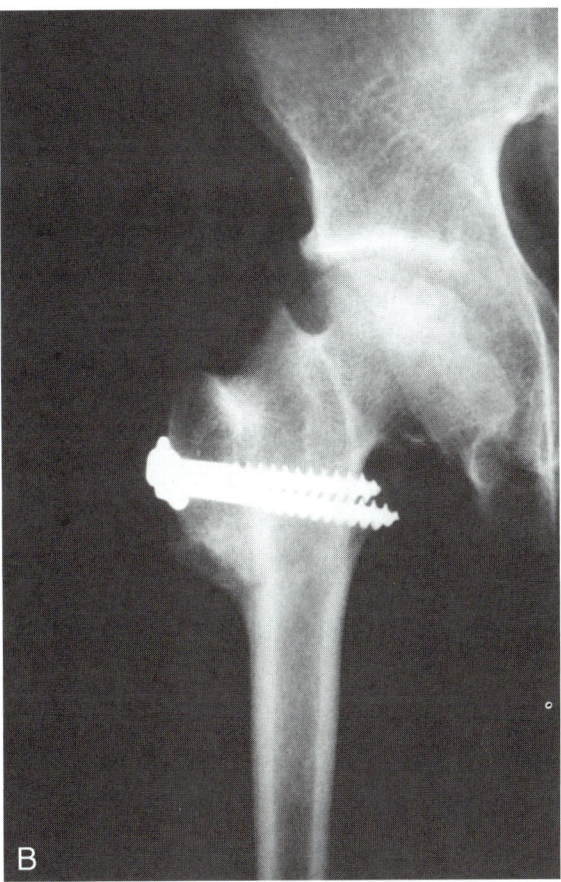

Figure 45.3. A. Overgrowth of the greater trochanter caused by damage of the capital femoral physis in infancy as a result of sepsis. **B.** Postoperative view of advancement of the greater trochanter.

ical (coxa plana) or may be too large for the acetabulum (coxa magna). Areas of subchondral collapse or chondritis may be present. With extensive head involvement, relative overgrowth of the greater trochanter may be present. Patients with incongruous joints may present with hip pain that seems to be out of proportion to the degree of joint space loss (21,22).

Skeletally mature patients with avascular necrosis usually have normal bone morphology in the early stages of the disease. Radiographs may be entirely normal, and the necrosis is detected only by bone or MRI scan. The femoral head is visualized in the AP and frog lateral views. The lateral view is especially important for assessing the degree of head involvement and/or subchondral bone collapse. Following head collapse (Ficat stage III), the hip may go onto arthritis, manifested by joint space loss (Ficat stage IV) (23).

Slipped Capital Femoral Epiphysis

Studies with instrumented hip arthroplasties have documented that the highest in vivo hip joint forces are found on the anterosuperior aspect of the femoral head (24). It is then no surprise that the majority of slipped capital

femoral epiphyses (SCFEs) have a deformity in which the head has fallen into varus and retroversion (25). The resultant deformity in adults is a pistol-grip appearance of the proximal femur seen on the AP radiograph (2,3). A bulge of bone is usually noted on the anterosuperior aspect of the femoral neck. The joint space may have a variable amount of narrowing; and osteophytes can be found on the neck, head, or rim of the acetabulum. Larger osteophytes may create impingement between the greater trochanter and the rim of the acetabulum as seen on an abduction film. The false profile view is the best method for assessing the posterior aspect of the joint for narrowing and osteophytes.

Posttraumatic Deformity

FRACTURES OF THE FEMORAL NECK

Femoral neck fractures in young patients are surgical emergencies that require open reduction and internal fixation (ORIF). Despite these efforts, young patients may go on to nonunion of the femoral neck and/or avascular necrosis of the femoral head. The risks are high due to the violent forces that are usually required to fracture the dense bone of younger patients. Femoral neck nonunion may be present after surgical fixation or may be noted for the first time weeks or months after trauma, if there is a delay in seeking medical attention. Tomograms of the femoral neck may be used in ambiguous cases to ascertain whether a nonunion is present. The status of the hardware should also be assessed (fatigue fracture, implant migration, intraarticular violation).

Avascular necrosis of the femoral head may be readily apparent on routine radiographs. If not, an MRI study should be obtained to rule out necrosis before surgical correction is performed. If necrosis is present, a joint-sparing procedure may no longer be indicated. The MRI scan also helps assess the status of the articular surfaces in the hip joint and the labrum, other potential sources of pain following trauma.

INTERTROCHANTERIC FRACTURES

Plain radiographs are used to assess whether intertochanteric fractures have gone onto union, supplemented with tomograms in equivocal cases. Malunions are readily apparent on plain radiographs. The condition and location of hardware should be noted. An MRI study should be obtained if there is any possibility of avascular necrosis, labral injury, or articular cartilage damage.

ACETABULAR FRACTURES

Patients may present de novo with neglected acetabular fractures or with pain following surgical correction. Plain radiographs (AP pelvis and frog lateral views) must be obtained along with the two Judet oblique views to ascertain if the fracture has healed and if the reduction achieved was acceptable. The condition of the joint space and the femoral head should be apparent. The location of hardware is critical to rule out intra-articular violation. CT scans help assess fracture and hip joint reduction, intra-articular hardware, and loose bodies. MRI scans may be obtained, even after hardware placement, to assess femoral head viability and the status of the articular cartilage and labrum (26).

IDIOPATHIC ARTHRITIS

On occasions, a young patient presents with arthritis that has no apparent underlying cause. Radiographic studies may reveal an inflammatory picture with diffuse joint space loss and synovitis. Some patients present with findings more typical of osteoarthritis, including asymmetric joint space loss and osteophyte formation.

TREATMENT

Nonoperative Treatment

Following the initial presentation, a course of nonoperative therapy is usually warranted. Activity modification, rest, physical therapy, and a course of nonsteroidal anti-inflammatories are all helpful, especially if there is any chance that the pain may be the result of bursitis, ten-

donitis, or synovitis. It is important to recognize the hip at risk, which occurs predominantly in the young patient with dysplasia or avascular necrosis. A wait-and-see attitude may lead to rapid, irreversible cartilage loss that might then preclude nonreplacement surgical options. This tenet is not as critical once advanced osteoarthritis is already present, including severe joint space loss and osteophyte formation. In these cases, operative intervention is usually limited to salvage procedures. If the only viable option is total hip arthroplasty, it is usually preferable to delay the procedure as long as possible, especially in the young patient.

Operative Treatment

Surgical options include intertrochanteric osteotomy of the femur, periacetabular osteotomy of the pelvis, advancement of the greater trochanter, arthrodesis, other salvage procedures (Chiari osteotomy of the pelvis), and total hip replacement. The selection depends on the patient's age, bone morphology and/or deformity, femoral head blood supply, and degree of arthritis (Clinical Table). We have found intertrochanteric osteotomy of the femur, periacetabular osteotomy of the pelvis, advancement of the greater trochanter, and arthrodesis to be extremely useful in the management of young patients. We rarely employ the Chiari osteotomy, since pain relief seems to be unpredictable and most patients can be managed with one of the other procedures. Primary total hip replacement is discussed in Chapters 41 and 42.

INTERTROCHANTERIC OSTEOTOMY OF THE FEMUR

The goal of the intertrochanteric osteotomy of the femur is to relieve pain and to improve hip function by altering the biomechanics of the joint. The osteotomy is usually made in the intertrochanteric region and may require any or all of the components of angulation, displacement, rotation, and length (Fig. 45.4). Pain relief and improved function can often be achieved by (a) replacing a weight-bearing eburnated and delineated area of the head with a head segment that still has remaining articular cartilage, (b) improving acetabular coverage of the femoral head, (c) moving an osteonecrotic segment out from under the acetabulum, (d) correcting the deformity and restoring a more sound biomechanical construct, and (e) improving the range of motion.

In coxa valga or dysplasia, an attempt is made to improve articular cartilage contact area and joint stability by placing the head deeper into the socket, usually with a varus osteotomy of the femur, with or without a pelvic osteotomy (18,19,27–30). Maistrelli et al. (31) described a valgus-extension osteotomy to improve joint congruency that uses the capital drop osteophyte.

Intertrochanteric osteotomy can be used for avascular necrosis, provided that a joint space remains (i.e., Ficat stage III or less) and the area of head involvement is small enough to allow viable bone and cartilage to be rotated

Clinical Table: Osteotomy and Arthrodesis of the Hip

Procedure	Indications	Technique	Anatomy	Pitfalls
Intertrochanteric osteotomy	• Coxa valga • Avascular necrosis • Femoral neck nonunion • SCFE • Femoral head lesion	• Preoperative planning • Lateral approach • Osteotomy above the lesser trochanter • Blade plate fixation	• Medial femoral circumflex vessels • Perforating vessels	• Poor planning • Malpositioned chisel • Femoral neck perforation • Insufficient bone bridge • Insufficient correction
Periacetabular osteotomy	• Acetabular dysplasia	• Smith-Petersen or ilioinguinal approach • Open capsule for labral tears • Cut through the ilium, ischium, and pubis • Screw fixation	• Femoral nerve • Lateral femoral cutaneous nerve • Femoral vessels • Obturator neurovascular bundle • Sciatic nerve • Superior gluteal vessels	• Nerve injury • Vascular injury and bleeding • Joint violation • Blind ischial cut • Poor acetabular mobilization • Insufficient correction
Greater trochanteric advancement	• Relative overgrowth of the trochanter • Impingement on the ilium • Abductor muscle weakness	• Lateral approach • Mobilize the trochanter • Screw fixation	• Medial femoral circumflex vessels	• Blood supply to femoral head • Insufficient mobilization of trochanter • Inadequate fixation
Hip arthrodesis	• Severe hip arthritis • Unilateral hip pathology	• Lateral or anterior approach • Spare the greater trochanter and abductors • Confirm the hip position • Plate fixation with supplemental screws	• Femoral nerve • Lateral femoral cutaneous nerve • Superior gluteal neurovascular bundle • Inadequate fixation	• Poor hip position • neurovascular injury • Bleeding • Blood supply to femoral head injured

into the weight-bearing zone with the osteotomy (Fig. 45.5). It has been suggested that the combined angles subtending the necrotic areas on an AP and lateral radiographs should be 200° or less (32–34). A flexion intertrochanteric osteotomy is frequently used for avascular necrosis, because most lesions are on the anterior section of the femoral head, and flexion of the shaft (and thus extension of the proximal fragment) moves the necrotic segment farther out the front of the hip joint. Flexion may be combined with either varus or valgus osteotomy, depending on location of the lesion. With more extensive areas of involvement, the entire head may be rotated up to 180° (35).

Valgus osteotomies are useful when a femoral neck fracture results in a nonunion. The nonunion is often vertically oriented (i.e., a high Pauwels angle), with high shear stresses at the interface. The goal of the valgus osteotomy is to stabilize the nonunion site and convert the shear stresses to compressive stresses by placing the nonunion site perpendicular to the resultant hip forces (36,37). A flexion intertrochanteric osteotomy that corrects the severe retroversion deformity following slipped capital femoral epiphysis has been described (38).

Technique

Preoperative planning is probably the most important step in the performance of any osteotomy, especially in the proximal femur when a three-dimensional correction is mandated (18,30). Functional radiographs simulate how the joint should appear after the osteotomy. Tracings should be made, detailing the steps involved, location of the osteotomy, manipulation of the fragments, and internal fixation type and location. An intraoperative image intensifier greatly facilitates the osteotomy, the placement of internal fixation, and the assessment of the degree of correction. It is important to understand the affect of a varus or valgus displacement on the mechanical axis of the leg and knee (Fig. 45.6). For this reason, medialization should occur with the varus osteotomy and lateralization should occur with the valgus osteotomy.

The patient is positioned supine on a fluoroscopy table with the involved extremity, flank, hip, and groin draped free. A straight lateral approach (Watson-Jones) to the hip is used. The fascia lata is opened longitudinally and extended proximally to expose the greater trochanter. The vastus lateralis is elevated off the lateral femur by incising the fascia just anterior to its insertion along the linea as-

Figure 45.4. Types of intertrochanteric osteotomies. Reprinted with permission from Schatzker J, ed. The intertrochanteric osteotomy. New York: Springer-Verlag, 1984.

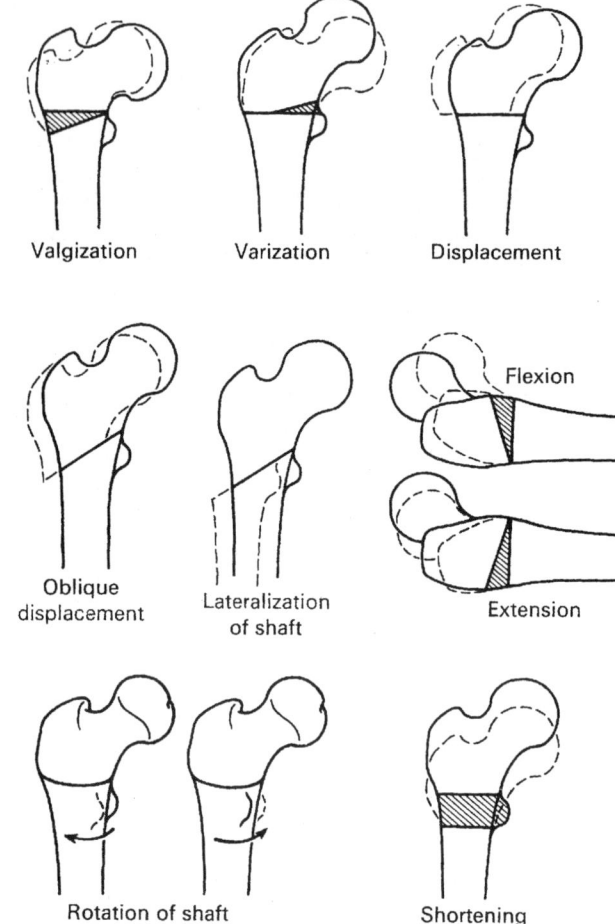

Valgization   Varization   Displacement

Oblique displacement   Lateralization of shaft   Flexion   Extension

Rotation of shaft   Shortening

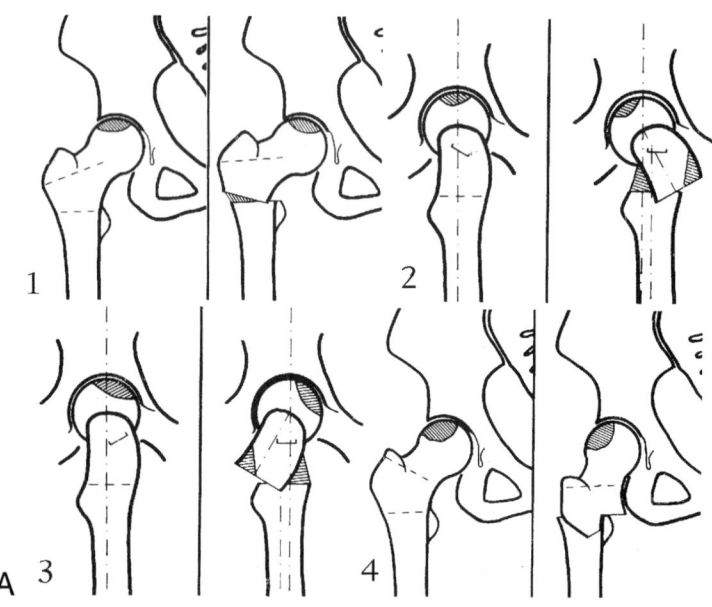

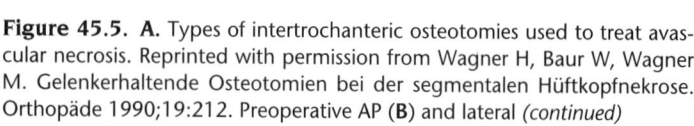

Figure 45.5. A. Types of intertrochanteric osteotomies used to treat avascular necrosis. Reprinted with permission from Wagner H, Baur W, Wagner M. Gelenkerhaltende Osteotomien bei der segmentalen Hüftkopfnekrose. Orthopäde 1990;19:212. Preoperative AP (**B**) and lateral *(continued)*

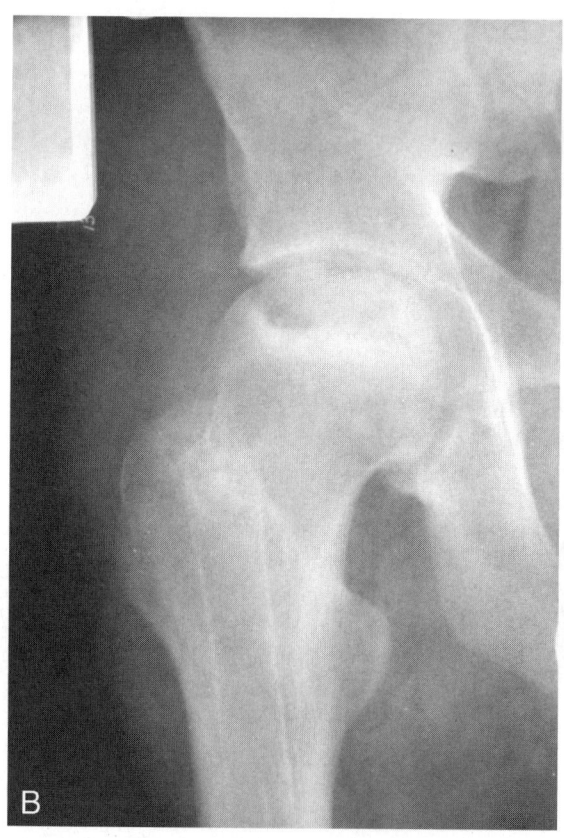

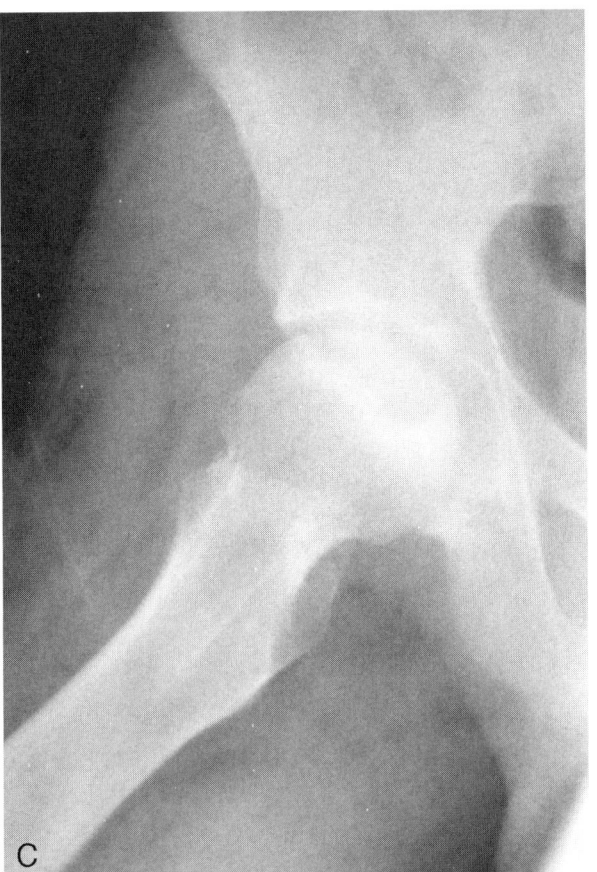

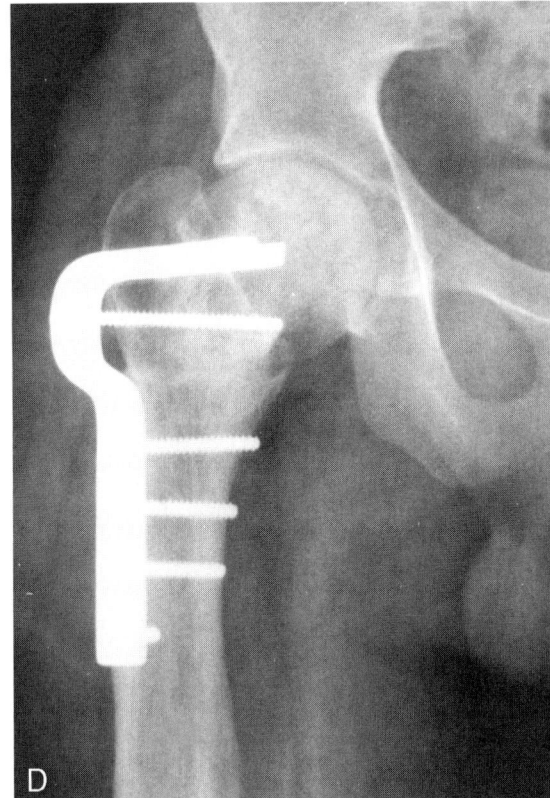

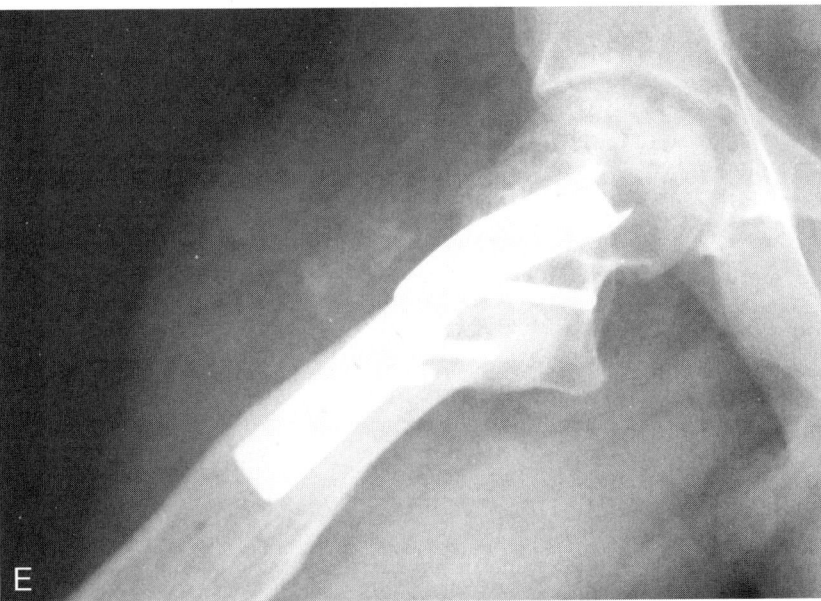

Figure 45.5. *(continued)* **(C)** views of a hip with avascular necrosis. AP **(D)** and lateral **(E)** views of a proximal femur, showing the results of the varus flexion intertrochanteric osteotomy, which moved the necrotic segment from the apex.

Figure 45.6. Effect of a varus intertrochanteric osteotomy on the mechanical axis of the leg and knee. Varus alone swings the mechanical axis into the medial compartment (**B**). Medial displacement alone places it into the lateral compartment (**C**). The shaft should be medialized with a varus osteotomy to maintain the axis in the center of the knee (**D**). The opposite is true for a valgus osteotomy. Reprinted with permission from Schatzker J, ed. The intertrochanteric osteotomy. New York: Springer-Verlag, 1984.

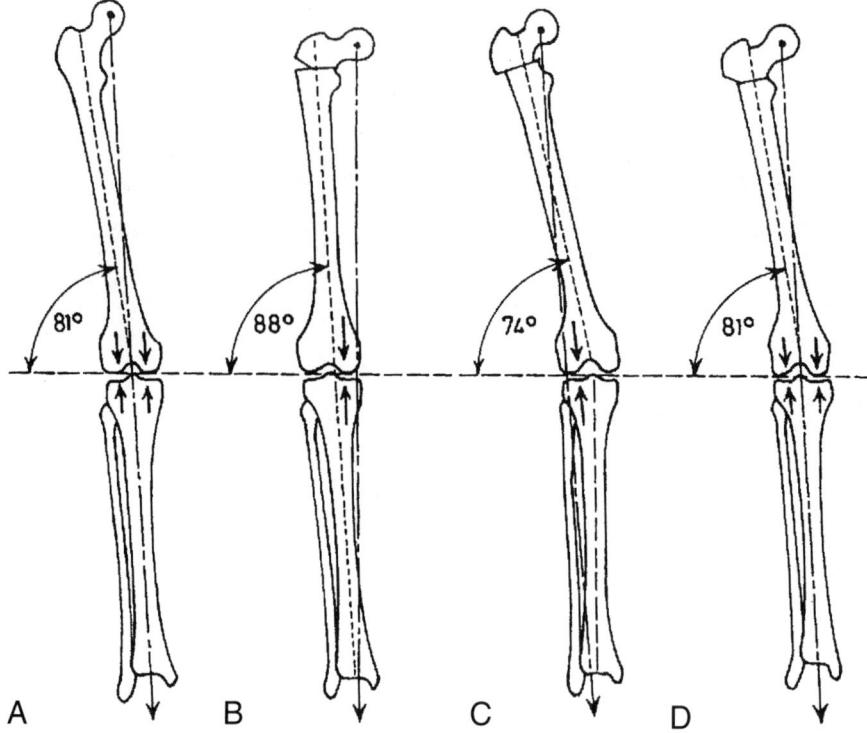

pera. Perforating vessels must be identified and coagulated. The vastus fascial incision is curved anteriorly as it is extended proximally, leaving a 1- to 2-cm cuff of the origin distal to the vastus ridge for reattachment. After sweeping the vastus lateralis anteriorly and medially, the shaft is exposed. If hip arthrotomy is required, the anterior capsule is exposed by elevating the anterior edge of the abductors.

The 90° osteotomy blade plate (Synthes; Paoli, PA) is used for varus osteotomies, since it permits 10°, 15°, or 20° of medial displacement of the shaft (Fig. 45.7). Blade lengths for the adult osteotomy plates are 50, 60, or 70 mm. The size is determined from the preoperative plan. For valgus osteotomies, the 110°, 120°, or 130° angled osteotomy blade plate is used. It may be helpful to plan with the 120° plate, since this may be switched to the 110° or 130° plate if it appears that there is either too much or too little correction. The most critical step in the intertrochanteric osteotomy is the insertion of the blade plate chisel. The point and angle of insertion (in both the sagittal and coronal planes) depends on the blade plate used and the amount of correction desired.

Guidewires are placed, and the positions are checked on the image intensifier (Fig. 45.8). One wire is placed along the anterior neck to assess femoral anteversion, one wire is placed at the proposed osteotomy, and one wire is placed in the femoral neck along the proposed chisel path. The angular triangles included in the blade plate set help orient the chisel in relation to the femoral shaft and the floor. For varus or valgus correction alone, the chisel is inserted without flexion or extension. If flexion or extension is to be performed, the handle of the chisel must be

flexed or extended the desired amount. Progress of the chisel is checked on fluoroscopy on the AP view, and the lateral view may be checked by frogging the leg and moving the image intensifier to an oblique angle. The chisel must be extracted a few millimeters after each centimeter of insertion to prevent entrapment in dense bone.

The osteotomy is usually transverse to the long axis of the shaft and is made at the upper border of the lesser trochanter. There should be at least a 2-cm bridge of bone between the chisel path and the osteotomy. Two parallel Kirschner (K) wires are inserted on either side of the proposed osteotomy. This is done to assess the degree of rotation, which may be difficult once the osteotomy is made. It is not necessary to remove a wedge of bone for a varus osteotomy; because the osteotomy is stabilized with impaction, healing is predictable and shortening is minimized. The predetermined angled osteotomy blade plate is then inserted, and the plate is clamped to the shaft, affecting the correction. For a valgus osteotomy, it is usually helpful to remove a lateral wedge from the distal fragment to enhance apposition. Additional wedges may be required if substantial flexion or extension has been performed. The distal fragment should be laterally displaced for a valgus osteotomy and medially displaced for a varus osteotomy. If the bone is dense, it may be necessary to remove the medial corner of the proximal fragment with the varus osteotomy to have sufficient apposition of the fragments.

The angled osteotomy blade plate is held to the shaft with Verbrugge clamps, and the articulated tensioning device is attached to the last screw hole. Large compressive forces can be generated across the osteotomy with the ar-

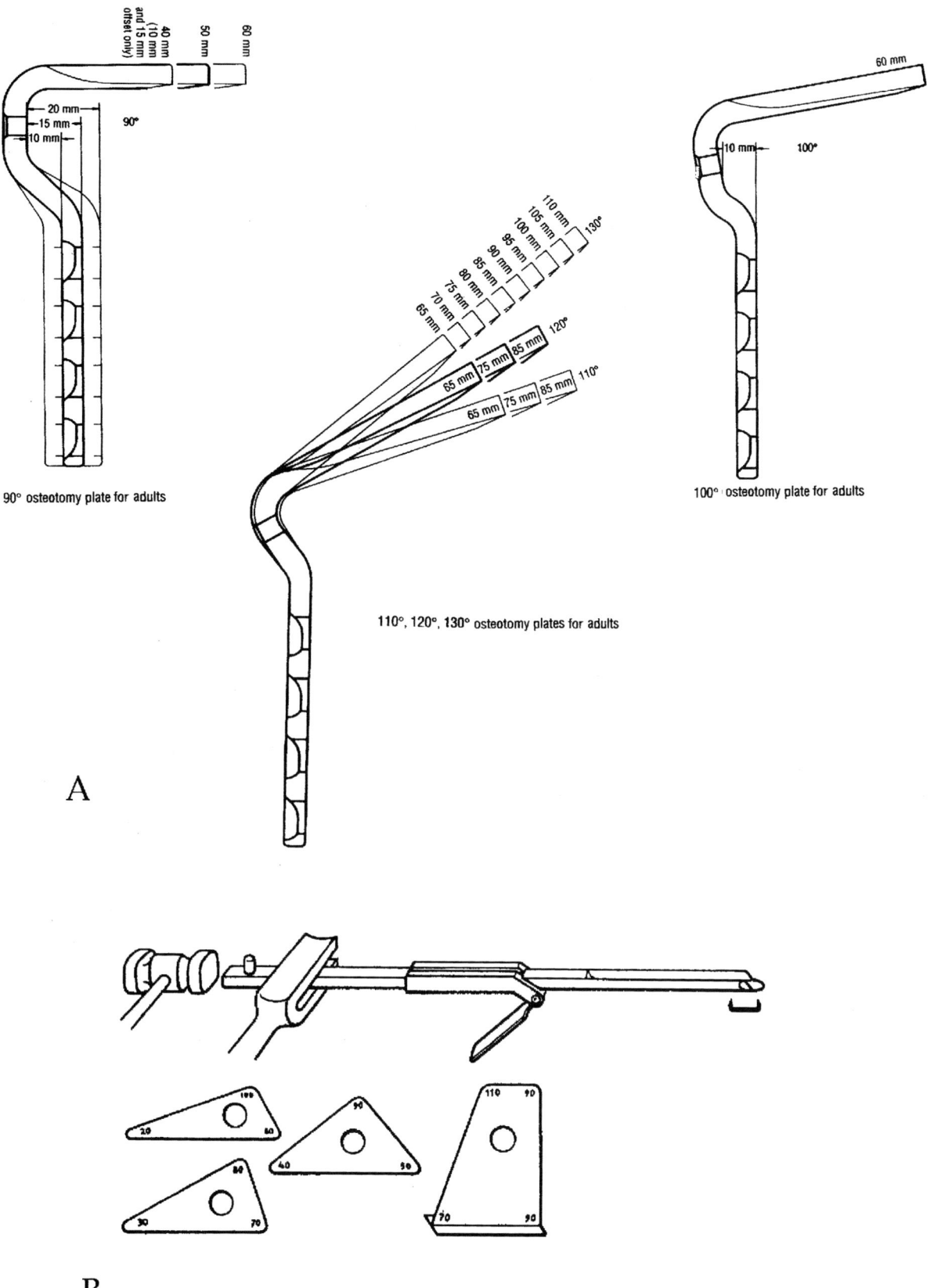

Figure 45.7. A. Plates used for intertrochanteric osteotomy. **B.** Blade plate instrument set. Reprinted with permission from Synthes, Paoli, PA.

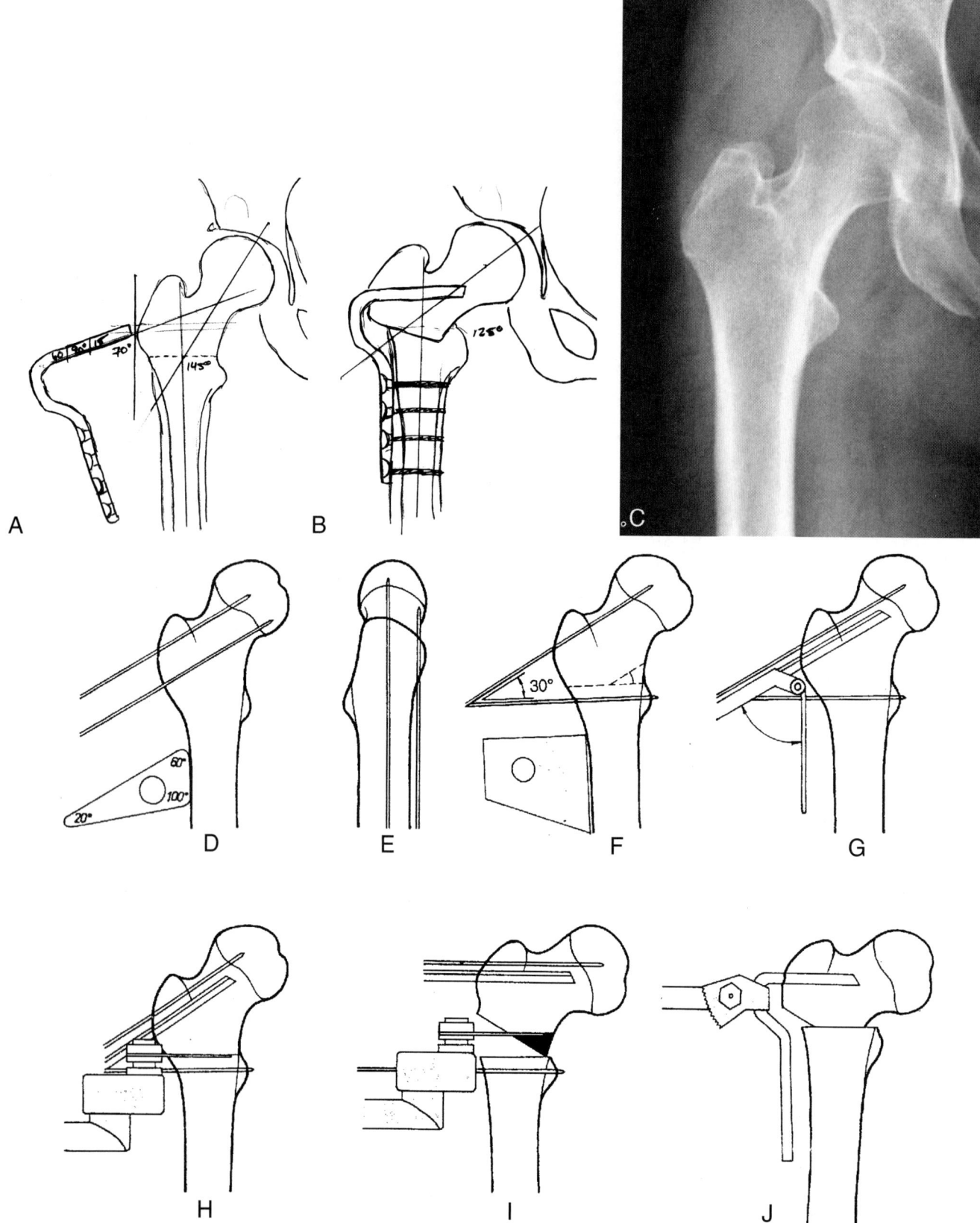

Figure 45.8. A and **B.** Preoperative plan for an intertrochanteric osteotomy of the femur. **C.** Preoperative view of a hip with coxa valga. **D–F.** K wires are placed along the proposed chisel path and osteotomy site. **G.** The chisel is inserted into the femoral neck. **H.** The osteotomy is performed. **I.** The medial corner of the proximal fragment is removed. **J.** The blade plate is inserted. *(continued)*

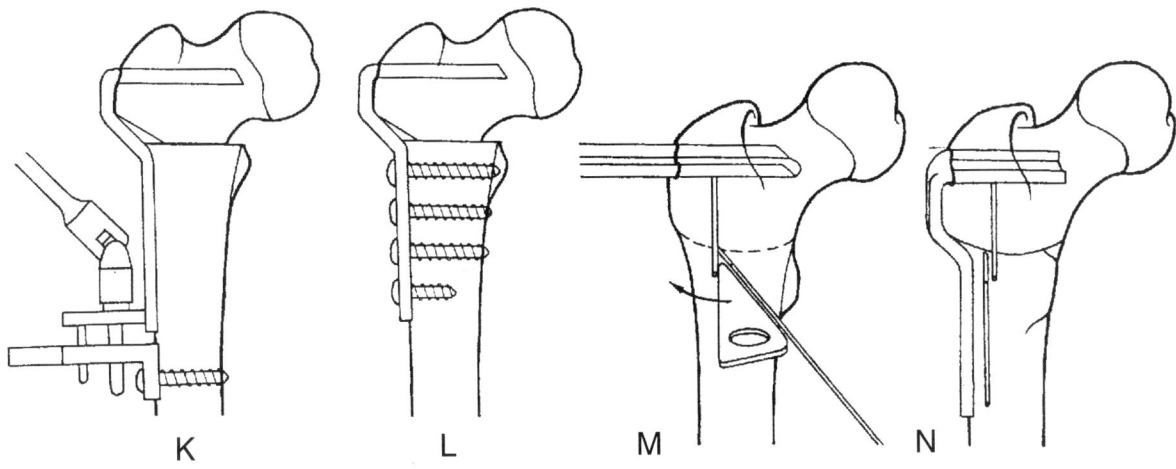

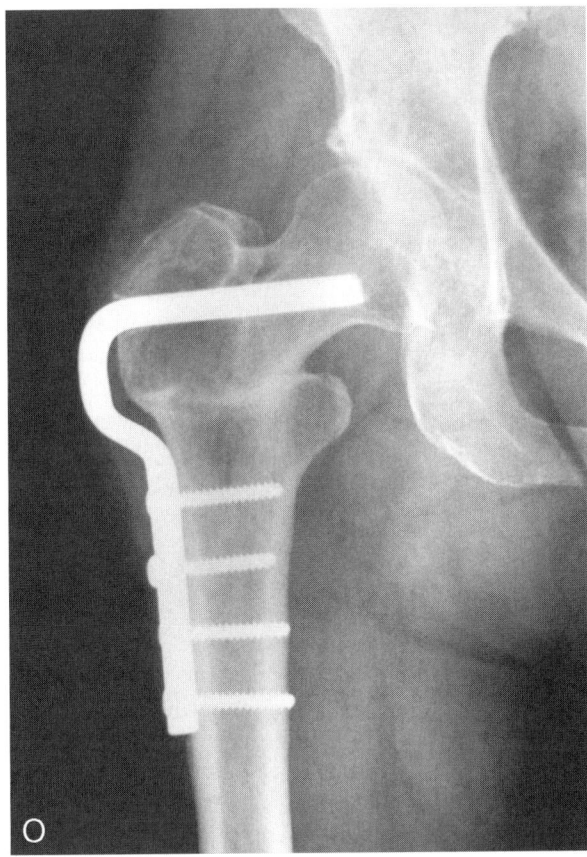

Figure 45.8. *(continued)* **K.** The blade plate is attached to the articulated tensioning device. **L.** Completion of osteotomy. **M** and **N.** Derotating the osteotomy. **O.** Postoperative view of the varus osteotomy. Reprinted with permission from Tonnis D. Congenital dysplasia and dislocation of the hip in children and adults. New York: Springer-Verlag, 1984.

ticulated tensioning device, and hence it should be anchored to the femoral shaft with a bicortical screw, distal to the plate. Care must be taken when tensioning a higher-angled valgus osteotomy blade plate, as the blade may slide out of the proximal fragment as a result of the oblique orientation of the blade relative to the applied compression forces. For the valgus osteotomy, a wedge of bone is usually removed to improve apposition and avoid excessive lengthening. A wedge of bone need not be removed with a varus osteotomy, as this will help minimize the shortening that the procedure produces. Drains are

placed, and the wounds are closed in layers with absorbable suture.

PERIACETABULAR OSTEOTOMY OF THE PELVIS

Certain conditions of hip dysplasia can be rectified by femoral osteotomy alone. If the femur is relatively normal and the problem is insufficient acetabular coverage, then a periacetabular osteotomy (PAO) should be performed. If there is both coxa valga and acetabular dysplasia, it may be necessary to perform a periacetabular and a femoral osteotomy. In hip dysplasia, the deficient coverage involves the roof of the acetabulum along with the supero-lateral and anterior walls. Not only is there inadequate contact between the femoral head and the acetabulum, but the acetabular roof is oblique, allowing the head to subluxate superiorly or laterally with weight bearing. A foreshortened roof places the labrum close to the apex of the femoral head where it is then subjected to unusual stresses. These stresses lead to labral tears, detachment, and ganglion formation. The goals of the PAO are to (a) stabilize the femoral head in the acetabulum; (b) increase the contact between the femoral head and acetabulum, thus stopping the inexorable progression of arthritis; and (c) move the labrum to a more peripheral location to prevent further labral deterioration and to decrease the accompanying mechanical symptoms.

To be a suitable candidate for a PAO, the patient should have sufficient hip joint space remaining and congruent joint surfaces. A preoperative AP x-ray with the hip abducted is useful to simulate the appearance after periacetabular osteotomy. Patients older than 50 years should opt for total hip arthroplasty as a less complicated alternative, because they are less likely to need future revision surgery.

Many pelvic osteotomies have been described. The majority are osteotomies that are made at a considerable distance from the acetabulum (39–42). The disadvantage with this type of osteotomy is that the correction may be more difficult to obtain in the adult patient, since most of the hemipelvis must be mobilized. The dense posterior pelvic ligaments and floor tether the fragment, and the sciatic nerve is at significant risk, because the sciatic notch is included and must be moved as well.

The alternative pelvic osteotomy is the juxta-articular spherical osteotomy (43–45). This procedure is technically demanding and has significant risks, including intra-articular osteotomy, chondrolysis, and devascularization of the acetabular fragment.

At our institution, we employ a procedure that is a compromise of the two, the PAO as described by Ganz et al. (46) (Fig. 45.9). The posterior column and greater sciatic notch are left intact, minimizing risk to the sciatic nerve. The posterior column ligamentous attachments and the pelvic floor are left intact, allowing extensive mobilization and correction. The osteotomies for the PAO are far enough from the joint so that intra-articular violation is unlikely; and the periacetabular blood supply, if the procedure is done carefully, is not violated.

Technique

The PAO is performed with the patient supine on a fluoroscopy table. It is preferable to use spontaneous electromyographic (EMG) monitoring during the procedure, to minimize the risk to the major nerves, especially the sciatic (47). Either the ilioinguinal or iliofemoral (Smith-Petersen) approach may be used (48). Patients should be warned that the lateral femoral cutaneous nerve is at risk and may be damaged during the operation. If the ilioin-guinal approach is used, the incision is placed 2.5 to 5 cm (1 to 2 in) farther distally than originally described. When combined with an osteotomy of the anterior superior iliac spine, easier access to the hip joint is possible (19).

Ilioinguinal approach. The incision for the ilioinguinal approach is made from the apex of the iliac crest to just lateral of the midline near the pubic symphysis. The external oblique muscle is opened to the level of the superficial ring, and the spermatic cord is protected with a Penrose drain. The anterior superior iliac spine is drilled and then osteotomized. The anterior superior iliac spine is mobilized in a medial and distal direction, with the inguinal ligament and sartorius reflected like an inverted U. The internal oblique and transversalis abdominal fascia are moved off the inguinal ligament to reveal the iliopsoas muscle and the femoral nerve. The lateral femoral cutaneous nerve is protected, if possible, but it may be severely stretched during the case. The iliopectineal fascia is isolated and incised along the pelvic brim to allow access to the quadrilateral plate through the middle window. The femoral vessels are identified medial to the iliopectineal fascia and may be isolated and protected with a Penrose drain or simply retracted medially. Access to the medial (third) window of this approach is usually not necessary. The straight head of the rectus femoris is released from the anterior inferior iliac spine, and the reflected head is released from the hip capsule. A capsulotomy is performed to inspect the joint if labrum pathology is suspected. If the labrum is intact but detached, it is repaired with nonabsorbable sutures through drill holes. If irreparable, it is resected.

Iliofemoral approach. An incision for the iliofemoral approach is made from the apex of the iliac crest and extended over the anterior hip joint and longitudinally into the upper thigh. Dissection is taken through the subcutaneous tissues down to the border between the tensor fascia lata laterally and the sartorius medially. Since the lateral femoral cutaneous nerve is usually in this interval, deeper dissection is extended through the fascia of the tensor fascia lata to expose the rectus. As with the ilioinguinal approach, the anterior superior iliac spine is drilled, osteotomized, and mobilized medially. The rectus is released in a similar fashion as described above.

The Osteotomies

The first osteotomy is made on the lateral surface of ischium below the acetabulum. This is a blind cut, which is made easier with a custom-designed forked osteotome with a 30° angle. The location and progress of the osteotome is followed with the image intensifier. The surgeon passes the osteotome between the medial hip capsule and iliopsoas tendon, after palpating the area with a finger. The hip must be flexed to allow relaxation of the iliopsoas. By tilting the image intensifier to either side, Judet oblique views are obtained to show the osteotome position on the ischial surface and the degree of penetration. Complete transection of the ischium is not necessary,

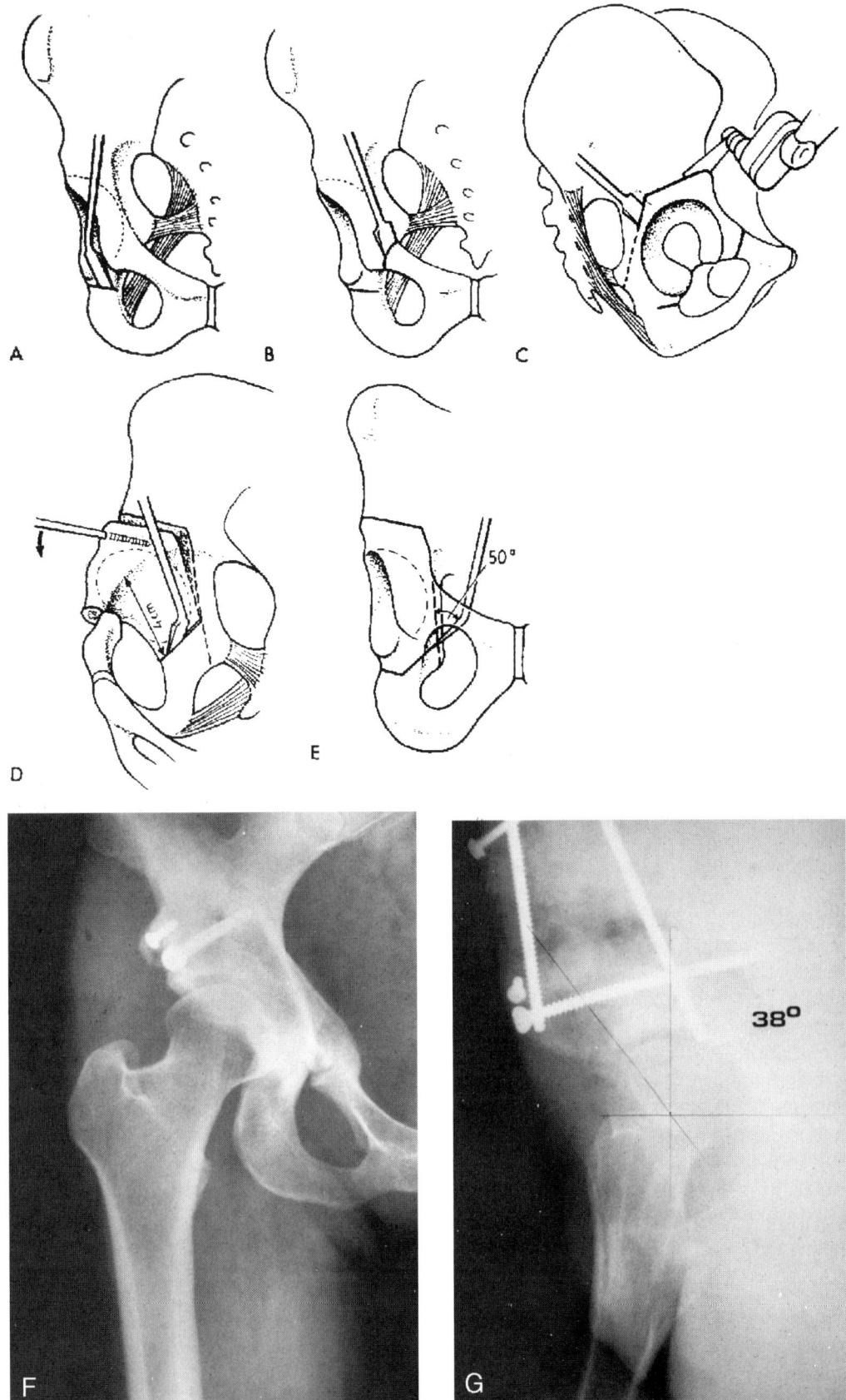

Figure 45.9. A. For a PAO, the ischial cut is made below acetabulum. **B.** Pubis cut. **C.** The iliac cut is made with oscillating saw and the posterior column cut is made with an angled osteotome. **D** and **E.** The ischial cut is completed below the quadrilateral plate with an angled osteotome. Reprinted with permission from Ganz R, Klaue K, Vinh TS, Mast JW. A new periacetabular osteotomy for the treatment of hip dysplasias. Technique and preliminary results. Clin Orthop 1988;232:26–36. AP (**F**) and false profile (**G**) views of the patient shown in Figure 45.1, taken at the 2-year follow-up.

but it must be scored sufficiently to allow for a controlled fracture once the acetabular fragment is mobilized.

A second cut is made through the superior pubic ramus medial to the iliopectineal eminence. This cut can be made through the middle window of the ilioinguinal approach or by retracting the iliacus muscle sufficiently (with maximal hip flexion) through the iliofemoral approach. Retractors protect the obturator neurovascular bundle lying beneath the superior pubic ramus. The osteotomy may be transverse or oblique, from proximal-medial to distal-lateral to increase the surface area for healing and to allow for unencumbered rotation of the acetabulum as it is redirected.

The third cut is made through the ilium, just above the anterior inferior iliac spine. This cut is made parallel to the acetabular roof; it is 4 to 5 cm long and stops 1 cm lateral to the pelvic brim. The iliacus muscle must have been mobilized earlier from the iliac fossa; and the abductor muscles are protected, lateral to the osteotomy, with a malleable retractor.

The fourth cut is made at a 120° angle to the iliac cut and is extended down the posterior column. Since this osteotomy is made between the dense bone of the greater sciatic notch and the posterior acetabulum, it tends to propagate distally to join up with the ischial cut that was made initially. The progression of this final cut may be followed with the image intensifier providing an iliac oblique view and is made with a nontoothed 30° angle osteotome.

A Schanz pin is placed into the anterior inferior iliac spine, and a lamina spreader is inserted into the iliac osteotomy. Mobility of the acetabulum is then assessed: It may be necessary to complete the ischial hinge with angled osteotomes that are placed inside the true pelvis 4 to 5 cm below the pelvic brim. The acetabulum should rotate when sufficiently free and not merely hinge out on the distal tether. To avoid undesired external rotation of the acetabular fragment, check the pubic ramus. With correction, the ends should be displaced approximately 100%, with the lateral end moving proximally and slightly posterior. The distal piece of the iliac osteotomy moves anteriorly with proper correction, jutting forward like a bow of a ship. The acetabular fragment is stabilized with Steinmann pins, and the correction is checked with the image intensifier. An AP pelvis radiograph should be obtained for a more precise assessment of the correction. There should be improved lateral and anterior coverage. The anterior coverage may be assessed on the iliac oblique view, which is an approximation of the false profile view. The acetabulum should not be lateralized but rotated to achieve correction.

Fixation of the acetabular fragment is provided with three 4.5-mm cortical screws, two of which are inserted antegrade from the iliac crest and the other inserted retrograde from just above the anterior roof directed toward the top of the greater sciatic notch. A final intraoperative AP pelvis radiograph is obtained, and the correction assessed. If adequate, the jutting portion of the ilium is removed to prevent impingement and may be used as bone graft. Additional graft may be taken from the inner table of the iliac crest, if necessary. The rectus origin is then repaired through drill holes, and the sartorius and inguinal ligament are repaired by reattaching the anterior superior iliac spine with a 3.5-mm cortical screw. The wound is closed in layers over drains; meticulous repair of the conjoined tendon and inguinal ligament prevents herniation in the ilioinguinal approach.

ADVANCEMENT OF THE GREATER TROCHANTER

Advancement of the greater trochanter is useful in the treatment of a high-riding trochanter, because it eliminates painful impingement in abduction and improves abductor muscle function and endurance (49,50). Wagner (51) considered the procedure to be "the most efficient joint-saving operation that may be performed about the hip." The advancement may be performed alone or in concert with other osteotomies, such as an intertrochanteric or periacetabular (Fig. 45.3).

Technique

For advancement of the greater trochanter, the patient is positioned supine on a fluoroscopy table. The direct lateral (Watson-Jones) approach to the hip is used, as for the intertrochanteric osteotomy. The vastus lateralis origin is released transversely just distal to the vastus ridge. Using image intensification, a K wire is placed along the proposed osteotomy, which is usually in line with the superior edge of the femoral neck. The osteotomy is performed with an oscillating saw and is stopped just short of the piriformis fossa. The osteotomy is then gently completed with a Lambotte osteotome. Great care is taken to minimize soft tissue disruption, especially the capsule and posterior tissues that provide vascularity to the femoral head. Soft tissue adhesions are released until the attached abductor muscles are "springy" and the trochanteric fragment can be advanced to its new location. The tip of the trochanter should now be even with the center of the femoral head.

The lateral cortex of the shaft is partially decorticated where the trochanter is to be placed to enhance bony healing. The trochanter is held in place with K wires; it may be necessary to abduct the leg to fully seat the trochanter. Two 4.5-mm cortical screws or 6.5-mm cancellous screws are placed with washers. The screw direction is proximal-lateral to distal-medial. After fixation, the hip is placed through range of motion to test the stability of the fixation. The screw heads are fully seated to avoid postoperative bursitis. The vastus origin is repaired with absorbable suture, and drains are placed deep to the fascia lata. The wound is then closed in layers.

ARTHRODESIS OF THE HIP

Femoral and periacetabular osteotomies work best when the joint surfaces are congruent and before the onset of arthritic changes. In certain situations, such as posttraumatic arthritis and septic arthritis, rapid irreversible damage may occur. The joint may have been destroyed before the initial presentation. In the older patient, total hip arthroplasty is the treatment of choice. The young patient, however, has a guarded long-term prognosis with a total hip arthroplasty. Other salvage reconstructive procedures include the Chiari pelvic osteotomy for dysplasia with joint incongruity; arthrotomy and osteophyte débridement, if the joint space remains and the patient has limited range of motion and true impingement pain; and arthrodesis of the hip.

Arthrodesis of the hip is indicated when there is advanced, disabling arthritis in a patient who is considered too young for total hip arthroplasty and in whom more conservative, reconstructive procedures are unlikely to work. Arthrodesis should provide pain relief by eliminating the grating of the eburnated joint surfaces. The arthritis must be limited to one hip. Arthrodesis is usually contraindicated for the inflammatory arthritides, because of the high incidence of bilateral hip disease and involvement of other joints. The same is true for avascular necrosis, unless the inciting event has been clearly documented and most likely will not occur in the contralateral hip. The contralateral hip should be examined by MRI scans to rule out silent avascular necrosis if the inciting event was thought to be the result of a systemic insult or disorder. The patient must also have a normal lumbar spine and ipsilateral knee. Patients with long-standing fusions are at risk for osteoarthritis in the contralateral hip, ipsilateral knee, and lumbar spine as a consequence of gait aberrations over time. A hip fused in a poor position may hasten this process and make the gait extremely awkward.

Arthrodesis is a good option for heavy patients and those who must perform strenuous labor. Low-demand patients with severe medical conditions may be better served with total hip arthroplasty. Patients have a difficult time understanding how it is possible to function with a fused hip and may benefit from meeting with a patient who has had a successful fusion. Although some activities, such as sitting or donning shoes may be awkward, patients are often surprised to see just how functional they can be with a hip arthrodesis.

Technique

A number of techniques have been described for hip arthrodesis (52). It is preferable to achieve rigid internal fixation to obviate the need for a cast immobilization in the postoperative period. A spica body cast may be required if fixation is inadequate or for the noncompliant patient. One of the more popular contemporary techniques is the lateral cobra-head plate procedure described by Schneider (53). An alternative is the anterior plate technique described by Matta et al. (54) (Fig. 45.10). The hip should be fused in 15° to 20° of flexion and 5° of external rotation. Leg position in the coronal plane is controversial. Adduction of 5° to 6° sets the mechanical axis of the leg perpendicular to the transverse pelvic axis (55). This posi-

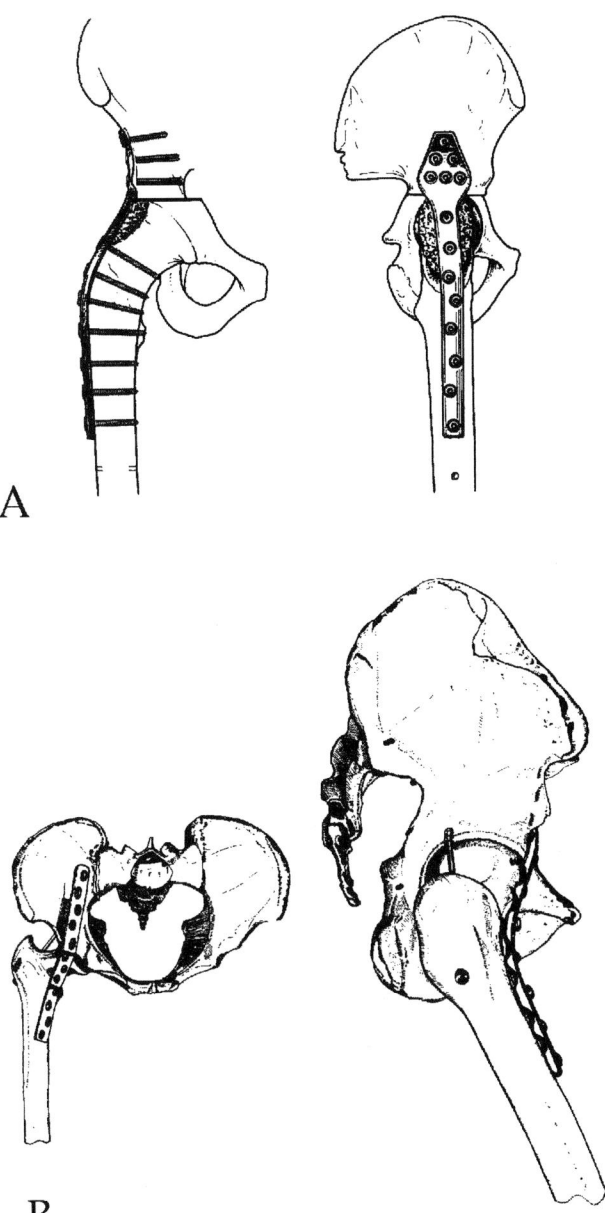

Figure 45.10. A. The Cobra plate technique for hip arthrodesis is performed through a lateral approach. Reprinted with permission from Lechti R. Hip arthrodesis and associated problems. New York: Springer-Verlag, 1978. **B.** Anterior plating technique for hip arthrodesis. Reprinted with permission from Matta JM, Siebenrock KA, Gautier E, et al. Hip fusion through an anterior approach with the use of a ventral plate. Clin Orthop 1997;337:129–139.

tion has also been recommended to minimize back and ipsilateral knee pain (56). Others report increased comfort with slight abduction (54). Anything in the range of 5° of abduction to 5° of adduction is probably acceptable.

Cobra plate technique. For the Cobra plate arthrodesis, the patient is positioned in a lateral decubitus position. The double-beanbag technique permits accurate positioning of the leg (57): One beanbag is positioned around the patient's torso, and the other is used to cradle the operative leg. An AP pelvis radiograph is obtained to assess the degree of abduction or adduction of the leg in the beanbag, and the position is adjusted as necessary. If internal fixation is subsequently applied with the leg in this position on the beanbag, the correct position in the coronal plane should be obtained. Hip flexion and rotation can then be assessed by noting the leg position in relation to the body.

A direct lateral (Watson-Jones) approach to the hip is used. As with the intertrochanteric osteotomy, the vastus lateralis is mobilized anteriorly. A trochanteric osteotomy is performed to expose the lateral ilium. An anterior arthrotomy is performed, and the hip is dislocated anteriorly. Acetabular reamers are used to remove the soft tissue from the socket, and femoral head reamers (from an old cup arthroplasty set) are used to denude the head of soft tissue. Alternatively, a high-speed, pneumatic burr may be used. The head is then reduced, and good bony apposition should be present. If not, morcellized iliac crest bone may be used to fill in the voids.

The Cobra plate is then contoured to the ilium, superior femoral neck, and lateral femoral shaft. The proximal screws are secured to the pelvis, and the articulated tensioning device is applied distal to the plate and used to compress the fusion site. An AP radiograph is checked to assess the position in the coronal plane; and if acceptable, the remainder of the femoral screws are applied.

The major criticism of this technique has been its destructive effect on the abductor musculature. This effect may be minimalized by mobilizing the abductor musculature and greater trochanter, which can then be applied over the plate. The greater trochanter is secured to the femur just anterior to the plate. If a total hip arthroplasty is later required, the greater trochanter may be osteotomized and the preserved abductor musculature elevated, thus providing a more predictable total hip arthroplasty.

Drains are inserted, the capsule and vastus fascia are repaired, and the wound is closed in layers with absorbable suture.

Anterior technique. For the anterior hip arthrodesis, the patient is positioned supine on a radiolucent table. The double-beanbag positioning technique may be used if desired. The iliofemoral approach (Smith-Peterson) is used, as described for the PAO; however, the femur must also be exposed. The tensor fascia lata is released from the lateral iliac crest, and the sartorius is released from the anterior superior iliac spine. The rectus is retracted medially, after its proximal release, as is the vastus lateralis. An anterior capsulotomy is performed, including joint débridement or dislocation as described above. A wide limited-contact dynamic compression titanium plate (Synthes; Paoli, PA) that is 12 to 14 holes long is contoured to the iliac fossa, anterior acetabular margin, and femoral neck and shaft. Care must be taken, as with all hip arthrodeses, to ensure proper hip flexion, external rotation, and abduction or adduction in the coronal plane. The proximal plate screws are inserted, and the articulated tensioning device is used to compress

the fusion site. While compression is maintained, the distal plate screws are inserted.

For additional fixation, two 7-mm cannulated screws are inserted from just below the greater trochanter, passing through the femoral neck and head and into the dense, supra-acetabular bone of the posterior column. Screw position is checked with the image intensifier. An intraoperative AP pelvis radiograph must be obtained. The capsule is repaired. The sartorius, tensor fascia lata, and rectus are repaired through drill holes with nonabsorbable sutures. The vastus fascia is repaired. The remainder of the wound is closed in layers with two subfascial drains: one in the iliac fossa and one along the femoral shaft.

PITFALLS

Intertrochanteric Osteotomy

Most pitfalls with the intertochanteric osteotomy can be prevented with careful preoperative planning, which is critical to a good result. The operation is merely the execution of this plan. Preoperative planning helps prevent intraoperative surprises and ensures that the proper implants are available. Furthermore, proper planning can prevent overcorrection or undercorrection. The use of the image intensifier and intraoperative radiographs also prevent malcorrection.

Another pitfall is the incarcerated blade plate chisel, which can be prevented by backing the chisel out after each centimeter of penetration, especially in young patients with dense bone. Chisel perforation of the cortical bone in the femoral neck can be prevented by placing a guidewire into the femoral neck first and following it with the chisel. The chisel's progress should be monitored with AP and lateral radiographic images. Fracture of the bone bridge between the osteotomy and blade can be avoided by keeping at least 2 cm of bone between the blade and the osteotomy site.

Periacetabular Osteotomy

For the PAO, an intra-articular osteotomy can be avoided by using the image intensifier to ensure that the chisel for the ischial cut is below the socket, that the pubic cut is medial to the socket, and that the posterior column osteotomy is between the greater sciatic notch and the articular surface. Inadequate mobility of the acetabular fragment can be prevented by checking all of the osteotomies to ensure that they have been completed. The culprit is usually the ischial cut, because it cannot be viewed directly.

It is important to make sure that there is sufficient mobility to permit rotation of the acetabular fragment. Lateralization of the acetabulum, which is caused by hinging the socket down and forward, should be avoided. External rotation of the fragment is caused by excessive pull on the Schanz pin. An intraoperative AP pelvic radiograph must be taken, even when an image intensifier is being used.

To avoid bleeding, induced hypotension is employed whenever possible. The nutrient vessel foramen entering the iliac fossa may need to be packed with bone wax. A corona mortis aberrant vessel may connect the iliac and obturator systems and is thus at risk with the ilioinguinal approach. The use of cell saver blood replacement is recommended. Arterial thrombosis can be prevented by avoiding any unnecessary retraction on the femoral vessels if the ilioinguinal incision is used.

Nerve injury is another pitfall. The sciatic nerve should be safe if the sciatic notch is kept intact. The lateral femoral cutaneous nerve may be damaged and may have to be sacrificed despite efforts for its preservation. The femoral nerve should be protected if it is maintained in continuity with the iliopsoas muscle. Retractors placed around the superior pubic ramus will help avoid injury to the obturator nerve.

Advancement of the Greater Trochanter

Avascular necrosis is a pitfall of the advancement of the greater trochanter. It can be prevented by making sure that the hip capsule is not violated and by avoiding excessive soft tissue dissection posteriorly in the piriformis fossa. Nonunion or loss of correction can be prevented by secure screw fixation of the trochanter to the femoral shaft. If fixation appears to be less than adequate or if the bone is osteopenic, a supplemental tension band wire may be used to counteract the pull of the abductor muscles.

Inadequate distalization can be avoided by making sure that the greater trochanter and abductor muscles are sufficiently free and have a springy feel when retracted distally. This is especially true if there has been previous surgery or scarring. Postoperative bursitis can be prevented by countersinking the screw heads into the greater trochanter to avoid excessive prominence.

Arthrodesis of the Hip

Malposition of the femur with arthrodesis of the hip can be avoided by using the double-beanbag position. An intraoperative AP pelvis radiograph should always be checked before final stabilization. The degree of hip flexion can be verified with the use of a sterile goniometer. Vascularity of the femoral head may already be compromised in cases of avascular necrosis. If the hip is to be dislocated for débridement of soft tissues, every attempt should be made to keep the posterior capsule and short extra rotators intact to maintain blood supply to the head.

The nerve most at risk of injury with the lateral Cobra plate technique is the superior gluteal nerve because of the proximal mobilization of the hip abductor muscles. With the anterior approach, the lateral femoral cutaneous nerve is at risk. The vastus lateralis muscle should be displaced medially to protect its femoral nerve supply.

Hip arthrodesis requires an extensive exposure and prolonged operating times; thus cell saver blood replacement should be used. With the anterior approach, the surgeon should watch for the nutrient vessel in the iliac fossa

as the iliacus is elevated and the lateral femoral circumflex branches in the rectus/vastus lateralis interval. With the Cobra plate technique, the superior gluteal artery is at risk as it exits the sciatic notch.

Inadequate fixation can be avoided by making sure the plate, whether the Cobra or anterior, is long enough to offer secure fixation into the pelvis (this is usually the weak link). The anterior approach has the advantage of providing excellent purchase in the sciatic buttress and allowing supplementation of the fixation with cannulated screws from the lateral aspect; thus there are two constructs at a 90° angle to each other. With either method, intraoperative attempts at mobilization of the femur should not demonstrate any motion at the fusion site.

REHABILITATION

Intertrochanteric Osteotomy

For the intertrochanteric osteotomy, secure internal fixation permits rapid mobilization. The patients begin toe-touch ambulation (9 kg; 20 lb) on postoperative day 1, along with range of motion and light strengthening exercises. After 6 weeks, partial weight bearing is maintained (25 to 50%) until 3 months after surgery. Full weight bearing is started at 3 months, if the osteotomy appears to be healed. Otherwise, partial weight bearing is maintained for an additional 1 to 2 months.

Periacetabular Osteotomy

Rehabilitation for PAO is similar to that for the intertrochanteric osteotomy. Partial weight bearing is routinely maintained for 3 to 5 months after surgery, depending on bone healing.

Advancement of the Greater Trochanter

The secure fixation of the greater trochanter with the advancement procedure obviates the need for cast immobilization and permits rapid mobilization. Partial weight bearing with crutches prevents undue stresses on the trochanter. Light strengthening exercises of the hip are permitted, except for active hip abduction. Restrictions are lifted after 6 weeks.

Arthrodesis of the Hip

If bone density is good and fixation is deemed to be adequate, no immobilization is required after hip arthrodesis. If fixation is less than adequate or if the patient is noncompliant, a spica cast is used for 6 weeks. In cases of obesity, a spica cast may be impractical, so 6 weeks of bed rest or bed to chair limitations are imposed. Full weight bearing is deferred until radiographic evidence of union is seen at 3 to 5 months and the fusion is solid by clinical examination.

RESULTS

Intertrochanteric Osteotomy

In carefully selected patients, intertrochanteric osteotomy will usually provide pain relief and improved function, although the results are not as spectacular as they are with total hip arthroplasty. Candidates for osteotomy, however, are usually considered to be too young for total hip arthroplasty, and it is hoped that an intertrochanteric osteotomy will either postpone or eliminate the need for total hip arthroplasty. As expected, the results are best if there are minimal arthritic changes before the osteotomy.

Morscher and Feinstein (58) noted that of the patients who had had intertrochanteric osteotomy one-third had long-lasting excellent results, one-third had less than excellent results but were satisfied, and one-third eventually required a total hip arthroplasty. Results were best with congruous joint surfaces, minimal osteoarthritis, and patients under the age of 40. The authors believed that if the total hip arthroplasty could be delayed 5 years or more, intertrochanteric osteotomy was worthwhile.

Pellicci et al. (29) reported the results of 56 hips in 48 patients who underwent intertrochanteric osteotomy for dysplasia. Average follow up was 8.6 years. Good to excellent results were obtained in 72% of patients, 5% had a fair result, and 23% eventually required a total hip arthroplasty. These authors stressed that the results were best if patients had minimal osteoarthritis before the osteotomy.

Perlau et al. (28) reported the results of intertrochanteric osteotomy in two groups of patients: those with osteoarthritis and those with arthritis associated with dysplasia. Results were best in both groups when the osteoarthritis was early. It was believed that patients who had a center edge angle of 15° or less should have a periacetabular osteotomy as well, since intertrochanteric osteotomy of the femur did not provide enough correction. The authors recommend intertrochanteric osteotomy in patients with grade I or II osteoarthritis only and thought that at least 10 years of success with the osteotomy was required to warrant its use.

Jacobs et al. (34) reported on 22 cases of intertrochanteric osteotomy of the femur for avascular necrosis. Of these, 16 had good to excellent results at an average follow-up of 5 years. Success was inversely proportional to the size of the femoral head lesion. Maistrelli et al. (33) reported on the results of intertrochanteric osteotomy on 106 hips with avascular necrosis. At the 2-year follow-up, 71% were satisfied with the outcome and 58% had good to excellent results. Approximately 24% required total hip replacement or fusion. Results were best in young patients and those with avascular necrosis from either trauma or idiopathic causes.

Marti et al. (37) reported the results of 50 patients with femoral neck nonunion treated with a valgus intertrochanteric osteotomy. Average follow-up was 7.1 years. A total of 43 patients (86%) went onto union; the other 7 required total hip replacement. There was evidence of avascular necrosis in 22 hips; only 3 of these required a replacement. The procedure was thought to be worthwhile even in the face of avascular necrosis, provided that the femoral head had not collapsed. Ballmer et al. (36) reported similar results: 12 of 17 cases went onto union (70%) after one osteotomy, 3 cases required a second procedure, and 2 cases with avascular necrosis required a total hip replacement.

Periacetabular Osteotomy

Trousdale et al. (13) reported on the use of PAO for acetabular dysplasia with osteoarthritis. A total of 42 patients underwent surgery. The results were good to excellent in 32 of 33 patients with grade I or II osteoarthritis. Out of the 9 patients with grade III osteoarthritic changes, 8 had fair or worse results; 6 patients required total hip arthroplasty. Periacetabular osteotomy was not recommended in cases of advanced osteoarthritis.

Advancement of the Greater Trochanter

Macnicol and Makris (50) reported the results in 26 patients (27 hips) at an average follow-up of 8 years. The average age at surgery was 14 years (range 8 to 39); the predominant cause was hip dysplasia, which accounted for 81.5% of cases. Pain relief and gait improvement was seen in 74%. Failures were attributed to progressive osteoarthritis of the hip.

Wagner (51) reported the results of 275 cases, broken into three groups: group I had no arthritis and did not initially require other reconstructive procedures (159 cases, average age 18.2 years, average follow-up 58 months), group II had the advancement done as part of more complex procedures, and group III already had osteoarthritis of the hip. In group I, 95% had no pain, 3% had mild pain, and 1% had worse pain. There was no limp in 77%, a mild limp in 22%, and a severe limp in 1%. The rate of reoperation for delayed union or loss of correction was 3%.

Arthrodesis of the Hip

Achieving a successful hip arthrodesis is not easy. The extremely long lever arm of the leg stresses the fusion site, often with resultant micromotion. As a result, nonunion rates are usually in the range of 10 to 25%, and even higher with femoral head avascular necrosis (52–54,59). Two long-term studies by Sponseller et al. (60) and Callaghan et al. (56) were reported at 38 and 35 years, respectively. Both studies showed that most patients were satisfied with the hip fusion. A total of 7 of 53 patients in the first study and 6 of 28 patients in the second study required total hip arthroplasty.

SUMMARY

The development of osteoarthritis of the hip is always tragic, but doubly so in the young patient. The surgeon should initially consider surgical options other than total hip arthroplasty, especially in the young patient. Osteotomies may be performed on the femur, acetabulum, or both, depending on deformity. It is important to recognize the hip at risk, since osteotomies are much more predictable in the early stages of osteoarthritis. Temporizing measures may allow the hip to deteriorate to the point at which an osteotomy is no longer practical.

For salvage procedures such as arthrodesis, the hip is already destroyed, and there is no harm in postponing the surgery until the patient is ready. Patients older than 40 with severe osteoarthritis are probably best served with total hip arthroplasty.

Preoperative planning and functional x-rays to simulate an osteotomy are crucial to determining if a patient meets the indications for a procedure and for the successful execution of the operation.

REFERENCES

1. Cooperman DR, Wallensten R, Stulberg SD. Acetabular dysplasia in the adult. Clin Orthop 1983;175:79–85.
2. Boyer DW, Mickelson MR, Ponseti IV. Slipped capital femoral epiphysis. Long-term follow-up study of one hundred and twenty-one patients. J Bone Joint Surg 1981;63A:85–95.
3. Harris WH. Etiology of osteoarthritis of the hip. Clin Orthop 1986;213:20–33.
4. Carney BT, Weinstein SL, Noble J. Long-term follow-up of slipped capital femoral epiphysis. J Bone Joint Surg 1991;73A:667–674.
5. Aronson J. Osteoarthritis of the young adult hip: etiology and treatment. Instr Course Lect 1986;35:119–128.
6. Wedge JH, Wasylenko MJ, Houston CS. Minor anatomic abnormalities of the hip joint persisting from childhood and their possible relationship to idiopathic osteoarthrosis. Clin Orthop 1991;264:122–128.
7. Goodman DA, Feighan JE, Smith AD, et al. Subclinical slipped capital epiphysis. Relationship to osteoarthrosis of the hip. J Bone Joint Surg 1997;79A:1489–1497.
8. Cornell CN, Ranawat CS. Survivorship analysis of total hip replacements. Results in a series of active patients who were less than fifty-five years old. J Bone Joint Surg 1986;68A:1430–1434.
9. Chandler HP, Reineck FT, Wixson RL, McCarthy JC. Total hip replacement in patients younger than thirty years old. A five-year follow-up study. J Bone Joint Surg 1981;63A:1426–1434.
10. Dorr LD, Luckett M, Conaty JP. Total hip arthroplasties in patients younger than 45 years. A nine- to ten-year follow-up study. Clin Orthop 1990;260:215–219.
11. Weinstein SL. Congenital hip dislocation. Long-range problems, residual signs, and symptoms after successful treatment. Clin Orthop 1992;281:69–74.
12. Klaue K, Durnin CW, Ganz R. The acetabular rim syndrome. A clinical presentation of dysplasia of the hip. J Bone Joint Surg 1991;73B:423–429.
13. Trousdale RT, Ekkernkamp A, Ganz R, Wallrichs SL. Periacetabular and intertrochanteric osteotomy for the treatment of osteoarthrosis in dysplastic hips. J Bone Joint Surg 1995;77A:73–85.
14. Lequesne M, de Seze S. La faux profil du bassin: nouvelle incidence radiographique pour l'etude de la hanche. Son utilite dans les dysplasies et les differentes coxopathies. Rev Rhum Mal Osteoartic 1961;28:643–652.
15. Wiberg G. Studies on the dysplastic acetabulum and congenital subluxation of the hip joint. Acta Chir Scand 1939;83:1–135.
16. Tonnis D. Congenital dysplasia and dislocation of the hip in children and adults. Berlin: Springer-Verlag, 1987.
17. Murphy SB, Kijewski PK, Millis MB, Harless A. Acetabular dysplasia in the adolescent and young adult. Clin Orthop 1990;261:214–223.
18. Schneider R. Intertrochanteric osteotomy in osteoarthritis of the hip joint. In: Schatzker J, ed. The intertrochanteric osteotomy. Berlin: Springer-Verlag, 1984:135–177.
19. Millis MB, Murphy SB, Poss R. Osteotomies about the hip for the prevention and treatment of osteoarthrosis. Instr Course Lect 1996;45:209–226.
20. Iwersen LJ, Kalen V, Eberle C. Relative trochanteric overgrowth after ischemic necrosis in congenital dislocation of the hip. J Pediatr Orthop 1989;9:381–385.
21. McAndrew MP, Weinstein SL. A long-term follow-up of Legg-Calve-Perthes disease. J Bone Joint Surg 1984;66A:860–869.
22. Stulberg SD, Cooperman DR, Wallensten R. The natural history of Legg-Calvé-Perthes disease. J Bone Joint Surg 1981;63A:1095–1108.
23. Ficat RP. Treatment of avascular necrosis of the femoral head. Paper presented at the Open Scientific Meeting of the Hip Society, 1983.
24. Davy DT, Kotzar GM, Brown RH, et al. Telemetric force measurements across the hip after total arthroplasty. J Bone Joint Surg 1988;70A:45–50.
25. Cooperman DR, Charles LM, Pathria M, et al. Post-mortem description of slipped capital femoral epiphysis. J Bone Joint Surg 1992;74B:595–599.
26. Potter HG, Montgomery KD, Heise CW, Helfet DL. MR imaging of acetabular fractures: value in detecting femoral head injury, intraarticular fragments, and sciatic nerve injury. AJR Am J Roentgenol 1994;163:881–886.
27. Poss R. The role of osteotomy in the treatment of osteoarthritis of the hip. J Bone Joint Surg 1984;66A:144–151.
28. Perlau R, Wilson MG, Poss R. Isolated proximal femoral osteotomy for treatment of residua of congenital dysplasia or idiopathic osteoarthrosis of the hip. Five to ten-year results. J Bone Joint Surg 1996;78A:1462–1467.
29. Pellicci PM, Hu S, Garvin KL, et al. Varus rotational femoral osteotomies in adults with hip dysplasia. Clin Orthop 1991;272:162–166.
30. Muller ME. Intertrochanteric osteotomy: indication, preoperative planning, technique. In: Schatzker J, ed. The intertrochanteric osteotomy. Berlin: Springer-Verlag, 1984:25–66.
31. Maistrelli GL, Gerundini M, Fusco U, et al. Valgus-extension osteotomy for osteoarthritis of the hip. Indications and long-term results. J Bone Joint Surg 1990;72B:653–657.
32. Wagner H, Baur W, Wagner M. Joint-preserving osteotomy in segmental femur head necrosis. Orthopäde 1990;19:208–218.
33. Maistrelli G, Fusco U, Avai A, Bombelli R. Osteonecrosis of the hip treated by intertrochanteric osteotomy. A four- to 15-year follow-up. J Bone Joint Surg 1988;70B:761–766.
34. Jacobs MA, Hungerford DS, Krackow KA. Intertrochanteric osteotomy for avascular necrosis of the femoral head. J Bone Joint Surg 1989;71B:200–204.
35. Sugioka Y, Hotokebuchi T, Tsutsui H. Transtrochanteric anterior rotational osteotomy for idiopathic and steroid-induced necrosis of the femoral head. Indications and long-term results. Clin Orthop 1992;277:111–120.
36. Ballmer FT, Ballmer PM, Baumgaertel F, et al. Pauwels osteotomy for nonunions of the femoral neck. Orthop Clin North Am 1990;21:759–767.
37. Marti RK, Schuller HM, Raaymakers EL. Intertrochanteric osteotomy for non-union of the femoral neck. J Bone Joint Surg 1989;71B:782–787.
38. Imhauser G. Late results of Imhauser's osteotomy for slipped capital femoral epiphysis. Z Orthop 1977;115:716–725.
39. Tonnis D, Behrens K, Tscharani F. A modified technique of the triple pelvic osteotomy: early results. J Pediatr Orthop 1981;1:241–249.
40. Salter RB, Hansson G, Thompson GH. Innominate osteotomy in the management of residual congenital subluxation of the hip in young adults. Clin Orthop 1984;182:53–68.
41. Steel HH. Triple osteotomy of the innominate bone. A procedure to accomplish coverage of the dislocated or subluxated femoral head in the older patient. Clin Orthop 1977;122:116–127.
42. Pemberton PA. Pericapsular osteotomy of the ilium for the treatment of congenitally dislocated hips. Clin Orthop 1974;98:41–54.
43. Eppright RH. Dial osteotomy of the acetabulum in the treatment of dysplasia of the hip. J Bone Joint Surg 1975;57A:1172.

44. Wagner H. Osteotomies for congenital hip dislocation. Paper presented at the Fourth Open Scientific Meeting of the Hip Society, 1976.

45. Ninomiya S. Rotational acetabular osteotomy for the severely dysplastic hip in the adolescent and adult. Clin Orthop 1989; 247:127–137.

46. Ganz R, Klaue K, Vinh TS, Mast JW. A new periacetabular osteotomy for the treatment of hip dysplasias. Technique and preliminary results. Clin Orthop 1988;232:26–36.

47. Helfet DL, Anand N, Malkani AL, et al. Intraoperative monitoring of motor pathways during operative fixation of acute acetabular fractures. J Orthop Trauma 1997;11:2–6.

48. Letournel E. The treatment of acetabular fractures through the ilioinguinal approach. Clin Orthop 1993;292:62–76.

49. Lloyd-Roberts GC, Wetherill MH, Fraser M. Trochanteric advancement for premature arrest of the femoral capital growth plate. J Bone Joint Surg 1985;67B:21–24.

50. Macnicol MF, Makris D. Distal transfer of the greater trochanter. J Bone Joint Surg 1991;73B:838–841.

51. Wagner H. Treatment of osteoarthritis of the hip by corrective osteotomy of the greater trochanter. In: Schatzker J, ed. The intertrochanteric osteotomy. Berlin: Springer-Verlag, 1984:179–201.

52. Liechti R. Arthrodesis and associated problems. Berlin: Springer-Verlag, 1974.

53. Schneider R. Hip arthrodesis with the Cobra head plate and pelvic osteotomy. Reconstr Surg Traumatol 1974;14:1–37.

54. Matta JM, Siebenrock KA, Gautier E, et al. Hip fusion through an anterior approach with the use of a ventral plate. Clin Orthop 1997;337:129–139.

55. Lindahl O. Determination of hip adduction, especially in arthrodesis. Acta Orthop Scand 1965;36:280–293.

56. Callaghan JJ, Brand RA, Pedersen DR. Hip arthrodesis. a long-term follow-up. J Bone Joint Surg 1985;67A:1328–1335.

57. Blasier RB, Holmes JR. Intraoperative positioning for arthrodesis of the hip with the double beanbag technique. J Bone Joint Surg 1990;72A:766–769.

58. Morscher E, Feinstein R. Results of intertrochanteric osteotomy in the treatment of osteoarthritis of the hip. In: Schatzker J, ed. The intertrochanteric osteotomy. Berlin: Springer-Verlag, 1984: 169–177.

59. Stewart MJ, Coker TP Jr. Arthrodesis of the hip. A review of 109 patients. Clin Orthop 1969;62:136–150.

60. Sponseller PD, McBeath AA, Perpich M. Hip arthrodesis in young patients. A long-term follow-up study. J Bone Joint Surg 1984; 66A:853–859.

Robert L. Buly and Michael J. Maynard

Arthroscopy of the Hip

Several factors—including the toughness of the hip joint capsule; the hemispherical bony morphology; and the fact that the joint lies beneath a relatively thick, muscular, and soft tissue envelope—combine to make the prospect of performing arthroscopic surgery on the natural hip joint a daunting technical challenge even to the most experienced arthroscopic surgeon. Traction is usually required for complete access to intra-articular structures. Therefore, it is not surprising that arthroscopic surgery has been performed and reported much less often for the hip joint than it has for the knee, ankle, shoulder, and elbow.

Hip arthroscopy is performed most often for abnormalities of the labrum and articular cartilage. The cartilage may degenerate with time from conditions such as Perthes disease, dysplasia, slipped capital femoral epiphysis, or idiopathic osteoarthritis. Catastrophic injury to the articular cartilage may occur with axial load or dislocation.

RELEVANT ANATOMY AND PATHOGENESIS

The labrum may undergo slow deterioration in conditions such as dysplasia where, at the anterosuperior margin of the acetabulum, it is situated close to the apex of the femoral head rather than in a more peripheral location (1,2). An otherwise normal labrum may be damaged acutely by trauma, even trauma that it is surprisingly trivial. Like the meniscus, the labrum is composed mainly of fibrocartilage. Although it does have innervation throughout, the blood supply is limited to the superficial layers (3), which helps explain why labral injuries may not heal spontaneously. Patients will often present with mechanical symptoms that have been present for years.

Loose bodies may be generated by trauma that leaves behind osteochondral fragments or by benign neoplastic disorders, such as synovial chondromatosis, that may liberate hundreds of loose bodies within the joint.

INITIAL FINDINGS, PHYSICAL EXAMINATION, AND DIAGNOSIS

Patients with hip disorders amenable to hip arthroscopy may present in a number of ways. Symptoms may arise after trauma, such as a fall on the ice, motor vehicle accident, or acetabular fracture. In many cases, the patient is unable to pinpoint a specific traumatic event. In degenerative conditions, the onset is usually insidious and progressive.

Tears of the labrum are usually along the anterosuperior portion of the rim (4–6). This may be due to the small anterior wall, which places the labrum close to the apex of the head. Nearly all patients complain of pain in the groin. Patients may also sense a clicking, catching, and even a locking sensation, which may worsen with increasing hip flexion, i.e., stair climbing, getting into a car, or stepping over an obstacle. It may difficult to distinguish labral disorders from tendonitis or iliopsoas bursitis. Unlike the last two, it is not unusual for symptoms to be present for years and to be refractory to anti-inflammatory medications and physical therapy. Symptoms can usually be reproduced by hip flexion and internal rotation or by bringing the hip into extension, as one would to check for a flexion contracture. Often a click may be felt or heard.

Patients with loose bodies often experience similar symptoms, though often in a more unpredictable fashion because the bodies shift position. The pain associated with articular cartilage damage is usually worse with weight bearing and may or may not have mechanical symptoms, such as locking or clicking. An intra-articular source for the pain can be confirmed by injecting local anesthetic into the joint. Patients with these conditions often report remarkable pain relief, lasting for several hours. Range of motion may not be limited unless there are advanced degenerative changes or osteophytes.

RADIOLOGIC STUDIES

Radiographs may be normal in patients with labral tears, chondral injuries, or loose bodies. Patients with pelvic or acetabular fractures may suffer from loose bodies, avascular necrosis (AVN), chondrolysis, and femoral head fractures that were not apparent previously. Areas of head collapse or flattening may indicate avascular necrosis. The joint space should be compared to that of the opposite side. It is important to ascertain whether dysplasia is present, i.e., a lateral or anterior center-edge angle of 25° or less on the AP and false profile views, respectively. This is important because labral abnormalities are common in dysplasia. An intra- or extra-articular ganglion may be associated with dysplasia and labral pathology. The intraosseous type is seen as a radiolucency at the superior osseous margin of the acetabulum. Synovial chondromatosis may be apparent if the cartilaginous bodies calcify.

Improved MRI techniques using a surface coil can provide wonderful documentation of intra-articular pathology. Although intra-articular contrast (saline or gadolinium) can be used to assess labral tears, it may mask articular cartilage lesions (7,8). We prefer to evaluate coronal and sagittal proton density-weighted, fast-spin echo sequences without contrast. Labral defects are detected easily (Fig. 46.1). Not only can cartilage defects be seen but their location on either the femoral or acetabular side can be ascertained (Fig. 46.2) (9). AVN, synovial chondromatosis, and pigmented villonodular synovitis are easy to diagnose on MRI studies. Bone scans may be positive when arthritis or AVN is present; however, MRI scans are more sensitive and specific. CT is best suited to assess bone defects and fractures.

TREATMENT

Nonoperative Treatment

The diagnosis of the hip abnormality is often difficult to ascertain. It helps to try a course of protected weight bearing, nonsteroidal anti-inflammatory medications, and physical therapy to rule out transient synovitis, bursitis, and tendonitis.

Patients with loose bodies do not seem to do well with nonoperative treatment; and the same holds true for those

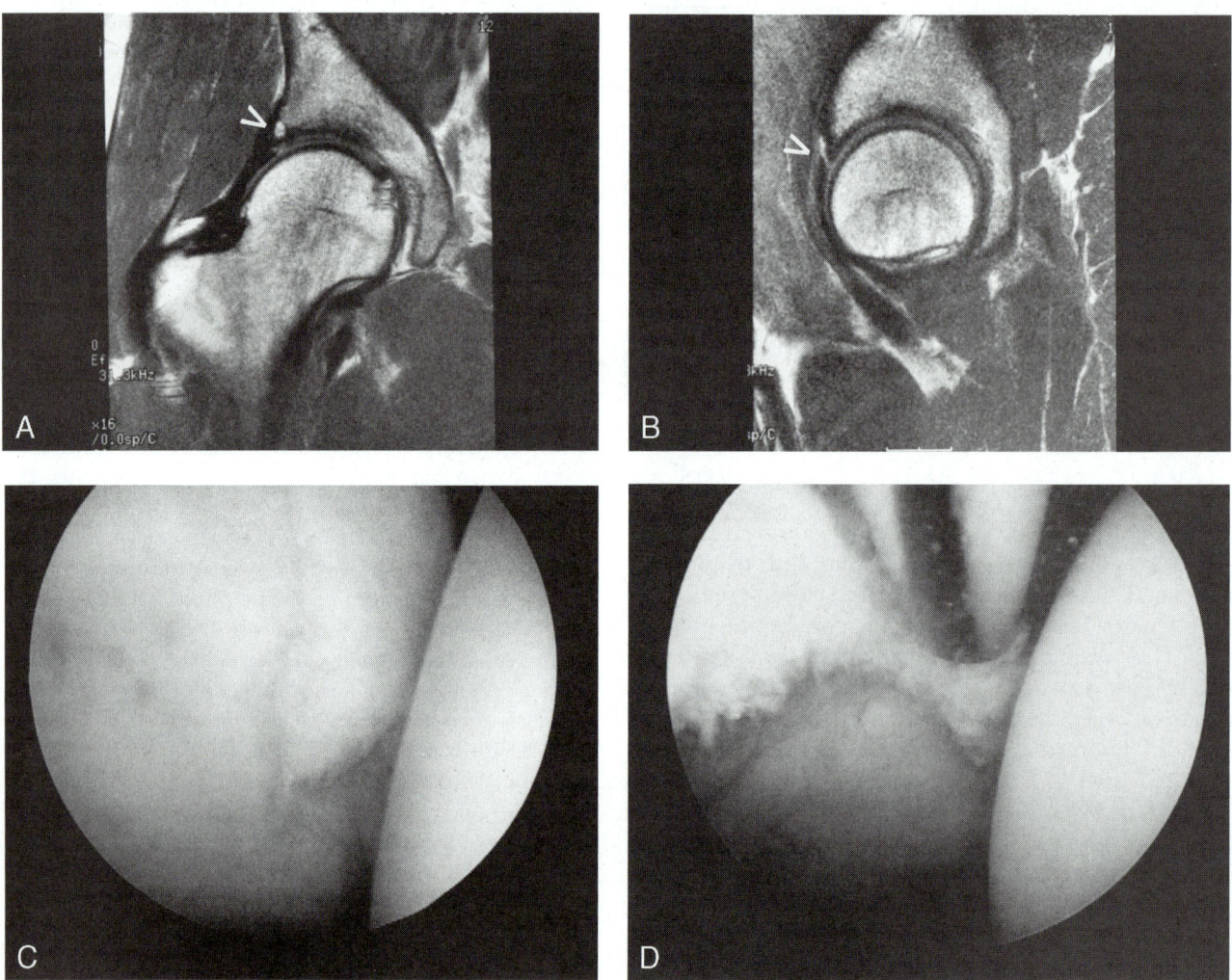

Figure 46.1. High-resolution coronal plane (**A**) and sagittal plane (**B**) MRI views showing a tear of the anterosuperior acetabular labrum and cyst formation (*arrow*). Intraoperative arthroscopic views of the labral tear before (**C**) and after (**D**) resection.

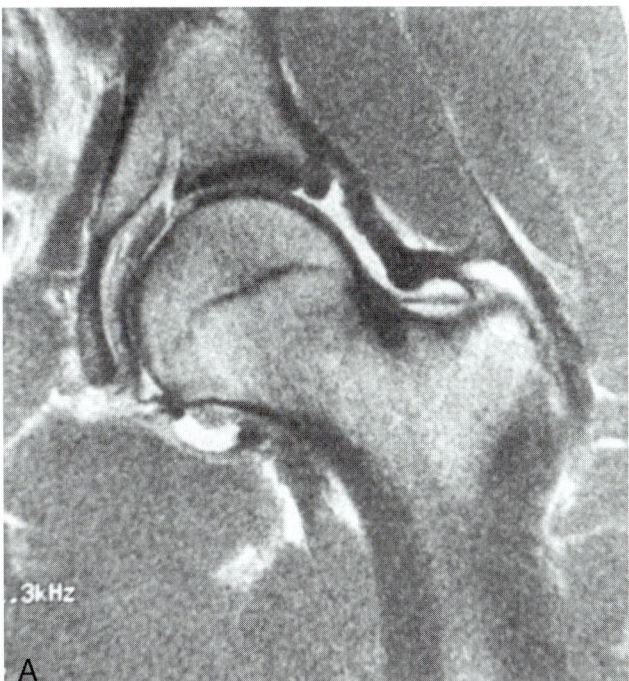

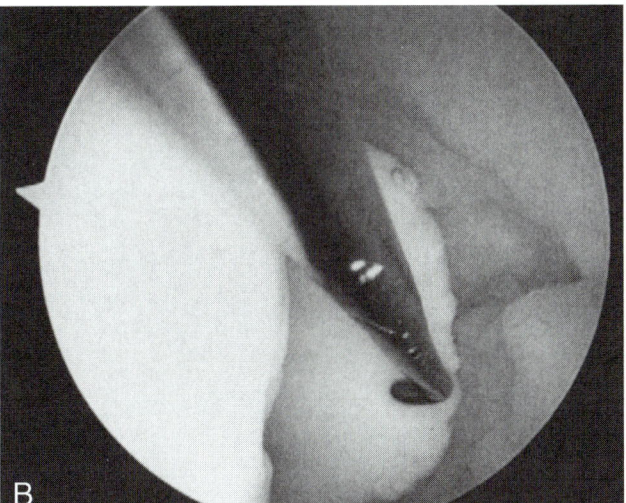

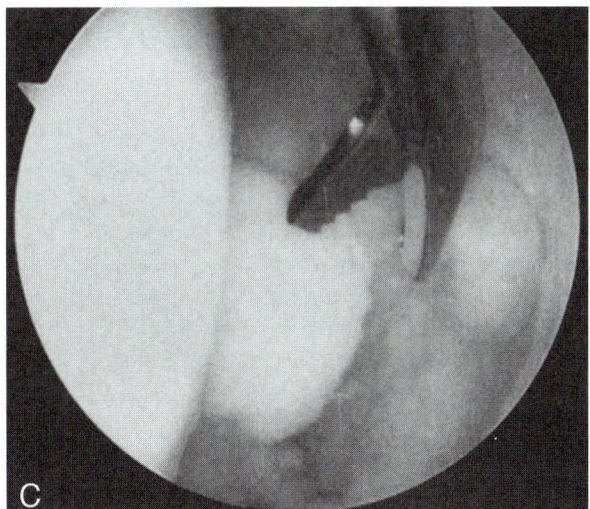

Figure 46.2. A. High-resolution coronal plan MRI view showing articular cartilage avulsion in a professional football player who sustained traumatic hip subluxation. Intraoperative arthroscopic views of the loose body before (**B**) and after removal (**C**) with an arthroscopic grasper.

with tears of the acetabular labrum, probably because of its deficient blood supply. As with other joints, chondral lesions do not heal spontaneously. Intra-articular injections, although useful for synovitis and diagnostic tests, relieve symptoms of chondral injuries only transiently, since they do not reverse the intra-articular pathology.

Operative Treatment

Burman (10) and Takagi (11) are generally credited with the first published reports concerning the application of arthroscopic surgical techniques to the evaluation and treatment of hip disorders. After these early reports, the next major advances in equipment and techniques were introduced by Watanabe (12) in the 1970s. Since then, numerous authors have reported their experience with

arthroscopic surgery of both the natural and artificial hip joint.

Both diagnostic and therapeutic objectives have been described as indications for arthroscopic surgery of the natural hip (Clinical Table). Some of the reported indications are (*a*) evaluation of the painful hip when the diagnosis is questionable after all diagnostic techniques have been exhausted; (*b*) evaluation of femoral and acetabular arthritic involvement as an adjunct to therapeutic osteotomy; (*c*) exploration and débridement of intra-articular debris after a fracture dislocation of the hip; (*d*) exploration and removal of foreign bodies; (*e*) débridement of torn acetabular labrum; (*f*) synovial and loose body débridement in synovial chondromatosis; (*g*) synovectomy for pigmented villonodular synovitis or inflammatory arthritis; (*h*) débridement of an impinging ligamentum

Clinical Table: Arthroscopy of the Hip

Procedure	Indications	Technique	Anatomy	Pitfalls
Hip arthroscopy	• Labral tears • Chondral injuries • Synovectomy • Débridement	• Lateral or supine position • Image intensifier • Special instruments • 30° and 70° scopes • Arthroscopic pump	• Femoral neurovascular structures • Lateral femoral cutaneous nerve • Superior gluteal neurovascular structures • Sciatic nerve	• Poor distraction • Instrument breakage • Cartilage scuffs • Neuropraxia
Scope-assisted arthrotomy	• Synovial chondromatosis • Inferior recess bodies • Poor mobility	• Expose the capsule • Maintain traction • Insert the scope	• Femoral neurovascular structures • Lateral femoral cutaneous nerve • Superior gluteal neurovascular structures • Sciatic nerve	• Blood supply to head with posterior approach

teres; (*i*) synovial biopsy; (*j*) evaluation of pediatric hip disorders, including congenital hip dislocation, Perthes disease, and slipped capital femoral epiphysis; and (*k*) evaluation of osteochondritis dissecans.

USE OF TRACTION

Eriksson et al. (13) reported an experimental study of hip distraction achieved with longitudinal traction applied to anesthetized and unanesthetized patients who were positioned supine on a fracture table. It was reported that a force of up to 900 N was required to achieve satisfactory distraction in an unanesthetized patient, compared to 300 to 400 N in a properly anesthetized patient. They suggested that a minimum of 7 mm of distraction must be achieved for successful arthroscopic evaluation of the hip and pointed out that the main forces resisting hip distraction are active muscular contraction, vacuum effect within the joint, and passive resistance of the periarticular and intra-articular soft tissues (Fig. 46.3). Glick (14), Johnson (15), Hawkins (16), and others have supported the use of traction for all hip arthroscopies; however, Klapper and Silver (17) and Dorfmann et al. (18) reported good results without traction.

SPECIALIZED EQUIPMENT

Most authors have reported using standard knee arthroscopy equipment for the performance of hip arthroscopy. Glick (14) advocated the use of longer cannulas and sheaths with a standard arthroscope and a reduced bridge length, which increases the effective useful length. Some authors reported good results with smaller arthroscopes or by using wider angles of vision, such as the 70° or 90° scope, in addition to the 30° scope. Cannulated arthroscopic obturators, which are introduced over 1.2-mm guidewires, are quite useful for placing the scope and cannulas within the joint (Fig. 46.4). The wires are placed through 17-gauge spinal needles, which are relatively easy to introduce into the joint at the onset of the procedure.

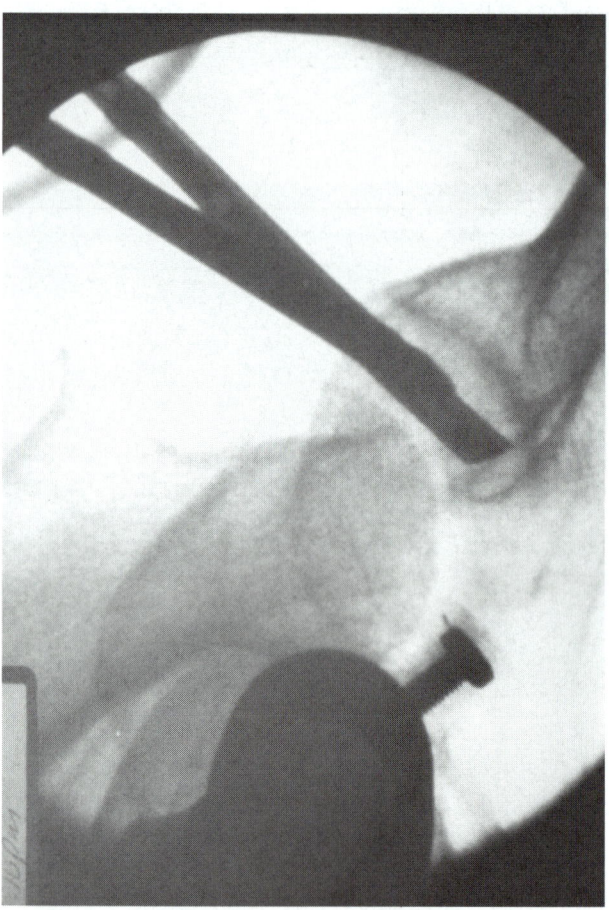

Figure 46.3. Fluoroscopic image showing the degree of distraction possible to allow easy introduction of the arthroscope and instruments.

PATIENT POSITION

Hip arthroscopy can be performed with the patient in either a supine or a lateral position (Fig. 46.5). A fracture table is used with a well-padded perineal post and padding around the foot and ankle to prevent nerve palsies. Specialized distraction equipment may also be

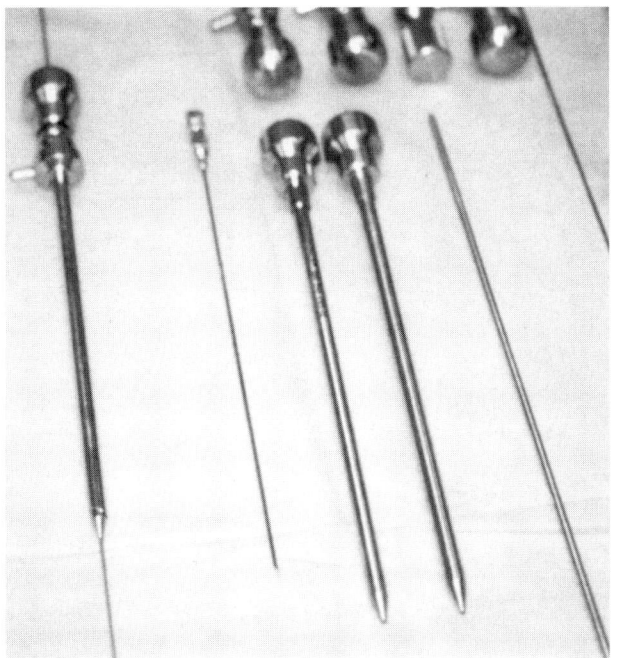

Figure 46.4. Cannulated obturators ease the insertion of instruments into the hip joint.

used that will monitor the amount of force generated during traction. Slight abduction of 20° to 40° will help relax the lateral soft tissues and facilitate scope and instrument manipulation. An image intensifier is used during the case to confirm the intra-articular location of equipment, and should be set up before draping to document clear imaging.

APPROACHES

The most versatile portals are the peritrochanteric portals. These are placed just slightly above the greater trochanter; one is slightly anterior and the other is slightly posterior. They should be far enough apart to avoid crowding of the instruments. An anterior portal may be used at the junction of the line extended vertically from the anterior superior iliac spine with one extended medially from the tip of the greater trochanter (Fig. 46.6). Care must be taken to avoid the femoral vessels and nerves located medially and the branches of the lateral femoral cutaneous nerve. A posterior portal may be used but should be combined with a mini arthrotomy to avoid damage to the sciatic nerve and the gluteal neurovascular structures. Gross (19) used a medial approach in a pediatric population.

A

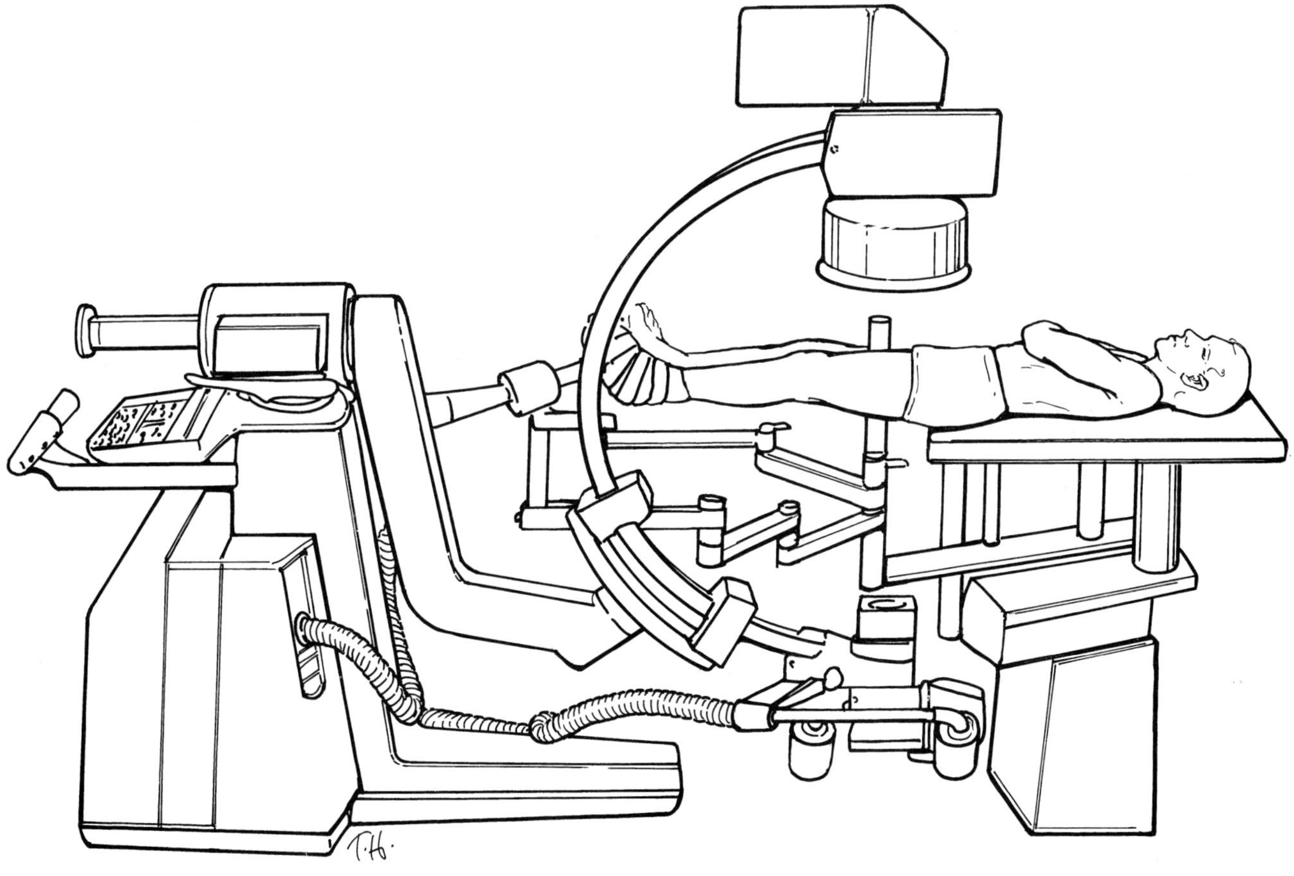

Figure 46.5. The patient may be in either the supine (**A**) or the lateral (**B**) position *(continued)*

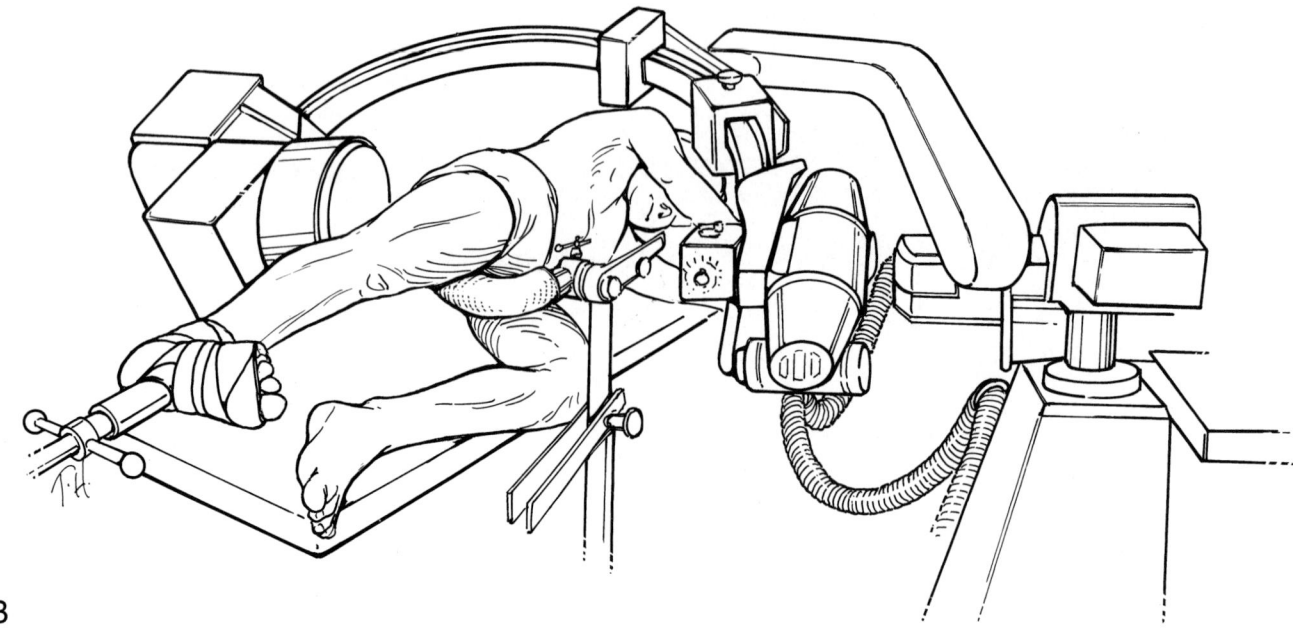

Figure 46.5. *(continued)* **B.** Lateral position.

A scope-assisted arthrotomy is helpful when the intra-articular process is so diffuse (i.e., synovial chondromatosis) that it is not possible to do a thorough débridement using the standard portals. This may also be necessary if there is extensive scarring from previous surgery or with loose bodies below the femoral neck. With this technique, an anterior or posterior approach is made to the level of the capsule. Traction is maintained for distraction, and the scope is introduced through the capsule. Mobility within the joint is markedly enhanced, including the inferior recess of the joint.

TECHNIQUE

After positioning the patient, the image intensifier is positioned to provide clear images of the hip joint. Before draping, preliminary traction is placed on the leg to assess the amount of distraction that is possible. The traction is then released and every effort is taken to release the traction during the procedure when not needed to avoid complications. The hip is then prepared and draped, and a sterile shower curtain is placed over the C arm of the image intensifier. The C arm can be tilted toward the patient's head or foot and then moved toward either end of the table when not in use.

Traction is then applied, and a 17-gauge, 15-cm (6-in.) spinal needle, is introduced into the joint under fluoroscopic guidance. A whoosh of air can often be heard as the vacuum seal of the joint is broken. Saline with epinephrine is then introduced into the joint, which should be easily aspirated back into the syringe. Much greater distraction should now be apparent on the image intensifier, and if need be, the traction can be diminished.

A 1.2-mm wire is introduced through the 17-gauge

spinal needle, and cannulated obturators (Dyonics; Smith and Nephew; Mansfield, MA) are used to establish both the scope and instrument portals. It should be possible to visualize most of the articular cartilage of the femoral head and acetabulum, the acetabular fossa, and the ligamentum teres and nearly all of the acetabular labrum. Synovium can be seen outside the labrum at the junction with the capsule, and the transverse acetabular ligament may also be seen. A 70° scope can be used to extend the field and see around corners. Care must be taken not to scuff the articular surfaces while introducing instruments or maneuvering in the joint. Large-bore shoulder cannulas may be used in the instrument portal to allow the introduction of a probe, shaver, grasper, or electrocautery device. Extra-long shavers (Dyonics) help the surgeon reach the acetabular fossa and allow the use of large-bore cannulas to maintain the instrument portal. An arthroscopic pump provides both the pressure and the flow rates necessary for visualization during the procedure.

ARTHROSCOPY AND TOTAL HIP ARTHROPLASTY

Shifrin and Reis (20), Nordt et al. (21), and Vikili et al. (22) have reported on arthroscopic procedures performed in total hip arthroplasties. Each of these procedures was performed to remove debris that prevented the concentric reduction of a prosthetic femoral head within a prosthetic acetabulum.

At the Hospital for Special Surgery, we have recently begun performing arthroscopic irrigation and débridement for a narrowly defined patient population who present with infected total hip arthroplasty (23). Our indications for this treatment option include (*a*) short duration of symptoms (less than 7 days), (*b*) a well-fixed prosthesis on

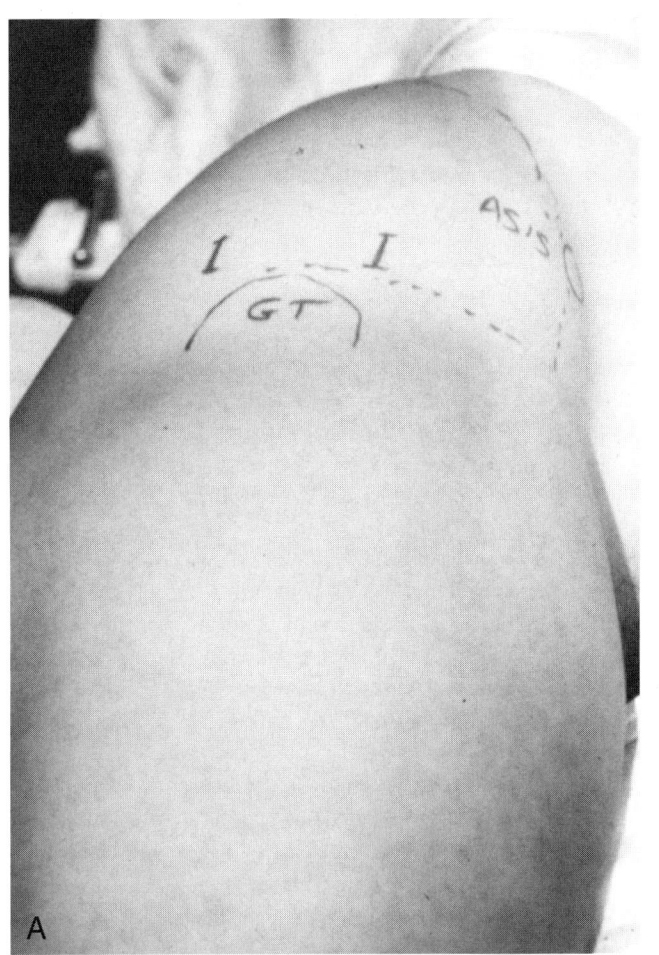

Figure 46.6. A. Arthroscopic portals for hip arthroscopy. **B.** Relevant anatomy in relation to arthroscopic portal location.

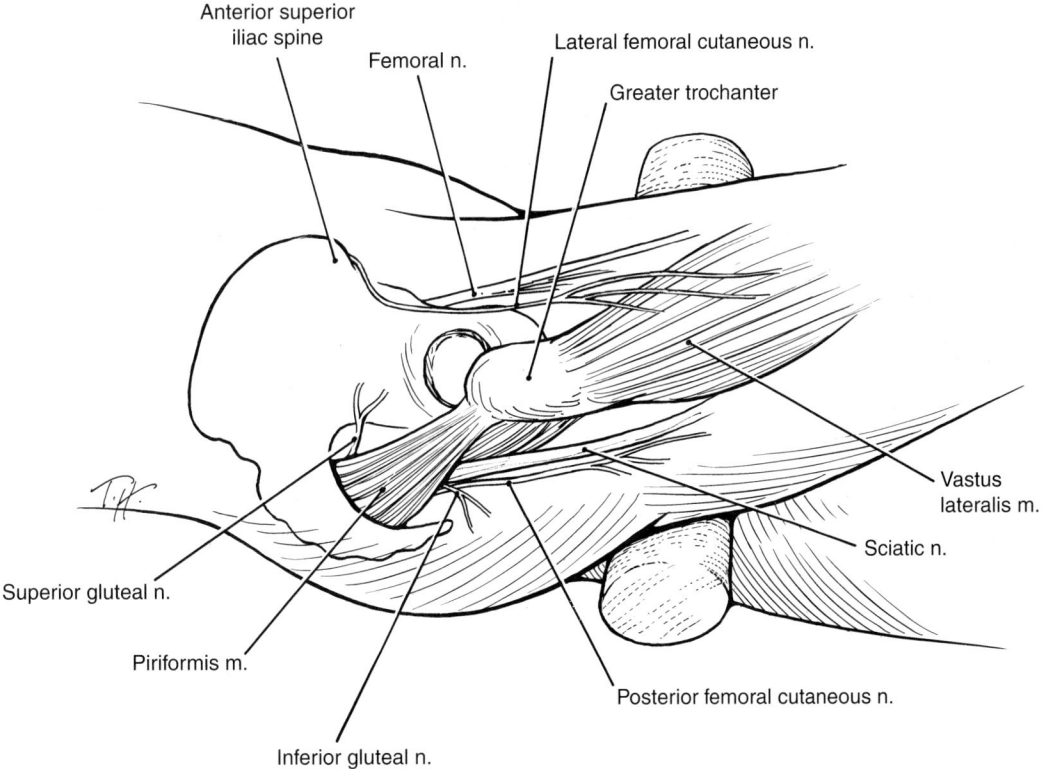

radiographic examination, (c) presence of a contraindication to extensive surgery (e.g., debilitated patient, patient with short life expectancy, well-fixed cemented long-stem prosthesis, multiple previous revisions), and (d) infectious agents sensitive to oral antibiotic treatment. Several patients have been entered into our series under these criteria. All patients have been treated with arthroscopic irrigation and débridement, and direct visualization of the prosthetic femoral head–acetabulum interface was achieved while a minimum of 12 L irrigation fluid was lavaged through the joint. Synovial débridement was carried out in all cases to some degree. All patients then received a 2- to 6-week course of intravenous antibiotic therapy followed by oral antibiotic therapy indefinitely. Six patients so treated have been able to retain their implants at an average follow-up of 39 months.

PITFALLS AND COMMON MISTAKES

Transient neuropraxia to both the pudendal and sciatic nerves has been reported (13,14,24,25). This may be minimized by ensuring that the perineal post is well padded and by keeping traction to a minimum, certainly less than 2 h total. Traction should be released whenever possible during the procedure to provide relief to the nerves. The position of neurovascular structures must be noted and kept in mind at all times.

A potential complication with arthroscopy of the hip is instrument breakage. This usually happens as a result of the significant torque generated by maneuvering the instruments in the thick tissue planes about the hip (14).

Cartilage injury can be avoided by using spinal needles and fine wires to establish the portals, which helps to minimize the chance of scuffing the articular surfaces. Fluoroscopy should be used to ensure that instruments do not impinge on either the acetabulum or the femoral head. Infection is a potential complication with any sur-

gical procedure, but it has not been reported in hip arthroscopy to our knowledge.

It may be difficult to maneuver within the hip joint, especially in large patients. It may be helpful to make the arthroscopy portals slightly larger than normal and to use an arthroscopic knife to open the capsule openings to allow more freedom of movement. Larger-angle scopes, such as the 70°scope, may help extend the field of vision.

REHABILITATION

Arthroscopy of the hip may be performed on an outpatient basis; however, because of the use of traction, it may be desirable for patients to remain overnight so their neurologic status can be monitored. Patients may start ambulation immediately; progression to full weight bearing occurs as hip tenderness subsides. Range of motion exercises and hip strengthening are then used to enhance return of function.

Hip patients will often experience greater postoperative pain than do those undergoing knee arthroscopy, because of traction and the depth of the joint. Patients with labral tear resection may have anterior hip tenderness for several weeks to months, despite resolution of their locking and clicking episodes. The cause is not clear, but it may be intra-articular in origin or due to tendonitis or bursitis over the anterior surface of the capsule. Patients with full-thickness cartilage loss may not have significant pain relief because of the inability to resurface the articular damage.

RESULTS

Arthroscopy can be used not only to diagnose intra-articular problems but also to provide therapeutic intervention. Fitzgerald (6) was able to treat a large series of patients with labral tears with arthrotomy and dislocation but recognized the usefulness of arthroscopy near the end of

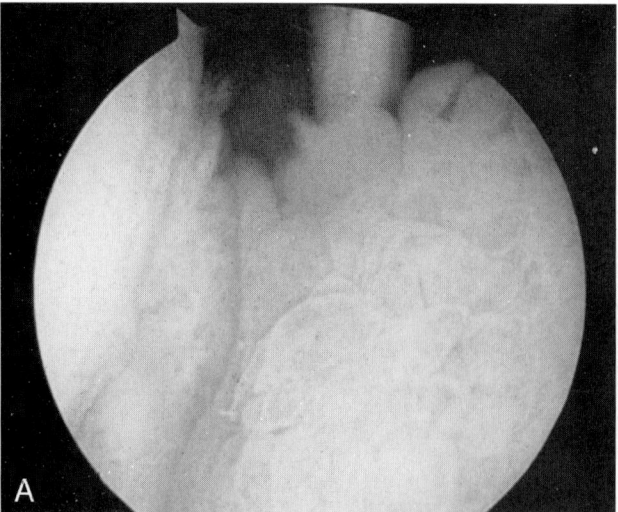
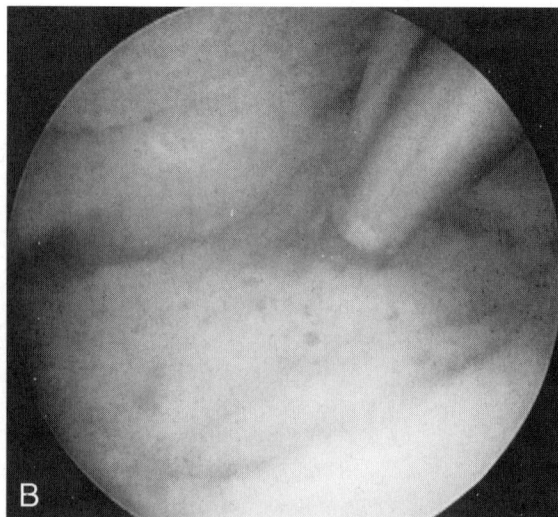

Figure 46.7. Hip synovitis before (**A**) and after (**B**) arthroscopic synovectomy.

that series. Other authors have had success treating patients with labral tears arthroscopically (5,14,26). Hip arthroscopy may provide some relief in patients with osteoarthritis, but its most significant role for osteoarthritis may be in diagnosis (13,16,26); although this use may be supplanted by MRI.

Other conditions that benefit from irrigation and synovectomy, such as juvenile rheumatoid arthritis (27), septic arthritis (28), and septic total hip replacement (23), may be significantly improved by minimally invasive hip arthroscopy (Fig. 46.7). Hip arthroscopy is especially useful for removing foreign bodies.

Certainly, few bridges are burned with hip arthroscopy. An arthrotomy can always be performed at a later date, or even combined at the same operative setting to complete the procedure.

SUMMARY

A relatively recent addition to the armamentarium of the operating orthopaedic surgeon is the arthroscopic evaluation and treatment of the hip joint. While a technically challenging operation, its use in treatment of symptomatic labral tears, chondral injuries, and synovial diseases makes it a valuable tool to evaluate and treat heretofore frustrating pathologies around the hip joint. In addition, it has an important role as an assist to hip arthrotomy in the treatment of more extensive synovial diseases, in removal of loose bodies in the more remote areas of the hip, and as an adjunct to the surgical treatment of the painful and stiff hip joint.

As surgeons become more familiar and comfortable with the anatomy and technical aspects of this procedure, its use and its value to the orthopaedic surgeon are certain to become more widespread to all surgeons treating muscloskeletal diseases.

REFERENCES

1. Dorrell JH, Catterall A. The torn acetabular labrum. J Bone Joint Surg 1986;68B:400–403.
2. Klaue K, Durnin CW, Ganz R. The acetabular rim syndrome. A clinical presentation of dysplasia of the hip. J Bone Joint Surg 1991; 73B:423–429.
3. Kim YT, Azuma H. The nerve endings of the acetabular labrum. Clin Orthop 1995;320:176–181.
4. McCarthy JC, Busconi B. The role of hip arthroscopy in the diagnosis and treatment of hip disease. Orthopedics 1995;18:753–756.
5. McCarthy JC, Day B, Busconi B. Hip arthroscopy: applications and technique. J Am Acad Orthop Surg 1995;3:115–122.
6. Fitzgerald RH Jr. Acetabular labrum tears. Diagnosis and treatment. Clin Orthop 1995;311:60–68.
7. Hodler J, Yu JS, Goodwin D, et al. MR arthrography of the hip: improved imaging of the acetabular labrum with histologic correlation in cadavers. AJR Am J Roentgenol 1995;165:887–891.
8. Petersilge CA, Haque MA, Petersilge WJ, et al. Acetabular labral tears: evaluation with MR arthrography. Radiology 1996;200: 231–235.
9. Buly RL, Potter HG, Connell D, et al. The diagnosis of labral and chondral injuries of the hip by high resolution MRI scanning: correlation with surgical findings. Paper presented at the summer meeting of the Hip Society, New York City, 1997.
10. Burman MS. Arthroscopy or the direct visualization of joints: an experimental cadaver study. J Bone Joint Surg 1931;13:669–695.
11. Takagi K. The classic: arthroscope. Clin Orthop 1982;167:6–8.
12. Watanabe M. Arthroscopy of small joints. 1971;45:908.
13. Eriksson E, Arvidsson I, Arvidsson H. Diagnostic and operative arthroscopy of the hip. Orthopedics 1986;9:169–176.
14. Glick JM. Hip arthroscopy. In: McGinty JB, ed. Operative arthroscopy. New York: Raven, 1991:663–676.
15. Johnson LL. Arthroscopic surgery principles and practice. 3rd ed. St. Louis: Mosby, 1986.
16. Hawkins RB. Arthroscopy of the hip. Clin Orthop 1989;249:44–47.
17. Klapper RC, Silver DM. Hip arthroscopy without traction. Contemp Orthop 1989;18:687–693.
18. Dorfmann H, Boyer T, De Bie B. Arthroscopy of the hip. Methods and values. Rev Rhum Ed Fr 1993;60:330-334.
19. Gross R. Arthroscopy in hip disorders in children. Orthop Rev 1977;6:43–49.
20. Shifrin LZ, Reis ND. Arthroscopy of a dislocated hip replacement: a case report. Clin Orthop 1980;146:213–214.
21. Nordt W, Giangarra CE, Levy IM, Habermann ET. Arthroscopic removal of entrapped debris following dislocation of a total hip arthroplasty. Arthroscopy 1987;3:196–198.
22. Vakili F, Salvati EA, Warren RF. Entrapped foreign body within the acetabular cup in total hip replacement. Clin Orthop 1980; 150:159–162.
23. Maynard MJ, Pellicci PM, Salvati EA, Sculco TP. Arthroscopic incision and drainage of the acutely infected total hip replacement. Paper presented at the summer meeting of the Hip Society, 1991.
24. Funke EL, Munzinger U. Complications in hip arthroscopy. Arthroscopy 1996;12:156–159.
25. Byrd JW. Hip arthroscopy utilizing the supine position. Arthroscopy 1994;10:275–280.
26. Villar RN. Hip Arthroscopy. Stoneham, MA: Butterworth-Heinemann, 1992.
27. Holgersson S, Brattstrom H, Mogensen B, Lidgren L. Arthroscopy of the hip in juvenile chronic arthritis. J Pediatr Orthop 1981; 1:273–278.
28. Blitzer CM. Arthroscopic management of septic arthritis of the hip. Arthroscopy 1993;9:414–416.

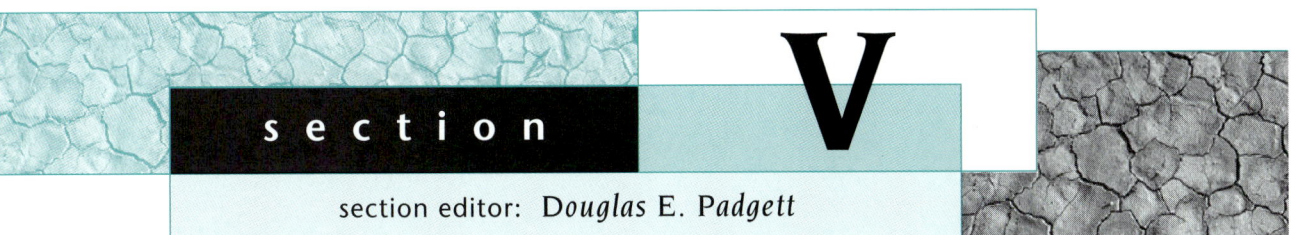

section **V**

section editor: *Douglas E. Padgett*

DEGENERATIVE KNEE

Geoffrey H. Westrich

Degenerative Joint Disease: Arthroscopy and Débridement

Great controversy exists concerning the role of arthroscopic débridement for the treatment of knee osteoarthritis (OA). The success of this procedure is variable and depends on several factors. Criteria that are useful for prognostic value include the degree of arthritis, the age of the patient, the patient's activity level, and the length of follow-up (1–4). Unfortunately, the impressive results of short-term follow-up have been tempered by the deterioration of pain relief and function seen on longer follow-up.

Knee arthroscopy has largely replaced open procedures for the treatment of knee disorders (1). Decreased morbidity and expedited return to a premorbid condition are noted with knee arthroscopy compared to the more extensive open procedures. Limited meniscal débridement or partial meniscectomy is now commonly performed by arthroscopy and is associated with little morbidity. In addition, arthroscopy may serve as a diagnostic tool and is useful for the assessment of degenerative knee arthritis.

RELEVANT ANATOMY AND PATHOGENESIS

The bony anatomy of the knee joint includes the distal femur, the proximal tibia, and the patella. The knee joint is a tricompartmental joint and consists of a patellofemoral articulation and medial and lateral femorotibial articulations. Ligaments about the knee include the collateral ligaments and the cruciate ligaments. The medial and lateral collateral ligaments prevent restraint to valgus and varus stresses, respectively. The anterior and posterior cruciate ligaments prevent anterior and posterior tibial translation on the femur and secondary restraint to rotation. A fibrocartilaginous medial and lateral meniscus provides stability and shock absorption, especially with axial loading in the knee.

Degenerative joint disease of the knee is characterized by wear and eventual loss of articular cartilage of the knee joint. Such degeneration may occur in any of the three joint compartments of the knee and can result in bone-on-bone contact. Patients with advanced arthritis of the knee joint complain of pain, swelling, decreased range of motion, and deformity. Such deformity can result in a valgus or varus knee, with or without a flexion contracture. Degeneration of the menisci (medial and/or lateral) frequently accompanies arthritis of the knee and may precede many of the bony and, therefore, radiographic changes.

INITIAL FINDINGS, PHYSICAL EXAMINATION, AND DIAGNOSIS

The most common complaint of patients with degenerative arthritis of the knee is pain. Initially, pain is of a mechanical-type and is exacerbated with motion of the knee. Eventually, patients may experience pain at rest; however, this is usually a more advanced finding. Swelling of the knee joint is also common with intra-articular knee disease and results from inflammation of the joint lining or synovitis. As the knee becomes inflamed, the normal range of motion is reduced, leading to fixed contractures of the knee. Bone loss from arthritis also exacerbates deformity in the knee and contributes secondarily to the development of soft tissue contractures.

The diagnosis of knee arthritis is based on the patient's history, the physical examination, and radiographic analysis of the knees. On physical examination, gross inspection of knee alignment, range of motion, ligamentous stability testing, and muscular strength assessment are all fundamental. Other physical signs, such as crepitus and joint effusion, are indicative of degenerative arthritis of the knee. Specific physical signs for meniscal disease are used to evaluate the integrity of the medial and lateral menisci; these signs include rotational and compressive tests, such as McMurray's, Steinmann's, and Apley's tests. A positive test is observed when pain is reproduced at the joint line with such maneuvers.

RADIOLOGIC STUDIES

To evaluate a patient with knee pain and presumed knee arthritis, the clinician should obtain standard radiographs. At the Hospital for Special Surgery, the knee clinic series consists of three views of the knee: a standing or weight-bearing AP view, a lateral view, and a Merchant view. Each film provides necessary information in regard to the anatomy of the knee joint. The weight-bearing AP radiograph allows visualization of the alignment of the knee with an axial load and is the best view for evaluating degenerative arthritis of the knee. Unweighted, supine AP radiographs can be misleading and should not be used. The lateral radiograph provides information about the anterior and posterior aspect of the knee, and the Merchant view allows visualization of the patellofemoral articulation.

Radiographs of a knee with degenerative joint disease demonstrate joint space narrowing, subchondral sclerosis, osteophyte formation, and bone loss. As such, the normal contour of the joint surfaces becomes misshapen, which contributes to further degeneration.

TREATMENT

Nonoperative Treatment

Early knee arthritis can be treated nonoperatively with some success, depending on the degree of degeneration. First, physical therapy with range of motion exercises, stretching, and strengthening can be helpful. Anti-inflammatory medications are also used and are the mainstay of nonoperative treatment, provided they are well tolerated by the patient. Unfortunately, patients with gastrointestinal problems may not be able to tolerate such medications. Intra-articular corticosteroid injections are also helpful and can provide significant pain relief. Note that much of the nonoperative treatment is directed at pain relief; the underlying disease of knee arthritis is unchanged and is usually progressive.

When patients fail nonoperative treatment, then it is necessary to consider operative intervention. Although total knee replacement remains the definitive treatment for advanced degenerative arthritis of the knee, the remainder of this chapter is directed toward less invasive treatment with arthroscopy and débridement. The success and failure, indications and contraindications will be discussed.

Operative Treatment and Indications for Surgery

HISTORICAL REVIEW

The concept of débridement of the knee joint for the treatment of arthritis was first introduced by Magnuson (5)

in 1941. He noted that "thorough removal of all mechanical irritating products of joint degeneration will, in a large percentage of cases, render the patient symptom free" (5). Magnuson performed a large arthrotomy with wide surgical exposure and removed a significant amount of bony tissue and damaged articular cartilage. Unfortunately, the procedure was associated with a painful, prolonged rehabilitation program before the patient regained motion and satisfactory ambulation. As such, the initial enthusiasm for this procedure slowly receded.

In 1959, Pridie (6) introduced the concept of drilling the osteosclerotic lesions of the osteoarthritic knee (6). This concept, as well as a thorough débridement, was also advocated by Insall (7,8). Once again, the enthusiasm waned, as the beneficial results were offset by the considerable extent of the operation and the postoperative rehabilitation.

The favorable effects of simple lavage of the knee without débridement were noted by several authors (2–4,9–11). It was observed that irrigation of the knee produced a large amount of debris, which was made up of joint fluid, fibrinous shreds, and cartilaginous fragments. Furthermore, it was postulated that the joint fluid contained irritants, such as prostaglandins, enzymes, and other chemicals (3,4). Débridement and abrasion chondroplasty were subsequently performed by Johnson (12) in 1981. He and others advocated abrasion of partial cartilaginous lesions to the level of the subchondral bone of the femur and tibia. At the time, it was thought that hyaline cartilage would fill in the defect; however, we now know that the new tissue is fibrocartilage (13). Although the ultimate fate of the fibrocartilaginous tissue is unknown, its mechanical properties are inferior to hyaline cartilage (14). As such, it is currently believed that fibrocartilage may be predisposed to subsequent degenerative disease and that abrasion chondroplasty should essentially be abandoned (15).

In 1991, Rand (15) compared arthroscopy with limited débridement to arthroscopy with abrasion chondroplasty. After a 3-year follow-up, he noted that "the results of abrasion arthroplasty are unpredictable" (15) and that little to no benefit is achieved with this technique. Furthermore, in a study of 126 patients, Bert and Maschka (16) noted that abrasion arthroplasty had a lower success rate than did débridement alone.

Novak and Bach (17) noted that the current trend is toward minimal débridement. They recommend removal of loose articular fragments, chondral flaps, osteophytes, and other debris that may cause impingement. In addition, removal of the fluid may also lessen the chemical irritant in the knee. With the advent of arthroscopy and newer arthroscopic equipment, these recommendations can be carried out expediently and with little morbidity.

DIAGNOSTIC ARTHROSCOPY

In 1986, an American College of Rheumatology subcommittee defined osteoarthritis as a "heterogeneous group

| table | 47.1 | The American College of Rheumatology's Classification of OA of the Knee |

Clinical and Laboratory	Clinical and Radiographic	Clinical Only

Knee pain
Plus at least 5 of the following 9:
  Age > 50 years
  Morning stiffness < 30 min
  Crepitus
  Bony tenderness
  Bony enlargement
  No palpable warmth
  ESR < 40 mm/h
  RF < 1:40
  Synovial fluid with OA signs[a]
	Knee pain
	Plus at least 1 of the following 3:
	  Age > 50 years
	  Morning stiffness < 30 min
	  Crepitus
	Plus osteophytes on x-ray
		Knee pain
		Plus at least 3 of the following 6:
		  Age > 50 years
		  Morning stiffness < 30 min
		  Crepitus
		  Bony tenderness
		  Bony enlargement
		  No palpable warmth

ESR, erythrocyte sedimentation rate; RF, rheumatoid factor.
[a]For example, clear viscus fluid with a white blood cell count < 2000/mL.

of conditions that lead to joint symptoms and signs which are associated with defective integrity of articular cartilage, in addition to related changes in the underlying bone and at the joint margins." The committee classified osteoarthritis into three categories: clinical and laboratory, clinical and radiographic, and clinical alone (18) (Table 47.1).

Overt knee arthritis is clearly visible on radiographic examination; however, more subtle knee degeneration may not be visible on plain radiographs. As such, knee arthroscopy may have a role in the evaluation of the painful knee in patients for whom osteoarthritis is part of the differential diagnosis. Several recent advances help support this opinion (1) (Fig. 47.1).

As noted, an American College of Rheumatology subcommittee refined the clinical definition of knee arthritis. The newer definition asserts that radiographic abnormalities are not the sine qua non for the diagnosis of OA and that the abnormalities in articular cartilage can be present in knees that have normal-appearing radiographs (1). With the advent of MRI and arthroscopy, significant abnormalities of intra-articular structures are now recognized in

symptomatic osteoarthritic knees. These abnormalities are complex and extensive and involve more than the usual triad of worn cartilage, reactive bone, and synovial proliferation/inflammation (1). The true impact of such abnormalities and their relation to knee symptoms and further degeneration remain unknown. Small arthroscopic units that are amenable for use in the office setting are now available. Such needle arthroscopes can provide useful diagnostic information at a substantially reduced cost by eliminating of the expense related to the surgical suite and anesthesia (1). Unfortunately, this technique is controversial and its use is limited in the current health care environment.

Presently, arthroscopy can aid in the differential diagnosis of the knee in five clinical settings (1):

A painful, swollen knee with normal radiographs and noninflammatory fluid;

Clinical and radiographic OA with pain that is out of proportion to the radiographic findings and is refractory to standard medical treatment;

Established chronic OA with an abrupt increase in symptoms;

OA with predominantly mechanical symptoms; and

OA with unexplained synovial fluid characteristics.

The Outerbridge grading system for articular cartilage degeneration can be used at the time of arthroscopy. Grade 1 changes include softening of an intact cartilage surface, grade 2 changes describe fissures or clefts in the cartilage surface, grade 3 changes include fibrillation of the cartilage, and grade 4 changes are characterized by visualization of bone (19).

SELECTION CRITERIA FOR KNEE ARTHROSCOPY

Although some selection criteria for knee arthroscopy in patients with degenerative knee arthritis have been elucidated, controversy still exists about the ideal surgical candidate, the timing of the surgical procedure, and the proposed surgical intervention (17). Knee arthroscopy for degenerative arthritis can be combined with arthroscopic lavage, débridement, or chondroplasty. Unfortunately, the

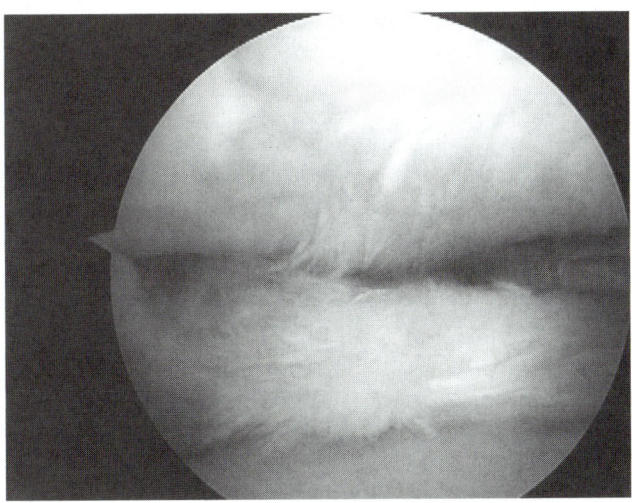

Figure 47.1. Arthritic knee with a torn medial meniscus.

literature is not replete with well-controlled studies that have long-term follow-up. Therefore, the surgeon must base his or her decision to perform a knee arthroscopy on selected clinical trials.

The establishment of absolute criteria for knee arthroscopy in the degenerative knee is next to impossible, based on the paucity of literature; however, relative indications and contraindications are available to help guide the orthopaedic surgeon. Several factors have been associated with a beneficial outcome (Table 47.2). Novak and Bach (17) conducted a literature review of knee arthroscopy for the osteoarthritic patient; they generated several conclusions that warrant discussion. Prospective factors that correlated with an improved outcome include normal limb alignment, history of mechanical symptoms, minimal radiographic degenerative findings, and short duration of symptoms. Criteria noted to correlate with a poor outcome include varus or valgus malalignment, loading symptoms, severe radiographic degenerative findings, previous surgeries, and chronic symptoms (Table 47.3).

Age

The role of arthroscopy for patients with degenerative knee arthritis has been evaluated by several authors. In a retrospective study, Lotke et al. (20) evaluated the late results of arthroscopic meniscectomy in a cohort of 66 patients. The average age was 55.6 years, but the authors stated that age alone did not influence the results of a traumatic meniscus tear in a normal joint treated with arthroscopy. Jackson and Rouse (21) reviewed 68 patients over 40 years of age who underwent arthroscopic meniscectomy and concluded that "patient's age at the time of meniscectomy did not adversely affect the eventual result." Using a subjective rating questionnaire of postoperative outcome after arthroscopy, Wouters et al. (22) determined that age did not have a statistically significant effect on outcome. In conclusion, advanced age, when considered as an independent variable, was clearly not a contraindication to arthroscopy.

table	47.2	Criteria for Knee Arthroscopy: Factors Associated with a Good Outcome

Normal limb alignment
History of mechanical symptoms
Minimal radiographic degenerative findings
Short duration of symptoms

table	47.3	Criteria for Knee Arthroscopy: Factors Associated with a Poor Outcome

Varus or valgus malalignment
Loading symptoms
Severe radiographic degenerative findings
Previous surgeries
Chronic symptoms

Chondrocalcinosis

Chondrocalcinosis describes cartilage that has calcified; it adversely effects the mechanical properties of articular cartilage and the menisci by producing a brittle and low-shock-absorbing material. In comparing the results of arthroscopic débridement in 12 knees that had chondrocalcinosis and 33 knees without chondrocalcinosis, Baumgaertner et al. (23) noted a trend toward more good and excellent results in patients with chondrocalcinosis. On the other hand, Ogilvie-Harris and Fitsialos (24) reviewed 51 patients with chondrocalcinosis who underwent arthroscopy and noted that only half of the patients with chondrocalcinosis had relief of symptoms. They concluded that chondrocalcinosis was a poor prognostic indicator. Although insufficient data exist to adequately evaluate the prognostic significance of chondrocalcinosis in the osteoarthritic knee, most surgeons exercise caution in proceeding with arthroscopic débridement in patients with chondrocalcinosis.

Duration of Symptoms

A long duration of symptoms before knee arthroscopy has been correlated with less satisfactory results (17). Lotke et al. (20) noted that patients who had preoperative symptoms for more than 1 year had much worse results following meniscectomy than patients who had symptoms of shorter duration. Patients with a longer duration of symptoms also had more degenerative disease than patients with a shorter duration of symptoms, thus precluding statistical analysis using duration of symptoms as an independent variable. In an analysis by Baumgaertner et al. (23), a similar trend was observed. In their series, 39% of patients with symptoms greater than 1 year experienced good to excellent results, whereas 72% of patients with symptoms less than 1 year had good to excellent results. Wouters et al. (22) noted that pain of less than 3 months' duration correlated with a beneficial score on subjective outcome assessments after knee arthroscopy. In summary, a shorter duration of symptoms has been associated with a better prognosis.

Previous Surgery

Previous surgery has been associated with a less favorable outcome following knee arthroscopy. Ogilvie-Harris and Fitsialos (24), noted that only 37% of patients with previous knee surgery had good results at a 3.9-year follow-up, whereas 53% of patients without previous surgery had good results at a 4.1-year follow-up. Similarly, Wouters et al. (22) determined that a history of previous knee surgery was statistically associated with a poor outcome after arthroscopy.

Limb Malalignment

Preoperative limb malalignment with varus or valgus angulation has been associated with a poor prognosis following arthroscopy for degenerative knee arthritis (17). Ogilvie-Harris and Fitsialos (24) found that 24% of valgus knees and 47% of varus knees had a good result after arthroscopy, in contrast to 61% of normal knees at a 4-year follow-up. Similarly, Baumgaertner et al. (23) reported good to excellent results after arthroscopic débridement in 26% of patients with varus knees and 52% of patients with normal alignment. In a study of 48 arthritic knees, Salisbury et al. (25) found that varus malalignment treated with arthroscopic débridement fared poorly; only 7% of patients with varus knees experienced 50% or better pain relief, and only 32% reported "acceptable" functional ratings. When arthroscopic abrasion arthroplasty was combined with high tibial osteotomy for the treatment of varus gonarthrosis in 21 patients, Fanelli and Rogers (26) observed that the arthroscopic abrasion arthroplasty "adds morbidity with no clear improvement in results." In conclusion, the literature does not support knee arthroscopy for the treatment of knee malalignment.

Severity of Degenerative Disease

The severity of degenerative disease in the knee is correlated with a negative result from arthroscopy (17). Patients with moderate to severe degenerative changes on plain radiographs have poor outcomes after knee arthroscopy. Using a questionnaire, Wouters et al. (22) found that patients' subjective outcomes had a negative correlation with the extent of knee arthritis. Lotke et al. (20) reported that patients with moderate to severe degenerative changes had only 21% good to excellent results following knee arthroscopy, whereas patients with normal knee radiographs had 90% good to excellent results. Ogilvie-Harris and Fitsialos (24) corroborated the results of the Wouters et al. study, concluding that the extent of radiographic disease also correlated with a negative outcome after knee arthroscopy. Baumgaertner et al. (23) noted the same finding, reporting only 33% good to excellent results in patients with severe degenerative changes on preoperative radiographs compared to 77% good to excellent results in patients with mild degenerative changes. Furthermore, Jackson and Rouse (21) studied partial arthroscopic meniscectomy and reported 80% good to excellent results in the presence of knee arthritis compared to 95% good to excellent results when no degenerative changes were observed (Fig. 47.2). In summary, the results of arthroscopy and arthroscopic débridement in patients with advanced degenerative arthritis are poor, and the clinician should seek alternative treatment.

Mechanical Symptoms

Mechanical symptoms, such as locking, clicking, popping, and joint effusion, are not uncommon in patients over 40 years old (17). Such physical findings are the result of torn menisci, loose bodies, or chondral injury. In this group of patients, arthroscopy tends to have a more favorable outcome. Jackson and Rouse (21) examined meniscal tears treated with arthroscopy and noted 95% good results

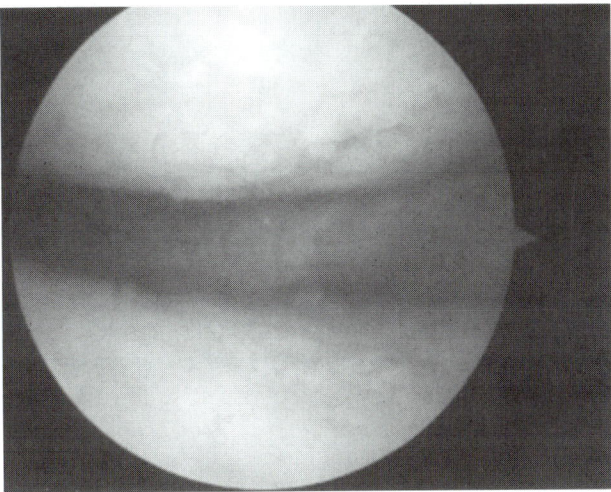

Figure 47.2. Arthritic knee after arthroscopy and débridement.

in patients with normal articular surfaces. When Baumgaertner et al. (23) stratified their patients into two groups—mechanical versus loading symptoms—and found 34% good to excellent results for patients with loading symptoms and 66% good to excellent results for patients with mechanical symptoms.

Lotke et al. (20) suggested that meniscectomy was useful in an elderly population for acute meniscus tears and when mechanical symptoms of a meniscus tear were observed. Ogilvie-Harris and Fitsialos (24) found that patients with unstable meniscal tears had the best results. A total of 96% of patients with acute tears treated arthroscopically experienced good to excellent results compared to 65% of patients with degenerative tears treated in the same manner. Thus the use of arthroscopy in patients with mechanical symptoms appears to be indicated.

SUMMARY

With the current advancement in technology, the arthroscope is useful not only in the treatment of the degenerative knee but also as a diagnostic tool when OA is part of the differential diagnosis for knee pain, including the following clinical scenarios: painful, swollen knee with normal radiographs and noninflammatory fluid; clinical and radiographic OA with pain out of proportion to the radiographic findings and refractory to standard medical treatment; chronic OA with an abrupt increase in symptoms; OA with predominantly mechanical symptoms; and OA with unexplained synovial fluid characteristics (1).

Arthroscopy of the knee is useful for treating knee arthritis; however, certain selection criteria are essential to the ultimate success or failure of the procedure. While absolute indications and contraindications are controversial, several criteria are available to guide the orthopaedic surgeon (Tables 47.1 and 47.2).

Further research with randomized, prospective studies using a large number of patients and long-term follow-up is necessary to establish definitive recommendations for arthroscopy in the treatment of knee arthritis.

REFERENCES

1. Ike RW. The role of arthroscopy in the differential diagnosis of osteoarthritis of the knee. Rheum Dis Clin North Am 1993; 19:673–696.
2. Jackson RW. The role of arthroscopy in the management of the arthritic knee. Clin Orthop 1974;101:28–35.
3. Jackson RW. Arthroscopic treatment of degenerative arthritis. In: McGinty JB, ed. Operative arthroscopy. New York: Raven, 1991:319–323.
4. Jackson RW, Marans HJ, Silver RS. The arthroscopic treatment of degenerative arthritis of the knee. J Bone Joint Surg 1988;70B:332.
5. Magnuson PB. Joint débridement, surgical treatment of degenerative arthritis. Surg Gynecol Obstet 1941;XX:73.
6. Pridie KW. A method of resurfacing osteoarthritic knee joints. J Bone Joint Surg 1959;41B:618.
7. Insall JN. Intra-articular surgery for degenerative arthritis of the knee. A report of the work of the late K. H. Pridie. J Bone Joint Surg 1967;49B:211–228.
8. Insall JN. The Pridie débridement operation for osteoarthritis of the knee. Clin Orthop 1974;101:61–67.
9. Burman MS, Finkelstein H, Mayer L. Arthroscopy of the knee joint. J Bone Joint Surg 1934;16:255–268.
10. Shahriaree H. O'Conner's textbook of arthroscopic surgery. Philadelphia: Lippincott, 1984:271–274.
11. Watanabe M, Takeda S, Ikeuchih H. Atlas of arthroscopy. Tokyo: Igaku Shoin, 1957.
12. Johnson LL. Diagnostic and surgical arthroscopy. St. Louis: Mosby, 1981.
13. Friedman MJ, Berasi CC, Fox JM. Preliminary results with abrasion arthroplasty in the osteoarthritic knee. Clin Orthop 1984; 182:200–205.
14. Green WT, Akeson WH, Mankin HJ. Can cartilage heal? Contemp Orthop 1981;3:157.
15. Rand JA. The role of arthroscopy in osteoarthritis of the knee. Arthroscopy 1991;7:358–363.
16. Bert JM, Maschka K. The arthroscopic treatment of unicompartmental gonarthrosis: a five-year follow-up study of abrasion arthroplasty plus arthroscopic débridement and arthroscopic débridement alone. Arthroscopy 1989;5:25–32.
17. Novak PJ, Bach BR Jr. Selection criteria for knee arthroscopy in the osteoarthritic patient. Orthop Rev 1993;22:798–804.
18. Altman R, Asch E, Bloch D. Development of criteria for the classification and reporting of osteoarthritis. Arthritis Rheum 1986; 29:1039–1049.
19. Outerbridge RE. The etiology of chondromalacia patellae. J Bone Joint Surg 1961;43B:752–757.
20. Lotke PA, Lefkoe RT, Ecker ML. Late results following medial meniscectomy in an older population. J Bone Joint Surg 1991; 63A:115–119.
21. Jackson RW, Rouse DW. The results of partial arthroscopic meniscectomy in patients over forty years of age. J Bone Joint Surg 1982; 64B:481–485.
22. Wouters RW, Bassett FH, Hardaker WT, Garett WE. An algorithm for arthroscopy in the over fifty age group. Am J Sports Med 1992; 20:141–145.
23. Baumgaertner MR, Cannon WD, Vittori JM. Arthroscopic débridement of the arthritic knee. Clin Orthop 1990;253:197–202.
24. Ogilvie-Harris DJ, Fitsialos DP. Arthroscopic management of the degenerative knee. Arthroscopy 1991;7:151–157.
25. Salisbury RB, Nottage VM, Gardner V. The effect of alignment on results in arthroscopic débridement of the degenerative knee. Clin Orthop 1985;198:268–272.
26. Fanelli GC, Rogers VP. High tibial valgus osteotomy combined with arthroscopic abrasion arthroplasty. Contemp Orthop 1989; 19:547–550.

Osteotomies About the Knee

Deformity about the knee associated with arthritis is a common presenting complaint to the orthopaedic surgeon. One of the standard operations in the orthopaedic armamentarium is the osteotomy to correct such deformity; the procedure has a long history in orthopaedics. The concept stems from the derivation of the term *orthopaedics*, which translates roughly from the Greek as "straight" (*orthos*) "child" (*paidion*). The term was first coined by Nicholas Andry in 1741.

Many orthopaedic procedures are available to help patients afflicted with deformities about the knee: arthroscopy, osteotomy, arthroplasty, and fusion in addition to observation and medication. This chapter deals with the use of the osteotomy to help correct the deformity and its associated symptoms.

RELEVANT ANATOMY AND PATHOGENESIS

A thorough understanding of normal knee alignment is needed before knee malalignment can be addressed. When standing, the standard knee bears 60% of the load through the medial aspect of the joint, and 40% through the lateral aspect of the joint. A line drawn from the center of the femoral head to the center of the ankle should pass just medial to the center of the knee in normal alignment (Fig. 48.1). This is the normal mechanical axis of the knee. Because the femur is offset by the femoral neck, an angle is created by the center of the shafts of the femur and tibia. The angle, or anatomic axis, is generally 6° to 8° of anatomical valgus (Fig. 48.2).

As deformity occurs about the knee, either from arthritic wear or malunion of a fracture, the manner in which the joint surfaces bear the load is altered, leading to overload. This may cause pain and progressive deformity. By correcting the deformity, the surgeon hopes to reverse the arthritic process and the progression of the disease, achieving an ideal mechanical solution to the problem.

The typical deformity is one of varus; overload occurs in the medial compartment, leading to degenerative changes. More concern is raised with the valgus deformity, because this is associated with rheumatoid patients, for whom osteotomy may be contraindicated. Each of these deformities is handled differently and will be discussed independently.

The classic high tibial osteotomy (HTO) for varus gonarthrosis was first mentioned by Jackson in 1958 and was later described by Jackson and Waugh (1). Wardle (2) noted that the operation has a history dating to Sir Robert Jones. At the turn of the century, the operation was performed distal to the tubercle, and the deformity was corrected but not overcorrected.

HTO was then championed by Coventry (3–6) during the 1960s and 1970s, when little else was available for the treatment of arthritis; the procedure is also known as the Coventry osteotomy. Coventry, using excellent follow-up, delineated the classic relative indications and contraindications along with the surgical approach and fixation. The key to the HTO is not the correction but the overcorrection of the deformity. The results deteriorate with incomplete correction and exuberant overcorrection of the deformity; unfortunately, there is a deterioration of outcome, despite adequate technical performance of the procedure.

Although the obvious source of pain relief is the correction of the deformity, microfracture and stiffness may also play roles. One concept is that the osteotomy decreases bony stiffness, thus decreasing pain as healing takes place (6). Another theory notes that osteotomy relieves the increased intraosseous pressure that is caused by the deformity (7). There is some support for all of these considerations, and each likely plays a role in the relief of pain after osteotomy.

The results of HTO must be viewed with an eye toward the reproducible and excellent outcomes of modern knee arthroplasty. Furthermore, revision of osteotomy to arthroplasty is generally believed to be more difficult than is primary arthroplasty (7). Today's sophisticated patient population may not accept the deformity created by HTO and is likely to opt for arthroplasty, which corrects the deformity instead of increasing it.

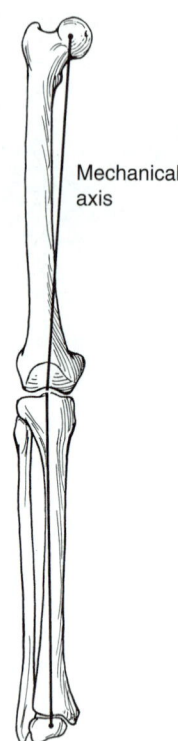

Figure 48.1. Mechanical axis of the knee. Note that the normal alignment of the femoral head with the center of the ankle falls in the center of the knee.

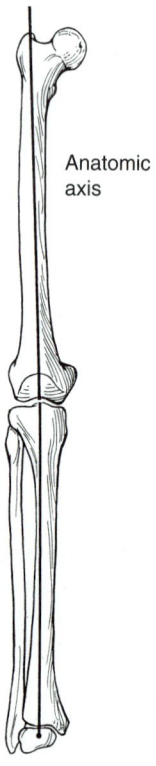

Figure 48.2. Anatomic axis of the knee. Note the valgus alignment created by the offset of the femoral neck.

INITIAL FINDINGS, PHYSICAL EXAMINATION, AND DIAGNOSIS

The degenerative changes after surgical meniscectomy were first described by Fairbanks in the 1940s. The classic findings are a squaring off of the compartment along with spurring of the joint surface. Progressive erosion and cystic changes are commonly seen in the more advanced stages. Typically, there is an increase of deformity, which lends itself to correction.

The patient usually presents with knee deformity and has had associated knee symptoms for several months or years. Pain is localized to the affected part of the knee; and the clinician should be wary of the valgus deformity, which is more common in the inflammatory arthritis population, for whom osteotomy is a relative contraindication. The history should reveal the progressive nature of the symptoms or perhaps trauma, with or without surgical intervention. The degree to which the patellofemoral region is involved should be evaluated, and any hip or back symptoms should be recorded.

The clinician should evaluate the knee joint thoroughly, noting the degree of swelling and the gross alignment of the limb in stance and at rest on the examination table. The degree of ligamentous laxity, particularly the degree of correction with stress on the joint, should be assessed. Active and passive range of motion should be evaluated, and the amount of crepitus about the affected side and the patellofemoral region should be documented. Any deformity remote from the site of the joint should be recorded. The clinician should evaluate the gait, looking specifically for a valgus thrust or adduction moment, in which the varus knee seems to wobble as it is weighted in the stance phase of gait. A complete correspondence of knee wobble with valgus thrust does not exist, as the gait laboratory will reveal. Evaluation of hip stiffness and the back should reveal any associated symptoms.

Typically, patients who are candidates for osteotomies should be in their fourth to sixth decade of life and wish to maintain an active lifestyle. An ideal candidate is a young laborer who anticipates years of significant joint loading; this is exactly the patient for whom arthroplasty is relatively contraindicated (6). An elderly patient may be considered a candidate for osteotomy; but arthroplasty, with its more reproducible outcome, is more strongly indicated. In addition, men are more likely to accept the necessary deformity created by the procedure than are women, who decline the operation because of it (8).

RADIOLOGIC STUDIES

Screening knee radiographs include a bilateral standing AP, lateral, and skyline views of the affected joint (6). Routine unweighted radiographs may miss significant disease. Although the short leg standing radiograph may show joint narrowing, the single view cannot accurately show overall limb alignment. Therefore, when contemplating an osteotomy, long leg standing films, from hip to ankle, are essential. Accurate evaluation of limb alignment made from these films guides the plan of treatment. The intramedullary canal allows an accurate evaluation for the anatomic axis.

The short leg films allow adequate evaluation of the involved compartment and the patellofemoral region. Significant involvement of additional compartments is a relative contraindication to the osteotomy. In addition, the radiographs can help screen for inflammatory components.

Bone scans and MRI studies are of little benefit; however, if there is concern over the intra-articular aspect of the knee, they may be helpful. Meniscal disease is not in and of itself a contraindication to osteotomy. Significant articular damage seen on the MRI studies may be of concern; however, these changes will likely be seen on the weighted radiographs. The classic patient will have a significant varus deformity with medial compartment changes and no significant changes in the lateral and patellar compartments. A valgus deformity may be amenable to correction if the other compartments are spared. These patients are routinely readily apparent on evaluation.

TREATMENT

Nonoperative Alternatives

Many patients may decide to observe and reevaluate their condition in 6 to 12 monthly intervals. The use of anti-

inflammatory medication on a running or as-needed basis may help alleviate symptoms. There are bracing options for unweighting the affected compartment, which may help the patient's symptoms; but many braces eventually become cumbersome, and the initial cost may be prohibitive. Orthotic management with medial or lateral shoe wedges can perform the same function as the brace and may be more cost effective. None of these options can truly alter the loading of the joint or the progressive nature of the degenerative arthritis.

In the classic presentation, the patient will have failed attempts at conservative care, and the opportunity for correction will have been presented. Patients whose lifestyles involve running or impact-loading activities may find the idea of osteotomy appealing, because arthroplasty requires that the joint experience only limited impact loading.

Operative Treatment

HIGH TIBIAL OSTEOTOMY

Indications

For patients with varus deformity and adequate motion, osteotomy about the metaphyseal region of the tibia, proximal to the tibial tubercle, to correct the deformity is considered (Fig. 48.3). The classic indications require minimal flexion contracture and an arc of motion of at least 80° (5,6) (Clinical Table). Patients do seem to lose some motion; thus markedly limited motion before surgery is a con-

---

Clinical Table: Osteotomies About the Knee

Procedure	Indications	Technique	Anatomy	Pitfalls
HTO	• Varus deformity • Adequate motion • Medial pain	• Closing wedge tibial metaphysis	• Tibiofibular joint • Peroneal nerve • Patellar tendon	• Undercorrection or overcorrection • Articular fracture • Nerve palsy • Delayed union or nonunion
Distal femoral osteotomy	• Valgus deformity • Adequate motion • Lateral pain	• Closing wedge femoral metaphysis	• Distal femur approach	• Fixation failure • Delayed union or nonunion
High tibial valgus osteotomy	• Valgus deformity • Lateral pain	• Closing wedge medially	• Tibial metaphysis • Patellar tendon	• Joint line angulation • Undercorrection or overcorrection • Articular fracture • Nerve palsy • Delayed union or nonunion
Combined HTO and ACL reconstruction	• Varus deformity • ACL deficient	• Closing wedge tibial metaphysis with arthroscopic ACL reconstruction	• Adductor patellar tendon • Intra-articular pathology	• Technically demanding
Dome osteotomy	• Varus deformity • Less leg length change than with wedge	• Dome saw blade in metaphysis	• Tibiofibular joint • Peroneal nerve • Patellar tendon	• Undercorrection or overcorrection • Articular fracture • Nerve palsy • Delayed union or nonunion

Figure 48.3. Lateral view of a typical preoperative varus deformity. Note the medial compartment narrowing. Reprinted with permission from Sulzer Orthopaedics, Inc., Austin, TX.

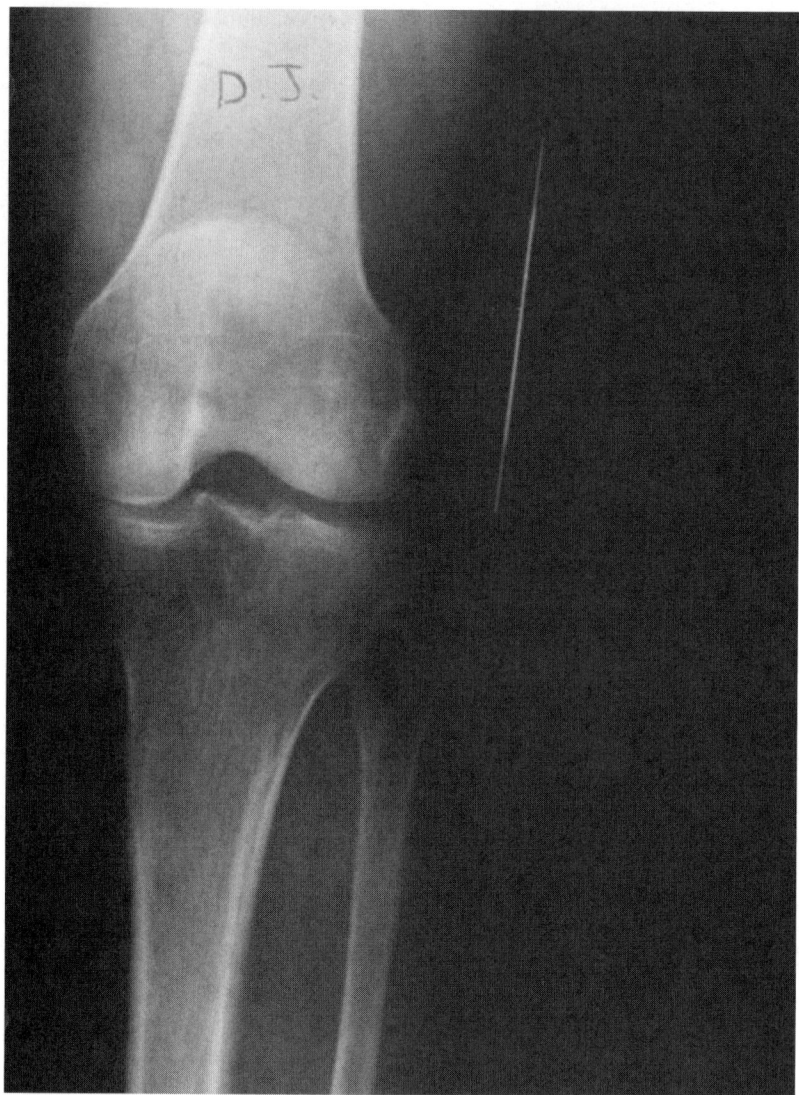

traindication. Significant degenerative change in the patellofemoral region is also a relative contraindication to the procedure.

The patient with a varus deformity but an otherwise stable knee who fits the criteria noted above is, therefore, a candidate for the procedure. A patient who has varus deformity and anterior cruciate ligament (ACL) deficiency may be treated with an ACL reconstruction in addition to the HTO. A technically demanding procedure, the HTO/ACL reconstruction addresses the underlying disorder and corrects the problems. Because it is not a routine procedure, it will not be discussed here.

Preoperative templating reveals the appropriate degree of correction; and several current guide systems are available to correct (or, rather, overcorrect) the deformity to provide the optimum outcome. The suggested overcorrection is an additional 3° to 6°, and the leg is returned to a neutral alignment (6).

Surgical Procedure

Under appropriate anesthesia, the leg is routinely prepped and draped with the use of a well-padded thigh-high tourniquet. Preoperative antibiotics are administered before the tourniquet is inflated. The patella, patellar tendon, and tibial tubercle are outlined. Fluoroscopic control is available for the procedure. A curvilinear incision is made along the lateral tibial crest, curving above the fibular region to create a flap. The tibiofibular joint is identified and disrupted with an osteotome; the medial portion of the fibular head is resected. Care is taken to avoid injury to the peroneal nerve as it winds around the fibular neck; many surgeons avoid fibular head resection for this reason. The anterior compartment musculature is identified and released from the tibial metaphyseal region, allowing access to the bone. At this time a sliding fasciotomy is performed to prevent the possibility of a postoperative compartment syndrome.

The medial and lateral compartments of the knee are then identified with the use of spinal needles under fluoroscopy; the medial side is felt through the skin, and the lateral side is found through the incision. These needles are used to help place the external guide for the proximal tibial pins. The placement of the pins is critical: approximately 1 cm distal to the tibial joint line and proximal to the tibial tubercle, with no tilt in the sagittal plane. Once the locations are confirmed with biplanar fluoroscopy, the pins are depth gauged to allow an adequate cut to be prepared. This placement prevents inadvertent fractures of the tibial plateau (as may occur with a more proximal and thinner cut) and allows the pins to be overdrilled and used as the proximal pins in a plate fixation system.

The anterior structures are protected with a thin, malleable retractor to prevent injury to the patellar tendon; the posterior neurovascular structures are likewise protected. The proximal tibial cut is made; the surgeon should take care to stop before completely transecting the tibia. The angular correction that will protect the proximal structures and will end the wedge-shaped osteotomy before complete transection of the tibia is chosen, using the angle-cutting guide. A thin osteotome is often needed to help remove the bone wedge, and a towel clip may also be useful. The idea that 1 mm equals 1° is true only for very small tibia (59 mm wide) and thus will lead to undercorrection in the majority of cases.

The plate is then placed by overdrilling and setting the large proximal cannulated screws. The plate is an assistive device for the specially designed clamp that closes down the osteotomy site, using the intact medial cortex as a hinge (Fig. 48.4). Perforation of the medial cortex with a drill will often assist in closing the osteotomy. The bone from the removed wedge is used as graft material for the stepoff that was created laterally and for any defect within the osteotomy surface; the plate is fixed with a standard technique. Other fixation methods, including step staples and external fixators, have been used; but the current technique using rigid internal fixation seems to allow early mobilization and encourage early healing. The wound is closed over a suction drain, and a bulky dressing is applied. The knee is placed in an immobilizer.

There are many intraoperative concerns and pitfalls. Adequate correction and overcorrection must be obtained. Protection of the peroneal nerve is necessary during both the procedure and the application of the postoperative dressing (9). The use of ribbon retractors posteriorly should protect the neurovascular bundle. The osteotomy should be performed slowly to allow the medial hinge to

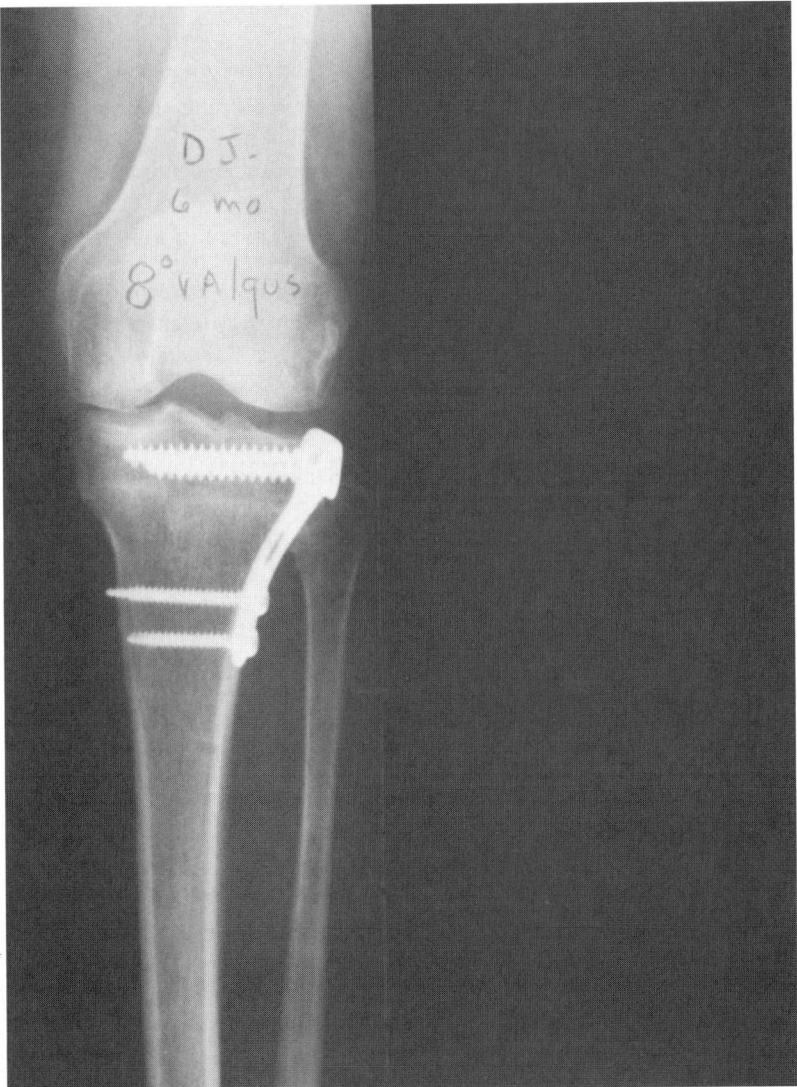

Figure 48.4. Lateral view of the typical postoperative appearance, 6 months after the procedure. Reprinted with permission from Sulzer Orthopaedics, Inc., Austin, TX.

remain intact. The osteotomy should be away from the joint line, to avoid inadvertent fracture of the tibial plateau. The routine concerns of superficial and deep infection should be addressed with perioperative antibiotics. Routine anticoagulation should be employed to avoid deep venous thrombus. Delayed union and nonunion are possible and may be treated with bone grafting, small wire fixation, or knee arthroplasty, on a case-by-case basis.

Postoperative care allows early weight bearing as tolerated and early range of motion exercises as limited by stiffness. Anticoagulation is prudent, as with all major limb procedures, during the period of high risk for clots. As Coventry noted, performing the osteotomy above the level of the tubercle ensures that the motion of the extensor mechanism applies a compressive force on the surgery site, encouraging healing. Routine follow-up imaging of the site to assess healing is done periodically. The patient returns to activities while using crutches and progresses to weight bearing based on clinical and radiographic assessment.

Other tibial osteotomy procedures have been recommended in specific situations by various authors. One procedure is the barrel-vault osteotomy, which has the advantage of not significantly altering leg length; another is the Maquet osteotomy, which allows anterior tubercle translation when associated with patellofemoral symptoms. Each of these procedures is somewhat more complex and difficult than the HTO and should be left to surgeons experienced in these settings.

DISTAL FEMORAL OSTEOTOMY

Indications

Patients with at least a 12° valgus deformity or a 19° joint line tilt and adequate motion, are candidates for distal femoral osteotomy. This operation is much less common than the HTO, because of the relative paucity of valgus knee in osteoarthritis and the still smaller number in the younger population. Although uncommon, the varus-producing femoral osteotomy may provide adequate results in a selected population. Fixation in this area is critical, and internal fixation with a blade plate or distal condylar screw is essential (10,11).

Surgical Procedure

Under appropriate anesthesia, the leg is routinely prepped and draped; a proximal tourniquet and control antibiotics are administered. A longitudinal incision is made over the medial femoral condyle, extending proximally; the standard midline incision may also be used, especially if a future arthroplasty is anticipated. The vastus medialis musculature is incised and elevated from the intermuscular septum, distally to the level of the joint line and proximally to allow appropriate fixation to be placed.

An osteotomy is then planned for the supracondylar region of the femur, using biplanar fluoroscopy. The fixation device is placed distally in the supracondylar region. A wedge of bone is then removed to allow the fixation device to rest snugly against the cortex, correcting the deformity by impacting the proximal fragment into the distal supracondylar region, where a stepoff is expected. The procedure requires significant preoperative planning and an intimate knowledge of the fixation device, either a Dynamic condylar screw or a blade plate. Routine fixation to the shaft of the femur is then secured using a standard technique. The bone wedge is used to graft the area about the stepoff. The wound is closed over suction drains, and the knee is placed in an immobilizer.

Early partial weight bearing based on the quality of the fixation and the patient's tolerance is allowed. Routine follow-up with radiographic evaluation is necessary to ensure adequate healing. Progression to normal activities may be expected over 3 months.

The most common complications include fixation failure and late fracture about the fixation device. Perioperative treatment methods common to all extremity wounds for preventing superficial or deep infection and postsurgery anticoagulation therapy minimize routine concerns. Delayed union and nonunion that require bone grafting have also been reported with osteotomies.

Coventry (12) described a varus tibial osteotomy as a sound counterpart to the more routine valgus-producing tibial osteotomy. In early series, a significant number of patients with valgus deformity were treated with this procedure; the results were acceptable and the procedures were considered routine HTOs. The varus-producing osteotomy, however, appears to produce some inherent difficulties with load transfer and may leave the joint line skewed; therefore, the distal femoral procedure should be performed for especially high valgus deformities (more than 10° of slope).

SUMMARY

HIGH TIBIAL OSTEOTOMY

Initial success and the lack of other surgical alternatives spurred on the early use of osteotomy. Long-term results are encouraging but clearly deteriorate with time. Furthermore, the results are related to the surgeon's attention to detail during the procedure. Coventry (8) reported that 67% of patients experienced pain relief at 4 years; but only 62% noted pain relief at 10+ years. These results correlate with the correction obtained at surgery and maintained during the postoperative period. Install et al. (8) achieved a success rate of 85% at 5 years, which deteriorated to 37% at 9 years. The strongest predictor of outcome in this series was time since the procedure. Healy and Riley (13) reported success rates from 92% at 2 years, 88% at 5 years, and 80% at 9 years. They suggested that adequate patient selection and careful operative technique accounted for their high rate of success over time.

The difficulties of revising osteotomy to arthroplasty must be tempered in light of the known failure rate. Gill et al. (7) noted that revision of an HTO to a total knee arthroplasty is technically demanding but appears to give good results. They wait 6.5 years before attempting the conversion. In addition, the outcomes surpass the results from the matched pair analysis of conversion from unicompartmental arthroplasty to total knee arthroplasty. Thus it is not surprising that Wright et al. (14) found that the HTO has been on the decline in the United States and Canada for about a decade. Most authors conclude that the operation may be best suited for young, active individuals for whom arthroplasty is best delayed.

DISTAL FEMORAL OSTEOTOMY

The success rates of one series of distal femoral osteotomies, based on Kaplan-Meier analysis, have been reported as 83% at 4 years and 64% at 10 years (15). Several of the early failures were related to poor patient selection, and significant degenerative changes were seen in the medial compartment before surgery. Late surgical failure was related to progressive changes in the knee joint at 7 to 9 years. In another study, the 4-year success rate was 86%, and none of the patients reported worsening symptoms (11). Thus as a palliative corrective procedure to delay arthroplasty, the distal femoral osteotomy appears to function as well as the HTO (16).

REFERENCES

 1. Jackson J, Waugh W. Tibial osteotomy for osteoarthritis of the knee. J Bone Joint Surg 1961;43B:746–751.
 2. Wardle E. Osteotomy of the tibia and fibula. Surg Gynecol Obstet 1962;115:61–64.
 3. Coventry M. Osteotomy of the upper portion of the tibia for degenerative arthritis of the knee. J Bone Joint Surg 1965; 47A:984–990.
 4. Coventry M. Osteotomy about the knee for degenerative and rheumatoid arthritis: indication, operative technique, and results. J Bone Joint Surg 1973;55A:23–48.
 5. Coventry M. Upper tibial osteotomy for gonarthrosis: the evolution of the operation in the last 18 years and long term results. Orthop Clin North Am 1979;10:191–210.
 6. Coventry M. Current concepts review: upper tibial osteotomy for osteoarthritis. J Bone Joint Surg 1985;67A:1136–1140.
 7. Gill T, Schemitsch E, Brick G, Thornhill T. Revision total knee arthroplasty after failed unicompartmental knee arthroplasty or high tibial osteotomy. Clin Orthop 1995;321:10–18.
 8. Insall J, Joseph M, Msika C. High tibial osteotomy for varus gonarthrosis. A long-term follow-up study. J Bone Joint Surg 1984; 66A:1040–1048.
 9. Wootton J, Ashworth M, MacLaren C. Neurological complications of high tibial osteotomy—the fibular osteotomy as a causative factor: a clinical and anatomical study. Ann R Coll Surg Engl 1995; 77:31–34.
10. Healy WL, Anglen JO, Wasilewski SA, Krackow KA. Distal femoral varus osteotomy. J Bone Joint Surg 1988;70A:102–109.
11. McDermott A, Finklestein J, Farine I, et al. Distal femoral varus osteotomy for valgus deformity of the knee. J Bone Joint Surg 1988; 70A:110–116.
12. Coventry M. Proximal tibial varus osteotomy for osteoarthritis of the lateral compartment of the knee. J Bone Joint Surg 1987; 69A:32–38.
13. Healy W, Riley L Jr. High tibial valgus osteotomy. Clin Orthop 1986;209:227–233.
14. Wright J, Heck D, Hawker G, et al. Rates of tibial osteotomies in Canada and the United States. Clin Orthop 1995;319:266–275.
15. Finkelstein J, Gross A, Davis A. Varus osteotomy of the distal part of the femur. A survivorship analysis. J Bone Joint Surg 1996; 78A:1348–1352.
16. Murray P, Rand J. Symptomatic valgus knee: the surgical options. J Am Acad Orthop Surg 1993;1:1–9.

Unicompartmental Knee Arthroplasty

One of the more difficult clinical situations that an orthopaedic surgeon may face is the problem of managing the patient with unicompartmental degenerative knee disease. Often these patients are young; and as such, their expectations are often great. All orthopaedic surgeons must have a clear understanding of the options available for treatment and the likelihood of success.

RELEVANT ANATOMY AND PATHOGENESIS

To understand unicompartmental knee disease, the surgeon must be familiar with knee mechanics. Overall alignment of the knee can be described in terms of the anatomic and mechanical axes (Fig. 49.1). The anatomic axis refers to the angle subtended between the shaft of the femur and the shaft of the tibia in the coronal plane. In the healthy individual without knee symptoms, the average angle of the anatomic axis is 5° to 7° of valgus. The mechanical axis refers to the angle drawn between a line intersecting the center of rotation of the femoral head to the center of the knee and a line drawn from the center of the knee to the center of the ankle. In an ideal setting, these lines would be colinear, yielding a mechanical axis of 0°; many knees actually fall in 1° to 2° of mechanical varus. Because of this relationship, investigators have shown that when the knee is loaded, such as in a single-leg stance, 55 to 60% of the load is borne by the medial compartment, while the remaining load is distributed on the lateral side. Knee alignment and its effect on load distribution are key to understanding unicompartmental disease.

Perhaps no single issue is as pertinent to the topic of degenerative knee disease than that of load distribution and the concept of load per unit area of contact. Articular cartilage has numerous outstanding properties, not the least of which is its ability to withstand impact loading. Unfortunately, when malalignment of the lower extremity significantly changes the distribution of load between the medial and lateral compartments, then load per unit area will increase. The capacity of the articular cartilage to withstand the elevated contact stresses is influenced by the load the cartilage bears (i.e., body weight) and the load shared by the contralateral compartment. With progressive malalignment, more load is shifted to a single compartment; hence the load per unit area is increased to the point at which it exceeds the remodeling capacity of the articular cartilage, leading to its degeneration. Once the protective layer of articular cartilage has been lost, direct contact of bone on bone produces pain and intra-articular particulate debris, which stimulates synovial fluid production, leading to warmth and swelling.

The cause of unicompartmental knee disease is often traced to mechanical factors. Patients with significant genu vara or valga may begin to manifest symptoms of knee disease as young adults or even as adolescents. Usually, the deformity is acquired either as a result of trauma or as a manifestation of postsurgical effects of meniscectomy. In the 1940s, Fairbank (1) recognized the effect of meniscectomy on the development of coronal plane malalignment and the predictable development of degenerative changes. Total meniscal resection leads to alterations in the distribution of load between compartments, creating a load per unit area that exceeds the capacity of articular cartilage and results in deterioration.

This chapter reviews the role of unicompartmental knee arthroplasty in the management of unicompartmental knee disease. The use of single compartment resurfacing and its role in the treatment of single compartment disease are discussed. The strict indications for the procedure's use in the setting of mechanical malalignment are emphasized, and the contraindications are noted. Although unicompartmental knee arthroplasty is a controversial procedure, I believe there is a clear role for it, if the

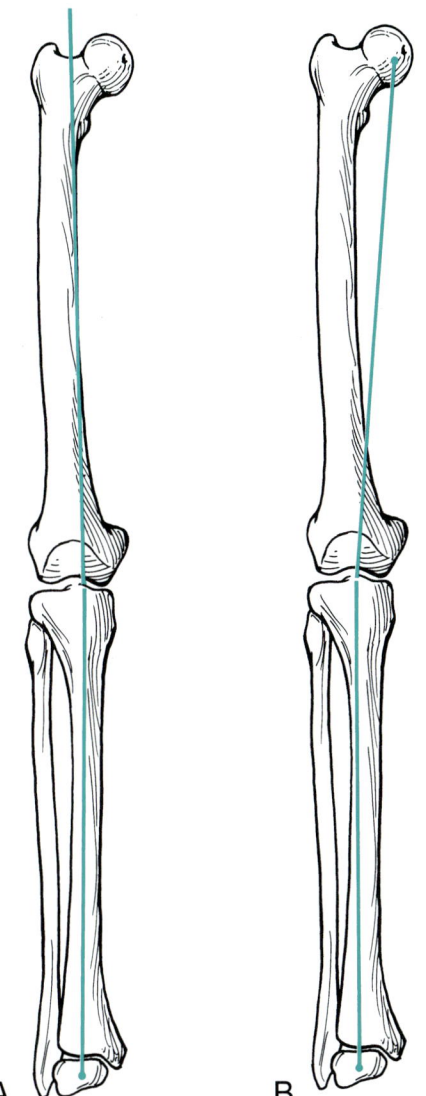

Figure 49.1. A. The anatomic axis of the knee is the angle subtended between a line drawn down the shaft of the femur and a line drawn down the shaft of the tibia. **B.** The mechanical axis of the knee is the angle between a line connecting the center of rotation of the hip to the center of the knee and a line drawn from the center of the knee to the center of rotation of the ankle.

surgeon understands the indications and pays careful attention to technique.

INITIAL FINDINGS, PHYSICAL EXAMINATION, AND DIAGNOSIS

The patient with unicompartmental knee disease presents with pain localized to either the medial or the lateral compartment. When recording the history, the clinician must discern between global (generalized) knee pain and pain that can almost be identified with the tip of one finger. In addition to the localization of pain, the quality of the pain must also be assessed. If the pain occurs at night

or at rest, then the clinician should suspect a more generalized process and perhaps an inflammatory component of the knee disease. The presence of other joint involvement may support a more generalized rheumatic process, and this information is crucial. Pain that is associated with weight bearing and loading is evidence of a mechanical origin. Obviously, it is important to note the onset of the pain and its relationship to trauma, prior surgery (e.g., meniscectomy), and any other sentinel event. Finally, the history should include the effect of rest that unloads the joint, the response to anti-inflammatory drugs, and the effectiveness of a cane or external support.

The physical examination of the patient who complains of unicompartmental knee disease begins with observing the gait. The patient should be dressed in shorts or a gown and asked to walk 6 to 9 m (20 to 30 ft). The examiner must pay particular attention to limb alignment and the single-leg stance. It is important to note any medial or lateral thrust and whether the knee shifts during stance, implying some degree of ligamentous laxity. The patient should be observed stepping up and down a single step to help define functional limitations and give insight into patellofemoral symptoms. Finally, the clinician should record the spinal and pelvic alignment and perform a cursory examination of each to ensure that the patient is not manifesting referred pain from above.

The effected knee should be inspected for the presence of any warmth or effusion. Passive motion should be evaluated, and the clinician should look for the presence and degree of flexion contracture and record the maximal flexion. The degree of varus or valgus alignment is recorded, as is the ability to passively correct the deformity. In general, more significant deformity tends to be fixed and application of varus or valgus stresses may not correct the malalignment. It is essential to test the ligamentous stability in both the anterior and the posterior directions. As will be discussed, ligamentous incompetence is a contraindication for unicompartmental arthroplasty.

RADIOLOGIC STUDIES

Radiographic evaluation is mandatory for determining the presence of unicompartmental knee disease. The standard four-view series developed by the Knee Service at the Hospital for Special Surgery (New York, NY) consists of a standing AP view, a flexed-knee lateral view, a notch view, and a Merchant view. The standing AP radiograph is an excellent initial screen for alignment problems, but it does not give complete information regarding mechanical alignment. If the patient's clinical picture and radiographs suggest isolated unicompartmental knee disease, then proceeding with a radiographic determination of the mechanical axis is indicated. Mechanical alignment must be assessed via a 1-m (3-ft) standing radiograph that includes the hip, knee, and ankle (Fig. 49.2). Based on these radiographs, the clinician determines the anatomic and mechanical axes.

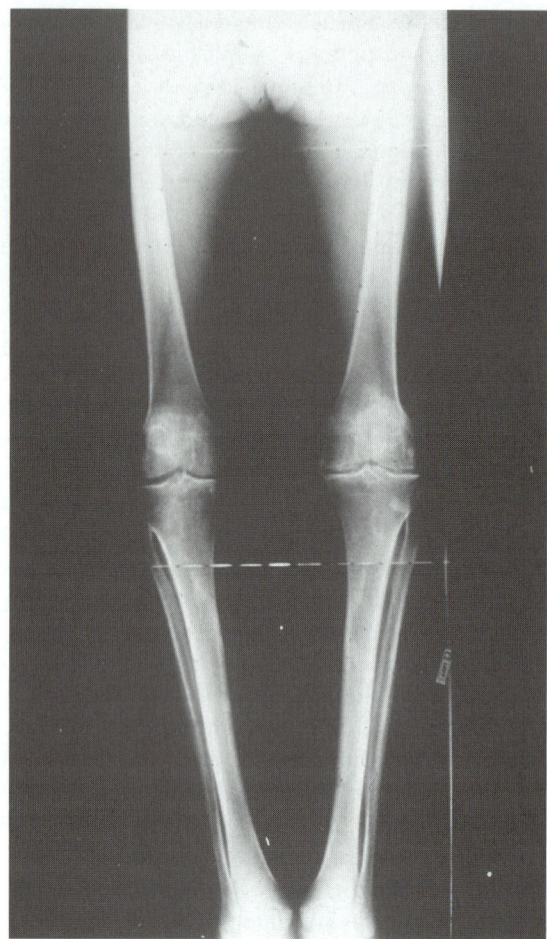

Figure 49.2. The anatomic and mechanical axes can be determined from the standing 1-m (3-ft) radiograph of the hip, knee, and ankle.

Additional Studies

Occasionally, a patient may present with isolated compartment complaints although the radiographs appear to be normal. The flexed-knee AP view, for which the patient stands in 45° of flexion, may be helpful (2). This radiograph can often demonstrate localized joint space narrowing that is not seen on the standard standing knee view. MRI is also useful in this setting and should be used as an adjunct to a thorough physical examination of the knee, not as a substitute.

Technetium bone scanning has been used to confirm the presence of isolated unicompartmental degenerative disease. Some authors have postulated that enhanced nuclide activity in the contralateral compartment or patellofemoral compartment suggests subclinical degenerative disease, which may turn the surgeon against isolated unicompartmental resurfacing.

Finally, the role of gait analysis in the evaluation of knee disease has been promoted by some authors as predictive of outcome, especially for tibial osteotomy. Gait laboratory analysis may provide the physician with data outlining the magnitude of loading forces about the joint. Based on prospective studies, Prodromos et al. (3) were able to define clear subgroups of patients with varus deformities based on the magnitude of adduction moments about the knee. They were able to predict which groups of patients undergoing tibial osteotomy were likely to have a successful outcome. Similar data on patients undergoing unicompartmental knee arthroplasty are being compiled, and it is hoped that this information may be used to predict the outcome of unicompartmental resurfacing.

TREATMENT

Indications for Surgery

The diagnosis of isolated unicompartmental knee disease is a synthesis of the patient's clinical symptoms, a supportive clinical examination, and radiographic confirmation. The treatment options for unicompartmental disease include conservative treatment with physical therapy and nonsteroidal anti-inflammatory drugs (NSAIDs), arthroscopic débridement, realignment osteotomy of the femur or tibia, unicompartmental resurfacing, and total knee arthroplasty.

RATIONALE FOR UNICOMPARTMENTAL ARTHROPLASTY

The main rationale for unicompartmental arthroplasty is that only the diseased part of the joint is resurfaced. To this end, proponents claim preservation of bone stock as a key feature. In addition, the retention of the anterior cruciate, posterior cruciate, and normal patellofemoral joint maintains a closer semblance to normal knee kinematics. Clinical series that have demonstrated knee motion approaching normal in many patients seem to support this claim. In addition, rehabilitation from unicompartmental arthroplasty appears to be faster than that from total knee arthroplasty, probably because of the more limited surgery involved. Finally, in the event of implant failure or the development of nonresurfaced compartment degenerative disease, conversion to total knee arthroplasty can be performed relatively easily and is easier than revision of a failed total knee arthroplasty.

INDICATIONS AND PATIENT SELECTION

It is imperative to remember that unicompartmental knee arthroplasty is similar in many ways to total knee arthroplasty. Therefore, relief of pain is the primary indication for unicompartmental arthroplasty. The patient must understand that joint arthroplasty may restrict his or her activity. The patient must avoid impact-loading activities to foster implant longevity. Therefore, the ideal candidate is older, somewhat sedentary, and unlikely to overuse the implant.

Experience has shown that some correction of deformity is possible with unicompartmental resurfacing, but the magnitude of correction is restricted to within 10° of neutral. Valgus or varus alignment exceeding 10° is difficult to correct with unicondylar resurfacing and should, therefore, be avoided. By design, unicompartmental resurfacing is a shared arthroplasty using both a prosthetic joint and the patient's remaining natural compartment. Its use is thus restricted to noninflammatory conditions.

CONTRAINDICATIONS FOR UNICOMPARTMENTAL KNEE REPLACEMENT

Conditions that preclude any joint arthroplasty can be applied to unicompartmental knee arthroplasty. These include inadequate bone stock, active sepsis, neuropathic joint, and neuromuscular conditions that yield inadequate motor control of the limb. The following are contraindications that are unique to unicompartmental arthroplasty.

1. *Excessive deformity.* Deformities greater than 10° of varus or more than 12° or 15° of valgus are not amenable to unicompartmental arthroplasty because of associated fixed contractures that may not be correctable.
2. *Inflammatory arthropathies.* Inflammatory conditions that compromise the load-bearing capacity of the articular cartilage are strict contraindications. These include all the rheumatic disease entities, such as rheumatoid arthritis; calcium pyrophosphate deposition disease; hemochromatosis; hemophilia; and ochronosis.
3. *Ligamentous incompetence.* Insufficiency of the cruciate ligaments or significant collateral ligament incompetence may cause abnormal loading and shear stress on the articulation, leading to material failure or premature implant loosening.
4. *Patellofemoral symptoms.* Although the extent of patellofemoral disease that can be accepted when performing unicompartmental arthroplasty is not known, the surgeon should avoid the procedure in patients with symptoms that suggest both unicompartmental disease and patellofemoral involvement.
5. *Patient expectations.* Return to vigorous activities is not recommended with unicompartmental arthroplasty. Assuming clinical criteria are met, younger patients with unicompartmental symptoms are better candidates for corrective osteotomy than for arthroplasty.

Operative Treatment

APPROACH

The operative approach to unicompartmental knee arthroplasty is similar to that of total knee arthroplasty: a midline anterior knee incision is recommended. Although Keblish (4) and others have used lateral arthrotomy for the total knee arthroplasty in valgus knees and when performing lateral unicompartmental arthroplasty, the medial parapatellar approach seems to be favored by most surgeons and affords ample visualization of the medial, lateral, and patellofemoral compartments.

Immediately on entering the joint, the surgeon should inspect the contralateral and patellofemoral compartments. Although Corpe and Engh (5) demonstrated that some degree of grade 3 or 4 change in the chondromalacia is acceptable in the patella and trochlea with unicompartmental knee arthroplasty, global loss of articular cartilage in the patellofemoral joint or loss on the weight-bearing surface in the contralateral compartment probably dictates a total knee arthroplasty instead. After inspection, the surgeon begins to correct the alignment. For the varus knee, a subperiosteal elevation of the superficial medial collateral ligament is performed. For the valgus knee, subperiosteal release of the iliotibial band off of Gerdy's tubercle is performed. Either of these is usually adequate to obtain a neutral mechanical axis. If ligamentous release and correction cannot be achieved, then total knee arthroplasty is recommended.

PROCEDURE

Bone resection is performed after the initial ligamentous balance is obtained and begins on the femoral side. Based on the preoperative assessment of the mechanical axis, the degree of femoral resection needed to allow a neutral axis is determined. Unlike osteotomy, for which overcorrection is acceptable, unicompartmental arthroplasty results are best when either a neutral axis or a slight undercorrection is obtained (6). The use of intramedullary rod systems for femoral resection has greatly improved the accuracy of bone resection, and most current unicompartmental systems employ them (Fig. 49.3).

Tibial bone resection is performed using extramedullary instrumentation (Fig. 49.4). It is imperative that the resection of the proximal tibia be performed perpendicular to the long axis. Care must be taken not to damage either the anterior or the posterior cruciate ligaments during bone resection. At this point, the surgeon assesses the gaps between the femur and the tibia in both flexion and extension. It is mandatory that full extension and full flexion (125°) be attained with no undue tightness. Tight flexion and extension gaps are achieved via additional proximal tibial bone resection. Space must be left for the 8-mm-thick polyethylene.

PITFALLS AND TECHNICAL MISTAKES

After the bone has been prepared with the chamfer cuts, trial reduction is performed. Pitfalls in component placement include (*a*) malrotation, especially internal rotation, of the femoral component; (*b*) residual varus placement of the tibial component; and (*c*) failure to juxtapose the tibial component with the tibial spines, which leads to either excess medial placement of medial unicompartmental knee or excessive materialization of a lateral unicompartmental knee arthroplasty. Once the component position is acceptable and full extension and flexion are obtained, the final implants are inserted (Fig. 49.5). Cementless unicompartmental knee arthroplasty has not performed well, and most surgeons advocate the use of bone cement for implant fixation.

Rehabilitation

The rehabilitation of a unicompartmental knee arthroplasty is similar to, but faster than, that of a total knee arthroplasty. Continuous passive motion is begun in the recovery room and is quickly progressed up to 90° by post-

Figure 49.3. The accuracy of distal femoral resection is greatly enhanced with the use of an intramedullary alignment device.

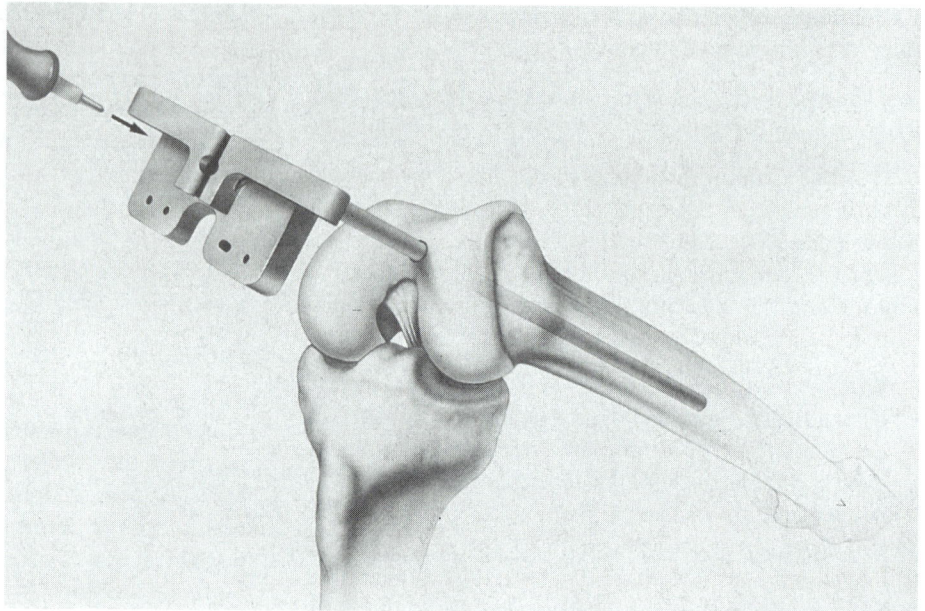

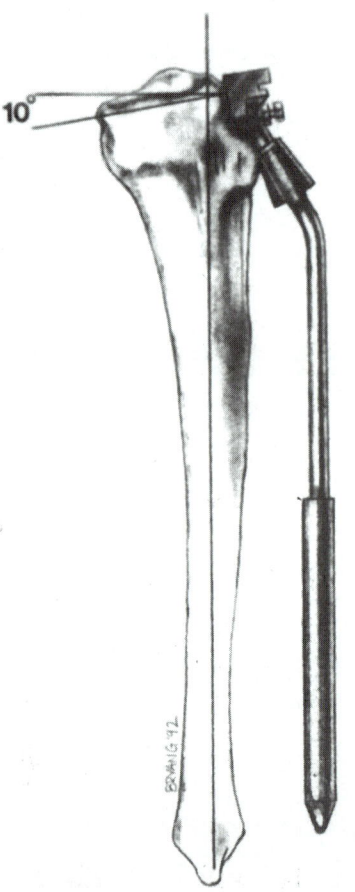

Figure 49.4. The extramedullary tibial resection guide is most commonly used for proximal tibial bone resection. The guide must be properly aligned not only for varus-valgus orientation but also for the appropriate degree of posterior slope. For unicompartmental arthroplasty, a posterior slope of 7° to 10° is desired.

operative day 3. Weight bearing as tolerated with the use of a walker or crutches is allowed. Quadriceps exercises to work on full extension are encouraged. The patient is usually independent by postoperative day 5 and is allowed to return home. Dangling with the knee bent at 90° for meals is encouraged, as are isometric quadriceps exercises for maintenance of extension. Following suture removal, patients are encouraged to use a stationary bicycle. Initially, the patient may find that it is easier to ride the bike with the seat elevated and to cycle in reverse; he or she should gradually lower the seat and begin to pedal forward to expedite recovery of flexion. Independent ambulation without aids is usually possible within several weeks, depending on the return of quadriceps function.

Clinical Results of Unicompartmental Arthroplasty

PRIMARY UNICOMPARTMENTAL ARTHROPLASTY

The design and instrumentation of unicompartmental knee arthroplasty have been evaluated. The initial results of unicompartmental replacement were far from uniformly successful. Success rates of only 62 to 75% have been reported (7–9). One of the main difficulties with the procedure was obtaining proper implant alignment. At the time of these reports, arthroplasty was performed almost freehand; thus predictable implant positioning was difficult. Unfortunately, implant failure due to component malposition was common. As a result of these poor results, the popularity of unicompartmental knee arthroplasty waned.

In the 1980s, however, second-generation implants were developed, improving the procedure (Fig. 49.6). The modern unicompartmental knee replacements yielded much improved clinical efficacy. Scott et al. (10) were able to show a 90% satisfaction rate at almost 10 years, using the Brigham unicompartmental knee replacement. These re-

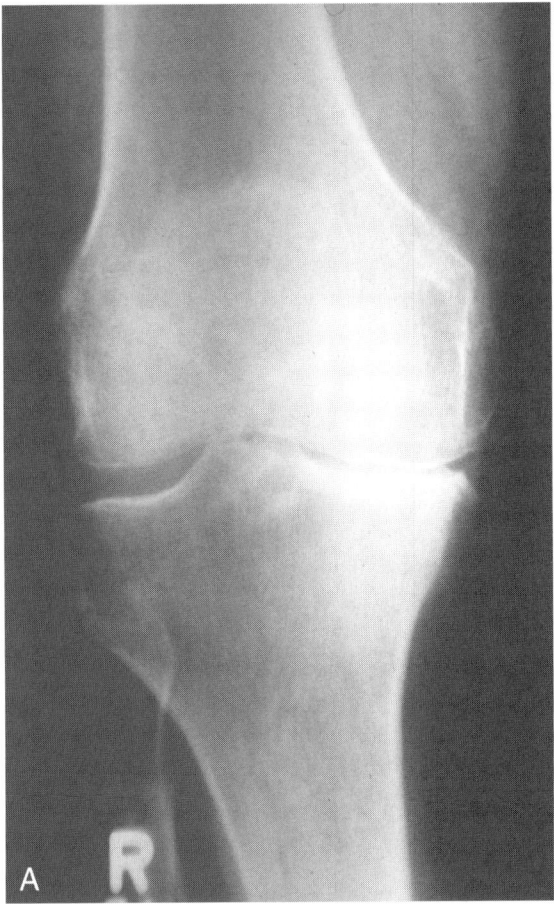
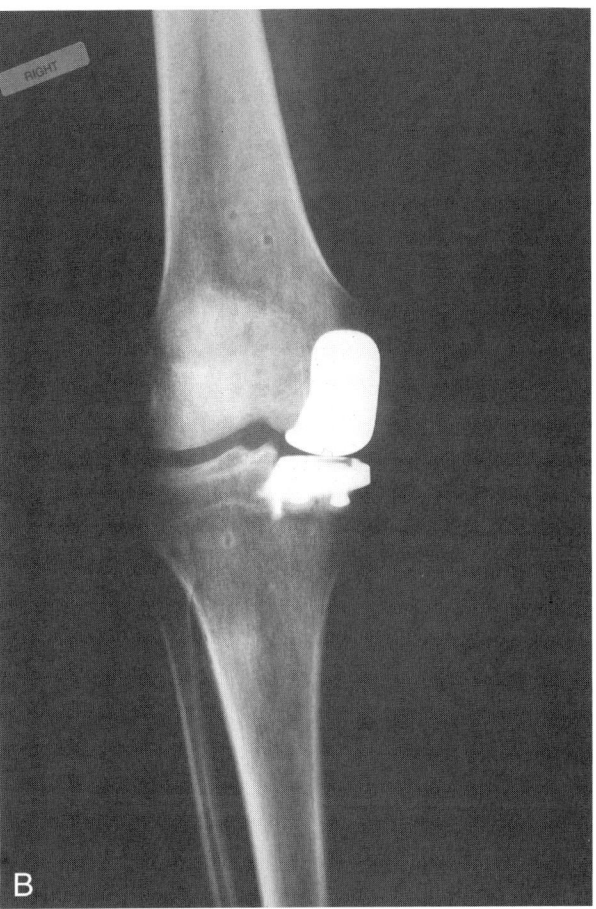

Figure 49.5. Preoperative (**A**) and postoperative (**B**) views of a patient with varus gonarthrosis (degenerative knee disease). For the long-term success of unicompartmental arthroplasty, it is imperative to avoid overcorrection of the varus deformity.

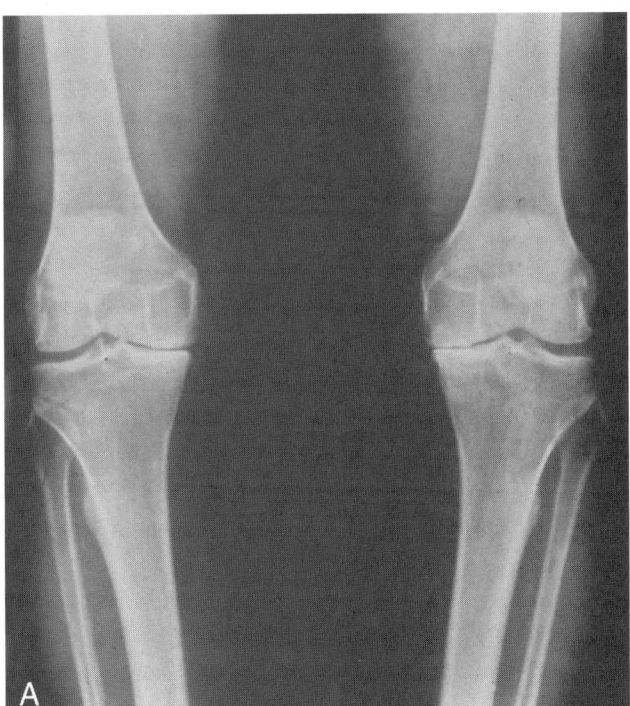
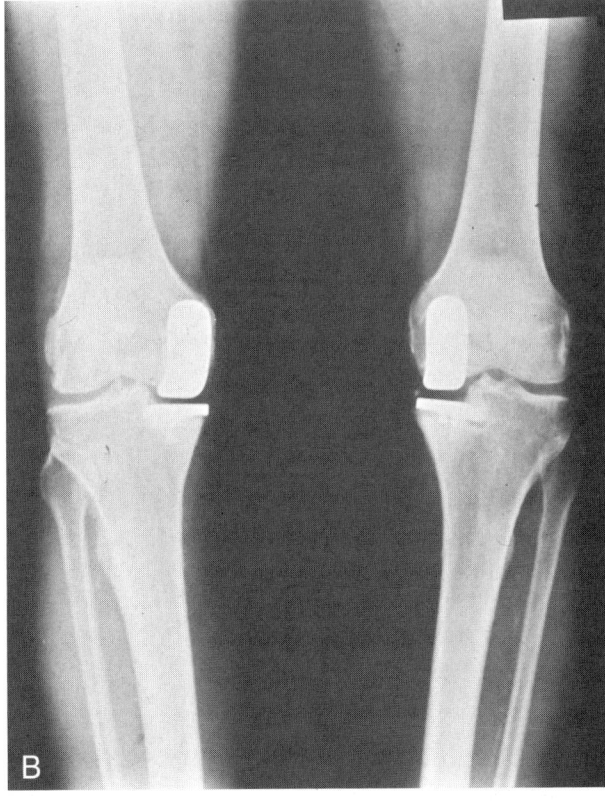

Figure 49.6. A. A 68-year-old sedentary male with isolated bilateral medial compartment degenerative changes. **B.** Single-stage bilateral medial unicompartmental knee arthroplasty was performed, resulting in complete pain relief and restoration of function.

| table | 49.1 | Unicompartmental Knee Disease: Quick Reference Chart |

Factor	Osteotomy	Unicompartmental Replacement
Age and lifestyle	Younger, active	Sedentary, low demand
Body habitus	Obesity not contraindicated	Close to ideal body weight preferred
Diagnosis	Osteoarthritis; mechanical malalignment	Noninflammatory, isolated condylar disease
Deformity	Within 10° of neutral axis	Within 10° of neutral axis
Ligament status	Intact anterior and posterior collateral ligament	Intact anterior and posterior collateral ligament
Subluxation	Contraindication	Not ideal
Motion	Full extension; flexion > 90°	Small flexion contracture acceptable
Common pitfall	Undercorrection	Overcorrection

sults were echoed by Stockelman and Pohl (11), who followed their patients for 12 years. In these studies, the authors were able to achieve satisfactory alignment of both the femoral and the tibial components, yielding loosening rates of less than 1% per annum. These studies seem to confirm that a well-aligned and well-cemented unicompartmental knee arthroplasty can give satisfactory clinical and radiographic results for at least 10 years.

Unfortunately, the experience with cementless unicompartmental knee arthroplasty has not been successful. This may be related to the more limited amount of porous surface available for biologic fixation or a function of the high stresses placed on the implant soon after surgery, resulting in suboptimal bone incorporation. Whatever the reason, the clinical results employing noncemented unicompartmental knee arthroplasty have not been predictably good; and at this time, their use cannot be supported.

REVISION OF UNICOMPARTMENTAL ARTHROPLASTY

One of the major premises of unicompartmental knee arthroplasty is that it is a relatively conservative arthroplasty in terms of bone resection. Because some failures are inevitable, the surgeon should evaluate the ease of revision to total knee arthroplasty before recommending unicompartmental knee arthroplasty. At the Hospital for Special Surgery, 76% of failed unicompartmental knee replacements that were revised to total knee replacements showed significant bone defects that required either a customized implant or bone grafting (12). In a parallel study from the Brigham and Women's Hospital, bone defects that required either customized implants or grafting were also encountered (13); however the authors did not believe that the defects compromised the results of revision. It is important to emphasize that many of these revised implants were of older designs that demanded extensive resection of the tibia and femur during unicompartmental implantation. Overall, these studies found that between 70 and 80% of patients undergoing revision of a failed unicompartmental knee arthroplasty noted a satisfactory outcome (12,13). Although these results are inferior to those of primary total knee arthroplasty, they are no worse than those of revision of a failed total knee arthroplasty. It is hoped that modern unicom-

partmental designs, which require minimal bone resection for implantation, will minimize bone loss, making revision arthroplasty easier.

SUMMARY

Unicompartmental knee arthroplasty is a useful procedure to consider when a patient presents with painful degenerative changes that affect only one compartment. Treatment options include tibial osteotomy, unicompartmental arthroplasty, and total knee arthroplasty (Table 49.1). Proper patient selection is the key to successful unicompartmental knee arthroplasty. The surgeon must adhere to the strict inclusion criteria and in particular recognize the contraindications to the procedure. Surgical technique is demanding, and knee alignment and soft tissue balance are crucial to success. Current systems, with appropriate cutting guides and jigs, have resulted in consistent reproduction of bone cuts; and their use is strongly encouraged. Although 10-year results appear promising, revision of some failed unicompartmental arthroplasties is inevitable. Anticipation of osseous defects on either the tibial or the femoral side at the time of revision and familiarity with the use of bone grafting techniques and modular implant systems to handle bone defects will result in a successful revision arthroplasty in most cases.

REFERENCES

1. Fairbank TJ. Knee joint changes after meniscotomy. J Bone Joint Surg 1948;30B:664–670.
2. Rosenberg TD, Paulos LE, Parker RD, et al. Forty-five degree posteroanterior flexion weight-bearing radiograph of the knee. J Bone Joint Surg 1988;70A:1479–1482.
3. Prodromos CC, Andriacchi TP, Galante JO. A relationship between gait and clinical changes following high tibial osteotomy. J Bone Joint Surg 1985;67A:1188–1194.
4. Keblish PA. The lateral approach to the valgus knee. Clin Orthop 1991;271:52–62.
5. Corpe RS, Engh GA. A quantitative assessment of degenerative changes acceptable in the unoperated compartments of knees undergoing unicompartmental replacement. Orthopedics 1990;13:319–324.
6. Kennedy WR, White RP. Unicompartmental arthroplasty of the knee: postoperative alignment and its influence on overall results. Clin Orthop 1988;221:278–284.
7. Laskin RS. Unicompartmental tibiofemoral resurfacing arthroplasty. J Bone Joint Surg 1978;60A:182–188.

8. Marmor L. Unicompartmental knee arthroplasty: 10–13 year follow-up study. Clin Orthop 1987;226:14–20.

9. Insall JN, Aglietti P. A five to seven year follow-up of unicondylar arthroplasty. J Bone Joint Surg 1980;62A:1329–1334.

10. Scott RD, Cobb AG, McQueary FG, Thornhill TS. Unicompartmental knee arthroplasty: eight to 12 year follow-up evaluation with survivorship analysis. Clin Orthop 1991;271:96–100.

11. Stockelman RE, Pohl KP. The long-term efficacy of unicompartmental arthroplasty of the knee. Clin Orthop 1991;271:88–95.

12. Padgett DE, Stern SH, Insall JN. Revision total knee arthroplasty for failed unicompartmental replacement. J Bone Joint Surg 1991;73A:186–189.

13. Barret WP, Scott RD. Revision of failed unicondylar unicompartmental knee arthroplasty. J Bone Joint Surg 1987;69A:1328–1335.

chapter 50

Steven H. Stern

Total Knee Replacement

Total knee arthroplasty (TKA) has become the definitive treatment for end-stage knee arthritis. The procedure has proven to be both reliable and durable (1–8). A successful total knee replacement allows the patient to resume almost all activities of daily living with minimal difficulty. In most cases, patients no longer require external aids or chronic medications. Finally, the TKA helps patients maintain their overall self-esteem, since their improved functional status permits a more independent lifestyle.

Modern total knee arthroplasty began during the 1970s, a decade that heralded the beginnings of a basic understanding of the principles of surgical instrumentation and ligament balance (9–11). During this time, bone cement (polymethyl methacrylate) was found to be a successful method for achieving prosthetic component fixation. Since then, both the operative technique and the prosthetic design have been improved. Modern instrumentation allows for more exacting bone cuts. Alternative modes of fixation have been developed, augmenting surgical options, and material property enhancement has increased the theoretical longevity of knee implants. Current research is focused on optimizing patellofemoral joint kinematics and maximizing the overall functional status of the patient with a knee replacement.

RELEVANT ANATOMY AND PATHOGENESIS

The knee is a hinge joint composed of three bones and three compartments. The bony anatomy is made up of the femur, tibia, and fibula. The compartments of the knee are medial (medial femoral condyle articulating with medial tibial plateau), lateral (lateral femoral condyle articulating with lateral tibial plateau), and patellofemoral (patella articulating with the trochlea grove of the femur.

The actual pathogenesis of osteoarthritis is not well understood and is probably multifactorial in nature. Although osteoarthritis (OA) is commonly referred to as

degenerative joint disease and thought by many authors to be a simple mechanical wearing of the articular surface, this is not clearly true. It is also not well understood what role, if any, is played by genetics or by metabolic or other forms of biologic failure. In general, OA is distinguished from other forms of arthritis chiefly by the lack of a significant inflammatory response (12).

INITIAL FINDINGS, PHYSICAL EXAMINATION, AND DIAGNOSIS

History

Patients with end-stage degenerative joint disease commonly complain of knee pain. The pain tends to be poorly localized, though some patients will pinpoint their maximum symptoms to the knee compartment with the most arthritic changes. Thus patients with medial knee degenerative joint disease may complain of more medial symptoms, whereas patients with severe patellofemoral arthritis may have more anterior knee symptoms. Patients tend to complain of increasing knee symptoms with increasing activity. Other complaints include knee stiffness or knee swelling (effusion), which may be present even though difficult to detect on examination.

Ambulation is commonly limited. This impediment to walking is normally most pronounced on uneven surfaces, hills, and stairs. Many patients are unable to reciprocate stairs normally, and some require a banister for support. Finally, many patients need an assistive device for walking. Routinely, patients with end-stage disease use a cane or even a walker to assist with their ambulation.

When obtaining the history, the clinician should ask about other musculoskeletal or medical complaints. Hip pain can occasionally radiate down the anterior thigh toward the knee. It is also important to document any pain or symptoms in the contralateral extremity or back. Active medical problems that could impact on a surgical procedure should be evaluated. Special attention should be paid to a history of diabetes, psoriasis, rheumatoid arthritis, or active infection. It is also important to ascertain if there have been any prior vascular, thrombophlebitic, or neurologic problems.

Physical Examination

Before doing any type of arthroplasty procedure, the clinician must perform a satisfactory examination of the involved extremity in a systematic fashion. Initially, inspection of the extremity and knee should be carried out, paying particular attention to any prior incisions or scars, as they will need to be dealt with during surgical exposure. Ideally, the skin should be free of any lesions.

Patients should be observed during walking, so that their gait can be evaluated and any limp or deficiency noted. Knee range of motion should be assessed and compared to the noninvolved side. Commonly, patients with arthritis will have decreased motion at the extremes of flexion and extension. Flexion deformities, in which the knee will not come to full extension, are commonly seen. Alignment of the extremity in either varus or valgus plane should be assessed. Normal limb alignment is approximately 7° of anatomic valgus. Patients with OA most commonly have varus malalignments of their extremities, although valgus deformities are seen. Finally, an appropriate musculoskeletal evaluation of the hips and lower back should be performed to ensure that there is no significant abnormality in these areas that would alter the surgical procedure.

The knee joint should be assessed for stability in both the AP and varus-valgus planes to ensure that the arthroplasty procedure will address any instabilities that are present. Alternations in the extensor mechanism should be evaluated, especially any evidence of an extensor lag, as this can lead to rehabilitation difficulties.

The distal neurovascular examination should include an evaluation of both the dorsalis pedis and the posterior tibial arterial pulses. Basic motor function of the lower extremity should be assessed. Occasionally, some degree of motor weakness is associated with OA secondary to disuse atrophy of the musculature; however, the overall neurologic examination is usually unremarkable in patients with degenerative arthritis. Nevertheless, patients may well have decreased peripheral pulses, because the age group that is at maximal risk for degenerative knee disease is also the group most commonly afflicted with arteriosclerosis.

RADIOLOGIC STUDIES

It is customary to obtain appropriate radiographic knee studies to further evaluate the extent and nature of arthritic changes within the joint. Commonly, three x-ray views of the extremity are obtained: standing AP, lateral,

and skyline (or Merchant). The standing AP radiograph allows the best evaluation of the femoral-tibial articulation. Occasionally, this is taken on a long film to best evaluate overall limb alignment (Fig. 50.1). Varus or valgus malalignments are best assessed on these views. The most common arthritic changes seen are joint space narrowing, articular cartilage deformity, and osteophyte formation. Subluxation of the knee on the AP plane can also be seen in patients with osteoarthritis. Finally, the presence of retained internal hardware from prior surgeries can be evaluated from the radiographs.

The lateral knee radiograph allows assessment of both the femoral-tibial and the patellofemoral compartments (Fig. 50.2). Osteophyte formation, especially in the patellofemoral joint, can commonly be seen on the superior or inferior pole of the patella. The lateral view also allows evaluation of posterior osteophytes or loose bodies within the posterior or suprapatellar knee compartments.

The skyline, or Merchant view, specifically addresses the patellofemoral compartment (Fig. 50.3). The patella's alignment within the trochlear groove can be assessed, including any propensity of the patella to subluxation or dislocation. Osteophyte formation of the patellar or trochlear grooves can also be seen.

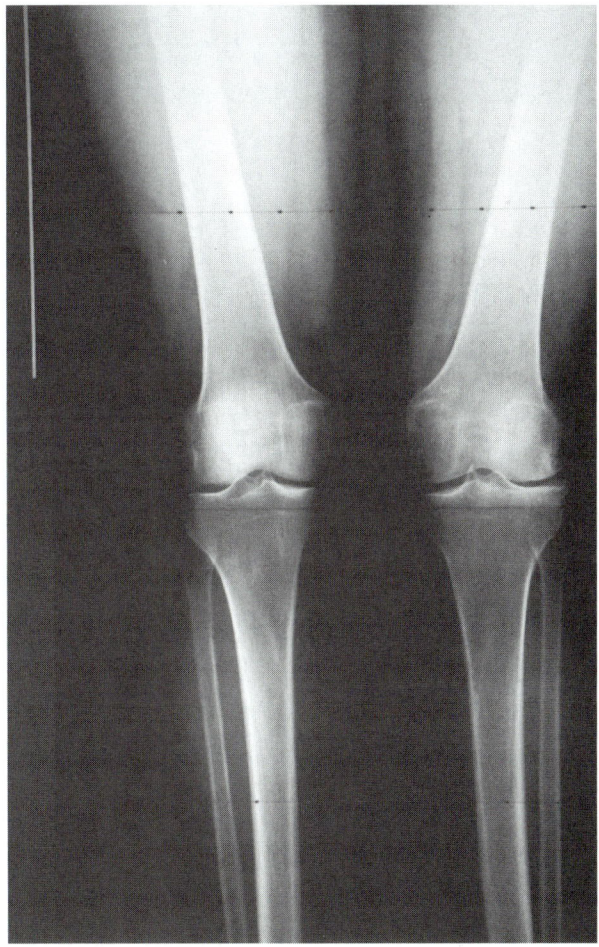

Figure 50.1. Standing AP view taken on a long cassette.

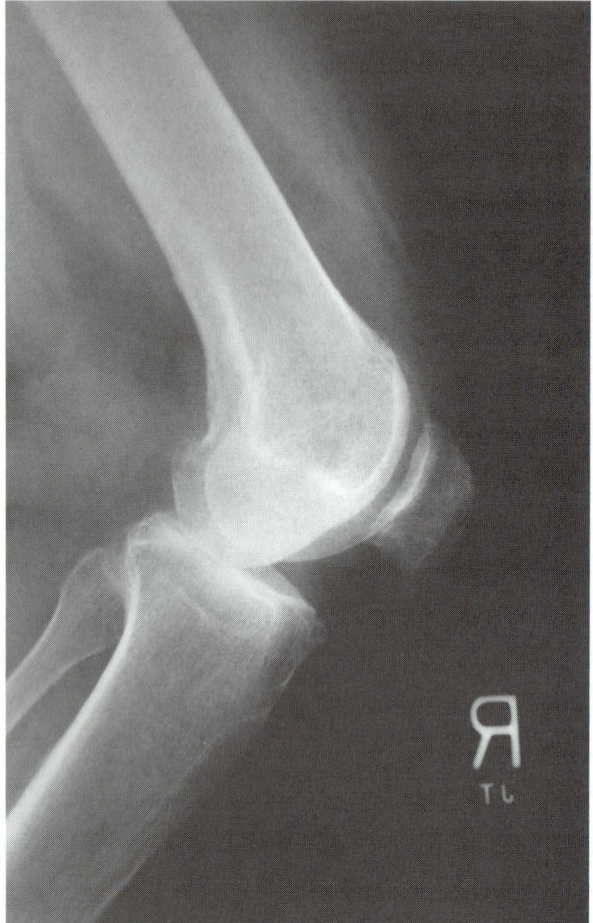

Figure 50.2. Lateral view of the knee showing space narrowing and osteophyte formation.

It is normally not necessary to proceed with any other diagnostic studies in the standard workup for OA or in preparation for knee replacement surgery. Nevertheless, some patients undergo MRI studies. Although MRI provides excellent information regarding soft tissue structures of the knee, it does not necessarily add any needed information regarding degenerative articular cartilage changes. In addition, meniscal or ligamentous pathology is so common that it is almost expected in patients with significant knee OA. Therefore, MRI evaluation of degenerative joint disease in preparation for TKA surgery is not generally required.

Preoperative nuclear medicine studies (e.g., bone scans) will reveal abnormalities consistent with arthritis. However, like MRI, they do not routinely yield information that is particularly valuable in evaluating a patient's degenerative knee joint pathology.

Preoperative vascular studies of the extremity are occasionally useful. In patients with a prior history of a thromboembolic disease, preoperative venous blood flow studies can rule out any active thrombophlebitic process and provide a baseline for later comparison, if necessary. In patients with decreased pedal pulses, an arterial vascular study may prove beneficial in certain instances. However,

this study is normally not performed if pedal pulses are either palpable or easily heard with a Doppler before surgery.

TREATMENT

Nonoperative Treatment and Indications for Surgery

Before proceeding with a TKA, patients should have exhausted a thorough nonoperative treatment protocol. Nonoperative treatment for degenerative joint disease falls into several broad categories.

MEDICATIONS

The most commonly used medications for degenerative joint disease are nonsteroidal anti-inflammatory drugs (NSAIDs). These are widespread medications in the United States, available either over the counter—ibuprofen, naproxen, ketoprofen—or via prescription—Feldene, Voltaren, Clinoril, Lodine. Common side effects of NSAIDs include gastrointestinal complaints, so these medications are normally taken with food. In addition, with chronic usage, changes in liver or kidney function can occasionally be seen. In patients who are not candidates for NSAIDs, acetaminophen is frequently used. Acetaminophen tends not to produce the same gastrointestinal side effects as NSAIDs, but can be effective in decreasing knee symptoms in patients with mild to moderate arthritis.

ACTIVITY MODIFICATION

Modification of patient activity can also be effective in decreasing knee complaints from degenerative joint dis-

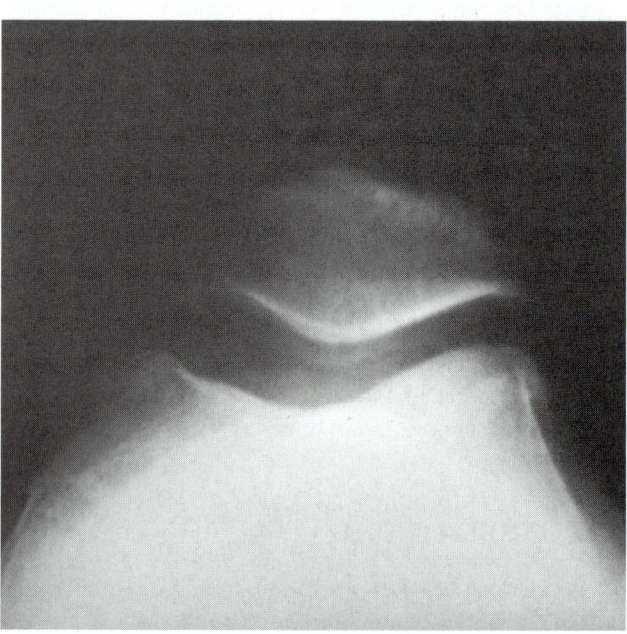

Figure 50.3. Skyline view of the patellofemoral compartment showing marginal and osteophyte formation.

ease. Many people with knee osteoarthritis will find that increased activities, especially impact exercises, will exacerbate their complaints. If these patients can modify their activity and attempt to avoid the endeavors that most aggravate their symptoms, they may notice an improvement in their symptoms.

ASSISTIVE DEVICE

As arthritic changes become more severe, patients may require the use of assistive devices, such as canes, crutches, and walkers. These aids will decrease the joint-reactive force in the affected extremity, decreasing pain in many cases. Patients should be taught to use the aid in the contralateral upper extremity.

Patients also may find a simple brace to be effective in decreasing a component of their symptoms; however, for most patients with degenerative arthritis, knee instability is usually not a significant problem. Therefore, large or formal braces are rarely indicated. Nonetheless, occasionally elastic or neoprene knee sleeves can be helpful in decreasing arthritic knee symptoms.

CORTISONE

Corticosteroid injections have been widely available and frequently used in the past for degenerative joint disease to decrease inflammation and, occasionally, pain. Unfortunately, it is now known that corticosteroids have a deleterious effect on chondrocytes and should be used only in moderation, and even then in patients who are not otherwise good candidates for surgical intervention because of their medical status. If possible, chronic use should be avoided.

EXERCISE

The role of exercise in the treatment of degenerative joint disease is perplexing. Exercise allows a patient with knee OA to remain as active as possible. It is beneficial for maintaining well-functioning cardiovascular and respiratory systems. In addition, exercise minimizes atrophy and rehabilitation of the lower extremity musculature. To a certain degree it can also help alleviate or decrease symptoms associated with arthritis. Conversely, increased exercise can cause further irritation, inflammation, and increased joint pain. Thus patients should be instructed to curtail any rehabilitation or exercise protocol that increases symptoms.

INDICATIONS FOR SURGERY

Indications for TKA include an appropriate history, physical examination, and radiographic changes consistent with significant arthritis. In general, the patient should have failed a nonoperative treatment protocol. The patient's medical condition should be reasonably conducive for proceeding with surgery, and he or she should be able to satisfactorily participate in postoperative rehabilitation. If these conditions are met, the option of a total knee replacement can be offered to the patient (Clinical Table). The patients should be apprised of the risks, options, benefits, and alternatives before making a decision regarding surgical intervention.

Clinical Table: Total Knee Replacement

Procedure	Indications	Technique	Anatomy	Pitfalls
Cruciate retaining	• Knee arthritis	• Preserve PCL • PCL is balanced with correct tension	• PCL	• PCL cut or too lax: instability • PCL too tight: seesaw effect
Cruciate substitution	• Knee arthritis	• Resect PCL from femoral insertion • PCL substitution mechanism built into prosthesis	• PCL	• Poor balance: prosthetic knee dislocation
Cemented TKA	• Knee arthritis	• Fixation of components achieved with the use of bone cement		• Cement debris • Cement can be difficult to remove in case of infection
Cementless TKA	• Knee arthritis • Younger patient	• Fixation of components achieved with Press-Fit, screws, and porous ingrowth surface		• Insecure fixation • Component loosening • Increased incidence of osteolysis
Metal-backed tibial component	• Knee arthritis			• Increased cost • Decreased polyethylene thickness
All-polyethylene tibial component	• Knee arthritis • Older patient			• Poor stress distribution • Possible early loosening

Operative Treatment

APPROACH

Adequate visualization of the relevant anatomical structures is as imperative for performing a total knee arthroplasty as it is for other procedures. Surgical exposure in total knee arthroplasty is especially important, because the surgeon is faced with the dual needs of obtaining adequate soft tissue coverage and wound closure while maximizing knee motion. Exposure must be adequate enough to allow for visualization but should minimize tension on the soft tissue envelope.

As a general rule, extensile approaches are favored. If necessary, visualization can be improved by extending the incisions either proximally or distally. It is widely accepted that prior transverse skin incisions can be crossed with a new longitudinal incision (13,14); however, prior vertical incisions should be incorporated into any current skin incision, if possible. Parallel incisions should be avoided; if they are necessary, as large an island of skin as possible should be maintained.

Before beginning the procedure and tourniquet elevation, the patient should receive appropriate preoperative antibiotics. Antibiotics should cover *Staphylococcus aureus* and can be optimized, depending on the particular institution's bacterial flora. Most TKA surgeries are done in a bloodless field, after limb exsanguination and tourniquet elevation. The patient's extremity should be prepped and draped in a routine sterile fashion. The skin incision is chosen as outlined above, and dissection is carried down to the extensor mechanism.

Most surgeons perform a medial retinacular arthrotomy, using a variety of retinacular incisions (Fig. 50.4). This allows for eversion of the patellar laterally and exposure of the joint. Insall (13,15) prefers a straight midline retinacular exposure, which is carried directly along the medial aspect of the patella and distally onto the anterior tibial cortex. The midline approach prevents a transection of the insertion of the medialis into the patella. Other surgeons advocate a medial parapatellar retinacular incision with dissection through the retinaculum medial to the patella. This allows for a thicker cuff of soft tissue for repair. Other authors use a midvastus approach (16), in which the proximal aspect of the retinacular excision is performed through the midportion of vastus medialis. Blunt dissection is used to separate the muscular fibers. This technique allows minimal disruption of the proximal quadriceps expansion. Engh et al. (16) noted the midvastus approach provides reproducible knee joint exposure and allows for close tracking of the patellar mechanism. Patellar tracking is believed to be improved because of the minimal disruption to the quadriceps mechanism.

Another surgical approach to the knee is the lateral approach (17). Theoretically, this is especially helpful for patients with a fixed preoperative valgus deformity, because dissection is carried directly onto the lateral structures. Most surgeons have more experience with the common medial techniques than with the lateral approach; thus they generally use the former technique, even for knees with preoperative valgus deformity.

Generally, with all of the common medial retinacular exposures, distal dissection is carried down along the medial aspect of the proximal tibia. The periosteum is normally sharply dissected off of the tibial bone. Care is taken to minimize stress to the extensor mechanism and patellar tendon region. The patella is everted and the knee is flexed, allowing exposure of the knee joint. In revision operations and in obese patients, it is occasionally difficult to fully evert the patella. In these instances, it may be possible to do the arthroplasty with just lateral retraction of the patella. If visualization is still not adequate, then the surgeon must consider either a proximal soft tissue technique

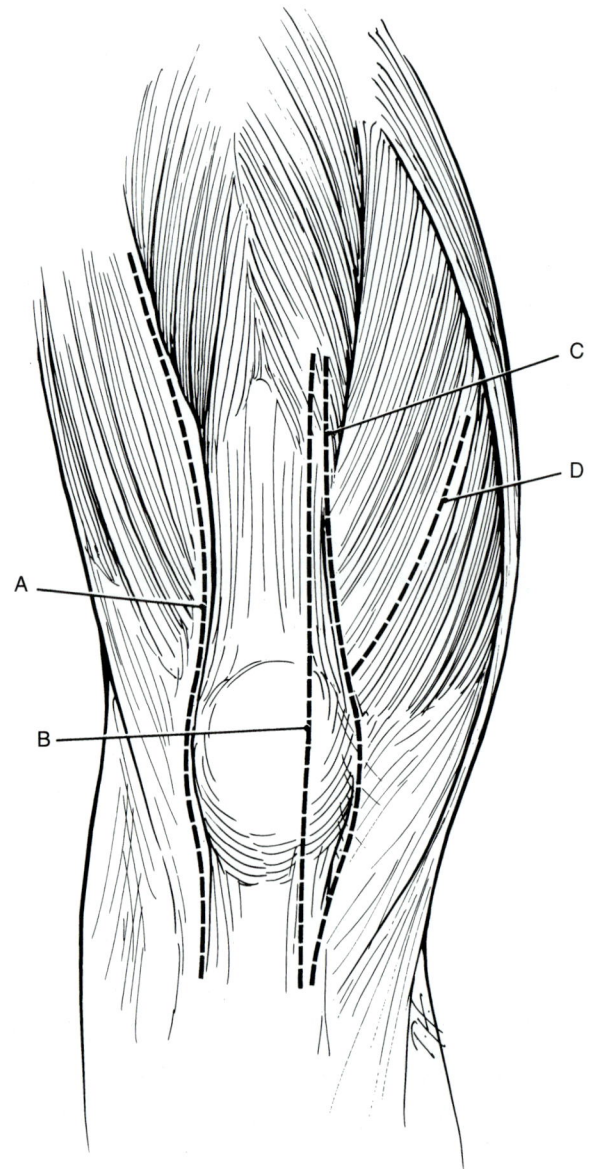

Figure 50.4. Lateral (*A*), straight midline retinacular (*B*), medial parapatellar retinacular (*C*), and midvastus (*D*) incisions.

(e.g., patellar turndown or rectus snip) (18–20) or a distal tibial tubercle osteotomy (21,22).

PROCEDURE

The actual order of bone cuts and the specific type of instrumentation used for a TKA are design specific and beyond the scope of this text. There are, however, some basic tenets that are usually followed. After adequate soft tissue exposure is obtained, the initial bone cuts can be performed on either the tibia or the femur. Tibial instrumentation and alignment guides are either extramedullary or intramedullary; the actual choice depends on the surgeon's preference. The proximal tibia is cut with an oscillating saw. This cut is usually done approximately 90° to the AP plane, although some surgeons advocate a slight varus (2° to 3°) cut. Depending on the prosthetic system used, the tibia is cut in the lateral plane either at 90° or with a slight posterior tilt. In general, systems that advocate sacrifice of the posterior cruciate ligament strive for a flat tibial cut in the sagittal plane, whereas those that recommend retention of the ligament normally aim for a slight posterior slope.

Intramedullary instrumentation is preferred for preparation of the femur. The femoral alignment guide is normally placed through a vented intramedullary hole to minimize intramedullary pressures and embolization (23). The order of the femoral cuts depends on the particular knee replacement system. When making the anterior femoral condyle cut, most surgeons take care to avoid notching the bone in the supracondylar region. The position of the distal femoral cut is usually referenced off the intramedullary canal. The purpose of this cut is to restore the mechanical axis to 0°, which normally necessitates an anatomical valgus cut of 5° to 8°.

In general, knees with a fixed preoperative valgus deformity are cut in less valgus, to decrease the propensity of the knee to return to a valgus orientation postoperatively. Further bone cuts, including the posterior condyles and chamfer cuts, are made with the oscillating saw, using the instrumentation as a guide. If the posterior cruciate ligament (PCL) is to be retained, care should be taken to preserve the structure throughout the surgical procedure. The stability, tension, and length of the PCL should be assessed before prosthetic implantation. If sacrifice or substitution of the PCL is desired, the ligament can be released from its femoral insertion.

No matter which technique is employed for dealing with the PCL, care should be taken to ensure that ligamentous balance is optimized as much as possible, with the knee in both flexion and extension. This is usually accomplished by releasing the structures on the concave, or tight, side of the knee. The medial collateral ligament (MCL) and semimembranosus tendon are released sharply off the proximal medial tibia in varus knees. In knees with a significant varus deformity, dissection is carried farther to release the expansion fibers of the MCL that insert distally along the medial tibia. Several methods of achieving ligamentous release in a valgus knee have been suggested (14,17,24). In general, the lateral structures to be released are the lateral collateral ligament, popliteus tendon, and lateral retinaculum. These can be resected either off the tibia or off the lateral femoral condyle.

Preparation of the patella can be performed at any time during the surgical procedure. Although not universally accepted, most surgeons believe in patellar resurfacing at the time of the knee replacement. This can be accomplished with either a resurfacing component or an inset-type of implant. The instrumentation used is up to the surgeon. No matter the method, it is beneficial to measure the patellar width before bone preparation to ensure that the bone–implant composite is not wider than the host patella.

After all of the components are implanted, the knee should be run through a range of motion to assess the stability of both the femorotibial articulation and the patellofemoral joint. The patella should track within the femoral groove, without any undo pressure being applied. Care should also be taken to assess the rotation of the femoral component during femoral bone preparation to ensure that it is aligned in either neutral or slight external rotation. Internal rotation of the patella leads to increased dislocation of the extensor mechanism.

Pitfalls and Common Technical Mistakes

MALALIGNMENT

Care should be taken to optimize alignment of the extremity in the frontal plane. Ideally, knee alignment should be between 4° and 10° of anatomical valgus to restore the mechanical axis to neutral (0°). Occasionally, because of a patient's preoperative ligamentous balance or obesity, this may be impossible to achieve. Malalignment of the components can result in joint instability and, depending on the component type, early wear of the plastic or component loosening. The femoral component should not be internally rotated, as this will lead to malalignment of the patellofemoral mechanism and predispose the patient to lateral dislocation or subluxation of the patella. This can be a significant problem, because patellar dislocations can significantly weaken the extremity.

LIGAMENT BALANCE

It is imperative that the knee be balanced as optimally as possible to give the joint adequate stability. Most primary knee arthroplasties, either PCL substituting or retaining, do not substitute the collateral ligamentous structures. It is, therefore, important that the biologic ligaments be optimally balanced to minimize instability with varus or valgus stress. Laxity or tightness can predispose the joint to early liftoff or early component wear.

For knees in which the PCL is to be retained, it is imperative that correct tension within the ligament be achieved. If the ligament is too lax, the knee may be prone to subluxate with flexion or during stair climbing. More troublesome, however, is a too tight PCL, which can limit flexion and cause excessive rollback. With excessive femoral component rollback, the polyethylene in the posterior tibial lip is exposed to significantly elevated stresses, which can exceed the failure threshold of the polyethylene. This can lead to early wear and failure of the tibial component. Excessive femoral component rollback can result in the so-called seesaw effect (25), which occurs when the rollback causes a tensile force or liftoff of the anterior aspect of the tibial component. Because the strength of the cement in tension is not as great as in compression, the seesaw effect can cause early loosening and failure. Finally, an excessively tight PCL can also make it difficult to achieve adequate arcs of flexion.

Because of the significant problems resulting from an overly taut PCL, this is a pitfall that should be avoided if at all possible. Advocates of PCL retention have recently suggested resection of the posterior ligament. In this technique, some of the fibers of the PCL are cut or resected from the femoral or tibial insertion. This helps minimize the chance of leaving the ligament too tight. Preliminary results have been encouraging (26,27).

WOUND PROBLEMS

To achieve a satisfactory arthroplasty, it is imperative that the soft tissue envelope heals satisfactorily. If the wound does not heal, the chances of an infection and a doomed arthroplasty significantly increase. Thus everything possible should be done to minimize wound problems and wound necrosis, including ensuring that the skin integrity is pristine before surgery. Intraoperatively, care must be taken to minimize skin flaps and minimize excess tension on the skin envelope. The wound should be copiously irrigated with an antibiotic solution and satisfactory hemostasis maintained. Wound closure should be meticulous. Finally, care should continue in the immediate postoperative period. If there is any question of a wound problem, flexion exercises of the knee can be deferred to take stress off the soft tissues and to maximize the chance of wound healing.

EXTENSOR MECHANISM PROBLEMS

Problems with the patellofemoral articulation and extensor mechanism continue are persistent areas of concern in knee replacement surgery. There is no clear-cut consensus on the most optimal method of dealing with these issues. Problems include subluxation and dislocation of the patella, patellar fractures, and avulsion of the tibial tubercle. Some surgeons suggest that the patella not be resurfaced to minimize the problems associated with bone fracture. There remains a concern, however, that the functional results of the arthroplasty will suffer if patellar resurfacing is not carried out.

The best treatment of extensor mechanism problems is prevention. Meticulous care of the extensor mechanism throughout the procedure will help minimize the chance of tibial tubercle avulsion. If excessive stress on the patellar tendon insertion is present, it is preferable to extend the surgical releases in a controlled fashion instead of allowing an uncontrolled failure at the tendon insertion site.

Fractures of the host patellar bone can be minimized in several ways. The bone should not be cut too thin; and if a lateral retinacular release is performed, care should be taken to preserve the geniculate vessels. This will help ensure adequate blood flow to the patellar and decrease the weakening of bone strength associated with patellar osteonecrosis. In addition, a careful intraoperative assessment of patellar tracking should be performed. If there is a question about lateral patellar subluxation, then a lateral retinacular release should be performed.

POLYETHYLENE WEAR

Recently, it has become apparent that polyethylene is the weak link in joint arthroplasty. The plastic is the material most prone to either catastrophic failure or overall wear degradation (28,29). Problems associated with the polyethylene can be minimized by ensuring that the plastic-bearing surface has an adequately sized contact area at the articulation points. In general, the larger the contact area between the components, the less the stress in the polyethylene and the less polyethylene wear. Furthermore, excessively thin plastic should be avoided, as this will also lead to significant increased stress within the material. Thus a thin, flat polyethylene insert should not be used, if at all possible.

Thicker and more conforming polyethylene inserts tend to be more forgiving and produce less wear and particulate debris. As in total hip arthroplasty, there is concern in TKA that articulate debris, especially from the polyethylene, can lead to osteolysis of the bone, which can result in implant failure. There is some evidence that this problem may be slightly more prevalent in uncemented designs (30) and heat-pressed plastics (31,32).

Rehabilitation

Theories about postoperative rehabilitation after a total knee replacement have undergone changes over the past few decades. Rehabilitation has evolved into a more aggressive and proactive process. Attempts are now made to achieve early knee motion, with early protected weight bearing. This seems to lead to improved early functional results without increased problems. Weight bearing normally starts with the use of an assistive device, such as a walker, cane, or crutch. This is continued for 4 to 6 weeks after surgery. With cemented knee replacements, the patient can bear weight as tolerated over this same 4- to 6-week period. With an uncemented replacement, the surgeon may recommend that the patient go slightly slower on the weight bearing to promote bony ingrowth.

More aggressive early range-of-motion protocols have recently come into vogue. If desired, knees can be started on a continuous passive motion (CPM) protocol or a drop-and-dangle rehabilitation technique immediately after surgery. My institution uses an early flexion protocol, and the knees are placed in a CPM device the day of surgery.

Initial motion is instituted between 50° and 100°. Jordan et al. (33) reported that knees that were maximally flexed the day of surgery tended to do well.

It is not imperative to use a CPM device as part of the rehabilitation protocol. Other authors have noted excellent results using an aggressive physical therapy and rehabilitation protocol, with no CPM device (34). By actively and aggressively bending knees early, patients can achieve excellent motion of the joint. It is much easier to achieve optimal motion in the first several weeks after an arthroplasty, then to regain motion later in a stiff knee. Most patients continue in some form of physical therapy for the first several weeks after surgery.

There is a subset of patients for whom overly aggressive therapy leads to increased inflammation and actually impedes flexion of the knee. These patients report increased pain and swelling after physical therapy and find that they have more difficulty bending the knee after they have done their exercises. In these cases, it is sometimes effective to decrease the formal physical therapy and allow the patients to more gently bend the knee on their own. The decreased formal exercise can reduce swelling and inflammation, thereby improving knee flexion. This possibility should be kept in mind in instances when the knee seems to be recalcitrant to bending.

SUMMARY

While no operation can be a guaranteed success, TKA has evolved into a relatively predictable orthopaedic operation. It allows the implant surgeon to decrease pain and improve function in the patient with an arthritic knee. Most patients achieve durable improvement over the long term. Of course, patients undergoing a prosthetic joint procedure are exposed to a degree of risk, which can only be minimized but never eliminated.

REFERENCES

1. Goldberg VM, Figgie MP, Figgie HE III, et al. Use of a total condylar knee prosthesis for treatment of osteoarthritis and rheumatoid arthritis. Long-term results. J Bone Joint Surg 1988; 70A:802–811.
2. Laskin RS. Total condylar knee replacement in patients who have rheumatoid arthritis. A ten-year follow-up study. J Bone Joint Surg 1990;72A:529–535.
3. Ranawat CS, Boachie-Adjei O. Survivorship analysis and results of total condylar knee arthroplasty. Eight- to 11-year follow-up period. Clin Orthop 1988;226:6–13.
4. Ritter MA, Campbell MS, Faris PM, Keating EM. Long-term survival analysis of the posterior cruciate condylar total knee arthroplasty. J Arthroplasty 1989;4:293–296.
5. Scuderi GR, Insall JN, Windsor RE, Moran MC. Survivorship of cemented knee replacement. J Bone Joint Surg 1989;71B:798–803.
6. Stern SH, Insall JN. Posterior stabilized prosthesis: results after 9–12 years follow-up. J Bone Joint Surg 1992;74A:980–986.
7. Vince KG, Insall JN, Kelly MA. The total condylar prosthesis: 10- to 12-year results of a cemented knee replacement. J Bone Joint Surg 1989;71B:793–797.
8. Wright J, Ewald FC, Walker PS, et al. Total knee arthroplasty with the Kinematic prosthesis. J Bone Joint Surg 1990;72A:1003–1009.
9. Insall JN, Ranawat CS, Aglietti P, Shine J. A comparison of four models of total knee-replacement prostheses. J Bone Joint Surg 1976;58A:754–765.
10. Insall JN, Ranawat CS, Scott WN, Walker P. Total condylar knee replacement. Preliminary report. Clin Orthop 1976;120:149–154.
11. Insall JN, Scott WN, Ranawat CS. The total condylar knee prosthesis. A report of two hundred and twenty cases. J Bone Joint Surg 1979;61A:173–180.
12. American Medical Association. Osteoarthritis of the knee and hip. Health Manage Bull 1997.
13. Insall JN. Total knee replacement. In: Insall JN, Windsor RD, Scott WN, et al., eds. Surgery of the knee. New York: Churchill Livingstone, 1984:587–696.
14. Stern SH. Surgical exposure in total knee arthroplasty. In: Fu FH, Harner CD, Vince KG, eds. Knee surgery. Baltimore: Williams & Wilkins, 1994:1289–1302.
15. Insall JN. A midline approach to the knee. J Bone Joint Surg 1971; 53A:1584–1586.
16. Engh GA, Parks NL, Ammeen DJ. The influence of surgical approach on lateral retinacular releases in TKA. Paper presented at the Knee Society Scientific Meetings, Atlanta, 1966.
17. Keblish PA. The lateral approach to the valgus knee: surgical technique and analysis of 53 cases with over two-year follow-up evaluation. Clin Orthop 1991;271:52–62.
18. Miller DV, Insall JN, Urs WK, Windsor RE. Quadricepsplasty in total knee arthroplasty. Paper presented at the American Academy of Orthopaedic Surgeons Meeting, Atlanta, 1988.
19. Trousdale RT, Hanssen AD, Rand JA, Cahalan TD. V-Y quadricepsplasty in total knee arthroplasty. Clin Orthop 1993;286:48–55.
20. Vince KG. Revision knee arthroplasty technique. Instr Course Lect 1993;42:325–339.
21. Whiteside LA, Ohl MD. Tibial tubercle osteotomy for exposure of the difficult total knee arthroplasty. Clin Orthop 1990;260:6–9.
22. Wolff AM, Hungerford DS, Krackow KA, Jacobs MA. Osteotomy of the tibial tubercle during total knee replacement. A report of twenty-six cases. J Bone Joint Surg 1989;71A:848–852.
23. Fahmy NR, Chandler HP, Danylchuk K, et al. Blood-gas and circulatory changes during total knee replacement. J Bone Joint Surg 1990;72A:19–20.
24. D'Ambrosio F, Scott WN. Ligament releases in the arthritic knee. In Scott WN, ed. The knee. St. Louis: Mosby-Year Book, 1994:1199–1210.
25. Insall JN. Historical development, classification, and characteristics of knee prostheses. In: Insall JN, Windsor RD, Scott WN, et al., eds. Surgery of the knee. 2nd ed. New York: Churchill Livingstone, 1993:677–717.
26. Hofmann AA, Pace TB. Cruciate ligament retention in total knee arthroplasty. In: Fu FH, Harner CD, Vince KG, eds. Knee surgery. Baltimore: Williams & Wilkins, 1994;1313–1320.
27. Ritter MA, Faris PM, Keating M. Posterior cruciate ligament balancing during total knee arthroplasty. J Arthroplasty 1988; 3:323–326.
28. Landy MM, Walker PS. Wear of ultra-high-molecular-weight polyethylene components of 90 retrieved knee prostheses. J Arthroplasty 1988;3(suppl 1):S73–S75.
29. Wright TM, Bartel DL. The problem of surface damage in polyethylene total knee components. Clin Orthop 1986; 205:67–74.
30. Peters PC, Engh GA, Dwyer KA, Vinh TN. Osteolysis after total knee arthroplasty without cement. J Bone Joint Surg 1992; 74A:864–876.
31. Wright TM, Rimnac CM, Stulberg SD, et al. Wear of polyethylene in total joint replacements: observations from retrieved PCA knee implants. Clin Orthop 1992;76:126–134.
32. Tsao AK, Mintz L, McCrae CR, et al. Severe polyethylene wear in PCA total knee arthroplasties. Paper presented at the Knee Society Scientific Meeting, Anaheim, CA, 1991.
33. Jordan LR, Siegel JL, Olivo JL. Early flexion routine: an alternative method of continuous passive motion. Clin Orthop 1995; 315:231–233.
34. Baldwin K, McPherson EJ, Dorr LD. Postoperative rehabilitation of TKR with CPM vs drop and dangle. Paper presented at the Knee Society Scientific Meeting, Atlanta, 1966.

chapter 51

Mathias P. G. Bostrom, and Steven B. Haas

Failed Knee Replacement: Revision Knee Arthroplasty

Although primary total knee arthroplasty has a low rate of failure, the number of revision total knee arthroplasty procedures is increasing (1). Indications for revision of primary total knee arthroplasties include aseptic loosening, infection, instability, malposition and malalignment, patellar dislocation, stiffness, massive polyethylene wear or failure, periprosthetic fracture, and unexplained pain (Table 51.1). The treatment for previous total knee arthroplasty is technically demanding, and its overall results have not compared favorably to those of primary total knee arthroplasties (1–12). This chapter discusses revision total knee arthroplasties with special emphasis on preoperative assessment and surgical techniques.

INITIAL FINDINGS, PHYSICAL EXAMINATION, AND DIAGNOSIS

The causes of failure of a total knee replacement are various; and before any treatment can be undertaken, it is imperative to establish the cause of failure. To do so requires a thorough evaluation of the patient's history, a physical examination, and radiographs.

As part of the history, it is essential to document previous operations, problems with surgery, and the postoperative course. Underlying medical conditions should also be carefully noted, especially if there is a history of diabetes mellitus or vascular disease. In addition, the nature of the pain should be defined, since activity-related pain may be potentially different from rest or night pain. The patient's functional status should also be assessed in regard to ambulatory ability, stair-climbing ability, need for assistive devices, and potential instability. Finally, the patient's expectations should be addressed.

When examining the patient, the clinician must assess not only the knee but also the spine, abdomen, and hips since knee pain can be associated with problems in these areas. Quality of the skin must be evaluated with special emphasis on the location and nature of the previous incision. The range of motion must be documented, and a careful examination of the extensor mechanism is critical. Any extensor lag or incompetence of the ligaments should be noted, as should any varus or valgus or rotational malalignment.

RADIOLOGIC STUDIES

Routine radiographs of the knee document not only the type of components used but also the position of the components. Any malposition of the components should be noted, as should the location of the joint line relative to the patella. The amount of polyethylene wear can sometimes be evaluated by radiograph. More important, loosening of the components can be determined from radiographs and is evident by either change in the position of the components or by progressive radiolucent lines. Comparison to old radiographs may be especially helpful. Special stress radiographs may be useful in assessing ligamentous instability. Radionucleotide studies are rarely useful, because increased activity remains in more than two-thirds of asymptomatic knees after 1 year.

CAUSES OF FAILURE

Since the treatment of an infected total knee arthroplasty differs from that of aseptic failure, the paramount aim in evaluating the cause of failure should be to establish the presence of infection. Knee infections can be characterized by constant pain (rather than activity-related pain), fever, knee effusion, erythema, and drainage; however, an infected total knee arthroplasty rarely displays all of these signs and symptoms. Often a high index of suspicion and multiple confirmatory studies are neces-

650

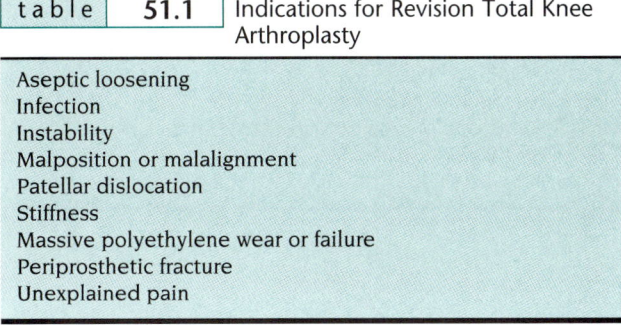

table	51.1	Indications for Revision Total Knee Arthroplasty

Aseptic loosening
Infection
Instability
Malposition or malalignment
Patellar dislocation
Stiffness
Massive polyethylene wear or failure
Periprosthetic fracture
Unexplained pain

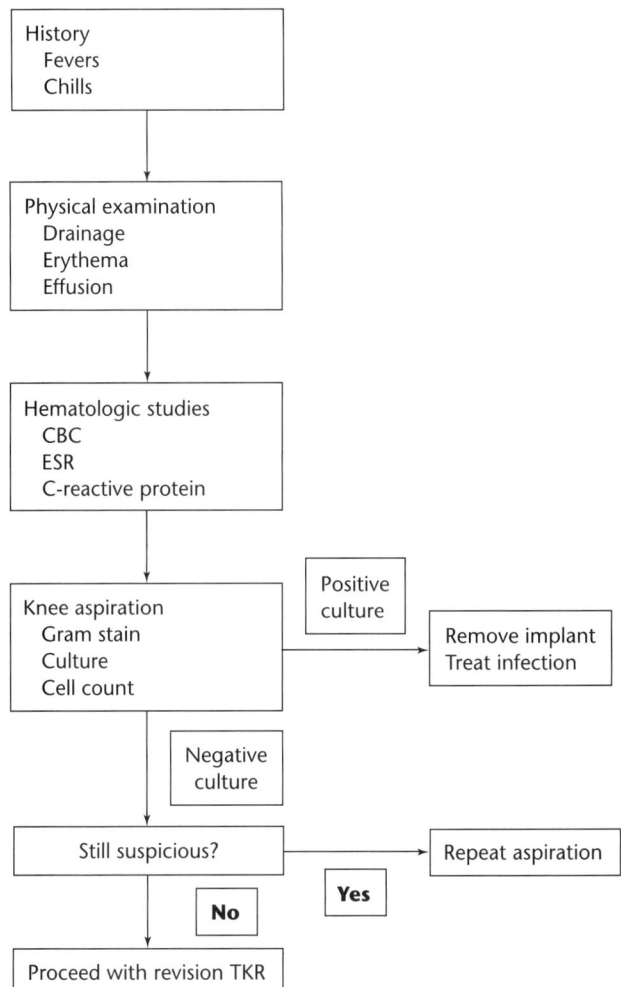

Figure 51.1. Diagnostic approach to total knee arthroplasty infection. *CBC,* complete blood count; *ESR,* erythrocyte sedimentation rate; *TKR,* total knee replacement.

sary to establish the correct diagnosis (Fig. 51.1.). A preoperative aspiration of the knee is strongly recommended. If infection is found to be the cause of the failure, then the prosthesis and all foreign material must be removed, the tissue aggressively débrided, and the appropriate antimicrobial regime instituted. Only when and if the infection is eradicated can the surgeon proceed with reimplantation of the prosthesis.

Reflex sympathetic dystrophy (RSD) is another problem that can lead to an unsuccessful outcome. In this entity, pain is out of proportion to other findings. These patients usually have a delayed postoperative recovery with limited flexion, cutaneous hypersensitivity, and temperature changes in the affected limb. The clinical impression is confirmed and treatment is initiated by a lumbar sympathetic block. Revising knees with RSD is not recommended, unless there is major mechanical failure of the total knee arthroplasty.

Mechanical failure of a total knee arthroplasty is characterized by activity-related pain that is relieved with rest. Aseptic loosening is the most common type of mechanical failure. It can be caused by instability, prosthetic wear, or malalignment. Loss of fixation can be confirmed radiographically by radiolucent lines greater than 2 mm or migration of the components.

Patellofemoral problems are also a major cause of unsuccessful total knee arthroplasties. Problems associated with the patellar component include subluxation, patellar fractures, avascular necrosis, patellar delamination (especially on metal back patellar prosthesis), and patellar clunk syndromes. Fortunately, not all of these require revision or operative treatment. Nondisplaced patellar fractures can often be treated conservatively, as can avascular necrosis. Patellar clunk syndromes most often associated with posterior stabilized total knee arthroplasties can be treated with arthroscopic débridement. Patellar subluxations may be treated conservatively but may require a lateral retinacular release or (rarely) a proximal realignment procedure. Failure of the polyethylene component (e.g., associated with delamination) does, however, require revision of the component.

Catastrophic failure of specific components, such as breakage of the metal tibial or femoral component or the posterior stabilizing cam, has been described but is becoming less prevalent with newer designs and metallurgy. Polyethylene wear remains a significant problem, leading to synovitis and an effusion. Although this process may be painless, the effusion and synovitis usually cause pain; and because of ligament relaxation, instability may be the presenting symptom. Postoperative stiffness, most often noted when getting in and out chairs and climbing stairs, can also be a problem with total knee arthroplasties. Inadequate flexion may be caused by a number of technical errors, such as leaving the flexion gap too tight, oversizing the femoral component, or cutting the tibia with an anterior tilt. These errors often require revision of some or all of the components. Contractures of the posterior cruciate ligament in posterior cruciate-retaining designs can also lead to inadequate flexion. Although an open arthrotomy with possible revision may be necessary, attempts at release of the posterior cruciate ligament arthroscopically may be worthwhile (13).

It is beyond the scope of this chapter to discuss all modes of failure and their treatment options; however, it is imperative to define the problem accurately before embarking on any treatment plan.

TREATMENT

Preoperative Planning

Before undertaking what may be a technically demanding procedure of revising a total knee arthroplasty, the surgeon must clearly understand the aims of the procedure. Before surgery, the surgeon must assess any special requirements of the case. This assessment should include technical aspects, such as method of exposure; the components to be revised, removal of the components, management of bone loss, the type of prosthesis to be implanted, soft tissue balancing, and the position of previous incisions. The possibility of sepsis should also be ruled out before the procedure via knee aspirations, hematologic studies, appropriate radiographic studies (if indicated), and in some cases exploration of the knee. In cases of early loosening, an infectious cause must especially be considered. An intraoperative Gram stain and frozen section should routinely be performed. Most important, the surgeon should attempt to clearly identify the mode of failure of the preceding arthroplasty, since revision without knowledge of a clear cause for failure will often lead to a second failure (8).

Surgical Technique

APPROACH AND EXPOSURE

Previous incisions should be carefully examined presurgery and should be used when possible. If these incisions are longitudinal and placed anteriorly, they can be reused during a revision procedure without significant risk of skin necrosis. On the other hand, if they are too medial or lateral, a new incision may be necessary, with a substantial increased risk of postoperative wound problems. Closely paralleled incisions and undermining of skin flaps, especially when new incisions are used, should be avoided, as they may lead to wound sloughing. If a new incision is used, the surgeon must maintain good tissue bridges. Consultation with a plastic surgeon is recommended, if there are multiple incisions and healing of the arthroplasty wound is questionable. To avoid wound-healing problems, some authors have recommended a trial incision, which is allowed to heal before the definitive procedure is undertaken (14). In some cases, muscle flap coverage or the use of tissue expanders to ensure proper coverage and healing of the arthroplasty wound may be necessary (9,15).

Exposure of the joint can be especially difficult during revision joint arthroplasty, especially if the joint is stiff (Table 51.2). A subperiosteal dissection of the proximal medial tibial is essential for obtaining proper exposure, although there is still a substantial risk of avulsing the tibial tubercle. To avoid this, an oblique incision of the proximal

table	51.2	Order of Exposure

Anterior skin incision
Medial parapatellar arthrotomy
Medial and lateral patellar recesses restoration
Lateral retinacular release
Rectus snip versus tibial tubercle osteotomy

quadriceps tendon—the so-called rectus snip—is often helpful. It is recommended that the rectus snip be performed early in the procedure (14). A full quadriceps turndown—or a tibial osteotomy—to gain exposure in difficult cases has also been recommended by some authors (16,17). Restoration of the medial and lateral patellar recesses and a complete synovectomy should be performed. An early lateral retinacular release is often useful for both obtaining exposure and everting the patella. If eversion of the patella is not immediately possible, then subluxating it laterally until the components have been removed may prove to be advantageous.

REMOVAL OF COMPONENTS

The removal of the failed components should take place with as little damage and loss to the remaining bone stock as possible. This can be quite challenging, especially when porous-coated implants were fixed with cement. With cemented components, the first principle is to separate the prosthesis from the cement. This can usually be accomplished with sharp osteotomes. A Gigli saw is helpful when freeing the anterior femoral bone–cement interface. All polyethylene tibial components can be removed by sawing beneath the component to divide the fixation peg or lugs. High-speed burrs may be of use in removing cemented stems and cement plugs. Once the cement–metal interface has been sufficiently compromised, a large slap hammer with a special attachment capable of grasping the metal prosthesis can be used to remove the implant. When using a slap hammer, it must be emphasized that the cement–metal interface must be sufficiently breached. In difficult cases, a diamond-tipped drill may be required to divide the metal implants in a piecemeal fashion, e.g., when removing cemented porous stems (18).

Although removal of all the cement from the joint is not as essential in nonseptic as it is in infected cases, an attempt should be made to remove as much cement as possible. This can usually be accomplished by using sharp osteotomes to create a mosaic pattern in the cement to facilitate its removal.

PATELLA REVISION

Removal of a well-fixed patella component may significantly compromise the bone stock; but in such cases, revision of the component may not be necessary. Indications for patellar revision include a loose patellar implant, an asymmetrically cut patella, and erosion of the polyethylene, which exposes metal backing. Of course, in infectious cases, even a well-fixed patella must be removed. Metal-backed patellar components with significant wear should also be revised.

All polyethylene patellar components can be removed by cutting across the flat surface of the patella at the plastic–cement interface; the lugs are subsequently removed with the cement. This procedure is difficult with inset-type patellae. Similarly, it can be difficult to remove metal-backed patellae without incurring significant bone loss. The procedure can be accomplished by using osteotomes to disrupt the bone–metal interface.

Many patellar components have a central fixation peg; revision of these components often leads to a large central defect. Fixation of a new patella can be accomplished with either a rectangular central fixation peg or a patellar component with three peripheral pegs. We have found the use of a biconvex patellar component helpful in cases with severe central bone loss (14,19). If the remaining patellar fragment is too fragile to accept a new component, then the patellar component can be omitted. A patellectomy is rarely needed and should generally be avoided.

The tracking and position of the patella are also critical. If a lateral release has not already been performed and patellar tracking is poor, lateral release should be carried out at this point. Rotational alignment of the tibial and femoral component should be evaluated. If severe patella infera is present, then reducing the size of the patella, placing the component superiorly, and omitting the patellar component are options.

Management of Bone Loss

Once the components are removed, the fibrous membrane on the bone surfaces and the synovium should be aggressively débrided to enhance fixation of the revision prosthesis and remove any debris that may cause third-body wear. Necrotic areas must be débrided back to viable bone before defect assessment can be made. Preparation of the bone surfaces should consist of manual débridement with curettes followed by the use of high-speed pulsating lavage. Sclerotic areas of bone should not be prepared with small drill holes, since this bone is often the only structurally sound bone available to support the prosthesis.

The amount of bone loss from the femur and tibia should be assessed by the use of spacers, which will also allow assessment of ligamentous integrity (14). As with primary total knee arthroplasty, the goal of a revision arthroplasty is to reconstruct the joint with emphasis on re-creating stability, axial alignment, and soft tissue balance. The components must be placed in the proper rotational alignment. The femoral epicondyles are often the most useful structures in ascertaining proper femoral rotation. The positions of the tibial tubercle, anterior tibia, and ankle joint are useful in obtaining proper tibial rotation. It is important, however, to use as many of these landmarks as available to achieve optimal restoration of the tibiofemoral and patellofemoral joint mechanics. The proper anteroposterior (AP) and mediolateral dimensions of the joint should be determined from the removed components and from preoperative radiographs or radiographs of the contralateral knee.

The bone defects can be addressed in a number of ways (Table 51.3). If the defects in the tibia are less than 5 mm, then the defect can be easily corrected by the use of cement alone. Peripheral defects greater than 5 mm and those involving an entire condyle are treated with metal wedges and augments (Fig. 51.2). When large half-wedges or full-wedges are used, fixation is supplemented with noncemented rods. The use of metal augments often helps replace lost bone and avoids elevating the joint line. Nonstructural contained defects are often suitably treated with bone autograft that is obtained either locally or from the iliac crest. Morcellizer allograft may also be used.

Bone grafting for peripheral cortical tibial defects greater than 5 mm has also been recommended by some authors (17). Such grafts can be secured with internal fixation, such as screws or pins. The incorporation of such grafts remains questionable in the compromised host environment of a failed total knee arthroplasty and has not generally been used at the Hospital for Special Surgery (New York).

Massive structural defects can also be treated with structural allografts fixed with plates and screws. Again, the long-term outcome of such grafts must be questioned, especially if the bone tumor surgery experience with such grafts is considered. For cases with massive defects, an alternative to allografts is the use of distal femoral or proximal tibial replacements with rotating hinge prostheses.

Choice of Implant

The choice of implants for revision total knee arthroplasty falls into four main categories: posterior cruciate ligament sparing, posterior cruciate ligament substituting, unlinked constrained, and linked constrained prostheses. As with primary total knee arthroplasty, posterior cruciate ligament-sparing implants can be used if the knee can be ligamentously balanced in both flexion and extension. Preserving the function of the posterior cruciate ligament may be difficult or impossible in revision cases, and it is recommended that the posterior cruciate ligament-substituting design be available. We routinely use a posterior cruciate ligament-substituting design in revision surgery.

table	51.3	Management of Bone Loss

Defect Size (mm)	Technique
<5	Cement
5–10	Bone graft versus cement
>10	Options:
	Metal augments or wedges
	Structural allografts
	Custom total knee replacement

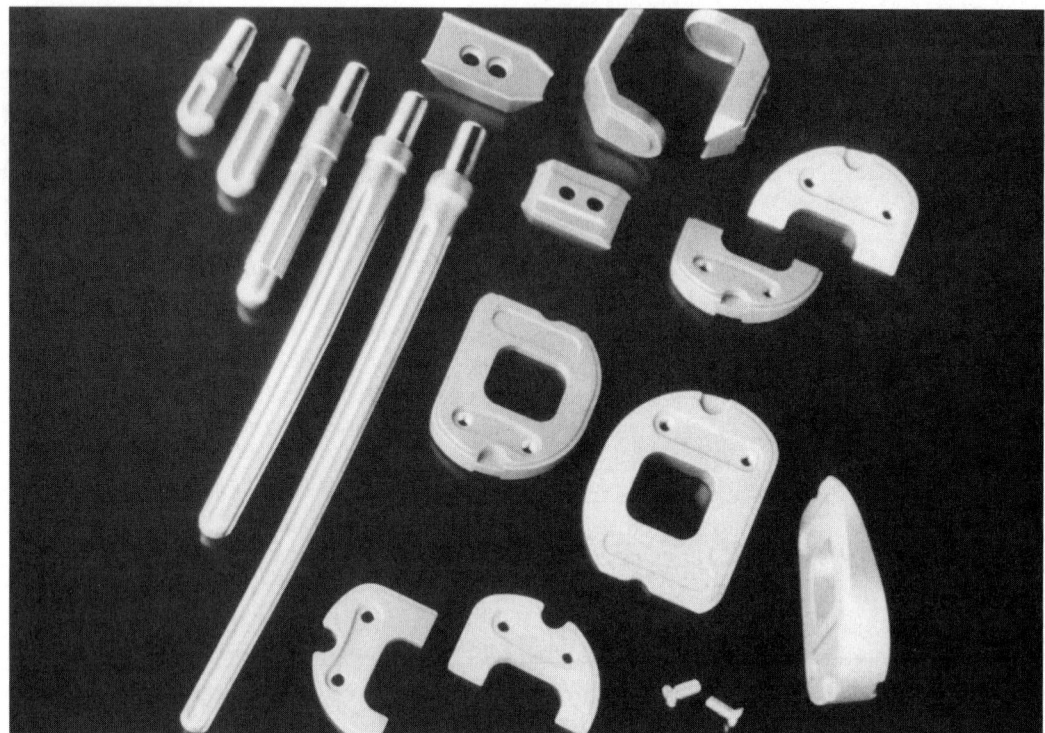

Figure 51.2. Several metal wedges and augments are available for the constrained condylar system.

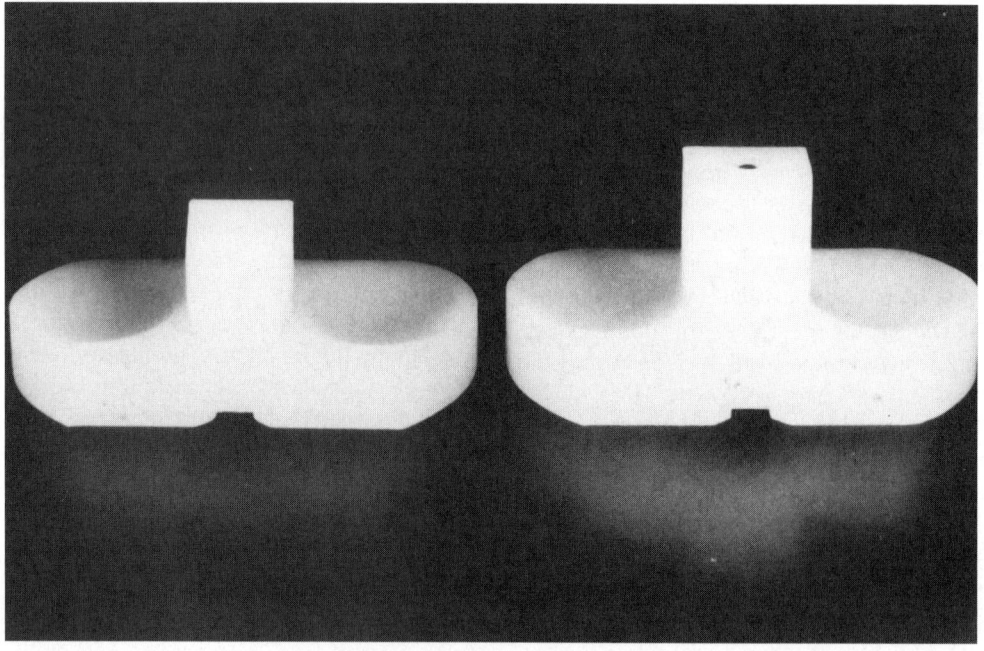

Figure 51.3. Posterior stabilized and constrained condylar tibial inserts. Note the increased height of constrained condylar central post.

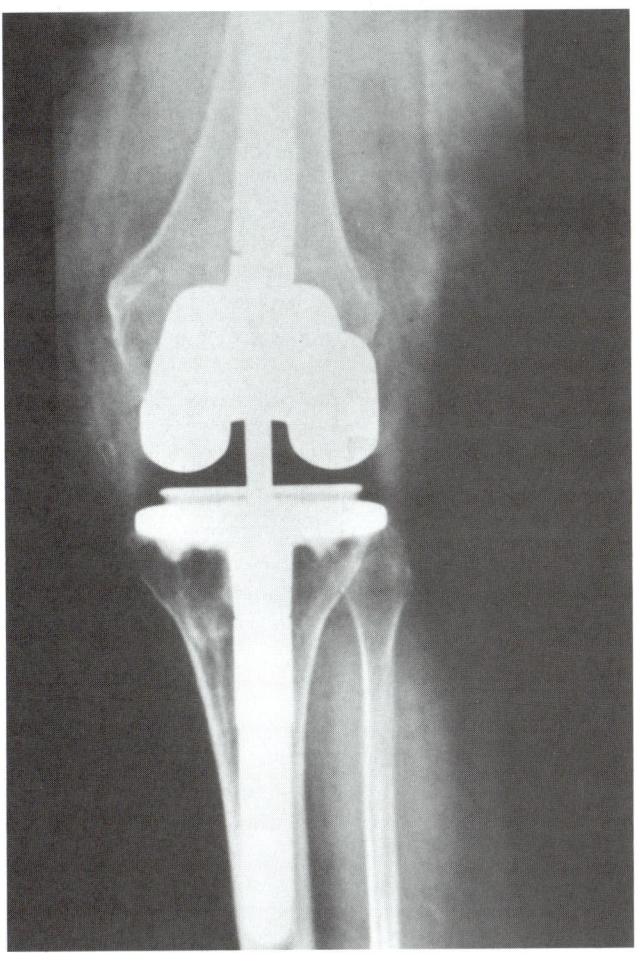

Figure 51.4. Postoperative AP view of a revision total knee arthroplasty that used intramedullary stems on both the femoral and tibial components. Note that the cement is present only on the cut bony surfaces, not on the intramedullary stems.

Posterior stabilized implants do not provide medial and lateral stability, and the collateral ligaments must be balanced. If ligamentous stability cannot be obtained, then a constrained condylar implant is used (Fig. 51.3). We recommend that noncemented rods be used routinely with constrained implants (Fig. 51.4). In cases with severe laxity, extensor mechanism incompetence, or massive bone loss, a rotating hinge-type implant may be necessary.

Although there are advocates of cementless fixation in revision total knee arthroplasty, the bone stock in revision cases is usually of poor quality and not ideally suited for cementless fixation. We chose to use cement fixation for all revision cases.

Reconstruction

We have found bone stock to be of poor quality in revision cases; therefore, we usually use noncemented rod to augment fixation. After removal of the components and appropriate débridement, the distal femur is usually ap-

proached first. Intramedullary rods are positioned by placing an 8-mm drill through the distal femoral metaphysis into the intramedullary canal. The canal is then reamed with a straight 10-mm reamer. Reamers are increased from 10 to 12 mm and then by 1-mm increments. Reaming is increased until the rod has achieved a clinical interference fit. Cortical contact is not obtained in most cases; and aggressive reaming is avoided, since it is believed that this leads to excessive bone loss. Reaming can often be performed by hand to obtain a proper interference fit.

After intramedullary reaming of the femur, the anterior and posterior femoral cuts are made with the appropriately sized template, adjusting rotation accordingly. The central bone of distal femur is then excised to allow for the femoral box and stem attachment of the revision prosthesis. Chamfer cuts can wait until the final seating of the components, as they may be unnecessary. Large medial and lateral condylar defects may be packed with bone graft.

The intramedullary reaming of the tibia is performed in the same manner as the femur. The location of the rod may displace the tibial component, usually anterior and medial to the optimal position. If overhang of the component is excessive, then downsizing of the component may be necessary. To avoid this problem, use of newer implants with offset tibial stems may be considered.

A trial fitting of the components, including the rods, is performed. A rod diameter that matches the largest reamer is chosen. The varus and valgus alignment of the tibial component is then assessed; the alignment block and rod are placed on the tibial component without the trial polyethylene insert. The rotation of the tibial component is determined using the tibial tubercle as the primary reference point.

Trial polyethylene inserts are then positioned. The soft tissues are meticulously balanced to equalize medial and lateral ligament constraint. The technique of soft tissue release differs little from standard techniques used in primary total knee arthroplasty. Both flexion and extension gaps must be balanced properly. Thicker tibial plastics or thicker femoral augments may be necessary to position the joint line appropriately. Flexion gap instability is often a problem. If insufficient ligament stability remains, a constrained condylar tibial insert is used.

The final components are then assembled. The bone surfaces are cleaned with pulsatile lavage. The femoral and patellar components are cemented in place, and care is taken to avoid introducing cement into the intramedullary canal. This is accomplished by cementing only the undersurface of the femoral component. The cement is applied in a dough state to avoid its leaking into the intramedullary canal; this significantly simplifies revision in cases of infection. The component is then gently impacted until it is firmly seated on the bony surface. After hardening of the femoral and patellar cement, the tibia is similarly cemented in place. Antibiotic impregnated cement is occasionally selected in cases thought to be at high risk for infection.

Postoperative Management and Rehabilitation

Postoperative management is similar to that of primary arthroplasty. Initially, patients are placed in splints until postoperative day 1, when active-assisted and continuous passive range of motion exercises are begun. If a quadriceps turndown was performed, a brace locked in extension is used for ambulation. Limited continuous passive motion may also be used. If a rectus snip was performed, no extra immobilization is required. Weight bearing is started on postoperative day 2.

Results of Revision Total Knee Arthroplasty

The initial reports of revision of resurfacing-type total knee arthroplasties were relatively poor. A total of 41% of cases that used a hinged-type prosthesis, such as the Guepar (Johnson & Johnson; Raynham, MA) or Herbert design, reported inadequate pain relief (1,5). Overall satisfactory results were as low as 37% in a series of 78 revisions (3). Cameron and Hunter (3) noted a correlation between the results and implant constraint: 48% of patients with semiconstrained prostheses noted satisfactory results, whereas only 21% of patients with hinged prostheses were satisfied. This trend of increased success with less-constrained revision prostheses was also noted in a review of the Mayo Clinic's experience with revision total knee arthroplasty (2,9–11). In that series of 427 revision cases, there was also a higher success rate for first revisions than for multiple revisions.

Many of the earlier studies were small, used diverse and older prostheses, included multiple surgeons, and had relatively short follow-up. Comparison between series is difficult due to the complex nature of revision operations, the different criteria used for inclusion in the studies, and the various rating systems employed.

More recent series using condylar knee designs show improvement of results. A 2-year follow-up of 116 revisions using a condylar prosthesis achieved 80% satisfactory results (6). Satisfactory results were also noted in 89% of 72 posterior stabilized prostheses (7). Rand and Bryan (10) reported satisfactory results in 76% of 51 revisions at the 5-year follow-up. In 28 failed total knee arthroplasties replaced with porous-coated anatomic components, good to excellent results were obtained in 68% of cases (8). The experience at the Brigham and Women's Hospital with 137 revision total knee arthroplasties showed a clinical success rate of 63% at 5 years for single revisions (20). The failure rate at 5 years was 5.8%. Other authors have had less encouraging results. Goldberg et al. (4) noted 42% poor results or failures using total condylar, posterior stabilized, total condylar III (Johnson & Johnson) and kinematic rotating hinge prostheses in 65 revision cases for mechanical failure.

The use of intramedullary stems in revision total knee arthroplasty appears to be justified both biomechanically and clinically. Using roentgen stereophotogrammetry, Albrektsson et al. (21) showed that the migration of the tibial component decreased with the use of a noncemented intramedullary rod. Bertin et al. (22) also showed radiographic evidence of load sharing of noncemented stems used for revision total knee arthroplasty. In another series, the use of constrained implants with uncemented rods had a high rate of aseptic loosening (23), and many of the failures had a previous history of infection.

We reported our experience with revision total knee arthroplasties using a contemporary modular system with noncemented rods (24). In this series of 76 revisions for aseptic failure, a prosthesis employing a metal-backed tibial tray, modular polyethylene inserts, and noncemented, Press-Fit, fluted, 75-mm-long intramedullary rods was used. Cement was placed in the cut surfaces of the femur and tibia in the metaphyseal region. Care was taken to avoid cement in the medullary canal. The types prostheses revised are shown in Table 51.4. The most common causes for revision were aseptic loosening, instability, and malalignment (Table 51.5).

If the patella was believed to be well fixed, it was not revised (49% of cases). In 10 cases, the patella was deemed too fragile to accept a component, and the patellar remnant was left in place. No patellectomies were performed

| table | 51.4 | Revised Prostheses |

Prosthesis	Manufacturer	Number
Total condylar	Howmedica (Rutherford, NJ)	20
Posterior stabilized	Zimmer (Warsaw, IN); Johnson & Johnson (Raynham, MA)	15
Townley	Depuy (Warsaw, IN)	7
Geometric	Howmedica ( )	5
PCA (noncemented)	Howmedica ( )	4
Guepar	Johnson & Johnson ( )	4
Custom posterior stabilized	Zimmer ( )	3
PCA (cemented)	Howmedica ( )	3
Total condylar III	Johnson & Johnson ( )	3
Freeman-Swanson	Howmedica ( )	2
Other	–	10

table	51.5	Revision Diagnosis

Diagnosis	Number (%)ᵃ
Loose tibial component	23(30)
Loose tibia and femur	21(28)
Instability	14(18)
Component failure (fracture)	5(7)
Loose femoral component	4(5)
Unexplained pain	3(4)
Tibial plateau fracture	2(3)
Supracondylar fracture	2(3)
Ankylosis	2(3)

ᵃDoes not equal 100% because of rounding.

during the revision procedures, although 3 knees had previous patellectomies. Autogenous bone grafts were used in 11 knees; and bony allograft, in 3 knees. A quadriceps-plasty as described by Coonse and Adams (16) was performed on 3 knees, and a rectus snip was performed on 2 knees to gain adequate exposure. No tibial tubercle osteotomies were performed.

A posterior stabilized insert was used in 73% of knees, and a constrained condylar polyethylene insert was used in 27% of knees. The posterior stabilized prostheses were condylar in design and had no inherent varus or valgus stability. The constrained condylar prostheses provide varus and valgus stability through a rectangular tibial post and high femoral box. Both prostheses require the resection of the posterior cruciate ligament and use a cam to allow for rollback of the femur during flexion and to provide posterior stability. Noncemented rods were used on both tibial and femoral components. A total of 25 tibial components had metallic wedges, and 23 femoral components had distal augments, posterior augments, or both.

Follow-up of these patients ranged from 2 to 9 years (mean 3.5 years). In general, the patients in this series showed marked improvement; 83% of cases had good to excellent clinical results. There were six failures: four resulting from infection and two resulting from aseptic loosening. Complete pain relief at rest was noted in 88% of patients; and 80% of patients reported pain-free ambulation. The predicted survivorship was 83% at 8 years (failure was defined as revision or recommended revision). Post-surgical pain relief was statistically significant. The majority of patients (59%) did, however, require external support for ambulation. Motion and knee stability were also improved after surgery. The results of first, second, and third revisions did not differ.

Radiographically, the tibiofemoral alignment changed from a mean of 2° of varus to 5° of valgus. All autografts and allografts incorporated. Multiple radiolucent lines were noted on postoperative radiographs; most were incomplete and nonprogressive. Only 3% of tibial components and 2% of femoral components had progressive radiolucencies. There was no correlation between radiolucencies and failure. Similarly, radiopaque lines developed around

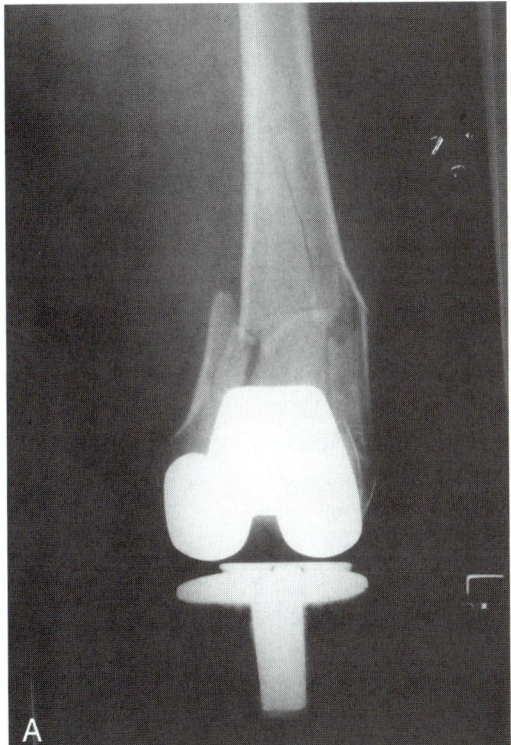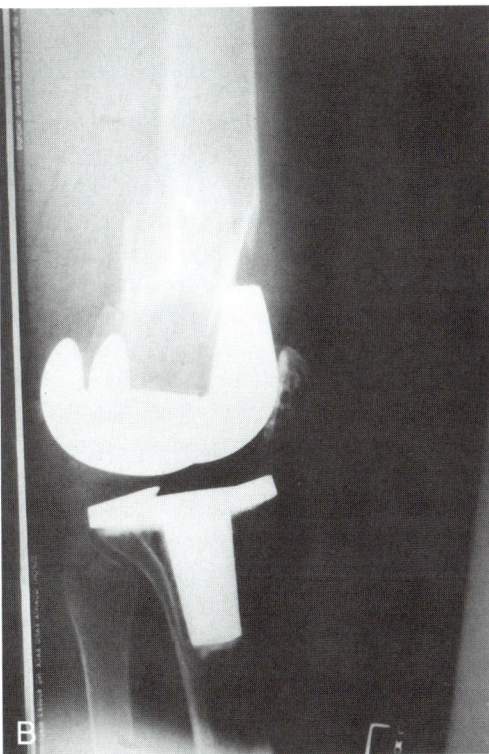

Figure 51.5. Preoperative AP (**A**) and lateral (**B**) views of a periprosthetic supracondylar femur fracture with a well-fixed total knee arthroplasty. *(continued)*

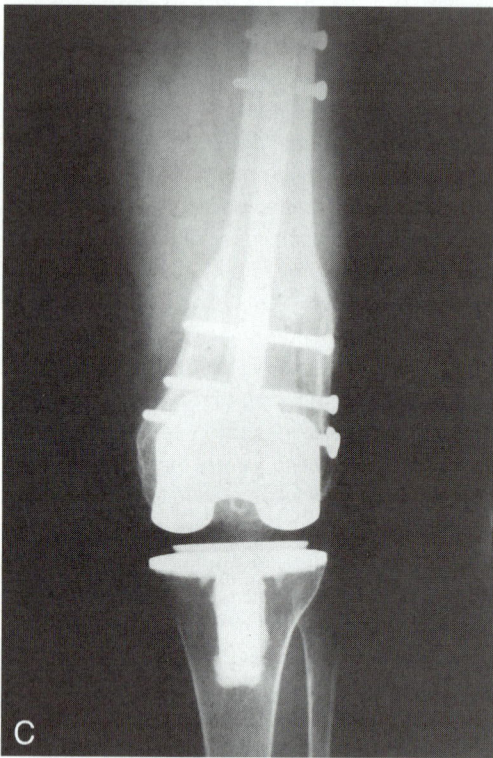
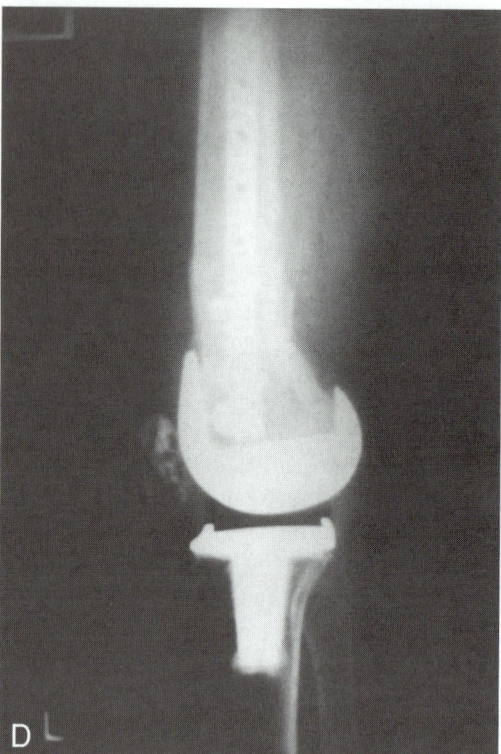

Figure 51.5. *(continued)* Postoperative AP (**C**) and lateral (**D**) views showing the interlocked intermedullary rod. Reprinted with permission from Smith, Nephew & Richards, Nashville, TN.

a small percentage of stems; but again there was no correlation between failure and these radiopaque lines.

Management of Periprosthetic Fractures

The management of periprosthetic fracture represents a difficult area in the field of total knee arthroplasty. If the implants are well fixed, the nondisplaced or minimally displaced fracture can be treated nonoperatively with traction or open reduction and internal fixation using plates and screws (25,26). In addition to standard methods, supracondylar femur fractures have been successfully treated using an intramedullary rod placed retrograde through the femoral component (Fig. 51.5) (23). We have found this new technique to be quite useful. Multiple Rush pins inserted in a retrograde manner have also been used; however, this method may be technically demanding and may provide less rigid fixation than plates and screws or intramedullary rod (27). More comminuted fractures can also be treated with either traction or internal fixation, but maintaining alignment with traction alone is difficult. In cases with severe loss of bone stock in the metaphysis, internal fixation devices may be inadequate. In these circumstances, treatment with a custom long-stem component to act as an intramedullary rod across the defect along with bone grafting is an alternative (28,29). This technique allows for the preservation of the soft tissue attachments to the metaphyseal fragment.

If the prosthesis is loose, the components must be removed, the bony architecture restored, and a new prosthesis (generally with a long intramedullary stem) implanted. If the bony architecture can be restored either with the use of an intramedullary rod or with plates and screws and the ligamentous integrity remains, then an unconstrained prosthesis can be used. If ligamentous stability cannot be obtained but bony architecture is restored, then a constrained condylar is used. In extremely severe cases where there is severe comminution and bone loss, rotating hinge devices that replace the distal femur or proximal tibia can be used.

SUMMARY

Revision total knee arthroplasty presents the surgeon with a variety of technical problems. The major problems include loss of bone stock and inadequacy of soft tissue constraints. Historically, these patients have done poorly; but when the problems are adequately addressed with the appropriate surgical technique and appropriate choice of implant, the results are quite good.

REFERENCES

1. Ahlberg A, Lunden A. Secondary operations after knee joint replacement. Clin Orthop 1981;156:170–174.
2. Bryan RS, Rand JA. Revision total knee arthroplasty. Clin Orthop 1982;170:116.
3. Cameron HU, Hunter GA. Failure in total knee arthroplasty: mechanisms, revisions, and results. Clin Orthop 1982;170:141–146.
4. Goldberg VM, Figgie MP, Figgie HE III, Sobel M. The results of revision total knee arthroplasty. Clin Orthop 1988;226:86–92.

5. Gross MS, Jaffe WL, Weinger EB. GUEPAR hinge knee arthroplasty: a five-year follow-up. Orthop Trans 1992;6:437.

6. Hood RW, Insall JN. Total knee revision arthroplasty: indications, surgical techniques, and results. Orthop Trans 1981;5:412.

7. Insall JN, Dethmers DA. Revision of total knee arthroplasty. Clin Orthop 1982;170:123–130.

8. Jacobs MA, Hungerford DS, Krackow KA, Lennox DW. Revision total knee arthroplasty for aseptic failure. Clin Orthop 1988;226:78–85.

9. Rand JA, Bryan RS. Revision after total knee arthroplasty. Orthop Clin North Am 1982;13:201–212.

10. Rand JA, Bryan RS. Results of revision total knee arthroplasties using condylar prostheses. A review of fifty knees. J Bone Joint Surg 1988;70A:738–745.

11. Rand JA, Peterson LF, Bryan RS, Ilstrup DM. Revision total knee arthroplasty. Instr Course Lect 1986;35:305–318.

12. Vince KG, Long W. Revision knee arthroplasty. The limits of Press-Fit medullary fixation. Clin Orthop 1995;317:172–177.

13. Williams RJ III, Westrich GH, Siegel J, Windsor RE. Arthroscopic release of the posterior cruciate ligament for stiff total knee arthroplasty. Clin Orthop 1996;331:185–191.

14. Insall JN. Revision of aseptic failed total knee arthroplasty. In: Insall JN, Windsor RE, Scott WN, et al., eds. Surgery of the knee. New York: Churchill Livingstone, 1995:935–957.

15. Kress KJ, Scuderi GR, Windsor RE, Insall JN. Treatment of nonunions about the knee utilizing custom total knee arthroplasty with Press-Fit intramedullary stems. J Arthroplasty 1993;8:49–55.

16. Coonse K, Adams JD. A new operative approach to the knee joint. Surg Gynecol Obstet 1943;77:344.

17. Whiteside LA. Cementless reconstruction of massive tibial bone loss in revision total knee arthroplasty. Clin Orthop 1989;248:80–86.

18. Windsor RE, Scuderi GR, Insall JN. Revision of well-fixed cemented, porous total knee arthroplasty. Report of six cases. J Arthroplasty 1988;3(suppl):S87–S94.

19. Rand JA. Revision total knee arthroplasty. In: Evarts CM, ed. Surgery of the musculoskeletal system. New York: Churchill Livingstone, 1990:3695–3689.

20. Friedman RJ, Hirst P, Poss R, et al. Results of revision total knee arthroplasty performed for aseptic loosening. Clin Orthop 1990;255:235–241.

21. Albrektsson BE, Ryd L, Carlsson LV, et al. The effect of a stem on the tibial component of knee arthroplasty: a roentgen stereophotogrammetric study of uncemented tibial components in the Freeman-Samuelson knee arthroplasty. J Bone Joint Surg 1990;72B:252–258.

22. Bertin KC, Freeman MA, Samuelson KM, et al. Stemmed revision arthroplasty for aseptic loosening of total knee replacement. J Bone Joint Surg 1985;67B:242–248.

23. Haas SB, Insall JN, Montgomery W III, Windsor RE. Revision total knee arthroplasty with use of modular components with stems inserted without cement. J Bone Joint Surg 1995;77A:1700–1707.

24. Culp RW, Schmidt RG, Hanks G, et al. Supracondylar fracture of the femur following prosthetic knee arthroplasty. Clin Orthop 1987;222:212–222.

25. Merkel KD, Johnson EW Jr. Supracondylar fractures of the femur after total knee arthroplasty. J. Bone Joint Surg 1986;68A:29–43.

26. Rolston LR, Christ DJ, Halpern A, et al. Treatment of supracondylar fractures of the femur proximal to a total knee arthroplasty. A report of four cases. J Bone Joint Surg 1995;77A:924–931.

27. Ritter MA, Stiver P. Supracondylar fracture in a patient with total knee arthroplasty. A case report. Clin Orthop 1985;193:168–170.

28. Cordeiro EN, Costa RC, Carazzato JG, dos Santos Silva J. Periprosthetic fractures in patients with total knee arthroplasties. Clin Orthop 1990;252:182–189.

29. Madsen F, Kjaersgaard-Andersen P, Juhl M, Sneppen O. A custom-made prosthesis for the treatment of supracondylar femoral fractures after total knee arthroplasty: report of four cases. J Orthop Trauma 1989;3:332–337.

chapter 52

James V. Bono and Steven R. Wardell

Salvage Knee Surgery: Arthrodesis and Resection Arthroplasty

Arthrodesis of the knee is an uncommon procedure and is rarely preformed primarily for arthritis. It is, however, a salvage procedure for unrevisable failed total knee arthroplasty (TKA) (1). Arthrodesis of the knee in the face of grossly deficient bone stock and ligamentous instability is difficult to achieve (2–5). In limb salvage surgery for malignant and potentially malignant lesions about the knee, resection arthrodesis using an intramedullary rod and local bone graft has been reported to be a successful primary procedure (6). When performed as a primary procedure after trauma, arthritis, or instability, solid fusion may not always occur at the reported union rates of 80 to 98%, depending on the method. Fibrous nonunion after attempted fusion is frequently painful (3,7–10), and rigid internal fixation promotes bony union. Using strict patient selection criteria, knee arthrodesis should be reserved as a salvage procedure for severe infection, bone loss, or instability primarily following failed TKA.

INDICATIONS

Unilateral Posttraumatic Osteoarthritis in a Young Patient

An arthrodesis should be recommended for a healthy, young laborer who has an isolated severely damaged knee (11). A successful fusion is more durable over time than any other reconstructive option; however, arthrodesis is often refused by men and is generally rejected unconditionally by women, which presents a dilemma for the surgeon. In the younger individual, a knee replacement is unlikely to endure a lifetime of hard use and will certainly require future revision.

The patient's decision to undergo arthrodesis should be made carefully, since conversion of a knee arthrodesis to successful arthroplasty is not easily performed (12). Fortunately, disabling unilateral, posttraumatic osteoarthritis in a young person is rare, and each case must be judged individually. Occasionally, joint débridement or realignment by osteotomy provides temporary symptomatic relief. Extensive preoperative discussion, including the risks, benefits, expectations, and alternatives to surgery help the patient decide whether to have surgery, postpone it, or avoid it altogether. Despite the long-term durability of fusion, the patient may still insist on TKA; such a patient should understand that the success of arthrodesis following unsuccessful arthroplasty may be less predictable.

Knee with Multiple Operations

Occasionally, there are patients who despite, or because of, multiple operations complain of a diffusely painful and usually unstable knee. The original insult may have been a ligament injury or patellar dislocation that resulted in reflex sympathetic dystrophy with or without subsequent operative intervention. Underlying emotional and psychiatric problems may be present. These patients are challenging to treat, and additional knee surgery of any kind may be unwarranted and inadvisable secondary to its poor outcome. Management should consist of simple conservative care: bracing, physical therapy, evaluation by a pain service, and (perhaps) psychiatric consultation. For a select few, arthrodesis may be the correct approach. In this situation, a preoperative trial with a cylinder cast will allow the patient to experience the functional limitations of knee arthrodesis.

Painful Ankylosis

Ankylosis of the knee is defined as a range of motion of not more than 10° to 20°. Patients who develop stiffness from rheumatoid arthritis or osteoarthritis may be successfully treated by total knee arthroplasty that uses quadriceps turndown or tibial tubercle osteotomy techniques, skeletonization of the femur, and reestablishment of the medial and lateral gutters by scar excision (13). Even in these cases, however, the likelihood of obtaining normal motion is small; the final outcome is often less than 90° of motion. In the ankylosed knee following sepsis or remote trauma, an arthroplasty may be either contraindicated or likely to produce a suboptimal result, particularly in terms of functional motion. Therefore, a painful ankylosis of the knee may benefit from an arthrodesis.

Paralytic Conditions

Currently, poliomyelitis is rare in the United States and western Europe where vaccination is widespread. Muscle weakness can usually be managed successfully by bracing, as these patients often have little pain. When associated with genu recurvatum, however, bracing is difficult and may not be successful. In this setting, arthroplasty is technically demanding (14). In paralytic conditions, arthrodesis adequately addresses the quadriceps weakness and angular deformity.

Neuropathic Charcot Joint

Arthrodeses of neuropathic knee joints have resulted in limited success and frequent nonunion. Thorough débridement of all bone detritus and complete synovectomy have been demonstrated to increase the rate of bony union (15). Drennan et al. (15) reported 10 cases of arthrodesis of a Charcot knee in nine patients. The best results were obtained after complete removal of the thickened, edematous synovium in these knees. When the Charcot knee is painless, bracing and conservative management is the treatment of choice. Some Charcot knees are painful and should be carefully selected for knee arthroplasty or arthrodesis. Variable results of TKA in Charcot joints have been reported (16,17). If TKA is performed, bone defects should be treated by implants with metal augments rather than by bone grafting; constrained posterior stabilized knee replacement designs are recommended.

Malignant and Potentially Malignant Knee Lesions

Certain potentially malignant and low-grade malignant tumors about the knee (e.g., aggressive giant cell tumor, chondrosarcoma, recurrent chondroblastoma) and carefully selected higher-grade malignant lesions may be satisfactorily controlled by adequate local resection of the lesion. Reconstruction of the defect created by such resection may be accomplished by (*a*) extremity shortening and arthrodesis, (*b*) arthrodesis with large intercalary bone grafts to preserve length, (*c*) arthroplasty with custom-made prosthetic replacements, and (*d*) allotransplantation of joints (18–29).

Local resection and arthrodesis for tumors about the knee was first described in 1907 by Lexer (19) and other authors (21,25,29,30). Success in controlling the tumor was frequently complicated by infection, nonunion, and late fatigue fracture. Enneking and Shirley (6) reported 20 patients with malignant or potentially malignant tumors (osteogenic sarcoma, giant cell tumor, synovial cell sarcoma, chondrosarcoma, and chondroblastoma) in the proximal tibia or distal femur. These patients were treated by local resection and arthrodesis using a customized fluted intramedullary rod and autogenous segmental cortical grafts obtained from the same extremity.

Failed Total Knee Arthroplasty

Currently, the most frequent indication for knee fusion and the most difficult circumstance in which to achieve union is the failed TKA. Mechanical failure of an arthroplasty can nearly always be better managed by revision. Two-stage reimplantation may be the best choice when the failure is caused by sepsis. Some cases of failed TKA with bone loss and infection can be managed only by resection arthroplasty and staged arthrodesis.

Arthrodesis as a salvage procedure for a failed septic knee replacement is indicated in the following circumstances: a patient (*a*) with persistent infection recalcitrant to repeated débridements and antibiotic regimen; (*b*) with disruption of the extensor mechanism; (*c*) with an infectious organism that is sensitive only to severely toxic antibiotic agents, such as *Candida albicans* and other fungi (31–33); and (*d*) who is young (or older and disillusioned) and does not wish to face possible future revision arthroplasties. Occasionally, fusion may be the best choice for an obese patient with a septic TKA. Although some patients insist on TKA reimplantation following sepsis, some do not want to risk recurrent infection and choose arthrodesis as definitive treatment.

Deficiency of the extensor mechanism is a compelling indication for arthrodesis when it occurs in the setting of an infected knee arthroplasty. The patient generally displays a profound extensor lag with poor results if reimplantation TKA is performed. Despite various reconstructive techniques, disruption of the extensor mechanism often yields a compromised result (34). The patient will never be able to adequately extend the knee and will generally display a profound extensor lag if reimplantation TKA is attempted. Repair of the extensor mechanism is often impossible because of extensive tissue destruction that occurs secondary to the infection. An extensor mechanism allograft may be needed to reconstruct the extensor deficit, but it is relatively contraindicated in the setting of previous sepsis.

ARTHRODESIS TECHNIQUES

Arthrodesis of the knee may be accomplished by one of four techniques: (*a*) compression arthrodesis with external fixation, (*b*) compression arthrodesis with compression plating (35,36), (*c*) intramedullary rod fixation, and (*d*) a combination of intramedullary rod fixation and compression plating (37) (Figs. 52.1–52.5).

A suitable cancellous surface on the femoral and tibial surfaces optimizes fusion. Bone shortening relaxes the hamstrings and increases flexibility at the hip joint, which is desirable if both knees must be fused (7). Charnley and Baker (7) reported that patients considered limb shortening advantageous for dressing and foot care. The desired alignment is 0° to 5° of valgus, with the knee flexed 10° to 15°. Less flexion can be accepted in the presence of marked bone loss. The patella can be left alone or used to augment the fusion mass.

When arthrodesis is indicated after failed total knee arthroplasty with bone loss, further host bone should not be resected; the surfaces must be roughly débrided and their irregular surfaces opposed to give the best possible contact. Intramedullary reamings and the patella can be used as graft to fill large defects.

Compression Arthrodesis

Compression arthrodesis using an external pin and frame technique was popularized by Key (38) and

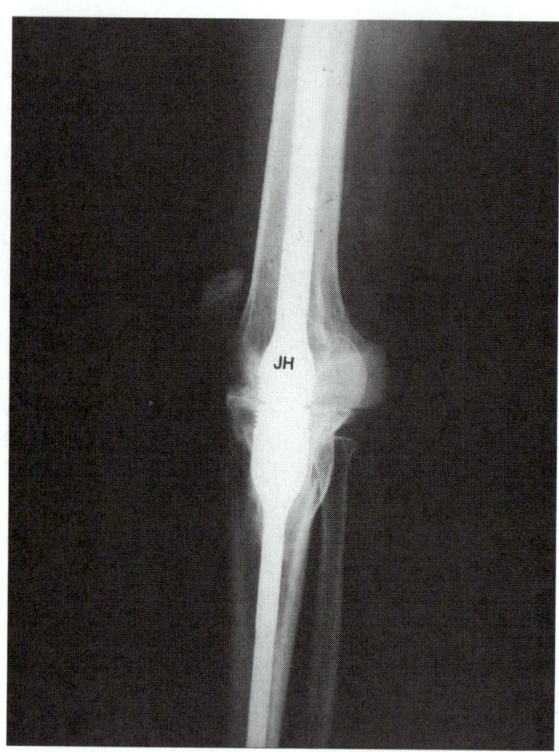

Figure 52.2. Postoperative lateral view of an intramedullary arthrodesis of the knee.

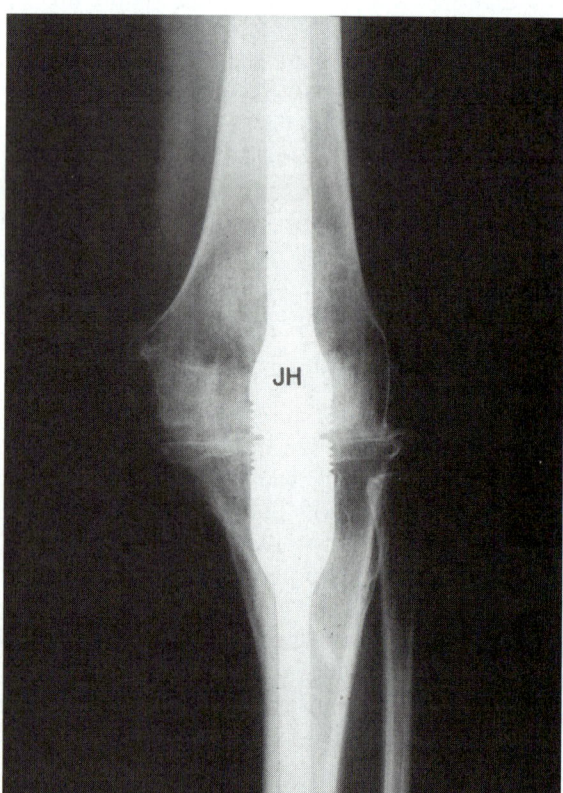

Figure 52.1. Postoperative AP view of an intramedullary arthrodesis of the knee.

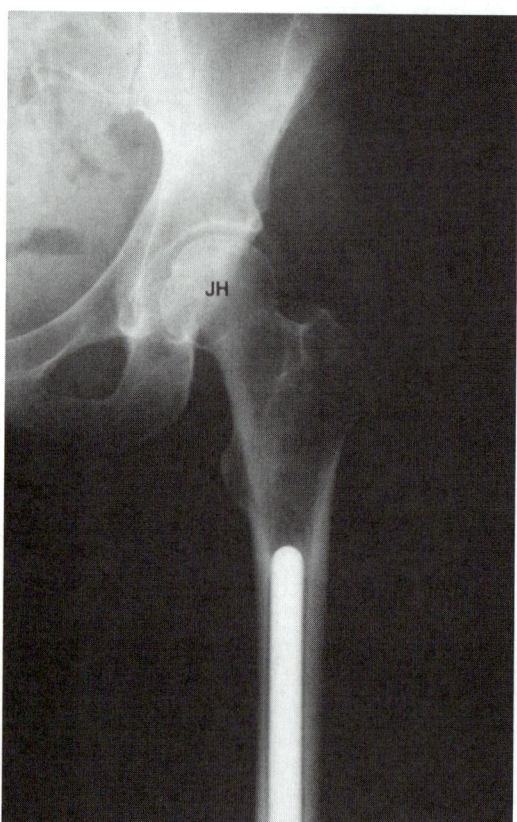

Figure 52.3. AP view of the hip showing the proximal extent of the intramedullary rod.

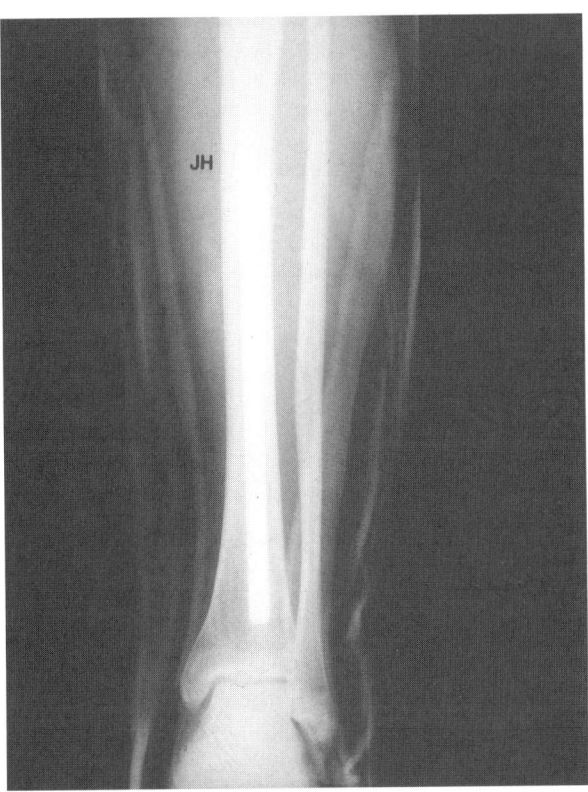

Figure 52.4. AP view of the distal tibia showing the distal extent of the intramedullary rod.

Charnley's group (7,8,39,40). Multiple transfixation pins are now used. Half-pins (6.5-mm Schanz screws) at right angles to the transfixation pins augment stability. Other configurations, such as triangular frames with half-pin fixation, result in a high degree of anteroposterior (AP) and mediolateral (ML) stability (9,41). Furthermore, success with Ilizarov external fixation systems have been achieved.

The advantages of external fixation are (*a*) stable compression across the fusion site (9,41), especially if half-pins are added anteriorly; (*b*) limb stabilization for management of extensive soft tissue infection; (*c*) technical ease of application and removal; and (d) dynamization and loading across the fusion site. The disadvantages include (*a*) external pin tract problems, (*b*) poor patient compliance, (*c*) frequent need for premature removal and cast immobilization, and (*d*) nonrigid fixation in cases of severe bone loss.

Success has been achieved with external fixation compression arthrodesis (7,8,38–41). Fusion rates of 50% occurred in series that included large numbers of failed hinged prostheses. In this situation, external fixation does not always provide the stability necessary for bone healing. Knutson et al. (42) reported 91 attempted fusions for failed knee arthroplasty. Fusions after surface replacement arthroplasties were much more successful than those after hinged prostheses. They believed that both intramedullary rod and external fixation methods were successful and that repeated attempts at fusion were worth-

while. External fixation devices must be in place for approximately 3 months; then cast immobilization is necessary until the arthrodesis is healed. One advantage of external fixation for treatment of septic knee replacements is that the device may be removed, leaving no retained hardware in the knee.

The use of compression plate fixation to achieve knee fusion has been described (35,36). Dual plate fixation has been recommended to achieve rigid biplanar fixation. Nicholas achieved solid fusion of 11 knees after failed TKA at an average of 5.6 months (42). A more extensive dissection is required; and the technique is demanding. especially in severely osteoporotic patients with significant bone loss for whom screw purchase may be compromised.

EXTERNAL FIXATION COMPRESSION ARTHRODESIS

Existing midline incisions are used for external fixation compression arthrodesis; transverse incisions that divide the quadriceps mechanism may be used in primary cases. Joint surfaces are prepared with a saw. Cutting jigs from a total knee arthroplasty tray are used to make accurate resections and obtain the correct alignment. Three parallel transfixation pins are passed through the distal femur, and three more through the upper tibia. If the knee demon-

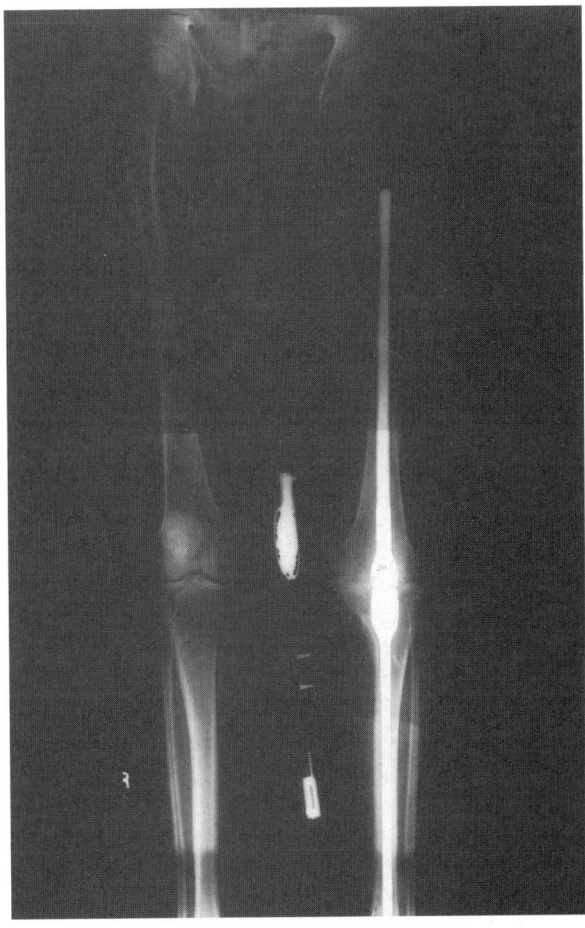

Figure 52.5. AP weight-bearing long-leg view showing excellent alignment in the coronal plane.

strates AP instability after the frame is applied, additional half-pins, three above and three below the knee, are inserted under radiographic control. The pins are connected to the frame, and compression is applied. Fixation is usually secure enough to allow weight bearing. Currently, the triangular frame configuration is popular; it uses 6.5-mm-diameter half-pins at a 45° angle to the AP and ML planes. This configuration yields rigid stability in both planes and is fairly tolerable.

Intramedullary Rod Arthrodesis

Intramedullary rod fixation has been reported to achieve union in a high percentage of patients (43–52) (Fig. 52.6). Knutson et al. (49) obtained fusion in 9 out of 10 knees treated with this method. Donley et al. (43) obtained an 85% fusion rate in 20 knees using intramedullary rod fixation and arthrodesis for the treatment of giant cell tumor, nonunion of a distal femur or proximal tibia fracture, aseptic loosening of a total knee replacement, and septic total knee replacement. Other authors have reported successful results using this technique (46,47,50). Wilde and Stearns (52), however, successfully fused only 6 of 9 knees with the intramedullary rod technique.

Advantages of the intramedullary rod technique include (a) immediate weight bearing and easier rehabilitation, (b) the elimination of problems associated with external transfixation pins and frames, (c) a high fusion rate, (d) the potential for dynamization and load sharing, and (e) increased stability in bone weakened by atrophy or osteopenia (with which screws or pins may pull out). The disadvantages include (a) the risk of proximal rod migration (requires removal), (b) difficulty achieving accurate alignment, (c) intramedullary dissemination of infection, (d) risk of fat embolism, and (e) potential incompatibility with ipsilateral hip arthroplasty.

After failure of a hinged arthroplasty, the femur and tibia may resemble hollow cones with little or no remaining cancellous bone. In this setting, external fixation devices cannot provide the stability required for arthrodesis. Cortical bone is often irregular, partially devascularized, or impregnated with metallic debris. Kaufer et al. (48) recommended an initial period of prolonged immobilization. If this results in a stable, painless, fibrous ankylosis, then no further treatment is indicated (53). After removal of the prosthetic components, a period of up to 1 year is allowed to pass before the formal arthrodesis is performed by intramedullary rod fixation.

Intramedullary arthrodesis has gained widespread favor for the salvage of severely infected knee replacements (Fig. 52.7). Most authors recommend performing the procedure in two stages, although Puranen et al. (51) reported single-stage arthrodeses in a few patients who were infected with organisms exquisitely sensitive to antibiotics. Donley et al. (43) and Kaufer et al. (48) recommended a curved nonmodular Küntscher rod (Biomet, Inc.; Warsaw, IN) that was cut down to an appropriate length during the procedure. In severe infections in which

a two-stage reimplantation of a new total knee replacement is not likely to succeed—e.g., infection with *Clostridium perfringens* (32) and *Candida albicans* (54)—arthrodesis has been successful. New, safer fungal-specific antimicrobial drugs may make salvage of the latter infection possible in the future. In our series, we reported the results of intramedullary arthrodesis of the knee after failed septic TKA (55). Union occurred in 16 out of 17 patients (94%) at an average of 16 weeks.

Stiehl and Hanel (37) reported eight cases of knee arthrodesis using combined intramedullary rodding and plate fixation. By adding a compression plate, intramedullary nail arthrodesis can be extended to situations in which bone loss requires a segmental allograft.

NONMODULAR INTRAMEDULLARY ROD

Our technique of intramedullary arthrodesis of the knee has been described (56). The original longitudinal incision is used whenever possible. The knee joint is exposed in a manner similar to that used in revision arthroplasty, and all scar tissue is resected. Cancellous bone is completely exposed on the distal femur and proximal tibia. An intramedullary ball-tip guidewire is introduced into the tibial shaft to the plafond of the ankle. The canal is sequentially reamed until the cortex is engaged at the tibial isthmus. This canal width determines the intramedullary rod diameter. The tibial length is measured using the guide rod as a reference.

The ball-tip guidewire is removed from the tibial canal and inserted into the femoral shaft until it contacts the piriformis recess. The femoral canal is reamed until it matches the size of the tibial reamer. The femoral length is measured using the guide rod at the piriformis fossa as a reference. The appropriate rod length is determined by subtracting 1 cm from the combined length of the femur and tibia measurements. The guidewire is tapped proximally through the piriformis recess with a mallet and is advanced until it can be easily palpated under the skin of the thigh, with the leg in an adducted position. An incision is made over the guidewire, and dissection is carried down through the gluteal musculature to the piriformis recess. The recess is reamed progressively to a size 1 mm larger than the tibial and femoral reamer size. After reaming, an arthrodesis nail of the appropriate length is selected. Alternatively, a 90-cm curved nonmodular Küntscher arthrodesis nail is cut to the appropriate length using a high-speed cutting tool. An extraction slot is made at the proximal end to allow later removal. The patella may be used to augment the fusion; two 6.5-mm cancellous screws are used for fixation at the level of the resection.

In the treatment of traumatic femoral shaft fractures, an intramedullary nail is inserted with its curve following the anterolateral bow of the femur. If the rod follows the anterolateral bow of the femur in intramedullary knee arthrodesis, however, it will create varus alignment. For this reason, the rod is inserted with the curve positioned anteromedially down the femoral shaft. The rod will then come through the tibia in valgus and slight flexion at the

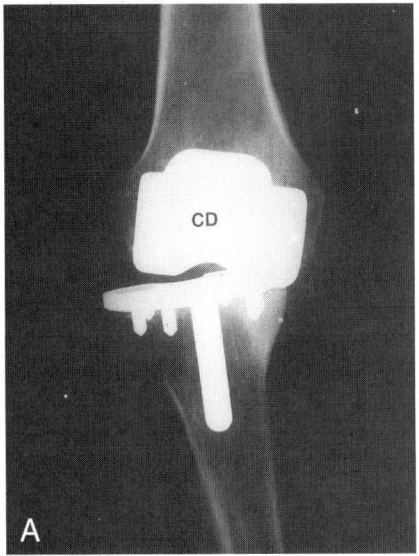
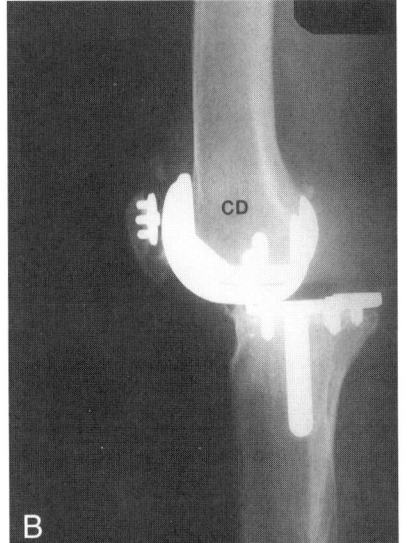
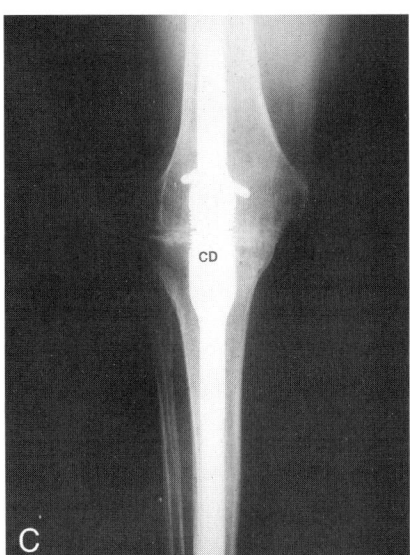

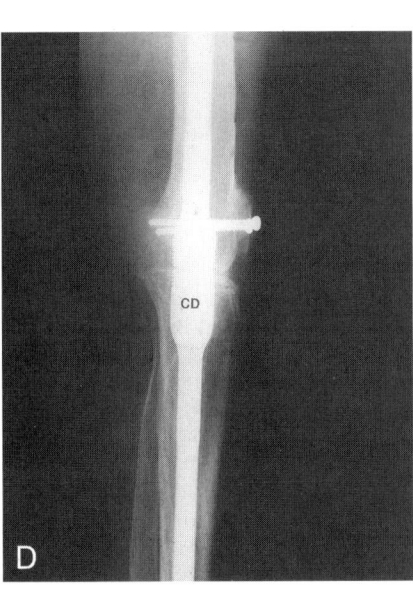
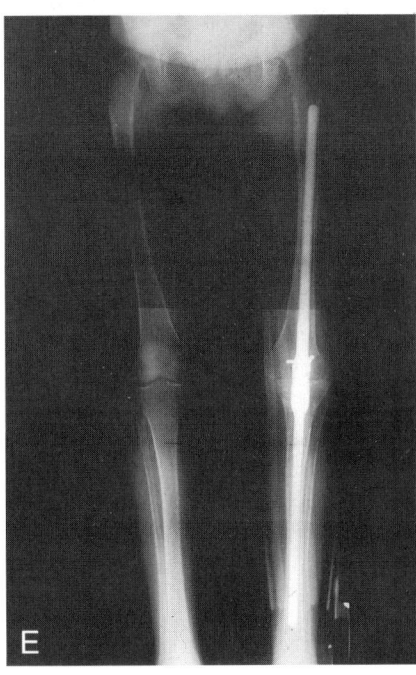

Figure 52.6. A. Preoperative AP view of 67-year-old female with a diagnosis of a failed right TKA. Note the coronal plane instability. **B.** Preoperative lateral view showing sagittal plane instability. Postoperative AP (**C**) and lateral (**D**) views following conversion to an intramedullary arthrodesis of the knee. **E.** Postoperative AP weight-bearing long-leg view showing excellent alignment in the coronal plane.

knee, which is a preferred position of arthrodesis. An axial load is placed on the proximal tibia against the distal end of the femur during rod insertion. Sometimes the rod forces the anterior tibial flare forward, making closure of the arthrotomy difficult. If this occurs, the surgeon may modify the anterior flare with a reciprocating saw. Resected bone and intramedullary reamings should be used as autograft, although some authors consider this unnecessary (43). Interlocking screws or wiring of the proximal portion of the rod has been recommended to prevent proximal migration (43,47).

MODULAR INTRAMEDULLARY NAIL

Intramedullary rodding may also be accomplished using the Neff femorotibial nail (Zimmer, Inc.; Warsaw, IN) or the Witchita nail (Stryker Howmedica Osteonics; Allendale, NJ), which is made up of independent femoral and tibial rods coupled at the knee joint (Fig. 52.8). Advantages of this technique include (a) the independent sizing of the femoral and tibial diaphyses, (b) the elimination of proximal or distal rod migration, (c) the elimination of a surgical incision about the hip, and (d) the ability to accommodate a future ipsilateral total hip arthroplasty.

The intramedullary canal is sequentially reamed until the cortex is engaged at the tibial and femoral isthmus. The canal widths of the tibia and femur determine the size of the tibial and femoral portions of the nail. The bony surfaces of the tibia and femur are prepared to maximize bony contact. The tibial and femoral lengths are measured using fluoroscopy. The appropriately sized tibial and femoral components are selected. Because the components have a fixed length, any shortening of the components is accomplished with a Midas Rex diamond-tipped cutting wheel (Fig. 52.9). After preparing the femoral and

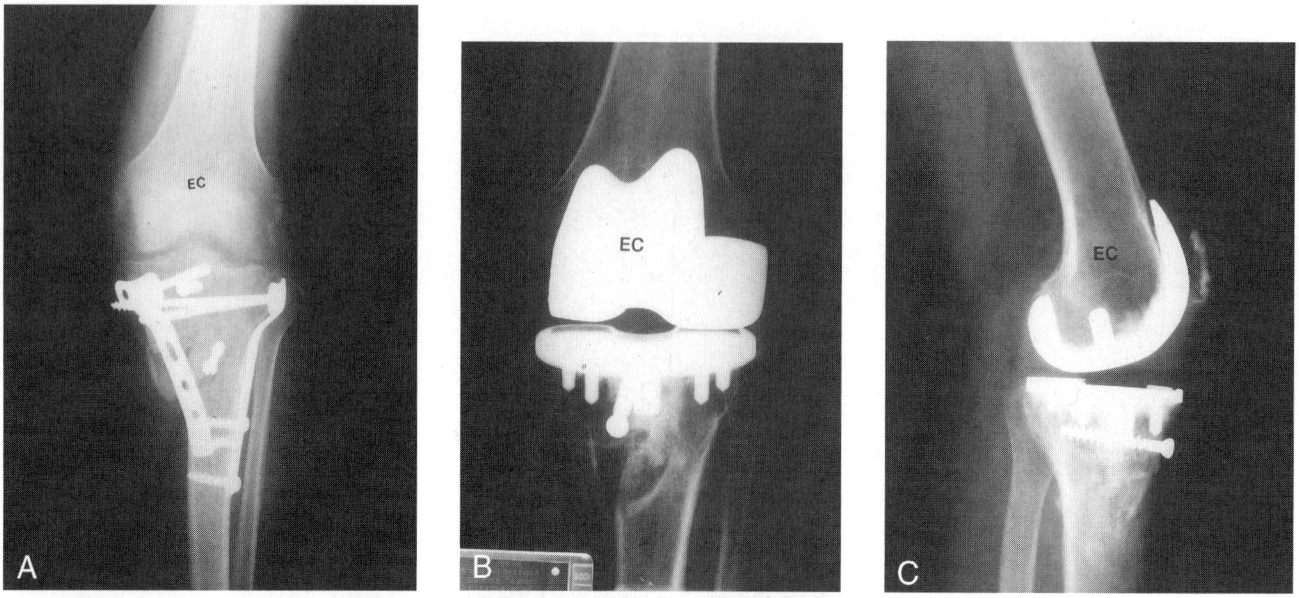

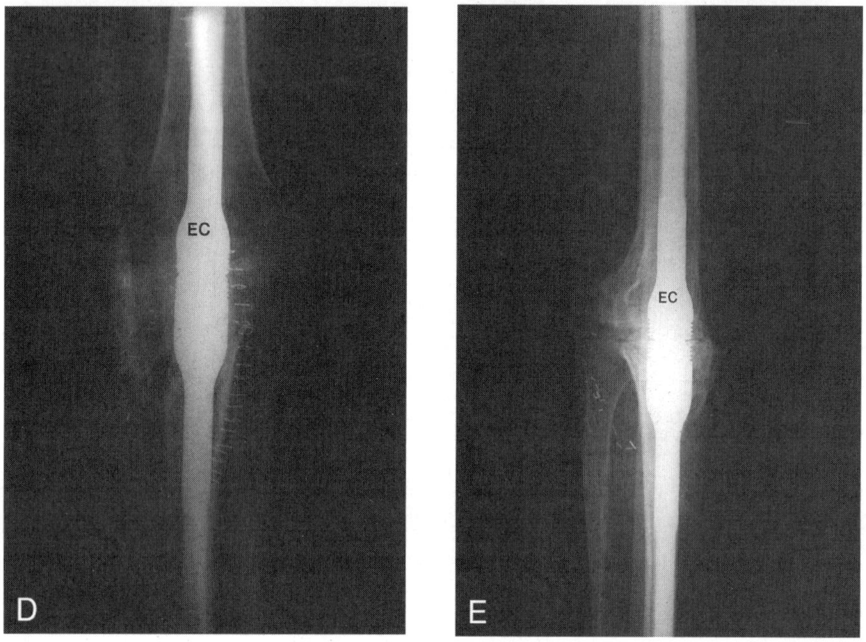

Figure 52.7. A. Postoperative AP view of a 33-year-old male who had complications following a proximal bicondylar tibial plateau fracture. Note the medial and lateral buttress plate internal fixation of the fracture. AP (**B**) and lateral (**C**) views following the total knee arthroplasty. AP (**D**) and lateral (**E**) views following a delayed knee arthrodesis.

Figure 52.8. Neff femorotibial nail.

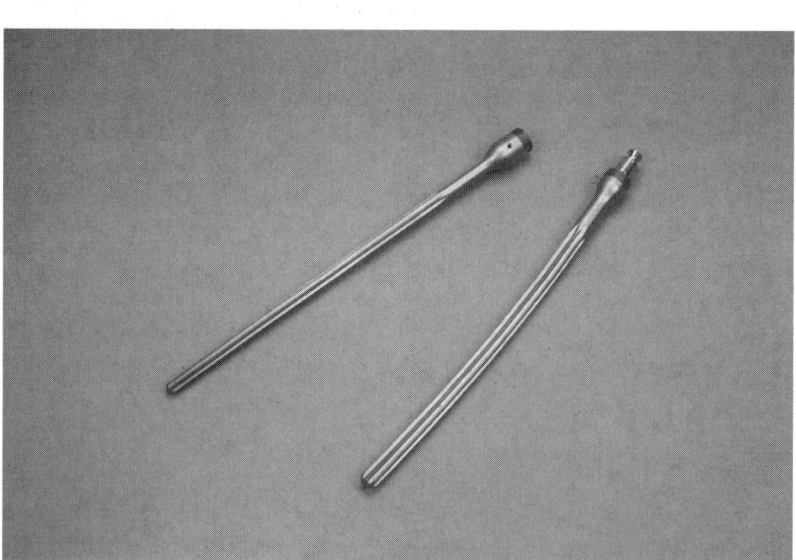

tibial metaphyses to accept the articulated portion of the nail, the components are inserted into the tibia and femur, respectively (Fig. 52.10). The male and female portions of the nail are coupled. Several blows to the heel secure compression of the Morse taper, which is then reinforced with two set screws (Fig. 52.11). Autologous bone from the intramedullary remains is then packed about the fusion site. The patella may be used as an additional source of autologous graft and is secured using two 6.5-mm cancellous screws (Fig. 52.12).

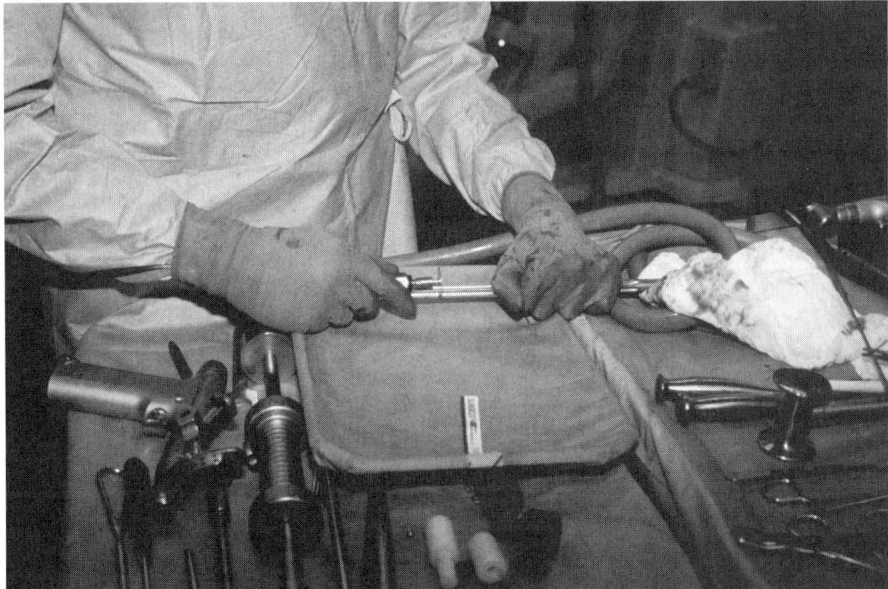

Figure 52.9. Shortening the Neff nail using a Midas Rex diamond-tipped cutting wheel.

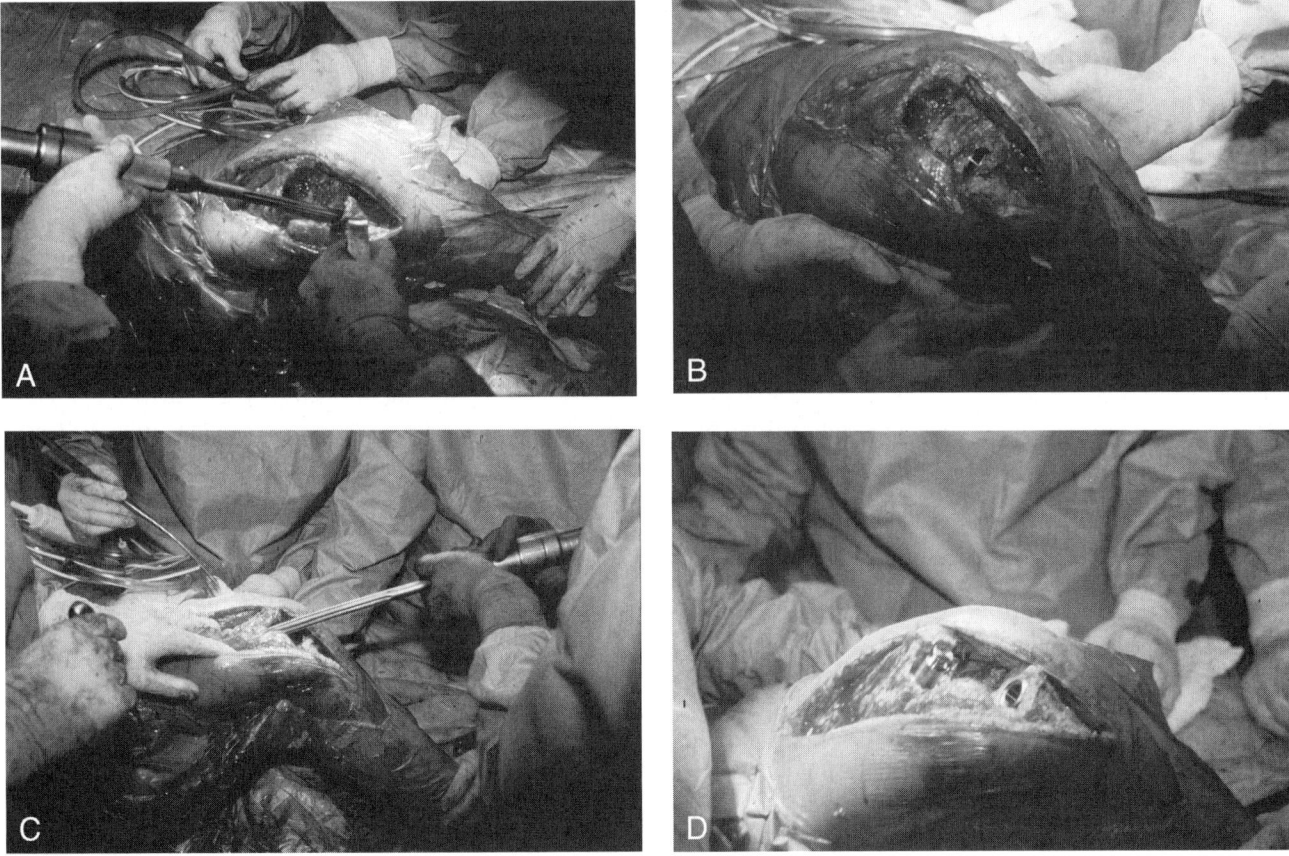

Figure 52.10. The tibial Neff nail is inserted (**A**) and seated (**B**). Then the femoral nail is inserted (**C**) and seated (**D**). The curve of the nail follows the anterior bow of the femur.

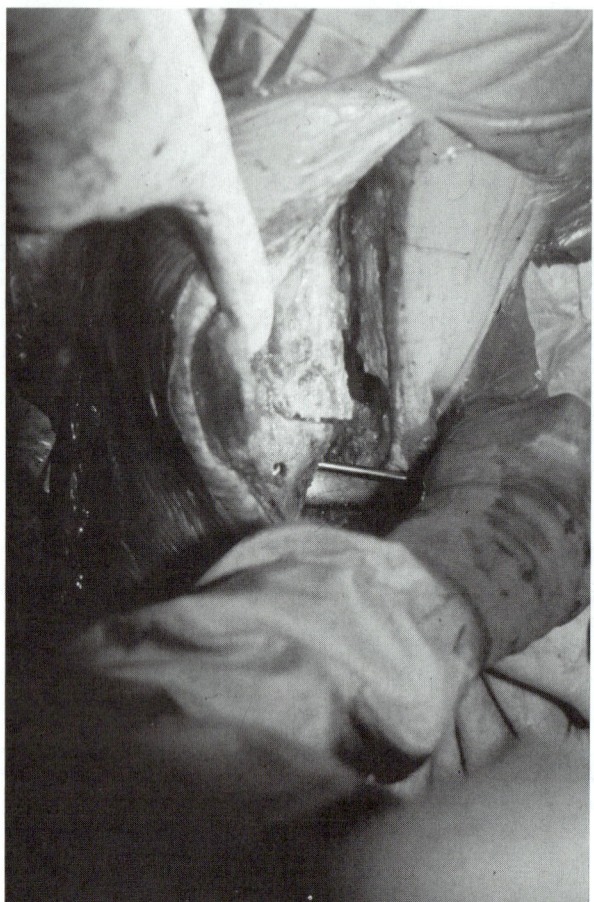

Figure 52.11. The Neff nail is coupled, and set screws are inserted to lock the modular nail together.

Complications of Arthrodesis

In our series of 17 intramedullary knee arthrodeses for the treatment of failed, septic TKA, complications occurred in 10 patients (55), including recurrent infection, nonunion with subsequent nail breakage, proximal migration of the nail, and perforation of the ankle joint. Regardless of the technique, union may not occur. If the resulting pseudarthrosis is painful, the arthrodesis should be revised. Failed intramedullary fusion with pseudarthrosis may eventually cause the rod to brake. Fatigue fracture of the rod occurs at or near the pseudarthrosis site. The arthrodesis may be revised using a larger intramedullary nail, supplemented by autologous bone grafting.

A successful arthrodesis may remain actively infected, particularly if foreign material or necrotic tissue remains. With external fixation, pin tract infections may require premature removal of the apparatus and can seed the intramedullary canal if followed by intramedullary rod fixation.

Hip pain can be related to proximal migration of an intramedullary nail. Femoral or tibial fractures can occur after successful arthrodesis secondary to increased forces generated from a large, single bone moment arm. Back

pain has been reported, and patient satisfaction is modest, even with the best arthrodesis. Shortening of the lower extremity by an average of 3 cm is common and must be discussed thoroughly with the patient before surgery. A stiff limb, although painless and functional, can be socially unacceptable. Furthermore, patients considering knee arthrodesis may benefit from a trial in a cylinder cast to allow them to understand the permanent disadvantages of a stiff limb.

Conversion of a solid knee arthrodesis to TKA has been reported (11). This procedure is relatively contraindicated for the following reasons: (*a*) collateral ligament integrity is compromised; (*b*) long-standing fusion may result in permanent contracture and scarring of the surrounding musculature, limiting knee flexion after conversion; (*c*) muscle atrophy may not be reversible and leaves a residual extension lag; (*d*) the new arthroplasty is at greater risk of infection or mechanical problems than routing knee replacements; and (*e*) if subsequent septic or aseptic failure occurs, there is probably a decreased chance of successful fusion.

Resection Arthroplasty

Resection arthroplasty is accomplished by excising the opposing articular surfaces of the distal femur and proximal tibia. Complete removal of scar tissue, synovium, and all foreign material (including metallic hardware, knee replacement components, and acrylic cement) is mandatory (53,57). This option is generally reserved for medically fragile patients who cannot tolerate a two-stage reimplantation protocol. It may also serve as an intermediate step for the patient who has reservations about arthrodesis.

Falahee et al. (53) reported on 28 knees that underwent resection arthroplasty for infected total knee arthroplasty. Of these, 6 patients with prior monarticular osteoarthritis found the resection arthroplasty unacceptable and underwent successful arthrodesis. In 3 patients, spontaneous bony fusion developed after the resection, with the knee in satisfactory alignment. Patients with more severe disability before the original knee arthroplasty were more likely to be satisfied with the functional results of the resection arthroplasty than were other patients. Conversely, patients with less disability originally were more likely to find the resection arthroplasty unacceptable. A total of 15 patients walked independently; 5 of which were able to stand and walk without external limb support. The other 10 patients used either a knee-ankle-foot orthosis or a universal knee splint. All 15 patients, however, required either a cane or walker and remained either moderately or severely restricted in their overall walking capacity.

Definitive resection arthroplasty is useful for the severely disabled sedentary patient. The procedure is least suitable for patients with relatively minor disability before their original total joint replacement. In the latter group, arthrodesis or reimplantation of a total knee replacement is recommended, if possible, depending on

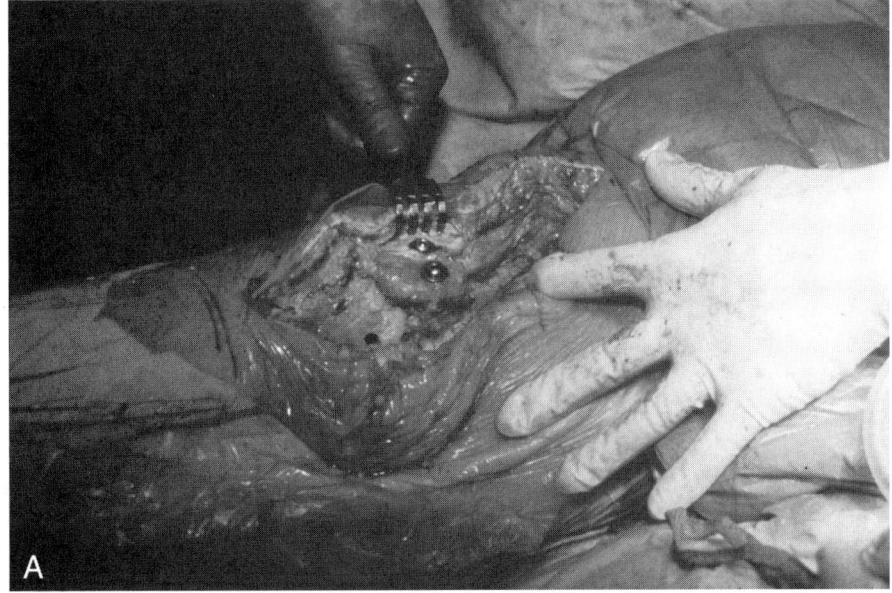

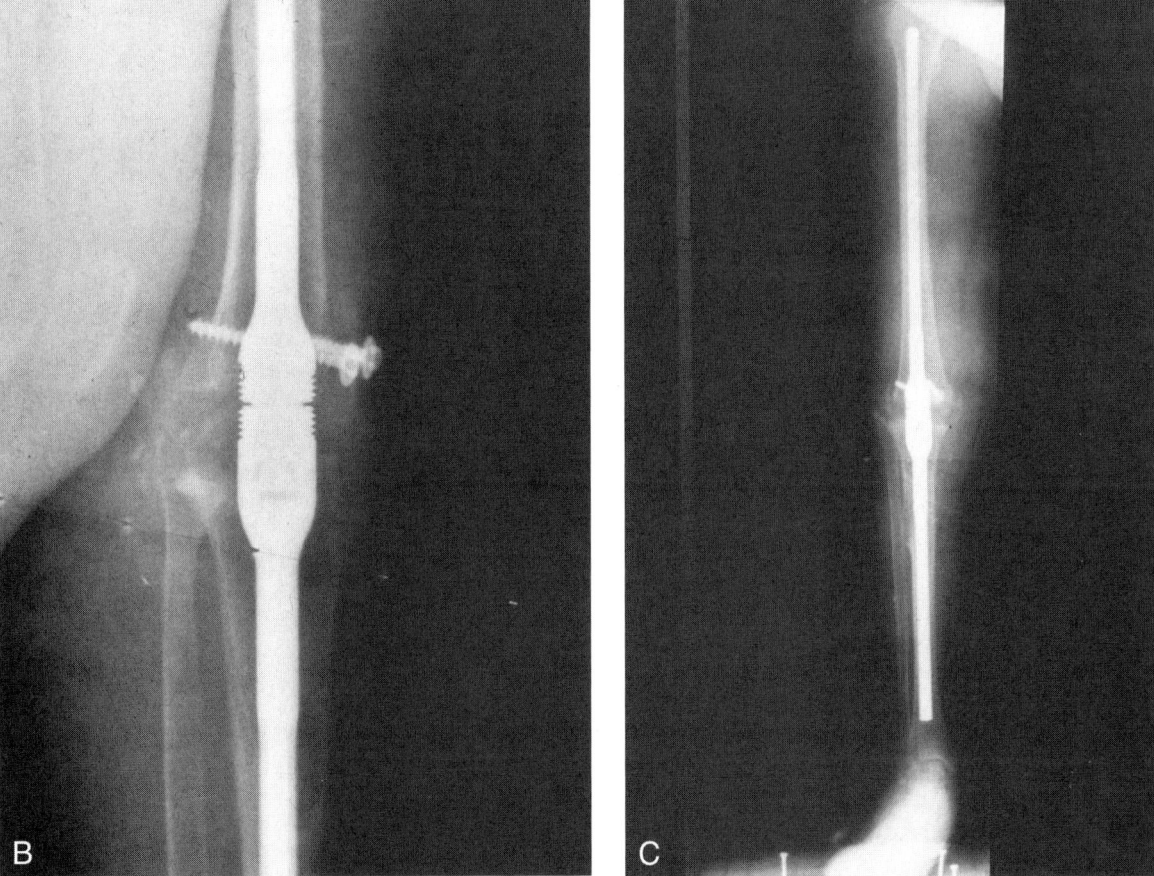

Figure 52.12. A. The patella, secured with 6.5-mm cancellous screws, is used as supplemental bone graft. **B.** AP view showing the completed arthrodesis. **C.** Postoperative AP (3-foot) standing view.

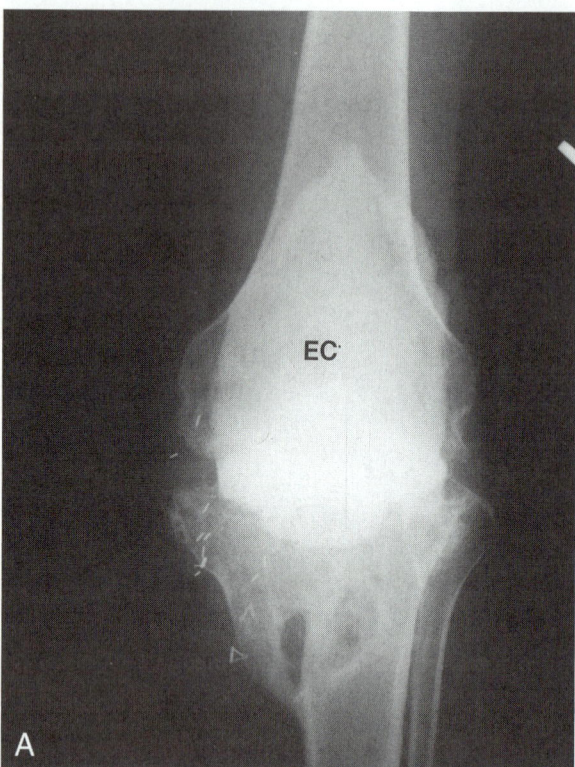
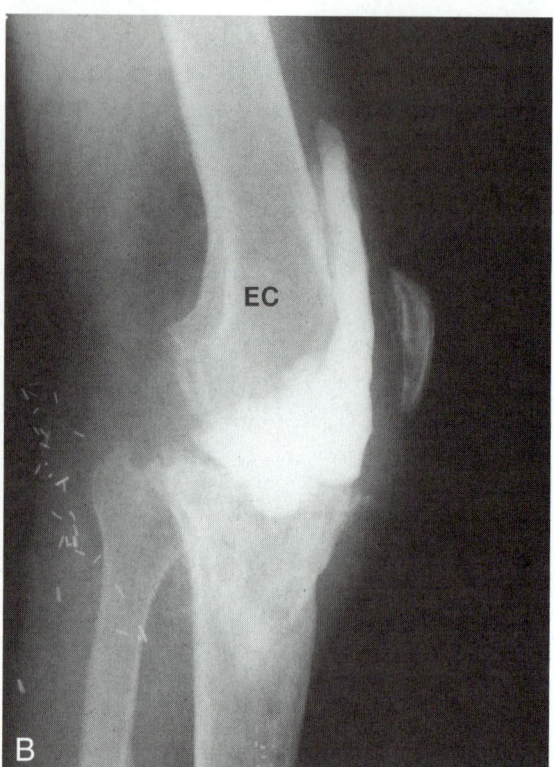

Figure 52.13. A. AP view showing a resection arthroplasty for TKA sepsis. Note the antibiotic-impregnated cement spacer. **B.** Lateral view showing the cement spacer.

the sensitivity of the organism and adequacy of the antibiotic treatment. The advantage of the resection arthroplasty is that some motion is preserved for sitting and transferring into and out of automobiles. The disadvantages are persistent pain and instability with walking.

A modified resection arthroplasty has been presented for problem cases with sepsis or excessive loss of bone stock in which exchange arthroplasty or arthrodesis is inadvisable or impossible (58). The space between the femur and tibia is filled with a bolus of heat-stable antibiotic-impregnated polymethyl methacrylate after implant removal (Fig. 52.13). The cement spacer improves initial stability and diminishes functional limb length discrepancy. Furthermore, the spacer maintains a potential area to ease reimplantation of a TKA after the spacer is removed (59–61).

SUMMARY

Arthrodesis as a salvage procedure remains a durable, time-proven technique for the treatment of sepsis, tumor, failed arthroplasty, and a flail limb. It should be performed selectively, especially in light of modern arthroplasty and the increasingly favorable results of two-stage reimplantation (62). Various techniques have been used, each of which has a role in these difficult salvage cases.

REFERENCES

1. Windsor RE, Bono JV. Infected total knee replacements. J Am Acad Orthop Surg 1994;2:44–53.
2. Broderson MP, Fitzgerald RH Jr, Peterson LFA, et al. Arthrodesis of the knee following failed total knee arthroplasty. J Bone Joint Surg 1979;61A:181–185.
3. Green DP, Parkes JC II, Stinchfield FE. Arthrodesis of the knee. A follow-up study. J Bone Joint Surg 1967;49A:1065–1078.
4. Hagemann WF, Woods GW, Tullos HS. Arthrodesis in failed total knee replacement. J Bone Joint Surg 1978;60A:790–794.
5. Stulberg SD. Arthrodesis in failed total knee replacements. Orthop Clin North Am 1982;13:213–224.
6. Enneking WF, Shirley PD. Resection-arthrodesis for malignant and potentially malignant lesions about the knee using an intramedullary rod and local bone grafts. J Bone Joint Surg 1977;59A:223–236.
7. Charnley J, Baker SL. Compression arthrodesis of the knee. A clinical and historical study. J Bone Joint Surg 1952;34B:187–199.
8. Charnley J, Lowe HG. A study of the end results of compression arthrodesis of the knee. J Bone Joint Surg 1958;40B:633–635.
9. Briggs B, Chao EY. The mechanical performance of the standard Hoffmann-Vidal external fixation apparatus. J Bone Joint Surg 1982;64A:566–573.
10. Siller TN, Hadjipavlou A. Arthrodesis of the knee. In: The American Academy of Orthopaedic Surgeons, eds. Symposium on reconstructive surgery of knee. St. Louis: Mosby, 1978:161.
11. Dee R. The case for arthrodesis of the knee. Orthop Clin North Am 1979;10:249–261.
12. Holden DL, Jackson DW. Considerations in total knee arthroplasty following previous knee fusion. Clin Orthop 1988;227:223–228.

13. Montgomery WH, Becker MW, Windsor RE, Insall JN. Primary total knee arthroplasty in stiff and ankylosed knees. Orthop Trans 1991;15:54–55.

14. Krackow KA, Weiss AP. Recurvatum deformity complicating performance of total knee arthroplasty. A brief note. J Bone Joint Surg 1990;72A:268–271.

15. Drennan DB, Fahey JJ, Maylahn DJ. Important factors in achieving arthrodesis of the Charcot knee. J Bone Joint Surg 1971; 53A:1180–1193.

16. Soudry M, Binazzi R, Johanson NA, et al. Total knee arthroplasty in Charcot and Charcot-like joints. Clin Orthop 1986;208:199–204.

17. Edmonson AS, Crenshaw AH. Campbell's operative orthopaedics. St. Louis: Mosby, 1980.

18. Higinbotham ML, Coley BL. The treatment of bone tumors by resection and replacement with massive grafts. Instr Course Lect 1950;XX:26–33.

19. Lexer E. Joint transplantations and arthroplasty. Surg Gynecol Obstet 1925;40:782–809.

20. Marcove RC, Lyden JP, Huvos AG, Bullough PB. Giant-cell tumors treated by cryosurgery. A report of twenty-five cases. J Bone Joint Surg 1973;55A:1633–1644.

21. Merle D'Aubigne R, Dejouany JP. Diaphyso-epiphyseal resection for bone tumor at the knee. With reports of nine cases. J Bone Joint Surg 1958;40B:385–395.

22. Ottolenghi CE. Massive osteoarticular bone grafts. Transplant of the whole femur. J Bone Joint Surg 1966;48B:646–659.

23. Ottolenghi CE. Massive osteo and osteo-articular bone grafts. Technique and results of 62 cases. Clin Orthop 1972;87:156–164.

24. Parrish FF. Treatment of bone tumors by total excision and replacement with massive autologous and homologous grafts. J. Bone Joint Surg 1966;48A:968–990.

25. Parrish FF. Homografts of bone. Clin Orthop 1972;87:36–42.

26. Tuli SM. Bridging of bone defects by massive bone grafts in tumorous conditions and in osteomyelitis. Clin Orthop 1972; 87:60–73.

27. Volkov M. Allotransplantation of joints. J Bone Joint Surg 1970; 52B:49–53.

28. Wilson PD Jr. A clinical study of the biomechanical behavior of massive bone transplants used to reconstruct large bone defects. Clin Orthop 1972;87:81–109.

29. Wilson PD, Lance EM. Surgical reconstruction of the skeleton following segmental resection for bone tumors. J Bone Joint Surg 1965;47A:1629–1656.

30. Lexer E. Substitution of whole or half joints from freshly amputated extremities by free plastic operation. Surg Gynecol Obstet 1908;6:601–607.

31. Iskander MK, Khan, MA. Candida albicans infection of a prosthetic knee replacement [Letter]. J Rheumatol 1988;15:1594–1595.

32. Koch AE. Candida albicans infection of a prosthetic knee replacement: a report and review of the literature. J Rheumatol 1988; 15:362–365.

33. Wilde AH, Sweeney RS, Borden LS. Hematogenously acquired infection of a total knee arthroplasty by Clostridium perfringens. Clin Orthop 1988;119:228–231.

34. Cadambi A, Engh GA. Use of a semitendinosus tendon autogenous graft for rupture of the patellar ligament after total knee arthroplasty. J Bone Joint Surg 1992;74A:974–979.

35. Lucas DB, Murray WR. Arthrodesis of the knee by double plasting. J Bone Joint Surg 1964;43A:795.

36. Nichols SJ, Landon GC, Tullos HS. Arthrodesis with dual plastes after failed total knee arthroplasty. J Bone Joint Surg 1991; 73A:1020.

37. Stiehl JB, Hanel DP. Knee arthrodesis using combined intramedullary rod and plate fixation. Clin Orthop 1993:294:238–246.

38. Key JA. Positive pressure in arthrodesis for tuberculosis of the knee joint. South Med J 1932;25:909.

39. Charnley JC. Positive pressures in arthrodesis of the knee joint. J Bone Joint Surg 1948;30B:478–486.

40. Charnley J. Arthrodesis of the knee. Clin Orthop 1960;18:37–42.

41. Knutson K, Bodelind B, Lindgren L. Stability of external fixators used for knee arthrodesis after failed knee arthroplasty. Clin Orthop 1984;186:90–95.

42. Knutson K, Hovelius L, Lindstrand A, Lindgren L. Arthrodesis after failed knee arthroplasty. A nationwide multicenter investigation of 91 cases. Clin Orthop 1984;191:202–211.

43. Donley BG, Matthews LS, Kaufer H. Arthrodesis of the knee with an intramedullary nail. J Bone Joint Surg 1991;73A:907–913.

44. Fern ED, Stewart HD, Newton G. Curved Küntscher nail arthrodesis after failure of knee replacement. J Bone Joint Surg 1989; 71B:588–590.

45. Figgie HE III, Brody GA, Inglis AE, et al. Knee arthrodesis following total knee arthroplasty in rheumatoid arthritis. Clin Orthop 1983;181:146–150.

46. Vander Griend R. Arthrodesis of the knee with intramedullary fixation. Clin Orthop 1983;181:146–150.

47. Harris CM, Froehlich J. Knee fusion with intramedullary rods for failed total knee arthroplasty. Clin Orthop 1985;197:209–216.

48. Kaufer H, Irvine G, Matthews LS. Intramedullary arthrodesis of the knee. Orthop Trans 1983;7:547–548.

49. Knutson K, Linstrand A, Lindgren L. Arthrodesis for failed knee arthroplasty J Bone Joint Surg 1985;67B:47–52.

50. Mazet R, Urist MR. Arthrodesis of the knee with intramedullary nail fixation. Clin Orthop 1960;18:43–52.

51. Puranen J, Kortelainen P, Jalovaara P. Arthrodesis of the knee with intramedullary nail fixation. J Bone Joint Surg 1990;72:433–442.

52. Wilde AH, Stearns KL. Intramedullary fixation for arthrodesis of the knee after infected total knee arthroplasty. Clin Orthop 1989; 248:87–92.

53. Falahee MH, Matthews LS, Kaufer H. Resection arthroplasty as a salvage procedure for a knee with infection after a total arthroplasty. J Bone Joint Surg 1987;69A:1013–1021.

54. Levine M, Rehm SJ, Wilde AH. Infection with Candida albicans of a total knee arthroplasty. Case report and review of the literature. Clin Orthop 1988;226:235–239.

55. Bono JV, Windsor RE, Sherman P, et al. Intramedullary arthrodesia following failed TKA. Orthop Trans 1995;19:336.

56. Windsor RE, Bono JV. Arthrodesis and resection arthroplasty. In: Fu F, Harner C, Vince K, eds. Knee surgery. Baltimore: Williams & Wilkins, 1994:1587–1595.

57. Lettin AW, Neil MJ, Citron ND, August A. Excision arthroplasty for infected constrained total knee replacements. J Bone Joint Surg 1990;72B:856–857.

58. Jones WA, Wroblewski BM. Salvage of failed total knee arthroplasty: "beefburger" procedure. J Bone Joint Surg 1989; 71B:856–857.

59. Booth RE Jr., Lotke PA. The results of spacer block technique in revision of infected total knee arthroplasty. Clin Orthop 1989; 248:57–60.

60. Cohen JC, Hozack WJ, Cuckler JM, Booth RE. Two-stage reimplantation of septic total knee arthroplasty. J Arthroplasty 1988; 3:369–377.

61. Wilde AH, Ruth JT. Two-stage reimplantation in infected total knee arthroplasty. Clin Orthop 1988;236:23–25.

62. Adelman R, Bono JV, Haas S, et al. Two-stage reimplantation for total knee arthroplasty salvage: Further follow-up and enlargement of cohort group. Paper presented at the 63rd Annual Meeting of the American Academy of Orthopaedic Surgeons, Atlanta, February 21–27, 1996.

53

Patellectomy/Patellar Resurfacing

The treatment of isolated patellofemoral degenerative disease is challenging. The patellofemoral joint degenerates slowly, and patients have usually undergone many conservative and operative therapeutic regimens before developing arthrosis. Patients are frustrated by the failures of those regimens and frequently have become pessimistic.

Osteoarthritis is defined as loss of articular cartilage, probably resulting from the progression of chondromalacia. Grade IV lesions are eroded to bone. This chapter focuses primarily on the surgical treatment of patients with isolated grade IV chondromalacia of the patellofemoral joint, also known as osteoarthritis or patellofemoral degenerative disease. The three most common causes of patellofemoral degenerative disease are chronic patellofemoral malalignment, trauma, and idiopathic osteoarthritis.

RELEVANT ANATOMY AND PATHOGENESIS

Grade IV chondromalacia, or degenerative arthritis, involves both sides of the joint. The exact location of the lesions depends on the cause of the disease. Patients with chronic patellofemoral malalignment usually have greater wear on the medial border of the patella and deformity of the lateral trochlea of the femur. Patients with traumatic or idiopathic disease usually present with central patellar and femoral groove involvement.

INITIAL FINDINGS, PHYSICAL EXAMINATION, AND DIAGNOSIS

The most common symptoms are pain and the catching of the patella on the femoral groove during knee motion. Patients have a severe pain behind the patella, which is exacerbated by activity; most patients cannot negotiate stairs without the aid of a banister. Swelling is frequently present. An audible grinding or crepitus is common, and patients frequently complain of the patella "getting stuck in the flexed position."

The most common signs of patellofemoral degenerative disease are tenderness in the retropatellar space and crepitus. Catching will be evident in advanced cases of degeneration. Lateral patellar maltracking will be present in many cases.

RADIOLOGIC STUDIES

Axial and lateral view radiographs are studied with special emphasis given to patellar height and alignment and patellofemoral congruity. The AP view must be taken to determine the degree of arthrosis of the femorotibial joint and the varus or valgus angulation. A bone scan is vital for evaluating the degree of degenerative change in the patellofemoral and femorotibial joints.

TREATMENT

Nonoperative Treatment

Nonoperative treatment consists of weight loss, quadriceps strengthening, nonsteroidal anti-inflammatory drugs (NSAIDs), and modification of activities.

Operative Treatment

Patellectomy, patellar resurfacing, and patellofemoral replacement are all salvage procedures and are reserved for patients with severe, isolated patellofemoral arthritis who have failed previous treatment (Clinical Table). The indications are among the strictest of all orthopaedic procedures. The patient must have intractable pain, palpable crepitus, extreme retropatellar tenderness on examination, radiographic evidence of severe patellofemoral degenerative dis-

Clinical Table: Patellectomy/Patellar Resurfacing

Procedure	Indications	Technique	Anatomy	Pitfalls
Miyakawa patellectomy	• Isolated patellar degenerative disease	• Midline • Excision of the patella	• Quadriceps tendon • Extensor mechanism	• Quadriceps weakness • Failure to address femoral groove
Compere patellectomy	• Isolated patellar degenerative disease	• Midline • Excision of the patella	• Quadriceps tendon • Extensor mechanism	• Quadriceps weakness • Failure to address femoral groove • Patellar tendon maltracking
Patellar resurfacing	• Isolated patellar degenerative disease	• Midline medial arthrotomy • Patellar resurfacing	• Extensor mechanism • Patellar surface	• Overstuff patellofemoral joint • Patellar maltracking
Noncustom patellofemoral replacement	• Combined patellofemoral degenerative disease	• Midline • Medial arthrotomy • Resurfacing of patellar and femoral grooves	• Extensor mechanism • Patellar and femoral groove surfaces	• Loss of femoral groove • Patellar impingement • Patellofemoral maltracking
Custom patellofemoral replacement	• Combined patellofemoral degenerative disease	• Midline • Medial arthrotomy • Resurfacing of patellar and femoral grooves	• Extensor mechanism • Patellar and femoral groove surfaces	• Mismatch of custom femoral groove prosthesis • Patellofemoral maltracking

ease, and (preferably) documented arthroscopic evidence of grade IV chondromalacia of the patellofemoral joint.

Patients with mild to moderate degenerative changes isolated to the patella and with evidence of lateral patellar malalignment are best treated by tibial tubercle elevation. Patients with isolated severe patellar degenerative disease are candidates for either patellectomy, patellar resurfacing, or patellofemoral replacement. Femoral groove osteoarthritis is a contraindication for tibial tubercle elevation, patellectomy, and patellar resurfacing.

Patellofemoral replacement is indicated in patients younger than 50 years who have severe osteoarthritis of the patella or severe osteoarthritis on both sides of the patellofemoral joint. Patients with degenerative changes in either the medial or the lateral compartments in addition to patellofemoral arthritis are best treated with a total knee replacement. Patients older than 50 years who have isolated patellofemoral degenerative arthritis are treated with a total knee replacement.

Operative Treatment

PATELLECTOMY

Patellectomy is a relatively old procedure but, nevertheless, continues to be controversial. The function of the patella is to increase the moment arm of the quadriceps tendon. A patellectomy will shorten the lever arm of the quadriceps tendon, and the function of these muscles will be compromised postoperatively. Clinical experience is varied; some authors report good to excellent results following patellectomy (1) and others report poor results (2), usually secondary to the combination of unrelieved pain and quadriceps weakness. Patients with femoral groove degenerative changes are at an increased risk for persistent pain and instability. In addition, a high failure rate in patients who have undergone total knee arthroplasty following patellectomy has been reported (3).

The goal of a patellectomy is to excise the degenerative patella to alleviate pain. A patellectomy is indicated only in patients with a badly comminuted patellar fracture, for which every effort at reduction and fixation has failed, and a relatively normal femoral groove. Patellectomy is also indicated in patients with patellofemoral arthrosis that is too severe to be treated with a tibial tubercle elevation and for whom a patellofemoral replacement of total knee replacement is either unacceptable or contraindicated secondary to chronic infection. The objectives of a patellectomy are to restore quadriceps strength and continuity, maintain or improve range of motion, maintain or improve patellar tendon tracking, and maintain the motor strength of the extensor mechanism. The creation of a soft tissue patella may be more cosmetically acceptable to the patient than the traditional patellectomy procedure. The Miyakawa's and Compere's techniques attempt to achieve these goals (1,4).

Miyakawa Patellectomy

For the Miyakawa procedure, a lateral parapatellar incision is begun 7.5 cm proximal to the patella and is completed at the tibial tuberosity (Fig. 53.1). A medial flap is developed; the quadriceps muscle and tendons and the patella are exposed. A medial arthrotomy is made, and the joint is inspected. Appropriate débridement is performed. The patella is removed by sharp dissection; the dorsal patellar aponeurosis is preserved. A superficial quadriceps flap is developed 1 cm above the patellar defect and extended proximally for 8 cm. This superficial flap is developed medially and laterally and is equal to the width of the patella. The flap is divided transversely at its proximal extension. The thickness of the flap is equal to one-half the thickness of the entire quadriceps tendon. The medial and lateral bases of the flap are supported by corner-reinforcing sutures. The flap is reflected distally and sutured into the patellar ligament through a rent developed in the patellar ligament and into the retinaculum. The length of the flap and the strength of fixation are tested by flexing the knee to 90°. If both flap length and fixation strength are adequate, the quadriceps tendon is sutured to retinaculum proximally to the base of the tongue of the quadriceps tendon.

The vastus medialis muscle is advanced laterally to the lateral margin of the defect in the quadriceps tendon. The vastus lateralis is advanced medially, and a mattress suture is placed into and through the advanced vastus medialis. It is important to incorporate the underlying quadriceps tendon with this mattress suture. The knee is again flexed to 90° to evaluate tension. The knee is flexed, and tension on the suture line is evaluated following each successive suture.

After surgery, a knee immobilizer is applied, and partial weight bearing is begun. Active-assisted and active range of motion exercises are started immediately. Active-assisted flexion greater that 110° is not allowed until 6 weeks after surgery.

Compere Patellectomy

For the Compere patellectomy, a transverse skin incision is made, and the patella is exposed (Fig. 53.2). A medial parapatellar arthrotomy is made; then a lateral parapatellar capsular incision is made parallel to the medial incision. The patella is everted and is removed by sharp dissection. The dorsal quadriceps aponeurosis is not violated. When the patella is removed, the medial edge of the quadriceps aponeurosis is folded underneath and sutured to the lateral edge of the expansion. This creates a tube of the quadriceps aponeurosis. The medial capsule is sutured to the tube, and the vastus medialis is advanced laterally and distally. The lateral capsule is not sutured to the tube. The knee is flexed to 90° so that tension on the suture line can be evaluated.

The postoperative care is identical to that of the Miyakawa patellectomy.

PATELLAR RESURFACING

The goal of patellar resurfacing, or patellofemoral hemiarthroplasty, is to resurface the degenerated patella with a dome-shaped patellar prosthesis. The femoral groove is left untouched. McKeever (5) introduced this concept and reported favorable short-term results. Other authors, however, have reported unsatisfactory long-term results (6–8). A patient with osteoarthritis of the patella severe enough to make him or her a candidate for patellar resurfacing invariably has changes in the femoral groove. Successful hemiarthroplasty in a patient with femoral involvement does not seem feasible. The indication for resurfacing is limited to patients with isolated patellar arthrosis who

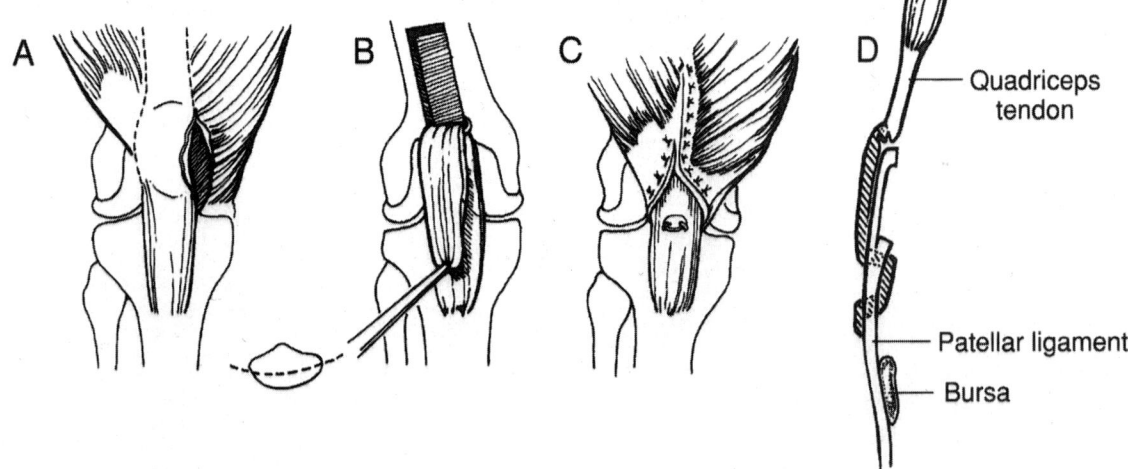

Figure 53.1. The Miyakawa patellectomy involves arthrotomy (**A**), fixation of the flap (**B**), and suturing of the quadriceps tendon (**C**). **D.** Lateral view of the procedure. Reprinted with permission from Fu F, Harner C, Vince K. Knee surgery. Baltimore: Williams & Wilkins, 1994.

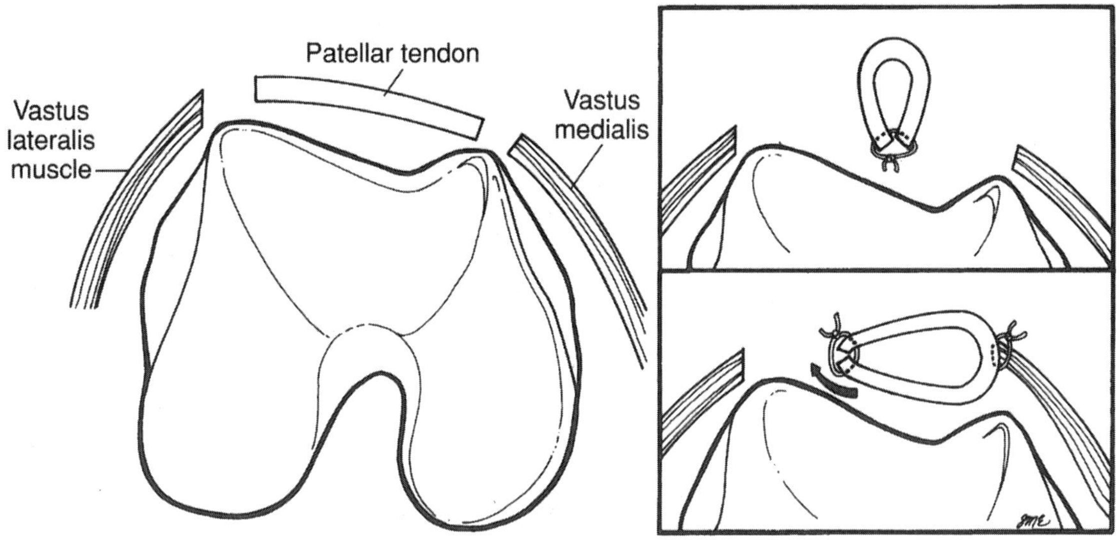

Figure 53.2. Compere patellectomy. Reprinted with permission from Fu F, Harner C, Vince K. Knee surgery. Baltimore: Williams & Wilkins, 1994.

have failed previous patellar surgeries. Patients with severe patellar degenerative disease combined with femoral groove involvement are candidates for a patellofemoral replacement. Younger patients with combined femorotibial arthrosis and older patients are candidates for total knee arthroplasty.

Technique

The goals of patellar resurfacing are to maintain proper patellar width, restore anatomic patellar tracking, maintain the integrity of the extensor mechanism, and resurface the degenerative patella with a standard dome-shaped polyethylene prosthesis that is cemented into position. The approach is a standard midline incision and medial arthrotomy. The patella is exposed and resurfaced in the standard fashion. A lateral release and/or proximal realignment is done to restore anatomic patellar tracking. The postoperative rehabilitation is the same as that for a total knee replacement.

PATELLOFEMORAL REPLACEMENT

The combination of unsatisfactory results in more conservative procedures for severe degenerative patellofemoral disease and the excellent long-term results of total joint replacement encouraged the development of patellofemoral replacement. Lubinus (9) introduced the patella glide replacement prosthesis in 1979 but did not report long-term results. Blazina et al. (10) designed a patellofemoral replacement with an anatomic patellar prosthesis combined with a deep, U-shaped retentive femoral trochlear design made of cobalt chrome. Arciero and Toomey (11) and Cartier et al. (12) reported 72 to 85% good to excellent results in selected patients.

The disadvantages of this prosthesis are twofold: It is technically demanding to insert, and it removes considerable bone stock. Creating a perfect match between the

patellar and femoral surfaces is extremely difficult, and clicking and catching are uncommon. Insall (13) and Scott (14) noted the difficulty of revision surgery of a failed patellofemoral replacement, particularly in younger patients.

Custom Patellofemoral Replacement

Blazina et al. (15) designed a custom patellofemoral replacement that avoids the disadvantages of the nonanatomic trochlear groove. A software program uses a CT scan to construct a three-dimensional model of the patient's own femoral groove. This is fabricated into a cobalt chrome custom prosthesis that fits exactly over the femoral groove and trochlear region. Three small fixation pegs on the trochlea lock the prosthesis in place, and it is cemented into position. In essence, a custom resurfacing prosthesis is made, which eliminates the need to remove bone stock from the femur. Impingement in flexion is reduced; and revision to total knee or patellectomy, if necessary, is facilitated.

Operative Technique

A standard anteromedial incision is made with a medial arthrotomy. A lateral release is performed, if indicated. The patella is retracted laterally, and the knee is flexed to 60°. Peripheral osteophytes are removed, and the custom femoral trial is placed on the femoral groove and held in position. The trial is outlined in methylene blue (Fig. 53.3). Gouges and curettes are used to remove the remaining articular cartilage, but no bone is removed at any time. The trial is reapplied to the decorticated femoral groove, and three drill holes are made in the appropriate slots in the trial (Fig. 53.4). These holes are countersunk, and the final implant is placed into position.

The patella is everted and resurfaced with an oscillating saw. A standard dome-shaped polyethylene patella is used, and the patellar surface is prepared in the usual

Figure 53.3. The femoral groove prosthesis is outlined with methylene blue. Reprinted with permission from Fu F, Harner C, Vince K. Knee surgery. Baltimore: Williams & Wilkins, 1994.

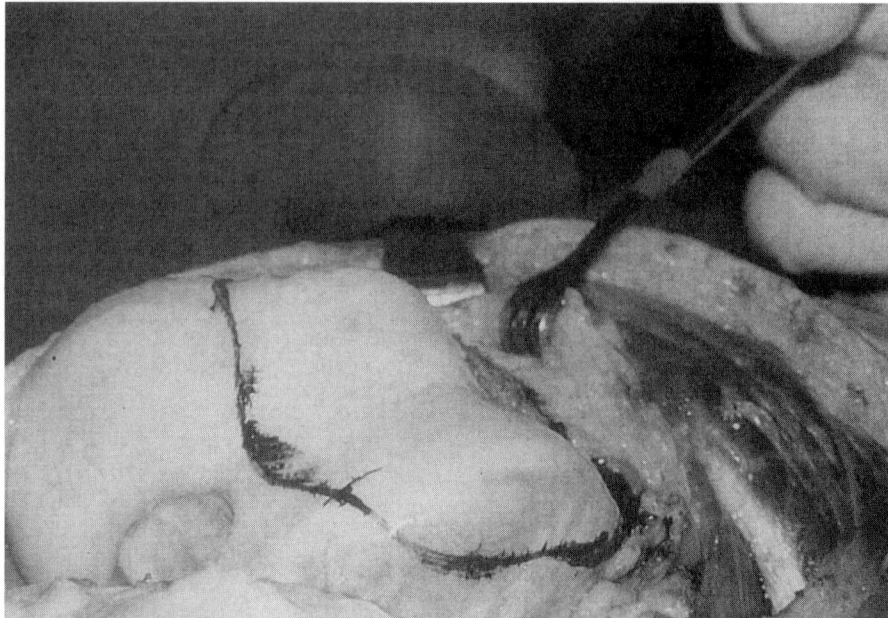

Figure 53.4. Holes to accept the prosthesis are drilled in the decorticated femoral groove. Reprinted with permission from Fu F, Harner C, Vince K. Knee surgery. Baltimore: Williams & Wilkins, 1994.

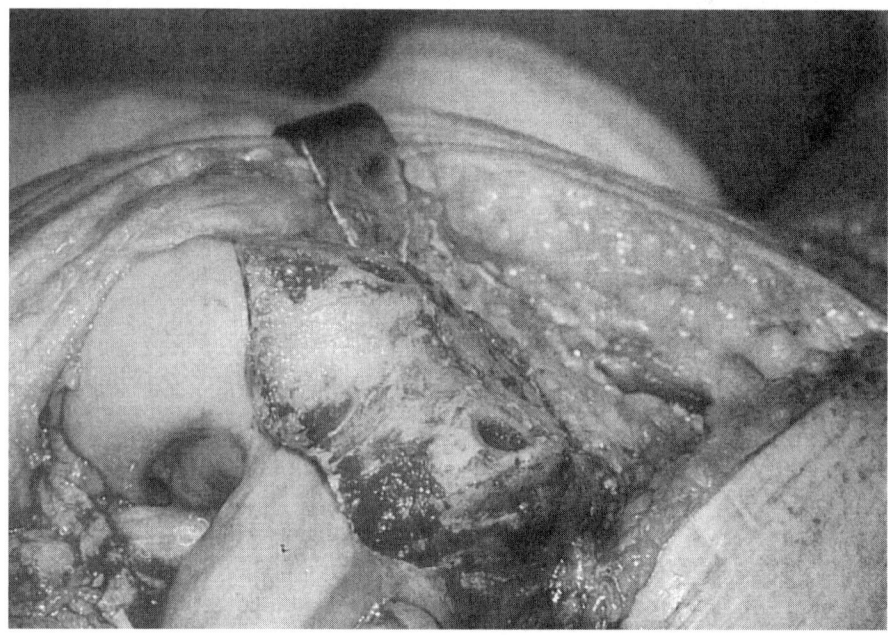

fashion. The trial patella and the custom implant are inserted; the knee is flexed fully and extended to 0°. Patellar tracking is assessed, and impingement of the inferior lip of the groove on the inferior pole of the patella is ruled out. The patella and femoral groove are cemented into position (Fig. 53.5).

Because the fixation of the components is solid and immediate, continuous passive motion with full range of motion is initiated after surgery. Full weight bearing is allowed immediately.

Results

Cook and I reported on 20 patients who underwent 23 (3 bilateral) custom patellofemoral arthroplasties (16). We noted 10 excellent, 10 good, and 2 fair results. Only 1 patient failed secondary to progressive osteoarthritis of the femorotibial compartments; this patient was revised to a total knee arthroplasty. There were no infections or systemic complications.

A patellofemoral arthroplasty can be effectively converted to a total knee arthroplasty in patients who develop progressive degenerative disease of the femoral and/or tibial articular surfaces. Cook and I reported on 18 patients with failed patellofemoral arthroplasties who underwent 20 (2 bilateral) revisions to total knee arthroplasties (17). We noted 14 excellent, 4 good, and 2 poor results. The 2 poor results included 1 patient with a rotating hinge total knee arthroplasty who had pain and tibial loosening

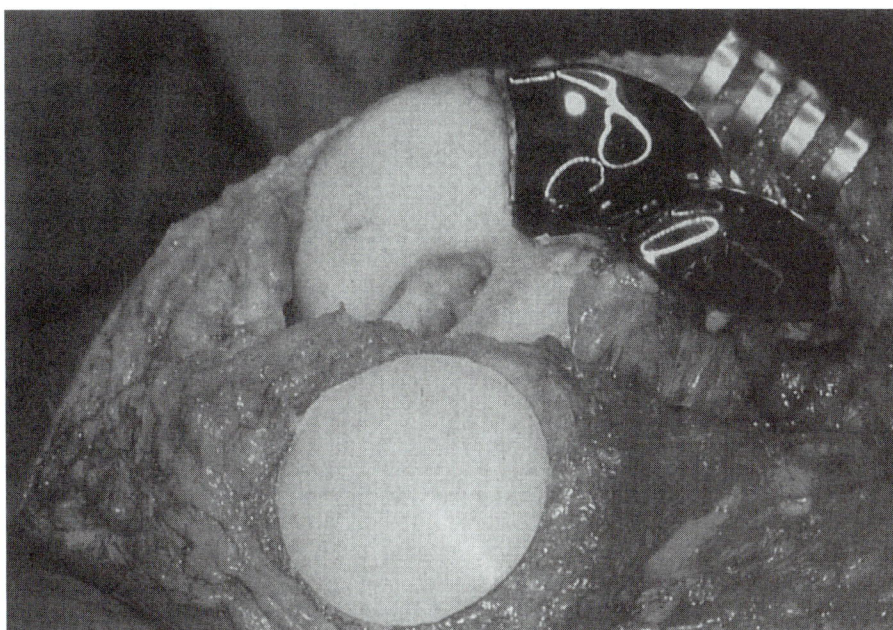

Figure 53.5. The custom femoral groove and patellar prostheses are cemented in place. Reprinted with permission from Fu F, Harner C, Vince K. Knee surgery. Baltimore: Williams & Wilkins, 1994.

17 years after the revision. The other poor result was a patient who developed an infection 17 months following revision; this patient underwent an exchange arthroplasty but still had persistent pain and disability. We concluded that patients with failed patellofemoral arthroplasties who are revised to posterior stabilized total knee arthroplasties have similar results to those patients who undergo a primary total knee arthroplasty. A failed patellofemoral arthroplasty does not compromise the result of a revision total knee arthroplasty at long-term follow-up.

SUMMARY

The operative treatment of patients with isolated, severe degenerative disease of the patellofemoral joint is challenging. Consistent good to excellent results can be obtained by rigidly following the indications for surgical intervention and selecting the appropriate procedure for each patient.

REFERENCES

1. Baker CL, Hughston JC. Miyakawa patellectomy. J Bone Joint Surg 1988;70A:1489–1494.
2. Ackroyd CE, Polyzoides AJ. Patellectomy for osteoarthritis. J Bone Joint Surg 1978;60B:353–357.
3. Lennox DW, Hungerford DS, Krackow KA. Total knee arthroplasty following patellectomy. Clin Orthop 1987;223:220–224.
4. Compere CL, Hill JA, Lewinnek GE, Thompson RG. A new method of patellectomy for patellofemoral arthritis. J Bone Joint Surg 1979;61A:714–719.
5. McKeever DC. Patellar prosthesis. J Bone Joint Surg 1955; 37A:1074–1084.
6. Insall JN, Tria AJ, Aglietti P. Resurfacing of the patella. J Bone Joint Surg 1980;62A:933–936.
7. Levitt RL. A long-term evaluation of patellar prostheses. Clin Orthop 1973;97:153–157.
8. Worrell RV. Resurfacing of the patella in young patients. Orthop Clin North Am 1986;17:303–309.
9. Lubinus. Patella glide bearing total replacement. Orthopedics 1979;2:119.
10. Blazina ME, Fox JM, Del Pizzo W, et al. Patellofemoral replacement. Clin Orthop 1979;144:98–102.
11. Arciero R, Toomey H. Patellofemoral arthroplasty: a three to nine year follow-up study. Clin Orthop 1988;236:60–71.
12. Cartier P, Sanouiller JL, Grelsamer R. Patellofemoral arthroplasty. J Arthroplasty 1990;5:49–55.
13. Insall JN. Disorders of the patella. In: Insall JN, Windsor RD, Scott WN, et al. eds. Surgery of the knee. New York: Churchill Livingstone, 1984:249.
14. Scott RD. Prosthetic replacement of the patellofemoral joint. Orthop Clin North Am 1979;10:129–137.
15. Blazina ME, Anderson LJ, Hirsh LC. Patellofemoral replacement: utilizing a customized femoral groove replacement. Tech Orthop 1990;5:53–55.
16. Sisto DJ, Cook DL. Custom patellofemoral replacement. Paper presented at the 63rd Annual Meeting of the American Academy of Orthopaedic Surgeons, Atlanta, February 26, 1996.
17. Sisto DJ, Cook DL. Total knee replacement in patients with a failed patellofemoral replacement. Paper presented at the 64th Annual Meeting of the American Academy of Orthopaedic Surgeons, San Francisco, February 14, 1997.

Fractures of the Knee

In this chapter, fractures of the knee are reviewed. The discussion includes a practical approach to fractures of the patella, tibial plateau, and distal femur. These fractures are quite prevalent, occurring in patients of all age groups. The mechanism of injury runs the gamut from low-energy community trauma to high-energy multitrauma.

In this practical approach to fractures of the knee, I discuss relevant anatomy and biomechanics, diagnosis, classification, nonoperative and surgical treatment options, indications for and techniques of surgery, pitfalls to be avoided, and rehabilitation.

I Fractures of the Patella

RELEVANT ANATOMY AND BIOMECHANICS

The patella is the largest sesamoid bone in the body and lies within the quadriceps tendon and extensor mechanism of the knee. It is a triangular-shaped bone, with its apex pointed distally. The proximal pole is thick and receives the insertion of the quadriceps tendon. The distal pole provides the origin of the patellar ligament, which inserts onto the tibial tubercle. These elements make up the extensor mechanism of the knee.

The patella improves the mechanical efficiency of the quadriceps muscle and the extensor mechanism by displacing the quadriceps tendon away from the axis of rotation, thereby increasing the moment arm. The principal function of the extensor mechanism is to maintain extension of the knee and the erect position. Maximal forces generated across the patella have been recorded at four to five times the standard body weight of 700 N (1).

The posterior articular surface is divided into medial and lateral facets separated by a vertical ridge, which articulates with the anterior distal femoral articular groove. The area of contact between the patella and the femur varies according to the position of the knee. The distal pole is nonarticular and comprises about 20% of the proximal to distal distance of the patella, as seen on a lateral x-ray of the knee.

A bipartite patella, which can be mistaken for a fracture, is the result of an accessory ossification center at the superolateral corner of the patella. Because this is most of-

ten a bilateral finding, comparison views of the contralateral knee are helpful in making the diagnosis. Also contributing to the extensor mechanism are the medial and lateral extensor retinacula, which are longitudinal fiber expansions that originate from the vastus medialis and vastus lateralis muscles. They combine with the fascia lata and bypass the patella and insert directly onto the proximal tibia. Together, the patellar retinaculum and the iliotibial band serve as auxiliary extensors of the knee.

The blood supply of the patella is from a plexus derived from the superior, middle, and inferior geniculate arteries. The primary blood supply enters at the distal pole and the anterior surface of the central portion of the patella.

INITIAL FINDINGS, PHYSICAL EXAMINATION, AND DIAGNOSIS

The diagnosis of patella fracture is made through history, physical examination, and x-ray. Patients often report a fall from a height, a direct blow to the kneecap, or a combination of these as the mechanism of injury.

On physical examination, a hemarthrosis is usually seen, unless the joint is decompressed through extensive retinacular tears. The skin should be carefully evaluated for the presence of an open fracture or open joint injury. The leakage of hematoma through a skin wound suggests an open fracture. A palpable defect of the kneecap suggests a displaced fracture. An inability to extend the knee implies a discontinuity of the extensor mechanism and a displaced fracture. Since pain can confound this important part of the examination, aspiration and injection of lidocaine under sterile conditions can be helpful. Note, however, that the ability to extend the knee does not rule out a patella fracture, since the reticulum may be assisting to perform this function.

Classification

Nondisplaced fractures can be defined by an articular surface displacement of less than 2 mm, and displaced fractures show displacement of greater than 2 mm. There are several types of fractures. First is the transverse fracture, which is manifest as a horizontal fracture line; a central transverse fracture is in the center of the patella; a polar transverse fracture is characterized by a small peripheral fragment of bone avulsed with either the quadriceps tendon (apical) or the patellar tendon (distal). Next is the comminuted fracture, or stellate pattern. The longitudinal fracture is generally in the lateral aspect of the patella and is usually nondisplaced. Finally, the osteochondral fracture occurs following a patellar dislocation.

RADIOLOGIC STUDIES

Radiographic examination should include AP, lateral, and Merchant views of the knee. The AP view can be confusing as a result of the overlap between the patella and the distal femur. The lateral x-ray usually shows a displaced transverse fracture rather dramatically, including fragment displacement and articular incongruity. Check the patellar height to rule out a patellar ligament rupture. An Insall-Salvati ratio (patellar length:patellar ligament length on the lateral x-ray) of less than 0.8 suggests patella alta and is consistent with a patellar ligament rupture. The Merchant view is helpful for diagnosing longitudinal fractures or osteochondral fractures. Although CT or bone scans are rarely necessary, they may be helpful in the diagnosis of occult fracture.

TREATMENT

The treatment options for fractures of the patella are (a) nonoperative, (b) open reduction and internal fixation, (c) indirect reduction and cerclage wiring, (d) partial patellectomy and tendon reconstruction, and (e) total patellectomy (Clinical Table).

Nonoperative Treatment

Nonoperative treatment is indicated for closed nondisplaced fractures of the patella with no disruption of the extensor mechanism of the knee. This consists of extension splinting in a cylinder cast or a brace in a reliable patient for 4 to 6 weeks. Immediate weight bearing may be started with the knee immobilized in extension. After evidence of

consolidation on x-ray at about 4 weeks, active range of motion may be started.

Operative Treatment

Surgical treatment is indicated for open fractures, fractures with articular displacement greater than 2 mm, and fractures associated with extensor mechanism disruption. Open fractures require urgent irrigation and débridement (I&D) as well as internal stabilization of the fracture. The management of the wound follows general guidelines of open fracture treatment. Although the wound should be left open after the initial I&D, the knee joint should be closed over drains. The patient should be returned to the operating room every 48 to 72 h until the wound is clean enough for delayed primary closure or flap coverage, depending on the soft tissue available for closure.

Open reduction and internal fixation (ORIF) is indicated for displaced fractures with no or minimal comminution. When technically feasible, this is the most preferred surgical option and can be performed through a longitudinal or transverse anterior approach. I prefer a longitudinal approach, as it is extensile and does not limit options for future knee surgery. The ideal indication for this approach is a simple displaced transverse fracture. The fracture should be exposed with minimal soft tissue stripping. The hematoma clot should be cleared and irrigated from the fracture site and the knee joint. The fracture can then be reduced with the knee in extension. A large pointed reduction forceps, such as a Weber clamp, can be used to maintain the reduction. The reduction may be checked with a C-arm fluoroscope in the lateral position or by palpation of the articular surface through a parapatellar retinacular tear or through a small parapatellar arthrotomy.

Next, partially threaded 3.5- or 4.0-mm cancellous screws (cannulated or noncannulated) can be used to stabilize the fracture. The surgeon should make sure that the treads completely cross the fracture site. The screws should be close to, but not violate, the articular surface. Intraoperative fluoroscopy in the lateral position is most helpful in this regard. Then an anterior tension band must be added to increase the strength of the construct and to provide dynamic compression of the fracture site with flexion of the knee (2–5). Either wire or heavy suture can be used to create the anterior tension band. It should run from the insertion site of the quadriceps tendon to the origin of the patellar tendon along the anterior surface of the patella, in either a figure eight or rectangular fashion (Fig. 54.1). Two strands of number 5 Ethibond or Tevdek suture can be used as an alternative to 18-gauge wire. Although the tension band often will eventually break as a result of cyclic loading, my impression is that broken suture is less likely to become symptomatic to the patient and less likely to require removal than will wire.

If ORIF is believed to have provided adequate stability, early active range of motion may be started. With the knee locked in extension, full weight-bearing ambulation may

Clinical Table: Fractures of the Knee

Procedure	Indications	Technique	Anatomy	Pitfalls
Fractures of the Patella				
ORIF with screws and tension band	• Displaced simple fracture, especially transverse	• 4.0-mm partially threaded screws • Anterior tension band	• Extensor mechanism • Parapatellar retinaculum	• Malreduction • Intra-articular screw placement • Loss of fixation
Indirect reduction and cerclage wiring	• Significant comminution ORIF not possible	• Cerclage wire • Indirect reduction • Anterior tension band	• Extensor mechanism • Parapatellar retinaculum	• Loss of fixation
Partial patellectomy and patellar tendon repair	• Comminution of the distal pole	• Excise bony fragment • Tendon repair with no. 5 suture	• Extensor mechanism • Parapatellar retinaculum	• Posterior tilt of patella
Total patellectomy	• Severe comminution		• Extensor mechanism • Parapatellar retinaculum	• Extension lag
Fractures of the Tibial Plateau				
ORIF with lag screws and buttress plate	• Schatzker types I–VI	• Arthrotomy • Elevate meniscus • Bone graft	• Meniscus • Coronary ligament	• Inadequate elevation of plateau • Wound problems
Indirect reduction with limited internal fixation	• Schatzker types I and III	• Ligamentotaxis • Cortical window • Bone graft • Fluoroscopy or arthroscopy		• Inadequate reduction • Compartment syndrome
External fixation	• Schatzker type VI	• Temporary external fixation across the knee • Hybrid external fixation	• Axial alignment of tibia	• Pin tract infection • Poor patient tolerance
Fractures of the Distal Femur				
ORIF with 95° blade plate	• AO/ASIF types A and C	• Lateral approach • Fluoroscopy • Blade parallel to joint • Fixed-angle device • Indirect reduction of metaphysis	• Valgus alignment of the distal femur • Distal femur trapezoidal • Relationship of condyles to shaft	• Flexion or extension of distal fragment
ORIF with 95° DCS	• AO/ASIF types A and C	• Cannulated compression screw • Fixed-angle device	• Valgus alignment of the distal femur • Distal femur trapezoidal • Relationship of condyles to shaft	• Distal fragment too small for device • Penetration of medial cortex
ORIF with condylar buttress plate	• AO/ASIF type C3 Blade and DCS cannot be used	• No fixed-angle device • Can be flexible with complex fractures	• Axial alignment of distal femur	• Drift into varus • Penetration of medial cortex
ORIF with lag screws and buttress plate	• AO/ASIF types B1 and B2	• Arthrotomy • Reduction • Fixation with 6.5-mm lag screws • Antiglide plate	• Restore joint surface anatomy	• Penetration into medial cortex
ORIF with screws	• AO/ASIF type B3	• Arthrotomy • Anterior to posterior lag screw fixation • 4.0-mm screws • Countersink screw heads	• Restore joint surface anatomy	• Avoid prominent intra-articular hardware
Intramedullary nailing	• AO/ASIF type A	• Retrograde	• Axial alignment of the distal femur	• Malalignment and malrotation of distal femur

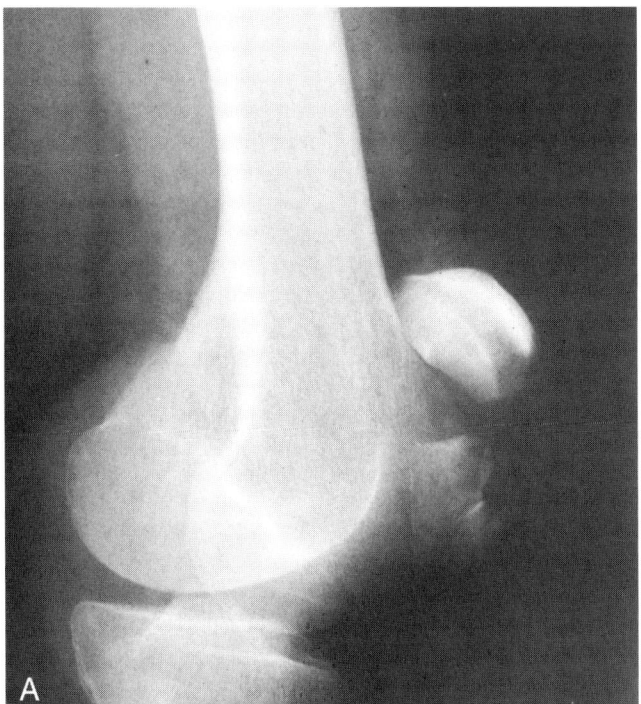

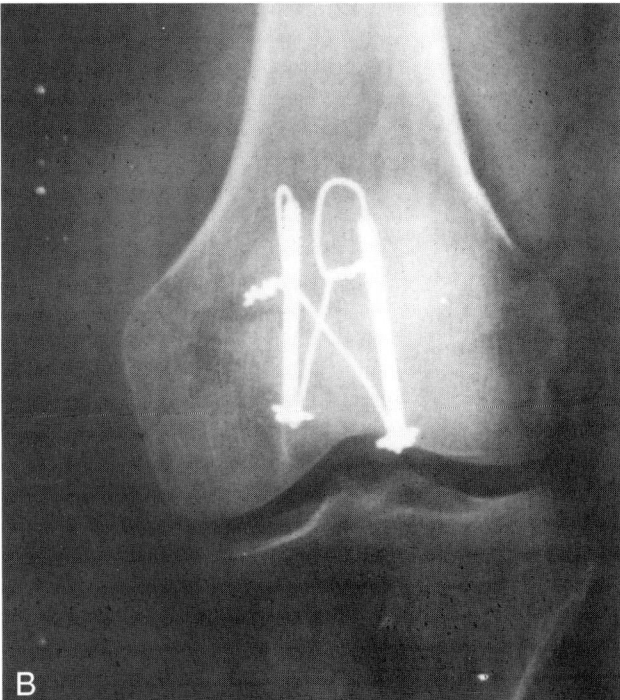

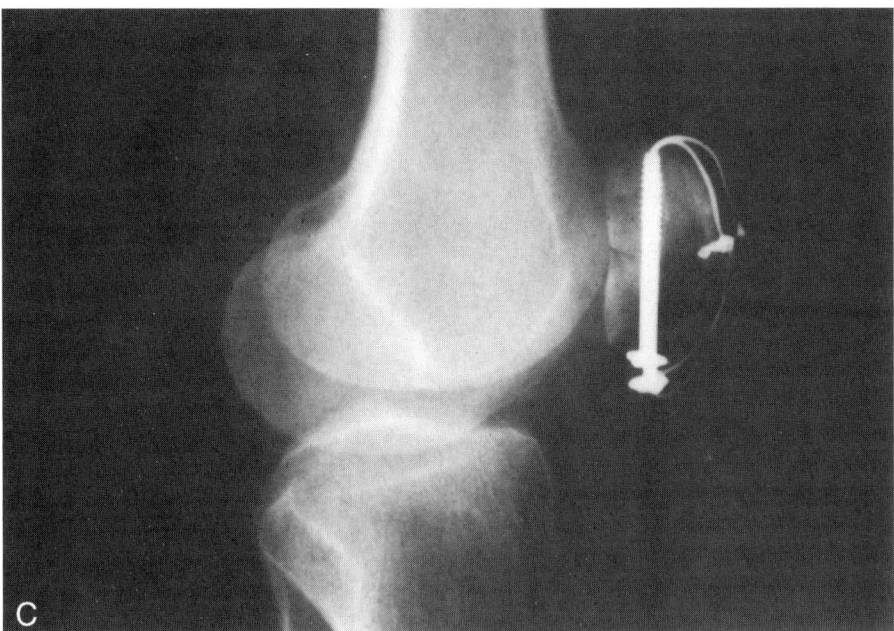

Figure 54.1. A. Lateral view of the knee showing a displaced transverse patella fracture. Postoperative AP (**B**) and lateral (**C**) views of the knee showing internal fixation of the patella fracture with two partially threaded 4.0-mm cannulated screws and an anterior tension band construct made of 18-gauge stainless-steel wire.

be started immediately after surgery. After 6 weeks, unprotected ambulation should be possible.

When treating comminuted fractures of the patella, the surgeon should try to reduce smaller fragments and fix them with a screw to create two larger fracture segments. If this can be accomplished, the above-described ORIF with partially threaded screws and an anterior tension band can be used.

If, on the other hand, the comminution is too great and involves a large part of the patella and if ORIF is not tech-

nically possible, then indirect reduction and cerclage wiring may be more appropriate. In this technique, an 18-gauge wire is passed around the patella through its junction with the quadriceps and patellar tendon and surrounding retinaculum. As the wire is tightened, fragments are manipulated into place. A reasonable reduction may be achieved with the assistance of fluoroscopy. An anterior tension band may then be added (1). Rehabilitation following this procedure depends on the degree of intraoperative stability achieved.

If the comminution is of the distal pole of the patella and the fragments are nonarticular, a partial patellectomy and patellar tendon repair is indicated. In this technique, the comminuted bony fragments are excised, and the patellar tendon is repaired to the distal patella (6). Two heavy nonabsorbable sutures, such as number 5 Ethibond, are used to hold the patellar tendon via a Bunnell or modified Kessler stitch. The four strands are then passed through three drill holes close to the articular surface of the main patellar fragment. By passing the sutures close to the articular surface, patellar tilt is avoided. This repair can then be neutralized with a tension band construct that runs from the quadriceps-patella junction to the tibial tubercle. In addition to all the above procedures, a meticulous repair of the retinaculum should be performed.

Immediate weight bearing may be started with the knee locked into extension in a brace. A safe range of motion zone is determined at the time of surgery.

Total patellectomy is a salvage procedure for the severely comminuted patella fracture for which there is no other surgical alternative. Its functional results are at best

compromised, and it is almost never indicated as a primary procedure (7).

Pitfalls to be avoided are as follows. Loss of fixation and displacement of the fracture can be avoided by adhering to the AO/ASIF principles of internal fixation, by making an accurate intraoperative assessment of the stability of the construct, and by forming an appropriate postoperative rehabilitation protocol. Posterior tilt of the patella after partial patellectomy and tendon repair is avoided by attaching the tendon close to the articular surface of the patella. Stiffness is caused by prolonged immobilization; of course, the period of immobilization must judged in view of the stability of the construct.

Although it is difficult to prevent the tension band from breaking, associated symptoms can be minimized by using suture rather than wire. The risks of nonunion and infection can be lessened by excising devascularized fragments and by minimizing soft tissue stripping of bony fragments during surgery. Patellofemoral arthritis can limited with restoration of the articular surface of the patella and the congruity of the patellofemoral joint.

II Fractures of the Tibial Plateau

RELEVANT ANATOMY AND BIOMECHANICS

The tibial plateau is the articular surface of the proximal tibia. It is composed of a medial plateau, which is convex upward, and a lateral plateau, which is concave upward, and a nonarticular intercondylar area in between. The articular surfaces of the plateaus are major weight-bearing areas; 3 mm of hyaline cartilage cover the medial plateau and 4 mm cover the lateral plateau. The bony articular surfaces slope about 10° inferiorly from the anterior to the posterior edge. The lateral plateau is higher than the medial plateau. This combined with their difference in shape helps the clinician distinguish the two on a lateral x-ray. The menisci cover the periphery of both plateaus and are attached to the tibial plateau at their peripheral edge by the meniscotibial or coronary ligament.

Other features of the proximal tibia include the tibial tubercle, which is the insertion site of the patellar tendon, and Gerdy's tubercle on the anterolateral surface of the lateral tibial flare, which is the insertion site of the iliotibial band. The fibula articulates with the tibia at the proximal tibiofibular joint, which is located posterolaterally on the tibial flare. The pes anserinus tendons and the medial collateral ligament insert on the proximal medial tibia, and the anterior cruciate ligament originates from the anterior intercondylar area.

The mechanism of injury is a varus or valgus stress that is often combined with an axial compressive force, resulting in a split and/or a depression of the plateau. The bony structure of the medial plateau is stronger than the lateral

side, and fracture of it is often the result of a high-energy injury; it is has a high association of soft tissue injury.

INITIAL FINDINGS, PHYSICAL EXAMINATION, AND DIAGNOSIS

When evaluating a patient with a tibial plateau fracture, it is important to distinguish between a high- and low energy injury. The history often includes a fall, ski injury, motor vehicle accident, or pedestrian–motor vehicle accident. The patient complains of pain and an inability to bear weight.

On physical examination, there is swelling, a hemarthrosis, and tenderness at the proximal tibia. A careful neurologic examination should be performed to rule out injury to the peroneal or tibial nerves. A careful vascular examination should be done to rule out a popliteal artery injury. If this is suspected, particularly in the context of a high-energy injury or a fracture of the medial tibial plateau, an arteriogram should be obtained.

Classification

Many classification systems of tibial plateau fractures have been proposed. A commonly used and reproducible classification is one popularized by Schatzker et al. (8). This system classifies fractures into six types and is helpful in planning surgical treatment.

Schatzker I is a wedge or split fracture of the lateral plateau. It does not have any depression or impaction of the articular surface and usually occurs in young people with strong bone.

Schatzker II is a split depression of the lateral plateau. It often occurs in older people in whom the cancellous bone of the proximal tibia is weak and cannot resist compression. The fracture involves an area of depressed or impacted articular surface in addition to a split or wedge fragment.

Schatzker III is a pure depression fracture of part of the articular surface of the lateral tibial plateau; there is no split.

Schatzker IV is a fracture of the medial tibial plateau. It is often the result of a high-energy injury that is associated with injuries of the lateral collateral ligament, peroneal nerve, popliteal artery, and cruciate ligaments.

Schatzker V is a fracture of both the lateral and medial tibial plateaus. The mechanism is likely an axial load imposed on an extended knee. Fractures that enter the knee joint in a nonarticular area are relatively more favorable and carry a better prognosis.

Schatzker VI is a metaphyseal fracture that extends into the diaphysis separating the articular surface from the diaphysis.

RADIOLOGIC STUDIES

Radiographic evaluation includes AP, lateral, and oblique views of the knee. The internal oblique x-ray helps with the evaluation of the lateral plateau, as does the external oblique with the medial plateau. A CT scan with coronal and sagittal reformatting or tomography is helpful if the surgeon requires additional information about the fracture pattern.

TREATMENT

The goals in the treatment of fractures of the tibial plateau are preservation of joint mobility, restoration of joint stability, restoration of the anatomy of the articular surface and joint congruity, restoration of axial alignment of the lower extremity, prevention of pain, and prevention of posttraumatic arthritis (9). The options for treatment include nonoperative treatment; ORIF, with bone grafting if necessary; indirect reduction, limited exposure, and internal fixation; limited internal fixation and application of a hybrid external fixator; and application of a bridging external fixator across the knee, delayed open reduction, and internal fixation (Clinical Table).

Nonoperative Treatment

Nonoperative treatment is indicated for nondisplaced fractures with no articular incongruity or significant varus or valgus instability. The treatment entails the use of a hinged knee brace, early range of motion, and strict avoidance of weight bearing for 6 weeks.

Operative Treatment

The indications for surgery are joint incongruity, joint instability in the coronal plane greater than 10° with the knee in full extension, articular stepoff greater than 2 mm, axial malalignment, open fracture, and fracture with a vascular lesion. The goal of surgical treatment is to restore the anatomy of the joint surface, restore axial alignment, and achieve adequate stability to allow early range of motion of the knee.

ORIF is the classic approach to all displaced tibial plateau fractures. There has been a trend toward less soft tissue stripping, limited dissection, and optimal rather than maximal internal fixation. Techniques may have to be modified or delayed, depending on the condition of the soft tissue envelope. Although the specific approach depends on the fracture type, some general principles can be outlined. A straight longitudinal incision should be used. The soft tissues should be handled with extreme care. The exposure of the joint surface is facilitated by flexing the knee and allowing it to hang, providing traction. Alternatively, a femoral distractor may be placed across the knee to provide assistance with exposure and reduction via ligamentotaxis. The meniscus is elevated after the coronary ligament is incised.

When possible, the surgeon should work on the articular surface through the split component of the fracture. The joint surface is reduced under direct vision. After elevation of a depressed articular fragment, there will be a metaphyseal bony defect. This should be grafted with iliac crest corticocancellous or cancellous bone, depending on the degree of structural support needed. The wedge fragment can then be reduced and held provisionally with a large pointed reduction clamp. Note that a stab wound can be made at the proximal medial tibia for placement of one arm of the clamp. The split fragment is fixed with partially threaded 6.5-mm cancellous screws and supplemented with a buttress plate. If a meniscal tear is noted, it can be repaired at this time.

Indirect reduction through a limited exposure and minimal internal fixation can be used to treat specific fracture types. With the assistance of arthroscopy and/or fluoroscopy to visualize the joint surface reduction, the surgeon can perform reduction and internal fixation of Schatzker I and III fractures percutaneously. Ligamentotaxis—the indirect reduction of displaced bony fragments by means of traction from the intact soft tissue attachments on those fragments—is a useful technique. For example, ligamentotaxis provided by a femoral distractor across the knee is particularly helpful for reducing the wedge fragment of a Schatzker I fracture. Percutaneous screws are then placed to stabilize the reduction. To reduce the articular depression of a Schatzker III fracture, a cortical window in the tibial flare should be made. Through it, a bone tamp can be used to elevate the depressed fragment. The reduction and the iliac crest bone graft can then be supported with two percutaneously placed partially threaded cancellous screws.

After surgery, the knee should be protected in a hinged knee brace for 6 weeks. Range of motion of the joint should be started immediately (10). The patient can use toe-touch weight bearing for the first 6 to 12 weeks, depending on the specific fracture and the intraoperative stability obtained following internal fixation. During this period, the quadriceps and hamstrings should be strengthened, and the range of motion should be optimized.

When the soft tissue swelling is severe, as in high-energy injuries and Schatzker VI fractures, care must be taken to avoid operating through these vulnerable areas. In these cases, I prefer to place a temporary external fixator across the knee to provide stability, gross reduction of the joint surface via ligamentotaxis, and proper axial alignment (11). Then, after the soft tissue swelling resolves, the fixator is removed and ORIF is performed. Alternatively, one can use a hybrid external fixator with skinny wires near the joint for these cases. The disadvantages include reported problems with pin tract infections and poor tolerance by patients.

Treatment of Specific Fracture Types

A Schatzker I simple wedge fracture of the lateral plateau can be reduced with traction. The reduction can be visualized with arthroscopy or fluoroscopy. Internal fixation with percutaneous partially threaded cancellous screws can then be performed. Alternatively, a formal ORIF can be performed through an arthrotomy. The meniscus is elevated, and the fracture is directly reduced. Internal fixation is achieved with partially threaded cancellous screws. For additional stability, a small buttress plate may be added.

A Schatzker II fracture of the lateral plateau should be treated with ORIF and bone grafting. After performing an arthrotomy and elevating the meniscus, the surgeon can visualize the joint surface. The wedge fracture is opened anteriorly with a small laminar spreader, like a book. By working through the fracture site, an excellent view of the depressed fragment is obtained. This is elevated and the metaphyseal defect is filled with iliac crest autograft. The wedge fragment is then reduced, provisionally held with a large Weber clamp and fixed with two partially threaded cancellous screws about 1 cm below the joint surface. The wedge fragment is then further supported by a buttress plate (Fig. 54.2).

A Schatzker III joint depression fracture of the lateral plateau requires restoration of the articular surface. In the absence of a wedge fragment, the joint depression should be elevated through a cortical window created on the under surface of the tibial flare. The reduction must be visualized, and this may be accomplished with an arthrotomy, arthroscopy, or fluoroscopy. The metaphyseal defect should then be grafted with an autogenous iliac crest bone graft. The elevated fragment and the bone graft should be supported with two large partially threaded cancellous screws. Because the thin lateral cortex of the plateau can

be further weakened by the cortical window, the use of a buttress plate is prudent despite the absence of a split fracture. My preference for these fractures is an open technique and miniarthrotomy to directly visualize the reduction and application a buttress plate. The shortcoming of the arthroscopic visualization is that the depressed area is often anterior and partially covered by the anterior horn of the meniscus, making excellent visualization difficult.

A Schatzker IV fracture of the medial plateau should be reduced and stabilized with a medial buttress plate. Reduction of these fractures is greatly assisted by the technique of distraction ligamentotaxis with a femoral distractor across the knee. The reduction of the articular surface can be visualized either directly or with fluoroscopy.

Schatzker V bicondylar fractures can be intra-articular or extra-articular. In the absence of articular comminution, reduction can often be achieved with distraction and ligamentotaxis. Although bilateral buttress plates are usually necessary to stabilize these fractures, most of the reduction and screw fixation can usually be done from the lateral side. The additional necessary medial stability can be achieved with a small medial plate through a limited exposure or even via a subcutaneous technique. Alternatively, a small external fixator can be placed medially to achieve the medial buttress without any surgical exposure. Overzealous dissection of both plateaus, such as that achieved with a Z-plasty of the patellar tendon or a tibial tubercle osteotomy should be avoided. The first requirement for a good result in these cases is avoiding wound slough and infection (11).

In Schatzker VI fractures, the metaphysis must be bridged to the diaphysis with proper alignment and the joint surface must be restored. A narrow 4.5-mm dynamic compression plate, a lateral tibial head buttress plate, or a fixed-angle blade plate from an AO/ASIF set can be used for this purpose. Note that the L and T buttress plates are not strong enough to bridge the metaphysis to the diaphysis. For fractures that are unstable and tend to shorten and when the soft tissues are too swollen for early surgery, a temporary bridging external fixator across the knee can be used until the swelling decreases. At a later date, an ORIF may be performed more safely. Alternatively, one can use a hybrid external fixator with skinny wires in the proximal tibia and standard Schanz screws in the diaphysis for these cases.

ASSOCIATED SOFT TISSUE INJURIES

Soft tissue injuries are often associated with fractures of the tibial plateau. These include meniscal tears, tears of the collateral ligaments, tears of the cruciate ligaments, and injuries to the popliteal artery and the peroneal nerve. At the time of arthrotomy, an accessible meniscal tear can be surgically repaired. Collateral ligament injuries can be managed nonoperatively, most often with a 6-week period in a hinged knee brace. It is difficult to diagnose and treat tears of the cruciate ligaments, unless a bony avulsion of the anterior cruciate ligament (ACL) is present,

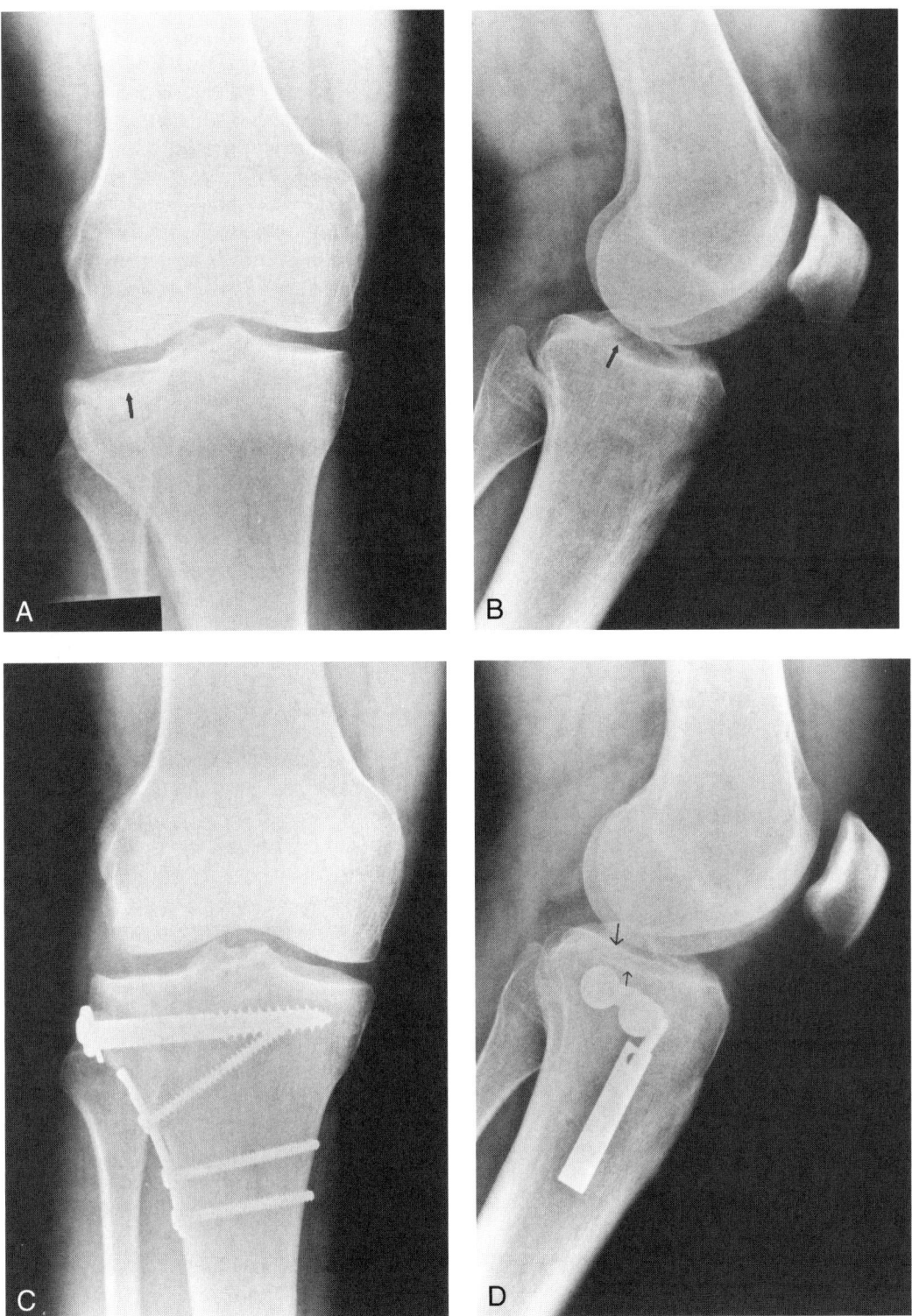

Figure 54.2. Preoperative AP (**A**) and lateral (**B**) views showing a depressed lateral tibial plateau fracture (*arrows*). Postoperative AP (**C**) and lateral (**D**) views showing a well-reduced lateral tibial plateau and internal fixation with two partially threaded 6.5-mm cancellous screws and a one-third tubular buttress plate. The lateral (*large arrow*) and medial (*small arrow*) plateaus are outlined on the lateral view.

which should be internally fixed at the time of surgery on the plateau fracture. Other cases of cruciate ligament injury should be approached at a later time, if the knee remains unstable and symptomatic. An examination of the tibial plateau fracture under anesthesia in the operating room immediately after ORIF can be helpful in the diagnosis of additional ligament injuries.

Vascular injuries should be diagnosed with a preoperative arteriogram, if there is a clinical suspicion. Vascular consultation should be obtained, and a coordinated approach to the vascular and orthopaedic injury should be undertaken. Closed injuries to the peroneal nerve are most often a neuropraxia and should be managed with supportive treatment and observation.

Possible complications include wound problems, failure of fixation, loss of articular reduction, malunion, and nonunion. Wound complications can be minimized by avoiding traumatic exposure through compromised soft tissue and by avoiding extensive soft tissue stripping of bone. Limited exposure and percutaneous screw placement are preferred, if the fracture can be sufficiently treated in this manner. Failure of fixation, loss of articular reduction, malunion, and nonunion can be avoided with careful surgical technique that achieves satisfactory reduction and stabilization of the fracture. I advise the liberal use of structural bone graft. An appropriate rehabilitation program must be prescribed.

III Fractures of the Distal Femur

RELEVANT ANATOMY

Understanding the bony anatomy of the distal femur is essential for the treatment of fractures in this area. In the coronal plane, the knee joint is parallel to the ground. The anatomic axis of the knee, or the femorotibial angle, is 6° to 9° of valgus. The mechanical axis of the knee joint is 3° of valgus from the vertical.

The femoral condyles are wider posteriorly than anteriorly. This is difficult to appreciate on plain x-ray because of overlap. A transverse cut through the condyle with a CT scan reveals a trapezoid with a 25% decrease in width from posterior to anterior. In the sagittal plane, the shaft of the femur is aligned with the anterior half of the condyles. The muscular anatomy includes the anterior compartment, which contains the quadriceps femoris, and the posterior compartment, which contains the hamstring group and the gastrocnemius muscle. The compartments are separated by the medial and lateral intermuscular septa.

After a fracture of the distal femur occurs, the bone fragments are deformed by the pull of the muscles. The quadriceps and hamstrings deform and shorten the femur. As a result of the pull of the gastrocnemius, the condyles become angulated with the apex posterior. If the fracture extends into the joint, the condyles can displace and rotate.

Important vascular anatomy of this region includes the superficial femoral artery, which is situated on the medial side of the distal femur and passes into the popliteal fossa to then become the popliteal artery at about 10 cm proximal to the knee joint through the adductor hiatus.

INITIAL FINDINGS, PHYSICAL EXAMINATION, AND DIAGNOSIS

The history is usually a direct trauma on a flexed knee, such as would occur from a fall in an older patient or an impact against the dashboard of a car in a younger patient.

The patient presents with swelling of the knee and supracondylar area. There is often visible deformity and tenderness on palpation. The clinician must carefully assess the vascular status and determine the possibility of compartment syndrome. A clinical suspicion of a vascular injury mandates an emergency arteriogram and vascular surgery consultation.

Classification

Although there are many classification systems described for fractures of the distal femur, the AO/ASIF classification is commonly used and is helpful for description, preoperative planning, and prognosis (13). There are three classes of distal femoral fractures, each of which is subdivided into three groups. Type A includes extra-articular supracondylar fractures. The proximal limit of the distal segment of the femur is determined by the square method, by which the side of the square is the same length as the widest part of the epiphysis. Type A fractures are further divided into simple (A1), wedge (A2), and comminuted (A3) fractures. Type B fractures are unicondylar intra-articular fractures of the distal femur. Type B1 is fracture of the lateral condyle in the sagittal plane, type B2 is fracture of the medial condyle in the sagittal plane, and type B3 is a coronal fracture of either condyle. Type C fractures are bicondylar intra-articular fractures. This group includes noncomminuted T or Y fractures (C1), fractures with supracondylar comminution (C2), and fractures with intra-articular comminution resulting in more than two joint fragments (C3). The subdivisions are more for the purposes of documentation and research than for clinical use.

RADIOLOGIC STUDIES

The standard radiographic evaluation includes AP and lateral views of the knee and femur. Careful evaluation of the joint surface of the distal femur and its alignment in relation to the femoral shaft is crucial. Oblique and femoral notch view x-rays and a CT scan may help delineate intra-articular fracture fragments. When severe comminution of the distal femur makes x-ray evaluation difficult, a traction x-ray will often help the surgeon better identify the fracture morphology (12).

TREATMENT

The goal of treatment is to restore the length, rotation, and axial alignment of the distal femur and its relation to the knee. For intra-articular fractures, the goal is an anatomic reconstitution of the articular surface.

The treatment options include casting, traction and delayed casting, and ORIF. Indications for surgical treatment include displaced intra-articular fractures, open fractures, fractures with vascular injury, floating knee (fracture of the distal femur and the proximal tibia), bilateral femoral fractures, polytrauma, associated ligamentous disruption of the knee, and extra-articular fractures in which reduction cannot be obtained or maintained (Clinical Table). Even in cases in which the position can be maintained with traction, surgery is useful to avoid prolonged immobilization and inevitable knee stiffness. In my judgment, there is little place for the closed treatment of these fractures, except when the patient cannot tolerate operative treatment or is a nonambulator or if the patient is elderly with an impacted minimally displaced fracture.

Operative Treatment

Surgical options include ORIF with a 95° condylar blade plate, a 95° Dynamic condylar screw (DCS), a condylar buttress plate, lag screws with or without a supplementary buttress plate, and an intramedullary nail. Specific fracture patterns may be best managed with a particular surgical approach.

The principles of surgical treatment include preoperative planning, timely surgery, and biologic surgical technique. Preoperative planning is essential to ensure that the surgeon has chosen the appropriately sized implant and has rehearsed the steps of the surgical procedure. Planning shortens the surgical time and, perhaps, avoids unexpected findings at surgery (11). Unless surgery is emergent as a result of an open fracture or vascular injury, it should be performed within the first 24 to 48 h. The surgeon should make certain that he or she has the adequate experience and resources to deal with these often difficult fractures.

The surgical technique is still evolving. Although anatomic reduction of the metaphyseal area was once considered a goal, it has become clear that the soft tissue stripping necessary to achieve this goal can lead to delayed healing and hardware failure. The principles of modern plating technique include careful handling of the soft tissues and indirect reduction techniques of the metaphysis to prevent soft tissue stripping of the fracture frag-

ments and to preserve as much vascularity as possible. Whereas anatomic reduction of the articular surface is mandatory, only restoration of the length, axial alignment, and rotation of the extra-articular area are needed. Stable internal fixation must be achieved to allow early active rehabilitation of the limb and the patient (11,14,14a).

The surgical exposure for plating of the distal femur is a lateral approach. The proximal extent of the incision is determined by the diaphyseal involvement. Distally, the incision may be extended to curve anteriorly beyond the knee joint to the lateral border of the tibial tubercle, if necessary. The iliotibial band is incised in line with the skin incision. The vastus lateralis is retracted anteriorly and is dissected from the lateral intermuscular septum. The superior geniculate artery must usually be ligated. The entire articular surface of the distal femur can often be visualized by placing a blunt Hohmann's retractor from lateral to medial across the joint surface. In unusual cases, additional exposure of the medial condyle can be achieved with either a tibial tubercle osteotomy or, preferably, an additional medial incision (12).

The 95° condylar blade plate is an excellent device for treating most AO/ASIF type A and C distal femur fractures. It is well suited for intra-articular and extra-articular fractures. It is not suited for the treatment of coronal fractures of the distal femur, unicondylar distal femur fractures, or fractures in which adequate purchase of the distal fragment cannot be obtained. The blade plate is technically demanding and requires attention to technical detail. When dealing with an intra-articular fracture, provisional fixation of the articular surface with Kirschner (K) wires should be obtained. Next, the insertion site of the blade must be planned before the insertion of 6.5-mm lag screws to stabilize the articular fracture. In extra-articular fractures, this additional concern is not necessary. The proper site for insertion of the blade is 1.5 to 2 cm proximal to the inferior articular surface in the middle third of the anterior half of the sagittal diameter of the condyles at their widest point. The 6.5-mm lag screws should then be inserted proximal to and out of the way of the blade insertion site.

The direction and rotation of the blade must be established carefully. The blade should be inserted both parallel to the distal articular surface and the anterior articular surface of the distal femur. (Recall the trapezoidal shape of the distal femur.) To accomplish this, two K wires should be placed parallel to each of these surfaces, and then a summation K wire should be inserted just distal to the planned blade site. Intraoperative fluoroscopy is helpful in this situation. Next, the rotation of the blade must be correct to avoid unwanted flexion or extension of the distal fragment. In young patients with hard bone, the blade tract should be predrilled with a triple drill guide before insertion of the seating chisel. The chisel should be disimpacted after every 1 cm of progression to avoid incarceration of the chisel. Be careful to maintain correct rotation, remain parallel to the summation K wire in both planes, and avoid penetration of the medial cortex.

The chisel is then removed and the blade plate is inserted in the same tract. Add one or two additional plate screws into the distal fragment. Next, reduce the proximal shaft fragment to the plate. Initial distraction and then compression can be achieved with a femoral distractor or an AO tensioning device; thus indirect reduction can be accomplished with minimal soft tissue stripping of the metaphyseal fragments. If the metaphyseal comminution is severe and there is no cortical contact, compression should not be performed. A long plate with a maximum of three screws in the proximal fragment and with good purchase should be used to achieve balanced fixation. If an interfragmentary lag screw can be inserted through the plate, this should be done.

Because the blade plate and the DCS are fixed-angle devices, the proper axial alignment is accomplished as long as the blade or lag screw of the DCS is parallel to the joint surface of the distal femur. Bone graft is usually not needed, if such a biologic approach to surgery is taken. With minimal soft tissue stripping, the metaphyseal comminution consolidates rather quickly. Early callus formation serves as a medial buttress to further enhance the stability of the construct (14) (Fig. 54.3).

The 95° DCS is similar to the blade plate and is indicated for the same assortment of fractures. It is technically easier, since it is a cannulated system and the insertion of the lag screw can be done directly over the summation guidewire (15,15a). The instruments are similar to the AO/ASIF Dynamic hip screw (DHS), which is commonly used for intertrochanteric hip fractures and is familiar to most orthopaedic surgeons. In addition, sagittal plane alignment can be adjusted before insertion of additional screws in the distal fragment. Another advantage when dealing with intra-articular fractures is that the large lag screw adds to the interfragmentary compression of the articular fragments. The disadvantages of this device are that a large amount of bone is removed for insertion of the lag screw and a larger distal fragment is necessary to achieve satisfactory purchase than is the case for the blade plate.

The condylar buttress plate is not a fixed-angle device. It does, however, offer greater versatility when treating complex fractures in which the blade or DCS lag screw cannot be inserted into the distal fragment as a result of the fracture morphology. It is helpful when treating AO/ASIF type C3 fractures with severe intra-articular comminution or coronal intra-articular fractures. Because the condylar buttress plate is not a fixed-angle device, achieving and maintaining satisfactory alignment are more challenging. There is a tendency for the distal fragment to drift into varus when there is severe metaphyseal comminution and the medial column is not supported. Consideration should then be given to an additional medial buttress plate and bone graft (12).

When treating type B1 or B2 unicondylar fractures, a medial or lateral approach should be used, depending on the fracture. The condyle should be reduced, and the surgeon must be sure that the articular surface of the distal femur is anatomic. The fracture should be stabilized with two 6.5-mm partially threaded interfragmentary lag screws and an antiglide buttress plate. The one-half tubular plate or the T buttress plate from the AO/ASIF large fragment set can be used for this purpose. Type B3 fractures, or coronal Hoffa fractures, should be exposed through a medial or lateral approach, depending on the condyle involved; the fractures are then reduced and stabilized with either 4.0- or 6.5-mm partially threaded lag screws in an anterior to posterior direction. If the screw must be inserted through the articular surface, it should be countersunk (12,16).

The intramedullary nail may be used to treat AO/ASIF type A extra-articular distal femur fractures. This is a technically demanding approach that requires a great deal of attention to prevent malposition of the distal fragment. A retrograde approach is preferable to anterograde, since it provides better control of the distal fragment. The insertion site of the nail into the distal femur and the direction determine the ultimate alignment of the distal fragment. This is done with the patient supine on a radiolucent table. A large bolster is placed under the knee, enabling approximately 45° of flexion. A 5-cm medial parapatellar arthrotomy is performed. Adequate retraction of the patella is necessary to gain access to the insertion site, 15 mm anterior to the femoral insertion of the anterior cruciate ligament, and to enable the surgeon to ream in the proper retrograde direction. Deviation from the proper starting point or direction will result in varus or valgus malposition. Fluoroscopic assistance is crucial for this part of the procedure.

Reduction is obtained with free-hand traction through the flexed knee. In addition, a Weber clamp can be placed percutaneously on the medial and lateral femoral condyles to manipulate the distal fragment. The reduction should be maintained during reaming and nail insertion. Following the retrograde insertion of the nail, rotation must be carefully checked before distal and proximal interlocking. I prefer the use of a specially designed retrograde nail because of low distal interlocking screws (15 mm from the tip of the nail) and the ability to place the free-hand proximal interlocking screws in an anterior to posterior direction. This is technically easier than a lateral to medial direction, which is used with a standard femoral nail placed in a retrograde fashion.

Postoperative rehabilitation is determined by the individual injury and the treatment rendered. If adequate stabilization has been achieved at surgery, then immediate active and passive range of motion of the knee should be started (10). Weight bearing, on the other hand, should be limited for the first 2 to 3 months after plating. Weight bearing and resistive exercises should be progressed as signs of fracture healing appear on radiographs. Solid union can usually be expected in 3 to 6 months. Earlier weight bearing can be allowed when an intramedullary nail is used, since it is a load-sharing device

Potential complications include infection, nonunion, malunion, loss of fixation, posttraumatic arthritis, and stiffness of the knee. The incidence of infection may be mini-

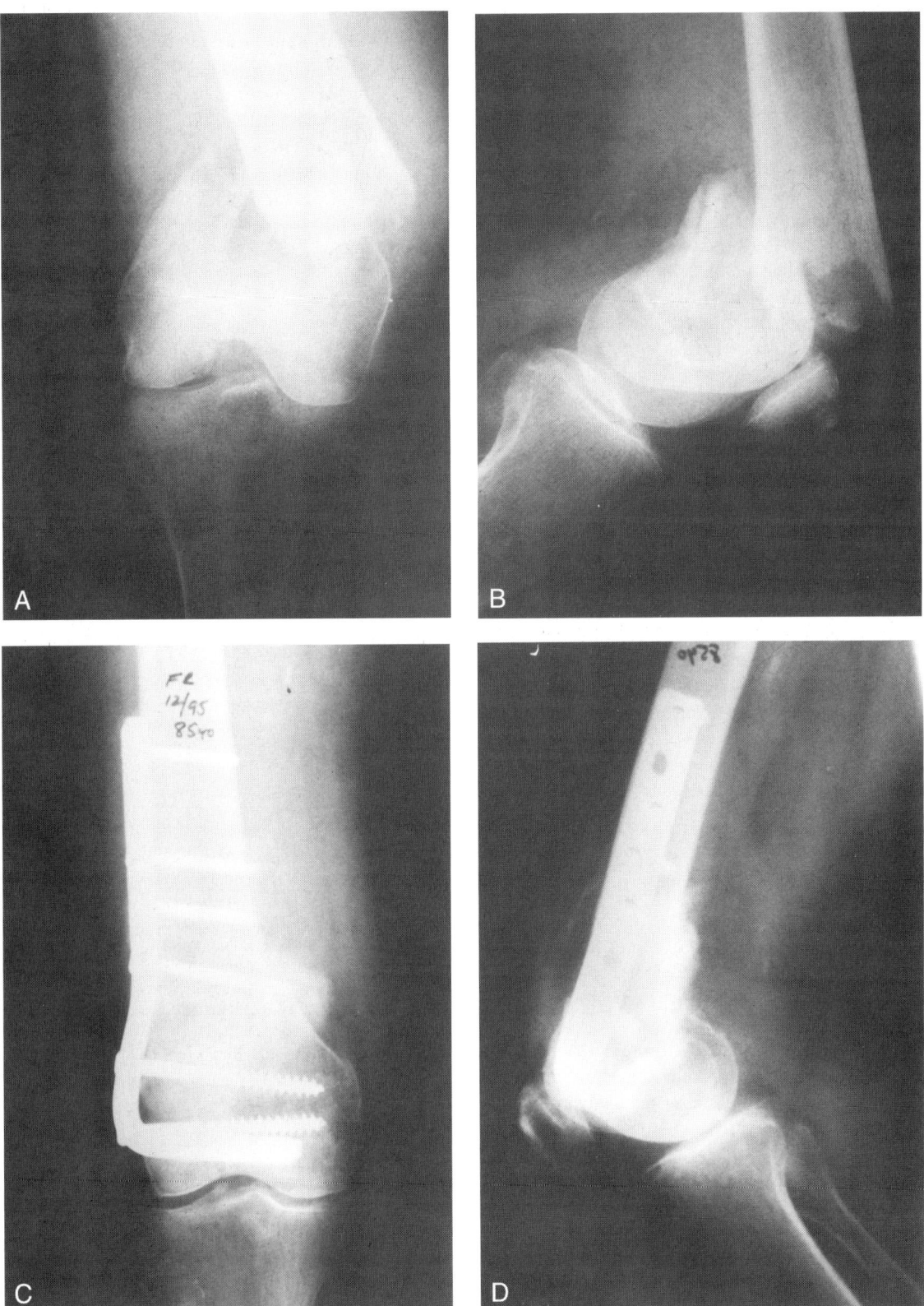

Figure 54.3. Preoperative AP (**A**) and lateral (**B**) views showing a supracondylar–intercondylar fracture (type C) of the distal femur. Postoperative AP (**C**) and lateral (**D**) views showing a well-reduced distal femur fracture and internal fixation with intercondylar 6.5-mm partially threaded cancellous lag screws and a 95° condylar blade plate.

mized by the proper handling of open fractures, careful handling of soft tissue, and avoidance of excessive dissection.

Nonunion usually occurs in the supracondylar region of the femur. Factors predisposing to this include high-energy injuries with extensive bony devascularization and the presence of a bony defect. The likelihood of nonunion may be decreased by avoiding excessive soft tissue stripping and by achieving adequate mechanical stability at surgery. An elegant way to achieve this is to use indirect reduction techniques and balanced fixation with a 95° condylar blade plate of adequate length (11). Although malunion is more common after nonoperative treatment than after surgery, it will occur if the distal femur is fixed in an improper position or if there is a loss of fixation and a gradual change in the position of the distal femur. The surgeon must be careful to restore the joint surface in an anatomic fashion and adequately stabilize the distal femur in the correct axial and rotational alignment. While this can be difficult, particularly if the distal fragment is small, attention to technical detail is the best method to prevent this complication.

Severe fracture comminution, osteopenic bone, infection, a small distal fracture fragment, delayed union, and poor patient compliance in regard to weight-bearing ambulation may lead to loss of fixation. This may be lessened by achieving adequate stability and by minimizing soft tissue stripping of bone at surgery to help promote bony union in a timely fashion. Balanced fixation of distal fractures may be technically challenging but can most often be accomplished with the 95° blade plate. In situations in which screw purchase is compromised by the presence of osteopenic bone, polymethyl methacrylate (PMMA) can be injected into the screw holes to achieve increased screw purchase.

Knee stiffness can be the result of a malreduction of the joint surface, intra-articular hardware, intra-articular adhesions, and capsular contracture. Stiffness can be minimized with an anatomic reduction of the articular surface of the distal femur, proper hardware placement, stable fixation, and the institution of early range of motion of the knee.

Posttraumatic arthritis is usually the result of articular damage at the time of injury or malunion. Both incongruency of the joint and abnormalities of axial alignment will predispose the patient to abnormal stress loading of the joint and subsequent arthrosis. A satisfactory reduction of the distal femur, which can usually be achieved with meticulous attention to technical detail, is the best method to prevent this outcome.

SUMMARY

For those who treat fractures of the knee, there are many choices to make. There are many different fracture types associated with different degrees of soft tissue injury and many different treatment options available.

A practical understanding of the anatomy, biomechanics, diagnosis, and fracture classification establishes a framework for choosing appropriate treatment options. The degree of soft tissue injury is an integral part of this decision-making process.

The role of nonoperative treatment, the indications for surgery, and practical points regarding surgical technique as well as pitfalls to be avoided have been discussed. With the rehabilitation protocol the surgeon should achieve a balance between adequate protection of the fracture during union and progressive mobility, range of motion, and muscle strengthening.

REFERENCES

1. Sanders R. Patella fractures and extensor mechanism injuries. In: Browner BD, Jupiter JB, Levine AM, Trafton PG, eds. Skeletal trauma. Philadelphia: Saunders, 1992:1685–1716.
2. Burvant JG, Thomas KA, Randall A, Harris MB. Evaluation of methods of internal fixation of transverse patella fractures: a biomechanical study. J Orthop Trauma 1994;8:147–153.
3. Hung LK, Chan KM, Chow YN, Leung PC. Fractured patella: operative treatment using the tension band principle. Injury 1985;16:343–347.
4. Muller ME, Allgower M, Schneider R, Willenegger H. Manual of internal fixation. Berlin: Springer-Verlag, 1992.
5. Weber MJ, Janeck, CJ, McLeod P, et al. Efficacy of various forms of fixation of transverse fractures of the patella. J Bone Joint Surg 1980;62A:215–220.
6. Saltzman CL, Goulet GA, McClellan RT, et al. Results of treatment of displaced patellar fractures by partial patellectomy. J Bone Joint Surg 1990;72A:1279.
7. Sutton FS, Thompson CH, Lipke J, Kettlekamp DB. The effect of patellectomy on knee function. J Bone Joint Surg 1976;58A:537–540.
8. Schatzker J, McBroom R, Bruce D The tibial plateau fracture. The Toronto experience. Clin Orthop 1979;138:94–104.
9. Schatzker J. Tibial plateau fractures. In: Browner BD, Jupiter JB, Levine AM, Trafton PG, eds. Skeletal trauma. Philadelphia: Saunders, 1992:1745–1769.
10. Salter R, Simmonds DF, Malcom BW, et al. The biological effects of continuous passive motion on healing of full thickness defects in articular cartilage: an experimental investigation in the rabbit. J Bone Joint Surg 1980;62A:1232–1251.
11. Mast J, Jakob R, Ganz R. Planning and reduction technique in fracture surgery. Berlin: Springer-Verlag, 1989.
12. Helfet DL. Fractures of the distal femur. In: Browner BD, Jupiter JB, Levine AM, Trafton PG, eds. Skeletal trauma. Philadelphia: Saunders, 1992:1643–1683.
13. Muller ME, Koch P, Nazarian S, Schatzker J. The comprehensive classification of fractures of long bones. Berlin: Springer-Verlag, 1990.
14. Ostrum RF, Geel C. Indirect reduction and internal fixation of supracondylar femur fractures without bone graft. J Orthop Trauma 1995;9:278–284.
14a. Chiron HS, Tremeoulet J, Casey P, Muller ME. Fractures of the distal third of the femur treated by internal fixation. Clin Orthop 1974;100:160–170.
15. Sanders R, Regazzoni P, Ruedi TP. Treatment of supracondylar-intracondylar fractures of the femur using the Dynamic condylar screw. J Orthop Trauma 1989;3:214–222.
15a. Neer CS, Grantham SA, Shelton ML. Supracondylar fracture of the adult femur. A study of one hundred and ten cases. J Bone Joint Surg 1967;49A:591–613.
16. Ostermann PA, Neumann K, Ekkernkamp A, Muhr G. Long term results of unicondylar fractures of the femur. J Orthop Trauma 1994;8:142–146.

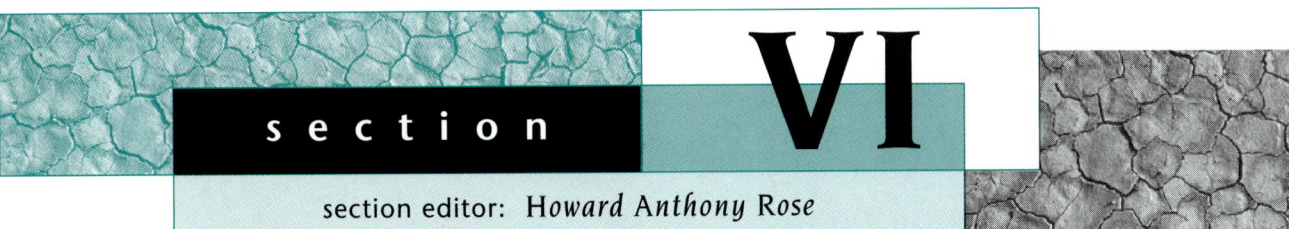

section VI

section editor: *Howard Anthony Rose*

ATHLETE'S KNEE

Patellofemoral Malalignment: Lateral Retinacular Release

Mark T. Wichman and Marc J. Friedman

There is perhaps no other area in orthopaedics more plagued by controversy and disagreement than in management of anterior knee pain when standard conservative management fails. A plethora of surgical procedures have been described, but the indications to perform these procedures vary widely among authors, which obviously complicates the surgeon's efforts to compare surgical results among studies. Thus young surgeons must master the concepts so that they may critically evaluate the literature and make intelligent decisions in caring for these challenging patients.

The lateral retinacular release (LRR) was initially described in the French literature in 1888 and was reported in the English literature shortly after. In 1970, Willner (1) was the first to present the lateral release as an isolated procedure. He described the technique of removing a 15- × 1.25-cm (6- × 0.5-in) strip of lateral fascia and capsule via an extensive anteromedial incision in seven patients with a history of recurrent patellar dislocation. Although isolated LRR is certainly not the current procedure of choice for recurrent patellar dislocation (Chapter 57), all seven patients in Willner's series were free of subsequent dislocations up to 2.5 years later.

The magnitude of the operation is large by today's standards but is relatively benign compared to the patellectomy, osteotomy, and realignment procedures that were available in the 1960s. In the 1980s, ease of the procedure combined with a perception of low morbidity led to empiric use of the lateral retinacular release to treat a variety of abnormalities. Unfortunately, it was realized that the procedure does have inherent risks and can indeed worsen a patient's problem or even create new ones (2–4). Since then, studies have evaluated results of the procedure, and rational indications for LRR have been formulated. Today, LRR is usually performed arthroscopically and often with electrocautery.

RELEVANT ANATOMY AND PATHOGENESIS

To perform a safe but adequate lateral retinacular release, the surgeon must understand the pertinent anatomy. The lateral retinaculum is composed of two distinct layers: the superficial oblique retinaculum and the deep transverse retinaculum. The superficial oblique retinacular fibers originate from the iliotibial tract and merge with the longitudinal fibers from the vastus lateralis and patellar tendon (Fig. 55.1). The deep transverse retinaculum runs from the deep portion of the fascia lata and inserts on the lateral patella. As seen in Figure 55.2, there are proximal and distal expansions of this layer: the epicondylopatellar and patellotibial bands, respectively. Note that these bands are actually ligaments, since they are anchored to bone on both sides. They tighten with knee flexion along with the iliotibial band and must be counterbalanced by competent medial structures to prevent lateral subluxation of the patella.

The surgeon must also be familiar with the vascular anatomy in this region, because hemarthrosis is a known complication of LRR that may be preventable. A ring-like anastomosis of vessels encircles the patella. As seen in Figure 55.3, the lateral superior geniculate artery is the most vulnerable vessel during LRR. Because of good collateral circulation, its sacrifice is generally well tolerated, unless trauma to the vessel goes unrecognized, which can lead to postoperative hemarthrosis.

The relationship between patellar malalignment and anterior knee pain has been recognized for almost three decades (5–7). Table 55.1 lists factors that contribute to patellar malalignment. These factors are often seen in combination, and contributions by each must be prioritized before surgical treatment is contemplated. Patients with a tight lateral retinaculum, patellar tilt, and a normal Q angle seem to respond most consistently to LRR. The

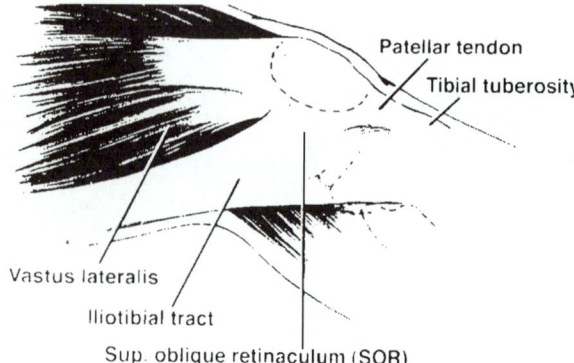

Figure 55.1. Extensor mechanism showing the superior oblique retinaculum interdigitating with the fibers of the vastus lateralis and patellar tendon. Reprinted with permission from Banas MP, Ferkel RD, Friedman MJ. Arthroscopic lateral retinacular release of the patellofemoral joint. Op Tech Sports Med 1994;2:291–296.

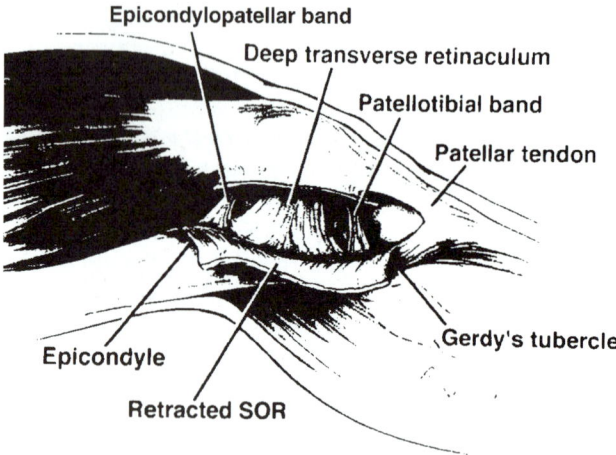

Figure 55.2. Deep transverse retinaculum with the epicondylopatellar and patellotibial expansions. *SOR,* superior oblique retinaculum. Reprinted with permission from Banas MP, Ferkel RD, Friedman MJ. Arthroscopic lateral retinacular release of the patellofemoral joint. Op Tech Sports Med 1994;2:291–296.

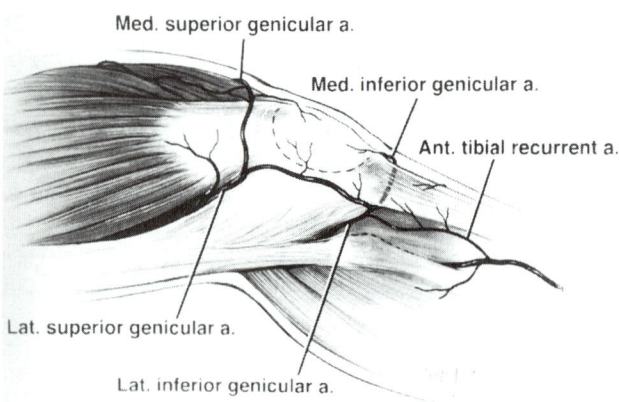

Figure 55.3. Vascular anatomy of the anterior knee. Reprinted with permission from Banas MP, Ferkel RD, Friedman MJ. Arthroscopic lateral retinacular release of the patellofemoral joint. Op Tech Sports Med 1994;2:291–296.

table	55.1	Factors That Contribute to Patellar Malalignment

Abnormal Q angle secondary to
  Excessive knee valgus
  Lateralization of tibial tubercle
  External rotation of the tibia
  Excessive femoral anteversion
Dysplasia of the femoral condyles
Patella alta
Insufficient vastus medialis obliquus
Tight lateral retinaculum
Generalized ligamentous laxity

Modified from Halbrecht JL, Jackson DW. Acute dislocation of the patella. In: Fox JM, Del Pizzo W, eds. The patellofemoral joint. New York: McGraw-Hill, 1993:124.

tight lateral retinaculum causes the patella to tilt laterally in the trochlear groove, which is one probable cause of anterior knee pain, originating from the compressed lateral facet of the patella or perhaps from the retinaculum itself.

The functional lateralization of the patella is called the lateral patellar compression syndrome (LPCS). The concept was first popularized by Ficat et al. (8) and was later modified to include the radiographic finding of lateral patellar tilt. The excessively tight retinaculum is thought to be the primary cause of the tilt. As the knee flexes, however, the patella is forced into a reduced position in the trochlear groove, which may stretch the tight lateral structures. The joint reaction force is increased across the lateral facet of the patella, which may lead to arthrosis. The result is inflammation and scarring, which further perpetuate the problem. This condition is also known as excessive lateral pressure syndrome (ELPS). LPCS and ELPS are similar, and ELPS is often used to describe the later stages of LPCS, when arthrosis develops (the origin of the terms is likely the result of differences in translation from the original French). LPCS and ELPS must be differentiated from subluxation of the patella, in which lateral instability is the primary disorder (Chapter 57). Although tilt and subluxation may coexist, it is important to evaluate these components separately. This chapter focuses on disorders that are amenable to isolated lateral retinacular release.

There is some confusion regarding the term *chondromalacia patellae* in the orthopaedic literature. It is an old term that is frequently misused as a diagnosis in patients with anterior knee pain. These patients are better served by a more specific diagnosis that is based on all the findings. Chondromalacia actually refers to the gross or histologic appearance of articular cartilage. It is not a diagnosis made by clinical evaluation, and we discourage the use of the term. Chondromalacia should be restricted to those patients with proven articular cartilage disease and no evidence of patellar malalignment.

Classification

Schutzer et al.'s (9) classification of patellofemoral malalignment brought attention to the important distinction between patellar tilt and subluxation. They distinguished three basic types of malalignment: patellar subluxation (type I), a combination of tilt and subluxation (type II), and patellar tilt (type III). Schutzer et al. described subtypes within each group that indicate the degree of patellofemoral arthrosis. The classic presentation of LPCS or ELPS is the patient with either normal alignment or type III malalignment. Several reports indicate that such patients respond most favorably and most predictably to lateral retinacular release (10–17). The majority of classic studies of LRR do not differentiate between tilt and subluxation. Frequently, all patellar pain disorders were lumped together as patellar subluxation. These disorders included everything from LPCS to chronic patellar dislocation; thus the results are difficult to interpret.

INITIAL FINDINGS, PHYSICAL EXAMINATION, AND DIAGNOSIS

Often the most important clinical information will arise from the patient's history. The history should address the following:

Onset and progression of instability and pain
Any incident of trauma
Previously documented dislocations
Characteristics of the pain
Any sensation of instability
Presence of swelling
Any other joint problems
Presence of generalized hyperlaxity
Previous treatment and results of such treatment

In classic LPCS, the pain is dull, poorly localized, and generally without traumatic origin. On the other hand, the patient may report a relatively trivial incident trauma. Pain in LPCS is aggravated by activities that load the patellofemoral joint, such as stair climbing, squatting, and even sitting for long periods of time (such as in a movie theater).

Even when the patient's history suggests a patellofemoral problem, the clinician should address other sources of knee complaints. The physical examination must first briefly rule out other infrequent but important causes of knee pain, such as referred pain from the hip or lumbar spine. Reflex sympathetic dystrophy is a rare but reported cause of knee pain and must also be evaluated.

Gait and standing alignment can be assessed as the patient walks into the room. It is critical that both lower extremities be well visualized, so findings such as excessive pronation of the feet or excessive tibiofemoral valgus can be noted. With the patient on the table, the clinician should first observe the muscle groups around the knee and measure thigh circumference for evidence of quadriceps atrophy. In particular, symmetry of the bulk of the vastus medialis should be noted.

The Q angle is measured with the patient supine (Fig. 55.4). This angle is formed by the intersection of a line drawn from the anterior superior iliac spine to the patella

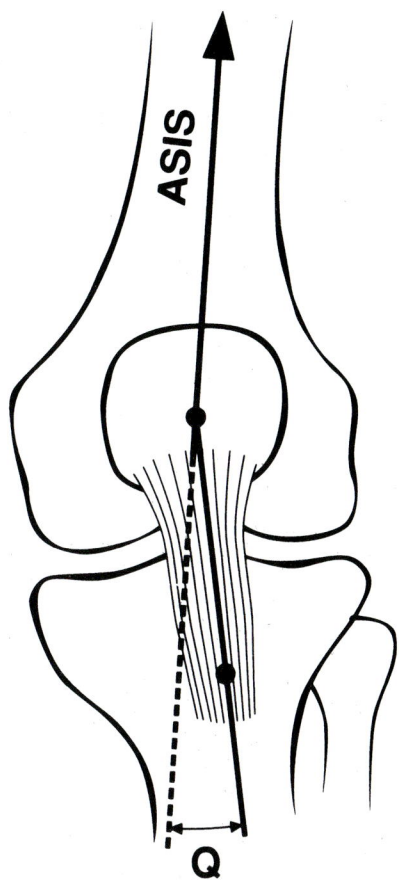

Figure 55.4. The Q angle is measured with the patient supine and knee extended. *ASIS,* anterior superior iliac spine. Reprinted with permission from Merchant AC. The lateral patellar compression syndrome. In: Fox JM, Del Pizzo W, eds. The patellofemoral joint. New York: McGraw-Hill, 1993:161.

and a line drawn from the patella to the tibial tubercle. A study of 150 normal knees found the average Q angle to be 15° (18). The average angle in men was 14°, and in women it was 17°. Based on this study, a normal Q angle should be 20° or less. Causes of an abnormal Q angle include excessive knee valgus, a lateral tibial tubercle, femoral anteversion, and external tibial torsion (Table 55.1).

It may be more helpful to measure the tubercle-sulcus angle, which is actually a fairly accurate measurement of the distal restraint vector (Fig. 55.5). It is measured with the knee flexed to 90°. In this position, the patella should be centralized within the sulcus. A vertical line is referenced by a midpoint in the patella and a midpoint in the tibial tubercle. This line should be perpendicular to a line through the transepicondylar axis. The normal angle is 0°, and an angle of 10° or more is considered to be abnormal.

The knee is then taken through a range of motion, while the clinician notes the presence of any crepitus. As the knee flexes, the patella should engage the trochlea smoothly at 30° of flexion, and an abnormal shift from a more lateral position into the trochlea should occur. This abnormal shift is known as the J sign. An effusion may indicate a recent dislocation or the presence of osteoarthri-

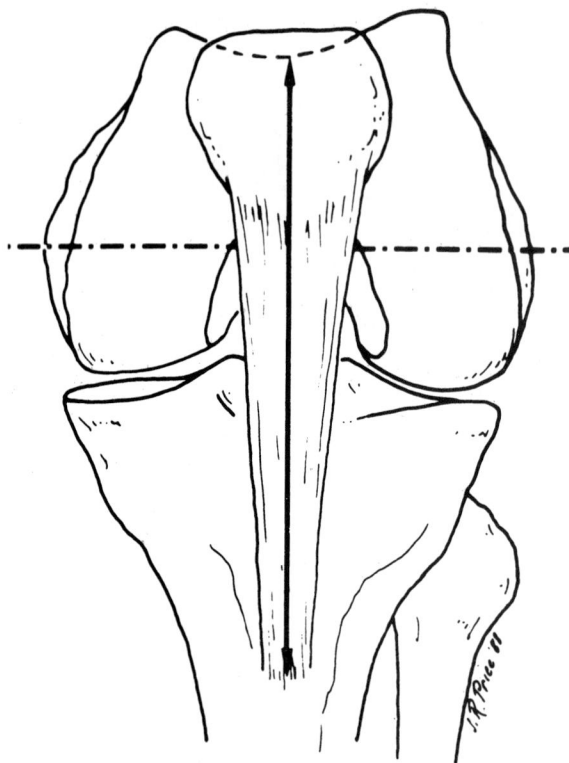

Figure 55.5. The tubercle-sulcus angle, which is normally 0°, is measured with the knee in 90° of flexion. Reprinted with permission from Kolowich PA, Paulos LE, Rosenberg TP, Farnsworth S. Lateral release of the patella. Am J Sports Med 1990;18:359–365.

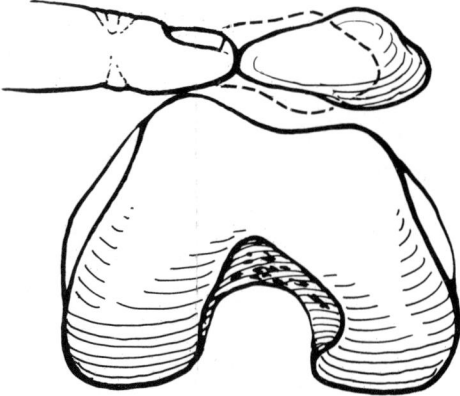

Figure 55.6. Patellar glide test performed with the patient supine and the knee flexed to 30°. Less than one quadrant of medial mobility indicates tight lateral restraints.

tis. Next, the clinician evaluates the collateral ligaments and cruciate ligament and palpates for joint line tenderness to screen for common problems such as anterior cruciate ligament (ACL) insufficiency and meniscal pathology. The techniques for this portion of the examination are covered in Chapter 61.

The patellar grind test is performed by placing gentle compression on the patella and asking the patient to contract the quadriceps. If pain is present, the test is positive and indicates the likelihood of articular cartilage defects contributing to the patient's problem. The medial and lateral retinacula are palpated to check for tenderness.

The patellar glide test is performed to assess integrity or tightness of the retinacular restraints (Fig. 55.6). With the knee flexed 20° to 30° and the quadriceps relaxed, the patella is longitudinally divided by imaginary lines into four quadrants. The patella is then passively displaced medially. Less than one quadrant of motion indicates a tight lateral restraint (also known as a positive Sage sign) (13). The clinician then displaces the patella laterally, noting the patient's level of anxiety during the maneuver. A sense of impending dislocation of the patella at this time describes the classic apprehension sign (19). A positive apprehension sign indicates that lateral displacement reproduces the patient's instability, which may be associated with pain. Up to two quadrants of lateral displacement may be normal, but three or four quadrants indicate deficiency in the medial restraint.

The patellar tilt test is performed next (Fig. 55.7). The patella is passively tilted with the examiner's thumb between the lateral femoral condyle and the lateral margin of the patella. Up to 15° of tilt is considered normal; a lateral retinacular tether is confirmed if the patella cannot be tilted past neutral.

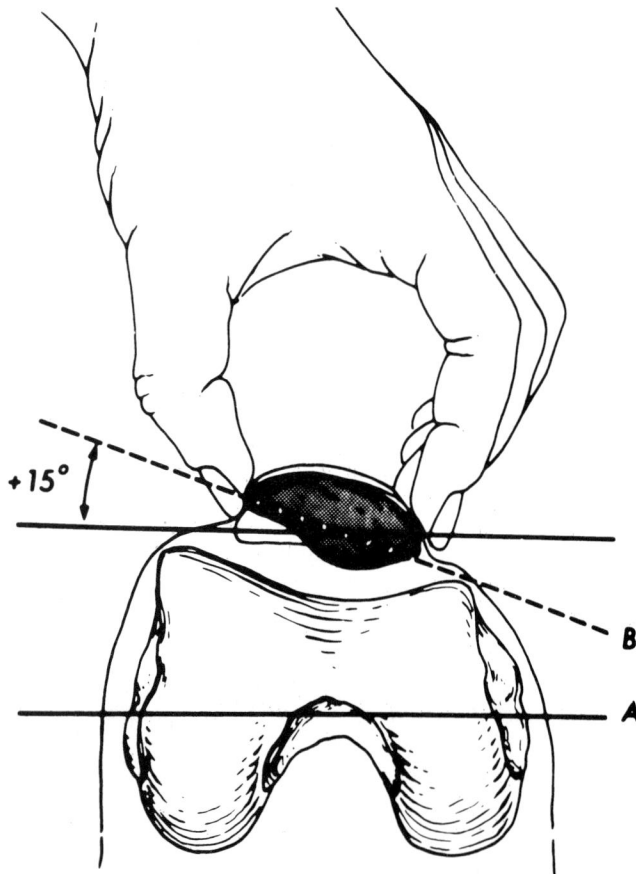

Figure 55.7. Passive patellar tilt test. Reprinted with permission from Kolowich PA, Paulos LE, Rosenberg TP, Farnsworth S. Lateral release of the patella. Am J Sports Med 1990;18:359–365.

The lateral pull sign analyzes the vector of quadriceps contraction. It is performed by observing the movement of the patella while the patient actively contracts the quadriceps with the knee in full extension and the muscles relaxed. If the patellar excursion is in a more lateral direction than in a straight superior position, there is a lateral quadriceps vector.

The examination for generalized ligamentous laxity is important, although commonly overlooked. The clinician assesses this by asking the patient to touch the forearm with his or her thumb. Checking for hyperextension of the elbows and knees also may be helpful. There is evidence to suggest that isolated LRR in patients with ligamentous laxity may have a less predictable outcome than LRR in other patients (20).

RADIOGRAPHIC EVALUATION

Standing AP, 30° flexion lateral, and Merchant views are obtained. The AP view is used to evaluate overall coronal alignment and to rule out other articular pathology. The lateral view is better suited for evaluation of the patellofemoral joint. The clinician should look for subchondral sclerosis and other evidence of degenerative joint disease. Patella alta and baja can be noted using Insall and Salvati's method (21) (Fig. 55.8). The length of the patellar tendon is divided by the length of the patella; the average ratio in Insall and Salvati's series was 1.02 (SD = 0.13). Thus the upper limit of normal for this ratio is estimated to be 1.2. It is helpful to remember that the inferior pole of the patella should be roughly at the level of Blumensaat's line (22), which is the radiographic roof of the intercondylar notch. This is noted on the lateral radiograph with the knee flexed at 30°.

The Merchant view is taken with the knee flexed to 45°; the x-ray beam is angled 30° caudal to the plane of the femur (6). This view can provide radiographic evidence of patellar subluxation. Using the technique illustrated in Figure 55.9, a positive number indicates that the patella is resting lateral to the bisector line. It is crucial to note the limitations of this x-ray. First, although tilt may be identified, there is no standardized way to quantify tilt from this radiographic view. In other words, the Merchant view is used to measure subluxation only. Second, this view gives information about the knee only at 45° of flexion. Even dramatic malalignment problems may sometimes be detected only at 15° or 30°; and by 45° of flexion, the patella may be relatively well seated in the trochlea.

A congruence angle of +16° or more was considered abnormal by Merchant et al. (6). This is a large number, considering the average congruence angle in their series was −6°. Aglietti et al. (18) found that the average congruence angle in 150 normal knees was −6° in men and −10° in women. In pathologic knees with patellar subluxation, however, the mean angle was +16°. For simplicity, we consider any positive congruence angle as a sign of possible malalignment. The greater the positive angle, the greater

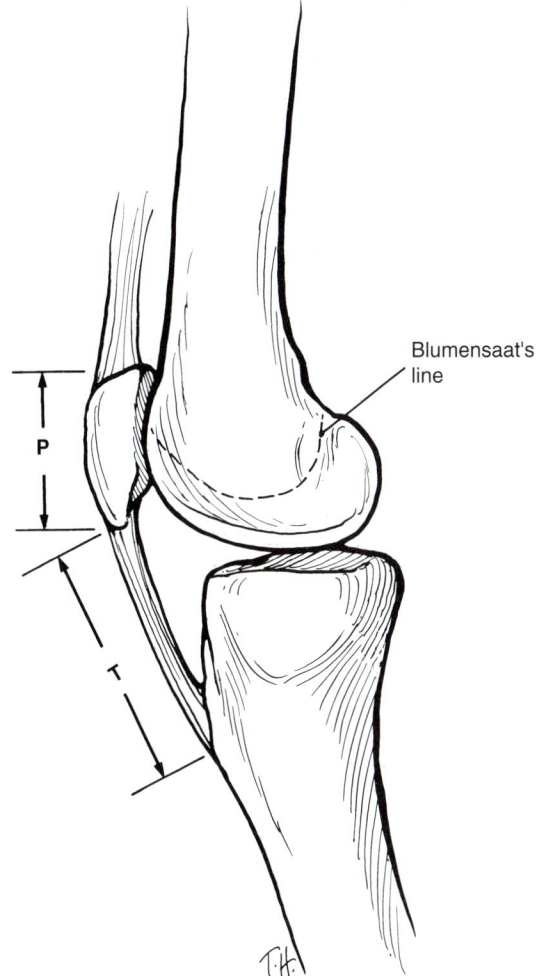

Figure 55.8. The Insall-Salvati ratio equals the length of the patellar tendon (*T*) divided by the length of the patella (*P*). The *T:P* ratio should equal 1; the upper limit of normal is 1.2. Note that the inferior pole of the patella is roughly at the level of the roof of the intercondylar notch.

the severity of lateral patellar subluxation. To assess patellar tilt, the clinician must obtain an additional film (the Laurin view) with the knee flexed to 20° (6). Patellar tilt is measured as illustrated in Figure 55.10. Normally, the lateral facet angle (α) will open laterally. Note that with a lateral patellar tether, this angle will be 0 or may even open medially.

A more exact method of measuring subluxation involves a CT or MRI scan. It is possible to obtain precise measurements of congruence at various amounts of knee flexion. Schutzer et al. (24) used CT to study the tracking of the patella in normal knees. They found that when the knee is in full extension, the patella is normally slightly lateralized, in terms of congruence angles (+2.5°). By 10° of flexion, however, the patella is normally well centered or even slightly medial. If the congruence angle remains positive beyond 10° of flexion, the patella may be considered subluxed. Patients with LPCS often have normal radiographs. CT or MRI studies can reveal the behavior of the

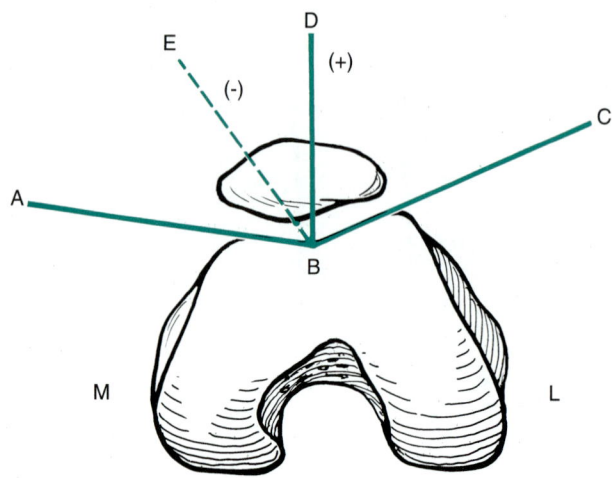

Figure 55.9. The sulcus angle is measured first by drawing lines *AB* and *BC,* which are tangential to the condyles. Line *BD* bisects the sulcus angle. Line *BE* runs through the medial ridge of the patella. Note that if the patella is centered medial to this line, a negative value is obtained, which indicates a normal patellofemoral relationship. *M,* medial; *L,* lateral.

patellofemoral joint between 0° and 45° of knee flexion. Fulkerson et al. (25) studied preoperative and post-LRR CT scans and demonstrated a much more dramatic postoperative change in tilt angle than in congruence angle (25). This was more pronounced in patients who had preoperative abnormal tilt (Schutzer et al. types II and III).

TREATMENT

Nonoperative Treatment and Indications for Surgery

Between 80 and 90% of patients with LPCS will respond to conservative treatment. The mainstay of this treatment is physical therapy, although there is a role for ice and anti-inflammatory medications if a significant inflammatory

component is present. Kowall et al. (27) seemed to question the benefits of patellar taping techniques, but we believe it still has a role in the rehabilitation protocol. Orthotics to control patellar tracking may also be useful in conservative management of patellofemoral malalignment problems.

Before recommending a specific rehabilitation program, the orthopaedist must clearly understand the structural abnormalities of the individual patient. Clearly, we do not have complete understanding how or why therapy is so successful for these problems. We do know, however, that of all the alignment abnormalities (e.g., normal Q angle, dysplasia of the femoral condyles, and torsional problems) the only elements amenable to rehabilitation are an atrophic vastus medialis obliquus (VMO) and possibly a tight lateral retinaculum. There are good exercise and stretching programs for these problems.

Therapy is aimed at quadriceps strengthening through progressive resistive exercises with the knee maintained near full extension. It is critical to understand that the joint reaction forces across the patellofemoral joint increase many-fold while doing standard knee extension exercises that begin with the knee in flexion. Stretching of the lateral retinaculum may also be useful, but the benefit is not as predictable. Other types of closed-chain exercises, such as the bicycle, treadmill, and cross-country ski machine, may be added to the rehabilitation program later.

To optimize surgical results it is imperative that the specific indications for performing LRR exist (Clinical Table). The history, physical examination, and radiographic information must all point to tight lateral restraints as the primary cause of the malalignment. Findings associated with the most successful outcomes include (*a*) normal lateral glide (fewer than two quadrants), (*b*) normal Q angle or tubercle-sulcus angle, (*c*) medial patellar glide at one to two quadrants, (*d*) negative or neutral patellar tilt, and (*e*) a superior or superolateral lateral pull test with no more than a 1:1 ratio of lateral:superior patellar migration (27). Note that these findings describe Schutzer et al. type

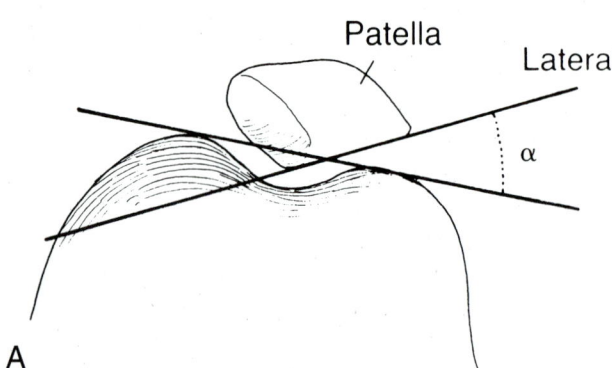

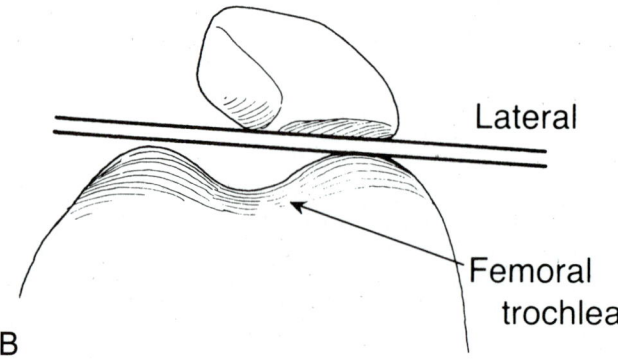

Figure 55.10. A. On the Laurin view of a normal knee, a line drawn across the femoral condyles intersects a line drawn through the lateral facet, forming angle α. **B.** In a knee with abnormal tilt, these lines are parallel; sometimes they intersect so that α opens laterally.

Reprinted with permission from Fulkerson JP. Patellofemoral pain disorders: evaluation and management. J Am Acad Orthop Surg 1994; 2:124–132. © American Academy of Orthopaedic Surgeons.

III and some type II malalignment patients. Good results can also be expected in well-selected patients with isolated patellar subluxation, as long as severe malalignment is not present (28).

Equally important is recognition of relative contraindications to isolated LRR. Other authors have attempted to identify factors associated with poor results following LRR (13,19); in general, our experience has been similar to theirs. These findings have been associated with less-than-optimal results in LRR: (a) deficient medial restraint, (b) patella alta, (c) small hypermobile patella, (d) major bony malalignment or abnormal tubercle-sulcus angle, (e) multiple patellar dislocations, and (f) greater than grade II cartilage changes. Mild degrees of arthrosis seem to have little effect on the results of LRR, but moderate to severe chondral injury seems to lead to less satisfactory results.

Operative Treatment

The patient is placed in the supine position and a general or regional anesthetic is administered. Although tourniquet is placed on the proximal thigh, it is generally used only if absolutely necessary for visualization. The use of an arthroscopic fluid pump almost eliminates the need for a tourniquet.

After the patient is prepared and draped in the standard fashion, a superomedial portal is made for fluid inflow. If a fluid pump is used, the diagnostic arthroscopy is begun by making an anterolateral portal for viewing. An anteromedial portal is made for fluid outflow (if using the pump) or for instrumentation. A standard diagnostic arthroscopy is performed, and other intra-articular abnormalities may be treated at this time. The patella is débrided, if necessary, by viewing through the anteromedial portal and shaving from the anterolateral portal.

Because the patella is sometimes tilted or subluxed laterally, this often provides the best angle for instrumentation. The lateral release is optimally performed last, since fluid extravasation is common after the retinaculum is incised.

The arthroscope is then introduced into the superomedial portal, and patellar tracking is evaluated. The electrosurgical instrument is placed into the joint through a nonconductive cannula in the anterolateral portal. Before beginning, the arthroscopic fluid must be changed to a nonconductive medium, such as glycine. After the surgeon verifies the settings on the generator (commonly 10 W), the LRR is performed.

Electrosurgery is best performed by activating the energy source while the tip of the instrument is approximately 1 mm from the tissue. A spinal needle is placed at the superior pole of the patella for orientation, and the release is performed from proximal to distal at about 5 mm from the border of the patella. The distal extent of the release is the inferior border of the anterolateral portal. Proximally, the surgeon should use caution to avoid violation of the vastus lateralis muscle or tendon. As the tissue is incised with the electrosurgical instrument, the depth of the release is constantly monitored. The release is performed from inside out, so the deep transverse retinaculum with proximal and distal expansion are incised first (Figs. 55.11 and 55.12). The superficial retinaculum is released next. The sight of subcutaneous tissue indicates that both layers of the retinaculum have been incised. Caution must also be used when completing the release distally around the anterolateral portal, since this is most vulnerable to thermal injury.

At the completion of the procedure, the surgeon repeats the passive patellar tilt test, or the turn-up test (Fig. 55.13). The surgeon should be able to tilt the patella 60° to

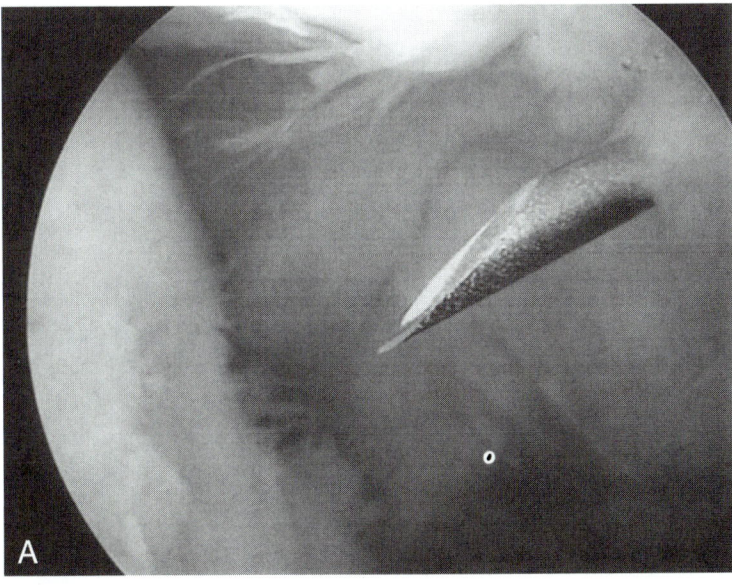

Figure 55.11. A. The arthroscopic lateral retinacular release begins at the level of the superior pole of the patella. *(continued)*

Figure 55.11. *(continued)* **B.** The deep transverse retinaculum is released. Reprinted with permission from Banas MP, Ferkel RD, Friedman MJ. Arthroscopic lateral retinacular release of the patellofemoral joint. Op Tech Sports Med 1994;2:291–296.

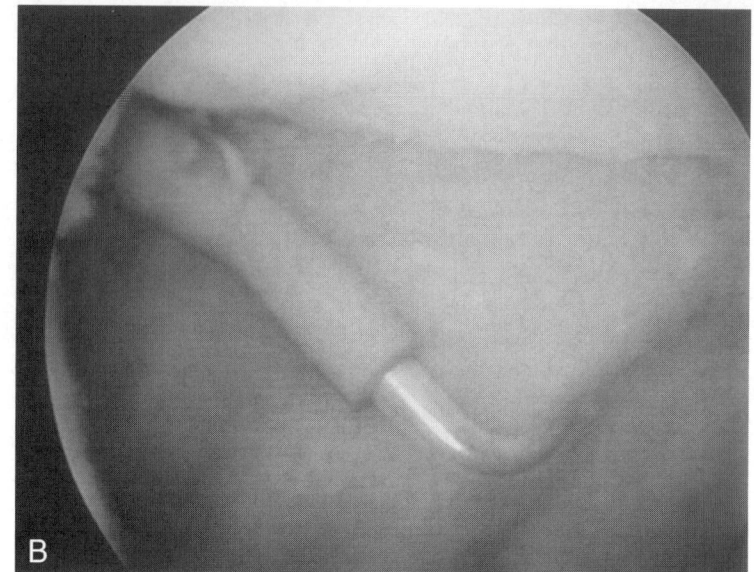

Figure 55.12. A. Release of the epicondylopatellar and patellotibial bands of the deep transverse retinaculum. **B.** Release of the superficial oblique retinaculum. Reprinted with permission from Banas MP, Ferkel RD, Friedman MJ. Arthroscopic lateral retinacular release of the patellofemoral joint. Op Tech Sports Med 1994;2:291–296.

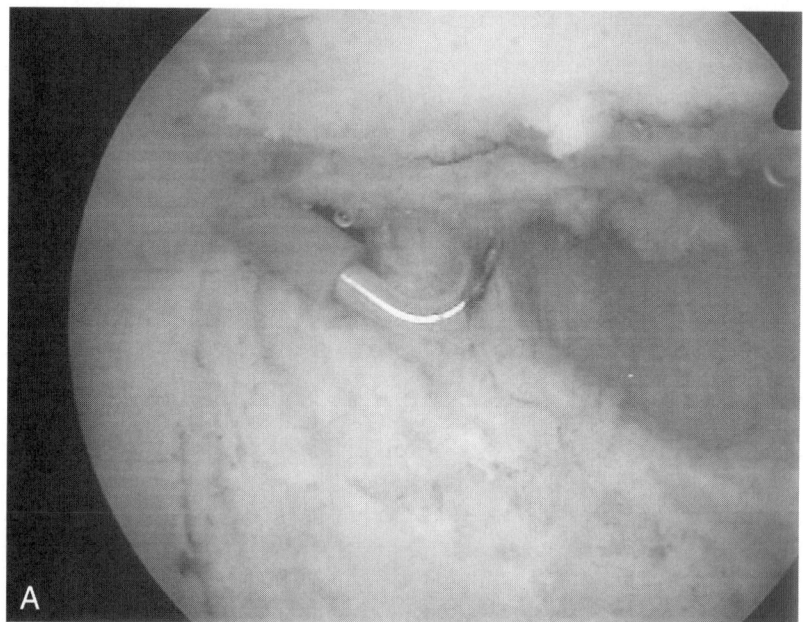

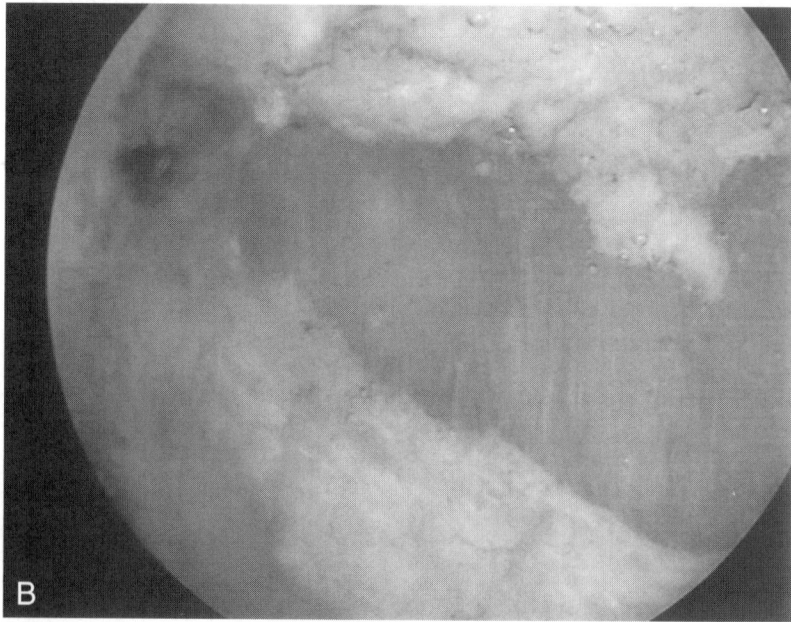

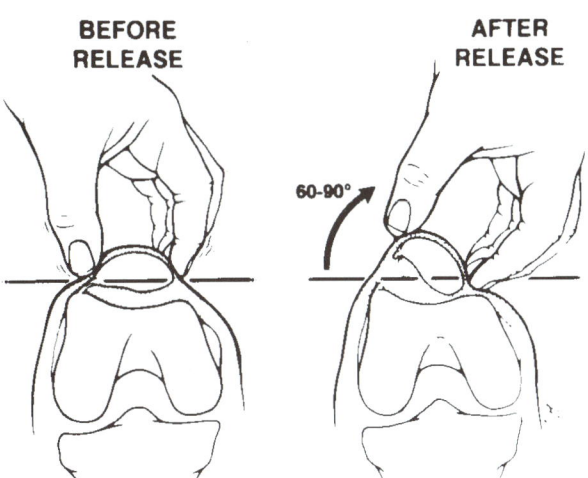

Figure 55.13. At the completion of the release, the turn-up test is performed to ensure 60° to 90° of tilt. Reprinted with permission from Banas MP, Ferkel RD, Friedman MJ. Arthroscopic lateral retinacular release of the patellofemoral joint. Op Tech Sports Med 1994;2:291–296.

90°, which should result in a final postoperative tilt of 30° to 45°. Hemostasis must be verified meticulously. If the surgeon uses a pump, the settings should be transiently lowered to identify additional bleeders. The arthroscopic fluid is then changed to Ringer's lactate to wash all the glycine from the knee. The wounds are closed with Steri-Strips, and dressings are held in place with a long-leg elastic support stocking. Postoperative drains are not used. A cold compression system is used whenever possible. Electrodes for electrical stimulation may be placed on the quadriceps, if desired.

PITFALLS AND COMMON MISTAKES

The greatest errors in performing LRR may occur secondary to poor patient selection and preoperative planning. For example, Hughston and Deese (3) noted the complication of medial subluxation following LRR in patients without malalignment. Nonetheless, the overall complication rate of the procedure is between 7 and 10% in most series. A multicenter study reported complications from 446 LRR procedures by arthroscopic surgeons (2). The overall complication rate was 7.2%. Hemarthrosis was the most common complication, and the most significant risk of complications was the use of a postoperative drain for 24 h or more. Higher complication rates were also noted when the surgeon used a tourniquet or an arthroscopically assisted technique, which involves making the release with scissors while viewing arthroscopically. There was no statistically increased risk of complications from the use of electrosurgical techniques.

The most common pitfalls of LRR surgery include inadequate release, sectioning the vastus lateralis tendon, and thermal injury. Errors in judging the extent of the release can be avoided by following the guidelines outlined above and by using a spinal needle to mark the superior

pole of the patella. In addition, good visualization is paramount and is facilitated by placing the arthroscope in the superomedial portal while performing the procedure.

After surgery, the patient may begin isometric exercises with active knee flexion. Crutches are used, but the patient may bear weight as tolerated. The dressings are changed after 48 h for showering. The elastic stocking is worn for approximately 1 week and changed; the patient wears a patellar brace when swelling is under control, at which time, a formal patellofemoral rehabilitation program is begun.

SUMMARY

Lateral retinacular release is a procedure that yields 80 to 90% good to excellent results when used judiciously. Poor results have been published repeatedly in the literature when patient selection failed to employ the principles outlined in this chapter. The attitude that it cannot hurt and can only help is no longer appropriate. The surgeon must have a clear mechanical sense of the patient's problems complemented by the history, physical examination, and radiographic findings. With adequate patient selection and surgical technique, lateral retinacular release is a relatively safe procedure with few complications, especially when performed with electrosurgical arthroscopic techniques.

REFERENCES

1. Willner P. Recurrent dislocation of the patella. Clin Orthop 1970; 69:213–215.
2. Small NC. An analysis of complications in lateral retinacular release procedures. Arthroscopy 1989;5:282–286.
3. Hughston JC, Deese M. Medial subluxation of the patella as a complication of lateral retinacular release. Am J Sports Med 1988; 16:383–388.
4. Nonweiler DE, DeLee JC. The diagnosis and treatment of medial subluxation of the patella after lateral retinacular release. Am J Sports Med 1994;22:680–686.
5. Hughston JC. Subluxation of the patella. J Bone Joint Surg 1968; 50A:1003–1026.
6. Merchant AC, Mercer RL, Jacobsen RH, Cool CR. Roentgenographic analysis of patellofemoral congruence. J Bone Joint Surg 1974;56A:1391–1396.
7. Insall J. Chondromalacia patellae: patellar malalignment syndrome. Orthop Clin North Am 1979;10:117–127.
8. Ficat P, Ficat C, Bailleau A. Syndrome d'hyperpression externe de la rotule (SHRF). Son intérêt pour la connaissance de l'arthpose. Rev Chir Orthop 1975;61:39–59.
9. Schutzer SF, Ramsby GR, Fulkerson JP. Computed tomographic classification of patellofemoral pain patients. Orthop Clin North Am 1986;17:235–248.
10. Fulkerson JP, Shea KP. Current concepts review. Disorders of the patellofemoral alignment. J Bone Joint Surg 1990;72A:1424–1429.
11. Kolowich PA, Paulos LE, Rosenberg TP, Farnsworth S. Lateral release of the patella. Am J Sports Med 1990;18:359–365.
12. Aglietti P, Pisaneschi A, Buzzi R, et al. Arthroscopic lateral release for patellar pain or instability. Arthroscopy 1989;5:176–183.
13. Gecha SR, Torg JS. Clinical prognosticators for the efficacy of retinacular release surgery to treat patellofemoral pain. Clin Orthop 1970;69:203–215.

14. Sherman OH, Fox JM, Sperling H. Patellar instability: treatment by arthroscopic electrosurgical lateral release. Arthroscopy 1987; 3:152–160.

15. Shea KP, Fulkerson JP. Preoperative computed tomography scanning and arthroscopy in predicting outcome of lateral retinacular release. Arthroscopy 1992;8:327–334.

16. Fulkerson JP. Patellofemoral pain disorders: evaluation and management. J Am Acad Orthop Surg 1994;2:124–132.

17. Fu FH, Moday ME. Arthroscopic lateral release and the lateral patellar compression syndrome. Orthop Clin North Am 1992; 23:601–612.

18. Aglietti P, Insall JN, Cerulli G. Patellar pain and incongruence. I: Measurements of incongruence. Clin Orthop 1983;176:217–224.

19. Dimon JH. Apprehension test for subluxation of the patella. Clin Orthop 1974;103:39.

20. Simpson LA, Barrett JP. Factors associated with poor results following arthroscopic subcutaneous lateral retinacular release. Clin Orthop 1984;186:165–171.

21. Insall J, Salvati E. Patella position in the normal knee joint. Radiology 1971;101:101–104.

22. Blumensaat C. Die lageabweichungen und verrenkungen der kniescheibe. Ergeb Chir Orthop 1938;31:149.

23. Deleted in proof.

24. Lauren CA, Dussault R, Levesque HP. The tangential x-ray investigation of the patellofemoral joint. Clin Orthop 1979;144:16–26.

25. Schutzer SF, Ramsby GR, Fulkerson JP. The evaluation of patellofemoral pain using computerized tomography—a preliminary study. Clin Orthop 1986;204:286–293.

26. Fulkerson JP, Schutzer SR, Ramsby GR. Computerized tomography of the patellofemoral joint before and after lateral release or realignment. Arthroscopy 1987;3:19–24.

27. Kowall MH, Kolk G, Nuber GW, et al. Patellar taping in the treatment of patellofemoral pain. A retrospective study. Am J Sports Med 1996;24:61–66.

28. Banas MP, Ferkel RD, Friedman MJ. Arthroscopic lateral retinacular release of the patellofemoral joint. Op Tech Sports Med 1994; 2:291–296.

29. Fabriciani C, Panni AS, Delcogliano A. Role of arthroscopic lateral release in the treatment of patellofemoral disorders. Arthroscopy 1992;8:531–536.

Richard A. Cautilli, Jr., and John P. Fulkerson

Patellar Malalignment: Distal Realignment*

The ideal state for the patellofemoral joint is one in which the retinacular structures are isometrically balanced both medially and laterally. In addition, the tracking vector of the patella should fall precisely into the femoral trochlea early in flexion and stay there as the trochlea deepens and the knee proceeds further into flexion. This should occur without undue pressure on the articular cartilage.

The purpose of this chapter is to review the concepts of distal extensor mechanism realignment. The relevant anatomy, pathogenesis, indications, and surgical techniques will be reviewed.

RELEVANT ANATOMY AND PATHOGENESIS

When patellar alignment is abnormal or unbalanced, an inappropriate increase in contact stress will occur. The most common malalignment patterns are patellar tilt and lateral subluxation. These patterns produce an overload of the lateral facet and late entry of the patella into the trochlea. The excessive lateral pressure causes shear stresses on the distal central and lateral aspects of the patella, leading to articular breakdown. In this alignment pattern the distal medial patellar articular surface may not have any contact, which generates a different type of articular change. Other patellar malalignment patterns may lead to subluxation and dislocation of the patella from the trochlea.

The tibial tubercle provides insertion for the patellar tendon and is the most anterior point on the tibia. The proximal epiphysis includes the proximal tibial plateau and the tibial tuberosity. The ossification nucleus of the proximal tibia is present at birth. The secondary ossification center of the tibial tubercle appears between the 9th and 14th year. By age 15 the upper epiphysis and the tu-

bercle are completely ossified. At 20 years, fusion with the tibial metaphysis is accomplished. Surgery at the tubercle before this time may lead to complications of recurvatum and distal migration (1).

Cross-sectional cuts through the tibia at the level of the tibial tuberosity demonstrate the triangular shape of the proximal tibia with the tuberosity at its apex. Therefore, the tibial tubercle can be transposed only a small distance medially before it produces an unwanted posterior displacement. Other osteotomies, however, can be performed to establish medialization and anteriorization, if additional anatomic features are kept in mind. It is important to note that the posterior lateral corner of the lateral limb of the triangular surface of the tibia is in close approximation to the anterior tibial artery, a terminal branch of the popliteal artery. The deep peroneal nerve, a terminal branch of the common peroneal also runs with the anterior tibial artery. This related anatomy is important when the osteotomy requires more anteriorization than medialization of the tibial tubercle such that a cut is made to the posterolateral tibia.

INITIAL FINDINGS, PHYSICAL EXAMINATION, AND DIAGNOSIS

The history and physical examination of the patient with patellofemoral malalignment are critical. In most cases, they reveal the diagnosis, and radiographic studies will be confirmatory. The key to understanding patellofemoral problems is to delineate instability patterns from articular problems of the patella. Making a specific diagnosis leads to the correct selection of an operative procedure.

In the history, questions about the onset of pain and previous dislocation or subluxation should be asked. The character (e.g., dull or lancinating) and onset (insidious or traumatic) of pain will help differentiate instability from articular problems. Patients with instability patterns may have prob-

---

*Parts of this chapter have been taken directly from Cautilli RA, Fulkerson JP. Operative treatment of patellofemoral disorders: distal realignment. Sports Med Arthosc Rev 1994;2:250–262, with permission.

lems with the knee giving way, especially with external rotation activities, because of quadriceps weakness. They may also complain of pain with prolonged sitting, e.g., during long car rides or at the theater. Patients with articular problems complain of cracking or crepitus with motion and especially with ascending stairs. These patients tend to complain of swelling and pain throughout the day.

The physical examination is an extension of the history. The examination begins with an evaluation of the patient in the standing position to assess varus and valgus alignment. The Q angle is determined by a line drawn from the anterior superior iliac spine through the center of the patella and then on to the tibial tubercle. This angle is normally 15° or less and is slightly higher in women than in men. A large Q angle and increased valgus are associated more with problems of instability. Signs of hyperelasticity of the joints, e.g., hyperextension of the knee, elbow, fingers, can indicate instability of the patella.

The knee is checked for range of motion and quadriceps tightness at extreme flexion. Palpation is then carried out to locate maximum areas of tenderness or tightness, especially of the lateral retinaculum. The patellar tendon and quadriceps tendon should also be palpated.

Patellar tilt is evaluated by lifting the lateral facet away from the femoral condyle. This test, which is performed while the patient is prone with the leg in extension, is normal if the patella is brought above the horizontal. Excessive lateral pressure syndrome with articular damage is common with patellae that do not tilt above the horizontal. While the knee is in extension, glide the patella both medially and laterally to evaluate retinacular tightness. Hold the patella medially and then abruptly flex the knee to check for medial subluxation. An apprehension test is performed at the end of lateral glide to assess patellar instability. Compression of the patella through a range of mo-

tion will also help differentiate articular problems from those of instability. Quadriceps and hamstring strength, tone, and girth should be evaluated. And while the patient is prone, quadriceps tightness and asymmetry of hip rotation should be examined.

RADIOLOGIC STUDIES

The radiologic evaluation of a patient with patellofemoral pain allows the clinician to confirm physical findings of malalignment. A standard radiologic series provides considerable information. A standing AP view quantifies varus and valgus deviation, height of the patella, and tubercle location. A true lateral view, which has the exact overlap of the femoral condyles, gives information on the shape of the femoral trochlea and indicates any dysplasia. The presence of patella alta or baja and tendon length can also be appreciated from these x-rays. A tangential view done with 20° to 30° of knee flexion gives additional information about the relationship of the patellofemoral joint to its static soft tissue restraints. A standard Merchant view with 30° or 45° of knee flexion is optimal. Knee flexion angles greater than this increase compression forces and force the patella into the trochlea (Fig. 56.1). In this view the rotation should be standardized. The congruence angle measures patellar subluxation and is determined from the tangential view (Fig. 56.2). This angle is formed by the perpendicular bisector of the trochlea angle and a line drawn from the posterior point of the patella to the center of the trochlea. If the angle lies medially, then medial subluxation exists; if it lies laterally, then lateral subluxation is present.

A CT scan of the patellofemoral joint can give additional information not appreciated on traditional radiographs. Midpatellar cuts at 15° to 20° of knee flexion allow the patellar tilt angle to be calculated (Fig. 56.3). Images may also be

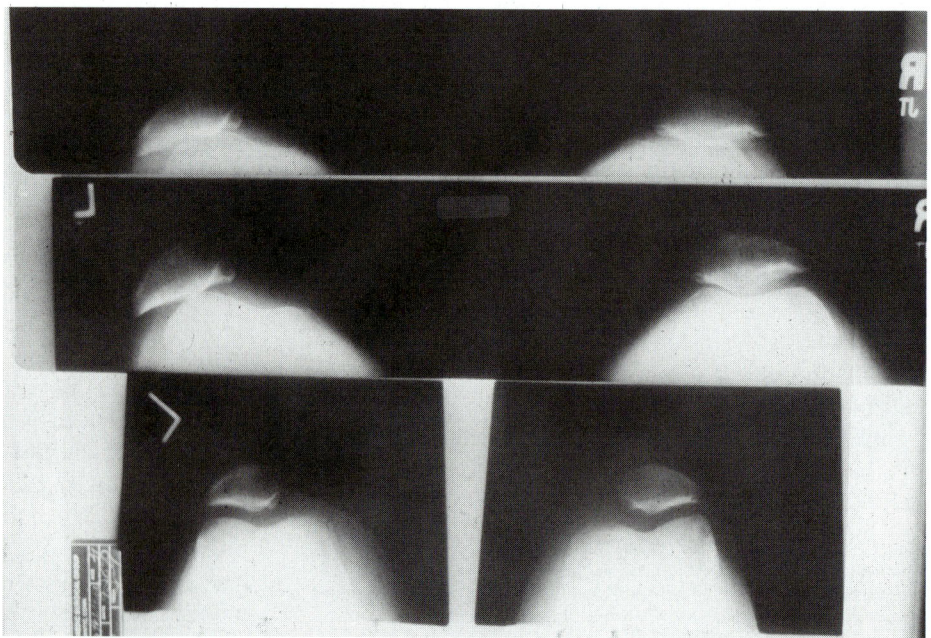

Figure 56.1. X-ray studies of the knee at increasing flexion angles from proximal to distal showing increasing compression forces pushing the patella into the trochlea.

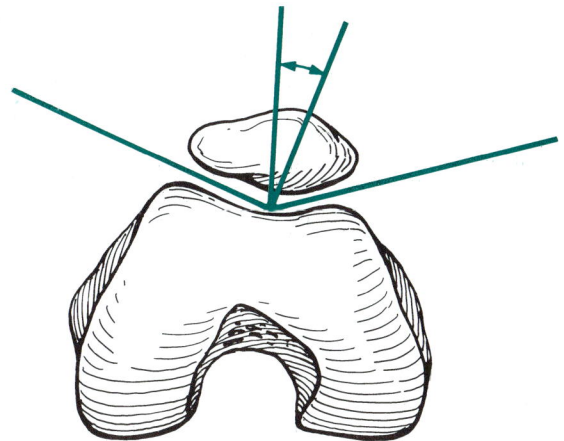

Figure 56.2. Congruence angle.

taken at 30° and 45° of knee flexion. Abnormal patellar tilt is indicated by the formation of an angle measuring less than 12° at the intersection of a line drawn from the lateral facet to the posterior femoral condyle. In addition, newer CT scanners can overlap images of the proximal and distal femur to allow measurement of femoral anteversion.

MRI provides much the same information as CT, because the patient is imaged in a similar supine position. The lack of bone detail is offset by the additional information obtained about the patellar articular cartilage. Controversy exists about the correlation of articular changes seen on MRI and the clinical symptomatology. MRI also allows visualization of medial and lateral retinacular structures but gives limited access to imaging at increasing knee flexion angles.

TREATMENT

Nonoperative Treatment

Conservative treatment of patellofemoral malalignment depends on the specific diagnosis, but several general principals are common to all nonoperative treatment programs. Initially, pain reduction must be accomplished. This can be done by rest, nonsteroidal anti-inflammatory

drugs (NSAIDs), injections, and analgesics. Once pain is controlled, the net phase of rehabilitation, which requires stretching the extensor mechanism, can be instituted. McConnell taping is effective in relieving pain during exercise in some patients and should be considered in the course of treatment.

Stretching is the second component of nonoperative treatment. Stretching of the tight structures round the knee aid greatly in pain reduction and return to function. Specific stretching of the lateral retinaculum and the iliotibial band, because of its attachment to the lateral retinaculum, is required in nonoperative treatment. Prone stretching of the quadriceps to achieve full flexion reduces compression forces on the patella. Closed-chain exercise, isometric exercises, and restricted range of motion (ROM) exercises allow strengthening of the extensor mechanism without significant increases in pain in many patients. Short arc quadriceps strengthening increases the strength in the atrophic vastus medialis obliquus (VMO) and may provide relief of symptoms. The progression to open-chain exercises and functional training complete the nonoperative treatment and return 85% of patients to their previous level of function.

Operative Treatment

There are two basic types of distal realignment procedures: those that involve distal soft tissue transfer and those that transfer the bony tibial tubercle (Clinical Table).

SOFT TISSUE PROCEDURES

The distal realignment procedures are always performed in conjunction with proximal soft tissue surgery. These include a lateral release and, if required, medial reefing. Soft tissue procedures are generally used for treating symptoms of instability, such as pain or giving way, rather than symptoms of patellofemoral pain. These procedures are most appropriate in patients who have not reached skeletal maturity. The primary soft tissue realignment procedures used today are the Galeazzi semitendinosus tenodesis, the Roux-Goldthwait patellar tendon transfer, and lateral release with medial imbrication.

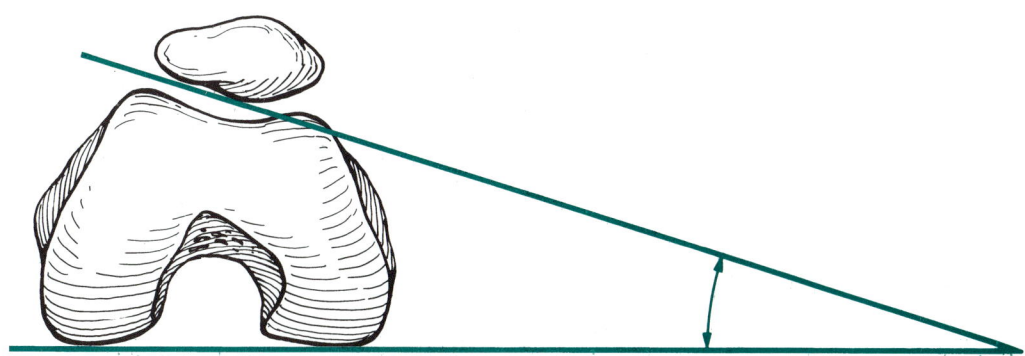

Figure 56.3. Patellar tilt angle.

Clinical Table: Patellar Malalignment: Distal Realignment

Procedure	Indications	Technique	Anatomy	Pitfalls
Galeazzi	• Skeletally immature • Instability	• Transfer of semitendinosus	• Semitendinosus • Vastus medialis obliquus • Patella	• Patellar fracture • Inadequate realignment • Chondral lesions
Roux-Goldthwait	• Skeletally immature • Instability	• Lateral patellar tendon transfer to medial side	• Patellar tendon • Tibial tubercle	• Tendon rupture • Inadequate realignment • Chondral lesion
Maquet	• Arthrosis • No malalignment	• Elevation of tibial tubercle • Interposed bone graft	• Vastus lateralis • Patellar tendon • Tibial tubercle	• Fracture of shingle • Difficulty with skin closure • Inadequate realignment • Neurovascular injury
Hauser	• None	• Distal and posterior tibial tubercle transfer	• Patellar tendon • Tibial tubercle	• Increase in contact stress leads to late arthrosis
Trillat	• Patellar instability • No chondrosis	• Medial tibial tubercle transfer	• Patellar tendon • Tibial tubercle	• Limited medial realignment
Anteromedialization	• Patellar malalignment • With chondrosis distally and laterally	• Anterior and medial shift of the tibial tubercle by oblique osteotomy	• Patellar tendon • Tibial tubercle	• Overtightening fixation reduces anteriorization • Trouble kneeling

Clinical Table: Patellofemoral Malalignment: Lateral Retinacular Release

Procedure	Indications	Technique	Anatomy	Pitfalls
LRR	• Patellar tilt	• Arthroscopic • Electrosurgery	• Lateral superior geniculate artery	• Medial subluxation • Hemarthrosis • Inadequate release • Sectioning of the vastus lateralis tendon

Galeazzi Semitendinosus Tenodesis

The semitendinosus tenodesis was initially detailed in 1921 by Galeazzi (2). This procedure involves detaching a split portion of the semitendinosus tendon proximal to its insertion while preserving its attachment to the pes anserinus. This slip of tendon is then passed through an oblique tunnel in the patella and then sutured to itself, which creates a passive medial and distal restraint to stabilize the patella in the trochlea. It is 81% effective in preventing dislocation but has poorer results with any degree of patella chondromalacia (3). A recent modification of the Galeazzi procedure uses a polyester ligament instead of the semitendinosus (4). This procedure, however, requires the use of a tunnel perpendicular to the long axis of the patella rather than an oblique tunnel. The polyester ligament is fixed to the medial femoral condyle by screw fixation and an interference knot at the lateral aspect of the patella. The modification has 95% good results in preventing dislocation.

These procedures have been criticized because they have no active realignment component. Poor results occur when there are chondral changes of the patella, and the tunnel may act as a stress riser where fractures of the patella can occur.

Roux-Goldthwait Patellar Tendon Transfer

Around the turn of the century, the patellar tendon transfer procedure was described independently by Roux and Goldthwait (5,6). In this procedure the lateral half of the patellar tendon is passed beneath the remaining tendon and sutured or stapled to the medial periosteum. Long-term studies show approximately 90% good to excellent results for recurrent dislocation only (7).

As with most distal soft tissue procedures, results were poor when there was severe chondromalacia or frank osteoarthritis of the patella (8). Furthermore, the Roux-Goldthwait procedure may create distal rotation and lateral tilt of the patella. Complications noted include patellar tendon rupture, loss of fixation, inadequate correction of malalignment, and the creation of patella baja or medial subluxation (9).

TIBIAL TUBERCLE PROCEDURES

Distal realignment procedures, using transfer of the tibial tubercle medially, anteriorly, or in combination, are most commonly used in skeletally mature patients. These procedures are always done in conjunction with lateral release and sometimes medial reefing. The direction in which the tibial tubercle is transferred depends on the specific pathologic condition to be addressed and the amount of incongruence seen radiographically. Although these procedures are effective in realigning the extensor mechanisms, some procedures, such as the Hauser, can cause problems.

Maquet's Procedure

Elevation with anterior displacement of the tibial tubercle was first described by Maquet (10). The procedure was devised to decrease the patellofemoral forces and provide an alternative to patellectomy in the patient with patellofemoral arthrosis and chondrosis. In the original description of the procedure, the osteotomy involved the tibial tubercle long with 12 cm of the tibial crest. A straight anterior elevation of 2 to 2.5 cm was achieved by interposing an iliac crest bone graft. Approximately 90% of patients reported good results in terms of pain relief and an increase in knee function (11).

Although this procedure is effective in relieving patellofemoral pain in 54 to 93% of patients, it has had a high complication rate, including skin necrosis, deep venous thrombosis (DVT), fracture of the crest, nonunion, and infection (12).

The Hauser Technique

The Hauser technique of tibial tubercle transfer strives to realign the patellar and extensor mechanism to prevent recurrent dislocation of the patella (13). In the original procedure, the patellar tendon insertion into the tibial tubercle was detached with a small piece of bone and transferred medially and distally. It was originally reattached with a screw, but this was later modified to a keyhole technique. In this modification, the bony fragment was trapped beneath the cortical bone by rotating it in place, obviating additional fixation. This bony transfer was combined with a lateral release and a vastus medialis advancement.

Although the Hauser procedure is effective in preventing dislocation, it increases the patellofemoral contract forces, which leads to late degenerative changes (14). This painful condition is noted on long-term follow-up and is the main reason that this procedure has fallen out of favor (15). Complications include compartment syndrome, infections, and peroneal nerve palsy. This procedure should not be done.

The Elmslie-Trillat Procedure

In 1964, Trillat et al. (16) described a procedure that involved tilting and medializing the tibial tubercle in combination with lateral release and medial reefing. The procedure is designed to align the extensor mechanism to prevent dislocation and subluxation, but it does not involve the distal advancement and tightening of the extensor mechanism of the Hauser operation (16). Cox (17) pop-ularized this procedure and found 88% good results in preventing recurrent dislocation at 2 years. Unfortunately, Cox noted that the results deteriorated over time, especially in the presence of interarticular pathology.

A review of the Trillat procedure noted that in some cases the results tend to be poor in patients with established patellofemoral articular abnormalities (18).

Anteromedialization

The anteromedialization procedure combines the best features of the Trillat procedure (i.e., correction of patellar tilt and lateral subluxation) with the anterior displacement concept of the Maquet procedure (19). In this procedure, an oblique osteotomy is performed from the medial aspect of the tibial tubercle and the lateral triangular surface of the proximal tibia. The osteotomized fragment is then displaced anteriorly and medially. The obliquity of the osteotomy determines whether the primary correction should be in the anterior or medial plane. The osteotomy is tailored to suit the degree of malalignment and articular damage seen in the patient. The correction is done without changing the volume within the soft tissues, and skin closure is done without tension. This aspect obviates the complication of skin slough that is so often seen with the Maquet procedure.

Patients with preoperative patellofemoral pain and moderate articular damage subjectively reported 93% good to excellent results; when objective criteria were used, 89% good to excellent results were noted (20). Patients followed for more than 5 years maintained this improvement. Anteromedialization can effect tubercle elevation of up to 1.7 cm without bone graft.

Complications include DVT and tibial tubercle fracture. Some surgeons believe that the procedure's disadvantages include difficulty in kneeling, hypesthesia around the scar, possible delayed union, and metal bursitis (21).

INDICATIONS FOR SURGERY

Cartilage deterioration and many patellofemoral pain problems are directly related to increased pressure on the articular cartilage; however, articular cartilage of the patella can also degenerate because of diminished contact stress as a result of extensor mechanism imbalance. The most common area affected is at the distal medial and/or central aspect of the patella. Ficat described this as the "critical zone." He noted that the cartilage of the distal pole of the patella was consistently softened or fibrillated in patients with lateral patellofemoral alignments. Presumably, the cartilage breaks down because of insufficient contact pressure to force nutrient synovial fluid into the cartilaginous cells.

The thrust of any well-done extensor mechanism realignment should be to restore stable patellofemoral tracking while minimizing or eliminating contact with deficient articular cartilage, which may be causing pain. The distal central region of the patella is particularly difficult to deal with because it is so commonly degenerated in patients with extensor mechanism malalignment. Consequently, procedures that might cause increased stress on this region of the patella can potentially create a painful articulation.

The distal central or medial critical zone is not the only region of the patella to consider when deciding what operation to choose. The surgeon must also recognize that patients who have sustained patellar dislocation commonly shear off articular cartilage medially at the time of patellar relocation. Consequently, the medial facet can be damaged because of deficient or abnormal shear stress distally and as a result of injury following patellar dislocation.

This background understanding of patellar articular lesion is of central importance in deciding whether to do proximal or distal realignment. When there is a significant lesion noted on the distal aspect of the patella related to the malalignment, the surgeon should consider distal realignment, with anteriorization of the tibial tubercle to diminish loading on the distal medial to central aspect of the patella. Similarly, anteriorization of the tibial tubercle to diminish contact stress on a deficient medial facet will minimize stresses to a deficient medial patella injured at the time of dislocation. Fortunately, many patients with patellar instability maintain good, intact articular cartilage at the proximal medial aspect of the patella. Again, anteromedial transfer of the tibial tubercle will shift contact stress onto this region and away from the distal and lateral aspects of the patella, where there are often articular lesions related to malalignment.

Proximal realignment and soft tissue procedures are most appropriate in the skeletally immature patient with lateral instability of the patella. Carefully performed, proximal realignment is also appropriate for skeletally mature patients who do not have patellar lesions or whose lesions are such that there will be no increased contact stresses.

SURGICAL TECHNIQUE

Basic Approach

The surgical approach to tibial tubercle realignment is similar for most patients. The surgeon should perform routine arthroscopy of the extensor mechanism with the patient supine on the operating table and should examine the patella from a superomedial or superolateral approach as well as from a distal approach. This allows confirmation of the preoperative impression regarding tracking and alignment. The arthroscopic assessment helps the surgeon choose the appropriate realignment procedure, moving the patella onto remaining intact articular cartilage and into a satisfactory alignment in regard to the femoral trochlea. At the time of the arthroscopic evaluation, the surgeon must also rule out other intra-articular problems, loose bodies, pathologic plica, and osteochondritis dissecans.

Although fragments of the articular lesion can be débrided arthroscopically, the surgeon should also look at the patella directly, whenever possible, to be sure that all lesions have been adequately treated. Open visualization of the patella through a lateral release incision sometimes reveals a significant articular lesion that was missed with the arthroscope.

Exposure for the tibial tubercle transfer should be through a vertical midline incision; depending on the specific osteotomy, it can be moved slightly to the medial or lateral side. The plane of the osteotomy is then determined based on the areas of damage to the articular cartilage and specific malalignment. The typical Trillat procedure requires a flat osteotomy in the coronal plane deep to the tibial tubercle. The osteotomy for an anteromedial tibial tubercle shaft will start just medial to the patellar tendon insertion and, depending on the relative amounts of anteriorization and medialization desired, be directed at a 10° to 15° angle from the coronal to sagittal plane.

If the surgeon desires straight anteriorization, a steep anteromedial tibial tubercle osteotomy plane is created. A bone graft can then be placed in the osteotomy site to offset the tibial tubercle laterally, thus giving straight anteriorization. To accomplish an anterolateral shift of the tibial tubercle (e.g., to salvage a failed Hauser procedure or overmedialization of the tibial tubercle), the osteotomy will be more shallow. In that case, the surgeon must remember that the medial tibial triangular surface is less steep than the lateral tibial surface, so the osteotomy plane created will permit less anteriorization.

Anteromedialization of the Tibial Tubercle

A straight midline or slightly anterolateral incision is made from the middle portion of the patella to 5 to 8 cm distal to the tuberosity. The previously described curvilinear incision from the lateral aspect of the patella may be modified to a standard longitudinal midline incision, if a total knee replacement may be required later. The surgeon performs the lateral retinacular release, making sure the vastus lateralis muscle is *not* released from the patella and that the fibers of the vastus lateralis oblique and those connecting the lateral retinaculum to the iliotibial band are released as necessary.

The anterior compartment is then opened with a Bovie knife, and subperiosteal dissection is used to carefully release the anterior musculature from the lateral aspect of the tibia. The anterior tibial artery and peroneal nerve are located at the posterolateral corner at this level and must be protected. The edges of the medial and lateral aspects of the patellar tendon must be precisely defined, especially at the insertion to the tuberosity. It is important to fully expose the medial aspect of the tendon because the closer to this the osteotomy is started, the steeper the osteotomy plane that may be obtained.

The longitudinal incision is carried down the crest and tapered distally, creating a wedge 3 to 4 cm wide proximally. The distal portion, which forms the hinge, is 5 to 8 cm distal to the tuberosity and is approximately 1 cm in width. A series of long 4-mm drill bits are placed in parallel, using the Hoffmann drill guide in a plane from the anterior medial aspect of the tibia to the posterior lateral aspect of the tibia. The Tracker guide system, which uses a cutting block fixed by pins (DePuy), may also be employed. The obliquity of the osteotomy is determined by the proximity of initial drill holes to the medial aspect of the patellar tendon. If the surgeon uses a curved AO or Tracker drill guide, he or she will be able to locate the exit point on the lateral cortex before beginning the drill hole. Care must be taken to not perforate the posterior cortex of the tibia with the drill and to keep the bits under direct vision to protect neurovascular structures. After the holes are made, the drill bits are maintained in only the most proximal and distal aspects of the drill guide.

A superior or proximal cut is made in the bone from the most superior and posterior drill hole on the lateral cortex to an anterior point proximal to the patellar tendon insertion. This defect relieves any tension and prevents extension of the osteotomy into the more proximal tibia. Next, the cortical bone medially and proximal to the tuberosity is cut. The guide is removed, and the main osteotomy is completed through the multiple drill holes with a 5-cm-wide (2-in-wide) osteotome (Fig. 56.4). The superior and inferior drill bits are kept in place as references for the proper cutting plane. If the Tracker system is used, the cut is made with an oscillation saw, using a cutting block fixed in the proper configuration with pins. When the osteotomy is completed and the bone pedicle is hinged distally, the proximal portion of the osteotomy is pushed anteriorly and medially up the incline.

Patellar tracking is then observed for congruence, and the tubercle is medialized until the extensor mechanism is centralized. Initially, two AO wires may be placed across the osteotomized bone to stabilize it; then two cortical screws are placed carefully into the posterior cortex. Anteriorization of 12 to 15 mm is routinely achieved without bone graft.

The tourniquet is released, and meticulous hemostasis is obtained with the Bovie electrocautery apparatus and by using Gelfoam-soaked thrombin (if necessary) before placing the suction drain. Closure of the subcutaneous tissue and skin is routine.

Postoperative care involves an ice and compression system and a drain for 24 h. A knee immobilizer is used for protective weight bearing with crutches. Quadriceps and ROM exercises are begun the following day to encourage cartilage nutrition and to prevent stiffness. Full ROM is desirable at 2 weeks. The immobilizer should be removed several times each day for ROM exercises. After 6 weeks, immobilization is discontinued and full range of motion is begun with weight bearing, as tolerated.

SUMMARY

Distal realignment procedures are associated with variable long-term results. These procedures are salvage techniques that offer pain relief, increased stability, and improved ability to carry out activities of daily living. The patient and surgeon must have realistic expectations. Best results are obtained when the realignment procedure ad-

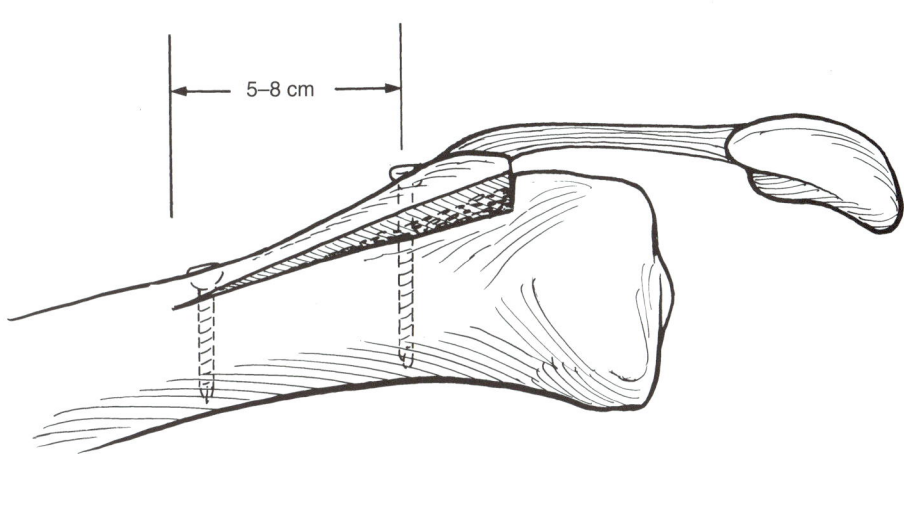

Figure 56.4. Osteotomy in antero-medialization. *L,* lateral; *M,* medial.

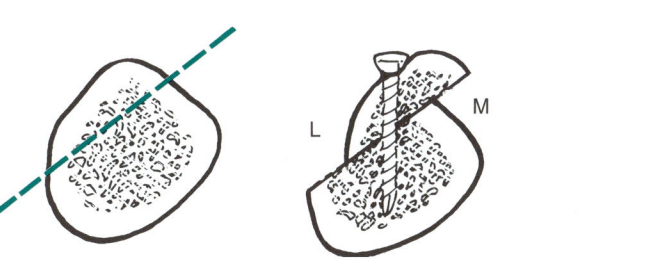

dresses the specific lesions found by clinical, radiographic, and arthroscopic studies.

REFERENCES

1. Fielding JW, Liebler WA, Tambakis A. The effect of tibial tubercle transplant in children on the growth of the upper tibial epiphysis. J Bone Joint Surg 1960;42A:1426–1434.
2. Galeazzi R. Nouve applicazioni di trapianto musculare e tendino. Arch Orthop 1922;38:4–7.
3. Baker RH, Carroll N, Bewar FP et al. The semitendinosus tenodesis for recurrent dislocation of the patella. J Bone Joint Surg 1972; 54B:103–109.
4. Gomes JL. Medial patellofemoral ligament reconstruction for recurrent dislocation of the patella: a preliminary report. Arthroscopy 1992;8:335–340.
5. Roux C. Luxation habituelle do la rotule: traitement operatoire. Rev Chir Paris 1988;8:682–689.
6. Goldthwait JE. Slipping or recurrent dislocation of the patella: with the report of eleven cases. Boston Med Surg J 1904; 150:169–174.
7. Christman OD, Snook GA, Wilson TC. A long-term prospective study of the Hauser and Roux-Goldthwait procedures for recurrent patellar dislocation. Clin Orthop 1979;1944:27–30.
8. Fondren FB, Goldner JL, Bassett FB. Recurrent dislocation of the patella treated by the modified Roux-Goldthwait procedure. J Bone Joint Surg 1985;67A:993–1004.
9. Templeman D, McBeath A. Iatrogenic patellar malalignment following the Roux-Goldthwait procedure corrected by dynamic intraoperative realignment. J Bone Joint Surg 1986;68A:1096–1098.
10. Maquet P. Advancement of the tibial tuberosity. Clin Orthop 1976:115:225.
11. Schmid F. The Maquet procedure in the treatment of patellofemoral osteoarthrosis. Clin Orthop 1993;294:254–258.
12. Radin EL, Pan HQ. Long term follow-up study on the Maquet procedure with special reference to causes of failure. Clin Orthop 1993;290:253–258.
13. Hauser EDW. Total transplant for slipping patella Surg Gynecol Obstet 1938;66:199–214.
14. Hampson WG, Hill P. Late results of transfer of the tibial tubercle for recurrent dislocation of the patella. J Bone Joint Surg 1975; 57B:209–213.
15. Barbari S, Raugstad TS, Lichtenberg N, et al. The Hauser operation for patellar dislocation. Acta Orthop Scand 1990;61:32–35.
16. Trillat A, Dejour H, Couette A. Diagnostic et traitement de subluxations recidivantes de la rotule. Rev Chir Orthop 1964; 50:813–824.
17. Cox JS. An evaluation of the Roux-Elmslie-Trillat procedure for knee extensor realignment. Am J Sports Med 1982;10:303–310.
18. Cerullo G, Paddu G, Conteduca F et al. Evaluation of the results of extensor mechanism reconstruction. Am J Sports Med 1988;16: 93–96.
19. Fulkerson JP. Anteromedialization of the tibial tuberosity for patellofemoral malalignment. Clin Orthop 1983;177:176–181.
20. Fulkerson JP, Meaney JA, Becker GJ, et al. Anteromedial tibial tubercle transfer without bone graft. Am J Sports Med 1990; 18:490–497.
21. Morshusis WS, Pavlov PW, DeRooy KP. Anteromedialization of the tibial tuberosity in the treatment of patellofemoral pain and malalignment. Clin Orthop 1990;255:242–250.

chapter 57

Mark T. Wichman and Marc J. Friedman

Patellar Instability: Proximal Realignment

Patellar instability may be simply defined as failure of the patella to track within the femoral sulcus. The two fundamental problems of patellar dislocation and patellar subluxation have far more similarities than differences. The difference between them is quantitative rather than qualitative. This chapter deals with the management of patients with a demonstrable patellofemoral malalignment (acute dislocation, recurrent dislocation, or chronic subluxation) for whom a lateral retinacular release alone is clearly insufficient. These are primarily patients with Schutzer-Fulkerson type I malalignment and some with type II.

RELEVANT ANATOMY AND PATHOGENESIS

Situated within the extensor mechanism of the knee, the patella is considered to be the largest sesamoid bone in the body. The patella receives insertions from the quadriceps muscle in three layers. The most superficial is from the rectus femoris. Some fibers actually continue over the patella to join the patellar tendon. The middle layer is the contribution from the vastus medialis and vastus lateralis. The vastus intermedius contributes to the deepest of the three layers of the quadriceps tendon. The vastus medialis is of particular interest here. There are two portions of the vastus medialis: the longus and the obliquus. The fibers of the vastus medialis obliquus (VMO) are oriented in the medial to lateral plane, making the muscle efficient at resisting lateral patellar translation.

The patella has five anatomic facets: lateral, medial, inferior, superior, and odd (Fig. 57.1). All but the inferior facet contact the trochlea in various degrees of knee flexion. In general, the contact area of the patella moves proximally as the knee flexes. Beyond 120° of flexion, the quadriceps tendon begins to contact the trochlea and "shares" the joint reaction force, which gets quite large during increased flexion. The patella withstands these large forces by virtue of its hyaline cartilage, which is the thickest in the body (up to 5 mm). The inferior one-fourth of the patella is devoid of articular cartilage and is nonarticular.

The shape of the patella is an important factor in patellar instability. Wiberg (1) and Baumgartl (2) described four types of patellar morphology (Fig. 57.2). For type I patellae, the medial and lateral facets are equal in size and are gently concave. Types II, III, and IV have progressively smaller medial facets with a flat or even convex shape. Type IV was described by Baumgartl (2) as having a "hunter's hat" appearance; it has almost no medial facet. Type II is the most common, followed by types I and III. The trend toward a dominant lateral facet is probably associated with patellar instability.

The trochlea contributes to the osseous stability of the patellofemoral joint. The lateral condyle is 9 mm high in normal controls but is only 4.7 mm in patients with patellar subluxation (3). The sulcus angle between the condyles is another major determinant of inherent bony stability. A flat sulcus angle has been implicated as a cause of patellar instability (4). These osseous variations combined with soft tissue findings (such as a tight lateral retinaculum, deficient VMO, and patella alta) may cause a predisposition to patellar subluxation or dislocation, especially when combined with an increased Q angle. Trauma alone is unlikely to cause a patellar dislocation in a knee with perfectly normal alignment.

INITIAL FINDINGS, PHYSICAL EXAMINATION, AND DIAGNOSIS

Patellar Dislocation

The examiner should take a comprehensive history from all patients who complain of knee problems (Chapter

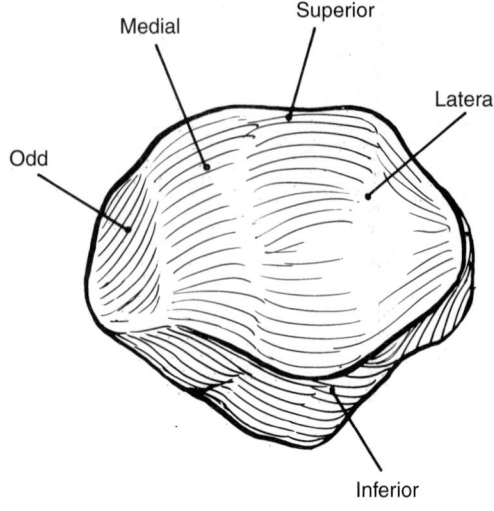

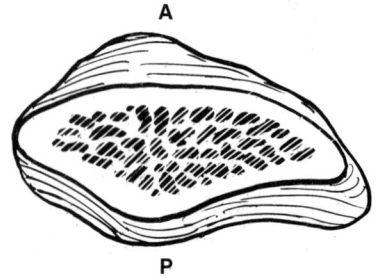

Figure 57.1. The five facets of the patella. Note that the inferior one-fourth is nonarticular.

55). A patient with acute patellar dislocation is often seen first in the emergency room; he or she describes acute knee pain that usually began after twisting (external rotation) the tibia on the femur combined with valgus and knee flexion. The patient often hears a pop or snap, after which the patella is displaced to the outside of the knee. Frequently, the patient will have manipulated the patella back into place or a spontaneous reduction occurred. This is commonly associated with considerable swelling, which is present almost immediately. Unfortunately, this classic history may not be available; if the clinician must rely on the patient's memory, he or she cannot be sure if a dislocation actually occurred. A patient with recurrent dislocations may not be able to provide an accurate account of the first dislocation. The patient may have, however, learned through experience which activities provoke symptoms, and often he or she has received nonoperative treatment from another orthopaedic surgeon.

If the patient has sustained an acute patellar dislocation, the complete knee examination may have to be modified because of swelling and pain. There is often an effusion, which may be aspirated to make the patient more comfortable. The apprehension test will be strongly positive, as will palpation of the medial retinaculum (the clinical may note a defect). The lateral retinaculum is often tender as well. Pain over the adductor tubercle, known as

Bassett's sign (5), is an indication of avulsion of the femoral insertion of the medial patellofemoral ligament. The clinician must attempt to rule out cruciate ligament injury via a standard instability examination. Rotatory instability that allows excessive external rotation of the tibia may exaggerate lateral tracking of the patella. The patient must also be able to perform an adequate straight leg raise, which rules out trauma to the extensor mechanism, such as a quadriceps or patellar tendon rupture.

The patient with recurrent patellar dislocations is examined as follows. The clinician should note both the patient's gait as he or she walks into the room and the patient's static standing alignment. After a brief screening for spine and hip problems, the clinician should check for abnormal hind foot pronation, since this can contribute to patellar malalignment. The precise mechanism of subtalar pronation that leads to patellofemoral problems is uncertain, but it is possibly due to compensatory internal rotation of the femur (6). The patient is placed on the examining table and the Q angle and tibiofemoral alignment are

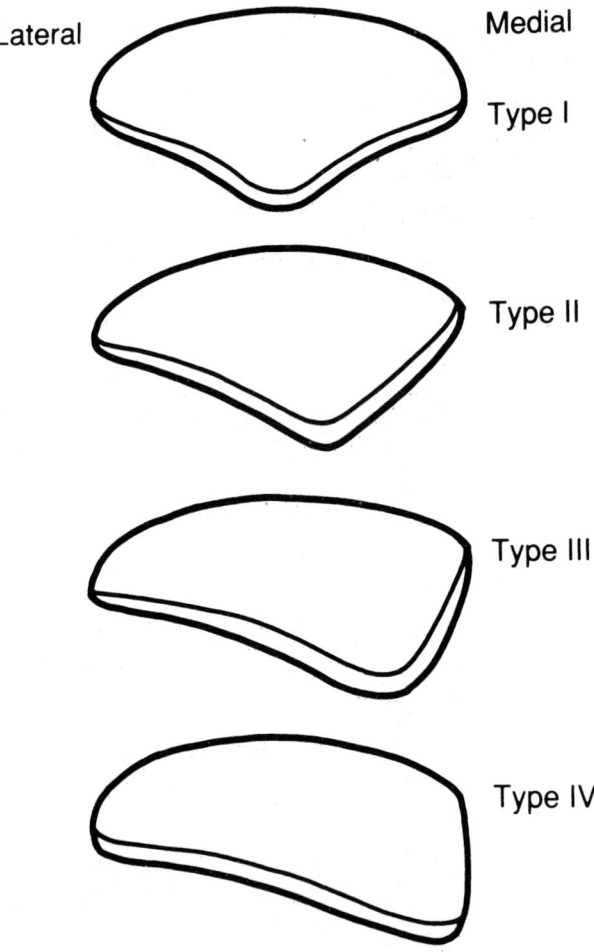

Figure 57.2. Classification of patella morphology according to Wiberg (1) and Baumgartl (2). Reprinted with permission from Aglietti P, Buzzi R, Insall JN. Disorders of the patellofemoral joint. In: Insall JN, Windsor RD, Scott WN, et al., eds. Surgery of the knee. 2nd ed. New York: Churchill Livingstone, 1993:242.

noted. The clinician should carefully evaluate the tracking of the knee, especially in early flexion, observing how the patella enters the sulcus. The patellar tilt test, glide test, and compression test are performed (Chapter 55). A screening for generalized hyperlaxity is also appropriate, because it is thought to be up to six times more common in patients with recurrent patellar dislocation than in people with normal knees. An atrophic VMO, positive apprehension and glide tests, and a positive history provide the diagnosis of a patient with recurrent patellar dislocation.

Patellar Subluxation

Patients with chronic subluxation of the patella often have anterior knee pain similar to those with lateral patellar compression syndrome. The pain is often poorly localized and is especially present after activities that load the patellofemoral joint. There may be a history of recent trauma, which is usually trivial.

As noted, the difference between patellar subluxation and dislocation is one of magnitude; thus the examination and physical findings overlap significantly. Therefore, the clinician uses a similar technique to examine both patients with chronic subluxation and patients with recurrent dislocations.

RADIOLOGIC STUDIES

Standard AP, lateral, and axial views are taken, along with oblique or notch views if an osteochondral fracture is suspected. If significant lower extremity alignment abnormalities are anticipated, a standing film from hip to ankle may be helpful. The degree of subluxation at 45° of flexion may be obtained by measuring the congruence angle on the axial view (Chapter 55). Since it is possible that a large effusion may cause a significant abnormality on axial imaging, we occasionally aspirate the hemarthrosis. Because decision making depends to some extent on the subluxation seen on the axial view, we do not want to draw erroneous conclusions based on a tense hemarthrosis that is altering the position of the patella. To measure the congruence angle, the sulcus angle must be first measured. A flat sulcus angle (150°) may be a predisposing factor to dislocation of the patella (3,4,7). The axial view also helps the clinician determine the patella's Wiberg-Baumgartl type. Patellar tilt may be qualitatively assessed, but a Lauren view is generally used to quantify the lateral patellofemoral angle (LPFA). The LPFA opens laterally in a normal knee without patellar tilt. The lateral view is used to rule out patella alta or baja and to screen for dysplasia of the femoral condyles. Both the lateral and the axial views help the clinician see changes consistent with patellofemoral arthrosis.

Sophisticated imaging studies, such as CT and MRI, are used in special cases. The use of CT to document patellar instability in the initial 30° of knee flexion is discussed in Chapter 55. Kinematic MRI scans have also been of use in these cases. Other indications for MRI studies are acute patellar dislocation with possible meniscal or cruciate ligament pathology, acute dislocation with incongruent reduction, and acute dislocation with point tenderness on the adductor tubercle (Fig. 57.3). In the latter situation, the patient will likely have sustained avulsion of the medial patellofemoral ligament (MPFL) (8,9). Conlan et al. (9) drew attention to this condition, and Sallay et al. (8) were quite successful in surgically addressing it. In the latter series, 87% of patients with acute patellar dislocation had this MRI finding, and 94% had the finding at the time of surgical exploration. Conlan et al.'s work elegantly described the medial soft tissue restraints, including the MPFL, which contributed the most restraint of any single anatomic structure to lateral displacement of the patella.

TREATMENT

Nonoperative Treatment

ACUTE PATELLAR DISLOCATION

In the absence of a large osteochondral fracture, we routinely manage acute patellar dislocations conservatively. There have been, however, some favorable reports of early surgery on these patients, especially those with anatomic predisposition to instability (8,10–12). Since many of these patients do well without surgery, we prefer not to routinely subject them to a surgical procedure, especially one of considerable magnitude. We do, however, operate early in high-performance athletes who cannot spare the time necessary for a trial of full conservative care. There is good evidence that patients who have had dislocations before age 20 or who have evidence of patellofemoral dysplasia in the opposite knee have a high rate of recurrent dislocation (15 to 44%) (10,13–16). It is thus important to tailor the treatment to each patient, taking into consideration the patient's physical demands, goals, and anatomy.

For patients with an acute patellar dislocation, we recommend the use of a knee immobilizer for 2 to 3 weeks. Ice and elevation are used in the first 3 to 4 days. We allow weight bearing as tolerated with the knee in extension. When the patient is comfortable, range of motion exercises and isometric quadriceps sets are begun. At this time, patellar taping is often initiated. Intensive quadriceps strengthening activity and generalized conditioning exercises are performed for 6 weeks. Criteria to return to athletic competition are absence of effusion, Cybex testing that demonstrates quadriceps strength at least 80% of the opposite side, minimal retinacular tenderness, and full range of motion.

CHRONIC SUBLUXATION AND RECURRENT DISLOCATION OF THE PATELLA

The conservative treatment of recurrent patellar instability is similar to that of the lateral patellar compression syndrome (LPCS). Although the anatomic variations may be different, there are only a few things that can be modified by

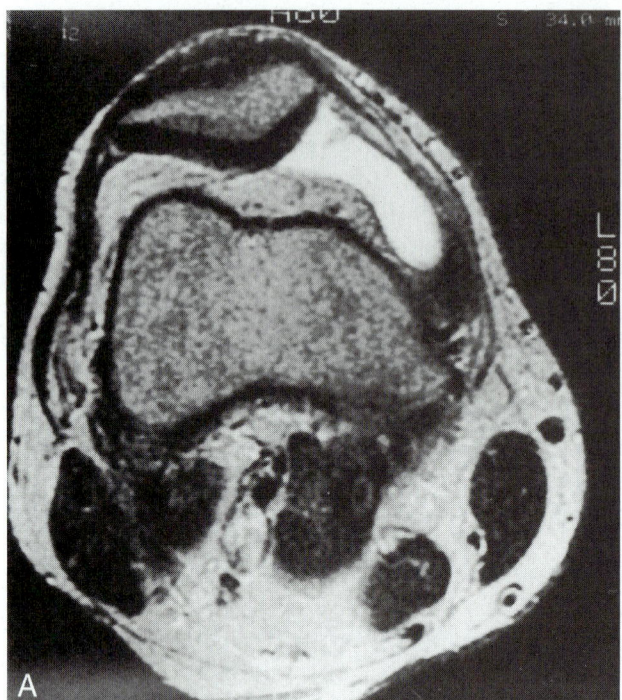
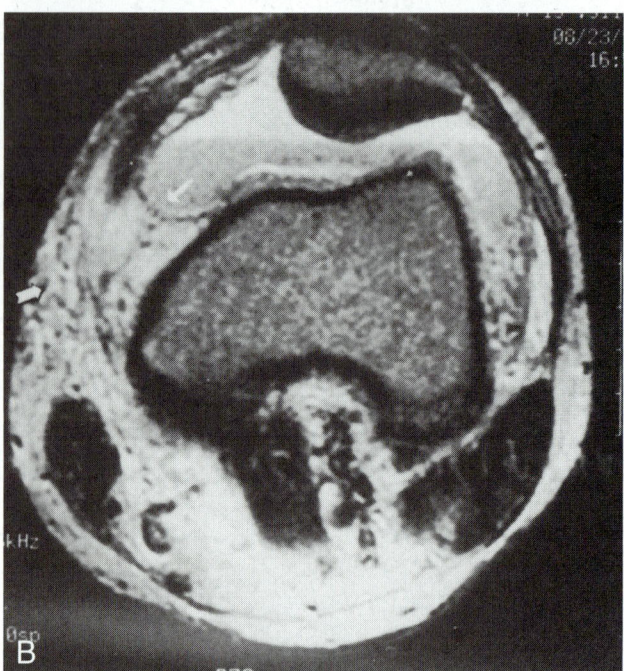

Figure 57.3. Patient with a chronic effusion in the right knee secondary to a meniscal tear (**A**) and a patella dislocation in the left knee (**B**). Note the torn medial patellofemoral ligament just off the adductor tubercle (*arrows*). Reprinted with permission from Sallay PI, Poggi J, Speer KP, Garrett WE. Acute dislocation of the patella. A correlative pathoanatomic study. Am J Sports Med 1996;24:55.

conservative measures. Quadriceps strengthening is the common denominator of most rehabilitation programs. The medial restraint (i.e., VMO) must be conditioned, and both the lateral retinaculum and iliotibial bands must undergo stretching. There is some evidence that physical therapy can improve the congruence angle in patients with LPCS (17), although this finding has not been reproduced. McConnell taping and patellofemoral knee bracing are other reasonable conservative treatment alternatives. From a biomechanical evaluation of a patellofemoral brace, Greenwald et al. (18) found that the brace had little effect on kinematic knee function, but subjectively it performed well. Approximately 75% of patients reported the main benefit of the brace was improved patellar stability, and most found some degree of pain relief.

After taking an adequate history and performing the physical examination, the clinician still lacks objective data for managing these patients. Based on Fithian et al.'s (19) work, objective information to guide rehabilitation or surgical decision making may soon be available. Their method involves instrumented measurement of patellar instability similar to the popular KT-1000 instrument used for anterior cruciate ligament (ACL) rupture. In summary, we do not fully understand the mechanisms of symptomatic relief from conservative treatment in these patients. Such treatment does work for patellar instability, however, and must be proven to fail before surgical treatment is recommended.

Operative Treatment

SURGICAL INDICATIONS

Acute Patellar Dislocation

The three primary indications for surgical management are osteochondral fracture, persistent lateral subluxation noted radiographically, and acute dislocation in a high-performance athlete (Clinical Table). We do not perform isolated lateral retinacular release for acute dislocations, as this has fared poorly in recent literature (20).

If surgery is based on radiographic evidence of persistent subluxation, it is important to repeat the x-ray after the knee is aspirated, if moderate hemarthrosis is present. The effects of hemarthrosis on x-ray interpretation of patellar subluxation are unpredictable. When performing surgery for an osteochondral fracture, the surgeon should assess the risk factors before attempting proximal realignment. These factors include an abnormal Q angle, dysplasia of the femoral condyles, a flat sulcus, and a patella with a dominant lateral facet (Wiberg-Baumgartl type III or IV). Tight lateral restraints and tilt in the opposite patella should also be considered. The surgeon should bear in mind the report of avulsion of the MPFL from the adductor tubercle as the "essential lesion" in patellar dislocation (7). Certainly, this finding on MRI combined with point tenderness at the adductor tubercle would make exploration reasonable. Since the MRI finding has yet to be reported in other centers, we have not included this in our current treatment algorithm.

Clinical Table: Patellar Instability: Proximal Realignment

Procedure	Indications	Technique	Anatomy	Pitfalls
Lateral release and proximal realignment	• Patellar subluxation or dislocation • Normal Q angle	• VMO advancement	• VMO	• Improper tensioning
Distal realignment	• Patellar subluxation or dislocation • Increased Q angle	• Anteromedialization of the tibial tubercle	• Tibial tubercle	• Nonunion • Hardware problems
Semitendinosus tenodesis	• Patellar dislocation • Skeletal immaturity	• Semitendinosus used as a patellar tether	• Pes anserinus tendon	• Nonanatomic reconstruction

Recurrent Patellar Instability

Recurrent patellar dislocation and chronic subluxation of the patella are both managed with conservative treatment for 3 to 6 months. In competitive athletes, however, we tend to be more surgically aggressive. Much of the decision making for these patients is done intraoperatively. Often the patients will have tight lateral restraints along with other pathologic anatomy. The result of lateral retinacular release (LRR) can be somewhat unpredictable, and surgical decisions begin at the time of the LRR; we will refer to the algorithm shown in Figure 57.4. Note that we have assumed skeletal maturity for the purposes of this discussion.

The assessment of lateral retinacular tightness is made preoperatively. The patient has Schutzer-Fulkerson type II malalignment, with both tilt and subluxation. An LRR is generally performed after a routine diagnostic arthroscopy of the knee (Chapter 55). At the next branch in the algorithm, the surgeon classifies the patellofemoral relationship as normal or abnormal. In this scheme, we consider abnormal to include two or more of the following characteristics (3):

Flat sulcus angle (150°)
Schutzer-Fulkerson type III or IV patella
Dysplasia of the femoral condyles
Patella alta
Patella hypermobility

The next variable to be assessed is the Q angle, which measures the degree of malalignment caused by the distal vector. We use a Q angle measured both with the knee in extension and with the knee in 90° of flexion (as a measurement of the tubercle-sulcus angle). If abnormal, we prefer to correct the distal vector first with a distal realignment. We then reassess patellar tracking, both grossly and arthroscopically, through a superomedial portal. If the patella is still lateralized, we perform a proximal realignment procedure. Distal realignment does not correct the congruence angle as reliably as does proximal realignment, and we do not hesitate to perform a combined procedure if necessary.

If the Q angle is normal, we proceed with a proximal realignment procedure first. If the tracking is not acceptable following proximal realignment, we refer back to the patellofemoral relationship for decision-making purposes

(Fig. 57.4). If the anatomy is normal, we simply re-tension our proximal realignment to optimize tracking. If the anatomy is abnormal, however, we first re-tension our repair and then may add a medial tether procedure, such as a semitendinosus tenodesis (Galeazzi's procedure) (21,22). In this procedure, the distal insertion of the semitendinosus is saved. The tendon is harvested proximally, fed through a drill hole in the patella, and sutured back on itself. This provides a tether to lateral subluxation or dislocation.

At this point, a brief discussion about proximal versus distal realignment is warranted. Some accomplished orthopaedic surgeons will perform only one or the other of these procedures. They have clinical results to support what they do. Insall popularized the proximal realignment, and Fulkerson contributed to the modern approach to distal realignment. We believe there are indications for each and a surgeon is best equipped with experience in both techniques. The proximal realignment seems to better centralize the patella within the sulcus; however, it can make the Q angle larger. Insall et al. (23) noted this but failed to show that it had an effect on their results. This adverse effect on Q angle is one rationale for performing a distal procedure first if the angle is abnormal. The distal realignment may normalize the Q angle but may not centralize the patella as predictably as will the proximal realignment. Aglietti et al. (24) noted no clinical difference in intermediate-term outcome for patients with chronic dislocation treated with proximal realignment, distal realignment, or a combined realignment procedure. Lateral release alone, however, gave an unacceptable (40%) rate of recurrent dislocation in this study. We attempt to first treat the most abnormal part of the patient's anatomy, whether it be proximal or distal.

SURGICAL TECHNIQUE

The classic and perhaps most reviewed technique is that of Insall's group (23–27). It combines an open LRR with an advancement of the VMO. The technique has been modified since it was first introduced. Initially, the lateral release was not described as extending proximally to detach the vastus lateralis tendon (27), but Insall et al. (23,28) later included full detachment of the vastus lateralis as an integral part of the procedure.

We, however, perform an arthroscopic lateral release

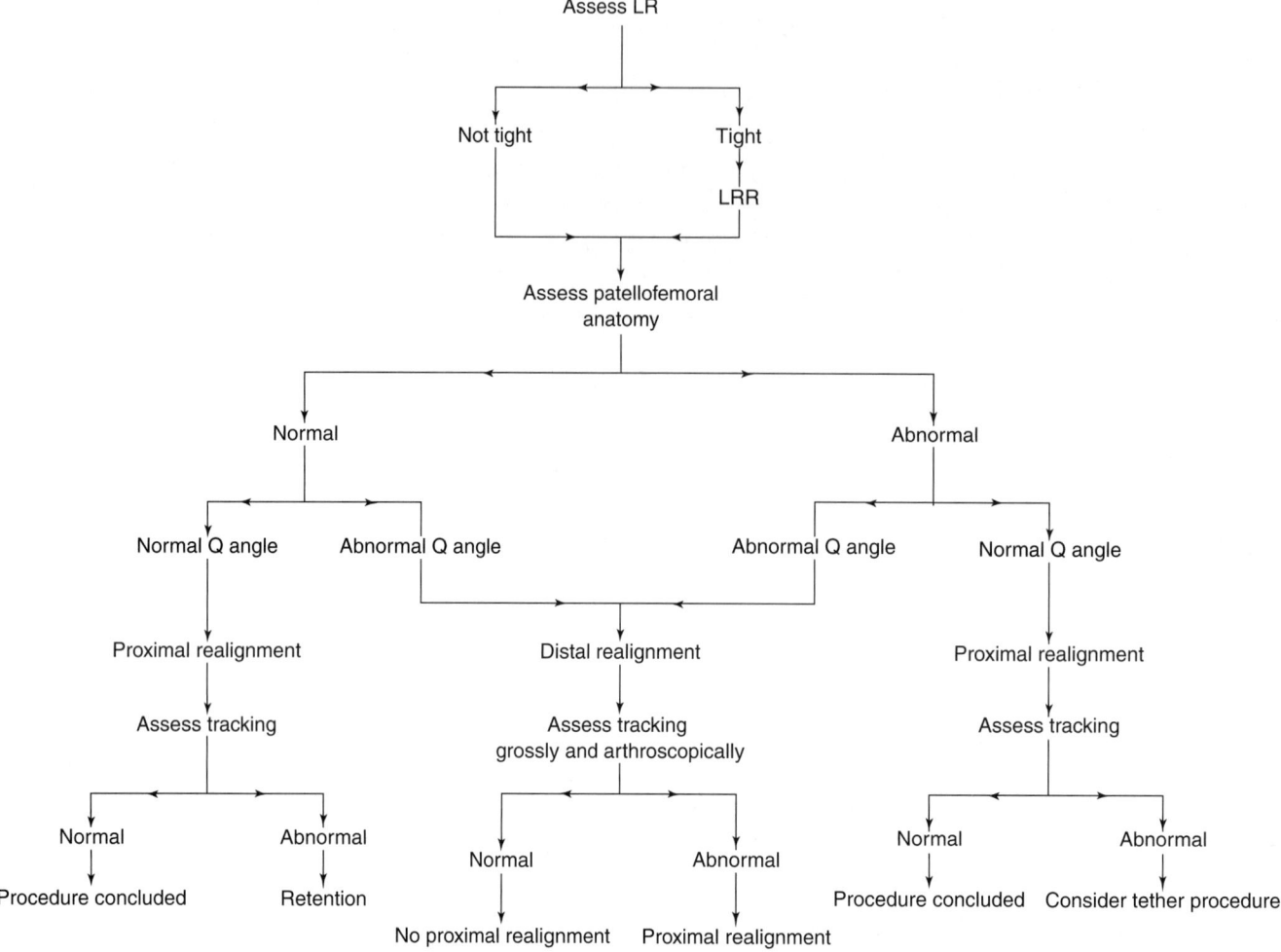

Figure 57.4. Intraoperative decision making for recurrent patellar instability. *LR,* lateral retinaculum.

(Chapter 55) followed by a proximal realignment. For completeness, we also describe three alternate techniques.

After LRR, the tracking and Q angle are rechecked both grossly and arthroscopically. We begin our proximal realignment with a 4- to 5-cm incision along the medial border of the patella. The adequacy of our LRR is checked with the turn-up test (Fig. 57.5) (Chapter 55). After making the incision through skin and subcutaneous tissue, the surgeon can see the fibers of the VMO entering the medial retinaculum. A medial parapatellar incision is made full thickness into synovium along the medial border of the patella, extending from 2 to 3 cm proximal to the superior pole down to the superomedial margin of the patellar tendon. The patellar tendon itself is not violated. We place sutures in the VMO tendon in a vest-over-pants fashion, suturing the tendon to the fascia on the patella. The VMO is advanced both medially and distally. Rarely, the fascia may be inadequate on the patella, and suture anchors will be necessary. After the first few sutures are placed, they are held snug while the knee is brought through a range of motion with flexion to 90° (Fig. 57.6). If satisfied with the tracking, we tie the knots of the sutures at this point (Fig. 57.7). If not satisfied, we re-tension the sutures or replace them to obtain the proper tension and tracking.

Intraoperative evaluation of patellofemoral tracking is an exercise of both science and art. We have two techniques that have served us well. The first is the arthroscopic evaluation of tracking while viewing through the superomedial portal (Fig. 57.8). This technique is then repeated following a surgical intervention, such as a lateral release (Fig. 57.9) and a proximal realignment (Fig. 57.10). The patient shown in Figures 57.8 to 57.10 had recurrent patellar dislocations. Note that the patellofemoral relationship was not adequately restored following the lateral release; it improved significantly after the proximal realignment. Patellar tracking is dynamic, and the knee must be taken through a range of motion so the surgeon can note the point at which the patella enters the sulcus. The alternative technique for evaluation of tracking is to place one thumb on the lateral femoral condyle while the knee is taken through a range of motion. The examiner notes the degree of lateral patellar displacement, if any. The patella should contact the thumb, but there should not be considerable pressure on the thumb keeping the patella within the sulcus.

After confirming adequate tracking, number 1 or 2 Ethibond (nonabsorbable) sutures are used for the closure of proximal realignment. We then oversew this with a

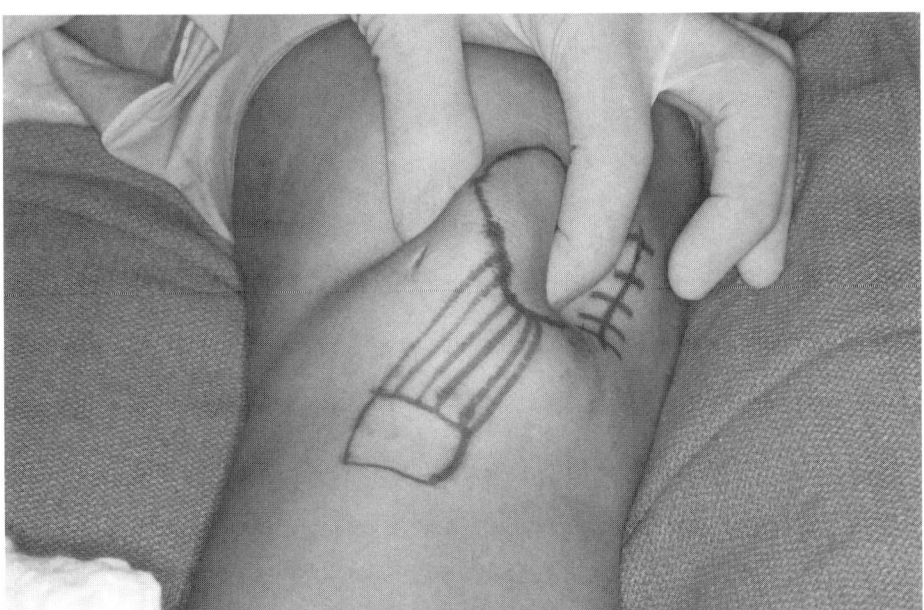

Figure 57.5. For the turn-up test, the patella is turned up to 90° to verify the adequacy of the lateral release.

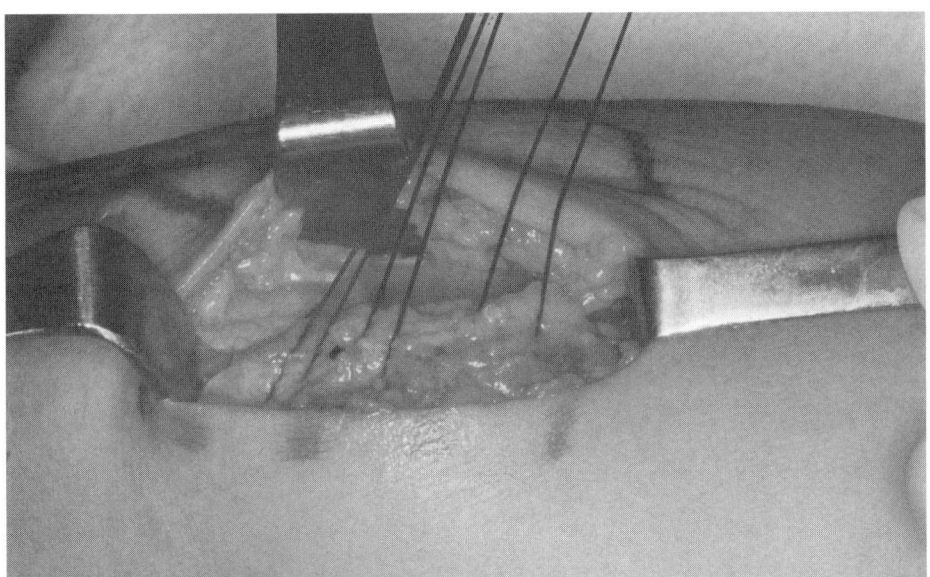

Figure 57.6. The sutures are held taut while the knee is taken through a range of motion from 0° to 90°.

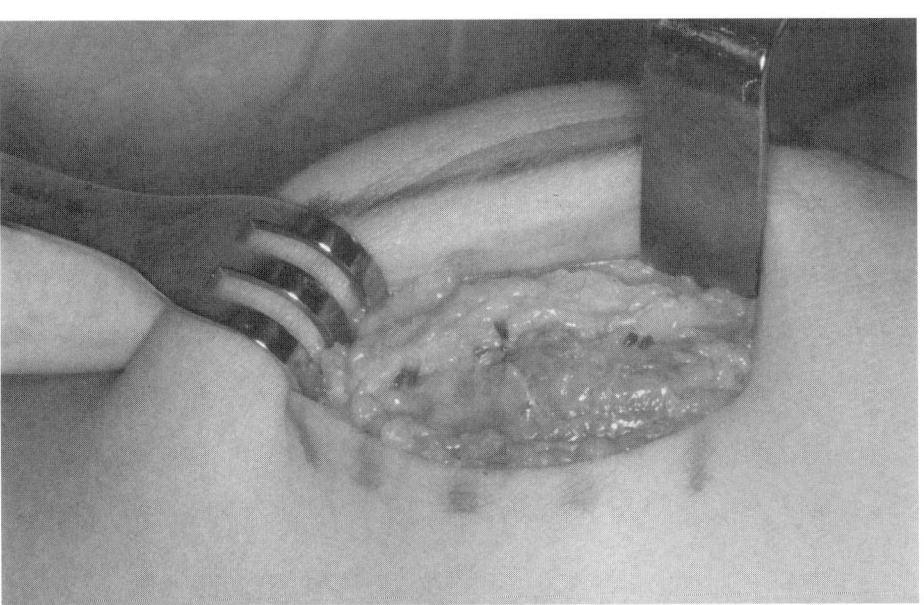

Figure 57.7. Completed repair with the advanced VMO fibers clearly in view.

Figure 57.8. Arthroscopic view of the patellofemoral articulation from the superomedial portal with the knee in 30° to 40° of flexion. The drainage cannula is entering from the anteromedial portal below. Note the severe lateral displacement of the patella.

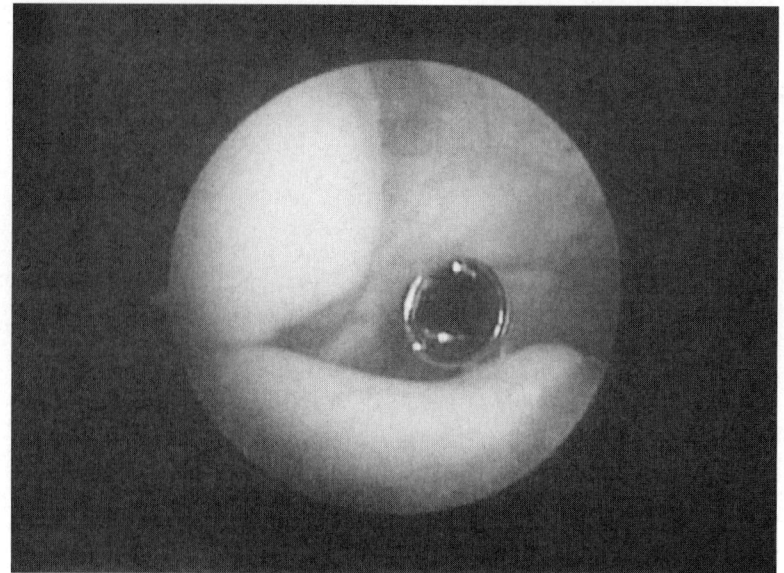

Figure 57.9. Arthroscopic evaluation of tracking following the LRR of the patient shown in Figure 57.8. Note that significant malalignment persists.

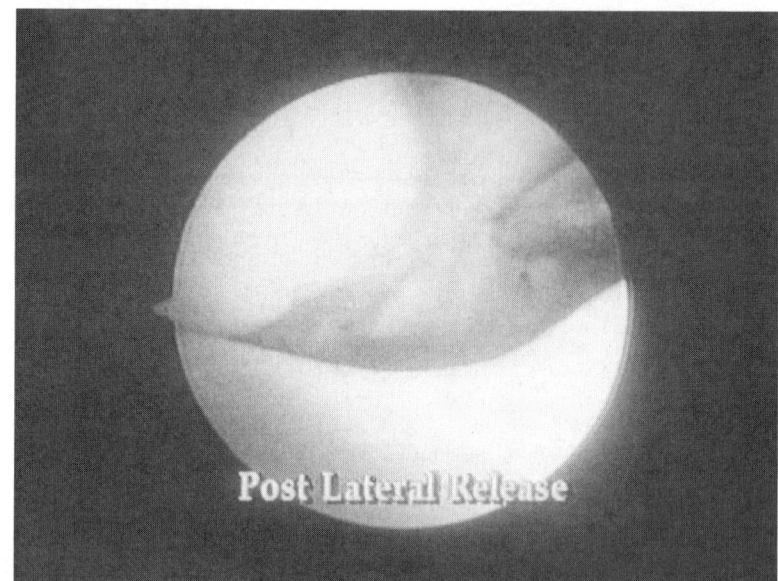

Figure 57.10. Arthroscopic evaluation of tracking following the LRR and proximal realignment of the patient shown in Figure 57.8. The patellofemoral relationship is now substantially improved.

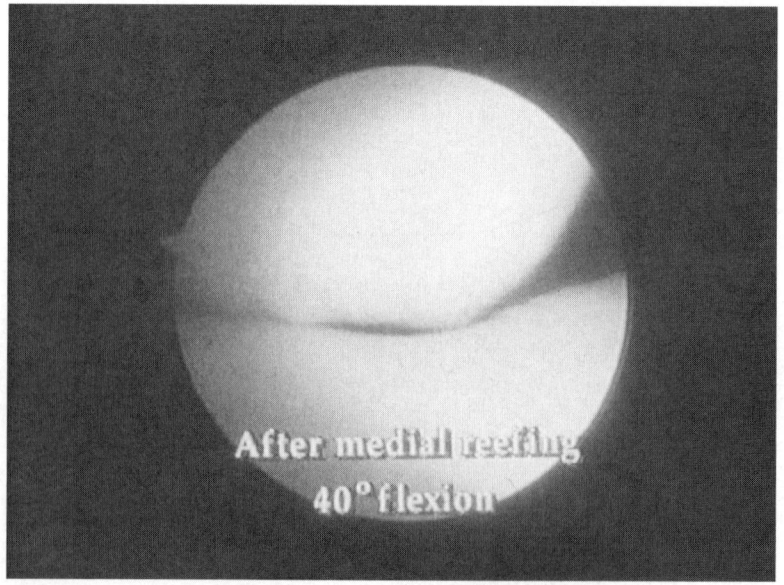

number 1 or 0 Vicryl (absorbable) suture to give added strength to the repair line and to reduce its profile. We try to cover the knots of the Ethibond sutures with tissue to avoid irritation in the subcutaneous region.

As noted in the algorithm (Fig. 57.4), the procedure is complete at this point unless the patient still demonstrates persistent subluxation and has patellofemoral dysplasia but a normal Q angle. In this case, Galeazzi's semitendinosus tenodesis is reasonable, which results in a distal "realignment" in that the tether is distally based using the anatomic insertion of the semitendinosus tendon. Using this procedure, we do not violate the tibial tubercle if the distal vector (Q angle) is normal. The tether procedure would also be an option in a skeletally immature patient, for whom tubercle surgery is contraindicated.

Alternative Techniques

There are three good alternative techniques for performing a proximal realignment. They will be briefly reviewed here.

Insall's proximal realignment. For Insall's proximal realignment, a 15-cm midline incision is made from several centimeters above the patella down to the tibial tubercle (29). The quadriceps tendon is exposed in its entirety, and an LRR is performed. Insall recommends that the proximal extent of the release should include the entire vastus lateralis tendon to allow an optimal change in the orientation of the quadriceps's pull on the patella. A medial parapatellar incision is made in the VMO and distally along the medial border of the patellar tendon. Both the medial and the lateral retinacular incisions should start from an equal point proximally. After thorough inspection of the joint, the surgeon sutures the medial flap over the patella, with distal and lateral advancement of the VMO (Fig. 57.11). The knee is carried through a range of motion at 90° of flexion without undue tension on the repair. More specific information is available (23,27–29).

Madigan's proximal realignment. Madigan's proximal realignment begins with a lateral release. For this procedure, the VMO tendon is isolated, with little proximal or

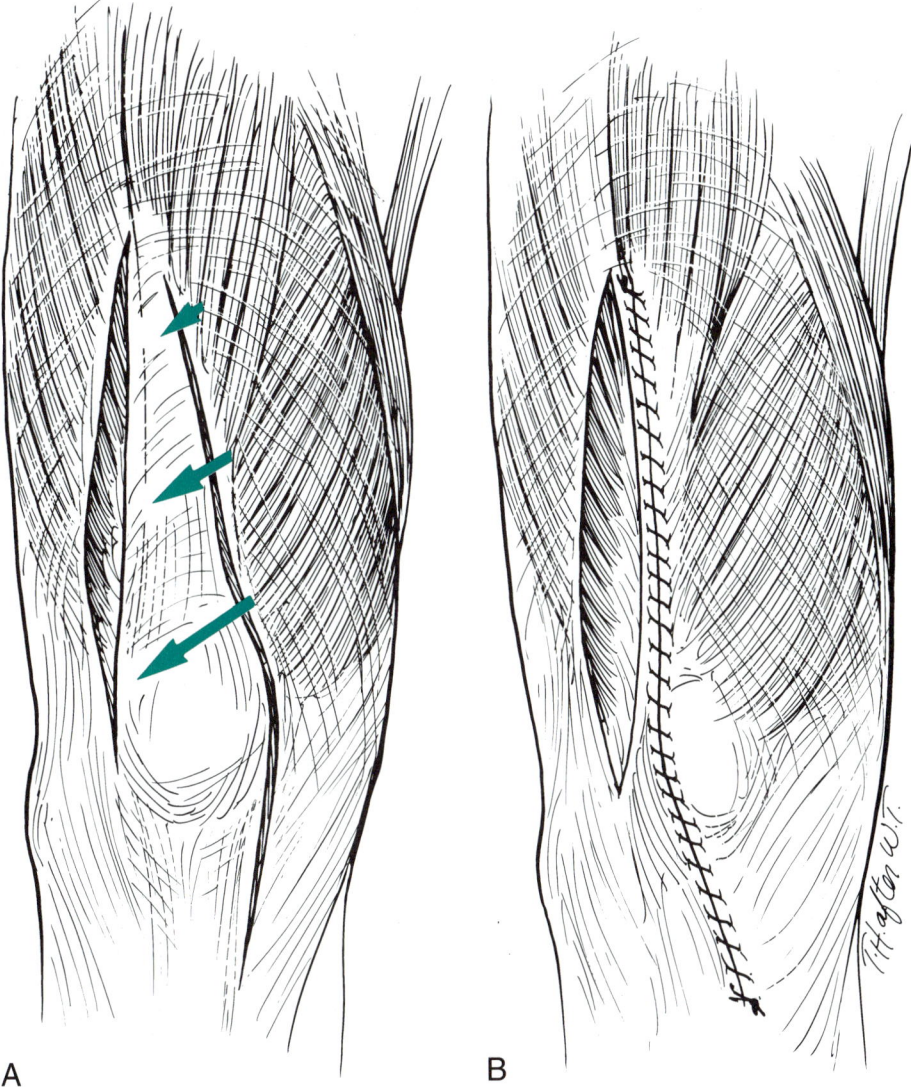

A   B

Figure 57.11. A. Note the direction of the advancement of the VMO in Insall's proximal realignment (*arrows*). **B.** The advancement is complete, and the lateral release should open widely.

distal exposure (30). The VMO is isolated back to the intermuscular septum and then advanced on the patella (Fig. 57.12). It is important to avoid abnormal rotational torques on the patella during this procedure.

Arthroscopic proximal realignment. Arthroscopic proximal realignment begins with an arthroscopic LRR. Next, the medial retinacular defect (if acute dislocation has occurred) is extended distally to the medial border of the

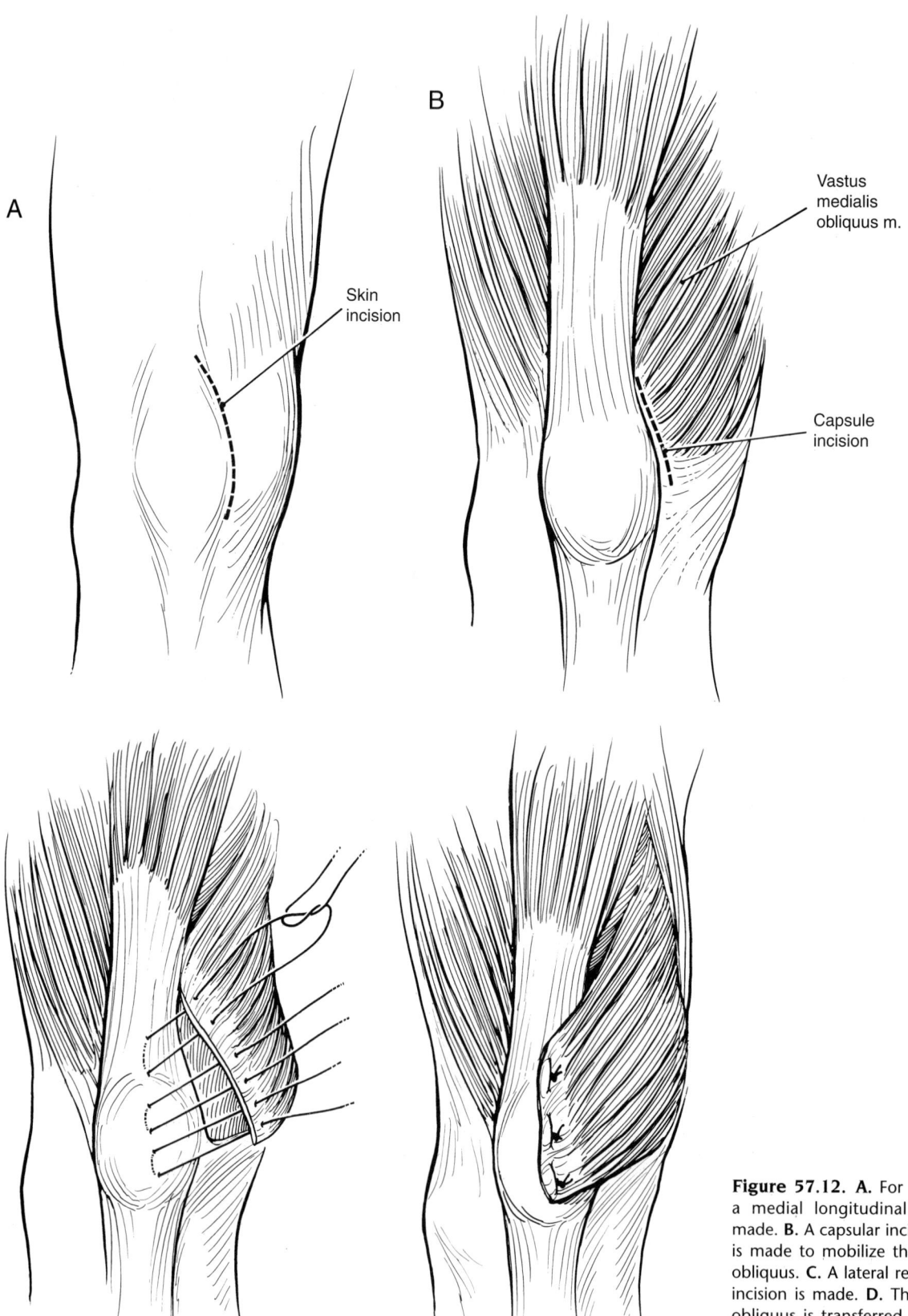

Figure 57.12. A. For quadricepsplasty, a medial longitudinal skin incision is made. **B.** A capsular incision (*dashed line*) is made to mobilize the vastus medialis obliquus. **C.** A lateral retinacular relaxing incision is made. **D.** The vastus medialis obliquus is transferred laterally and distally and is sutured in place.

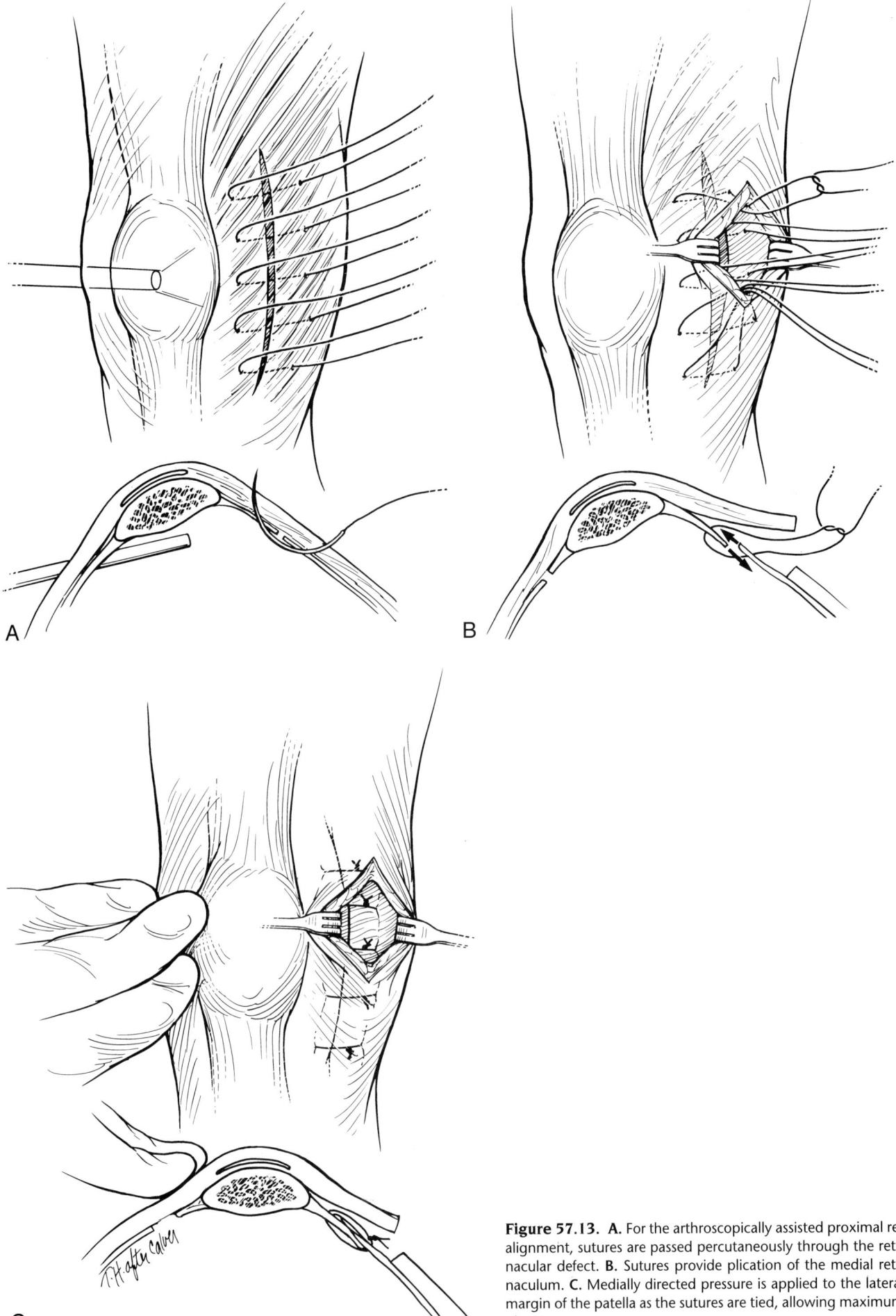

Figure 57.13. A. For the arthroscopically assisted proximal realignment, sutures are passed percutaneously through the retinacular defect. **B.** Sutures provide plication of the medial retinaculum. **C.** Medially directed pressure is applied to the lateral margin of the patella as the sutures are tied, allowing maximum plication.

patellar tendon and then proximally to expose 2 to 3 cm of the vastus medialis tendon (31,32). Several number 2 monofilament sutures are placed as shown in Figure 57.13, and blunt dissection is used through a 2-cm skin incision to retrieve the sutures. These are then tied to allow medial plication to occur. Techniques that require only a medial puncture wound for knot tying have also been described (Fig. 57.14) (32). In addition, medial imbrication with new thermal shrinkage techniques may have some role in the future.

POSTOPERATIVE CARE

We routinely perform the proximal realignment on an outpatient basis. The patient is placed in a knee immobilizer with cryotherapy (ice therapy) and electrical stimulation of the quadriceps via surface electrodes. Weight bearing is permitted as tolerated when the patient is wearing the knee immobilizer. At 2 to 3 weeks after surgery, gentle, active quadriceps exercises are started. At this time, the immobilizer is removed and a neoprene patellar sleeve is used for comfort. When quadriceps strength is 80% of that of the other side, the patient may resume full sports participation. This is typically 3 to 4 months after surgery but depends on the patient's motivation and degree of underlying abnormality.

RESULTS

Relatively few studies have reviewed the results of proximal realignment. Most large studies focused a modification of Insall's technique (23–26). Between 79 and 91% good to excellent results using these techniques have been reported. Because the exact source of pain has not been elucidated in these disorders, we do not know which factors are absolutely crucial for success. Several generalizations can be made, however, in light of the clinical studies available: (a) radiographic centralization of the patella seems to correlate with good results (23,26); (b) the degree of chondromalacia does not correlate well with results, and the outcome for these patients may not hold up over time (25); (c) there may be a tendency for younger age and male sex to correlate with better results (26); and (d) surgery is more successful for treating dislocation than for treating pain.

Madigan et al. (30) reported 58% good to excellent results with their technique and noted inferior results for patients with genu valgum greater than 15° and those with symptomatic chondromalacia patellae. Small et al. (31) reported 92.5% good to excellent results in 27 knees treated with an arthroscopically assisted technique. Approximately half of this group had acute dislocations, and the other half was a mixture of patients with chronic dislocation and chronic subluxation.

COMMON PITFALLS

The surgical procedures as outlined here are straightforward; thus surgical complications are infrequent. Errors

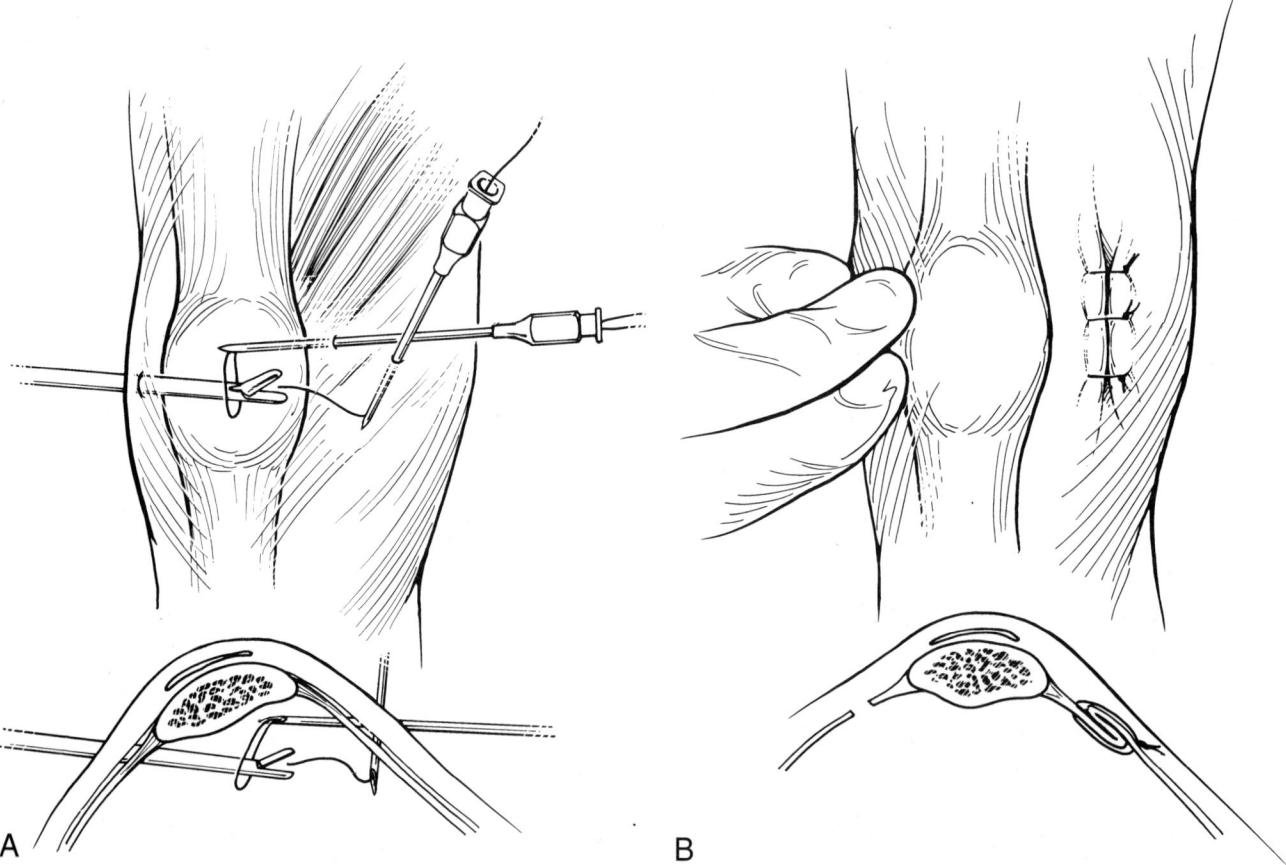

Figure 57.14. A. For an essentially all-arthroscopic proximal realignment, the suture is passed and retrieved with a wire loop. **B.** The knot is tied through a small skin portal with a knot pusher.

are generally due to either too much or too little surgery. An inadequate lateral release, for example, may preclude a good result with proximal realignment. An overaggressive medial tightening may cause a poor result because of medial patellar subluxation. The surgeon must be cautious, especially in the case of an extremely hypermobile patella. These patients often have patella alta, and proximal realignment may make them worse.

SUMMARY

Patellar instability is a continuum of disorders, all characterized by abnormal patellar tracking. Several anatomic variations may contribute to the problem and must be sought out. Conservative management of these patients is the mainstay of treatment, but surgery is effective in well-selected patients. The surgery must address the pathologic structures and be proportional to the magnitude of the disorder. We would like to stress that both proximal and distal realignment have good, predictable results when applied to the appropriate patient, with a success rate of 80 to 90%. Furthermore, proximal realignment is a safe procedure with few complications. Quadriceps rehabilitation is a crucial element in the postoperative care. Return to sports is usually achieved within 3 to 4 months, depending on the motivation of the athlete.

REFERENCES

1. Wiberg G. Roentgenographic and anatomic studies on the patellofemoral joint with special reference to chondromalacia patella. Acta Orthop Scand 1941;12:319–410.
2. Baumgartl F. Das kniegelenk. Berlin: Springer-Verlag, 1944.
3. Aglietti P, Insall JN, Cerulli G. Patellar pain and incongruence I: measurements of incongruence. Clin Orthop 1983;176:217–224.
4. Malahan J, Maldague B. Depth insufficiency in the proximal trochlear groove on lateral radiographs of the knee: relation to patellar dislocation. Radiology 1989;170:507–510.
5. Bassett FH. Acute dislocation of the patella, osteochondral fractures and injuries to the extensor mechanism of the knee. Inst Course Lect 1976;25:40–49.
6. Tiberio D. The effect of excessive subtalar joint pronation on patellofemoral mechanics: a theoretical model. J Orthop Sports Phys Ther 1987;9:160–165.
7. Kujala UM, Osterman K, Kormano M, et al. Patellofemoral relationships in recurrent patellar dislocation. J Bone Joint Surg 1989; 71B:788–792.
8. Sallay PI, Poggi J, Speer KP, Garrett WE. Acute dislocation of the patella. A correlative pathoanatomic study. Am J Sports Med 1996;24:52–60.
9. Conlan T, Garth WP, Lemons JE. Evaluation of the medial soft-tissue restraints of the extensor mechanism of the knee. J Bone Joint Surg 1993;75A:682–693.
10. Hawkins PJ, Bell RH, Anisette G. Acute patellar dislocation. The natural history. Am J Sports Med 1986;14:117–120.
11. Vainionpaa S, Laasonen E, Silvennoinen T, et al. Acute dislocation of the patella. A prospective review of operative treatment. J Bone Joint Surg 1990;72B:366–369.
12. Boring TH, O'Donoghue DH. Acute patellar dislocation: results of immediate surgical repair. Clin Orthop 1978;136:182–185.
13. Cofield R, Bryan R. Acute dislocation of the patella: results of conservative treatment. J Trauma 1977;17:526.
14. McManus F, Rang M, Heslin DJ. Acute dislocation of the patella in children: the natural history. Clin Orthop 1979;139:88.
15. Larson E, Laundson F. Conservative treatment of patellar dislocation: influence of evident factors in the tendency to redislocation and the therapeutic result. Clin Orthop 1982;171:131.
16. Cash JD, Hughston JL. Treatment of acute patellar dislocation. Am J Sports Med 1988;16:244–249.
17. Doucette SA, Golde EM. The effect of exercise on patellar tracking in lateral patellar compression syndrome. Am J Sports Med 1992;20:434–440.
18. Greenwald MS, Bagley AM, France EP, et al. A biomechanical and clinical evaluation of a patellofemoral knee brace. Clin Orthop 1996;324:187–195.
19. Fithian DC, Mishra DK, Balen PF, et al. Instrumented measurement of patellar mobility. Am J Sports Med 1995;23:607–615.
20. Dainer RD, Barrack RL, Buckley SL, Alexander AH. Arthroscopic treatment of acute patellar dislocations. Arthroscopy 1988; 4:267–271.
21. Galeazzi R. Nuove applicazion del trapianto muscolare e tendineo (XII Congress Societa Italiana di Ortopedia). Arch Ortopedia 1922:38.
22. Baker RH, Carroll N, Dewar FP, Hall JE. The semitendinosus tenodesis for recurrent dislocation of the patella. J Bone Joint Surg 1972;54B:103–109.
23. Insall JN, Aglietti P, Tria AJ. Patellar pain and incongruence II: clinical application. Clin Orthop 1983;176.225–232.
24. Aglietti P, Buzzi R, DeBiase P, Giron F. Surgical treatment of recurrent dislocation of the patella. Clin Orthop 1994;308.8–17.
25. Abraham E, Washington E, Huang TL. Insall proximal realignment for disorders of the patella. Clin Orthop 1989;248:61–65.
26. Scuderi G, Cuomo F, Scott N. Lateral release and proximal realignment for patellar subluxation and dislocation. A long term follow up. J Bone Joint Surg 1988;70A:856–861.
27. Insall JN, Falvo KA, Wise D. Chondromalacia patellae. J Bone Joint Surg 1976;58A:1–8.
28. Insall J, Bullough PG, Burstein AH. Proximal "tube" realignment of the patella for chondromalacia patellae. Clin Orthop 1979; 144:63–69.
29. Aglietti P, Buzzi R, Insall JN. Disorders of the patellofemoral joint. In: Insall JN, Windsor RD, Scott WN, et al., eds. Surgery of the knee. 2nd ed. New York: Churchill Livingstone, 1993:329–334.
30. Madigan R, Wissinger HA, Donaldson WF. Preliminary experience with a method of quadricepsplasty in recurrent subluxation of the patella. J Bone Joint Surg 1975;57A:600–607.
31. Small NC, Glogau AI, Berezin MA. Arthroscopically assisted proximal exterior mechanism realignment of the knee. Arthroscopy 1993;9:63–67.
32. Henry JE, Pflum FA. Arthroscopic proximal patella realignment and stabilization. Arthroscopy 1995;11:424–425.

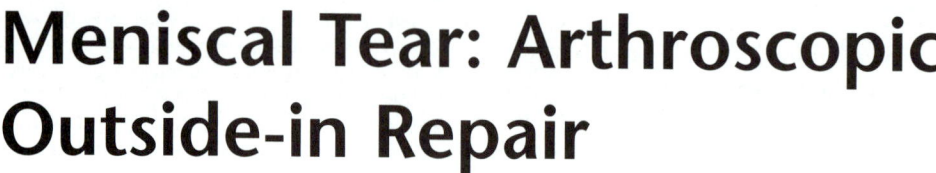

Meniscal Tear: Arthroscopic Outside-in Repair

Meniscal injury or tearing is a common source of knee pain, disability, limitation of function, and interference with athletic and recreational pursuits. The torn meniscus encompasses virtually all age groups, and the nonoperative or operative approach to the problem must take into consideration factors such as patient age, activity level, associated injury of the knee, potential for soft tissue healing, and judicious and expeditious return to work, sports, and other recreational pursuits.

Many types of meniscal repair are included in the orthopaedic armamentarium. The benefits of the outside-in technique include better visualization, better access, flexibility of placement, simplicity, and safety (1).

RELEVANT ANATOMY AND PATHOGENESIS

The menisci are semilunar-shaped fibrocartilaginous structures located at the periphery of the knee joint between the tibial and femoral surfaces. The anterior and posterior horn attachments are directly to bone, and the remainder of the meniscus is attached to the adjacent capsule via the coronary ligaments (also called the meniscofemoral and meniscotibial ligaments). The medial meniscus is more C-shaped and has a wider diameter than the lateral meniscus, which is circular. In addition, the lateral meniscus is free of capsular attachment at the popliteal hiatus.

The meniscus is 70% water by total weight; and dry weight components consist primarily of type I collagen, proteoglycans, and elastin. The type I collagen fibers are arranged in both a circumferential and a radial fashion; they convert compressive vertical load into circumferential stresses (hoop stresses). The proteoglycans maintain meniscal hydration and viscoelasticity.

The blood supply to the meniscus is via vessels from the perimeniscal capsular and synovial tissues; penetration into the meniscus is 10 to 30% (2). These vessels are branches of the superior and inferior medial and lateral geniculates. The inner 66 to 75% of the inner margin of the meniscus is essentially avascular and receives its nutrition via substrate diffusion from the synovial fluid. Thus the meniscus is commonly divided into red-red, red-white, and white-white zones, which reflect the relative blood supply (Fig. 58.1). Adequate blood supply is critical to meniscal healing after a repair, because meniscal healing, as for other connective tissues, involves vascular invasion, the formation of fibrovascular scar tissue, and subsequent remodeling. Clinically, tears in the white-white zone yield significantly poorer results than do tears in the other zones.

Once thought to be insignificant vestigial structures, the medial and lateral menisci are currently recognized as being critical structures within the knee joint. Clinical and basic science research have demonstrated that the menisci serve a number of important biomechanical functions: joint stability, joint lubrication, and load bearing or shock absorption during routine and recreational activity. The menisci improve joint stability by increasing the congruency between the tibial plateau and femoral condyles. This stabilizing function is of particular importance when the major ligamentous stabilizers of the knee, specifically the anterior cruciate ligament (ACL), are torn and incompetent. With ACL deficiency, there is increased anterior translation of the tibia relative to the femur, and the medial meniscus becomes a critical secondary restraint to further increases in translation.

The load-bearing function of the menisci has been demonstrated in vivo, and multiple studies have shown that even partial meniscectomy increases the contact stresses on the articular cartilage. The intact medial meniscus transmits approximately 50% of the contact force, whereas the lateral meniscus transmits greater than 50% of the force across the lateral compartment of the knee. With loss of a portion or all of the meniscus, the con-

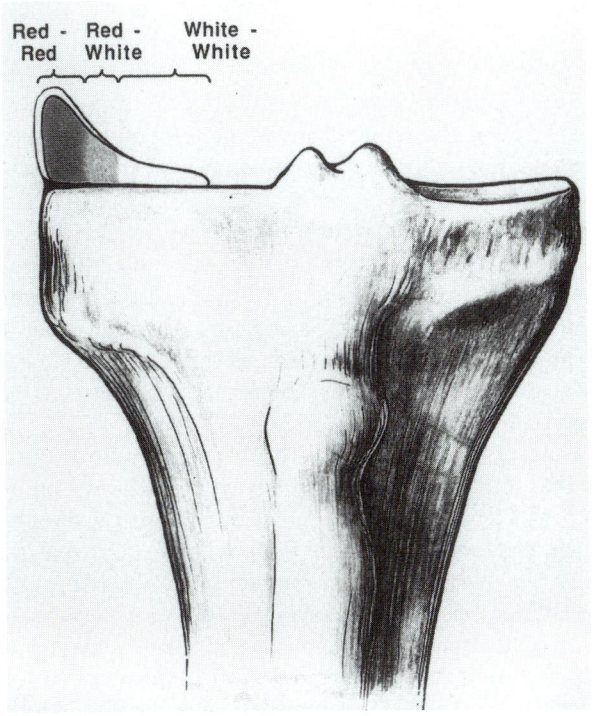

Figure 58.1. Vascular zones of the meniscus. Reprinted with permission from Miller MD, Ritchie JR, Harner CD. Meniscus surgery: indications for repair. Op Tech Sports Med 1994;2:164–171.

tact area between the femur and tibia decreases. Thus the compressive load across the joint is distributed across a smaller articular surface area, resulting in an increase in the contact stress on the articular cartilage. If only 16 to 34% of the meniscus is removed, joint surface contact forces can increase up to 350% (3,4).

The clinical consequences of a complete or partial meniscectomy are the development of degenerative changes and associated symptoms (5,6). The amount of degeneration is often proportional to the amount of meniscus removed. It is now well recognized that even a partial meniscectomy is not a benign procedure, but one that can result in significant intra-articular degeneration, with associated functional limitation. Therefore, the current approach to treating a torn meniscus includes attempts at preservation or repair, if possible. Current technical options for repair include open repair and arthroscopic outside-in, inside-out, and all-inside techniques (7–12). This chapter focuses on the arthroscopic outside-in technique.

INITIAL FINDINGS, PHYSICAL EXAMINATION, AND DIAGNOSIS

Meniscal tears can occur as a result of acute injury or age-related degeneration. Meniscal tears in young patients are most commonly longitudinal (vertical) tears that result from acute flexion or rotational injury. By contrast, degenerative tears in the older patients can result from

acute injury or from minimal to no identifiable trauma. Such tears are frequently complex, showing both radial and horizontal cleavage components.

The diagnosis of a meniscus tear can be made by history and examination in the majority of patients. A history of an acute fall or twisting injury to the knee followed by pain and mild to moderate swelling that develops over several hours or is noted the next day is fairly common. Occasionally, an acute pop or snap, perhaps with an immediate episode of locking, is described. Massive, immediate swelling or hemarthrosis after an injury should raise suspicion for a ligamentous or osteochondral injury. Following the acute injury, intermittent recurrent pain and swelling with activity are common. The pain will typically be localized to the medial or lateral side of the knee and is also felt posteriorly, particularly with knee flexion. Episodes of knee locking, most commonly after deep flexion, or snapping and clicking along the joint line with activity strongly suggest the presence of a meniscal tear.

The physical examination should include an assessment of quadriceps atrophy, swelling, and joint line pain. Muscle atrophy is common following acute injury or the presence of recurrent symptoms with periods of activity restriction. Effusion is present in more than half of patients, particularly in those presenting for evaluation within the first several days of injury. Pain to palpation along the medial or lateral joint line is believed to be the most sensitive indicator of meniscal pathology on examination. This is especially true of posterior joint line tenderness, as the collateral ligaments overlie the menisci in the midmedial and lateral aspect of the knee, and injury to these structures can yield joint line tenderness. Varus and valgus stress testing can help clarify the status of the collateral structures. Physical examination in all patients should evaluate the possibility of coexisting collateral, cruciate, or patellofemoral injury.

Provocative tests can be used to specifically assess the status of the meniscus, such tests include squatting and the McMurray, Apley grind, and Steinmann tests. Joint line or posterior pain that prohibits a full squat is often present when there is a meniscal tear. The examiner should clarify the location of the pain with squatting, because anterior patellofemoral pain may also limit a patient's ability to squat. The patient is in the supine position for the McMurray test; the knee is placed in maximal flexion and the hip is flexed to 90°. The examiner imparts combinations of internal-external and varus-valgus rotational stresses while the knee is brought into extension. For the Apley grind test, the patient is placed prone, with the knee flexed 90°. Axial compression is placed along the tibia, while the leg is forcefully internally and externally rotated. For the Steinmann test, the patient is supine or sitting with his or her leg flexed comfortably over the table. Quick, mildly forceful, internal and external rotation is imparted to the tibia by grasping the foot and ankle. For all tests, localizing joint line pain or clicking strongly suggests a meniscal tear.

RADIOLOGIC STUDIES

As noted, the diagnosis of meniscus tear is typically made on the history and physical examination. Plain radiographs (standing AP or PA flexed, lateral, and infrapatellar or sunrise views) should be obtained for all patients. Following acute injury, it is critical to rule out a fracture. For all patients, the presence of osteoarthritis should be evaluated by assessing joint space narrowing and/or spur formation. Although the presence of minimal to mild arthritic change on plain radiography does not exclude the potential of a meniscal tear being the source of the patient's symptoms, it may change the initial course of treatment; well-established degenerative changes will affect the course of treatment.

MRI is not clinically indicated for all patients, but it is useful if the diagnosis remains in question. The reported overall accuracy rate for identifying tears in the menisci ranges from 90 to 96%. Although it has not been clearly demonstrated in clinical practice, MRI has the potential to demonstrate preoperatively the size and location of a meniscus tear, allowing the surgeon to determine if a repair is indicated or possible. Unfortunately, there are significant cost implications for the routine use of MRI for suspected meniscal tears. The surgeon should be prepared to repair the meniscus if such a procedure is indicated at the time of surgery.

TREATMENT

Nonoperative Treatment

Meniscal tears are treated symptomatically. Following acute injury, protected weight bearing, ice, nonsteroidal anti-inflammatory drugs (NSAIDs), and activity modification are used. A similar program, particularly ice and NSAIDs, is recommended for patients who have an established history of recurrent symptoms and who were not treated at the time of the initial evaluation. Surgery is considered and offered if the patient remains symptomatic despite nonoperative measures.

Two situations, however, may require immediate surgical intervention. A patient who presents with a locked knee should be operated on acutely to restore knee motion. In this situation, a displaced bucket handle tear is usually present and should be addressed with early surgery. When the history and examination of a young athlete suggest a meniscal tear, immediate surgery may be indicated. This is especially true if transient locking has occurred. In this situation, it is possible that recurrent catching or transient locking may cause further damage to the torn meniscus, rendering it more difficult or even impossible to repair. In addition, waiting more than 8 weeks from the time of injury to attempt repair may diminish the expected healing rate. In this case, an MRI study may help determine the size and location of the tear. The treating physician must choose an expectant or surgical treatment plan on a case-to-case basis.

Operative Treatment

INDICATIONS FOR SURGERY

The following factors are important for determining whether meniscal repair is an option: location and size of the tear, anatomy of the tear (simple or complex; radial, longitudinal/vertical, or horizontal), age of the tear, the presence of associated injury, and the age and activity demands of the patient. Tears should be evaluated for tissue quality, with consideration of the potential for altered shape or contraction in chronic cases. Although there is continued debate or controversy in the literature regarding each of these variables, some generalizations can be made.

Tears within the red-red or red-white zones are more favorable for repair than are tears within the white-white zone, which have a high rate of failure following attempted repair. The use of a fibrin clot placed into the site of white-white tears may improve subsequent healing rates, but it has not been clearly established (13–15). Tears less than 1 to 1.5 cm long and those involving less than half the thickness of the meniscus are generally stable and do well if left alone. Synovial abrasion can be done along with rasping of the edge of the tear to stimulate a healing response. Suture fixation is not generally indicated. Stability at the site of a tear can be demonstrated and is best evaluated by direct probing at the time of arthroscopy. If it is possible to evert the edge of the meniscus or to displace it 3 mm or more under or anterior to the femoral condyle, suture repair is done. Generally, tears longer than 2 cm are unstable and should be considered for repair, although healing rates generally diminish as the size of the tear increases.

Radial and horizontal flap tears are less amenable to repair than are vertical (longitudinal) tears, as they typically involve the white-white zone of the meniscus. Similarly, complex tears, in addition to being technically difficult, may yield a higher failure rate as the result of extension into the white-white zone of the meniscus.

The age or chronicity of the tear is significant when the fragment becomes deformed or displaced, making an anatomical reduction impossible at the time of surgery. This can be a particular problem with chronic, large, bucket-handle tears. Some authors have noted that smaller or less complex tears that are older than 8 weeks have a higher failure rate than do more acute injuries, although this has not been the experience of all authors. Some of the discrepancy may be due to the difficulty in identifying the exact time of injury in many cases.

The age and activity level of the patient should also be evaluated. Although no study has definitively demonstrated that healing rates decrease with age, partial meniscectomy may be a reasonable option for middle-aged or older patients, because activity demands usually decline with age. Similarly, degenerative tears or tears associated with preexisting arthritic change should be carefully considered before repair is attempted, as these circumstances (poor meniscal tissue and an unfavorable mechanical environment) may not be conducive to successful healing.

The presence of associated cruciate injury has a significant affect on the healing potential of the meniscus. Meniscus tears done simultaneously with cruciate reconstruction have higher healing rates than do isolated meniscal repairs. This is likely due to the presence of postoperative hemarthrosis, which may contribute exogenous factors to the site of the repair that improve the healing response. Conversely, repair of only the meniscal tear in the presence of coexisting anterior cruciate insufficiency leads to a high rate of failure: the repair is not able to withstand the forces placed on it by the abnormal joint kinematics present in the face of cruciate deficiency. Therefore, both the meniscus and the cruciate ligament should be addressed at surgery (16).

Overall, the suggested ideal candidate for meniscal repair is a young individual with a 2-cm-long vertical acute tear of the lateral meniscus that is located in the red-red zone. A corresponding ACL reconstruction should be done at the same time as the repair. For all patients, each of the above factors should be considered, and the decision to repair or excise the meniscus should be made on an individual basis.

APPROACH

A routine arthroscopic setup is used. The surgeon positions the patient to allow access to both sides of the knee joint. The leg can be free or placed into a thigh-holding device. Access to the medial side of the knee may be improved if the legs are allowed to flex over a break in the foot of the table. Alternatively, the nonoperative extremity can be placed into a well-leg holder and flexed and abducted away from the operative field. A routine diagnostic arthroscopy is performed. If a tear is identified, the decision to repair or to excise it is made. If a coexisting ACL tear will be reconstructed, the meniscal repair sutures are placed, as described below, but not tied until after completion of the ligament reconstruction. This avoids undue stress on the ligament reconstruction during the subsequent meniscal repair that may impart a valgus external rotation force across the knee, especially with tears of the medial meniscus.

The use of a joint distractor may improve visualization and passage of sutures. Skeletal pins are placed into the tibia and femur and are used to increase and maintain the amount of varus or valgus joint space opening during the repair. Although more commonly described in medial meniscus repair, use of the joint distractor is often not necessary for adequate visualization but, in tight or difficult knees, could be considered.

PROCEDURE

Outside-in meniscal repair basically involves passing sutures from outside the knee joint and across the tear site. The sutures are then secured in one of two basic fashions: (a) multiple internal mulberry knots with externally tied ad-

jacent sutures or (b) a vertical or horizontal mattress suture placed (with a suture retrieval system) across the tear site with externally tied individual knots. For both techniques, multiple suture fixation points are necessary. Generally, sutures should be placed at 3- to 5-mm intervals, and the tear should be reapproximated in as anatomic a position as possible. The sutures should be placed perpendicular across the tear to increase the ability of the tear to resist shear and tensile forces. To achieve stable anatomic reapproximation, a combination of sutures placed through both the femoral and the tibial surfaces of the meniscus is often required. Of potential suture materials, only PDS, or nonabsorbable, sutures have been found to yield enough long-term strength for repair. Although there is a concern about the potential for surface wear caused by nonabsorbable suture, this has not been clearly demonstrated in clinical practice. Nonetheless, PDS remains perhaps the most commonly used suture, likely due to its ease of passage and handling at the time of surgery.

Once a tear has been identified as repairable, it is prepared for the procedure. The perimeniscal synovium is rasped to incite a vascular ingrowth and healing response. The torn surface or edges of the meniscus are also rasped or gently shaved to remove any fibrous or cellular overgrowth and to incite a healing response. Attention is then directed to passing the meniscal repair sutures.

A vertical, or longitudinal, incision can be made along the joint line at the site of the tear before suture passage, or the sutures can be passed and then retrieved into one or multiple small incisions just before tying the external knots. Making an initial vertical incision is a more predictable technique and avoids entrapment of adjacent neurovascular structures (saphenous nerve and vein medially; peroneal nerve laterally). The location of the incision can be determined by transilluminating the joint line from inside-out with the arthroscope and passing an 18-gauge spinal needle from outside-in at the site of the tear. For long tears, a single long transverse incision or multiple small vertical incisions may be required to span the entire course of the tear.

On the medial side, it is critical to protect the saphenous neurovascular structures, which lie deep and at the posterior aspect of the sartorius muscle proximal to the joint line. The infrapatellar branch penetrates the sartorius to become superficial and subcutaneous to the fascia at a variable distance from the joint line. A 1- to 2-cm medial vertical skin incision should be made, followed by an incision along the anterior edge of the sartorius. A retractor placed in this interval will protect the saphenous structures posterior; but care should be taken to look for and protect the infrapatellar branch, if its course places it into the operative field. Keeping the knee relatively flexed will also allow the nerve to fall back into a more posterior location. The position of the knee during repair, however, is often dictated by the size and location of the tear; tears on the medial side typically require a position of relative extension for adequate visualization and access.

On the lateral side, the peroneal nerve is at less risk, as it lies posterior to the biceps femoris tendon with the knee in flexion. Because this is typically the position of greatest visualization on the lateral side, the nerve can be easily avoided if all needles enter the joint anterior to the biceps femoris tendon.

Sutures can be passed either with standard 18-gauge spinal needles or with commercially available needles and retrievers. Using standard spinal needles, the needle is passed (with the stylet intact) across the meniscus; and following removal of the stylet, a number 0 or 1 PDS suture is fed through the needle into the joint. To facilitate passage of the needle across the meniscus, it may be necessary to hold the meniscus reduced with a probe or blunt introducer placed via an anterior portal. Once passed, the end of the suture is grasped with an arthroscopic grasper and delivered out through the anterior portal. The needle should be withdrawn once the end of the suture is grasped, but before the suture is delivered anteriorly, to avoid accidental transection of the suture by the edge of the needle. A large mulberry knot is tied into the suture via multiple throws (three to four, generating a 2-mm knot) and is pulled back into the joint. The knot will lie against the surface of the meniscus and reduce the tear. This process is repeated until adequate fixation is achieved. Multiple sutures are passed, and external knots are fashioned by tying together adjacent suture tails (Fig. 58.2). All required sutures are passed before the external knots are tied. This helps avoid inadvertent transection of sutures by subsequent needle passage. It also allows for easy removal if a suture is placed in an unacceptable position.

Another option is to pass two adjacent needles across the meniscus, and deliver two sutures simultaneously via the anterior portal. The sutures can be tied to each other, creating a single mulberry knot that lies against the surface of the meniscus, yielding a mattress-type suture (Fig. 58.3). Alternatively, the two sutures can be tied together

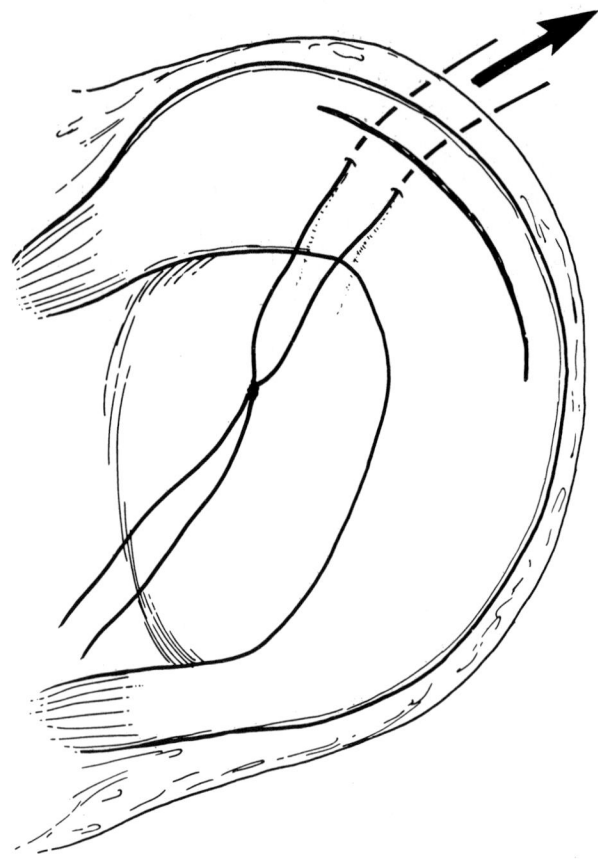

Figure 58.3. The tails of two adjacent sutures may be tied together to create a single intra-articular knot and a mattress-type suture. Reprinted with permission from Cooper DE. Arthroscopic meniscal repair: "outside-in" technique. Op Tech Sports Med 1994;2:190–200.

with a small knot; then one of the sutures is used to retrograde the other (and the knot) back through the meniscus. The result of this technique is a traditional simple mattress suture (Fig. 58.4).

Figure 58.2. Outside-in meniscal repair using a spinal needle and a mulberry knot suture technique. Reprinted with permission from Miller MD, Ritchie JR, Harner CD. Meniscus surgery: indications for repair. Op Tech Sports Med 1994; 2:164–171.

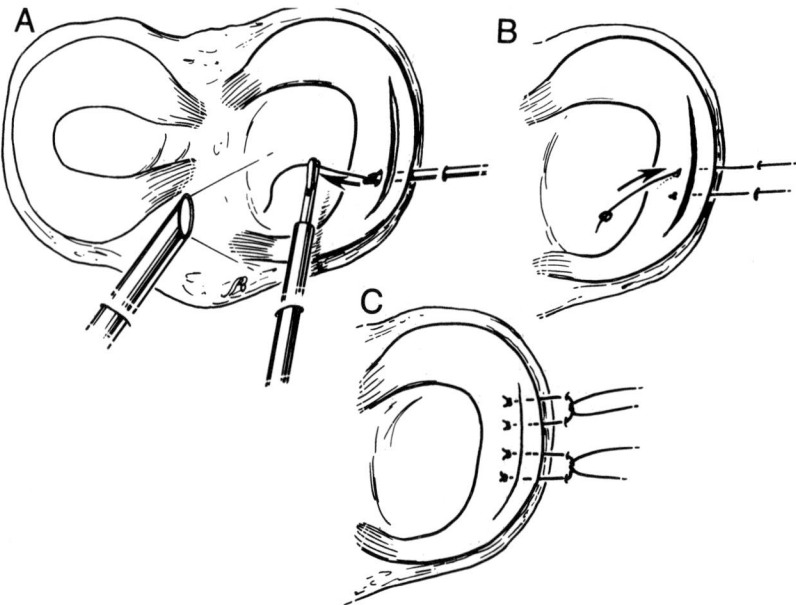

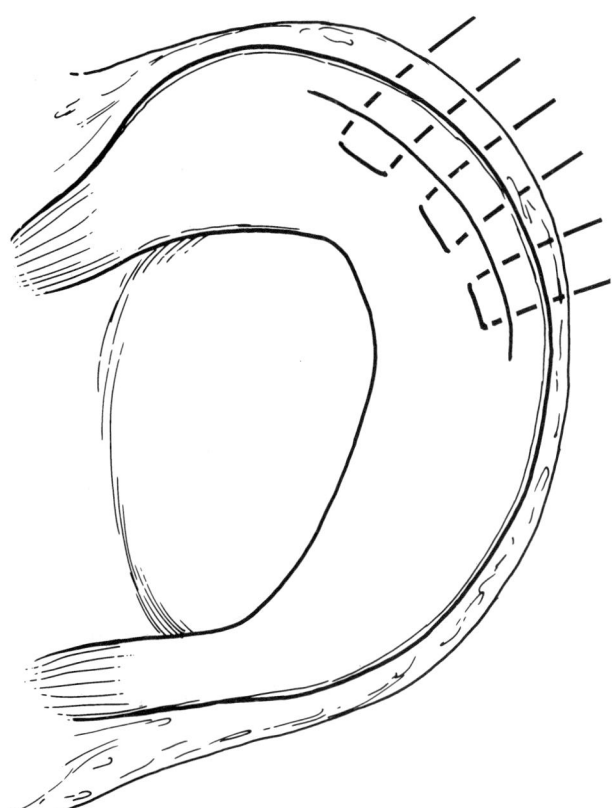

Figure 58.4. A traditional mattress suture can be created from two adjacent sutures by using the intra-articular end of one suture to retrograde the intra-articular end of the other back across the meniscus. Reprinted with permission from Cooper DE. Arthroscopic meniscal repair: "outside-in" technique. Op Tech Sports Med 1994;2:190–200.

Commercially available suture sets typically consist of straight and curved needles. Wire snares and stylets allow for intra-articular retrieval of the suture to create simple mattress sutures. With these systems, retrieval of the suture out the anterior portal is eliminated. Two needles are passed across the meniscus from outside in. A suture is delivered into the joint via one of the needles, while a snare is passed through the other needle. A retriever or grabber is delivered via the anterior portal and through the loop of the snare to grab the end of the intra-articular suture (Fig. 58.5). The suture end is then pulled through the snare and, finally, retrograded back across the meniscus to complete the creation of a mattress suture.

After the sutures are passed, tension is held across them so the adequacy of the repair can be assessed. The meniscus should be anatomically reapproximated and show no tendency to invert or buckle. In addition, the repair should be stable to probing. If the placed sutures are inadequate, they should be removed and replaced or additional sutures added. If ligament reconstruction is to be performed, clamps are placed on the suture tails (maintaining identification of associated tails for mattress sutures), and the external knots are tied after the ligament reconstruction is complete. If a fibrin clot is to be added to the repair site, it is carefully placed just before the meniscal sutures are tied.

When tying the sutures, the surgeon must be careful to maintain adequate tension so the meniscus can be approximated. It is critical to check and ensure that neurovascular structures are not caught between the suture tails before the knots are tied. After the sutures are sequentially tied, the meniscal repair is reassessed for acceptable anatomic position and stability.

PITFALLS AND COMMON TECHNICAL MISTAKES

Besides the potential neurovascular complications discussed above, one of the greatest potential complications of the outside-in repair is inadvertent damage to the articular surface when passing the spinal needles. Great care must be taken when placing these needles; the surgeon should use the associated instrumentation to avoid gouging or lacerating the chondral surface during the repair.

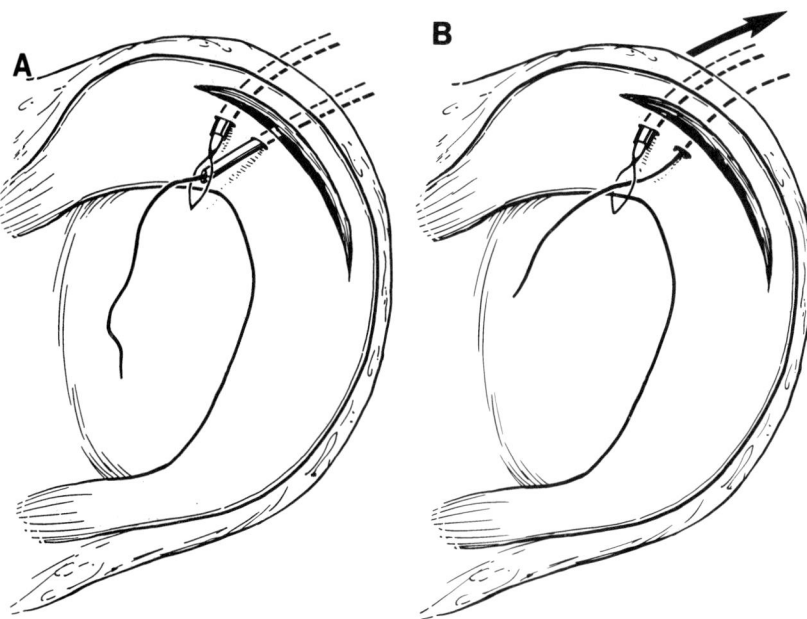

Figure 58.5. Using a suture snare, a mattress suture is created by retrograding the intra-articular tail of the suture back across the meniscus. Reprinted with permission from Cooper DE. Arthroscopic meniscal repair: "outside-in" technique. Op Tech Sports Med 1994;2:190–200.

Another potential pitfall of the outside-in repair is difficult access to posterior horn tears. To ensure optimal tear approximation and fixation, sutures should be passed as perpendicular to the line of the tear as possible. As the tear progresses posteriorly, the sutures tend to become more obliquely oriented to the tear, especially with vertical tears. Occasionally, oblique sutures may create buckling or suboptimal apposition of the torn segments of the meniscus. Although a more posterior incision may improve access to the posterior horns for needle passage, it places the neurovascular structures at increased risk. Fortunately, the use of curved needles in these situations can improve access to the posterior horn and allow passage of the sutures in most cases (Fig. 58.6).

REHABILITATION

Surgeons use a wide variety of rehabilitation protocols following meniscal repair. Although early protocols were fairly conservative, advocating casting or other forms of immobilization and allowing no weight bearing, current protocols are relatively aggressive. These accelerated programs have shown no adverse effect on healing rates. Most surgeons allow partial to full weight bearing in extension

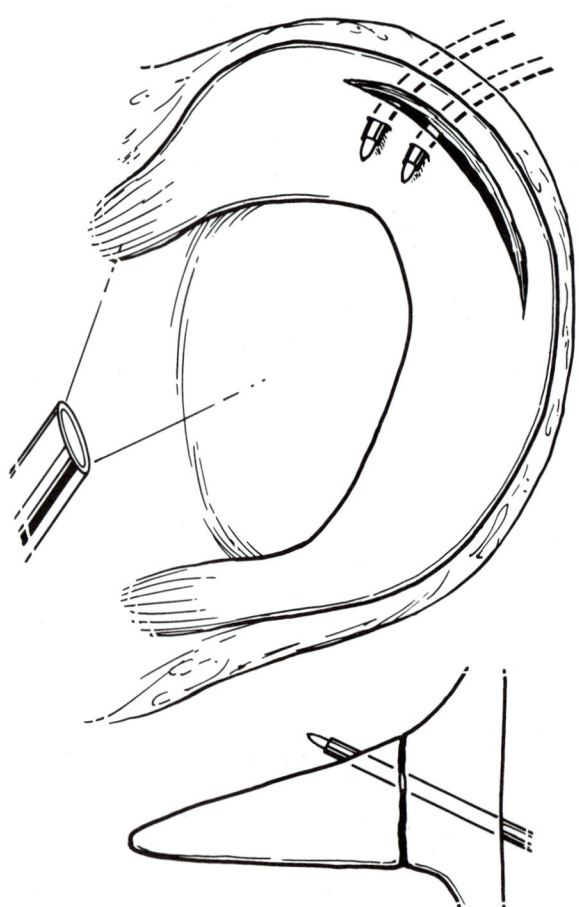

Figure 58.6. Access to the posterior horn may be obtained by using curved needles. Reprinted with permission from Cooper DE. Arthroscopic meniscal repair: "outside-in" technique. Op Tech Sports Med 1994;2:190–200.

immediately following surgery. Some authors believe that the compressive load and generated hoop stresses may maintain apposition of the repair site during weight bearing in extension. Isometric hamstring and quadriceps exercises and straight-leg exercises are initiated immediately after surgery.

The range of motion allowed following surgery is more variable and controversial; some surgeons allow full immediate motion and others follow a graduated program of increasing motion. Flexion beyond 90° has the potential to place increased stress on the posterior meniscus; however, patients who followed an accelerated rehabilitation program (particularly in the presence of a concomitant ACL reconstruction) demonstrated no solid evidence of poor meniscal healing rates. Regardless, hyperflexion and squatting are usually discouraged for the first 4 to 6 months, as is participation in most athletic activities, except for swimming and jogging.

RESULTS

Healing rates for arthroscopic-assisted meniscal repair have been quite good; success rates range from 78 to 95%, with an average failure rate of 10 to 15%. The increased rates of healing reported in more recent studies likely represent improved techniques and patient selection for repair. The clinical success rate is typically higher than the absolute rate of healing as determined by second-look arthroscopy, arthrography, or MRI. Some tears remain unhealed but clinically asymptomatic. Although overall healing rates are high, the long-term success of meniscal repair in terms of its ability to prevent or diminish subsequent degenerative change remains under investigation.

SUMMARY

Once thought to be vestigial and functionless, the menisci are now recognized as vital and integral components of normal knee function. Meniscal repair is currently considered an alternative to meniscectomy in some patients, as meniscectomy has been shown to be associated with a significant risk of long-term degenerative changes within the knee. Besides having knowledge of and familiarity with the available techniques, the surgeon must be able to identify the tears that are favorable for repair and healing. These factors are summarized in Table 58.1. Although all of these factors are important to consider, there remains some controversy in the literature, and a general consensus regarding all potential variables is lacking. Most surgeons support the concept that the ideal candidate for repair is a young patient with an acute, 2-cm-long vertical peripheral (red-red) tear of the lateral meniscus. Best results are achieved when a concomitant ACL reconstruction is performed.

At the time of repair, adequate visualization and preparation of the tear are mandatory. Sutures must be placed to ensure stable anatomic reapproximation of the torn segments, and care must be taken to protect the neu-

| table | 58.1 | Identifying the Potential for Repair |

Characteristic	Good Potential for Repair	Poor Potential for Repair
Vascularity	Red-red; red-white	White-white
Type of tear	Vertical (longitudinal)	Horizontal; radial; complex; degenerative
Age of tear	Acute	Chronic (>8 weeks)
Size of tear	<2.0–2.5 cm	>2.5 cm
Ligamentous injury	Torn ACL (simultaneous repair)	ACL intact (or no reconstruction of a torn ACL)

rovascular structures and articular surfaces from iatrogenic injury. Recommended rehabilitation protocols vary, but the trend is toward accelerated protocols that allow immediate weight bearing in extension and progressive range of motion exercises. Hyperflexion and squatting are initially avoided, and return to full athletic activity is generally delayed until the 4th or 6th month after surgery. Overall rates of healing are between 78 and 95%; the average failure rate is 10 to 15%. It is hoped that a successful repair will preserve meniscal function and prevent subsequent degenerative articular changes within the knee.

REFERENCES

1. Johnson LL. Meniscus repair. The outside-in technique. In: Jackson DW, ed. Reconstructive knee surgery. New York: Raven, 1995:51.
2. Arnoczky SP, Warren RF. Microvasculature of the human meniscus. Am J Sports Med 1982;10:90–95.
3. Seedhom BB. Transmission of the load in the knee joint with special reference to the role of the menisci. Part I: Anatomy, analysis, and apparatus. Eng Med 1979;8:207–219.
4. O'Meara PM. The basic science of meniscus repair. Orthop Rev 1993;22:681–686.
5. Fairbank TJ. Knee joint changes after meniscectomy. J Bone Joint Surg 1948;30B:664–670.
6. Johnson RJ, Kettlekamp DB, Clark W. Factors affecting late results after meniscectomy. J Bone Joint Surg 1974;56A:719–729.
7. Diment MT, DeHaven KE, Sebastianelli WJ. Arthroscopy: current concepts in meniscal repair. Orthopedics 1993;16:973–977.
8. O'Meara PM. Surgical techniques for arthroscopic meniscal repair. Orthop Rev 1993;22:781–790.
9. Cooper DE, Arnoczky SP, Warren RF. Meniscal repair. Clin Sports Med 1991;10:529–548.
10. Morgan CD. The "all-inside" meniscus repair. Arthroscopy 1991; 7:120–125.
11. Warren RF. Arthroscopic meniscal repair. Arthroscopy 1985; 1:170–172.
12. Marzo JM, Warren RF, Arnoczky SP, Nicholas SJ. Arthroscopic meniscal repair: review of the outside-in technique. Am J Knee Surg 1991;4:164–172.
13. Arnoczky SP, Warren RF, Spivak JM. Meniscal repair using an exogenous fibrin clot: an experimental study in dogs. J Bone Joint Surg 1988;70B:1209–1217.
14. Rodeo SA, Warren RF, Arnoczky SP. Meniscal repair using an exogenous fibrin clot. Tech Orthop 1993;8:113–119.
15. Rodeo SA, Warren RF. Indications and techniques for use of a fibrin clot in meniscal repair. Op Tech Sports Med 1994;2:217–222.
16. Warren RF. Meniscectomy and repair in the anterior cruciate ligament-deficient patient. Clin Orthop 1990;252:55–63.

chapter 59

Arthroscopic Meniscus Repair: Inside-out Technique

Marc H. Rubman and Thomas N. Lindenfeld

The menisci of the human knee are structures vital to the long-term preservation and function of the knee. As a result of their collagen orientation and proteoglycan matrix, the menisci can decrease the stresses to the articular surfaces by distributing the forces associated with weight bearing. They also function as shock absorbers, secondary stabilizers to anterior subluxation, and lubricators of the knee (1). Loss of meniscus function, either through tearing, degeneration, or surgical excision, has been shown to decrease the tibiofemoral contact area and greatly increase the contact stresses (2,3). Long-term follow-up of patients who underwent total meniscectomies showed rapid degeneration of the joint with joint space narrowing, flattening of the femoral condyle, erosion of the articular cartilage, and osteophyte formation (4,5). These studies underscore the biomechanical importance of the menisci.

Unfortunately for many young active patients, up until the late 1970s the standard treatment for meniscal tears was total meniscectomy. Partial meniscectomy, a procedure that became technically feasible with the advent of arthroscopy, provided the surgeon with an alternative to complete removal of the meniscus. However, follow-up studies showed that retaining a portion of the meniscus did not protect the knee from the rapid degeneration of the articular surfaces that was seen with total meniscectomy (2,6–8).

In an attempt to preserve meniscus function, meniscus repair was introduced to eliminate the symptoms associated with a torn meniscus without loss of meniscus tissue. First introduced as open procedures, arthroscopically assisted meniscal repair techniques were developed as the technical abilities of arthroscopic surgeons kept pace with the development of smaller and more precise instrumentation. Numerous studies have been published that outline the techniques and modifications (9–14). Our preferred method for meniscal repair is the arthroscopically assisted inside-out method in which, under arthroscopic control, the suture needles are directed through the meniscus and then out through the posteromedial or posterolateral corner of the knee. A second incision is used in the posterior corner for needle retrieval and knot tying. This method allows an accurate reduction and stable repair of the meniscus tear, which are not possible with the other commonly employed methods.

RELEVANT ANATOMY AND PATHOGENESIS

The menisci, or semilunar cartilages, are interposed between the femoral condyles and the tibial plateau in the knee. One meniscus is located in each tibiofemoral compartment. Although they are firmly affixed to the peripheral tissues and tibial plateau, there is a normal amount of excursion or motion associated with them. This motion allows the meniscus to conform to the changing shape of the femoral condyle during knee flexion and extension. The lateral meniscus has greater excursion and motion than the medial meniscus. This is the reason for a decreased incidence of lateral meniscal tears.

The menisci are composed primarily of type I collagen arranged circumferentially to allow for stress reduction during weight bearing and knee motion. The remainder of the meniscus is composed of water, mucopolysaccharides, and proteoglycans. Its composition assists greatly in its role to reduce tibiofemoral contact stresses.

Vascularity in the meniscus changes with age. At birth, the meniscus is almost entirely vascularized. By age 9 months, the inner one-third has lost its vascular supply, and by age 10 years, the meniscus resembles the adult meniscus with vessels penetrating only to the peripheral one-third (15). In the adult meniscus the outer one-third is classified as the "red" zone, while the inner one-third is considered avascular and referred to as the "white" zone.

Meniscal tears can occur as a result of acute trauma, age-related changes to the tissues, or a combination of both. Tear patterns have been described previously (16). Tear pattern and location are critical issues in the success of a meniscal repair, regardless of the method employed.

INITIAL FINDINGS, PHYSICAL EXAMINATION, AND DIAGNOSIS

Eliciting a careful history and completing a comprehensive physical examination are usually all that is necessary to diagnose a torn meniscus. Associated injuries to the soft tissues and articular surfaces may be present as well and need to be differentiated from the meniscal injury. The patient will usually describe an acute twisting injury with associated pain in either compartment and the posterior aspect of the knee. Locking may be present, and there is pain with deep flexion or squatting and usually on weight bearing. The patient may describe increased pain when descending steps.

The important components of the physical examination include range of motion testing, palpation of the joint line with special attention to the posterior aspect of the respective compartment, and provocative maneuvers to elicit symptoms. The patient may have loss of extension as a result of a displaced meniscal fragment into the anterior aspect of the joint or increased pain with deep flexion as the posterior horn of the meniscus is compressed by the posterior aspect of the femoral condyle. Careful palpation along the entire joint line, including the posterior aspect of the compartment, will usually elicit pain as a result of the inflammatory reaction of the synovium and neuroreceptors within the meniscus. Provocative maneuvers, such as the McMurray test, can aid in the diagnosis of the tear by displacing it and re-creating the pain.

RADIOLOGIC STUDIES AND DIAGNOSTIC TESTS

Plain radiographs should be performed for any acute injury to the knee to rule out a fracture involving the articular surface; but they may not reveal any information about soft tissue injuries, such as a meniscus tear. Before the routine use of noninvasive diagnostic testing such as MRI, arthrography was used to either diagnose or confirm the diagnosis of a meniscal tear. This method was shown to be both sensitive and specific to meniscal tears and to have an accuracy approaching that of arthroscopy (17–22). MRI, perhaps the best noninvasive diagnostic method for evaluating soft tissues, has all but replaced arthrography as the test of choice in diagnosis of meniscal tears; and recent studies show its sensitivity to equal that of arthroscopy (23). MRI however, is limited in its ability to accurately determine the pattern of the tear and is an expensive examination. In most cases, a detailed history and careful physical examination are all that is required to make the

diagnosis, and diagnostic testing should be reserved for only the most unusual or difficult cases.

TREATMENT

Nonoperative Treatment

Conservative treatment of meniscal tears is based on the symptoms and limitations that the patient is experiencing. If the symptoms are mild and the patient is able to perform activities of daily living (ADLs), then nonsteroidal anti-inflammatory drugs (NSAIDs) and a simple knee rehabilitation program to restore full range of motion and strengthen the knee flexors and extensors may be initiated. Meniscal tears that are not repaired have a low potential for healing. Tears at the meniscal–synovial junction or 1 to 2 mm central to this region in the vascular portion of the meniscus may heal spontaneously. Other tears may become asymptomatic over time, but will be unlikely to heal on their own.

If the patient is disabled by the severity of the symptoms and has loss of knee motion, the conservative approach should be rejected in favor of arthroscopic examination and, if indicated, meniscal repair. A locked knee should never be treated conservatively because of the potential for significant long-term damage to the meniscus or the joint surfaces and possible permanent motion loss.

Operative Treatment

Operative indications for arthroscopy when a meniscal tear is diagnosed include locked knee, pain and inability to perform ADLs following an acute injury after concomitant soft tissue swelling has subsided, and pain that lasts longer than 3 or 4 months despite a conservative treatment program (Clinical Table). In the majority of cases when instability of the knee is present from an anterior cruciate ligament rupture, reconstruction should be performed if the patient has an active lifestyle and participates in activities that require jumping, cutting, or twisting. At the time of reconstruction, any meniscal disorder should be addressed and any repairable tear should be treated.

Repair of a meniscal tear is based on five factors: tear pattern, quality of meniscal tissue, location of the tear, ability to reduce the tear, and the patient's age. The surgeon should carefully visualize and probe the menisci during arthroscopic examination to identify the tear pattern. All tear patterns are potentially repairable, but single longitudinal tears have higher healing rates than do other more complex tear patterns. The quality of the meniscal tissue is an important consideration. Menisci that have marked tissue degeneration may not be able to hold the sutures and thus are not amenable to repair.

Tears within the peripheral one-third of the meniscus are vascular and have been shown to have highest rates of both arthroscopic healing and clinical success (24–29). Tears within the avascular portion of the meniscus (red-

Clinical Table: Arthroscopic Meniscus Repair: Inside-out Technique

Procedure	Indications	Technique	Anatomy	Pitfalls
Medial meniscus repair	• Repairable tear that causes joint symptoms	• Arthroscopically assisted using an inside-out technique	• Accessory incision to the posteromedial corner of the knee • Arthroscopic placement of sutures	• Poor-quality meniscal tissue • Infrapatellar branch of the saphenous nerve • Postoperative motion loss
Lateral meniscus repair	• Repairable tear that causes joint symptoms	• Arthroscopically assisted using an inside-out technique	• Accessory incision to the posterolateral corner of the knee • Arthroscopic placement of sutures	• Poor-quality meniscal tissue • Peroneal nerve • Postoperative motion loss
Arthroscopic partial meniscectomy	• Meniscal tear that is not amenable to repair • Tibiofemoral joint symptoms	• Arthroscopic hand instruments and suction shaver	• Standard arthroscopic portals • Accessory portal may be used if needed • Meniscus is trimmed to a stable edge, leaving as much tissue as possible remaining	• Loss of even a small percentage of meniscus may lead to degenerative changes

white and white-white) are amenable to repair in select cases and, when possible, should be repaired to preserve meniscal function (15,16,25,30). The surgeon must be able to reduce the tear and firmly repair the inner fragment to the rim. The two sides of the tear must be brought into direct apposition and any gaps or clefts must be eliminated. In chronic tears, the displaced segment of the meniscus may have undergone degeneration, shortening, or deformation; and in these cases, a partial meniscectomy may be needed to trim any portion that cannot be reduced. Again, the meniscal tissue must be strong enough to support the sutures needed for repair.

The age of the patient is a consideration; however, the decision to repair should not be made solely on this criterion. A recent study has shown that age does not have a significant influence on healing (29). In young patients, every effort must be made to preserve meniscal function; and repair should always be attempted in amenable tears. Older individuals who have active lifestyles should also be considered candidates for repair if the above criteria are met.

Once the decision has been made to repair the meniscus, the first two steps—rasping the parameniscal synovium and tear edges and making the approach to the posteromedial or posterolateral capsule—must be performed. Rasping of the synovium creates an inflammatory reaction that promotes bleeding along the meniscosynovial junction and into the tear. This inflammatory reaction has been shown to improve healing rates of tears repaired with the inside-out method (31). A ball-tipped or similar rasp is used to abrade the parameniscal synovium and the tear edges. Abrasion of the tear removes any fibrinous debris that may have accumulated on the edges in the interval between injury and repair. This allows direct apposition of the meniscal tissue and improves healing potential.

The patient should be positioned supine on the operating table with the operative knee flexed to 90°. The table may be tilted so the appropriate aspect of the knee is brought up into view. The operative extremity should be exsanguinated to allow a bloodless field, and the surgeon may choose to sit for this portion of the procedure.

MEDIAL APPROACH

The approach to the posteromedial corner of the knee requires careful dissection to avoid the infrapatellar branch of the saphenous nerve; but it is a direct approach that, once mastered adds only several minutes to the procedure time. Before making an incision, the surgeon should identify the medial collateral ligament (MCL), the joint line, and the semimembranosus tendon. The 3-cm incision is made obliquely, from posterior-superior to anterior-inferior, parallel to the anterior fibers of the sartorius fascia, one-third above the joint line and two-thirds below it (Fig. 59.1A). The incision proceeds through the subcutaneous fat down to the first layer: the sartorius fascia. The infrapatella branch of the saphenous nerve runs in an oblique direction along the surface of the sartorius fascia, roughly parallel to its fibers. At the anterior margin of the incision, the surgeon opens the fascia in line with its fibers, taking care to avoid aiming posteriorly (Fig. 59.1B). The fascia is retracted and bluntly dissected through the fatty tissue. The semimembranosus tendon should be palpable in the center of the wound, surrounded by its sheath. The interval is sharply opened just superior to the tendon's insertion onto the tibia, and the surgeon bluntly enlarges this opening. The medial gastrocnemius tendon is palpated; and with blunt dissection, the surgeon opens the interval just anterior to this, between the gastrocnemius tendon and the posteromedial capsule (Fig. 59.1C). The joint line and the corresponding femoral condyle and

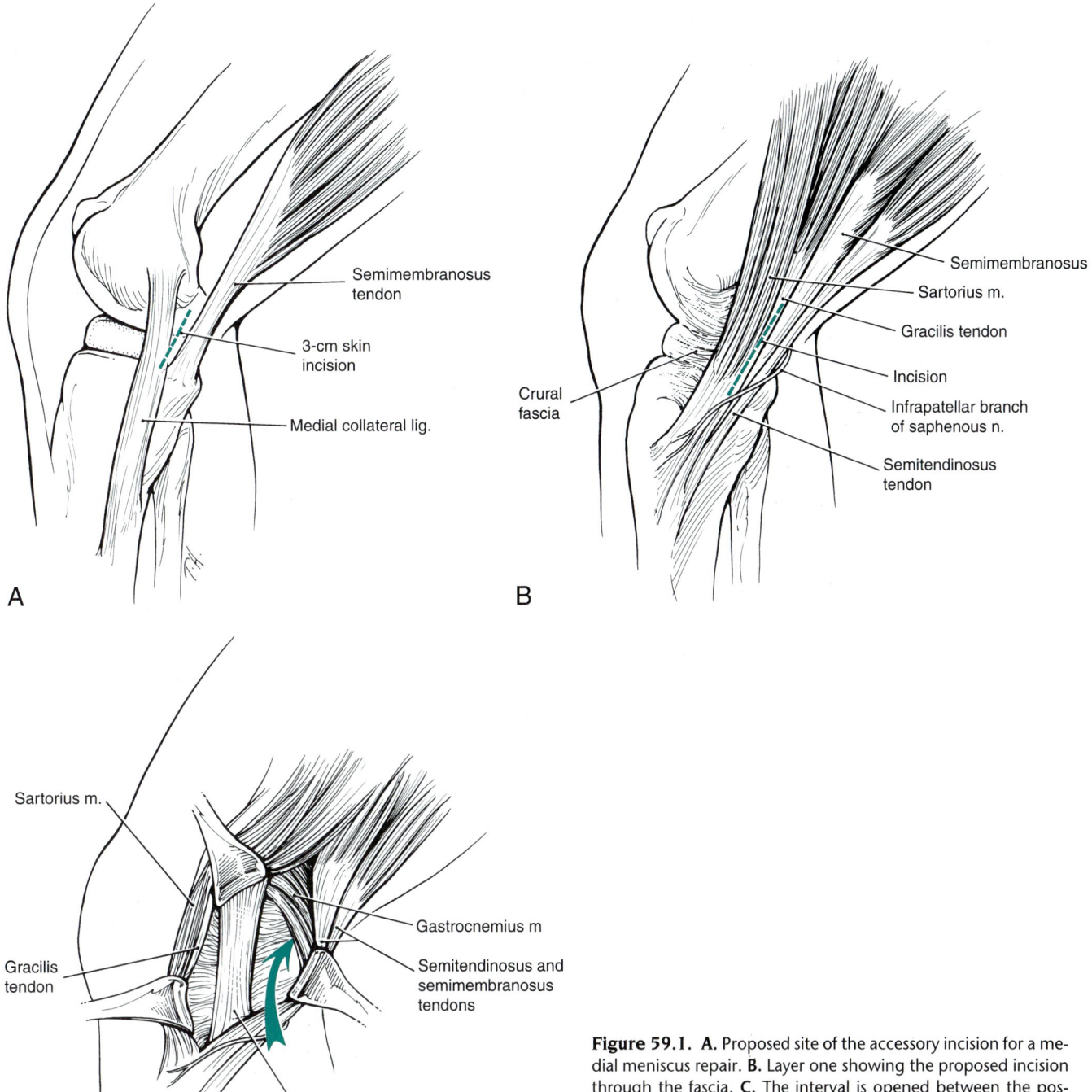

Figure 59.1. A. Proposed site of the accessory incision for a medial meniscus repair. **B.** Layer one showing the proposed incision through the fascia. **C.** The interval is opened between the posteromedial capsule and the gastrocnemius, just proximal to the semimembranosus tendon (*arrow*).

tibial plateau are palpated. This interval is opened to allow easy passage of a popliteal retractor.

LATERAL APPROACH

The corresponding approach to the posterolateral corner is performed for repair of a lateral meniscus. In these cases, care is taken to avoid the peroneal nerve, which is posterior to the working area. The surgeon identifies the fibula head, the lateral collateral ligament (LCL), and the joint line. A 3-cm incision is made obliquely posterior to the LCL, parallel to the posterior edge of the iliotibial band (ITB) and the anterior edge of the biceps tendon

(Fig. 59.2A). The incision is carried through to the subcutaneous tissue until the ITB is identified. The surgeon clears any overlying subcutaneous tissue off of the ITB and identifies its posterior edge and the musculotendinous junction of the biceps femoris. The biceps tendon can be palpated down to the fibula head. The interval between the ITB and the biceps is opened, and the biceps is brought posterior and inferior (Fig. 59.2B). The peroneal nerve is posterior and medial to the biceps at this level. By placing an Army-Navy retractor on the biceps and gently pulling it posterior and inferior, the surgeon can protect the peroneal nerve. The superior lateral geniculate ves-

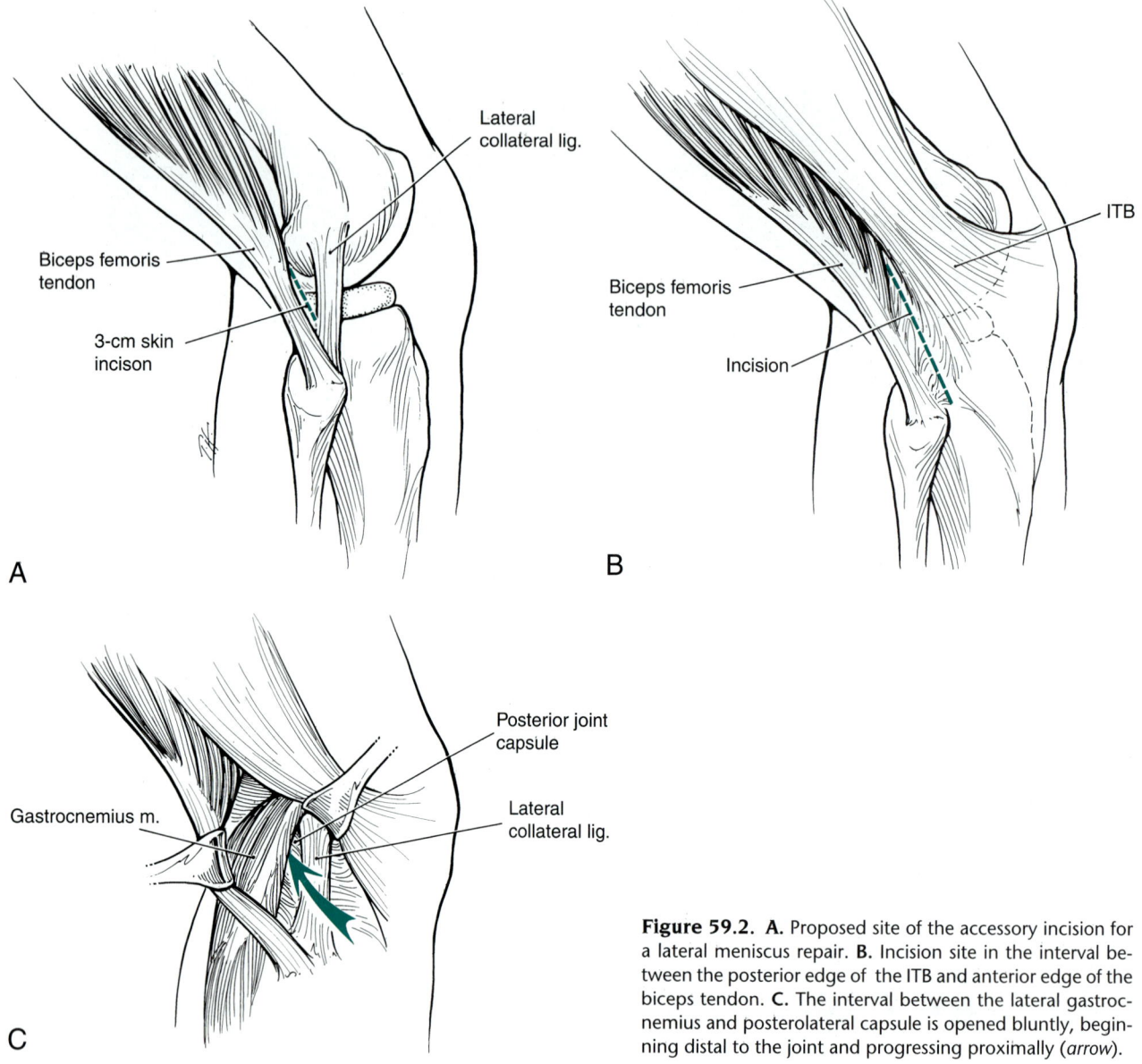

A

B

C

Figure 59.2. A. Proposed site of the accessory incision for a lateral meniscus repair. **B.** Incision site in the interval between the posterior edge of the ITB and anterior edge of the biceps tendon. **C.** The interval between the lateral gastrocnemius and posterolateral capsule is opened bluntly, beginning distal to the joint and progressing proximally (*arrow*).

sels course through this area and, if encountered, may be coagulated and transected. The surgeon enlarges this interval and palpates the lateral gastrocnemius tendon. The lateral gastrocnemius tendon inserts closer to the epicondyle than does the medial gastrocnemius tendon, which inserts posterior, almost on the distal metaphysis of the femur. The interval between the gastrocnemius and the posterior capsule is identified at the level of the musculotendinous junction, which is just inferior to the joint line and the meniscus. The surgeon opens this interval bluntly to the level of the meniscus and joint line so a popliteal retractor can be easily inserted into this area (Fig. 59.2C).

ARTHROSCOPICALLY ASSISTED MENISCAL REPAIR TECHNIQUE

After the accessory incision has been completed, the surgeon can reinitiate arthroscopy. For both medial and lateral meniscal repairs, we begin with our arthroscope in the inferolateral portal and our needle cannula in the inferomedial portal (Fig. 59.3). Zone-specific cannulae are available and can be helpful in certain situations. Occasionally, it is necessary to switch portals to access a tear with the needle cannula. If during the approach to the posteromedial or posterolateral corner the capsule was torn, it should be oversewn with a 2–0 absorbable suture. This prevents fluid extravasation and allows an improved view of the needle tip when it enters the popliteal retractor.

We use a single-barrel needle cannula because it allows accurate placement of the sutures across the tear. Double-barrel cannulae, in our opinion, do not separate the arms of the suture sufficiently or allow the suture to be placed into the best tissue. We use 2–0 monofilament absorbable polydioxanone suture (PDS II; Ethicon, Sommerville, NJ) and 2–0 braided nonabsorbable polyester suture

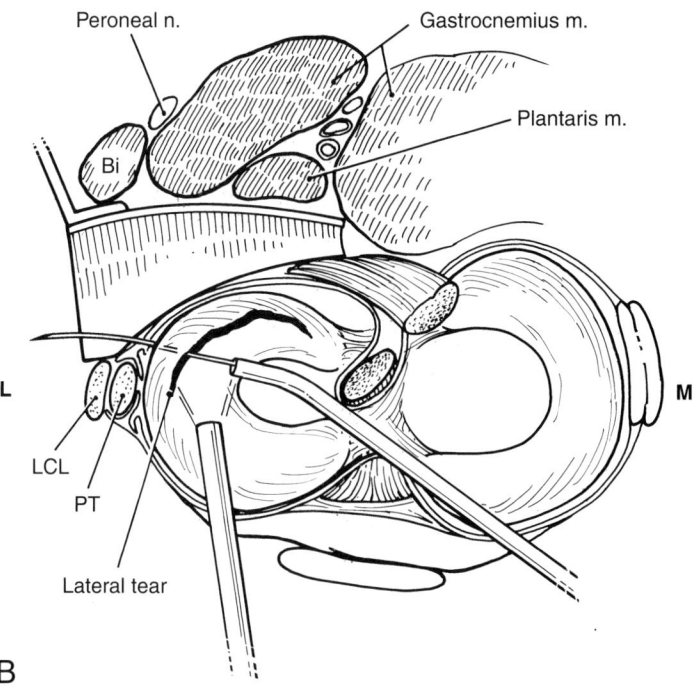

Figure 59.3. Top view of the joint with arthroscope, needle cannula, and popliteal retractor in place for a medial meniscus repair (**A**) and a lateral meniscus repair (**B**). *PT,* posterior tendon; *Bi,* biceps.

(Ethibond; Ethicon) double-armed with a 25-cm trocar-point needles, alternating between suture type. Sutures are placed in a double-stacked vertical arrangement and are placed through both the superior and the inferior surfaces (Fig. 59.4). Sutures are placed every 3 to 4 mm to ensure a tight repair.

Our first stitch is always into the peripheral rim of the superior surface, followed by a stitch into the central fragment, also on the superior surface (Fig. 59.5). This allows for approximation of the tear edges. If the first throw is placed into the central fragment with the meniscus in a displaced position, the tear edges will not be approximated (Fig. 59.5D). If the initial stitch is placed into the inferior (tibial) surface, the central fragment may again be

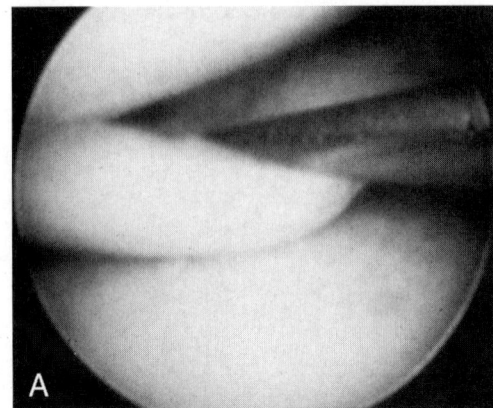

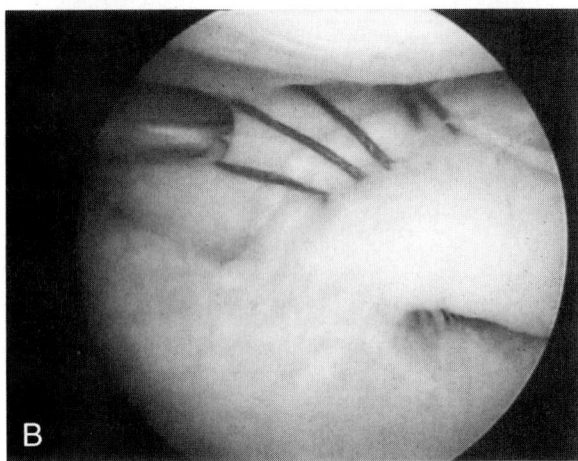

Figure 59.4. A. Arthroscopic evaluation of a longitudinal meniscus tear. Note the displacement into the tibiofemoral joint. **B.** The double-stacked vertical sutures have been placed. Note the reduction of the tear.

secured in a displaced position. The reduction of the meniscus must be checked after the first set of sutures are placed and tied.

A popliteal retractor is used at all times during needle passage to prevent injury to the neurovascular structures of the posterior knee. An assistant is seated on the appropriate side of the leg and retrieves the sutures, then firmly ties each one as they are passed. A headlight may be necessary to illuminate the depths of the wound. We no longer clamp each pair of sutures and tie them at the end of the procedure. Once the first throws of the suture are placed, tension in the knot is checked arthroscopically.

Once the sutures have been placed, tied, and checked arthroscopically, the meniscus is probed to ensure that the repair is stable. Any portion that can be displaced must be either repaired or excised. If the repair is holding, any other procedure that may need to be performed can be addressed. The accessory incision is copiously irrigated and the deep structures are closed with absorbable 2–0 sutures (Vicryl; Ethicon); 4–0 absorbable sutures (PDS; Ethicon) are placed in subcuticular fashion for the skin. Care must be taken when placing the medial sutures in the deep layer to avoid the infrapatellar branch of the saphe-

nous nerve. Sutures that put tension on this nerve may cause neuritis.

PITFALLS, COMPLICATIONS, AND COMMON MISTAKES

The complications most frequently encountered in arthroscopic meniscal repairs are nerve injury or irritation, arterial injury, infection, and limitation of postoperative knee motion. The neurovascular structures are at risk during the approach to the posteromedial or posterolateral capsule, suture passage, and suture tying. Small (32) reported that the rate of complications from arthroscopic meniscal repairs was lower than that found in arthroscopic partial meniscectomies.

Nerve injuries in meniscal repair can occur from either direct trauma or traction-type injury. They are most likely to occur during the approach to the posteromedial or posterolateral corner of the knee but can also occur as a result of suture passage or knot tying. To limit damage to the nerves, the surgeon must be familiar with the course of the saphenous and common peroneal nerves (33,34). Because of its anatomic variability on the medial side, the surgeon

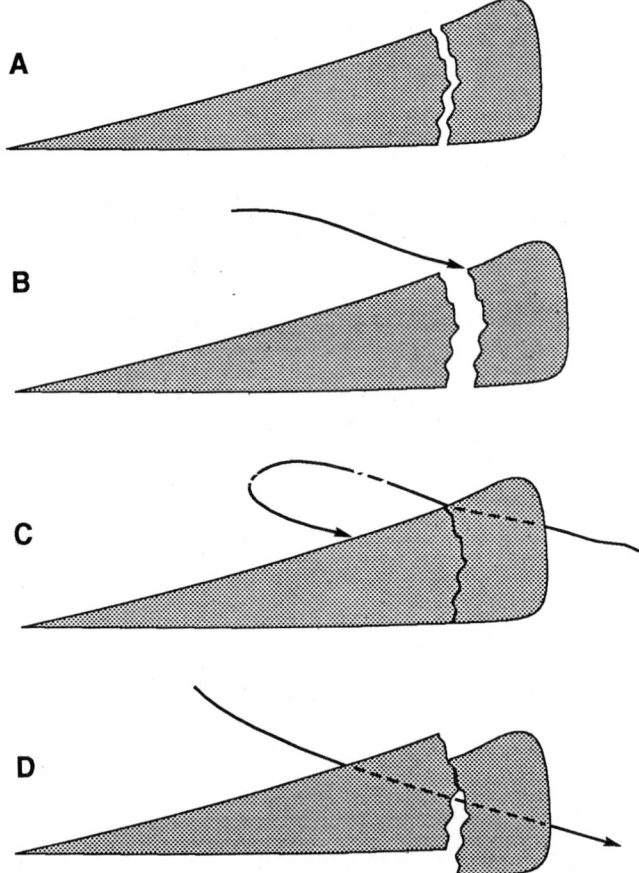

Figure 59.5. A. A tear in the meniscus is identified. **B.** Our preferred technique of repair is to place the first throw into the superior corner of the meniscal rim. **C.** The second throw reduces the central fragment to the rim in an anatomic position. **D.** An incorrectly placed first stitch goes into the central fragment, which will leave the meniscus in a displaced position.

must identify the infrapatellar branch of the saphenous nerve during the approach to avoid injury. Maintaining knee flexion at 90° during the approach will shift the saphenous nerve posterior to the incision. Injury to this nerve, by either direct trauma or traction, can result in pain or paresthesias and may initiate sympathetically mediated saphenous neuritis. On the lateral side, the peroneal nerve lies posterior to the biceps tendon and, therefore, should be posterior to the incision and dissection. The surgeon should limit the distal extension of the incision to the proximal border of the fibula head and keep the knee flexed to 90° during the approach to avoid injury to this structure.

Vascular injury is a rare occurrence in arthroscopic meniscal repair; however, it can occur if care is not taken during suturing and needle passage. The popliteal artery runs through the popliteal space; and although it is a safe distance from the posterior corner of the knee, the artery (and the tibial nerve) is at risk if the surgeon crosses the midline during the approach. During needle passage, the surgeon must be aware of the position of the needle tip and the bend in the cannula to avoid directing the needle tip toward the midline.

Meniscal repair using the inside-out technique requires a second posteromedial or posterolateral incision, which can increase the risk of infection. As with any surgical procedure, maintenance of a sterile field, meticulous soft tissue technique, and copious irrigation will decrease the incidence of infection, as will the use of perioperative antibiotics.

Postoperative limitation of motion from intra-articular scarring is a potential complication of any operative procedure of the knee (35). A rehabilitation program that emphasizes early motion can be instituted if the meniscal repair is stable (36,37). Many meniscal repairs are performed in conjunction with anterior cruciate ligament (ACL) reconstructions, and early motion programs have been shown to not adversely affect meniscal healing (25). Early identification of motion problems will allow the surgeon and therapist to initiate a specific program designed to improve the range of motion.

REFERENCES

1. Mow VC, Ratcliffe A, Chern KY, Kelly MA. Structure and function relationships of the menisci of the knee. In: Mow VC, Arnoczky SP, Jackson DW, eds., Knee meniscus: basic and clinical foundations. New York: Raven, 1992:37–57.
2. Baratz ME, Fu FH, Mengato R. Meniscal tears: the effect of meniscectomy and of repair on intraarticular contact areas and stress in the human knee. Am J Sports Med 1986;14:270–275.
3. Seedhom BB, Hargreaves DJ. Transmission of the load in the knee joint with special reference to the role of the meniscus. Eng Med 1979;8:220–228.
4. Fairbank TJ. Knee joint changes after meniscectomy. J Bone Joint Surg 1948;30B:664–670.
5. Johnson RJ, Kettelkamp DB, Clark W, Leaverton P. Factors affecting late results after meniscectomy. Bone Joint Surg 1974;56A:719–729.
6. Ferkel RD, Davis R, Friedman MJ, et al. Arthroscopic partial me-

7. Jackson RW, Rouse DW. The results of partial arthroscopic meniscectomy in patients over 40 years of age. J Bone Joint Surg 1982;64B:481–485.
8. Lynch MA, Henning CE, Glick KR Jr. Knee joint surface changes. Long-term follow-up meniscus tear treatment in stable anterior cruciate ligament reconstructions. Clin Orthop 1983;172:148–153.
9. Barber FA, Stone RG. Meniscal repair. An arthroscopic technique. J Bone Joint Surg 1985;67B:39–41.
10. Henning CE. Arthroscopic repair of meniscus tears. Orthopedics 1983;6:1130–1132.
11. Jakob RP, Staubli HU, Zuber K, Esser M. The arthroscopic meniscal repair. techniques and clinical experience. Am J Sports Med 1988;16:137–142.
12. Lindenfeld TN. Arthroscopically aided meniscal repair. Sports Med 1987;10:1293–1296.
13. Morgan CD, Casscells SW. Arthroscopic meniscus repair: a safe approach to the posterior horns. Arthroscopy 1986;2:3–12.
14. Warren RF. Arthroscopic meniscus repair. Arthroscopy 1985;1:170–172.
15. Rubman MH, Noyes FR, Barber-Westin SD. Technical considerations in the management of complex meniscus tears. Clin Sports Med 1996;15:511–530.
16. Henning CE, Clark JR, Lynch MA, et al. Arthroscopic meniscus repair with a posterior incision. Instr Course Lect 1988;37:209–221.
17. Bonamo JJ, Shulman G. Double contrast arthrography of the knee. A comparison to clinical diagnosis and arthroscopic findings. Orthopedics 1988;11:1041–1046.
18. Ekstrom JE. Arthrography—where does it fit in? Clin Sports Med 1990;9:561–566.
19. Farley TE, Howell SM, Love KF, et al. Meniscal tears: MR and arthrographic findings after arthroscopic repair. Radiology 1991;180:517–522.
20. Gillies H, Seligson D. Precision in the diagnosis of meniscal lesions: a comparison of clinical evaluation, arthrography, and arthroscopy. J Bone Joint Surg 1979;61A:343–346.
21. Ireland J, Trickey EL, Stoker DJ. Arthroscopy and arthrography of the knee. J Bone Joint Surg 1980;62B:3–6.
22. Manco LG, Berlow ME. Meniscal tears—comparison of arthrography, CT, and MRI. Crit Rev Diag Imaging 1989;29:151–179.
23. Kimori K, Suzu F, Yamashita F, et al. Evaluation of arthrography and arthroscopy for lesions of the posteromedial corner of the knee. Am J Sports Med 1989;17:638–643.
24. Arnoczky SP, Warren RF. Microvasculature of the human meniscus. Am J Sports Med 1982;10:90–95.
25. Buseck MS, Noyes FR. Arthroscopic evaluation of meniscal repairs after anterior cruciate ligament reconstruction and immediate motion. Am J Sports Med 1991;19:489–494.
26. Horibe S, Shino K, Nakata K, et al. Second-look arthroscopy after meniscal repair. Review of 132 menisci repaired by an arthroscopic inside-out technique. J Bone Joint Surg 1995;77B:245–249.
27. Morgan CD, Wojtys EM, Casscells CD, Casscells SW. Arthroscopic meniscal repair evaluated by second-look arthroscopy. Am J Sports Med 1991;19:632–638.
28. Rosenberg TD, Scott SM, Coward DB, et al.. Arthroscopic meniscal repair evaluated with repeat arthroscopy. Arthroscopy 1986;2:14–20.
29. Tenuta JJ, Arciero RA. Arthroscopic evaluation of meniscal repairs. Factors that effect healing. Am J Sports Med 1994;22:797–802.
30. Scott GA, Jolly BL, Henning CE. Combined posterior incision and arthroscopic intra-articular repair of the meniscus: an examination of factors affecting healing. J Bone Joint Surg 1986;68A:817–861.
31. Henning CE, Lynch MA, Clark JR. Vascularity for healing of meniscus repairs. Arthroscopy 1987;3:13–18.
32. Small NC. Complications in arthroscopic meniscal surgery. Clin Sports Med 1990;9:609–617.

dial meniscectomy: an analysis of unsatisfactory results. Arthroscopy 1985;1:44–52.

33. Hunter LY, Louis DS, Ricciardi JR, O'Connor GA. The saphenous nerve: its course and importance in medial arthrotomy. Am J Sports Med 1979;7:227–230.

34. Seebacher JR, Inglis AE, Marshall JL, Warren RF. The structure of the posterolateral aspect of the knee. J Bone Joint Surg 1982; 64A:536–541.

35. Noyes FR, Wojtys EM, Marshall MT. The early diagnosis and treatment of developmental patella infra syndrome. Clin Orthop 1991; 265:241–252.

36. DeMaio M, Noyes FR, Mangine RE. Principles for aggressive rehabilitation after reconstruction of the anterior cruciate ligament. Orthopedics 1992;15:385–392.

37. McLaughlin J, DeMaio M, Noyes FR, Mangine RE. Rehabilitation after meniscus repair. Orthopedics 1994;17:463–471.

Meniscal Tear and Cyst: Arthroscopic Meniscectomy

Once thought of as vestigial, the menisci are now known to play an important role in shock absorption, joint lubrication, and load distribution (1). Injuries to the menisci can, therefore, affect not only the underlying joint congruity but also the joint's essential stability. Management of patients with meniscal injuries requires both an appreciation of the pathologic process and natural history of the problem and an understanding of the crucial biomechanical role played by the menisci.

RELEVANT ANATOMY AND PATHOGENESIS

An examination of meniscal anatomy reveals that the medial meniscus is C-shaped and wider posteriorly than anteriorly (Fig. 60.1). It attaches posteriorly to the posterior intercondylar fossa just medial to the tibial attachment of the posterior cruciate ligament (PCL) and anteriorly to the tibia in front of the anterior cruciate ligament (ACL). It covers approximately 30% of the medial tibial surface. The transverse ligament connects the medial and lateral menisci anteriorly. The medial meniscus is attached medially to the capsule, most firmly in the area in which it blends with the deep medial ligament (Fig. 60.2).

The lateral meniscus is more circular than the medial meniscus and provides greater coverage to the lateral tibial plateau (70%). Its anterior attachment is somewhat more posterior than that of the medial meniscus, and it blends with the tibial attachment of the ACL. Posteriorly, the meniscus attaches to the intercondylar fossa just anterior to the attachment of the medial meniscus. The lateral meniscus is also attached to the medial femoral condyle through the ligament of Humphrey (anterior to the PCL) or the ligament of Wrisberg (posterior to the PCL). Rarely are both ligaments found. Laterally, the meniscus is attached to the capsule, except at the area of the popliteal hiatus.

Despite these firm attachments, the menisci are fairly mobile, primarily in the AP plane. The medial meniscus

moves as much as 6 mm during knee flexion, and the lateral meniscus moves up to 12 mm (2) (Fig. 60.3).

The unique orientation of the collagen matrix—mainly circumferentially directed fibers connected by a smaller number of radially organized ones—increases the ability of the meniscus to resist the large shear and compression forces applied to it (3) (Fig. 60.4). The patterns of meniscal tears are more easily understood if this anatomy is appreciated.

The vascular anatomy of the menisci has been well described elsewhere (4) and has been shown to arise primarily from the lateral and medial geniculate arteries, which arborize at the level of the meniscus-capsular attachment. This plexus is principally oriented circumferen-

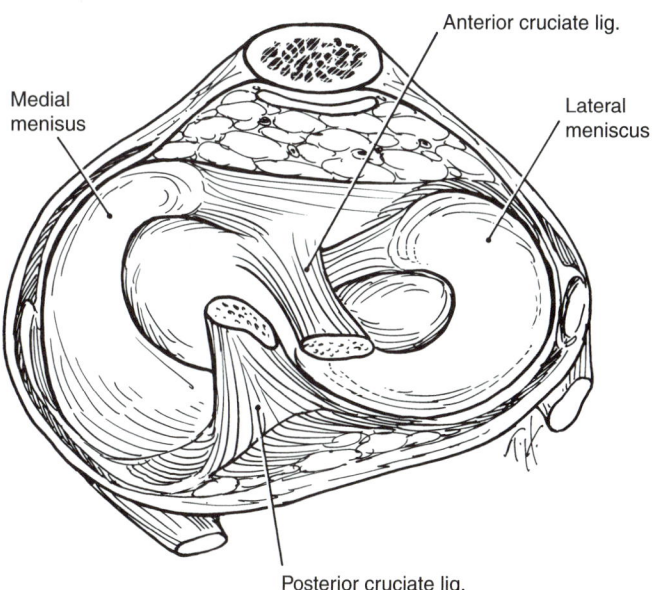

Figure 60.1. Superior view of tibia showing the position of the menisci relative to the cruciate ligament attachments.

Figure 60.2. Coronal view of the knee showing the relationship of the capsule to the peripheral meniscus.

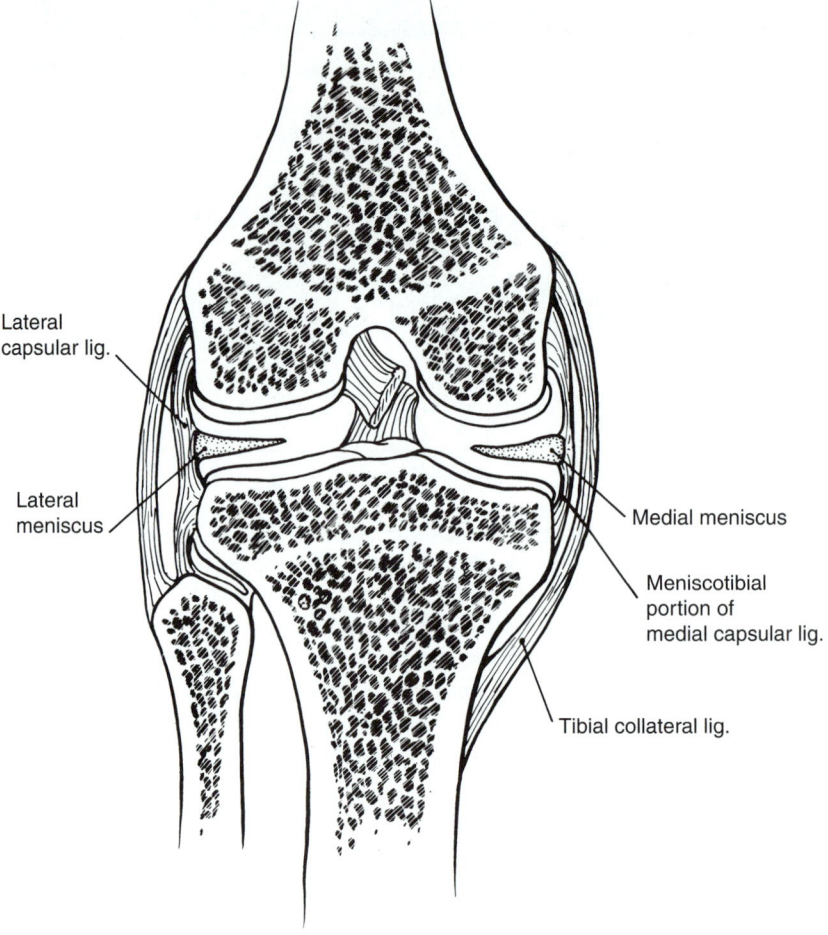

Lateral capsular lig.

Lateral meniscus

Medial meniscus

Meniscotibial portion of medial capsular lig.

Tibial collateral lig.

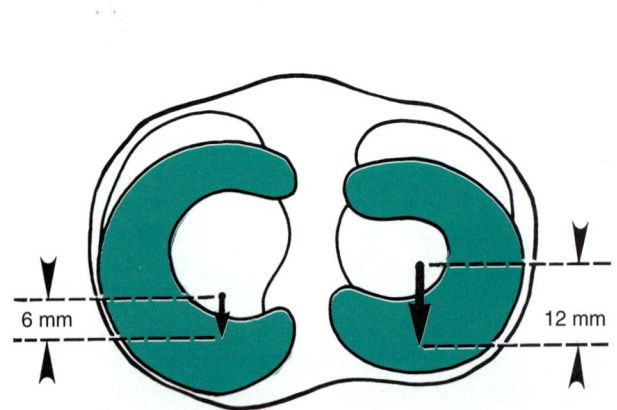

6 mm

12 mm

Figure 60.3. Maximum movement of the medial and lateral menisci.

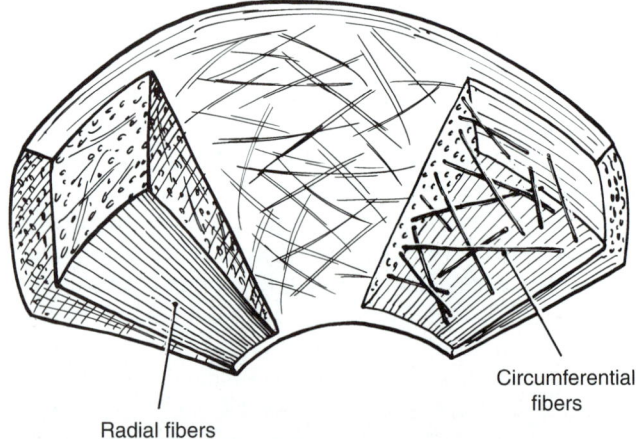

Radial fibers

Circumferential fibers

Figure 60.4. Microstructure of the meniscus showing radial and linking circumferential fibers.

tially, but it sends radial branches into the meniscus for 10 to 30% of its width. Thus at least 70% of the meniscus can be considered to be avascular (Fig. 60.5).

Biomechanics

The menisci perform an important role in force distribution in the knee and are responsible for the transmission of up to 90% of the joint force with the knee in flexion. Injury or removal of a meniscus can lead to markedly increased peak stresses and subsequent joint degeneration (5). The menisci also act as shock absorbers, lessening by as much as 20% the stress waves that pass through the knee during activity. The menisci play an important role in joint lubrication: Under loading, fluid is extruded into the joint, lubricating it. Loss of this weeping lubrication after meniscectomy may contribute to joint degeneration (1).

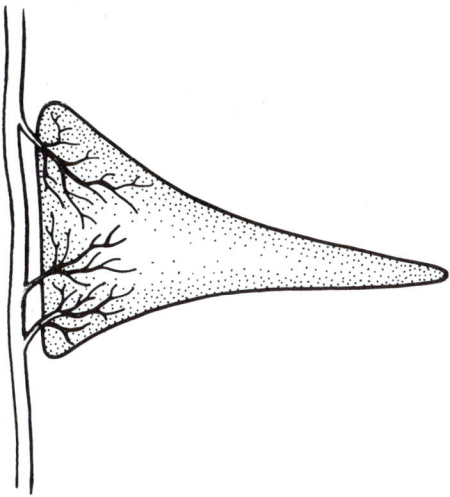

Figure 60.5. Approximately 30% of the meniscus is vascularized.

I   Meniscal Tears

CLASSIFICATION

Meniscal tears can occur in an unlimited number of patterns, but most acute tears can be classified into four anatomic types. Longitudinal tears include the common bucket-handle tears that are often found in association with ACL injuries (Figs. 60.6 and 60.7) Flap tears are seen in both menisci and are common in the posterior two-thirds of the meniscus. Radial tears are frequently seen in the lateral meniscus and rarely extend to the periphery (Fig. 60.8). Horizontal, or cleavage, tears are most often seen in conjunction with vertical tears or as part of a com-

plex degenerative tear, and they are closely associated with the development of meniscal cysts (Fig. 60.9).

Acute meniscal tears are most commonly the result of compression or shear stresses applied to the knee in flexion and rotation, but they may occur with hyperextension or hyperflexion (6). In otherwise stable knees, these forces often are great (e.g., as seen in vigorous cutting or leaping), but in the unstable knee (e.g., one with an ACL deficiency), tears may develop with significantly less force. Degenerative tears, often found in the older population, are associated with degenerative changes in the articular cartilage of the joint and are not always linked with an acute event (Fig. 60.10). They are often complex tears and likely develop secondary to ongoing abnormal forces in an arthritic or otherwise traumatized knee.

INITIAL FINDINGS, PHYSICAL EXAMINATION, DIAGNOSIS

The most common symptoms of a meniscal tear are pain, intermittent locking, swelling, and giving way (or buckling). Patients often report that they have trouble squatting. Most patients can relate the onset of symptoms to a specific incident and will identify the pain as being either lateral or medial and along the joint line. Often patients report or are able to demonstrate reduction maneuvers used when the knee locks. Chronic, mild effusions with intermittent pain is a common pattern of presentation. Pain is activity related unless the patient has degenerative joint disease, in which case there is often night pain. Patients with degenerative changes complain of a long history of aching, secondary to degenerative joint

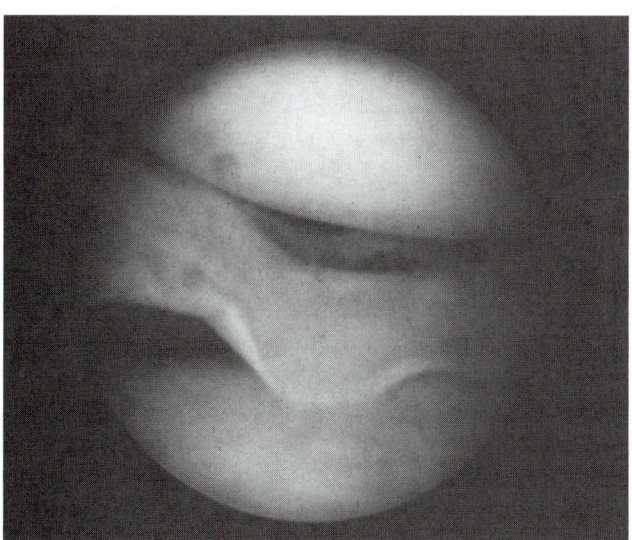

Figure 60.6. Longitudinal meniscal tear.

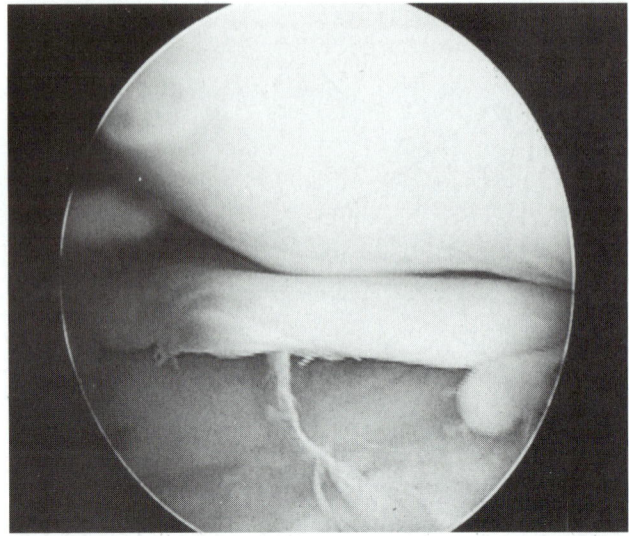

Figure 60.7. Displaced bucket-handle tear of the medial meniscus.

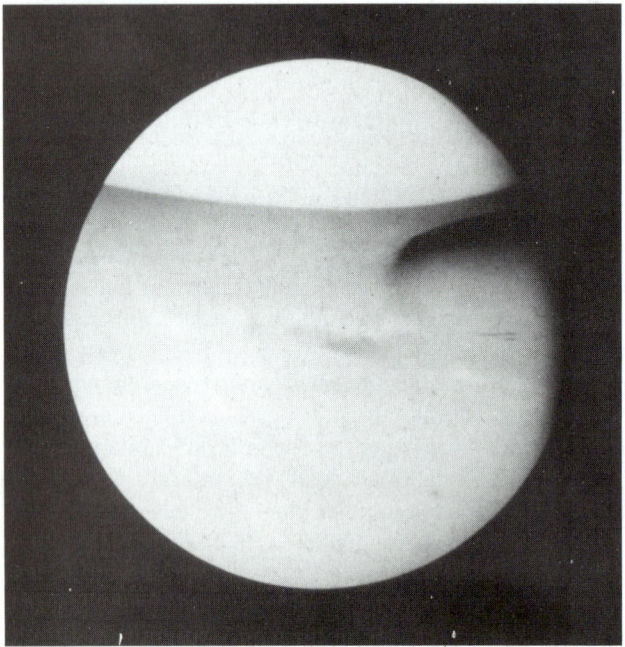

Figure 60.8. Radial meniscal tear.

Tenderness is the most common finding in patients with meniscal pathology. The Steinmann and McMurray tests should be performed while the examiner notes any signs of discomfort or abnormal clunk. The Apley grind test is occasionally useful. Ligamentous stability of the knee should be determined to rule out associated injuries.

Systematic examination of both knees should provide a diagnosis in a majority of cases. Diagnosis can sometimes be difficult immediately after an acute injury if the patient has a lot of pain or swelling. Such patients are best managed with compression, icing, elevation, and protected weight bearing until the swelling has subsided and a more complete examination is possible.

RADIOLOGIC STUDIES

A trauma series of radiographs of the knee is important to rule out fractures, significant degenerative disease, osteochondritis, and loose bodies. This series should include AP, lateral, and notch views along with a tangential

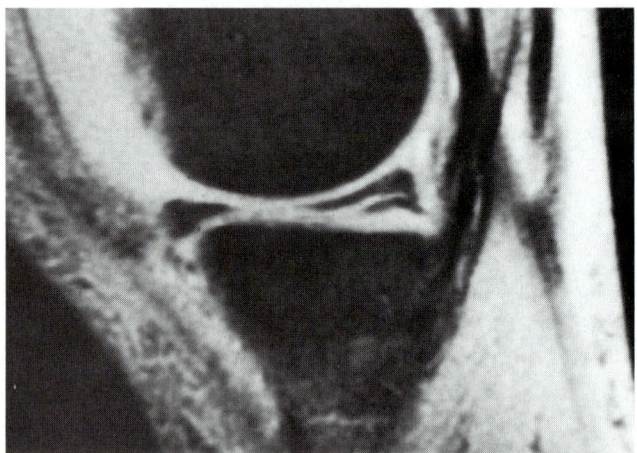

Figure 60.9. Cleavage tear of the medial meniscus.

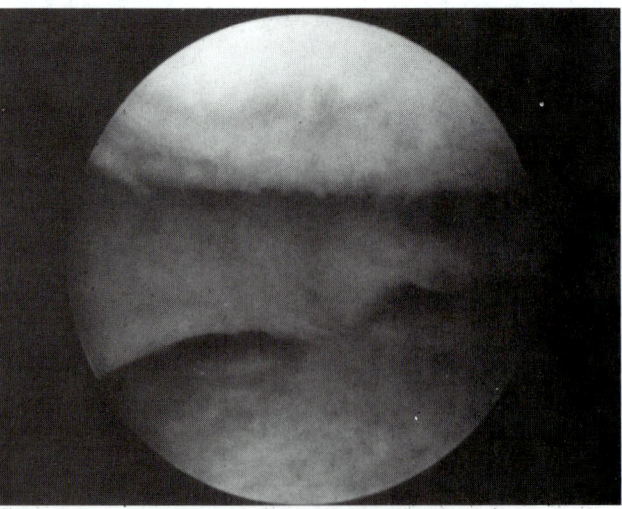

Figure 60.10. Degenerative meniscal tear. Note the degenerative changes on the femoral and tibial articular surfaces.

changes; intermittent sharp discomfort; and mechanical symptoms in the knee believed to be meniscal in origin.

The physical examination of these patients should always begin with an analysis of gait; the clinician should specifically look for an antalgic pattern or a flexion contracture. Sharp pain can be induced if the patient does a deep knee bend, squats, or performs a "duck walk." Examination of range of motion will often reveal pain in the extremes of flexion and sometimes hyperextension. Loss of full flexion is common with posterior horn tears, whereas pain in hyperextension is seen with anterior horn tears and bucket-handle tears. With the patient supine, the clinician should seek an effusion and palpate the joint lines for tenderness in both flexion and extension.

view in 30° to 40° flexion. Weight-bearing films in full extension are used to evaluate alignment, and weight-bearing 45° PA films reveal joint space narrowing in a functional position. The routine use of arthrography has all but disappeared since the introduction of MRI, but it remains useful for patients for whom MRI is contraindicated or in institutions not serviced by MRI. The accuracy of double-contrast arthrography is 78% (7) (Fig. 60.11).

The use of MRI studies of the knee is common, and the high degree of accuracy (90 to 98%) of MRI has made it a useful tool. Both enhanced and nonenhanced scans can provide nearly complete views of a meniscal tear. MRI evaluation of all knees with a suspected meniscal tear is not indicated, however, because most diagnoses can be made by history and physical examination. We reserve MRI studies for patients (a) who require a rapid return to sport or activity, (b) with complex multiligamentous injuries that complicate management, (c) with symptoms that suggest meniscal injury but whose physical examination is inconclusive, (d) who have failed a trial of conservative management, and (e) in whom avascular necrosis is suspected.

TREATMENT

Nonoperative Treatment and Indications for Surgery

Unless they are experiencing true locking, significant effusion, or marked pain, patients with a history suggesting a meniscal tear should undergo a trial of conservative management. Nonoperative treatment involves the use of range of motion exercises, icing, and graduated return to full activity. To prevent the development of marked weakness and patellofemoral symptoms, the patient should perform quadriceps strengthening exercises from the outset. Many patients thus treated quickly return to full function, implying either a small, stable tear or a healed peripheral tear. Patients who present with a locked knee,

who have unresolving effusion with joint line tenderness, or who have failed conservative management are candidates for surgery.

Operative Treatment

The techniques of operative arthroscopy are well documented and beyond the focus of this chapter. Nonetheless, some details of technique are worth review. Although office arthroscopy is advocated by some authors, we have no experience with it and perform all operative cases under sterile conditions in the operating room. Anesthesia can be general, spinal, or local. The patient is positioned supine; and a lateral thigh post is used, allowing the leg to be flexed over the side of the bed.

We prefer the standard use of a superomedial inflow portal and use the anterolateral portal for arthroscopy, but other portals are widely used (Fig. 60.12). The use of a pressure pump is not advocated for routine arthroscopy, but a tourniquet is customarily applied although not always inflated.

A complete examination of the knee should be performed in a routine, thorough manner so that all areas of the knee are seen and disorders in all compartments can be identified. In particular, the posterior aspect of the knee should be assessed for meniscal displacement. This may require a posterior medial portal or the use of a 70° arthroscope, but normally a 30° scope through the notch is sufficient. An anteromedial portal should then be made, and a probe introduced into the knee. Each meniscus should be probed on both the femoral and tibial surfaces, to completely delineate any abnormality.

After identification of a meniscal tear, the surgeon is faced with the decision to débride and resect, repair, or leave the tear alone. This choice is based on the position and size of the tear and its chronicity. Techniques of meniscal repair are discussed elsewhere in this book.

It is generally accepted that unstable tears that produce mechanical symptoms of locking or recurrent giving way or that cause recurrent effusion and pain are best treated with arthroscopic partial meniscectomy (Clinical Table). The tear should be well visualized before resection to ensure that all unstable portions of the meniscus are removed and to prevent unnecessary resection. Removal should be performed with sharp instruments to allow the creation of an even, stable rim. The meniscal shaver is a useful adjunct to arthroscopic scissors and punches for making a sculpted, smooth leading edge.

A longitudinal or bucket-handle tear is initially reduced so the surgeon can completely visualize the tear pattern; the tear is then sharply resected (Fig. 60.13). The posterior pole is first detached using a sharp punch, which allows the meniscus to float into the notch, attached only by its anterior pole. The anterior horn is then examined, and the meniscus is detached gently and removed through the anteromedial portal. Care should be taken to provide a large enough portal to remove the meniscal fragment and prevent it from becoming stuck in the anterior soft tissues.

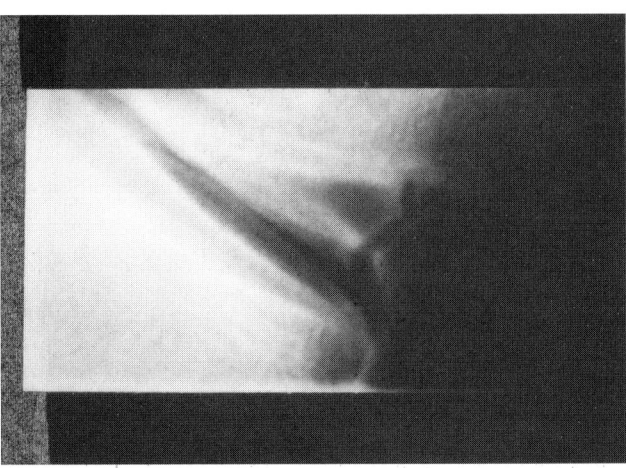

Figure 60.11. Arthrogram of a peripheral meniscal tear.

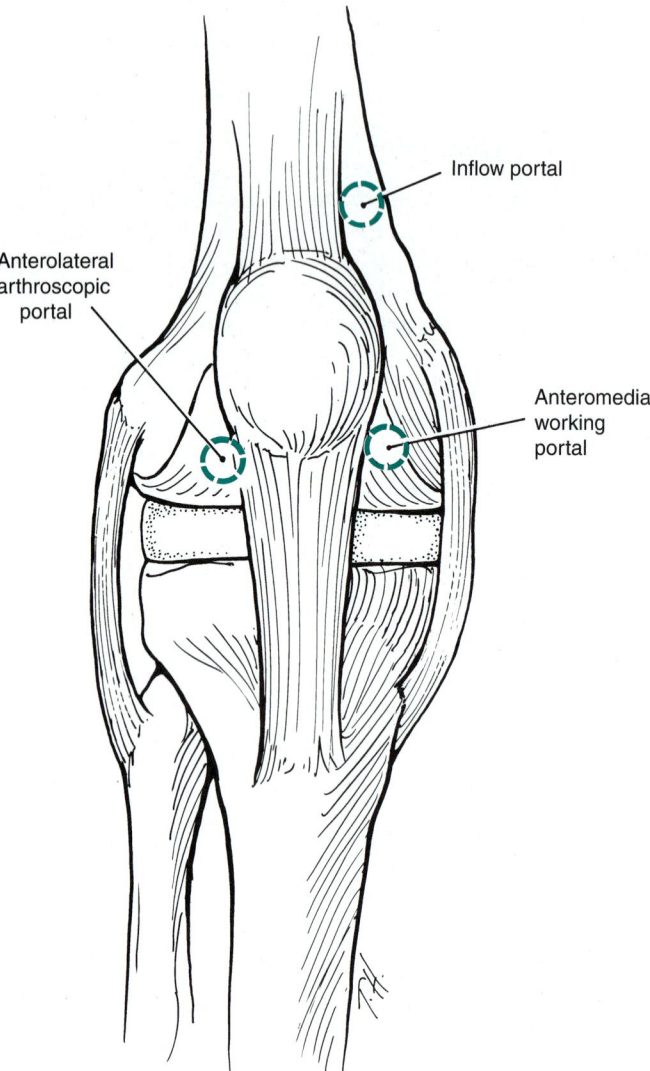

Figure 60.12. Commonly used anterior arthroscopy portals.

Simple radial tears should be addressed by removing a portion of the normal meniscus anterior and posterior to the defect, producing a smooth, stable edge (Fig. 60.13). Some controversy exists concerning the débridement of stable small radial tears, and some authors prefer not to débride tears less than 5 mm deep. We routinely débride such small tears, taking care to probe the meniscus carefully to ensure that there is no other significant tear posteriorly.

Cleavage tears can initially be débrided with a meniscal shaver and then resected back to a stable rim by using a punch or angled beaver blade. These tears should be carefully probed to assess stability of the superior and inferior aspects of the rim, and resected as much as necessary to ensure stability. These tears are often complex and are associated with degenerative joint disease, which may necessitate débridement before the meniscal resection can be performed.

The use of lasers in knee arthroscopy has become rela-

tively common since the late 1980s, as technology has improved the instrumentation and lowered its cost. Advantages of lasers in meniscal surgery include improved access to confined areas of the knee, improved ability to sculpt meniscal resection edges, and easier resection of ossified tissue. The ability to control tissue cutting depth with pulsed laser delivery systems has prevented overheating and necrosis of tissue (8). Laboratory and clinical research continues to find new applications for this exciting technology.

POSTOPERATIVE REHABILITATION

Postoperatively, wounds are closed with Steri-Strips or with a single stitch, and the knee is dressed in a bulky dressing. Cryotherapy and elevation are prescribed for the first few days, to rapidly decrease the inevitable effusion. Weight bearing is encouraged as tolerated, with crutches if necessary; range of motion exercises are prescribed. Quadriceps setting exercises are started immediately, followed as tolerated with quadriceps strengthening and cycling. A pain-free knee with full range of motion and no effusion is considered essential before return to sports.

PITFALLS AND COMMON MISTAKES

Portal Problems

A common problem with arthroscopic meniscectomy is inferior placement of the arthroscope and operating portals. The anterolateral arthroscope portal should be placed no lower than the inferior pole of the patella to allow adequate visualization of all areas of the joint. Similarly, a low medial portal makes instrumentation difficult. Access to the lateral compartment for resecting a lateral meniscus is relatively easy if the medial portal is placed with the leg in the figure 4 position. If an inflow portal is used, it should be far enough from the patella so that inflow does not cause a problem when the knee is in flexion.

Inadequate Visualization

Inability to fully visualize the meniscal tear, particularly posteriorly, is a common problem that can result in the retention of unstable fragments. Care must be taken to ensure that the entire meniscus is well seen and probed carefully. The use of a lateral traction post or a leg holder facilitates access to the posterior aspect of the medial and lateral compartments. The surgeon must be careful not to injure the collateral ligaments with excessive traction.

Inadequate Meniscal Resection

Failure to remove an adequate amount of meniscus can lead to a persistence or recurrence of symptoms. All areas of meniscus that are deemed unstable to probing must be removed.

RESULTS

Multiple studies have documented the acceleration of degenerative changes in knees that have undergone a complete medial or lateral meniscectomy (9). In theory,

Clinical Table: Meniscal Tear and Cyst: Arthroscopic Meniscectomy

Procedure	Indications	Technique	Anatomy	Pitfalls
Arthroscopic meniscectomy	• Failed conservative management • Persistent effusion • Locked knee • Joint line tenderness	• Anterolateral scope portal • Anteromedial working portal	• Meniscus • Patellofemoral alignment	• Portal placement • Inadequate visualization • Inadequate resection
Arthroscopic meniscal cyst decompression	• Painful cystic swelling • Persistent effusion	• Arthroscopic meniscectomy and cyst decompression	• Anterolateral position of the cyst	• Inadequate decompression
Open meniscal cyst decompression	• Failed arthroscopic decompression • Large, multiloculated cyst	• Arthroscopic meniscectomy and open lateral approach	• Lateral collateral ligament • Lateral joint capsule • Lateral geniculate artery	• Recurrence • Lateral geniculate artery bleeding

preservation of a rim of meniscus will permit more normal joint forces and delay or prevent the development of degenerative changes. Although long-term studies that compare partial meniscectomy with total meniscectomy are unavailable, it appears that over the short term, conservation of a stable rim leads to better overall results. At the 5-year follow-up, McGinty et al. (10) showed better overall results with patients who had partial meniscectomies than with patients who underwent complete resection. Similar findings were documented by other studies (11,12).

There is compelling evidence to support arthroscopic over open meniscectomy. Initial morbidity is lower, patients return to work or sports more quickly. Overall cost is significantly decreased with the use of outpatient surgery.

Overall, good to excellent results have been reported in 84 to 97% of patients with simple excision of bucket-handle or flap tears. Results in older age groups with degenerative changes are somewhat worse, but Jackson and Rouse (13) reported good results in 80% of older patients. For older patients, arthroscopic meniscectomy offers a safe and easy method of resection, although it provides no real improvement in the degenerative process.

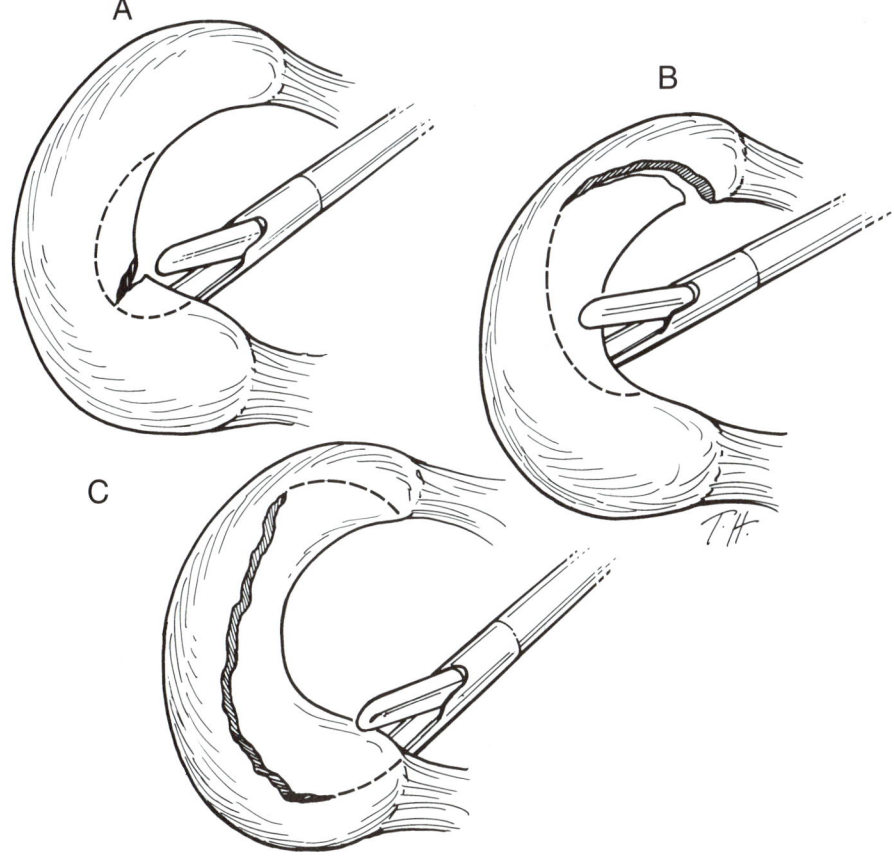

Figure 60.13. Surgical excision margins for small radial (**A**), bucket-handle (**B**), and parrot beak (**C**) meniscal tears.

II Meniscal Cysts

Meniscal cysts were first described by Ebner (14) in 1904, but it was not until 1923 that Phemister (15) proposed meniscectomy as a treatment. In 1943, Ghourmly (16) described myxoid degeneration in the menisci adjacent to the cysts, and in 1979, Barrie (17) proposed that horizontal tears of the menisci provide access to synovial fluid and promote the formation of synovial cysts (Fig. 60.14). Barrie's concept provides the basis for our understanding of the pathophysiologic process of meniscal cysts. The incidence of meniscal cysts has been repeated as being between 2 and 22% of the general population; men are affected three times as often as women. Lateral meniscal cysts are much more common than medial cysts.

INITIAL FINDINGS, PHYSICAL EXAMINATION, AND DIAGNOSIS

Patients with meniscal cysts often complain of a dull ache in the knee and a localized swelling along the medial or lateral joint line. Trauma to the knee is only sporadically recalled, and many patients present with no history of mechanical symptoms. Pain tends to be insidious, worse at night and aggravated by exercise. Some patients do present with mechanical symptoms, and effusions are not uncommon.

The physical examination of the affected knee often reveals joint line swelling, which is seen best with the knee at 20° to 30° of flexion. Medial cysts, when present, are frequently larger than those seen on the lateral side. Although joint line tenderness is common, range of motion is usually good. Serial examinations will occasionally reveal that the cyst varies in size, often increasing in size with exercise. Careful examination of the popliteal space should be performed to rule out a cyst in that area.

RADIOLOGIC STUDIES

Routine x-rays should be obtained for all patients with a suspected meniscal cyst. The radiographs should be examined carefully for evidence of degenerative joint disease, loose bodies, and tumors. The routine use of arthrography has largely been supplanted by MRI, which

Figure 60.14. Lateral meniscal cyst and its relationship to the lateral joint capsule.

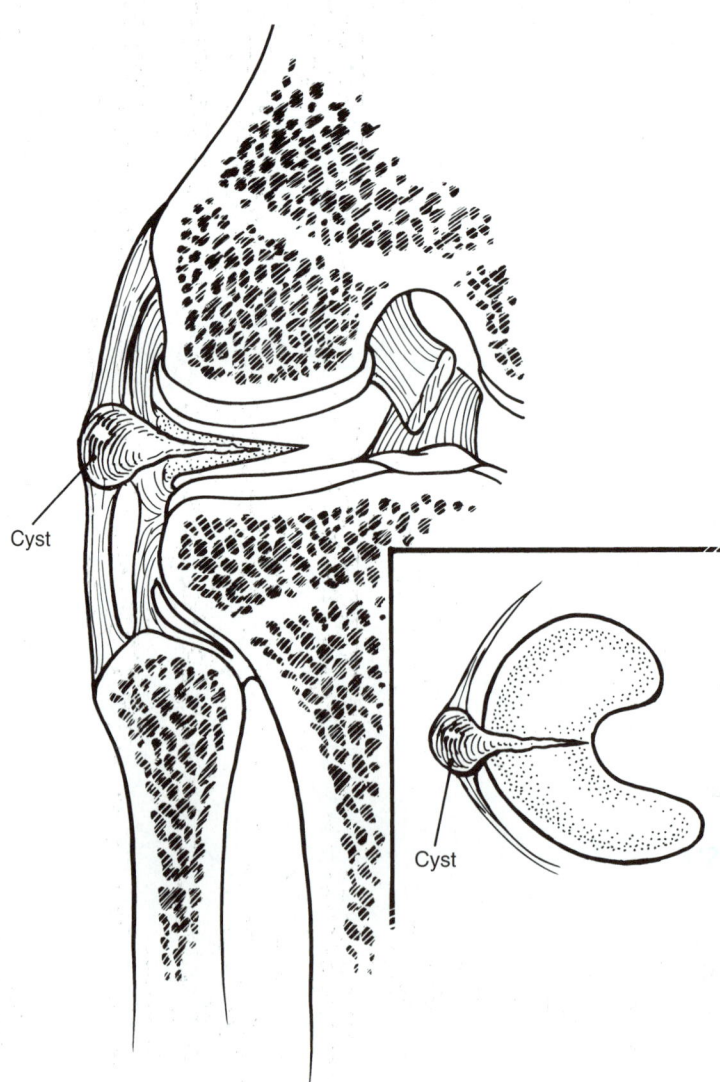

gives an excellent view of the meniscus and related cysts, in most cases.

TREATMENT

Most authors agree that small, asymptomatic cysts can be observed. Aspiration and injection with corticosteroids has been described for selected patients (18). Most symptomatic cysts, however, are successfully treated with excision, either open or arthroscopically.

Arthroscopic treatment begins with a routine inspection of the joint using standard portals and instrumentation. A meniscal tear will almost universally be found on the symptomatic side of the joint (19). Débridement of the tear may reveal a punctate opening into the cyst, which often spontaneously decompresses into the joint. If this does not occur, placement of a probe or spinal needle into the cyst will allow complete decompression. A spinal needle can also be used percutaneously into the knee and through the cyst.

In cases in which arthroscopic débridement and attempted decompression fail or when a large multiloculated cyst is present open decompression is advised. This is accomplished through a lateral incision directly over the cyst. The cyst is completely excised down to the meniscus. Suturing of the peripheral edge of the meniscus to the meniscosynovial edge of the capsule has been recommended (20).

Pitfalls and Common Mistakes

Failure to completely remove the unstable portions of the torn meniscus or to adequately decompress the cyst can lead to persistence of symptoms. If decompression is inadequate after arthroscopic manipulation and partial meniscectomy, the cyst should be removed through an open procedure.

Postoperative Rehabilitation

After surgery to decompress a cyst, patients are treated as described for partial meniscectomy patients. If open excision and suturing of the meniscus are required, partial weight bearing should be maintained for 2 to 3 weeks.

Results

Appropriate arthroscopic meniscal débridement and cyst decompression led to good to excellent results in up to 89% of patients in one study (19). Similar results were achieved for medial meniscal cysts (21).

SUMMARY

Meniscal injuries are commonly encountered in orthopaedic practice, and management depends on careful history taking and physical examination. When conservative management fails, arthroscopic resection of the torn portions of meniscus is recommended. Adequate removal requires good visualization, careful probing of the tear, and sharp débridement of all unstable fragments. Excellent results in the majority of patients can be expected.

Meniscal cysts are most commonly found laterally and can often be managed conservatively. When symptomatic, they are best treated with arthroscopic débridement and decompression of the cyst, although occasional cysts may require open resection if arthroscopic treatment fails. Overall results of arthroscopic treatment of meniscal cysts are good.

REFERENCES

1. Woo SL-Y, An KN, Arnoczky SP. Anatomy, biology and biomechanics of tendon, ligament, and meniscus. In: Simon HE, ed. Orthopaedic basic science. Rosemont, IL: American Academy of Orthopaedic Surgeons, 1994.
2. Kapandji IA. The menisci and their function. In: The physiology of the joints. Vol. 2. Baltimore: Williams & Wilkins, 1970:98–99.
3. Bullough PG, Munuera L, Murphy J, Weinstein AM. The strength of the menisci of the knee as it relates to their fine structure. J. Bone Joint Surg 1970;52B:564–567.
4. Arnoczky SP, Warren RF. Microvasculature of the human meniscus Am J Sports Med 1982;10:90–95.
5. Johnson RJ, Kettelkamp DB, Clark W, Leaverton P. Factors affecting late results after meniscectomy. J Bone Joint Surg 1974;56A:719–729.
6. Nicholas JA, Hershman EB. The lower extremity and spine in sports medicine. St. Louis: Mosby, 1986.
7. DeHaven KE, Collins HR. Diagnosis of internal derangement of the knee. The role of arthroscopy. J Bone Joint Surg 1975;57A:802–810.
8. Trauner K, Nishioka N, Patel, D. Pulsed holmium:yttrim-aluminium-garnet (Ho-YAG) laser energy on adult articular cartilage in vitro. Arthroscopy 1992;8:36–42.
9. Fairbank TJ. Knee joint changes after meniscectomy. J Bone Joint Surg 1948;30B:664–670.
10. McGinity JB, Geuss LF, Marvin RA. Partial or total meniscectomy. J Bone Joint Surg 1977;59A:763–766.
11. Northmore-Ball MD, Dandy DJ, Jackson RW. Arthroscopic, open partial, and total meniscectomy. J Bone Joint Surg 1983;65B:400–404.
12. Hershman EB, Nisonson B. Arthroscopic meniscectomy: a follow up report. Am J Sports Med 1983;11:253–257.
13. Jackson RW, Rouse DW. The results of partial meniscectomy in patients over 40 years of age. J Bone Joint Surg 1982;64B:481–485.
14. Ebner A. Ein fall von ganglion am kniegelenksmeniskus. Munchen Med Wochenschr 1904;51:1737–1739.
15. Phemister DB. Cysts of the external semilunar cartilage of the knee. JAMA 1923;80(9).
16. Ghormley RK. Cystic myxomatous tumors about the knee: their relation to cysts of the menisci. J Bone Joint Surg 1943;25A(2).
17. Barrie HJ. The pathogenesis and significance of meniscal cysts. J Bone Joint Surg 1979;61B:184–189.
18. Muddu BN, Barrie JL, Morris MA. Aspiration and injection for meniscal cysts. J Bone Joint Surg 1992;74B:627–628.
19. Glasgow MM, Allen PW, Blakeway C. Arthroscopic treatment of cysts of the lateral meniscus. J Bone Joint Surg 1993;75B:299–302.
20. Sisk TD. Knee injuries. In: Crenshaw AH, ed. Campbell's operative orthopaedics. 7th ed. Toronto: Mosby, 1987:2321–2323.
21. Mills CA, Henderson IJ. Cysts of the medial meniscus. J Bone Joint Surg 1993;75B:293–298.

Endoscopic Anterior Cruciate Ligament Reconstruction Using Autograft Patellar Tendon Substitution

The mid-1980s witnessed remarkable advancements in the treatment of anterior cruciate ligament (ACL) deficiency. Advances in arthroscopic skills, technology, and instrumentation allowed surgeons to perform arthroscopic-assisted ACL reconstruction with patellar tendon autograft, allograft, or hamstring tissues. In the late 1980s, further advances in instrumentation allowed ACL reconstruction with patellar tendon tissue via a single incision or endoscopic technique. Until 1991, I almost exclusively used the middle third bone-tendon-bone patellar tendon substitution for ACL deficiency via a two-incision arthroscopic-assisted technique; then I switched to endoscopy (1,2). Although clinical studies demonstrated high satisfaction and stability at an average follow-up of 3 years (3,4), the single-incision technique promised lower surgical morbidity, early enhanced recovery of motion, and improved rehabilitation via an outpatient procedure. This chapter describes the technique of endoscopic, single-incision ACL reconstruction with patellar tendon autograft (Clinical Table).

RELEVANT ANATOMY AND PATHOGENESIS

The ACL is one of two cruciate ligaments in the knee. It runs in an anterior direction from the superolateral femur to the anteromedial tibia. Its most important function is to prevent anterior displacement of the tibia on the femur. Its origin on the medial surface of the lateral femoral condyle is somewhat semicircular.

The ACL changes in its histology from flexible ligamentous tissue to rigid bony attachment, and this transition is mediated by a transition zone of fibrocartilage and mineralized cartilage. This zone reduces stress at the attachment site by allowing a gradual change in stiffness.

Much has been written about the described bundles or bands of the ACL that are anatomically separate. These bands may be more functionally separate than actually anatomically separate. These bands allow variable tension among the fibers within the ligament throughout its range of motion. For example, with the knee in extension, the entire ACL is taut, and all fibers lie parallel. As the knee flexes, the anterior fibers continue to remain taut and cross over the posterior fibers, which gradually become loose. It appears that the anterior medial band of the ACL is tighter in flexion and the posterolateral band is tighter in extension. These two precise bands often are not clearly demarcated, but the transition may be more gradual between the fascicles as the knee undergoes its range of motion.

Surrounding the entire ligament is paratenon, which blends with epitenon. Synovium then covers the ligament. Thus the ligament is extrasynovial.

The predominant blood supply of the ACL is the middle geniculate artery. This artery exits the popliteal artery, piercing the posterior capsule. There may also be some blood supply from the fat pad via the inferior medial and lateral geniculate arteries. There does not appear to be a significant amount of evidence that osseous attachments of the ACL contribute to its vascular supply.

The innervation of the ACL probably shares innervation with the posterior cruciate ligament (PCL) from the popliteal plexus of nerves. The popliteal plexus is derived

Clinical Table: Endoscopic ACL Reconstruction Using Autograft Patellar Tendon Substitution

Procedure	Indications	Technique	Anatomy	Pitfalls

ACL reconstruction	• ACL injure
	• Failure with bracing
	• Recurrent instability (>3 times/year)
	• Associated multiligament injury
	• Repairable meniscus
	• Sports activity > 5 h/week
	• KT1000 MMD > 5 mm
	• Category 1 sports
	• Elite-level athlete
		• Single incision
		• Patellar tendon autograft
		• Notch preparation
		• Notchplasty
		• Tibial tunnel
		• Femoral tunnel
		• Phase two notchplasty
		• Graft passage
		• Push-in technique
		• Hyperflex pin
		• 7 × 25 mm interference screw
		• Tibial fixation in extension
			• Patellar tendon
			• Intercondylar notch
			• Over the top
			• PCL
			• Pes anserinus tendons
			• Neurovascular bundle
				• Graft harvest
				  – Too narrow
				  – Too wide
				  – Bone plug fracture
				  – Patellar fracture
				• Improper tibial tunnel
				  – Too horizontal
				  – Nonanatomic
				  – Notch impingement
				• Inadequate notchplasty
				  – Graft abrasion
				  – PCL impingement
				  – Notch impingement
				• Improper femoral tunnel
				  – Too anterior
				  – Posterior blowout
				• Graft passage
				  – Graft delamination
				• Graft fixation
				  – Inadequate fixation
				  – Bone quality
				  – Screw divergence
				  – Graft laceration
				  – Construct mismatch

MMD, maximum manual difference.

mainly from the posterior articular surface of the knee, a branch of the posterior tibial nerve. The mechanoreceptors of the cruciate ligament seem to be arranged more toward the subsynovial surface of the ligament.

INITIAL FINDINGS, PHYSICAL EXAMINATION, AND DIAGNOSIS

The initial history is often an accurate indicator of an ACL tear. Many patients will feel a pop in the knee accompanied by sharp pain after landing "in an awkward manner" while engaging in athletic or even innocuous activity. Frequently, when the patients are engaged in an athletic activity, they are unable to continue playing and rapidly develop swelling in the knee. Patients frequently will comment that the knee almost immediately feels unstable to them.

Often patients will describe a feeling of the knee "slipping" out of place. The injury may be described as either a twisting or a funny landing to the knee and may initially be thought of as having a sprain or some other minor injury to the knee.

While ACL injuries frequently occur in direct contact sports, perhaps the most common mechanism of injury is noncontact twisting or deceleration in sports such as skiing, basketball, football, or soccer.

Not infrequently, the patient will have a history of a prior knee injury that at the time may have been considered to be minor and that subsequently resolved. This may represent a partial tear of the ligament, which later goes on to a complete tear with a more

significant injury, or may even represent the initial phase of an ACL injury, which subsequently becomes well compensated.

After the initial injury subsides and the symptoms become more chronic, the patient often will give a history of episodes of the knee going out, giving way, buckling, or feeling unstable, particularly with activities such as running, gliding, or cutting. Many patients will actually twist their fists together to describe more graphically the knee going out or giving way. This giving way episode may be accompanied by repeated episodes of swelling that can subsequently resolve.

The history of giving way or instability is quite characteristic of ACL injuries and frequently is distinguished by the patient from other painful episodes of the knee that may accompany other anatomic abnormalities. A history of giving way or instability must be sought after by the clinician and specifically tested for in evaluation and examination.

Not infrequently, other injuries may accompany ACL tears, particularly tears of the meniscus, collateral ligaments, or posterolateral corner of the knee.

The differential diagnosis of an acute hemarthrosis of the knee in addition to a major ligamentous tear would include meniscal tear or patellar dislocation or osteochondral fracture.

On clinical examination, an acute injury to the ACL is frequently very different from that of a chronic ACL-insufficient knee. When seen acutely, patients will often have a significant hemarthrosis, a limitation of motion, and guarding that may make examination difficult. Spasm of the quadriceps and hamstring muscles can make initial evaluation more dependent on the characteristic history than adequacy of various ACL stress maneuvers. Frequently, orthopaedic examination after the initial swelling subsides is important to establish the diagnosis. Aspiration of hemarthrosis and installation of local anesthesia may make initial examination easier and may assist in the diagnosis if frank hemarthrosis is encountered. Examination of the normal knee provides a control in order to identify what is the baseline knee laxity for each individual patient.

A patient may have tenderness both on the anterior and posterior aspects of the knee and on either the lateral or medial aspect of the knee if accompanying injuries to the collateral ligament or menisci occur.

The knee should be examined and tested for varus-valgus instability to identify associated meniscus tear. These injuries frequently accompany ACL injuries.

A number of tests have been designed to test ACL integrity. These frequently are more able to be elicited in the chronic setting or after the initial pain, swelling, and muscle spasm of an acute injury have subsided. The Lachman test is one of the best examinations to evaluate ACL injury. The Lachman test consists of two components: the amount of translation in the tibia anteriorly in relation to the femur, and the sense of end point. The examiner, while stabilizing the femur with one hand, moving the tibia anteriorly in a slight flexion, identifies the degree of anterior tibial translation. With an intact ACL, there will often be a solid or sudden end point as well as limitation to the amount of anterior tibial translation. With a torn ACL, there is not only an excessive amount of anterior translation but also a "soft" end point due to the loss of ACL restraint. Of the two components, the amount of translation appears to be a critical determinant of ACL integrity. The second test that appears to be quite important is the "pivot shift." In the pivot shift test, the tibia is rotated slightly externally with the knee in near-full extension. This maneuver allows the distal femur to subluxate posteriorly with regard to the tibia. The tibia is held at a slight valgus in extension. As flexion of the knee is performed, the tibia suddenly reduces in relation to the femur with a palpable shift, jump, or transient lock in the motion of the knee. The flexion-rotation drawer test is a similar test to evaluate ACL integrity. In this test the clinician holds the tibia in neutral rotation while the femur drops posteriorly and rotates externally. As the knee is reduced with gentle flexion and push on the tibia, reduction is felt, and the knee jumps into the reduced position. The hallmark of all ACL evocative tests is the ability to evaluate the pathologic tibial rotation course caused by a torn ACL. A familiarity with all of these tests and comfort with one will prove adequate in most clinicians' hands.

RADIOLOGIC STUDIES

Every knee that is suspected of ACL damage should be evaluated with plane radiographs. This should consist of an AP view, lateral view, and patellofemoral projection. A tunnel view in addition may be helpful. Plain radiographs may reveal osteochondral fractures or ligamentous avulsion of small pieces of bone. The Segond fracture or lateral capsular sign, seen in the lateral edge of the tibia on the AP view, is pathognomonic of ACL tear. Avulsion from fibula head or femur may indicate associated collateral ligament injury.

In more chronic ACL injuries, there may be interchondral eminence spurring or hypertrophy, patellar facet osteophyte formation, and joint space narrowing with marginal osteophytes.

It is particularly important in skeletally immature patients to have plain radiographic assessment. This is because there is frequently a ligamentous avulsion in this age group.

MRI may offer additional clinical information to plain radiography. Frequently the MRI is helpful to assess additional ligamentous or meniscal damage. With an acute injury, MRI may reveal an associated bone bruise. MRI findings consistent with ACL injury include actual disruption in the ligament, an irregular or wavy anterior margin, significant increased signal in the T_2-weighted image, and a buckled PCL suggesting anterior translation of the tibia. It must be emphasized that a high-quality MRI scan is important to visualize the ACL. An image in the incorrect plane may make visualization of the ACL difficult.

The bone bruise has recently been identified as an important MRI indicator accompanying ACL injury. Speer et al. (5) found that 83% of patients with ACL tears had an osseous injury directly over the lateral femoral condyle sulcus terminalis. Of those, 96% had evidence of posterolateral injury to either the tibia or soft tissue.

Rosen et al. (6) in evaluating ACL injuries with MRI showed that 85% had occult bony lesions such as bone bruises and 80% had demonstrated lesions of the lateral tibial plateau or lateral femoral condyle. It has been suggested that bone impaction site detection by MRI in the posterolateral tibia and lateral femoral condyle suggests an acute ACL tear, although the long-term significance of these bone bruise lesions are not clear at this time.

TREATMENT

Indications for Surgery

ACL reconstructive surgery is considered for patients who have torn a ligament. Candidates for surgery are young and have high expectations in regard to their activity levels. Surgical treatment is more commonly recommended for patients who are involved in category 1 activities (e.g., basketball and volleyball) than for those involved in category 3 activities (linear). Reconstructive surgery is also recommended for individuals who participate in more than 5 h of athletic activities a week (7). A maximum manual difference greater than 5 mm, measured by a KT1000 arthrometer, is associated with a poor prognosis for conservative care (7). Concomitant repairable meniscal tears are considered a relative indication for ACL reconstructive surgery.

Patients with generalized ligamentous laxity are at high risk for repeated episodes of instability, yet this group is also at a high risk for graft attenuation. Skeletally immature patients present a different dilemma. Individuals with a skeletal age of 14 years and females who have been menstruating at least 2 years will experience minimal skeletal growth at the knee; thus ACL reconstructive surgery can be safely performed.

The good results and reduced morbidity associated with modern ACL reconstruction techniques have encouraged an increasing number of active middle-aged patients to seek treatment. Currently, approximately 8% of ACL reconstruction patients seen by my group are aged 35 years or older; 2% are aged 40 years or older. Although age is a consideration, activity level is more important. Patients with chronic ACL deficiency who experience repeated episodes of instability even when using an orthosis are candidates for reconstructive surgery.

Surgical Technique

PATIENT POSITIONING

The patient's knees should be examined before positioning him or her in the arthroscopic leg holder, because the leg holder may eliminate the clinician's ability to accurately assess the pivot shift test (8). Knee flexion is more important with the endoscopic technique than with the double-incision arthroscopic technique. A padded thigh tourniquet is placed on the patient's leg before it is put into the leg holder. The waist and foot of the table are flexed to minimize hyperlordosis of the spine and to allow at least 110° of knee flexion. The opposite leg is placed in a well-padded gynecologic leg holder; the hip and knee are flexed to protect the common peroneal nerve.

GENERAL CONSIDERATIONS

Routinely, 1g first-generation cephalosporin is administered before surgery. The tourniquet is not inflated unless necessary. I have found that approximately 90% of surgeries can be conducted without inflating the tourniquet. A pump inflow system is used, as much of the procedure is performed with the knee flexed to 70° to 80°.

From May 1994 to May 1996, my group performed nearly 150 outpatient endoscopic surgeries; there were no readmissions or emergency room visits. Perioperative management of pain and nausea by the anesthesia team is critical. Before surgery, 60 mg IM ketorolac tromethamine (Toradol; Syntex Laboratories, Palo Alto, CA) is administered; 30 mg IV is administered at the conclusion of the

procedure. Oral ketorolac tromethamine is not used after surgery. Propofol (Diprivan; Stuart Pharmaceuticals, Wilmington, DE) is routinely used as an anesthetic agent. The majority of my patients undergo a general endotracheal anesthetic. A dilute 1:300,000 epinephrine solution is used at the beginning of the surgery, and 0.25% Marcaine (Sanofi Winthrop, New York, NY) is injected into the knee joint, arthroscopic portals, and surgical access region. At the conclusion of the procedure, 0.25% Marcaine is liberally injected into the donor site and intra-articular area. A Hemovac is infrequently used.

DIAGNOSTIC ARTHROSCOPY

Diagnostic arthroscopy is performed along with any necessary meniscal débridement or repair. Attention is directed toward partial-thickness tears; displaced bucket-handle tears; and the status of the articular surfaces, including the patellofemoral joint. A superomedial portal is used for pump inflow. The surgeon must confirm that the cannula is placed intra-articularly at the beginning of the procedure, because marked soft tissue fluid extravasation can quickly occur with the pump inflow system. An inferolateral portal is established at the level of the distal patellar pole, slightly lateral to the lateral edge of the patellar tendon. A similar level in regard to the patella is used for the inferomedial portal. Following diagnostic arthroscopy, graft procurement is performed. In selected patients who have an obvious pivot shift phenomenon and no significant radiographic degenerative joint disease, the middle-third patellar tendon graft may be harvested before the diagnostic arthroscopy is performed.

GRAFT HARVEST

Although mini incisions have been popular for endoscopic ACL reconstruction, I use a 7.5- to 8.75-cm (3.0- to 3.5-in) longitudinal incision placed slightly medial to the midline. This incision extends from the distal pole of the patella to 2.5 cm (1 in) below the tibial tubercle. The skin is incised and infiltrated with 1:300,000 epinephrine; then the dissection is carried through the subcutaneous tissue down to the transverse fascial fibers. The subcutaneous tissue is mobilized proximally, distally, medially, and laterally. The fascia is incised in the middle portion of the patellar tendon and extended proximally and distally with Metzenbaum scissors. The fascia is initially retracted medially and laterally with Senn retractors and subsequently with larger rake retractors.

The distal portion of the patellar tendon is measured and noted in the operative report. A right angle (Army-Navy) retractor may be placed proximally to allow visualization of the distal portion of the patella. The distal pole of the tibial tubercle in the central portion is marked with a sterile marking pen as a reference point. A middle third bone-tendon-bone graft is outlined with a scalpel (Fig. 61.1). A provisional cut is made on the bone, extended down through the patellar tendon, and directed along the

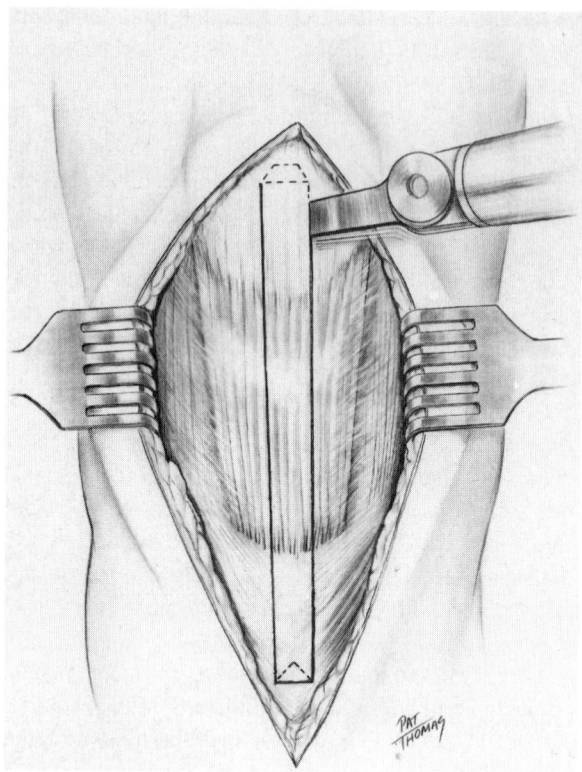

Figure 61.1. A construct length of 90 to 100 mm is usually obtained along the middle third of the patellar tendon. Note that the patellar bone plug has a trapezoidal profile, which minimizes the depth of the cut on the patella; the tibial tubercle site has a triangular profile.

plane of the fibers toward the tibial tubercle region. Care must be taken not to converge or diverge this incision. A 10-mm-wide osteotome is used as a template to allow accurate procurement of the graft.

Once the graft has been sharply outlined, a Micro-Aire oscillating saw blade (number 238) is used to harvest the bone plug. The blade is initially directed toward the tibial tubercle, and a triangular bone plug profile is obtained. The saw blade should be started at the tendo-osseous junction and moved distally on the tibial tubercle plug; on the patella, it should move from the tendo-osseous junction proximally to lessen the chance of violating any patellar tendon tissue. The bone plug should be harvested to create a trapezoidal profile on the patella and should be no more than 5 to 6 mm thick. Once the plug has been outlined with the number 238 oscillating saw blade, 0.63- and 0.94-cm (0.25- and 0.375-in) curved osteotomes are used to gently tap and remove the graft. The graft should not be levered because it may fracture. The tibial tubercle plug is held with a sterile sponge, and dissection from the fat pad is performed with Metzenbaum scissors from distal to proximal.

As noted, the patellar tendon may be harvested before arthroscopic placement if the surgeon has documented a pivot shift phenomenon and is convinced that there is insufficient articular injury to preclude ACL reconstruction.

GRAFT PREPARATION

The graft is prepared at the back table by an assistant, who shapes it generally for a 10-mm sizing tube for the femoral drill hole and an 11-mm tube for the tibial tunnel; the graft should slide relatively easily through the tubes. With an endoscopic technique, it is advisable to use the longer bone plug, which usually comes from the tibial tubercle, on the femoral side to reduce the likelihood of graft–tunnel mismatch. The tendo-osseous junctions are marked with a sterile marking pen to facilitate visualization when the graft is passed (Fig. 61.2). Three 0.062 Kirschner (K) wire drill holes are placed parallel to the cor-

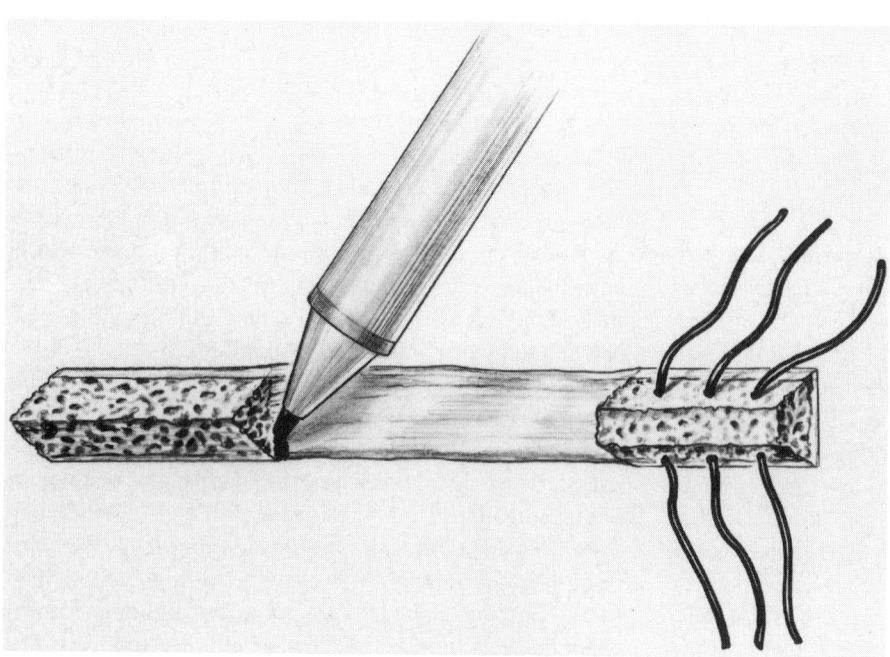

Figure 61.2. The tendo-osseous junction is marked with a sterile marking pen, providing a visual demarcation of this interval and helping the surgeon judge the depth of graft placement on the femoral side.

tical edge of the bone plug for the placement of number 5 Ticron sutures. Alternatively, the surgeon could place an 18-gauge wire through the drill hole to minimize the likelihood of suture laceration caused by interference from the screw placement. The graft is placed on a moist sponge and set aside. All intraoperative personnel should be aware of the graft's location.

While the graft is being prepared, an osteoperiosteal window is opened at the medial metaphyseal flare of the tibia. The surgeon should take care not to violate the superficial medial collateral ligament (MCL), pes anserinus, and remaining third medial patellar tendon. The window is a 2.5-cm^2 (1-in^2), medially based, trapdoor osteoperiosteal flap. A plexus of vessels is routinely encountered and should be meticulously electrocoagulated.

INTERCONDYLAR NOTCH PREPARATION AND NOTCHPLASTY

The arthroscope is reinserted through the inferolateral portal, and the surgeon prepares for the notchplasty. A motorized shaver is placed through an inferomedial portal and used to débride residual tissue (Fig. 61.3). Before using the shaver, the surgeon may create tissue access channels with a combination of arthroscopic scissors and an arthroscopic osteotome to débride and morcellize the remnant ACL tissue. The arthroscopic osteotome may also be used to peel off residual tissue from the lateral wall of the intercondylar notch. The tissue may then be aggressively débrided with an arthroscopic shaver (Fig. 61.3). The over-the-top position must be confirmed with an arthroscopic probe; remember that approximately two-thirds of the way posteriorly along the lateral wall there is a ridge that may be confused as the over-the-top position.

Notchplasty is performed with a round 5.5-mm burr; the surgeon works from the anterior aspect of the inter-

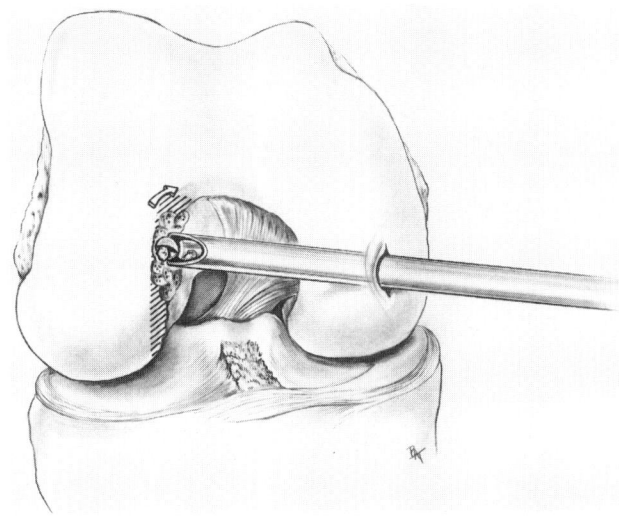

Figure 61.4. Notchplasty is performed with a 5- to 6-mm round motorized abrader to expand the wall, minimizing graft abrasion postsurgery and allowing arthroscopic visualization of the over-the-top region.

condylar notch posteriorly and from distal to proximal (Fig. 61.4). In general, expand the notch so it is approximately 20 mm wide; there should be at least 10 mm between the lateral edge of the PCL and the lateral wall of the intercondylar notch. This expansion allows improved visualization and makes it easier to remove intercondylar osteophytes, when necessary. The notch architecture should be assessed; it may be necessary to create a more trefoil-appearing notch apex in some individuals. Some patients may have a low intercondylar roof, requiring elevation of the roof arthroscopically. At this point attention may be focused on tibial tunnel placement.

TIBIAL TUNNEL PLACEMENT

A variety of tibial aiming devices are commercially available. The tibial tunnel should be placed so that the graft is not impinged by the roof of the intercondylar notch and should reside within the middle third of the former ACL insertion site. Remember that on the tibia there is a fairly wide insertion of approximately 3 cm of ACL tissue. General guidelines include placing the provisional pin at the posterior edge of the anterior horn of the lateral meniscus within the former ACL insertional footprint. A similar site position can be achieved by splitting the difference between the posterior edge of the anterior horn of the medial meniscus and the anterior edge of the PCL coming from the tibia. Finally, once the pin is positioned it must be posterior to the intercondylar apex by approximately 4 mm with the knee in extension.

With the endoscopic technique, tibial tunnel insertion placement is critical (Fig. 61.5). If the tunnel is placed too horizontally (e.g., 45°), a graft tunnel mismatch may occur, necessitating distal graft fixation with staples or a screw

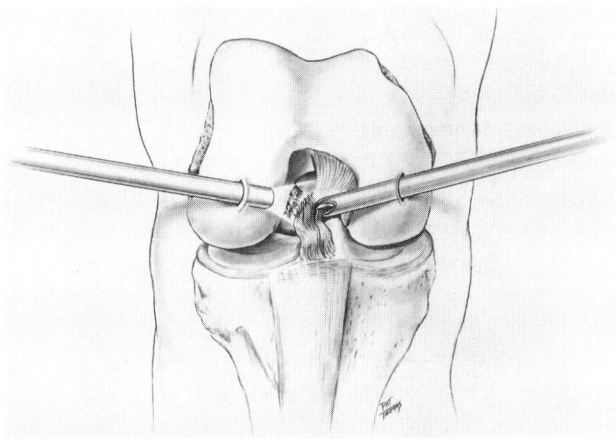

Figure 61.3. The arthroscope is placed in the inferolateral portal for intra-articular débridement of the remnant ACL tissue. Attention is directed to débriding tissue on the insertion site and along the intercondylar wall.

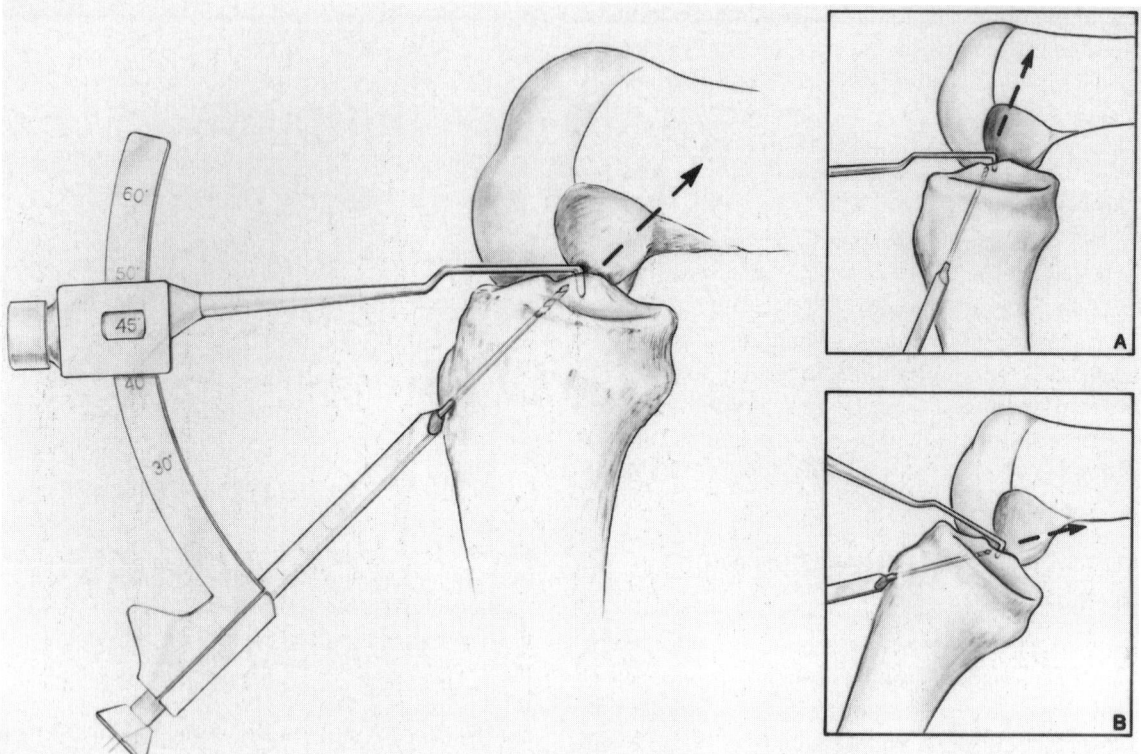

Figure 61.5. The knee flexion position and orientation of the tibial pin are critical. **A.** If the tibial tunnel is too steep, the femoral tunnel placement may be made too anteriorly when the knee is flexed at 90°. A steep tibial tunnel may necessitate less knee flexion at the risk of posterior cortex violation. **B.** If an appropriate tibial tunnel angle is selected (50° to 55°), but the knee is inadequately flexed, posterior cortical blowout may occur.

and post. The angle of inclination should be in the 50° to 55° range, resulting in a tibial tunnel that is long enough to facilitate interference screw fixation. Using this principle, my group uses tibial interference screws in more than 95% of our patients.

The entrance site on the tibial metaphyseal flare is also important and can be achieved by swinging the entrance site medially. With the knee in flexion, place a K wire superficially over the knee to estimate the angle of the tibial tunnel in relation to the femoral tunnel. A tibial tunnel placed in the sagittal plane results in a fairly vertically oriented graft on the femoral tunnel, which may control AP translation but not rotation. Optimally, the surgeon should obtain an 11-o'clock (right knee) or 1-o'clock (left knee) position on the femur.

In patients with patella alta, a distally placed accessory anterior medial portal may facilitate further distalization of the tibial tunnel, allowing a longer tibial tunnel and subsequent tibial interference screw fixation. Slight modifications in the tibial pin placement may be performed using a parallel guide device. I prefer to use a parallel pin system and grasp the pins with two Kocher clamps. This allows rotation in any plane and provides for accurate adjustments of the tibial pin.

Once the pin has been drilled and visualized intra-articularly, the tibial-aiming device is removed. The knee is brought into extension so the surgeon can assess the pin's position in relation to the intercondylar apex. It should clear the intercondylar apex by 4 mm. After appropriate positioning of the 0.23-cm (³/₃₂-in) threaded Steinmann pin, it is overreamed with a 10- or 11-mm reamer. The bone fragments should be collected during tibial reaming, and if the inflow system is turned off immediately before penetration of the intra-articular region, the surgeon can more easily control the collection of fragments. These shavings are used for subsequent grafting of the distal patellar and tibial tubercle defects. While the knee is dry, the intra-articular area of the tunnel entrance can be cleared of debris.

An arthroscopic shaver is placed through an inferomedial portal and used to smooth the intra-articular entrance. The shaver could also be placed through a midpatellar portal or placed retrograde through the tibial tunnel. An arthroscopic grasper may be used to remove tissue from the tibial entrance site. A chamfer reamer and arthroscopic hand rasp can be used to smooth the tibial tunnel posteriorly and posterolaterally (Fig. 61.6).

After the tibial tunnel is placed, the knee is reirrigated, and an outflow diaphragm is used to minimize fluid loss. The knee is copiously suctioned and attention is directed toward visualization of the over-the-top region and femoral tunnel placement.

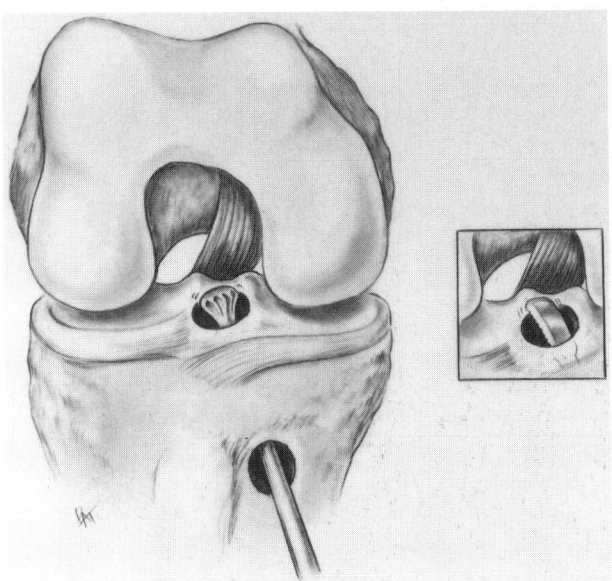

Figure 61.6. A motorized shaver is placed retrograde through the tibial tunnel to smooth the opening posteriorly and posterolaterally. **Insert.** An arthroscopic rasp is used to smooth the posterior region of the tibial tunnel.

FEMORAL TUNNEL PLACEMENT

While the knee is dry, a femoral aiming device may be used for accurate placement of the femoral guidepin. A freehand technique can be used, but commercially available femoral aiming devices make placement of the femoral pin considerably easier (Fig. 61.7). A 7-mm endoscopic femoral aimer is used for this purpose (Fig. 61.8); because the radius of a 10-mm-diameter reamer is 5 mm,

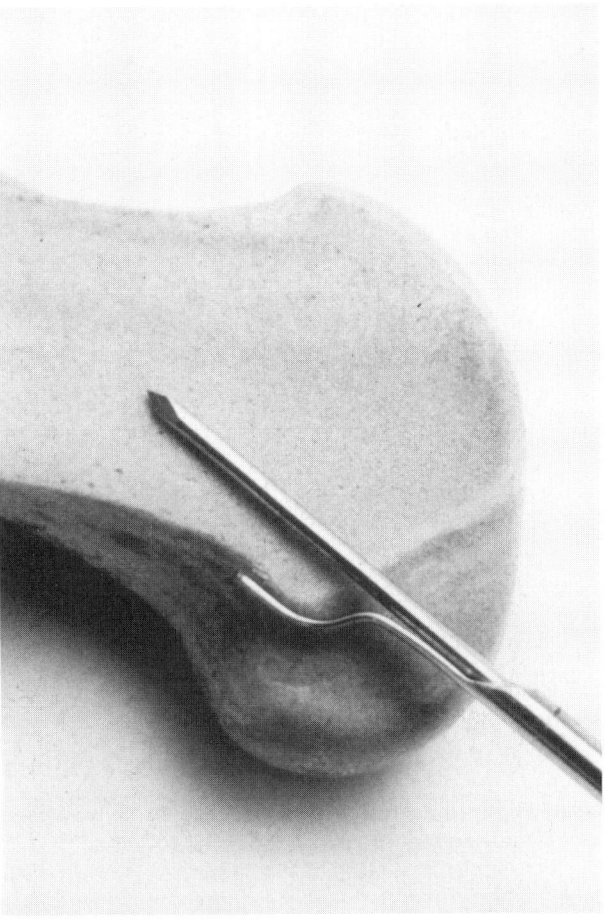

Figure 61.8. A commercial femoral pin placement guide sets the femoral pin 7 mm from the over-the-top location. Reprinted with permission from Arthrex Inc., Portsmouth, NH.

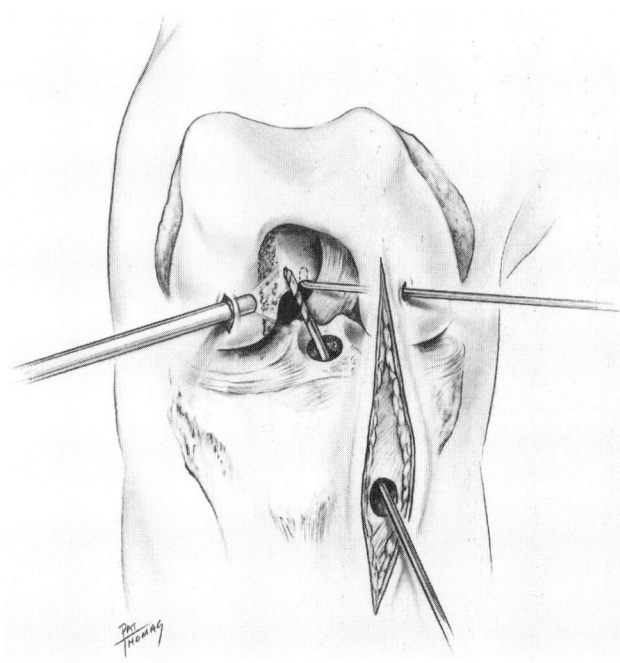

Figure 61.7. Freehand technique for placing the femoral pin, which will be overreamed with a cannulated reamer.

a 2-mm cortical bridge will be left when the aimer is properly positioned. The tongue of the aiming device hugs the over-the-top position, and once the device is placed and oriented—in the 11-o'clock (right knee) or 1-o'clock (left knee) position—the knee should be flexed between 80° and 90°. The pin is then drilled to a depth of 3.75 cm (1.5 in) (Fig. 61.9). In most cases, the flange of the offset guide may be placed in its position without altering the knee flexion position. Occasionally, the surgeon may slightly extend the knee (5° to 10°) to slide the guide into position. Pin placement may be fine-tuned by subtle rotation of the guide. Drilling and reaming should be performed with the knee in 80° to 90° of flexion. The aiming device is then removed.

At this point, knee flexion should not be altered to avoid bending the femoral guidepin. A 10-mm endoscopic reamer is then passed retrograde (Fig. 61.10) to smooth the posterior entrance of the tibial tunnel and is manually slid up to the femoral tunnel position. The reaming may be performed with the knee wet or dry. A provisional footprint is created to a depth of 8 to 10 mm to allow the surgeon to accurately assess the posterior cortex. A 1- to 2-mm cortical rim should be maintained, which can be as-

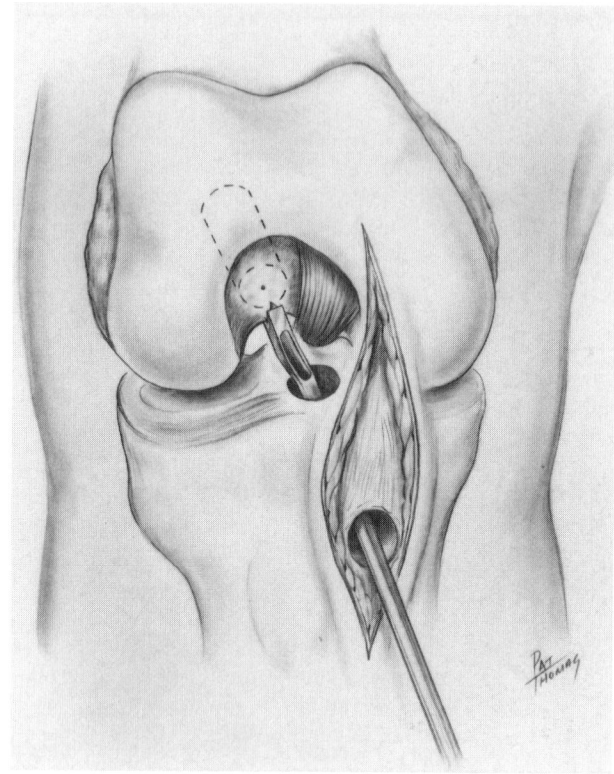

Figure 61.9. The tongue of the aimer must slip over the posterior cortex. The knee is usually flexed between 75° and 90°.

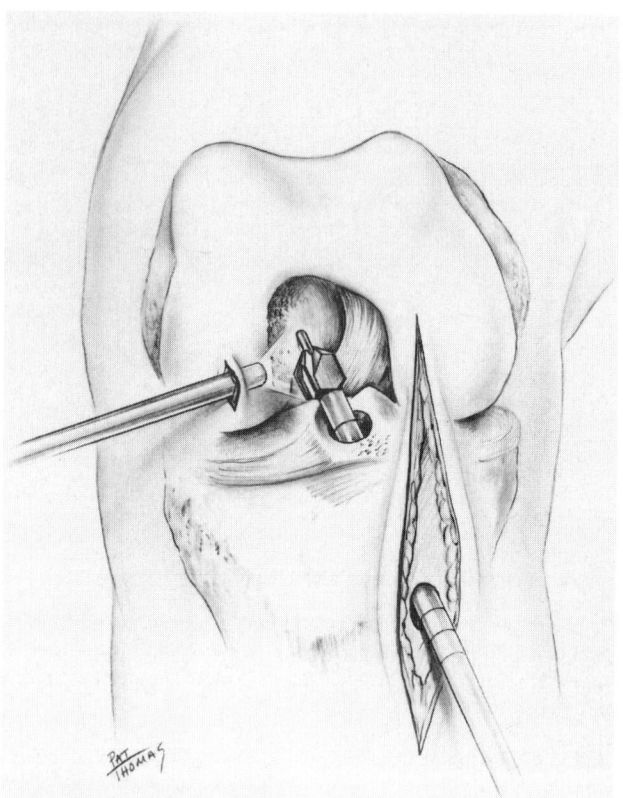

Figure 61.10. A 10-mm endoscopic reamer is manually inserted retrograde through the tibial tunnel up to the femoral region.

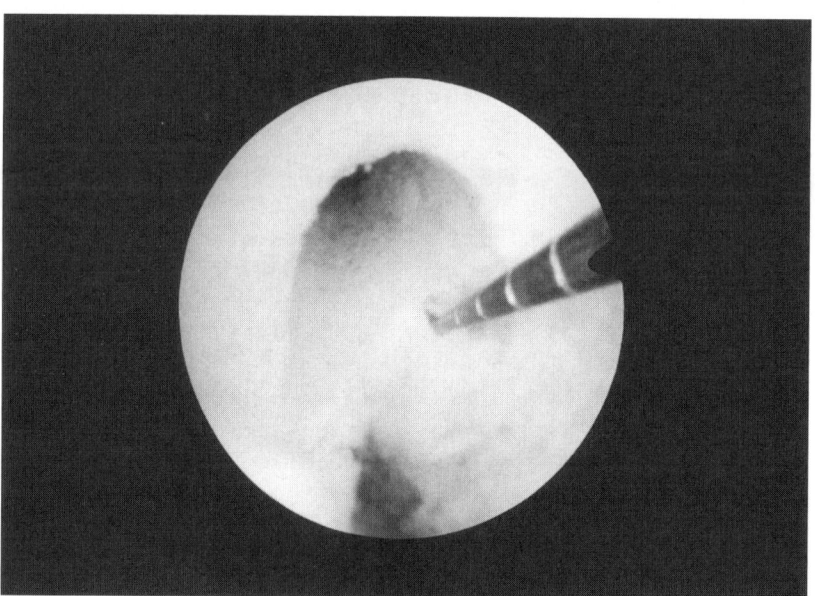

Figure 61.11. After femoral tunnel reaming, an arthroscope probe is used to confirm that the posterior cortical has been maintained. The arthroscope can be placed in either the inferomedial portal or retrograde via the tibial tunnel.

sessed with an arthroscopic probe (Fig. 61.11). Reaming may then be completed to a depth of 5 to 10 mm longer than the bone plug that will be placed on the femoral side. In general, the tunnel is 30 to 35 mm.

Once reaming is completed, the area is copiously irrigated and suctioned to remove the bone fragments. The arthroscope is passed retrograde through the tibial tunnel into the femoral tunnel. Rotation of the arthroscope will

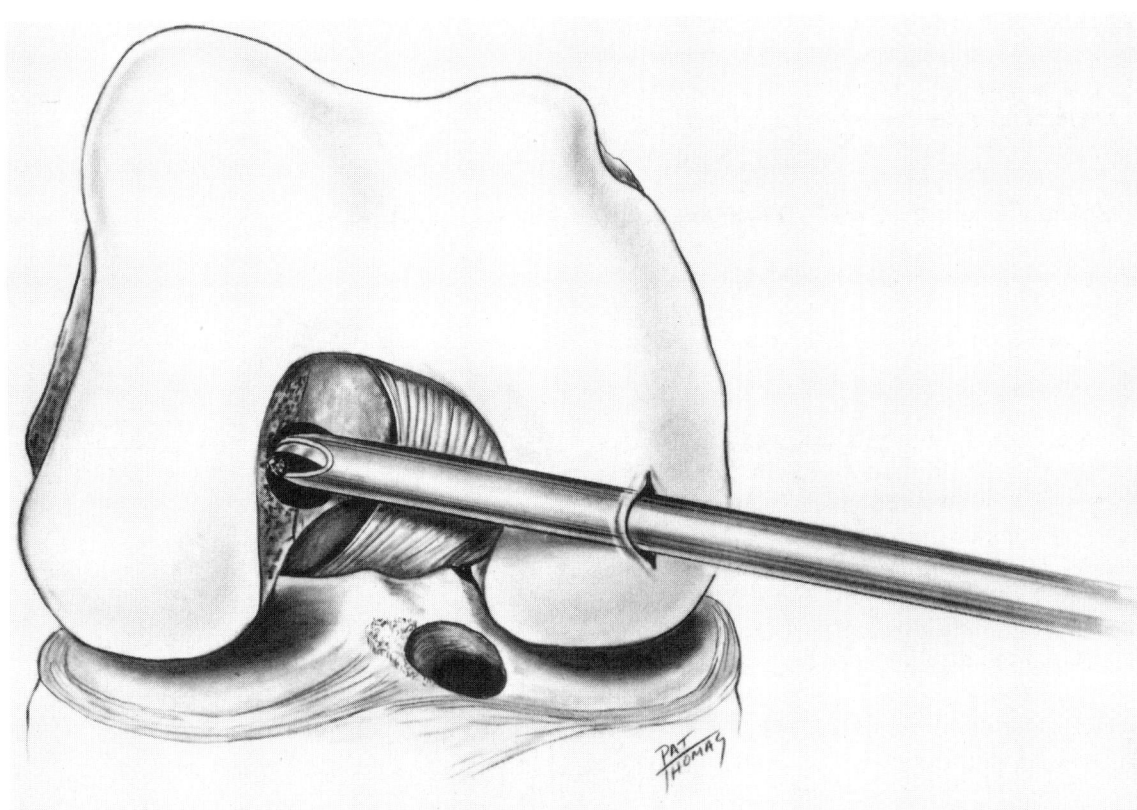

Figure 61.12. After reaming the femoral tunnel, the surgeon performs phase two notchplasty. The inner edge of the femoral tunnel is smoothed.

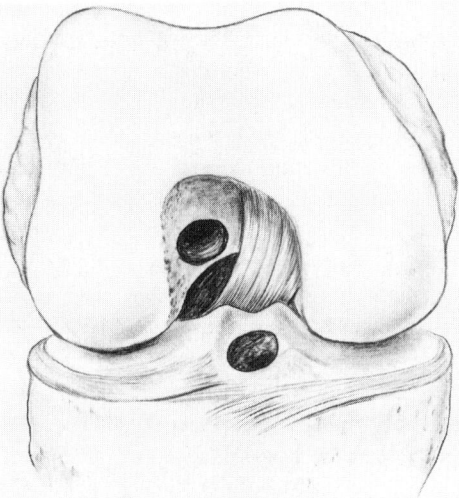

Figure 61.13. Femoral tunnel after reaming has been completed. The anterolateral quadrant may be shaped into an ellipse to facilitate graft and screw passage.

confirm that there has been no intratunnel or posterior cortical blowout and allows the surgeon to wash out any remaining shavings. The arthroscope is repositioned through the inferolateral portal, and the surgeon reassesses the intercondylar notch region. Phase two notchplasty is completed at this time (Fig. 61.12). The lateralization of the notch may be fine-tuned (Fig. 61.13). I shape the anterolat-

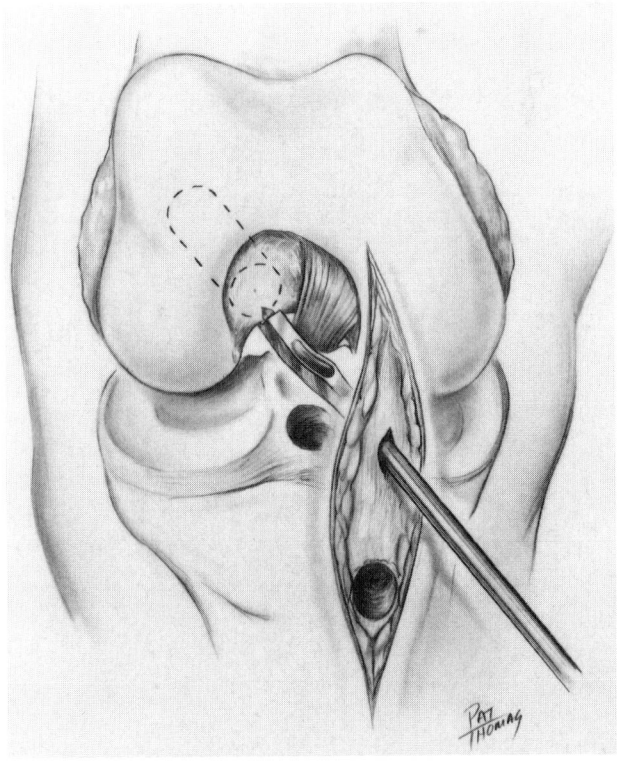

Figure 61.14. An alternative approach is through an accessory inferomedial portal instead of retrograde through the tibial tunnel.

eral quadrant of the femoral tunnel entrance into an ellipse to facilitate screw positioning and minimize graft abrasion.

An alternative approach to femoral tunnel placement is to slide the femoral offset guide through an accessory inferomedial portal (Fig. 61.14) (9). The flange of the guide is positioned in the same location. Using this modification, the surgeon must hyperflex the knee (110°) before drilling the Steinmann pin. The reamer is passed over this wire through the portal, and reaming is completed. The potential advantage of this technique is that parallel interference screw placement is fairly consistent (9).

GRAFT PLACEMENT

For the two-incision technique, the graft is oriented on the femoral side and the bone plug is in the sagittal plane. To minimize the possibility of soft tissue injury by the interference screw, endoscopic ACL surgery places the graft in the coronal plane. The cortex of the femoral bone plug is oriented posteriorly. A push-in technique has been used since 1991 as an alternative to the Beath needle pull-through or two-pin passer technique (Fig. 61.15).

Graft positioning should be performed with the knee dry, because a wet environment may result in edema of the graft, making screw placement difficult. The graft is pushed in with a two-pronged pusher and is grasped through the inferomedial portal with a hemostat or arthroscopic grasper, which may be used to slide the bone plug

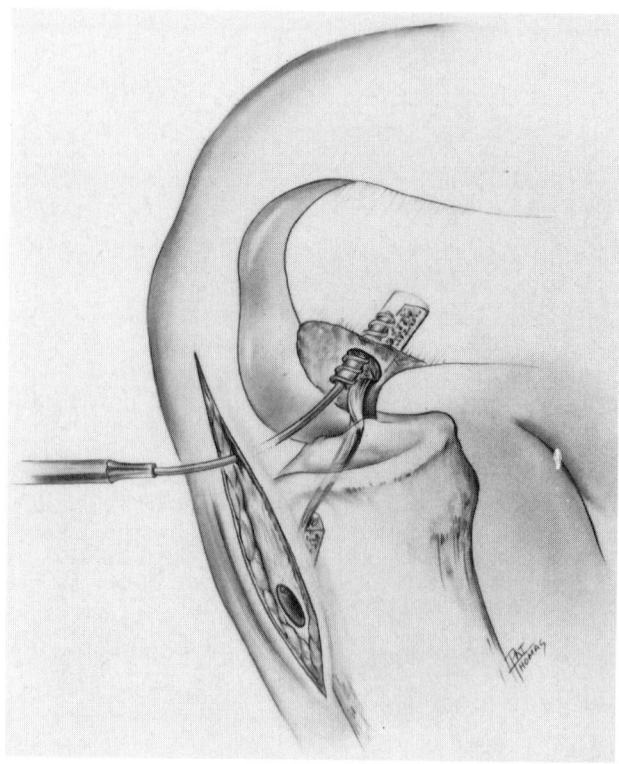

Figure 61.16. A flexible 35-mm Nitinol pin passed through an accessory parapatellar tendon portal eases the interference screw placement.

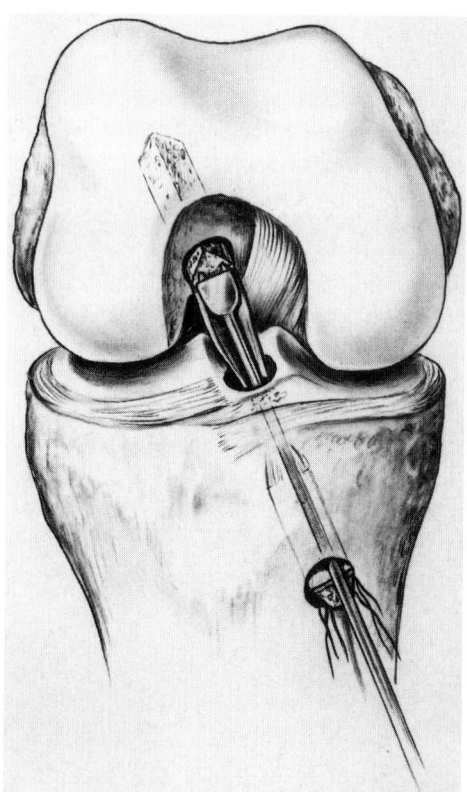

Figure 61.15. The graft is pushed retrograde through the tibial tunnel, the intra-articular space, and, in some situations, directly into the femoral tunnel. If the cortical edge of the graft is placed posteriorly, graft injury is less likely to occur during screw placement.

into the femoral blind-end tunnel. The graft should slide easily through the tibial tunnel, which is why I use an 11-mm tibial tunnel for a 10-mm graft. If there is difficulty in passing the graft retrograde through the tibial tunnel, the surgeon must be careful that the soft tissue is not delaminated from its bony plug. Fine-tuning of the femoral plug rotation should occur before complete seating of the graft, because it is difficult to execute once the graft has been positioned within the tunnel. During graft preparation, the tendo-osseous junction is routinely marked with a sterile marking pen (Fig. 61.2) as a reference point for graft placement. The tendo-osseous junction should be placed at the femoral tunnel entrance. Occasionally, the length of the graft construct requires that the graft be slightly deeper, but this increases the possibility of graft tissue injury.

GRAFT FIXATION

A 35-cm (14-in) hyperflex Nitinol pin (Concept, Inc., Largo, FL) is passed through the inferomedial portal and oriented at approximately the 11:45 (right knee) to 12:15 (left knee) position. This is provisionally seated at several millimeters, and the knee is hyperflexed an additional 15° to 20° (Fig. 61.16). The pin is then advanced between the bone plug and the tunnel. This takes into account the difference in angle between the inferomedial portal and the tibial tunnel in reference to the femoral tunnel. The pin should slide relatively easily and should not be forced. If there are difficulties, the bone plug should be pulled an-

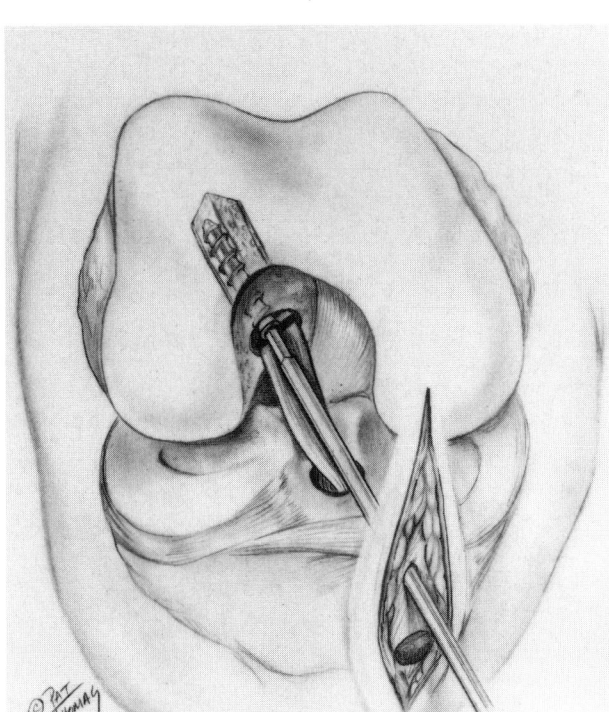

Figure 61.17. After the screw has been secured to half its length, the Nitinol pin is removed. The screw is then advanced to the articular margin or is slightly recessed.

tegrade a few millimeters to act as a skid for the pin. If the bone plug is slightly prominent intra-articularly once the pin has been seated, an arthroscopic pusher may be used to adjust its position.

Testing indicates that there is relatively little difference in the biomechanical pullout characteristics of 7- versus 9-mm interference screws on the femoral side. A 7- × 25-mm cannulated interference screw is used for femoral graft fixation. For osteopenic bone, the surgeon may select a 9-mm-diameter interference screw, but this is not often required. With the endoscopic technique, the femoral bone block is positioned so that the cortical edge of the bone plug is oriented posteriorly. The interference screw is placed anteriorly on the cancellous surface, which reduces the possibility of graft tissue injury. Provisional dilation of the soft tissue portal with a hemostat or screwdriver may facilitate screw passage. The knee is maintained in a position of hyperflexion, 100° to 110°, and the interference screw is introduced and secured (Figs. 61.17 and 61.18).

The surgeon should note any rotation of the graft, which may suggest that the graft tissue is being injured during screw placement. Once the screw has been engaged halfway, the Nitinol pin should be removed. The screw may then be completely seated. This is preferably performed with the knee dry.

Once the femoral graft has been secured, manual ten-

sion is placed on the graft via the tibial bone plug sutures. The knee is cycled several times; and under direct arthroscopic visualization, a rock test is performed to assess fixation: Sufficient force is applied by manually tugging on the tibial plug sutures to oscillate or rock the patient on the operating table. If there is any question about the graft's fixation, a Nitinol pin should be slid up through the cannulated lumen of the screw; the screw is removed and replaced with a 9-mm-diameter screw. Until the surgeon is completely comfortable with this technique, an intraoperative radiograph is advisable.

After cycling the knee, gross isometry may be assessed by placing tension on the external tibial tunnel and bringing the knee out into complete extension. Generally, there is a 1- to 2-mm change in the terminal 30° of extension that mimics the anatomic behavior of the normal ACL. On the tibial side, an interference screw is placed on the bone plug cortex and oriented anteriorly. If this screw is placed posteriorly to the bone plug and extends beyond the tendo-osseous junction, fraying of the graft may occur with flexion and extension of the knee. If the screw is placed anteriorly, graft injury is unlikely to occur, unless marked convergence of the screw has occurred. This also facilitates screw removal, if necessary.

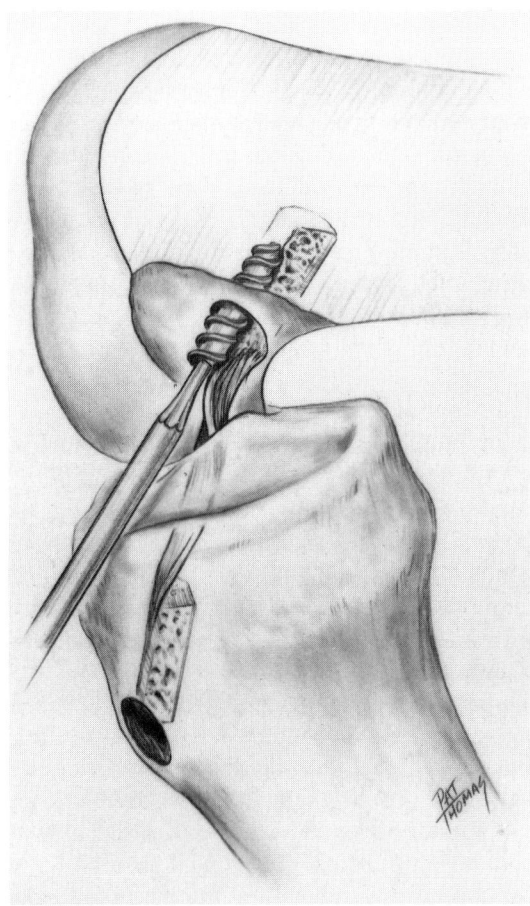

Figure 61.18. Lateral view showing the relationship of the cannulated interference screw and the bone plug. Note that the femoral bone plug has been oriented with its cortex posterior to minimize soft tissue injury.

Since 1987, I have performed tibial screw fixations with the knee in complete extension. Although many surgeons secure the tibial screw with the knee flexed at 20° to 30° and apply a posterior Lachman test, the rigid fixation afforded by interference screws has convinced me to secure the graft in complete extension. The rationale for this technique takes into consideration the change in graft tension during terminal extension. If a patient develops a postoperative knee flexion contracture, the surgeon may have captured the knee with the graft secured in flexion.

On the tibial side, the graft is rotated with the cortex facing anteriorly and in the coronal plane with occasional slight rotational variations. A hyperflex Nitinol pin is repositioned, and a 9- × 20-mm cannulated interference screw is generally positioned.

When there is extrusion of less than 50% of the tibial bone plug, I create a small trough posterior to the graft; this often allows me to use an interference screw for graft fixation instead of a screw and post or staple fixation. If a short tunnel or long graft construct has resulted in significant graft–tunnel mismatch (more than 50% of the bone plug length), a double-barbed staple fixation system, instead of sutures tied over a screw and post, provides excellent fixation.

Once the graft has been secured, the knee is cycled several times and the Lachman, anterior drawer, and pivot shift tests are performed. The graft should be inspected arthroscopically and assessed for tension and orientation. Remember that because the knee is generally in 70° to 80° of flexion throughout the procedure, the graft may initially look slightly lax. The knee should be brought out to approximately 30° of flexion and the graft reassessed by probe palpation. The surgeon must fine-tune the intercondylar notch at this point, if necessary. The knee is copiously irrigated and suction dried. Attention is now directed toward closure.

WOUND CLOSURE

The Hemovac drainage system is selectively used. Until 1994, my group exclusively placed one limb intra-articularly and one within the surgical wound region; since then, we have seldom used the Hemovac drainage system.

Before closing, the graft harvest site is copiously injected with 0.25% Marcaine. The 0.25% Marcaine is also used intra-articularly.

The patellar tendon rent is closed with interrupted absorbable sutures with the knee in flexion. Collected bone reamings are packed into the distal patellar defect, and the first layer is closed with inverted absorbable sutures (10). The osteoperiosteal window over the tibial metaphyseal region is also closed with an absorbable suture. Before closing, any areas of protruding tibial bone plug may be smoothed with a motorized burr. Subcutaneous tissues are closed with inverted absorbable sutures. The skin is closed with a running subcuticular nylon pullout suture.

Loosely applied Steri-Strips without benzoin are placed over the wound, along with Owen's gauze, unclipped sponges, Kerlix dressing, and a cryotherapy device. An Ace bandage and a drop-lock extension brace are used.

Postoperative Management

Patients undergoing single-incision endoscopic reconstruct have been prospectively followed since October 1991. An accelerated rehabilitation protocol is used that allows weight bearing in extension, full weight bearing as tolerated, immediate prone extension hangs, and immediate use of the quadriceps. A drop-lock extension brace is used during the first 6 weeks to protect the donor site during weight bearing; it may be removed for all flexion and range of motion activities. The brace is worn when the patient is sleeping to enhance extension. The accelerated rehabilitation protocol popularized by Shelbourne and Nitz (11) has been a cornerstone of my group's recommended rehabilitation treatment.

CLINICAL OBSERVATIONS

We have conducted a clinical review of endoscopic ACL reconstruction patients. Presently, 108 patients (96%) have been evaluated at a minimum follow-up of 2 years after surgery. A high stability rate, determined by negative pivot shift tests, has been observed in approximately 90% of patients. KT1000 maximum manual side-to-side differences are less than 3 mm in greater than 90% and more than 5 mm in less than 5% of patients. Reoperation rates for symptomatic knee flexion contracture has been less than 5%. Patient satisfaction has been extremely high; more than 95% of patients report being completely or mostly satisfied.

My group has performed single-incision endoscopic ACL reconstructions on an outpatient basis since May 1994. Overall, the long-term results of this technique may not be different from those of the two-incision arthroscopic-assisted technique, which we employed between 1987 and 1991 (3,4). The endoscopic single-incision technique is demanding and should be performed by seasoned arthroscopic surgeons who have had extensive experience with ACL reconstructions. Although there are pitfalls specific to the endoscopic technique, the single-incision technique has a low risk of surgical morbidity and allows ACL surgery to be performed on an outpatient basis without sacrificing clinical outcome.

REFERENCES

1. Bach BR Jr. Arthroscopy assisted patella tendon substitution for anterior cruciate ligament insufficiency: surgical technique. Am J Knee Surg 1989;2:3–20.
2. Hardin GT, Bach BR Jr, Bush-Joseph J, Farr J. Endoscopic single incision ACL reconstruction using patellar tendon autograft-surgical technique. Am J Knee Surg 1992;5:144–155.
3. Bach BR Jr, Jones GT, Sweet F, Hager CA. Arthroscopic assisted

ACL reconstruction using patellar tendon substitution: two-year follow-up study. Am J Sports Med 1994;22:758–767.

4. Bach BR Jr, Jones GT, Hager CA, Sweet F. Arthrometric aspects of arthroscopic assisted ACL reconstruction using patellar tendon substitution. Am J Sports Med 1995;23:179–185.

5. Speer KP, Spritzer CE, Bassett FH III, et al. Osseous injury associated with acute tears of the anterior cruciate ligament. Am J Sports Med 1992;20:382–389.

6. Rosen MA, Jackson DW, Berger PE. Occult osseous lesions documented by magnetic resonance imaging associated with anterior cruciate ligament ruptures. Arthroscopy 1991;7:45–51.

7. Daniel DM, Stone ML, Dobson BE, et al. Fate of the ACL-injured patient. A prospective outcome study. Am J Sports Med 1994; 22:632–644.

8. Bach BR Jr, Warren RF, Wickiewicz TL. Observations on the effects of the hip and foot position on the pivot shift phenomenon: results and description of a modified clinical test for ACL insufficiency. Am J Sports Med 1988;16:571–576.

9. O'Donnell JB, Scerpella TA. Endoscopic anterior cruciate ligament reconstruction: modified technique and radiographic review. Arthroscopy 1995;11:577–584.

10. Daluga D, Johnson JC, Bach BR Jr. Primary bone grafting following graft procurement for ACL insufficiency. J Arthroscopy 1990;6: 205–208.

11. Shelbourne KD, Nitz P. Accelerated rehabilitation after anterior cruciate ligament reconstruction. Am J Sports Med 1990;18: 292–299.

chapter 62

K. Donald Shelbourne and Ferdinand J. Liotta

Anterior Cruciate Ligament Reconstruction: Two-Incision Miniarthrotomy Technique

Numerous techniques are used for anterior cruciate ligament (ACL) reconstruction. This chapter describes a two-incision miniarthrotomy technique. Using this method, we have been successful in achieving excellent stability, full range of motion, and predictable satisfactory results for our patients while allowing them to participate in an aggressive rehabilitation program that facilitates a rapid return to sports (1). The goal of ACL reconstruction is to perform a predictably successful surgery at the best possible time to obtain long-term stability and a normal-functioning knee. Our miniarthrotomy technique offers our patients these reproducible excellent results and is, therefore, our method of choice for ACL reconstruction.

Our preferred source for an ACL graft is an autogenous bone-patellar tendon-bone construct. We have found it to be ideal for the restoration of predictable normal stability. Because the bone-patellar tendon-bone graft has been found to be constantly viable (2) and has ability to positively respond to early stress, patients can participate in an aggressive rehabilitation program and return to sports rapidly (1,3).

RELEVANT ANATOMY AND PATHOGENESIS

The ACL is the main stabilizing structure that controls rotational stability in the knee. As we have gained a better understanding of knee anatomy, our ability to make the diagnosis and to perform diagnostic physical examination tests has become more reliable. In addition, our understanding of the mechanism for ACL injury has become clearer.

The patient with an ACL injury typically describes the injury by saying, "I planted my foot to change directions. My knee twisted, and I felt a "pop" and fell down. I could

not walk well, and my knee was swollen by a couple hours after the injury." There are variations to this description. Sometimes, the patient feels like the knee hyperextended. Sometimes, the patient does not have a lot of swelling. Most of the time, however, the patient feels that a major injury has occurred, and the physician can know, or at least be suspicious, that the ACL is injured when the typical history is reported.

INITIAL FINDINGS, PHYSICAL EXAMINATION, AND DIAGNOSIS

When the orthopaedist sees a patient with an acute ACL tear, the patient either is walking with a bent-knee gait or is using crutches for ambulation. The patient has pain when extending the knee fully, either from a bone bruise from the injury or because the stump of the ACL gets impinged between the femur and the tibia with full extension. A hemarthrosis is usually present but can be of varying degrees, depending on the severity of the force during injury.

The physical examination can confirm the diagnosis in most cases, and it should be done with ideal circumstances. It is best if the patient has on a pair of shorts that amply expose the knee for the physical examination. To facilitate relaxation, the examination table should be long enough to support the patient's head and heels. The best physical test to determine ACL laxity is the Lachman test. Performing a Lachman test on the patient's normal knee first helps the patient relax and gain confidence in the testing procedure. The patient's leg muscles must be totally relaxed for the examination to be accurate. Grasp the patient's thigh just above the knee and externally rotate the patient's hip to relax the hip flexor muscles while supporting the knee in slight flexion. The physician can feel with the hand on the thigh whether the patient's leg is relaxed. The physician's other hand is placed on the tibia. A firm motion that pulls the tibia forward while pushing the femur backward can determine the amount of translation and the quality of an endpoint.

The flexion-rotation drawer test is a gentle test that can be performed on the patient with an acute knee injury. While cradling the calf and flexing the knee from 20° to 30°, the examiner can apply gentle posterior pressure to the tibia. If the ACL is torn, this pressure will cause the tibia to reduce and the femur to rotate internally. The result of this test must be compared with that of the contralateral normal knee because some patients may have mild physiologic pivot shift that is normal for them.

The pivot shift and anterior drawer tests are difficult to perform when the injury is acute. Furthermore, the tests are not usually needed to establish the diagnosis. If the Lachman and flexion-rotation drawer tests are not conclusive, it is very easy to treat the initial symptoms and have the patient come back for another physical examination a few days later. We do not routinely recommend the use of magnetic resonance imaging for making the diagnosis of an ACL tear because the physical examination is diagnostic in greater than 95% of the cases.

RADIOLOGIC STUDIES

We obtain routine radiographs before the ACL surgery is performed. The standing posteroanterior weight-bearing view (4) provides a way of evaluating the joint space between the femur and tibia. It also allows for a measurement of the intercondylar notch width, which is important for predictive values for ACL tears (5). The patellar tendon length and height are measured on the lateral radiographic view. If the patellar tendon is used for the graft, the 60° flexed lateral view can give an accurate measurement of the patellar tendon length, which allows for surgical technique changes. The Merchant's radiographic view (6) not only shows the joint space between the femur and patella but also helps to determine whether the patient has patellofemoral malalignment.

TREATMENT

Preoperative Preparation

Success with the miniarthrotomy technique begins before the surgical procedure. We have found that patients who come to surgery with a normal-appearing knee (full range of motion, including hyperextension equal to that of the opposite normal leg, minimal swelling, normal gait and leg control) have the best chance for a smooth postoperative course, without the complications of arthrofibrosis and quadriceps muscle weakness (3). Patients are educated about the surgery and their expected rehabilitation

goals and have their minds focused on a full positive recovery from the reconstruction.

Procedure

After an examination under anesthesia confirms the preoperative diagnosis, a full arthroscopic evaluation is performed under tourniquet control on all patients before the ACL reconstruction is undertaken. If a meniscal lesion is encountered, it is left in situ, repaired, or partially removed as indicated.

MEDIAL ARTHROTOMY

At completion of the arthroscopy, a wedge is placed under the thigh, and the leg is redraped. The tourniquet remains inflated from the arthroscopy; it does not present a problem because average total procedure time is under 60 min.

A 4- to 6-cm incision is made from the inferior medial border of the patella proximally (beginning at the inferomedial portal) to the level of the medial tibial tubercle distally. The length of the incision depends on the preoperative patellar tendon length, as measured on a 60° lateral radiograph. The incision is continued sharply to the level of the peritenon and joint capsule. Blunt and sharp dissection are used to develop a plane proximally into and through the prepatellar bursa and between capsule and subcutaneous tissue medially, laterally, and distally. This dissection allows easy retraction of the skin for graft harvest while maintaining a small incision.

Using electrocautery, the surgeon creates a flap of periosteum approximately 4 cm distal to the joint line, superior to the pes anserinus tendon insertion, and medial to the patellar tendon and tibial tubercle. This allows for a tibial tunnel that will be 30 to 40 mm in length. An elevator is used to complete the flap, which is conserved to close over the tibial tunnel and fixation button upon completion of the reconstruction. Using this technique, we have essentially eliminated painful tibial hardware (0.6% tibial button removal in the last 1229 patients). The medial arthrotomy is made with electrocautery from the anterior horn of the medial meniscus to the insertion of the vastus medialis into the patella. This exposure affords a superior view of the intercondylar notch without dislocating the patella (Fig. 62.1).

LATERAL INCISION

The surgical table is elevated while the foot is lowered completely, allowing 90° of flexion at the knee. The distal lateral femoral cortex is exposed by making a 2.5-cm oblique incision in Langer's lines, 2.5 cm proximal to the superior pole of the patella at the level of the iliotibial (IT) band (Fig. 62.2). Blunt dissection is used to expose the IT band. The leg is extended, and the IT band is split longitudinally. Blunt digital dissection is used to strip the vastus lateralis from the intermuscular septum and retract it anteriorly to expose the lateral femoral cortex. A Slocum

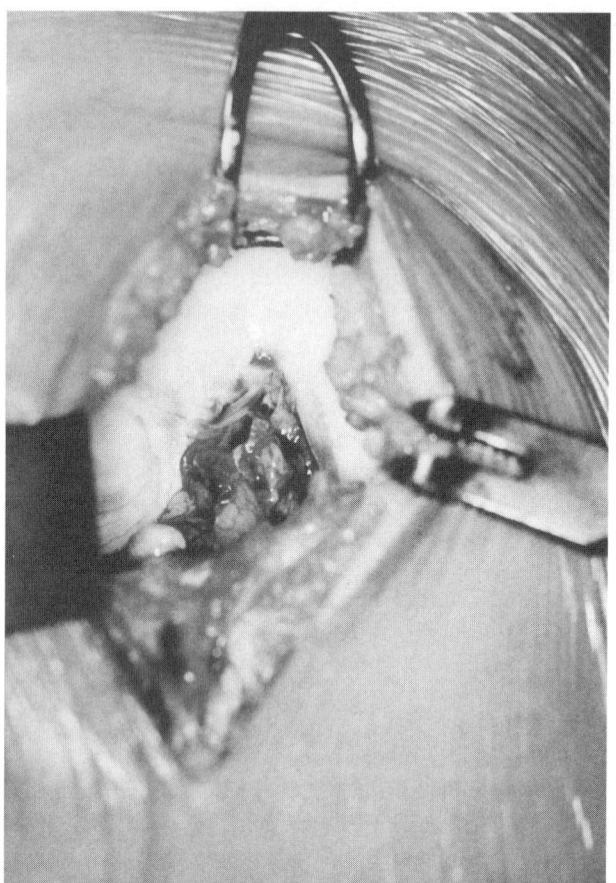

Figure 62.1. Superior view of the intercondylar notch.

retractor is placed over the anterior femur to hold the vastus lateralis anteriorly. A Cushing retractor holds the IT band posteriorly. Branches of the lateral geniculate artery and vein are usually found along the metadiaphyseal area of the lateral femoral cortex; these are cauterized. The periosteum along the lateral femoral cortex is split in T fashion, and the flaps are elevated. The periosteal dissection coincides with the ideal exit point for the femoral tunnel, which is 5 cm proximal to the articular surface and on the flat surface of the distal diaphysis of the lateral femur.

NOTCHPLASTY

A Slocum retractor is placed posterior to the fat pad in the anterior joint and around the lateral femoral condyle to retract the patellar tendon laterally without dislocating the patella. Using a Cushing retractor, the surgeon retracts vastus medialis obliquus (VMO) and uses a two-pronged rake to retract the fat pad medially. This exposure provides an excellent view of the tibial plateau and intercondylar notch. The ligamentum mucosum and any fat pad that impedes visualization are removed with electrocautery. After identifying the lateral border of the posterior cruciate ligament (PCL), the surgeon completely cleans the lateral notch of all soft tissue, which consists of the old ACL and fibrofatty tissue. The over-the-top position is completely visualized in the posterolateral notch.

The width of the intercondylar notch and the width from the lateral border of the PCL to the lateral wall of the notch (the space for the previous ACL) are measured and recorded. A number 4 curette is used to enlarge the space from the PCL to the lateral wall of the notch to 11 mm, to accommodate the 10-mm graft and avoid lateral notch impingement (Fig. 62.3). The complete visualization of the entire lateral notch is crucial for placement of the femoral tunnel. Attention is now turned to the femoral and tibial tunnels.

CREATION OF FEMORAL AND TIBIAL TUNNELS

The exact anatomic placement of the tibial and femoral bone tunnels is paramount to the successful outcome from this procedure. By using independent placement of the bone tunnels, we can repeatedly obtain exact anatomic placement of each tunnel. The exposure offered by the miniarthrotomy simplifies this effort.

The tibial footprint of the ACL is large, which makes the tibial bone tunnel relatively more difficult to find. The ideal graft placement is a position that is posterior enough so that when the knee is hyperextended the graft lies just posterior and parallel to the roof of the intercondylar notch. In the past, anterior placement of the tibial tunnel was emphasized to avoid problems in achieving full range of motion (7). We, and others (8), have found that the anterior placement of the tibial tunnel leads to restriction of hyperextension, impingement of the graft with the possibility of graft failure, and hindrance of obtaining a perfect graft notch fit in full hyperextension.

The tibial tunnel is drilled first. To identify the position of the tibial tunnel, the medial tibial plateau is visualized as a clock face (Fig. 62.4). Set the 9-o'clock position as the center of the plateau for a right knee and the 3-o'clock for the left knee, the appropriate position for the guidepin will be 5 mm lateral to the articular surface and at the 9-o'clock position. Drilling outside to inside, a 0.094 ($^3/_{32}$-in) Steinmann pin is passed from the anteromedial tibia into the knee joint to exit at the previously planned spot on the

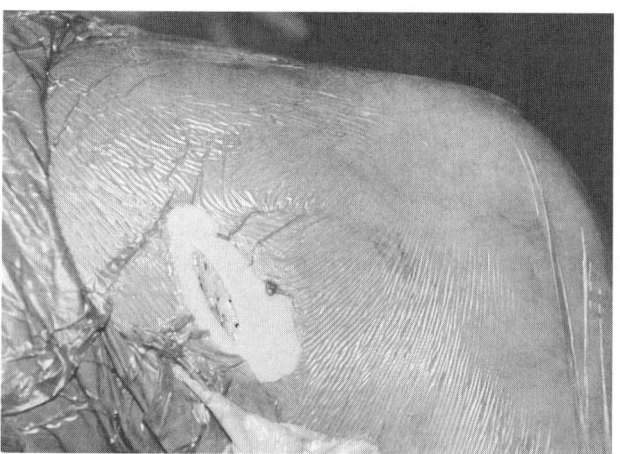

Figure 62.2. Lateral skin incision.

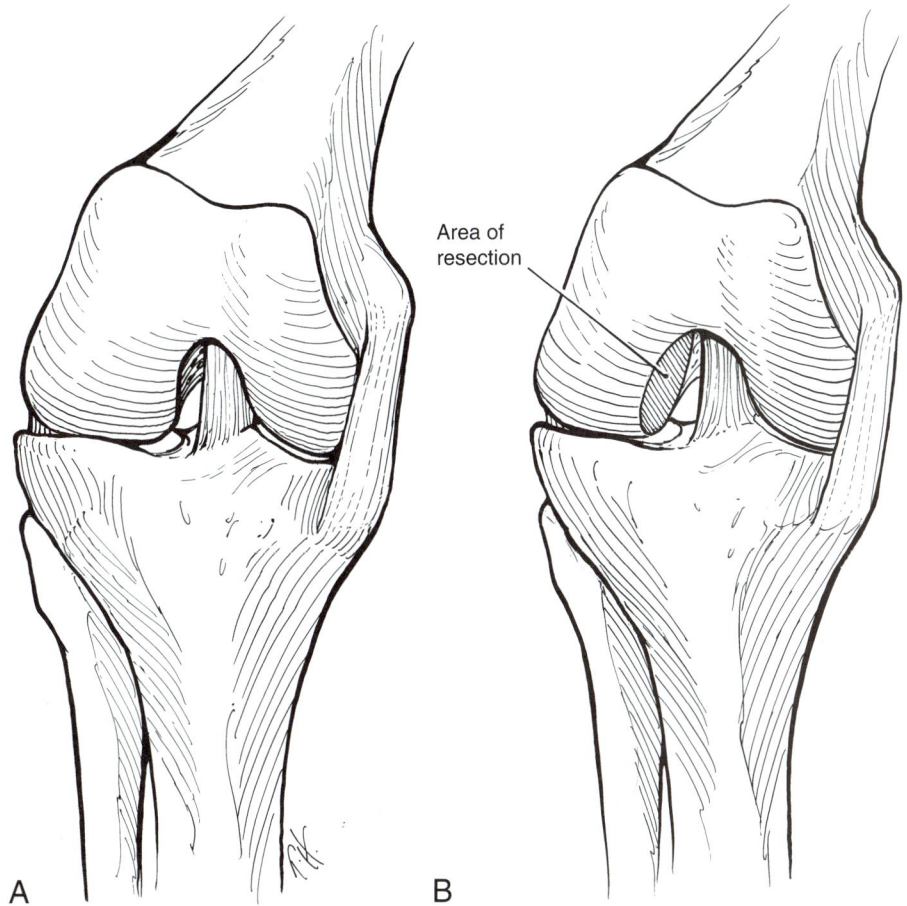

Figure 62.3. A. Intercondylar notch view showing the space for the ACL before the lateral notchplasty has been performed. **B.** Area of resection of the lateral femoral condyle.

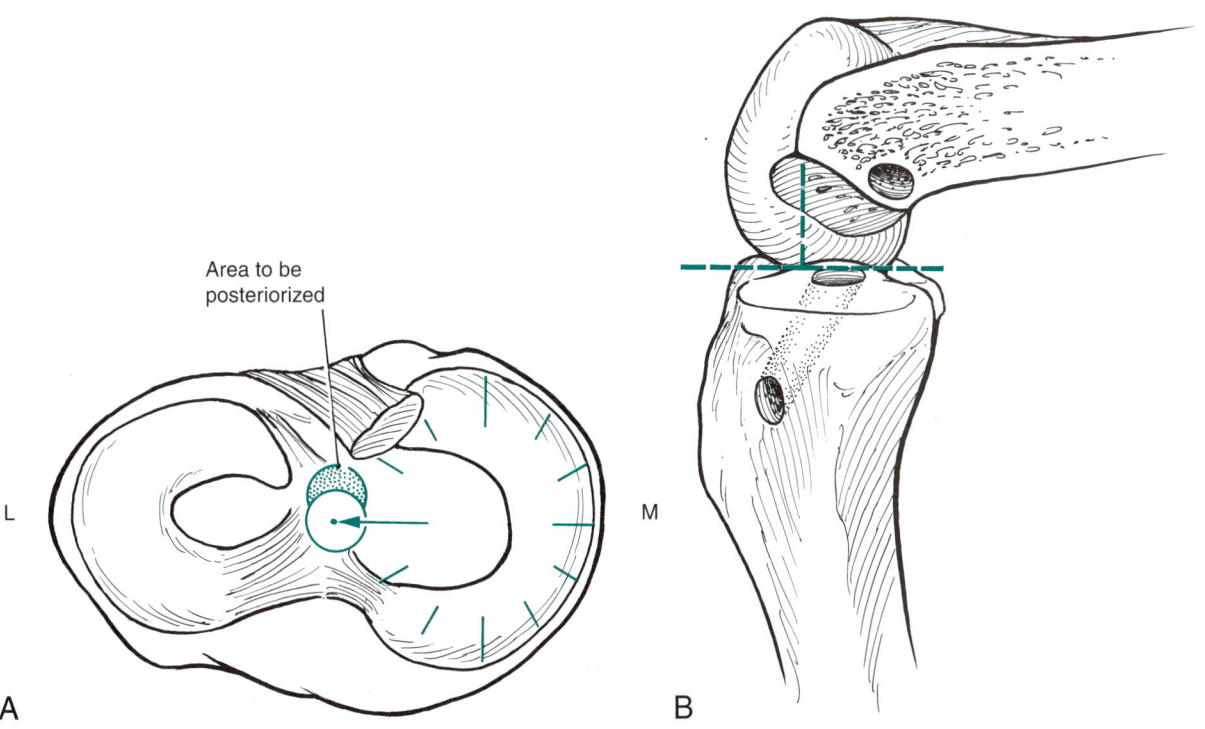

Figure 62.4. A. A clock face is visualized on the medial tibial plateau to show the ideal placement of the tibial tunnel. **B.** Lateral view of the knee showing the tibial tunnel placement posterior to a perpendicular line drawn from the anterior opening of the intercondylar roof.

plateau. The starting point for drilling the tibial tunnel is 10 mm medial to the tibial tubercle and superior to the pes anserinus tendon, coinciding with the periosteal flap and 3 to 4 cm distal to the joint line. This configuration should ensure a tibial tunnel of 30 to 40 mm and position the tunnel medial to the tibial tubercle, allowing a flat seating of the fixation button.

Perfect positioning on the first pass of the guidepin is difficult. Because the guidepin is small, repositioning is easy should it be necessary. A 9-mm cannulated reamer is used to make the tunnel, once the guidepin has been correctly placed. The bone removed during reaming is saved for bone grafting the patella and tibial bone plug defects.

The soft tissue is removed sharply from the floor of the tibial tunnel after the reaming is complete. Because the patellar tendon is 4 mm thick, the back wall of the tunnel is posteriorized to place the tendon 3 to 4 mm posterior to the 9-o'clock position. The posteriorization is performed starting with a number 5 (9-mm) curette and increasing to a number 6 (11-mm) curette. Delaying the patellar tendon harvest until the tunnels are made allows for appropriate sizing of the bone plugs. This modification of the tunnel makes its shape conical, permitting a press fit of the bone plug. The usual length of the tibial tunnel is 30 to 40 mm.

Femoral tunnel placement is the most difficult but possibly the most important aspect of this procedure. In our opinion, inaccurate placement of the femoral tunnel is the most common cause of ACL reconstructive failure. Once the tibial tunnel has been drilled, there should be a straight-line orientation with the femoral tunnel. Because of the excellent visualization of the notch afforded by the miniarthrotomy, the femoral tunnel can be drilled by beginning from inside the notch; thus the surgeon can make a complete and accurate assessment of the notch anatomy to ensure proper anatomic placement of the tunnel. This visualization of the entire notch anatomy offers a distinct advantage over the close-up view provided by the arthroscope. The keys to successful femoral tunnel placement are (a) to place the femoral tunnel as posterior as possible in the notch, leaving a 1- to 2-mm bony bridge anterior to the over-the-top position; (b) to align the tunnel so it lies adjacent to the PCL; and (c) to allow a straight-line orientation of the graft with the tibial tunnel when the knee is in 30° of flexion.

With the notch completely prepared and the above considerations in mind, the knee is placed in a figure-four position. A 0.094 (³/₃₂-in) Steinmann pin is placed on the lateral border of the PCL and passed a few millimeters out the back of the notch. This helps orient the posterior portion of the notch. The guidepin is brought forward into the notch 6 to 7 mm and placed 2 to 3 mm laterally, establishing the center of the femoral tunnel. With the appropriate starting point for the guidepin identified, the pin is directed to the previously made periosteal window on the lateral femoral cortex with the knee held in greater than 90° of flexion. Once the pin has penetrated the lateral cortex, it is palpated beneath the vastus lateralis to ensure it

is in the appropriate position. The guidepin should exit on the lateral wall of the femur in the area previously prepared. If the position is not appropriate, the guidepin is redirected from the same starting point in the notch.

Once the guidepin is in the correct position, it is overdrilled with an 10-mm reamer. The completed tunnel should have a 1- to 2-mm-thick posterior cortical bony bridge, and the medial wall of the tunnel should lie just posterior to the lateral border of the PCL. The reamings are retrieved for future bone grafting. The femoral tunnel usually measures 50 to 80 mm in length. The lateral cortex is visualized to ensure that the tunnel opening is clear of soft tissue.

To confirm the tunnel placement, the knee is flexed to 30°. A straight measuring rod should easily pass from the tibial tunnel through the knee and femoral tunnel, exiting laterally. If the rod does not pass easily, it means the tibial tunnel is too anterior. This can be remedied by using a curette to further posteriorize the tunnel. Since the graft has not yet been harvested, the bone plugs can be sized to fit the tunnels. The individual tunnel lengths and the entire tunnel length are measured to ensure appropriate graft harvest length.

HARVEST OF THE BONE-PATELLAR TENDON-BONE GRAFT

A Metzenbaum scissors is used to enter the peritenon. The plane between the peritenon and the patellar tendon is developed. The peritenon is split longitudinally to the tibial tubercle distally and over the patella proximally. The medial and lateral borders of the tendon are dissected free, preserving the peritenon flaps for later closure with the tendon defect. The width of the tendon is measured at the joint line. A 10-mm bone-patellar tendon-bone graft is harvested from the central portion of the tendon. Outlines of the bone plugs are made with a scalpel over the tibial tubercle and patella. An osteotome is used to score the proximal end of the patellar bone plug and the distal end of the tibial bone plug. An oscillating saw is used to harvest a 10 or 11 by 25-mm bone plug. The size of the bone plug harvested depends on the size of the tunnel.

The patellar bone plug is harvested first. It is removed from its bed and contoured to tightly fit the tibial tunnel. Three drill holes are made from the cancellous surface out in the bone plug with a 1.6-mm (¹/₁₆-in) drill. A number 2 Ethibond suture is placed through each of the drill holes. The bone plug is left in the patellar defect, and the ends of the suture are secured to the drapes to avoid inadvertent dropping of the graft. The tibial bone plug is harvested next and is contoured to fit a 10-mm sizer. The sutures are placed through drill holes in the same way as the patellar bone plug.

Once the three sutures are placed in the tibial bone plug, the patellar tendon's soft tissue attachments and fat pad are removed sharply. The graft is inspected and débrided of soft tissue and excess fat on the back table (Fig. 62.5). The graft length, width, and thickness are mea-

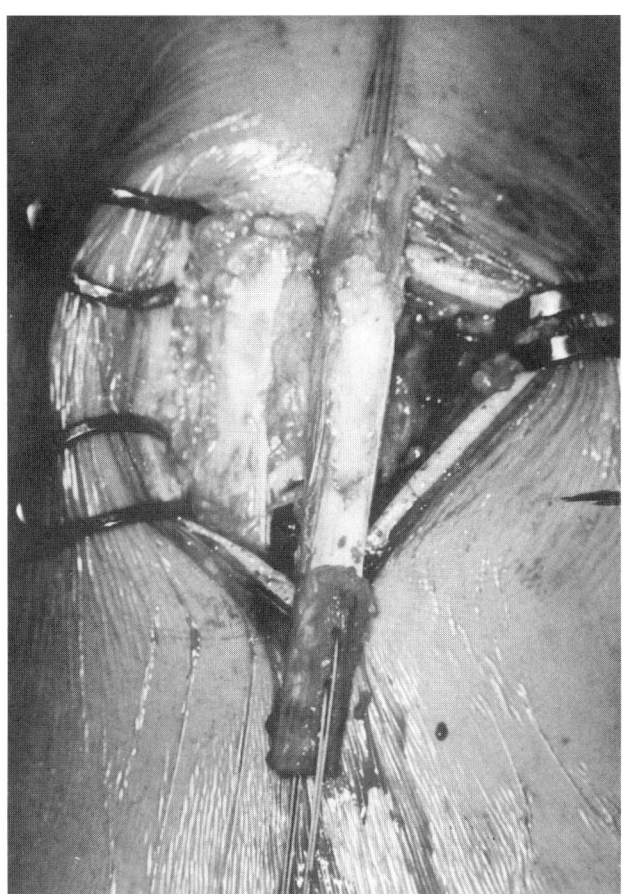

Figure 62.5. Prepared graft before insertion into the knee.

sured and recorded. The overall length of the graft is always longer than the native ACL. We have found the graft length to vary from 34 to 72 mm, whereas the native ACL length varies from 20 to 32 mm. The extra length of the graft can be easily accommodated, since the femoral tunnel can vary from 40 to 90 mm in length. The two-incision technique ensures that there will never be a graft–tunnel mismatch.

PLACEMENT OF THE GRAFT INTO THE BONE TUNNELS

Passage of the graft is a simple matter, because of the tunnels' straight-line orientation and the open, inside to outside graft placement. The patella bone plug is passed into the tibial tunnel, and the tibial bone plug is passed into the femoral tunnel. A suture passer is placed from the outside into the joint through the tibial tunnel. The patellar bone plug sutures are brought out of the tibial tunnel with a suture passer. The patellar bone plug is oriented so the tendon is facing posterior and the cancellous bone is facing anterior. It is guided into place with a pair of forceps while tension is placed on the sutures. A tight press fit of the patellar bone plug is obtained. Once the desired snug fit is achieved and the bone plug is below the articular surface of the tibial plateau, the sutures are tied to a 19-mm polyethylene button on the medial tibial cortex. This se-

cures the bone plug into the tibial tunnel. Only two throws of the suture are made at this point to allow for easy untying if further retensioning is required.

The tibial bone plug sutures are placed into a suture passer and are passed through the femoral tunnel, exiting laterally. The sutures are held laterally and pulled taunt, and the tibial bone plug is guided into the femoral tunnel with the tendinous portion facing posterior and the cancellous bone facing anterior. A snug fit of the bone plug in the femoral tunnel is ensured by the appropriate sizing of the plug at harvest. The sutures are pulled tightly, seating the bone plug into the femoral tunnel while accommodating the extra graft length. The sutures are tied tightly with five throws over a 19-mm polyethylene button on the lateral cortex of the femur (Fig. 62.6). The button now lies flush on the lateral femoral cortex.

GRAFT TENSIONING

The goal of ACL reconstruction is to provide a stable knee with full range of motion. With button fixation, adjustments in graft tension can be easily made to ensure that these goals are met. All adjustments are made in 30° of flexion, which is the position in which the graft is most lax. The tibial sutures are again tightened, in an attempt to overtension the graft. The knee is put into full hyperextension and full flexion. Because of the flexibility in the suture–button fixation, the graft will find its "isometry" when put through a full range of motion. If the graft is too tight before the knee is ranged, the sutures on the button will loosen. This loosening allows enough graft laxity to achieve a full range of motion without capturing the joint and while maintaining stability. After ranging the knee, the surgeon returns it to 30° of flexion and pulls on the tibial sutures. If the button can be lifted off the tibia, the sutures are retightened, and the knee is put through another full range of motion. The tibial sutures are again pulled to evaluate how far the button comes off the tibial cortex. If the tunnels are placed appropriately, the button should remain tight on the tibia. When the button has the appro-

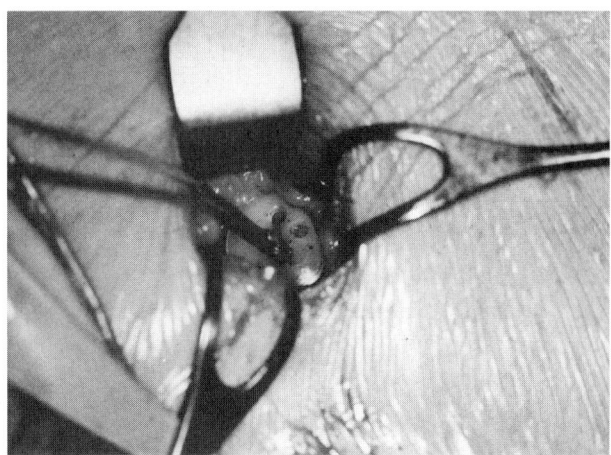

Figure 62.6. The button is placed on the lateral femoral condyle.

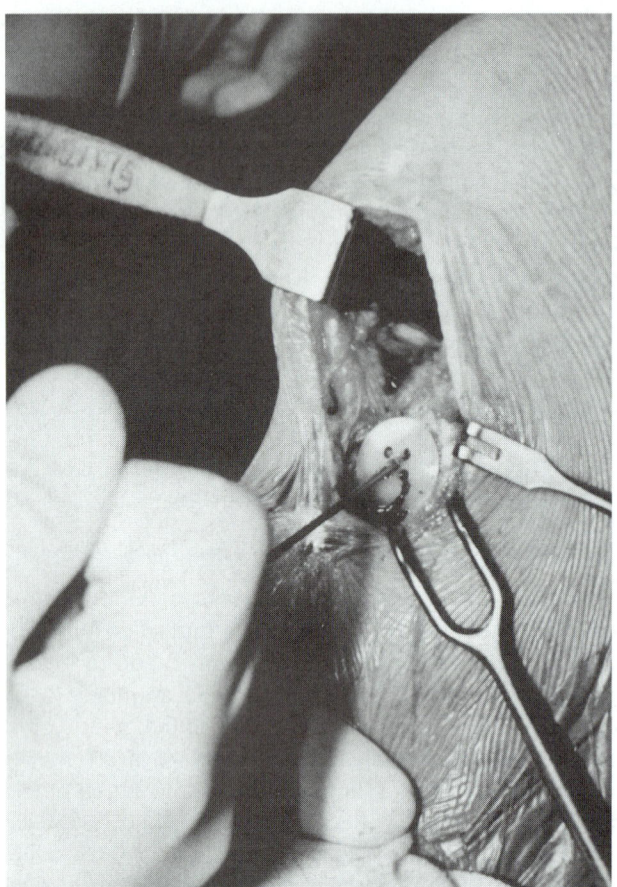

Figure 62.7. Confirming the tibial button placement and appropriate graft tension.

priate give, three more throws are placed in the sutures to lock the graft in place (Fig. 62.7).

COMPLETION OF THE OPERATION

The intra-articular portion of the graft is inspected after the knee has demonstrated a full range of motion and the buttons are tight. The graft is inspected at full hyperextension to ensure that there is no superior notch impingement. There should be a perfect fit of the graft in the notch in full hyperextension, if the tibial tunnel is correctly placed. If the tibial tunnel is slightly anterior, there may be a minor impingement in full hyperextension. If impingement occurs, the superior roof can be enlarged with a number 4 curette. Once there is full, unimpinged hyperextension, the tourniquet is released. Hemostasis is achieved with electrocautery. Both wounds are copiously irrigated with an antibiotic solution (bacitracin). The wounds, fat pad, and deep structures are infiltrated with 0.25% Marcaine with epinephrine.

The patellar tendon defect is loosely closed with the peritenon using a running absorbable number 1–0 suture. Bone graft collected during tunnel reaming is packed into the patella defect, and the peritenon is sutured over it to keep the bone graft in the defect. The tibial defect is similarly packed. The miniarthrotomy is closed with inter-

rupted number 1–0 absorbable sutures in a figure-eight fashion. A medium ConstaVac drain (Stryker; Kalamazoo, MI) is placed in the subcutaneous space in both wounds. The IT band is closed with a number 2–0 absorbable interrupted suture. The skin and subcutaneous tissue are closed in a standard fashion. An Exu-Dry (Exu-Dry Wound Care Products; Bronx, NY) is placed over both wounds, which are then covered with a square of Plastizote (Fillauer; Chattanooga, TN) to provide local wound edema control and to diminish wound-healing problems. The leg is placed in a long leg TED hose (Kendall; Mansfield, MA). A Cryo/Cuff (Aircast; Summit, NJ) is applied snugly and is then filled with ice-cold water to provide cold and compression. The patient is sent to the recovery room with this dressing in place. Once the patient arrives in his or her room, the knee is placed in a continuous passive motion machine with the Cryo/Cuff in place.

SUMMARY

We believe that the miniarthrotomy technique using an autogenous central third bone-patellar tendon-bone graft has distinct advantages over other procedures.

1. The miniarthrotomy approach allows excellent visualization of the tibial plateau and deep into the intercondylar notch.
2. Drilling the femoral tunnel from inside out allows for a predictable, reproducible anatomic position of the femoral graft site, straight-line graft placement, and enough length to accommodate any size patellar tendon graft with a standard 30- to 40-mm long tibial tunnel.
3. The independent drilling of the tunnels lessens the chance for error and avoids the problems caused by one tunnel being less than ideal and affecting the placement of the subsequent tunnel.
4. Patella harvest that occurs after tunnel construction permits variable graft sizing to achieve a snug fit in the respective bone tunnels.
5. Independent inside-out placement of the bone plugs into each tunnel, instead of pulling the graft completely through the knee, allows press fit fixation, which enhances bone plug incorporation.
6. Tight bone plug fit and button fixation allows the surgeon to adjust the tension intraoperatively to ensure postoperative full range of motion and sufficient strength for unlimited rehabilitation.
7. Button fixation avoids prominent, painful hardware and leads to early healing of the bone plugs in the tunnels. It also makes revision reconstruction easy if needed, since redrilling of the bone tunnels is not compromised by hardware.
8. Clinically, button fixation has not failed in more than 2100 ACL reconstructions.

The miniarthrotomy technique with an autogenous patellar tendon graft using suture and button fixation is a

Clinical Table: Two-Incision Procedure

Procedure	Technique	Anatomy	Advantages
Creation of the periosteal flap	• Electrocautery; elevator	• 4 cm distal to joint line; superior to pes anserinus tendon insertion; medial to patellar tendon and tibial tubercle	• Protection from soreness with kneeling
Exposure	• 5-cm medial arthrotomy	• Anterior horn of medial meniscus to the insertion of the vastus medialis	• Superior view overall of intercondylar notch and tibia for tunnel placement without distortion; constant bone tunnel orientation and length, since extra length of tendon graft will go into the femoral tunnel
Notchplasty	• Measure current space from lateral border of PCL to lateral femoral condyle; curette lateral wall of notch to accommodate 10-mm graft	• Intercondylar notch of the femur	• Complete visualization of the entire lateral notch; allows for exact placement of femoral tunnel; new notch size to fit new ligament size; new ligament graft must fit into new notch in full extension
Independent femoral and tibial tunnel placement	• Freehand placement of pen tip in center of desired tunnel	• Place tunnels where anatomy dictates, not through the other tunnel	• Exact placement of tunnels
Harvest of the patellar tendon (immediately before fixation)	• Outline of bone plugs scored with scalpel; osteotome scores proximal and distal ends; oscillating saw	• Central portion of the patellar tendon; consistent 10-mm piece; thickest portion of patella least likely to fracture	• Bone plugs sized to fit tunnels perfectly; theoretical advantage of the short amount of time the graft is away from a natural environment; better graft viability
Graft fixation	• Sutures tied over buttons	• Lateral femur; proximal tibia	• Strong enough to allow rehabilitation as tolerated without fixation failures; complete bone to bone healing within bone tunnels without hardware; flexible fixation; low rate of hardware removal (<1%) and easy revision if necessary
Graft tensioning	• Range the knee from full hyperextension to flexion with the heel of the foot to the buttocks		• Allows bone plugs to position themselves into the bone tunnels; allows for full range of motion without capturing the joint

simple, reproducible technique that has minimal morbidity and offers predictable, excellent results (Clinical Table).

REFERENCES

1. Shelbourne KD, Klootwyk TE, Wilckens JH, et al. Ligament stability two to six years after anterior cruciate ligament reconstruction with autogenous patellar tendon graft and participation in accelerated rehabilitation program. Am J Sports Med 1995;23:575–579

2. Rougraff B, Shelbourne KD, Gerth PK, et al. Arthroscopic and histologic analysis of human patellar tendon autografts used for anterior cruciate ligament reconstruction. Am J Sports Med 1993; 21:277–284.

3. Shelbourne KD, Wilckens JH, Mollabashy A, De Carlo M. Arthrofibrosis in acute anterior cruciate ligament reconstruction: the effect of timing of reconstruction and rehabilitation. Am J Sports Med 1991;19:332–336.

4. Rosenberg TD, Paulos LE, Parker RD, et al: The 45-degree posteroanterior flexion weight-bearing radiograph of the knee. J Bone Joint Surg 1988;70A:1479–1483.

5. Shelbourne KD, Davis TJ, Klootwyk TE. The relationship between intercondylar notch width of the femur and the incidence of anterior cruciate ligament tears. A prospective study. Am J Sports Med 1998;26:402–408.

6. Merchant A: Patellofemoral malalignment and instabilities. In: Ewing JW, ed. Articular cartilage and knee joint function: basic science and arthroscopy. New York: Raven Press, 1990:79–91.

7. Clancy WG Jr, Nelson DA, Reider B, Narechania RG. Anterior cruciate ligament reconstruction using one-third of the patellar ligament, augmented by extra-articular tendon transfers. J Bone Joint Surg 1982;64A:352–359.

8. Howell SM, Clark JA. Tibial tunnel placement in anterior cruciate ligament reconstructions and graft impingement. Clin Orthop 1992; 283:187–195.

chapter 63

George A. Paletta, Jr., and Carl L. Stanitski

Anterior Cruciate Ligament Injury in Patients with Open Physes: Diagnosis and Treatment

Isolated tears of the anterior cruciate ligament (ACL) in skeletally immature individuals were once thought to be rare (1). Such injuries are now being more frequently recognized and reported (2–11). The increasing frequency of diagnosis is the result of increased participation of children in sports, enhanced awareness that children sustain ligamentous injuries of the knee similar to those adults sustain, and increased proficiency in physical diagnosis of such injuries. Recognition of ACL injuries in the skeletally immature patient has highlighted the lack of an effective and reliable management plan to treat these patients. This chapter focuses on treatment alternatives for ACL injuries in individuals with open distal femoral and proximal tibial physes.

The true incidence and prevalence of acute and chronic ACL injuries in the skeletally immature are unknown. Recent studies that have addressed skeletally immature patients have suffered from design flaws, including lack of documentation of skeletal maturity and of specificity of diagnosis. Nevertheless, it is clear that ACL injuries in children are being more frequently diagnosed than they were in the past. Early studies reported tibial eminence avulsion injuries to be much more common than midsubstance ACL ruptures (1,12). More recent reports document significant numbers of skeletally immature individuals who have sustained partial or complete intraligamentous ACL injuries independent of tibial eminence fractures. It is now thought that midsubstance ACL tears occur more frequently than do tibial eminence fractures (2–11). Bony avulsion of the ACL at its femoral insertion is extremely rare. Only one documented case has been reported.

The incidence of acute ACL tears in female athletes, including adolescent girls, has increased fourfold to sixfold. Theoretical explanations for this include generalized ligamentous laxity, morphologic differences in the femoral notch, and differences in the quadriceps:hamstrings strength ratio. The exact cause of the increased frequency of injury in females remains undetermined.

Partial tears of the ACL are common in skeletally immature individuals. Stanitski et al. (13) reviewed arthroscopic findings in 70 children with hemarthrosis. Approximately 45% of the preadolescents (aged 7 to 12 years) had ACL tears, of which 58% were partial tears. A total of 65% of the adolescents (aged 13 to 18) had ACL tears, of which 60% were partial.

A tibial eminence fracture is a special type of injury to the ACL complex. The classification system described by Zaricznyj (14) is based on the morphology and amount of displacement of the fracture fragment (Fig. 63.1).

RELEVANT ANATOMY AND PATHOGENESIS

The tibial attachment of the ACL is just anterior and lateral to the anterior tibial spine. In children, this attachment site is a perichondral epiphyseal cuff, which, with maturity, progresses to the fibrocartilage–bone attachment seen in adults. In addition to the perichondral cuff attachment, there is a slip of ligament that attaches to the lateral meniscus anterior horn. Before closure of the proximal tibial physis, the intercondylar eminence is less resistant to traction forces than is the ligament. This relative strength disparity can explain the purported propensity in

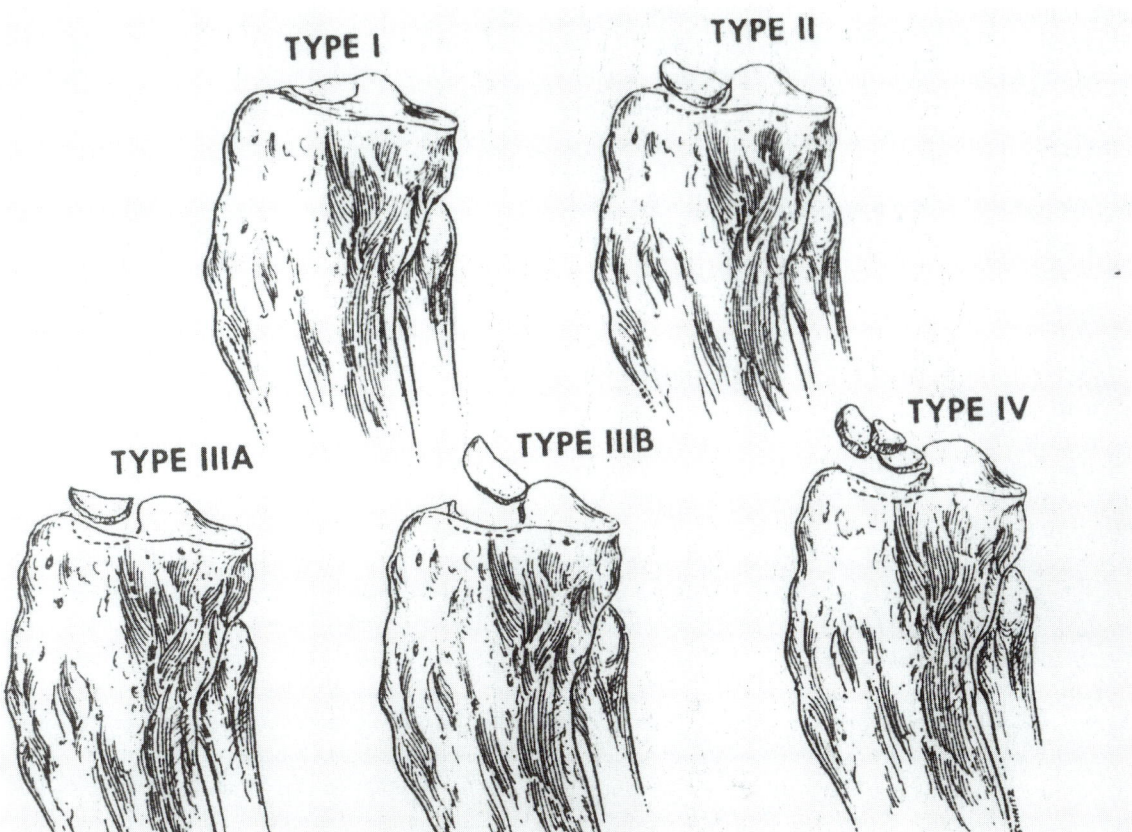

Figure 63.1. Zaricznyj classification of tibial eminence fractures: type I is nondisplaced, type II is hinged with some displacement, type IIIA is completely displaced, type IIIB is completely displaced and rotated, and type IV is displaced and comminuted.

children for tibial eminence avulsions rather than intrasubstance ACL ruptures. Despite this weak link, the ACL does undergo irreversible plastic deformation, elongation, and attenuation before chondroepiphyseal failure.

Juvenile knee ligaments experience the same pathodynamics of disruption as adult ligaments. Skak et al. (12), among others, demonstrated that ligament–bone junction injuries occur with high-energy, slow-loading events, whereas midsubstance ligament injuries occur with low-energy, rapid-loading events.

Natural History

There have been few natural history studies of isolated ACL injury in skeletally immature patients (3–5). Most early reports suffered from a multitude of deficiencies in study design, including small patient numbers, mixed ages and genders, varied athletic demands and treatment protocols, inadequate definition of mechanism of injury and duration of ligament insufficiency, varied evaluation criteria, and poorly defined control groups. The principal deficiencies have been lack of rigid criteria to define skeletal immaturity and lack of diagnostic specificity with respect to primary and associated injuries. It appears that the natural history of ACL deficiency in the skeletally im-

mature patient is similar to that in the adult (5). Thus, to extrapolate from the adult data, children who fail to modify their activities and continue to participate in demanding acceleration-deceleration athletic activity are likely to experience recurrent giving-way episodes with increased risk for meniscal tears and premature degenerative osteoarthritis (4). A number of small short-term follow-up series lend support to this conclusion (4,5).

The natural history of fractures of the tibial eminence is more clearly understood. A displaced tibial eminence fracture that remains unreduced can act as a mechanical block to knee extension; and most patients with eminence fractures demonstrate evidence of some residual ACL laxity in the sagittal plane, as indicated by either Lachman or anterior drawer testing. Baxter and Wiley (15) reviewed 45 patients with a history of tibial eminence avulsion fractures. Fractures that had been partially or completely displaced were associated with ACL laxity. Overall, 51% of patients had clinical and arthrometric evidence of positive Lachman or anterior drawer tests. No patient complained of instability; and none had a positive pivot shift test, which suggests that the secondary restraints were intact.

The fate of the adolescent knee with a partial tear of the ACL is a subject of debate. Buckley et al. (3) reviewed a series of 35 young adults with arthroscopically documented partial ACL tears. All were treated with a program of protected weight-bearing, early range of motion, and strengthening exercises to restore the quadriceps:hamstrings strength ratio. At mean follow-up of 41 months, 86% were minimally symptomatic, and 40% had returned to their preinjury level of performance. Buckley et al. concluded that patients with minimal anterior translation, no rotatory instability, and low demand or performance expectations after partial ACL injury appear to do well at 3 to 4 years after injury.

INITIAL FINDINGS, PHYSICAL EXAMINATION, AND DIAGNOSIS

DeLee and Curtis (1) divided anterior cruciate laxity patients into two groups. The first group is characterized as having nontraumatic anterior cruciate laxity. The second group has posttraumatic anterior cruciate ligament deficiency. This recognition of two groups of patients with anterior cruciate laxity underscores the importance of the initial history and physical examination.

Children with nontraumatic anterior cruciate laxity in the sagittal and rotatory planes usually have generalized nonpathologic ligament laxity or congenital absence of the ACL. Excessive physiologic knee laxity may erroneously suggest ACL insufficiency. Examination of both knees reveals symmetry of laxity. Findings may include positive anterior drawer and Lachman tests and a physiologic pivot shift sign. Pathologic states such as benign hypermobility and Ehlers-Danlos syndrome should be considered.

Congenital absence of the ACL is rare and is usually associated with other congenital anomalies of the involved limb, including congenital knee dislocation, proximal focal femoral deficiency, congenital short femur, fibular hemimelia, and other leg length discrepancies. In cases of congenital absence of the ACL, plain radiographs show tibial intercondylar eminence aplasia and flattening of the intercondylar notch. The association of major limb abnormalities with diminished functional demands usually renders the ACL absence asymptomatic. With current enhanced limb equalization techniques and resultant normalization of function, such previously unstressed knees may become symptomatic.

Studies of children with acute knee injuries show that the best attempts at accurate diagnosis by careful history and thorough physical examination correlate poorly with the correct diagnosis documented by arthroscopy. Nonetheless, the importance of a careful history and physical examination cannot be overemphasized. The history will usually relate a specific injury, the experience of a "pop," and the inability to return to play. Stanitski (10) characterizes the mechanism of injury and its severity based on whether there has been contact and whether there is a deceleration or rotation component to the injury. In general, injuries without an element of contact, deceleration, or rotation are less likely to be associated with an ACL injury. It must be kept in mind that acute patellar in-

stability can also be produced by deceleration-rotation mechanisms. Varus or valgus stress on the knee may suggest collateral ligament, femoral physeal injury, or (less likely) tibial physeal injury. Knee effusion from hemarthrosis occurs rapidly, usually within several hours of acute injury, and heralds major intra-articular injury.

In a chronic ACL-insufficient knee, the patient may complain of recurrent giving-way episodes, particularly with activities that require pivoting on the affected limb. Recurrent effusion with each giving-way episode is common. These episodes result in meniscal tears and produce meniscal symptoms of joint line pain, locking, or catching. It is important to determine the extent of previous knee trauma and the treatment and course of recovery that followed.

Physical examination of the acutely injured knee is difficult because of patient apprehension and limited cooperation. The examination is usually more easily done on patients with chronic ACL insufficiency. Examination of the whole extremity, especially the hip, and the unaffected limb is essential. Knee pain in the skeletally immature patient is assumed to be hip pain until proven otherwise. The presence of an effusion should be noted, and range of active and passive motion documented. The presence of any tenderness at the collateral ligaments, joint line, and femoral and tibial physes should be recorded. The patellofemoral joint, including the patellar retinaculum at the peripatellar area, and the quadriceps–adductor junction are examined to rule out an acute patella dislocation, which can present as a history similar to acute ACL rupture.

Physiologic laxity, which may be significant in children, must be assessed in all planes. The motion and laxity of the opposite knee are used as a baseline for comparison if there has not been previous injury to that knee. Translational tests, such as the anterior drawer and Lachman, are usually positive in the ACL-deficient knee. Both the magnitude of translation and the quality of the end point are considered. Children with physiologic laxity may have abnormal anterior translation but a distinct, firm end point. In the acute setting, rotation tests (e.g., pivot shift) are often difficult to perform because of muscle spasm and pain. The pivot shift sign is usually easily detected in the chronic ACL-insufficient knee. Use of instrumented arthrometers may provide baseline sagittal plane laxity information and side-to-side comparison, but age-adjusted normal values are not available. Limb length and girth constraints may invalidate arthrometer testing in small-stature patients.

RADIOLOGIC STUDIES

Imaging evaluation of the knee should include a routine radiographic four-view series: AP, lateral, tunnel, and skyline views. In the acute injury setting, routine radiographs are assessed for presence of fracture, including tibial eminence avulsion. Comparison and stress views may be required if a tibial or femoral physeal fracture is suspected.

Stress radiographs can be used to distinguish physeal separation from ligament disruption (11). Malformation of the tibial spine and/or femoral notch suggests congenital absence of the ACL. The extent of physeal closure can also be assessed on routine radiographs. CT or MRI can be used to assess the degree of epiphyseal closure if skeletal maturity is in question.

MRI can provide valuable information about the location of the ACL tear, presence of associated meniscal or bony injury, and status of maturity of the femoral and tibial epiphyses. Visualization of the ACL with MRI can be difficult and depends on proper patient positioning and specificity, and thickness of the individual imaging slices. A common MRI finding associated with acute ACL tears is the so-called bone bruise. These occult bony lesions most commonly involve the subchondral bone of the lateral femoral condyle and/or lateral tibial plateau and occur in the majority of patients with acute ACL injury. The clinical significance and long-term sequelae of these lesions are unknown because most resolve spontaneously within 6 to 8 months. This subchondral injury may cause pain in the lateral compartment, which suggests the erroneous clinical diagnosis of a lateral meniscal tear. Although MRI may suggest associated meniscal injury, it usually cannot accurately determine meniscal lesion size and stability.

MRI has had a significant affect on knee injury diagnosis, but false-positive and false-negative studies are not uncommon, especially when the clinician is inexperienced with pediatric musculoskeletal MRI assessment. The history and physical examination findings must be correlated with the MRI studies. MRI cannot substitute for a complete history and physical examination.

TREATMENT

Tibial Eminence Avulsion

Treatment of tibial eminence avulsion injuries depends on the displacement of the fracture. Type I and II injuries are treated with closed reduction and immobilization with the knee in extension for 4 to 6 weeks. Closed reduction is best achieved by maximally extending the knee; as the final 5° to 10° of extension are reached, the femoral condyles impinge on the fragment and reduce it. Type II fractures that cannot be anatomically reduced by closed means and type IIIA, IIIB, and IV fractures are treated with open reduction and internal fixation (ORIF), which can usually be done arthroscopically through standard portals. The fracture is reduced anatomically and fixed with sutures, pins, or screws (Fig. 63.2). Regardless of the type, the fixation should be confined to the proximal tibial epiphysis and not violate the tibial physeal plate. Postoperative rehabilitation is similar to that outlined below for intrasubstance ACL reconstruction; but the time to full activity participation is usually shorter, because of rapid osseous union.

Intrasubstance ACL Injuries

Treatment of intrasubstance ACL injuries in the child and young adolescent remains controversial. No consensus has been reached because of the paucity of accurate, objective data of sufficient follow-up length. An ACL injury is not a surgical emergency. An accurate initial diagnosis is imperative so that proper treatment can be outlined to produce a predictable outcome. With a combination of

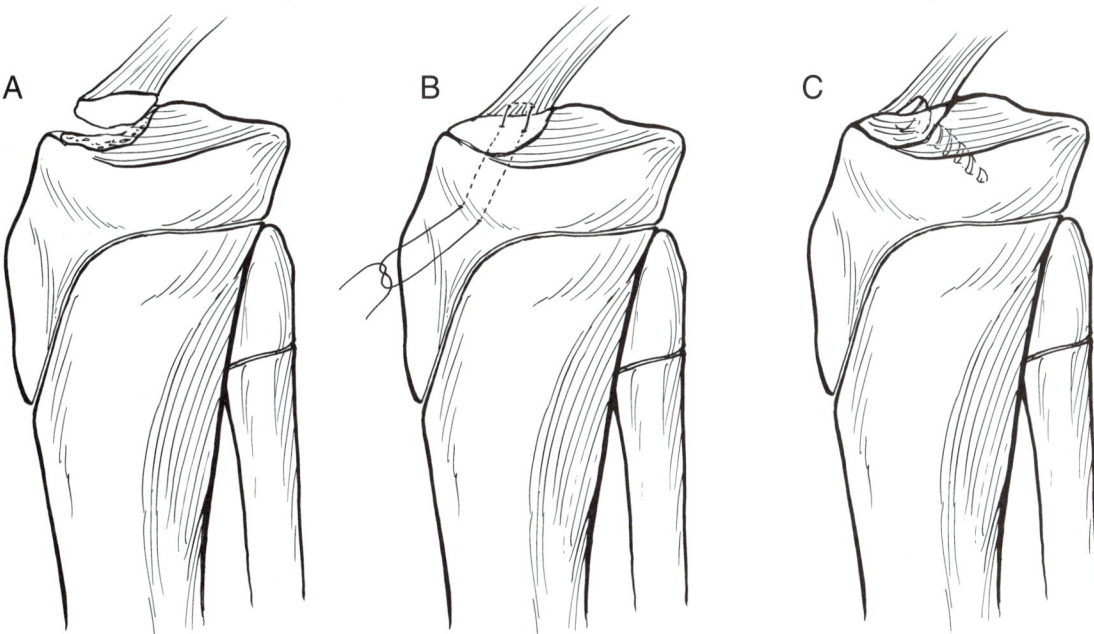

Figure 63.2. Repair of a type III tibial eminence avulsion fracture (**A**) with suture fixation (**B**) and screw fixation (**C**).

data from the history, physical examination, and imaging studies, an informed decision can usually be made. If the diagnosis is in doubt, arthroscopy may be necessary. Once a specific diagnosis is made, a specific treatment program can be determined. Patients and their families must understand that rehabilitation, no matter what the treatment, requires time and effort. The treatment plan must take into consideration assessment of the patient's physical maturity; the level of functional instability; and the vocational and avocational demands on the knee, which may not be clear for the adolescent.

ASSESSMENT OF MATURITY

Assessment of skeletal maturity has important implications for potential treatment. The adolescent nearing physeal closure with limited skeletal growth remaining differs markedly from the prepubescent juvenile with wide-open physes and significant remaining skeletal growth. Physical maturity is a dynamic process. The path of skeletal growth toward physeal closure is individual and varies in time of onset, duration, rate, and magnitude. Maturity is evaluated on chronologic, physiologic, and radiologic bases.

Tanner and Davies (16) reported on normal growth curves in North American children. They noted that the adolescent growth spurt begins, on average, at age 10.5 in girls and 12.5 in boys. Peak height velocity was reported to occur at age 11.5 in girls and 13.5 in boys. Cessation of changes in shoe size is a useful indicator of growth deceleration, since feet reach approximately 95% of their adult size by age 12.5 in girls and 14 in boys. Menarche is an excellent predictor of growth deceleration. Onset of menses is preceded by the period of peak height velocity, with rapid diminution of growth rate following menarche. Physical maturity can be assessed via the Tanner grading scale of development based on secondary sexual characteristics. Development of pigmented pubic and axillary hair in boys is approximately equivalent physiologically to the onset of menarche in girls.

Because of the wide range of normal values the use of imaging techniques to establish maturity suffers from potential inaccuracies. This is especially true for bone age determination because the standards are based on measures made almost 50 years ago on a fairly uniform population. It is unknown whether those standards hold true for today's multicultural American society.

FUNCTIONAL INSTABILITY

Functional instability is defined as repeated giving-way episodes with activities of daily living and/or sports participation. Functional instability does not imply functional limitation, as these children may continue to participate fully in athletics. Children with complete ACL insufficiency typically fall into one of two groups based on the significance of their functional instability. Members of the first group demonstrate no functional instability and are able to carry out activities of daily living and participate in sports without giving-way episodes. Children in the second group have varying degrees of instability with such activities.

Although classification of functional instability is important when formulating a treatment plan, it is impossible at the time of the initial acute injury to accurately predict which child will have such instability. In an effort to determine the level of functional instability, a trial of nonoperative treatment may be warranted in the prepubescent child with an acute ACL injury. It is essential to inform the patient and parents that each giving-way episode puts the menisci and articular cartilage at risk for injury. In the prepubescent child with chronic ACL insufficiency and functional instability, treatment should be instituted to limit the risk of damage to the menisci and articular cartilage. In the postpubescent adolescent with limited skeletal growth remaining, determination of functional instability is less crucial to formulating a treatment plan, because the treatment options are less constrained. Such children can essentially be treated as adults.

Nonoperative Treatment and Indications for Surgery

As detailed above, the natural history of the unreconstructed isolated ACL-deficient knee in children is one of recurrent episodes of instability and development of meniscal tears (3–5). Such a history should not, however, serve as condemnation of nonoperative treatment of ACL insufficiency in the skeletally immature patient. A trial of nonoperative treatment is indicated in children with isolated acute ACL injuries who are determined to be truly skeletally immature with significant growth remaining. Such children include boys and premenarcheal girls of Tanner stages 1 and 2. Nonoperative treatment is indicated in individuals who have contraindications to or refuse consideration of surgery. The goal of nonoperative treatment of ACL insufficiency is to prevent recurrent episodes of giving way, with their sequelae of meniscal injury, intra-articular damage, and premature degenerative arthritis.

Nonoperative management of acute ACL tears consists of a three-phase program. Phase 1 includes early crutch-protected walking with progressive weight bearing as tolerated; early, active-assisted and passive range of motion exercises; and use of a knee immobilizer for comfort. The emphasis of this phase is on regaining full, pain-free knee motion. Phase 1 usually lasts 7 to 10 days. During this phase the patient and parents are counseled about the treatment options, including the need for activity modification and reduction or elimination of sports that place high demands on ACL function. Progression to phase 2 occurs when the goal of full, pain-free knee motion has been achieved.

Phase 2 is an objectively monitored and documented rehabilitation effort to restore normal muscle balance to the lower extremity. Emphasis is on regaining and maintaining quadriceps strength and on normalizing the quadriceps:hamstrings strength ratio. This phase usually lasts up to 6 weeks.

Phase 3 is a graduated return to functional activities and continued maintenance rehabilitation. Return to low- and moderate-demand sports is allowed when lower-extremity strength approaches that of the uninjured side. Progression to more high-demand sports and competitive levels of participation is allowed as the patient demonstrates no functional instability at lower levels of activity.

The role of functional braces to control instability following ACL injury is still debated. There is no unanimity of opinion on the timing or use of these devices. The mechanism of brace efficacy is unknown. Improved proprioceptive feedback while wearing an orthotic device has been suggested. Proper fit of a functional brace is often difficult in children because of their relatively small leg length and girth. Customized braces may be required, but the high cost may make their use prohibitive. Use of a functional brace in conjunction with a comprehensive rehabilitation program may allow temporization until the patient reaches skeletal maturity. If functional instability remains, a surgical reconstruction is considered. Understanding that no current consensus for their use exists in adults or children, we recommend functional bracing during sports participation.

Surgery is indicated for any patient who demonstrates functional instability with activities of daily living or who refuses to comply with activity modification to prevent recurrent giving-way episodes. Surgical reconstruction of the ACL is also indicated for patients who are near skeletal maturity and who have associated knee injuries that require surgical treatment, especially meniscal tears. For patients who are physically immature and have associated meniscal injury, arthroscopy allows accurate assessment of intra-articular pathology, especially meniscal stability and tear location and size. All reasonable attempts should be made to preserve the menisci if the tear pattern is amenable to repair. If the menisci are repairable, we recommend surgical stabilization of the knee.

The surgical procedure of choice is determined by the physical maturity of the patient (Clinical Table). We currently recommend physis-sparing procedures for Tanner stage 1 patients who fail nonoperative treatment and have persistent functional instability with activities of daily living. Reconstruction with partial (tibia only) transphyseal technique is used for Tanner stage 2 patients who fail nonoperative treatment and have persistent functional instability with activities of daily living. Complete transphyseal reconstructions are done for patients who are approaching skeletal maturity (Tanner stage 3 adolescents, postmenarcheal girls, boys who demonstrate pigmented axillary and

Clinical Table: ACL Injury in Patients with Open Physes

Procedure	Indications	Technique	Graft Tissue	Fixation	Pitfalls
Tibial eminence avulsion repair	• Type II fractures if not anatomic: closed reduction; all types III and IV fractures	• Arthroscopic		• Epiphyseal suture or screw; do not violate the tibial physis	• Physeal plate violation; nonanatomic reduction with resultant extension block; residual ACL laxity; arthrofibrosis
Nontransphyseal reconstruction	• Tanner stage 1 with persistent functional instability or associated meniscal injury	• Arthroscopic assisted: two incisions, over the front of the tibia; over the top of the femur	• Autograft patella tendon; autograft hamstrings; graft tissue remains attached to proximal tibial insertion (i.e., tibial tubercle or pes anserinus)	• Tibia graft remains attached; femur suture to periosteum; screw and washer sutures tied to post	• Nonanatomic, non-isometric; femoral physeal injury; questions about the effect of continued skeletal growth on neoligament and on adequate graft size
Partial transphyseal reconstruction (tibia only)	• Tanner stage 2 with persistent functional instability or associated meniscal injury	• Arthroscopic assisted: two incisions; central tibial drill hole; over the top of the femur	• Autograft hamstrings; may be harvested as free grafts or left attached to the pes anserinus at proximal tibia	• Tibia graft remains attached; if detached fix with staple or sutures tied to post; femur suture to periosteum; screw and washer sutures tied to post	• Nonanatomic, nonisometric (but better than nontransphyseal); femoral physeal injury; questions about the effect of continued skeletal growth on neoligament and adequate graft size
Complete transphyseal reconstruction	• Postmenarcheal girls or Tanner stage 3–4 boys with persistent functional instability or associated meniscal injury	• Arthroscopic assisted; two incisions or endoscopic	• Autograft bone-patella tendon-bone; autograft hamstrings; harvested as free grafts	• Tibia interference screw; sutures tied to post; staple; femur interference screw; extracortical button	• Questions about the need for hardware removal

pubic hair and who have had no significant change in shoe size for 6 months). Patients at any Tanner stage who have associated meniscal pathology with the ACL tear undergo surgical treatment for both lesions. Meniscal treatment depends on tear morphology, location, and stability.

Operative Treatment

Many surgeons have been reluctant to attempt intra-articular isometric ACL reconstruction (such as is achieved in adults using a bone-patella tendon-bone graft) in skeletally immature patients because of possible growth retardation and angular deformity associated with violation of the tibial and femoral physes. Guzzanti et al. (17) presented experimental data on the effects of intra-articular ACL reconstruction on physeal growth in a rabbit model. They used a semitendinosus tendon placed through 2-mm tibial and femoral tunnels in skeletally immature rabbits. Histologic examination of a physeal specimen 6 months after the operation showed no epiphysiodesis. The mean area of involvement of the femoral physis was 11% in the frontal plane and 3% in cross section, but there was no alteration in longitudinal growth or axial deviation. On the tibial side, the mean area of physeal involvement was 12% in the frontal plane and 4% in cross section. Two tibiae developed varus angulation, and one was shortened.

Stadelmaier et al. (18) examined the effects of transphyseal drilling on physeal growth in a dog model. In their study, they used a fascia lata graft for ACL reconstruction that was placed across transphyseal tibial and femoral bone tunnels. Histologic and radiographic follow-up demonstrated no evidence of bony bridge formation, physeal arrest, longitudinal growth disturbance, and angular deformity. The dogs' quadruped posture may have affected these results.

Unfortunately, initial clinical results from recent small series of patients with limited follow-up do not clarify the treatment of choice in the truly skeletally immature individual with ACL insufficiency (6–9). Surgical options remain restricted in such patients because of concern about physeal violation. The threshold ratio of physeal area:graft tunnel size that is safe is currently unknown.

A number of surgical procedures have been attempted to stabilize the skeletally immature ACL-deficient knee. Operative management options include primary repair, intra-articular reconstruction, intra-articular plus extra-articular procedures, and extra-articular reconstruction. Of these options, primary repair of a midsubstance rupture and isolated extra-articular reconstruction are not recommended. Both primary repair of intrasubstance tears and extra-articular reconstructions have resulted in poor long-term functional stability (19). One exception is for bony avulsion injuries with a large bone fragment, which may undergo primary repair.

Intra-articular reconstructions include physis-sparing and partial or complete transphyseal procedures. The choice of graft tissue is determined in part by the reconstructive procedure itself. The principal choices include bone-patellar tendon-bone autograft, hamstrings (semitendinosus/gracilis) autograft, and allograft (2). Because of concerns of pathologic viral transmission, we do not recommend the use of allograft tissue for routine cases; fur-

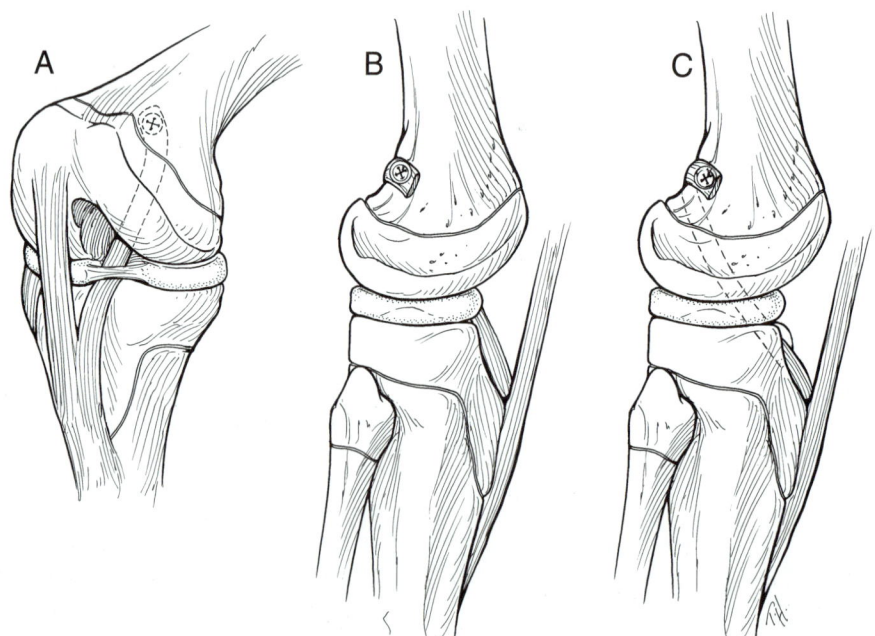

Figure 63.3. A. Oblique view of a nontransphyseal ACL reconstruction using a patellar tendon autograft that is left attached to the tibial tubercle. Here, the graft passes underneath transverse meniscal ligament. **B.** Lateral view showing a graft that passes in the over-the-front position on the tibia. **C.** A modification in which a groove is created in the proximal tibial epiphysis above the level of the physis. The graft passes through the groove to closely approximate the anatomic tibial insertion site of the ACL.

thermore, we do not recommend synthetic grafts and ligament augmentation devices (LAD) for pediatric knee reconstruction, as their use remains controversial.

Several questions concerning surgical reconstruction remain unanswered. The ability of uniplanar transplanted tissue to act in the same manner as the normal ACL, with its multifunctional bundle orientation, has not been fully determined. Long-term follow-up may be able to reveal the knee's tolerance of the lack of isometry caused by various reconstruction procedures. The effects of youth and diminished graft size on the maturation rate of the transferred neoligament are unclear. A 6- or 7-mm graft may be appropriate and proportional for the patient's size at the time of the reconstruction; as the patient matures, however, it is unknown whether the intra-articular segment of the graft will assume the size and mechanical properties of an adult ACL and be able to withstand long-term vocational and avocational demands.

NONTRANSPHYSEAL RECONSTRUCTION

Nontransphyseal, or physeal-sparing, reconstruction can be accomplished using an arthroscopic-assisted technique with autograft tendon augmentation. Autograft patella tendon or hamstrings may be selected as graft tissue (Fig. 63.3 and 63.4). After standard arthroscopic preparation of the intercondylar notch, including notchplasty if necessary, an anteromedial incision is used to harvest the selected autograft tissue and provide access to the anterior tibial epiphysis. The graft tissue may be left attached

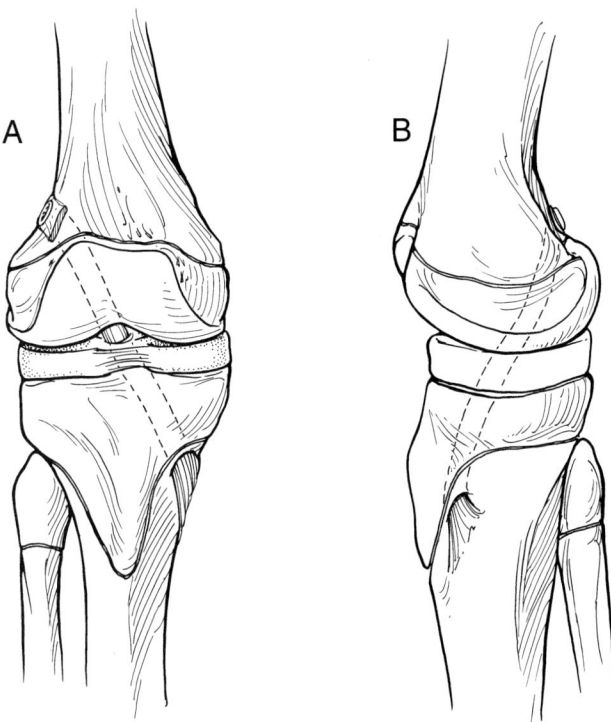

Figure 63.5. A partial transphyseal ACL reconstruction using autograft hamstring tendons, which may be left attached to the pes anserinus at the proximal tibia (as shown) or harvested as a free graft. Note the central tibial drill hole and the over-the-top femoral position.

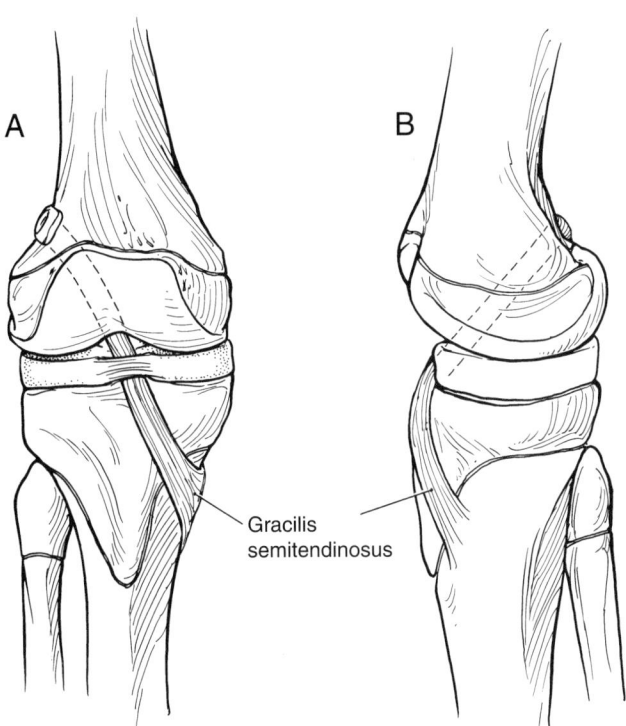

Figure 63.4. A nontransphyseal ACL reconstruction using a hamstring tendon autograft that is left attached to the pes anserinus at the proximal tibia. Note the over-the-front and over-the-top positions of the graft.

Gracilis
semitendinosus

to the proximal tibia (tibial tubercle for patella tendon; pes anserinus for hamstrings). A second incision is made at the lateral femur at the level of the metaphyseal flair. The graft is passed in continuity over the front of the tibia, beneath the transverse meniscal ligament, through the intercondylar notch, and over the top of the femur. This eliminates physeal violations.

A trough can be created in the anterior tibial and posterior lateral femoral epiphyses in an effort to more closely approximate the anatomic insertion sites of the ACL (Fig. 63.3C). The graft can be fixed to the lateral femur by directly suturing to the periosteum, using a screw and washer, using a staple, or tying a suture around a screw post. Disadvantages of these physis-sparing procedures include the creation of a nonanatomic, nonisometric graft position and the risk of femoral physeal injury. Furthermore, as noted earlier, the effect of continued skeletal growth on the biologic maturation of the neoligament and the adequacy of the graft size are unknown.

PARTIAL TRANSPHYSEAL RECONSTRUCTION

Partial transphyseal reconstruction is accomplished using an arthroscopic-assisted technique with autograft or allograft tendon augmentation. Autograft hamstring tendon is the preferred graft tissue. Autograft patella tendon is typically not used as a graft because violation of the tibial tubercle in the skeletally immature patient may lead to genu recurvatum. Allograft tissue should be reserved for cases with a contraindication to autograft tissue use.

After standard arthroscopic preparation of the inter-condylar notch, including notchplasty if necessary, an an-teromedial incision is used to harvest the selected auto-graft tissue and provide access to the anterior tibial metaphysis. Autograft hamstring graft tissue may be left attached to the pes anserinus at the proximal tibia or har-vested as a free graft. The graft should be prepared using large nonabsorbable suture at the free ends.

In partial transphyseal reconstructions, the tendon graft is passed through a drill hole in the center of the tibial ph-ysis and placed in an over-the-top femoral position. A 6- to 8-mm tunnel, depending on the size of the graft tissue, is drilled in the tibia. A second incision is made at the lateral femur at the level of the metaphyseal flair. The graft is passed through the tibial drill hole and intercondylar notch to the over-the-top position of the femur, which eliminates eccentric violation of the femoral physis (Fig. 63.5). A trough can be created in the posterior lateral femoral epiphysis to place the graft in a more isometric position. The graft can be fixed to the lateral femur by su-turing directly to the periosteum, using a screw and washer, or tying the suture around a screw post. If the graft is harvested as free tissue, fixation to the tibia can be ac-complished using staples or sutures tied to a screw post. Disadvantages of the partial transphyseal procedure are similar to those listed for the nontransphyseal technique.

COMPLETE TRANSPHYSEAL RECONSTRUCTION

Complete transphyseal reconstructions require place-ment of graft tissue through tibial and femoral bone tun-nels and can be performed using an arthroscopic-assisted technique with autograft or allograft tendon augmentation (Fig. 63.6). Autograft patella tendon or hamstrings may be selected as graft tissue. Allograft tissue should be re-served for cases with a contraindication to autograft tissue.

After standard arthroscopic preparation of the inter-condylar notch, including notchplasty if necessary, an an-teromedial incision is used to harvest the selected tissue as a free graft and provide access to the anteromedial tib-ial metaphysis. The graft should be prepared using large, nonabsorbable suture at both ends. Hamstring tendons may be doubled or even quadrupled. Depending on the size of the graft tissue, an 8- to 10-mm tibial bone tunnel is drilled. A matched-size femoral drill hole is made using an

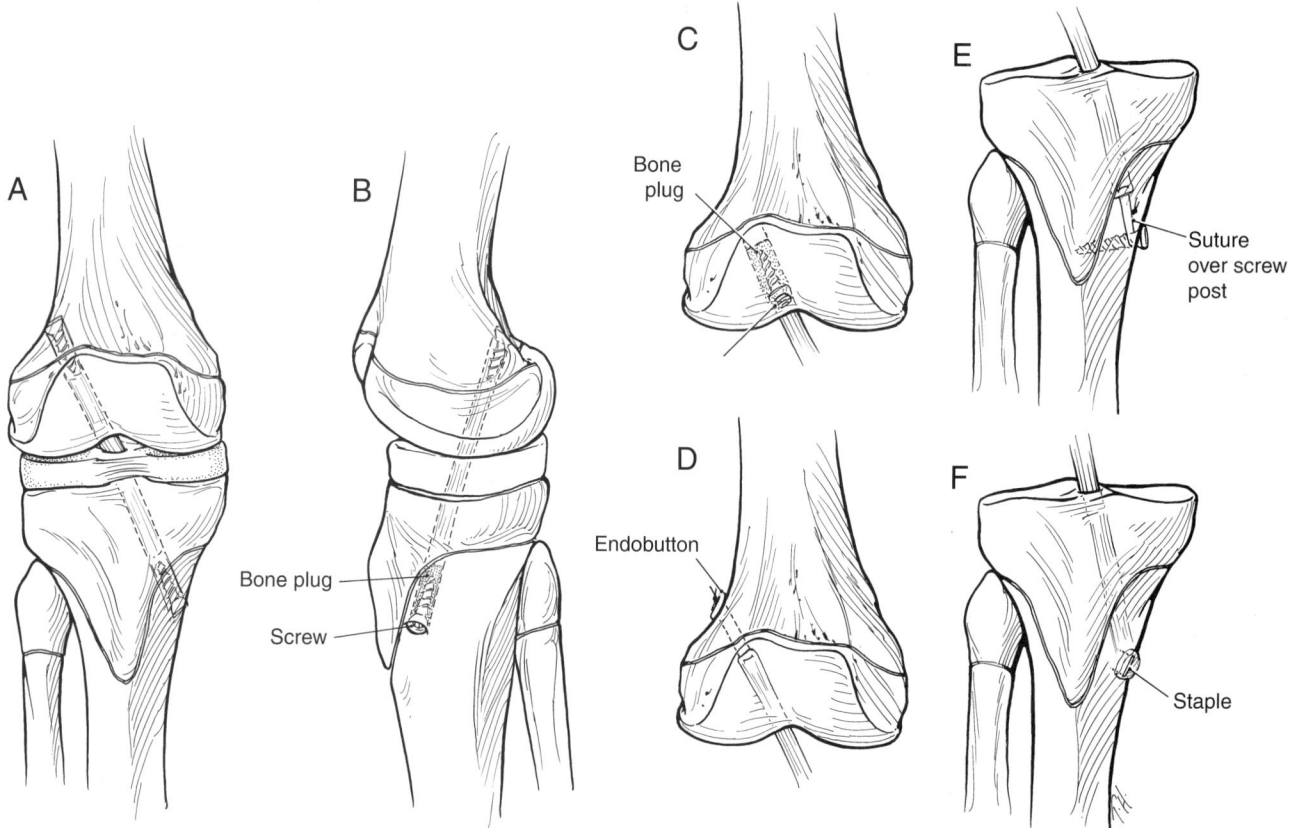

Figure 63.6. A and **B.** In a complete transphyseal ACL reconstruc-tion, the autograft patella tendon is placed through the tibial and femoral tunnels with interference screw fixation. The femoral screw is placed from outside in, using the two-incision technique. Alternative femoral fixations include the use of an endoscopic inter-ference screw (**C**) and the use of an endoscopic technique and an ex-tracortical fixation device (Endobutton), which may be used with a patella tendon or hamstrings graft (**D**). Alternative tibial fixations in-clude the use of sutures tied around a screw post, which may be used with a patella tendon or hamstrings graft (**E**), and the use of a staple for a hamstrings tendon graft (**F**).

endoscopic technique or an outside-in technique, which requires a second incision at the lateral femur (as described above). The tibial and femoral drill holes should be placed in the anatomic positions to optimize graft isometricity. The graft is passed through the tibial tunnel, intercondylar notch, and femoral tunnel.

Fixation at the femur can be accomplished using an interference screw placed either endoscopically or from outside-in. Newer femoral fixation techniques include extracortical devices, such as the Endobutton (Acufex, Boston, MA), which eliminates the risk of transecting the graft when placing an interference screw. Fixation at the tibia is best accomplished using an interference screw. Staples or sutures tied to a screw post can also be used.

The complete transphyseal reconstruction allows for anatomic, isometric placement of the graft. Disadvantages include the technical demands of the procedure (especially femoral tunnel placement), the risk of pain at the tibial screw site, and the risk of partial or complete transection of the graft with endoscopic interference screw placement.

Rehabilitation

Current rehabilitation programs after ACL reconstruction incorporate the biologic principle of progressive, physiologically tolerable stress by allowing early motion, weight bearing, and muscle strengthening to prevent the sequelae of disuse, misuse, and abuse. Emphasis on regaining strength and endurance of the entire lower extremity through isometric, isotonic, and closed- and open-chain isokinetic exercises (both concentric and eccentric) contributes to rapid rehabilitation. The program should be customized to accommodate the patient's size and the availability of rehabilitation equipment.

The graduated rehabilitation program places early emphasis on regaining full knee motion and quadriceps control. Early strengthening emphasizes co-contraction of the hamstrings and quadriceps and limited arcs of motion by avoiding active-resisted knee extension beyond $-30°$. Progression of the rehabilitation program with gradual return to full activity is allowed only as full motion is achieved and restoration of the normal quadriceps:hamstrings strength ratio occurs. The preparticipation phase incorporates sport-specific tasks performed at full speed, followed by the return to full sports participation.

Complications

Complications of ACL reconstruction in children are similar to those in adults: motion loss (especially extension), arthrofibrosis, infrapatellar fat pad contractures, anterior knee pain, infection, and graft harvest site morbidity. Complications unique to the skeletally immature patient are potential limb length inequality and angular and rotational deformities. The prevalence of these complications is unknown because few truly skeletally immature patients have undergone long-term follow-up.

SUMMARY

ACL injury in children is being recognized with greater frequency because of improved diagnostic techniques and heightened awareness of the condition. Unfortunately, the diagnosis is still missed because the attitude persists that children do not suffer ligament injuries. Hemarthrosis must be considered an indication of a significant intra-articular injury. Since the late 1980s, ACL reconstruction has developed into a reproducible technique with low morbidity. Aggressive rehabilitation programs allow accelerated return to activity while allowing the biology of graft maturation to progress.

The basic principle of diagnosis and the treatment goals in the skeletally immature patient are the same as those in the adult patient. The diagnostic approach to ACL injury in children must, however, also include evaluation of skeletal maturity, since it plays a major role in treatment decisions. Maturity is evaluated on the basis of chronologic age; various physiologic factors, such as family height, patient's projected height, and estimation of sexual development; and radiographic findings in the knee, pelvis (Risser's sign), or hand and wrist (bone-age study). Because of the special characteristics of the skeletally immature patient, the orthopaedic surgeon must act as a knee counselor by attempting to identify at-risk patients, particularly those who engage in activities that abuse their knees.

The nonoperative treatment principles are the same as those for adult patients. Consideration of surgical treatment must take into account assessment of skeletal maturity. If questions remain about the status of the femoral and tibial physes, polytomography or MRI is used to assess the extent of physeal closure. The more skeletally mature the patient, the fewer reservations the surgeon should have about performing a transphyseal reconstruction.

REFERENCES

1. DeLee JC, Curti, R. Anterior cruciate ligament insufficiency in children. Clin Orthop 1983;172:112–118.
2. Andrews M, Noyes FR, Barber-Westin SD. Anterior cruciate ligament allograft reconstruction in the skeletally immature athlete. Am J Sports Med 1994;22:48–54.
3. Buckley SL, Barrack RL, Alexander AH, et al. The natural history of conservatively treated anterior cruciate ligament tears. Am J Sports Med 1989;17:221–225.
4. Graf BK, Lange RH, Fujisak CK, et al. Anterior cruciate ligament tears in skeletally immature patients: meniscal pathology at the time of presentation and after attempted conservative treatment. Arthroscopy 1992;8:229–233.
5. Kannus P, Jarvinen M. Knee ligament injuries in adolescents. Eight year follow-up of conservative treatment. J Bone Joint Surg 1988;70B:772–776.
6. Lipscomb AB, Anderson AF. Tears of the anterior cruciate ligament in adolescents. J Bone Joint Surg 1986;68A:19–28.
7. McCarroll JR, Shelbourne KD, Porter DA, et al. Patella tendon graft reconstruction for midsubstance anterior cruciate ligament rupture in junior high school athletes: an algorithm for management. Am J Sports Med 1994;22:478–484.

8. McCarroll JR, Rettig AC, Shelbourne KD. Anterior cruciate ligament injuries in the young athlete with open physes. Am J Sports Med 1988;16:44–47.

9. Parker AW, Drez D Jr, Cooper JL. Anterior cruciate ligament injuries in patients with open physes. Am J Sports Med 1994; 22:44–47.

10. Stanitski CL. Anterior cruciate ligament injury in the skeletally immature patient: diagnosis and treatment. J Am Acad Orthop Surg 1995;3:146–158.

11. Sullivan JA. Ligamentous injuries of the knee in children. Clin Orthop 1990;255:44–50.

12. Skak SV, Jensen TT, Poulsen TD, et al. Epidemiology of knee injuries in children. Acta Orthop Scand 1987;58:78–81.

13. Stanitski CL, Harvell JC, Fu FH. Observations on acute hemarthrosis in children and adolescents. J Pediatr Orthop 1993; 3:506–510.

14. Zaricznyj B. Avulsion fracture of the tibial eminence: treatment by open reduction and pinning. J Bone Joint Surg 1977;59A:1111–1114.

15. Baxter MP, Wiley JJ. Fractures of the tibial spine in children: an evaluation of knee stability. J Bone Joint Surg 1988;70B:228–230.

16. Tanner JM, Davies PS. Clinical longitudinal standards for height and weight velocity for American children. J Pediatr 1985; 107:317–329.

17. Guzzanti V, Falciglia F, Gigante A, et al. The effect of intra-articular ACL reconstruction on the growth plates of rabbits. J Bone Joint Surg 1994;76B:960–63.

18. Stadelmaier DM, Arnoczky SP, Dodds J, et al. The effect of drilling and soft tissue grafting across open growth plates. a histologic study. Am J Sports Med 1995;23:431–435.

19. Engebretsen L, Svenninginsen S, Benum P. Poor results of anterior cruciate ligament repair in adolescents. Acta Orthop Scand 1988; 59:684–686.

chapter 64

Marc H. Rubman and Frank R. Noyes

Varus Angulation with Chronic Ligament Deficiency: The Role of High Tibial Osteotomy

Younger patients with varus angulation and unicompartmental arthrosis secondary to meniscectomy, articular fracture, joint instability, or injury pose a difficult challenge to orthopaedic surgeons. These patients wish to remain active and, because of their age, are not candidates for total knee arthroplasty. Anterior cruciate ligament (ACL) insufficiency and associated deficiency of the lateral and posterolateral ligamentous structures add another level of complexity to the varus-angulated knees. Patients who have such combined abnormalities often experience pain, swelling, giving way, and functional limitations that are disabling. In symptomatic knees, many questions arise concerning treatment recommendations and the role of high tibial osteotomy (HTO).

Valgus-producing osteotomy of the tibia is indicated when medial tibiofemoral arthrosis and associated pain lead to functional limitations. HTO must restore a valgus alignment to the lower extremity and redistribute the tibial plateau forces toward the lateral compartment of the knee to provide a satisfactory clinical result (1). If narrowing and obliquity of the medial tibiofemoral joint have progressed far enough to prevent closure of the lateral tibiofemoral joint, HTO is contraindicated (2).

RELEVANT ANATOMY AND PATHOGENESIS

The degree of medial joint line pain does not necessarily correlate with the extent of medial compartment arthrosis (3). In the early stages of medial compartment arthrosis, patients usually complain of medial pain with sports activity but rarely with activities of daily living (ADLs). When pain occurs with ADLs, there is a strong probability that extensive articular cartilage damage with exposed subchondral bone exists. Previous loss of medial meniscus function is a major risk factor for arthritic progression of the medial compartment (4,5). It is possible that preoperative medial joint line pain will remain after HTO and ACL reconstruction, particularly for patients who engage in athletic activities.

We have identified two distinct groups of young, athletically active patients for whom the goals of osteotomy differ (6). Symptoms and the articular surface damage present on arthroscopic examination differentiate the groups. The first group of patients has significant medial tibiofemoral arthrosis and moderate to severe symptoms of pain and swelling with ADLs. The goal of osteotomy for group 1 patients is to diminish their symptoms, not to return them to athletics. Patients of group 2 do not have advanced arthrosis. Their symptoms occur with activity and are of recent onset. The majority of these patients have an ACL deficiency with varus alignment, and ligament reconstruction is often necessary. Data are not available, however, to determine whether returning group 2 patients to their previous sports activity levels will accelerate arthritic progression. Large in vivo loading occurs with athletics, and patients are advised to use common sense and avoid activities that cause pain and swelling. An osteotomy allows an active lifestyle in the short term, but in the long term, such activities may not be possible (6).

To devise a rational treatment program, the clinician must first correctly diagnose all abnormalities of the knee joint. We defined the terms *primary*, *double*, and *triple varus knee* to simplify the task of logically assessing abnormal alignment and ligamentous deficiencies (7). A primary varus knee refers to the tibiofemoral osseous alignment, including increased varus alignment resulting from loss of the medial meniscus and medial tibiofemoral articular cartilage.

As the overall tibiofemoral weight-bearing line (WBL) shifts into the medial compartment, greater medial compressive loads are expected. Eventually, the lateral tibiofemoral joint will tend to separate during standing and walking activities. As a result, excessive tensile forces develop in the lateral ligaments, iliotibial tract, and other lateral soft tissue structures. This tensile stress can lengthen the lateral tissues, leading to lateral condylar liftoff (the separation of the lateral tibiofemoral joint) with activity. This condition is termed the double varus knee because lower-limb varus alignment is the result of two factors: tibiofemoral osseous alignment and abnormal separation of the lateral tibiofemoral compartment (because of insufficiency of the lateral ligamentous structures).

The active and passive structures on the lateral side that resist lateral joint line opening include the iliotibial tract, biceps femoris, gastrocnemius, and quadriceps muscles. In some circumstances, however, they may not be able to restrain lateral joint line opening. This condition results in excessive tensile forces in passive ligamentous structures, with added injury to the posterolateral structures (popliteus and arcuate complex, in addition to the lateral collateral ligament). A varus recurvatum position of the limb may then occur (8). This is termed a triple varus knee because the varus alignment is the result of three factors: tibiofemoral osseous and geometric alignment, lateral tibiofemoral compartment separation because of lateral collateral ligament (LCL) damage, and added varus angulation because of a varus recurvatum position (increased hyperextension and external tibial rotation). There is involvement of the entire posterolateral ligament complex and usually ACL rupture. The decision-making process for treatment must consider the associated ligamentous injuries in addition to the osseous varus alignment.

INITIAL FINDINGS, PHYSICAL EXAMINATION, AND DIAGNOSIS

Subjective symptoms of pain, swelling, and recurrent giving way with activity are well-known sequelae of the chronic ACL-deficient knee (9,10). What is unique to the varus-angulated, ACL-deficient knee is that there may be two or three different knee subluxations that produce the giving-way symptoms. These subluxations may be the result of anterior tibial subluxation, lateral tibiofemoral joint separation on walking (varus thrust), posterior subluxation of the lateral tibial plateau (particularly with flexion), excessive hyperextension or varus recurvatum, or a combination of these subluxations. It is incumbent on the clinician to take a careful history to determine all symptomatic subluxations that are present. The presence of a varus thrust on walking and the presence of a varus tibiofemoral osseous alignment are indications for a valgus-producing osteotomy because an ACL reconstruction alone will not eradicate the varus thrust instability. A

varus recurvatum, or back-knee symptom of giving way, usually characterizes a triple varus knee, indicating the need to reconstruct insufficient lateral and posterolateral ligamentous structures.

Physical Examination

The most important factors that must be determined on physical examination are the abnormal motion limits (the subluxations that occur to the medial and lateral tibial plateaus), the flexion angle at which they occur, and the anatomical deficiencies that explain the abnormal motion limits and subluxations. This topic has been described in detail elsewhere (9,11,12). Terms such as *posterolateral rotatory instability* may be used generally; however, all abnormal motion limits (e.g., posterior subluxation of the tibial plateau at 30° and 90°, increased lateral joint opening at 0° and 30°, posterior translation, hyperextension, and varus recurvatum) and specific ligamentous deficiencies should be specified (12,13). Each ligament and motion restraint in the knee should be isolated, if possible, and tested at various flexion angles to determine its function. Only then can a diagnosis and treatment plan be determined.

Particular attention must also be given to patellofemoral abnormalities, including any extensor mechanism malalignment that is accentuated by increased external rotation of the tibia and posterolateral tibial subluxation. Furthermore, the clinical examination should note medial tibiofemoral crepitus on varus loading as an indicator of early articular cartilage damage before the presence of radiographic changes, palpate to detect inflammation of the lateral soft tissue supporting the structures, and detect gait abnormalities (14).

RADIOLOGIC STUDIES

Radiographic assessment of lower-limb alignment is based on an examination of full standing radiographs. Separation of the lateral tibiofemoral compartment may occur, preventing correct assessment of true tibiofemoral osseous alignment. We recommend double-stance, full-length AP radiographs that show both lower extremities from the femoral heads to the ankle joints. We also look for the teeter effect described by Kettelkamp et al. (15), in which simultaneous contact of the medial and lateral tibiofemoral compartments is impossible because of tibial obliquity and bone loss of the medial tibiofemoral joint. This finding indicates that overall limb alignment will probably remain in a varus position after HTO, since tibiofemoral contact cannot be reestablished in the lateral compartment.

The steps for making a valid assessment of alignment by radiographic means have been described (16). No matter what technique is used for full standing radiographs, it is imperative that medial and lateral tibiofemoral contact occurs (or that the appropriate calculations are made to subtract the lateral compartment

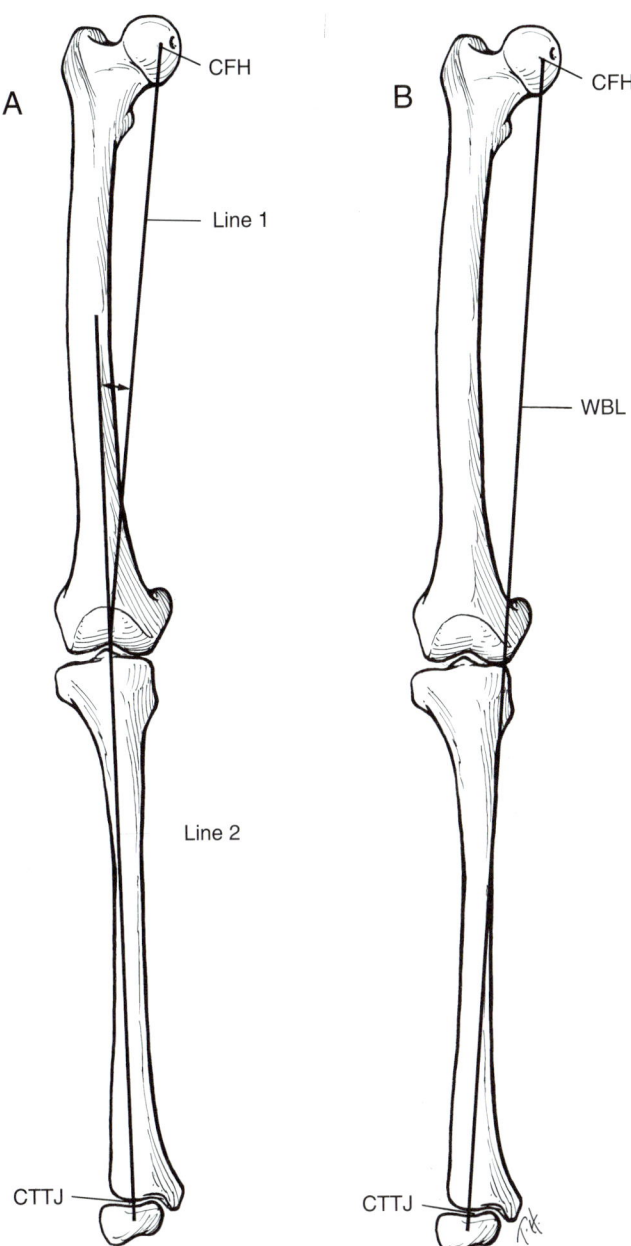

Figure 64.1. A. The radiographic measurement of the tibiofemoral mechanical axis is determined by the angle between a line drawn from the center of the femoral head (*CFH*) to the center of the intercondylar notch (*Line 1*) and a line drawn from the center of the intercondylar notch to the center of the tibiotalar joint (*CTTJ; Line 2*). **B.** The WBL is determined by a line drawn from the CFH to the CTTJ. The point of intersection at the tibial plateau is measured.

opening), so that the true osseous tibiofemoral alignment can be determined. The radiographic measurements include the tibiofemoral mechanical axis and the tibiofemoral WBL (Fig. 64.1). We believe that the position of the WBL on the tibia is the most accurate method for determining angular alignment and the angular correction required at osteotomy. Lateral radiographs are examined for any abnormal tibial slope, such as an excessive poste-

rior sloping of the tibial surface, which is an unusual occurrence.

TREATMENT

Preoperative Assessment for Gait Abnormalities

It is important to recognize and correct gait abnormalities before conducting any surgical procedure (14,17). The patient's gait is inspected to determine the presence of a noticeable varus thrust or hyperextension varus thrust (recurvatum) during the stance phase of gait. Frequently, the patient will walk with a back-knee gait, and there will be little or no observable quadriceps muscle contraction. Before surgery, the patient must be taught to reestablish a normal stance-phase flexion of the knee during gait; i.e., the patient must be instructed to walk slowly while maintaining 5° of knee flexion during the stance phase, voluntarily contracting the quadriceps muscle and preventing knee hyperextension. The patient is also instructed to push off with the forefoot and to lift the heel sooner in the stance phase to limit the chance for a back-knee gait to occur.

Preoperative gait testing may be used in select cases to determine the adductor moment (a medially directed torque acting on the knee that increases the varus angulation) and to calculate the tensile forces within the lateral ligamentous structures. A markedly high adductor moment correlates with high medial tibiofemoral compartment pressures, a poor prognosis, and the likelihood for a gradual return to a varus angulation. The excessive tensile forces on the lateral and posterolateral ligamentous structures, with a possible gradual lengthening and stretching of these tissues, also play a role (14).

Preoperative Planning

The most common method of preoperative planning for a closing-wedge osteotomy of the proximal tibia involves determining the wedge angle, which is equal to the amount of varus deformity, and adding the amount of overcorrection desired. The correction should shift the WBL on a standing x-ray to just lateral of the center of the joint. The tibial plateau is measured at the joint line from the medial to the lateral edge. The standing x-ray allows for calculation of the location of the WBL, which is expressed as a percentage of the total width of the plateau (Fig. 64.2). The optimal correction shifts the WBL to 62 to 66% of the plateau.

The method we use to determine the angle of the correction wedge involves cutting the full-standing radiograph horizontally through the line of the upper tibial osteotomy cut (Fig. 64.3). A vertical cut of the lower tibial

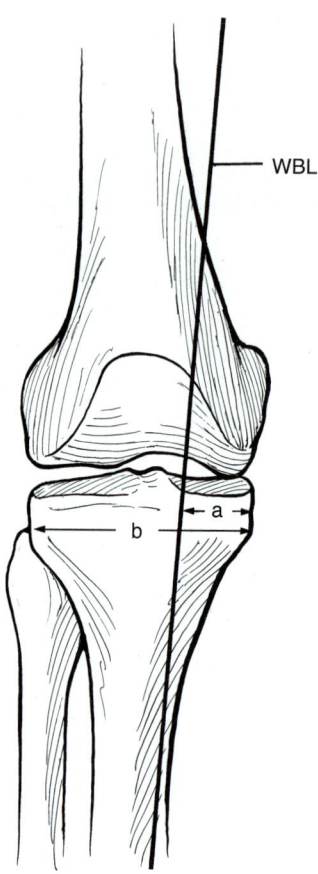

Figure 64.2. The width of the tibial plateau (*b*) and the distance from the medial edge to the WBL (*a*) are measured from a standing full-length radiograph. The location of the WBL is expressed as a percentage of the entire width of the plateau (*a*/*b* × 100%).

segment converges with the first cut at the level of the medial cortex. The distal portion of the radiograph is rotated until the center of the femoral head, the selected WBL coordinate point on the tibial plateau, and the center of the tibiotalar joint are aligned; the radiograph is taped in that position. The angle of the wedge formed by the overlap of the two radiographic segments is measured; it represents the angle of the correction wedge that must be removed at the time of surgery. The mechanical axis is measured to determine the final alignment and the angular correction needed. Although rarely used, an opening medial wedge osteotomy may be performed in knees with associated medial collateral ligament slackness with increased medial joint opening. Our overall preference, however, is for a laterally based closing wedge osteotomy (Clinical Table).

Operative Treatment

Arthroscopy is usually performed immediately before HTO to fully evaluate the articular surfaces of the medial

and lateral tibiofemoral compartments and patellofemoral joint. Cartilage grading is important for both prognosis and minor adjustments in the angle of correction of the osteotomy cut (18). A moderate lateral compartment arthrosis might require less shifting of the WBL so that correction might be planned with the WBL between 50 and 62%. ACL-deficient patients often have associated meniscus tears that require repair or partial removal. Abrasion of the subchondral exposed areas is controversial but may diminish the patient's pain. The increase in lateral joint line opening on standing adds to the varus angulation (approximately 1 degree per mm) and must be subtracted at the time of the HTO.

The entire lower extremity is prepped and draped free. A sterile tourniquet is inflated before the skin incision is made. An oblique incision is made from the fibula head to the anterior crest of the tibia, 2 cm distal to the tibial tubercle (Fig. 64.4A). The subcutaneous tissues are incised down to the fascia of the anterior tibialis muscle. A dome-shaped fascial incision is made from the lateral aspect of the tibial tubercle to slope up proximally to the distal aspect of the Gerdy tubercle and is then extended distally and laterally to the anterior bare area of the fibula (Fig. 64.4B). The bare area of the fibula is an important landmark and indicates the area of the fibular head and neck that can be safely exposed. The LCL and peroneal nerve are safely avoided when the surgeon carefully identifies the bare area.

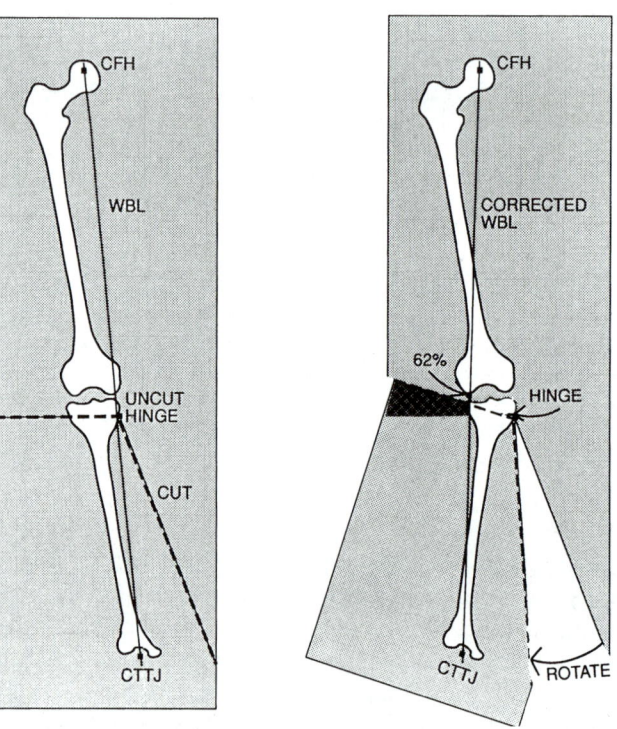

Figure 64.3. Preoperative determination of the wedge angle.

Clinical Table: Varus Angulation with Chronic Ligament Deficiency: The Role of High Tibial Osteotomy

Procedure	Indications	Technique	Anatomy	Pitfalls
High tibial osteotomy	• Varus angulation • High medial tibiofemoral compartment pressures	• Laterally based closing wedge osteotomy • Osteotomy of the fibula	• Subperiosteal dissection • peroneal nerve • Adequate width of proximal tibial fragment	• Inadequate correction • Overcorrection • Nonunion • Peroneal nerve injury • Patella infera • Postoperative loss of correction
Proximal advancement of lateral and posterolateral ligamentous structures	• Ligamentous insufficiency • Abnormal lateral joint opening • Increased external rotation of the tibia	• Proximal advancement of the femoral origin of the LCL and popliteal-arcuate complex	• Lateral epicondyle of femur • Peroneal nerve	• Insufficient tissue integrity • Inadequate correction of varus angulation
Reconstruction of lateral and posterolateral ligamentous structures	• Ligamentous insufficiency • Poor tissue integrity	• Autograft or allograft reconstruction of the LCL and popliteal-arcuate complex		• Inadequate correction of varus angulation
ACL reconstruction	• Abnormal anterior translation of tibia with activity	• Intra-articular reconstruction of the ACL with autograft tissues	• Tibial plateau • Medial wall of the lateral femoral condyle	• Anterior tibial or femoral tunnel placement • Weak graft tissue
PCL reconstruction	• Abnormal posterior translation of tibia with activity • Increased tibial external rotation	• Intra-articular reconstruction of the PCL with autograft tissues	• Tibial plateau • Lateral wall of the medial femoral condyle	• Proximal tibial tunnel placement • Femoral tunnel location • Weak graft tissue

Subperiosteal dissection on the tibia is performed sharply with a scalpel, starting just distal to the Gerdy tubercle, followed by dissection with a Cobb elevator. Subperiosteal dissection is also continued just lateral to the patellar ligament. Dissection should be performed cleanly with a relatively bloodless field, preventing damage to the muscle tissue. Recurrent vessels usually must be coagulated. The patellar ligament is retracted anteriorly using an Army-Navy retractor. Subperiosteal dissection is also continued anteriorly. It is may be necessary to release a few millimeters of the patellar tendon attachment distally if the osteotomy wedge is large. Subperiosteal dissection is continued posteriorly on the tibia. Because of the close proximity of the neurovascular structures it is important to remain in the subperiosteal plane. Dissection is completed across the width of the tibia in one location and then is carefully extended proximally and distally in this safe subperiosteal plane.

FIBULAR OSTEOTOMY

The three options for the fibula when performing an HTO are proximal slide, proximal fibula osteotomy, and distal fibula osteotomy. Maquet (19) described tibial osteotomy over the middle third of the fibula, but we do not recommend this osteotomy location because of the close proximity of the nerve to the extensor hallucis longus and thus the risk of nerve injury.

If the proximal tibiofibular joint is entered, the fibular head will slide proximally and further slacken the lateral ligaments. We, therefore, strongly discourage the use of a proximal slide-type procedure, particularly in an ACL-deficient knee. A distal fibula osteotomy with a step cut can be performed at the junction of the middle and distal thirds of the fibula through a 3-cm vertical incision. In this case, the proximal tibiofibular joint is preserved. The peroneal tendons are retracted anteriorly. The medial cortex of the proximal fibula is preserved. Approximately 10 mm of lateral cortex is resected so that the medial cortex of the proximal fibula segment can be displaced medially to maintain bony contact and promote union. One problem with fibular osteotomy in this location is an apparent increase in the rate of nonunion. Bone graft from the tibial osteotomy site is recommended.

Our procedure of choice is a proximal fibula osteotomy through the head and neck region, with a subperiosteal dissection of the tissues that protect the peroneal nerve (Fig. 64.4C). The posterior cortex is removed with curettes and a Kerrison punch. Meticulous surgical technique and protection and palpation of the peroneal nerve are essential. The wedge height removed is 2 to 3 mm less than the computed size of the tibial wedge, to allow compaction of the distal fibula into the cancellous fibula head. The lateral and posterior periosteal sleeve is carefully preserved and not retracted under tension, to protect the peroneal

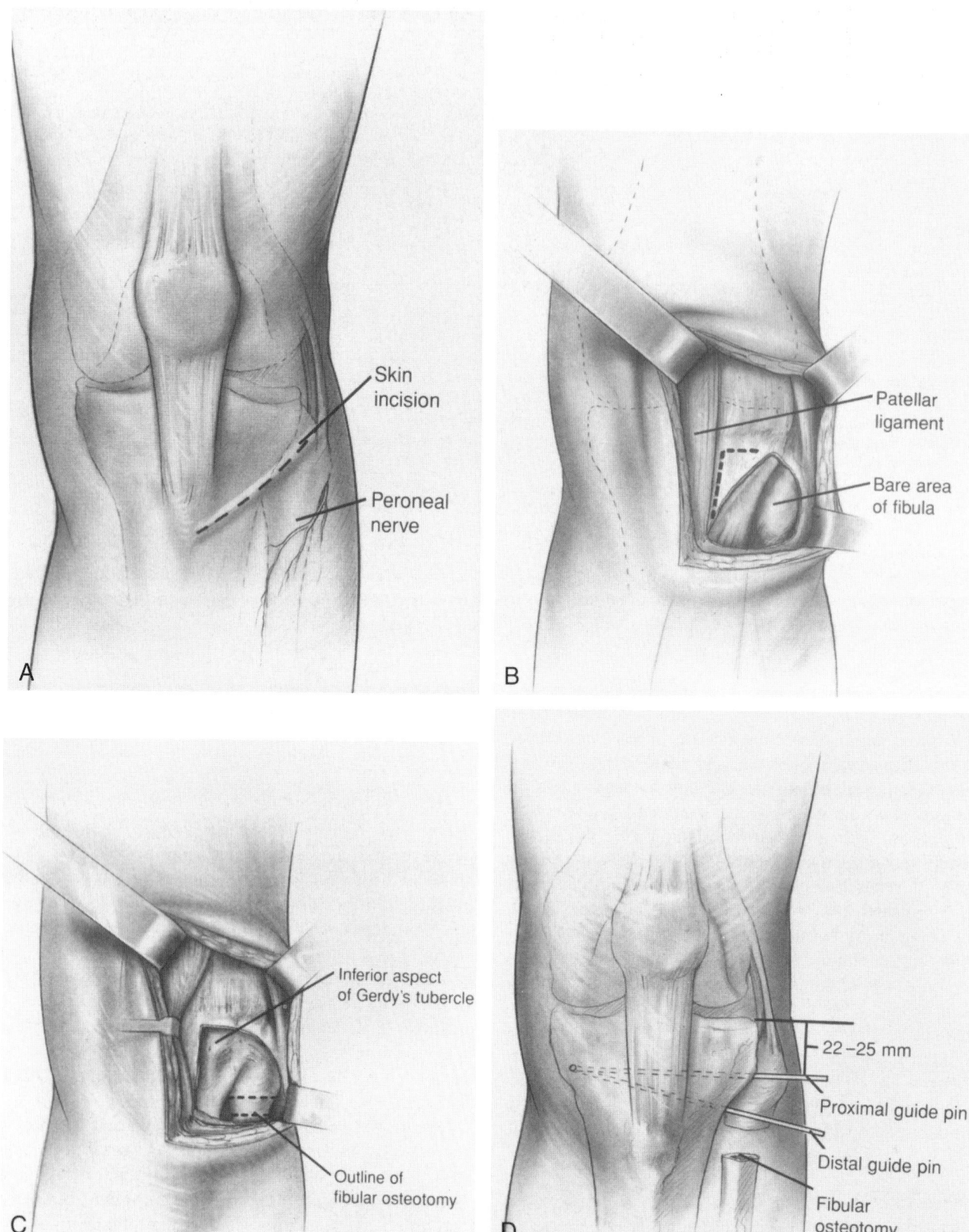

Figure 64.4. **A.** An incision is made from the proximal aspect of the fibular head obliquely to the distal aspect of the tibial tubercle. **B.** Anterior compartment musculature is dissected subperiosteally from the tibial crest down to the bare area of the fibular head. **C.** Subperiosteal dissection continues up to the Gerdy tubercle and around to the fibular neck; a 6- to 8-mm osteotomy is performed. **D.** A K wire (the proximal guidepin) is inserted 22 to 25 mm below and parallel to the tibial plateau and is checked by fluoroscopy. The second K wire (the distal guidepin) is inserted distal to the first wire and is checked by fluoroscopy.

nerve. Excellent bony apposition is achieved when the osteotomy gap is closed; it is usually not necessary to add bone graft to enhance bone healing.

TIBIAL OSTEOTOMY WEDGE MEASUREMENT AT SURGERY

A smooth Kirschner (K) wire is placed transversely just through but not beyond the medial cortex, 25 mm distal to the joint line under image intensifier control (Fig. 64.4D). It is critical to perform the osteotomy by leaving 22 to 25 mm of proximal tibia to avoid a fracture into the tibial plateau. The length of the K wire is measured to determine the width of the proximal tibia. The method described by Slocum et al. (20) uses the angle of the wedge (calculated before surgery) and the tibial width to determine the width of the tibial bone to be removed and the entry point of the second K wire. The tangent of the correction angle θ is multiplied by the tibial width (in millimeters), which equals the width of the wedge at the lateral cortex (in millimeters) to be removed:

$$\text{Tan } \theta \times \text{Tibial width} = \text{Wedge width}$$

It is helpful to estimate the tibial width and calculate this value before surgery. Intraoperative measurement of tibial width verifies the preoperation calculation. The second K wire is inserted into the lateral cortex at the calculated distance distal to the first wire and directed toward the tip of the first wire. Again, the proper positioning of the wires is confirmed with the image intensifier. The K wires are essentially used as an external jig to guide the osteotome across the tibia. As an alternative, the location of the bone cuts can be determined and carried out using a commercial external jig.

We prefer to use a microoscillating saw to cut only the outer cortex; we complete the osteotomy with a thin, wide osteotome. A saw can wander in the cancellous bone and potentially change the correction angle. A malleable retractor is placed posteriorly. The lateral half of the wedge is removed as a single piece; the remaining medial wedge fragments are dislodged after the osteotome is used. A small curette is useful for removing the medial cancellous bone, but the medial 10 mm of the wedge should not be disturbed. The medial cortex and periosteum are preserved to provide stability, to prevent medial or lateral translation of the tibia, and to prevent varus recurrence. Three to four perforations of the medial cortex with a K wire are often required before the osteotomy gap can be closed with a gentle valgus force. Apposition of the bony surfaces should be visualized and inspected. A large single staple may be placed across the lateral tibial osteotomy site for provisional fixation.

An alignment guide rod (a 1-m-long, rigid, 3- to 4-mm-diameter rod) is positioned over the center of the femoral head (determined by image intensifier) and the center of the tibiotalar joint to determine the newly corrected WBL intersection at the tibial plateau. During this procedure the lower limb is axially loaded to maintain contact and closure of both tibiofemoral compartments. The knee is kept at 5° to 10° of flexion with no hyperextension. The alignment guide rod represents the new WBL, which should agree with the preoperative calculations. If necessary, more bone may be removed from the osteotomy cuts to adjust the WBL, as required.

Rigid fixation of the osteotomy is achieved using an L-shaped, five-hole buttress plate (Fig. 64.5). Two 6.5-mm cancellous screws are placed in the proximal tibia, and two or three cortical screws are placed distal to the osteotomy. If needed, a short-threaded 6.5-mm cancellous screw can be placed in a lag fashion from proximal to distal across the osteotomy site and into the medial aspect of the proximal tibial bone for additional compression of the medial aspect of the osteotomy. The final WBL determination is made, using the alignment guide rod.

The tourniquet is released, and hemostasis is obtained. The fascia of the anterior compartment musculature is reattached to the anterolateral aspect of the tibial border. The anterior compartment fascia is routinely released distally over the mid-muscle belly over a distance of 15 cm (6 in) to prevent an anterior compartment syndrome. A Hemovac drain may be used, although we do not routinely use one. If a drain is used, place it superficial in the wound (not next to the osteotomy site), followed by routine wound closure.

We currently perform HTO on an outpatient basis; the patient leaves the hospital 12 to 23 h after surgery. Deep venous thrombosis prophylaxis is maintained by the use of antithrombotic stockings, sequential compression boots (begun during surgery and continued after surgery until discharge from the hospital), and warfarin. The warfarin is started the night before surgery and is continued after surgery on a total joint arthroplasty protocol.

ASSOCIATED PROCEDURES

Any further surgical procedures that are needed to correct laxity in the lateral ligamentous structures are performed at this time. Such procedures are necessary only in cases of gross instability, since a valgus postoperative position may lead to subsequent adaptive shortening of the lateral and posterolateral ligamentous structures. The oblique incision may be extended proximally, or a single vertical incision may be used for both the osteotomy and the advancement or reconstruction of the posterolateral structures. In knees selected for posterolateral reconstruction, the LCL and the popliteal–arcuate complex may be intact but abnormally slack, requiring only the proximal advancement of the femoral origin (21). If the lateral and posterolateral tissues are significantly stretched or of poor quality, a reconstructive approach using an autograft or allograft may be required (22).

Postoperative Rehabilitation

Immediate, continuous passive motion is begun in the 0° to 90° range. Quadriceps isometric exercises are initi-

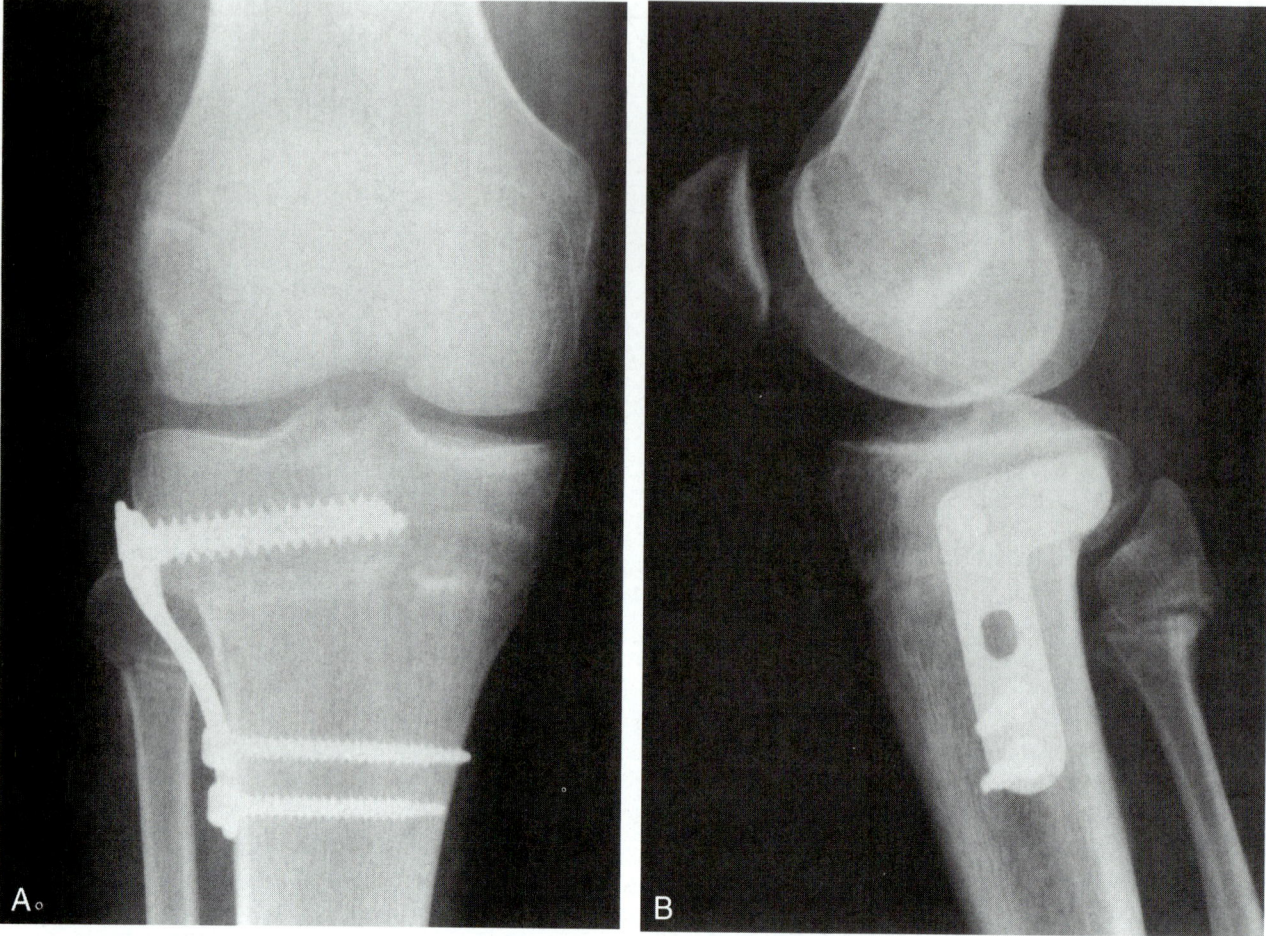

Figure 64.5. Postoperative radiographs showing fixation with an L-shaped plate and cortical- and cancellous-type screws. Note the compression at both the tibial and the fibular osteotomy sites.

ated hourly, and straight-leg raises are begun on postoperative day 1. Patellar mobilization and proximal-distal patellar glides are performed daily to diminish the likelihood of peripatellar soft tissue contractures and developmental patella infera, a complication reported after tibial osteotomy (23).

Toe-touch weight bearing only is permitted for the first 4 weeks after surgery. We remain concerned that settling at the osteotomy site and loss of the desired correction could occur in younger patients if aggressive weight bearing is allowed before healing. Weight bearing is increased to $\frac{1}{4}$ body weight at 4 to 6 weeks, to $\frac{1}{2}$ body weight at 6 to 8 weeks, and to full weight bearing by 12 weeks after surgery. Weight bearing is advanced beyond $\frac{1}{2}$ body weight only if radiographs show evidence of early healing and maintenance of the osteotomy position. Radiographs are taken at 2, 4, 8, and 20 weeks to assess tibiofemoral alignment.

Timing of ACL Reconstruction

ACL reconstruction is usually performed as an arthroscopically assisted procedure after the osteotomy has healed, although it may be performed simultaneously in select cases. The additional surgery, the increased opera-

tive time, and the complexity of performing both procedures at once may increase the complication rate.

Several technical points arise with ACL reconstruction in the knee after HTO. First, the tibial screws of an osteotomy plate often prevent drilling of the tibial tunnel. If the osteotomy is healed, the hardware should be removed at the time of ACL reconstruction. ACL reconstruction at the time of osteotomy requires that the osteotomy be performed first and the osteotomy position be maintained by shorter and carefully placed proximal cancellous screws. Alternatively, staple fixation of the osteotomy site can be used, although staples provide less rigid fixation than does a buttress plate with multiple screws. For an endoscopic ACL reconstruction, the tibial valgus overcorrection makes it difficult to obtain a proper orientation for the drilled femoral hole, requiring medial placement of the tibial tunnel (up to 12 mm medial of the tibial tubercle).

Complications

The most common complications after HTO are inadequate or overcorrection of lower limb alignment, delayed union or nonunion, peroneal nerve injury or palsy, arthrofibrosis and patella infera, and loss of correction of lower-limb alignment.

Inadequate or overcorrection of lower-limb alignment has been reported (3,24,25). Careful preoperative planning is necessary to avoid an inadequate correction and begins with the calculation of the mechanical or anatomic axis on full-length standing radiographs. Calculations to determine the amount of bone to be resected should be made well before the osteotomy. During surgery, confirmation of adequate correction (WBL at 62 to 66%) should be accomplished using image intensification. If there is an unnoticed lateral opening on the standing radiographs, a larger wedge than necessary will be removed, and the knee will be in an overall excessive valgus position. After surgery, the lateral joint assumes a contact position, resulting in overcorrection.

Nonunion and delayed union can occur after HTO. Jackson and Waugh (26) reported that 19 of 226 (8%) patients undergoing operation had a delayed union; 14 of these patients were immobilized for more than 12 weeks before union was achieved, and the remaining 5 required bone grafting. The occurrence of healing difficulties can be reduced by several technical details. First, placing the osteotomy proximal to the tibial tubercle increases the amount of cancellous bone surface contact, which will enhance healing and increase inherent stability. The two surfaces should be cut in a manner that will maximize the amount of surface area that will be in opposition. Internal fixation is also believed to enhance healing, particularly when loss of the medial cortex has occurred.

A delayed union can be treated, if the overall alignment is acceptable, by electric stimulation. If the overall alignment is lost, the surgeon must reoperate and use bone grafting to obtain the desired alignment. Patients should be strongly discouraged from using tobacco after surgery because of its potentially deleterious effects on tibial healing (27).

Jackson and Waugh (26) reported 27 of 226 (12%) cases of partial or complete injury to the peroneal nerve during osteotomy. There was a higher incidence of injury from dome-type osteotomies located below the tibial tuberosity. Other authors have noted an incidence of postoperative peroneal dysfunction of less than 1% (28,29). Peroneal nerve palsy has several causes; the most common is a cast or bandage that is applied too tightly after surgery. Internal fixation makes casting unnecessary. There is increased risk to the peroneal nerve if the osteotomy is performed in the proximal third of the fibula, where the nerve is close to the fibular neck. If osteotomy of the fibular head is necessary, dissection of the peroneal nerve may be considered if difficulty is encountered during subperiosteal dissection and exposure. Fibular osteotomy in the middle portion of the fibula may injure the peroneal nerve innervation to the extensor hallucis longus.

Arthrofibrosis and developmental patella infera after knee surgery require prompt recognition and treatment (23,30,31). The development of adhesions and the development of scar tissue surrounding the patellar ligament are important factors in the development of patella infera. The patella infera condition may develop after surgery as a result of quadriceps weakness and concomitant contracture of peripatellar tissues. If unrecognized, developmental patella infera can rapidly progress to a permanent patella infera and disabling patellofemoral arthrosis. We reviewed the vertical height of the patella and determined that a diagnosis of patella infera is established when there is a decrease in the vertical height ratio of the patella of 11 to 15%, either from preoperative measurements or from the opposite knee, depending on the method used (23). After surgery, lateral radiographs may be used to detect any decrease in the patellar vertical height ratio. These radiographs can be repeated for any patient who shows early and persistent signs of developmental patella infera, e.g., inability to perform a strong quadriceps contraction, decreased patellar mobility, decreased palpable tension in the patellar ligament and failure of the patella to displace proximally on quadriceps contraction, and distal malposition of the involved patella compared with the opposite side.

Loss of axial alignment postoperatively is a well-known complication and may be attributed to several factors, including lack of or inadequate internal fixation and collapse of the distal fragments settling into the cancellous bone of the plateau. Late drifting into a varus position may be due to a progressive loss of the medial osteochondral cartilage complex or to stretching of the lateral soft tissue structures. Patients with a high adduction moment measured by preoperative gait analysis are at risk of losing the correction that was obtained at surgery and must be closely followed to ensure that correction is maintained.

Clinical Results

We reviewed the short-term results of HTO in a group of 41 younger patients with varus alignment and chronic ACL deficiency (6). All patients underwent an osteotomy, 14 in conjunction with an iliotibial band extra-articular reconstruction and 16 with a delayed intra-articular allograft reconstruction. All patients returned for follow-up at a mean of 58 months (range: 23 to 86 months). Before surgery, 30 patients (73%) had pain with ADLs and all sports activities. At follow-up, 32 patients (78%) had no pain with ADLs or light sports. Patient satisfaction was excellent; 36 patients (88%) reported that they would have the surgery again, and 32 patients (78%) reported that their knee had improved. We concluded that HTO should be performed early in the disease process for younger athletes who experience symptoms with activity. It may be unrealistic to expect continuation of sports beyond the light recreational level, given the joint arthrosis that is usually present and the high in vivo joint loading that athletes endure.

SUMMARY

HTO, when performed in conjunction with indicated ligamentous reconstruction or advancement procedures, is a safe, predictable procedure that allows return to normal ADLs with a marked reduction in pain and symptoms in the varus-angulated, ACL-deficient knee. The success of the procedure depends on correct diagnosis of the ligamentous insufficiencies, preoperative planning, and a meticulous surgical technique. The patient who undergoes correction of a varus-angulated knee with a valgus-producing osteotomy must be closely followed to avoid any complications and to ensure maintenance of the correction and relief of symptoms. Patients with associated joint damage must have realistic expectations about their postoperative activity levels.

REFERENCES

1. Coventry MB, Ilstrup DM, Wallrichs SL. Proximal tibial osteotomy. A critical long-term study of eighty-seven cases. J Bone Joint Surg 1993;75A:196–201.
2. Morrey BF. Upper tibial osteotomy for secondary osteoarthritis of the knee. J Bone Joint Surg 1989;71B:554–559.
3. Hernigou P, Medevielle D, Debeyre J, Goutallier D. Proximal tibial osteotomy for osteoarthritis with varus deformity. A ten to thirteen-year follow-up study. J Bone Joint Surg 1987;69A:332–354.
4. Fairbank TJ. Knee joint changes after meniscectomy. J Bone Joint Surg 1948;30B:664–670.
5. Noyes FR, Mooar LA, Matthews DW, Butler DL. The symptomatic anterior cruciate deficient knee I: The long-term functional disability in athletically active individuals. J Bone Joint Surg 1983; 65A:154–162.
6. Noyes FR, Barber SD, Simon R. High tibial osteotomy and ligament reconstruction in varus angulated, anterior cruciate ligament-deficient knees. A two- to seven-year follow-up study. Am J Sports Med 1993;21:2–12.
7. Noyes FR, Munns SW, Andriacchi TP, Mayhall MT. The double-varus and triple varus anterior cruciate insufficient knee: gait analysis and surgical correction. Trans Am Orthop Soc Sports Med 1985;11:41.
8. Hughston JC, Jacobson KE. Chronic posterolateral rotatory instability of the knee. J Bone Joint Surg 1985;67A:351–359.
9. Noyes FR, Grood ES. Diagnosis of knee ligament injuries: five concepts. In: Feagin J, ed. The crucial ligaments. New York: Churchill Livingstone, 1988.
10. Noyes FR, Barber SD, Mooar LA. A rationale for assessing sports activity levels and limitations in knee disorders. Clin Orthop 1989;246:238–249.
11. Wroble RR, Grood ES, Cummings J, et al. The role of the lateral extraarticular restraints in the anterior cruciate ligament-deficient knee. Am J Sports Med 1993;21:257–263.
12. Noyes FR, Stowers SF, Grood ES, et al. Posterior subluxations of the medial and lateral tibiofemoral compartments. An in vitro ligament sectioning study in cadaveric knees. Am J Sports Med 1993;21:407–414.
13. Grood ES, Stowers SF, Noyes FR. Limits of movement in the human knee. Effect of sectioning the posterior cruciate ligament and posterolateral structures. J Bone Joint Surg 1988;70A:88–97.
14. Noyes FR, Schipplein OD, Andriacchi TP, et al. The anterior cruciate ligament-deficient knee with varus alignment. An analysis of gait adaptations and dynamic loadings. Am J Sports Med 1992; 20:707–716.
15. Kettelkamp DB, Leach RE, Nasca R. Pitfalls of proximal tibial osteotomy. Clin Orthop 1975;106:232–241.
16. Dugdale TW, Noyes FR, Styer D. Pre-operative planning for high tibial osteotomy: the effect of lateral tibiofemoral separation and tibiofemoral length. Clin Orthop 1991;271:105–121.
17. Noyes FR, Dunworth LA, Andriacchi TP, et al. Knee hyperextension gait abnormalities in unstable knees. Recognition and preoperative gait retraining. Am J Sports Med 1996;24:35–45.
18. Noyes FR, Stabler CL. A system for grading articular cartilage lesions at arthroscopy. Am J Sports Med 1989;17:505–513.
19. Maquet P. Valgus osteotomy for osteoarthritis of the knee. Clin Orthop 1976;120:143–148.
20. Slocum DB, Larson RL, James SL, Grenier R. High tibial osteotomy. Clin Orthop 1974;104:239–243.
21. Noyes FR, Barber-Westin SD. Surgical restoration to treat chronic deficiency of the posterolateral complex and cruciate ligaments of the knee joint. Am J Sports Med 1996;24:415–426.
22. Noyes FR, Barber-Westin SD. Surgical reconstruction of severe chronic posterolateral complex injuries of the knee using allograft tissues. Am J Sports Med 1995;23:2–13.
23. Noyes FR, Wojtys EM, Marshall MT. The early diagnosis and treatment of developmental patella infera syndrome. Clin Orthop 1991;265:241–252.
24. Insall JN, Joseph DM, Msika C. High tibial osteotomy for varus gonarthrosis. A long-term follow-up study. J Bone Joint Surg 1984; 66A:1040–1048.
25. Matthews LS, Goldstein SA, Malvita TA, et al. Proximal tibial osteotomy. Factors that influence the duration of satisfactory function. Clin Orthop 1988;229:193–200.
26. Jackson JP, Waugh W. The technique and complications of upper tibial osteotomy. A review of 226 operations. J Bone Joint Surg 1974;56B:236–245.
27. Schmitz MA, Finnegan MA, Champine J, Jones AL. Effect of smoking on the clinical healing of tibial shaft fractures. Paper presented at the 62nd Annual Meeting of the American Academy of Orthopaedic Surgeons, Orlando, FL, February 18, 1995.
28. Coventry MB. Upper tibial osteotomy for gonarthrosis. The evolution of the operations in the last 18 years and long term results. Orthop Clin North Am 1979;10:191–210.
29. Bauer GC, Insall J, Koshino T. Tibial osteotomy in gonarthrosis (osteo-arthritis of the knee). J Bone Joint Surg 1969;51A: 1545–1563.
30. Scuderi GR, Windsor RE, Insall JN. Observation on patellar height after proximal tibial osteotomy. J Bone Joint Surg 1989;71A: 245–248.
31. Noyes FR, Wojtys EM. The early recognition, diagnosis and treatment of the patella infera syndrome. Instr Course Lect 1991;40: 233–237.

chapter 65

John A. Bergfeld and Charles J. Gatt, Jr.

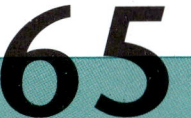

Posterior Cruciate Ligament: Arthroscopic and Open Reconstruction

In contrast to the anterior cruciate ligament (ACL), the posterior cruciate ligament (PCL) has historically received little attention in the orthopaedic literature. Recently, however, the PCL has entered the limelight, owing to the increased awareness of athletic and other nonvehicular trauma injuries to the PCL and to the exhaustive amount of information available on ACL injuries. Because the results of ACL reconstruction are reproducibly good to excellent, orthopaedic surgeons have set their sights on improving the results of PCL reconstruction. Better biomechanical testing techniques, modern surgical techniques, and more critical knee evaluations should produce the data necessary to improve the current inconsistent results obtained from PCL reconstruction.

RELEVANT ANATOMY AND PATHOGENESIS

The femoral attachment of the PCL is a broad semicircle located on the medial femoral condyle (Fig. 65.1). The average anterior to posterior dimension of this insertion is 32 mm (1). At the most distal aspect of the femoral insertion site, the fibers of the PCL are quite close to the articular cartilage of the medial femoral condyle. The PCL tapers in its midsubtance to a minimal diameter of 11 mm. This is approximately 1.5 times the diameter of the ACL (1). The tibial attachment site, for which the PCL is named, is located approximately 1 cm below the articular surface of the tibia. The site is a depression on the posterior aspect of the tibia; and at this level, the ligament averages 13 mm in diameter. The average length of the PCL is 38 mm.

The PCL is generally thought to consist of two bands or fiber regions: a thick anterolateral portion and a less-substantial posteromedial portion. Functionally, the anterolateral band is tight in flexion and the posteromedial band is tight in extension. Biomechanical testing has demonstrated that the anterolateral bundle is six times stronger than the posteromedial bundle (2). The average ultimate strength of the anterolateral portion of the PCL is approximately 1600 N, and its modulus of elasticity is significantly greater than that of the posterolateral portion (3). Because of the mechanical superiority of the anterolateral bundle, most reconstructive techniques aim to replicate the anatomy and mechanics of this portion of the PCL.

The meniscofemoral ligaments play a role in the functional anatomy of the PCL. Although their existence may be variable, studies in our laboratory have proven the presence of both the anterior meniscofemoral ligament of Humphrey and the posterior meniscofemoral ligament of Wrisberg in 88% of knees studied (DeMeo P, personal communication). It has been noted that the meniscofemoral ligaments represent 22% of the bulk of the PCL (5). As is discussed later, these two ligaments serve as secondary restraints against posterior tibial translation.

The blood supply to the PCL is primarily from the middle geniculate artery. It is important to realize that the PCL has a significant synovial sheath that also contributes to the rich vascularity of the ligament. The distal portions of the ligament receive additional vascular supply from the inferior geniculate and popliteal arteries. The PCL receives innervation from a branch of the posterior tibial nerve and from the terminal portions of the obturator nerve. Histologic studies have confirmed the presence of Ruffini corpuscles, Pacini corpuscles, and free nerve endings in the substance of the PCL (6). The ligament is composed of type I collagen with variable amounts of elastin and reticulin. Microscopic evaluation of the collagen fibers demonstrates the typical crimp pattern.

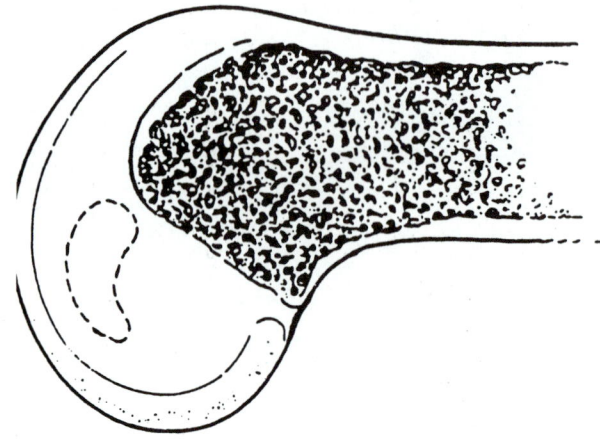

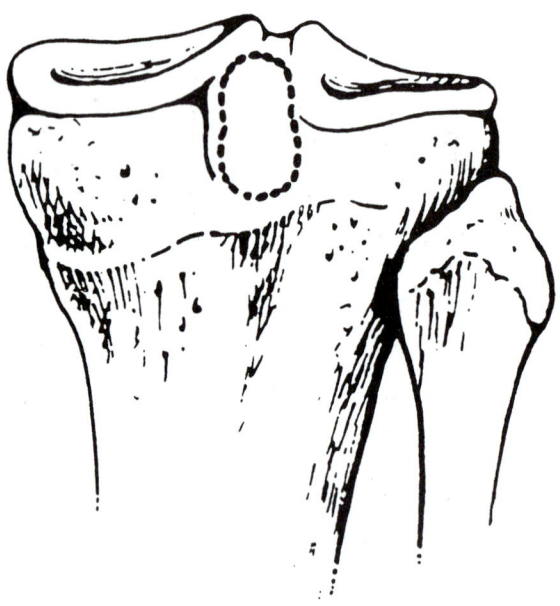

Figure 65.1. Femoral and tibial insertions of the PCL. Reprinted with permission from Miller MD, Harner CD, Koshiwaguchi S. Acute posterior cruciate ligament injuries. In: Fu FH, Harner CD, Vince KG, eds. Knee surgery. Baltimore: Williams & Wilkins, 1994;1:749–767.

Stress in the PCL accounts for 85 to 100% of the resistance to posterior tibial translation at 90° of knee flexion but only 45 to 55% at 30° of flexion. Isolated sectioning of the PCL results in increased posterior tibial translation at all angles of knee flexion; the maximum excursion occurs at 90°. The PCL also serves as a secondary restraint to varus angulation and tibial external rotation (7). The meniscofemoral ligaments also serve as restraints to posterior tibial translation. Selective cutting studies have demonstrated that the meniscofemoral ligaments may account for up to 38% of posterior resistance when posterior tibial translation exceeds 15 mm. Finally, it has been suggested that isolated cutting of the PCL leads to in-

creased contact pressures in the medial compartment of the knee (8).

Epidemiology

The most common cause of PCL injury is motor vehicle accidents. These account for 50% of injuries to the PCL. Athletic-related injures account for approximately 44% of PCL injuries and 6% are the result of other causes. In a review of 1098 acute knee injuries evaluated at San Diego Permanente, the incidence of PCL injury was 2.2% compared to 17.5% for ACL injuries. Because the isolated PCL injury syndrome is relatively benign and has often gone unrecognized, there is a large group of individuals with asymptomatic functionally stable knees with posterior laxity. At the annual National Football League predraft physical, approximately 2% of the athletes have isolated posterior laxity.

The mechanism of injury is most commonly a fall onto a flexed knee with further hyperflexion. The foot is usually plantarflexed, which allows the tibia, rather than the patella, to strike the ground (Fig. 65.2). In the case of motor vehicle accidents, the proximal tibia is forced posteriorly on impact with the dashboard. In addition, hyperextension has been described as a mechanism for PCL injury. Hyperextension injuries may also affect the ACL.

INITAL FINDINGS, PHYSICAL EXAMINATION, AND DIAGNOSIS

The posterior drawer test is the most useful test for diagnosing injury to the PCL. The examination is performed

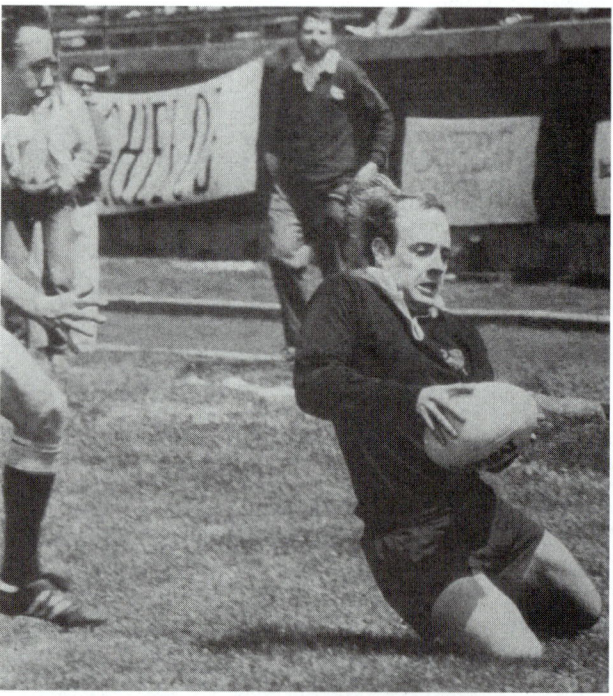

Figure 65.2. Mechanism of injury for the rupture of the PCL.

with the patient supine and the knee flexed 90°. Initially, the examiner should palpate the relationship between the anterior tibia and the femoral condyle. In the uninjured knee, the anterior tibial condyles should be approximately 10 mm anterior to the femoral condyles. Then a posterior force is applied to the proximal tibia, and the amount of posterior translation is compared to that of the uninjured knee. The presence of a firm or soft end point should be recorded. If increased posterior tibial translation is detected, the examination should be repeated with the tibia held in internal rotation; the amount of posterior translation should be compared to that obtained with the tibia in neutral rotation.

If posterior sag is present—the tibia is posteriorly subluxated with the knee at 90°—a quadriceps active test will demonstrate the presence of PCL insufficiency. In this test, the patient is supine and the knee is held in 90° of flexion. In a PCL-deficient knee, the active quadriceps contraction will cause the proximal tibia to move anteriorly; in an uninjured knee, the quadriceps contraction will result in a slight posterior translation of the tibia relative to the femur. The dynamic posterior shift test is positive when a posteriorly subluxated tibia suddenly reduces as the flexed knee is passively extended while the hip is flexed to 90°.

The complete examination should also include tests for increases in varus and valgus rotations along with internal and external tibial rotations for identification of multiple ligament injuries.

RADIOLOGIC STUDIES

Initial radiologic studies should include a standard radiographic knee series that would include AP, lateral, and some view toward identifying the patellofemoral articulation. A standard radiograph can identify associated bony injuries, such as a fracture, and small pieces of bone that may have avulsed from the PCL attachment site. In addition, radiographic studies may identify abnormalities of the patellofemoral joint, as patellofemoral pain may be associated with reconstruction of the PCL, and it is important to get a baseline assessment of the initial appearance of the patellofemoral joint.

MRI scan is an excellent imaging test to identify both partial and complete disruptions of the PCL. The MRI can identify the site of the disruption of the PCL and will often identify associated injuries to meniscus, collateral ligament, or articular cartilage of the knee joint.

TREATMENT

Nonoperative Treatment

Although recently questioned, successful nonoperative treatment of isolated PCL injuries has been well established in the orthopaedic literature. Parolie and Bergfeld (9) reported on a 6.2-year follow-up of isolated PCL injuries treated nonoperatively. Approximately 80% of pa-

tients were satisfied with the result, and 84% had returned to their previous sport. For this study, return of quadriceps strength correlated with a successful result. Several other studies have disputed these results; however, we believe that the diagnostic criteria for an isolated injury of the PCL are strict and must be met for successful nonoperative treatment.

With the knee in 90° of flexion and the tibia in neutral rotation, posterior translation should not exceed 10 mm. When the posterior drawer test is performed with the tibia in internal rotation, the posterior translation should decrease at least 4 mm. With the knee flexed 30°, there should be no more than 5° of abnormal external or internal tibial rotation. Finally, there should be no increased varus or valgus laxity compared to the uninjured knee.

At the Cleveland Clinic, cadaveric cutting studies have provided anatomical and biomechanical evidence of the examination findings of decreased posterior translation with internal rotation of the tibia. It was hypothesized that the meniscofemoral ligaments were responsible for this finding. Selective cutting demonstrated, however, that although the meniscofemoral ligaments did provide secondary restraint to posterior tibial translation they were not responsible for the decrease in translation with internal tibial rotation. A subsequent study indicated that an intact superficial medial collateral ligament (MCL) may be responsible for this finding. After cutting the PCL and MCL, no decrease in posterior tibial translation occurred when the posterior drawer test was performed with the tibia in internal rotation (Fig. 65.3).

Operative Treatment

The most widely used technique for PCL reconstruction is an arthroscopic technique using drill holes in the femur and tibia through which the PCL graft is placed (Clinical Table). After diagnostic arthroscopy has confirmed the rupture of the PCL and associated meniscal pathology has been attended to, the remnant of the PCL is resected with a motorized shaver. It is wise to leave the femoral footprint of the PCL as a guide for femoral tunnel placement. Resection of the tibial stump is best performed through a posteromedial portal while visualizing with a 70° arthroscope through the intercondylar notch.

The arthroscope is then transferred to the posteromedial portal; then the PCL tibial drill guide is inserted through the intercondylar notch, and the tip is placed distal and lateral to the center of the anatomic insertion of the PCL (8). A guidewire is then drilled through the anteromedial tibia to the tip of the drill guide at a 45° to 55° angle to the long axis of the tibia (Fig. 65.4). This should be performed under arthroscopic visualization. An intraoperative lateral radiograph should be obtained to confirm proper placement of the guidewire. Once confirmed, the guidewire is overreamed to an appropriate diameter. Placing a curved curette over the tip of the guided wire will prevent inadvertent injury to posterior neurovascular

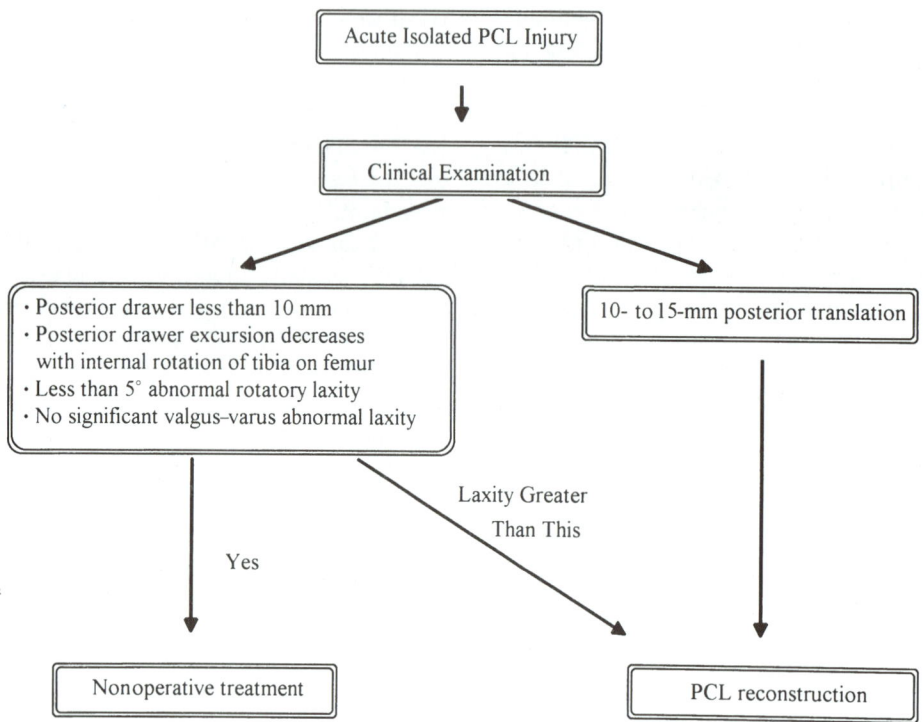

Figure 65.3. PCL injuries in the athlete can be classified into two clinical entities: (*a*) isolated abnormal posterior laxity and (*b*) posterior abnormal laxity associated with other capsuloligamentous injury.

Clinical Table: PCL: Arthroscopic and Open Reconstruction

Procedure	Indications	Technique	Anatomy	Pitfalls
Open repair PCL avulsion	• PCL avulsion with bone fragment	• Posterior or posteromedial approach for tibial avulsion • Parapatellar arthrotomy for femoral avulsion	• Posterior neurovascular bundle	• Failure to address midsubstance injury
Arthroscopic PCL reconstruction	• Posterior tibial translation of >10 mm that does not decrease with internal rotation of the tibia	• Anterior to posterior tibial tunnel *or* • Anatomic fixation of bone block to posterior tibia	• Posterior neurovascular bundle	• Tibial tunnel placement not in proper anatomic location

structures. Creation of the tibial drill hole may also be safely accomplished through a posteromedial arthrotomy.

Next, the femoral tunnel is prepared. The tip of the femoral drill guide is placed in the anterior aspect of the PCL footprint and approximately 8 mm from the articular surface. Through a small anteromedial incision, the articular surface of the medial femoral condyle is visualized; the guidewire is inserted distal to the vastus medialis obliquus, again approximately 8 mm from the articular surface through the condyle to the intra-articular tip of the PCL femoral drill guide (Fig. 65.5). The femoral tunnel is then created with a cannulated reamer of appropriate size.

Graft selection and fixation techniques are primarily based on the preference of the surgeon. The relative strengths of graft materials and fixation techniques have been discussed in the literature. The graft is usually inserted in a proximal to distal direction and initially fixed to the femur. With the knee in 70° of flexion and anterior drawer force applied to the tibia, the graft is fixed to the tibia.

The results of arthroscopic PCL reconstruction have not been as good as those of arthroscopic ACL reconstruction. Subjectively, the results are acceptable; however, the persistence of abnormally increased posterior laxity after reconstruction has plagued the objective outcomes. In a review of 30 patients by Maday et al. (10), only 50% of patients were converted from 3+ laxity to 1+ laxity. Although Lipscomb et al. (11) reported optimistic subjective results in 28 patients, they concluded that the procedure inconsistently limited posterior abnormal laxity and, therefore, could not be recommended.

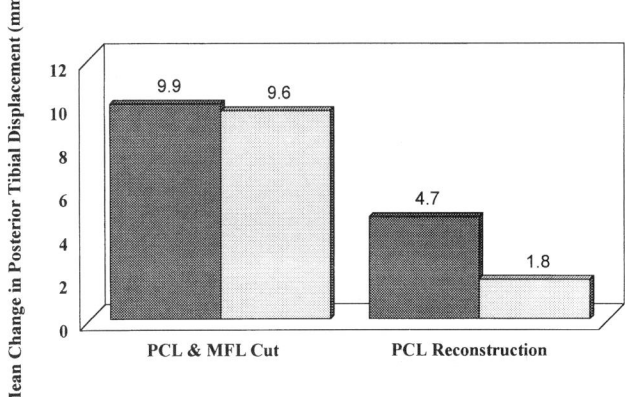

Figure 65.6. A comparison of the mean change in posterior tibial displacement after transection of the PCL and meniscofemoral ligaments (*MFL*), followed by PCL reconstruction performed with the tibial tunnel technique (*dark bars*) or the anatomic fixation technique (*light bars*). Reprinted with permission from Edelson R, Bergfeld JA, Katchis S, et al. Biomechanical effects of an alternative tibial attachment site in bone-patellar tendon-bone reconstruction of the PCL. Paper presented at the 62nd Annual Meeting of the American Academy of Orthopaedic Surgeons, AOSSM specialty day, February 19, 1995.

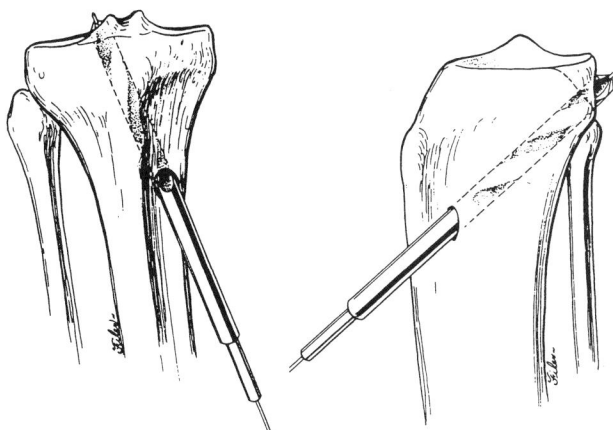

Figure 65.4. The placement of the tibial drill hole is performed over a guidewire. If performed arthroscopically, care must be taken to avoid injury to the posterior neurovascular structures. Reprinted with permission from Miller MD, Harner CD, Koshiwaguchi S. Acute posterior cruciate ligament injuries. In: Fu FH, Harner CD, Vince KG, eds. Knee surgery. Baltimore: Williams & Wilkins, 1994;1:749–767.

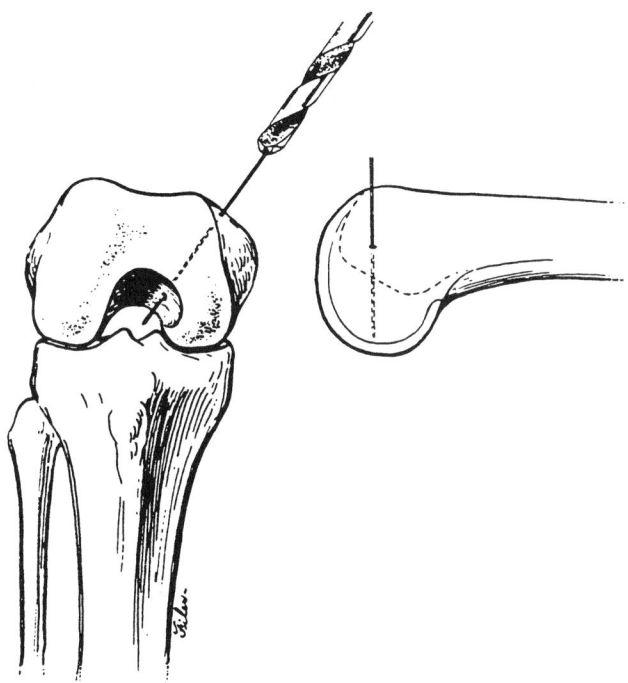

Figure 65.5. The placement of the femoral drill hole is performed over a guidewire. Both the entrance and the exit holes are quite close to the articular surface. Reprinted with permission from Miller MD, Harner CD, Koshiwaguchi S. Acute posterior cruciate ligament injuries. In: Fu FH, Harner CD, Vince KG, eds. Knee surgery. Baltimore: Williams & Wilkins, 1994;1:749–767.

At the Cleveland Clinic, attention has been turned to a more anatomic tibial fixation of the PCL graft. The inconsistent results obtained with the tibial tunnel may be owing to the acute turn the graft makes around the posterior tibial articular surface and into the tibial tunnel. As a result, a technique for fixing the tibial bone block to the posterior aspect of the tibia has been studied biomechanically and is now being used clinically. The fixation technique involves direct screw fixation of the bone block into a vertically oriented trough created on the posterior surface of the tibia at the anatomic origin of the PCL. Laboratory studies revealed that this technique resulted in an average of 2.9 mm less posterior displacement of the tibia at the time of reconstruction than did the standard tibial tunnel technique (12) (Fig. 65.6). An additional finding was that the new technique created more normal appearing posterior drawer force displacement curves than did the standard tibial tunnel technique.

The Cleveland Clinic technique is now being used clinically. The procedure starts arthroscopically, with débridement of the PCL remnant and identification of the PCL femoral footprint. The patient is then turned to the prone position, and the posterior surface of the tibia is exposed through an approach described by Burks (13). This is basically a posteromedial approach performed deep and medial to the medial head of the gastrocnemius. By retracting the medial head laterally, the posterior neurovascular structures are protected. If necessary, the femoral origin of the medial head of the gastrocnemius may be released to improve exposure. The patellar tendon graft is set into a trough created in the posterior cortex of the tibia and secured with a 6.5 AO cancellous screw and washer. The patient is then turned to a supine position, and the graft is passed through the femoral tunnel and secured with an interference screw. The preliminary results have been promising; and as longer follow-up data are obtained, this technique should provide improved and more reproducible objective results for PCL reconstructions.

Postoperative Rehabilitation

Since the weight of the leg tends to stress the newly fixed graft when the patient is in the supine position, early rehabilitation usually involves a period of immobilization (1 to 4 weeks) with the knee braced in full extension. During that time, isometric quadriceps contractions and straight leg raises are performed. Full weight bearing is allowed with the knee in full extension. After about 2 months, hamstring exercises are added to the rehabilitation program. The patient should do these exercises in the prone position and with little knee flexion, to minimize the stress on the graft. At 6 weeks, closed-chain exercises such as minisquats, bicycling, and leg presses may be performed safely because of cocontraction of the quadriceps and hamstrings muscles. In addition, the axial load on the joint results in increased stability and less stress on the graft. Jogging may be started at 24 weeks after surgery. Patients return to unrestricted activity between 9 and 12 months after surgery.

SUMMARY

The improvement of arthroscopic surgical instrumentation and techniques has recently lead to a more aggressive surgical approach to injuries of the PCL. In properly selected patients, however, nonoperative management remains the treatment of choice (Fig. 65.7): (a) Patients should have an isolated injury to the PCL; those with associated collateral ligament injuries, especially posterolateral complex injuries should be considered candidates for early repair and/or reconstruction. (b) The extent of increase in the posterior drawer should be evaluated; translation should not exceed 10 mm. When the posterior drawer test is performed with the tibia in internal rotation, the posterior translation should decrease by an average of 4 mm. Patients with these findings are candidates for nonoperative treatment, and the long-term result is usually good to excellent.

For patients who are surgical candidates, the optimal surgical technique remains uncertain. Although the subjective results of PCL reconstruction with the graft fixed in a tibial tunnel have been good, the objective results have not been consistently satisfactory. Newer techniques, such as anatomic fixation of the graft to the posterior surface of the tibia, may provide more reproducible and acceptable objective results for PCL reconstruction.

REFERENCES

1. Miller MD, Johnson DL, Harner CD, Fu FH. Posterior cruciate ligament injuries. Orthop Rev 1993;22:1201–1210.
2. Race A, Amis AA. The mechanical properties of the two bundles of the human posterior cruciate ligament. J Biomechanics 1994;27:13–24.
3. Miller MD, Harner CD. The anatomic and surgical considerations for posterior cruciate ligament reconstruction. Instr Course Lect 1995;44:431–440.
4. Deleted in proof.
5. Harner CD. Rosemont, IL: American Orthopaedic Society of Sports Medicine, 1996.
6. Covey DC, Sapega AA. Injuries of the posterior cruciate ligament: current concepts review. J Bone Joint Surg 1993;75A:1376–1385.
7. Gollehon DL, Torzilli PA, Warren RF. The role of the posterolateral and cruciate ligaments in the stability of the human knee: a biomechanical study. J Bone Joint Surg 1987;69A:233–242.
8. Schulte KR, Harner CD. Management of isolated posterior cruciate ligament injuries. Oper Tech Orthop 1995;5:270–275.
9. Parolie JM, Bergfeld JA. Long-term results of nonoperative treatment of isolated posterior cruciate ligament injuries in the athlete. Am J Sports Med 1986;14:35–38
10. Maday MG, Harner CD, Miller MD, et al. Posterior cruciate ligament reconstructions using fresh-frozen Achilles tendon allograft: indications, techniques, results, and controversies. Paper presented at the 60th Annual Meeting of the American Academy of Orthopaedic Surgeons, San Francisco, February 1993.
11. Lipscomb AB Jr, Anderson AF, Norwig ED, et al. Isolated posterior cruciate ligament reconstruction. Long-term results. Am J Sports Med 1993;21:490–496.
12. Edelson R, Bergfeld JA, Katchis S, et al. Biomechanical effects of an alternative tibial attachment site in bone-patellar tendon-bone reconstruction of the PCL. Paper presented at the 62nd Annual Meeting of the American Academy of Orthopaedic Surgeons, AOSSM specialty day, February 19, 1995.
13. Burks RT, Schaffer JJ. A simplified approach to the tibial attachment of the posterior cruciate ligament. Clin Orthop 1990;254:216–219.

Suggested Reading

Fanelli GC. Posterior cruciate ligament arthroscopic evaluation and treatment [Review]. Arthroscopy 1994;106:673–678.

- Abnormal posterior laxity < 10 mm
- Abnormal laxity decreases with internal rotation of the tibia
- No abnormal rotatory laxity > 5–10°
- No significant varus or valgus abnormal laxity

Figure 65.7. Patients outside this examination envelope are candidates for surgical reconstruction.

John C. L'Insalata, Christopher D. Harner, Jon J. P. Warner

Posterolateral Instability: Operative Treatment

Injuries of the lateral knee structures are uncommon and have received much less attention in the orthopaedic literature than have medial and cruciate ligament injuries. Most injuries involving the posterolateral corner are associated with combined injuries of the anterior cruciate ligament (ACL) and/or the posterior cruciate ligament (PCL) (1–3). This undoubtedly has added confusion to the diagnosis and treatment of posterolateral corner injuries, frequently resulting in multiple operations, insufficient stabilization procedures, and poor outcome (1). Proper treatment of injuries to the posterolateral corner requires an understanding of the anatomy, biomechanical principles, clinical findings, and treatment options.

RELEVANT ANATOMY

The lateral compartment of the knee extends from the PCL posteriorly to the lateral border of the patellar tendon anteriorly (4). Seebacher et al. (5) organized the structures of the lateral knee into three layers. The most superficial layer (layer I) includes (a) the iliotibial band (ITB) and its expansion anteriorly and (b) the superficial portion of the biceps and its expansion posteriorly. The peroneal nerve lies deep to layer I, posterior to the biceps tendon. Layer II consists of the quadriceps retinaculum anteriorly; posteriorly, this layer is incomplete and consists of the two patellofemoral ligaments and the patellomeniscal ligament. The deepest layer (layer III) consists of the lateral capsule, including the coronary ligament, which is the capsular attachment to the lateral meniscus. This layer divides into two laminae: The superficial encompasses the lateral collateral ligament (LCL) and the fabellofibular ligament (short external or short collateral ligament); and the deeper lamina forms the coronary ligament, the hiatus for the popliteus tendon and arcuate ligament. The inferior lateral geniculate artery runs between these two laminae.

Some authors have questioned the clinical practicality of a detailed anatomic division of the posterolateral corner and have referred to these structures as a single functional tendoligamentous complex called the arcuate ligament complex (2,4). This complex consists of the LCL, the arcuate ligament, the aponeurotic and tendinous portions of the popliteus muscle, and the lateral head of the gastrocnemius muscle. The LCL originates proximally on the lateral femoral epicondyle and inserts distally on the fibular head. It is described as the primary static restraint to varus stress although clinically, isolated injury of the LCL is rare (6).

The popliteus muscle originates from the posterior tibia and runs obliquely, deep to the LCL to insert anterior and distal to it on the lateral femoral condyle. The popliteofibular ligament arises from the posterior part of the fibula, posterior to the biceps insertion, and joins the popliteus tendon just proximal to its musculotendinous junction (7). The arcuate ligament, a condensation of fascia over the posterior surface of the popliteus muscle, runs with the fabellofibular ligament from the apex of the fibular styloid to the lateral head of the gastrocnemius, where they are joined by the oblique popliteal ligament of Winslow (5). These structures are variable and poorly defined. Seebacher et al. (5) noted that the arcuate ligament alone was present in 13% of knees, the fabellofibular ligament alone was present in 20%, and both were present in 67% (5).

The final static stabilizer of the lateral knee is the capsular layer, which is often divided into anterior, middle, and posterior thirds. The anterior third is reinforced by lateral expansion of the quadriceps retinaculum, and the posterior third is reinforced by the arcuate ligament. The middle third (lateral capsular ligament) consists of the meniscofemoral and meniscotibial portions and is a secondary restraint to varus stress. Injury of this structure may be observed radiographically as a lateral capsular avulsion (Segond fracture), usually associated with an ACL tear.

The biceps femoris muscle inserts primarily on the fibular head but also sends strong attachments to the iliotibial tract, the Gerdy tubercle, LCL, posterolateral capsule, and the posterolateral tibia. It acts together with the popliteus and ITB as a strong lateral stabilizer and powerful external rotator of the tibia (4).

The ITB has been described as having three insertions. Proximally, it is conjoined with the intermuscular septum at its insertion into the supracondylar tubercle of the femur. More distally, there is an insertion into the patella and patellar tendon and a separate insertion into the Gerdy tubercle. It has been suggested that the ITB acts as an accessory anterolateral ligament in stabilizing the knee (8). In flexion, the ITB moves posteriorly and becomes taut, exerting an external rotation and posterior force on the tibia. In extension it moves forward and is thus usually spared in most cases of varus and posterolateral injury.

Most injuries of the posterolateral corner are associated with injuries of the ACL and/or the PCL (1–3). All injuries are caused by trauma resulting most commonly from a motor vehicle accident or sports injury. For isolated posterolateral instability, DeLee et al. (4) reported that 9 of 12 patients had a direct blow to the anteromedial tibia during sports or a motor vehicle accident. In series including combined injuries, the most common mechanisms have been hyperextension with or without an external rotation force, a posterolaterally directed blow to the proximal tibia in an extended or, less commonly, flexed knee, and noncontact, twisting injuries of the knee (1–3).

Biomechanics

Using selective ligament sectioning studies, the contributions of the lateral and posterolateral knee structures to knee stability have been determined (6,9,10). These studies have shown that the LCL and arcuate–capsular ligament complex (arcuate ligament complex plus posterolateral capsule) are the primary restraints to varus rotation (adduction) in all degrees of knee flexion, whereas the ACL and PCL are secondary stabilizers that significantly contribute to stability only after the posterolateral structures are cut.

The posterolateral structures are the principal restraints to primary and coupled (with posterior force) external rotation in all degrees of knee flexion; the maximal increase in external rotation occurs at 30° of flexion. Subsequent cutting of the PCL produces significantly increased primary and coupled external rotation at 90° of flexion. Subsequent cutting of the ACL produces increased coupled external rotation in all angles of flexion but decreased primary external rotation while increasing primary internal rotation (10).

Isolated cutting of the posterolateral structures increases primary posterior translation between 0° and 30° flexion, similar to that observed after isolated PCL cutting. At larger flexion angles, cutting the PCL causes progressively greater posterior translation. Combined sectioning of the PCL and posterolateral structures causes significantly greater posterior translation than that observed after cutting either structure alone. The PCL is the only structure that provides initial restraint to posterior translation at all angles of flexion.

INITIAL FINDINGS, PHYSICAL EXAMINATION, AND DIAGNOSIS

The clinical assessment of posterolateral instability begins with the history, with particular attention paid to symptoms and the mechanism of injury as previously described. In acute injuries, patients most commonly complain of pain in the posterolateral aspect of the knee. It is important to ask about any weakness or numbness, which may signal injury of the peroneal nerve. With chronic posterolateral instability, patients most frequently complain of instability with the knee in extension. They often report difficulty in ascending or descending stairs or slopes because of inability to lock the knee in full extension and may note improved stability when wearing higher-healed shoes, which tend to maintain the knee in slight flexion during the stance phase of gait. When pain is present with chronic instability, it is most often located along the medial joint line. Patients often also report symptoms related to associated injuries.

The physical examination of the acutely injured knee should include evaluation of the posterolateral aspect of the knee for swelling, ecchymosis, and tenderness. The anteromedial tibia should be inspected for abrasions or ecchymosis, which may indicate a mechanism of direct contact. A neurovascular examination should be performed; particular attention should be directed to the peroneal nerve, which DeLee et al. (4) reported to be injured in 2 of 12 patients and Baker et al. (2) reported to be injured in 2 of 17 patients. The presence of an occult knee dislocation should be considered if there are multiple acute ligament instabilities and proper vascular assessment performed. Gait should be observed, particularly for patients with chronic instability who may have a varus (lateral) or varus hyperextension thrust during the stance phase. Hughston and Jacobson (1) believed this is analogous to a positive external rotation recurvatum test and represents external rotation of the tibia in full extension and not true tibia vara. A flexed-knee gait with a variable degree of internal rotation may also be present as a compensatory means of avoiding posterior subluxation of the lateral tibial condyle relative to the lateral femoral condyle. The standing alignment of the knees should be observed, particularly in chronic instability in which loss of coaptation of the lateral compartment may occur as a result of laxity of the arcuate ligament complex causing significant varus alignment.

Ligament Stability Testing

Ligament stability testing is performed, with specific attention directed to potential associated injuries of the ACL and PCL, and the results should always be compared to those from testing of the contralateral normal knee. This testing may be limited in the acute setting, in which guarding related to pain, anxiety, and muscle spasm may be present. In these conditions, examination under anesthesia should be considered. Evaluation consists of assessment of anterior and posterior translation, varus-valgus rotation, tibial external rotation, the external rotation recurvatum test, the posterolateral drawer test, and the true and reverse pivot shift tests.

ANTERIOR-POSTERIOR TRANSLATION

The techniques for the Lachman and the anterior and posterior drawer tests have been described elsewhere. Increased anterior translation with a solid end point should raise the suspicion for PCL or arcuate ligament complex injury, thus making it important to evaluate the starting point of the tibia in relation to the femur. Furthermore, DeLee et al. (4) suggest that a markedly positive anterior drawer test with the knee in internal rotation indicates an injury of the PCL. Increased posterior translation greater at 90° than at 30° of flexion indicates injury of the PCL, whereas increased posterior translation greater at 30° than at 90° of flexion suggests a rare isolated injury of the arcuate ligament complex (6). The posterior drawer test should be performed in neutral, internal, and external rotation; a posterior drawer test more marked in external rotation and less marked in internal rotation indicates an intact PCL with isolated injury of the arcuate ligament complex (11,12).

TIBIAL EXTERNAL ROTATION

Forced external rotation of the tibia on the femur using the medial border of the foot as a reference should be measured and compared with that of the opposite knee at 30° and 90° of knee flexion; 10° of increased external rotation is considered clinically significant. In addition, the tibial plateaus are palpated to determine their relative positions in relation to the femoral condyles. In posterolateral instability, external rotation causes the lateral tibial plateau to subluxate posteriorly, whereas in anteromedial instability, external rotation causes the medial tibial plateau to move anteriorly. These two can be further differentiated by associated physical findings, including varus-valgus stability.

Based on the results of biomechanical testing, the degree of external rotation can be used to predict the injured structure(s) (6,9). With isolated injury of the arcuate ligament complex, there is increased external rotation at all angles of knee flexion, which is greatest at 30° flexion and less increased at 90° flexion. Significantly increased external rotation that is similar at both 30° and 90° of flexion indicates a combined injury of the PCL and arcuate ligament

complex. Veltri et al. (10) noted that with combined injury of the ACL and the arcuate ligament complex increased external rotation is not a reliable finding. They suggested that increased total (combined internal and external) rotation should be used with an assessment of increased anterior-posterior translation and varus rotation to detect combined injuries of the ACL and the arcuate ligament complex.

VARUS-VALGUS ROTATION

Varus rotation is tested at full extension and at 30° of knee flexion. Increased laxity at 30° flexion compared with that of the opposite knee indicates injury of the arcuate ligament complex. Isolated injury of the PCL or ACL does not clinically increase varus rotation. DeLee et al. (4) found this to be the most sensitive indicator of isolated posterolateral instability, present in 12 of 12 knees with this diagnosis. Hughston and Jacobson (1) and Baker et al. (2) confirmed the clinical sensitivity of this test. Increased varus laxity with the knee in full extension indicates a combined injury of the arcuate ligament complex, the PCL, and possibly the ACL.

POSTEROLATERAL DRAWER TEST

The posterolateral drawer test is a posterior drawer test performed with the tibia in 15° of external rotation (11). The patient is supine with the hip flexed 45° and the knee flexed 80°. The foot is secured to the table by the examiner's thigh, and the hamstrings must be relaxed. The test is considered positive when the lateral tibial condyle rotates posteriorly while the medial tibia does not change position. Cooper (13) found the interpretation of this test to be subjective and believed that a grossly positive result required concomitant injury of the PCL. He found no false-positive results in 100 normal knees examined under anesthesia. Baker et al. (2,3) reported a sensitivity of 71% in acute posterolateral instability, which increased to 77% with combined injury of the PCL. DeLee et al. (4) reported sensitivities of 33% for office examination of acute isolated posterolateral instability and 75% during examination under anesthesia.

EXTERNAL ROTATION RECURVATUM TEST

For the external rotation recurvatum test, the legs of the supine patient rest on the examining table. The examiner then grasps the great toes of both feet and lifts the legs off the table. With posterolateral instability, there will be relative hyperextension of the lateral side of the knee, external rotation of the tibia, and the appearance of relative tibia vara (11). Hughston and Norwood (11) stated that the uninjured ACL will not allow this test to be positive and that neither this test nor the posterolateral drawer test alone can make the diagnosis of posterolateral instability. Cooper (13) found this test was normal in 100 knees examined under anesthesia, but he and others have questioned the sensitivity of the test for isolated injury of the arcuate ligament complex (4,12). Although

Baker et al. (2) report a positive external rotation recurvatum test in 16 of 17 patients with acute posterolateral instability, 11 of these knees had concomitant injury of the ACL. DeLee et al. (4) reported a sensitivity of only 33% for isolated posterolateral instability during examination under anesthesia.

REVERSE PIVOT SHIFT TEST

The reverse pivot shift test is performed by bringing the knee from a position of 80° flexion to full extension with the tibia in external rotation while a valgus and axial load is applied to the knee (12). With a positive test, the lateral tibial plateau begins in a posteriorly subluxated position and at approximately 20° flexion will reduce with a palpable jerk-like shift. This test may be positive in up to 35% of normal knees (13). Thus, as Jakob et al. (12) suggested in their initial description, this test should be considered clinically significant only when it is unilateral, painful, reproduces the patient's symptoms, and is accompanied by other signs of posterolateral instability.

RADIOLOGIC STUDIES

Plain radiographs are routinely obtained to look for associated fractures of the tibial plateau or fibula, osteochondral fractures, and a Segond fracture. DeLee et al. (4) reported 5 fibular head fractures, 1 Segond fracture, and 1 displaced medial tibial plateau fracture in 12 patients with acute posterolateral instability. In chronic injuries, radiographs may demonstrate osteoarthritis and should include a 45° PA flexion weight-bearing view and a long cassette view to quantify the degree of varus alignment if present. Stress views under anesthesia may help define the degree and direction of instability and should also be considered when there are open physes. MRI can be helpful in determining the status of the cruciate ligaments, LCL, and popliteus tendon.

TREATMENT

Nonoperative Treatment and Indications for Surgery

Most reported series of posterolateral knee instability deal with the surgical treatment of acute and chronic injuries with moderate to severe instability, frequently in association with cruciate ligament tears. In contrast, there are few reports dedicated to the nonoperative treatment of these injuries. Baker et al. (2) treated 14 patients with mild (1+) posterolateral instability nonoperatively, with cast immobilization. They reported that all patients returned to their preinjury level of activity and none required subsequent reconstructive surgery. DeLee et al. (4) performed acute stabilization if varus instability at 30° of flexion was 2+ or greater or if the posterolateral drawer or external rotation recurvatum test was positive.

Isolated injury of the LCL is uncommon and is best classified as a straight lateral instability rather than posterolateral instability. Ellsasser et al. (14) reported 95% success of nonoperative treatment of these injuries using supportive bracing with protected motion and functional rehabilitation. Kannus (15) noted good results at the 8-year follow-up in 9 of 11 patients with grade II straight lateral instability treated with 2 to 5 weeks of immobilization followed by a supervised rehabilitation program. However, of 12 patients with grade III instability, only 1 was asymptomatic, and 50% had clear evidence of osteoarthritis. It is likely that grade III varus laxity represents a combined injury that involves the posterolateral corner structures and possibly the cruciate ligaments and does not represent an isolated injury of the LCL.

Most patients with chronic posterolateral instability have associated instabilities and severe laxity. In these cases, we agree with other authors that it is important to surgically address all associated ligament injuries (3,7).

Operative Treatment

Several surgical techniques have been described for the treatment of acute and chronic posterolateral knee instability. These include primary ligament repair, recession, advancement, augmentation, and reconstruction (Clinical Table). Several reports have suggested that results are improved following treatment of acute rather than chronic posterolateral instabilities, and most authors recommended acute treatment within 2 to 3 weeks of injury. Arthroscopy is routinely performed to assess the articular cartilage, cruciate ligaments, and menisci. Peripheral meniscal tears are repaired; and associated ACL or PCL injuries are reconstructed arthroscopically using techniques described elsewhere. We pass the ACL or PCL graft and fix it to the femur before beginning the posterolateral procedure. After the sutures or grafts for the posterolateral reconstruction are placed, the tibial portion of the cruciate graft(s) is fixed (PCL fixed first in 90° flexion, ACL fixed next in extension) followed by graft fixation or tying of the final sutures at the posterolateral corner.

If there is varus knee alignment and a varus thrust during the stance phase of gait, a corrective proximal tibial osteotomy should be performed before posterolateral reconstruction. Uncorrected excessive varus alignment causes a distraction force on the posterolateral structures and will lead to failure of a posterolateral reconstruction. With posterolateral instability, we usually perform a medial opening wedge osteotomy to avoid creating further laxity of the lateral structures. If a lateral closing wedge osteotomy is performed, a longitudinal incision should be used, and the ITB with its bony attachment at the Gerdy tubercle is advanced distally and fixed with a cancellous screw. The osteotomy may be performed in conjunction with posterolateral reconstruction or in a staged manner. If staged, osteotomy alone may improve the symptoms of posterolateral instability in some patients. Posterolateral reconstruction can then be performed later in those with persistent symptoms.

Clinical Table: Posterolateral Instability: Operative Treatment

Procedure	Indications	Technique	Anatomy	Pitfalls
Advancement and recession of the LCL	• Stretched but intact	• Advance and repair at the anatomic femur insertion	• ITB • LCL • Popliteus • Inferior lateral geniculate artery	• Isometric placement at the femur
Biceps tendon augmentation	• Complete tear of the LCL or popliteofibular ligament	• Tendon (one-third width) pedicled at the fibula • Attach to the anatomic femur insertion	• ITB • LCL • Popliteus • Inferior lateral geniculate artery • Biceps femoris • Peroneal nerve	• Isometric placement at the femur
LCL reconstruction	• Chronic LCL tear • Sever acute injury	• Achilles tendon allograft • Bone block at the fibula • Tension native LCL	• ITB • LCL • Popliteus • Inferior lateral geniculate artery • Biceps femoris • Peroneal nerve	• Protect the peroneal nerve • Isometric placement at the femur
Popliteofibular ligament reconstruction	• Chronic popliteus tear • Severe acute injury	• Semitendinosus tunnel in the fibula and femur • Graft deep to the LCL	• ITB • LCL • Popliteus • Inferior lateral geniculate artery • Biceps femoris • Peroneal nerve	• Protect the peroneal nerve • Isometric placement at the femur • Avoid intra-articular drilling across the femur

SURGICAL TECHNIQUES

The patient is placed supine on the operating table with a tourniquet applied to the proximal thigh and the knee flexed at 90°. A curvilinear incision is made beginning midway between the fibular head and the Gerdy tubercle, continuing proximally to the lateral femoral epicondyle, and paralleling the posterior edge of the ITB for a total length of approximately 15 cm. The peroneal nerve is identified proximally, posterior to the biceps tendon, and is dissected distally to the point at which it enters the anterior tibial muscular compartment. If hematoma is present, particularly with acute injuries, the epineurium is released.

Dissection is continued between the posterior edge of the ITB and the biceps tendon, and the ITB is split longitudinally at the level of the lateral femoral epicondyle, allowing it to be retracted anteriorly and posteriorly for further exposure of the posterolateral structures. A vertical capsular incision is then made at the posterior border of the LCL, providing visualization of the popliteus tendon and lateral meniscus. The inferior lateral geniculate vessels are typically encountered and cauterized. Each of the structures of the posterolateral corner is then systematically evaluated for injury. Evaluation of the popliteus includes assessment of its tendinous insertion onto the femur; the musculotendinous junction, which is a frequent site of injury; its tibial origin; and its insertion into the fibular via the popliteofibular ligament.

With acute injury, we attempt direct repair of all injured structures to their anatomic locations using nonabsorbable suture (Fig. 66.1). Structures that are stretched but intact, such as the popliteus or LCL, are advanced and recessed at their anatomic insertion into the femur. For complete tears of the LCL, popliteus tendon, or popliteofibular ligament, the repair may be augmented with a strip of biceps tendon left attached to the fibula (8). The arcuate ligament and fabellofibular ligament are then advanced and used to anchor sutures to tighten the posterolateral repair (2–4). For severe injuries, a ligament reconstruction is performed, as described below for chronic injuries.

With chronic injuries, some form of reconstruction is usually performed. Associated varus malalignment and cruciate ligament injuries are addressed first. We generally do not advocate advancement of the common insertion of the popliteus-LCL on the femur or biceps tenodesis because these do not restore the normal anatomy, are nonkinematic, and may be prone to stretching (1,8,16). Biceps tenodesis also removes an important dynamic lateral stabilizer, and its failure may exacerbate patients' symptoms and make subsequent reconstruction more difficult. Noyes and Barber-Westin (17) performed LCL reconstruction for chronic posterolateral instability using an Achilles tendon allograft looped through fibular and femoral bone tunnels with advancement of redundant posterolateral structures. They reported satisfactory out-

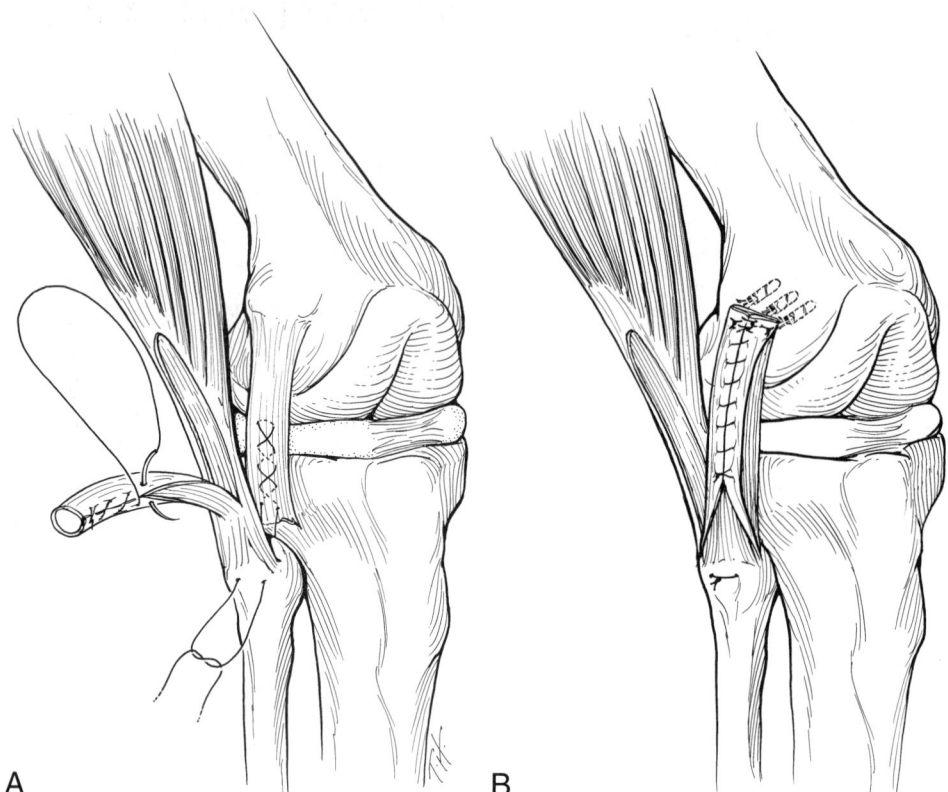

A   **B**

Figure 66.1. A. The LCL is primarily repaired using nonabsorbable sutures, and a central slip of biceps tendon is pedicled distally and tubularized. **B.** Biceps tendon slip is tensioned and anatomically at-tached at the lateral femoral epicondyle, using suture anchors. The tendon graft is sutured to the native LCL.

comes in 76% of patients. Veltri and Warren (7) recom-mended reconstruction of the tibial and fibular attach-ments of the popliteus using a split Achilles or patellar tendon allograft and LCL reconstruction using a strip of bi-ceps tendon. Jakob and Warner (8) recommended a "small popliteal plasty" in which a strip of biceps tendon pedi-cled distally is directed under the LCL into a bone tunnel at the popliteus insertion, exiting behind the LCL, and is augmented with artificial tissue.

We do not believe that a static graft reconstruction of the popliteus musculotendinous unit can restore the dy-namic function of this nonisometric structure, and we have thus placed our primary emphasis on reconstruction of the LCL with plication of the arcuate and fabellofibular liga-ments, as described above. We reconstruct the LCL using Achilles tendon allograft with a 7- to 8-mm bone block fixed at the fibula with an interference screw (Fig. 66.2). The LCL is incised and elevated at its distal insertion, and the allograft tendon is fixed at the lateral femoral epi-condyle with suture anchors or transosseous sutures tied over a button medially. The native LCL is then tensioned and sutured to the graft.

If the popliteus is torn, its static component via the popliteofibular ligament is reconstructed with a semi-tendinosus autograft (Fig. 66.3). The double-limbed graft is fixed anatomically on the femur into a bone tunnel with an Endobutton (Acufex, Boston, MA) set at the medial

femoral condyle. It is passed deep to the LCL through a tunnel in the fibula, from posterior to anterior, where it is sutured to the soft tissues. Alternatively, a single strand of semitendinosus autograft may be looped through the fibula tunnel, with the posterior limb directed anteriorly deep to the LCL and the anterior limb directed posteri-orly, crossing superficial to the LCL. A cancellous screw with a soft tissue washer is inserted at the anatomic femoral insertion of the popliteus tendon, and both limbs of the graft are looped around the screw and fixed at the femur forming a figure eight.

Following reconstruction or repair, the knee is brought through a range of motion from 0° to 90° of flexion. The tourniquet is released and hemostasis is obtained. The wound is closed over suction drainage.

PITFALLS

The peroneal nerve lies directly posterior to the biceps tendon and may be injured by excessive retraction of the tendon or by misguided drilling at the fibula. The per-oneal nerve should be identified before beginning the re-pair and reconstruction procedures.

With chronic posterolateral instability, associated liga-mentous instability and malalignment are frequently pre-sent. The arcuate ligament complex, ACL, and PCL are intimately related in stabilizing the knee against anterior-posterior translation, varus-valgus rotation, and internal-

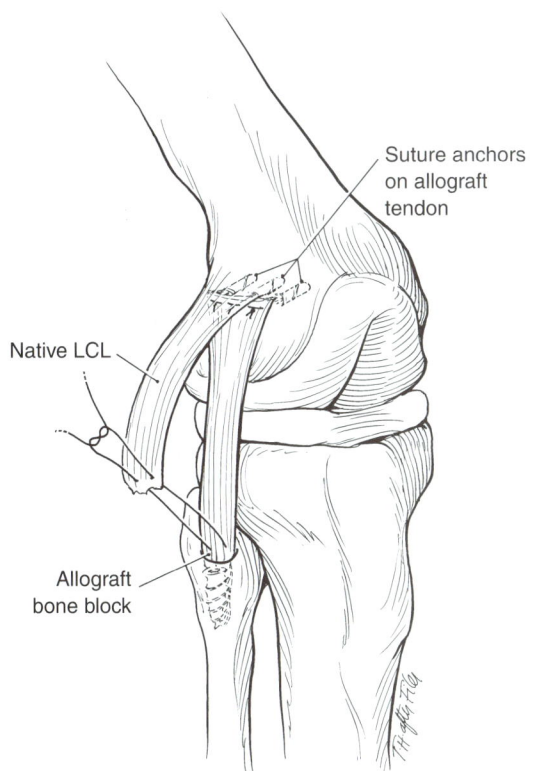

Figure 66.2. For the reconstruction of the LCL using an Achilles tendon allograft, the LCL is detached and elevated from its distal insertion. The allograft bone block is fixed in a tunnel at the fibula with an interference screw. The allograft tendon is then tensioned and repaired at the lateral femoral epicondyle with suture anchors. The native LCL is then tensioned and repaired to the graft.

external rotation, whereas varus deformity places increased stress on the arcuate ligament complex during gait. Varus deformity and associated ACL or PCL instability should be corrected before or with posterolateral reconstruction to prevent recurrent instability.

The goal of surgical repair or reconstruction is to restore the normal anatomy as best as possible. As such, proper graft placement on the femur is important. Nonanatomic graft placement cannot restore normal kinematics and will likely lead to graft stretching. After placement of the fibular portion of the graft, the proper site for graft placement on the femur is determined by using normal anatomic landmarks if present (e.g., stretched LCL or popliteus). Placement may be further guided by the use of a small pin at the selected insertion site and by observation of the tensioned graft in relation to this pin during knee range of motion to determine the most isometric position.

REHABILITATION

Immediately after surgery the knee is placed in full extension in a hinged knee brace, and quadriceps isometric exercises are begun. The knee is maintained in full extension for 4 weeks to allow graft healing; then range of motion is begun and progressed as tolerated. Patients ambulate with no weight bearing with the brace locked in full extension for 4 weeks. The brace may then be unlocked for am-

bulation, but the patient remains non-weight bearing for a total of 3 months. Active hamstring exercises are avoided for 4 months to prevent posterior translation and external rotation stresses. Postoperative rehabilitation may need to be modified, based on associated cruciate ligament injuries.

SUMMARY

Posterolateral instability is frequently associated with cruciate injury. Proper treatment requires an accurate diagnosis with attention directed toward detection of varus laxity; increased external rotation; the posterior drawer with the tibia in external rotation; and the posterolateral drawer, reverse pivot shift, and external rotation recurvatum tests. Acute injuries should be treated within 3 weeks of injury and may provide better results than chronic reconstruction. All injured structures and associated injuries should be repaired or reconstructed; emphasis should be placed on the LCL and the fibular attachment of the popliteus via the popliteofibular ligament. Postoperative rehabilitation emphasizes restoration of quadriceps strength while protecting the posterolateral structures by avoiding hyperextension and varus, posterior, and external rotation stresses.

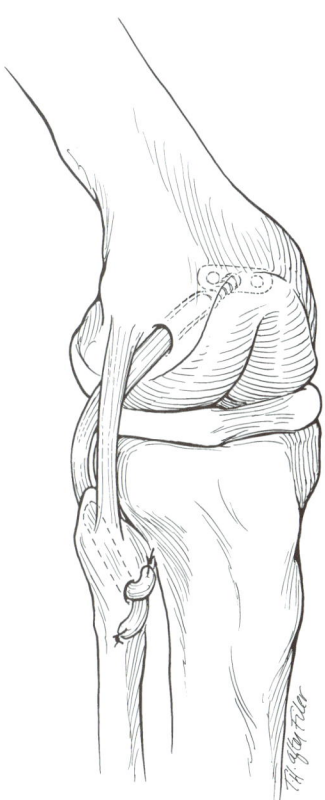

Figure 66.3. For the reconstruction of the popliteofibular ligament using a double-looped semitendinosus graft, the graft is anatomically fixed within a tunnel in the lateral femoral condyle with an Endobutton set at the medial femoral condyle. The graft is brought deep to the LCL and through a tunnel in the proximal fibula, from posterior to anterior, where the graft is sutured to the soft tissues.

REFERENCES

1. Hughston J, Jacobson K. Chronic posterolateral rotatory instability of the knee. J Bone Joint Surg 1985;67A:351–359.
2. Baker C, Norwood L, Hughston J. Acute posterolateral rotatory instability of the knee. J Bone Joint Surg 1983;65A:614–618.
3. Baker C, Norwood L, Hughston J. Acute combined posterior cruciate and posterolateral instability of the knee. Am J Sports Med 1984;12:204–208.
4. DeLee J, Riley M, Rockwood C. Acute posterolateral rotatory instability of the knee. Am J Sports Med 1983;11:199–206.
5. Seebacher JR, Inglis AE, Marshall JL, Warren RF. The structure of the posterolateral aspect of the knee. J Bone Joint Surg 1982;64A:536–541.
6. Grood E, Stower, S, Noyes, F. Limits of movement in the human knee. J Bone Joint Surg 1988;70A:88–97.
7. Veltri D, Warren R. Posterolateral instability of the knee. Instr Course Lect 1995;44:441–453.
8. Jakob R, Warner J. Lateral and posterolateral rotatory instability of the knee. In: DeLee J, Drez D Jr, eds. Orthopaedic sports medicine: principles and practice. Philadelphia: Saunders, 1994:1275–1312.
9. Gollehon D, Torzilli P, Warren R. The role of the posterolateral and cruciate ligaments in the stability of the human knee. J Bone Joint Surg 1987;69A:233–242.
10. Veltri D, Deng X, Torzilli P, et al. The role of the cruciate and posterolateral ligaments in stability of the knee. Am J Sports Med 1995;23:436–443.
11. Hughston J, Norwood L Jr. The posterolateral drawer test and external rotational recurvatum test for posterolateral rotatory instability of the knee. Clin Orthop 1980;147:82–87.
12. Jakob R, Hassler H, Staeubli H. Observations on rotatory instability of the lateral compartment of the knee. Acta Orthop Scand 1981;191(Suppl):1–32.
13. Cooper D. Tests for posterolateral instability of the knee in normal subjects. J Bone Joint Surg 1991;73A:30–36.
14. Ellsasser J, Reynolds F, Omohundro J. The nonoperative treatment of collateral ligament injuries of the knee in professional football players. J Bone Joint Surg 1974;56A:1185–1190.
15. Kannus P. Nonoperative treatment of grade II and III sprains of the lateral ligament compartment of the knee. Am J Sports Med 1989;17:83–88.
16. Clancy W Jr, Shelbourne K, Zoellner G, et al. Treatment of knee joint instability secondary to rupture of the posterior cruciate ligament. Report of a new procedure. J Bone Joint Surg 1983;65A:310–322.
17. Noyes FR, Barber-Westin SD. Surgical reconstruction of severe chronic posterolateral complex injuries of the knee using allograft tissues. Am J Sports Med 1995;23:2–12.

chapter 67

Peter T. Simonian, Claude T. Moorman III, and Thomas L. Wickiewicz

Knee Dislocation: Operative Repair and Reconstruction

Knee dislocation is a potentially devastating injury. This injury is generally the result of high-energy trauma with a high incidence of neurovascular injury. The initial management is centered on limb salvage and viability. Stabilization of ipsilateral fractures is the second priority. Finally, ligamentous knee stability is addressed.

Knee dislocation is defined as a complete disruption in the articulation of the tibia with the femur. These injuries are relatively unusual; the reported incidence is one per year at two major institutions (1,2). Some trauma centers experience more than eight per year (3). This discrepancy may represent a higher index of suspicion with improved recognition, rather than an actual increase in incidence. These injuries often spontaneously reduce or are reduced at the scene, resulting in a relatively benign appearance on presentation at the medical center. Information has been disseminated that enables clinicians to have a high suspicion for knee dislocation based on the history, multiplanar knee instability, and/or vascular compromise.

Most knee dislocations are the result of high-energy trauma; 20 to 30% are open injuries and the amputation rate ranges from 0 (low-velocity dislocation) to 85% (ischemic time more than 8 h) (1,4). Fracture of the ipsilateral extremity is reported in 32 to 40% of patients (5,6). Nerve injury is reported in 30 to 40% of patients, most commonly involving the peroneal nerve (6,7). Vascular injury generally involves the popliteal artery and is present in one-third of patients (range 4.8 to 64%) (1,8,9).

These injuries can be classified by the position of the tibia relative to the femur (directional) or by the energy level of the injury (low versus high velocity) (4,10). In the directional classification, anterior is the most common (31%) and is typically the result of a hyperextension mechanism. Posterior dislocation is seen in 25% of cases and occurs as posterior force is applied to the anterior tibia

with the knee flexed. Posterior dislocations are believed to require the greatest force. Lateral and medial dislocations are less common (13 and 5%, respectively) and are the result of valgus and varus forces, respectively. Combination rotary and directional forces make possible any number of additional injury patterns. Posterolateral dislocation is worthy of mention because of an anatomic feature affecting treatment. This is also known as the irreducible dislocation because of the tendency of the medial femoral condyle to buttonhole through a characteristic vertical tear in the capsule, resulting in a trap-door effect (11–14).

The incidence of associated injuries is also linked to the mechanism of injury. Anterior and posterior dislocations have a significantly increased incidence of vascular injury and are implicated in 39 to 50% of vascular injuries (2,15). The vascular injury pattern is usually an intimal tear in anterior dislocations and a complete transection in posterior dislocations (2,15). Peroneal nerve injury is highest in lateral and posterolateral dislocations.

Classification is also possible by energy level. A recent increase in dislocation secondary to athletic trauma has given rise to the term *low-velocity dislocation*, as distinct from the more devastating high-velocity dislocation associated with falls from a height and motor vehicle and industrial accidents (4). As would be expected, the incidence of associated injuries is less in the low-velocity group. The prognosis for recovery is likewise better.

It has been noted recently, in contrast to traditional opinion, that both cruciate ligaments do not have to be torn to permit dislocation. Several reports now detail the presence of an intact posterior cruciate ligament in completely dislocated knees. This has been noted in two series with a predominance of anterior dislocation. Anterior cruciate ligament integrity has been noted in three of eight patients sustaining posterolateral dislocations (16–18).

RELEVANT ANATOMY AND PATHOGENESIS

Knee dislocation can result in injury to the anterior cruciate ligament, the posterior cruciate ligament, the medial collateral ligament, the lateral collateral ligament, the posterolateral complex, the capsule, the extensor mechanism, the menisci, and the articular surface. Multiple ligament reconstructions require a thorough understanding of the regional anatomy.

The tibial insertion of the anterior cruciate ligament is a broad, irregular, diamond-shaped area located directly in front of the intercondylar eminence of the tibia. The femoral attachment of the ligament is a semicircular area on the posteromedial aspect of the lateral femoral condyle. It is about 33 mm in length and 11 mm in diameter. It is composed of two bundles: the anteromedial, which tightens in flexion, and the posterolateral, which tightens in extension.

The posterior cruciate ligament inserts in a sulcus posteriorly, below the articular surface of the tibia, and originates in a broad half-moon or crescent-shaped area anterolaterally on the medial femoral condyle. It is approximately 38 mm in length and 13 mm in diameter. It also is composed of two bundles: the anterolateral, which tightens in flexion, and the posteromedial, which tightens in extension.

The lateral collateral ligament is a cord-like structure that originates on the lateral femoral epicondyle, posterior and superior to the popliteus tendon, and inserts on the lateral aspect of the fibular head. Because it is posterior to the axis of rotation, it is tightest in full extension and loosens in flexion. Lateral structures of the knee have been described in three layers: (a) lateral fascia, iliotibial tract, and biceps tendon; (b) patellar retinaculum and patellofemoral ligament; and (c) capsule, arcuate ligament, and fabellofibular ligament. Anatomic variations exist with both the arcuate and the fabellofibular ligament; both are present 67% of the time, the fabellofibular alone 20% of the time, and the arcuate alone 13% of the time. If a fabella is present, then typically there is a large fabellofibular ligament. If the fabella is absent, then typically there is a large arcuate ligament. The posterolateral part of the capsule is divided into two laminae that encompass the lateral collateral, the fabellofibular, and the arcuate ligament (19). The popliteus serves as a primary restraint to external rotation; it has both a static and a dynamic role. The popliteofibular ligament, a static restraint that attaches from the popliteal tendon to the fibular head, has recently been found to contribute to posterolateral stability (20).

The medial collateral ligament is a broad, flat ligament composed of separate superficial and deep portions. The superficial ligament is deep to the semitendinosus and gracilis tendons and fascia. It originates at the medial femoral epicondyle and inserts distally into the periosteum of the proximal tibia; its primary insertion is deep to the pes anserinus. The anterior fibers tighten during the first 90° of flexion, and the posterior fibers tighten in extension. The medial structures have been described in three layers: (a) sartorius and sartorius fascia; (b) superficial medial collateral ligament, posterior oblique ligament, and semimembranosus; and (c) deep medial collateral ligament and capsule.

The vascular anatomy of the knee plays an important role in determining the sequelae of arterial injury in knee dislocation. The popliteal artery, the direct continuation of the femoral artery, is tethered proximally to the femur in the adductor hiatus and distally to the fibula by the fibrous bands of the soleus fascia (1) (Fig. 67.1). Both of these points serve as tethers and are common sites of injury. Of 10 arterial injuries in one series, 2 (20%) occurred at the proximal tether, 5 (50%) occurred distally, and 2 (20%) occurred between these two points (8). The five genicular arteries arise from the artery within the popliteal space, though they provide for poor anastomotic channels through the superficial femoral and anterior tibial arteries. These anastomoses generally do not provide adequate flow to ensure limb survival; amputation rates in acute injury without revascularization approach 75% (21).

Neurologic injury is often an associated injury in knee dislocation. The common peroneal nerve descends first along the lateral side of the popliteal fossa, overlapped by the medial margin of the biceps femoris; then it passes be-

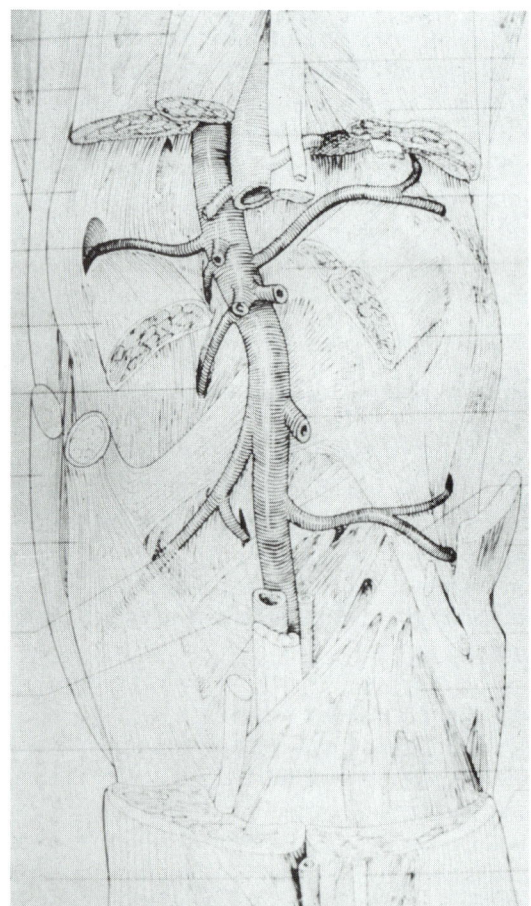

Figure 67.1. Popliteal artery.

tween the biceps tendon and the lateral head of the gastrocnemius muscle to reach the back of the fibular head. Finally, it winds around the back of the neck of the fibula between the two heads of the peroneus longus muscle and divides into the superficial and deep peroneal nerves. Peroneal nerve injury is the most common, though injury may be seen in any of the distal peripheral nerves (4).

INITIAL FINDINGS, PHYSICAL EXAMINATION, AND DIAGNOSIS

Management of the patient with a knee dislocation is initiated in the same manner as for any multitrauma patient. This begins with ensuring an adequate airway, breathing, and cardiac output. The clinician should also consider obtaining trauma series radiographs—lateral cervical spine, AP chest, and AP pelvis—if the injury was the result of high energy. The next priority is extremity perfusion and viability. This is assessed first by palpation of the dorsalis pedis and posterior tibial pulses. Neurologic evaluation is also crucial, both before and after reduction. If the knee is dislocated on presentation, reduction is generally possible with gentle traction. If the vascular supply has been compromised for a period of time, the clinician must be vigilant of compartment syndrome after the extremity is revascularized. The skeletal and soft tissue integrity must be evaluated. The ipsilateral hip and ankle joints must also be carefully evaluated.

With the airway, breathing, and cardiac status stabilized and the secondary survey completed, the vascular status of the limb becomes the primary focus. Arteriography is justified in all cases of knee dislocation, even if pulses are normal. Physical examination should initially focus on evaluation of pulses. Normal pulses do not rule out injury (15,22). Significant injury to the popliteal artery has been reported in 10 to 50% of patients with palpable distal pulses (15,22). A warm but pulseless foot should not be observed (1,15,22). Absent pulses should likewise not be attributed to spasm, since diminished or absent pulses in knee dislocations almost always result from a true injury to the vessel (1). Even with perfusion of the skin and superficial tissue, the metabolic demands of the muscle are great, and necrosis can occur. The need for reperfusion within 6 h of a compromised extremity is recognized.

As noted, neurologic injury is often associated injury in knee dislocation, and the peroneal nerve is the most commonly affected nerve (4). Injury to the peroneal nerve is present in about one-third of patients; the reported range is 10 to 43% (4,6,13). Injury to this nerve has a particularly grave prognosis, and axonal injury occurs in 50% of cases. Less than half will recover nerve function (2,6,7). Results of nerve decompression and/or repair are not predictable (2,6,7). Peroneal nerve injuries appear to be more common in lateral and posterolateral dislocations.

After the vascular and neurologic statuses have been addressed, ipsilateral fractures about the knee are stabilized next. Care must be taken to avoid traction on vascular repairs during stabilization. Fractures and concomitant dislocation of the ipsilateral extremity round out the triad of commonly associated injuries in knee dislocation (5,6). The incidence of associated avulsion (ligament), plateau, or diaphyseal fracture of the femur or tibia is high in knee dislocation. Patellar fractures have also been reported. The incidence of associated fracture appears to be between 30 and 40% (5,6). Fractures must be stabilized to allow for a scaffold for ligament reconstruction. In the case of ligament avulsion, ligamentous stability can be restored simply with reduction and fixation of the avulsed bone (6).

Physical examination of the anterior cruciate ligament is best done with the Lachman test, at 30° of flexion. Both the amount of excursion and the end point are evaluated. The examiner should also be suspicious of posterior cruciate insufficiency when doing the Lachman test. Significant anterior excursion with a firm end point may indicate that the starting point was subluxated posteriorly, incriminating an injury to either the posterior cruciate ligament, the posterolateral complex, or both. The pivot shift and pivot jerk tests may also be used. The posterior cruciate ligament is best evaluated by the posterior drawer test, at 90° of flexion, compared with the drop back of a typical tibial tubercle with respect to the opposite knee flexed at 90°. The quadriceps active test done in 70° of flexion and the posterior sag sign can help confirm a posterior cruciate injury. The reverse pivot shift may also be used. In the multiligament injured knee, the pivot and reverse pivot shift tests may not be helpful because both require a stable medial hinge (the superficial medial collateral ligament), which may be disrupted.

Evaluation of the lateral and posterolateral corner is performed by stressing the knee into varus in extension and 30° of flexion and by subjecting the tibia to external rotation at 30° and 90° of flexion. The primary restraint to varus stress is the lateral collateral ligament. Injury to only this structure and an intact popliteal complex will not lead to significant increases in the joint opening to varus stress. The posterolateral complex (i.e., the lateral collateral ligament and popliteus) resists external rotation of the tibia with respect to the femur. In isolated injuries, the amount of excursion is maximal at 30° of flexion, without significant increases at greater degrees of flexion. The posterolateral drawer test can also indicate an injury to the posterolateral complex. A positive posterolateral drawer test would demonstrate increased varus and hypertension with internal tibial rotation while both heels are held in the air.

The external rotation recurvatum test can also be used to evaluate posterolateral instability. A positive test demonstrates increased varus and hyperextension with internal tibial rotation while both heels are held in the air. Combination injuries with the posterior cruciate ligament demonstrate increased rotation with increased knee flexion. Isolated posterior cruciate ligament injuries with an intact posterolateral corner do not lead either to an increase in external rotation or to a positive reverse pivot shift test.

Stability of the medial side is evaluated both in extension and in 30° of flexion. The primary restraint is the superficial medial collateral ligament. Instability in extension, whether to varus or valgus stress, incriminates disruption to the cruciate ligaments.

RADIOLOGIC STUDIES

Diagnostic studies begin with plain radiographs, which identify frank dislocation; however, frank dislocation should be reduced immediately based on the initial clinical examination, before radiographs are obtained, especially when vascular compromise is evident. Radiographs also identify subluxation of the knee, associated fractures about the knee, and effusion. Dislocation of ipsilateral joints is an unusual phenomenon, which has been reported with increasing frequency in the recent literature. These dislocations may involve the ankle, the hip, or the proximal tibiofibular joint (23–26). The importance of radiographic evaluation of the joint above and below the knee is emphasized to avoid overlooking these injuries.

Additional Studies

Further workup of arterial injury beyond examination is controversial, particularly in the case of normal pulses. Some researchers have advocated serial examination and Doppler evaluation with calculation of ankle-brachial indices and comparisons with the opposite side. Concern with this approach centers on a report of 16% false-negative results with Doppler ankle-brachial indices as a screening tool (27). Many authors have recommended arteriography in all cases of knee dislocation (24,28–30). In the case of diminished or absent pulses following reduction, some authors have advocated immediate exploration without the delay inherent in proceeding with arteriography (1,6,31). This philosophy stems from amputation rates of greater than 80% when revascularization is delayed more than 8 h (1). Snyder (32) noted treatment time nearly doubled (6.5 h versus 3.7 h) when surgery was delayed for arteriography. Other authors have suggested intraoperative arteriography as a means of obtaining the same information more expeditiously (8,31). Intraoperative arteriography can be carried out with injection of 45 mL contrast through an 18-gauge catheter with a single-film exposure (8). Communication among the orthopaedic surgeon, general surgeon, vascular surgeon, and the radiologist is critical in developing a workable philosophy for making these decisions at each institution.

MRI can also be used to help operative planning. MRI has been shown to better predict the extent of soft tissue injury than does physical examination alone for the knee with multiple ligament injuries. An exception was decreased MRI visualization and accuracy of predicting injury to the lateral collateral ligament and the posterolateral capsule (33).

TREATMENT

Nonoperative Alternatives and Indications for Surgery

Management of ligamentous disruption in knee dislocation has been controversial. Reported series are small in number and have different management protocols, minimal follow-up, and different evaluation criteria (5,6,8,12,23,24,34–36). Several studies, however, support the role for nonoperative management. The majority of nonoperative treatments have included periods of immobilization and cast braces. Taylor et al. (35) reported good results in 26 patients treated nonoperatively and poor results in 13 patients treated surgically. They concluded that nonoperative treatment is as good as or better than operative treatment. The major problem with this work was patient selection. The group treated surgically often had more severe or associated injuries. We concur that a direct comparison between the two groups was not possible and that nonoperative treatment is preferred for dislocation in the absence of complications. Reckling and Pelteir (12) reported a series of 15 cases with good results of nonoperative treatment in anterior and posterior dislocations. Thomsen et al. (36) reported 10 patients and concluded that good knee function was achievable with either operative or nonoperative treatment. Almekinders et al. (34) support nonoperative treatment.

Operative Treatment

The majority of authors believe that operative management is the treatment of choice for multiple ligament injuries after knee dislocation (2,3,5,6,8,9,13,23,24). Before surgical intervention, a thorough examination under anesthesia should be done.

APPROACH

The philosophy for ligament reconstruction is based on two principles: Early motion and mobilization are the common denominators of success, and stabilization of all instability patterns provides the optimal platform for early motion. The surgical approach, whether open or arthroscopic, is dictated by the pathology and the comfort level of the surgeon (Clinical Table). Within a few days, capsular structures will form a seal to allow arthroscopy. The arthroscopic approach facilitates intra-articular reconstruction, including the anterior and posterior cruciate ligaments, and management of chondral and meniscal injuries. Accessory incisions can be used medial and lateral for collateral ligament surgery. When an open approach is used, the entire reconstruction may be done through a single utilitarian incision.

PROCEDURE

When an open approach is chosen, a utility incision that crosses distally over the anterior aspect of the knee in a medial direction is made proximally and laterally so that

Clinical Table: Knee Dislocation: Operative Repair and Reconstruction

Procedure	Indications	Technique	Anatomy	Pitfalls
		Anterior Cruciate Ligament		
Repair	• Bone avulsion	• Open reduction and internal fixation • Sutures to bone	• Anterior cruciate ligament insertion and origin	• Failure • Ligament stretched
Augmentation	• Partial injury • Support repair	• Autologous tissue: hamstrings	• Anterior cruciate ligament insertion and origin	• Failure • Ligament stretched
Reconstruction	• Complete disruption	• Autologous tissue: hamstrings	• Two bundles	• Anterior femoral tunnel
		Posterior Cruciate Ligament		
Repair	• Bone avulsion	• Open reduction and internal fixation • Sutures to bone	• Popliteal vessels • Tibial and peroneal nerves	• Failure • Ligament stretched
Augmentation	• Partial injury • Support repair	• Autologous tissue: hamstrings • Allograft tissue: Achilles tendon	• Popliteal vessels • Tibial and peroneal nerves	• Failure • Ligament stretched
Reconstruction	• Complete disruption	• Autologous or allograft tissue: patella • Allograft tissue: Achilles tendon • 1 or 2 femoral tunnels	• Popliteal vessels • Tibial and peroneal nerves • Two bundles	• Acute turns of graft in tunnels
		Lateral Collateral Ligament		
Repair	• Acute injury • Good tissue	• Open reduction and internal fixation • Sutures to bone	• Peroneal nerve • Tightest in extension	• Failure • Ligament stretched
Augmentation	• Partial injury • Support repair	• Biceps aponeurosis • Iliotibial band	• Peroneal nerve • Tightest in extension	• Posterior to axis of rotation
Reconstruction	• Complete disruption • Poor tissue	• Autologous tissue: hamstrings • Allograft tissue: Achilles tendon	• Peroneal nerve • Tightest in extension	• Posterior to axis of rotation
		Posterolateral		
Repair	• Acute injury • Good tissue	• Sutures to bone	• Peroneal nerve • Three layers	• Failure • Unrecognized damage to structures
Augmentation	• Partial injury • Support repair	• Autologous tissue: hamstrings • Allograft tissue: Achilles tendon	• Peroneal nerve • Three layers	• Failure • Unrecognized damage to structures
Reconstruction	• Complete disruption • Poor tissue	• Allograft tissue: Achilles tendon	• Peroneal nerve • Three layers	• Failure to understand anatomy
		Medial Collateral Ligament		
Repair	• Acute injury • Good tissue	• Sutures to bone	• Superficial and deep • Deep to pes anserinus	• Failure • Ligament stretched
Augmentation	• Partial injury • Support repair	• Autologous tissue: hamstrings • Attach distally	• Femoral isometric point • Three layers	• Isometry
Reconstruction	• Chronic injury • Poor tissue	• Autologous tissue: hamstrings • Attach distally	• Femoral isometric point • Three layers	• Isometry

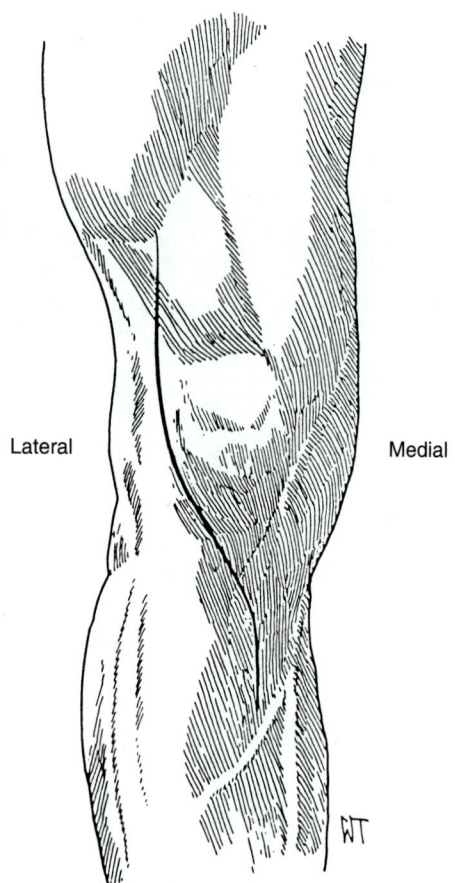

Lateral   Medial

Figure 67.2. Incision for the open approach. Reprinted with permission from Insall JN, ed. Surgery of the knee. New York: Churchill Livingstone, 1984.

the incision crosses between the patella and the tibial tubercle, allowing for ligament reconstruction of both cruciate ligaments and approaches to both the medial and the lateral side of the knee through one incision (Fig. 67.2). This does necessitate elevation of skin flaps. This approach allows access to the anteromedial tibia for anterior cruciate or posterior cruciate ligament drill hole preparation and to the posterolateral corner of the knee for repair and augmentation procedures. With the knee exposed in this manner, access to the cruciate ligaments is similar to that during arthroplasty. The tibia may be subluxated anteriorly to allow for easier exposure to the posterior tibia for tunnel placement.

Graft options are another consideration. Primary repair should be considered in the proper situation. These include avulsions to the cruciate ligaments with good bulk or bone, injuries to the medial side, lateral side avulsions from the femur or fibula, and avulsions of the iliotibial band. Injury patterns to the popliteus may be repaired, but it can be difficult to predict the degree of injury at the muscle tendon junction, and thus the repair may fail.

After repair, augmentation is often reasonable. The hamstring tendons are an excellent source of collagen for medial side injuries, repaired cruciate ligaments, and the popliteal ligament complex (Fig. 67.3). Augmentation of the lateral collateral ligament can use the aponeurosis of the biceps femoris, which can be harvested, left attached to the fibula, and brought to the femoral origin (Fig. 67.4). The iliotibial band may also be used, but we do not favor it.

Reconstruction is the third option and can be done with autologous and allograft tissue (Fig. 67.5). Autogenous reconstructions are performed with the central third bone-patellar tendon-bone or hamstrings from the injured and/or contralateral extremity. Allograft reconstructions use predominantly patellar or Achilles tendon with their respective bone blocks. If the patient will not allow the use of allograft material, then a typical reconstruction includes hamstring autograft for the anterior cruciate ligament, patellar tendon autograft for the posterior cruciate ligament, repair and augmentation of the posterolateral structures with biceps fascia and/or hamstring tendons, and direct repair of the medial side. If the tissue graft sources are unlimited, we prefer to reconstruct the cruciate ligaments with patellar and Achilles tendon allografts. The medial side is directly repaired and is augmented with autologous hamstrings. The lateral side is repaired when possible, and the popliteal complex is augmented with autologous hamstrings or allograft Achilles tendon.

Individual ligament reconstructions are done in standard fashion. Regarding the anterior cruciate ligament, endoscopic fixation techniques can be used arthroscopically. When using an open technique, the surgeon can use endoscopy, or the femoral tunnel can be drilled using an outside-in technique. Similarly, the posterior cruciate ligament can be reconstructed with either an endoscopic or an open technique. Access to the posterior tibia is often present with multiligament reconstructions; in these cases, fixation of the tibial portion of the posterior cruciate ligament into a slot in the tibia, thus eliminating the acute angles needed in the conventional tibial tunnels, should be considered. The fixation in the slot is augmented with a screw. If this technique is used, the tibial portion of the graft must be secured first in an anatomic location. Reconstruction then proceeds to either one or two tunnels in the femur. When tensioning the grafts, the knee is placed in extension to maximize the stability of the bone contours of the joint.

SUMMARY

Knee dislocation is a potentially devastating injury that requires surgeon and therapist skills and patient motivation to achieve a functional outcome. The initial management focuses on vascular, neurologic, and bony injury. Management of the complex ligament injuries is best accomplished after arterial repair and skeletal stabilization. Motion is started immediately after reconstruction. Recovery is slow, and return to normal activities may be prolonged.

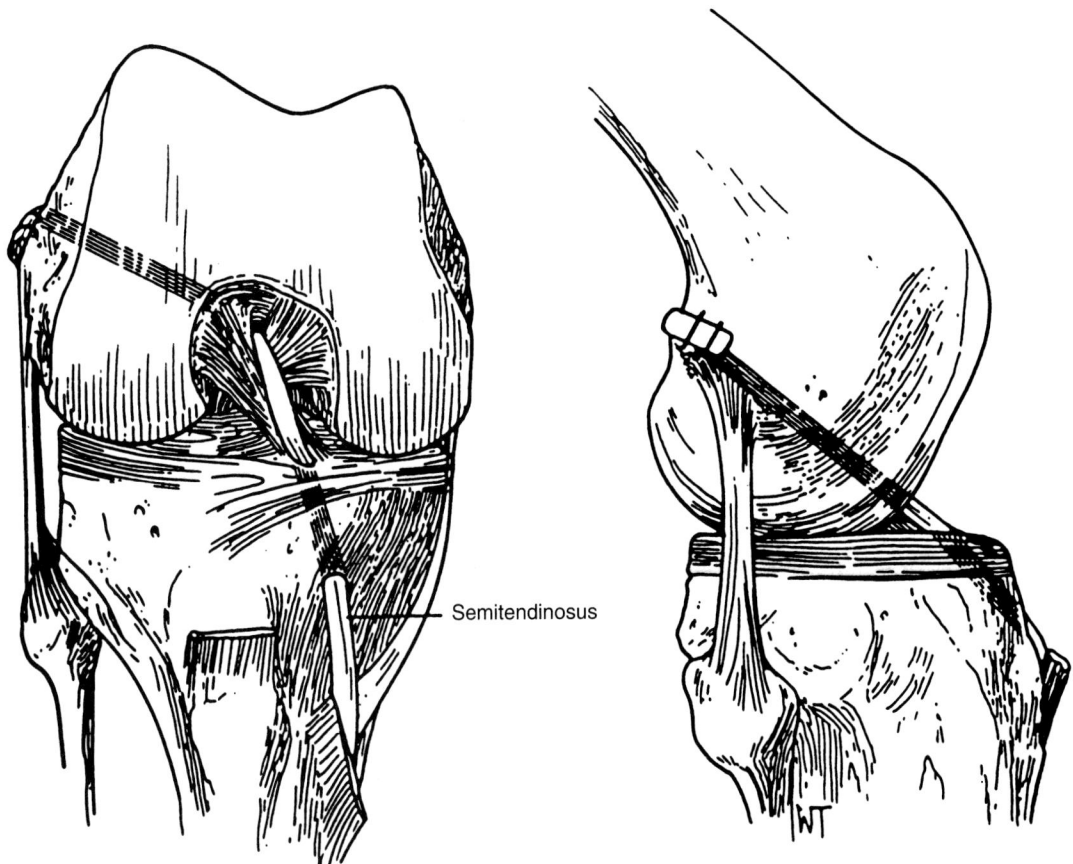

Figure 67.3. Repaired cruciate ligaments. Reprinted with permission from Insall JN, ed. Surgery of the knee. New York: Churchill Livingstone, 1984.

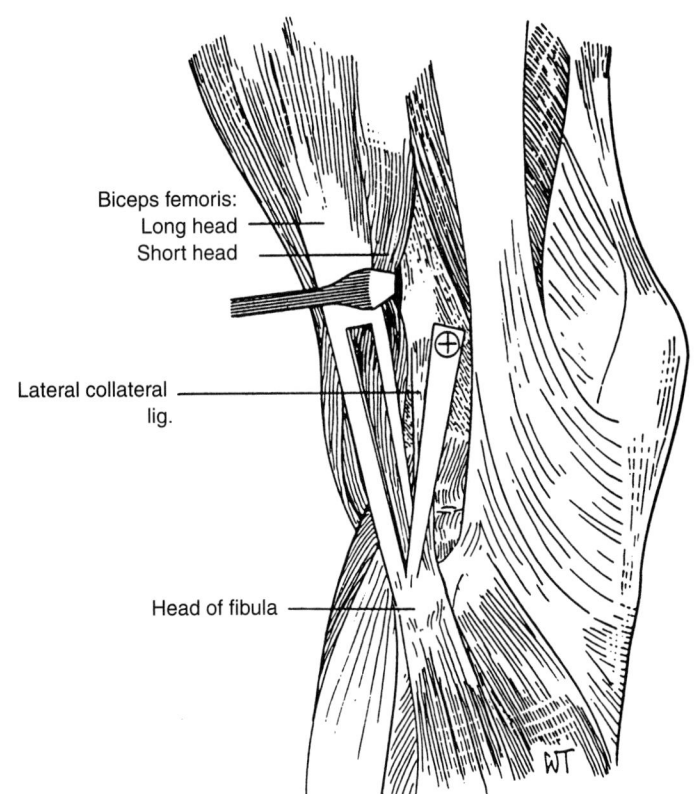

Figure 67.4. Augmentation of the lateral collateral ligament with the aponeurosis of the biceps femoris. Reprinted with permission from Insall JN, ed. Surgery of the knee. New York: Churchill Livingstone, 1984.

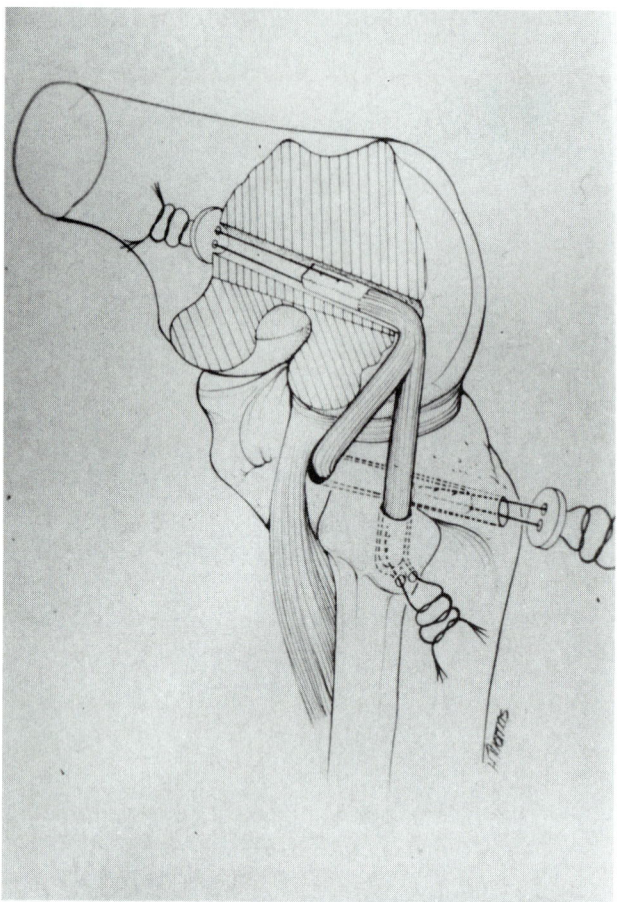

Figure 67.5. When the popliteus is irreparable, substitution with graft material is the preferred technique. Reprinted with permission from Bowen MK, Warren RF, Cooper DE. In: Insall JN, ed. Surgery of the knee. New York: Churchill Livingstone, 1993:505–554.

REFERENCES

1. Green NE, Allen BL. Vascular injuries associated with dislocation of the knee. J Bone Joint Surg 1977;59A:236–239.
2. Shields L, Mital M, Cave EF. Complete dislocation of the knee: experience at the Massachusetts General Hospital. J Trauma 1969;9:192–215.
3. Meyers MH, Moore TM, Harvey JP Jr. Traumatic dislocation of the knee joint. J Bone Joint Surg 1975;57A:430–433.
4. Shelbourne KD, Porter DA, Clingman JA, et al. Low-velocity knee dislocation. Orthop Rev 1991;20:995–1004.
5. Jones RE, Smith EC, Bone GE. Vascular and orthopedic complications of knee dislocation. Surg Gynecol Obstet 1979;149:554–558.
6. Sisto DJ, Warren RF. Complete knee dislocation. A follow-up study of operative treatment. Clin Orthop 1985;198:94–101.
7. Marks PH, Harner CD. The anterior cruciate ligament in the multiple ligament-injured knee. Clin Sports Med 1993;12:825–838.
8. Frassica FJ, Sim FH, Staeheli JW, Pairolero PC. Dislocation of the knee. Clin Orthop 1991;263:200–205.
9. Meyers MH, Harvey JP Jr. Traumatic dislocation of the knee joint. A study of eighteen cases. J Bone Joint Surg 1971;53A:16–29.
10. Montgomery JB. Dislocation of the knee. Orthop Clin North Am 1987;18:149–156.
11. Nystrom M, Samimi S, Ha'Eri GB. Two cases of irreducible knee dislocation occurring simultaneously in two patients and a review of the literature. Clin Orthop 1992;277:197–200.
12. Reckling FW, Pelteir LF. Acute knee dislocations and their complications. J Trauma 1969;9:181–191.
13. Roman PD, Hopson CN, Zenni EJ Jr. Traumatic dislocation of the knee: a report of 30 cases and literature review. Orthop Rev 1987;16:917–924.
14. Samimi S, Shahriaree H. Arthroscopic view of an irreducible knee dislocation. Arthroscopy 1993;9:322–326.
15. Welling RE, Kakkasseril J, Cranley JJ. Complete dislocations of the knee with popliteal vascular injury. J Trauma 1981;21:450–453.
16. Bratt HD, Newman AP. Complete dislocation of the knee without disruption of both cruciate ligaments. J Trauma 1993;34:383–389.
17. Cooper DE. Tests for posterolateral instability of the knee in normal subjects. Results of examination under anesthesia. J Bone Joint Surg 1991;73A:30–36.
18. Shelbourne KD, Pritchard J, Rettig AC, et al. Knee dislocations with intact PCL. Orthop Rev 1992;21:607–611.
19. Seebacher JR, Inglis AE, Marshall JL, Warren RF. The structure of the posterolateral aspect of the knee. J Bone Joint Surg 1982;64A:536–541.
20. Maynard MJ, Deng X, Wickiewicz TL, Warren RF. The popliteofibular ligament. Rediscovery of a key element in posterolateral stability. Am J Sports Med 1996;24:311–316.
21. DeBakey M, Simeone F. Battle injuries of the arteries in World War II. Ann Surg 1946;123:534–579.
22. Peck JJ, Eastman AB, Bergan JJ, et al. Popliteal vascular trauma. A community experience. Arch Surg 1990;125:1339–1343.
23. Fallon P, Virani NS, Bell D, Hollinshead R. Delayed presentation: dislocation of the proximal tibiofibular joint after knee dislocation. J Orthop Trauma 1994;8:350–353.
24. Freedman DM, Freedman EL, Shapiro MS. Ipsilateral hip and knee dislocation. J Orthop Trauma 1994;8:177–180.
25. Manaster BJ, Andrews CL. Fractures and dislocations of the knee and proximal tibia and fibula. Semin Roentgenol 1994;29:113–133.
26. Millea TP, Romanelli RR, Segal LS, Lynch CJ. Ipsilateral fracture-dislocation of the hip, knee, and ankle: case report. J Trauma 1991;31:416–419.
27. Bishara RA, Pasch AR, Lim LT, et al. Improved results in the treatment of civilian vascular injuries associated with fractures and dislocations. J Vasc Surg 1986;3:707–711.
28. Kremchek TE, Welling RE, Kremchek EJ. Traumatic dislocation of the knee. Orthop Rev 1989;18:1051–1057.
29. McCoy GF, Hannon DG, Barr RJ, Templeton J. Vascular injury associated with low-velocity dislocations of the knee. J Bone Joint Surg 1987;69B:285–287.
30. McNeil JW, McGee GS. Popliteal artery injury in a lumberjack. South Med J 1994;87:958–960.
31. Merrill KD. Knee dislocations with vascular injuries. Orthop Clin North Am 1994;25:707–713.
32. Snyder W. Vascular injuries near the knee: An updated series and overview of the problem. Surgery 1982;91:502–506.
33. Twaddle BC, Hunter JC, Chapman JR, et al. MRI in acute knee dislocation. J Bone Joint Surg 1996;78B:573–579.
34. Almekinders LC, Logan TC. Results following treatment of traumatic dislocations of the knee joint. Clin Orthop 1992;284:203–207.
35. Taylor AR, Arden GP, Rainey HA. Traumatic dislocation of the knee. A report of forty-three cases with special reference to conservative treatment. J Bone Joint Surg 1974;54B:96–102.
36. Thomsen PB, Rud B, Jensen UH. Stability and motion after traumatic dislocation of the knee. Acta Orthop Scand 1984;55:278–283.

chapter 68

Dale J. Federico

Tendinopathies of the Knee

Tendons are an integral portion of the muscle–tendon unit, connecting muscle to bone and assisting in both dynamic and static function of the joint. By far the most common tendon injuries are a response to overuse or trauma. Approximately 30% of all sports-related injuries in the United States are associated with overuse (1), and close to 33% of all outpatient sports injuries are related to the knee. Males have a significantly higher incidence of tendon injuries than do females (4 to 7 times greater) (2). These overuse injuries are affected by both intrinsic and extrinsic factors (3) (Table 68.1).

Treatment of these injuries depends on the extent of the injury, the quality of the structure, the amount of displacement, and the amount of residual function available (Table 68.2). Complete tendon ruptures require surgical repair. Incomplete ruptures and partial tendon injuries that do not respond to nonoperative care can be treated with operative intervention. Operative treatment for chronic tendinitis, without evidence of tear, can be performed based on lack of improvement in pain or performance, despite appropriate nonoperative care (4). Surgery for chronic overuse tendinopathies is usually considered as a last resort. Tendinopathies of the knee include extensor tendon injuries (patellar and quadriceps tendon) and flexor tendon injuries (hamstrings and popliteal tendon). This chapter discusses extensor tendon injuries.

PATHOPHYSIOLOGY

Tendons are relatively avascular, containing approximately 68% water, 30% collagen, and 2% elastin (5). They are deformable and strong and are able to sustain great tensile stresses. The wavy configuration of tendons noted via electron microscopy disappears at approximately 2% of stretch. The elastic quality of tendons is lost at greater than 4% of stretch; and cross-linkages within the fiber fail, and microfibril failure begins, between 4 and 8% of stretch. Maximum load to failure and tear resistance decrease with age and in the presence of preexisting injuries (e.g., recur-

rent tendinitis) and intrinsic problems (e.g., collagen-vascular diseases) (6).

Patellar Tendon Injuries

Patellar tendinitis, patellar ruptures, and patellar avulsions usually occur in patients younger than 40 years. Patellar tendinitis, or jumper's knee, is a condition that affects athletes involved in repetitive activities, such as jumping and running, and is related to overuse of the quadriceps. The mechanism of these tendon injuries occurs primarily with eccentric loading of the knee. The high tension generated during eccentric activity (lengthening of the muscle fibril while it is contracting) leads to failure of the tendon fibers. This failure can occur at the microscopic or macroscopic level.

Patients usually complain of tenderness and pain at the inferior pole of the patella. On occasion, they describe tenderness near the insertion of the tibial tubercle or within the substance of the tendon. Localized swelling can be seen in the tender area. Occasionally, a palpable defect can be felt. Patients may have pain with resistive activities of the quadriceps musculature, which can be tested by physical examination. Symptoms may be present during the activity, immediately after the activity, or at some time after the activity. With tendonitis the onset of pain is usually gradual and insidious, whereas with partial or complete tendon ruptures the onset of pain is acute and significant.

The differential diagnosis should include Sinding-Larsen-Johansson syndrome (apophysitis of the inferior pole of the patella) and Osgood-Schlatter disease (apophysitis of the tibial tubercle). Fractures of the patella and the tibial tubercle are also included in the differential diagnosis.

As noted, tendon ruptures are accompanied by immediate and significant pain. Patients with complete ruptures classically describe the pain as similar to having been kicked in the tendon (sharp, distinct, and acute). On physical examination a distinct palpable defect can be felt directly inferior to the patella. Leg extension is limited, if not absent.

Radiographic examination may be normal with acute or chronic tendinopathies. Ossicles or bone spurs may be seen within the substance of the tendon, usually near its origin or insertion. Patellar fractures and tibial tubercle avulsion injuries will be evident on plain radiographs. In patients with tendon ruptures, the patella may be high riding, increasing the Insall-Salvati index (7). Ultrasonography helps in the evaluation of tendinopathies, especially in the presence of tendon sheath swelling or intrasubstance degeneration.

MRI is extremely helpful for the evaluation of soft tissue injuries. MRI can differentiate intrasubstance tears, degeneration, and peritenon swelling. A MRI study is indicated if there is a question about the diagnosis and in chronic situations when the patient is not improving. MRI studies are not necessary for making the diagnosis of an acute rupture

For the patients who have tendinopathies and not true distinct tendon ruptures, conservative treatment should be used. Anti-inflammatories, rest, elevation, compression bandage, and ice can help decrease the patient's symptoms. Once the symptoms have decreased enough to allow the patient to function, a course of physical therapy to strengthen the knee is beneficial. Other modalities, such as ultrasound, ionophoresis, and photophoresis, may also be useful.

Surgical treatment is reserved for patients with acute ruptures, patients who have not had significant improvement with conservative measures, and those with intrasubstance degeneration of a tendon.

Osgood-Schlatter Disease

Osgood-Schlatter disease primarily affects athletically active adolescents and preteens. It is usually found at the level of the tibial tubercle and has been described as an apophysitis, not a tendinitis. In Osgood-Schlatter patients, repetitive tensile strength from the quadriceps musculature results in avulsions at the secondary ossification site

table	68.1	Overuse Tendon Injuries

Intrinsic	Extrinsic
Management	Training errors
Excessive pronation	Distance
Femoral anteversion	Intensity
Limb length discrepancy	Hill work
Muscular imbalance	Technique
Muscular insufficiency	Fatigue
	Surfaces
	Environmental conditions
	Footwear and equipment

Modified from Renstrom P, Johnson RJ. Overuse injuries in sports: a review. Sports Med 1985;2:316–333.

table	68.2	Tendinopathies of the Knee

Injury	Pathophysiology	Physical Examination	Treatment	Technique	Pitfalls
Patellar tendon rupture	<40 years old Eccentric loading Sharp, distinct, acute pain	Palpable defect No active extension	Surgery	Midline approach Débride mucoid tissue and frayed tendon ends	Inadequate repair Patella infera ends
Patellar tendinitis	Repetitive eccentric loading activities Gradual onset	Localized swelling Pain with resistive extension	Symptomatic NSAIDs Rest Physical therapy	Débride unhealed lesion Reinforce tendon	Inadequate débridement Weaken tendon Secondary rupture Surgery if failed treatment
Osgood-Schlatter disease	Adolescent or preteen Tibial tubercle apophysitis or avulsion	Local tenderness Ossicle may be present	Symptomatic Rest Cast if severe Surgery if tubercle avulsion or adult with painful ossicle	Midline approach Shell out ossicle	Damage to tendon
Sinding-Larsen-Johansson syndrome	Adolescent or preteen Inferior patellar pole	Local tenderness Pain with resistive extension	Symptomatic Rest Cast if severe Surgery if patellar occlusion or adult with painful ossicle	Midline approach Shell out ossicle	Damage to tendon
Quadriceps tendon rupture	>40 years old Eccentric loading Systemic disease or degenerative joint disease Sharp severe pain	Palpable defect No active extension	Surgery	Midline approach Repair retinaculum Débride defect Evaluate intra-articular extent	Intra-articular damage

NSAIDs, nonsteroidal anti-inflammatory drugs.

of the immature tibial tuberosity (8). This apophysitis is an acute and inflammatory response and may result in fragmentation of cartilage and/or bone. The fragmentation may develop into an ossicle that can be seen on radiographs. In severe situations, the apophysitis may present as a fracture of the tibial tubercle, leading to displacement of the fragment.

Initial treatment consists of symptomatic relief of pain. Ice, rest, anti-inflammatory medications, and quadriceps stretching exercises can decrease the pain. Protective pads can also be used to limit the amount of direct impact to the prominent tibial tubercle. Complete resolution of symptoms usually occurs within 1 to 2 years of apophysis closure. Occasionally, a patient may continue to have symptoms despite conservative measures and time. These patients usually have persistent pain from an ununited ossicle within the patellar tendon. Excision of this ossicle can alleviate the symptoms entirely; this procedure can be performed before skeletal maturity without adverse physeal effects.

In the mature patient, the prominence of the tibial tubercle makes it vulnerable for injury and pain. Symptomatic treatment (e.g., the use of kneepads and job and lifestyle modification) can be used. The indications for ossicle removal include failure of adequate conservative treatment and the presence of pain with point tenderness. The goal of surgical removal of the ossicle is to alleviate pain, not to eliminate the bump. Rarely does this condition lead to tendon disruption.

Sinding-Larsen-Johansson Syndrome

Sinding-Larsen-Johansson syndrome affects the inferior pole of the patella. Its mechanism of injury is similar to Osgood-Schlatter disease: Repetitive traction creates an apophysitis and a partial avulsion of the patellar tendon off the inferior pole of the patella. The typical patient is a preteen male who has activity-related knee pain. Patients with Sinding-Larsen-Johansson syndrome usually have tenderness at the inferior pole of the patella and pain with resistive knee extension.

The treatment is similar to Osgood-Schlatter disease, although Sinding-Larsen-Johansson syndrome is usually self-limited. Symptomatic relief and lifestyle modification are usually all that needs to be done. Rarely, surgery may be necessary to remove a discrete calcified mass that is causing the symptoms.

Quadriceps Tendon Injuries

Quadriceps tendon ruptures or avulsions usually occur in patients who are older than 40 and who have systemic disease or degenerative osteoarthritis. The systemic diseases commonly seen in these patients are collagen-vascular diseases such as lupus erythematosus and rheumatoid arthritis, diabetes mellitus, hyperthyroidism, gout, and pseudogout; obesity may also play a role.

Quadriceps tendinitis occurs at the insertion of the quadriceps into the patella. It is rarer than patellar tendinitis. Patients usually complain of pain at the proximal pole of the patella and often describe an achy feeling that is associated with training. Acute ruptures usually present with a sharp, severe onset of pain. As with patellar tendon ruptures, patients describe the pain as similar to having been kicked in the tendon (sharp, distinct, and acute).

Patients with tendinitis usually note tenderness to direct palpation of the central portion of the quadriceps tendon and pain on resistive extension. Patients with chronic tendinitis usually splint the extensor mechanism and note tightness of the quadriceps mechanism. This can be detected with a passive femoral stretch test. With tendon ruptures, a palpable defect can be detected that is exaggerated with the knee in flexion.

Plain radiographs may show calcification within the tendon, especially for chronic injuries. Unlike patellar tendon ruptures, quadriceps ruptures may not affect the position of the resting patella. MRI studies may be useful in chronic situations but are usually not necessary in the acute setting.

Treatment options depend on the severity, extent, and location of the injury and the age of the patient. Symptomatic treatment and rehabilitation are useful in most cases of extensor mechanism trauma. Surgical treatment is indicated for patients who do not improve after adequate conservative care, those who have chronic tendinitis with heterotopic calcifications, and patients with complete ruptures of the tendon. Complete tendon ruptures will need surgical intervention urgently to prevent an extension loss. Partial tendon ruptures can be treated nonoperatively if the patient has full function and if his or her lifestyle does not place high demands on the knee.

TREATMENT

Surgical Principles

Surgical repair creates a stable extensor mechanism, provides an environment in which adequate healing can occur, and prevents shortening of the extensor mechanism. It also allows for early mobilization of the knee joint to prevent contracture formation and to obtain normal function and motion. An essential initial process of surgical treatment for tendinopathy—whether it involves the quadriceps tendon, distal pole of the patella, patellar tendon, or the tibial tubercle insertion—is the identification of the degenerative process. Surgery for mucoid degeneration or microtear is done to remove the defect and to obtain healing. For complete ruptures, surgical treatment is usually required. The repair technique depends on the severity of the injury, the chronicity of the injury, and the quality of the tissue that remains. Acute spontaneous ruptures that occur within the substance of the tendon can usually be treated with direct end-to-end repair. If the rupture occurs at the level of the tendon-bone interface, both the tendon and the bone must be prepared for adequate healing before a fixation method is used. If an excessive amount of tendon is removed, patellofemoral mismatch will occur.

Acute tendon ruptures are usually accompanied by a disruption of the retinacular fibers (especially the patellar tendon); thus, at time of surgery, evacuation of the intra- and extra-articular hematoma needs to be done. During the examination of the intra-articular involvement of the tendon rupture, visualization of the articular surface of the patella and trochlea can be done. It is important to document the existence and extent of the condyle damage present, so an accurate assessment of the patient's long-term outcome can be made.

Surgical Technique

The patient is placed in a supine position, adequate anesthesia is provided, and a tourniquet is usually placed on the patient's thigh. It is important to remember that if retraction of the muscle has occurred, the tourniquet can jeopardize the repair by encompassing the muscle and holding it down. In this situation a tourniquet may not be required.

A midline incision is usually used, which allows adequate visualization of both sides of the tendon origin and insertion to the patella and the patellar tendon. A transverse incision has been described, but this can compromise future incisions if the patient should require total knee replacement. I prefer a vertical incision, because it is most extensive and does not compromise any future incisions. Once the skin is incised, the surgeon identifies the tendon, rupture, or fracture and assesses the amount of retinacular damage that has occurred. Visualization of the intra-articular extension of the rupture is important. Because the amount of articular damage can affect the outcome, it is important to describe the damage at the time of surgery. This information will be important when the surgeon instructs the patient in the proper care of the wound and for determining the long-term outcome.

For patients with mucoid degeneration or intrasubstance tears, a vertical incision is usually made into the tendon substance to identify the intratendinous degeneration. With isolated intratendinous degeneration or a mucoid-type lesion, simple curettage of the mucinous fluid down to normal tendinous structure is usually all that is necessary. An insult can be created in the bone next to the tendon to encourage bleeding and scar formation and thus promote healing (9) (Fig. 68.1). When the mucoid degeneration is quite extensive, reinforcing sutures may be used to protect the remaining portion of the tendon during the healing and rehabilitation process.

In acute ruptures, after the hematoma is evacuated, the ends of the tendon need to be débrided of all necrotic tissue and frayed irregular ends. For avulsion-type injuries in which the tendon has pulled off the bone (usually the patella), the bone is prepared to ensure adequate heal-

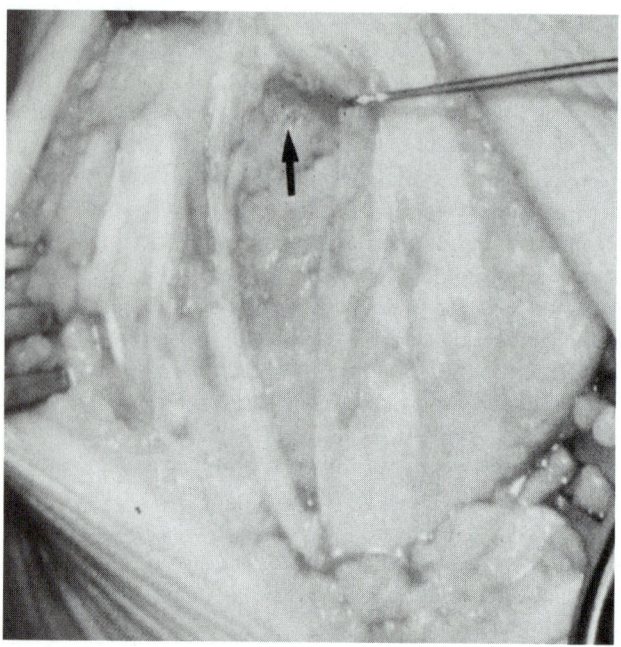

Figure 68.1. After abnormal tendon débridement, any bone at the tip of the patella that has been incidentally exposed (*arrow*) is rongeured back to a raw bleeding surface. Reprinted by permission from Krumins P, Reider B. Operative treatment of disorders of the patella tendon. Op Technol South Med 1994;2:303–307.

ing. I prefer to make a trough in the distal pole of the patella for patellar tendon ruptures and in the proximal pole of the patella for quadriceps ruptures to increase the healing surface area, before placing the fixation devices. I secure the tendon with a heavy nonabsorbable suture (number 2 and 5 Ethibond) and use the Krackow suture technique (10). Vertical holes are then drilled in the patella for placement of heavy nonabsorbable sutures, which are tied on the opposite pole (Fig. 68.2). Care is taken to maintain reduction of the tendon–bone interface before securing the knots in the sutures. For tibial tubercle tendinous avulsion injuries, anchoring devices allow for good fixation and are sometimes easier to use than sutures through drill holes. Anchoring devices have also been used to reattach the tendon to the patella.

For patients with a complete disruption of the tendon, it is important to adequately reduce the tendon disruption to its anatomical position. Judicious débridement of a tendon is necessary so that the patellofemoral mechanism is not affected once healing has occurred. If extensive débridement occurs or is performed, patella infra or patella baja may be a factor, leading to a long-term patellofemoral pain syndrome.

Some surgeons prefer a supplemental repair in addition to the vertical placement of the tendon sutures. This repair uses circumferential implanted or pullout wire sutures to reinforce the tendon repair. It is important to close the retinacular defects to ensure a watertight seal of the capsule. Before closure, I usually put the knee through a gentle range of motion, depending on the security of the

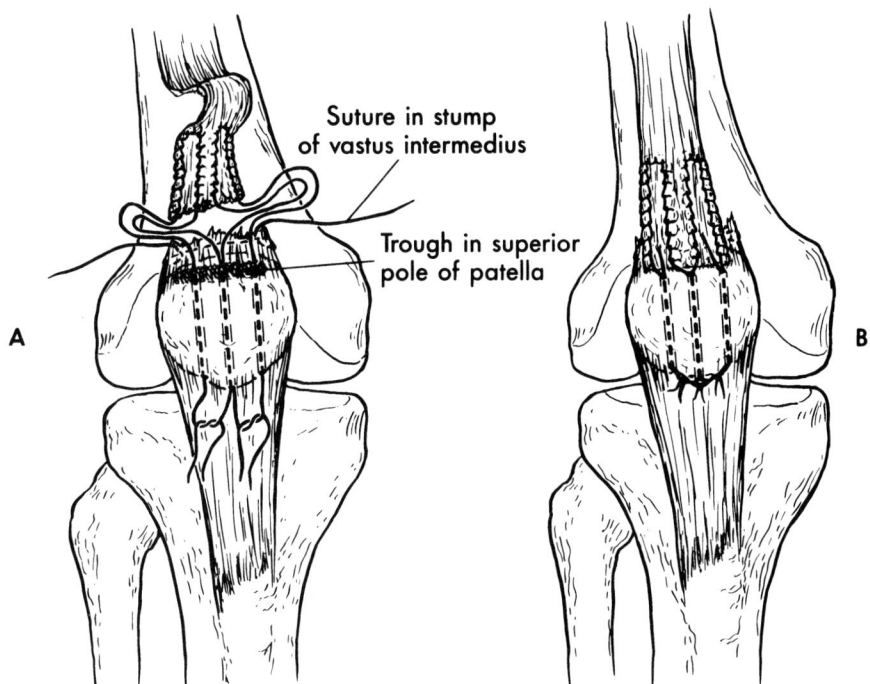

Figure 68.2. Repair of a fresh quadriceps femoris tendon rupture using Krackow sutures, a trough in the superior pole of the patella, and vertical patellar drill holes. Reprinted with permission from Phillips BB. Traumatic disorders. In: Crenshaw AH, ed. Campbell's operative orthopaedics. St. Louis: Mosby-Year Book, 1992:1919.

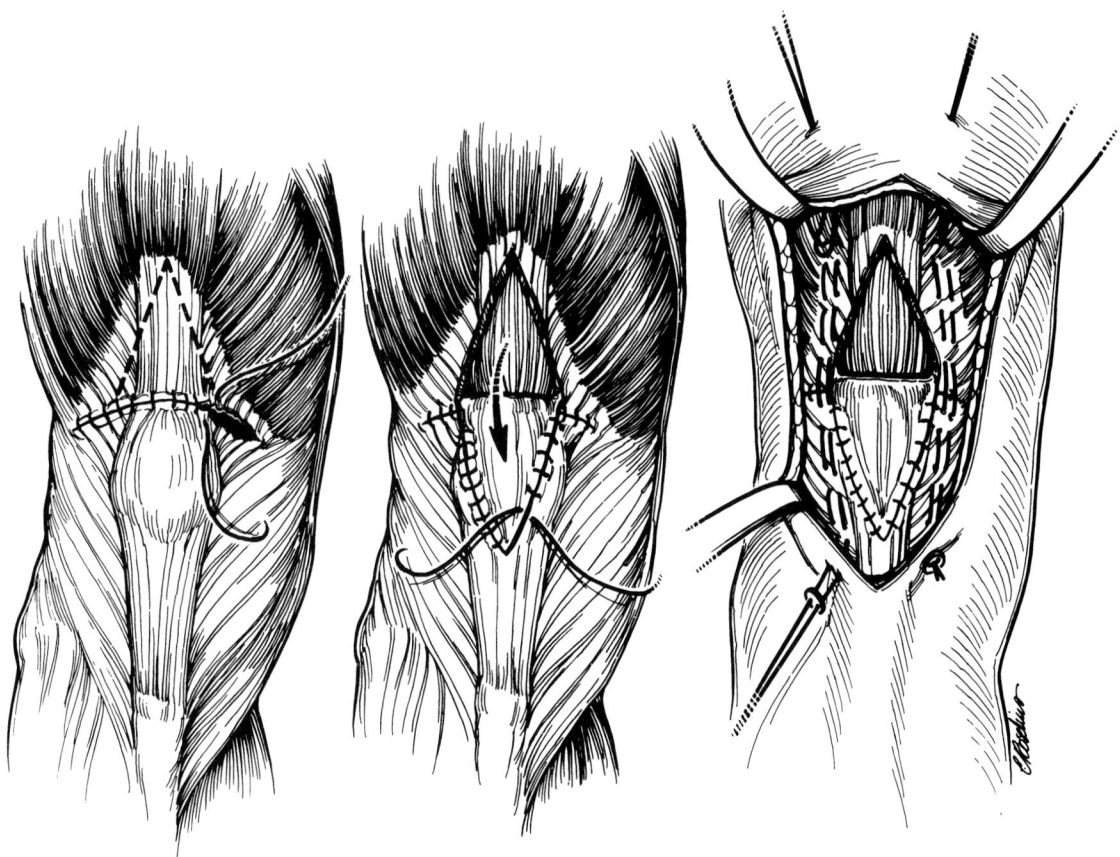

Figure 68.3. In chronic situations, this turndown procedure provides length to the quadriceps tendon so the rupture defect can be closed. Reprinted with permission from Scuderi G. Ruptures of the quadriceps tendon: study of twenty tendon ruptures. Am J Surg 1958;95:626–635.

repair, to determine the degree of flexion that puts tension on the repair.

Postsurgery, the patient is placed in a cylinder cast or extension brace for 2 to 3 weeks. Depending on the fixation method, gentle passive range of motion can then be initiated; initially, the range of motion does not usually exceed the degree of flexion determined at the end of the surgical repair. Weight bearing in a cylinder cast or extension brace at the 3- to 4-week interval depends on the quality of the tendon and repair that was achieved. If the repair is precarious, longer immobilization may be necessary to ensure adequate healing. In this situation, the patient avoids weight bearing for 4 to 6 weeks. Gentle range of motion is initiated both actively and passively at the 4- to 6-week interval. The patient is maintained in a limited-arch-of-motion brace for a total of 6 to 8 weeks.

In chronic situations and when tendon or muscle retraction has occurred, direct end-to-end repair may not be possible. In these situations, a turndown technique involving the quadriceps mechanism (rectus femoris tendon) can be used (11) (Fig. 68.3). Preoperative skeletal traction has been advocated for patients with quadriceps muscle contracture and chronic patellar tendon ruptures. The traction bow is applied to a traverse pin from the patella, and traction is applied. One- and two stage traction methods have been described. If an end-to-end repair can be achieved, then it is performed.

If an end-to-end repair is not amenable because of the extent of the contracture, the surgical possibilities available include releasing a portion of the quadriceps musculature to gain length of the patellar tendon (12) or of the quadriceps tendon (13) and to interpose a tendon graft (14) to work as an extensor mechanism. The tissues that have been used include fascia lata, semitendinosus, and even gastrocnemius rotation flaps. It is important that the patient is aware that these types of grafts provide only fair to good results; supplemental procedure are usually necessary to unload the repaired tissue.

SUMMARY

Lower-extremity abnormalities and/or injuries can be devastating. Since we as humans stand erect and spend a significant amount of time on our feet, any problems to our hips, knees, or ankles can severely limit our lifestyle and activity level. By far the most common joint and soft tissue problems for humans are the knee and the extensor mechanism of the knee. Extensor mechanism tendinopathies

can occur throughout life from adolescence through adulthood.

Tendon injuries about the knee can occur either proximal or distal to the knee joint. Treatment of these injuries depends on the location and extent of the lesion. Symptomatic intrasubstance lesions in continuity can be débrided and reinforced with sutures to prevent rupture while healing occurs. Tendon ruptures need to be repaired surgically to maintain knee function. Débridement of nonviable tissue is usually necessary prior to repair. There are numerous techniques for repairing either patellar or quadriceps tendon ruptures. After surgery, early rehabilitation is initiated. The physician must be confident in the stability of the repair prior to initiating rehabilitation. On occasion, injuries that occur near the origin or insertion of the tendon can heal with osseous union. These ossicles can be painful, as they are prominent. Excision is sometimes necessary if the pain cannot be relieved with pads or lifestyle modification.

REFERENCES

1. Renstrom P. Sports traumatology today: a review of common current sports injury problems. Ann Chir Gynaecol 1991;80:81–93.
2. Kannus P, Niittymaki S, Jarvinen M. Recent trends in women's sports injuries. J Sports Traumatol 1990;3:161.
3. Renstrom P, Johnson RJ. Overuse injuries in sports: a review. Sports Med 1985;2:316.
4. Clancy WG. Tendon trauma and overuse injuries. In: Leadbetter WB, Buckwalter JA, Gordon SL, eds. Sports-induced inflammation: clinical and basic science concepts. Park Ridge, IL: American Academy of Orthopaedic Surgeons, 1990:609.
5. Borynsenko M, Beringer T. Functional histology. 3rd ed. Boston: Little, Brown, 1989.
6. O'Brien M. Functional anatomy and physiology of tendons. Clin Sports Med 1992;11:505–520.
7. Insall J, Salvati E. Patella position in the normal knee joint. Radiology 1971;101:101–104.
8. Ehrenborg G, Lagergrenn C. Roentgenologic changes in the Osgood-Schlatter's lesion. Acta Chir Scand 1961;121:315–327.
9. Krumins P, Reider B. Operative treatment of disorders of the patella tendon. Op Technol South Med 1994;2:303–307.
10. Krackow KA, Thomas SC, Jones LC. A new stitch for ligament-tendon fixation. J Bone Joint Surg 1986:68A:764–766.
11. Scuderi G. Ruptures of the quadriceps tendon: study of twenty tendon ruptures. Am J Surg 1958;95:626–635.
12. Mandelbaum BR, Bartolozzi A, Carney B. A systematic approach to reconstruction of neglected tears of the patellar tendon. Clin Orthop 1988;235:268–271.
13. Scuderi C, Schrey E. Ruptures of quadriceps tendon. Arch Surg 1950;61:42–54.
14. Kelikian H, Riashi E, Gleason J. Restoration of quadriceps function in neglected tear of the patellar tendon. Surg Gynecol Obstet 1957;104:200–204.

chapter 69

Wayne J. Sebastianelli and William A. Lohrer

Arthroscopic Treatment of Osteochondral Lesions of the Knee

The development and recent advances of arthroscopy have had a significant impact on the treatment of the athlete's knee, including the treatment of osteochondral lesions, such as osteochondritis dissecans and osteochondral fractures.

Osteochondritis dissecans (OCD) is a focal separation of a segment of subchondral bone and/or hyaline cartilage from the underlying bone. The lesion may be purely chondral or osteochondral, depending on the level of the plane of separation relative to the subchondral bone. The lesion may initially be nondisplaced with maintenance of articular surface congruity. Joint surface incongruity and cartilage degeneration may occur with time; and the lesion may become partially detached, completely detached, or loose within the joint.

Paré first removed loose bodies from the knee joint in 1558. Such bodies were originally thought to be of traumatic origin. In 1854, Broca proposed the theory that spontaneous necrosis was responsible for the loosening of fragments that were subsequently deposited in the knee joint. In 1879, Paget agreed that "quiet necrosis" was the initial cause and subsequent trauma led to fragment displacement. In 1888, Konig (1) first used the term *osteochondritis dissecans* to describe these lesions. Konig's terminology was thought to be inappropriate and was a source of considerable controversy in the medical community; although his has since become well established, there remains controversy over the incidence, cause, and treatment of this condition.

RELEVANT ANATOMY AND PATHOGENESIS

The four most common theories for the origin of OCD are trauma, ischemia, abnormal ossification, and genet-

ics. Trauma remains the most popular of the proposed causes. Osteochondral fractures have been created in both cadaver and animal models by repetitive microtrauma. Proposed indirect mechanisms, such as contact of the anterior tibial spine with the lateral aspect of the medial femoral condyle with forced internal rotation of the tibia, have received more support than have direct mechanisms, because the most common sites of occurrence are well protected from direct trauma. Proponents of the ischemia theory note that end-artery thrombosis results in avascular necrosis of subchondral bone and subsequent formation of an osteochondrotic lesion. Not all lesions, however, contain necrotic bone, and some contain little if any bone at all. Irregularities of the distal femoral epiphysis occur commonly in normal children and can be difficult to distinguish radiographically from OCD. It has been postulated that trauma to such irregularities may cause an accessory bone nucleus, or locus minoris resistentiae, to develop into an osteochondrotic lesion. Although a genetic predisposition has been noted, studies have failed to demonstrate a hereditary basis for the condition.

It may be that the cause for the lesion known as osteochondritis dissecans is multifactorial. The primary pathology most likely involves cumulative cyclic stress to the subchondral bone. Subchondral injury leads to vascular compromise and a bone nucleus of variable viability, initially covered with intact articular cartilage. With motion and lack of underlying support, the cartilage may deform, fissure, fibrillate, or even enlarge as the cartilage remains nourished by the surrounding joint fluid. Continued microtrauma may lead to fragment displacement.

The anatomic location of lesions within the knee varies, and lesions of the distal femur predominate (Fig. 69.1).

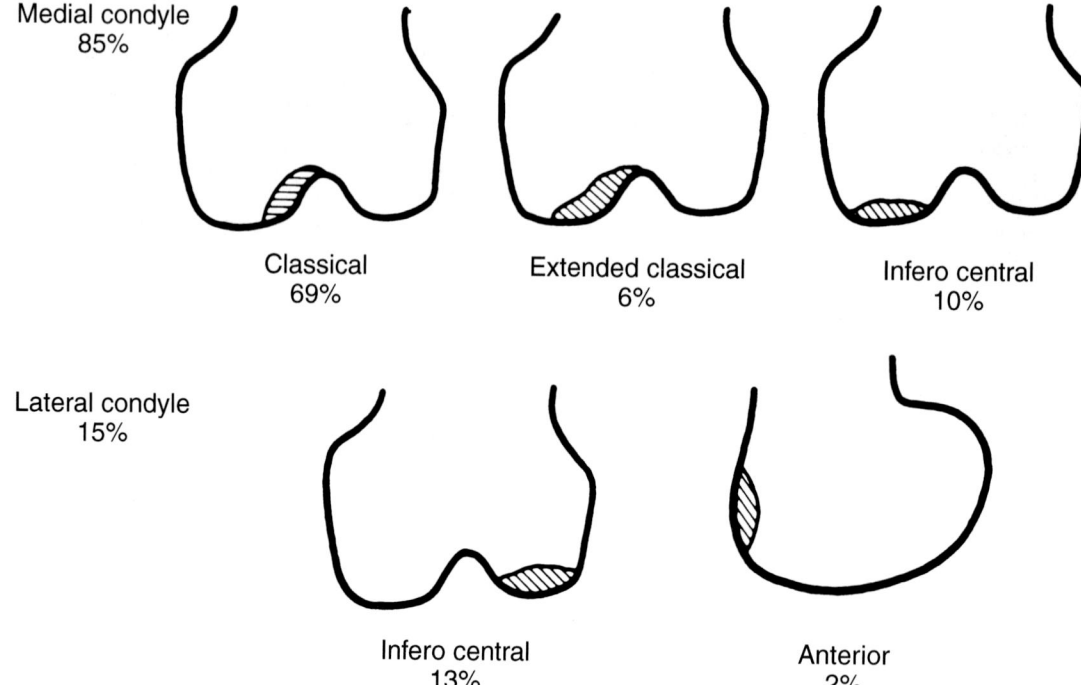

Figure 69.1. Sites and frequency of osteochondrotic lesions of the distal femur. Reprinted with permission from Aichroth P. Osteochondritis dissecans of the knee. J Bone Joint Surg 1971;53B: 440–447.

Among distal femoral lesions, the most common, or classical, location involves the lateral aspect of the medial femoral condyle (69%). The more central weight-bearing aspect of the medial femoral condyle may be involved either alone or as an extension of the classical lesion (16%). Lesions of the lateral femoral condyle (15%) are often larger and more posterior than medial condylar lesions. Lesions involving the patella and tibial plateau are relatively rare.

OCD typically presents in the second decade of life, but the condition may become symptomatic any time in the first six decades. It has been suggested that the growing popularity of organized school-age athletic competition has been responsible for a progressively younger age at presentation in recent years (2). Males outnumber females 2 to 3:1 and the condition has been noted bilaterally in as many as 30 to 50% of patients.

Multiple classification systems have been proposed. Lesions can most simply be classified by location and size, both of which influence prognosis. Pappas (3) staged the disease by patient age. The distinction between juvenile osteochondritis dissecans (JOCD) and OCD, based on skeletal maturity, is important because of the prognostic significance of physeal closure in the treatment of patients with such lesions. Classification systems based on scintigraphic, MRI, and arthroscopic appearance of the lesion exist as well.

Although OCD is most likely secondary to cyclic cumulative stresses, a single traumatic episode can produce osteochondral lesions in the form of chondral or osteo-chondral fractures. Komer first reported a chondral fracture of the knee in association with a patellar dislocation in 1904. The traumatic cause of such fractures may be exogenous (because of direct impact) or endogenous (because of rotational, compressive, or shearing forces between adjacent articular surfaces). Sites of injury include the patella, the medial and lateral femoral condyles, and (rarely) the tibial plateau. Fractures frequently involve tangential endogenous forces associated with lateral patellar subluxation or dislocation. When the patella dislocates, it is trapped by the lateral edge of the lateral femoral condyle. The osteochondral fracture can occur with either dislocation or reduction, and the location of the fracture depends on the degree of knee flexion. Recently, the endogenous forces associated with ligamentous injuries of the knee, specifically anterior cruciate ligament injuries, have been increasingly recognized as an additional cause of chondral and osteochondral fractures.

Osteochondral fractures occur predominantly in adolescent and young adults before the appearance of the histologic tidemark. In the skeletally immature, the chondral layer is firmly attached to the underlying bone. Shear forces are transmitted deep to the osteochondral junction; and the fracture occurs through the weaker subchondral cancellous bone, leaving the osteochondral junction undisturbed. In the skeletally mature, the same forces lead to purely chondral fractures, because the fracture occurs at the tidemark, the junction of calcified and uncalcified cartilage.

Chondral and osteochondral fractures can be classified by the age (acute or chronic), size, depth (superficial, partial thickness, full thickness, or osteochondral), and location of the lesion. Purely chondral lesions have been classified by fracture geometry (linear, stellate, flap, crater).

INITIAL FINDINGS, PHYSICAL EXAMINATION, AND DIAGNOSIS

As noted, OCD typically presents in the second decade of life. Symptoms may initially be vague or nonspecific. Early on, pain may predominate and is frequently related to the level of activity. Physical examination may be normal or findings may be limited to tenderness over a condylar lesion, elicited by flexing the knee and palpating just adjacent to the patellar tendon. Wilson (3a) described a test to elicit pain in patients with the classic lesion. The knee is flexed to 90°, and the tibia is internally rotated. As the knee is extended to 30°, pain is elicited as the anterior tibial spine impacts the medial femoral condyle. Relief is noted upon external rotation of the tibia. Although a positive test may be present in association with the classic lesion, a negative test is of little value in ruling out OCD as the cause of the patient's symptoms.

With time, the patient's lesion may become partially detached and displaced. Pain is then more likely to be associated with the presence of an effusion. Mechanical symptoms, such as catching or locking, may occur. Rarely, with complete separation and displacement, a loose body may be palpable. If mechanical symptoms are present at the time of initial evaluation, OCD must be differentiated from meniscal pathology as the source of the patient's symptoms.

With acute chondral and osteochondral fractures, the predominant signs and symptoms are typically those associated with the mechanism of injury. With a patellar dislocation, medial retinacular tenderness may predominate, and the patient may be unable to activate the

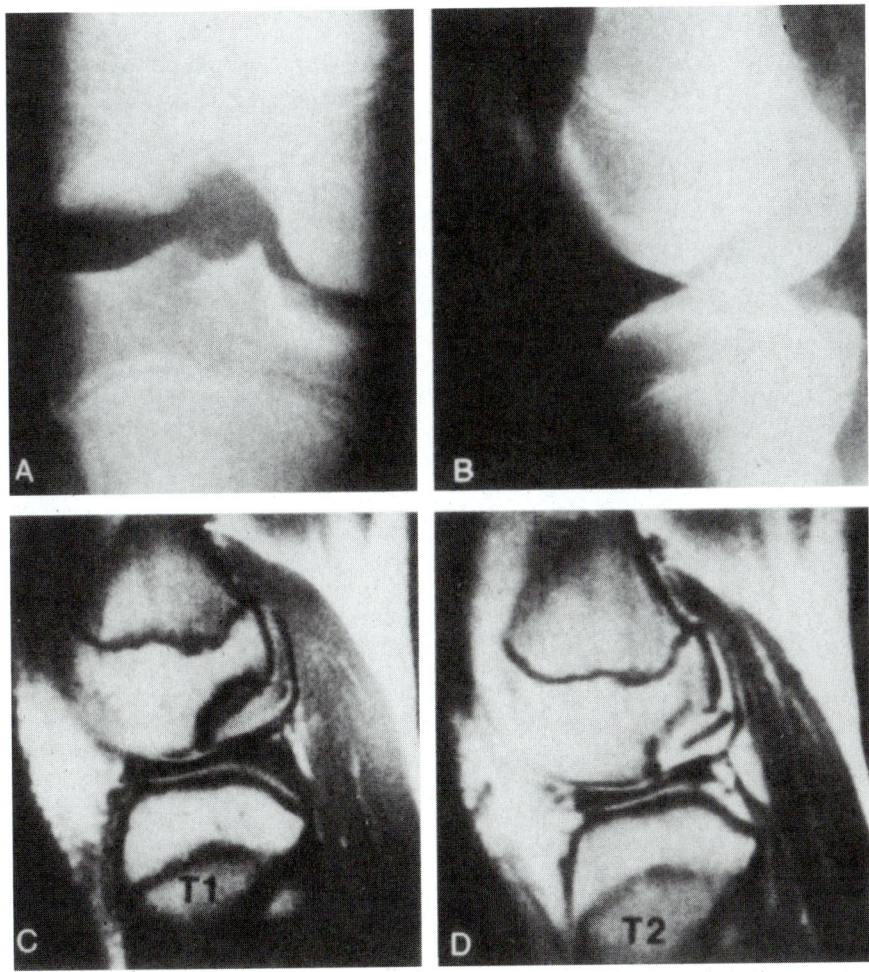

Figure 69.2. AP (**A**) and lateral (**B**) views showing a large osteochondrotic lesion of the lateral femoral condyle with a thick sclerotic margin, which indicates that the lesion is loose. **C.** T₁-weighted image showing the discontinuity of the hyaline cartilage and the displacement of the fragment. **D.** T₂-weighted image showing the bright signal from the fluid at the interface of the lesion. Note the increased signal intensity from the margin of the fragment and parent bone. Reprinted with permission from Mesgarzadeh M, Sapega AA, Bonakdarpour A, et al. Osteochondritis dissecans: analysis of mechanical stability with radiography, scintigraphy, and MR imaging. Radiology 1987;165: 775–780.

quadriceps mechanism. With anterior cruciate ligament tears, the physical examination may be most remarkable for the pathologic laxity associated with the ligament injury. With or without associated injury, a snap may be felt or heard with the sudden onset of pain. Osteochondral fractures are accompanied by a rapidly developing hemarthrosis. Aspiration can confirm the presence of a hemarthrosis with associated fat droplets. The swelling may be minimal with nondisplaced fractures and may be nonexistent with purely chondral fractures. Tenderness may be present at the fracture site, if it is accessible to palpation.

If displaced fractures present late, symptoms may be those associated with loose bodies. Persistent pain is accompanied by recurrent effusions and intermittent catching and locking, symptoms typically also associated with meniscal pathology. Chondral or osteochondral fractures need to be considered in the differential diagnosis when such symptoms persist, especially in the absence of focal meniscal signs such as joint line tenderness. Chronically, it may be difficult to differentiate such fractures from degenerative lesions or OCD. A nondisplaced femoral fracture fragment may undergo necrosis and attempted repair and be radiographically indistinguishable from OCD,

a finding cited in support for the traumatic cause of OCD. In summary, a high level of suspicion for such fractures, either as isolated entities or in conjunction with other pathology, is essential for early diagnosis so that the opportunity for reduction and fixation as treatment options is not lost.

RADIOLOGIC STUDIES

Radiographic evaluation of patients suspected to have OCD should begin with standard x-rays consisting of AP, lateral, tunnel, and patellofemoral views. The lesion in the classic location is typically better identified on the tunnel projection. On the lateral view, the lesion is typically located in a triangular area defined by the roof of the intercondylar notch and an imaginary extension of the posterior femoral cortex. The lesion appears as one or more bony fragments sitting in its bed with an intervening radiolucency. A radiodense appearance of the lesion can be the result of necrotic subchondral bone, new bone formation secondary to repair, or calcification of degenerated cartilage.

Radiographs should be assessed for skeletal maturity; and the lesion should be examined for size, sclerosis, and

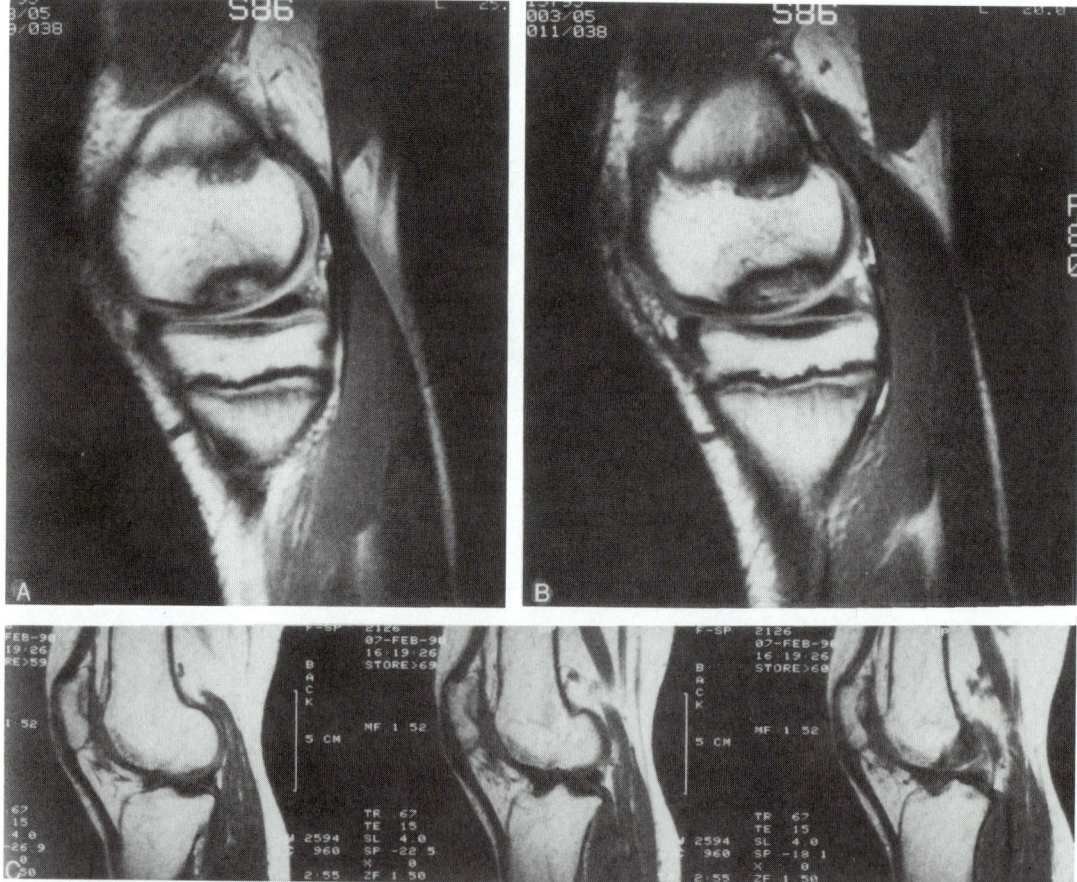

Figure 69.3. **A** and **B.** Sagittal view MRI studies of a large osteochondrotic lesion of the medial femoral condyle. Note that the articular cartilage is intact. **C.** MRI studies showing a nondisplaced osteochondrotic lesion of the patella. Reprinted with permission from

Sebastianelli WJ, DeHaven KE. Chondral fractures and intra-articular osteochondroses. In: DeLee JC, Drez D, eds. Orthopaedic sports medicine: principles and practice. Vol. 2. Philadelphia: Saunders, 1994:1444–1467.

degree of displacement. In a partially separated lesion, the thickness of the bony component should be quantified. In the case of completely separated and displaced lesions, the bed may be empty.

For osteochondral fractures, high-quality radiographs are essential. Films must be examined carefully, and should be "bright lighted," because an osteochondral fracture fragment may appear as a narrow, wafer-thin, irregular radiodense line. Oblique views may also be helpful. Films should be examined for both an osteochondral fragment and a donor site. Distal femoral fractures may appear as a double density along the articular surface. Patellar views in differing degrees of flexion may be required to identify a patellar fracture. Osteochondral fractures of the patella are typically located inferomedially, as opposed to bipartite patellar lesions, which are more typically located superolaterally. Purely chondral fractures present with normal radiographs.

Other Diagnostic Studies

Arthrography in evaluation of OCD is of historical interest only. Tomography and CT can be helpful in assessing the lesion. MRI has, in large part, replaced these studies as the test of choice for further workup of such lesions. MRI will accurately identify defects in the integrity of the articular cartilage and has also proved useful in the assessment of lesion stability (4) (Figs. 69.2 and 69.3). A heterogeneous area of mixed higher and lower signal intensity behind the lesion indicates a stable fibrous attachment. Unstable lesions demonstrate a homogeneous high-intensity signal on T_2-weighted images, which indicates a loss of articular surface integrity and fluid between the lesion and underlying subchondral bone. MRI is somewhat less useful in completely displaced lesions and in osteochondral fractures. Although it may accurately identify the donor site, it is a poor technique compared to high-quality conventional radiographs or CT for identifying loose bodies.

Bone scintigraphy has also been advocated as a predictor of lesional stability in OCD, and Cahill et al. (5) developed a classification system based on the scintigraphic appearance of the lesion (Fig. 69.4). They defined four stages based on the degree of activity of the femoral condyles and adjacent tibial plateau. The greatest usefulness of scintigraphy, however, may be in monitoring OCD lesions for healing via serial scans. Although changes in a lesion are often apparent at 6 to 8 weeks, repeat scanning can be performed at 3- to 4-month intervals.

For any type of osteochondral pathology, arthroscopic evaluation represents the ultimate diagnostic tool. In OCD, it allows for definitive evaluation of articular surface integrity and lesion stability for staging purposes. Evaluation should include both visualization and probing of the lesion. Arthroscopy offers the opportunity for a full

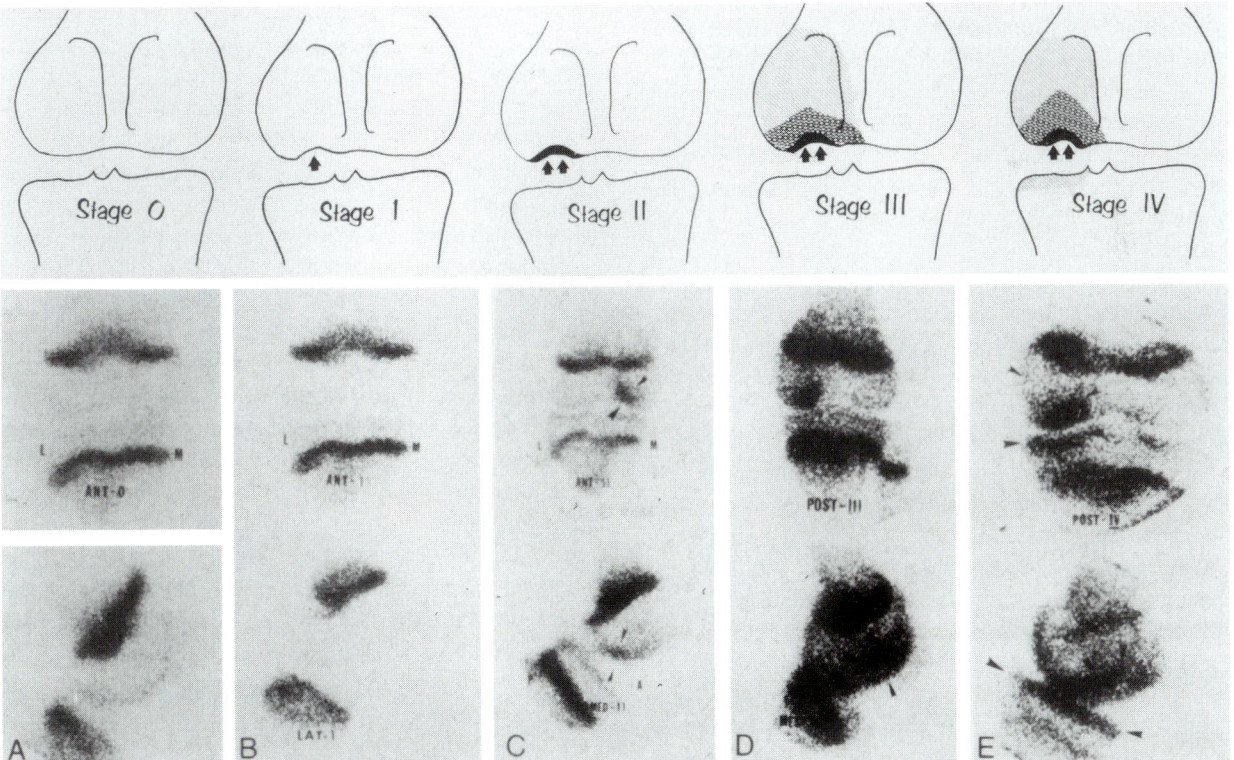

Figure 69.4. Scintigraphic evaluation of OCD. **A.** Normal knee. **B.** Stage I disease is characterized by a normal bone scan, despite some abnormalities on the radiograph. **C.** In stage II disease, abnormalities appear on both the radiograph and the bone scan. **D.** In stage III disease the defect is usually outlined. **E.** Stage IV disease includes an abnormal juxta-articular tibial plateau. Reprinted with permission from Cahill B, Berg B. 99m-Technetium phosphate compound joint scintigraphy in management of juvenile osteochondritis dissecans of the femoral condyles. Am J Sports Med 1983;2:331–333.

assessment of the knee joint, permitting detection and treatment of coincidental intra-articular pathology. When the decision is made to proceed with arthroscopy, a complete arthroscopic examination of the knee is always indicated and is especially important in the case of suspected osteochondral fractures. The search for loose bodies should include examination of the suprapatellar pouch, medial and lateral gutters, and the popliteal hiatus, sites where such bodies typically come to rest. A 70° arthroscope is helpful for evaluation of the posteromedial and posterolateral compartments.

The arthroscope, although a valuable diagnostic tool, can frequently be used for definitive treatment of these conditions during the same procedure. The indications for proceeding to arthroscopic evaluation and treatment are discussed below.

TREATMENT

Nonoperative Treatment and Indications for Surgery

For OCD, the goals of treatment are eliminating the symptoms, restoring the congruous joint surface, healing the fragment, and avoiding long-term degenerative changes. Treatment protocols have been based on lesion size, location, stability, and symptoms. Studies of treatment results have produced confusing data from a host of retrospective studies involving mixed age groups and stages of lesions. Patient age is a critical factor in the decision to proceed with nonoperative treatment for OCD. Although not uniformly successful, nonoperative treatment has generally been limited to patients with open physes. The prognosis for nonoperative treatment is temporally related to skeletal maturity and the vascular alterations that occur with physeal closure.

Pappas (3) categorized patients with OCD lesions by patient age, noting an excellent prognosis for nonoperative treatment of patients in childhood through early adolescence. Cahill et al. (5) reported an approximately 50% chance of healing of stable lesions in 10 to 18 months for this population and recommended a trial of conservative treatment, even within 6 to 12 months of physeal closure. The favorable prognosis in skeletally immature patients is related to rapid epiphyseal articular cartilage overgrowth and necrotic fragment remodeling. Therefore, initial nonoperative treatment is recommended for in situ, MRI-stable lesions in the skeletally immature population.

For MRI-unstable or displaced lesions and for mechanical or worsening symptoms, operative treatment is recommended. Renewal and repair is unlikely after physeal closure, and there is little role for nonoperative treatment of OCD in the symptomatic adult. Of course, there is significant overlap between these populations, because some patients with open growth plates who are initially treated nonoperatively may fail to heal. Most adult OCD represents juvenile cases that failed to heal, although true adult onset OCD exists and can begin anytime up to age 50.

Nonoperative treatment options include observation, relative rest with or without protected weight bearing, and immobilization. Observation is appropriate for the asymptomatic youth in whom OCD is discovered as an incidental finding. For symptomatic patients, the principles of relative rest usually begin with elimination of recreational and competitive athletic participation so that activities of daily living (ADLs) can be performed symptom free. If symptoms persist after 6 weeks, use of crutches and/or a knee immobilizer can be instituted. Cast immobilization is rarely required. Once the patient is symptom free, the crutches and/or knee immobilizer can be discarded. As healing progresses clinically and radiographically, nonimpact activities such as cycling and swimming can be added; activity progression thereafter is based on symptoms. Although advocated by some authors, the role of pulsed electromagnetic fields for treatment of OCD is still undefined.

Plain radiographs are relatively insensitive with respect to early healing; and as noted, bone scintigraphy is the most sensitive way to evaluate healing. Most patients present with stage III or IV scintigrams, and healing is generally indicated on subsequent scans by a decrease in activity (to stage II levels). Scans can be repeated at 3- to 6-month intervals with the understanding that low-level activity may persist for up to 1 year after healing.

Many patients present for treatment after experiencing at least 6 months of symptoms. Both the patient and parents are often disappointed with the recommended conservative approach, seeking a more immediate solution to permit return to full function, including athletic participation. Parents should be reassured in regard to the duration of symptoms at presentation and informed of the favorable prognosis for healing before physeal closure. Patients should know that operative treatment entails a restriction from athletic participation similar to that associated with nonoperative treatment.

Nonoperative treatment can be considered for small nondisplaced osteochondral fractures; however, operative intervention is standard for large and displaced lesions. Remember that a larger area may be involved than is apparent by plain x-ray workup. Size and location are best judged arthroscopically; therefore, operative treatment is indicated for the majority of osteochondral fractures. A delay in treatment may make it difficult or impossible to reduce and fix the fracture fragment.

Indications for operative treatment of OCD include failed nonoperative treatment with persistent symptoms in a compliant patient, advanced lesions with detachment and instability, and skeletal maturity. Operative treatment is indicated for all but the smallest nondisplaced osteochondral fractures.

Operative Treatment

The operative approach to both OCD and osteochondral fractures begins with a complete arthroscopic examination of the knee, including visualization and probing.

Clinical Table: Arthroscopic Treatment of Osteochondral Lesions of the Knee

Procedure	Indications	Techniques	Pitfalls
Drilling	• Stable lesions with intact cartilage in the skeletally immature • Internal fixation of unstable lesions in the skeletally immature	0.062 K wire	• Use of drill bit • K wire misdirection or breakage
Bone peg fixation	• Large, unstable in situ lesions in the skeletally mature	• Best performed open • 2.5-mm drill bit • Proximal tibial matchstick grafts • Countersink grafts	• Inability to obtain compression • Donor site morbidity • Graft displacement • Lesion fragmentation
Pin fixation	• Unstable wafer-thin or comminuted lesions • Osteochondral fractures	• Bed preparation • 0.062 K wires • Smooth vs. threaded • Commercial ACL guides • Retrograde pin removal at 6–10 weeks	• Pin migration or breakage • Less rigid fixation than screws
Cannulated screw fixation	• Unstable lesions • Osteochondral fractures with salvageable fragments	• Bed preparation • 3.5-mm cannulated screws • Decision to countersink • Screw removal at 6–10 weeks	• Guidewire impingement or breakage • Lesion articular surface damage with countersinking • Lesion fragmentation • Immobilization vs. risk of opposing articular surface damage • Need for screw removal
Herbert screw fixation	• Unstable lesions • Osteochondral fractures with salvageable fragments	• Bed preparation • Cannulated screws available • Countersink screws	• Guidewire impingement or breakage • Lesion fragmentation
Retrograde bone grafting	• In situ lesions with intact articular cartilage in the skeletally mature (with or without internal fixation)	• Commercial ACL guides • 5- to 10-mm cannulated reamer • Iliac crest or proximal tibial donor site vs. allograft	• Donor site morbidity • Graft misplacement or displacement
Fragment removal with drilling and abrasion	• Multiple small fragments • Inadequate bone for fixation • Pure chondral lesions	• Fragment removal • Trephination of lesion • Abrasion with motorized burr • Drilling with 0.062 K wire	• Inability to locate loose bodies • Excessive depth of abrasion
Osteochondral allografts	• Large lesions of the weight-bearing portion of the lateral femoral condyle • Salvage following failed procedure	• Age and skeletal size match • Specially designed cylindrical cutting instruments for donor and recipient • Herbert screw fixation	• Donor availability • Risk of disease transmission • Donor-recipient graft mismatch • Technically demanding

ACL, anterior cruciate ligament.

The lesion should be assessed for size, location, stability, depth of attached bone, and condition of the overlying cartilage. Lesions may be classified by the condition of the overlying cartilage as intact, early separation, partially detached, or completely detached or loose; the latter three classifications indicate an unstable lesion (6).

In OCD, the goals for stable in situ lesions are to enhance vascularization of the fragment and encourage union. For unstable displaced lesions, the goals are reduction for anatomic restoration of the joint surface, stabilization of the fragment (preferably with rigid internal fixation to permit early joint motion), and enhancement of revascularization to encourage union. For completely displaced loose lesions, the goals are to replace and stabilize the lesion when possible.

For loose lesions, arthroscopic examination should include inspection of the suprapatellar pouch, the medial and lateral gutters, the popliteal hiatus, and the postero-medial and posterolateral compartments, sites at which loose bodies commonly come to rest. Every effort should be made for reduction and internal fixation of loose bodies and long-standing partial detachments, especially of weight-bearing areas, as the long-term results of removal are poor. The same principles apply to the treatment of osteochondral fractures; reduction and stabilization should be performed whenever possible.

In cases for which reduction and stabilization of osteochondral lesions are not possible, removal and débridement are performed. In addition to the treatment of osteochondral fractures, any concomitant ligamentous injuries and patellar instability must be addressed.

PROCEDURES

Based on the findings at the time of diagnostic arthroscopy, several arthroscopic and open treatment options are available. Indications and surgical techniques for the most commonly performed operative procedures are detailed below (Clinical Table).

Antegrade Drilling

Drilling of osteochondritis dissecans lesions may be performed as an isolated procedure or in association with internal fixation (Fig. 69.5) (6,7). Drilling as an isolated

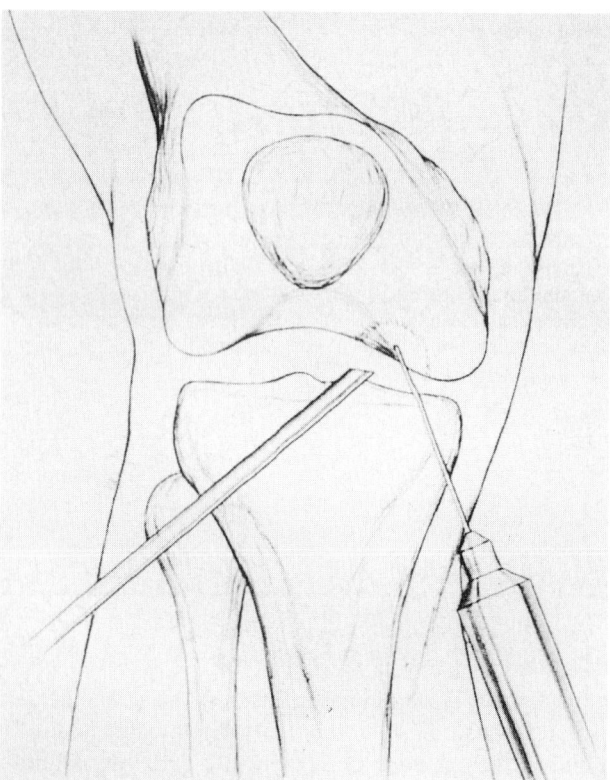

Figure 69.5. For the medial approach to arthroscopic drilling of a lesion on the femoral condyle, the arthroscope is placed in the anterolateral portal. Reprinted with permission from Guhl JF, Johnson RP, Stone JW. The impact of arthroscopy on osteochondritis dissecans. In: McGinty JB, ed. Operative arthroscopy. New York: Raven, 1991:297–317.

treatment is indicated for stable lesions with intact cartilage and has been most successful in skeletally immature patients. Its purpose is to allow blood vessels to traverse the drilled holes and revascularize the fragment.

Drilling is generally performed arthroscopically, based on triangulation techniques; sometimes, because of the location of the lesion, the drilling may be performed as an open procedure. Antegrade drilling is performed with a 0.062 Kirschner (K) wire, which creates less articular surface trauma than does a comparably sized drill bit. A soft tissue guide sleeve from an internal fixation tray or a small-diameter arthroscopic cannula can be used to protect the soft tissues at the level of the arthroscopic portal. Three to four holes are recommended per square centimeter of lesion.

For larger lesions, drilling all the holes through a single portal may cause the K wire to be too tangential with respect to the articular surface. The arthroscope and K wire can be exchanged among several portals so that all holes can be drilled perpendicular to the surface and the wire can penetrate the vascular cancellous bone. Other authors advocate drilling multiple bone holes, at varying angles, through a single cartilage hole to minimize articular surface damage. Satisfactory depth and orientation of the drilled holes are confirmed by observing the flow of blood from the holes after deflating the tourniquet and decompressing the joint.

The advantages of this technique over retrograde drilling through the femoral metaphysis include more accurate placement of the holes, no need for proximal incisions, no violation of the growth plate, and no risk of displacing the fragment. The disadvantage of violating the articular surface has not been associated with identifiable long-term problems. Since motion interferes with revascularization and healing, isolated drilling for the treatment of OCD should be reserved for intact stable lesions in skeletally immature patients.

Bone Peg Fixation

Although less commonly used than other forms of fixation, bone pegs can be used for the fixation of OCD lesions (Fig. 69.6) (8–10). Bone peg fixation is indicated for the treatment of large, unstable in situ fragments in skeletally mature patients. Its purpose is to stabilize the fragment, and it has the potential physiologic benefit of providing autogenous bone graft to promote healing.

The procedure is technically demanding and is best performed open rather than arthroscopically. An anteromedial or anterolateral incision is used, depending on the location of the lesion. A 2.5-mm drill bit is used to create two to three holes perpendicular to the lesion through the fragment and into the underlying bone. Through a small separate longitudinal incision, the proximal tibia is exposed subperiosteally just distal and medial to the tibial tubercle. Two or three matchstick-sized grafts (35 × 2.5 × 2.5 mm) are harvested. They are trimmed to size and used to internally fix the fragment.

Arthroscopic pin fixation can be carried out under these principles.

If partial or complete detachment provides access to the bed of the lesion, fibrous tissue is débrided from the interface of the lesion. The subchondral bone of the crater can be drilled to ensure the presence of bleeding bone. The fragment is then reduced, ensuring the presence of a congruous joint surface. If the surface is not congruous, which requires either extensive fragment débridement or cancellous bone grafting, a limited open approach may be advisable.

Once the fragment is reduced, 0.062 K wires are drilled antegrade through the lesion and the condyle and then advanced to the metaphysis of the femur. Multiple wires are used in larger fragments. Comminuted lesions are anatomically reduced; each fragment is fixed with its own K wire. Smooth K wires tend to migrate and should be crossed on insertion. An alternative for improved fixation involves bending the articular end of a smooth pin 90°, 1 mm from its end. Threaded K wires are less likely to migrate but are more difficult to remove and more

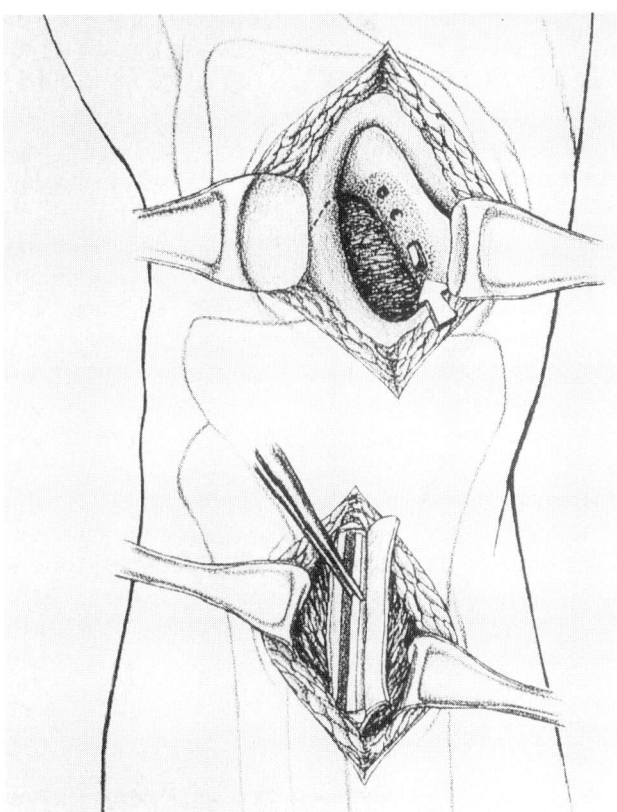

Figure 69.6. Bone peg fixation of a lesion on the medial femoral condyle. Reprinted with permission from Guhl JF, Johnson RP, Stone JW. The impact of arthroscopy on osteochondritis dissecans. In: McGinty JB, ed. Operative arthroscopy. 2nd ed. Philadelphia: Lippincott-Raven, 1996:389.

Fixation is based on an interference fit of square pegs in round holes. The pegs need to be well spaced to avoid fragmentation of the lesion. The pegs can be countersunk 2 mm below the articular surface with a small punch; care is taken not to countersink them so deeply that fixation is lost. Bone peg fixation can be supplemented by drilling in larger lesions, if care is taken to avoid fragmentation of the lesion.

The advantages of bone peg fixation include no risk of hardware migration and failure, ability to countersink the fixation device, and no need for a second procedure for hardware removal. The disadvantages of the technique include the potential for donor site morbidity, lack of a congruent surface in some healing lesions, inability to obtain compression, and the need for external immobilization if less-than-rigid internal fixation is achieved.

Pin Fixation

Pin fixation is indicated for unstable OCD lesions and osteochondral fractures, especially for unstable wafer-type lesions for which the use of a screw could risk comminution of the fragment (Fig. 69.7) (11,12). Open pin fixation techniques emphasize meticulous preparation of the fragments and supplemental cancellous bone grafting to ensure a vascularized bed and a congruous joint surface.

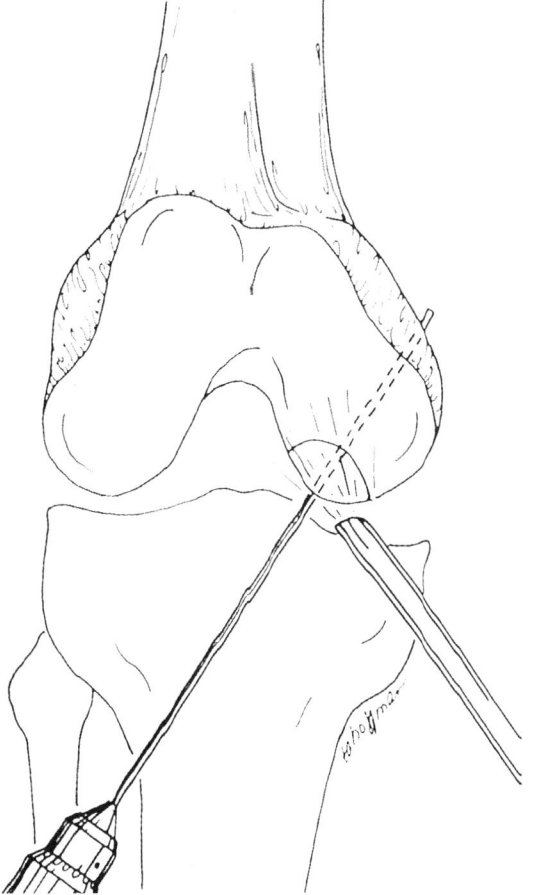

Figure 69.7. For arthroscopic pin fixation, a partially threaded 0.062 K wire is inserted through the anterolateral portal, and the arthroscope is placed in the anteromedial portal. Reprinted with permission from Guhl JF, Johnson RP, Stone JW. The impact of arthroscopy on osteochondritis dissecans. In: McGinty JB, ed. Operative arthroscopy. 2nd ed. Philadelphia: Lippincott-Raven, 1996:378.

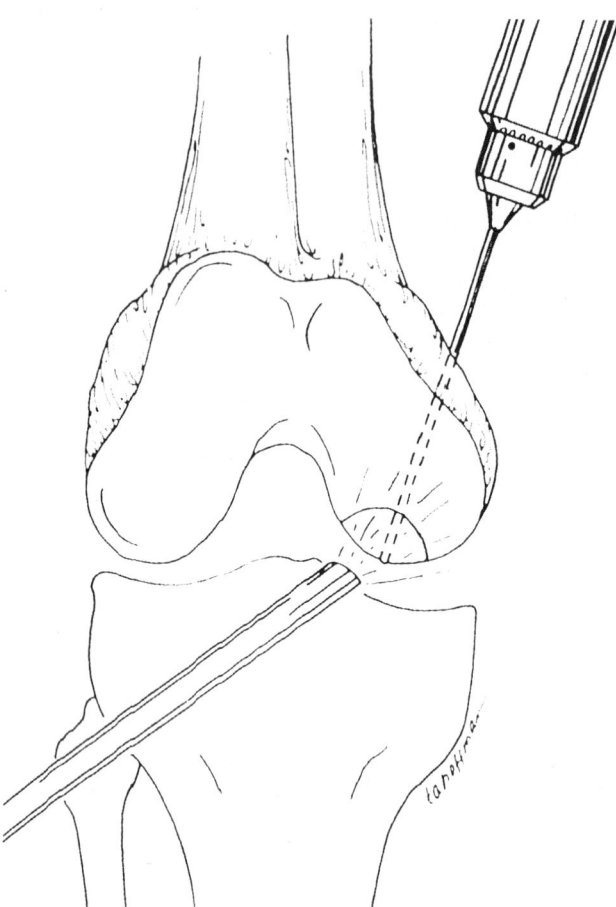

Figure 69.8. The wire is removed with the drill in the proximal position. Reprinted with permission from Guhl JF, Johnson RP, Stone JW. The impact of arthroscopy on osteochondritis dissecans. In: McGinty JB, ed. Operative arthroscopy. 2nd ed. Philadelphia: Lippincott-Raven, 1996:378.

likely to break. The wires are inserted through a small cannula or soft tissue guide. Once the wires have penetrated the metaphysis, they are advanced proximally through small medial or lateral skin incisions. The drill is changed from the distal to proximal end of the wire, and the wire is withdrawn under arthroscopic guidance until the distal (or threaded) end just disappears beneath the articular surface, securing the lesion in place (Fig. 69.8). If a smooth bent pin is used, a clamp and small slap hammer can be used proximally to seat the bent distal end over the last few millimeters into the subchondral bone. The protruding proximal ends of the wires are cut so that they can be easily palpated beneath the skin. The pins are removed in a retrograde manner 6 to 12 weeks later, depending on clinical and radiographic criteria for healing. Smooth K wires can be removed in the office under local anesthesia; some authors recommend general anesthesia for removal of threaded K wires.

This technique of pin insertion may require excessive knee flexion, and determination of the proximal exit point can be difficult and unpredictable. The use of commer-

cially available arthroscopic anterior cruciate ligament (ACL) reconstruction guides may eliminate these problems (Fig. 69.9). The tip of the guide can be inserted through the appropriate portal and placed over the lesion, securing it in place during drilling. A pin can then be inserted through the metaphysis via a limited skin incision and advanced to the articular surface until it is just visible arthroscopically. It is then withdrawn a few millimeters, securing the lesion in place. Multiple pins can be placed with this technique; they are cut to the appropriate length as described above.

One advantage of pin fixation is that a second arthroscopic procedure is not required for hardware removal. The disadvantages of pin migration and breakage and less rigid fixation than achieved by other techniques limit its use to small, thin, or comminuted lesions.

Biodegradable pins have been used for fixation of osteochondral lesions. Although obviating the need for hardware removal, their insertion is complicated by their lack of rigidity, and they too lack the compressive qualities of other internal fixation devices.

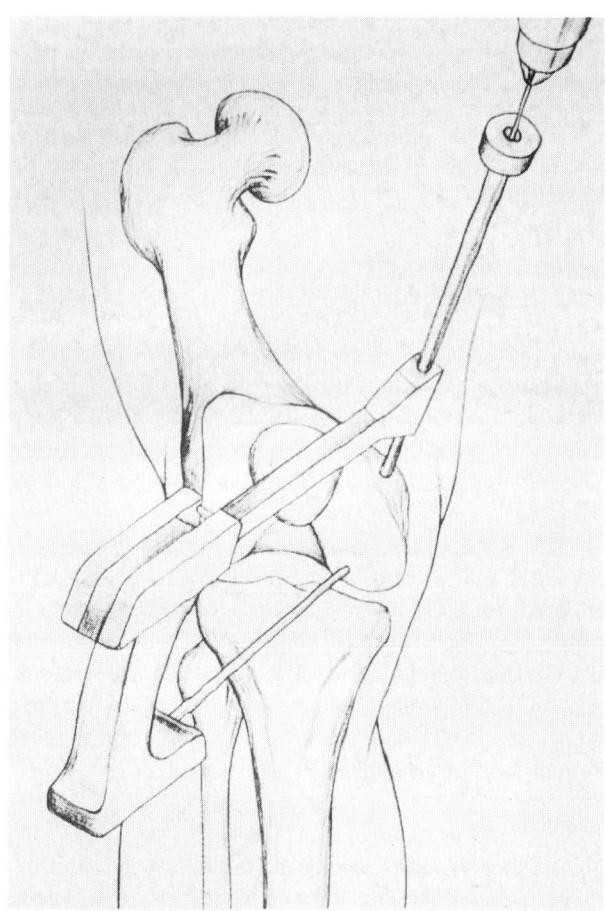

Figure 69.9. An ACL guide facilitates pin placement. Reprinted with permission from Guhl JF, Johnson RP, Stone JW. The impact of arthroscopy on osteochondritis dissecans. In: McGinty JB, ed. Operative arthroscopy. 2nd ed. Philadelphia: Lippincott-Raven, 1996:378.

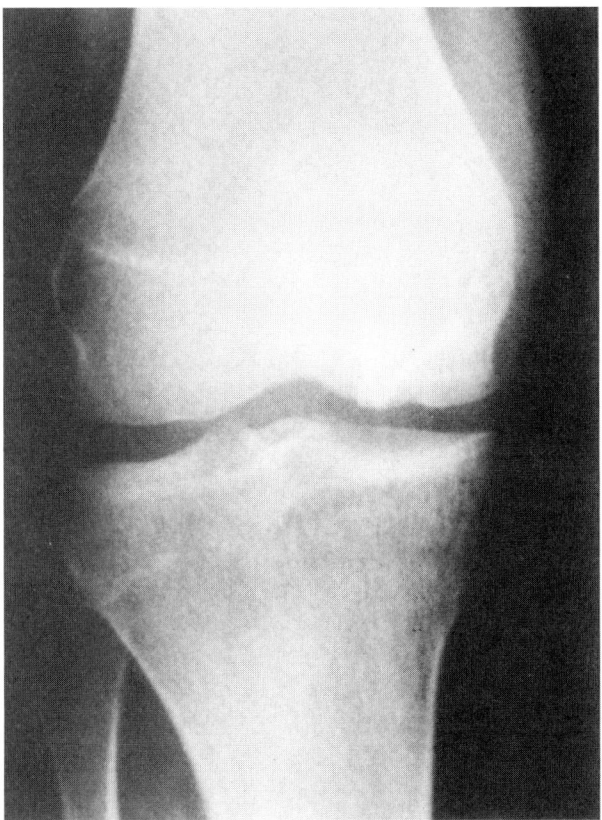
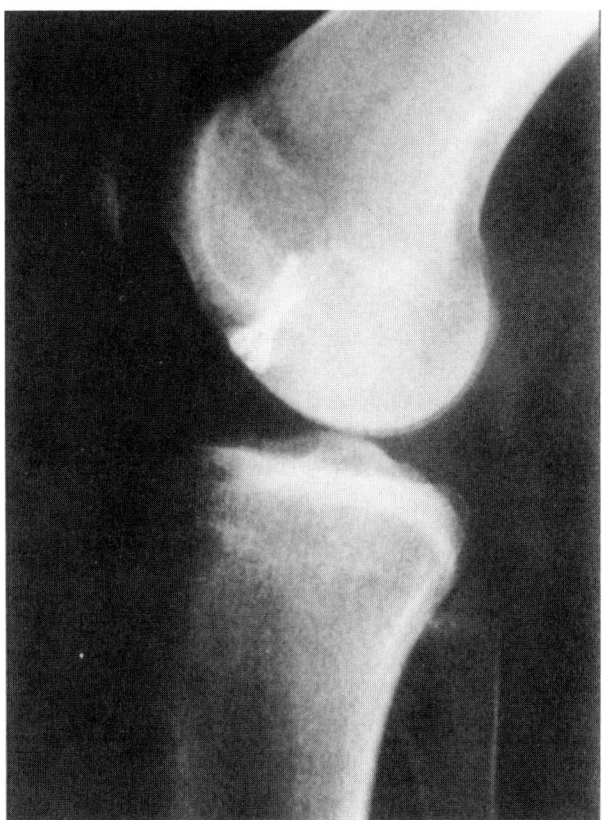

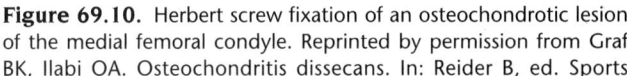

Figure 69.10. Herbert screw fixation of an osteochondrotic lesion of the medial femoral condyle. Reprinted by permission from Graf BK, Ilabi OA. Osteochondritis dissecans. In: Reider B, ed. Sports medicine: the school age athlete. 2nd ed. Philadelphia: Saunders, 1996:284.

Screw Fixation

Screw fixation for the treatment of osteochondral lesions is applicable to both OCD and osteochondral fractures (Fig. 69.10) (13–16). In OCD, screw fixation is indicated for unstable lesions with salvageable fragments, whether intact, partially detached, or loose. For osteochondral fractures, screw fixation is indicated if the fragment is large enough, there is enough bone, and the procedure is performed before deformation of the fragment precludes open reduction and internal fixation. The procedure can be performed arthroscopically, although the size and/or location of the lesion may dictate the need for arthrotomy. This is frequently the case with osteochondral fractures, many of which involve patellar, trochlear, and posterior condylar sites. Retrograde arthroscopic fixation (anterior to posterior) of patellar OCD lesions has been reported as an alternative to arthrotomy.

Options for screw fixation of OCD lesions include the use of cannulated screws and Herbert screws. For intact lesions, fixation can be supplemented by drilling the lesion (younger patients) or by retrograde bone grafting (older patients). In partially detached and loose lesions, the base of the lesion is prepared by curettage, abrasion, and drilling. For partially detached lesions, the hinge should be preserved, because it may be a blood supply to the fragment. In loose OCD lesions and displaced frac-

tures, the nonarticular surface of the fragment should be similarly prepared. Fibrous tissue removal can be accomplished with rongeurs, rasps, curettes, and motorized instruments.

Initial experience with screw fixation of OCD lesions involved use of cannulated screws. Following preparation, the fragment is reduced. Provisional fixation is accomplished with accompanying guidewires. The wires are typically of small diameter and are prone to bending or breaking, necessitating great care during their insertion. Following drilling and depth gauging, the screws are inserted over the guidewires; care is taken to follow their course. Divergence of the drill or screw and the wire will cause the guidewire to impinge or break. Use of an image intensifier to ensure proper screw placement can be quite helpful. If the guidewire bends, it should be removed and replaced before screw fixation is performed. Buried broken wires can be left in place, despite aesthetically displeasing postoperative radiographs. Protruding broken wires require removal and may necessitate an arthrotomy.

Use of multiple screws is indicated for fixation and control of rotation in larger lesions. Screw heads can be countersunk, permitting early motion; however, countersinking increases the area of articular cartilage damage. If the screws are not countersunk, immobilization is required until the screws are removed, typically between 6 and 10 weeks. Note that damage to the opposing articular surface has been reported, even with countersinking of cannulated screws.

Herbert screws fixation is an alternative to the use of cannulated screws for OCD lesions and osteochondral fractures. Herbert screws are headless, are threaded at both ends, and have a proximal core shaft diameter of 2.5 mm, resulting in relatively little damage to the articular surface. The differential pitch of the two sets of threads permits compression, and the headless design permits the screw to be completely buried beneath the articular surface in the subchondral bone of the fragment. A cannulated Herbert screw is available and is accompanied by instrumentation designed for arthroscopic insertion; as with cannulated screws, however, an open approach is sometimes advisable.

The principles for Herbert screw fixation are similar to those described for cannulated screws. Reduction and fixation are preceded by bed and fragment preparation and are supplemented by drilling and/or bone grafting as indicated. The screws are inserted over guidewires, for which the same concerns apply as those noted for cannulated screws. The number of screws used is determined by the size of the lesion. In skeletally immature patients, shorter screws can be used to avoid crossing the physeal plate. Screw lengths generally vary from 22 to 30 mm. The trailing end of the screw is countersunk beneath the articular surface, permitting early postoperative mobilization. As the screw is seated, fragment compression can be observed arthroscopically. Some authors advocate screw removal at 6 to 8 weeks, although routine removal is not required. Healing fibrocartilage will eventually cover the screw; if screw removal is to be performed, this cartilage must be débrided so the screwdriver can be properly aligned. Screw removal is usually performed by the same approach used for insertion (whether open or arthroscopic).

The advantages of screw fixation include more consistent compression of the fragment and more rigid fixation than can be accomplished with pins, K wires, or pegs. The disadvantages of prominent screw heads and the need for a second anesthesia for hardware removal are avoided with the use of Herbert screws.

Bone Grafting

The development of techniques for screw fixation has limited the indications for isolated bone grafting for treatment of OCD in recent years (17,18). Bone grafting remains indicated, either alone or in association with pin or screw fixation, for in situ lesions with intact articular cartilage in skeletally mature patients. Bone grafting is preferable to isolated drilling in this population and is most applicable to large lesions with sclerotic borders. Corticocancellous grafting may involve the use of autograft (from an iliac crest or proximal tibial source) or allograft bone. Arthroscopic grafting may be performed by direct or retrograde methods.

Grafting in a retrograde manner is carried out using

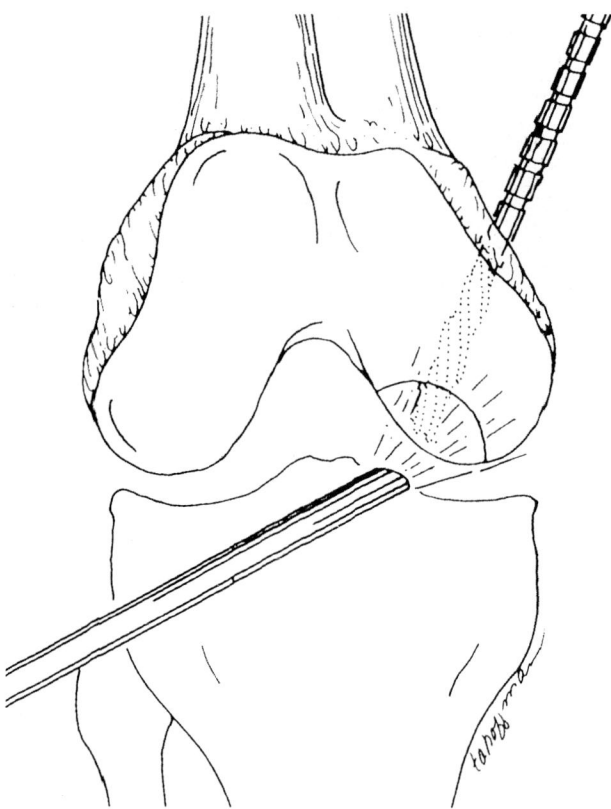

Figure 69.11. A reamer can be used for grafting by the retrograde method. Reprinted with permission from Guhl JF, Johnson RP, Stone JW. The impact of arthroscopy on osteochondritis dissecans. In: McGinty JB, ed. Operative arthroscopy. 2nd ed. Philadelphia: Lippincott-Raven, 1996:386.

commercially available arthroscopic ACL reconstruction guides (Fig. 69.11). A guidewire is inserted as described for retrograde K wire pinning. A 5- to 10-mm cannulated reamer is inserted over the guidewire; the reamer size is determined by the size of the lesion. The reamer is advanced until the lesion vibrates or "chatters." The canal is then packed with corticocancellous graft from above. Intraoperative use of the image intensifier may be of assistance in reaming the canal and in ensuring delivery of the graft to the lesion.

Direct or antegrade arthroscopic grafting is the arthroscopic equivalent to the open bone peg fixation described above (Fig. 69.12). Following the antegrade placement of a guidewire, a 4- to 5-mm-diameter canal is drilled through the articular surface and underlying bone. Grafts of a corresponding diameter are inserted through the cannulas with the aid of grasping instruments. The grafts are advanced up the canal and countersunk by tamping; care is taken to avoid advancing the grafts too far. Practically, large lesions requiring more than one to two such grafts are best treated by open techniques.

With bone grafting, the preparation of the tunnel breaks the sclerotic edges of the lesion. The retrograde approach, unlike the direct technique, delivers the graft to the bed without violating the articular surface. Depressed frag-

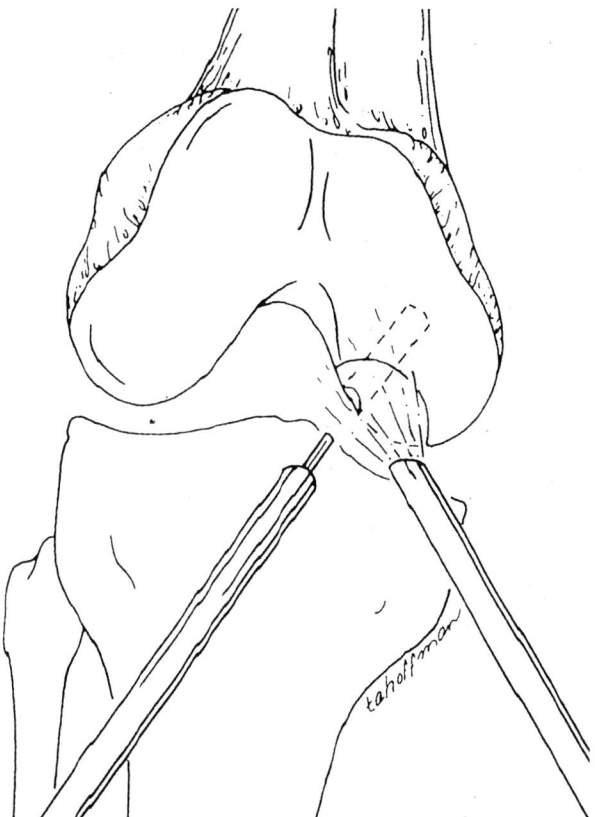

Figure 69.12. For antegrade grafting of a lesion of the medial femoral condyle, the cannula is placed through the anterolateral portal and the arthroscope is placed in the anteromedial portal. Reprinted with permission from Guhl JF, Johnson RP, Stone JW. The impact of arthroscopy on osteochondritis dissecans. In: McGinty JB, ed. Operative arthroscopy. 2nd ed. Philadelphia: Lippincott-Raven, 1996:387.

ments can also be elevated by this approach. Although few problems have been reported, the use of an autograft holds the potential for donor site morbidity. The decision to combine bone grafting by either technique with pin or screw fixation should be based on lesion stability.

Fragment Removal with Drilling and Abrasion

In OCD and osteochondral fractures, removal of loose bodies or unstable lesions by drilling and/or abrading the bed eliminates mechanical symptoms, resulting in short-term improvement (7,19,20). Removal of small free fragments has a favorable prognosis. When large lesions that involve a significant portion of the weight-bearing surface, where degenerative changes are expected to occur, are removed, long-term results are likely to be less satisfactory. Removal should be reserved for lesions not appropriate for one of the previously discussed forms of treatment. Removal is indicated in the case of multiple small fragments, especially if they have been displaced for more than a few weeks. Removal is also indicated for large fragments with inadequate bone for fixation and for pure chondral lesions. If removal is indicated, it is better done early than late. The goal of the procedure is to change the

local environment from one of exposed bone to one that will stimulate cartilage repair.

The fragment to be removed can be retrieved with arthroscopic grasping instruments through standard or accessory arthroscopic portals. A scalpel should be used for portal enlargement as necessary to avoid entrapment of the fragment in the subcutaneous tissue. Attention is next directed to the bed of the lesion. Overhanging cartilage is removed or trephined until a stable hyaline cartilage rim is created. Although cartilage can be débrided with motorized instruments, it is better removed with a small curette to create side walls perpendicular to the chondral surface and limit damage to the cartilage being left behind.

How much cartilage should be removed? Any undermined cartilage with no attachment to bone should be removed. If the cartilage is not separated and has bony support, it should be left in place, to avoid creating a larger defect. The base of the defect is then abraded and drilled (Fig. 69.13). Abrasion is performed systematically over the entire lesion to remove dead surface osteons and to provide a surface for blood attachment. Abrasion is a superficial débridement, best performed with a motorized burr. The depth of abrasion rarely exceeds 1 to 2 mm. Drilling should also be performed; the number of holes and the depth of drilling is determined as previously described. Satisfactory abrasion and drilling is confirmed by evidence of blood flow with tourniquet deflation and joint decompression. If a large weight-bearing lesion must be removed, an osteotomy to realign the weight-bearing axis may be indicated.

If successful, abrasion and drilling result in regrowth of fibrocartilaginous reparative tissue. Histologically, the fibrocartilage substitute lacks the type II collagen content that would be found in hyaline cartilage, although drilling may increase the content of type II collagen. The fibrocartilage substitute is less resistant to weight-bearing stresses than is hyaline cartilage; however, it is better than

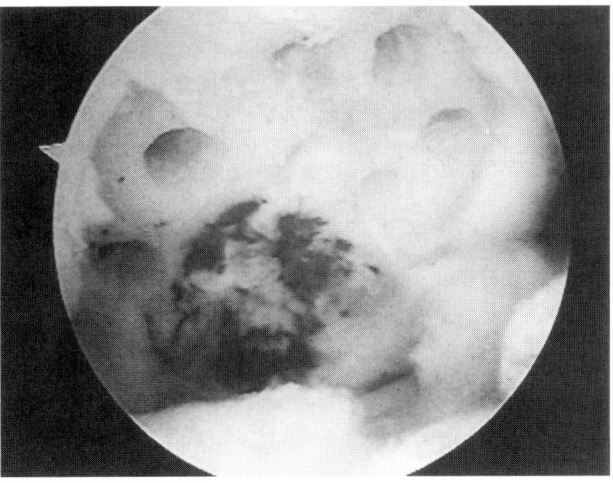

Figure 69.13. A 1- × 1-cm lesion of the lateral femoral condyle has been abraded and drilled with a 0.062 K wire.

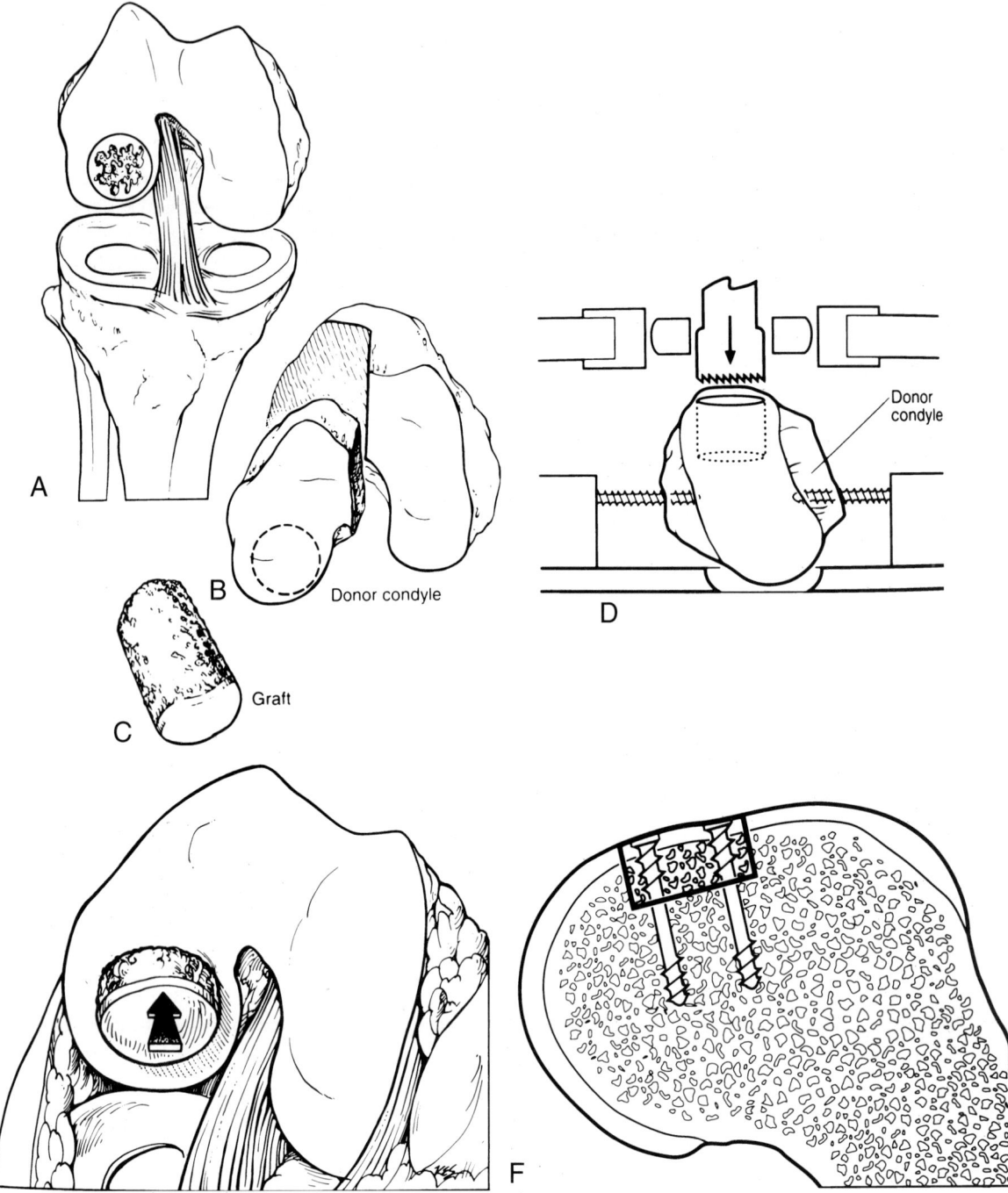

Figure 69.14. A. A defect is identified in the condyle of a possible osteochondral allograft recipient. **B.** The defect is matched to the donor condyle. **C.** A cylindrical graft of articular cartilage and underlying bone is taken. **D.** The transplant condyle is placed in a jig and oriented to the articular surface with a hand-powered cutter. **E.** The donor plug graft is placed in the recipient condyle defect. **F.** Herbert screws are used to fix the osteochondral allograft. Reprinted by permission from Garret JC. Osteochondral allografts for reconstruction of articular defects. In: McGinty JB, ed. Operative arthroscopy. 2nd ed. Philadelphia: Lippincott-Raven, 1996:387.

the joint incongruity associated with a persistent defect filled with fibrous tissue.

Osteochondral Allografts and Autografts

Osteochondral allografts are used for reconstruction of large defects around the knee (21,22). In addition to their use following en bloc tumor excision, they have been used in osteoarthritis and osteonecrosis. Allografts have also been advocated for smaller defects, such as OCD lesions and osteochondral fractures that are at least 2 cm in diameter.

Use of osteochondral allografts is indicated for large OCD lesions of the weight-bearing portion of the lateral femoral condyle. These lesions are prone to fragmentation, making previously discussed treatment options less applicable. Their use may also be indicated for patients younger than 40 years who have persistent symptoms and disability following failure of a previous procedure, such as abrasion arthroplasty.

An osteochondral allograft is used to restore normal joint architecture and mechanics. Such a graft replaces the defect in the articular surface with a structural graft of normal articular cartilage securely anchored to subchondral bone. Success of the procedure depends on immunologic survival of the transplant and congruous restoration of the joint surface. Because of the immunologically privileged nature of cartilage, rejection has not been a large problem, obviating the need for immunologic suppression of recipients. Cryopreservation is deleterious to the grafts' chondral layers, making implantation of fresh grafts the procedure of choice.

The technique involves harvest of an entire knee from a suitable deceased donor, matched with the recipient for age and for skeletal size (Fig. 69.14). Potential recipients are on a waiting list and must be available within hours. Following harvest, the osteochondral allograft and recipient site are prepared simultaneously. A hole centered over the lesion is drilled in the recipient condyle, resulting in a 4- to 5-mm-deep defect with viable bone at the base. The defect is replaced with an osteochondral donor plug of similar dimensions. Specially designed instruments are used to obtain a graft to match the condylar contour in both planes. The donor plug is internally fixed with countersunk Herbert screws.

Other methods of graft fixation have been used, including interference fit, K wires, cannulated screws, bone pegs, and bioabsorbable implants. Successful results have also been reported with autogenous osteochondral grafts from patellar and non–weight-bearing medial femoral condylar sources using similar techniques. Recently developed techniques for chondrocyte replantation may play a role in the treatment of these types of lesions in the future.

Use of osteochondral allografts is occasionally indicated as the primary treatment for OCD and osteochondral fractures, in addition to its use as a salvage procedure following failure of other treatment options. Risk of disease transmission remains a concern, although improved screening procedures have substantially decreased the risks. It is an exacting and technically demanding procedure. Although its application and use may become more common, osteochondral allograft should presently be performed by surgeons specifically trained in and familiar with these techniques.

PITFALLS AND COMPLICATIONS

Each of the procedures described here has potential pitfalls and complications.

When drilling a lesion, the surgeon should use a K wire instead of a drill bit to minimize articular surface damage. K wires are prone to misdirection and breakage, especially the small guidewires associated with cannulated screw systems. Broken wires may remain buried in bone or may become loose within the joint. In either case, an arthro-

tomy may be required for retrieval. The availability of a C-arm for intra-operative images can be invaluable for avoiding and dealing with these problems.

K wires used for pinning are susceptible to migration. All hardware used for internal fixation, whether pins or screws, are subject to failure under weight-bearing loads over time. Bone grafts are subject to misplacement and displacement and, like hardware, can become loose within the joint when inserted by the direct approach.

Searching for loose bodies in OCD or osteochondral fractures and attempting to retrieve lost or broken grafts or hardware can be frustrating. A systematic arthroscopic approach to joint examination is essential. Arthroscopic examination should include sites that frequently harbor loose and foreign bodies: the suprapatellar pouch, the gutters, the popliteal hiatus, and the posteromedial and posterolateral compartments. Loose bodies occasionally come to rest beneath the menisci, where they may be missed on inspection without probing. When a loose or foreign body is encountered, the inflow should be turned off to prevent migration. The fragment can then be retrieved with grasping instruments through a standard or accessory portal.

Selection of the implant for internal fixation of lesions is based on size and location. Although proper selection of the implant can minimize the problem, internal fixation may be complicated by comminution or fragmentation of the lesion. When this occurs, removal of the lesion may be required.

Careful preoperative workup and planning include anticipating intraoperative equipment needs; aiding in the ultimate assessment of the lesions; and determining the final treatment, which is made at the time of diagnostic arthroscopy. The surgeon should avoid the situation in which a patient who is under anesthesia cannot be treated as desired because the equipment or instrumentation required for the procedure is either unavailable or inadequate.

Arthroscopic treatment for osteochondral lesions about the knee is technically demanding, requiring attention to detail for a successful result. In many cases, lesion size, location, and fragment–bed mismatch are formidable obstacles to definitive arthroscopic treatment, even for the most experienced arthroscopist. In such cases, arthrotomy is indicated. Failure to proceed to open treatment when indicated can lead to malreduction, lesion fragmentation, hardware breakage, and less-than-satisfactory end results. While the benefits of arthroscopy with respect to cost, cosmesis, and morbidity are well documented, it should be remembered that a well-performed open procedure is superior to a poorly performed arthroscopic technique.

REHABILITATION

The literature is replete with reports on the operative treatment of OCD in which patients were treated with 6 or more weeks of postoperative immobilization. The deleterious effects of joint immobilization on articular cartilage are well known. Therefore, postoperative immobilization should be avoided whenever possible. The goal of operative treatment for both OCD lesions and osteochondral fractures should be rigid internal fixation to permit early joint mobilization with protection of weight-bearing stresses. Treatment options not compatible with early joint mobilization are less desirable.

Following fixation of OCD or osteochondral fractures, the patient can be placed in a supportive dressing; cryotherapy may be prescribed. Use of a hinged rehabilitative brace permits motion while providing some support and protection for the knee. Intermittent active range of motion exercises are begun immediately. Salvageable lesions for which rigid internal fixation cannot be obtained can be treated with limited range of motion exercises in a hinged brace, allowing protection of the affected area as an alternative to full immobilization. Use of continuous passive motion (CPM) is rarely indicated; internal fixation of osteochondral allografts is an exception. The patient is instructed in quadriceps setting exercises and straight leg raises to minimize muscle atrophy.

Crutches are used for non–weight-bearing ambulation for the first 6 to 8 weeks. Thereafter, weight bearing is progressed; and lightweight progressive resistance exercises (PREs) are added, depending on clinical (i.e., pain, effusion) and radiographic criteria for healing. Radiographs may demonstrate bony trabeculae bridging the lesion, although radiographic evidence for early union may be difficult to determine. As noted, bone scintigraphy is a more sensitive method of following healing. For lesions of the weight-bearing surfaces, protection from rotational stresses is continued for at least 3 months. Time to healing averages 5 months for OCD lesions, although healing may occur sooner for acute osteochondral fractures. Progres-

sion of activity and return to athletic participation is permitted once healing has been documented.

When a lesion requires removal with curettage and débridement, postoperative treatment includes early motion and protected weight bearing. For large lesions of the weight-bearing surface, postoperative use of CPM can be considered. Active range of motion exercises are sufficient for smaller lesions. Non–weight-bearing crutch ambulation is continued for 8 weeks after surgery. Weight bearing and activity are progressed thereafter, although the prognosis for long-term function of substitute fibrocartilage under athletic levels of weight-bearing stresses is poor.

SUMMARY

OCD lesions are likely the result of cyclic cumulative stresses to the subchondral bone. With time, the subchondral stress fracture may become associated with an overlying cartilage lesion. The literature provides support for a variety of treatment options (Table 69.1). Note that radiographic healing does not always correlate with a satisfactory subjective or functional result. The goals of treatment, as for other intra-articular fractures, are to obtain a congruous reduction, improve vascularity for healing, and provide stability with internal fixation as necessary to allow for early motion. Review of the literature and application of these principles allow the surgeon to develop an algorithm for the treatment of OCD lesions.

Initial evaluation should include a clinical assessment and plain radiographs. Based on the initial assessment, a distinction should be made between JOCD and OCD. MRI evaluation to assess lesion stability can be performed, if indicated.

table 69.1	Results of Treatment of OCD				
Treatment	Number of Patients	Average Follow-up	Results[a]	Average Time to Healing	Reference
Nonoperative	92	4.2 years	51% success; healed		5
	22	9.4 years	82% good to excellent		23
	18	4.5 years	95% excellent; healed		24
Drilling	16	4.7 years	100% success; healed	4.9 months	7
	15	3 years	93% good to excellent; 100% healed	5 months	6
Bone pegs	10	2.9 years	80% good to excellent		10
	18	3.2 years	94% good to excellent; 100% healed	4.6 months	8
	20	5 years	75% G/E; 100% healed	6 months	9
Pin fixation	17	5–7 years	65% good to excellent; 94% healed	8 months	11
	8	9 years	88% good to excellent		12
Cannulated screws	29	3.5 years	88% good to excellent; 88% healed		14
	15	1 year	93% good to excellent		13
Herbert screws	18	4–30 months	89% success; healed		15
	11	1.3 years	82% good to excellent; 73% healed		16
Retrograde bone grafting	3	7 months	100% success; healed		18
	3	3–8 years	100% success; healed		17
Removal; abrasion; drilling	29	2.9 years	72% good to excellent		19
	10	3 years	78% good to excellent		6
Osteochondral allograft	40	1–6 years	98% success		21
	2	2–6 years	100% success		22

[a]Healed radiographic healing.

In JOCD, stable lesions should initially be treated non-operatively, with the expectation that 50 to 80% will heal. JOCD lesions that fail to progress to healing as skeletal maturity approaches, unstable JOCD lesions, and all OCD lesions merit operative treatment.

Operative treatment begins with an assessment of lesion's stability by arthroscopy. Stable lesions with intact cartilage can be treated by isolated drilling (JOCD) or isolated bone grafting (OCD). Stable lesions of large size or with associated cartilage defects are at risk of becoming unstable, and initial operative treatment should include internal fixation and drilling (JOCD) or bone grafting (OCD). The optimal device for internal fixation has not been agreed on; the options include pins, bone pegs, and screws. We prefer Herbert screw fixation of appropriate lesions because of the ability to provide rigid internal fixation while avoiding some of the problems associated with other devices.

Unstable lesions, whether loosened, partially detached, or completely detached, are categorized as either salvageable or unsalvageable. Salvageable lesions should be treated with internal fixation and supplemented with drilling (JOCD) or bone grafting (OCD), depending on the lesion's size. Internal fixation devices that provide compression assist with the reduction of the elevated fragments. Supplemental bone grafting can be used for elevation of depressed fragments.

Treatment of unsalvageable lesions is based on size. Small lesions can be débrided, abraded, and drilled, with the expectation of satisfactory results. Osteochondral allografts should be considered for large lesions, which typically involve weight-bearing surfaces, to avoid degenerative changes that may follow débridement. Osteochondral allografts can also be considered for salvage procedures after other procedures have failed. Osteochondral autografts and replantation of chondrocytes may have increasing roles in the treatment of OCD in the future.

A high level of clinical suspicion is required for the diagnosis of acute osteochondral fractures. They should be treated by adhering to the principles of treatment for intra-articular fractures as well. Every effort should be made to attempt open reduction and internal fixation. Removal, abrasion, and drilling can be considered for small lesions. Osteochondral allograft should be considered for large unsalvageable lesions.

Arthroscopy is an invaluable tool for the assessment and treatment of osteochondral lesions. When lesion size, lesion location, or the technical demands of the procedure dictate, it is prudent to proceed to open techniques for definitive treatment.

REFERENCES

1. Konig F. Ueber freie korper in den gelenken. Dtsch Z Chir 1888; 27:90–109.
2. Linden B. Osteochondritis dissecans of the femoral condyles. A long-term follow-up study. J Bone Joint Surg 1977;59A:769–776.
3. Pappas AM. Osteochondritis dissecans. Clin Orthop 1981;158: 59–69.
3a. Wilson JN. A diagnostic sign in osteochondritis dissecans of the knee. J Bone Joint Surg 1967;49A:477–480.
4. Mesgarzadeh M, Sapega AA, Bonakdarpour A, et al. Osteo-chondritis dissecans: analysis of mechanical stability with radiography, scintigraphy, and MR imaging. Radiology 1987;165:775–780.
5. Cahill BR, Phillips MR, Navarro R. The results of conservative management of juvenile osteochondritis dissecans using joint scintigraphy. A prospective study. Am J Sports Med 1989;17: 601–606.
6. Guhl JF. Arthroscopic treatment of osteochondritis dissecans. Clin Orthop 1982;167;65–74.
7. Aglietti P, Buzzi R, Bassi PB, Fioriti M. Arthroscopic drilling in juvenile osteochondritis dissecans of the medial femoral condyle. Arthroscopy 1994;10:286–291.
8. Gillespie HS, Day B. Bone peg fixation in the treatment of osteochondritis dissecans of the knee. Clin Orthop 1979;143:125–130.
9. Lindholm S, Pylkkanen P, Osterman K. Fixation of osteochondral fragments in the knee joint. A clinical survey. Clin Orthop 1977; 126:256–260.
10. Slough JA, Noto AM, Schmidt TL. Tibial cortical bone peg fixation in osteochondritis dissecans of the knee. Clin Orthop 1991; 267:122–127.
11. Anderson AF, Lipscomb AB, Coulam C. Antegrade curettement, bone grafting, and pinning of osteochondritis dissecans in the skeletally mature knee. Am J Sports Med 1990;18:254–261.
12. Lipscomb PR Jr, Lipscomb PR Sr, Bryan RS. Osteochondritis dissecans of the knee with loose fragments. J Bone Joint Surg 1978; 60A:235–240.
13. Cugat R, Garcia M, Cusco X, et al. Osteochondritis dissecans: a historical review and its treatment with cannulated screws. Arthroscopy 1993;9:675–684.
14. Johnson LL, Uitvlugt G, Austin MP, et al. Osteochondritis dissecans of the knee: arthroscopic compression screw fixation. Arthroscopy 1990;6:179–189.
15. Thompson NL. Osteochondritis dissecans and osteochondral fragments managed by Herbert compression screw fixation. Clin Orthop 1987;224:71–78.
16. Rey Zuniga JJ, Sagastibelza J, Lopez Blasco JJ, Martinez Grande M. Arthroscopic use of the Herbert screw in osteochondritis dissecans of the knee. Arthroscopy 1993;9:668–670.
17. Johnson RP, Aaberg TM Jr. Use of retrograde bone grafting in the treatment of osseous defects of the lateral condyle of the knee: a preliminary report of three knees in two patients. Orthopaedics 1987;10:291–297.
18. Lee CK, Mercurio C. Operative treatment of osteochondritis dissecans in situ by retrograde drilling and cancellous bone graft. A preliminary report. Clin Orthop 1981;158:129–136.
19. Ewing JW, Voto SJ. Arthroscopic surgical management of osteochondritis dissecans of the knee. Arthroscopy 1988;4:37–40.
20. Johnson LL. Arthroscopic abrasion arthroplasty. In: McGinty JB, ed. Operative arthroscopy. New York: Raven, 1991:341–360.
21. Garrett JC. Osteochondritis dissecans. Clin Sports Med 1991; 10:569–593.
22. Yamashita F, Sakakida K, Suzu F, Takai S. The transplantation of an autogeneic osteochondral fragment for osteochondritis dissecans of the knee. Clin Orthop 1985;201:43–50.
23. Hughston JC, Hergenroeder PT, Courtenay BG. Osteochondritis dissecans of the femoral condyles. J Bone Joint Surg 1984; 66A:1340–1348.
24. Green WT, Banks HH. Osteochondritis dissecans in children. J Bone Joint Surg 1953;135A:26–47.

Suggested Readings

Aichroth P. Osteochondritis dissecans of the knee. J Bone Joint Surg 1971;153B:440–447.
Cahill BR. Osteochondritis dissecans of the knee. J Am Acad Orthop Surg 1995;3:237–247.
Clanton TO, DeLee JC. Osteochondritis dissecans—history, pathology, and current treatment concepts. Clin Orthop 1988;167:50–64.

Graf BK, Lange RH. Osteochondritis dissecans. In: Reider B, ed. Sports medicine: the school age athlete. Philadelphia: Saunders, 1991:240–254.

Guhl JF, Johnson RP, Stone JW. The impact of arthroscopy on osteochondritis dissecans. In: McGinty JB, ed. Operative arthroscopy. New York: Raven, 1991:297–317.

Hohl M, Larson RL, Jones DC. Fractures and dislocations of the knee. In: Rockwood CA, Green DP, eds. Fractures in adults. Philadelphia: Lippincott, 1984:1429–1592.

Kennedy JC, Grainger RW, McGraw RW. Osteochondral fractures of the femoral condyles. J Bone Joint Surg 1966;48B:436–440.

O'Donoghue D. Chondral and osteochondral fractures. J Trauma 1966; 6:469–481.

Sebastianelli WJ, DeHaven KE. Chondral fractures and intra-articular osteochondroses. In: DeLee JC, Drez D, eds. Orthopaedic sports medicine: principles and practice. Philadelphia: Saunders, 1994: 1444–1467.

Smillie IS. Treatment of osteochondritis dissecans. J Bone Joint Surg 1957;39B:248–260.

Sweeney HJ. Chondral and osteochondral fractures of the knee. In: McGinty JB, ed. Operative arthroscopy. New York: Raven, 1991: 285–295.

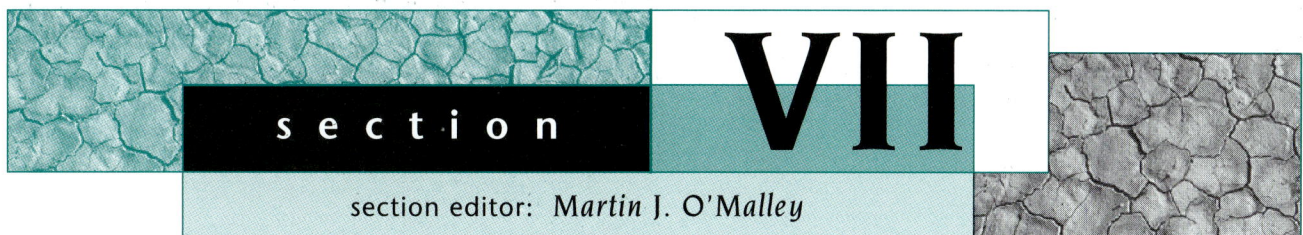

FOOT AND ANKLE

Fractures of the Ankle

Ankle fractures are one of the more commonly treated fractures in orthopaedics. Understanding the anatomy of the normal and the fractured ankle is necessary to adequately restore the function of the joint after a fracture. Treatment decisions are based on clinical history, physical examination, and radiographic evaluation of the fracture pattern and amount of displacement. The principle of treatment is to restore the normal tracking of the talus in the ankle mortise by providing an anatomical reduction of the fracture and by maintaining the reduction by either closed treatment or open treatment with internal fixation.

RELEVANT ANATOMY AND PATHOGENESIS

The ankle is a highly congruent saddle-shaped joint with an articulation between the superior aspect of the talus, the distal aspect of the tibia, and the distal aspect of the fibula. The tibial plafond and the fibula together form the ankle mortise with which the talus articulates. The medial facet of the talus articulates with the medial malleolus of the distal tibia, and the lateral facet of the talus articulates with the lateral malleolus of the distal fibula. The lateral malleolus is posterior to the medial malleolus. The distal aspect of the lateral malleolus is distal to the distal tip of the medial malleolus. The talus is wider anteriorly than it is posteriorly and it is wider medially than it is laterally.

The syndesmotic ligament complex maintains the integrity of the distal tibia and fibula to form the ankle mortise (Fig. 70.1). This complex is made up of the distal anterior tibiofibular ligament, the distal posterior tibiofibular ligament, the transverse tibiofibular ligament, and the interosseous ligament. The anterior and posterior distal tibiofibular ligaments attach to the inner aspect of the tibia and proceed laterally and downward to attach to the fibula. Because the posterior ligament is stronger than the anterior ligament, a torsional force in the area will usually result in an avulsion fracture off the posterior tibia and a rupture of the anterior ligament. The interosseous ligament is the key transverse stabilizer of the tibiofibular ar-

ticulation. The interosseous membrane is located between the entire length of the tibia and fibula and the fibers run from superior medially to inferior laterally. This membrane stabilizes the fibula and serves as an additional attachment site for the lower leg muscles.

The normal range of motion of the ankle joint has been estimated to be 12° of dorsiflexion to 56° of plantar flexion in the unloaded state (1). The ankle joint is not a pure hinge-type joint. The normal motion of plantar flexion and dorsiflexion is a combination of sliding and rolling. Ankle dorsiflexion and plantar flexion are associated with rotation along the vertical axis. Plantar flexion causes between 4° and 8° of internal rotation of the talus, and this rotation is thought to be the result of tethering of the medial aspect of the talus by the deltoid ligament. Dorsiflexion and plantar flexion of the ankle cause motion of the fibula. With dorsiflexion, the fibula moves in a medial to lateral direction and externally rotates as much as 2°.

During weight bearing with the ankle in normal alignment, 80 to 90% of the load to the talus is transmitted from the tibial plafond (1). The remainder of the load is transmitted from the fibula. The tibiotalar articulation is not flat but has two shallow condylar projections from the talus, which articulate with matching depressions in the tibial plafond. This configuration helps the talus remain in the most congruent position of the joint when it is loaded. The joint reaction force in the ankle has been measured to be almost four times body weight in the stance phase of gait.

When the ankle is fractured, the bones and the ligaments about the ankle are injured. The mechanism and force of the injury determines the fracture pattern and the extent of the ligamentous injury. The static and dynamic congruency of the joint is determined by the fracture pattern and the displacement of the fragments. A statically incongruent ankle joint has an articular step-off in the weight-bearing area. Although radiographs of ankle fractures do not commonly reveal an articular step-off in the weight-bearing areas, studies have shown that more than

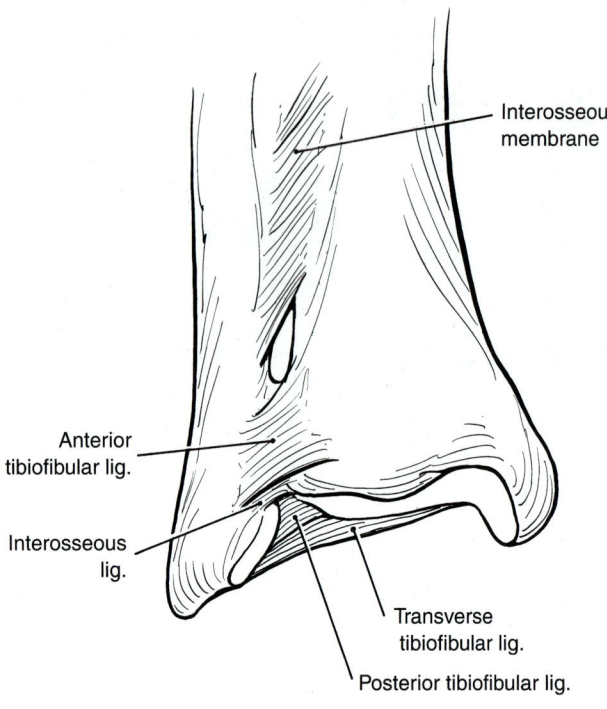

Figure 70.1. Syndesmotic ligaments of the ankle.

Interosseous membrane

Anterior tibiofibular lig.

Interosseous lig.

Transverse tibiofibular lig.

Posterior tibiofibular lig.

40% of ankle fractures that have undergone operative fixation have demonstrable cartilage injury (usually on the talar side) (2). With dynamic incongruity, also known as instability, there is a derangement of the alignment of the bony structures of the ankle, which leads to abnormal motion of the ankle. The abnormal kinematics can lead to premature arthritis.

In a bimalleolar ankle fracture, the talar displacement usually follows the lateral malleolus in. If the lateral malleolus fractures, the dynamic congruity of the joint is maintained as long as the medial deltoid ligament and the medial malleolus are intact. If the deltoid ligament or the medial malleolus is disrupted, anterolateral rotatory instability results, and the contact area of the joint is diminished. The goal of treatment for all ankle fractures is to establish a statically and dynamically congruous joint.

Classification

Ankle fracture classification systems are used to determine the most appropriate treatment for the fracture. The two most widely used classification systems for fractures about the ankle are the Weber AO classification and the Lauge-Hansen classification. The Lauge-Hansen classification was developed as a guide for the closed treatment of these fractures. It is based on the mechanism of injury and

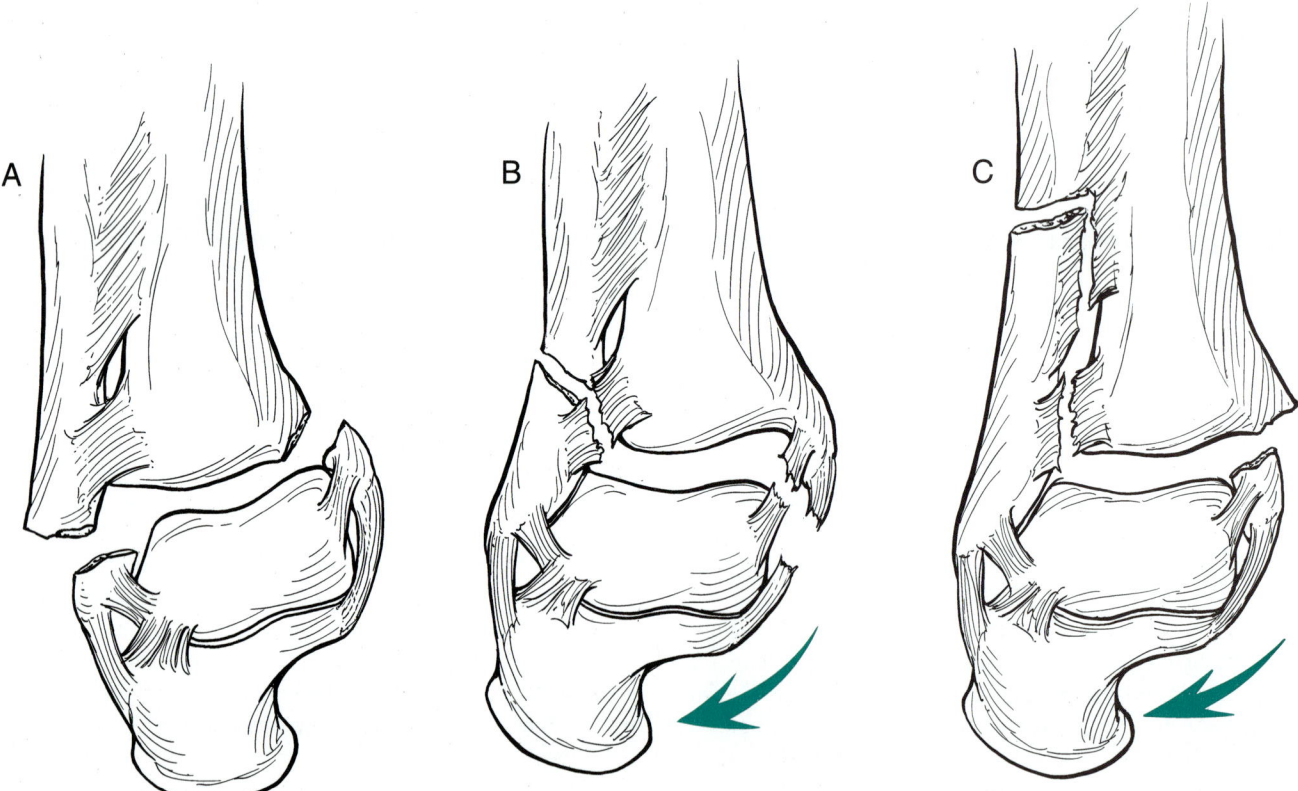

Figure 70.2. Weber classification system for malleolar fractures.

suggests that ankle fractures can be reduced by reversing that mechanism. The Weber classification system is a much simpler than the Lauge-Hansen system; however, the Weber system does not consider medial injuries (Fig. 70.2). This is a particular problem with type B injuries, for which the presence of a medial injury can significantly influence the treatment plan. Neither classification system has been found to be prognostic (3).

INITIAL FINDINGS, PHYSICAL EXAMINATION, AND DIAGNOSIS

Patients with a fractured ankle usually give a history of twisting the ankle. The injury is usually followed by imme-

diate pain and swelling. Patients may complain that the ankle feels loose or unstable. Patients with stable fractures may be able to bear weight on the injured limb; but with unstable injuries, walking is rarely possible.

On physical examination, the ankle is often swollen and may be ecchymotic. It is important to note if there was a medial injury, because this determines the method of treatment. The entire length of the fibula should be checked for tenderness to rule out a more proximal fracture. If there is any suspicion of a proximal fracture, x-rays of the entire fibula should be ordered to rule out a syndesmotic injury with a proximal fibular fracture. After completing the physical examination, the examiner should have an idea if the lateral side, the medial side, or both are

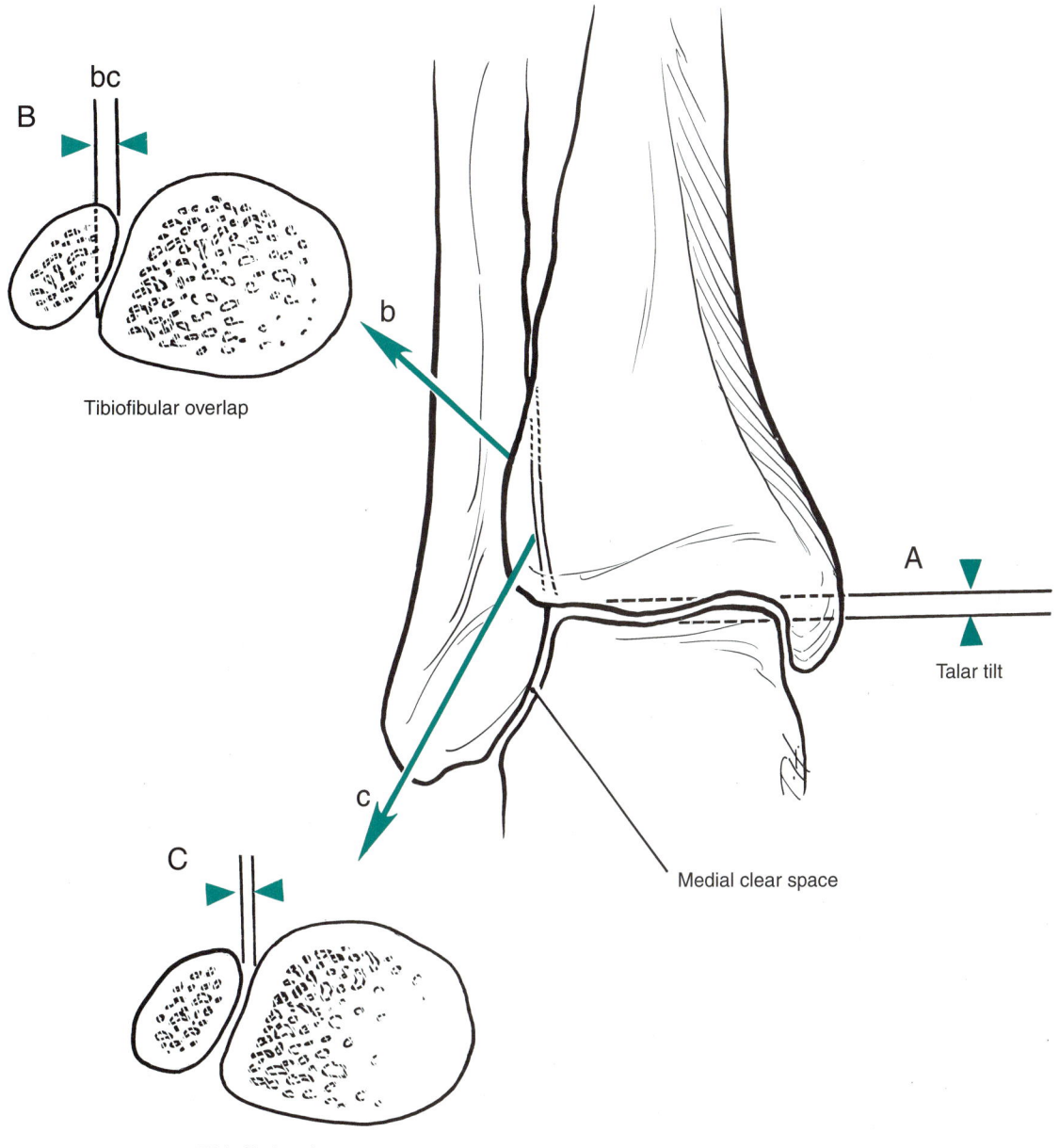

Figure 70.3. A. Talar tilt measure should produce parallel lines. **B.** Tibiofibular overlap should be at least 10 mm; a distance of less than 10 mm indicates a syndesmotic injury. **C.** Tibiofibular clear space should be less than 5 mm. *b*, incisura of tibia; *c*, medial wall of fibula.

injured and whether x-rays of the full fibula are necessary to rule out a proximal fracture.

RADIOLOGIC STUDIES

With ankle fractures, most treatment decisions are based on the radiographic examination of the ankle. Standard radiographs include AP, lateral, and mortise (15° internal oblique) views. A recent study showed a 95% accuracy of diagnosis of ankle fractures using only the mortise and lateral views (4).

From the radiographs, the clinician should determine the extent of soft tissue swelling, the pattern of fractures, and the alignment of the joint. On the AP view, the articular congruity, the relative malleolar length, the syndesmotic integrity, and the extent of the talar shift should be assessed. The lateral view is used to determine the alignment of the ankle and the congruity of the articular surface. The mortise view demonstrates the alignment of the joint, the fibular length, the extent of the talar shift, and the talocrural angle. If there is a question of syndesmosis injury, the clinician should make several important measurements on the AP view: talar tilt,

tibiofibular overlap, and tibiofibular clear space (Fig. 70.3).

The external rotation of the distal fibular fragment seen on standard radiographs is more apparent than real. CT studies of ankle fractures have shown that the relationship of the distal fibular fragment and the talus is unchanged and that the proximal fibula is actually internally rotated on the distal fibular fragment. Proximal migration of the distal fibular fragment (fibular shortening) can be measured by the talocrural angle; however, this measurement has not been found to be reproducible.

TREATMENT

Nonoperative Treatment

About 85% of fractures of the lateral malleolus are not associated with substantial medial injuries. Clinical studies limited to isolated lateral malleolus fractures have shown no advantage of operative treatment over closed treatment of these injuries (5). Recent studies of ankle fracture mechanics that allow for unconstrained motion of the ankle during testing have demonstrated that an isolated lateral

Clinical Table: Fractures of the Ankle

Procedure	Indications	Technique	Anatomy	Pitfalls
Casting	• Nondisplaced Weber A or B fractures without medial injury • Nondisplaced medial malleolus fractures below the level of the joint line	• Short leg cast, ankle in neutral dorsiflexion/ plantar flexion, foot in a plantigrade position		• Loss of reduction
Open reduction and internal fixation	• Lateral malleolus fractures with medial injury • Bimalleolar and trimalleolar fractures or equivalent • Medial avulsion fracture at the joint line or sheer fracture	• Lateral fracture: lateral or posterior fibular plate; lateral approach • Medial fracture: screws, pins, or tension band; medial approach • Posterior fracture: if <25% of the joint surface or >2 mm of displacement, then direct or indirect reduction with the ankle dorsiflexed after the fibula is fixed; posterior lateral approach	• Lateral fracture: superficial peroneal nerve • Medial fracture: saphenous nerve	• Wound infection • Failure of fixation • Inadequate reduction • Iatrogenic nerve injury
Syndesmosis fixation	• Widening of the syndesmosis or ankle mortise	• Screw from the fibula to the tibia through 3 or 4 cortices, parallel to the tibial plafond; the screw should be directed about 30° anteriorly; when the screw is tightened, the ankle should be held in approximately 10° to 15° of dorsiflexion	• Superficial peroneal nerve	• Wound infection • Failure of fixation • Inadequate reduction • Iatrogenic nerve injury

MMD, maximum manual difference.

injury does not lead to abnormal mechanics or kinematics of the joint. Furthermore, the amount of displacement of the fibula does not determine talar displacement when the ankle is axially loaded. For lateral malleolar fractures without a medial injury, dynamic incongruity cannot be demonstrated experimentally. CT studies have shown that the apparent external rotation deformity of the lateral malleolus is actually an internal rotation of the proximal aspect of the fibular shaft, which occurs after the fracture, and that the position of the lateral malleolus in relation to the talus is unchanged.

Isolated lateral malleolar fractures (Weber type A or B fractures) should be treated in a cast or brace. Weight bearing can begin as soon as the patient feels comfortable, as weight bearing is not associated with further displacement of these stable fractures. Isolated fractures of the medial malleolus are rare and can be treated nonoperatively if they are not displaced, if they involve the portion of the malleolus below the joint line, or if they can be anatomically reduced by closed reduction.

A closed reduction is obtained by reversing the mechanism of injury. Once the reduction is achieved and a short leg cast applied, radiographs are obtained to determine the adequacy of the reduction. For cases with a great deal of swelling, a splint should initially be used. Once the swelling subsides, a cast may be applied.

Stable fractures are treated in a short leg walking cast or fracture brace for about 6 weeks. For unstable fractures, a long leg cast is necessary for 6 weeks; then a short leg cast or fracture brace can be used. For about 4 weeks after the reduction of an unstable fracture, radiographs of the ankle are checked weekly to identify and correct any loss of reduction.

Operative Treatment

Once operative intervention has been decided on, surgery should either be performed before maximal swelling of the ankle occurs or be delayed until after the swelling has subsided. The timing of the surgery depends on the patient's overall condition, the condition of the soft tissue, and the amount of swelling. Upon presentation, the ankle should be gently reduced and immobilized in a well-padded splint. Immobilizing the fracture helps prevent further soft tissue damage, and elevation of the injured extremity helps decrease the swelling (Clinical Table).

BIMALLEOLAR ANKLE FRACTURES

Bimalleolar ankle and lateral malleolus fractures with a medial deltoid disruption (the bimalleolar equivalent) result in the loss of the ankle's medial and lateral supports; thus these fractures are unstable (Fig. 70.4). Experiment-

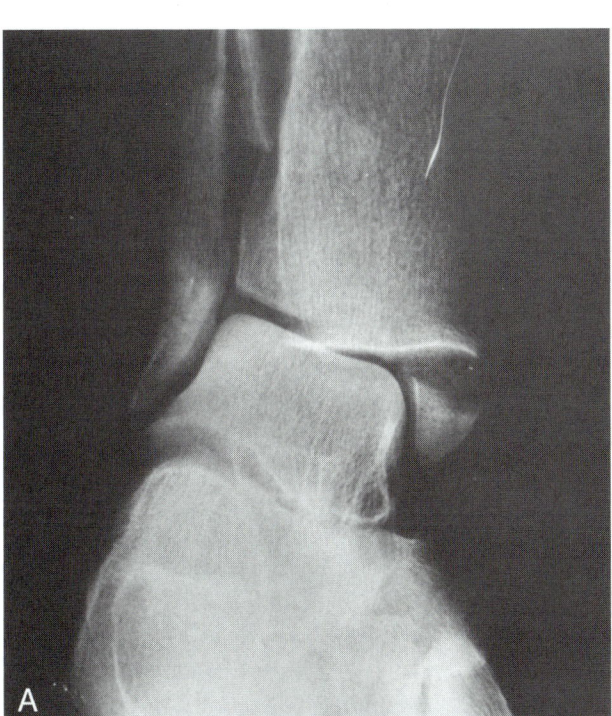
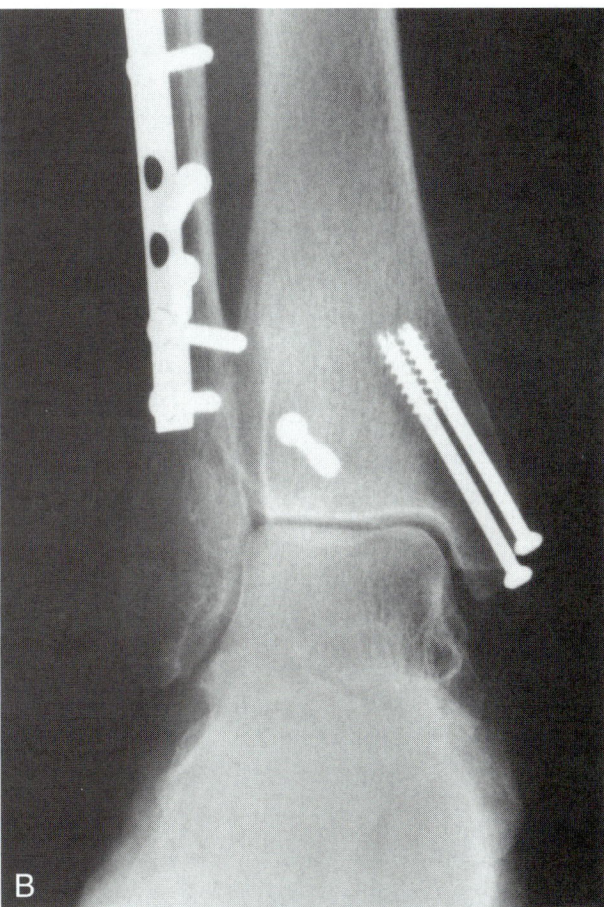

Figure 70.4. Preoperative (**A**) and postoperative (**B**) AP views showing a bimalleolar ankle fracture.

ally, both the deltoid disruption and the medial malleolus fracture lead to changes in the tibiotalar contact area and in the kinematics of the joint. For bimalleolar or bimalleolar equivalent ankle fractures, the best results are obtained with surgical anatomic reduction and fixation. Between 85 and 90% of patients who undergo an anatomic reduction of these fractures can expect good to excellent results at 3 years or longer (1).

Diagnosing a deltoid injury with a lateral malleolar fracture is difficult. The presence of medial tenderness and more than 5 mm of space between the medial malleolus and the talus in either initial or stress radiographs allows the presumptive diagnosis of a substantial medial deltoid ligament injury (Fig. 70.5). When the lateral malleolus is fractured and the deltoid is disrupted, it is not necessary to repair the deltoid ligament (1). In these cases, anatomic reduction with fixation of the lateral malleolus fracture and treatment with a short leg cast provide satisfactory results. The only indication for opening the medial side is a failure to reduce the talus medially with a wide medial clear space. In such cases, the medial side is explored to remove the ligament, which may have flipped into the ankle joint. The ligament does not need to be sutured back into

place. In fact, patients who have undergone primary repair of the deltoid ligament have poorer results than those who did have the repair.

The decision for surgery should not be based on the age of the patient. Studies have shown that older patients who have undergone open reduction and internal fixation of bimalleolar fractures have improved clinical results, compared with those who have been treated nonoperatively. The major concerns with operative fixation in older patients are a higher rate of wound complications and, because of osteopenic bone, difficulty obtaining stable fixation. This latter concern can be treated by placing an antiglide plate on the posterior aspect of the fibula.

For surgery, the patient should be positioned with a bump under the ipsilateral buttock to improve exposure of the lateral malleolus. The incision to access the distal fibula is either anterolateral or posterolateral to the subcutaneous aspect of the lateral fibula. The distal aspect of the incision may be curved, if additional exposure is needed. If the incision is carried proximally, the deeper interval is between the peroneus tertius anteriorly and the peroneus longus and brevis posteriorly. The superficial peroneal nerve passes from posterosuperior to anteroin-

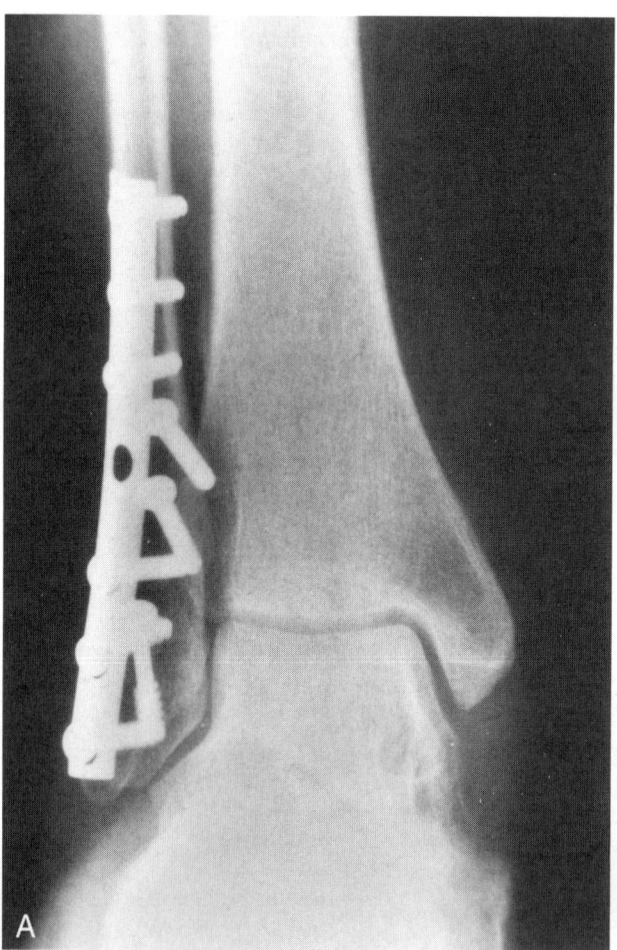
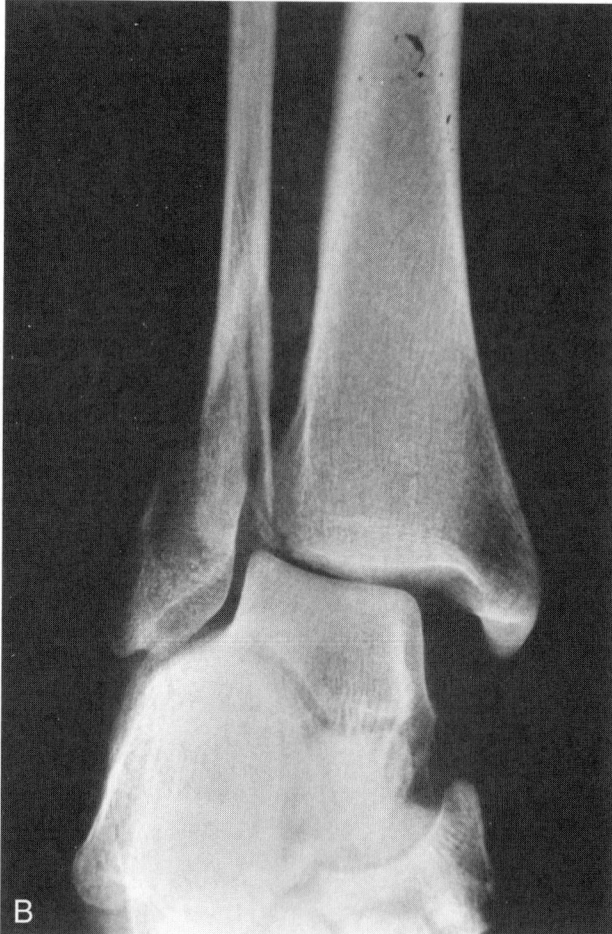

Figure 70.5. Preoperative (**A**) and postoperative (**B**) AP views showing a medial deltoid injury with a fibula fracture.

ferior and can be encountered beneath the fascia at various levels. It should be protected during dissection, fracture fixation, and closure of the wound.

After reducing the fibula fracture, a clamp is used to hold the bone while at least one 3.5-mm lag screw is placed perpendicular to the fracture line. If the oblique portion of the fracture is longer than two times the diameter of the fibula, lag screws alone can be used to hold the fracture reduced. In the majority of cases, however, a lateral neutralization plate is used to obtain rotational and axial stability. Usually, the one-third tubular plate is used, because it has a low profile and is fixed to the fibula with 3.5-mm cortical screws. Distally, in the area of the ankle joint, cancellous screws can be used to engage the lateral cortex and the cancellous bone. The medial cortex should not be engaged, so that the fibular talar joint is not entered.

Alternatively, the plate may be placed posteriorly on the fibula as an antiglide plate. This is especially helpful in patients with osteoporotic bone; some surgeons prefer this placement because the plate is not subcutaneous. To place the plate posteriorly, the incision should be made over the posterior aspect of the fibula. The peroneal tendons are retracted posteriorly from the posterior fibula. After the fracture is reduced, screws are placed through the plate into the proximal fragment; one screw is just proximal to the tip of the fracture site. A lag screw is placed from posterior to anterior through the plate and across the fracture site. Screws may be placed in the distal fragment if the surgeon prefers.

Comminuted fractures of the fibula often result from high-energy injuries and make it difficult to judge rotation and length. Before beginning surgical reduction of these fractures, it is often helpful to have an x-ray of the uninjured fibula and ankle to use as a template for the reduction. Indirect reduction techniques are used to preserve the soft tissue attachments of all the fracture fragments. To perform an indirect reduction, a plate is fixed to the distal fragment, then the plate is pulled or pushed distally to distract the fracture site. With this technique, the tension on the soft tissue helps reduce the fragments, and the position of the fragments and the distal fibula are confirmed radiographically before the plate is secured to the proximal fragment.

There are several common pitfalls and technical mistakes that are made during operative fixation of distal fibula fractures. When placing a lag screw from anterior to posterior in a Weber type B fracture, the starting point on the anterior aspect of the fibula and drill should be aimed posteriorly and slightly laterally to engage the posterior fragment. When placing an antiglide plate on the posterior aspect of the fibula, it is important to aim the drill anteriorly to pass through cancellous bone of the fibula and engage the anterior cortex. If the drill is not aimed anteriorly enough, it will pass through the medial cortex of the fibula, and the second cortex encountered will be the tibia. To al-

low room for the drill to be aimed anteriorly it is helpful to place a sterile bump under the calf with the leg on the edge of the operating table, or if a medial incision will not be necessary, the patient can be positioned in the lateral decubitus position.

SYNDESMOTIC INJURIES

Fibular fractures that begin proximal to the tibial plafond (Weber type C) are assumed to include an injury to the syndesmosis. If there is more than 5 mm of space between the distal aspects of the tibia and the fibula on the mortise x-ray, then the syndesmosis is considered widened. If the syndesmosis is disrupted, it must be stabilized to restore the stability of the ankle mortise. Depending on the fracture pattern, the syndesmosis can be stabilized in a variety of ways. A syndesmosis screw is not necessary if the disruption extends more than 3 cm proximal to the tibial plafond and there is an associated medial malleolar fracture that can be stabilized without residual displacement of the fibula. A syndesmotic screw is necessary if the deltoid ligament is disrupted and the syndesmotic injury extends more than 3 cm proximal to the tibial plafond. In either case, the fibula fracture should be reduced (6).

The surgical approach to the fibula was described above. The syndesmosis screw should be placed after the lateral malleolus fracture is reduced and stabilized. The screw is placed from the lateral fibula into the tibia and should engage three or four cortices. It should be placed parallel to the tibial plafond to avoid displacing the fibula superiorly or inferiorly. Since the fibula lies at the posterior aspect of the tibia, the screw should be aimed about 30° anteriorly from the lateral cortex of the fibula. To avoid compressing the ankle mortise and restricting ankle motion, the syndesmosis should not be placed with the lag technique, and the ankle should be held in 10° to 15° of dorsiflexion. If the ankle is positioned in more plantar flexion when the screw is placed, the mortise will be overtightened and will not be able to accommodate the wide portion of the talar dome; therefore, dorsiflexion range of motion will be diminished.

POSTERIOR MALLEOLAR (TRIMALLEOLAR FRACTURES)

Trimalleolar fractures occur when the posterior ankle injury includes a fracture of the posterior lip of the tibia. This fracture is an avulsion fracture of the tibia from the posterior tibiofibular ligament at its attachment. Treatment depends on both the size and the displacement of the fractured fragment. Reduction and fixation of the associated fibula fracture frequently reduces the posterior malleolus fragment. Open reduction and internal fixation of these fragments is generally recommended for fragments that involve more than 25% of the articular surface as measured on the lateral radiograph and for fractures that are displaced more than 2 mm (2).

Stabilization of the fragment can be approached either directly or indirectly. The fragment may be stabilized directly via a posterior approach. After stabilizing the fibula through an incision placed closer to the posterior aspect of the fibula, direct access to the posterior tibia is gained via the interval between the peroneal tendons and the flexor halluces longus muscle. The external edges of the fracture and x-ray are used as a guide for the reduction of the fragment. The one or two lag screws are placed from posterior to anterior to fix the fragment.

Alternatively, after internally fixing the fibula, a stab incision can be made anteriorly over the tibia, and a lag screw can be placed from anterior to posterior after the posterior fragment is reduced. Dorsiflexing the ankle can reduce the fragment by a ligamentotaxic effect from the posterior capsule. In addition, the fragment can be reduced digitally from the lateral incision and held in place with a reduction clamp.

There are several important points to remember when trying to reduce and fix posterior malleolus fractures. The lateral malleolus must be reduced first, which helps in the reduction of the posterior malleolar fragment. The incision over the fibula should be placed posteriorly to allow access to the posterior malleolar fragment, either directly or indirectly. When placing the screws from anterior to posterior, the fragment should be held securely so the reduction is not lost. If the posterior fragment does not need to be fixed, the ankle should be immobilized in dorsiflexion after surgery to help maintain the position of the posterior malleolus.

MEDIAL MALLEOLAR FRACTURES

Operative fixation of a medial malleolus fracture is indicated if the fracture occurs in conjunction with a lateral malleolus fracture, if the fracture involves the medial malleolus at or above the level of the tibial plafond, or if the fracture is displaced and not reducible. The fracture can be fixed with one or more cancellous screws, with a combination of a screw and wire, or with a tension-band technique. To access the medial malleolus, a longitudinal incision centered over the medial malleolus can be used. The incision can be curved distally, if needed for exposure. Depending on the surgeon's preference, the incision may be shifted anteriorly or posteriorly. The saphenous nerve and the long saphenous vein are just anterior to the medial malleolus and must be protected, especially if a fairly anterior incision is used. The posterior tibial tendon runs in a groove in the posterior tibia and medial malleolus, and this tendon should be protected during exposure and fixation of the fractured fragment.

Once the fracture is reduced, it is provisionally held with Kirschner (K) wires or 2-mm drill bits that are placed perpendicular to the fracture line. Then each K wire or drill bit is removed and replaced with a 4-mm cancellous screw that is long enough to allow the tip to end in metaphyseal bone. It is not necessary to engage the opposite cortex. If the fragment is too small for two screws, then one screw and a K wire can be used. If a K wire is used, the distal end should be bent and buried in the bone and soft tissue.

REHABILITATION

The postoperative management of ankle fractures depends on the surgeon's preference. Ideally, once the fracture is fixed operatively, early mobilization of the ankle should begin to restore function and motion; however, concerns about loss of fixation and patient compliance to avoid weight bearing lead many surgeons to immobilize the ankle until there is evidence of fracture healing. Most studies have not demonstrated a difference between ankles treated with early motion and those immobilized for 3 to 6 weeks (7). As long as there is no syndesmosis injury, many surgeons allow patients to engage in partial weight bearing in a cast or fracture brace, if the fixation of the fracture is adequate. Studies have also demonstrated that weight bearing does not effect either the time to recuperation or the clinical results in operatively and nonoperatively treated ankle fractures. The hardware should be removed if it causes symptoms. The literature generally supports leaving asymptomatic hardware in place, but the final decision is up to the surgeon and the patient.

When a syndesmosis screw has been placed, controversy exists about when to allow weight bearing after surgery (8). Concern that the screw will break with weight bearing causes some authors to advocate removing the syndesmosis screw before permitting weight bearing, although there have been few reports of screw breakage with weight bearing. If the screw engages only three cortices, the normal motion of the fibula is probably not affected with weight bearing and the radiolucency around these screws seen after weight bearing demonstrates that motion between the tibial and fibula will occur. Removing the syndesmosis screw before 6 to 8 weeks should be avoided, because early removal is associated with redisplacement of the fibula and widening of the syndesmosis.

SUMMARY

Accurate diagnosis and appropriate treatment are necessary to optimally restore the function of the ankle after a fracture. Regardless of the method employed, the goal of ankle fracture treatment is to maximize the long-term function of the joint by providing and maintaining an adequate reduction of the fracture.

REFERENCES

1. Michelson JD. Current concepts review. Fractures about the ankle. J Bone Joint Surg 1995;77A:142–152.
2. Vander Griend RA, Savoie FH, Hughes JL. Fractures of the ankle. In: Rockwood CA, Green DP, Bucholz RW, eds. Fractures in adults. 3rd ed. Philadelphia: Lippincott, 1991:1983–2039.
3. Broos LO, Bisschop APG. Operative treatment of ankle fractures in adults: correlation between types of fractures and final results. Injury 1991;22:403–406.
4. Vangsness CT, Carter V, Hunt T, et al. Radiographic diagnosis of an-

kle fractures: are three views necessary? Foot Ankle Int 1994; 15:172–174.

5. Bauer M, Bergstrom B, Hemborg A, Sandegard J. Malleolar fractures: nonoperative versus operative treatment. A controlled study. Clin Orthop 1985;199:17–27.

6. Boden SD, Labropoulos PA, McCowin P, et al. Mechanical consid- erations for the syndesmosis screw. A cadaver study. J Bone Joint Surg 1989;71A:1548–1555.

7. Tropp H, Norlin R. Ankle performance after ankle fracture: a ran- domized study of early mobilization. Foot Ankle Int 1995;16:79–83.

8. Amendola A. Controversies in diagnosis and management of syn- desmosis injuries of the ankle. Foot Ankle 1992;13:44–49.

Ankle and Hindfoot Arthritis: Fusion Techniques

Arthrodesis remains the treatment of choice for end-stage ankle and hindfoot arthritis that is unresponsive to conservative care. The durability and predictable good functional results following these arthrodeses have been well documented. Historically, hindfoot arthritis was typically treated with a triple arthrodesis of the talocalcaneal, talonavicular, and calcaneocuboid joints (1). Current recommendations have evolved to preserve as many joints as possible to prevent additional stresses on adjacent joints and subsequent degeneration of those joints. This chapter outlines the decision processes for determining which joints require fusion and the techniques to achieve those fusions.

RELEVANT ANATOMY AND PATHOGENESIS

Ankle function is intimately associated with the hindfoot joints. The hindfoot joints include the talocalcaneal, talonavicular, and calcaneocuboid joints. The motion of the hindfoot joints is interrelated, which led to the historical tendency to fuse all three of these joints if any of them were arthritic. Recent biomechanical studies have demonstrated the marked differences between the functional motions of these joints.

The tibiotalar joint essentially allows for only plantar flexion and dorsiflexion. The subtalar or talocalcaneal joint allows for a gliding, complex motion of inversion and eversion, with an axis of rotation oriented obliquely across the joint from distal medial to proximal lateral. The talonavicular joint, through its gliding and rotational motion, allows for inversion-eversion, abduction-adduction, and plantar flexion-dorsiflexion. Fusion of this single joint essentially locks the entire hindfoot, including the calcaneocuboid and subtalar joints. The calcaneocuboid joint, with its large, flat articulation allows for relatively limited motion. Recent biomechanical studies have demonstrated that fu-

sion of this joint limits hindfoot inversion-eversion by only approximately one-third. Fusion of the subtalar joint precludes inversion and eversion; however, it does not interfere with plantar flexion and dorsiflexion through the transverse tarsal joints (talonavicular and calcaneocuboid). Therefore, since residual motion will persist with isolated fusions of the calcaneocuboid or subtalar joints, attempts should be made to preserve as many hindfoot joints as possible, especially the talonavicular joint.

Ankle and hindfoot arthritis is most often secondary to degenerative arthritis. Other degenerative conditions, such as posterior tibial tendon rupture and inflammatory arthritis; congenital problems, such as residual clubfoot deformities; and tarsal coalitions necessitate many other ankle or hindfoot fusions. Each of these origins of arthritis leads to painful, arthritic joints and at least some degree of deformity. The ultimate surgical goal of treatment of all these problems, however, remains a stable, plantigrade, painless foot and ankle.

INITIAL FINDINGS, PHYSICAL EXAMINATION, AND DIAGNOSIS

Patients presenting with ankle and hindfoot arthritis complain initially of pain with weight-bearing activities. Generally, the pain develops gradually and becomes progressively worse over months to years. Initially, nonoperative measures, such as anti-inflammatories and bracing, may be successful in providing some relief of symptoms. Patients with ankle arthritis will complain of pain with essentially any weight-bearing activity and especially when walking up or down hills. Patients with hindfoot arthritis likewise have pain with weight-bearing activities but complain of trouble walking on uneven surfaces. With progression of the arthritis, many patients complain of pain at night or at rest.

Upon physical examination, these patients demonstrate tenderness over the affected joints. Ankle tenderness is generally most pronounced along the anterior joint line. It is exacerbated with range of motion, especially at the extremes of plantar flexion and dorsiflexion. With inflammatory arthritis, a boggy edema may be palpable along the anterior aspect of the ankle joint.

With hindfoot arthritis, tenderness is also localized over the affected joint. The talonavicular and calcaneocuboid joints are generally tender over the subcutaneous locations. Tenderness over the subtalar joint is generally localized over the sinus tarsi, just inferior and distal to the lateral aspect of the ankle joint. Pain with inversion and eversion of the subtalar joint is also present.

RADIOLOGIC STUDIES

Evaluation of the ankle should include AP and lateral standing radiographs of the ankle. Specific factors to be evaluated include the presence of arthritis in the ankle and adjacent hindfoot joints. Varus or valgus bony defects and any other posttraumatic bone deformities should be noted. The presence of a sclerotic body of the talus may suggest avascular necrosis, which could affect surgical treatment. Bone density, especially in patients with rheumatoid arthritis, should be evaluated to anticipate fixation needs at the time of surgery.

Evaluation of patients with hindfoot arthritis should include AP and lateral standing radiographs of the foot. The presence of degenerative changes in the subtalar, talonavicular, and calcaneocuboid joints should be assessed individually. If any question exists regarding the ankle joint or if a significant varus or valgus hindfoot deformity exists, an AP x-ray of the ankle should also be obtained. The alignment of the hindfoot should also be assessed on the standing radiographs, including specifically the presence of talonavicular sag or other alteration in the alignment of the hindfoot bones.

TREATMENT

Nonoperative Treatment and Indications for Surgery

Before fusion, patients should receive nonoperative treatment, which can include any or all of the following: nonsteroidal anti-inflammatory drugs (NSAIDs); intra-articular steroid injections; use of an ambulatory aid, such as a cane; and ankle or hindfoot support. Support devices include lace-up or wrap-around ankle supports, ankle-foot orthoses, and a walking boot.

Patients who have failed a course of conservative treatment can be offered a fusion as a surgical option. Determining which joints require fusion can be challenging (Clinical Table). Many patients will have isolated arthritis of the ankle with tenderness over only the ankle joint, pain with range of motion of the ankle joint, and radiographic evidence of isolated ankle arthritis. No further evaluation is required in such patients, and the surgeon can proceed with a fusion of the ankle joint and expect predictable results.

Many patients, however, present with varying degrees of degenerative changes in the adjacent joints, such as the ankle and subtalar joints. These patients may have tenderness over both the ankle and the sinus tarsi. In such cases, the use of differential blocks can be particularly helpful in selecting which joints are symptomatic and require fusion. A small amount of a local anesthetic can be injected into the ankle joint, and the amount of pain relief can be evaluated. During a subsequent examination, the subtalar joint can be injected, and the amount of relief obtained there is assessed. If the patient has near complete relief of pain with the block of either joint, then only that joint need be fused. If the patient has partial relief of pain after each of the two injections, then a combined fusion should be considered.

Before surgery, all patients must have a complete medical evaluation. Medical problems such as diabetes should be under optimal control. Patients with rheumatoid arthritis or other inflammatory arthritis should be under the supervision of a rheumatologist. Methotrexate should be discontinued 1 week before surgery and not resumed until at least 2 weeks after surgery, to minimize the risk of wound-healing problems. Prednisone doses of 7.5 mg or more per day can lead to relatively high rates of infection and to wound-healing problems, but this is often an unavoidable medication (2).

Both dorsalis pedis and posterior tibialis pulses should be palpable. If not, a Doppler ankle-arm index or possibly a vascular surgical consultation is in order. A careful sensory examination should be performed to rule out any pre-existing nerve injuries from old trauma or peripheral neuropathy. In addition, the skin should be examined, and old surgical scars should be assessed to aid in planning the surgical approach. Alignment and range of motion of all the joints in the lower extremity—hip, knee, ankle, subtalar joint, and forefoot—should be assessed. The contralateral extremity should be examined to assess for the normal alignment of the foot, including specifically the rotational alignment of the foot.

Operative Treatment

ANKLE FUSION

All patients should receive appropriate intravenous antibiotic prophylaxis in the preoperative room. A general or spinal anesthetic is used. A bump is placed under the ipsilateral hip, and a thigh tourniquet is applied. The lower extremity is prepped and draped above the level of the knee to allow for intraoperative evaluation of alignment.

A lateral, transfibular approach to the ankle is used. The incision is generally 12 to 15 cm long, extending over the distal aspect of the fibula and curving gently and anteriorly to end over the sinus tarsi. The distal fibula is exposed

Clinical Table: Ankle and Hindfoot Arthritis: Fusion Techniques

Procedure	Indications	Technique	Anatomy	Pitfalls
Ankle fusion	• Isolated symptomatic end-stage ankle arthritis.	• Transfibular approach • Parallel cuts in the tibia and talus • Cancellous screws	• Superficial peroneal nerve branches	• Improper positioning • Medial abutment • Inadequate fixation
Triple arthrodesis	• End-stage arthritis of the hindfoot joints • Severe fixed hindfoot deformity	• Joint surface resection and decortication • Two incisions • Internal fixation with screws and staples	• Superficial peroneal nerve branches	• Improper positioning, especially forefoot supination • Inadequate bony apposition • Inadequate preparation of concave surfaces • Inadequate fixation of the TN joint
Subtalar fusion	• Isolated arthritis of subtalar joint • Fixed valgus deformity following posterior tibial tendon rupture	• Moldable bone graft technique with iliac crest graft • Joint surface resection and decortication	• Superficial peroneal nerve branches	• Inadequate correction of deformity
TN arthrodesis	• Isolated arthritis of the TN joint	• Joint surface resection and decortication • Two incisions • Internal fixation with screws and staples	• Saphenous vein	• Inadequate preparation of concave surface • Varus deformity without use of bone graft
Double arthrodesis (TN and CC joints)	• Isolated arthritis of one or both joints • Chronic posterior tibial tendon rupture with fixed deformity	• Joint surface resection and decortication • Two incisions • Internal fixation with screws and staples	• Saphenous vein • Sural nerve	• Inadequate correction • Inadequate internal fixation
Tibiotalocalcaneal fusion	• Arthritis of the ankle and subtalar joints • Especially in the presence of avascular necrosis of the talus	• Transfibular approach • Internal fixation with screws • Extra-articular fusion • Copious iliac crest bone graft • Intramedullary nail can be useful	• Superficial peroneal nerve branches • Sural nerve	• Inadequate positioning of fusion • Inadequate fixation, especially if using cancellous screws alone
Pantalar fusions	• Rarely indicated • For extensive arthritis of ankle and hindfoot joints	• A combination of the techniques for ankle fusion and triple arthrodesis	• Superficial peroneal nerve branches • Sural nerve	• Inadequate positioning • Inadequate fixation • High risk of nonunion

TN, talonavicular; *CC,* calcaneocuboid.

subperiosteally, and an oblique osteotomy is performed at the syndesmosis. The distal fibula is excised and saved for possible use as bone graft.

Subperiosteal dissection is performed across the anterior and posterior aspects of the distal tibia and to the neck of the talus. Retractors are placed both anterior and posterior to the tibia. A tibial osteotomy is then performed using a 2.5-cm-wide oscillating saw perpendicular to the shaft of the tibia, immediately above the level of the subchondral bone of the ankle joint. When the cut has reached the medial aspect of the plafond, it may be possible to crack the remaining bridge of the bone with a large straight osteotome. If this is not possible, an anteromedial approach along the ankle joint approximately 3 cm in length is made, and a narrow straight osteotome can be used to complete the tibial osteotomy and resect the medial malleolus.

The talar cut is performed next. An assistant holds the foot in a properly aligned position (5° of hindfoot valgus, neutral flexion, and approximately 10° of external rotation) while the surgeon makes a cut across the dome of the talus with the oscillating saw, parallel to the surface of the tibia. It should then be possible to oppose the two, well-vascularized cancellous surfaces to allow for assess-

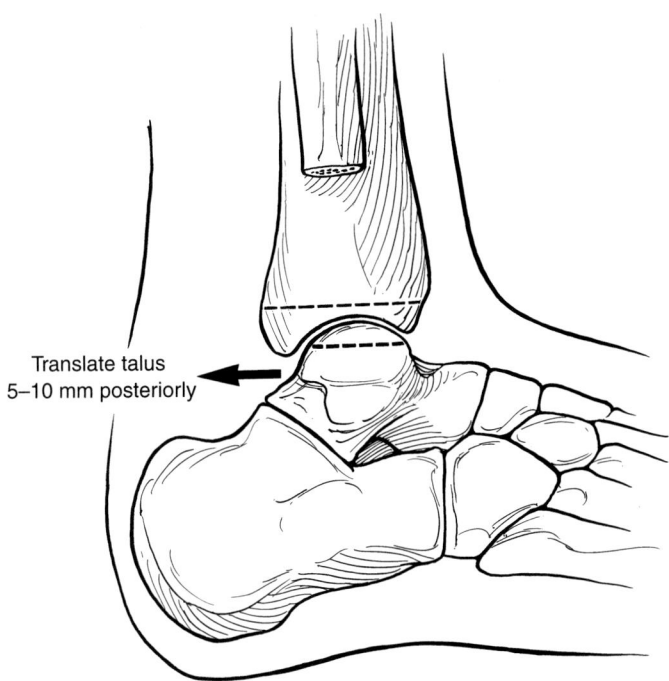

Figure 71.1. Lateral view of the ankle showing the level of the fibular, tibial, and talar osteotomies made to prepare the arthrodesis site.

ment of the alignment (Fig. 71.1). If medial abutment between the tip of the malleolus and medial aspect of the talus is encountered, then the medial malleolus must be resected. Proper position of the foot includes apposition of the two bony surfaces and translation of the foot posteriorly, approximately 5 to 10 mm (thus shortening the forefoot).

An assistant holds the foot in a properly aligned position, while the surgeon secures the arthrodesis site with two or three cancellous screws. The screws can be inserted from the anteromedial and anterolateral aspects of the tibia into the body of the talus (Fig. 71.2). In addition, a screw can be inserted through the sinus tarsi into the talus, engaging the posteromedial cortex of the tibia. If noncannulated screws are used, the first drill bit can be left in place while the first screw is placed. The drill bit can subsequently be removed and exchanged for a second cancellous screw. Otherwise, cannulated, large cancellous screws are an acceptable method of fixation. After placing two large cancellous screws, no motion should be visible when stressing the fusion site. If any question exists regarding the stability of the arthrodesis site or if motion is grossly evident, a third screw should be used.

If stability remains questionable after three screws have been placed, the distal fibula can be used as an onlay graft. The fibula should be hemisected with an oscillating saw in the sagittal plane. The proximal end of the fibula should be secured to the distal tibia with a transverse 4.5-mm cortical screw and with a distal 6.5-mm cancellous screw into the talus. Intraoperative radiographs should be obtained to assess bony apposition and screw length and to rule out penetration of the subtalar joint with a screw (Fig. 71.3).

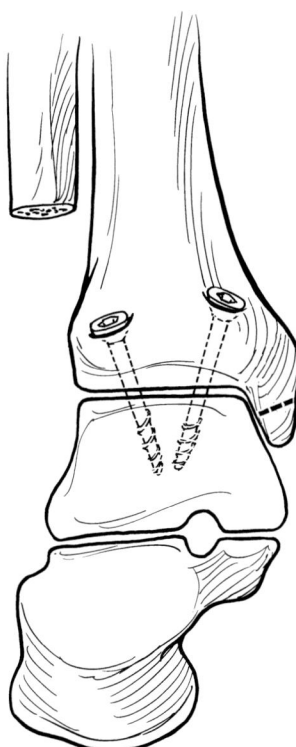

Figure 71.2. Anterior view of the arthrodesis site showing the position of two tibiotalar screws. *Dashed line,* level of resection if medial abutment occurs when attempting to oppose the arthrodesis site or if further narrowing of the ankle is desired.

Figure 71.3. Preoperative AP (**A**) and lateral (**B**) views of a 65-year-old male with osteoarthritis. Postoperative AP (**C**) and lateral views (**D**) showing the solid fusion with cancellous screws.

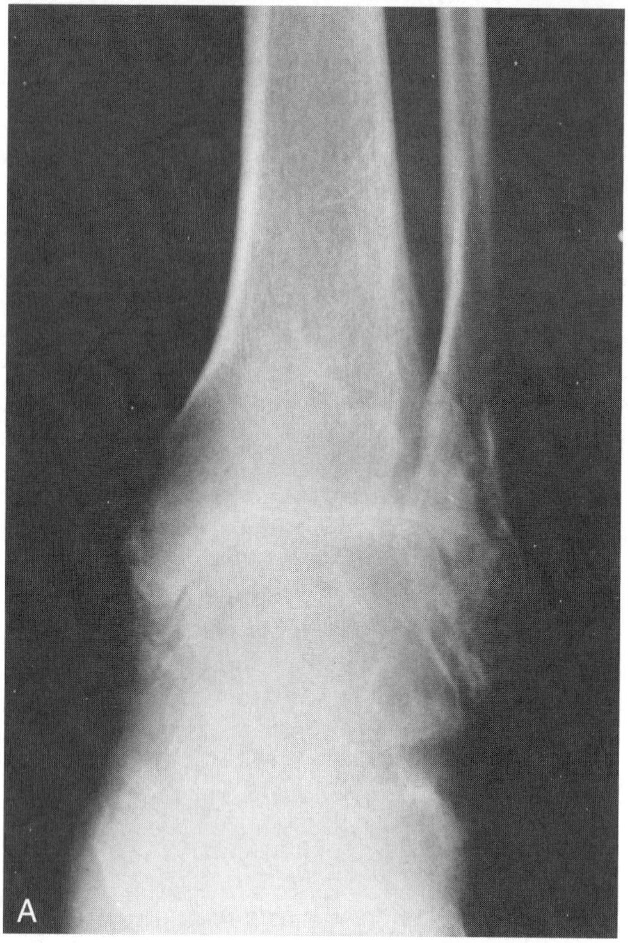

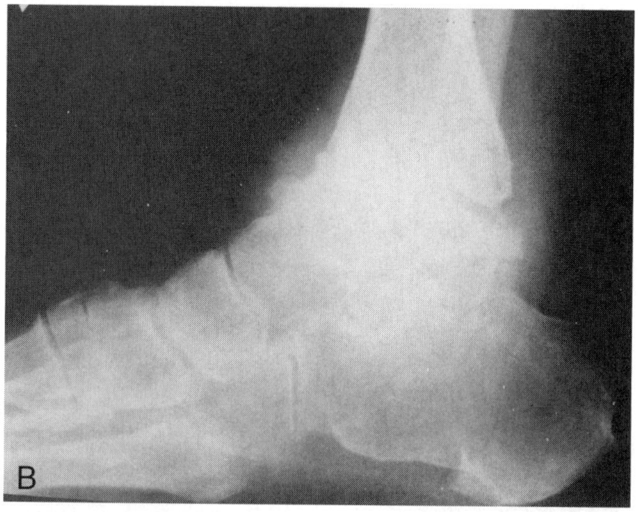

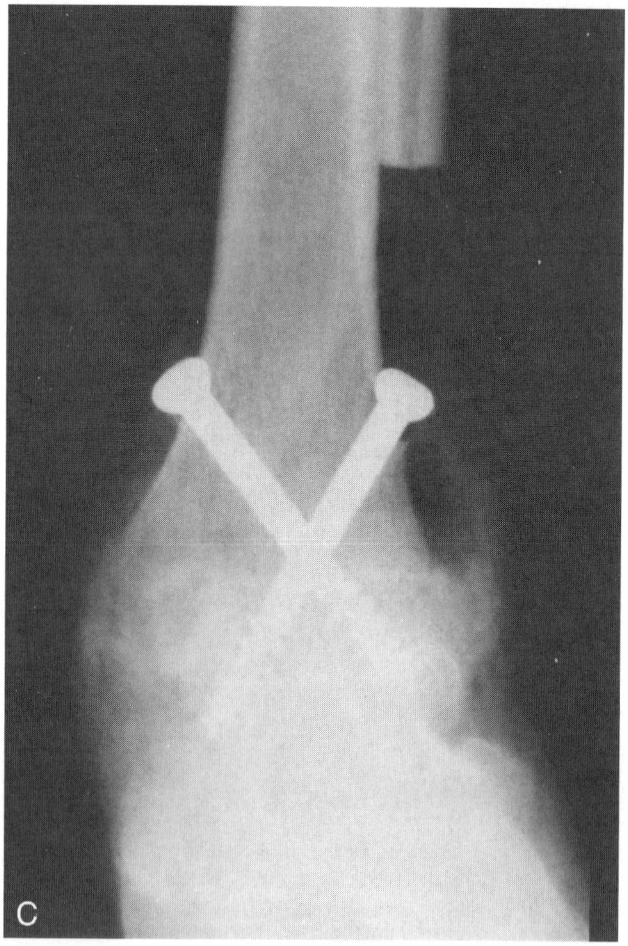

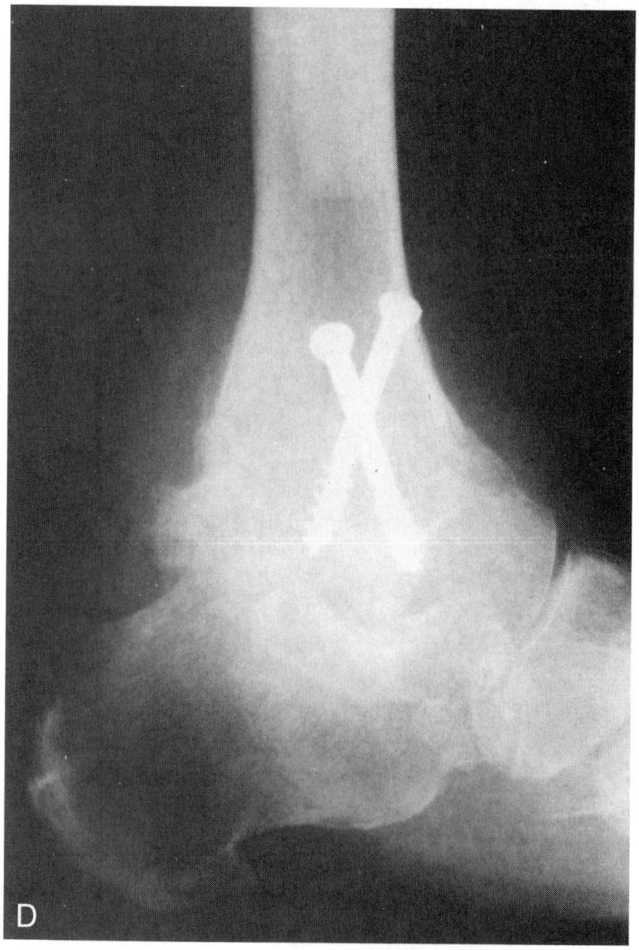

A running or interrupted layer of absorbable subcutaneous sutures and a simple or mattress nonabsorbable suture are used for skin closure. The tourniquet is generally deflated after skin closure to minimize blood loss. A well-padded posterior splint is applied in the operating room, and intravenous antibiotics are used for the first 24 to 48 h after surgery. A short leg cast is placed before the patient is discharged from the hospital.

The patient is seen 10 to 14 days after the surgery to remove the sutures and to reapply the non–weight-bearing cast. At 6 weeks, radiographs are assessed and a short leg walking cast is applied. The patient then advances weight bearing as tolerated. If the patient has been ambulating pain free and there is evidence of radiographic consolidation, the cast can be removed at 12 weeks. If the patient has had pain with ambulation or if there is no evidence of radiographic fusion, the patient is kept in a short leg walking cast for at least 4 more weeks.

TRIPLE ARTHRODESIS

Triple arthrodesis is the surgical fusion of the talocalcaneal, talonavicular, and calcaneocuboid joints. Historically, these joints were fused together when any one of them was arthritic, since their function is interrelated. Today, attempts are made to preserve as many joints as possible to decrease the stresses on adjacent joints and to maintain mobility. Triple arthrodesis is performed only as a salvage procedure in the presence of arthritis or a deformity involving all three joints. The technique presented follows Ryerson's (1) initial description.

The patient is placed in a supine position with a bump under the ipsilateral hip. A pneumatic tourniquet is placed on the thigh. Generally, an iliac crest bone graft is not required except in cases with large posttraumatic defects; therefore, the iliac crest is not routinely prepped. The ankle should passively dorsiflex to neural with the hindfoot in neutral position. If this is not possible, then a percutaneous tendo-Achilles lengthening should be performed before the arthrodesis portion of the case.

The subtalar and calcaneocuboid joints are approached through a lateral incision from the anterior aspect of the distal fibula toward the base of the fourth metatarsal. The extensor digitorum brevis muscle is identified and incised along its inferior margin and reflected superiorly. Sharp dissection into the sinus tarsi is then performed, and the posterior facet of the subtalar joint is visualized. The lateral joint capsule of the subtalar joint is stripped with a periosteal elevator, and a curved retractor is placed along the lateral aspect of the subtalar joint. A lamina spreader, with the handle directed anteriorly, is placed into the depths of the sinus tarsi and used to distract the subtalar joint. It is then possible to gain access to the entire posterior facet. Any remaining articular cartilage is removed with a sharp Cobb periosteal elevator. Care must be taken to remove the cartilage from both the calcaneal and talar surfaces of the posterior facet.

After the articular cartilage has been removed, it should be possible to correct any varus or valgus hindfoot malalignment by properly rotating the calcaneus beneath the talus. In cases of hindfoot valgus, the anterior calcaneus must be rotated beneath the head of the talus to correct the deformity. If the deformity cannot be corrected, then additional soft tissue release and stretching with a lamina spreader must be performed. Generally, bone resection is unnecessary to correct hindfoot deformities.

The calcaneocuboid joint is identified along the anterior aspect of the calcaneus in the distal aspect of the wound. It is distracted with a lamina spreader, and the remaining articular cartilage from both sides of the joint is removed with a Cobb elevator. The lateral aspect of the talonavicular joint can also be exposed through this incision. Any articular cartilage exposed in the lateral aspect of the talonavicular joint should be removed.

A second, longitudinal incision over the superomedial aspect of the talonavicular joint is made along the medial aspect of the tibialis anterior tendon. Branches of the saphenous vein are identified and cauterized. The subcutaneous tissue is incised sharply down to the bone; and the joint capsule is stripped dorsally, medially, and in a plantar direction with a periosteal elevator. A lamina spreader is used to distract the joint, and the remaining articular cartilage is removed from the convex head of the talus and the concave surface of the navicular with a combination of curettes and small sharp periosteal elevators. The concavity of the navicular is the most difficult surface to adequately prepare in this fusion.

After the articular cartilage has been removed from the three joints, it should be possible to position the foot into 5° to 7° of hindfoot valgus and neutral pronation and supination of the forefoot.

Once the soft tissue releases are achieved to allow for proper position of the foot, the subchondral bone of the three joints on both sides is decorticated with a narrow straight or curved osteotome, as needed. When good apposition of the bony surfaces can be achieved and the decorticated bone is used as bone graft, additional harvesting of bone graft is generally unnecessary.

Internal fixation of the arthrodesis sites is now performed. The first joint stabilized is the subtalar joint. A 6.5-mm cancellous screw can be inserted through the medial wound through the dorsomedial aspect of the neck of the talus into the body of the calcaneus (Fig. 71.4). The surgical assistant must hold the foot in a correctly aligned position while the screw is drilled and placed. Optimally, the drill should cross the subtalar joint perpendicular to the joint surfaces to allow for maximum compression. The screw can also be inserted through a stab incision from the posteroinferior calcaneus into the talus.

Next, attention should be directed to the talonavicular joint. After securing the subtalar joint in proper alignment, the surgeon should assess forefoot pronation and supination. The forefoot must be placed in neutral pronation and supination to allow for a plantigrade foot. For patients who have had long-standing hindfoot valgus, the surgeon often

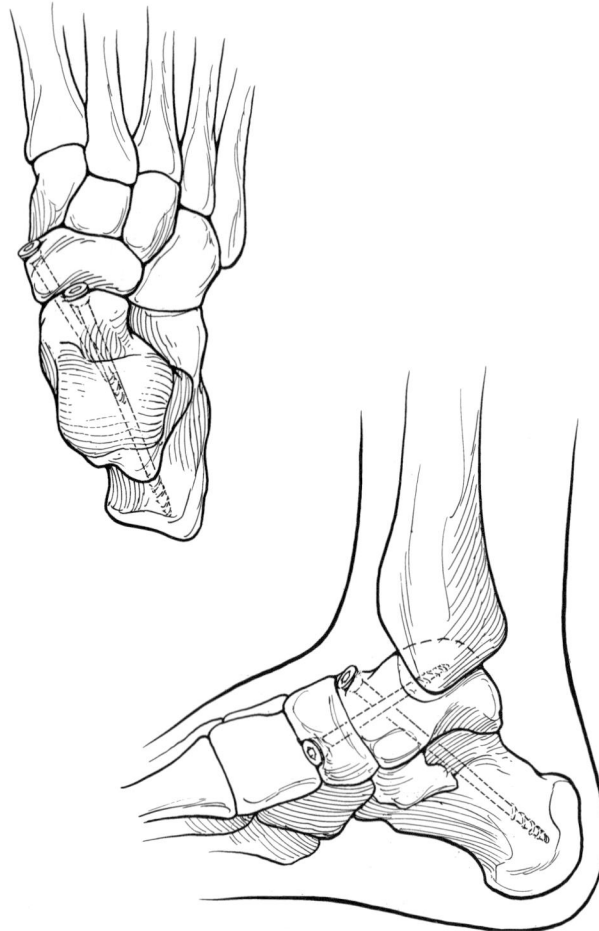

Figure 71.4. Proper screw positions for the subtalar and talonavicular joints.

The skin is closed with interrupted nonabsorbable mattress sutures, and the leg is placed in a posterior splint. Use of a drain is optional. The patient is generally discharged 2 days following surgery and is placed in a non–weight-bearing short leg cast before discharge.

After surgery, the patient is prevented from weight bearing in a short leg cast for 6 weeks. If radiographs at that time demonstrate early consolidation of the fusion sites, the patient is placed in a short leg walking cast and allowed to bear weight, as tolerated, for 6 weeks. If the patient is able to ambulate without pain at the end of the second 6-week period, the cast is removed. If the patient continues to have pain, the walking cast is maintained for an additional 4 weeks or more.

SUBTALAR FUSION

Patients may have isolated arthritis in the subtalar joint following trauma, such as a calcaneus fracture. A fixed valgus deformity can develop secondary to a chronic posterior tibial tendon rupture (3). Most patients, however, require only an isolated, in situ fusion of the subtalar joint, owing to isolated degenerative changes. The fusion can be

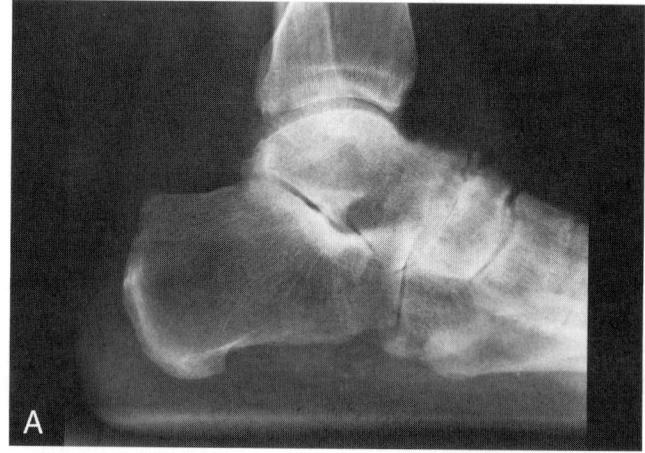

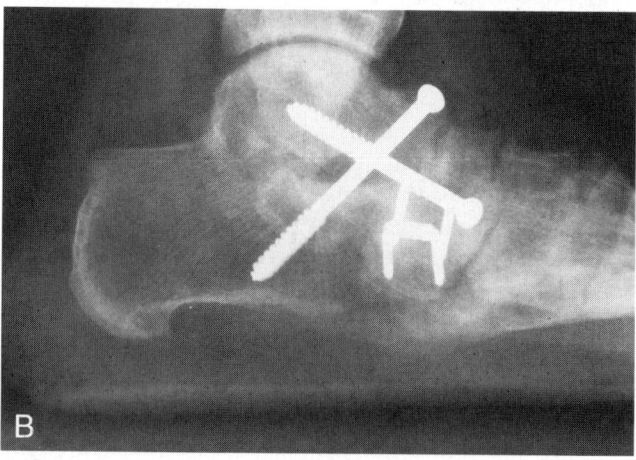

Figure 71.5. A. Preoperative lateral view of a 35-year-old with rheumatoid arthritis. Note the narrow joint spaces and cysts in the hindfoot. **B.** Postoperative lateral view showing the solid fusion of the talonavicular, subtalar, and calcaneocuboid joints.

must "desupinate" the forefoot, which requires depressing the navicular on the head of the talus while securing the talonavicular joint. The talonavicular joint can be secured with a single large cancellous screw inserted from the distal aspect of the navicular and inserted obliquely and laterally into the body of the talus. To minimize the risk of fracturing the navicular while inserting the screw, the drill should be placed at the level of the naviculocuneiform joint. The drill must be directed slightly cephalad, since the talus is inclined toward the first metatarsal. If the screw is inserted parallel to the plantar aspect of the foot, the screw will pass beneath the talus.

The calcaneocuboid joint is secured last. Although a large cancellous screw can be used to fix this joint, it is generally easier and just as successful to use bone staples. After properly positioning the calcaneocuboid joint (which in cases of forefoot supination requires placing a dorsally directed pressure on the plantar aspect of the cuboid), the calcaneocuboid joint is secured with two or three bone staples. The foot should then be visually inspected again with the ankle in the neutral position to confirm alignment of the forefoot. Intraoperative AP and lateral x-rays are obtained to confirm apposition of the three arthrodesis sites and proper placement of the hardware (Fig. 71.5).

performed in the same manner as the triple arthrodesis. The correct rotational alignment of the calcaneus must be achieved, especially in cases of hindfoot valgus when the calcaneus has externally rotated from beneath the talus. Another satisfactory method of performing an isolated subtalar fusion is the moldable bone graft technique described by Russotti et al. (3). More aggressive subchondral bone excision is performed and a morsellized iliac crest bone graft is routinely used.

For a severe calcaneus fracture with marked deformity, the surgeon should perform a distraction arthrodesis of the subtalar joint. In cases such as these, a tricortical iliac crest graft is inserted into the subtalar joint to help reestablish calcaneal morphology and function. The technique is beyond the scope of this chapter (4).

TALONAVICULAR AND DOUBLE ARTHRODESIS

An isolated talonavicular arthrodesis or a double arthrodesis of the talonavicular and calcaneocuboid joints can be performed in a manner similar to that of the triple arthrodesis. An isolated fusion of the talonavicular joint requires an iliac crest bone graft to preserve the length of the medial column of the foot more often than for the lateral column of the foot. Otherwise, a similar incision, approach, preparation, and fixation technique can be employed for these fusions. These arthrodeses can be performed for isolated arthritis of these joints or to correct a fixed deformity after a chronic rupture of the posterior tibial tendon.

TIBIOTALOCALCANEAL FUSION

A tibiotalocalcaneal fusion is often used as a salvage procedure for significant posttraumatic arthritis of the ankle and hindfoot and in cases of failed ankle fusion with loss of talar bone stock. It can be used in the presence of combined ankle and subtalar arthritis or in patients with avascular necrosis of the talus following a talar neck fracture. The fusion can be performed via the transfibular approach, as described for ankle fusion; the incision is extended distally to allow for preparation of the subtalar joint. Long cancellous screws can be used to fix the joint. In patients with deficient bone stock or with bony defects, the arthrodesis can be performed with a short intramedullary rod or with external fixation. Discussion of these techniques, which are used relatively infrequently, is beyond the scope of this text (5).

PANTALAR FUSION

A pantalar fusion includes fusion of the ankle joint and the three joints of the hindfoot (talonavicular, talocalcaneal, and calcaneocuboid). As a single procedure, this operation is now rarely performed, since studies indicated that as many functional joints as possible should be preserved. More frequently, a patient who has previously undergone a triple arthrodesis or ankle fusion develops arthritis in the adjacent joint, owing to added stress or ongoing inflammatory arthritis, and requires a conversion

from either an ankle or triple arthrodesis to a pantalar fusion. The surgical technique for the extension of the fusion is the same as that employed for an isolated ankle fusion or triple arthrodesis. The same position of the arthrodesis should be employed in the pantalar fusion as for any of the component portions of this extended arthrodesis: neutral ankle flexion, 5° of hindfoot valgus, and plantigrade forefoot.

PITFALLS AND COMMON ERRORS

Ankle Fusion

Difficulties encountered in performing an ankle fusion can generally be grouped into problems with preparation and apposition of the fusion site and fixation problems. When preparing the joint surfaces for arthrodesis using an oscillating saw, the surgeon must make certain that two flat cancellous surfaces exist to allow for bony apposition. A ridge of bone left on the far side of the osteotomy will distract the entire fusion site. Following resection of the tibial and talar articular surfaces, the medial aspect of the fusion site may not appose secondary to impingement between the medial malleolus and medial aspect of the talus or tethering of the medial side through the deltoid ligament. In such case, a separate medial incision must be made to resect the tip of the medial malleolus. Care must be taken to prevent the foot from translating anteriorly owing to pressure on the posterior aspect of the calcaneus during the case. A bump must be kept beneath the distal aspect of the tibia to allow the foot to hang free and thus not put pressure on the posterior aspect of the calcaneus. In addition, a significant degree of precision is required in making the bone cuts to ensure that the ankle is placed in a neutral position of dorsiflexion and to prevent excessive hindfoot varus or valgus.

Care must be taken while placing the screws to allow for adequate fixation. One potential problem occurs in patients who have had an excessive amount of the dome of their talus resected. In this situation, the body of the talus is not large enough to allow fixation without having threads cross the arthrodesis site, which prevents adequate compression. In addition, screws can be inserted too obliquely, which causes them to miss the talus distally. If motion is still evident at the arthrodesis site with gentle stress after placing two screws from the anteromedial and anterolateral aspects of the tibia into the talus, a third screw must be placed. The easiest screw to supplement an unstable fusion site can be placed through the sinus tarsi and into the posteromedial tibia (6).

Triple Arthrodesis

The most common problems encountered while performing a triple arthrodesis involve position of the fusion. Many patients undergoing a triple arthrodesis will have some type of hindfoot and/or midfoot deformity. Care must be taken to properly rotate the calcaneus beneath the head of the talus in cases of hindfoot valgus.

When correcting a valgus hindfoot, the forefoot will

supinate as the heel is brought into a more neutral position. This forefoot supination must be corrected through the talonavicular and calcaneocuboid joints, which involves depressing the navicular on the head of the talus before fixation and dorsally displacing the cuboid on the calcaneus before securing the calcaneocuboid joint. Failure to correct a forefoot supination deformity that occurred secondary to the correction of hindfoot valgus results in a supinated forefoot with overloading of the fifth ray.

The talonavicular joint presents the greatest fixation challenge in a triple arthrodesis. A screw must be inserted at the level of the naviculocuneiform joint. If the screw is inserted through the midportion of the navicular tuberosity instead of through its distal edge, the bridge of bone of the navicular will frequently fracture as the screw is tightened. In addition, if the screw is not angled slightly cephalad, the tip of the screw can be placed into the talocalcaneal fusion site.

Subtalar Fusion

The most common problem encountered while performing a subtalar fusion is inadequate correction of the deformity as described for triple arthrodesis. Another common problem encountered when performing a subtalar fusion is failure to inspect the calcaneofibular space in patients who have suffered a previous calcaneus fracture. If any impingement of the space exists, a lateral wall decompression should be performed (3). This is easily performed through the anterior incision over the sinus tarsi by stripping the soft tissues off the lateral aspect of the calcaneus. A large straight osteotome can then be used to remove a portion of the lateral wall of the calcaneus that is impinging beneath the fibula and irritating the peroneal tendons.

RESULTS

Following a successful hindfoot or ankle fusion, most patients can expect good to excellent pain relief from the involved joint (1–7). Most large series of ankle fusions report fusion rates in 90% or more patients (6,7). Triple arthrodesis rates are typically as successful; however, some studies note 10% or more patients with radiographic evidence of talonavicular nonunion (1). Subtalar fusions typically have an even greater rate of fusion (2). Patients must be warned preoperatively that the full benefit of the surgery will not be appreciated for 6 to 12 months.

Although patients should have a durable, functional result from an ankle or hindfoot fusion, some problems do exist after these fusions. Because the hindfoot motion is limited, patients who have undergone a triple arthrodesis or subtalar fusion complain of difficulty walking on uneven or slanting ground. In addition, cutting-type sports are also

limited, since the hindfoot will not be able to accommodate to the ground with rapid changes in direction. Since the hindfoot can no longer act as a shock absorber at heel strike by allowing for hindfoot eversion, many patients develop radiographic evidence of ankle arthritis after a hindfoot fusion.

A well-positioned ankle fusion can function quite well. Most patients maintain approximately 30% of the sagittal plane motion of their foot through their transverse tarsal joints (talonavicular and calcaneocuboid joints). In normal gait, it is frequently difficult to determine which ankle has been fused. Many patients continue to complain of mild to moderate pain after prolonged standing or walking or after lifting of heavy objects, such as that encountered in a heavy labor job.

SUMMARY

Arthritis pain of the foot and ankle region that has failed to respond to conservative care is generally best treated by arthrodesis. Since recent studies have demonstrated that the added stress on adjacent joints for fusion can lead to arthritic changes, as few joints as possible are included in any foot or ankle fusion.

The optimum biomechanical function of the foot should be maintained after each fusion. Each joint has an ideal position of fusion, which is detailed in this chapter. Fusion is achieved by resecting any remaining articular cartilage and as little bone as possible and by placing rigid internal fixation. After each fusion, a patient is protected initially with a period of non-weight bearing and subsequently has protected weight bearing and some type of immobilization to allow consolidation of the fusion. The results of fusion are durable and generally lead to good to excellent pain relief from the afflicted joint.

REFERENCES

1. Ryerson EWP. Arthrodesis operations on the feet. J Bone Joint Surg 1923;5A:453.
2. Cracchiolo A, Cimino WR, Lian G. Arthrodesis of the ankle in patients who have rheumatoid arthritis. J Bone Joint Surg 1992;74A:903–909.
3. Russotti GM, Cass RJ, Johnson KA. Isolated talocalcaneal arthrodesis: a technique using moldable bone graft. J Bone Joint Surg 1988;70A:1472–1478.
4. Carr JB, Hansen ST, Benirschke SK. Subtalar distraction bone block fusion for late complications of os calcis fractures. Foot Ankle 1988;9:81–86.
5. Johnson KA. Tibiotalocalcaneal arthrodesis. In: Johnson KA, ed., Master techniques in orthopaedic surgery—the foot and ankle. New York: Raven, 1994:483–496.
6. Mann RA, VanMannen JW, Wapner K, Martin J. Ankle fusion. Clin Orthop 1991;268:49–55.
7. Morgan CD, Henke JA, Bailey RW, Kaufer H. Long-term results of tibiotalar arthrodesis. J Bone Joint Surg 1985;67A:546–550.

72

William G. Hamilton

Ankle Instability: Surgical Reconstruction

RELEVANT ANATOMY AND PATHOGENESIS

The sprained ankle is the most common injury in sports that involves running and jumping. Lateral (inversion) sprains occur roughly 80 to 90% of the time, compared with the medial (eversion) sprains. Surgical treatment for acute ankle sprains is rarely, if ever, indicated because the majority of sprains will heal well with conservative treatment and rehabilitation. However, symptoms may reoccur in up to 30% of ankle sprains. A thorough knowledge of the anatomy and pathomechanics involved in these injuries will help in their management. In this chapter we cover the anatomy, pathogenesis, biomechanics, physical examination as well as diagnosis and treatment choices, both surgical and nonsurgical, for a sprained ankle.

The ankle joint is shaped like a carpenter's mortise, formed by the medial malleolus, the tibial plafond, and the lateral malleolus, which contains the dome of the talus. Normally, the ankle joint has 15° to 20° of dorsiflexion and 35° to 40° of plantar flexion. This motion is highly variable, depending on the shape of the talar dome (arched or flat) and the presence of a large posterior process. The mortise is held together by the syndesmosis (the anterior and posterior tibiofibular ligaments), which keeps the fibula in the sigmoid notch of the tibia. The dome of the talus within the mortise is shaped like the segment of a cone with its apex on the medial side; it is wider anteriorly and laterally. This makes the medial ligament complex (the deltoid ligament) compact and relatively stable but leaves the lateral ligament complex—the anterior talofibular ligament (ATFL), calcaneofibular ligament (CFL), and posterior talofibular ligament (PTFL)—radiating outward from the lateral malleolus like the spokes of a wheel, potentially unstable (Fig. 72.1). The critical angle between the ATFL and the CFL is quite variable (70° to 140°) (1). This, along with generalized ligamentous laxity and the cavovarus foot, makes some ankles more potentially unstable than others.

The medial anatomic structures around the ankle include the deltoid ligament, the posterior tibial tendon, the neurovascular bundle, the flexor digitorum longus, and the flexor hallucis longus (mnemonic: Tom, Dick, and Harry). The lateral structures are the lateral ligament complex, the peroneus brevis and longus tendons, and the sural nerve. The anterior structures are the anterior tibial tendon, the extensor hallucis longus, the neurovascular bundle, the extensor digitorum longus, and the peroneus tertius (mnemonic: Tom, Harry, and Dick). The posterior anatomic structures include the Achilles tendon, the flexor hallucis longus, and the posterolateral (Stieda) process of the talus (if separate, the os trigonum).

In the subtalar joint, the talus rides sidesaddle on the os calcis beneath it. The longitudinal axis of the talus is in line with the first web space of the foot, and that of the os calcis is in line with the fourth web space. The ligaments stabilizing the subtalar joint are the deep deltoid ligament medially; the CFL, the lateral branches of the extensor retinaculum, the cervical ligament, the lateral talocalcaneal ligament, and the interosseus talocalcaneal ligament laterally; the talonavicular and calcaneocuboid joints and their ligaments anteriorly; and the posterior talocalcaneal ligament posteriorly.

In 80% of people, the subtalar joint is helical (1), so motion here occurs in three planes: eversion to inversion, anterior glide to posterior glide, and internal rotation to external rotation. Therefore, instabilities involving the subtalar joint (grade III ankle sprains) are complex and triplaner.

Biomechanics

The tibiotalar (talocrural) joint, subtalar joint, midtarsal joints, and their ligaments must be considered as one bone–ligament complex that works in concert. The

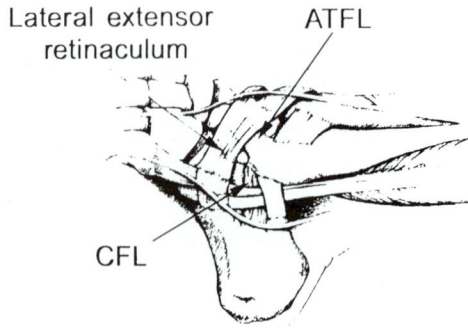

Lateral extensor retinaculum ATFL

CFL

Figure 72.1. Lateral anatomy of the ankle.

subtalar joint is the key to the biomechanics of the foot and ankle (2). It must evert at heel strike to unlock the foot–ankle complex, making it flexible to absorb energy. It must invert at toe-off to lock the joints for rigidity and efficient transfer of power from the Achilles mechanism through the ankle and forefoot. This motion is limited (8° of eversion and 18° of inversion), but it is absolutely essential for normal function, especially in high-performance athletics. Anything that interferes with or reduces this motion, such as arthritis, a tarsal coalition, or arthrofibrosis, will cause dysfunction of the entire foot–ankle complex. This loss of motion should be looked for carefully during the physical examination.

INITIAL FINDINGS, PHYSICAL EXAMINATION, AND DIAGNOSIS

Tibiotalar Instability

Chronic ankle sprains are usually categorized as functional or mechanical (3). Functional instability is motion beyond voluntary control but not exceeding the physiologic range of motion of the joint, i.e., subjective "giving way." Mechanical instability is motion beyond the physiologic range, i.e., objective looseness. Greater than 50% of functionally unstable ankles are also mechanically unstable (4). Grade I ankle sprains do not usually result in significant instabilities. Grade II injuries with rupture of the ATFL result in mildly increased anterior, rotatory, and inversion laxity, but if peroneal strength is normal, recovery is usually complete. The CFL is an important stabilizer of the subtalar joint, and when it is torn (grade III sprain), a combined tibiotalar and subtalar instability results. In addition, rotatory laxity is present and can be symptomatic in turning athletes (dancers, gymnasts, and skaters).

Subtalar Instability

The CFL is a major stabilizer of the subtalar joint; and when it is stretched or attenuated, a combined tibiotalar and subtalar instability occurs. In the majority of lateral ankle sprains, the inversion occurs in plantar flexion, tearing the ATFL first and the CFL second. In the rare incidence

when the ankle is dorsiflexed and then inverted, the CFL can be torn, leaving the ATFL intact and resulting in a pure subtalar instability. It is characterized by apparent functional instability (giving way in an ankle with a minimal anterior drawer sign).

In this case, the true nature of the mechanical instability will not be apparent on physical examination, and the standard talar tilt x-rays may be normal. The diagnosis can be made from a stress Broden view (5) of the subtalar joint. In this view, the subtalar joint under stress should open only a few millimeters at most. Any more than that is abnormal. Subtalar instability is multiplanar: varus-valgus, anterior-posterior, and rotational. Any operative procedure to correct subtalar instability must restore the anatomic integrity of the CFL.

Lateral Ankle Sprain

The sprained ankle is the most common injury in sports that involve running and jumping. By definition, an injury to a ligament is a *sprain*; an injury to a tendon or muscle is a *strain*. Ankle sprains occur at a rate of 1/10,000 people/day and make up 25 to 50% of injuries from running sports. Between 10 and 30% of sprains develop chronic symptoms (6). Ligament injuries are classified into three grades (7): A grade I injury is a minor tear that causes no instability, a grade II injury involves a partial tear and moderate instability, and a grade III injury is characterized by a complete tear with gross instability (Table 72.1). Roughly 90% of ankle sprains are lateral; the rest are medial.

Lateral ankle sprains usually occur when the ankle is plantar flexed, during loading or unloading. The ankle is 80% stable with all ligaments sectioned when it is loaded in the neutral position. In plantar flexion, the ATFL is vertical, under tension, and usually the first ligament damaged. If the stress continues, it tears completely and is followed by rupture of the CFL. Isolated tears of the CFL can result if the inversion stress occurs when the ankle is dorsiflexed, but such injuries are rare (Fig. 72.2).

The physical examination will usually reveal swelling, ecchymosis, and tenderness around the lateral malleolus, which may not necessarily correlate with the extent of the injury. The examiner should always begin at the proximal fibula and look for a Maisonneuve fracture, which may not be evident on x-ray of the ankle below. The midshaft of the

table	72.1	Classification of Lateral Ankle Sprains

Grade	Injury	Diagnosis
I	Partially torn ATFL	Normal drawer sign and talar tilt
II	Torn ATFL; intact CFL	Drawer sign 2+ (<5mm); mild talar tilt (<10°)
III	Torn ATFL and CFL	Drawer sign 3+ (>10 mm); talar tilt 3+ (>15°)

Modified from O'Donoghue DH. Treatment of injuries to athletes. 4th ed. Philadelphia: Saunders, 1975.

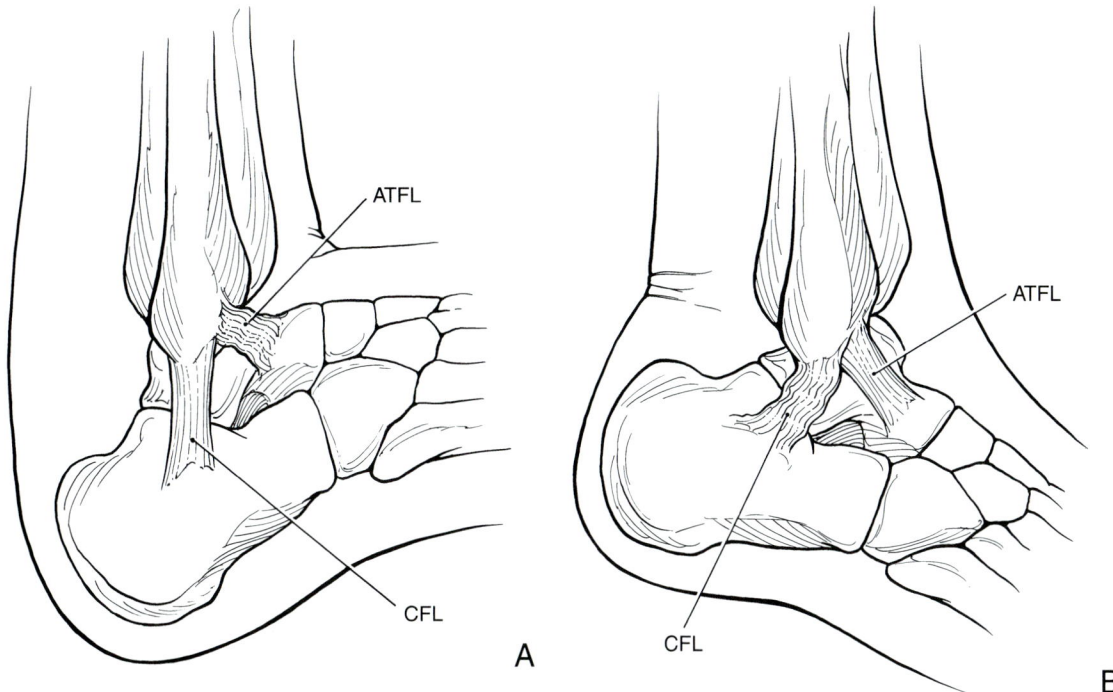

Figure 72.2. Lateral ligaments in dorsiflexion (**A**) and plantar flexion (**B**).

fibula should be squeezed (the West Point sign for syndesmosis injury). The anterior syndesmosis should be palpated for evidence of a high ankle sprain. The sinus tarsi and anterior lateral malleolus should be checked for ATFL damage. It is important to check the anterior process of calcaneus for an avulsion fracture at the origin of the extensor digitorum brevis and extensor hallucis brevis.

The exact location of the tenderness is important because it indicates which structures have been injured. Tenderness directly on the lateral malleolus or epiphysis may indicate a fracture instead of a sprain. The tip of malleolus will be tender when the CFL is injured or when an avulsion fracture is present. Tenderness posterior to the lateral malleolus may indicate a Shepherd fracture of the posterior process or peroneal subluxation. Tenderness at the base of the fifth metatarsal may indicate a tubercle fracture.

A plantar flexion test for a Shepherd fracture should be performed. The drawer sign, done in 15° of plantar flexion, is extremely useful for evaluating the degree of ligament injury. The following radiographic studies should be obtained: standard AP, mortise, and lateral views. If indicated from the physical examination, an AP view of the foot may be required. Stress x-rays are optional. The talar tilt x-ray taken in plantar flexion reveals laxity of the ATFL, while the talar tilt x-ray taken in dorsiflexion shows laxity of the CFL.

Syndesmosis Sprain

A "high" ankle sprain is a partial tear of the anterior tibiofibular ligament. Patients present with tenderness over the anterior syndesmosis and pain on external rotation of the tibia with the ankle in dorsiflexion. If there is a possibility that significant injury has taken place, then weight-bearing x-rays and stress films in dorsiflexion and external rotation should be taken (which may require a local anesthetic). Patients should be warned that this injury could take much longer to heal than a "regular" ankle sprain. Sometimes this injury fails to heal (persists for more than 3 months) and thus may require a corticosteroid injection or even exploratory surgery; synovial hernias through the anterior tibiofibular ligament have been reported (8). If the entire syndesmosis has been disrupted, then open reduction and internal fixation (ORIF) should performed. A lag screw is placed just above the syndesmosis while the ankle is held in slight dorsiflexion so that the mortise is not closed too tightly.

Failure to Heal

Most sprains (even grade III injuries) will heal uneventfully with rehabilitation. The degree of the injury usually governs the healing time. Symptoms that persist for more than 3 months can be a diagnostic challenge. The clinician should look for residual peroneal weakness (common), peroneal tendon pathology (e.g., subluxation, rents, partial tears), rotatory instability (especially in patients who engage in turning activities), and subtalar instability. Other possible causes of failure to heal are posterior impingement on the os trigonum, trigonal (Stieda) process, or soft tissue (the posterior pseudomeniscus); a Shepherd fracture; and flexor hallucis longus tendonitis. The clinician should consider pathology around the tip of the fibula, such as soft tissue entrapment (the meniscoid lesion) (9), an avulsion fracture (usually the insertion of the CFL), a troublesome os subfibulare, a congenital defect that was asymptomatic before the injury, a fracture of the lateral process of the talus (snowboarder's fracture), a fracture of the anterior process of the os calcis, and sinus tarsi syndrome. Osteochondritis dissecans of the talus, chronic anterior lateral pain caused by a talar dome fracture, scar tissue and synovitis in the anterior lateral gutter (Ferkel's phenomenon) (10), and an abnormal slip of the distal anterior tibiofibular ligament that is draped over the lateral talar dome (Bassett's ligament) (11) will also cause failure to heal.

Medial Ankle Sprains

Deltoid ligament injuries are rare (10%) compared with lateral injuries, because the deltoid ligament is much stronger and more compact than the lateral ligament. Complete disruption requires massive trauma and is usually associated with fractures or dislocations. The diagnosis can usually be made on the basis of the physical examination. If disruption is suspected, standing x-rays and a reverse talar tilt stress film can be obtained to determine the presence of significant instability. Before performing this study, the clinician should be sure that there are no fractures present and should look for associated injuries (e.g., medial talar dome lesions).

Medial ankle sprains are valgus–external rotation injuries and result in tenderness and ecchymosis around the medial malleolus. Treatment is similar to that of lateral sprains. Grade I and II injuries should be protected, and patients should undergo early rehabilitation. Grade III injuries should be immobilized for 6 to 8 weeks; rarely do such injuries require open repair.

Medial injuries that fail to heal may be caused by talar dome lesions, posterior tibial tendon injuries or subluxations, medial malleolar pathology (e.g., bone fragments), and chronic laxity.

TREATMENT

Nonoperative Treatment

The standard of treatment for acute ankle sprains remains RICE—rest, ice, compression, and elevation. Unless contraindicated, the patient should be encouraged to begin weight bearing as tolerated with support (via an air stirrup or cam walker, cane, or crutches), as necessary. Early active use of the ankle should be encouraged with controlled stress. Cast immobilization (in slight dorsiflexion) is rarely used, except for some grade III injuries.

The overall prognosis is good, even with grade III sprains. Open repair of acute grade III sprains is usually not indicated. Most patients do well without surgery;

those that do not do well can undergo reconstruction later. Physical therapy speeds up the healing process considerably and is essential for professional and high-performance athletes. Range of motion exercises, weight bearing as tolerated with taping or support, toe raises, and peroneal strengthening (in full plantar flexion) are progressed as tolerated. Return to sports occurs when pain and swelling are minimal and the peroneals are strong.

Operative Treatment

Traditional operations for chronic lateral instability involve taking all or half of the peroneus brevis tendon and reconstructing the ATFL and CFL, either by weaving the graft through drill holes in the talus and calcaneus (Watson-Jones, Elmslie, and Chrisman-Snook procedures) (12–14) or by creating a tenodesis by connecting the peroneus brevis to the tip of the fibula (Evans and Larsen procedures) (15,16) (Clinical Table). These operations are difficult and have significant complications, including sural nerve injuries and subtalar joints locked in eversion. Studies comparing these operations have shown similar results regardless of the type of surgery used (17). Since the mid-1980s, a new approach to this problem has been developed that is much simpler than the traditional weaving procedures.

MODIFIED BRÖSTROM PROCEDURE

In 1966, Bröstrom (18) described an anatomic repair of attenuated ATFL and CFL for the correction of chronic instability. The ligaments are shortened to their physiologic lengths and sutured to their anatomic locations, thus preserving isometricity and a full range of motion. The operation assumes that the ATFL lies within the capsule of the lateral ankle joint, similar to the anterior glenohumeral ligaments of the shoulder. The ligament is in place but has been stretched out. The operation simply restores the original anatomy by shortening the lax ligament. The procedure has proven effective for the correction of laxity in the ATFL but does not address CFL laxity and subtalar instability.

In 1980, Gould et al. (19) modified the Bröstrom procedure by mobilizing the lateral portion of the extensor retinaculum and suturing it to the tip of the lateral malleolus over the repaired ligaments. This accomplishes three things: (a) reinforces the repair, (b) limits inversion (the position of danger for reinjury), and (c) helps correct the subtalar component of the instability. The CFL is an important stabilizer of the subtalar joint; when it is injured, as in most grade III sprains, a combined tibiotalar and subtalar instability is usually present.

INDICATIONS AND CONTRAINDICATIONS

Of course, no operative intervention is indicated until conservative treatment has failed. Insufficient rehabilitation is a common source of residual ankle symptoms after

Clinical Table: Ankle Instability: Surgical Reconstruction

Procedure	Indications	Technique	Anatomy	Pitfalls
Watson-Jones	• Chronic lateral instability	• Peroneus brevis into neck of talus, then into fibula	• Sural nerve • Lateral superficial peroneal nerve	• Only replaces ATFL • Sural nerve injury
Elmslie	• Chronic lateral instability	• ATFL and CFL are replaced with fascia lata graft	• Sural nerve • Lateral superficial peroneal nerve	• Difficult procedure • Requires graft • Stiffness • Sural nerve injury
Chrisman-Snook	• Chronic lateral instability	• A half peroneus brevis into fibula • CFL replaced	• Sural nerve • Lateral superficial peroneal nerve	• ATFL not addressed • Sural nerve injury • Can lock subtalar joint
Evans	• Chronic lateral instability	• Peroneus brevis rerouted through tip of lateral malleolus • Acts as a vector between ATFL and CFL	• Sural nerve • Lateral superficial peroneal nerve	• May not correct subtalar instability • Nonanatomic repair • Sural nerve injury
Larsen	• Chronic lateral instability	• Similar to the Evans procedure • The proximal end of the peroneus brevis is sutured into the os calcis	• Sural nerve • Lateral superficial peroneal nerve	• Nonanatomic repair • Sacrifices peroneus brevis • Sural nerve injury
Bröstrom	• Chronic lateral instability	• Anatomic repair of ATFL and CFL • Can restore normal anatomy	• Sural nerve • Lateral superficial peroneal nerve	• May not correct subtalar instability • CFL may be too badly damaged to repair • Sural nerve injury

sprains, specifically, residual peroneal weakness. In my experience, the most common cause of rolling over in the ankle is not instability but is residual peroneal weakness. Many athletes with positive stress films will not need surgery if the peroneals are strong. These muscles should be exercised in full plantar flexion rather than in the neutral position.

The modified Bröstrom operation is ideal for high-performance athletes, such as ballet dancers, gymnasts, and figure skaters, who have chronic instability unresponsive to conservative therapy. These athletes need to have the stability restored but must also maintain full dorsiflexion, plantar flexion, and peroneal strength.

Other than the usual surgical precautions, such as poor circulation and infection, there are few absolute contraindications. If there is neurologic weakness of the peroneal muscles, an Evans tenodesis and correction of any heel varus are necessary. If there is advanced arthritis of the ankle joint, an ankle fusion may be a more appropriate procedure.

The heavy athlete (a lineman in football) who needs stability more than motion can also benefit from operative repair. In such cases, I supplement the Bröstrom repair by performing an Evans-type procedure over it, using half of the peroneus brevis.

In patients with fixed heel varus, any soft tissue repair will fail if the heel is not brought out of the varus position. In this situation, a lateral closing-wedge calcaneal osteotomy should be performed along with the reconstruction.

Technique

The modified Bröstrom operation is performed as an outpatient procedure. The patient is put under general or spinal anesthesia and is placed in the semilateral decubitus position. A thigh tourniquet is set over cast padding. A small incision is made along the anterior border of the distal fibula and is carried down to the peroneal tendons. The lateral portion of the extensor retinaculum is identified running parallel to the skin incision and is mobilized for use later (Fig. 72.1). A capsular incision is then made; a cuff is left on the fibula for reattachment. The ATFL is usually seen as a thickening in this capsule. The CFL is identified deep to the peroneal tendons at the distal end of the incision and is also divided; a stump is left on the tip of the fibula for reattachment after the ligament has been shortened. I believe that leaving these attachments on the fibula is important for maintaining the isometricity of the repair, similar to anterior cruciate ligament reconstructions in the knee (Fig. 72.3).

The capsule and ligaments are then shortened to their normal lengths and sutured to their anatomic locations with permanent sutures. The extensor retinaculum is then

Figure 72.3. Postoperative view of the ATFL and CFL.

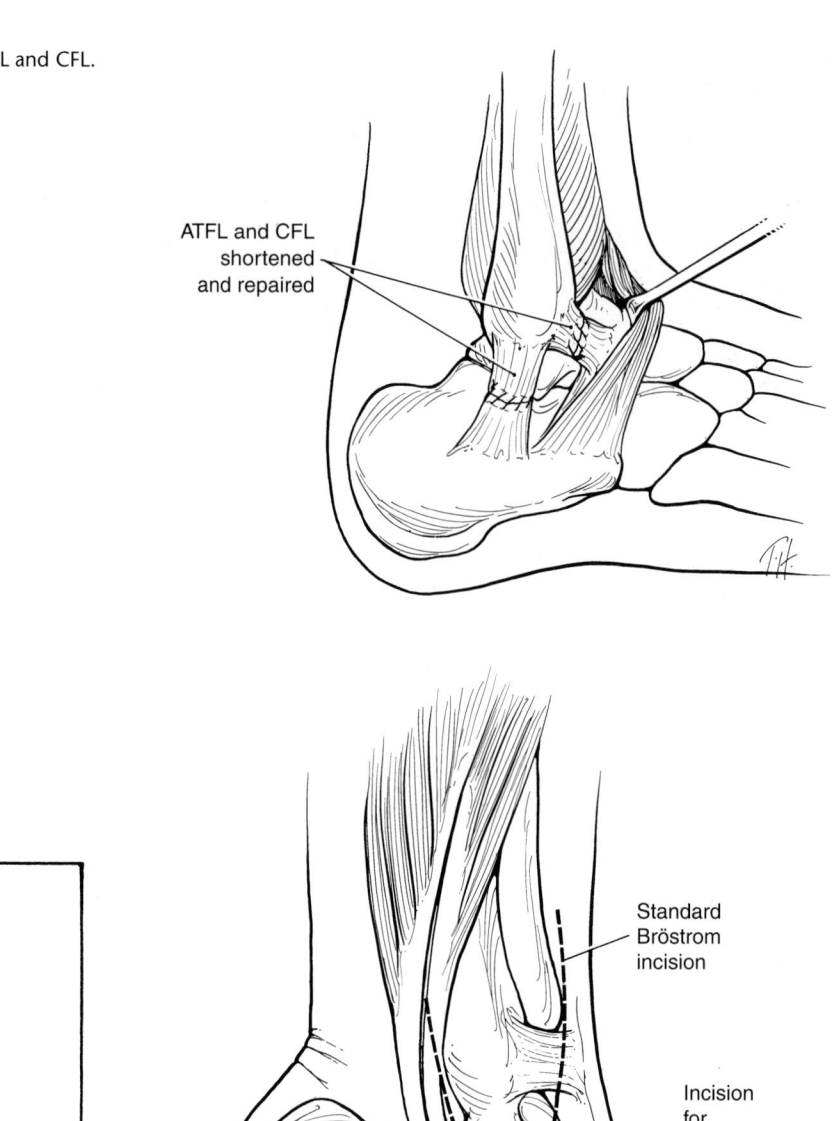

ATFL and CFL
shortened
and repaired

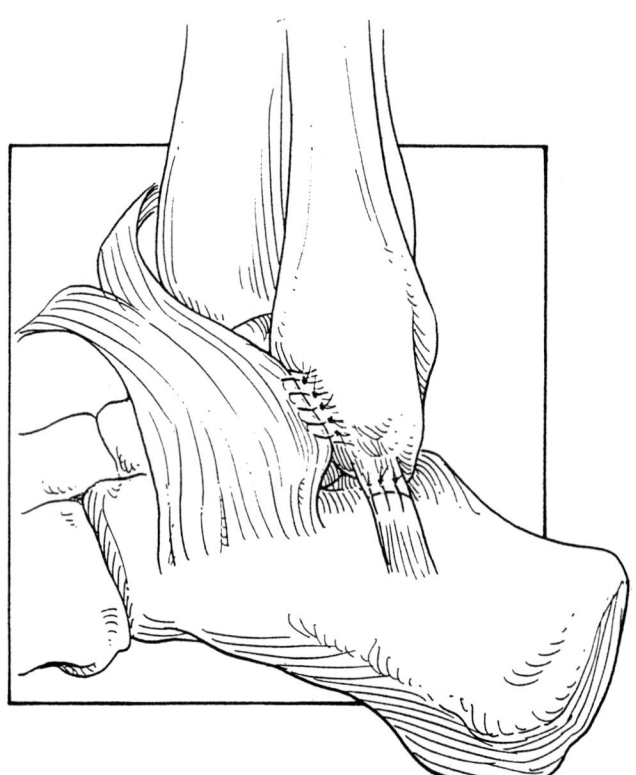

Figure 72.4. The extensor retinaculum has been sutured in place.

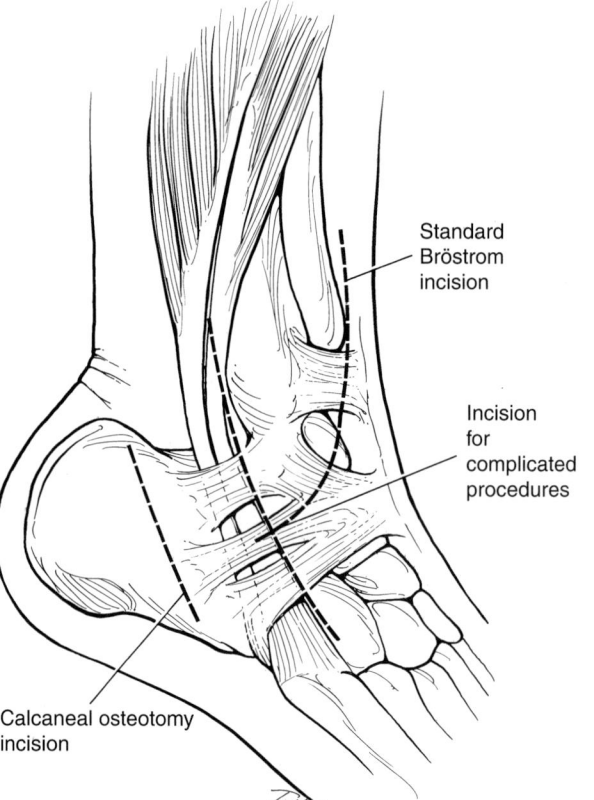

Standard
Bröstrom
incision

Incision
for
complicated
procedures

Calcaneal osteotomy
incision

Figure 72.5. Possible incision sites.

pulled up over the tip of the fibula and sutured to the periosteum with chromic catgut (Fig. 72.4). The ankle is checked for stability and taken through a full range of motion.

A subcuticular closure is performed with an absorbable suture and sterile strips. The ankle is placed in anterior-posterior plaster splints, and the patient is sent home on crutches. No weight bearing is permitted.

The Alternate Incision

A different incision site should be used for very large patients, patients with suspected peroneal rents or tears, and patients with heel varus who require a lateral closing wedge osteotomy. The longitudinal incision should run across the tip of the fibula and be directed toward the base of the fourth metatarsal (Fig. 72.5). This incision is less cosmetic, but more useful.

Postoperative Regimen

Between 4 and 7 days after surgery, a short leg walking cast or walking boot is applied and worn for 3 to 4 weeks. After the cast is removed, the ankle is protected with an airsplint for 6 to 8 weeks. Physical therapy and swimming are begun when the cast is removed. Inversion should be avoided, but range of motion, toe raises, and peroneal exercises (in full plantar flexion) are begun. Running and jumping are allowed at 7 to 8 weeks after surgery, and return to full activity begins when the peroneals are strong, usually by 8 to 12 weeks after surgery.

RESULTS

Many authors have reported good results with the modified Bröstrom technique. In 1993, my group reported on a series of 28 patients (20). The series now includes 75 patients; of these, 95% have experienced good to excellent results over a 16-year period. Approximately 50% of patients in the series are professional athletes (dancers, skaters, hockey players, basketball players, football players). One patient sustained a significant reinjury and underwent a second operation. I routinely use the modified Bröstrom technique on all patients who need a ligament reconstruction. There have been no significant complications in this series of patients.

SUMMARY

In this chapter we have tried to give the clinician a working knowledge of the anatomy and pathomechanics of this injury so that it can be managed either by surgery or by rehabilitation to restore the patient to his or her preinjury level of function. Fortunately, the overall prognosis is quite good. If surgery is necessary, research has shown a 90% success rate regardless of the surgical method used.

REFERENCES

1. Inman VT. The joints of the ankle. Baltimore: Williams & Wilkins, 1976.
2. Mann RA. Biomechanics of the foot and ankle. In: Mann RA, Coughlin MA, eds. Surgery of the foot and ankle. St. Louis: Mosby, 1993:19–23.
3. Freeman MAR. Treatment of ruptures of the lateral ligament of the ankle. J Bone Joint Surg 1965;47B:661–668.
4. Freeman MAR. Instability of the foot after injuries to the lateral ligament of the ankle. J Bone Joint Surg 1965;47B:669–677.
5. Broden B. Roentgen examination of the subtaloid joint in fractures of the calcaneus. Acta Radiol 1949;31:85–91.
6. Garrick JG, Requa RK. The epidemiology of foot and ankle injuries in sports. Clin Sports Med 1988;7:29–36.
7. O'Donoghue DH. Treatment of injuries to athletes. 4th ed. Philadelphia: Saunders, 1975.
8. McLaughlin HL. Trauma. Philadelphia: Saunders, 1959.
9. Wolin I, Glassman F, Sideman S, Leventhal D. Internal derangement of the talofibular component of the ankle. Surg Gynecol Obstet 1950;91:193–200.
10. Ferkel RD, Karzel RP, Del Pizzo W, et al. Arthroscopic treatment of anterolateral impingement of the ankle. Am J Sports Med 1991;19:440–446.
11. Bassett FH, Gates HS, Billys JB, et al. Talar impingement by the anterior-inferior tibiofibular ligament. J Bone Joint Surg 1990;72A:55–59.
12. Watson-Jones SR. Fractures and joint injuries. 4th ed. Baltimore: Williams & Wilkins, 1955;2:821–823.
13. Elmslie RC. Recurrent subluxation of the ankle. Ann Surg 1934;100:364–367.
14. Chrisman OD, Snook GA. Reconstruction of lateral ligament tears of the ankle. An experimental study and clinical evaluation of seven patients treated by a new modification of the Elmslie procedure. J Bone Joint Surg 1969;51A:904–912.
15. Evans GA, Hardcastle P, Frenyo AD. Acute rupture of the lateral ligament of the ankle. To suture or not to suture? J Bone Joint Surg 1984;66B:209–212.
16. Larsen E. Tendon transfer for lateral ankle and subtalar joint instability. Acta Orthop Scand 1988;59:168–172.
17. St. Pierre R, Allman F, Bassett F. A review of lateral ankle ligamentous reconstructions. Foot Ankle 1982;3:114–123.
18. Bröstrom L. Sprained ankles. Acta Chir Scand 1966;132:551–565.
19. Gould N, Seligson D, Gassman J. Early and late repair of the lateral ligament of the ankle. Foot Ankle 1980;1:84–89.
20. Hamilton WG, Thompson, FM, Snow SW. The modified Bröstrom procedure for chronic lateral ankle instability. Foot Ankle 1993;14:1–7.

chapter 73

Louis S. Mezman and Paul J. Hecht

Arthroscopic Surgery of the Ankle

Since the early 1980s, ankle arthroscopy has become recognized as a new and important advance in orthopaedic surgical technique. Ankle arthroscopy is now the technique of choice for many procedures that would previously have required arthrotomy or perhaps would not have been done at all. Familiarity with this technique is an important part of the orthopaedic surgeon's area of expertise.

The Japanese literature contains much of the preliminary work involving ankle arthroscopy and arthroscopy in general. The long pauses in progress in this area correspond to pauses in technologic advancement. Each advancement created new opportunities in arthroscopy, which eventually allowed the explosion of work in ankle arthroscopy seen in the 1980s and 1990s. Drez et al. (1) published a report on techniques and indications for ankle arthroscopy in 1982 that was an important contribution to the American literature on this subject. Guhl (2) published the first reports of his techniques of ankle distraction in 1988. This was another landmark in the evolution of ankle arthroscopy.

RELEVANT ANATOMY

A thorough knowledge of the extra-articular and intra-articular anatomy of the ankle is vital for limiting the number of avoidable complications associated with this surgical technique. Arthroscopy was originally performed via two standard anterior portals (anteromedial and anterolateral), but anterocentral, posteromedial, and posterolateral portals have also been used

The anteromedial portal is at or just above the level of the joint line, just medial to the tibialis anterior tendon (Fig. 73.1). The structures at risk are the saphenous vein (average distance 9 mm; range 3 to 16 mm), and the saphenous nerve (average distance 7.4 mm; range 0

to 17 mm) (3). This is the safest portal and so is placed first.

The anterolateral portal is at or just above the joint line, just lateral to the tendon of the peroneus tertius. Care must be taken to avoid the branches of the superficial peroneal nerve (average distance 6.2 mm, range 0 to 24 mm). If necessary, the portal can be placed just to the medial side of the peroneus tertius (1,3). Occasionally, it will be necessary to place an accessory portal adjacent to the anteromedial or anterolateral portal.

The anterocentral portal is mentioned for completeness sake only, because a recent study (3) noted that the neurovascular bundle was in contact with or perforated by the arthroscope in 5 of 18 cases. It is placed just lateral to the tendon of the extensor hallucis longus. Branches of the superficial peroneal nerve can also be injured when placing this portal.

The posterolateral portal is used with relative frequency (Fig. 73.2). It is placed just lateral to the Achilles tendon at the level of the joint line, 1 to 2 cm proximal to the tip of the lateral malleolus. A spinal needle, placed from inside out, can aid in locating this portal, because the subtalar joint should not be entered at this level. The small saphenous vein (average distance 9.5 mm; range 2 to 18 mm) and sural nerve (average distance 6.0 mm; range 0 to 12 mm) can be injured during placement of this portal (1,3). The posteromedial portal is placed just medial to the Achilles tendon. It is a dangerous and little-used portal and is thus not recommended.

The trans-Achilles or posterocentral portal is placed through the Achilles tendon and is little used because of the fear of morbidity to the tendon. Transmalleolar portals are drilled under arthroscopic and fluoroscopic visualization via small incisions over the malleoli, often with a cannulated drill. The start hole is 2 to 3 cm above the joint line.

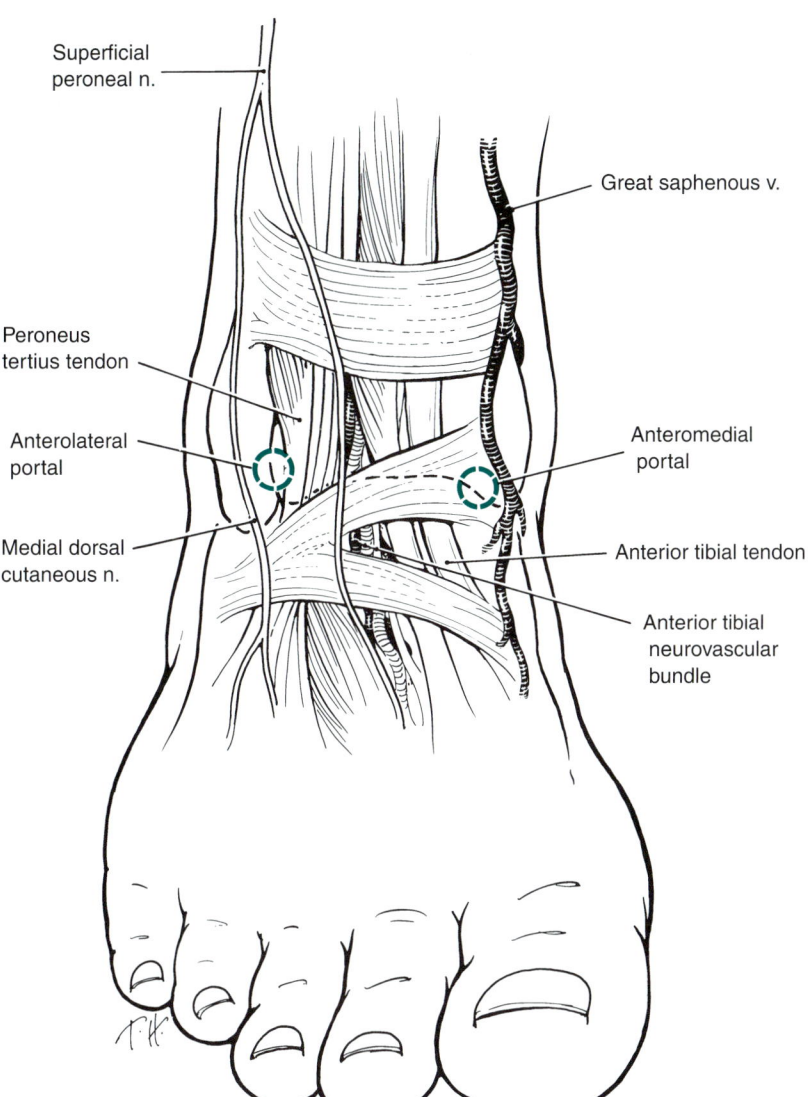

Figure 73.1. Anatomy of the anterior ankle. Note the anteromedial and anterolateral portals.

Superficial peroneal n.

Great saphenous v.

Peroneus tertius tendon

Anterolateral portal

Anteromedial portal

Medial dorsal cutaneous n.

Anterior tibial tendon

Anterior tibial neurovascular bundle

TREATMENT

Indications for Surgery

Arthroscopy can be a valuable diagnostic tool when other tools are inconclusive, especially for cartilage and soft tissue injuries; loss of motion; persistent pain, swelling, or stiffness; hemarthrosis; abnormal snapping sensations; and instability (4–6). Operative indications include débridement of injuries to the cartilage and soft tissues, anterolateral impingement, bony impingement, osteochondral lesions of the talus, instability, fractures, plafond lesions, synovitis, arthrofibrosis, septic arthritis, and loose bodies. Among the contraindications are infection of the overlying skin, moderate or severe degenerative arthritis, severe edema, reflex sympathetic dystrophy, and poor vascular status.

Surgical Instrumentation

A 2.7-mm 30° arthroscope is used most frequently for procedures about the ankle, but sometimes 2.7-mm 70°

and 4.0-mm arthroscopes are needed. Flow can be either via gravity or via an arthroscopy pump set for 50 to 70 mm Hg. Devices providing both invasive and noninvasive distraction are available. We use a multimode distractor and have had no occasion to use it in the invasive distraction mode, because of the excellent results possible with noninvasive distraction.

We find that small joint instruments are best for ankle arthroscopy and use a small joint shaver, 3.5-mm ring curettes, small cervical curettes, a 1.5-mm probe, assorted 2.9-mm graspers and baskets, suction punches, and small banana knives. A number 11 blade is used to make the skin incisions; and a mosquito clamp is used to dissect down to the capsule, which is pierced with a blunt trocar. The knee is supported with a standard urology leg holder, and a thigh tourniquet is placed. Also needed are a minidriver, Kirschner (K) wires, pituitary forceps, a small joint golden retriever for removing broken instruments, intra-articular aiming devices, a number 18 spinal needle, ankle arthroscopy drapes, and (possibly) fluoroscopy equipment.

Figure 73.2. Anatomy of the posterior ankle. Note the posteromedial, postero-lateral, and trans-Achilles portals.

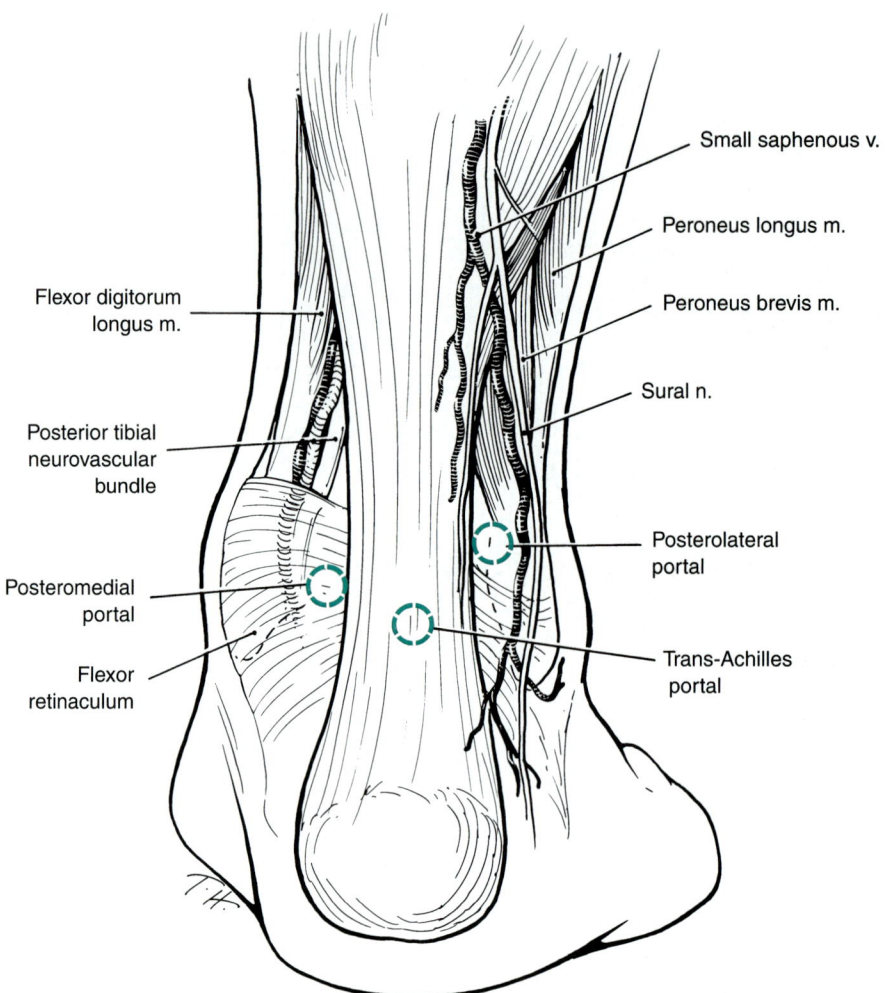

Flexor digitorum longus m.

Posterior tibial neurovascular bundle

Posteromedial portal

Flexor retinaculum

Small saphenous v.

Peroneus longus m.

Peroneus brevis m.

Sural n.

Posterolateral portal

Trans-Achilles portal

General Surgical Technique

Patients are given a spinal or general anesthesia to relax the muscles about the ankle and allow for the use of a thigh tourniquet. An 18-gauge, 3.75-cm (1.5-inch) needle is used to inject 10 mL 0.5% bupivacaine hydrochloride (Marcaine) with 1:200,000 epinephrine into the ankle via the anteromedial portal. A urology leg holder is padded and placed just proximal to the popliteal fossa (to avoid injury to the neurovascular bundle there); the hip is flexed to 40°. The leg is prepped to just below the knee. Draping commences with placement of a 7.5- to 10-cm (3- to 4-inch) stocking net, an impervious U drape, and then the arthroscopy drape.

The pertinent anatomic landmarks are palpated and marked: the dorsalis pedis artery, the tendons of the tibialis anterior and the peroneus brevis, the branches of the superficial peroneal nerve, and the saphenous vein. The branches of the superficial peroneal nerve can be seen and palpated by placing the foot in a plantar-flexed and inverted position.

The distractor is assembled and clamped to the Clark rail through the drapes. The strap is placed about the ankle and affixed to the distractor with a moderate amount of manual traction.

Both portals are injected subcutaneously with 0.5% bupivacaine hydrochloride with epinephrine via a 23-gauge needle; then the medial portal is created. Using a number 11 blade, the surgeon incises only the skin longitudinally for 8 to 10 mm. A mosquito clamp is used to spread the tissues down to the joint capsule, which is entered with a blunt trocar placed through the camera cannula. Removal of the trocar should give a return of fluid if it is placed in the correct location. Ankles with anterior scarring can be difficult to enter. The camera, already assembled, is placed into the cannula; and inflow is attached and opened. We use an arthroscopy pump, set at 50 to 70 mm Hg. The camera is used to transilluminate the antero-lateral corner of the joint. The anterolateral portal is then established using the identical technique; the surgeon must take care to avoid injury to the branches of the superficial peroneal nerve.

The tourniquet is inflated only if necessary, and occasionally increasing the pressure on the arthroscopy pump will allow adequate visualization. The addition of 1 mL 1:1000 epinephrine to each 3-L bag of irrigation solution can decrease intra-articular bleeding. The distractor is adjusted to yield 7 or 8 mm of distraction and can be maintained for up to 60 min (5,6). When we have had to maintain distraction for longer periods of time, no untoward effects

effects were noted. The viscoelastic properties of the ligaments can be exploited by applying additional tension after some time has passed.

In general, optimal visualization of a lesion is obtained when the arthroscope is placed on the same side of the joint as the lesion. The arthroscopist should develop a routine that he or she is comfortable with and that allows a systematic, consistent, and thorough examination of all portions of the joint, including the anterior pouch; the medial gutter; the joints between the medial malleolus and the talus and between the talus and the lateral malleolus; the talar dome; the lateral gutter; the anterior talofibular ligament; the anterior, central, and posterior aspects of the syndesmosis; the plafond; and the posterior tibiotalar joint.

Placement of a posterolateral portal may allow for better outflow (we have not found this to be necessary when using an arthroscopy pump). In unusual situations, this portal allows the arthroscope or instruments to have access to areas otherwise out of reach. We use the posterolateral portal in about 5% of cases.

Following completion of the procedure, it is important to again visualize the joint to be sure no debris is left behind. Portals are closed with nylon suture, and a bulky compression dressing is placed. Extra care is needed for the soft tissue closure because of the thinness of coverage on the anterior ankle. The surgery is done on an outpatient basis.

DISTRACTION

When Guhl (2) first reported the distraction technique, he used 0.1875 threaded pins placed unicortically into the tibia and calcaneus. Complications associated with this technique include fractures, nerve injuries, infections, and hardware failure. With the availability of noninvasive distraction techniques, we have found no reason to use invasive distraction.

The noninvasive distraction device provides excellent visualization of the joint, and to date we have had no complications with it. A disposable padded figure-eight strap is placed over the ankle, and tension is applied by hand or by a threaded knob. The hip is held in a flexed position by a urology leg holder, which allows countertraction to be applied and elevates the leg so it is free posteriorly in case a posterior portal must be created. Other methods of distraction that may not be as optimal but are more readily available include the use of a gauze roll placed in clove hitch fashion, gravity by flexing the knee and allowing the leg to hang off the bed, and manual distraction.

Specific Surgical Technique

SYNOVITIS AND SOFT TISSUE IMPINGEMENT

Localized synovitis of the ankle joint is not uncommon and generally occurs at the anterolateral aspect of the joint. It known by a variety of terms, including meniscoid lesion, anterolateral corner compression syndrome, synovial impingement, and anterolateral impingement (6–8).

Wolin et al. (8) first used the term *meniscoid* to describe a soft tissue mass they found on arthrotomy in a series of nine patients with chronic anterolateral ankle pain. Excellent results were noted following excision of the meniscoid, and the authors hypothesized that, after an inversion injury, tears occurred in the anterior talofibular and calcaneofibular ligaments. This resulted in hemorrhage into the joint, which usually resolved; sometimes, it organized and persisted as a mass in the talofibular recess, where it is repeatedly pinched, producing recurrent pain and swelling (7).

Stetson and Ferkel (6) hypothesized that an inversion sprain tears the anterior talofibular and calcaneofibular ligaments and that repeated motion of the ends of these ligaments leads to chronic inflammation, synovial reaction, and scarring. Impingement of this accumulated mass of tissue at the junction of the tibia, talus, and fibula creates a cycle of irritation, pain, and further inflammation. Histologically, moderate synovial hyperplasia and subsynovial capillary proliferation are noted, with or without the presence of fibrosis or hyalinization.

Patients often present with a history of an inversion injury and subsequent pain that may have resolved and then recurred. Swelling is noted, often localized; and the patient experiences pain, especially while negotiating stairs and during other activities that require dorsiflexion. A minority of patients complain of clicking or the sensation of instability. Examination may reveal anterolateral joint line tenderness, tenderness with forced dorsiflexion and eversion, anterolateral swelling, and joint effusion.

Impingement is poorly defined by imaging modalities, although MRI studies can occasionally be helpful. It is a diagnosis of exclusion and has an extensive differential diagnosis, including fracture of the anterior process of the calcaneus, fracture of the lateral process of the talus, fracture of the lateral aspect of the cuboid, osteochondral lesion of the talus, peroneal tendonitis or subluxation, sinus tarsi pain, lateral or syndesmotic ligament instability, and early degenerative joint disease.

In multiple series of patients with chronic anterolateral ankle pain treated by arthroscopic débridement, good to excellent results range from 75 to 90% (6,7,9,10). Bassett et al. (7) described talar impingement by a separate distal fascicle of the anterior inferior tibiofibular ligament, which was débrided with excellent results (3). Impingement by soft tissue can occur posterolaterally as well, and it is important to visualize this area arthroscopically during the operative procedure. This lesion occurs via a similar mechanism to that with anterolateral impingement, but the tears occur in the posterior inferior tibiofibular ligament, the transverse tibiofibular ligament, and the transverse slip.

The synovectomy and débridement are performed with the 2.9- or 3.5-mm full-radius resector (Clinical Table). Care must be taken in the region of the anterior capsule to avoid injury to the neurovascular bundle. If the postero-

Clinical Table: Arthroscopic Surgery of the Ankle

Procedure	Indications	Technique	Anatomy	Pitfalls
Synovectomy débridement	• Synovitis • Anterolateral corner compression • Synovial impingement • Anterolateral impingement	• Tourniquet • Distraction • Pump • Appropriate portals • 2.9- to 3.5-mm full-radius resector • 2.7-mm arthroscope	• Neurovascular bundle • Anterior capsule • Talus • Calcaneus • Inferior tibiofibular ligament • Anterior tibiofibular ligament • Posterior tibiofibular ligament • Superficial peroneal nerve • Articular surface of the talus	• Neurovascular injury • Poor visualization • Bleeding
Osteochondral lesion treatment	• OCD lesion of talus	• Excise for grade 1 • Internally fix large fragment	• Same as for synovectomy débridement	• Loss of fixation • Poor control of fragment
Débridement of chondral lesion	• Talar dome degenerative changes	• Anterior approach • Débride fibrinous cartilage • Débride flaps of cartilage • Drill exposed subchondral bone • Early range of motion	• Same as for synovectomy débridement	• Poor exposure
Débridement of arthritis	• Symptomatic loose bodies • Symptomatic arthrofibrosis • Symptomatic osteophytes • Small chondral defects	• Small full-radius resector • Synovectomy in rheumatoid arthritis	• Same as for synovectomy débridement	• Poor exposure
Osteophyte removal	• Impingement of tibial and talar osteophytes	• Anteromedial portal • Anterolateral portal • Direct blade resector away from neurovascular bundle • Burr osteophyte • Early range of motion • Possible miniarthrotomy	• Same as for synovectomy débridement	• Neurovascular injury • Loose bodies created • Incomplete resection of osteophytes
Loose body removal	• Symptomatic loose bodies • Synovial chondromatosis	• Anterior anteromedial anterolateral portal • Posterior portal for inflow, flushing, or pushing loose bodies anterior	• Same as for synovectomy débridement	• Incomplete visualization • Incomplete retrieval of loose bodies
Open reduction and internal fixation	• View and reduce articular surface as adjunct for percutaneous fixation • Pilon fracture • Plafond fracture • Posterior malleolus fracture	• View anteriorly • Allow percutaneous fracture fixation	• Same as for synovectomy débridement	• Neurovascular injury • Incomplete reduction • Poor internal fixation

Clinical Table: Arthroscopic Surgery of the Ankle *(Continued)*

Procedure	Indications	Technique	Anatomy	Pitfalls
Irrigation and débridement	• Infection	• Portals same as above • Débride necrotic tissue • Culture • Large-quantity irrigation • Necrotic synovium only removed	• Same as for synovectomy débridement	• Incomplete débridement • Continued infection • Cartilage injury during débridement
Arthrodesis	• Tibiotalar arthrosis • Good bony stability	• Challenging • All portals utilized • Remaining cartilage removed • Bony surfaces decorticated • Appropriate fixation methods	• Same as for synovectomy débridement	• Visualization difficult with distorted anatomy • Incomplete preparation of tibial and talar surfaces

lateral portion of the joint cannot be reached anteriorly, a posterolateral portal can be created. We begin our procedure without the use of the tourniquet, but will inflate it if needed. The use of an arthroscopy pump allows us to increase the intra-articular pressure to gain some control of bleeding that would otherwise obscure visualization of the operative field; the addition of epinephrine to the irrigation solution can be helpful as well.

OSTEOCHONDRAL LESION OF THE TALUS

Since Alexander Monro first reported the finding of loose osteocartilaginous bodies in the ankle, many terms have been used to describe this disease process, including osteochondritis dissecans (OCD), flake fracture, transchondral fracture of the talar dome, and osteochondral lesion of the talus (OLT). One reason for the presence of so many terms is the controversy over the cause of the lesion: trauma (transchondral fracture) or ischemia (OCD). Berndt and Harty's classic 1959 report (11) established a clear role for trauma in the cause of OLT, especially for the lateral lesions (Fig. 73.3). They were able to produce these lesions experimentally in cadavers. Canale and Belding (12) reported on a series of 29 patients, noting that lateral lesions were associated with inversion or inversion and dorsiflexion, were shallower, and were more likely to displace and cause persistent symptoms. It has been noted that 10 to 20% of patients will have contralateral lesions (4,7).

The Berndt and Harty classification of lesions, based on radiographic evidence, is as follows:

Stage 1: Compression fracture
Stage 2: Incomplete avulsion of the fragment
Stage 3: Complete separation without displacement
Stage 4: Avulsed fragment displaced in the joint

This classification was the basis for many treatment protocols. Canale and Belding (12) used this scheme when recommending nonoperative treatment of stage 1 and 2 lesions, operative treatment of lateral stage 3 and all stage 4 lesions, and a trial of nonoperative treatment for medial

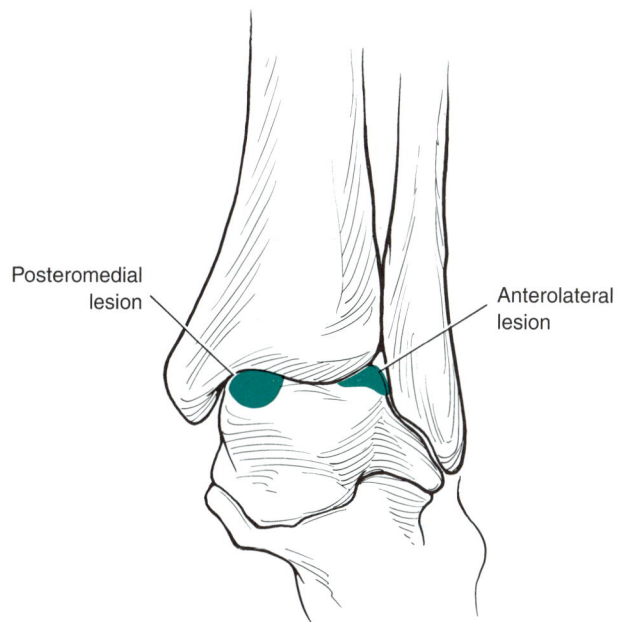

Figure 73.3. Locations of the anterolateral and posteromedial osteochondral lesions of the talus

stage 3 lesions. Many published reports based treatment recommendations on fairly small numbers of patients within each stage of lesions. In addition, Pritsch et al. (13) noted no correlation between the radiologic classification and the appearance of the lesion on arthroscopy. They believed that the arthroscopic appearance, and not the appearance on x-ray films, should decide the treatment. Bone scans, CT scans, and MRI studies can be used in the workup of OLT; the indications for each of these modalities are presently poorly defined.

Patients with OLT usually present after an acute ankle sprain or later with persistent pain after an ankle sprain. They may or may not have received appropriate treatment at presentation. Patients note pain that is frequently localized to a specific point, intermittent swelling, catching, and sensations of instability. Physical examination usually does not confirm the instability, but often there is a specific point of tenderness at the talar dome. For the posteromedial lesion, pain may be elicited on palpation just posterior to the medial malleolus with the ankle in dorsiflexion.

When an OLT is identified, initial treatment has historically been based on the Berndt and Harty classification; surgical treatment is generally recommended for stage 3 and 4 lesions (Fig. 73.4). Berndt and Harty noted 84% good to excellent results with operative treatment, compared to only 17% good to excellent results with conservative care (11). Pritsch et al. (13) reported 93% good to excellent results with arthroscopic curettage of arthroscopic grade 3 lesions; grade 1 lesions were not surgically manipulated, and three of the four patients noted good to excellent results.

Our treatment protocol involves initial nonoperative care, unless the fragment is causing mechanical symptoms or the patient has already failed an appropriate course of conservative treatment. Nonoperative treatment is usually immobilization in a cast or cast boot and some form of restricted weight bearing. The cast is worn for 6 to 12 weeks, and weight bearing is protected for a somewhat shorter period of time. Next the patient undergoes a rehabilitation program. If the patient is not satisfied with the ankle after rehabilitation, arthroscopy is considered.

Generally, all lesions can be approached via the two standard anterior portals, and the posterior placement of instruments is usually not necessary for a posteromedial OLT. The lateral lesions are more easily reached through the anterior portals than the medial lesions are. We have not had the need to perform a malleolar osteotomy; we usually excise lesions that remain symptomatic through the anterior portals.

Recommendations for treatment of specific lesions are varied and are based on several different classification systems. For an arthroscopic grade 1 lesion, we believe excision of the lesion via curettage is the most appropriate treatment (Fig. 73.5). This treatment is recommended for most other OLTs as well. There is no evidence to suggest that drilling of such a lesion will allow it to attain the theoretical goal of healing with preservation of the cartilage, and only occasionally do we drill a lesion.

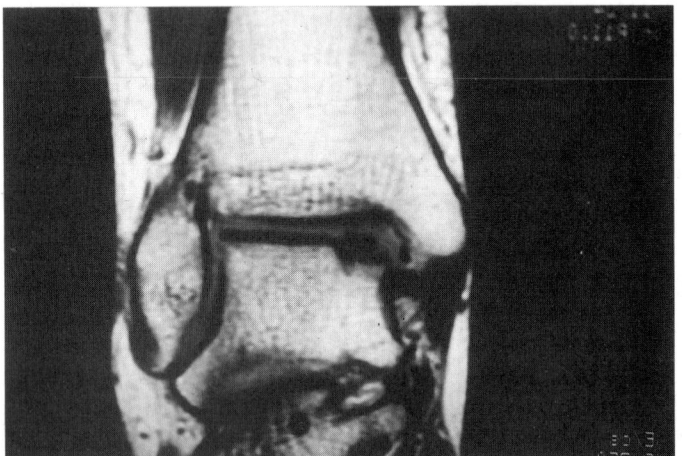

Figure 73.4. MRI study of a stage 3 posteromedial lesion.

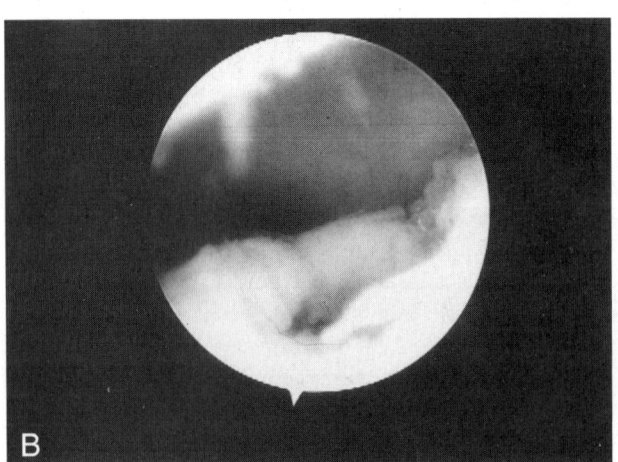
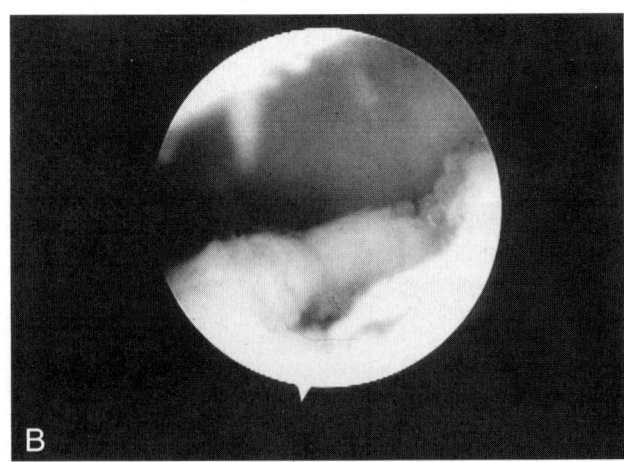

Figure 73.5. A. Stage 3 lesion. **B.** After débridement and drilling.

Rarely is a bony fragment large enough for the surgeon to entertain the idea of internal fixation. But when that does occur, a resorbable pin, a Herbert screw, or K wires can be used. A bone graft may be needed to support such a lesion; and in this case, reduction and fixation should probably be reserved for younger patients with acute lesions, because these patients have the best chance to heal. Stone (14) discussed the retrograde drilling of lesions via the sinus tarsi using an endoscopic drill guide. A similar technique was used to place bone graft. Because lesions so rarely required reduction and fixation, with or without bone grafting, there are no studies available to evaluate the efficiency of these treatments. OLT in the adult has a lower potential for healing than in the skeletally immature patient, and this must be kept in mind when deciding on the length of time to try conservative care.

The postoperative routine depends on the surgical procedure performed. If the lesion was excised or drilled, a period of non-weight bearing will allow for healing; range of motion exercises can be started at 1 week. If internal fixation or a bone graft was used, then immobilization will be needed to avoid displacement of the lesion. Eventually, weight-bearing and strengthening exercises are allowed, and rehabilitation commences. We place patients who have had excision or drilling of a lesion into a cast boot and let them begin range of motion at 7 days. Weight bearing is delayed for 6 weeks, which allows fibrocartilage to grow into the base of excised lesions and some healing (bony or fibrous) of the drilled lesions.

CHONDRAL LESIONS

For patients with a chronically painful ankle who have no findings on imaging studies (MRI studies may detect cartilage lesions), an intra-articular injection of local anesthetic and steroid may be administered. If this provides only temporary relief, arthroscopy can be performed and may reveal a chondral lesion, usually at the talar dome. Treatment involves gently débriding the fibrinous cartilage and any flaps of cartilage. If subchondral bone is exposed, it should be drilled in an attempt to promote formation of a fibrocartilaginous surface.

After surgery, early range of motion provides a stimulus to the cartilage. If subchondral bone was exposed, weight bearing is delayed for 6 weeks.

ARTHRITIS

The results of arthroscopic treatment of degenerative joint disease have been disappointing. Specific lesions, however, that frequently coexist with degenerative joint disease (osteophytes, loose bodies, arthrofibrosis, and small chondral defects) can be treated with good results. Early range of motion is encouraged in the postoperative regimen.

Occasionally, the ankle joint of a patient with rheumatoid arthritis will be affected with a severe synovitis that has not been responsive to more conservative treatments.

An arthroscopic synovectomy may be performed. For a complete synovectomy, a posterolateral portal may be needed. A 2.7- or 3.5-mm full-radius resector is used, and special care must be taken around the anterior capsule to avoid injury to the neurovascular bundle, because the capsule in this area may be quite thin. An Ho:YAG laser can be used to provide synovectomy with concurrent hemostasis.

Osteophytes

Osteophytes can be found in the ankle after fracture healing, but are most commonly found following repetitive dorsiflexion trauma, without fracture. These osteophytes project inferiorly from the anterior lip of the tibia, and a kissing lesion occasionally rises to meet it from the adjacent neck of the talus. The lesion is seen with relative frequency in soccer players, although dancers, jumpers, and runners are also susceptible. A lateral plain film taken with the ankle in dorsiflexion will show the bony contact. The spur results in impingement, with lesser and lesser amounts of dorsiflexion.

Patients generally complain of anterior ankle pain, especially with athletic activity, stair climbing, and forced dorsiflexion. Examination reveals tenderness along the anterior joint line and loss of dorsiflexion. A bone scan shows activity in this region, and the spur is easily seen on plain films.

Generally, if the area is acutely painful, a period of rest, nonsteroidal anti-inflammatory drugs (NSAIDs), and perhaps an injection of corticosteroids should be tried. If the spur remains symptomatic or precludes return to sports, it can be removed arthroscopically.

Anteromedial and anterolateral portals are created, and a full-radius resector is used to débride the synovium from the anterior aspect of the osteophyte. The blade of the resector should always be kept in view and directed away from the neurovascular bundle. A bur is used to resect the osteophyte, although a small osteotome could also be used. An increase in dorsiflexion of approximately 10° can be expected, along with significant improvement in pain, swelling, stiffness, and limping. Patients should be able to return to sports activity, and spurs rarely recur (3).

After surgery, patients are placed in a bulky compression dressing and a postoperative shoe. Range of motion and strengthening exercises are begun immediately.

Loose Bodies

Intra-articular loose bodies of the ankle joint can be traumatic or atraumatic in origin. Traumatic causes include OLTs, acute fractures, fractures of osteophytes, and (rarely) foreign bodies. The principal atraumatic cause is synovial chondromatosis. The ossicles seen around the malleoli following avulsion injuries are generally extra-articular, as they are attached to the collateral ligaments.

Symptoms of these lesions include the general problems associated with intra-articular ankle pathology, such as swelling, pain, sensations of giving way, locking, and crepitans. Lesions that have an ossified component can usually be seen on plain films, but purely chondral lesions cannot (which is usually the case). Both MRI studies and arthrograms can be useful in imaging these lesions. It is important to try to determine the origin of the loose body to determine if is intra-articular in origin and thus amenable to arthroscopy.

Arthroscopic treatment is directed at removal of all loose bodies, so the inspection of the joint must reach all corners and recesses. Treatment must also address the source of the loose bodies. The posterolateral portal is especially useful here because inflow can be established at this portal, flushing the loose bodies toward the scope and the outflow. Instruments can be placed posteriorly to grasp the loose bodies or to push them anteriorly, where they are removed with a suction punch. If the cause of the loose bodies is synovial chondromatosis, synovectomy should be performed.

FRACTURES

Ankle arthroscopy can be of value in viewing and reducing the articular surface of the plafond after a pilon fracture, allowing for percutaneous fixation. Holt (15) reported on the use of this technique in posterior malleolus fractures. These fractures should be fixed if they involve more than one-quarter to one-third of the weight-bearing surface of the joint and are displaced following reduction of the lateral malleolus. Surgical approaches for open reduction can be extensive, and much stripping of the bone and soft tissue trauma can be avoided with reduction under arthroscopic visualization and percutaneous fracture fixation.

SEPTIC ARTHRITIS

Arthroscopic treatment of an infected ankle joint is an efficient method of treatment. Débridement of necrotic tissues, retrieval of synovium for culture, and irrigation with large quantities of fluid can be easily accomplished. Removal of necrotic synovium only is indicated; the synovium has phagocytic properties, and its removal is an unnecessary trauma to the joint. Drains are placed and removed within 48 h.

ARTHRODESIS

Many techniques are available for surgical treatment of the symptomatically arthritic ankle joint; one is arthroscopic arthrodesis. We find that open fusion of the ankle joint yields extremely satisfactory results. Even with careful patient selection, the results of arthroscopic fusion at best match that of a procedure performed on a much less carefully selected group of patients. That being said, it must be acknowledged that—at least in the group of patients in whom this procedure gives its best results—there is a theoretical advantage to the minimal dissection needed with the arthroscopic technique: less devascularization of the bone, resulting in quicker healing; lower infection and nonunion rates; and less postoperative pain, resulting in shorter hospital stays. The trade-offs for the smaller dissection are that there is less ability to thoroughly prepare the joint surfaces and bony alignment problems cannot be readily corrected. The appropriate patient for this procedure is one with little or no bony deformity in whom the contours of the joint are such that there will be adequate bony apposition for fusion after the remaining cartilage and subchondral bone are removed.

The procedure is fairly technically demanding, and, as mentioned, is limited in its applicability. In the appropriately selected patient, the results are roughly equivalent to those of open techniques. Myerson and Quill (16) reported a 94% fusion rate for the arthroscopic procedure and a 100% fusion rate for the open procedure in a retrospective review. Ogilvie-Harris et al. (17) reported on 19 arthroscopic ankle arthrodeses and noted a nonunion rate of 11%. They were impressed by the minimal amount of postoperative pain and swelling experienced by patients and noted a decreased hospital stay compared to open procedures. They recommended arthroscopy for fusion in situ of the ankle with symptomatic osteoarthritis and good bony stability.

Complications

The complication rate with arthroscopic surgeries in general can be difficult to access. The 1986 report of the Committee on Complications of the Arthroscopy Association of North America (18) showed an overall complication rate of 0.56%. Of 4478 ankle arthroscopies, no nerve or vascular injuries were noted and only 1 case of infection was reported. The committee did not feel it appropriate to editorialize on the results of the survey (18).

Ferkel et al. (19) reported a 10% complication rate in their first 518 cases, noting that a learning curve is present. Neurologic injury accounted for approximately 50% of these complications, and injury to the superficial peroneal nerve was the most common. Martin et al. (20) noted a 15% complication rate in 58 ankle arthroscopies.

Potential complications include nerve or vascular injuries, infection, instrument breakage, tendon and ligament injuries, and scuffing of articular cartilage. Other complications are caused by the tourniquet, distraction, and anesthesia. Postoperative hemarthrosis, fractures (acute or stress), reflex sympathetic dystrophy, and painful scars are other complications. Stetson and Ferkel (6) noted an apparent association of postoperative wound infections with the closeness of adjacent portals, the use of tapes for closure of wounds, and early mobilization.

The use of cannulas and distraction should reduce the risk of instrument breakage and intra-articular cartilage damage; transillumination of the portals along with careful attention to surface landmarks can help reduce the risk of injury to nerve or vascular structures. The use of prophylactic antibiotics before surgery is recommended. After surgery, we place a bulky dressing that restricts joint motion somewhat, but we do not formally restrict joint motion.

SUMMARY

Arthroscopy of the ankle is one of the most rapidly advancing fields in orthopaedic surgery. Progress in the field shows no sign of slowing. Both technology and technique continue to mature, allowing orthopaedic surgeons to help patients who otherwise would have gone undiagnosed or untreated.

REFERENCES

1. Drez D Jr, Guhl JF, Gollehon DL. Ankle arthroscopy. Techniques and indications. Clin Sports Med 1982;1:35–45.
2. Guhl JF. New techniques for arthroscopic surgery of the ankle: preliminary report. Orthopedics 1986;9:261–269.
3. Feiwell LA, Frey C. Anatomic study of arthroscopic portal sites of the ankle. Foot Ankle 1993;14:142–147.
4. Ferkel RD, Scranton PE. Arthroscopy of the ankle and foot. J Bone Joint Surg 1993;75A:1233–1242.
5. Stetson WB, Ferkel RB. Ankle arthroscopy. I: Technique and complications. J Am Acad Orthop Surg 1996;4:17–23.
6. Stetson WB, Ferkel RB. Ankle arthroscopy. II: Indications and results. J Am Acad Orthop Surg 1996;4:24–34.
7. Bassett FH III, Gates HS III, Billys JB, et al. Talar impingement by the anteroinferior tibiofibular ligament. J Bone Joint Surg 1990; 72A:55–59.
8. Wolin I, Glassman F, Sideman S, Levinthal DH. Internal derangement of the talofibular component of the ankle. Surg Gynecol Obstet 1950;91:193–200.
9. Meislin RJ, Rose DJ, Parisien JS, Springer S. Arthroscopic treatment of synovial impingement of the ankle. Am J Sports Med 1993;21:186–189.
10. Pritsch M, Lokiec F, Sali M, Velkes S. Adhesions of distal tibiofibular syndesmosis. Clin Orthop 1993;289:220–222.
11. Pritsch M, Horoshovski H, Farine I. Arthroscopic treatment of osteochondral lesions of the talus. J Bone Joint Surg 1986;68: 862–865.
12. Canale ST, Belding RH. Osteochondral lesions of the talus. J Bone Joint Surg 1980;62:97–102.
13. Berndt AL, Harty M. Transchondral fractures (osteochondritis dissecans) of the talus. J Bone Joint Surg 1950; 41A:988–1020.
14. Stone JW. Osteochondral lesions of the talar dome. J Am Acad Orthop Surg 1996;4:63–73.
15. Holt ES. Arthroscopic visualization of the tibial plafond during posterior malleolar fracture fixation. Foot Ankle 1994;15:206–208.
16. Myerson MS, Quill G. Ankle arthrodesis: a comparison of an arthroscopic and an open method of treatment. Clin Orthop 1991; 268:84–95.
17. Ogilvie-Harris DJ, Liebermann I, Fitsialos D. Arthroscopically assisted arthrodesis for osteoarthritic ankles. J Bone Joint Surg 1993; 75A:1167–1174.
18. Committee on Complications of the Arthroscopy Association of America. Complications in arthroscopy, the knee and other joints. Arthroscopy 1986;2:253–258.
19. Ferkel RD, Guhl J, Van Buecken K, et al. Complications in ankle arthroscopy: analysis of the first 518 cases. Orthop Trans 1992; 16:726–727.
20. Martin DF, Baker CL, Curl WW, et al. Operative ankle arthroscopy. Am J Sports Med 1989;17:16–23.

Achilles Tendon Ruptures

Achilles tendon ruptures were recognized by Hippocrates, who believed a bruised or cut tendon led to acute fevers, choking, derangement of the mind, and eventually death (1). The first accurate clinical description of Achilles tendon rupture was made by Paré (2) in 1575, who published his findings in 1633. Rupture of the Achilles tendon is a serious injury and, if not diagnosed and treated appropriately, can cause long-term problems.

Achilles tendon rupture occurs infrequently, although it is the third most common major tendon disruption; rotator cuff and extensor mechanism ruptures are first and second (3). Although no epidemiologic studies estimate the incidence of Achilles tendon ruptures, an increasing number of publications discuss the injury and treatment options. This interest may be secondary to physicians' greater awareness of this injury or to the general population's growing participation in physical activities.

The Achilles tendon is one of the strongest tendons of the body, withstanding loads up to 400 kPa (4). Acute ruptures most commonly occur 2 to 3 cm proximal to the insertion site on the calcaneus. The typical patient is a man between 30 and 50 years old who holds a sedentary job but who is physically active. Proper diagnosis is straightforward but can be easily missed on examination by the unaware physician. Missed diagnoses have been estimated to be as high as 25% (5). Treatment can be operative or nonoperative. Regardless of approach, the basic goal of treatment is to return the Achilles tendon complex to its normal length and tension.

Chronic Achilles tendon ruptures are more complex than acute ruptures. They can result from a long-term degenerative or overuse process, a missed diagnosis, or inadequate treatment of an acute rupture. Treatment of chronic Achilles ruptures tends to be more difficult than that of acute ruptures.

RELEVANT ANATOMY AND PATHOGENESIS

The Achilles tendon, also known as the triceps surae or gastrocsoleus tendon, gets its name from the Greek hero of Homer's *Iliad*, who was vulnerable only in his right heel. The tendon receives contributions from both the gastrocnemius and the soleus muscle. The gastrocnemius is composed of a lateral head and larger medial head, which arise from facets above their respective femoral condyles. The soleus originates from the oblique line of the tibia, from the middle third of the internal border of the tibia, from the back of the head of the fibula, and from the upper third of the shaft of the fibula. The aponeuroses of both muscles combine to form the Achilles tendon.

The tendon is 10 to 15 cm in length and inserts onto the middle third of the posterior of the calcaneus. Two bursa exist: between the tendon and the superior portion of the calcaneus and superficial to the tendon below the skin near its insertion. The Achilles tendon is surrounded by a paratenon, which helps supply blood to the tendon.

Acute Achilles tendon ruptures occur through direct and indirect mechanisms of injury. Direct injuries result in rupture less often than do indirect injuries; rupture can be the result of either a closed or an open injury. Closed injuries are the result of a direct blow to the tendon, which is usually under mild tension when ruptured. Open injuries are the result of sharp lacerations or severe open crush-type injuries.

Indirect rupture of the Achilles tendon is a result of tension overload to the tendon. The Achilles tendon follows a typical S-shaped stress–strain curve. Ultimate strain levels have been reported to range from 7 to 15, and tensile strength has been reported to be as high as 400 kPa with static loading of the tendon (4,6). As a result of the rapid loading rates that occur in most acute ruptures, the modulus of elasticity of the collagenous tissue increases, and the tendon behaves as a stiffer material. This would imply that these values underestimate the ultimate stresses and strains at rupture.

Indirect Achilles tendon ruptures occur from any event that stretches or places tension on the Achilles tendon. Athletic activities that require jumping and pushing off have been notorious for causing ruptures. Ruptures may also occur from falls that result in rapid, forced dorsiflexion of the ankle. Arner and Lindholm (7) described three types of indirect loading mechanisms: (a) pushing off with the weight-bearing forefoot while simultaneously extending the knee; (b) sudden unexpected dorsiflexion of the ankle accompanied by a strong contraction of the Achilles tendon, as when falling forward; and (c) violent dorsiflexion of the plantar-flexed foot. Although most mechanisms require rapid loading of an already taut tendon, ruptures may also occur with normal walking or running.

Chronic tears of the Achilles tendon may be the result of inadequately diagnosed or treated acute ruptures. In this situation there is rapid tendinous degeneration along with retraction of the proximal tendon stump, resulting in a large gap in the tendon. Secondary contraction and fibrosis of the Achilles tendon complex may occur. Chronic ruptures may also be the result of an overuse syndrome or a slow degenerative process. Partial ruptures, or micro tears, from cumulative trauma and scarring can result in lengthening of the tendon and insufficiency of the Achilles tendon complex.

Because of the presence of prerupture Achilles tendon pain, researchers have investigated the role of inflammation in ruptures of this tendon. Arner et al. (8) found distinct histologic inflammatory and degenerative changes in 74 specimens of Achilles tendons treated surgically from a few hours to 8 months after rupture. Puddu et al. (9) similarly concluded that rupture was secondary to degenerative changes that could be found in both symptomatic and asymptomatic patients. Other authors disagree with the idea that degenerative changes lead to rupture. Hooker (10) noted degenerative changes in only 1 of 5 tendons examined histologically.

Investigations into the vascular distribution of the Achilles tendon have also shed light onto the cause of tendon rupture. Lagergren and Lindholm (11) note that the vascularity of the Achilles tendon is poorest in the segment most commonly ruptured (2 to 6 cm proximal to its insertion) and suggest that this increases susceptibility to rupture. Schmidt-Rohlfing et al. (12) found poor vascularization in both the middle and the distal part of the tendon. Since Achilles ruptures occur in the middle part of the tendon and rarely in the distal part, they could not confirm a direct relationship between blood supply and the frequency of ruptures.

Systemic diseases that require chronic steroid therapy have been associated with Achilles tendon rupture. Steroid injections around the area of the Achilles tendon may predispose patients to tendon rupture. Other diseases associated with Achilles tendon ruptures are syphilis and gout.

INITIAL FINDINGS, PHYSICAL EXAMINATION, AND DIAGNOSIS

Acute Ruptures

The diagnosis of acute Achilles tendon rupture can be made quite simply from a good history and physical examination. As noted, the typical patient is a 30- to 50-year-old male who was participating in an athletic activity. Usually, the patient recalls a pop or snap, which may have been audible, after jumping, pushing off, or landing after a jump, resulting in sudden pain in the calf posterior to the ankle. Many patients feel as if they had been struck in the back of the ankle or calf when the rupture occurred. Patients generally present with complaints of pain, weakness, ecchymoses, swelling, and/or difficulty walking. The intensity of the pain is variable, and patients who experience little or no pain may wait before seeing a physician.

For ruptures that do not occur during athletic activity—e.g., from falls, missteps, or slips—the clinician should determine the mechanism of injury. If the patient reveals a rapid or sudden dorsiflexion force, as might occur in slipping on stairs or a ladder, Achilles tendon rupture should be suspected.

Patients who are ambulatory will walk with a limp or abnormal gait. Inspection of the injured calf will reveal edema and ecchymosis. On palpation, a defect in the tendon can be appreciated. There is usually some tenderness around the area of rupture. Weakness or absence of active plantar flexion may be present; but owing to the action of the tibialis posterior and flexor digitorum longus, plantar flexion may be maintained and appear normal.

The most reliable test used in the diagnosis of Achilles tendon rupture is the Thompson and Doherty test (13). The patient should lie in the prone position on the examination table with the feet hanging over the edge of the table or with the knees bent at a 90° angle. The clinician should squeeze the calf just distal to its maximum circumference: when the tendon is intact, passive plantar flexion will be noted. This is considered a negative Thompson and Doherty test. A positive test results in no plantar flexion, indicating a complete rupture of the Achilles tendon.

Chronic Ruptures

Patients with a chronic Achilles tendon rupture present with complaints of persistent pain and/or weakness. They may reveal a history of an acute injury after which the symptoms began, possibly indicating a missed or untreated acute rupture. Gradual onset of symptoms may occur when overuse or degenerative changes lead to rupture. In runners, a history of transient or repeated episodes of pain in the area of the tendon may indicate a partial rupture.

On examination the patient may walk with a limp, and weakness is usually present with plantar flexion. There is usually tenderness to palpation over a palpable nodule or fusiform swelling within the tendon. A defect in the tendon may or may not be appreciated. The Thompson and Doherty test may be negative with chronic ruptures, because partial healing and scarring make the tendon continuous, and with partial ruptures, because some tendon fibers remain intact.

RADIOLOGIC STUDIES

Since the diagnosis of acute Achilles tendon rupture is usually made with the history and examination, radiologic studies for these injuries are rarely necessary. There have been some recent studies on the value of ultrasound and MRI in the diagnosis of Achilles tendon injuries. Maffulli et al. (14) noted that on ultrasound the path of the tendon may disappear and that hematoma formation may be seen. MRI can accurately depict acute Achilles tendon ruptures and may be of value in equivocal cases, in the presence of severe edema or massive soft tissue swelling (15).

MRI is useful for the diagnosis of chronic Achilles ruptures because of its ability to show the extent of damage to the tendon. It can differentiate between complete and partial tears and can identify areas of intrasubstance degeneration that is not palpable on examination.

TREATMENT

After the diagnosis of Achilles tendon rupture has been made, the physician must decide on treatment. As with many orthopaedic diagnoses, controversy exists concerning the best course of management. Achilles ruptures can be treated nonoperatively or operatively. With each approach, the goal is to return the tendon to its normal anatomy and function, while minimizing the potential for complications.

Nonoperative Treatment

The nonoperative approach to acute Achilles tendon ruptures has its theoretical foundation in basic science experiments that demonstrated the regenerative capacity of the Achilles tendon. Using a rat model, Lipscolmb and Wakim (16) excised the Achilles tendon from its musculotendinous junction to its insertion. Complete regeneration of the tendon occurred in 12 weeks. In addition, when the tendon was sectioned at its insertion, looped back on itself, and tied, reconstitution across the resulting gap also occurred.

Nonoperative treatment for Achilles tendon ruptures typically consists of casting. Either a short or long leg cast in gravity equinus has been advocated. *Gravity equinus* refers to the relaxed position the foot assumes when the patient is sitting on a table with his or her knees flexed over the edge. No plantar flexion force is applied to the

foot. The patient is kept immobilized for 8 to 12 weeks. During the first 4 weeks the patient is kept non-weight bearing. After the cast is removed, a 2.5-cm heel lift is used for an additional 4 weeks. The most common complications with nonoperative treatment are rerupture and lengthening of the tendon.

Lea and Smith (17) and Nistor (18) were early proponents of nonoperative treatment and obtained favorable results with simple casting. These authors concluded that conservative treatment is an easily justifiable method of treatment, despite the high frequency of rerupture. The treatment method of both studies consisted of short leg casts; however, because the gastrocnemius spans the knee joint, a long leg cast may be biomechanically advantageous, since it would tend to relax this muscle.

Whether to use a short or a long leg cast is not entirely clear. There have been no prospective randomized studies comparing the two techniques. Several authors have used long leg casts with good results (19–22). Studies of patients treated in non–weight-bearing, long leg equinus casts reported excellent functional results and a relatively low rate of rerupture (19,20). The low rerupture rate was thought to be related to the support given to the gastrocnemius muscle. The use of a long leg cast is our preferred method for closed treatment.

Operative Treatment

ACUTE RUPTURE

Successful treatment of acute Achilles tendon ruptures can be achieved through surgical repair. Surgical options include open and percutaneous techniques (Clinical Table). Numerous open procedures have been described, including simple end-to-end suture, plantaris weave reinforcement, peroneus brevis reinforcement, fascial augmentation, and pullout wire techniques.

Regardless of the surgical technique, patients require a general or spinal/epidural anesthetic. The surgical procedure is traditionally performed with the patient in the prone position, but it may be done with the patient supine. A medial or lateral incision can be used. The medial approach has the advantage of avoiding the sural nerve and providing easy access to the plantaris tendon. With either approach the incision should be taken straight down to the paratenon, creating full-thickness skin flaps. The paratenon is then incised along the line of the incision. Dissection between the subcutaneous tissue and the paratenon should be avoided, because it can increase the chance of wound problems.

The ends of the tendon are débrided, and any hematoma is cleared out. Several suturing techniques have been advocated. We prefer to use the Kessler technique with number 3 cottony Dacron and to oversew with a vertical locking circumferential suture of number 1 cottony Dacron (Fig. 74.1). We bury all knots on the deep side of the tendon. The paratenon is closed next, and the subcutaneous tissue and skin are carefully reapproximated.

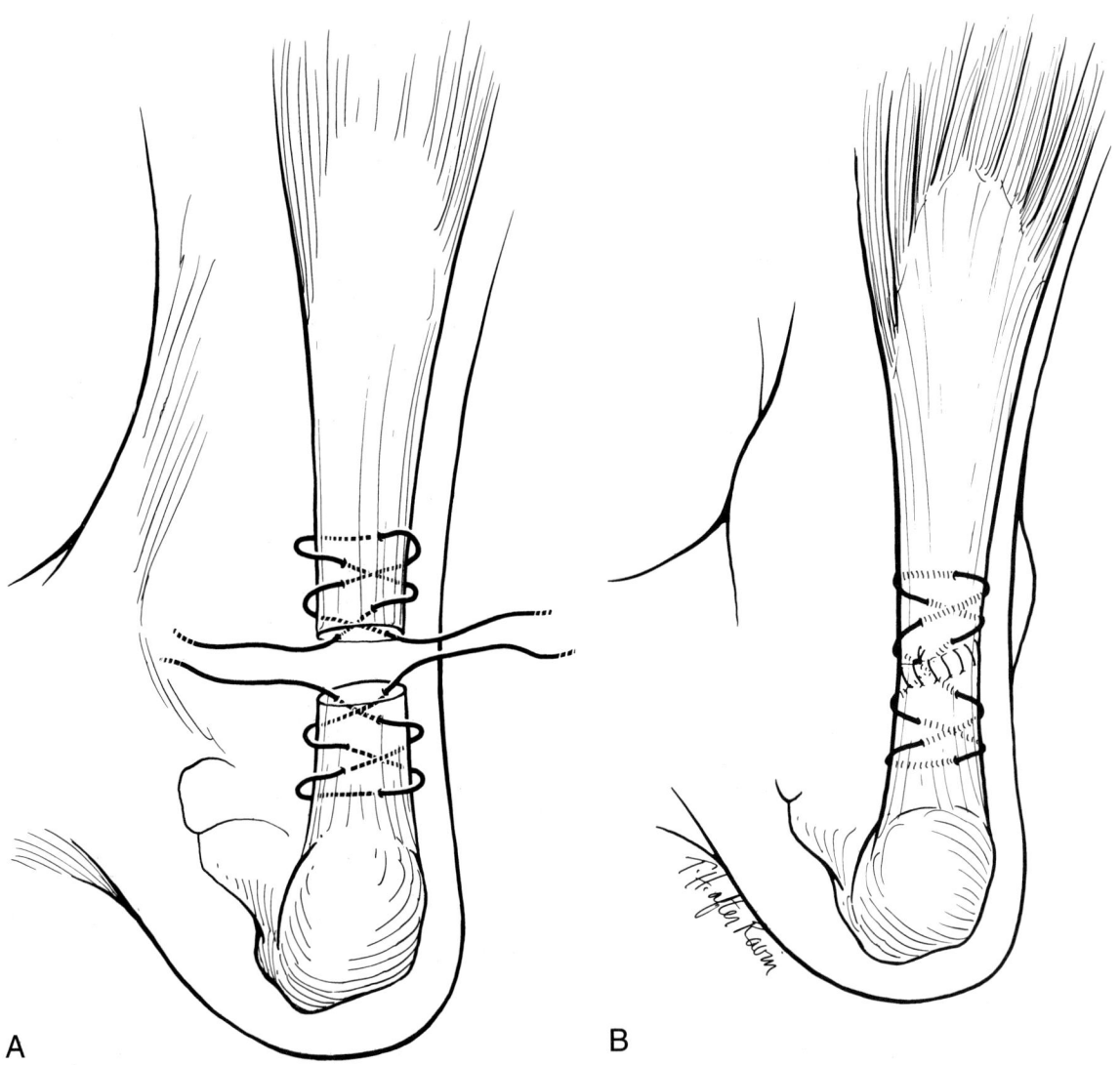

Figure 74.1. Suturing the tendon.

The patient is then placed in a short leg cast in gravity equinus for 6 to 8 weeks. For the first 4 weeks, the patient must not bear weight on the repaired tendon. After casting, a small heel lift may be used for 3 to 4 weeks.

Complications from surgical treatment include infection, skin slough, rerupture, and sural nerve injury as well as risks associated with receiving anesthetic. The advantages of surgery include relatively low rerupture rates and good postoperative strength. Several clinical studies have examined operative versus nonoperative treatment of acute Achilles rupture. Nistor (23) reviewed 105 patients randomly assigned to surgical and nonsurgical treatment. Of 60 nonsurgically treated patients, 5 experienced rerupture (8%). Of the 45 surgically treated patients, 2 experienced reruptures (4%) and 2 developed infections. Average follow-up was 2.5 years. Cybex II testing of plantar flexion strength found only minor differences between the two groups. Nistor concluded that conservative treatment offers advantages over surgical treatment.

In a more recent prospective randomized study, 7 of 55 patients treated nonoperatively sustained reruptures (13%) (24). Of the 56 patients treated surgically, 3 sustained reruptures (5%) and 2 developed infections. The follow-up for this study was 1 year. The surgically treated patients had a higher rate of resuming sports at their preinjury level, had decreased calf atrophy, regained better motion, and noted fewer complaints.

To minimize the rerupture rate and surgical complication rate, Ma and Griffith (25) introduced the technique of percutaneous Achilles tendon repair. They noted excellent results with minimal complications.

One study that compared the percutaneous and open repair techniques noted that 2 of 12 patients treated percutaneously experienced rerupture by the 1.8-year follow-up (26). There were no complications in the 15 patients treated with the open technique. Both groups of patients were satisfied with the results, and there were no significant differences on Cybex II testing. The authors recommend percutaneous repair for recreational athletes and patients concerned with cosmesis. Open repair was recommended for high-caliber athletes. Another study concluded that percutaneous repair offered excellent results for patients under 50 years old (27). Of the 14 patients treated with percutaneous repair, none experienced rerupture, infection, or delayed wound healing. Sural nerve injury occurred in 1 patient.

Postoperative management after surgical repair of the Achilles tendon has typically consisted of rigid casting for 6 to 8 weeks. Although casting provides excellent protection of the repair, there has been increasing enthusiasm for beginning early protected range of motion exercises. Several studies have found favorable results with this regimen, reporting improved ankle range of motion with no increased risk of rerupture (28,29). Special mobile casts and dorsiflexion blocking orthoses have been used as part of this postoperative management regimen.

Chronic Rupture

The treatment of chronic Achilles tendon ruptures is more difficult than that of acute ruptures (Clinical Table). Because the tendon has usually healed in a way that makes it longer than normal or that leaves a large fixed gap, the chance of improving function of the tendon with conservative treatment is poor. Patients who do not want surgery generally obtain adequate pain relief with a polypropylene ankle-foot orthosis (AFO) that relieves the pressure on the tendon. Typically, surgery is needed to restore function of the Achilles tendon complex.

During the surgery, the scarred and fibrosed portion of the tendon is excised, which leaves a defect in the tendon.

End-to-end suture of the tendon is usually impossible, and it is necessary to either bridge the gap or perform a tendon transfer. We recommend tendon transfer; favorable results have been obtained by using the flexor hallucis longus (FHL) to reconstruct chronic Achilles tendon ruptures (30). Harvesting of the FHL tendon is done through an incision made along the medial border of the foot just above the abductor hallucis from the navicular to the first metatarsal head (Fig. 74.2). The abductor and the flexor hallucis brevis are reflected plantar to expose the deep midfoot anatomy. The FHL and flexor digitorum longus (FDL) tendons are identified, and the FHL is divided as far distally as possible (Fig. 74.3). The distal limb of the FHL is then sewn into the FDL with all five toes in a neutral position.

A second incision is made posteriorly along the medial aspect of the Achilles tendon from the level of its musculotendinous junction to 2.5 cm below its insertion on the calcaneus (Fig. 74.2). Dissection is carried down sharply to the paratenon, where it is opened longitudinally to expose the Achilles tendon. The fascia overlying the posterior compartment of the leg is then opened longitudinally, and the FHL is identified. Its tendon is brought proximally from the midfoot into the posterior incision.

A transverse hole is drilled just distal to the insertion of the Achilles tendon, halfway through the calcaneus from medial to lateral. A second vertical drill hole is made just deep to the insertion to meet the first hole. A towel clip can be used to help interconnect the two holes. The FHL is brought down the tunnel from proximal to distal and woven through the Achilles tendon from distal to proximal (Fig. 74.4).

Clinical Table: Achilles Tendon Ruptures

Procedure	Indications	Technique	Complications	Advantages
		Acute Ruptures		
Casting	• Poor operative candidate; patient refuses surgery	• Non-weight-bearing long leg cast for 4–6 weeks; then short leg cast for 4–6 weeks	• Relatively high rerupture rate; delayed rehabilitation	• Avoids potential operative complications
Surgery	• Rapid rehabilitation necessary; patient refuses long leg casting	• Medial incision; primary suture; short leg cast: non-weight bearing for 4 weeks; then full weight bearing for 4 weeks	• Potential wound problems	• Relatively low rerupture rate; early rehabilitation and return to activity
		Chronic Ruptures		
Bracing	• Poor operative candidate; patient refuses surgery	• Molded polypropylene AFO	• Skin irritation from brace; no rehabilitation	• Avoids potential operative complications
Surgery	• Potential for rehabilitation; patient refuses long-term bracing	• Transfer of FHL tendon; short leg cast: non-weight bearing for 4 weeks; then full weight bearing for 4 weeks	• Potential wound problems	• Potential for rehabilitation and return to normal activity

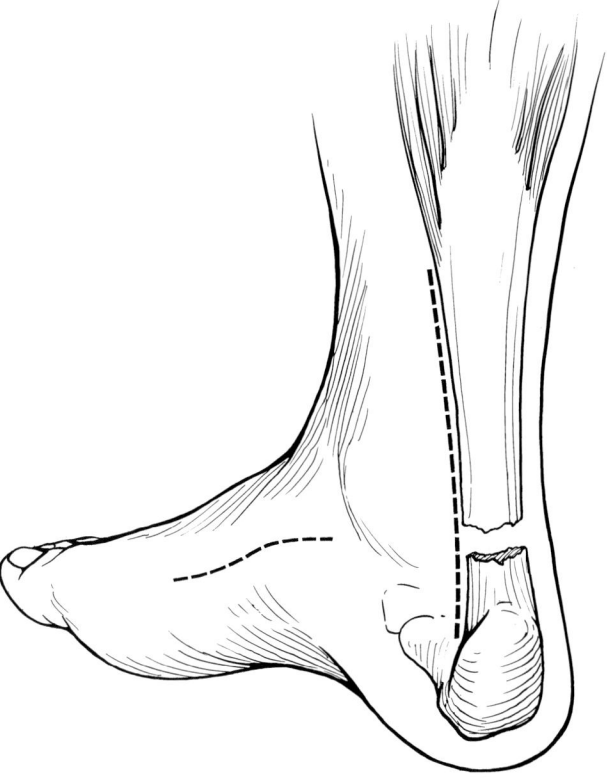

Figure 74.2. Incision sites for treating chronic Achilles tendon rupture.

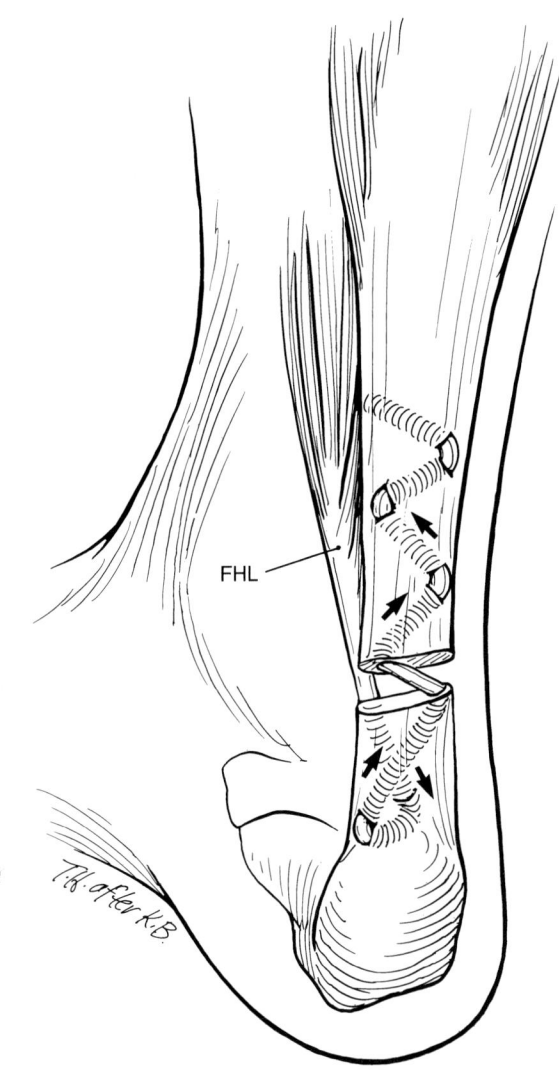

Figure 74.4. The FHL is woven through the remaining portion of the Achilles tendon to secure fixation and to supplement the tendon. *Arrows,* direction of the transfer.

FHL

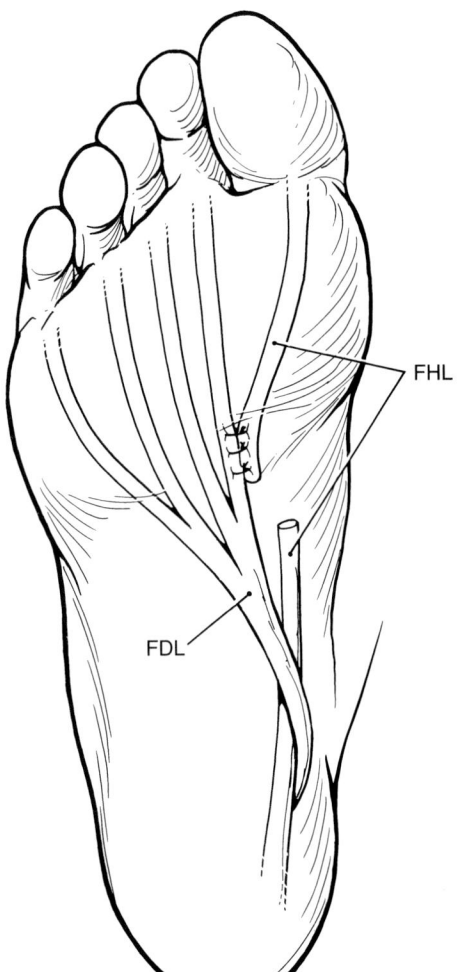

FHL

FDL

Figure 74.3. The distal portion of the FHL is anastomosed into the FDL.

CONCLUSION

Acute Achilles tendon ruptures are serious injuries that can easily be diagnosed from the history and physical examination. They tend to occur in 30- to 50-year-old men during athletic activity. Treatment options include both surgical and nonsurgical techniques, and both types of treatment can provide excellent results. Before deciding on treatment, it is important to discuss the options with the patient. Each case must be handled on an individual basis. The patient should be made aware of the advantages and possible complications of each type of treatment and should take an active role in the final decision. We currently recommend surgical treatment for very active patients regardless of their age (31). Cast treatment is reserved for patients who are not good surgical candidates and for those who do not have an active lifestyle.

Chronic ruptures can be treated for pain relief with an AFO. Some patients become pain free and can be weaned out of their brace after 6 months. These patients must be warned that they have a high risk for recurrent symptoms or complete rupture. Repair can be accomplished surgically, which usually requires augmentation. We currently recommend FHL transfer for this purpose (30).

REFERENCES

1. Carden DG, Noble J, Chalmers J, et al. Rupture of the calcaneal tendon. J Bone Joint Surg 1987;69B:416–420.
2. Paré A. Les oeuvres. 9th ed. Lyon: Rigard & Obert, 1633.
3. Weiner AD, Lipscolmb PR. Rupture of muscles and tendons. Minn Med 1956;39:731–736.
4. Stucke K. Uber das elastische verhalten der Achillessehne im belastngsversuch. Arch Klin Chir 1950;265:579.
5. Inglis AE, Scott WN, Sculco TP, Patterson AH. Ruptures of the tendo Achillis. An objective assessment of surgical and non-surgical treatment. J Bone Joint Surg 1976;58A:990–993.
6. Barfred T. Achilles tendon rupture. Aetiology and pathogenesis of subcutaneous rupture assessed on the basis of the literature and rupture experiments on rats. Acta Orthop Scand Suppl 1973;152: 3–126.
7. Arner O, Lindholm A. Subcutaneous rupture of the Achilles tendon. Acta Chir Scand Suppl 1959;239:1–51.
8. Arner O, Lindholm A, Orell SR. Histological changes in subcutaneous rupture of the Achilles tendon. Acta Chir Scand 1959; 116:484–490.
9. Puddu G, Ippolito E, Postacchini F. A classification of Achilles tendon disease. Am J Sports Med 1980;8:244–249.
10. Hooker CH. Rupture of the tendo calcaneus. J Bone Joint Surg 1963;45B:360–363.
11. Lagergren C, Lindholm A. Vascular distribution in the Achilles tendon: an angiographic and microangiographic study. Acta Chir Scand 1958–59;116:491–495.
12. Schmidt-Rohlfing B, Graf J, Schneider U, et al. The blood supply of the Achilles tendon. Int Orthop 1992;16:29–31.
13. Thompson TC, Doherty JH. Spontaneous rupture of tendon of Achilles: a new clinical diagnostic test. J Trauma 1962; 2:126–129.
14. Maffulli N, Dymond NP, Capasso G. Ultrasonographic findings in subcutaneous rupture of Achilles tendon. J Sports Med Phys Fitness 1989;29:365–368.
15. Marcus DS Reicher MA, Kellerhouse LE. Achilles tendon injuries: the role of magnetic resonance imaging. J Comput Assit Tomogr 1989;13:480–486.
16. Lipscolmb PR, Wakim KG. Regeneration of severed tendons: an experimental study. Mayo Clin Proc 1961;36:271–276.
17. Lea RB, Smith L. Non-surgical treatment of tendo achillis rupture. J. Bone Joint Surg 1972;54A:1398–1407.
18. Nistor L. Conservative treatment of fresh subcutaneous rupture of the Achilles tendon. Acta Orthop Scand 1976;47:459–462.
19. Fruensgaard S, Helmig P. Riis J, et al. Conservative treatment for acute rupture of the Achilles tendon. Int Orthop 1992;16:33–35.
20. Keller J, Rasmussen TB. Closed treatment of Achilles tendon rupture. Acta Orthop Scand 1984;55:548–550.
21. Stein SR, Leukens CA. Closed treatment of Achilles tendon ruptures. Orthop Clin North Am 1976;7:241–246.
22. Stein SR, Luekens CA. Methods and rationale for closed treatment of Achilles tendon ruptures. Am J Sports Med 1976; 4:162–169.
23. Nistor L. Surgical and nonsurgical treatment of Achilles tendon rupture. J Bone Joint Surg 1981;63A:394–399.
24. Cetti R, Christensen S, Ejsted R. Operative versus nonoperative treatment of Achilles tendon rupture. A prospective randomized study and review of the literature. Am J Sport Med 1993; 21:791–799.
25. Ma GW, Griffith TG. Percutaneous repair of acute closed ruptured Achilles tendon: a new technique. Clin Orthop 1977;128:247–255.
26. Bradley JP, Tibone JE. Percutaneous and open surgical repairs of Achilles tendon ruptures. A comparative study. Am J Sports Med 1990;18:188–195.
27. Fitzgibbons RE, Hefferon J, Hill J. Percutaneous Achilles tendon repair. Am J Sports Med 1993;21:724–727.
28. Cetti R, Henrikson LO, Jacobsen KS. A new treatment of ruptured Achilles tendons. A prospective randomized study. Clin Orthop 1994;308:155–165.
29. Solveborn SA, Moberg A. Immediate free ankle motion after surgical repair of acute Achilles tendon ruptures. Am J Sports Med 1994;22:607–610.
30. Wapner KL, Pavlock GS, Hecht PJ, et al. Repair of chronic Achilles tendon rupture with flexor hallucis longus tendon transfer. Foot Ankle 1993;14:443–449.
31. Wapner KL. Acute repair of the Achilles tendon. In: Johnson KA, ed. Master techniques in orthopaedic surgery. New York: Raven, 1994.

Posterior Tibial Tendon Dysfunction

Posterior tibial tendon dysfunction (PTTD) has been recognized with increasing frequency. It is associated with a progressive painful deformity of the foot that causes significant disability. With progression of pain and deformity, walking becomes difficult. It is best recognized and treated early before progressing to a severe and painful deformity.

RELEVANT ANATOMY AND PATHOGENESIS

The posterior tibial muscle and tendon perform a critical function for the foot. The tendon with its muscle is the dynamic stabilizer of the arch. When contracted, the muscle inverts the subtalar joint and, through insertions into the midfoot and metatarsals, adducts and plantar flexes the forefoot. The muscle early in stance phase, when the heel is in eversion, is active from heel rise to full inversion. The posterior tibial muscle helps allow the successful progression of the foot from its everted flexible position to the relatively stiff supinated position for forward propulsion. Although the muscle mass of the gastrocnemius–soleus complex is well over six times that of the posterior tibialis, the posterior tibial muscle, owing to its medial insertion on the navicular, has a superior mechanical advantage (lever arm) for initiating inversion. Without the posterior tibial muscle inversion strength is severely compromised (1).

The posterior tibial muscle originates from the posterior surfaces of the tibia, interosseous membrane, and fibula; passes directly behind the medial malleolus; and gives rise to several insertions. The main insertion is to the navicular and medial cuneiform, with branches onto the spring ligament complex and sustentaculum talus of the calcaneus. Other insertions are the remaining cuneiforms and metatarsals two, three, and four. Because of the multiple insertions, pull on the tendon behind the

medial malleolus inverts the heel and adducts the forefoot, resulting in elevation of the medial longitudinal arch. It is well known, however, that in the standing position, activity in the posterior tibial muscle is not necessary to maintain the normal height of the arch, because it is statically held by the bony architecture and supporting ligaments.

The cause of PTTD is multifactorial (2). The condition is also known as posterior tibial tendon insufficiency or rupture or lateral peritalar subluxation. PTTD is more common in women than in men. Some patients, but by no means the majority, note a particular traumatic incident, which is usually superimposed on an already degenerated tendon. Obesity and hypertension have been noted more frequently in those with PTTD than in the general population, and in my experience obesity or recent weight gain is quite common in these patients. Although not a proven cause of degeneration, decreased vascularity has been noted in the tendon at and distal to the level of the medial malleolus (3), the latter of which is the most common site of rupture. Finally, many patients believe that they had a flatfoot before the disorder (although the flatfoot may have increased). Unfortunately, there seems to be no one factor uniting all patients with posterior tibial tendon dysfunction.

INITIAL FINDINGS, PHYSICAL EXAMINATION, AND DIAGNOSIS

Patients in the early stages of PTTD have pain over the course of the posterior tibial tendon, most frequently distal to the medial malleolus. Late in the course of the disease, the pain over the ruptured tendon disappears. Patients are left with a poorly functioning tendon and muscle imbalance that promotes an increasing valgus deformity of the foot and the likelihood of lateral pain from bony impingement.

Physical examination reveals tenderness and swelling over the posterior tibial tendon early in the course of the disease. This is most commonly noted in between the medial malleolus and the navicular, although the tenderness can be proximal to the malleolus. Muscle testing shows weakness in the posterior tibial tendon–muscle complex when the tendon has become dysfunctional but not necessarily fully ruptured. The muscle testing must be done carefully. The most sensitive method is to have the patient invert and simultaneously plantar flex the uninvolved foot from an everted position when sitting or with the foot hanging down; the patient does this against the resistance of the examiner's hand. Repeat the sequence on the symptomatic side. The patient with PTTD will not be able to strongly go from the everted position to one of inversion and plantar flexion. It is important to do this test with the ankle in plantar flexion to prevent recruitment of the anterior tibialis.

The standing alignment of the patient's feet should be noted. The amount of sag in the medial longitudinal arch, usually a combination of forefoot abduction and heel valgus, should be recorded. Heel valgus is best observed from the posterior view; the examiner notes the amount of valgus of the calcaneus in relation to the tibia. This valgus is usually at this level of the joints below the talus but can also be from malalignment in the ankle mortise. Patients with PTTD have difficulty going into a single-stance heel rise, i.e., going up on their toes when the asymptomatic foot is already off the ground. This will be painful, and with considerable dysfunction of the tendon, the normal inversion of the heel will be decreased. Heel rise may not be possible if the foot is too painful. This test is not pathognomonic for PTTD. Arthritis in the midfoot, a stiff flatfoot, or a deformity from another cause can give a positive single-stance heel rise test.

The range of motion of the hindfoot and midfoot (triple-joint complex) is assessed while the patient is seated. The calcaneus is grasped, and the amount of inversion and eversion that can be achieved underneath the talus is estimated and compared to the opposite foot. Patients with long-standing PTTD frequently have contractures and deformity that cause decreased inversion and increased eversion from the neutral position of 5° of heel valgus. The clinician should assess the alignment of the forefoot versus the hindfoot, which is measured by placing the heel in the neutral position and pressing up on the fifth and first metatarsal heads. If there is greater than 10° of elevation on the medial side of the forefoot from the plane parallel to the plantar aspect of the calcaneus, significant forefoot varus is present from ligamentous laxity or deformity along the medial column. Using standing lateral x-ray and assessing the instability in the dorsiflexion–plantar flexion plane, the examiner should try to determine if the deformity is from the first metatarsal-tarsal, talonavicular, and/or naviculocuneiform joint.

RADIOLOGIC STUDIES

Routine x-rays for assessing PTTD include the following views: standing AP of the foot, standing lateral of the ankle, and supine oblique of the foot. The standing AP and lateral views of the foot can be used to assess the location of the deformity in the arch. On the AP view, the clinician should look for lateral subluxation of the navicular on the talar head at the lateral end points of the articular surfaces and should note the amount of uncovered medial talar head. On the lateral view, the clinician should determine if sag is present at the talonavicular, naviculocuneiform, or talometatarsal joint or at a combination of these joints, which can be seen as plantar angulation.

Measurements of the flatfoot deformity can be made by noting the talonavicular coverage angle on the AP view and the talometatarsal and talocalcaneal angles and the medial cuneiform to ground distance on the lateral view (4). The measurements are most useful when done by the same observer, to assure consistency in technique. Because arthritis and other causes of flatfoot deformity can increase these measurements, they should not be used to diagnose posterior tibial tendon dysfunction.

The standing AP view of the ankle is particularly useful for patients with considerable deformity. Valgus deformity of the heel can be the result of deformity of the subtalar joints and midfoot joints and or from valgus tilting of the talus within the ankle mortise. It is, therefore, important to identify any ankle subluxation, so treatment can include this deformity.

MRI and CT scans are not necessary for the diagnosis of posterior tibial tendon insufficiency. The diagnosis of PTTD is made primarily from the clinical examination and history. Patients can have good strength in the posterior tibial tendon and be asymptomatic, even though MRI studies show some degeneration in the posterior tibial tendon. MRI can be used to exclude pathology within the tendon and may be able to identify those few patients who could benefit from a tenosynovectomy rather than a more extensive procedure.

TREATMENT

Nonoperative Treatment

PTTD is likely to progress, even if the patient wears orthotics and braces. Orthotics are, therefore, best used to provide symptomatic relief in those who, although aware of the progressive nature of the disease, opt for conservative treatment. The rate of progression can be difficult to predict. Orthotics with medial posting at the heel and accommodation of forefoot varus may give some symptomatic relief. Care should be taken to avoid hard and high posting against the navicular, which makes the orthotics too uncomfortable to wear. Restrictive orthoses, such as a UCBL model, can provide some correction of the heel but generally are poorly tolerated by adults. For severe deformities, an ankle-foot orthosis (AFO) may give symptomatic relief, but this devise has not been proven to halt the collapse of the arch.

Operative Treatment

Operative treatment of PTTD depends on the associated deformity (Clinical Table). The patient may present with no deformity, considerable collapse of the arch with good motion remaining, or fixed deformity. Although surgeons need a procedure that corrects the deformity and maintains maximum function, no existing technique restores the full strength of the muscle and tendon or completely corrects different degrees of deformity while retaining normal range of motion. Surgical treatment of PTTD is, therefore, still evolving. The tendon used for transfer is usually the flexor digitorum longus (FDL) or possibly the flexor hallucis longus (FHL), neither of which has more than half the muscle mass of the posterior tibial muscle. Ligament reconstructions for the deformity in the longitudinal arch have not been shown clinically to be successful, at least when used without a bony procedure.

Although staging systems have been proposed for MRI findings of posterior tendon dysfunction, no clinical grading system for directing treatment has been universally accepted. Both Johnson and Myerson (4) have presented the most common grading system; a modification of these systems will be presented here. In stage I disease, there is swelling and tenderness in the tendon with some difficulty in heel rise but no deformity in the foot. Most patients already have significant degeneration of the tendon when they seek medical treatment. For patients who have only synovitis and minimal degeneration—determined by MRI studies and direct inspection—a tenosynovectomy should be considered, followed by 4 to 6 weeks of casting (5).

Stage II disease is characterized by considerable tendon degeneration or tear and some flexible deformity. A tendon transfer should be considered for these patients, although the procedure is not necessarily performed alone (6). Since the tendon transfer does not correct the deformity and may still allow progression, surgeons are now combining the transfer with bony procedures to correct the deformity while retaining good motion. For example, some surgeons perform a medial slide calcaneal osteotomy to correct the static valgus alignment and shift the Achilles tendon force (7). There is evidence that this procedure corrects the deformity, although data from long-term follow-up are not yet available. I recommend the me-

Clinical Table: Posterior Tibial Tendon Dysfunction (PTTD)

Procedure	Indications	Technique	Anatomy	Pitfalls
FDL transfer	• Degeneration or tear without deformity or contracture	• Drill hole in navicular; connect to posterior tibial tendon proximally	• Medial plantar nerve	• Questionable whether full strength is restored; may supplement with osteotomy
Calcaneal osteotomy	• Flexible, mild to moderate deformity (<50% talonavicular uncoverage on AP view)	• 1-cm medial slide fixed with screw; done with tendon transfer	• Sural nerve	• Does not correct severe deformity
Evans	• Flexible, moderate to severe deformity with forefoot abduction and heel valgus	• 8–10 block; 1–2cm proximal to the calcaneocuboid joint	• Sural nerve	• Calcaneocuboid arthritis
Calcaneocuboid fusion	• Flexible, moderate to severe deformity with forefoot abduction and heel valgus	• 8–12 block; staple or H plate	• Sural nerve	• Nonunion; stiffness with lateral discomfort; risk of overcorrection or undercorrection
Subtalar fusion	• Moderate deformity with heel valgus without forefoot vulgus	• 1–2 screws across the joint	• Sural nerve	• Stiffness; cannot correct forefoot abduction or varus without risk of excessive lateral weight bearing
Double or triple arthrodesis	• Fixed deformity with heel valgus and forefoot abduction	• Screws, staples for calcaneocuboid joint	• Sural nerve • Saphenous nerve	• Considerable loss of motion; salvage operation only

dial slide calcaneal osteotomy for mild to moderate calcaneal valgus.

Other surgeons prefer lateral column lengthening, in which a bone block is added to the lateral side of the foot (the calcaneus) to correct heel valgus and forefoot abduction (8). This can be performed either at the level of the anterior process of the calcaneus or through the calcaneocuboid joint. Arthritis of the calcaneocuboid joint has been noted after correction at the anterior process of the calcaneus, although not commonly when a medial slide posterior osteotomy has been conbined with the anterior process (Evans) procedure. Clinical follow-up of adults treated with lateral column lengthening is just becoming available. Considerable correction of the arch has been noted, but long-term follow-up data have not been reported. In general, lateral column lengthening can be used for moderate to severe flexible deformity when there is considerable abduction of the forefoot and heel valgus.

Deformity at the first metatarsal tarsal joint can often be seen as widening at the plantar aspect of the joint on the standing lateral radiograph. Instability at this joint, which is considered stage II disease, can be identified by stabilizing the second metatarsal and pushing dorsally and plantarly on the first metatarsal head. Considerable instability at this joint can be eliminated with a fusion; the surgeon must take care to leave the first metatarsal not dorsiflexed or plantiflexed with respect to the second metatarsal. Fortunately, motion at this joint is not critical to the function of the foot.

Note that all stage II procedures include the tendon transfer. Because the tendon transfer cannot be expected to work against contracture, a prerequisite for the procedure is the presence of near normal passive inversion motion. Patients with stage II PTTD can be treated with a subtalar fusion, which leaves some motion in the midfoot, but is not the author's preference. This fusion significantly limits patients' participation in sports and ability to walk on uneven ground.

Stage III disease is characterized by contracture that prevents the inversion of the subtalar and talonavicular joints. This is most often seen in severe, long-standing deformity. When such deformity and contractures are noted, a major arthrodesis (subtalar, double, or triple) is necessary. Effort is made to avoid these procedures in nonelderly patients because of the significant postoperative limitation of motion.

Patients with PTTD often have contracture of the Achilles tendon, which can be severe in stage III disease. Therefore, if the Achilles contracture does not allow the foot to be placed in the neutral position, percutaneous lengthening is usually performed at the beginning of the operative procedure. When the talus tilts within the ankle mortise, in addition to the deformity in the midfoot and hindfoot, there is no good restorative procedure. Fusions and corrective procedures are staged to try to avoid a pantalar fusion, and fusions can be combined with a brace for the talar tilt. It is better to treat patients with PTTD early in the course of the disease and thus avoid such severe deformities.

TENOSYNOVECTOMY

Although rare, some patients with swelling, tenderness, and pain on attempted single-stance heel rise will have tenosynovitis of the posterior tibial tendon with no considerable degeneration. Indications for a tenosynovectomy are tenosynovitis of the posterior tibial tendon and failure of conservative therapy, which often includes the use of a cast for 4 to 6 weeks. Contraindications include significant tear or degeneration of the posterior tibial tendon. If carefully inspected, most patients with posterior tendon complaints have considerable tendon degeneration (more than one-third to one-half the tendon in cross section).

Technique

For the tenosynovectomy, the patient is placed in the supine position, and a thigh tourniquet is applied. An incision is made from the inferior aspect of the medial malleolus to the navicular, and the tendon sheath is incised. The tendon is inspected on both its medial and lateral sides; the surgeon should note any longitudinal tears. If tenderness is present above the medial malleolus, the tendon is also inspected at this level. Between 1 and 2 cm of the tendon sheath is left intact along the posterior border of the malleolus to prevent subluxation of the tendon. The inflamed synovium is excised, and the tendon sheath is not repaired. After wound closure, the patient is kept in a cast for 4 to 6 weeks. Progressive weight bearing is allowed.

FLEXOR TENDON TRANSFER

For the flexor tendon transfer, the surgeon makes the incision described for the tenosynovectomy. The tendon is inspected on both its medial and lateral sides, and the surgeon notes any enlargement of the tendon; longitudinal tears; or loss of normal tendon fibers, indicating significant tendon degeneration and failure. Even with tendon continuity, the presence of symptomatic degeneration of 50% of the tendon without fixed deformity is an indication for a tendon transfer, which is now commonly used with other procedures, as described below.

Once the decision to do the transfer has been made, the incision is extended along the posterior border of the tibia up to 6 cm above the ankle joint. If there is good excursion of the posterior tibial tendon, it is sutured to the FDL just above the level of the ankle joint. The incision is then lengthened along the medial border of the foot, distally to the level of the base of the first metatarsal; and the abductor muscle is reflected down (3). At the level of the talar head, inferior to the spring ligament complex, the sheath of the flexor digitorum is entered. The FDL tendons of the FHL and FDL are located and followed to the level of the base of the first metatarsal. With the patient's toes in a neutral position, the surgeon exposes the tendons of the FHL and FDL and sews them together or harvests the digitorum proximal to any interconnection between the tendons. The FDL is brought into the wound at the talar head level and is placed through a 1-cm (0.375-in) drill hole in the navicular from plantar to dorsal (Fig. 75.1). The patient's foot is placed in near maximum inversion, and the tendon is pulled halfway between no and full tension and sewn to itself and/or to the old posterior tibialis insertion.

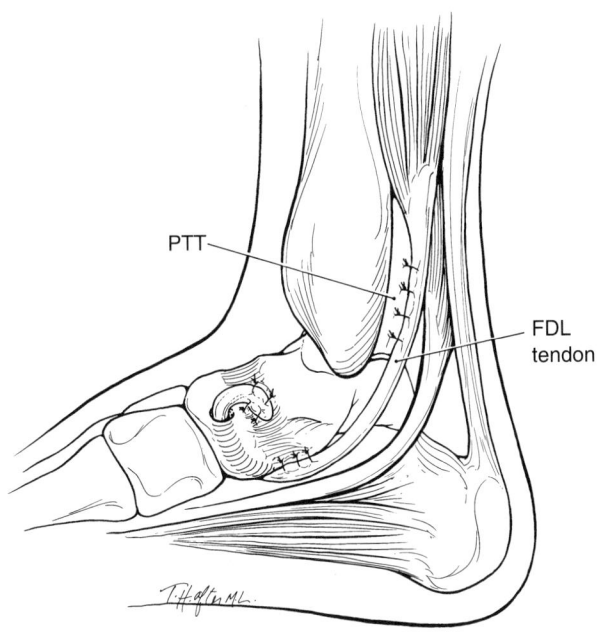

Figure 75.1. The FDL is transferred through a drill hole in the navicular.

NEWER PROCEDURES

The two procedures discussed here will likely continue to be used to treat PTTD. Note that long-term follow-up of these procedures when used with the tendon transfer has not yet been obtained; readers are encouraged to study these data when they become available.

Medial Slide Calcaneal Osteotomy

To perform a medial displacement calcaneal osteotomy, the patient is placed supine with a large bolster underneath the hip to provide access to the lateral heel. An oblique incision is made behind the peroneal tendons, just posterior to the level of the sural nerve (9). An oblique osteotomy is made well anterior to the superior tuberosity of the calcaneus and inferior medial lateral tuberosities of the calcaneus. When first performing this procedure, the surgeon should use fluoroscopy in the operating room to make sure that the osteotomy is made at the correct level. The osteotomy cut is made with a sagittal saw, and an elevator and laminar spreader are used to free up the periosteum medially and inferiorly.

The distal fragment is then slid 1 cm medially and pinned; a cannulated screw is placed percutaneously from the posterior fragment across the osteotomy site (Fig. 75.2). The screw should be directed proximally so that it stays within the calcaneus rather than deviating medially out into the soft tissues and neurovascular bundle. Once the screw is placed, good fixation of the osteotomy should be noted, and the heel alignment should be checked for complete connection of excessive heel valgus.

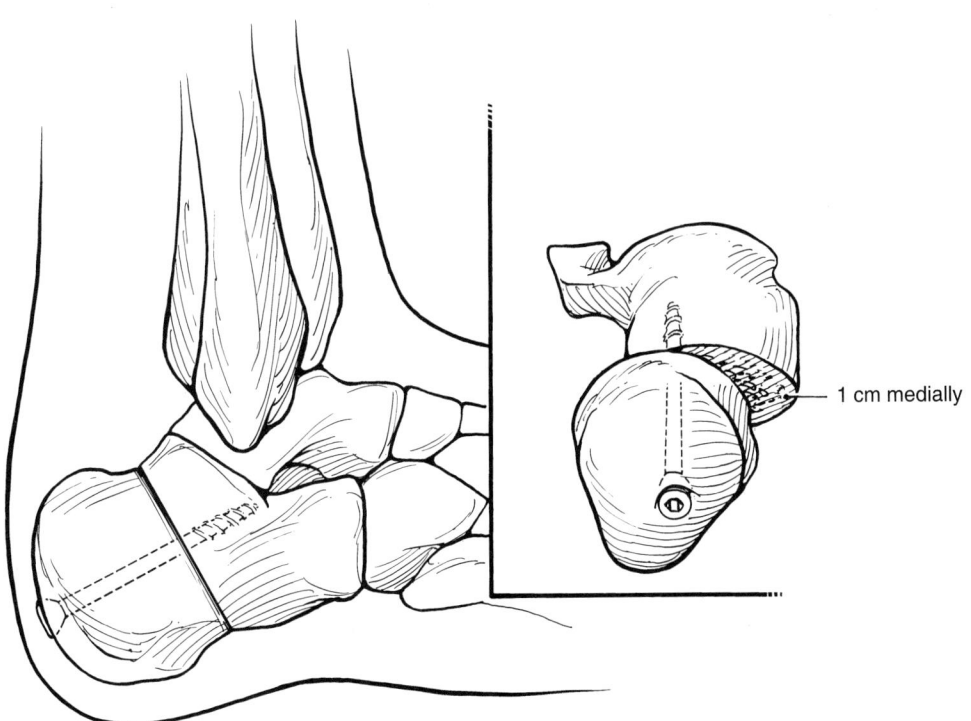

Figure 75.2. For a medial slide calcaneal osteotomy, the fragment should be moved 1 cm medially **(insert)**.

Lateral Column Lengthening

Lateral column lengthening is made through an incision dorsal to the peroneal tendons from the sinus tarsi to the midportion of the cuboid. The proximal portion of this exposure can be used for the Evans procedure, which is an osteotomy made approximately 12 mm proximal and parallel to the calcaneocuboid joint (8). The Evans procedure has been performed along with the medial osteotomy.

Because of the incidence of calcaneocuboid arthritis in adults after an Evans procedure, many surgeons perform the lateral column lengthening with a distraction arthrodesis of the calcaneocuboid joint (10). Two flat cuts in the joint perpendicular to the plantar aspect of the foot are made, taking just the joint surfaces and subchondral plate. A laminar spreader is then used. The amount of distraction provided by the tricortical graft should correct but not overcorrect the deformity (Fig. 75.3). Originally, the fusion was fixed with screws, but because of difficulty in healing these fusions, surgeons are using a cervical H plate with screws to improve fixation.

The tendon transfer is performed with both the medial slide calcaneal osteotomy and the lateral column lengthening procedures, but the tendon is not tied down until after fixation is completed. It is the author's preference to correct deformity with a conbined medial slide and Evans procedure and not fuse the calcaneocuboid joint.

FUSIONS

When any hindfoot fusion is performed, the patient will experience limitation of function. Therefore, it is important for the surgeon to discuss expectations and the outcome of the procedure with the patient and for the patient to be aware that participation in sports, such as running and tennis, will not usually be possible.

Subtalar Arthrodesis

A subtalar arthrodesis is performed through a sinus tarsi incision from the distal tip of the fibula to the anterior process of the calcaneus above the level of the peroneal tendons. The posterior facet is débrided, exposing cancellus bone; and the middle facet is curetted. The surgeon must properly align the heel in the normal 5° to 10° of valgus before fixation. Guidepins for the cannulated screws are used to temporarily fix the subtalar joint so the alignment of the forefoot can be assessed. The anterior portion of the calcaneus and the medial talar head are grasped, and subluxation is reduced by pressing them together and lifting the talar head back up toward the calcaneus. The surgeon must not overcorrect, which leads to forefoot varus. Forefoot varus of 10° or more is unacceptable, as the patient would bear weight excessively on the lateral side of the foot, which leads to lateral pain. Two partially threaded large cancellous screws are used for the fixation; one screw is placed percutaneously from the posterior in-

Figure 75.3. Lateral column lengthening through the calcaneocuboid joint with a tricortical iliac crest bone graft.

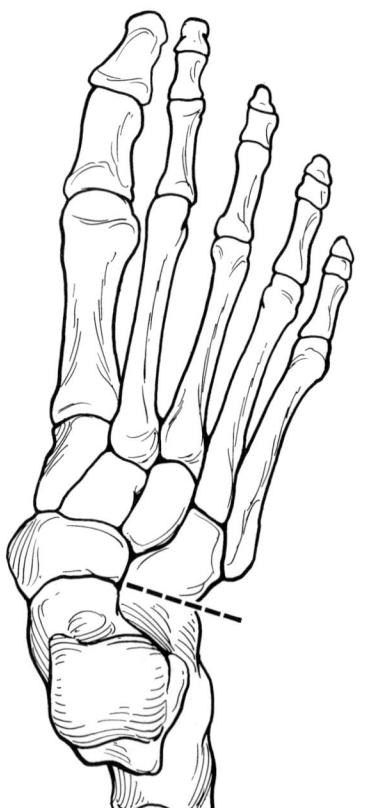
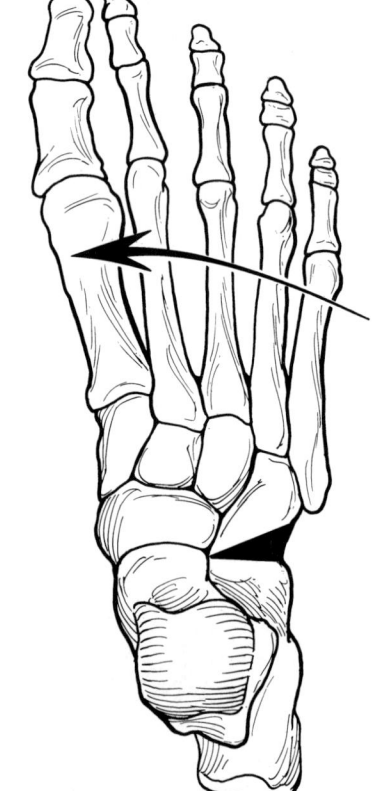

ferior heel close to perpendicular to the posterior facet for compression and the other similarly placed or run from the dorsal talar neck across the joint.

Double Arthrodesis

A double arthrodesis is performed through a longitudinal incision over the calcaneocuboid joint, as described for the lateral column lengthening, and an oblique incision anteromedially just medial to the anterior tibialis tendon. Through these two incisions, the calcaneocuboid and talonavicular joints are exposed and débrided. Care is taken when débriding the talonavicular joint to retain the spherical surfaces of the joint; to perform adequate débridement the surgeon should use curved osteotomies and remove minimal bone.

Once the joints are down to cancellus bone, the position of the fusion is assessed. Rather than lengthening the lateral column, it is possible to shorten the medial column by removing slightly more bone medially, thereby correcting the forefoot abduction. Fixation of the talonavicular joint can be obtained with either screws or staples. Two screws can be used, but the surgeon should care not to fracture the medial tuberosity of the talus. Whatever the fixation, the most important aspect is the position of the foot when the fixation is placed. The aim is to achieve a plantigrade foot with the corrected alignment of the heel and without excessive forefoot varus or valgus.

If fixed subluxation of the subtalar joint is noted before the procedure or if it is not possible to place the foot in a good plantar-flexed position during the procedure, extension to a triple arthrodesis can be performed using the lateral wound. Triple arthrodesis is necessary for treating the severest deformities. Fixation of the subtalar joint can be done with a single screw, as the talonavicular fixation helps immobilize the subtalar joint. Fixation of the calcaneocuboid joint is most easily done with staples.

PITFALLS AND COMMON MISTAKES

A common error with tenosynovectomies is to perform the procedure in a patient with significant tendon degeneration. Such a patient will experience failure of the tendon, which leads to deformity and symptoms. Care should be taken to inspect the tendon medially and laterally for longitudinal tears, which may not be apparent from the one view.

For the tendon transfer, a common error is to select a patient with fixed or progressive deformity. The patient should have nearly full passive inversion of the foot to benefit from a tendon transfer. Because a tendon transfer cannot address deformity, the procedure should not be performed alone in a patient with deformity. Finally, it is important that the patient undergo physical therapy, once the tendon has healed, to strengthen the transfer.

For the medial slide, it is important to slide the distal fragment a full centimeter. In my experience, patients with large amounts of forefoot abduction should be excluded

from this procedure alone. For lateral column lengthening, there is the possibility of overcorrection or undercorrection; the calcaneocuboid arthrodesis may prove difficult to heal. The position of the foot should be carefully assessed. The patient should not be left with excessive forefoot varus; in such a case, additional arthrodesis or change of position of the arthrodesis is necessary.

The worst error to make in any of these fusions is malposition. In subtalar fusions, it is possible to both undercorrect and leave excessive valgus or to overcorrect into a heel and forefoot varus that results in excessive lateral weight bearing in the foot. The same is true for a double or triple arthrodesis. It is important that the patient have a plantigrade foot with even tripod weight bearing between the heel, fifth metatarsal, and first metatarsal. If the surgeon finds that after full correction of the talonavicular joint, there remains a forefoot varus greater than 10°, subluxation at the first metatarsal tarsal or naviculocuneiform joints should be sought. There could also be malpositron of the talonavicular fusion. Consideration can be given to allow some increased heel valgus in the correction to avoid excessive forefoot varus; however, too much remaining heel valgus can lead to lateral impingement and promote deltoid ligament failure after a triple arthrodesis or subtalar arthrodesis.

POSTOPERATIVE REHABILITATION

Tenosynovectomy patients are placed in a cast for 4 to 6 weeks, after which they may try a shoe with an arch support. Patients are not put on a strengthening program but should practice range of motion exercises, gradually building up a walking tolerance for 3 months after surgery.

Postoperative rehabilitation is particularly important for a tendon transfer. Without a good physical therapy program, the tendon transfer can fail, because patients do not strengthen the muscle–tendon complex. The program should begin approximately 10 weeks after surgery. For the first 6 weeks after the operation, patients are in a cast with limited weight bearing; and for the next 4 to 6 weeks, patients will be in a removable cast or weight-bearing cast. After any other procedures performed on the foot have healed, gentle range of motion exercises can be started at 2 months. Full aggressive strengthening is not begun until 4 months. Patients should continue the strengthening exercises, at home if necessary, for at least 6 months after the operation.

Although a calcaneal osteotomy is well healed by 6 weeks after the operation, the fusions are not. In general, weight bearing is begun on a subtalar double or triple arthrodesis when x-rays show evidence of fusion, and it progresses to full weight bearing by 10 weeks, depending on healing. If the x-rays show full healing at the fusion site, casting is discontinued at 12 weeks; patients are placed in a supportive shoe and possibly in an ankle support. It is important for patients to understand that full improvement is not reached until 8 to 9 months after the operation. Physical therapy is most often not necessary in these patients but can be done once the fusion has consolidated.

RESULTS

Johnson reported that 16 of 19 patients with stage I PTTD who underwent synovectomy noted considerable relief of their discomfort at an average 30-month follow-up (5). By his grading system, these patients had minimum secondary deformity. Note that the minimum follow-up for this study was 12 months; owing to the progressive nature of posterior tibial tendon dysfunction, further follow-up is needed.

Mann reported initial satisfactory results in patients who received a tendon transfer but noted that the results declined after 60 months (6). This tendency may be partially explained by the inclusion of patients with more deformity than were admitted in the early part of the study. Today, the tendon transfer is combined with a bony procedure if deformity is present.

The addition of a medial slide calcaneal osteotomy to the tendon transfer showed significant improvement in the radiographic parameters of the arch at a minimum of 12 months after the procedure (7,9). Consistent improvement in the arch had not been noted with the use of the tendon transfer alone. Lateral column lengthening also gave significant improvement in the radiographic parameters of the arch, even in those with considerable deformity (8). Although some initial loss of correction has been noted, radiographic improvement of the arch after lateral column lengthening can be impressive.

The results of triple arthrodesis in adults have shown a satisfaction rate of approximately 70%, with some discomfort remaining. In a study of subtalar arthrodesis for posterior tibial tendon dysfunction, 17 of 21 patients had no or mild pain, but 7 of 21 complained of difficulty walking on uneven ground (11). The functional results of the patients receiving subtalar arthrodesis seem better than the results of patients receiving triple arthrodesis; the former experienced less pain and better maneuverability. Based on biomechanical studies, it would be expected that results of subtalar arthrodesis would be functionally different from those of a triple, talonavicular, or double arthrodesis, because up to half the motion can remain in the transverse tarsal joint (12). After lateral column lengthening with calcaneocuboid fusion, half the motion can remain in the talonavicular joint and more can remain in the subtalar joint, leaving greater motion overall. The best treatment

for the patient is to successfully treat the disorder before fusion of any joints is necessary (9).

SUMMARY

PTTD often requires surgery because of persistent symptoms and/or progressive deformity. Although conservative treatment with an orthotic, bracing or casting is an option, inversion weakness, particularly combined with deformity, makes progression likely. Progression occurs at variable rates. It can occur slowly over years or months, depending on the condition of the tissues, the amount of deformity, and the weight of the patient. Since fusion causes stiffness and discomfort, the best treatment avoids fusion of the hindfoot. The condition is therefore best treated when the deformity is still flexible and mild to moderate. Both the bony malalignment and inversion weakness should be corrected for the best results.

REFERENCES

1. Mann RA. Biomechanics of the foot and ankle. In: Mann RA, Coughlin MJ, eds. Surgery of the foot and ankle. 6th ed. St. Louis: Mosby, 1993:3–44.
2. Holmes GB, Mann RA. Possible etiologic factors associated with rupture of the posterior tibial tendon. Foot Ankle 1992;13:70–79.
3. Mann RA. Flatfoot in adults. In: Mann RA, Coughlin MJ, eds. Surgery of the foot and ankle. 6th ed. St. Louis: Mosby, 1993:767–780.
4. Myerson, MS. Adult acquired flatfoot deformity. J Bone Joint Surg 1996;78A:780–792.
5. Teasdall RD, Johnson KA. Surgical treatment of stage I posterior tibial tendon dysfunction. Foot Ankle 1994;15:646–648.
6. Mann RA, Thompson FM. Rupture of the posterior tibial tendon causing flat foot. Surgical treatment. J Bone Joint Surg 1985;67A:556–561.
7. Myerson MS, Corrigan J, Thompson F, Schon LC. Tendon transfer combined with calcaneal osteotomy for posterior tibial tendon insufficiency: a radiological investigation. Foot Ankle 1995;16:712–718.
8. Sangeorzan BJ, Mosca V, Hansen ST. Effect of calcaneal lengthening on relationships among the hindfoot, midfoot, and forefoot. Foot Ankle 1993;136–141.
9. Myerson MS, Corrigan J. Treatment of posterior tibial tendon dysfunction with flexor digitorum longus tendon transfer and calcaneal osteotomy. Orthopedics 1996;19:383–388.
10. Sands A, Grujic L, Sangeorzan B, Hansen ST Jr. Lateral column lengthening through the calcaneo-cuboid joint alternative to triple arthrodesis for correction of flatfoot. Paper presented at the annual meeting of the American Orthopaedic Foot and Ankle Society, Orlando, FL, February 19, 1995.
11. Kitaoka HB, Patger G. Clinical results of subtalar rotational arthrodesis for posterior tibial tendon dysfunction and flatfoot deformity. Paper presented at the specialty day of the American Orthopaedic Foot and Ankle Society, Atlanta, February 1996.
12. Astion DJ, Deland JT, Otis JC, Kenneally S. Motion of the hindfoot after simulated arthrodesis. J Bone Joint Surg 1997;79A:241–246.

Plantar and Posterior Heel Pain

Heel pain is one of the most common foot problems seen in an orthopaedic practice, and it can be one of the most frustrating problems encountered by the orthopaedic surgeon. The terms used to describe this condition are often confusing. *Heel pain* has been described as plantar fasciitis, heel spur, Achilles spur, Haglund deformity, pump bump, retrocalcaneal bursitis, subcalcaneal pain, and posterior heel pain. One reason for the confu-sion may be the lack of a standardized nomenclature for this disease entity in the literature. Another contributing factor is that the cause of heel pain often is unclear. When the term *heel pain* is used, it is important to specify whether the pain is on the posterior, plantar, medial, or lateral aspect of the heel. This chapter focuses on plantar and posterior heel pain, which are the two most common types of heel pain.

I Plantar Heel Pain

RELEVANT ANATOMY AND PATHOGENESIS

Understanding the anatomy around the plantar heel is the key to diagnosing and treating different types of plantar heel pain (1). The heel pad is specifically designed to function as a shock absorber. The skin around the heel pad is approximately 10 times thicker than the skin on the dorsum of the foot. Deep to the skin is a layer of adipose tissue, which is compartmentalized into microchambers (superficial) and macrochambers (deep) by fibrous septa. The microchambers also contain a superficial venous network. Both chamber systems contribute to the absorption of the compressive and torsional forces exerted on the heel.

The next structure encountered is the plantar fascia (Fig. 76.1). It originates from the medial-plantar tubercle of the posterior calcaneus tuberosity and inserts into the plantar aspect of the flexor tendon sheaths and the base of the proximal phalanges. Dorsal to the plantar fascia is the most superficial layer of the plantar muscle layers: abductor hallucis (AbH), flexor digitorum brevis (FDB), and abductor digiti quinti (AbDQ). They all originate from the calcaneus; the FDB and AbDQ also arise from the plantar fascia. If an inferior calcaneal spur is present, it is the ori-gin of FDB, not the plantar fascia, that is attached to the spur.

The medial and lateral plantar nerves, which are branches of the posterior tibial nerve, travel dorsal to the superficial muscle layer. The first branch of the lateral plantar nerve is the nerve to AbDQ (Baxter nerve), which can be compressed between the deep fascia of AbH and quadratus plantae (QP). The posterior tibial nerve courses posterior to the tibialis posterior and flexor digitorum longus, travels around the medial malleolus, and divides into the medial calcaneal branch and the medial and lateral plantar nerves. This division occurs within the tarsal tunnel in 93% of cases. The medial calcaneal branch of posterior tibial nerve, which provides sensation to the posterior-medial aspect of the heel, sometimes can be irritated and cause plantar heel pain.

The most common cause of plantar heel pain is proximal plantar fasciitis. For reasons that are still not fully understood, degeneration and inflammation can occur in the plantar fascia at its medial-plantar insertion on the calcaneus (2). One theory is that chronic microtears of the fascia can create a chronic inflammatory response. Surgical specimens of the excised portion of the fascia often reveal degeneration, metaplasia, or calcification of the collagen tis-

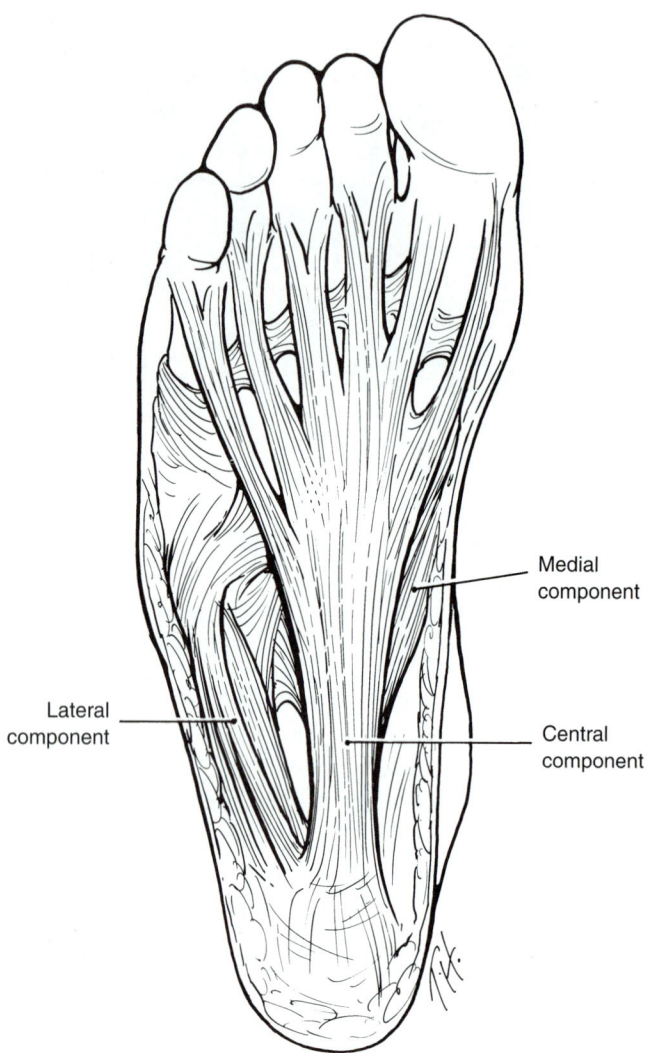

Figure 76.1. Plantar fascia.

Lateral component

Medial component

Central component

physical activities, such as marathon runners and military recruits.

INITIAL FINDINGS, PHYSICAL EXAMINATION, AND DIAGNOSIS

The most common type of plantar heel pain is proximal plantar fasciitis. Pain is usually worst in the morning, as the patient takes his or her first few steps. As the day progresses, the pain tends to decrease. The theory is that during sleep, the foot rests in a plantar-flexed position and the plantar fascia contracts. When taking the first few steps, as the contracted plantar fascia is being stretched, significant pain is experienced. The onset of symptoms is usually insidious and is seldom associated with trauma. Occasionally, there is a history of overuse or intense physical exercise. Most patients are middle-aged or older. The general consensus is that females and males are affected equally. Bilateral involvement occurs in 8 to 13% of patients with this problem.

In bilateral heel pain, seronegative spondyloarthropathies or inflammatory arthritides should be ruled out. On physical examination, the point tenderness is most frequently localized to the insertion of the plantar fascia on the plantar-medial tubercle of the posterior calcaneal tuberosity. Rarely, point tenderness is central or lateral. Passive dorsiflexion of the ankle and toes may enhance the pain at the insertion site, but this is not a reliable test. Other physical findings that have been observed in some patients with plantar fasciitis are tight heel cord and pes planus, which are present in many asymptomatic people.

In heel pain caused by nerve compression, the quality of pain may be more achy or burning in nature. The location usually follows the course of the nerve, and maximum pain is felt at the area of entrapment more medially on the calcaneus. A positive Tinel sign may be present. There are two potential sites for compression of the nerve to abductor digiti quinti: One is between the fascia of the AbH and medial border of the QP; and the other is around the heel spur, if present, and insertion site of the FDB and plantar fascia. In tarsal tunnel syndrome, the tenderness is usually located slightly inferior to the medial malleolus. The pain may be aggravated with weight bearing.

Stress fracture of the calcaneus can be diagnosed by a history of overuse, pain exacerbated by weight bearing, swelling around the hindfoot region, and tenderness to medial and lateral compression of the calcaneus. Finally, heel pad atrophy is a diagnosis of exclusion. After all other diagnoses have been excluded, the diagnosis of heel pad atrophy can be made if the pain is gradual in onset and nonradiating and if most of the tenderness is located at the center of the heel.

RADIOLOGIC STUDIES

Because the various diagnoses of plantar heel pain are usually made on clinical grounds, radiographic studies

sue. Some systemic inflammatory disease (Reiter syndrome, psoriasis, ankylosing spondylitis, systemic lupus erythematosus, gout, and rheumatoid arthritis) may also contribute to the development of plantar fasciitis. In general, the heel spur (where the FDB inserts) does not cause heel pain. There is, however, a higher association between the amorphous type of heel spur and the heel pain caused by seronegative spondyloarthropathies.

Other common causes of plantar heel pain include rupture of the plantar fascia, compression of the nerve to AbDQ (the first branch of the lateral plantar nerve), tarsal tunnel syndrome, heel pad atrophy, and stress fracture of the calcaneus. Plantar fascia can rupture acutely, especially after multiple steroid injections into the heel near the fascia insertion. Heel pad atrophy is usually idiopathic but can be associated with aging or poorly placed steroid injections. Histologic studies have shown that the atrophy is the result of the failure of the fibrous septi, loss of resilience in the collagen and elastin, and loss of water content. Stress fractures of the calcaneus usually occur in those who have experienced intense

should be obtained only to rule out other causes of heel pain, such as tumor, infection, subtalar arthritis, and stress fractures. The lateral x-ray of the foot is the most cost-effective and useful view. The presence of a heel spur (at the origin of the FDB) is associated with plantar heel pain in 50% of patients; conversely, only 15% of asymptomatic patients demonstrate spurs. Thus an exact relationship between plantar heel pain and calcaneal spurs has not been established (2). Stress fracture of the calcaneus may not be apparent on x-ray until 2 to 3 weeks after the initial injury.

Technetium bone scans have a limited role in the work-up of plantar heel pain, since such studies were found to be positive in up to 97% of cases (2). In a typical patient with plantar fasciitis, the early dynamic phase involves hyperemia at the heel, and blood pool images show increased blood flow to the area of the inflamed soft tissue. The delayed phase may reveal an increased uptake as a result of periosteal reaction. Bone scans may reveal a calcaneal stress fracture that cannot be detected on plain radiographs.

MRI is also not used routinely in the work-up of plantar heel pain; but it may be useful in ruling out other causes of heel pain, such as infection or tumor. It can help in the evaluation of the integrity of the plantar fascia, if a partial or complete rupture of the plantar fascia is suspected. The typical appearance of the inflamed plantar fascia is a thickening of the fascia and increased signal intensity within the substance of the fascia (Fig. 76.2).

TREATMENT

Nonoperative Treatment and Indications for Surgery

The majority of the patients with plantar heel pain will improve with nonoperative treatment; thus the treatment plan should begin with patient education. Patients need to understand the pathogenesis of the disease process, which should help them understand the chronic nature of their problem.

The nonoperative treatment options for plantar fasciitis include nonsteroidal anti-inflammatory drugs (NSAIDs), heel pad or cup, orthosis, short leg cast, night splint, physical therapy, steroid injections, shoe modification, activity modification, weight reduction, ice, heat, and rest. A heel pad is used to absorb shock. The purpose of a plastic heel cup is to increase padding on the weight-bearing surface. The two types of orthoses that are occasionally used for the treatment of plantar fasciitis are a three-quarter length orthosis and a UCBL insert. Both attempt to unload the plantar fascia during weight bearing.

A short-leg walking cast can be placed for 4 to 6 weeks to keep the plantar fascia and the Achilles tendon in a stretched position, preventing their contraction. For recalcitrant plantar fasciitis, a night splint may be used as an adjunct to other treatment methods (3).

Steroid injections should be used judiciously, as multiple (more than three) injections into this region can cause a rupture of the plantar fascia and fat necrosis of the plantar fat pad. One study showed that 41% of patients noted continued pain relief 5 months after one steroid injection (4). Shoe modification, such as a steel shank with a rocker bottom or raised heel, may also help improve the symptoms.

Almost all patients with plantar fasciitis will respond to a combination of the conservative modalities, assuming high compliance (5). Complete resolution of symptoms may take several months to more than 1 year, with occasional flare-ups. The only indication for surgical intervention for the treatment of plantar fasciitis is the failure of conservative therapy for at least 1 year.

In patients with a clear diagnosis of compression of the nerve to AbDQ or tarsal tunnel syndrome, treatment should begin with an orthosis with heel cushion and medial arch support to relieve pressure on the nerve. Nonsteroidal anti-inflammatory drugs, and a steroid injection into the site of maximal tenderness (for entrapment of the nerve to AbDQ only) may decrease the inflammation around the nerve. The only indication for surgery is the failure of conservation treatment for at least 6 months, and preferably for 12 months.

The pain from heel pad atrophy can be treated with a heel cushion as a shock absorber or a plastic heel cup to centralize the natural heel pad. There is absolutely no role for surgery or steroid injection. The treatment for a stress fracture of the calcaneus is rest, heel cushioning, and casting if the patient notes moderate to severe pain with weight bearing.

Operative Treatment

The key to successful results of surgical treatment for plantar heel pain is to perform the correct operation on the

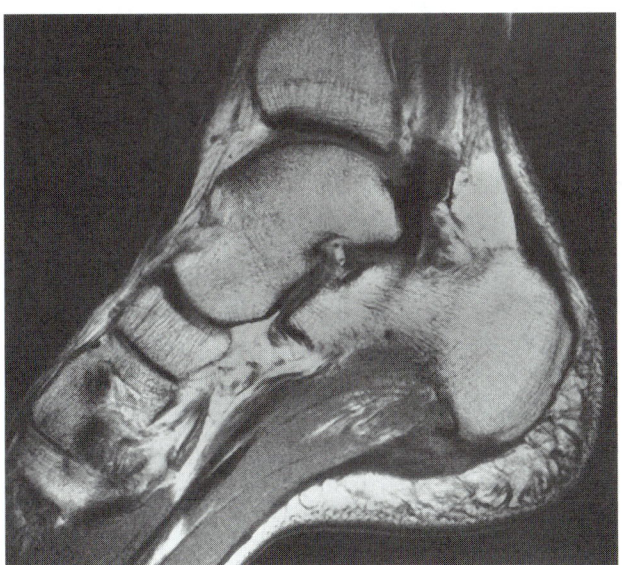

Figure 76.2. MRI study of an inflamed plantar fascia.

Clinical Table: Plantar and Posterior Heel Pain

Procedure	Indications	Technique	Anatomy	Pitfalls
Open plantar fascia release	• Recalcitrant plantar fasciitis	• Oblique medial incision • Release of medial third of fascia • Excise spur • Explore nerve	• Nerve to the AbDQ • FDB	• Release too much fascia • Fail to explore nerve to the AbDQ
Endoscopic plantar fascia release	• Recalcitrant plantar fasciitis	• Medial and lateral portals • Endoscope medial; blade lateral • Release medial third of fascia	• Nerve to AbDQ • Medial and lateral plantar nerve • FDB	• Injury to plantar nerve • Cannot explore nerve to the AbDQ • Cannot excise spur
Nerve to AbDQ release	• Entrapment of the nerve to the AbDQ	• Oblique medial incision • Release fascia of AbH • Excise spur • Release medial third of fascia	• Nerve to the AbDQ • AbH	• Injury to nerve to the AbDQ
For posterior heel pain	• Recalcitrant posterior heel pain	• Choice of incision • Excise the retrocalcaneal bursa, superior calcaneus, and spur	• Sural nerve • Medial calcaneal branch	• Skin necrosis • Injury to sural nerve • Injury to medial calcaneal branch • Inadequate bone resection

right patient for the correct diagnosis (Clinical Table). It is beyond the scope of this chapter to list every surgical approach described in the literature for the treatment of plantar fasciitis. The most commonly used surgical procedure is open plantar fascia release with excision of the subcalcaneal spur and exploration of the nerve to the AbDQ. The results of this technique are often quoted to be around 70% (6). A new controversial technique, endoscopic plantar fascia release, will also be discussed, although it has not gained wide acceptance in the orthopaedic field.

OPEN PLANTAR FASCIA RELEASE

To perform a plantar fascia release, the patient is positioned supine on the operating table, and an ankle block is usually used with an ankle Esmarch. An oblique medial incision extending into the plantar arch distal to the weight-bearing surface of the heel pad or an oblique plantar incision just distal to the heel pad away from the weight-bearing surface is made with a number 15 scalpel blade (Fig. 76.3) The medial calcaneal branch of the posterior tibial nerve is preserved by careful dissection (the nerve should not be encountered if a plantar incision is used). The plantar fascia is identified, and the medial one-third of the fascia should be released. Studies have shown that complete release of the plantar fascia can cause flattening of the longitudinal arch and lateral foot pain (7).

If a heel spur is present, some of the FDB insertion can be dissected off, and excision of the spur is made using a rongeur or a small osteotome (remember that the nerve to AbDQ runs just superior to the spur). An attempt to visu-

alize and explore the nerve to AbDQ should be made by dividing the fascia of the AbH and QP. If a tourniquet is used, it should be released and hemostasis obtained. The wound is irrigated and closed in a routine fashion. A sterile dressing and well-padded posterior splints are applied.

Postoperative Care

The patient should be placed in a short leg cast, weight-bearing cast, or a walking brace on the first postoperative visit. After 3 weeks, the patient may start wearing wide shoes, which will accommodate the residual swelling. Full activity is permitted 6 weeks after surgery or later, depending on the patient's recovery.

Pitfalls and Helpful Hints

If too much plantar fascia is released, flattening of the longitudinal arch and lateral foot pain may ensue. Meticulous attention to the wound helps eliminate the wound problems that often accompany this procedure.

ENDOSCOPIC PLANTAR FASCIA RELEASE

For endoscopic plantar fascia release, the patient is positioned supine on the operating table. An incision (through the skin only) for the first portal is made 1 cm distal to and in line with the medial calcaneal tubercle with a number 15 scalpel blade. A hemostat is used to bluntly dissect the subcutaneous tissue down to the plantar fascia. A blunt probe is inserted to locate the medial and lateral extent of the fascia (the probe should be directly on the fascia to avoid injuring other structures).

A 5-mm dilator is passed plantar to the fascia to create a potential space. The slotted channel is inserted plantar to the plantar fascia, and a stab wound is made laterally for the slotted channel to exit. The endoscope is then placed into the slotted channel medially, with the probe laterally, to estimate the width of the fascia. The endoscopic blade is then placed laterally, and the fascia is cut from medial to lateral with the ankle dorsiflexed (the surgeon should attempt to cut only the medial third). The muscle belly of the FDB will be visualized after the fascia is released.

After surgery, a soft dressing is used along with a night splint for 1 week. A night splint only is used for an additional month.

Pitfalls and Helpful Hints

The endoscopic plantar fascia release has not been widely accepted by most orthopaedic surgeons, and this procedure should still be considered somewhat experimental. Many structures are located near the plantar fascia (e.g., the medial and lateral plantar nerve, the nerve to the AbDQ, and the FDB) that could be at risk during this procedure (8). Endoscopic plantar fascia release does not allow for the excision of the spur or the exploration of the nerve to the AbDQ; if part of the heel pain is owing to the compression of this nerve, then the patient may have residual postoperative heel pain.

NERVE TO THE ABDQ RELEASE

To release the nerve to the AbDQ, the patient is placed supine on the operating table. A generous oblique medial incision is made centered over the course of the nerve with a number 15 scalpel blade (the medial calcaneal branch of the nerve should be proximal to this incision). The fascia of the AbH is incised in line with the muscle fibers, and the muscle is retracted superiorly. A deep fascia near the inferior border of the AbH is identified, and the portion of the fascia where the nerve is being compressed (between the deep fascia and the QP) should be excised. For better exposure of the nerve, the medial plantar fascia may need to be released slightly. The heel spur should be excised, if present (remember that the nerve runs just superior to the spur). The medial third of the plantar fascia should also be released if inflammation is present.

Postoperative Care

The patient is kept non-weight bearing while in the postoperative dressing and splints. After the dressing has been changed after the first office visit, the patient may start wearing wide sneakers with a heel cushion. Full activity may begin after 4 weeks or later, depending on the patient's recovery.

Pitfalls and Helpful Hints

Compression of the nerve to the AbDQ is often missed in chronic plantar heel pain. The success of this procedure depends on making the correct diagnosis.

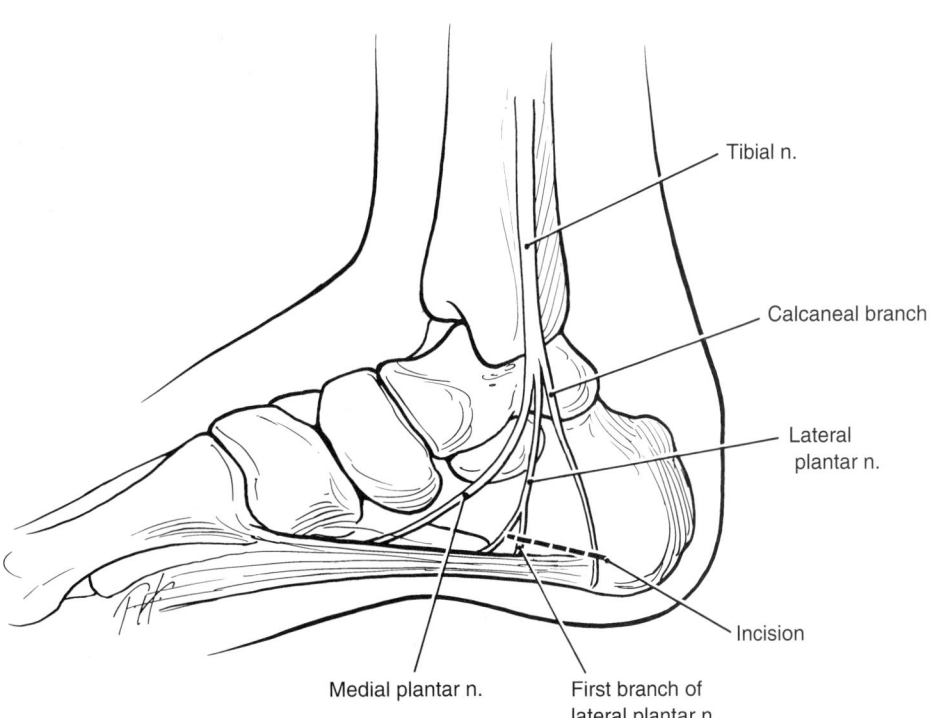

Figure 76.3. Incision site for an open plantar fascia release.

II Posterior Heel Pain

RELEVANT ANATOMY AND PATHOGENESIS

The anatomy of the posterior heel region is much simpler than the anatomy around the plantar heel. The posterior calcaneal tuberosity is marked by the most superior insertion of the Achilles tendon. The terms *superior calcaneal tuberosity* and *superior calcaneal prominence* are synonymous and describe the bony projection above the posterior calcaneal tuberosity, which can take on various shapes. There is always a bursa (retrocalcaneal bursa) located between the Achilles tendon and the superior calcaneal tuberosity. Occasionally, a more superficial bursa exists between the skin and the Achilles tendon.

INITIAL FINDINGS, PHYSICAL EXAMINATION, AND DIAGNOSIS

Patients with pain in the back of their heel often are afflicted with multiple problems in this region. Starting from the most superficial layer, the bursal lining between the skin and the Achilles tendon can be inflamed as a result of chronic irritation from the top of the shoe counter. This is often referred to as the "pump bump." On physical examination, the tenderness is superficial and posterior or posterolateral to the Achilles tendon. Sometimes, the skin is also inflamed.

The Achilles tendon is the next layer of problem. In insertional Achilles tendinitis, there is tenderness and crepitus to palpation at the insertion site, especially with plantar flexion and dorsiflexion of the foot. Retrocalcaneal bursitis can be diagnosed by tenderness to simultaneous medial and lateral compression of the retrocalcaneal bursa, which is anterior to the Achilles tendon. This pain may be aggravated by dorsiflexion of the foot. If the patient is a runner, posterior heel pain that increases when running uphill suggests the diagnosis of retrocalcaneal bursitis. Often, posterior heel pain is caused by all these possibilities; the term used to describe this entity is *Haglund syndrome* (9).

RADIOLOGIC STUDIES

A lateral radiograph of the foot can be obtained to evaluate the size and shape of the superior calcaneal prominence and the size and shape of the spur at the tendon insertion. One method of estimating the size of the superior calcaneal tuberosity is by using the parallel pitch lines (PPLs) described by Heneghan and Pavlov (9) (Fig. 76.4). The lower parallel pitch line (PPL$_2$) connects the anterior tuberosity and medial tuberosity of the calcaneus. The upper parallel pitch line (PPL$_1$) is parallel to the PPL$_2$ and runs from the posterior talar articular facet. A normal-sized superior calcaneal tuberosity falls below the PPL$_1$. If it extends above the PPL$_1$, it is considered prominent. Note

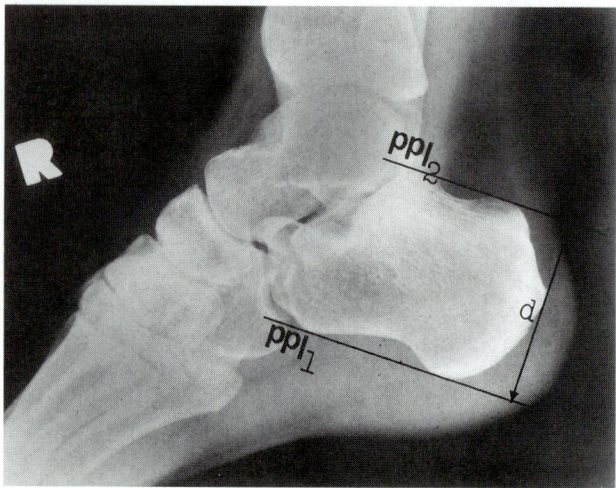

Figure 76.4. Parallel pitch line method of estimating the size of the superior calcaneal tuberosity (*d*).

that not all people with a prominent superior calcaneal tuberosity will have symptoms in the posterior heel region.

Recently, some foot and ankle surgeons have started using CT scans for evaluating the extent of the Achilles spur. The only other imaging study that might be useful is MRI, which can delineate the extent of the bursitis and demonstrate the area of tendinitis.

TREATMENT

Nonoperative Treatment and Indications for Surgery

The same nonoperative treatment modalities can be used for all types of posterior heel pain. The goals of conservative therapy are to remove the external source of irritation, decrease local inflammation, and immobilize the affected area if symptoms are persistent. A 1- to 1.25-cm (0.375- to 0.5-in) heel cushion will elevate the inflamed area above the shoe counter and decrease the stress on the bursa and tendon insertion. Another method of relieving pressure in this region is to soften the shoe counter itself or to place padding between the shoe counter and the affected area. This can be accomplished by placing the cushioning device either directly on the skin or on the inside of the shoe counter.

Inflammation may be reduced by NSAIDs or, in the case of recalcitrant retrocalcaneal bursitis, a steroid injection into the bursa only (avoiding the Achilles tendon). The possibility of tendon rupture should be discussed with the patient before the injection is administered. A short leg, weight-bearing cast can also be used in refractory cases of posterior heel pain. For high-performance athletes, reduction in activity should be recommended. Consideration for surgical treatment can be made after 6 to 12 months of conservative measures.

Operative Treatment

The general indication for surgical treatment of posterior heel pain is a failure of adequate conservative therapy for 6 to 12 months (Clinical Table). Surgery is almost never required for patients with superficial bursitis alone. During preoperative discussion with the patient, the prolonged course of postoperative care and rehabilitation should be emphasized. It may be 6 to 12 months before the patient can resume full activity.

After spinal, epidural, or general anesthesia, the patient should be placed into either the prone or the lateral decubitus position for better exposure of the posterior aspect of the heel (10). A thigh tourniquet is optional. Several incisions have been used: medial only, lateral only, medial and lateral, posterior, and J-type para-Achilles longitudinal. A recommended method is to make the first para-Achilles longitudinal incision on the side that is most tender. A second para-Achilles longitudinal incision can always be made later if more exposure is needed.

Soft tissue dissection is performed, down to the Achilles tendon sheath. Skin necrosis can be prevented if the surgeon avoids making a skin flap. Care should be taken to protect the sural nerve and medial calcaneal branch during this dissection. The Achilles tendon is retracted posteriorly with the foot in plantar flexion. The inflamed retrocalcaneal bursa is excised. The superior calcaneal tuberosity is osteotomized from the top of the Achilles insertion to approximately 1 cm anterior to the tuberosity. A generous piece of bone should be removed to prevent persistence of symptoms. If any evidence of residual prominence is present (either by palpation, by direct visualization, or under fluoroscopy) a second para-Achilles longitudinal incision should be made for better exposure to the other side.

After completion excision of the superior tuberosity bony prominence, all sharp edges, especially at the Achilles insertion, need to be smoothed down. The Achilles tendon is inspected. Any fibrosis or necrotic tendon should be excised. If a spur is present, it should be removed. Depending on the amount of excision and dissection that was done to the diseased tendon, either primary repair of the tendon itself or repair of the tendon through drill holes into the bone may be required. The wound is irrigated aggressively to remove all bony debris. The incision is closed in the usual fashion.

Sterile dressings and well-padded splints are placed with the foot in plantar flexion.

POSTOPERATIVE CARE

After surgery, the patient is non-weight bearing until the dressing and splints are removed. The type and the length of postoperative immobilization depend on the extent of the surgery on the Achilles tendon:

- *No or minimal tendon excision*: short leg walking cast for 3 to 4 weeks, followed by a heel lift for 3 to 4 weeks

- *Extensive tendon excision and repair*: short leg, non–weight-bearing cast with the foot in plantar flexion for 4 to 6 weeks, followed by a short leg walking cast for 4 weeks, followed by a heel lift for 4 weeks

Physical therapy with strengthening and range of motion exercises can start after the patient comes out of the cast. Return to full activity, include jogging and sports, may take 6 to 12 months.

PITFALLS AND HELPFUL HINTS

It is crucial to warn patients that it may take as long as 1 year before they can resume their full activities, including sports. The surgeon must be gentle with the soft tissue to prevent skin necrosis. The skin incision(s) should be made so that the shoe counter will not irritate the wounds. The sural nerve and medial calcaneal branch of the posterior tibial nerve are at risk for injury. The surgeon must remove a generous piece of the superior calcaneal tuberosity prominence. Underresection with residual symptoms is a common complication. Aggressive irrigation is necessary to remove all bony debris and to prevent heterotopic ossification. It is important to excise the diseased portion of the Achilles tendon and to repair the tendon to prevent residual symptoms and postoperative rupture of the tendon.

SUMMARY

Heel pain is best described based on the location of the pain. The two most common sites of heel pain are the plantar heel and the posterior heel. The etiology of pain is different in each area. For plantar heel pain, the most common cause is proximal plantar fasciitis. For posterior heel pain, symptoms are usually due to a combination of retrocalcaneal bursitis, Achilles tendinitis, and a prominent superior calcaneal tuberosity. Nonoperative treatment is often successful for both types of heel pain. Surgery is indicated when nonoperative treatment fails to resolve the symptoms after 6 months.

REFERENCES

1. Sarrafian SK. Anatomy of the foot and ankle. 2nd ed. Philadelphia: Lippincott, 1993.
2. Mann RA, Coughlin MJ. Surgery of the foot and ankle. 6th ed. St. Louis: Mosby, 1993.
3. Wapner KL, Sharkey PF. The use of night splints for treatment of recalcitrant plantar fasciitis. Foot Ankle 1991;12:135–137.
4. Dreeben S. Heel pain. In: Lutter L, Mizel M, Pfeffer GB, eds. Foot and ankle. Orthopaedic knowledge update series. Rosemont, IL: American Academy of Orthopaedic Surgeons, 1994:179–193.
5. Wolgin M, Cook C, Graham C, Mauldin D. Conservative treatment of plantar heel pain. Foot Ankle 1994;15:97–102.

6. Baxter DE, Pfeffer GB. Treatment of chronic heel pain by surgical release of the first branch of the lateral plantar nerve. Clin Orthop 1992;279:229–236.

7. Daly PJ, Kitaoka HB, Chao EYS. Plantar fasciotomy for intractable plantar fasciitis: clinical results and biomechanical evaluation. Foot Ankle 1992;13:188–195.

8. Hofmeister EP, Elliott MJ, Juliano PJ. Endoscopic plantar fascia release: an anatomical study. Foot Ankle 1995;16:719–723.

9. Heneghan MA, Pavlov H. The Haglund painful heel syndrome. Clin Orthop 1984;187:228–234.

10. Schepsis AA, Leach RE. Surgical management of Achilles tendinitis. Am J Sports Med 1987;15:308–315.

11. Keck SW, Kelly PJ. Bursitis of the posterior part of the heel. J Bone Joint Surg 1965;47A:267–273.

12. Jones DC, James SL. Partial calcaneal ostectomy for retrocalcaneal bursitis. Am J Sports Med 1984;12:72–73.

chapter 77

Craig L. Levitz and Enyi Okereke

Nerve Disorders of the Foot: Tarsal Tunnel Syndrome and Interdigital Neuroma

Systemic factors, compression by anatomic inflammation or space-occupying lesions, repetitive trauma, and neuropathy are some of the more common causes of nerve entrapment in the foot and ankle. Patients usually present with activity-related pain, though altered sensation and paresthesias can occur, depending on the stage of injury. On the cellular level, compressed nerves exhibit progressive demyelination that may progress to axonotmesis if left untreated for a long period of time. A detailed knowledge of the anatomy of the posterior tibial nerve is necessary to understand the pathophysiology, to diagnose, and to treat the two most common nerve entrapment syndromes in the foot and ankle: tarsal tunnel syndrome and interdigital (Morton) neuroma.

RELEVANT ANATOMY

The posterior tibial nerve, a branch of the tibial portion of the sciatic nerve, travels distally along the posterior medial tibia to cross the ankle joint just posterior to the medial malleolus within the tarsal tunnel. The tarsal canal is formed by the flexor retinaculum behind and distal to the medial malleolus. The tarsal tunnel is a fibro-osseous structure created by the retinaculum passing over the tibia, the posterior process of the talus, and the calcaneus. The nerve runs posterior to the posterior tibialis tendon, the flexor digitorum longus tendon, and the posterior tib-

ial artery. It runs anterior to the flexor hallucis longus tendon. Just distal to the malleolus and proximal to the superior border of the abductor hallucis, the posterior tibial nerve divides into the medial and lateral plantar nerves and the medial calcaneal nerve (Fig. 77.1). Although the medial and lateral planter nerves arise from within the tunnel in 93% of people, there may be some variation in the branching of the calcaneal nerve (1).

The medial plantar nerve runs along the medial plantar border of the foot under the fascia of the abductor hallucis and deep to the knot of Henry at the talonavicular joint. It runs beneath the crossing of the flexor hallucis longus and flexor digitorum. This nerve gives rise to the interdigital nerve between the first and second metatarsals and the second and third metatarsals on the plantar aspect of the foot (2,3).

The lateral plantar nerve courses deep to the deep fascia of the abductor hallucis brevis muscle and then passes transversely, superficial to the quadratus plantae. The lateral plantar nerve also gives rise to the interdigital nerve between the fourth and fifth metatarsals. The interdigital nerve between the third and fourth metatarsals, the common digital nerve, arises from a branch from both the medial and lateral plantar nerves. This nerve passes plantar, beneath the transverse metatarsal ligament before bifurcating to form the digital nerves at the level of the metatarsal heads (1–3).

I Tarsal Tunnel Syndrome

PATHOGENESIS

The posterior tibial nerve may be compressed behind the medial malleolus, which leads to radicular pain and

tingling on the plantar aspect of the foot. The causes include systemic diseases that may decrease the volume of the canal, such as rheumatoid arthritis (4). Diabetes, hy-

Figure 77.1. The four branches of the tibial nerve in the tarsal tunnel.

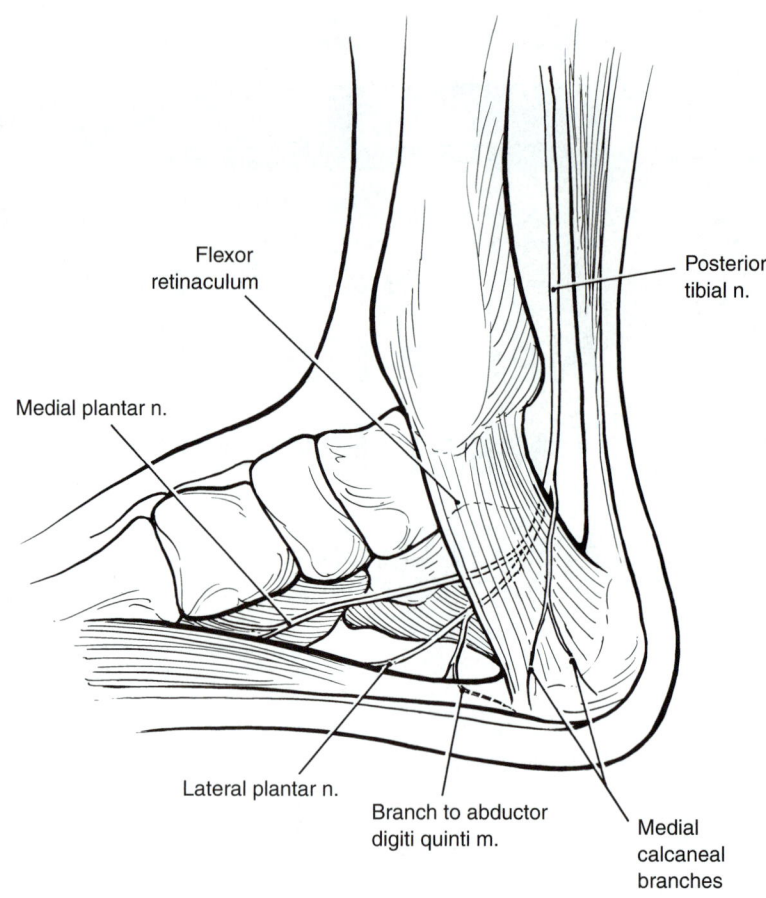

Flexor retinaculum

Posterior tibial n.

Medial plantar n.

Lateral plantar n.

Branch to abductor digiti quinti m.

Medial calcaneal branches

pothyroidism, and pregnancy have been reported to be associated with tarsal tunnel syndrome (3,5,6). Synovitis of the flexor tendons that run alongside the nerve can also result in nerve compression. Excessive pronation may stretch the nerve and reduce the relative volume of the tarsal tunnel, causing relative nerve compression. A prominence on the posterior medial talus and/or a large os trigonum may directly compress the nerve. Trauma, such as fractures of the distal tibia, calcaneus, or talus, can cause exostoses, which may impinge on the nerve. Ganglia, lipomas, and anomalous muscles are less common causes of direct compression of the posterior tibial nerve (3,5–7).

INITIAL FINDINGS, PHYSICAL EXAMINATION, AND DIAGNOSIS

Tarsal tunnel syndrome is characterized by diffuse and often nonspecific pain on the plantar aspect of the foot. It is described as burning or numbing in nature and is worse with activity and relieved with rest. Some patients report paresthesias. A small subset of patients has been reported to have pain at night, which is relieved with activity. One-third report proximal radiation along the medial aspect of the leg (3,5,8).

Physical examination should include percussion of the path of the posterior tibial nerve and its branches to elicit a percussion sign. Pressure with the thumb or thenar eminence over the tarsal tunnel may elicit pain or paresthesias. A thickening or swelling of the nerve may be palpable. Atrophy in the abductor hallucis or digiti quinti is rarely noted when comparing both feet. Sensory and motor examinations are usually normal. Occasionally, diminished sensation in the distribution of the medial or lateral plantar nerves is noted.

RADIOLOGIC AND OTHER DIAGNOSTIC STUDIES

Routine radiographs of the feet should be obtained, although these are usually normal. Evidence of a space-occupying lesion is an indication for MRI. It is our current practice to obtain electrodiagnostic testing (electromyelography and nerve conduction studies) on all patients in whom we have clinical suspicion of tarsal tunnel syndrome to confirm the diagnosis. These tests are reported to be only 90% accurate, and the results must be viewed in the context of a strongly suggestive history and physical examination. Electrodiagnostic studies do not correlate with surgical outcome.

TREATMENT

Nonoperative Treatment

Conservative treatment consists of relative rest, heel cord stretching, medial longitudinal arch support, casting, contrast baths, anti-inflammatory medications, and night splints. The use of a longitudinal arch support to prevent excessive pronation, if it is the cause of nerve compression, has shown good results. Corticosteroid injections can be useful as an adjuvant to orthotic management. If conservative treatment fails after 10 to 12 months, surgical treatment should be considered. Conservative treatment can be bypassed if a space-occupying lesion is identified.

Operative Treatment

A local nerve decompression can be performed through a 10-cm longitudinal incision over the tarsal tunnel that parallels the course of the tibial nerve (Clinical Table). The incision is placed approximately 2 cm posterior to the tibia. The tibial nerve is identified proximal to the flexor retinaculum. A wide release of the nerve should be per-

formed if no specific pathology is found. Distally, the medial and lateral plantar nerves should be decompressed by releasing the deep fascia of the abductor hallucis. It is important to always identify the medial calcaneal nerve and the first branch of the lateral plantar nerve. If compression is the result of a posterior medial prominence or large os trigonum, the bony prominence may have to be removed.

When the tourniquet, if used, is released, the nerve should appear vascularized. Hemostasis is obtained, and the wound is closed. The retinaculum should not be repaired. A compression dressing and posterior splint is applied.

After surgery, the patient is immobilized for 3 weeks and kept non-weight bearing. After the 3rd week, weight bearing is allowed and active and passive motions are started. The patient may return to normal activities as tolerated after 3 weeks.

Common pitfalls of surgery include inadequate distal release of the medial and lateral plantar nerves. Success rates of operative treatment vary; some authors report significant improvement of symptoms in more than 90% of patients. The results are best with the removal of a space-occupying lesion (6,8–10).

II   Interdigital Neuroma

PATHOGENESIS

Morton neuroma results from compression of the interdigital nerve at the level of the metatarsal head, deep to the transverse metatarsal ligament. It has been hypothesized that the interdigital nerve to the third interspace is subject to trauma and neuroma formation secondary to its increased thickness as a result of receiving branches from the lateral and medial plantar nerve. Accessory branches of the plantar nerves have been reported to pass beneath the metatarsal head to join the common digital nerve and may be the cause of recurrent neuromas.

A neuroma may develop in the common digital nerve from direct trauma or extrinsic pressure against the nerve. As the medial three metatarsals are fixed to the metatarsal-cuneiform joints and the fourth and fifth metatarsals articulate with the more mobile cuboid, there is increased motion between the third and fourth ray. This mobility may result in trauma to the nerve or development of a reactive bursa, which may place pressure on the nerve (3).

Excessive hyperextension of the metatarsophalangeal joint results in plantar flexion of the metatarsal heads, which can expose the nerve to increased trauma. The nerve may also be tethered across the transverse meta-

tarsal ligament. This mechanism may explain the increased incidence in females, whose footwear often hyperextends the metatarsal phalangeal joints (5,7).

Pressure on the digital nerve may result from thickening of the metatarsal ligament or an aberrant band of the ligament. Ganglions or synovial cysts arising from the metatarsophalangeal joint and formation of a plantar lipoma may lead to nerve compression.

INITIAL FINDINGS, PHYSICAL EXAMINATION, AND DIAGNOSIS

Interdigital neuromas most commonly occur in women. The majority of Morton neuromas occur in the third metatarsal interspace, although many occur in the second interspace as well. Neuromas occur bilaterally in 15% of cases (7).

The most common presentation is that of pain localized to the plantar aspect of the foot between the metatarsal heads. It is a burning pain that frequently radiates to the digits. A sensation of something moving or getting caught has been described. Symptoms are aggravated by activity in a shoe and by high-heeled shoes. Pain is relieved with rest and removal of shoes. Numbness, cramping, and extensive distal and proximal radiation of pain have been described.

The physical examination may reveal fullness in the metatarsal interspace. Atrophy of the plantar pad and synovitis of the joint should be ruled out. Pain should be reproduced with palpation of the metatarsal interspace. Pain with radiation to the toes produced on metatarsal interspace palpation is highly suggestive of a neuroma. The Mulder sign consists of a crunching or clicking associated with reproduction of pain when medial lateral pressure is applied to the metatarsal interspace. This is a rare finding. A mass may be palpable in the interspace. Sensory examination is usually normal (3).

Reevaluation may prove to be the most useful diagnostic tool. Injection of the web space with lidocaine and a compatible injectable steroid mixture is a useful diagnostic and therapeutic adjunct. Although radiographic and electrodiagnostic studies have not proved to be useful, a standing radiograph of the foot should be obtained to rule out any osseous abnormality. Ultrasound and MRI have been described, but are usually not necessary.

TREATMENT

Nonoperative Treatment

Treatment of interdigital neuromas consists of a soft metatarsal bar or pad just behind the metatarsal heads to decrease the traction on the nerve. A wide and soft shoe is also helpful. Elevated heels should be avoided, resulting in less hyperextension of the joint and less pressure in the head region, If not successful, injection with corticosteroid can be attempted. Up to 80% of patients may improve with conservative treatment and steroid injections, although only 30% report acute improvement. Mann (3) reported 60 to 70% of patients go on to surgical treatment. He noted that, although patients usually improve with conservative treatment, they rarely improve enough to wear high-heeled shoes. This leads many patients to choose surgery, even though the pain could be controlled with conservative measures (3).

Operative Treatment

If conservative therapy fails to provide adequate pain relief, nerve excision through a dorsal incision with release of a portion of the intermetatarsal ligament should be considered (Clinical Table). A longitudinal incision is made, starting in the involved web space and extending 3 cm proximal to the level of the metatarsal head. Failure to remain in the midline risks injury to the dorsal digital nerves. The incision is carried through soft tissue to the level of the metatarsal heads (Fig. 77.2). A self-retainer is placed between the metatarsal heads to spread them and place the deep transverse metatarsal ligament under tension.

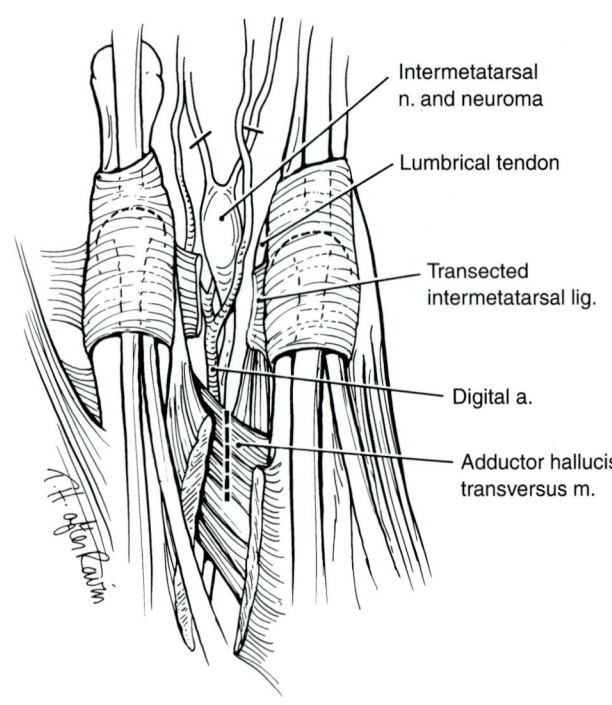

Intermetatarsal n. and neuroma

Lumbrical tendon

Transected intermetatarsal lig.

Digital a.

Adductor hallucis transversus m.

Figure 77.2. View of the third and fourth metatarsal heads showing the position of the interdigital nerve in relation to the surrounding structures.

Clinical Table: Nerve Disorders of the Foot

Procedure	Indications	Technique	Anatomy	Pitfalls
Tarsal tunnel release	• Failure of conservative care	• Decompress tarsal tunnel • Release flexor retinaculum (lacinate ligament) • Excise space-occupying lesions	• Medial and lateral plantar nerves • Medial calcaneal nerve • Branches of the tibial nerve	• Inadequate distal release of medial and lateral plantar nerves
Excision of Morton neuroma	• Failure of conservative care	• Release intermetatarsal ligament through dorsal medial approach • Plantar approach for recurrence	• Perineural fibrosis of the interdigital nerve is not a true neuroma	• Wrong diagnosis • Failure to release the plantar branches of the interdigital nerve, preventing retraction of the stump

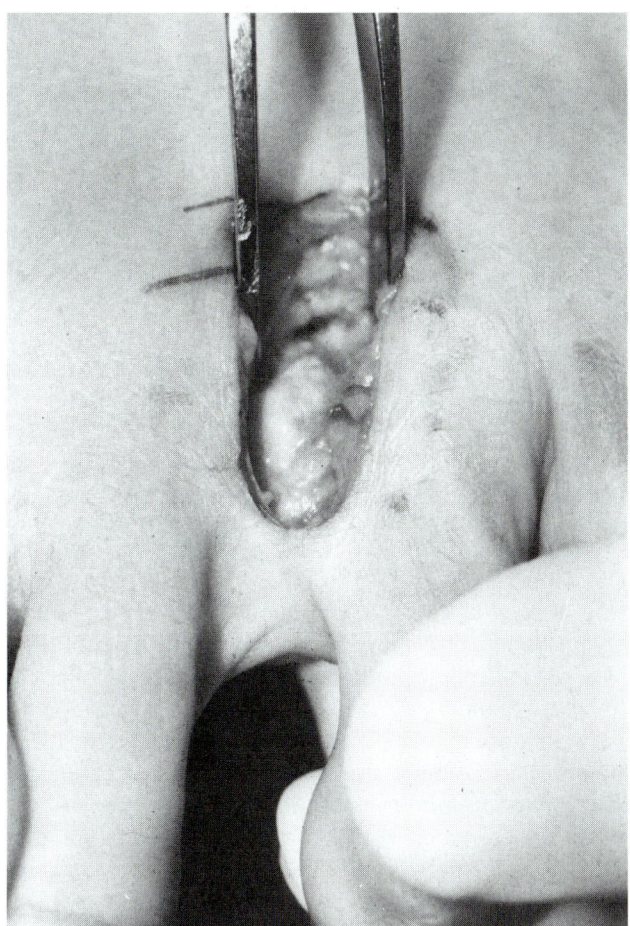

Figure 77.3. Interdigital neuroma.

The transverse metatarsal ligament is divided. Retractors are adjusted so the surgeon can visualize the common digital nerve, which is traced distally to its bifurcation. The nerve frequently exhibits fusiform swelling (Fig. 77.3). The common digital nerve is cut proximal to the metatarsal head and then excised with the neuroma distal to the bifurcation. The interspace should be explored for any accessory nerve branches.

After surgery, the patient is allowed to ambulate in a postoperative shoe for 3 weeks, after which time activity can be gradually increased.

Mann (3) reported a success rate of approximately 80% with nerve excision. A recurrent neuroma owing to either inadequate resection or adherence of the nerve beneath the metatarsal head may occur in a small percentage of patients. The treatment regimen previously described should be repeated; more extensive excision and exploration are necessary if the symptoms warrant surgical treatment. Some authors recommend a plantar approach with redirection of the nerve into intrinsic muscles if a neuroma recurs (9).

SUMMARY

The two most common nerve disorders in the foot and ankle are tarsal tunnel syndrome and interdigital neuromas. The etiologies of these disorders include compression of nerves at anatomically constant fibrous or fibro-osseous tunnels, systemic factors, space-occupying lesions, repetitive trauma, and neuropathy. Patients typically present with activity-related pain. Altered sensation and paraesthesias can occur, depending on the stage of injury to the involved nerves.

Treatment can be conservative initially with the use of specific foot orthosis and corticosteroid injections. With failure of conservative treatment, surgery in carefully selected patients usually yields good results with both disorders.

REFERENCES

 1. Hazel PE, Ebrahim NA, Clark SE, et al. Tibial nerve branching in the tarsal tunnel. Foot Ankle 1988;9:117–119.
 2. Jones JR, Klenerman L. A study of the communicating branch between the medial and lateal plantar nerves. Foot Ankle 1984;4:313–315.
 3. Mann R. Static nerve diseases. In: Mann RA, Coughlin MJ, eds. Surgery of the foot and ankle. St. Louis: Mosby, 1993:544–559.
 4. Baylan SP, Paik SW, Barner AL, et al. Prevalence of the tarsal tunnel syndrome in rheumatoid arthritis. Rheumatol Rehabil 1981; 20:148–150.
 5. Baxter DE, Zingas C. The foot in running. J Am Acad Orthop Surg 1995;3:136–145.
 6. Cimino WR. Tarsal tunnel syndrome. A review of the literature. Foot Ankle 1990;11:47–52.
 7. Baxter DE. Functional nerve disorders in the foot. In: Mann R, ed. Surgery of the foot and ankle. St Louis: Mosby, 1993:559–568.
 8. Keck C. The tarsal tunnel syndrome. J Bone Joint Surg 1962; 44A:180–182.
 9. Baxter DE, Thigpen CM. Heel pain: Operative results. Foot Ankle 1984;5:16–25.
10. Pfeiffer WH, Cracchiolo A III. Clinical results after tarsal tunnel decompression. J Bone Joint Surg 1994;76A:1222–1230.

chapter 78

Hallux Valgus

Walter Pedowitz

Hallux valgus is a common forefoot disorder that includes medial deviation and axial rotation of the first metatarsal phalangeal joint and causes pain, difficulty with normal shoe wear, and loss of the biomechanical integrity of the forefoot in locomotion.

RELEVANT ANATOMY AND PATHOGENESIS

Stability, range of motion, and weight transfer across the first metatarsophalangeal (MTP) joint are provided by the interplay of the capsular ligamentous sling and the intrinsic shape of the joint itself (Fig. 78.1). The metatarsal head of the joint, however, has no actual muscle insertions. Failure of the supporting structures may, therefore, lead to deviation. Initial stability is maintained through strong fan-shaped collateral ligaments from the head of the metatarsal to the base of the proximal phalanx medially and laterally. Similar ligaments also extend from the metatarsal head to the medial and lateral sesamoids.

The sesamoids, located within the split tendon of the flexor hallucis brevis, articulate with the inferior surface of the metatarsal head on either side of the cresta and are further stabilized medially by the abductor hallucis and laterally by the adductor hallucis. These attachments coalesce under the MTP joint to form the strong plantar plate, which inserts into the base of the proximal phalanx. The flexor hallucis longus passes just inferior to the plantar plate toward its insertion on the distal phalanx. The extensor hallucis brevis and longus are stabilized dorsally by the foot alignment of the MTP joint and insert into the proximal phalanx and distal phalanx, respectively. The shapes of the first MTP joint and first metatarsocuneiform joint help determine stability as well. Opposing flat surfaces are inherently stable, whereas rounder joints are more easily deviated (1,2).

Hallux valgus may result from a multitude of causes, which are divided into extrinsic and intrinsic events. The principal extrinsic cause is related to shoes. The incidence of hallux valgus has shown to be higher in shoe-wearing societies than in populations that do not wear shoes. Women's shoe wear is often implicated as the cause of the high preponderance of hallux valgus found in females. In general, the outline of men's feet is comparable to the outline of men's shoes, resulting in no constriction or compression of the forefoot. Women's shoes, however, do not conform to the outer dimensions of the foot and are, on average, 1.2 cm narrower than the forefoot. In addition, as the height of the heel rises, the forefoot force increases exponentially, driving the hallux into the narrow toe box of the shoe, leading to lateral deviation of the great toe (3–6).

Hypermobility of the first ray at the metatarsal cuneiform joint, metatarsus primus varus, and abnormal metatarsal length are intrinsic causes of hallux valgus formation. Hyperpronation and/or a relatively tight Achilles tendon leads to pronation of the first ray, causing stress on the medial aspect of the toe during normal gait.

With valgus deviation of the great toe, the pull of the adductor hallucis muscle causes lateral deviation of the base of the proximal phalanx on the metatarsal head, which pushes the first metatarsal into increased varus. The medial capsule is attenuated, and the lateral structures contract. The transverse metatarsal ligament anchors the sesamoids to the second metatarsal; thus the sesamoids stay in place while the head of the first metatarsal moves medially, flattening the cresta. The result is a mechanical derangement of the first MTP joint, including a prominent medial eminence, lateral subluxation of the base of the proximal phalanx, dissociation of the first metatarsal sesamoid complex, pronation of the hallux, and an increased angle between the first and second metatarsals.

Pronation of the hallux varies with axial rotation of the first metatarsal. With increasing pes planus pronation, the first metatarsal rotates longitudinally, the orientation of the MTP joint becomes oblique in relation to the floor, great toe function markedly decreases, and weight bearing is transferred laterally. Some bunion deformities involve congruent joints, meaning that there is a lateral de-

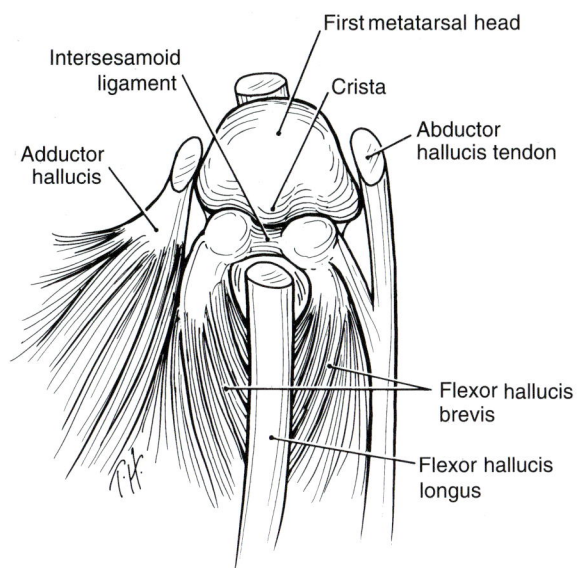

Figure 78.1. Anatomy of the first MTP joint.

viation of the articular surfaces of the first MTP joint without sesamoid displacement, hallux rotation, or sequential progression of the hallux valgus. Any attempt to move the proximal phalanx around on the articular surface of the metatarsal head would disrupt the normal joint relationship.

Lateral deviation of the great toe may also take place at the interphalangeal (IP) joint and is referred to as hallux valgus interphalangeus. The condition may be an isolated entity or exist in conjunction with deviation at the MTP joint. All bunion deformities, therefore, are not the same; and a clear understanding and assessment of the underlying pathologic anatomy is critical to patient assessment (1,2).

INITIAL FINDINGS, PHYSICAL EXAMINATION, AND DIAGNOSIS

The bunion patient will complain of swelling, redness, and pain on the inner side of the foot at the level of the MTP joint. Pain will be especially pronounced when wearing shoes, but will diminish while walking barefoot. Patients note that they have difficulty in finding shoes that fit.

This is a dynamic deformity, and the patient should be evaluated both in weight-bearing and non–weight-bearing phases. While the patient is standing, the degree of forefoot spread, angulation of the great toe, and deformity of the lesser toes should be noted. The clinician must determine whether the great toe and lesser toes purchase the floor in the standing position. The position of the hindfoot and longitudinal arch should be assessed both while the patient is standing and during normal gait.

Special attention is given to the first MTP joint. Axial rotation, angular deformity, and dorsiflexion are carefully

measured. Normal dorsiflexion at the first MTP joint is 70°. Any metatarsophalangeal arthritis, as noted by pain on range of motion of the joint associated with limited dorsiflexion, should be recorded. In general, patients with hallux valgus have pain when walking while wearing shoes but no pain when the shoes are removed. Patients with degenerative arthritis at the MTP joint have pain when walking, with the shoes on and off (7).

Instability at the first metatarsocuneiform joint is difficult to evaluate. Examination is carried out by holding the first MTP joint with one hand and the second MTP joint with the other hand. The first metatarsal is then moved in a dorsomedial and plantar lateral direction and compared to the opposite side. Loss of weight bearing under the first metatarsal head may also be signaled by a callus under the second metatarsal head. The prevalence of clinically significant hypermobility at the metatarsocuneiform joint is still subject to debate. Definite reproducible measuring techniques for metatarsocuneiform instability are not yet available.

RADIOLOGIC STUDIES

Radiographs should be taken in the weight-bearing position, and several measurements should be taken (Fig. 78.2). The hallux valgus angle is subtended by lines that

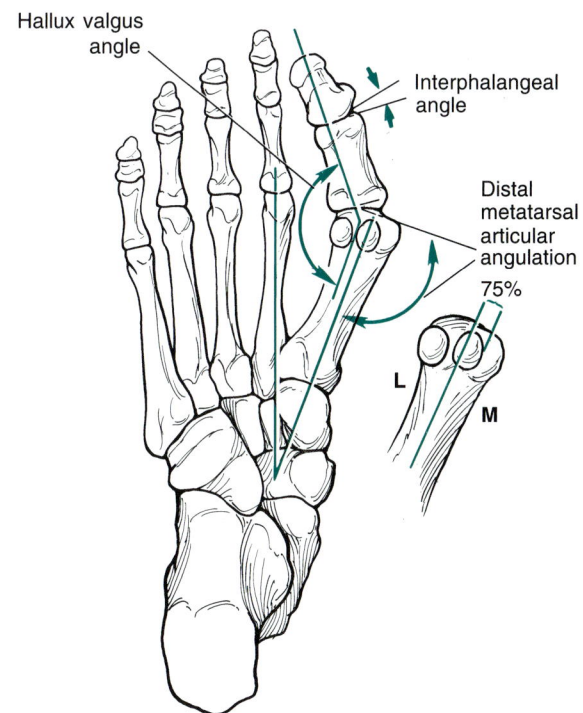

Figure 78.2. Angles of deformity seen from the plantar aspect. The tibial sesamoid is considered medial if 75% of its width is medial to the central line, and it is considered lateral if 75% of its width is lateral to the central line. Otherwise, the sesamoid is considered to be centrally located. *L,* lateral; *M,* medial. Reprinted with permission from Pedowitz W. Bunion deformity. In: Pfeffer G, Frey C, eds. Current practice in foot and ankle surgery. New York: McGraw-Hill, 1993:219–242.

bisect the first metatarsal and the proximal phalanx. The angle between the first and second metatarsals is subtended by lines that bisect the longitudinal axis of these bones. The hallux valgus interphalangeus angle is defined by lines that bisect the proximal and distal phalanxes. The distal metatarsal articular angulation (DMAA) is determined by a line that transversely connects the proximal edge of the articular surface and a line that bisects the long axis of the first metatarsal. Other measures are the lengths of the first and second metatarsals, the angulation of the first metatarsocuneiform joint, the amount of arthritis at the first MTP joint, and assessment of the generalized metatarsus adductus. Sesamoid location should also be assessed. The hallux valgus interphalangeal angle as measured on a radiograph may be relatively normal because of toe pronation (clinical examination is often required to detect this abnormality).

Radiologic assessment of the first metatarsocuneiform joint is difficult. AP weight-bearing radiographs, with and without the forefoot wrapped tightly in an elastic bandage, may give clues to the stability of the joint. An increased slope to the metatarsal cuneiform articulation may indicate instability.

It is well documented that measurements taken from radiographs can vary from examiner to examiner; and slight deviations in the angle of the beam, placement of the cassette, and rotation of the foot can significantly affect accuracy. Radiologic indices, therefore, should be used as clinical guides and not as absolute indications for any specific surgical procedure (8,9).

TREATMENT

Nonoperative Treatment

Initial treatment should always be conservative. With mild deformity, a patient who is willing to compromise with a properly fitting, low-heeled, extra-depth or combination last shoe, augmented with a good-quality cushioned insole, has a good chance of finding comfort. With more significant deformity, a bunion-last shoe that has a broad toe box made of soft leather and a flexible sole will often relieve symptoms. Continued pain after the failure of conservative management, split-size shoe requirements (i.e., one must be significantly wider than the other), and deformity that greatly interferes with the patient's lifestyle are appropriate reasons to operate. Cosmesis is a poor indicator, and the risk:benefit ratio needs to be assessed carefully.

A frank, realistic discussion with the patient, including the expectations, surgical outcome, and possible pitfalls and complications, is an absolute prerequisite to good surgical planning. One-third of patients who have surgery do not return to a complete range of shoe wear, and previous levels of athletic activity may be diminished after surgery (10). The goal of foot surgery, in general, is to create a painless, plantigrade, shoeable foot. The bunion op-

eration should correct all elements of the deformity, produce no residual deficits, maintain a normal weight pattern, maintain a flexible first MTP joint, and (if the procedure fails) retain an easy route to salvage.

Hallux valgus has been classified into three degrees of severity. The normal intermetatarsal angle (i.e., the angle between first and second metatarsals) is up to 9°, and the normal hallux valgus angle is up to 15°. In mild deformity, the hallux valgus angle is less than 20° and the intermetatarsal angle is less than 11°. In moderate deformity, the hallux valgus angle is 20° to 40° and the intermetatarsal angle is 11° to 18°. In severe hallux valgus, the hallux valgus angle is greater than 40° and the intermetatarsal angle is greater than 18°. Patients can be grouped by the condition of their joints: congruent joints, incongruent joints, and joints with degenerative disease. Figure 78.3 is an algorithm for treatment (1,7).

Operative Treatment

DISTAL SOFT TISSUE PROCEDURE

The distal soft tissue procedure (DSTP), or the modified McBride procedure, corrects all soft tissue components of the MTP joint deformity and, when combined with a proximal crescentic osteotomy, corrects moderate to severe deformity (Fig. 78.4). This procedure is contraindicated for a congruent joint with an increased distal metatarsal articular angulation, because rotation of the base of the proximal phalanx around the articular surface of the metatarsal head would disrupt the normal joint relationship. Use of the DSTP is also unacceptable in the presence of degenerative joint disease and spasticity (e.g., head injury, cerebral palsy, cerebrovascular accident).

Through a dorsal incision between the first and second metatarsals, the lateral capsule is released, and the metatarsosesamoid portion of the joint capsule is cut so that the metatarsal head can be recentralized. The adductor hallucis is removed from its attachment to the base of the proximal phalanx and transferred to the soft tissues between the neck of metatarsals one and two. The transverse metatarsal ligament is then cut, completing the release of the major restraints on the lateral MTP joint. Care must be taken to protect the intermetatarsal neurovascular bundle.

Through a medial incision, the bunion eminence is removed by a cut made just medial to the sulcus and parallel to the metatarsal shaft, to prevent excessive metatarsal head excision. Management of the medial capsule through a central longitudinal incision, an L-shaped cut, or a distally based flap sewn down to a hole in the neck of the metatarsal works well.

Because the distal soft tissue realignment can be expected to correct the intermetatarsal angle approximately 5°, a proximal first metatarsal osteotomy is indicated when the intermetatarsal angle is greater than or equal to 15°. This osteotomy is also indicated for patients who have less

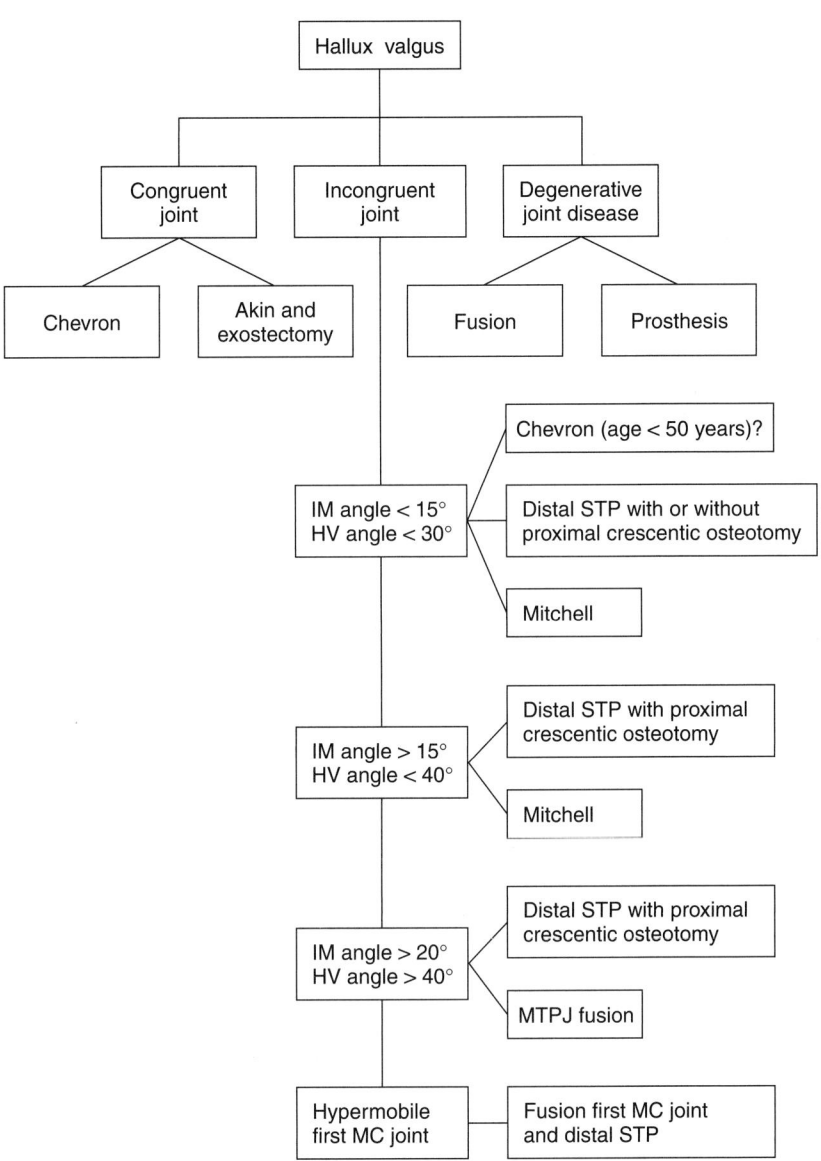

Figure 78.3. Algorithm for treatment decisions. *IM,* intermetatarsal; *HV,* hallux valgus; *STP,* soft tissue procedure, *MTPJ,* metatarsophalangeal joint; *MC,* metatarsocuneiform. Modified from Mann RA. Decision-making in bunion surgery. Instr Course Lect 1990;39;3–13.

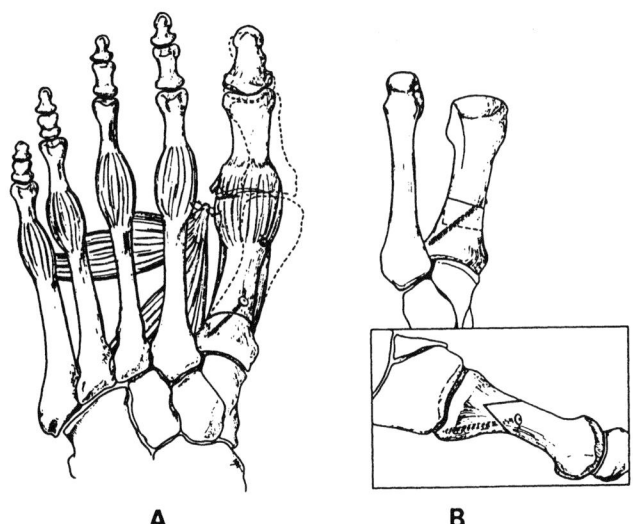

Figure 78.4. A. DSTP with a proximal crescentic osteotomy. **B.** Proximal chevron osteotomy. Reprinted with permission from Pedowitz W. Bunion deformity. In: Pfeffer G, Frey C, eds. Current practice in foot and ankle surgery. New York: McGraw-Hill, 1993:219–242.

angulation if the surgeon finds significant rigidity when attempting to manually close the ankle between metatarsals one and two (e.g., when a lateral facet at the base of the first metatarsal prevents correction).

The crescentic osteotomy is oriented so that the concavity is directed toward the heel. This orientation allows for adequate correction but prevents excessive medial displacement of the osteotomy, leading to a negative angle between metatarsals one and two. This osteotomy is done through a dorsal incision over the proximal third of the metatarsal; the plane of the osteotomy is halfway between perpendicular to the first metatarsal and the bottom of the foot (approximately 120°). By maintaining this plane, excessive dorsiflexion or plantar flexion is avoided.

Instead of the crescentic osteotomy, a proximal chevron, or V, osteotomy can be performed through a medial incision. This procedure is biomechanically stable and increases cancellous bone contact (Fig. 78.4).

Through the combined use of a DSTP and a proximal crescentic osteotomy, overall length is maintained, the sesamoids are centralized, and potential devascularization of the metatarsal head is avoided. This combined procedure does, however, have a high morbidity with increased swelling and pain and a longer recovery period than found with a distal chevron osteotomy (average of 4 months to return to normal shoe wear). In the presence of a complex deformity, however, it is the procedure of choice.

Concern about the long-term postoperative stability of the metatarsocuneiform joint after a proximal osteotomy is still discussed, but long-term results indicate maintenance of the postoperative angle between metatarsals one and two (11). The main postoperative complication is hallux varus, which is a result of medial displacement of the proximal osteotomy. Hallux varus can be avoided by directing the crescentic cut with the concavity oriented proximally.

DISTAL CHEVRON OSTEOTOMY

The distal chevron osteotomy involves resection of the medial eminence combined with a transverse V osteotomy in the coronal plane and lateralization of the head of the first metatarsal (Fig. 78.5). This procedure relaxes the lateral soft tissues and allows correction of the hallux valgus and intermetatarsal angle without significant shortening, joint stiffness, or pain (Clinical Table). Its indications include mild to moderate hallux valgus deformity with an intermetatarsal angle of 14° or less, a hallux valgus angle up to 30°, and no significant sesamoid subluxation or great toe pronation.

In patients over 50 years of age who have poor bone stock secondary to osteoporosis, fixation may be difficult,

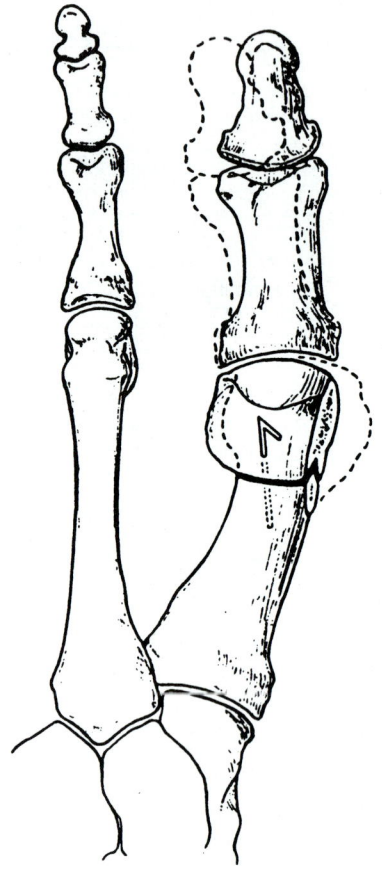

Figure 78.5. With a chevron osteotomy, lateral displacement of the metatarsal head allows the proximal phalanx to be corrected. Reprinted with permission from Pedowitz W. Bunion deformity. In: Pfeffer G, Frey C, eds. Current practice in foot and ankle surgery. New York: McGraw-Hill, 1993:219–242.

Clinical Table: Hallux Valgus

Procedure	Indications	Technique	Anatomy	Pitfalls
Distal chevron	• IM angle <15°; minimal sesamoid subluxation	• 60° chevron cut 1 cm proximal to joint surface	• Long extensor, dorsal nerve • Long flexor, plantar nerve	• Excess lateral translation; avascular necrosis; poor fixation
Proximal first metatarsal osteotomy	• IM angle >15°; rigid first metatarsal	• Fix with screws or pin to prevent migration	• Long extensor • Long flexor, dorsal pedal artery, deep peroneal nerve	• Negative IM angle; hallux varus; elevation of first metatarsal
Akin procedure	• Hallux valgus interphalangeus; congruent joint	• Crack through lateral cortex; fix; preserve soft tissues	• Long extensor • Long flexor	• Overcorrection; nonunion; cut flexor hallucis longus
MTP joint fusion	• Arthritis; severe hallux valgus deformity	• Internally fix; maximize bleeding bone contact	• Dorsal nerve • Plantar nerve • Long extensor • Long flexor	• Excess dorsiflexion or plantar flexion; varus or valgus
Keller procedure	• Impending skin breakdown; low-demand lifestyle	• Resect the base of the proximal phalanx; fix with pin; remove after 6 weeks	• Dorsal nerve • Plantar nerve • Long extensor • Long flexor	• Overresection leading to toe migration; poor push-off; deformed foot

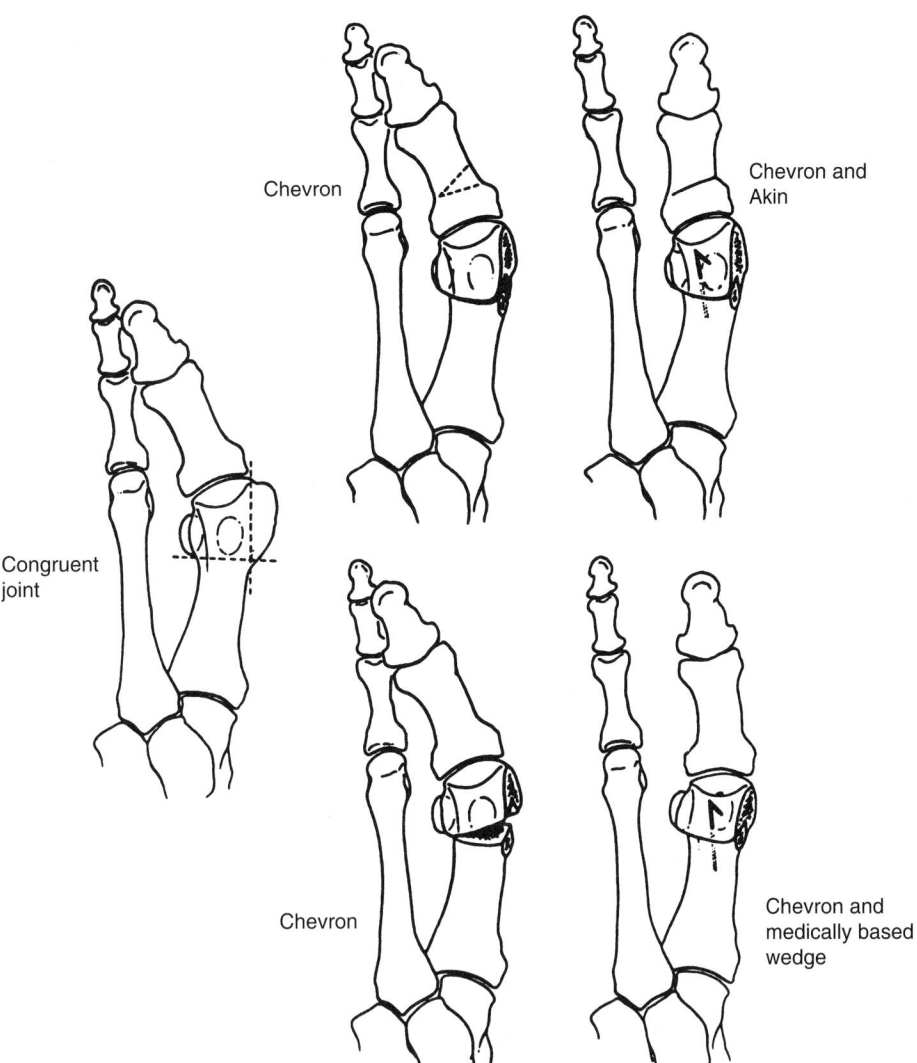

Figure 78.6. Management of the congruent joint with a chevron osteotomy combined with the Akin procedure and of a chevron osteotomy combined with a medial wedge. Reprinted with permission from Pedowitz W. Bunion deformity. In: Pfeffer G, Frey C, eds. Current practice in foot and ankle surgery. New York: McGraw-Hill, 1993:219–242.

and the surgeon may encounter increased incidence of stiffness and pain around the MTP joint. A chevron osteotomy should be placed 1 cm proximal to the articular surface of the metatarsal head with the V angle at 50° to 60°. The capital fragment is laterally displaced 4 to 5 mm and manually impacted. One degree of intermetatarsal angle correction can be expected for each millimeter of lateral displacement of the metatarsal head. Plication of the medial capsule is carried out in a slightly overcorrected position to centralize the sesamoids underneath the metatarsal head. Fixation is enhanced by a Kirschner (K) wire that is passed dorsomedial to plantar lateral. Interfragmentary screws or absorbable polyglycolide pins can also be used. A plaster cast may by used after surgery for 3 to 4 weeks if fixation in uncertain (12).

The distal chevron osteotomy is also helpful for patients with incongruent joints. When the distal metatarsal articular angle (DMAA) must be corrected, a small medial wedge is removed from the osteotomy site. This procedure creates a biplane chevron, which realigns the metatarsal head. Another technique combines the chevron osteotomy with an Akin procedure to correct the deformity without disturbing the congruent joint (Fig. 78.6).

Improper displacement of the capital fragment or excessive shortening through the osteotomy site can lead to transfer metatarsalgia. This problem is usually avoided by internal fixation. Postoperative arthritis and arthrofibrosis can be prevented by ensuring that the inferior limb of the osteotomy site remains extra-articular so that it does not interfere with sesamoid motion. Osteonecrosis is rare, but it may occur.

AKIN PROCEDURE

The Akin procedure corrects the angular deformity of the first ray by reorienting the longitudinal axis of the proximal phalanx (Clinical Table). It is the procedure of choice for hallux valgus interphalangeus and can be used in conjunction with a distal or proximal metatarsal osteotomy in the presence of a congruent joint. The procedure is also helpful for mild recurrent bunion deformity and mild painless hallux valgus with an overriding second toe, but it cannot be used to correct a significantly subluxated MTP joint.

A medially based wedge is taken out of the proximal phalanx about 8 mm distal to the articular surface. The wedge is removed up to but not including the lateral cortex. Enhanced stability is obtained by gently cracking through the lateral cortex manually. When internally fixed (with a wire and/or sutures through drill holes) and maintained in neutral position, the osteotomy heals rapidly, causes minimal morbidity, and maintains a congruent articular surface. When the osteotomy is performed through the middle or distal portion of the proximal phalanx, complications, such as inadvertent cutting of the flexor hallucis longus tendon and stiffness of the IP joint, have been observed.

MITCHELL PROCEDURE

The Mitchell procedure is a complex biplane, double-step-cut osteotomy through the neck of the first metatarsal. It is indicated for moderate hallux valgus deformity with a subluxated MTP joint. By shortening and laterally displacing the distal first metatarsal, the forefoot is narrowed and the soft tissues causing lateral deviation of the great toe are relaxed. This is a technically demanding operation and too much shortening or dorsal displacement of the distal first metatarsal may result in lateral transfer metatarsalgia. Therefore, it is imperative to plantar flex the metatarsal head fragment to the appropriate level. This procedure is contraindicated in the presence of a short first metatarsal or a congruent joint. Salvage is difficult when this procedure fails.

ARTHRODESIS

Arthrodesis of the first MTP joint is a time-tested, reliable, long-lasting procedure that is especially well suited to the management of severe deformity (Fig. 78.7). Indications include hallux valgus and degenerative joint disease, severe hallux valgus deformity, severe deformity with a short first metatarsal, neuromuscular instability, and salvage for current deformity or previous infection. With the proximal phalanx positioned in 15° to 20° of valgus and 10° to 15° of dorsiflexion from the plantar aspect of the foot, a stable MTP joint is created, which maintains metatarsal length, decreases lateral metatarsalgia, protects the lesser toes from further deformity, and preserves hallux valgus strength. Although normal shoes can usually be worn, this procedure is chosen more frequently by men than by women because it limits heel height to about 3.75 cm (1.5 in) and shortens the great toe. Relative contraindications include arthrosis of the IP joint distally and the metatarsocuneiform joint proximally or the presence of an insensate foot.

Screws and plates enhance stability, and fusion rates of

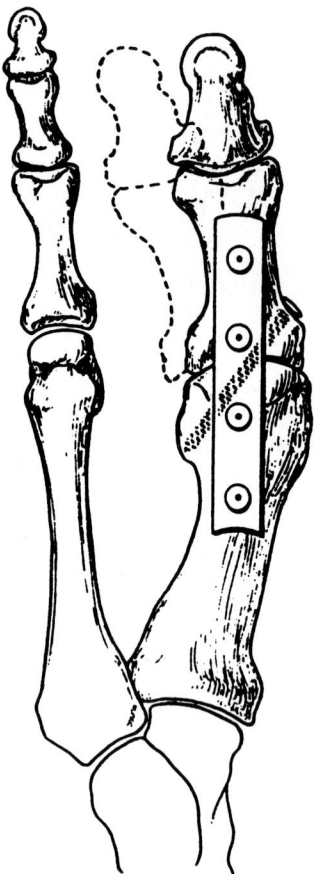

Figure 78.7. MTP joint arthrodesis.

90 to 95% can be expected. In osteoporotic bone, however, multiple longitudinal or oblique pin fixation seems to work best. Fibrous unions, if encountered, often are pain free and give an acceptable clinical result. If not, a revision with a bone graft is necessary.

METATARSOCUNEIFORM FUSION

First metatarsocuneiform fusion corrects metatarsus primus varus at the apex of the deformity (Fig. 78.8). It is a technically demanding procedure because the joint is irregular and multiplanar. There can be prolonged morbidity, and 4 to 6 months are often required to achieve fusion. This procedure produces significant rigidity to the medial side of the foot, and even slight rotation or dorsiflexion of the first metatarsal is not well tolerated. It is critical that the fusion be done in slight plantar flexion and lateral deviation to prevent lateral transfer metatarsalgia. Indications include severe hypermobile metatarsus primus varus, first metatarsocuneiform arthritis, and selected revision. The fusion can be combined with a distal soft tissue realignment to correct the hallux valgus (10). Contraindications include adolescents with open epiphyses and moderate deformity in the absence of first ray hypermobility. The procedure should not be done when a better alternative is available.

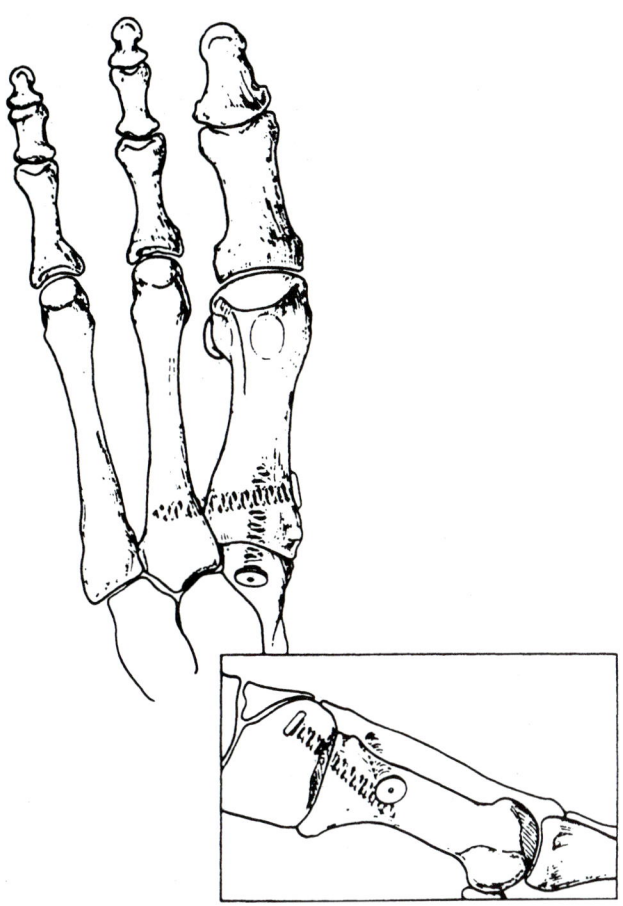

Figure 78.8. Metatarsocuneiform arthrodesis. Reprinted with permission from Pedowitz W. Bunion deformity. In: Pfeffer G, Frey C, eds. Current practice in foot and ankle surgery. New York: McGraw-Hill, 1993:219–242.

KELLER PROCEDURE

Resection of the base of the proximal phalanx with removal of the medial eminence, the Keller procedure, has been widely used for many bunion deformities but now has more limited indications (Clinical Table). Large series continue to demonstrate excellent pain relief and patient satisfaction when the procedure is done for hallux rigidus. Resulting diminished toe function, however, has led many orthopaedic surgeons to seek other procedures when available. Despite attempts to reestablish flexor hallucis brevis continuity and techniques to create a stronger arthrofibrosis, the patient is left with a shortened toe, decreased strength on push-off, and an increased incidence of lateral transfer metatarsalgia. A cock-up toe deformity may also occur.

In addition to hallux rigidus, this procedure is indicated for low-demand patients with hallux valgus and as a salvage procedure for bunion surgery in older patients in whom the joint has been damaged (in a younger patient, a fusion would be indicated). Reattachment of the plantar plate to the base of the proximal phalanx

through several drill holes and suturing the plantar aponeurosis to the flexor hallucis longus tendon have recently been advocated as methods to help reestablish flexor function.

MEDIAL EMINENCE RESECTION

Simple resection of the medial eminence (with or without lateral capsule release and adductor tenotomy) is reserved for elderly patients with vascular compromise and impending ulceration, as well as some cases in which the medial eminence is the primary problem. It is a quick procedure that has limited morbidity and preserves MTP motion. When used for anything more serious than the mildest deformities, however, it has a high dissatisfaction rate because of recurrence of the deformity.

IMPLANTS

The use of a flexible, double-stemmed, Silastic implant in the first MTP joint is quite controversial. Made of the same material as breast implants, which have been recalled by the Food and Drug Administration, these implants are subject to acute inflammatory reaction, local bone resorption, Silastic wear with synovitis, bone invasion, proximal lymphatic involvement, and wear and fracture. Although they may provide motion and adequate weight-bearing support, the risk:benefit ratio is uncertain. An implant is clearly not indicated for active individuals who put significant demands on the forefoot.

SUMMARY

Operative intervention can provide a reliable long-lasting correction of a hallux deformity (Fig. 78.9). Morbidity, shoe wear expectations, return to sports, and possible complications must be discussed fully with the patient.

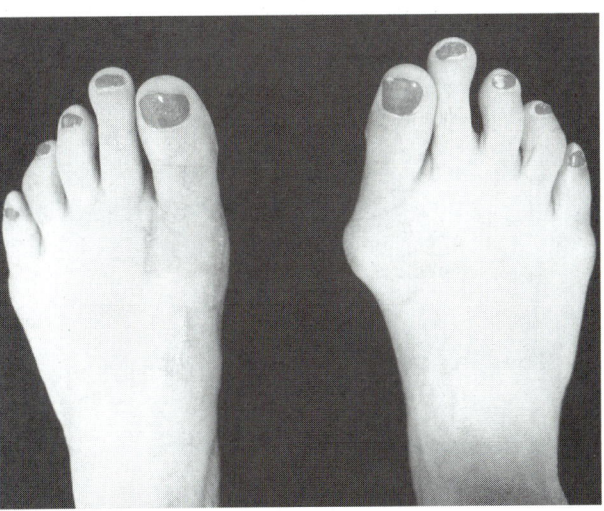

Figure 78.9. Results of a DSTP and proximal crescentic osteotomy performed on the left foot.

REFERENCES

1. Mann RA. Decision-making in bunion surgery. Instr Course Lect 1990;39;3–13.
2. Bordelon RL. Evaluation and operative procedures for hallux valgus deformity. Orthopaedics 1987;10:38–44.
3. Coughlin MJ, Thompson FM. The high price of high-fashion footwear. Instr Course Lect 1995;44:371–377.
4. Frey C, Thompson F, Smith J, et al. American Orthopaedic Foot and Ankle Society women's shoe survey. Foot Ankle 1993; 14:78–81.
5. Frey CC. Trends in women's shoewear. Instr Course Lect 1995; 44:385–387.
6. Seale KS. Women and their shoes: unrealistic expectations? Instr Course Lect 1995;44:379–384.
7. Pedowitz W. Bunion deformity. In: Pfeffer G, Frey C, eds. Current practice in foot and ankle surgery. New York: McGraw-Hill, 1993:219–242.
8. Johnson KA. "What's a foot surgeon to believe?" [Editorial]. Foot Ankle 1992;13:508.
9. Scott G, Wilson DW, Bentle G. Roentgenographic assessment in hallux valgus. Clin Orthop 1991;267:143–147.
10. Lillich JS, Baxter DE. Bunionectomies and related surgery in the elite female middle-distance and marathon runner. Am J Sports Med 1986;14:491–493.
11. Drecben S, Mann RA. Advanced hallux valgus deformity: long term results utilizing the distal soft tissue procedure and proximal metatarsal osteotomy. Foot Ankle 1996;17:142–144.
12. Johnson KA. Surgery of the foot and ankle. New York: Raven, 1989.

Hallux Rigidus

Hallux rigidus, or osteoarthritis of the first metatarsophalangeal (MTP) joint, was first described by Davies-Colley in 1887 (1). The gradual onset of pain and limitation of motion, especially dorsiflexion, characterize this condition, which occurs in approximately 1 in 40 adults (2). This chapter outlines the pathogenesis and current treatment modalities and emphasizes surgical treatment options.

RELEVANT ANATOMY AND PATHOGENESIS

The first metatarsophalangeal (MTP) joint is a diarthrodial joint that has its greatest motion in the sagittal plane. Normal motion range of motion has been estimated to be from 30° of plantar flexion to nearly 90° of dorsiflexion. The convex metatarsal head articulates with the concave proximal phalanx to allow this motion. The sesamoids are found plantar to the metatarsal head in the grooves but are rarely involved in the disease process of hallux rigidus. It has been estimated that 60° of dorsiflexion are required for pain-free conduction of normal activities of daily living (3).

The cause of hallux rigidus is secondary to degenerative arthritis. Although adolescents can have hallux rigidus of the first MTP joint as a result of osteochondritis dissecans, this condition is exceedingly rare. The cause of the arthritis has been greatly debated; multiple theories have been proposed, including trauma (intra-articular fracture), compression of the joint surfaces (turf toe), and a long or elevated first metatarsal (3,4). The overwhelming majority of cases, however, have an unknown cause, which is probably the result of an imperfect ball-and-socket joint and altered joint kinematics, leading to early compressive forces during dorsiflexion (5). Radiographically, this is manifested by a flattened metatarsal head that articulates with the curved articular surface of the proximal phalanx.

INITIAL FINDINGS, PHYSICAL EXAMINATION, AND DIAGNOSIS

The hallmark of the physical examination of patients with hallux rigidus is restricted active and passive dorsiflexion, which reproduces the patients' pain. Initially, synovitis is present; but the articular surface of the metatarsal head undergoes variable but progressive degeneration, especially in the dorsal half (Fig. 79.1). As the process continues, osteophytes develop above the dorsal, medial, and lateral metatarsal head. Osteophytes and cartilage loss may develop secondarily along the proximal phalanx but are never as severe as on the metatarsal head. A loose body is often present, which is an intra-articular fracture, usually off the dorsal aspect of the proximal phalanx.

As the osteophytes enlarge, a mechanical barrier to dorsiflexion is created, leading to a stiff, painful toe (Fig. 79.2). This impingement causes jamming instead of gliding of the proximal phalanx on the metatarsal head. As the mechanical block increases, difficulty with push-off occurs, and patients find themselves walking on the lateral border of the foot to avoid pushing off through the first MTP joint.

On examination, the pain is reproduced by forced dorsiflexion of the first MTP joint. The dorsal prominence and often the dorsolateral ridge are painful on palpitation. Plantar flexion can cause pain secondary to stretching of the capsule and extensor hallucis longus (EHL) over the osteophytes. Neuritic symptoms can occur because of pressure over the dorsal medial nerve to the great toe.

RADIOLOGIC STUDIES

Radiographs of the foot are consistent with degenerative arthritis. Joint-space narrowing is best evaluated on the lateral view, which will reveal the extent of dorsal ex-

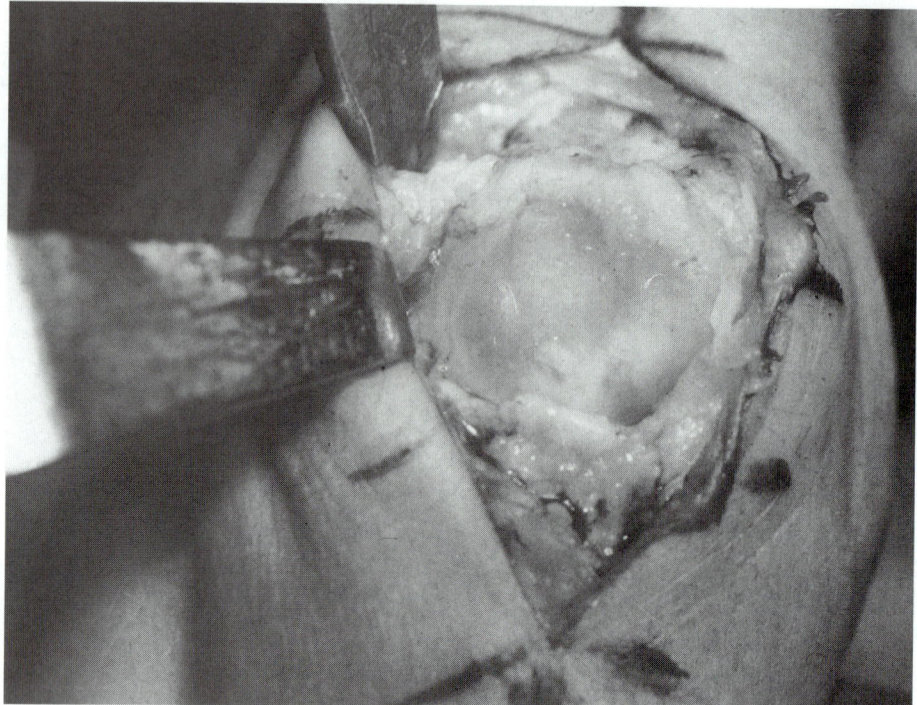

Figure 79.1. Intraoperative view of a patient with hallux rigidus. Note the complete loss of cartilage on the dorsal half of the metatarsal head.

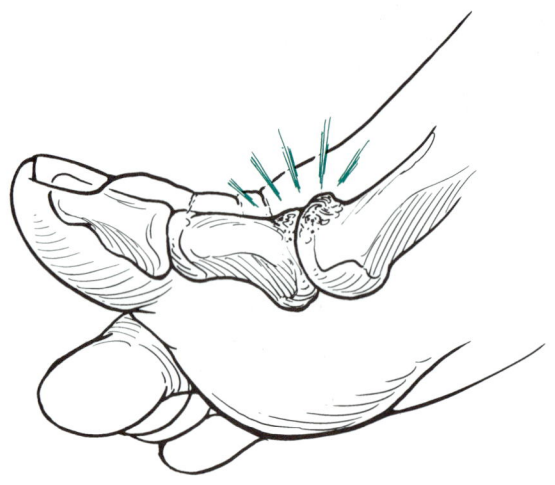

Figure 79.2. Dorsal impingement.

ostosis, the width of the joint space, and the presence of a loose body (Fig. 79.3). The plantar joint space is most often maintained, whereas the dorsal half may be absent on the lateral view. An exostosis on the dorsal half of the proximal phalanx and/or a fracture may be present. The joint space may be difficult to determine on the AP view, because of the overlap from the dorsal osteophyte but it usually shows squaring off of the metatarsal head. Special notice of lateral osteophytes should be taken, as these are often seen early in the disease process.

Classification

A classification system based on plain radiographs has been proposed and consists of three grades. Grade I hallux rigidus is characterized by minimal narrowing with dorsal osteophytes. In grade II disease, there is more extensive joint-space narrowing, and only the plantar joint is preserved. In grade III disease, there is complete joint-space narrowing and severe arthritis (6).

TREATMENT

Nonoperative Treatment

Conservative care for patients with hallux rigidus consists mainly of orthotic and footwear modifications to decrease stress across the first MTP joint. A stiff-soled shoe to decrease the dorsiflexion across the MTP joint is recommended for work shoes. For athletics, a rocker sole insert across the MTP joint can be used with a commercial sneaker, providing a relatively good cosmetic result. Custom orthotic inserts with a Morton's extension can also provide relief if the forefoot part of the orthotic is made of rigid material. Since all orthotic devices occupy space in the toe box, the shoe must be big enough to accommodate the enlarged MTP joint as well as the orthotic device. An extra-depth shoe will alleviate this problem, but most are not cosmetically acceptable. Most commercially available running and walking shoes will have sufficient depth in the toe box to accommodate the orthotic device; thus I rarely prescribe custom shoes.

Operative Treatment

If the pain becomes too disabling and the patient has failed conservative therapy, surgical intervention may be considered. The decision for surgery is based on the patients' complaints, age and activity requirements and on the radiographic classification. Occasionally, the specific procedure can be chosen during surgery, after the articular cartilage of the metatarsal head has been evaluated (Clinical Table). There are two broad categories of operations: joint preserving (cheilectomy, ostectomy of the proximal phalanx) for milder cases and joint sacrificing (resection arthroplasty, interposition arthroplasty, implant arthroplasty, and arthrodesis) for more advanced disease.

CHEILECTOMY

As a general rule, cheilectomy should be considered as the initial operation for most patients with hallux rigidus (7). It is relatively simple, has a short recovery, and does not eliminate any further operations. The indication for cheilectomy is early hallux rigidus with dorsal impingement (grade I or II). If the patient has some joint space left, as seen on the lateral radiograph, especially on the plantar half of the joint, then a cheilectomy has a good chance of success. The cheilectomy eliminates the dorsal impingement, removes any loose bodies, improves dorsiflexion, and decreases the bulk of the joint. I have had success with cheilectomy in older patients with severe degenerative arthritis, no joint space, and large dorsal

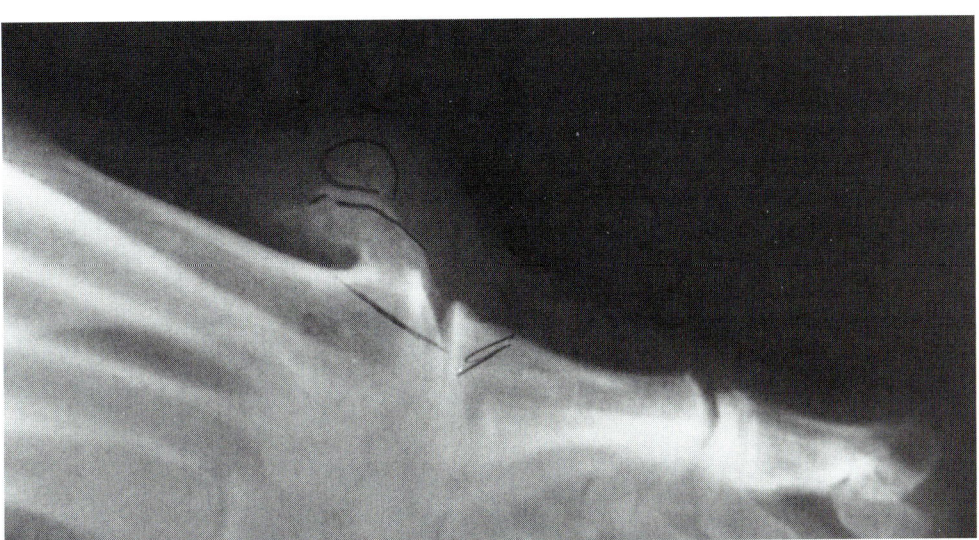

Figure 79.3. Lateral view showing a large dorsal osteophyte, soft tissue swelling, and loss of joint space.

Clinical Table: Hallux Rigidus

Procedure	Indications	Technique	Anatomy	Pitfalls
Cheilectomy	• Early DJD • Dorsal spur	• Dorsal third metatarsal head • Dorsal proximal phalan	• Dorsal medial nerve	• Too little bone removed • Advanced DJD
Moberg procedure	• Young, active patient	• Extension osteotomy • 25° to 30° of extension • Crossed K wires	• Dorsal medial nerve	• Poor fixation • Inadequate elevation
Interposition arthroplasty	• Older patient • Advanced DJD • First and second metatarsals are of equal length	• Dorsal capsule • EHB • Limited Keller procedure • One-quarter of proximal phalanx	• Dorsal medial nerve	• Short first metatarsal • Too much bone removed
Implant arthroplasty	• Advanced DJD	• Hemiarthroplasty • Meal of Silastic	• Dorsal medial nerve	• Silastic wear • Metal wear
Arthrodesis	• Advanced DJD	• Crossed 3.5-mm screw • Dorsal third plate • 15° of dorsiflexion	• Dorsal medial nerve	• Malposition • Nonunion • Arthritis

DJD, degenerative joint disease.

osteophytes, making shoe wear difficult. Again, if cheilectomy fails, all other procedures are still available to the patient.

Technique

A dorsal approach just medial to the extensor hallucis longus is standard. The capsule is dissected off the dorsal osteophyte and around the metatarsal head to free the capsule, exposing the medial and lateral aspects of the joint. The proximal phalanx is plantar flexed to completely expose the metatarsal head. The amount of bone resection depends on the amount of cartilage destruction on the metatarsal head. I usually start just above the point at which the articular cartilage has been lost and make my first resection from distal to proximal, using an oscillating saw and removing at least the dorsal third of the metatarsal head (Fig. 79.4).

Next, I will remove the lateral osteophyte in the line with the metatarsal shaft and round off the edges of the metatarsal head. The dorsal quarter of the proximal phalanx is then removed. The toe is placed through passive range of motion; if 90° of motion are obtained, then adequate bone has been resected. If not, a gentle plantar capsule release is performed and/or more dorsal bone is resected to reach a range of motion of 90°. A transverse groove across the dorsum of the metatarsal head can also be made to further increase the dorsiflexion. The edges of the metatarsal head are smoothed with a rasp, and the capsule is closed in layers.

A postoperative shoe with dressing is used for 2 weeks, until the wound heals. The patient should wear a sneaker for an additional 4 to 6 weeks. Range of motion exercises are started after a few days; if the patient fails to reach at least 60° of motion, a manipulation in the office under an ankle block is preferred.

MOBERG PROCEDURE

A Moberg procedure can be used in addition to a cheilectomy in younger patients who need more range of motion for athletics (8) This procedure increases the degree of dorsiflexion by resecting a dorsally based wedge of

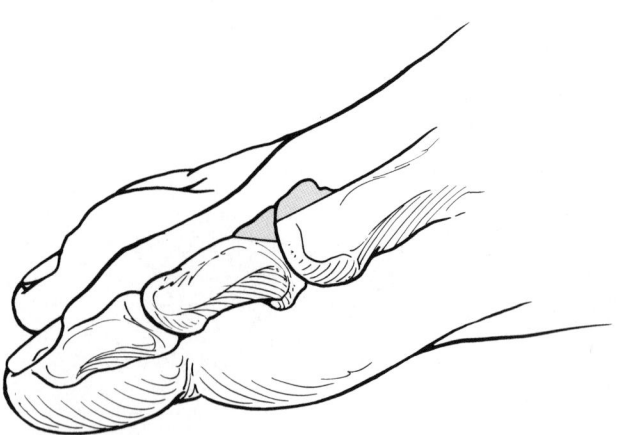

Figure 79.4. Bone resection for a cheilectomy.

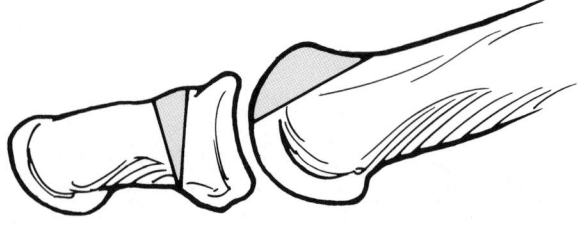

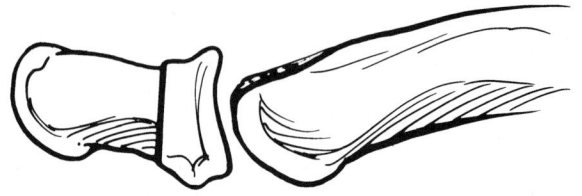

Figure 79.5. Moberg procedure.

the bone from the proximal aspect of the proximal phalanx. The absolute range of motion remains the same, but it starts at a greater degree of dorsiflexion. The ideal candidate is a younger patient who has adequate joint space but has difficulty with running sports because of limited dorsiflexion. This procedure is performed at the same time as a cheilectomy; thus range of motion exercises must be delayed until the osteotomy has healed.

Technique

A medial incision along the proximal phalanx is used. The surgeon carefully dissects down to the bone. A dorsal-based wedge approximately 5 mm wide is removed to place the toe in 25° to 30° of extension in relation to the metatarsal shaft (Fig. 79.5). Crossed 0.45-mm Kirschner (K) wires are used to fix the osteotomy. They are removed at 4 weeks, if the osteotomy has healed.

MODIFIED KELLER PROCEDURE

The Keller procedure (resection of the proximal half of the proximal phalanx) can be used for older, sedentary patients with hallux rigidus. Problems with transfer metatarsalgia, shortening of the hallux, and weakness in push-off make it a less than desirable alternative for more active patients (6). Hamilton et al. (7) reported the results of a modified Keller procedure with interposition of the dorsal capsule and extensor hallucis brevis (EHB) for patients with severe hallux rigidus. They achieved good results in 24 of 25 patients and noted no evidence of transfer metatarsalgia. The ideal candidate for this procedure is 50 to 60 years old, has severe hallux rigidus (grade II to III) that is too advanced for cheilectomy, and wishes to retain some motion at the MTP joint. The Keller procedure is an alternative to arthrodesis and results in about 40° of dorsiflexion, which allows some variation in the heel height of the shoe. A contraindication is a short first metatarsal, because of the risk of transfer metatarsalgia.

Technique

A medial approach is employed, and the medial capsule is incised along with the skin incision. A number 15 blade is used to free the soft tissues (attachment of the capsule, EHB dorsally, some fibers of the flexor hallucis brevis (FHB), and the plantar plate). A dorsal cheilectomy of the metatarsal head is performed. A sagittal saw is then used to resect 25% or less of the proximal phalanx. The EHB is cut proximal on the dorsum of the foot to prevent the tendon from retracting as a result of contraction of the EHB (Figs. 79.6 and 79.7). The EHB and dorsal capsule are sutured to the FHB with number 2 nonabsorbable suture. A 0.62-mm K wire is placed across the joint (through the interpositional tissue) and left in place for 3 weeks.

Gentle passive range of motion is begun at 3 weeks. The patient is allowed to wear sneakers at 6 weeks.

IMPLANT ARTHROPLASTY

Silastic implant arthroplasty gained wide popularity with the use of single-stem hemiarthroplasty during the mid-1980s. Most orthopaedists, however, have abandoned this use because of poor results owing to silicone wear, osteolysis, foreign body reaction, and fractures of the implant (9). The use of grommet liners and a double-stem implant can be used in the rheumatoid population with good results. Townley and Taranow (9) reported results with a nonconstrained, metal-resurfacing arthroplasty to replace the articular surface of the proximal phalanx. Long-term findings show good to excellent results in more than 95% of patients.

Technique

The techniques for the Silastic and metatarsal hemiarthroplasty are the same and are performed through a dorsal incision with careful release of the soft tissues off the proximal phalanx. An oscillating saw is used to remove the articular cartilage of the proximal phalanx in a flat plane; sufficient bone is removed to accommodate the thickness of the articulating plate of the implant. The surgeon must avoid prosthetic oversizing and excessive joint

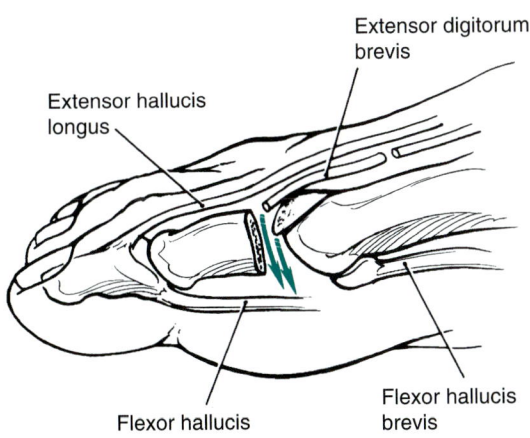

Figure 79.6. Interposition capsular arthroplasty. *Arrows,* dorsal capsule.

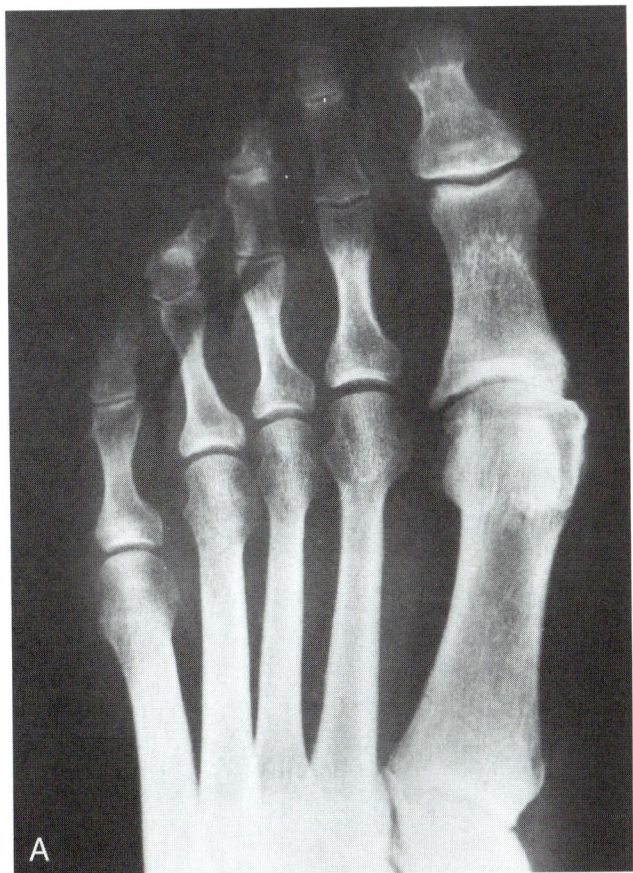

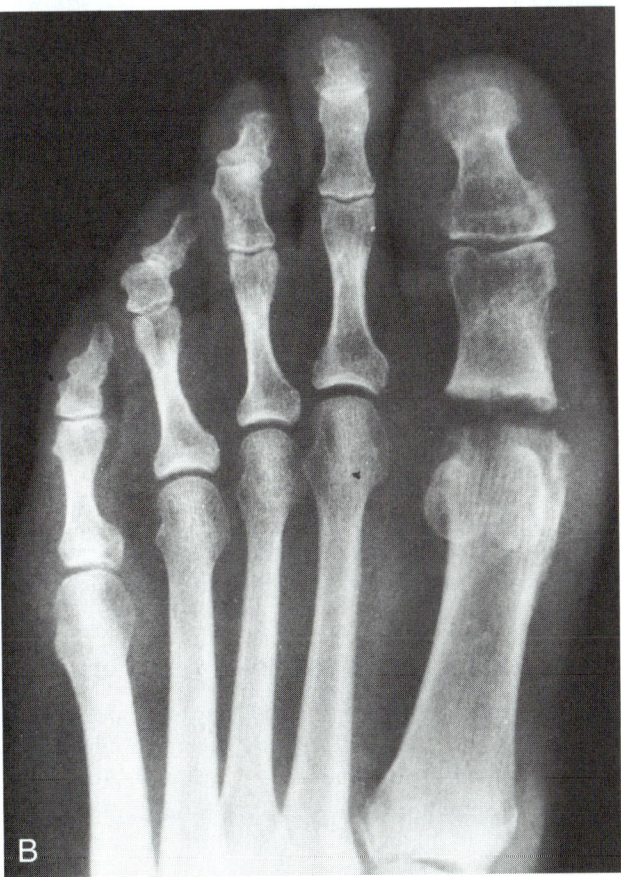

Figure 79.7. Preoperative (**A**) and postoperative (**B**) AP views showing an interposition capsular arthroplasty.

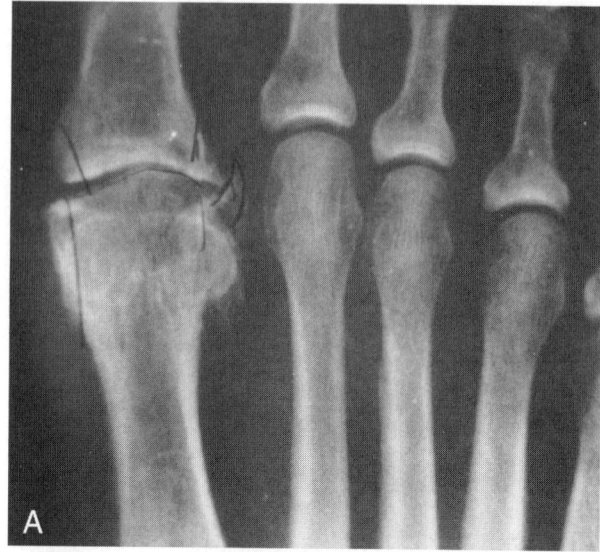

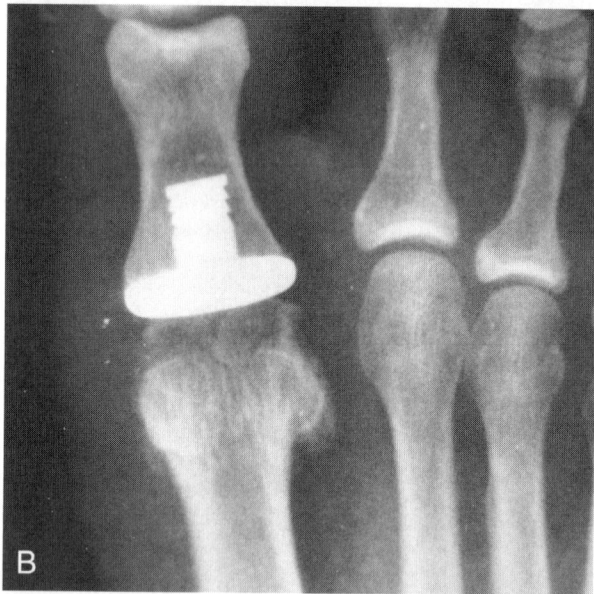

Figure 79.8. Preoperative (**A**) and postoperative (**B**) AP views showing a metal hemiarthroplasty.

tension. A 6-mm burr is used to core out the proximal phalanx to accept the implant. When the implant is properly seated, some play in the joint and full dorsiflexion should be present (Fig. 79.8). The capsule and skin are closed in layers. The patient is allowed to ambulate in a postoperative shoe.

FIRST METATARSOPHALANGEAL JOINT ARTHRODESIS

For patients with severe arthritis (grade III) of the first MTP joint, an arthrodesis can provide predictable pain relief but at the sacrifice of motion (10). After an arthrodesis, a patient should be able to walk fast, ride a bike, and play golf; but he or she will have difficulty running and must limit heel height and shoe wear (2). A successful arthrodesis depends on bony union in a satisfactory alignment. Many techniques have been described for arthrode-

sis of this joint: All rely on internal fixation to achieve stable apposition of the bony surfaces. Internal fixation should permit reliable and consistent maintenance of the chosen MTP alignment during bony consolidation and ultimate fusion. Remembered that some correction of the intermetatarsal angle will occur with a MTP arthrodesis; thus a metatarsal osteotomy is usually not required when the patient has both severe hallux rigidus and severe hallux valgus. The two most commonly used techniques are crossed screws and a dorsal plate.

Technique

Crossed screws. For the crossed-screws technique, a dorsal approach is used, and the joint is opened medial to the EHL tendon. The collateral ligaments are cut, the toe is flexed down, and 5 to 8 mm of the metatarsal head is removed. Commercially developed conical reamers that produce a convex metatarsal head and reciprocally shaped concave proximal phalanx can be used but are not necessary. I use an oscillating saw to remove the cartilage off the metatarsal head and to create a rounded surface. The proximal phalanx is flexed down and a power burr is used to remove the cartilage on the proximal phalanx. The joint is reduced in 15° of dorsiflexion with respect to the ball of the foot (30° to the metatarsal shaft) and 10° to 15° of valgus; it is provisionally fixed with crossed 0.62-mm K wires.

The position is checked with a small fluoroscopy unit and by simulating weight bearing of the foot on a metal tray. As a rough guide, it should be possible to slide a finger under the proximal phalanx. Two crossed cortical 3.5-mm cannulated screws (use 2.7-mm screws if the metatarsal head is small) or one screw and one K wire can be used to prevent rotation (Fig. 79.9).

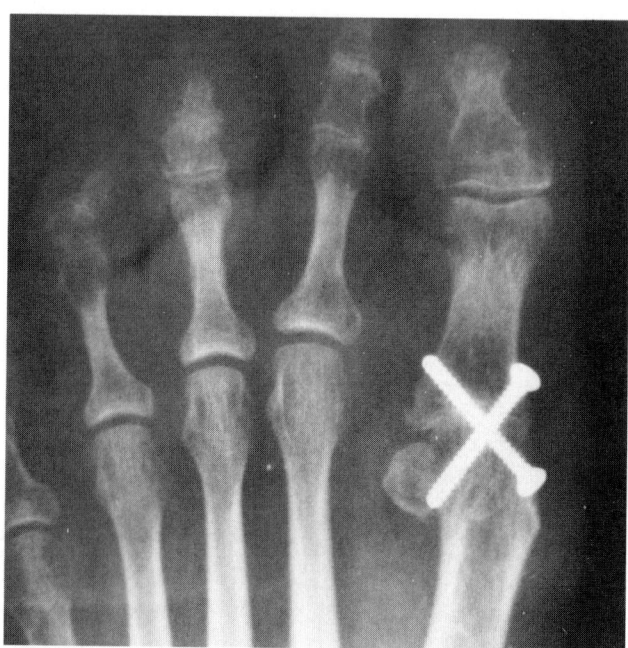

Figure 79.9. Crossed-screws technique for an MTP joint arthrodesis.

Dorsal plate. For the dorsal plate technique, a dorsal approach is used, and the surfaces are prepared in a manner similar to the crossed-screws technique with provisional 0.62-mm K wire fixation. A one-third tubular, five-hole plate is placed on the dorsal surface. Although this is the compression side, the forces applied across the joint do not seem to be of sufficient magnitude to disrupt the fixation. The plate must be bent slightly into dorsiflexion at the first MTP joint. The plate is fixed to the bone with 3.5-mm screws. The two screws in the proximal phalanx are placed first. Alternatively, one crossed screw plus a one-third tubular, three-hole plate may be used.

The patient is allowed to ambulate immediately in a wooden shoe. Degenerative changes of the interphalangeal joint of the great toe develop in 30 to 40% of patients who have undergone an arthrodesis, but it is rarely of clinical significance.

SUMMARY

Although hallux rigidus is a degenerative arthritic condition of the first MTP joint, its occurrence in the younger and middle-aged athletic population can be particularly disabling. Although it is known that hallux rigidus is secondary to degenerative arthritis, precise factors leading to the unique degeneration of the joint are debated and presently unknown.

Nonoperative treatment may be effective if particular attention is paid to modification of footwear in order to diminish the motion through the first MTP joint.

Surgical treatment, whether a cheilectomy or a Moberg procedure, is designed predominantly to increase range of motion, particularly in dorsiflexion. The use of the Keller procedure or implant arthroplasty may be considered in selected patients, in particular the older population with severe degenerative changes who wish to maintain motion. Arthrodesis may be considered, as successful union predictably eliminates pain at the expense of lost motion through this joint.

REFERENCES

1. Davies-Colley N. Contraction of the metatarsophalangeal joint of the great toe (hallux flexus). Br Med J 1887;1:728.
2. Mann RA. Disorders of the first metatarsophalangeal joint. J Am Acad Orthop Surg 1995;3:34–40.
3. Pfeffer G. Cheilectomy. In: Johnson KA, ed. Master techniques in orthopaedic surgery: foot and ankle. New York: Raven, 1994: 119–134.
4. Shereff MJ, Bejjani FJ, Kummer FJ. Kinematics of the first metatarsophalangeal joint. Bone Joint Surg 1986;68A:392–398.
5. Moberg E. A simple operation for hallux rigidus. Clin Orthop 1979; 142:55–56.
6. Love TR, Whynot A, Farine I, et al. Keller arthroplasty: a prospective review. Foot Ankle 1987;8:46–54.
7. Hamilton WG, O'Malley MJ, Thompson FM. Capsular interposition arthroplasty for severe hallux rigidus. Foot Ankle 1997;17:62–65.
8. Shereff M, Jahss M. Complications of Silastic implant arthroplasty in the hallux. Foot Ankle 1981;1:95–101.
9. Townley CO, Taranow WS. A metallic hemiarthroplasty resurfacing prosthesis for the hallux metatarsophalangeal joint. Foot Ankle Int 1994;15:575–580.
10. Coughlin M, Mann RA. Arthrodesis of the first metatarsophalangeal joint as a salvage for failed Keller procedure. J Bone Joint Surg 1987;69A:68–72.

Fractures of the Calcaneus and Talus

I   Calcaneus Fractures

The calcaneus is an integral part of the complex and biomechanically sound foot. It provides a sound base for weight bearing, particularly during the heel-strike phase of gate and, through its articulations with the talus, navicular, and cuboid bones, participates in the complex motion of the foot during ambulation. Fractures of the calcaneus have been recognized for their potential to lead to significant long-term disability. These fractures have been described for centuries; and early attempts at treatment, including both nonoperative and operative management, were often fraught with complications and associated with poor functional outcome and chronic pain. Operative complications include wound dehiscence, soft tissue infections, osteomyelitis, septic arthritis, and nerve injury. The poor functional outcome associated with nonoperative management results from the residual deformity in which posttraumatic arthritis develops within the unreduced joint. Although a better understanding of calcaneus fractures and the surrounding soft tissues has led to a decrease in the number of operative complications, considerable controversy still exists regarding their best management.

RELEVANT ANATOMY AND PATHOGENESIS

The calcaneus is the largest of the tarsal bones, and as such it plays an integral function in locomotion. It is responsible for weight bearing, particularly during the heel-strike phase of ambulation. Through its articulation with the talus, cuboid, and navicular, the calcaneus provides

the hindfoot with inversion and eversion. The calcaneus also provides a point for insertion for the Achilles tendon, acting as a lever for plantar flexion of the foot during the stance and toe-off phases of ambulation.

The calcaneus has three surfaces that are designed to articulate with the undersurface of the talus, forming the complex subtalar joint. These include the posterior (largest), middle, and anterior facets. The anterior aspect of the calcaneus contains a facet that articulates with the cuboid, forming the calcaneocuboid joint.

Because of the complex anatomy of the calcaneus, its multiple points of attachment for ligaments and tendons, and the different forces applied to it, it is subject to a host of different fracture patterns. The pattern that has received the most attention, because of its complex nature and potential for morbidity, is the joint-depression intraarticular fracture.

Joint-depression fractures of the calcaneus are commonly a result of axial compression of the hindfoot (1). This axial compression often occurs after a fall from a height, in which the individual lands directly on one or both heels, or from a motor vehicle accident, in which the floorboard compresses the heel of the foot that is applying the brakes. In both scenarios, the lateral process of the talus comes in direct contract with the lateral aspect of the calcaneus; and acting as a wedge, the talus drives the calcaneus apart. The primary fracture line created runs from the area of the crucial angle of Gissane posteriorly and medially, dividing the calcaneus into two major fragments: an anteromedial fragment and a posterolateral fragment. The final fracture pattern and the amount of displacement of the fracture fragments depend on the position of the calcaneus and talus at the time of impact and the amount and direction of the impact load. This force not only results in a disruption of the bony calcaneus but also causes injury to the ligaments and articular cartilage, all of which may directly influence the patient's final clinical outcome, regardless of how the calcaneus is ultimately treated.

INITIAL FINDINGS, PHYSICAL EXAMINATION, AND DIAGNOSIS

The initial findings for a patient with an acute calcaneal fracture include pain localized to the hindfoot and generalized swelling of the foot and ankle, which may be massive in some cases. Hindfoot deformity is also common, with shortening, angulation, and widening. Shortly after the fracture occurs, ecchymosis of the hindfoot, ankle, and lower leg usually develops. In patients who have sustained high-energy fractures, superficial and deep blisters may ensue, particularly along the medial aspect of the foot and ankle. Because of the pain associated with this injury, patients may not complain of pain associated with injuries to other parts of the body. Thus it is important to thoroughly examine any patient who has sustained a calcaneus fracture—especially as the result of a fall. The clinician should evaluate the contralateral foot and lower lumbar spine and, if indicated, obtain x-rays.

The incidence of open wounds associated with fractures of the calcaneus is essentially unknown. These wounds are, however, most commonly associated with high-speed motor vehicle accidents or falls from a great height. The open wound is commonly found along the medial aspect of the hindfoot and may range in size from small to 4 to 5 cm in length. The wound is typically created as the calcaneal tuberosity shortens and displaces laterally through the primary fracture line: The sharp tip of the sustentaculum fragment pierces the medial soft tissues and skin.

Swelling and bleeding that occur at the time of fracture can result in elevated compartment pressures within the foot, particularly in the deep calcaneal compartment, and may lead to a compartment syndrome. It is important to remember that this can occur in both closed and open calcaneus fractures. The signs and symptoms of a compartment syndrome of the foot are the same as those in other areas of the body. The most common symptom is pain; and although most of these patients will have pain associated with the fracture, the pain associated with a compartment syndrome is generally more intense and commonly involves the entire foot and lower leg, not just the calcaneus. Compartment syndrome generally develops within the first 36 h after the fracture occurs (2).

Patients suspected of having a fracture of the calcaneus, particularly those who were involved in a fall from a significant height or high-speed motor vehicle accident, should undergo a thorough musculoskeletal examination.

Particular attention must be paid to the lower lumbar spine and contralateral hindfoot, because 5 to 10% of patients with a calcaneal fracture will have a concomitant lumbar spine compression fracture and 5% will have a contralateral calcaneus fracture. A thorough neurologic and vascular examination of the lower extremities must, of course, be carried out also.

The clinician should carefully examine the heel for any breaks in the skin, particularly along the medial aspect of the foot and ankle. A skin wound in the presence of a displaced calcaneal fracture indicates that the fracture is open; thus the injury should be treated emergently, with serial irrigation and débridement, intravenous antibiotics, fracture stabilization, and early soft tissue coverage.

RADIOLOGIC STUDIES

The diagnosis of a calcaneus fracture can generally be suspected based on the history and physical examination. Nevertheless, to confirm the presence of a calcaneus fracture and to characterize the fracture, a thorough radiographic evaluation must be undertaken. Radiographic evaluation in the emergency room includes AP, lateral, and oblique views of the foot and ankle, a mortise view of the ankle, and a Harris view of the heel. This series is generally sufficient to make the diagnosis of a calcaneus fracture. To confirm the presence of extension of the fracture into the posterior, middle, or anterior facets or the calcaneocuboid joint and to evaluate the displacement of the fracture fragments, additional radiographs are necessary. Broden views allow visualization of the posterior facet at several points. These views are taken with the patient supine, the ankle in neutral, and the leg internally rotated 45°.

Fractures of the calcaneus have long been recognized on radiographs, and important functional landmarks and relationships among them have been thoroughly described. The tuber joint angle of Böhler (the Böhler angle) is determined by measuring the intersection of two lines drawn on the lateral radiograph (Fig. 80.1). The first line is drawn from the anterior process of the calcaneus to the highest point of the posterior facet. The second line is drawn from the posterior-superior point of the tuberosity

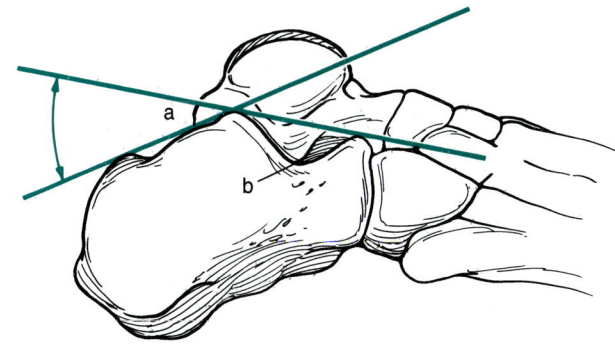

Figure 80.1. Böhler angle (a) and crucial angle of Gissane (b).

to the highest point of the posterior facet. The Böhler angle is the complement of the obtuse angle formed by these lines. A normal Böhler angle is 25° to 40° and is usually equal to the contralateral side. The Böhler angle represents the height of the calcaneus and typically approaches 0° in joint-depression calcaneal fractures.

The crucial angle of Gissane is also seen on the lateral radiograph and is determined by drawing two intersecting lines along the cortical struts visible beneath the lateral process of the talus. This angle is disrupted in intra-articular, joint-depression calcaneus fractures (3).

CT is commonly used to assess a fractured calcaneus. Images are usually taken in two planes (the axial and coronal planes) and 2-mm cuts through the articular surfaces are required (Fig. 80.4A). CT scans obtained in this fashion allow a complete assessment of the articular surfaces and morphology of the fractured calcaneus. The contralateral calcaneus can be scanned for comparison (4–7).

Classification

Numerous classification systems have been presented to describe calcaneus fractures. Such schemes have suffered from a lack of both accurate data and extensive intraoperative experience. Most of these systems are based on plain radiographs, which include a lateral view of the hindfoot, Broden views, and an axial view of the heel. A classification scheme based on CT studies of the fracture is being used widely in North America (5). Although this system is an improvement over those used in the past, it has

shortcomings. For example, the classification is based on CT studies taken in two distinct planes, thus the anterior process, the middle and anterior facets, and the anterior calcaneocuboid facet are not addressed. (4).

The classification scheme of Sanders et al. (5) is based on the coronal section, which is the widest undersurface area of the posterior facet of the talus (Fig. 80.2). Once this section is identified, the complementary surface of the posterior surface of the calcaneus is inspected. According to the Sanders classification, type I fractures are nondisplaced, regardless of the fracture pattern and number of fragments. Type II fractures are characterized by two fracture fragments that are at least 2 mm displaced. There are three subtypes, identified by the location of the primary fracture line (types IIA, IIB, and IIC). Type III fractures have three fracture fragments, each of which are at least 2 mm displaced. There are three subtypes, identified by the location of the primary fracture lines (types IIIAB, IIIAC, and IIIBC). Type IV fractures have more than two primary fracture lines and separate the posterior facet into four or more displaced fragments.

TREATMENT

Nonoperative Treatment and Indications for Surgery

Extra-articular fractures (e.g., anterior process fractures, fractures of the calcaneal tuberosity) and nondisplaced intra-articular fractures of the calcaneus can usually be

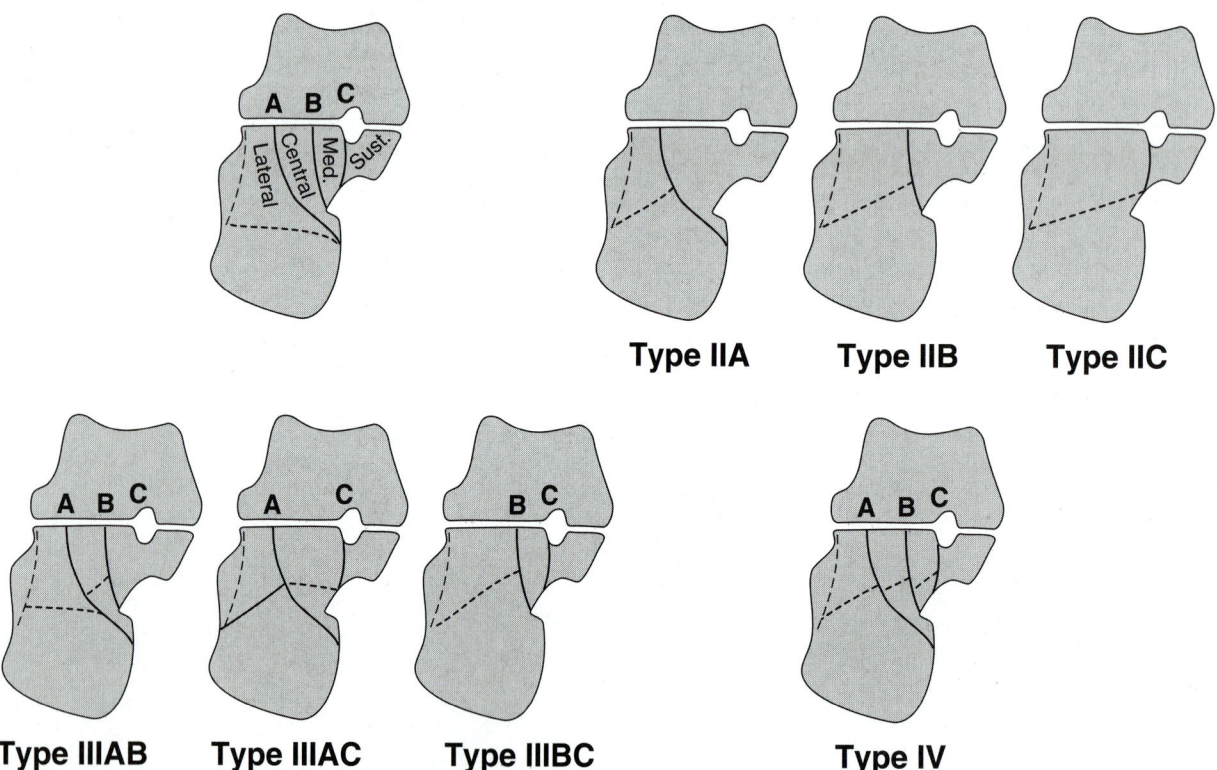

Figure 80.2. The Sanders classification of calcaneus fractures.

treated nonoperatively. This generally means early motion of the foot and ankle but protected weight bearing for 6 to 8 weeks. Symptomatic nonunion of anterior process fractures is not uncommon and may ultimately require operative stabilization or excision. Displaced calcaneal tuberosity fractures that contain a portion or all of the Achilles tendon attachment and those that tent the overlying skin posteriorly should be operatively stabilized to avoid ulceration, once soft tissue conditions permit.

Nondisplaced intra-articular calcaneal fractures (Sanders type I) can and should be treated nonoperatively. The initial assessment and management is the same as that described earlier and includes the application of a well-padded posterior U splint, with the ankle and foot in neutral position and alignment. The patient should be trained in the use of crutches and kept to toe-touch weight bearing. The patient should be informed of the possibility of a compartment syndrome and, if reliable, can be sent home from the emergency department. Once the initial discomfort has subsided, approximately 7 to 10 days after injury, the splint can be replaced with a removable walking boot, and a program of early ankle and subtalar motion should be initiated. The patient should maintain toe-touch weight bearing (20% body weight) for 6 weeks and then advanced to partial weight bearing (50% body weight) while continuing hindfoot and ankle motion. Muscle strengthening and proprioception training should be started at the time of partial weight bearing. Full weight bearing can begin at 12 weeks, if radiographs demonstrate bony union.

Nonoperative management of displaced intra-articular fractures of the calcaneus should be seriously considered for medically unfit patients and patients unwilling to accept the risk associated with open reduction and internal fixation (ORIF).

Surgical intervention is indicated for the treatment of displaced intra-articular calcaneal fractures in healthy individuals who, after being informed of the risks and benefits of both nonoperative and operative intervention, are willing to undergo ORIF. Some clinicians still find this statement controversial, even though ORIF, instead of nonoperative management, is indicated for almost all other intra-articular fractures of weight-bearing joints. ORIF is relatively contraindicated for patients who are unwilling to refrain from smoking during the postoperative period (smoking leads to healing problems) and patients with significant peripheral vascular disease (also compromises wound healing). Surgical management is absolutely contraindicated for patients who, because of other injuries or medical infirmity, are unable to tolerate surgical intervention; patients whose swelling does not resolve within 3 weeks after the injury; patients who have full-thickness blisters in the path of the proposed surgical incision; and patients who have persistent wounds or ulceration of the ankle and hindfoot areas.

Surgical indications include the presence of displaced intra-articular fractures of the posterior, middle, anterior, or calcaneocuboid facets; and the presence of significant lateral wall deformity, particularly when impingement of the peroneal tendons is obvious (on CT studies) or can be reasonably expected. Surgery is indicated when there is a loss of calcaneal height and length, which causes the talus to dorsiflex, resulting in impingement of the talus on the anterior tibia; furthermore, loss of calcaneal length can weaken the Achilles tendon plantar flexion mechanism. Without operative intervention, these deformities may result in considerable compromise of function and chronic pain. Late, salvage-type operative reconstruction of the calcaneus and hindfoot to correct these deformities after nonoperative treatment has failed is technically demanding and considerably more difficult than a subtalar arthrodesis in an otherwise normally shaped calcaneus (2,8).

Operative Treatment

Operative intervention for the displaced calcaneal fracture is designed to restore not only the articular surface(s) but also the normal calcaneal width, height, length, and alignment. The postoperative rehabilitation regimen should be designed to help restore motion of the subtalar and ankle joints. Motion is initiated after the incision appears to be healing without complication (Clinical Table: Calcaneus Fractures).

OPEN REDUCTION AND INTERNAL FIXATION

The timing of surgery is critical. Calcaneus fractures are associated with considerable soft tissue swelling and blister formation. Before operative intervention can be undertaken, the surrounding soft tissues must be given a chance to recover from the injury. Surgical intervention should be delayed until a significant decrease in the swelling and wrinkling of the skin of the foot and ankle has begun, usually within 5 to 7 days after the injury. Efforts should be made to operate within 21 days of the injury, beyond which surgical reconstruction is more difficult and results are not as reliable.

A radiolucent table is used with the patient in the lateral decubitus position with the uninjured side down. The contralateral hip and knee are flexed to keep the contralateral foot out of the x-ray field, and extra padding is placed beneath the proximal fibula to prevent peroneal nerve injury. The ipsilateral iliac crest and leg are also prepped and draped after a pneumatic tourniquet to the proximal thigh is applied.

Exposure of the posterior facet of the calcaneus is facilitated by placing a bump of rolled sheets beneath the medial malleolus, allowing the hindfoot to fall into varus. An L-shaped incision is made, half a finger's breadth anterior to the Achilles tendon and carried distally to the junction of the lateral and planar skin. It is then carried anteriorly along the line of demarcation between the lateral and plantar skin, to the level of the calcaneocuboid joint; it fin-

Clinical Table: Calcaneus Fractures

Procedure	Indications	Technique	Anatomy	Pitfalls
Nonoperative treatment	• Anterior process fractures • Tuberosity fractures • Extra-articular fractures • Nondisplaced intra-articular fractures (Sanders I)	• Short-term immobilization (7–10 days) • Limited (20% TTWB) weight bearing (6 weeks) • Early range of motion foot and ankle • Partial weight bearing (50%) after initial 6 weeks • Muscle strengthening, proprioceptive training • Full weight bearing begins at 12 weeks	• Anterior calcaneal process • Tuberosity • Anterior, middle, and posterior talocalcaneal articular facets	• Malalignment of fracture fragments
Open reduction and internal fixation	• Displaced (>2 mm) fractures of calcaneal facets, calcaneocuboid joint • Deformity of lateral calcaneal cortex • Varus alignment • Excessive shortening/flattening of calcaneus	• Lateral decubitus position • L-shaped lateral incision • Subperiosteal full-thickness flap • "No touch" technique • Reduction of articular fractures • Correction of alignment, length, height, width • Stable internal fixation plates and screws (small fragment and/or minifragment) • Meticulous soft tissue closure • Short-term immobilization (2 weeks)	• Lateral calcaneal artery • Sural nerve • Peroneus brevis tendons • Posterior tibial artery • Tibial nerve • Flexor hallucis longus	• Considerable learning curve • Soft tissue complications • Infection • Sural neuroma
Percutaneous osteosynthesis	• Relative articular congruity • Early treatment (<48°) • Severely compromised soft tissues Able to correct nonarticular deformity closed	• Distraction of fracture fragments (external fixator) • Reduction of articular fracture • Compression of lateral and medial walls • Correction of alignment • Percutaneous fixation (cannulated screws, wire)	• Sural nerve • Peroneus brevis tendons • Posterior tibial artery • Tibial nerve	• Considerable learning curve • Nonrigid fixation

TTWB, toe touch weight bearing.

ished by curving it dorsally. A full-thickness flap is maintained by subperiosteally elevating the soft tissues off the lateral aspect of the calcaneus.

Single and double skin hooks should be used to facilitate exposure, and the surgeon must refrain from grabbing the skin with pick-ups. A no-touch retraction technique, involving three 2.0-mm Kirschner (K) wires, is used. The first K wire is placed beneath the peroneal tendons (without exposing them) and driven up into the distal fibula, the second K wire is passed through the sinus tarsi and into the neck of the talus, and the third K wire is passed beneath the peroneal tendons, near the insertion of the brevis and into the cuboid. These three wires are then bent dorsally to allow retraction of the flap and exposure of the lateral surface of the calcaneus.

Further dissection is necessary to expose the anterior

process of the calcaneus to the calcaneocuboid joint. The lateral wall of the calcaneus is elevated and reflected posteriorly, leaving it hinged posteriorly, or is removed altogether and placed in saline on the back table (Fig. 80.3A). Once the lateral wall has been reflected, the impacted portions of the articular fragments of the posterior facets are visible. The organizing hematoma is removed from the subtalar joint and from between the articular fragments with a pituitary rongeur.

A 4.5- or 5.0-mm Schanz screw is placed in the inferior posterior corner of the tuberosity fragment and is used to draw the tuberosity out of varus, restore its length, and translate it medially (Fig. 80.3A). The tuberosity fragment can also be temporarily stabilized in this corrected posi-

tion by passing two K wires (1.62 mm) percutaneously from the tuberosity across the subtalar joint and up into the talus (Fig. 80.3B). The residual bony defect beneath the posterior facet must be assessed, and consideration should be given to the placement of a bone graft.

The articular fragments are reduced sequentially from medial to lateral and stabilized with 1.6-mm K wires to the medial sustentacular fragment. These wires should be positioned to allow placement of the interfragmentary lag screws (Fig. 80.3C). The adequacy of the reduction is assessed by using intraoperative fluoroscopy, including Broden views.

When the surgeon is satisfied with the reduction of the posterior facet, attention is turned to the anterior process

Figure 80.3. A. ORIF of a calcaneal fracture. *Numbers* indicate the steps for correction of the tuberosity displacement: *(1)* First, restore length; *(2)* second, correct varus alignment, and *(3)* correct lateral displacement. *Arrows* explain which way to pull the Schanz screw within the tuberosity. **B.** Temporary stabilization of calcaneal tuberosity in corrected position. *(continued)*

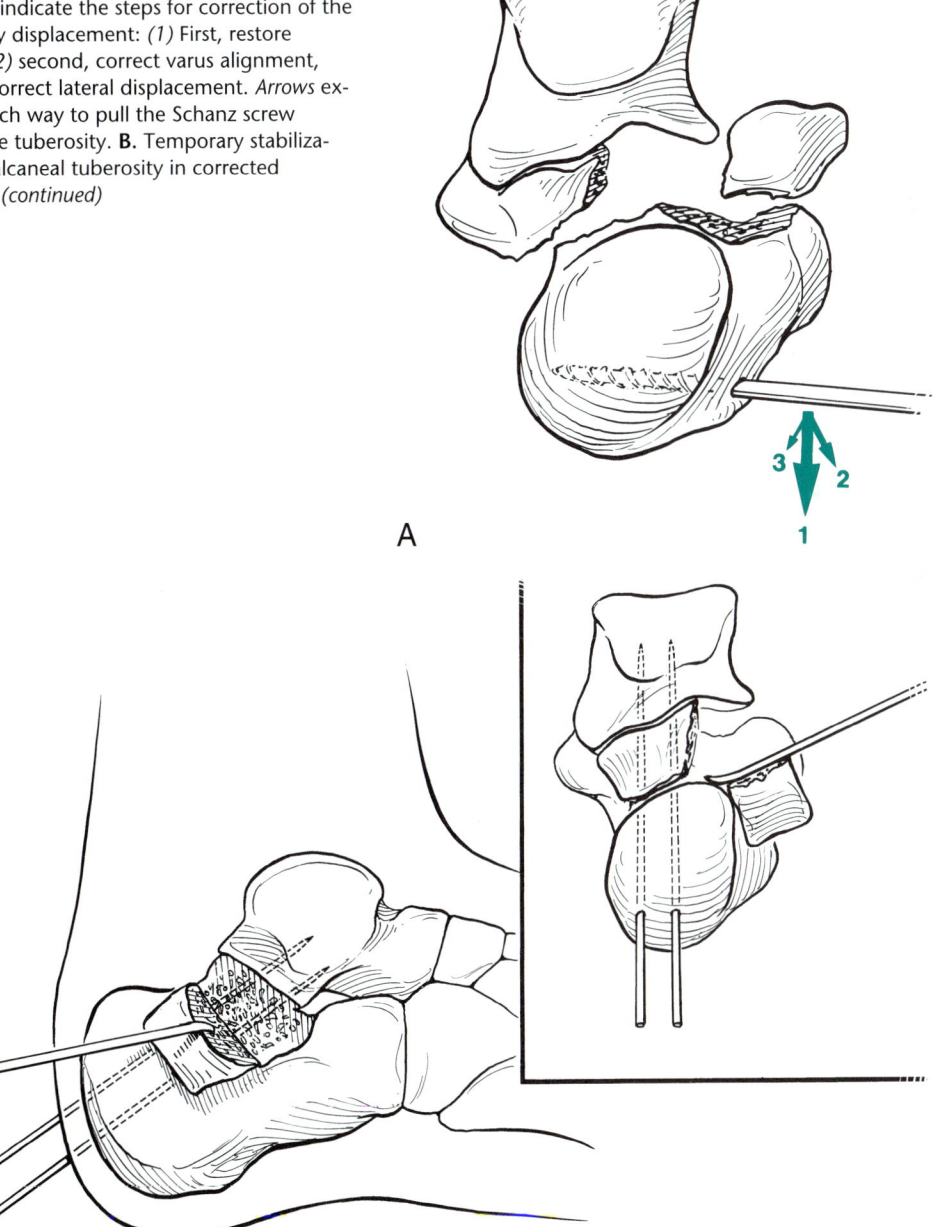

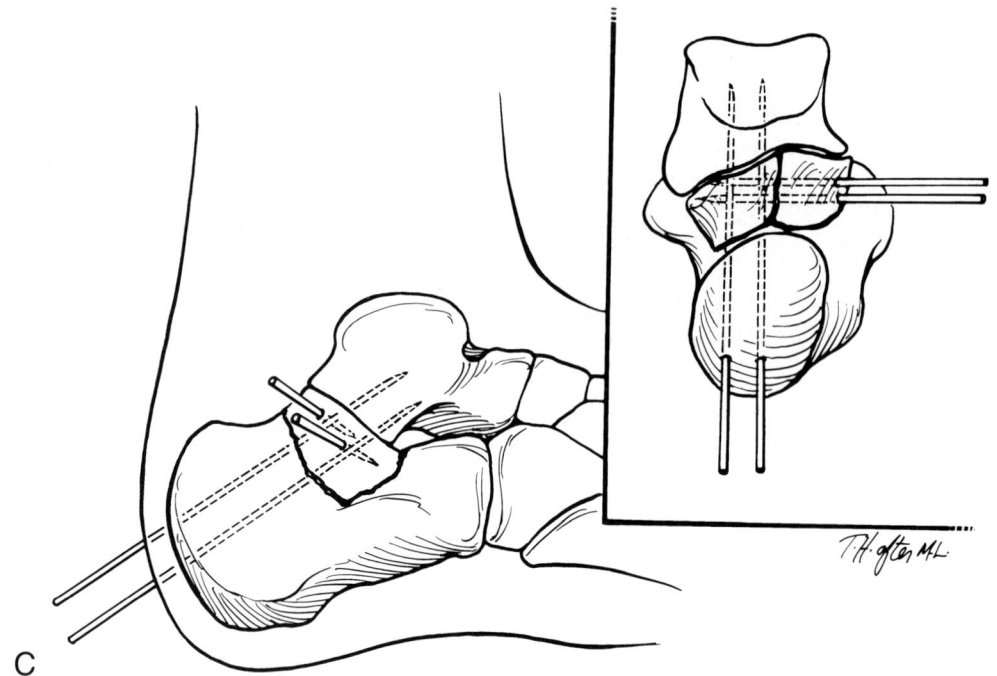

C

Figure 80.3. *Continued.* **C.** Temporary stabilization of anatomically reduced posterior calcaneal facet.

and tuberosity. The anterior process is usually manipulated with a dental pick or Weber reduction forceps (Synthes; Paoli, PA), until the angle of Gissane is reduced. This fragment is then temporarily stabilized to the "constant" medial fragment with a K wire.

The wound is copiously irrigated, the bone graft is placed, the lateral wall is replaced, and the implant is chosen. There are several available implants, including the anterior cervical spine plate, calcaneal plate, 3.5-mm pelvic reconstruction plate, and minifragment plate, all of which can be used alone or in combination. The design of the plate is probably of little clinical significance and attention should remain on the anatomic restoration of the articular surface and correction of the deformity. The calcaneus is securely fixed with a plate, and bicortical screws are placed along the lateral aspect of the calcaneus. The surgeon must take care when drilling to avoid injuring the medial neurovascular structures.

The wound is thoroughly irrigated, and bleeding vessels within the muscle are carefully cauterized. The wound is closed over a drain. A two-layered closure is performed with 2-0 absorbable suture for the subcutaneous tissue and 3-0 nylon for the skin. The Allgower modification of the Donati stitch with the knots on the inferior aspect of the incision minimizes soft tissue trauma.

After final plain radiographs are taken, a well-padded posterior U or trilaminar splint is applied with the ankle in neutral dorsiflexion. For the first 48 h, the patient receives intravenous antibiotics, and the drain remains in place. The wound is assessed at 72 h. The patient is placed in a removable cast or cast boot and taught toe-touch weight bearing with crutches. The sutures are left in place for 2 to 3 weeks, and active and active-assisted range of motion

exercises of the foot and ankle are started at the time of suture removal. The patient is kept toe-touch weight bearing for 6 weeks and then advanced to partial weight bearing for 6 weeks. Full weight bearing is generally allowed at 3 months (9).

PERCUTANEOUS OSTEOSYNTHESIS

To avoid the soft tissue complications associated with formal ORIF of displaced calcaneal fractures, techniques involving closed reduction and percutaneously placed internal fixation have been developed. It is important to perform the closed reduction within the first 48 h after the injury, before the hematoma begins to organize, which will prevent the fragments from moving. One of the more commonly used techniques involves reduction of the tuber-joint angle first by gradually applying distraction between the calcaneal tuberosity, the talus, and the cuboid with Schanz screws and an external fixator-like triangular device that is placed laterally. The reduction is achieved by distraction and is confirmed with intraoperative fluoroscopy. The lateral wall deformity is approached by using a Böhler clamp to compress the medial and lateral walls of the calcaneus, thus narrowing the heel and correcting the alignment. The reduction is achieved by inserting a thick K wire through a small laterally placed skin incision and levering the displaced lateral fragment until it is reduced to the medial fragment. The joint fragments are then fixed with percutaneously placed screws, gaining intrafragmentary compression. Once the entire calcaneus is reduced and the articular facet is stabilized, the rest of the calcaneus is fixed by means of long screws placed through small stab incisions over the heel and passed up into the body of the calcaneus (10).

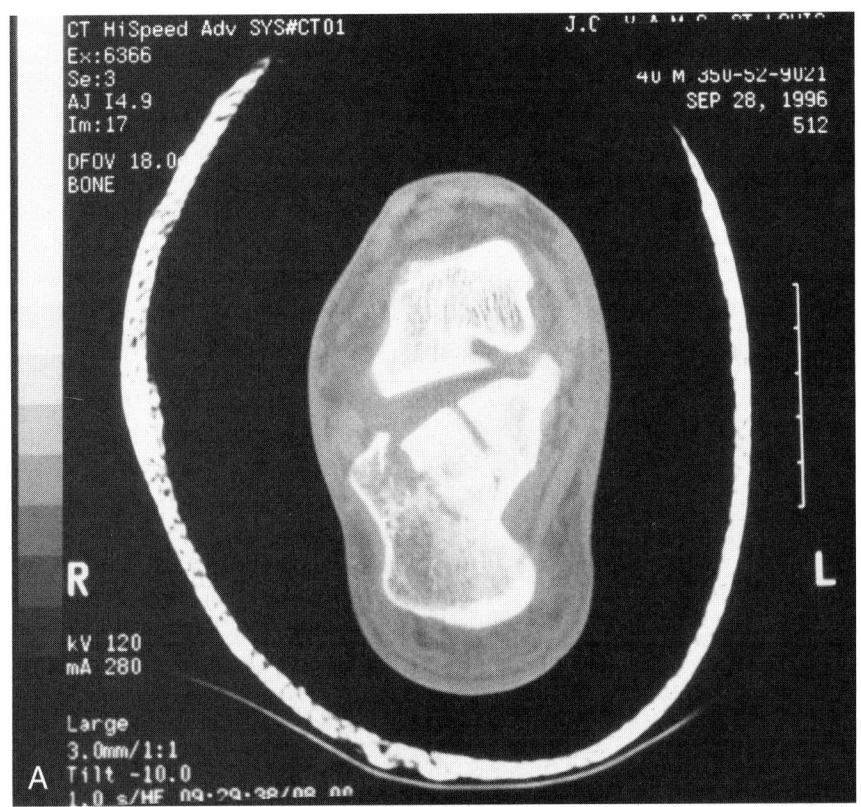

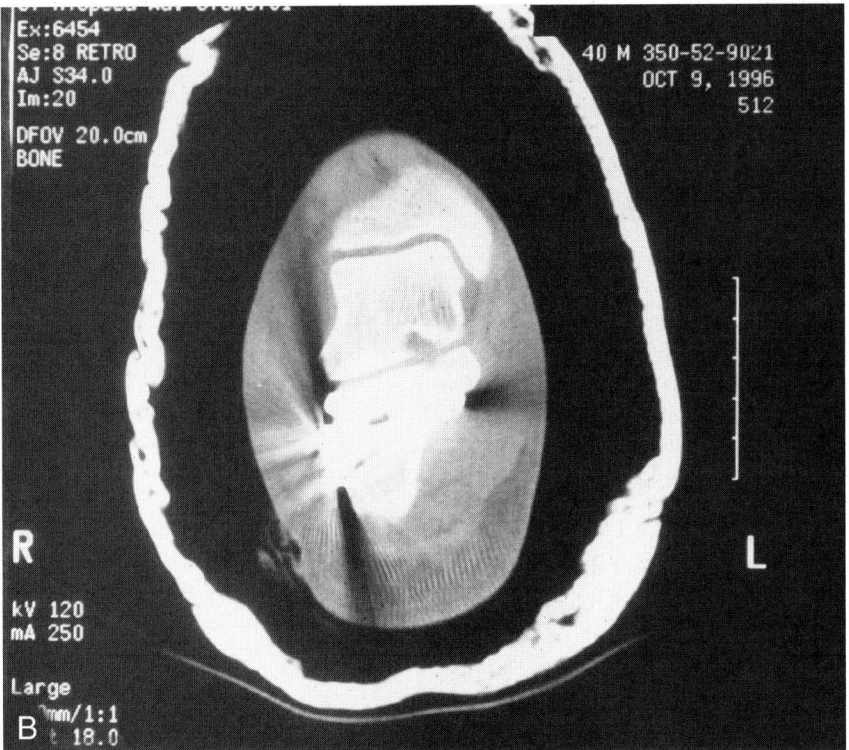

Figure 80.4. Preoperative (**A**) and postoperative (**B**) CT studies showing the restoration of the posterior facet of the subtalar joint.

EXTERNAL FIXATION

In the presence of an open calcaneal fracture, temporary stabilization can be obtained by applying a medially placed external fixator, with three medullary-placed Schanz screws, one each in the first metatarsal, the tuberosity of the calcaneus, and the medial distal tibia. This triangular frame allows distraction of the major fracture fragments and provides stability while the soft tissues are being managed. Calcaneal fractures have also been managed with thin wire external fixators, which have lead to inconsistent results.

PRIMARY SUBTALAR ARTHRODESIS

A technique that is gaining more widespread use and acceptance for the treatment of the severely comminuted and displaced calcaneal fracture is the primary subtalar fusion. This acceptance is the result of an honest evaluation of the long-term results of successful ORIF of these difficult fractures. This procedure is indicated for a Sanders type IV calcaneal fracture. The calcaneus undergoes ORIF with concomitant subtalar arthrodesis. The most common technical mistake is failure to restore the height and alignment of the calcaneus. Preliminary results of this procedure are encouraging (11,12).

SALVAGE

Salvage procedures for late collapse and/or subtalar arthrosis include in situ subtalar fusion and bone-block distraction subtalar arthrodesis. Because most patients lose a significant amount of subtalar motion after intra-articular calcaneal fractures, they often tolerate subtalar arthrodesis well.

COMPLICATIONS

Compartment syndrome occurs in up to 10% of cases and may lead to clawing of the toes or other foot deformity (2). Complications of nonoperative treatment include peroneal tendon impingement, stiffness, subtalar arthrosis, late collapse, and hindfoot varus. Complications related to operative management of calcaneus fractures include wound breakdown and sural and cutaneous nerve injury. Wound breakdown may lead to osteomyelitis if not caught early. The incidence of wound problems has been significantly reduced with the use of the no-touch lateral L-shaped incision, described above. Nevertheless, even this incision may be vulnerable to wound breakdown at the angle of the incision. Stiffness, late-collapse and subtalar arthritis may occur after either nonoperative or operative management of displaced intra-articular calcaneal fractures.

RESULTS

Nonoperative methods for the treatment of intra-articular calcaneal fractures have been used for many years and continue to make up a mainstay of management of these fractures around the world and in the United States.

Recently, several authors reported their results with nonoperative treatment of displaced intra-articular calcaneal fractures. The combined experience implies that the fractures with the least displacement and deformity are best treated with nonoperative techniques; when displaced and deformed calcaneal fractures are treated nonoperatively, persistent deformity, decreased function, and chronic pain are often seen.

Recently, the results of operative stabilization for the treatment of intra-articular calcaneal fractures have been reported. Bézes et al. (13) reported the results of 257 operatively treated intra-articular fractures of the calcaneus. They used an incision that extended from the base of the fifth metatarsal to close beneath the lateral malleolus. The peroneal tendon sheath was entered, and the tendons, sural nerve, and lesser saphenous vein were retraced proximally. The fracture fragments were reduced through this window and stabilized with small fragment tubular plates. With an average of 3.25 years of follow-up for 205 cases, the functional results were considered good to excellent in 85% of cases; the infection rate was just 2.7%, and only 6 patients required a late subtalar arthrodesis. Letournel (14) noted that most patients lost at least half of their subtalar motion.

Zwipp et al. (9) looked at the operative results of displaced intra-articular fractures of the calcaneus in 123 patients. They found 61% of patients experienced good to excellent results, 8.3% developed superficial wound necrosis, 1.9% became infected, 1.3% experienced nonunion.

As discussed earlier, Sanders et al. (5) reported results of a prognostic CT scan classification system for 120 displaced intra-articular calcaneal fractures. They were able to restore heel height in 98% of cases, heel length in 100% and heel width in 100%. These authors reported anatomic radiographic reduction of type II fractures for 85% of patients. The clinical outcome for type II fractures was 77% good to excellent, 10% fair, and 13% poor. For type III fractures, the authors noted only 60% radiographic reduction, and the clinical results were 70% good to excellent, 10% fair, and 20% were poor. No anatomic reductions were reported for type IV fractures, and only 9% of patients noted good to excellent results. A total of 18% of cases had a fair result, and 73% had poor results. The authors concluded that anatomic reduction was needed to obtain a good or excellent result and that results deteriorated as the number of fracture fragments increased.

SUMMARY

Fractures of the calcaneus are often the result of high-energy trauma and, as such, are associated with significant concomitant injuries. A high level of suspicion for soft tissue injury and compartment syndrome must be maintained when managing these fractures acutely. Calcaneus fractures are best managed with thorough radiographic delineation and immobilization while the soft tissues recover and a preoperative plan is formulated. The classification of the fracture and the indications for surgery should be clear to the surgeon. The risks and benefits of surgical intervention should be explained to the patient. The operative goals are anatomic restoration of the articular surface and restoration of calcaneal height, width, and length. Respect for the soft tissues is of paramount importance before, during, and after surgery.

II   Talus Fractures

The talus plays an important role in the motion and transmission of forces in the hindfoot. Fractures of the talus have been recognized for hundreds of years; and because of their associated morbidity, these fractures are among the most dreaded by orthopaedists (15–17). Because more than 60% of the talus is covered with articular cartilage, fractures of the talus often lead to substantial loss of motion and posttraumatic arthritis (17–19). These fractures may be further complicated by disruption of the talus's tenuous blood supply and the development of avascular necrosis (AVN) (20). Fortunately, fractures of the talus are relatively uncommon, making up only about 0.32% of all fractures and 3.4% of all foot fractures (21–23).

This section reviews the anatomy, mechanism, classification, treatment options, and methods used for fractures of the talus. The common treatment pitfalls and possible complications following fractures of the talar head, neck, and body are also discussed.

RELEVANT ANATOMY AND PATHOGENESIS

The talus may be conveniently divided into three distinct areas, each with its own important contribution to the function of the ankle, subtalar, and talonavicular joints. The head of the talus is positioned anteriorly and medially; it is covered almost entirely with articular cartilage. This cartilage articulates with the navicular anteriorly and the calcaneonavicular ligament and anterior facet of the calcaneus inferiorly.

The neck of the talus lies posterior and lateral to the head. It serves as a point of attachment for the talonavicular joint capsule anteriorly, the ankle joint capsule posteriorly, the talonavicular ligaments medially, the extensor retinaculum laterally, and the talocalcaneal interosseous ligament inferiorly. Each of these structures contributes to the stability of the talus. The neck of the talus forms the roof of the sinus tarsi and tarsal canal and is perforated by numerous nutrient vessels.

The body, or dome, of the talus lies posterior to the neck and articulates with the tibial plafond superiorly and the calcaneus, through the posterior facet, inferiorly. The talar dome is wider anteriorly than posteriorly. Dorsiflexion of the talus places the body snugly within the ankle mortise. Plantar flexion, however, positions only the relatively narrow portion of the talus in the ankle mortise, resulting in increased motion between the talus and tibia. Laterally, the body articulates with the distal fibula and serves as a point of attachment for the talocalcaneal ligament and for the anterior and posterior talofibular ligaments. Medially, the talus articulates with the medial malleolus and has several foramina for penetration of nutrient vessels. It is at the posteromedial aspect of the talus that the deep portion of the deltoid ligament attaches. Posteriorly, the talus has two tubercles that form a sulcus through which the flexor hallucis longus tendon travels; the posterolateral tubercle is the larger of the two; it may be in continuity with the inferior articular facet and may be found in association with an os trigonum.

The blood supply of the talus has been studied extensively because of the high incidence AVN following fractures and dislocations of the talus (24). The talus gets its blood supply from each of the three prominent vessels in the lower extremity: the anterior and posterior tibial arteries and the peroneal artery. Branches of the anterior tibial artery (dorsalis pedis) and the medial tarsal artery penetrate the superior neck of the talus directly. The lateral malleolar artery, a branch of the dorsalis pedis artery, anastomoses with a perforating branch of the peroneal artery to become the artery of the tarsal sinus. The peroneal artery also contributes to the blood supply of the talus through branches that join the calcaneal branches of the posterior tibial artery to form a vascular plexus over the posterior tubercles of the talus. The artery of the tarsal canal, a branch of the posterior tibial artery that originates approximately 1 cm proximal to the take-off of the medial and lateral plantar arteries, gives rise to the deltoid branch, which passes to the medial aspect of the talus.

The artery of the tarsal canal (from the posterior tibial artery), the artery of the sinus tarsi (from the dorsalis pedis artery), and the medial periosteal vessels (from the posterior tibial artery) are believed to be the most important contributions to the blood supply of the talus. The interosseous blood supply, and its disruption with fractures and dislocations, is also thought to have an influence on the development of avascular necrosis.

INITIAL FINDINGS, PHYSICAL EXAMINATION, AND DIAGNOSIS

Patients with fractures of the talus complain of pain and swelling in the area of the hindfoot and ankle. They are almost always unable to bear weight on the affected foot. On physical examination there is typically significant swelling, ecchymosis, and deformity. The overall appearance of the foot and ankle depend on the displacement of the fracture fragments and direction of the dislocation. If the body of the talus is dislocated anteriorly, it is often palpable just beneath the skin in the area just anterior to the distal fibula. It is in these cases that the typical open fracture-dislocation occurs. If closed, early reduction is necessary to avoid local ischemia of the skin and significant soft tissue compromise. In posterior fracture-dislocations, the body of the talus dislocates medially or laterally to the Achilles tendon. With a posteromedial fracture-dislocation, the long toe flexors may be tented over the dislocated talus, resulting in a fixed flexion deformity of the toes. The posteromedial neurovascular structures may also be compromised, resulting in paresthesias distally.

Open fracture-dislocations are relatively common, are easily diagnosed, and may represent as many as 44% of all major fracture-dislocations of the talus (21). Because of the significant risk of infection, AVN, and nonunion, these injuries represent an extreme emergency. Prompt open reduction, thorough irrigation and débridement, internal fixation, and early soft tissue coverage should be undertaken.

Concomitant musculoskeletal injuries are common with fracture-dislocations of the talus. Associated fractures of the medial malleolus are common, particularly with displaced fractures of the talar neck (25%). Some authors believed that a concomitant fracture of the medial malleolus is beneficial, in that the deltoid ligament branch of the posterior tibial artery is often uninjured, thus preserving some blood supply to the talar body.

RADIOLOGIC STUDIES

The initial radiographic evaluation of talus fractures includes an AP view, a mortise or oblique view, and a lateral view of the ankle. Broden views to evaluate the subtalar joint, may be helpful in preoperative planning and for assessing reduction. The AP and mortise views usually demonstrate the talus within the mortise, vertical fractures of the body, and ankle subluxation or dislocation. Fractures of the medial malleolus are clearly visualized on the AP and mortise views. The lateral view of the ankle images talar neck or head fractures. The lateral film should be carefully inspected to assess subluxation of the subtalar and tibiotalar joints. Even the most minimally displaced fracture of the talar neck may be associated with subluxation of the subtalar joint. This subluxation and displacement must be corrected to restore the normal mechanics of the subtalar joint and to minimize the chance of posttraumatic arthritis.

CT studies can assess the pattern of fractures of the head, neck, and body of the talus, as well as the congruity of the subtalar joint. CT allows a more detailed evaluation of the articular surfaces. Three-dimensional reconstructions of the CT scans may help the surgeon further understand the fracture geometry and fracture fragment orientation.

Classification

Classification of fractures of the talus is based on the anatomic location of the fracture and the degree of fracture displacement.

TALAR HEAD FRACTURES

Talar head fractures account for 5 to 10% of all talus fractures (21). They generally result from axial compression or impingement of the talar head on the anterior aspect of the distal tibia with forced dorsiflexion of the foot. These fractures are often associated with midfoot instability, including instability of the calcaneocuboid and subtalar joints. There is no commonly used classification of talar head fractures. Treatment of these injuries is based primarily on the size, number, and displacement of the fracture fragments and the presence of associated injuries and instability.

TALAR NECK FRACTURES

Fractures of the talar neck represent 50% of all fractures of the talus. Approximately 65% are associated with other musculoskeletal injuries, and 16 to 44% are open fractures (20–22). Fractures of the talar neck are three times more common in men than in women. They most commonly occur when the ankle is forcibly dorsiflexed, causing the vulnerable neck of the talus to impinge against the anterior lip of the distal tibia. Axial injury is a less common mechanism. The most widely used classification scheme considers displacement of the fracture along with subluxation or dislocation of the talocalcaneal, tibiotalar, and talonavicular joints (Fig. 80.5) (Table 80.1). This classification system, developed by Hawkins (20) and later modified by Canale and Kelly (18), not only provides a guide for treatment but is also somewhat prognostic (19,21).

Hawkins type I fractures are generally low-energy, closed injuries in which the talar neck has been fractured but has remained nondisplaced. The actual amount of displacement of the fracture fragments at the time of injury is essentially unknown but it is probably safe to say that the fragments probably did not travel much farther than they appear on the initial radiographs. The vascular leash around the neck of the talus may have been disrupted, however; and this may account for the approximately 10% incidence of avascular necrosis that has been reported with this type of injury.

Although the overall prognosis of type I injuries is good, radiographs and CT scans must be scrutinized for the presence of any subluxation of the surrounding joints, particularly the subtalar joint. If subluxation of the subtalar joint is present, it is assumed that the talar neck fracture has some degree of displacement or that instability of the hindfoot or midfoot is present. Rotation of the head fragment may have occurred, resulting in malposition of the

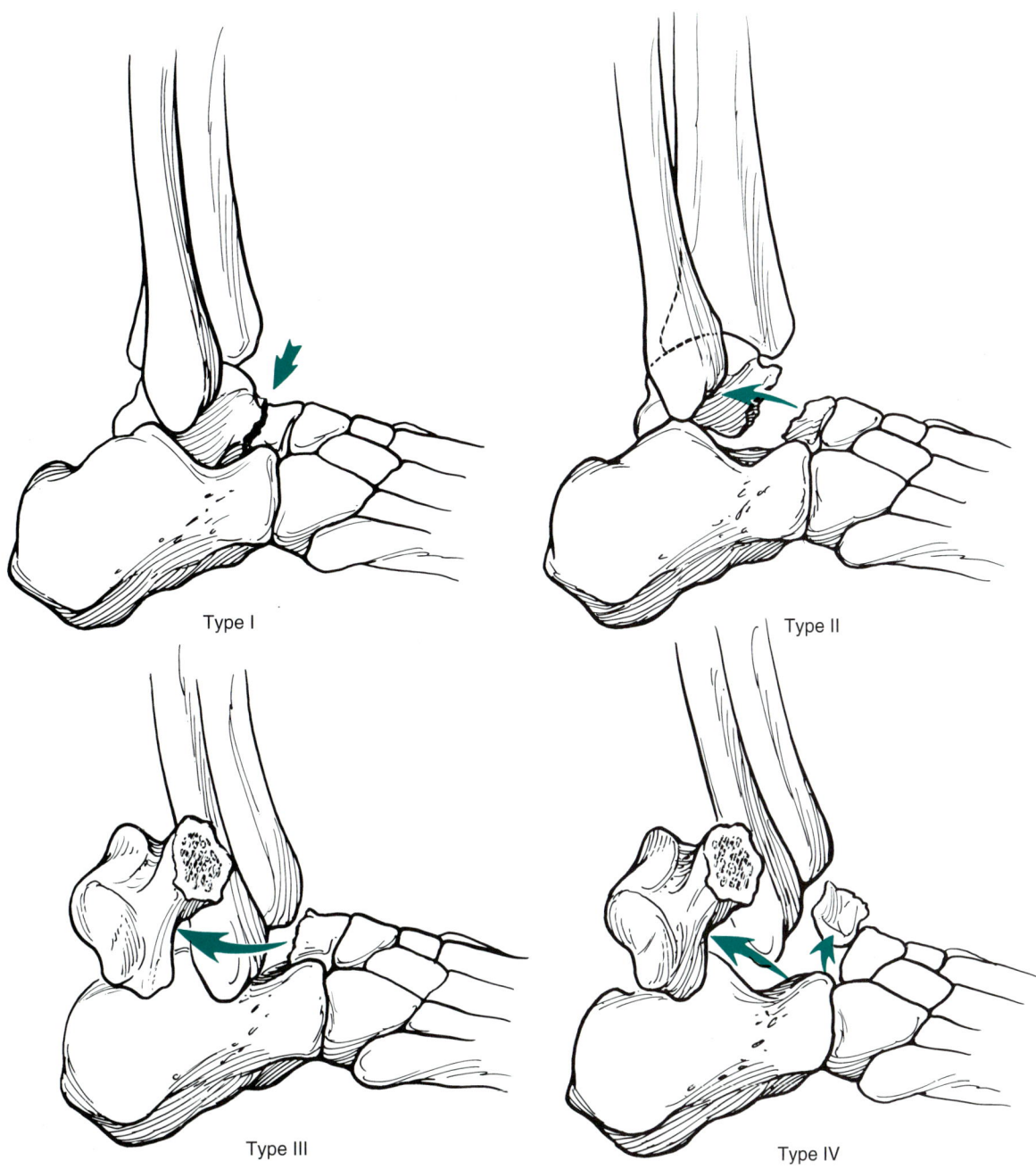

Figure 80.5. Classification of talar neck fractures.

table	80.1	Talar Neck Fractures

Type	Description
I	Nondisplaced; neck vessels disrupted
II	Subtalar subluxation or dislocation; normal ankle joint; anastomosis sinus tarsi disrupted (neck and tarsal canal vessels)
III	Subtalar and tibiotalar subluxation or dislocation; neck, tarsal canal, and medial deltoid vessels injured
IV	Subtalar, tibiotalar, and talonavicular joint subluxation or dislocation

hindfoot, even though the fracture does not appear displaced. This malrotation can be better evaluated on the oblique view of the foot, as described by Canale and Kelly (18). This view can also help evaluate the presence of talar head fractures.

Type II fractures include a displaced fracture of the talar neck and an associated subluxation or dislocation of the subtalar joint. In this fracture pattern, the tibiotalar joint remains intact with no evidence of injury. These fracture-dislocations are easily seen on plain radiographs, particularly on the lateral view; but the entire series must be scrutinized to identify the presence of concomitant injuries, most particularly those of the ankle (medial malleolus fractures) and midfoot joints. CT scans are commonly employed to further evaluate these injuries and to better assess comminution and articular involvement. Type II injuries are generally associated with significant disruption of both the extraosseous and intraosseous blood supplies and as such have been associated with AVN rates as high as 20%. These fracture-dislocations should be treated emergently to minimize ischemia of the talus and the risk of avascular necrosis of the body of the talus.

Type III fractures are characterized by displaced fractures of the talar neck with subluxation or dislocation of both the tibiotalar and subtalar joints. Radiographic evaluation of these fractures is generally all that is necessary, as the AP and mortise views of the ankle clearly demonstrate the tibiotalar dislocation, and the lateral view demonstrates the talar neck fracture and the disruption of the subtalar joint. These radiographs should be scrutinized for the presence of other skeletal injuries. Again, CT scans are helpful, but not always necessary. Because type III fractures significantly compromise the extraosseous and intraosseous blood supply of the talus, and possibly the posteromedial neurovascular structures and overlying skin, emergent reduction and internal fixation of the subtalar and tibiotalar joints should be performed. The AVN rate following these injuries is between 70 and 100%.

Type IV fractures, as described by Canale and Kelly (18), include displaced fractures of the talar neck and dislocation of the tibiotalar, subtalar, and talonavicular joints. These fractures are relatively uncommon and are particularly difficult to manage because of the significant instability of the fracture fragments and the near complete disruption of the intraosseous and extraosseous blood supply. Type IV fractures are easily visualized on the initial radiographs and must undergo emergent reduction and stabilization to minimize ischemia of the talus (18).

FRACTURES OF THE TALAR BODY

Fractures of the body of the talus make up 13 to 23% of all talus fractures (21). The rate of avascular necrosis is lower than with fractures of the talar neck and has been correlated with the degree of soft tissue injury and fracture pattern. Fractures of the talar body include fractures of the articular surface, the talar body itself, the posterior tubercles, and the lateral process. These fractures have been classified by Sneppen et al. (25) (Table 80.2). Sneppen type I fractures are transchondral fractures of the talar dome; and type II fractures are coronal, sagittal, or horizontal fractures of the talar dome. Type III fractures are fractures of the posterior tubercle (20%), and fractures of the lateral process are type IV fractures (24%). Type V fractures are crush fractures of the talar dome.

Transchondral fractures of the talar body commonly occur in the anterolateral aspect of the dome after a dorsi-

table	80.2	Talar Body Fractures
Type		Description
I		Transchondral (osteochondral lesions)
II		Coronal, sagittal, and horizontal shear
III		Posterior tubercle
IV		Lateral process
V		Crush

flexion and inversion injury and occasionally occur with ankle sprains (6.5%) (26). Posteromedial transchondral fractures, which occur with plantar flexion and inversion, may be visualized on plain radiographs but are best visualized by MRI or CT scans.

TREATMENT

Nonoperative Treatment and Indications for Surgery

After the physical examination and radiographic assessment are performed and a diagnosis of talar fracture is made, a definitive treatment plan can be developed. Talar head fractures, type I talar neck fractures, and minimally displaced fractures of the talar body are usually immobilized in a splint, and the patient is admitted to the hospital. The limb is elevated, and the patient is observed for any evidence of a compartment syndrome.

Nonoperative treatment includes a short leg cast, which is applied once swelling has subsided. Toe-touch weight bearing (approximately 9 kg) should be initiated. Patients may be advanced to partial weight bearing (22.5 kg) at about 6 weeks after injury. At that time, a removable cast/boot is applied. Active-assisted and passive range of motion exercises of the foot and ankle should be initiated. Patients are advanced to full weight bearing at approximately 3 months, at which time aggressive range of motion and muscle strengthening are begun.

Displaced intra-articular fractures of the talus should be treated in a similar manner as other intra-articular fractures of weight-bearing joints. If the displaced (more than 2 mm) articular fragments are large enough for stable internal fixation with available implants, they should be reduced and fixed. If the articular fragments are too small for stable internal stabilization, they should be excised.

Isolated type I fractures of the talar neck can be treated nonoperatively as long as care is taken to ensure there is no displacement or malrotation of the fracture or subluxation of the subtalar joint. The ankle should be immobilized in a short leg cast, and the patient should begin toe-touch weight bearing. Types II, III and IV fractures of the talar neck are usually treated with emergent ORIF. Theoretically, the sooner the fracture fragments are reduced and the blood supply restored, the less the chance of AVN and other complications. An anatomic reduction of the talar neck must be obtained to ensure reduction of the subtalar and ankle joints, which is necessary to restore normal joint mechanics of the hindfoot.

Other indications for ORIF are open fractures (following a thorough irrigation and débridement) and neurologic or vascular injury. In cases of neurovascular compromise, the fracture should be reduced and stabilized to protect any vascular repair and to avoid further injury.

Treatment of fractures of the talar body and dome can be quite challenging. Nevertheless, these fractures should be approached as other intra-articular fractures: When there is more than 2 mm of displacement, ORIF should be attempted. Transchondral fractures can often be treated with excision and drilling or freshening of the bed to stimulate the ingrowth of fibrocartilage into the defect. This can often be accomplished arthroscopically but may require an arthrotomy.

Operative Treatment

Displaced intra-articular talar head fractures, Hawkins types III and IV fractures, and crush or comminuted fractures of the talar body are typically treated operatively. In most cases, active and active-assisted range of motion of the foot and ankle are started about 48 h after surgery, although weight bearing is prohibited for 6 to 12 weeks. Early range of motion is begun to avoid arthrofi-

brosis and permanent loss of motion (Clinical Table: Talus Fractures).

TALAR HEAD FRACTURES

The approach for ORIF of fractures of the talar head is usually dictated by the location and size of the fracture fragments and the local anatomy. If the fracture comprises the medial aspect of the head of the talus, an anteromedial approach is performed to allow direct visualization and anatomical reduction and internal fixation of the fracture fragments. On the other hand, fractures of the lateral aspect of the talar head are approached through the sinus tarsi, similar to the one used for subtalar lesions. Fracture fragments are reduced and stabilized, preferably with screws. The smallest fragments should probably be excised, but care should be taken to assess the talonavicular joint stability before aggressive débridement of a talar head fracture is undertaken.

TALAR NECK FRACTURES

Type I talar neck fractures are typically treated nonoperatively and are at low risk for displacement or complication. The primary goals of operative stabilization of types II, III, and IV fractures are anatomic reduction of the talar neck; anatomic reduction of the subtalar, tibiotalar, and talonavicular joints; and stable fixation of the fracture to allow early motion of the ankle and hindfoot. As the degree

Clinical Table: Talus Fractures

Procedure	Indications	Technique	Anatomy	Pitfalls
Open reduction and internal fixation	• Displaced intra-articular fractures • Displaced talar neck fractures • Fracture dislocations of the talus	• Medial and lateral approaches • Osteotomy of medial malleolus • Stable internal fixation (small fragment screws, cannulated screws)	• Superficial peroneal nerve • Toe extensor tendons • Anterior tibialis	• Wound complications • Avascular necrosis • Nonunion • Posttraumatic arthritis
Nonoperative management	• Avulsion fractures • Nondisplaced talar head fractures • Type I talar neck fractures	• Well-padded splint • Ice, elevation, observation • Short-leg toe-touch weight-bearing cast • Close radiographic follow-up • Advance to partial weight bearing cast at 6 weeks • Range of motion, muscle strengthening, weight bearing as tolerated at 3 months	• Talar head • Talar neck • Talar body • Capsular ligaments	• Ankle stiffness • Avascular necrosis • Nonunion • Posttraumatic arthritis

of displacement of the fracture fragments increases, the need for emergent reduction and stabilization of the talus increases.

The fractured talus can be approached, reduced, and stabilized via an anterolateral (sinus tarsi) and/or antero-medial approach. The anteromedial approach, however, may further compromise the already vulnerable vascularity and does not allow for optimal screw placement and orientation for compression across the fracture site. The posterolateral approach minimizes the risk to the already attenuated blood supply and allows the screws to be placed perpendicular to the fracture and into the talar head.

The patient is placed in the lateral position on the operating table, with the uninjured side down, with the foot and ankle extending slightly beyond the edge of the table. Types III and IV fractures may require calcaneal pin traction to provide adequate distraction for the reduction of the tibiotalar joint. Reduction of type II fractures is achieved by plantar flexion to align the talar head and neck with the plantar flexed body. Eversion tends to bring the fracture out of varus alignment. The reduction is checked with fluoroscopy in the anteroposterior and lateral planes, as well as with live fluoroscopy.

A 6- to 8-cm incision is made lateral to the Achilles tendon, extending distally to the calcaneal tubercle. The sural nerve is identified and retracted laterally, and the flexor hallucis longus is retracted medially. The lateral process of the talus is palpable lateral to the flexor hallucis longus. Two 2.0-mm guidepins are drilled from the posterolateral body of the talus, across the fracture site, and into the talar head; the position of these pins is confirmed with fluoroscopy. The appropriate screw length is determined, and the pins are sequentially replaced with cannulated, short-threaded, 4.5-mm cancellous screws. Titanium screws allow for better visualization on MRI than do stainless steel pins; MRI is used to assess the development of postoperative AVN.

A drain is placed, and the skin is closed with nylon suture. A well-padded trilaminar splint is placed with ankle in the neutral position. Patients are kept non-weight bearing so the talar neck can heal without collapsing. The stability of the fixation should allow for early range of motion without weight bearing.

FRACTURES OF THE TALAR BODY

The approach for ORIF of fractures of the talar body is dictated by the type and location of the fractures. Sneppen types II and IV talar body fractures are best treated through an anterior or anteromedial extensile approach to permit direct visualization of the fracture fragments. An osteotomy of the medial malleolus is preferred to disruption of the deltoid ligament in order to maintain the integrity of the deltoid branch of the posterior tibial artery. The primary goals of surgery should be reduction of the talar articular surface and stable internal fixation with repair of the medial malleolus.

Internal fixation can be obtained from a host of implants, including small-fragment screws (3.5 mm), minifragment screws (2.0, 2.7 mm), Herbert or Herbert-Whipple screws, and absorbable pins. Small-diameter smooth K wires can be used to maintain the reduction of the osteochondral fragments during operative stabilization; but these smooth pins cannot be used to gain interfragmentary compression, and therefore, their use should be limited. Countersinking the screw heads is important when the screws are placed on the articular surface.

Débridement of the small unreconstructable cartilage fragments is often necessary. In addition to the reduction of the articular surfaces, an anatomical reduction of the subtalar and ankle joints must also be obtained. Finally, the osteotomized medial malleolus must be anatomically reduced and fixed to allow early range of motion of the ankle joint.

A lateral sinus tarsi approach can be used if the fracture involves the lateral aspect of the talar body and/or the lateral process of the talus. The lateral aspect of the talar body can also be treated with an osteotomy of the lateral malleolus through a direct lateral approach. We do not recommend this approach, however, because the anterior tibiofibular ligaments and a portion of the interosseous membrane or ligament must be taken down to allow the distal fibula to be booked open.

PITFALLS AND COMMON TECHNICAL MISTAKES

Because of the high-energy nature of these injuries and subsequent swelling, the soft tissues around the foot and ankle are compromised at the time of injury. Therefore, the soft tissues must be treated with great respect and patience to avoid surgical disasters. Thus the timing of the surgery, the approach chosen, and the soft tissue handling during the surgery and closure must be done with the utmost of care. Open fractures or dislocations of the talus and closed Hawkins types III and IV fractures require immediate operative intervention, even though further soft tissue compromise is possible, which may delay soft tissue coverage. For closed fractures of the talar head and body, when there is no tenting of the skin by the fracture fragments, operative stabilization should be performed within 4 to 6 h of the injury or delayed until the surrounding soft tissues have had the opportunity to recover.

REHABILITATION

Protected weight bearing while maintaining range of motion is the mainstay of the postoperative regimen. Patients are generally kept toe-touch weight bearing for 6 weeks, but the highest-energy fractures are protected for up to 12 weeks. Toe-touch weight bearing is often followed by a 4- to 6-week period of partial weight bearing, if radiographic evidence of healing is present. At 12 weeks, patients are usually advanced to full weight bearing, if radiographic evidence of healing is present, if there has been

table	80.3	Incidence of Avascular Necrosis by Type of Talar Neck Fracture[a]

Hawkins Type	Incidence of AVN (%)
I	0–13
II	20–50
III	80–100

[a]Overall incidence = 50%.

no change in the reduction or position of the implants, and if revascularization has occurred.

Results

Outcome following fractures of the talar head, neck, and body are variable and are influenced by the fracture pattern, the associated injuries, the adequacy of the treatment, and any complications. The crescent sign, a subchondral lucency seen on plain radiographs at 6 to 8 weeks after injury, indicates revascularization. Nonunion or delayed union of fractures of the talus occur in 0 to 10% of cases, depending on the energy of the trauma at the time of fracture and the subsequent development of avascular necrosis.

A clear correlation between the development of AVN and the type of talar neck fracture has been established (20) (Table 80.3). Hawkins type I talar neck fractures have an incidence of 13%; type II fractures, 50%; and type III fractures close to 100%. When present, AVN does not necessarily involve the entire body of the talus, nor is it necessarily clinically relevant. The distribution of the avascular segment reflects the injury to the nutrient vessels and the pattern of revascularization. Most surgeons recommend protecting the avascular talus until revascularization begins in an effort to avoid collapse of the talar body. this may necessitate prolonged periods of protected weight bearing and ultimately may not prevent the talus from ultimate collapse and the development of posttraumatic arthritis. Remember that the amount of involvement may be variable, and most likely depends on the nutrient vessels that remain patent following the fracture.

The most common position for a malunion of the talus is varus and dorsiflexion. This position causes a loss of accommodation through the midtarsal joints and alteration in weight-bearing forces within the subtalar joint. Subtalar arthrosis has been reported to occur in almost 50% of patients when talar varus is allowed to persist. The full effects of varus malunion on forefoot and hindfoot motion have been investigated in a cadaver model (27).

SUMMARY

Fractures of the talus can take many different forms. Typically, fractures that occur as a result of high-energy trauma are the most difficult to treat and are associated with the greatest number of concomitant injuries and complications. To restore blood supply after a fracture-dislocation of the talar neck, prompt reduction of the fracture fragments is necessary to avoid AVN and posttraumatic arthritis. ORIF of displaced fractures of the talar head, neck, and body is becoming routine. The proper respect must be accorded to the soft tissues in regard to both the timing of surgery and the intraoperative handling. A postoperative protocol must be developed to allow early range of motion of the ankle and subtalar joints while the fractures are healing. Posttraumatic arthritis is initially treated nonoperatively with orthotics and shoe modification. If this fails to relieve symptoms, arthrodesis of the degenerative joints should be considered.

REFERENCES

1. Essex-Lopresti P. The mechanism, reduction technique and results in fractures of the os calcis. Br J Surg 1952;39:395–419.
2. Manoli A II, Weber TG. Fasciotomy of the foot: an anatomical study with special reference to release of the calcaneal compartment. Foot Ankle 1990;11:54–55.
3. Hall RL, Shereff MJ. Anatomy of the calcaneus. Clin Orthop 1993;290:27–35.
4. Broden B. Roentgen examination of the subtaloid joint in fractures of the calcaneus. Acta Radiol 1949;31:85–91.
5. Sanders R, Fortin P, DiPasquale T, Walling A. Operative treatment in 120 displaced intraarticular calcaneal fractures. Results using a prognostic computed tomography scan classification. Clin Orthop 1993;290:87–95.
6. Koval KJ, Sanders R. The radiographic evaluation of calcaneal fractures. Clin Orthop 1993;290:41–46.
7. Martinez S, Herzenberg JE, Apple JS. Computed tomography of the hindfoot. Orthop Clin North Am 1985;16:481–496.
8. Benirschke SK, Sangeorzan BJ. Extensive intra-articular fractures of the foot: surgical management of calcaneal fractures. Clin Orthop 1993;292:128–134.
9. Zwipp H, Tscherne H, Thermann H, Weber T. Osteosynthesis of displaced intra-articular fractures of the calcaneus. Clin Orthop 1993;290:76–86.
10. Forgon M.. Closed reduction and percutaneous osteosynthesis: technique and results in 265 calcaneal fractures. In: Tscherne H, Schatzker J, eds. Major fractures of the pilon, the talus, and the calcaneus. Current concepts of treatment. New York: Springer-Verlag, 1993:207–214.
11. Hall MC, Pennal GF. Primary subtalar arthrodesis in the treatment of severe fractures of the calcaneum. J Bone Joint Surg 1960;42B:336–343.
12. Myerson MS. Primary subtalar arthrodesis for the treatment of comminuted fractures of the calcaneus. Orthop Clin North Am 1995;26:215–227.
13. Bézes H., Massart P, Delvaux D, et al. The operative treatment of intra-articular calcaneal fractures. Clin Orthop 1993;290:55–59.
14. Letournel E. Open treatment of acute calcaneal fractures. Clin Orthop 1993;290:60–67.
15. Grob D, Simpson LA, Weber BG, Bray T. Operative treatment of displaced talus fractures. Clin Orthop 1985;199:88–96.
16. Kuner EH, Lindenmaier HL, Munist P. Talus fractures. In: Tscherene H, Schatzker J, eds. Major fractures of the pilon, the talus, and the calcaneus. Current concepts of treatment. New York: Springer-Verlag, 1993:71–86.
17. Szyszkowitz R, Reschauer R, Seggl W. Eighty-five talus fractures treated by ORIF with five to eight years of follow-up study of 69 patients. Clin Orthop 1985;199:97–107.
18. Canale ST, Kelly FB. Fractures of the neck of the talus. J Bone Joint Surg 1978;60A:143–156.

19. Comfort TH, Behrens F, Gaither DW, et al. Long term results of displaced neck fractures. Clin Orthop 1985;199:81–86.

20. Hawkins LG. Fractures of the neck of the talus. J Bone Joint Surg 1970;52A:991–1002.

21. Adelaar RS. Fractures of the talus. Instr Course Lect 1990; 39:147–156.

22. Kenwright J, Taylor RG. Major injuries to the talus. J Bone Joint Surg 1907;52B:36–48.

23. Kleiger B, Ahmed M. Injuries of the talus and its joints. Clin Orthop 1976;121:243–262.

24. Gelberman RH, Mortensen WW. The arterial anatomy of the talus. Foot Ankle 1983;4:64–72.

25. Sneppen O, Christensen SB, Krogsoe O, et al. Fracture of the body of the talus. Acta Orthop Scand 1977;48:317–324.

26. Canale ST, Belding RH. Osteochondral lesions of the ankle joint. J Bone Joint Surg 1956;38A:857–861.

27. Daniels TR, Smith JW. Talar neck fractures. Foot Ankle 1993; 14:225–234.

Suggested Readings

Buckley RE, Meek RN. Comparison of open versus closed reduction of intra-articular calcaneal fractures: a matched cohort in workmen. J Orthop Trauma 1992;6:216–222.

Jarvholm U, Korner L, Thoren O, Wiklund LM. Fractures of the calcaneus. A comparison of open and closed treatment. Acta Orthop Scand 1984;55:652–656.

Pozo JL, Kirwan EO, Jackson AM. The long-term results of conservative management of severely displaced fractures of the calcaneus. J Bone Joint Surg 1984;66B:386–390.

Stephenson JR. Treatment of displaced intra-articular fractures of the calcaneus using medial and lateral approaches, internal fixation, and early motion. J Bone Joint Surg 1987;69A:115–130.

chapter 81

Bruce E. Cohen and Robert B. Anderson

Injuries to the Midfoot and Forefoot

Over the last several years there have been significant advances made in describing the classification, treatment, and prognosis of injuries of the midfoot and forefoot. In patients with multiple trauma, these injuries have historically been given lesser importance than their associated long bone fractures. A neglected fracture of the midfoot or forefoot, however, may result in chronic disability, pain, and deformity. This chapter reviews the clinical aspects of each of these injuries and the tools that are available to improve outcome.

I The Midfoot

RELEVANT ANATOMY AND PATHOGENESIS

The midfoot consists of the tarsals—navicular, cuboid, and three cuneiforms—and the tarsometatarsal joints. This complex obtains stability from its own architecture and from dense interosseous ligaments. As a result of this stability, the midfoot is relatively rigid. The majority of motion in this area occurs through the transverse tarsal joints (Chopart joint), which represent the combined motion of the talonavicular and calcaneocuboid joints. These joints are primarily involved with the motion planes of supination and pronation and have a negligible effect on dorsiflexion and plantar flexion. The remaining midfoot joints participate in limited degrees of abduction, adduction, dorsiflexion, and plantar flexion. The most lateral tarsometatarsal joints provide a greater freedom of plantar flexion and dorsiflexion, thereby providing a compensatory function to the midfoot (1).

The tarsometatarsal joints, composed of the bases of the five metatarsals and the corresponding cuneiforms and cuboid, have been called the Lisfranc joint. The keystone to this joint's stability is the second metatarsal base, recessed within the medial and lateral cuneiforms. A large oblique ligament extends from the plantar base of the second metatarsal to the medial cuneiform (Lisfranc ligament). Interosseous ligaments join the bases of the second through fifth metatarsals, each strongest on the plantar aspect. On cross section, the midfoot forms a transverse plantar arch composed of asymmetrically shaped bones. The second and third metatarsal bases are wedge shaped and widest dorsally. The bony architecture and ligamentous support provide a mortise configuration to the midfoot, which supports the weight-bearing forces. Secondary stabilizers to the transverse arch include the plantar fascia, intrinsic muscles, and extrinsic tendons. The interrelationships among these structures account for associated injuries distal and proximal to the injured Lisfranc joint (2–5).

Isolated injuries of the midfoot are rare. Typically, a high-energy force is required to disrupt the complex. Several fracture patterns occur and usually involve more than one structure. Fracture-dislocations are frequently seen. These injuries may be subtle radiographically but can lead to late collapse and deformity.

After careful clinical examination of the foot, injuries of the midfoot are best evaluated by AP, lateral, and oblique radiographs. If possible, the AP and lateral radiographs are performed standing to help accentuate collapse deformities secondary to ligamentous disruption. CT or MRI studies can be used to help identify subtle injuries or intra-articular fractures.

Basic principles of treatment of midfoot injuries involve restoring and maintaining the stability of the medial and

Clinical Table: Injuries to the Midfoot

Injury	Procedure	Indications	Technique	Anatomy	Pitfalls
Navicular fracture—acute	• ORIF	• >1-mm displacement	• Anteromedial lag screws • External fixation if unstable	• Anterior tibialis	• Comminution • Medial column length
Navicular fracture—stress	• Cast • ORIF	• No displacement • Displacement	• Non-weight bearing • Screw fixation	• Anterior tibialis	• Early weight bearing • Early weight bearing
Cuboid fracture	• Cast • ORIF	• No displacement • Displacement • Bone loss	• Walking cast • External fixation • Bone grafting	• Calcaneocuboid joint	• Shortened lateral column length
Lis franc fracture	• Pinning • ORIF	• Nondisplaced fracture • Displacement	• K wires, percutaneous • Dorsal approach • 2 incisions • K wires with bone injury • Screws with ligamentous injury	• Second metatarsal base • Dorsalis pedis artery • Deep peroneal nerve	• Nonanatomic reduction • Entrapped anterior tibialis, peroneus longus • Shortened lateral column
Compartment syndrome	• Fasciotomy	• Elevated pressure • Severe swelling	• 2 dorsal incisions or 1 plantar, medial	• Dorsalis pedis artery • Deep peroneal nerve • Abductor hallucis	• Failure of diagnosis • Claw toe

lateral columns of the foot (Clinical Table: Injuries to the Midfoot).

NAVICULAR ACUTE FRACTURE

Fractures of the navicular bone are classified into four types: dorsal lip (cortical avulsion), tuberosity, body, and stress. The most common type, which is usually insignificant, is the fracture of the dorsal lip. This fracture results from a twisting injury with inversion forces and can be managed symptomatically.

Avulsion fractures of the tuberosity are the result of a contraction of the posterior tibial tendon against resistance. Significant displacement is rare as a result of the broad insertion of this tendon and the attachments of the deltoid ligament and talonavicular joint capsule to the tuberosity. Associated fractures of the cuboid should be considered. An accessory navicular bone can be mistaken for fractures of the tuberosity (12% occurrence, 64% bilateral) (3).

The most potentially disabling fracture of the navicular is one of the body, which involves the talonavicular and naviculocuneiform joints. Failure to recognize and properly treat this fracture may result in severe deformity and posttraumatic arthritis.

Three types of navicular body fractures have been described (Fig. 81.1). In type I fractures, the primary fracture line is transverse in the coronal plane and involves less than 50% of the body. Type II fractures are the most common type; the fracture extends from a dorsal-lateral position to a plantar-medial position. The dorsal-medial fragment is the larger one, and the plantar-lateral fragment is often comminuted. Type II fractures may be associated with adduction of the forefoot. Type III fractures involve central or lateral comminution. The major fragment is medial, and there is often disruption at the naviculo-cuneiform joint. There may be associated calcaneocuboid joint subluxation, fracture of the cuboid, or fracture of the anterior process of the calcaneus. The foot displaces laterally (6–8).

TREATMENT

Avulsion fractures are initially managed with splint immobilization, which minimizes the pain and swelling. When symptoms allow, a short leg walking cast is applied and maintained for 4 to 6 weeks. The cast should be well molded in the arch and maintain a neutral to slightly supinated posture. If a nonunion occurs, it is rarely symptomatic. Historically, the prognosis for navicular body frac-

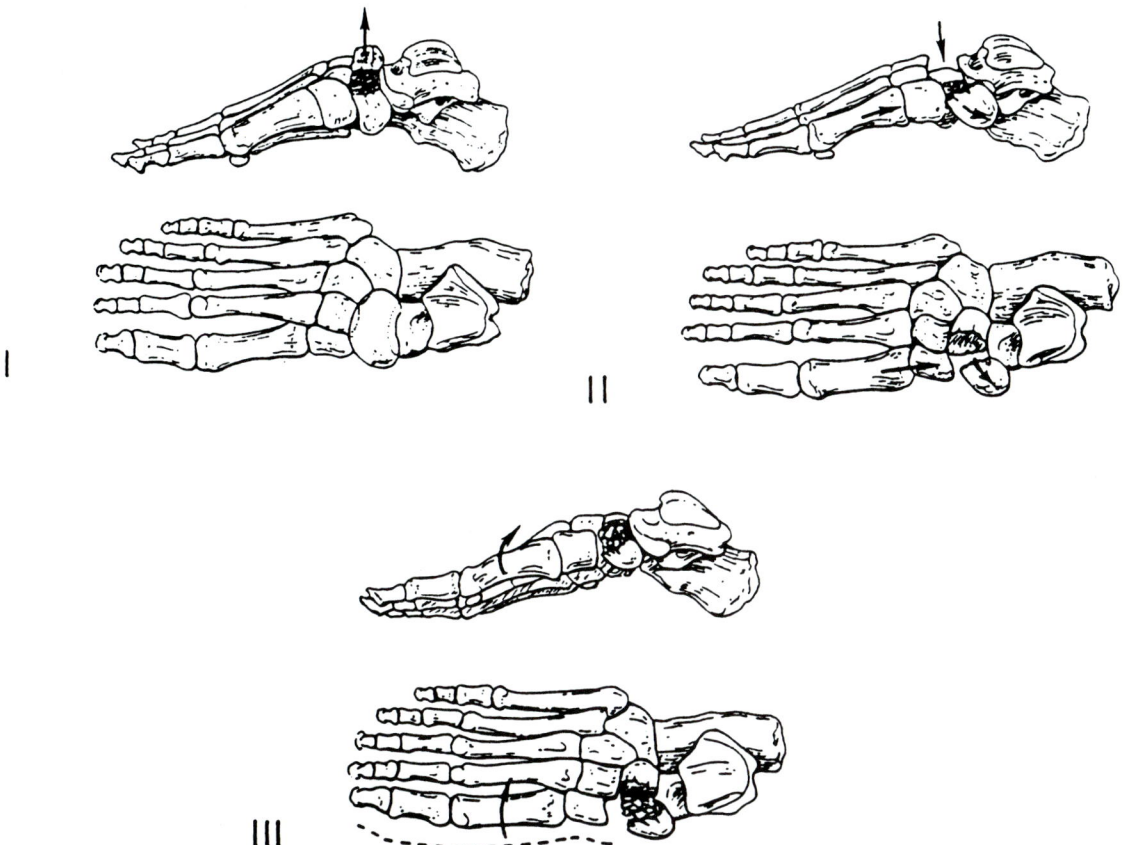

Figure 81.1. Classification of navicular body fractures. *Arrows,* direction of displacement.

tures has been poor. For this reason, even minimally displaced fractures (>1 mm) of the body require open reduction and internal fixation (ORIF) (7,8).

Operative treatment involves an anteromedial approach, medial to the anterior tibialis tendon. Type I fractures can be stabilized with lag screws from dorsal to plantar. In type II fractures, if the lateral fragment is large, a lag screw may be used from the medial to the lateral aspect of the navicular. If severe comminution is present (i.e., types II and III), fixation to the naviculocuneiform joints may be necessary. For comminuted fractures, it is important to preserve medial column length and restore a neutral alignment to the forefoot. This may require placement of a medial external fixator and interpositional bone graft (7,8).

NAVICULAR STRESS FRACTURE

Stress fractures of the navicular are most common in athletes involved in repetitive stress activities, such as running. The average time to diagnosis is 4 months. A failure to diagnose this injury and treat it aggressively may result in chronic disabling pain. Stress fractures of the navicular generally occur as partial or complete fractures in the sagittal plane and occur in the central third of the navicu-

lar bone. It is important to obtain a prompt diagnosis to minimize the incidence of nonunion and posttraumatic arthritis. A bone scan can aid in localizing the lesion in patients with nonspecific midfoot pain. A CT or tomogram may help secure the diagnosis of a stress fracture (9,10).

TREATMENT

For patients with nondisplaced fractures, good results have been achieved with a non–weight-bearing cast for 6 to 8 weeks. Displaced fractures require ORIF followed by 6 weeks of non-weight bearing in a cast. Early unprotected weight bearing has been implicated in the development of nonunion. Tomography is recommended to verify bony union before allowing patients to begin unrestricted weight bearing. The possibility for refracture has been described and should be considered in cases of recurrent pain. With misdiagnosis or failure to adequately treat, delayed union and nonunion can occur. In such cases, an inlay bone graft is recommended.

CUBOID INJURIES

The majority of cuboid injuries are minimally displaced avulsion fractures that may be seen as flecks along the lateral aspect of the calcaneocuboid joint on AP radiographs. These injuries are typically the result of an inversion strain and can be treated symptomatically, usually with 4 weeks of a weight-bearing cast.

The most important fracture of the cuboid to recognize—and one that is frequently overlooked—is the nutcracker fracture. This compression injury occurs as a result of abduction forces with lateral subluxation of the forefoot. These high-energy injuries may not only compress the cuboid, decreasing the lateral column length, but also can cause extrusion of bone in a plantar direction. Long-term complications include arthritis at the calcaneocuboid joint and, to a lesser extent, at the tarsometatarsal joint. The foot may tend to assume a position of forefoot abduction. A painful plantar prominence may develop (3,6).

TREATMENT

Nondisplaced or minimally displaced fractures of the cuboid can be treated with a short leg walking cast for 4 to 6 weeks. Displaced fractures require ORIF. Fractures resulting in significant comminution or loss of bone frequently require external fixation and/or autogenous bone graft to restore the lateral column length. Restoration of forefoot alignment and the longitudinal arch are important for minimizing late deformity. A calcaneocuboid arthrodesis is performed for symptomatic arthritis. An effort should be made to avoid an arthrodesis for arthritis at the cuboid-metatarsal joint, because this joint provides significant compensatory mobility to the forefoot. Nonunion is common when an arthrodesis of this joint is attempted (6,11).

CUNEIFORM INJURIES

Like the cuboid, isolated cuneiform injuries are uncommon and will generally result from direct trauma only. A majority of fractures and dislocations that occur at the cuneiform level usually do so in association with other high-energy injuries. The most common occurrence is with Lisfranc fracture-dislocations. The force transmitted through the tarsometatarsal joint in this injury can propagate proximally into the cuneiform region and exit out through the naviculocuneiform joint. These injuries may be occult and are frequently overlooked. Unprotected weight bearing after injury may result in late deformity and pain. A bone scan helps identify these subtle injuries, and CT or tomography can assist in identifying areas of diastasis or intra-articular disruption.

TREATMENT

Because a number of these injuries are primarily ligamentous in nature, a long period of immobilization is required for healing. In the event of displacement, ORIF is recommended, followed by a period of non–weight-bearing immobilization (8,12).

LISFRANC FRACTURE-DISLOCATION

The Lisfranc fracture-dislocation is the most important midfoot injury. It may be subtle or initially appear insignificant, only to progress to severe deformity and chronic pain.

PATHOGENESIS

The mechanism for the development of Lisfranc fractures extends along a spectrum from a low-velocity compression and twisting force to a high-energy crush injury. The prevalence rate of this injury has been increasing, primarily because of clinicians' heightened awareness of the injury's subtleties, severity, and poor prognosis. The injury pattern can be caused by a direct force, typically moving in a plantar direction, with associated comminution of the metatarsal bases and the cuneiforms or severe soft tissue injury. Open fractures and compartment syndromes are not uncommon.

The indirect mechanism for injury is more common and is caused by an axial load applied to a plantar-flexed foot. As the forefoot hyper–plantar flexes, the weak dorsal tarsometatarsal ligaments rupture. With progression of the injury, the plantar aspect of the metatarsal bases fracture or the plantar capsule ruptures, allowing for dorsal displacement of the metatarsals. Occasionally, the forces of injury can dissipate proximally through the midtarsal joints, resulting in further injury. Severe abduction and lateral displacement of the metatarsals can lead to a compression fracture (nutcracker) of the cuboid. Avulsion of the base of the second metatarsal by the strong Lisfranc ligament is common. Associated injuries of the forefoot include metatarsophalangeal joint dislocation and metatarsal neck fractures (1,2,4,66,11).

INITIAL FINDINGS, PHYSICAL EXAMINATION, AND DIAGNOSIS

It is important to diagnose a Lisfranc fracture at the onset. Standard radiographs must be carefully evaluated for soft tissue swelling, joint diastasis, and associated forefoot injuries. Avulsion fractures of the second metatarsal base and compression fractures of the cuboid are pathognomonic.

Spontaneous reduction may occur, even after severe injury; thus the joint relationships may appear normal on radiographs. In cases of appreciable trauma, the diagnosis of midfoot sprain should not be made until stress radiographs are obtained. Under adequate anesthesia or sedation, abduction and adduction forces are applied to the forefoot, and any displacement or alteration of alignment is noted.

RADIOLOGIC STUDIES

Instability patterns can be detected by fluoroscopic imaging, but the final determination of a Lisfranc fracture rests on the plain radiographs in three views. In a normal foot, a consistent relationship exists between the medial margin of the second metatarsal base and the medial margin of the middle cuneiform on the AP view. On the internal oblique view, there is an unbroken line along the medial base of the fourth metatarsal and medial margin of the cuboid. On the lateral view, there exists an unbroken line (although not necessarily a straight line) along the dorsum of the first and second metatarsals and their corresponding cuneiforms. Any loss of these normal alignments should alert the clinician to the possibility of a Lisfranc injury.

Weight-bearing AP and lateral radiographs, if feasible, may reveal a subtle injury, reflected in the loss of longitudinal arch height or subluxation of the tarsometatarsal joints. CT scans, with splay-view reconstruction, can help assess fracture patterns and detect subtle injuries. When all radiographic evaluations of the foot are normal, but pain persists at the midfoot level, technetium bone scan imaging may be diagnostic. Pinhole images are recommended and provide confirmation of the specific location of uptake (2,3,13).

TREATMENT

The goal of treating tarsometatarsal joint injuries is to obtain and/or maintain precise anatomic reduction. If typical fracture patterns are identified but anatomic reduction is preserved, short leg cast immobilization is recommended for 6 weeks. Weight bearing is initiated when the patient is free of pain. Percutaneous Kirschner (K) wire fixation can be used in patients with nondisplaced injuries identified by stress radiographs.

The majority of displaced Lisfranc fracture-dislocations should be managed with ORIF to ensure anatomic reduction and rigid stabilization. It is mandatory that the second metatarsal base be reduced, occasionally requiring débridement of avulsed bone fragments. Interposition of the anterior tibial tendon and peroneus longus tendon has been implicated in irreducible injuries. The entrapment of these soft tissue structures occurs within the Lisfranc joint, which is often involved with the fracture fragments of the second metatarsal base. Generally, after the tarsometatarsal joint has been reduced, the associated forefoot injuries will spontaneously correct. Lateral column length restoration may be necessary with nutcracker injuries. When severe comminution is present, an external fixation device and interposition bone graft can be considered (4,14).

In cases in which the primary injury pattern is ligamentous and open reduction is necessary, screw fixation across the involved joints is recommended. A dorsal approach using a single longitudinal incision or two parallel incisions is advocated. Debris and soft tissue interposition between the first and second metatarsal bases are removed, and anatomic reduction is achieved. Fully threaded 3.5-mm cortical screws are used for the medial joints and, if necessary, K wire fixation is used for the more mobile lateral joint complex (Fig. 81.2) (14).

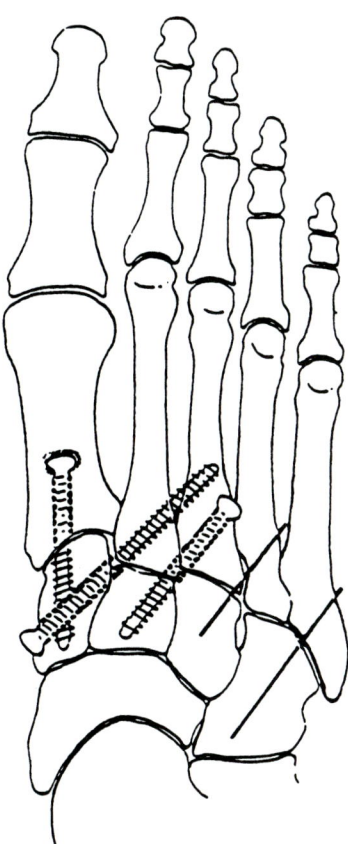

Figure 81.2. Screw placement for Lisfranc fracture-dislocation.

When the injuries are primarily bony (which require less time to heal than ligamentous injuries), K wire fixation is adequate. Wires can be removed at 6 weeks, followed by protected weight bearing. When screw fixation is used, unprotected weight bearing is not recommended until the screws are removed at 10 to 12 weeks after injury. Longitudinal arch support devices are recommended for months thereafter.

Complications

Late reductions (7 to 8 weeks after injury) are associated with a poor prognosis, and a primary reduction arthrodesis should be considered. The arthrodesis should be limited to the medial column joints in an effort to maintain motion at the fourth and fifth tarsometatarsal joints, which provide a compensatory function. Despite timely treatment and precise reduction, the long-term sequelae of a Lisfranc injury may include posttraumatic arthritis and fixed deformity. Arthrodesis, either in situ or with reduction, can be used as salvage procedure for a painless, stable, and plantigrade foot (2,4,5,14,15).

COMPARTMENT SYNDROME

Compartment syndrome of the foot is now a well-recognized entity. Certain injuries are predisposed to its development: crush injuries, Lisfranc or midtarsal fracture-dislocations, and injury patterns involving multiple metatarsal fractures.

RELEVANT ANATOMY AND PATHOGENESIS

Historically, the foot was divided into four fascial compartments: medial, central, lateral, and interosseous. Each has distinct boundaries and contents. A fifth compartment, the calcaneal, has recently been described. It lies deep within the hindfoot and includes the quadratus plantar muscle. Injection studies have identified at least nine compartments of the foot as well as a communication between the calcaneal compartment of the foot and the deep posterior compartment of the leg. This communication follows neurovascular and tendinous structures through the retinaculum posterior to the medial malleolus.

INITIAL FINDINGS, PHYSICAL EXAMINATION, AND DIAGNOSIS

Unlike its counterpart in the leg or forearm, there are no classical signs of compartment syndrome in the foot. Pain on passive stretch, dysesthesia, and diminished pulses are not reliable findings. Tense swelling may be suggestive. Therefore, a high index of suspicion is necessary and should increase when certain fracture patterns are present. When the diagnosis for a compartment syndrome is entertained, evaluation by invasive catheterization techniques is mandatory. Pressure measurement of all major compartments is required (16–18).

TREATMENT

After the diagnosis is made, expedient release of the involved compartments is necessary. Numerous fasciotomy techniques have been described. When associated with multiple metatarsal fractures or Lisfranc injuries, which require internal fixation, the double dorsal incision method is recommended. Incisions are made along the axes of the second and fourth metatarsal bones, followed

by blunt dissection to release the remainder of the compartments. If associated with hindfoot trauma, a separate medial incision near the origin of the abductor hallucis muscle may be necessary to decompress the calcaneal compartment. For midfoot injuries that do not require open repair and for cases with isolated hindfoot trauma, a single longitudinal plantar medial incision may be used. This incision follows the course of the abductor hallucis muscle and first metatarsal. The incision may be extended proximally to allow for decompression of the tarsal tunnel (16–18).

Fasciotomy incisions are left open initially. A delayed primary closure of the wound can usually be performed at 5 to 7 days. Split-thickness skin grafts can be used if necessary.

Complications

Late contractures may occur as a result of a foot compartment syndrome. The most common deformity associated with these contractures is the claw toe. A cavus posture to the compromised foot is also recognized. Injury to the intrinsic musculature has been implicated in the development of these deformities. Because of the communication between the foot and leg, it is possible that these contractures may arise from an isolated deep posterior compartment syndrome. Differentiating the two causes can be difficult. A tenodesis effect of the extrinsic tendons to the foot seen with ankle plantar flexion and dorsiflexion may implicate the calf as the site of injury (16,18).

SUMMARY

Many significant injuries to the midfoot require close attention. Prompt diagnosis and treatment are imperative. Most midfoot injuries are usually the result of high-energy trauma, and variable fracture patterns occur. Basic treatment of midfoot injuries involves restoring and maintaining the stability of the medial and lateral columns of the foot, as well as stabilizing the soft tissue injury.

II | The Forefoot

Fractures of the forefoot are frequently managed by primary care physicians, ancillary health care personnel, or patients themselves. This site of injury accounts for the greatest percentage of fractures in the foot. The orthopaedist may become involved only in cases complicated by soft tissue damage, delayed or nonunion, or malunion that results in pain and shoe fitting problems (Clinical Table: Injuries to the Forefoot).

METATARSAL FRACTURES

Fractures of the metatarsals generally result from direct trauma, frequently from a heavy object dropped onto the

dorsum of the forefoot. Avulsion and stress fractures may also occur. The outcome of these fractures depends on maintaining a normal distribution of weight-bearing forces.

TREATMENT

The majority of isolated metatarsal shaft and neck fractures can be treated nonoperatively. It is important that lateral radiographs be carefully evaluated for displacement in the sagittal plane. A metatarsal that is allowed to heal with significant plantar displacement will result in isolated areas of increased weight-bearing load, with a potential to develop a painful plantar keratosis. Metatarsal

Clinical Table: Injuries to the Forefoot

Injury	Procedure	Indications	Technique	Anatomy	Pitfalls
Metatarsal fracture	• ORIF	• >10° angulation • >3- to 4-mm displacement	• Dorsal incision • K wires, plates	• Anterior tibialis	• Plantar keratosis • Interdigital neuromas
Fifth metatarsal fracture— avulsion	• Nonoperative	• All tuberosity fractures	• Cast, shoe	• Peroneus brevis	
Fifth metatarsal fracture— Jones	• Nonoperative • ORIF	• Acute fracture • Stress fracture • Nonunion • Athlete	• Non-weight bearing, 6–8 weeks • 4.5-mm screw, intramedullary • Fluoroscopy	• Diaphyseal fracture • Intramedullary sclerosis • Watershed area	• Stress fracture, athlete • Poor screw placement • Cortical perforation
Lesser toe fracture	• Closed reduction • ORIF	• Displaced fracture • Displaced articular fracture • Open fracture	• Reduction • Buddy taping • K wires	• Phalanx fractures • Displaced condyle	• Joint subluxation • Arthritis
Lisfranc fracture	• Pinning • ORIF	• Nondisplaced fracture • Displacement	• K wires, percutaneous • Dorsal approach • 2 incisions • K wires with bone injury • Screws with ligamentous injury	• Second metatarsal base • Dorsalis pedis artery • Deep peroneal nerve	• Nonanatomic reduction • Entrapped anterior tibialis peroneus longus • Shortened lateral column
Compartment syndrome	• Fasciotomy	• Elevated pressure • Severe swelling	• 2 dorsal incisions or 1 plantar, medial	• Dorsalis pedis artery • Deep peroneal nerve • Abductor hallucis	• Failure of diagnosis • Claw toe

fractures displaced in the transverse plane are generally well tolerated. However, excessive medial or lateral angulation may cause mechanical impingement and interdigital neuromas. Lateral displacement of the fifth metatarsal or medial displacement of the first metatarsal will result in difficult shoe fitting and subsequent soft tissue irritation. Multiple displaced metatarsal shaft fractures, like metacarpal fractures of the hand, are unstable and generally require ORIF. Longitudinal incisions are made over the appropriate intermetatarsal spaces and fixation can be obtained with crossed K wires or plates and screws (19).

Overprotection and overtreatment of the nondisplaced metatarsal fracture should be avoided. Prolonged immobilization and non-weight bearing may result in osteopenia, disuse atrophy, and reflex sympathetic dystrophy. Early weight bearing with the protection of a rigid-soled device such as a sandal or cast is recommended for nondisplaced or minimally displaced fractures. In general, displaced fractures refractory to closed reduction require more invasive treatment. Specific indications for operative treatment of metatarsal fractures have not been described in the literature. One author has suggested that an attempt

at reduction should be performed if angulation of the distal fragment in any plane is greater than 10° or displacement is greater than 3 to 4 mm (19).

A metatarsal shaft or neck fracture that requires reduction can be managed with longitudinal traction and manipulation. A short leg cast is recommended for 4 to 6 weeks, and weight bearing is initiated when tolerated. Multiple displaced metatarsal neck fractures can often be reduced with longitudinal traction and remain stable thereafter. This obviates the need for ORIF, although weight bearing should be withheld for approximately 3 weeks while the patient is immobilized in a short leg cast.

Metatarsal head fractures are rare and require careful evaluation. They usually result from direct trauma, and it is important to rule out proximal metatarsal or tarsometatarsal joint injuries. The intra-articular fragment is usually displaced plantar and lateral. A subtle osteochondral fracture pattern of the metatarsal head has been described that occurs as a shear injury, resulting from a dorsal dislocation of the metatarsophalangeal joint. Gentle traction and manipulation may achieve a stable reduction. Open reduction may be necessary in fractures void of soft tissue attachments. If the injury is unstable after reduction, interosseous wire or K wire fixation should be used. Stiffness and traumatic arthritis may complicate the final result (20). Surprisingly, avascular necrosis has not been described.

FIFTH METATARSAL FRACTURES

An avulsion fracture of the base of the fifth metatarsal occurs commonly. Its cause is a sudden inversion, when the peroneus brevis contracts to prevent further inversion of the foot. The fracture fragment varies in size but should not be mistaken for a failure of the apophysis to fuse. Even with considerable displacement (>1 cm) these fractures can be managed symptomatically. Wooden-soled shoes, casts, splints, and soft wraps have all been successfully used. Although ORIF of these widely displaced fractures can be considered in the highly competitive or professional athlete, there is no literature available to support a quicker recovery or an improved prognosis in this group. Clinical union generally occurs by 3 weeks, and radiographic union at 6 to 8 weeks. Although significantly displaced fractures may result in nonunion, they are rarely symptomatic. The few symptomatic nonunions that do occur can be managed with excision of the proximal fragment with reattachment of the peroneus brevis tendon (21).

Special consideration and attention is given to fractures of the fifth metatarsal diaphysis. Although confusion still exists in regard to terminology, a fracture at the proximal part of the diaphysis, distal to the tuberosity, is generally termed the Jones fracture (Fig. 81.3). Although both a direct and a indirect mechanism for injury have been noted, the majority occur as a result of repetitive stress in athletes. There is a surprisingly high incidence in basketball players. Often, there is a history of discomfort along the lateral border of the foot 2 weeks or so before the occurrence of the injury itself. Changes in the vascularity at the site of this fracture, with a watershed area at the proximal diaphysis, have been implicated in its occurrence (22).

Two classification systems have been described for these fractures. Torg et al. (23) based their classification on the presence and amount of intramedullary sclerosis. The fracture is described as acute in the absence of sclerosis,

as a delayed union when sclerosis is present, and as nonunion when the sclerosis completely obliterates the medullary canal. Delee et al. (22) described the injuries as acute or stress fractures, based on the presence of prodromal symptoms and intramedullary sclerosis.

TREATMENT

In the acute fracture, a non–weight-bearing short leg cast is the treatment of choice. Immobilization is maintained until radiographic union has been obtained, usually at 8 weeks, and is then followed by 6 weeks of limited activity (21). Operative indications are controversial but generally include a stress fracture, delayed union or nonunion, refracture, or failure of conservative treatment. Operative fixation should be considered in highly competitive athletes who will find it difficult to comply with inactivity and for whom refracture is common.

Intramedullary screw fixation is currently recommended for operative treatment (22). Under fluoroscopic guidance, a 4.5-mm malleolar screw is placed with its entry at the proximal tuberosity of the metatarsal. Exposure of the fracture site is not necessary. A gradual return to weight-bearing activity is begun after 2 weeks. Patients are allowed to return to competitive sports when pain and tenderness have resolved. Delayed unions and nonunions may also be managed with the intramedullary screw technique. When intramedullary sclerosis is present, however, open curettage and bone grafting are recommended (22,23).

SUMMARY

Most forefoot injuries are initially treated by nonorthopaedic health care personnel. The management of these injuries requires recognition of the injury and/or deformity and appropriate treatment. Complications that may require orthopaedic attention include malunion, nonunion, plantar keratosis, interdigital neuroma, and generalized shoe-fitting problems.

REFERENCES

1. Anderson RB. Injuries to the midfoot and forefoot. In: Lutter LD, Mizel MS, Pfeffer GB, eds. Orthopaedic knowledge update foot and ankle. Rosemont, IL: American Academy of Orthopaedic Surgeons, 1996:255–268.
2. Anderson RB. Lisfranc's fracture-dislocation. In: Pfeffer GB, Frey CC, eds. Current practice in foot and ankle surgery. New York: McGraw Hill, 1993:129–159.
3. Heckman JD. Fractures and dislocations of the foot. In: Rockwood CA, Green DP, Bucholz RW, eds. Fractures in adults. Philadelphia: Lippincott, 1991:2132–2151.
4. Myerson MS, Fisher RT, Burgess AR, et al. Fracture dislocations of the tarsometatarsal joints: end results correlated with pathology and treatment. Foot Ankle 1986;6:225–242.
5. Sangeorzan BJ, Veith RG, Hansen ST. Salvage of Lisfranc's tarsometatarsal joint by arthrodesis. Foot Ankle 1990;4:193–200.
6. Main BJ, Jowett RL. Injuries of the midtarsal joint. J Bone Joint Surg 1975;57B:89–97.

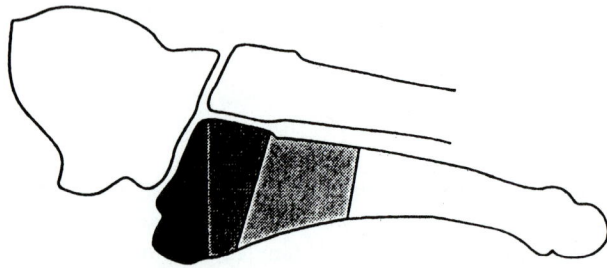

Figure 81.3. Fracture zones of the proximal fifth metatarsal. *Solid area,* tuberosity avulsion fracture; *dark stippled area,* Jones fracture; *light stippled area,* diaphyseal stress fracture.

7. Sangeorzan BJ, Benirschke SK, Mosca V, et al. Displaced intra-articular fractures of the tarsal navicular. J Bone Joint Surg 1989;71A:1504–1510.

8. Schiller MG, Ray RD. Isolated dislocation of the medial cuneiform bone—a rare injury of the tarsus. J Bone Joint Surg 1970;52A:1632–1636.

9. Khan KM, Fuller PJ, Brukner PD, et al. Outcome of conservative and surgical management of navicular stress fracture in athletes. Am J Sports Med 1992;20:657–666.

10. Torg, JS, Pavlov, H, Cooley, LH, et al. Stress fracture of the tarsal navicular. J Bone Joint Surg 1982;64A:700–712.

11. Dewar FP, Evans DC. Occult fracture-subluxation of the midtarsal joint. J Bone Joint Surg 1968;50B:386–391.

12. Holstein A, Joldersma RD. Dislocation of first cuneiform in tarsometatarsal fracture-dislocation. J Bone Joint Surg 1950;32A:419–421.

13. Adelaar RS. The treatment of transmetatarsal fracture-dislocation. Instr Course Lect 1990;39:141–145.

14. McClain EJ, Grue, GS, Hanse. ST. Fracture-dislocation of the tarsometatarsal joint. Open reduction and internal fixation with screw fixation. In: Heckman JD, ed. Perspective in orthopaedic surgery. St. Louis: Quality Medical, 1991:35–44.

15. Johnson JE, Johnson KA. Dowel arthrodesis for degenerative arthritis of the tarsometatarsal (Lisfranc) joints. Foot Ankle 1986;6:243–253.

16. Manoli A. Compartment syndromes of the foot: current concepts. Foot Ankle 1990;10:340–343.

17. Manoli A. Fasciotomy of the foot: an anatomical study with special reference to release of the calcaneal compartment. Foot Ankle 1990;10:267–274.

18. Shereff MJ. Compartment syndrome of the foot. Instr Course Lect 1990;39:127–132.

19. Shereff MJ. Complex fractures of the metatarsals. Orthopedics 1990;13:875–882.

20. Dutkowsky J, Freeman BL. Fracture-dislocation of the articular surface of the third metatarsal head. Foot Ankle 1989;10:43–44.

21. Zogby RG, Baker BE. A review of nonoperative treatment of Jones' fracture. Am J Sports Med 1987;15:304–307.

22. Delee JC, Evans JP, Julian J. Stress fracture of the fifth metatarsal. Am J Sports Med 1983;11:349–353.

23. Torg JS, Balduini FC, Zelko RR, et al. Fractures of the base of the fifth metatarsal distal to the tuberosity. J Bone Joint Surg 1984;66A:209–214.

Lesser Toe Deformities

Deformities of the lesser toes can present a considerable challenge to the orthopaedic surgeon. Treatment of lesser toe deformities should aim to restore function to the lesser toes, to alleviate pain, and to allow the use of a reasonable variety of footwear. With careful evaluation and treatment, these goals are attainable in most patients with lesser toe deformities. This chapter provides an overview of the anatomy and pathophysiology of lesser toe deformities as well as their surgical treatment.

RELEVANT ANATOMY AND PATHOGENESIS

The lesser toes are each made up of three phalanges: proximal, middle, and distal. The proximal phalanx is the longest and has two plantar tubercles at the base for the insertion of the interossei. In 37% of the population the middle phalanx is fused to the distal in the fifth toe giving the radiographic appearance of a two-boned fifth toe (1). The middle phalanx serves as the insertion of the long extensor dorsally and the flexor digitorum brevis (FDB) plantarly. The distal phalanx is the insertion of the terminal extensor tendon dorsally and the flexor digitorum longus (FDL) on the plantar aspect. The proximal interphalangeal (PIP) and distal interphalangeal (DIP) joints allow up to 65° of flexion without any extension.

The extensor mechanism of the lesser toes is formed by the centrally located extensor digitorum longus (EDL) tendon, receives contributions laterally from the extensor digitorum brevis (EDB) tendon, and then divides into three slips (Fig. 82.1A). There is no fifth extensor digitorum brevis tendon. The central slip inserts on the base of the middle phalanx; the two lateral slips extend distally over the dorsolateral aspects of the middle phalanx until they reunite and together with the fibers of the lumbricals form the terminal tendon, which inserts into the base of the distal phalanx (Fig. 82.1B). The central tendons are held in place by a fibroaponeurotic extensor sling that extends from the metatarsophalangeal (MTP) joint level over the proximal phalanx. This sling originates on the long extensor and inserts plantarly into the plantar plate, flexor tendon sheath, and deep transverse metatarsal ligament. More distally, the extensor hood is composed of fibers from the plantar interossei and lumbricales. Together these fibers suspend the proximal phalanx without any real extensor tendon insertions onto the bone. The extensor apparatus functions to dorsiflex the proximal phalanx. The PIP is extended by this only when the proximal phalanx is flexed or held in a neutral position.

The flexor system is more straightforward. The FDB (an intrinsic muscle, originating in the foot itself) originates on the medial tubercle of the calcaneus and inserts on the middle phalanx, causing flexion at the PIP. The FDL (an extrinsic muscle, originating outside of the foot) inserts on the base of the distal phalanx flexing the DIP. Note that there is no flexor insertion on the proximal phalanx, minimizing the flexion force at the MTP.

The lumbricals and interossei (both intrinsic muscles) exert the remaining forces on the lesser toes. The lumbricals take their origin from the long flexor tendons and insert onto the medial sides of the toes and the extensor mechanism, as discussed above. Their function is to flex the MTP and extend the PIP and DIP joints. The dorsal interossei insert into the lateral aspects of the proximal phalanges and the extensor expansions. The plantar interossei insert into the medial sides of the third, fourth, and fifth proximal phalanges and extensor expansions. With the lumbricals, they flex the MTP and extend the PIP and DIP joints (because of their position, which is plantar to the MTP and dorsal to the PIP and DIP axes of motion). The interossei, however, as a result of their scant insertion into the extensor mechanism, are weak extensors of the interphalangeal joints compared to the lumbricals. Alone, they function to adduct and abduct the lesser toes and to bring the toes together during weight bearing.

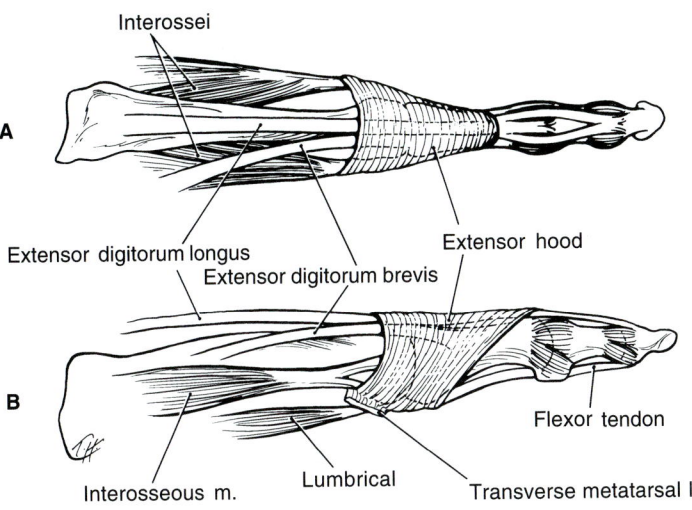

Figure 82.1. Dorsal (**A**) and lateral (**B**) views of the lesser toe extensor mechanisms.

The final structures to be considered in the anatomy of the lesser toes are the static constraints. These include the capsules, collateral ligaments, and plantar plates. The joints are stabilized in the sagittal (flexion/extension) plane by the plantar plates, which are formed from the plantar capsule and the proximally originating plantar aponeurosis. This structure is the major stabilizer of the MTP joint to extension. The joints are stabilized in the coronal plane by the medial and lateral collateral ligaments.

I   Hammer Toes, Claw Toes, and Mallet Toes

Hammer toes, claw toes, and mallet toes are most commonly acquired deformities caused by prolonged use of shoes with constricting narrow toe boxes. For this reason they usually develop over time and with increasing age. They frequently occur in the second toe, which in most Americans is the longest ray (2). These deformities occur most commonly in women (5.7:1). Discomfort usually occurs as the dorsal surface of the toe strikes the top of the shoe at the affected joint, and a corn can develop (Fig. 82.2). Painful calluses can form as the tip of the toe strikes the ground.

INITIAL FINDINGS, PHYSICAL EXAMINATION, AND DIAGNOSIS

The clinician should determine if the deformities are flexible or rigid. Flexible deformities are passively correctable as the patient stands, whereas a rigid deformity cannot be passively corrected to a neutral position. The severity of the deformity must also be assessed. Mild deformities have only a few degrees of flexion, and severe deformities involve complete rigid flexion at the involved joint. Any associated forefoot abnormalities should be noted, for example, hallux valgus (which may require correction to make room for the corrected adjacent toe), multiple toe involvement, and abnormal alignment of the adjacent lesser toes (which may preclude normal positioning). Painful corns or calluses must be recorded. Evaluation should also include prior methods of treatment, including any forms of surgical intervention that might make the approach to correction more difficult.

RADIOLOGIC STUDIES

Standing radiographs in the AP, lateral, and oblique planes should be obtained. Associated bony abnormalities, such as degeneration, should be noted. Abnormalities in joint alignment, including subluxation or dislocation and varus or valgus malalignment of the toes should be recorded (Fig. 82.3).

HAMMER TOE

A hammer toe is a PIP flexion deformity. The middle phalanx is flexed on the proximal phalanx, and the MTP and DIP are uninvolved. Poorly fitting footwear with constricting narrow toe boxes worn over many years is the most common cause. Neuromuscular disease, with its associated muscle imbalance, may also be the cause, as is the case for Charcot-Marie-Tooth disease, cerebral palsy, Friedreich ataxia, myelodysplasia, and multiple sclerosis. Compartment syndrome can be the underlying pathology, as can neuropathies associated with diabetes mellitus and Hansen disease. A painful corn can develop over the dorsal surface of the PIP.

TREATMENT

Nonoperative Treatment

Initial treatment of a hammer toe should be conservative and aimed at shoe modification to provide ample toe box space to accommodate the deformity. Avoiding high

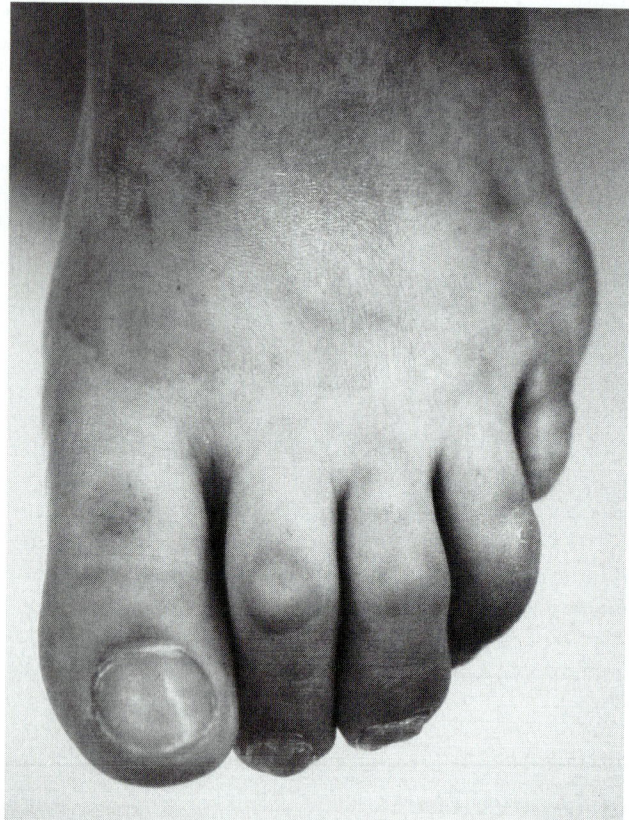

Figure 82.2. Multiple fixed hammer toes with associated PIP corn development.

heels helps prevent toe buckling. Elastic splints, which exert plantar pressure on the proximal phalanx, can be used for flexible deformities (Fig. 82.4). Small felt pads may be worn under the toe to prevent the toe tip from striking the ground, and some authors advocate stretching exercises to keep the deformity flexible.

Operative Treatment

Surgical management is reserved for patients who fail conservative treatment and is determined by the nature of the deformity (Clinical Table). A flexible hammer toe may be treated by a percutaneous FDL tenotomy but usually requires a Girdlestone-Taylor flexor-to-extensor transfer (3). Dorsal and plantar approaches are necessary. A small transverse incision is made in the MTP flexion crease, the flexor sheath is opened, and the FDL (the most central tendon with a midline raphe) is brought out of the wound with a hemostat. The FDL is released from its distal insertion at the distal phalanx percutaneously. The tendon is pulled proximally and brought out of the wound where it is split down its raphe, and each limb is tagged with a suture. A longitudinal incision is made over the proximal phalanx to reveal the extensor tendons. A hemostat is passed from dorsal to plantar next to the proximal phalanx, under the neurovascular bundle, and superficial to the extensor mechanism. Each limb of the FDL is passed

dorsally and sutured to the extensor mechanism with the toe in 20° of flexion. A 0.045 Kirschner (K) wire may be used to stabilize the repair.

Rehabilitation is begun with immediate weight bearing in a wooden postoperative shoe. The K wires and sutures are removed at 3 weeks and toe taping is done for 6 weeks. Passive manipulation is begun 6 weeks after surgery to maintain flexibility.

A fixed deformity is addressed with a DuVries arthroplasty. An elliptical incision is made over the PIP and is carried down to bone. The collateral ligaments are released, and the head of the proximal phalanx is resectioned. Bone is resected until there is no longer tension at the PIP. If necessary, a release of the FDL is performed through the plantar capsule. Some surgeons prefer to resect the articular surface of the base of the middle phalanx; but this is not required, as a fibrous union usually develops postoperatively with approximately 15° of residual motion. Alignment is temporarily held with a 0.045 K wire across the DIP or vertical mattress sutures of 3–0 nylon tied

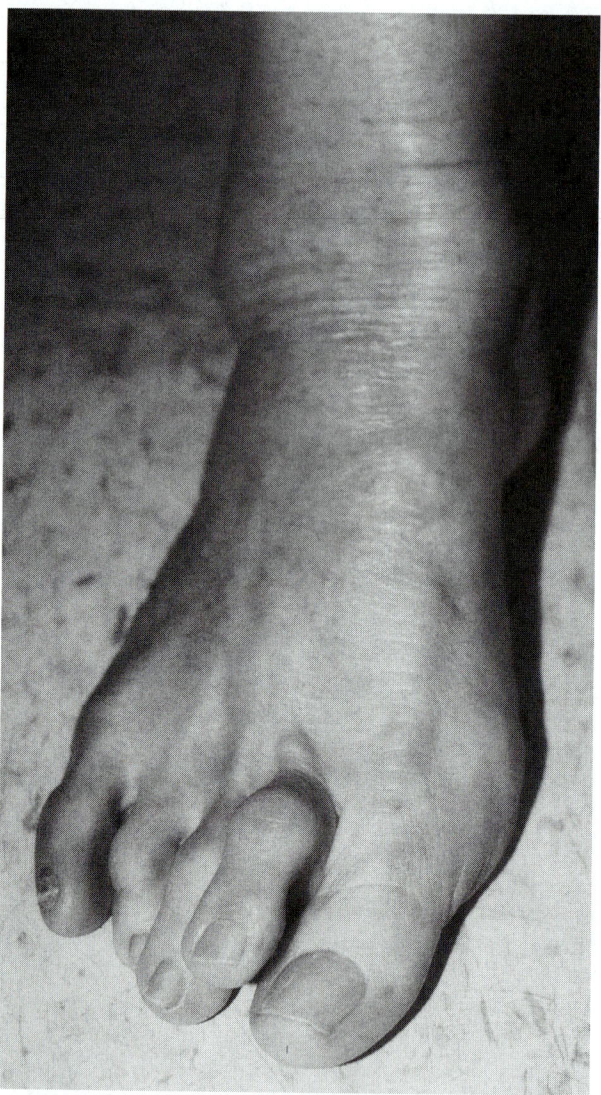

Figure 82.3. Dislocated second MTP joint and hammer toe.

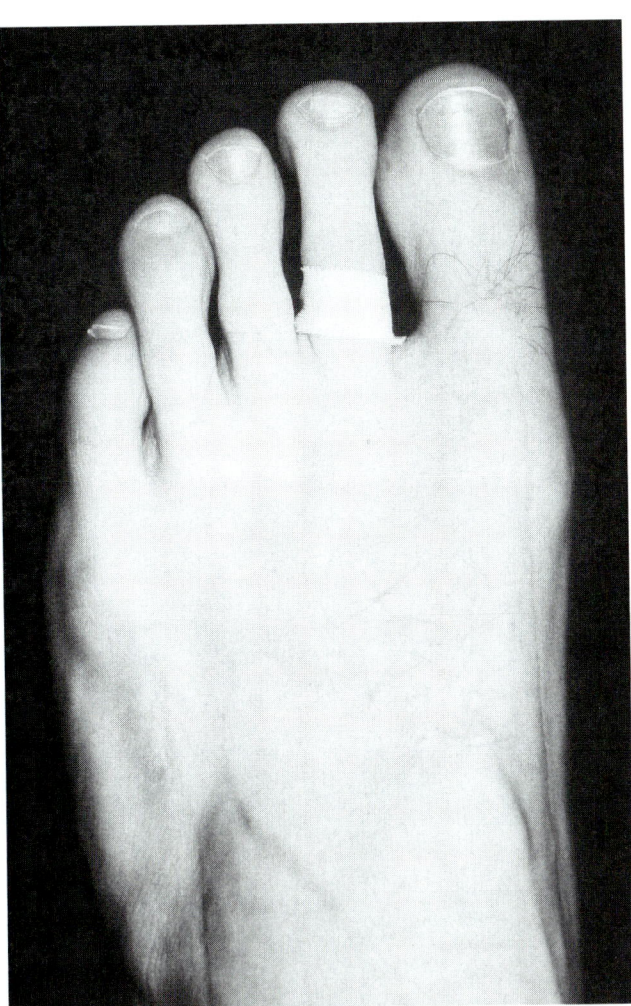

Figure 82.4. Hammer toe splint.

over Telfa bolsters (Kendall Healthcare Products, Mansfield, MA).

Rehabilitation consists of immediate weight bearing followed by removal of the bolsters at 1 week and removal of the K wire and sutures at 3 weeks. Toe taping is then instituted for 4 to 6 weeks.

TECHNICAL ERRORS AND COMPLICATIONS

Technical errors with the flexor-to-extensor transfer include inadequate correction and using the K wire to maintain the correction (deformity will recur when the K wire is removed). Failure to recognize any hyperextension at the MTP and address these with extensor lengthening or tenotomies and capsule releases leads to inadequate correction.

Problems with the DuVries arthroplasty occur when the surgeon fails to recognize MTP contracture and fails to perform adequate release at this joint. Inadequate correction can occur when the head of the proximal phalanx is inadequately resected. Shortening occurs but is allowed for joint decompression and realignment. Complications include recurrence and swelling for up to 6 months after surgery.

CLAW TOE

A claw toe is a hammer toe deformity combined with a hyperextension at the MTP joint, often resulting in metatarsalgia and possible plantar ulceration (Fig. 82.3). It develops from the same conditions as does the hammer toe, including spinal cord injury, multiple sclerosis, myelodysplasia, polio, lumbar disc disease, compartment syndrome, and tibial fracture. Claw toes are frequently bilateral, involve multiple toes, and can be associated with cavovarus foot deformities. Weakness of the intrinsic muscles, which cause muscle imbalance, can be responsible. Evaluation begins with an accurate diagnosis of the underlying cause, if at all possible. The deformity is classified based on its flexibility or rigidity and the degree of deformity at the MTP and PIP joints.

TREATMENT

Conservative treatment is aimed at symptom relief and is similar to that for a hammer toe. Surgical treatment for a claw toe is similar to that for a hammer toe at the PIP joint but must also address the MTP joint (Clinical Table). The surgical approach is through a dorsal longitudinal incision centered over the MTP and carried down to the extensor tendons. The EDB is tenotomized, and the EDL is Z-lengthened or tenotomized. The capsule is released medially, dorsally, and laterally 1 cm plantar; and the collateral ligaments are released. The toe is stabilized with a 0.45 or 0.62 K wire that crosses the MTP joint. Rehabilitation is similar to that for hammer toe repair. Pitfalls are the same as those for hammer toe repair. Undercorrection of the MTP extension contracture can lead to recurrence.

MALLET TOE

A mallet toe is a deformity whereby the distal phalanx is flexed on the middle phalanx. It is usually acquired from shoes with constricting, narrow toe boxes. Discomfort occurs when the dorsal surface of the DIP strikes the ground.

TREATMENT

Surgical treatment is determined by the nature of the deformity (Clinical Table). In the case of a flexible mallet toe, a percutaneous FDL tenotomy may adequately address the deformity. A fixed deformity is addressed with a DuVries arthroplasty of the DIP, with temporary wire fixation across the DIP only or Telfa bolsters. Pitfalls include recurrence as a result of inadequate decompression or failure of FDL release. Rehabilitation is similar to that for a hammer toe.

CURLY TOE

A curly toe is one in which the middle phalanx is flexed on the proximal phalanx and the distal phalanx is flexed on the middle phalanx, causing flexion deformities at both the PIP and the DIP joints. There is often also an element

Clinical Table: Lesser Toe Deformities

Procedure	Indications	Technique	Anatomy	Pitfalls
Girdlestone-Taylor	• Flexible hammer toe • Subluxation at the MTP joint	• FDL split • Dorsal flexor-to-extensor transfer • Suture into extensor	• Digital arteries • Digital nerves	• Inadequate correction • Failure to recognize and correct MTP hyperextension
Du Vries arthroplasty	• Fixed hammer toe • Fixed mallet toe	• Collateral ligament release • Appropriate phalangeal head resection • May include FDL tenotomy • K wire or Telfa bolsters	• Digital arteries • Digital nerves	• Inadequate phalangeal resection • Inadequate collateral ligament release • Failure to recognize MTP hyperextension
MTP release	• Claw toe • Dislocated MTP joint • Crossover second toe • Fifth toe cock-up	• EDB tenotomy • EDL Z-lengthening • Capsular release • K wire stabilization	• Medial interosseous muscle • EDB tendon	• Inadequate release
Synovectomy	• MTP synovitis • Type I Freiberg disease	• Extensor tendon retraction • Dorsal capsulotomy • Synovectomy	• Plantar plate	• Inadequate synovectomy • Failure to release interdigital nerve adhesions • Failure to resect neuroma
Arthroplasty of the MTP joint	• Dislocated MTP joint • Crossover second toe • Type III Freiberg disease	• MTP release • Partial metatarsal head resection	• Plantar plate • Collateral ligaments	• Inadequate release • Excessive metatarsal head resection
Chevron osteotomy	• Bunionette without plantar or plantar-lateral callus	• Inverted L capsular incision • Lateral eminence resection • Horizontal proximally based 60° chevron osteotomy • Medial head translation • Fixation • Lateral eminence resection	• Dorsolateral cutaneous nerve	• Excessive head resection • Inappropriate head translation • Used when plantar or plantar-lateral callus was present
Oblique midshaft osteotomy	• Bunionette with plantar or plantar-lateral callus	• Inverted L capsular incision • Lateral eminence resection • Horizontal proximally based 60° chevron osteotomy • Medial head translation • Lateral eminence resection • Dorsal proximal to plantar distal osteotomy • Fixation with screw or K wire	• Dorsolateral cutaneous nerve	• Excessive head resection • Inappropriate head translation medially
Ruiz-Mora	• Fifth toe cock-up	• Elliptical plantar incision • FDL tenotomized • Total or subtotal proximal phalanx resection		• Excessive resection of proximal phalanx • Instability

of rotation. A curly toe can be congenital and is often asymptomatic.

TREATMENT

Curly toes that are symptomatic can usually be addressed by a tenotomy of the contracted FDL tendon, which is responsible for the deformity. The approach for FDL tenotomy is through a plantar oblique incision centered under the middle phalanx. Temporary fixation of the PIP and DIP joints can be achieved with a K wire, which is removed at 3 weeks. After surgery, immediate weight bearing is allowed, and the toe is taped for 4 to 6 weeks after the pins are removed.

II Metatarsophalangeal Deformities

MTP SYNOVITIS

Synovitis at the MTP joint most commonly affects the second toe but can be found in other digits (4). Possible causes include inflammatory arthritides, infection, and acute injury; however, idiopathic synovitis of the MTP joint has been found to occur. Inflammation occurs at the MTP, which can lead to swelling and thickening of the joint. If persistent, the capsule and surrounding soft tissues stretch; the plantar plate attenuates; and subluxation dorsally can occur, which increases the pain.

INITIAL FINDINGS, PHYSICAL EXAMINATION, AND DIAGNOSIS

Initial evaluation may demonstrate only swelling and tenderness of the joint with pain on palpation. The joint may be warm, and passive range of motion can be painful. Flexion is usually limited, but as the surrounding soft tissues become incompetent joint instability can occur. A hammer toe deformity may be associated with MTP synovitis. Evaluation requires determination of the stability of the MTP joint and the nature of the hammer toe deformity. Radiographs can be completely normal, demonstrate widening of the MTP, or reveal dorsal subluxation.

TREATMENT

Failure of conservative care necessitates early operative intervention (Clinical Table). The MTP joint is approached through a dorsal incision centered over the joint. The extensor tendons are retracted, and a dorsal capsulotomy is made. An aggressive synovectomy is then performed. The interdigital nerve is released from any adhesion to the capsule; and if a neuroma has developed, it is resected. Immediate weight bearing in a postoperative shoe is begun, and at 3 weeks the patient is allowed to wear roomy shoes and resume normal activities. Pitfalls of surgery include a less than adequate synovectomy and failure to recognize and address MTP joint instability.

MTP INSTABILITY

INITIAL FINDINGS, PHYSICAL EXAMINATION, AND DIAGNOSIS

Instability of the MTP occurs most commonly at the second toe. In its earliest form, it manifests as a subluxation in which the proximal phalanx moves dorsally during toe-off, causing synovitis and pain. With time, a crossover toe (discussed below) or frank dorsal dislocation of the proximal phalanx dorsally over the metatarsal head can develop. Instability occurs as a result of plantar plate attenuation and stretch of the joint capsule.

Physical examination may reveal only pain with vertical stress of the joint. The vertical stress test (the Lachman test) is performed by stabilizing the metatarsal head with one hand while attempting to translate the base of the proximal phalanx dorsally (Fig. 82.5). Laxity (which can be graded) and pain are indicative of a positive test. Standing radiographic evaluation may be normal, since the proximal phalanx may undergo subluxation only with toe-off. In the case of frank dislocation, the joint may be irreducible; and radiographs reveal that the proximal phalanx is dislocated dorsally. A hallux valgus deformity is often associated with dislocation, and patients may develop a painful callus under the depressed metatarsal head. As the toe undergoes subluxation and eventually dislocates, flexion contractures develop at the PIP joint and a hammer toe deformity develops.

TREATMENT

Surgical management is tailored to the nature of the deformity (Clinical Table). If the deformity is a reducible MTP subluxation, then surgical intervention is to approach the MTP dorsally either longitudinally or with a zigzag incision. If no contractures are present in the extensor mechanism, the tendons are retracted, the joint is entered through a dorsal capsulotomy, and a synovectomy is performed (described earlier). A Girdlestone-Taylor flexor-to-extensor transfer is then performed. If a fixed hammer toe deformity is present, a DuVries arthroplasty is added; but if the hammer toe is flexible, the Girdlestone-Taylor procedure will address

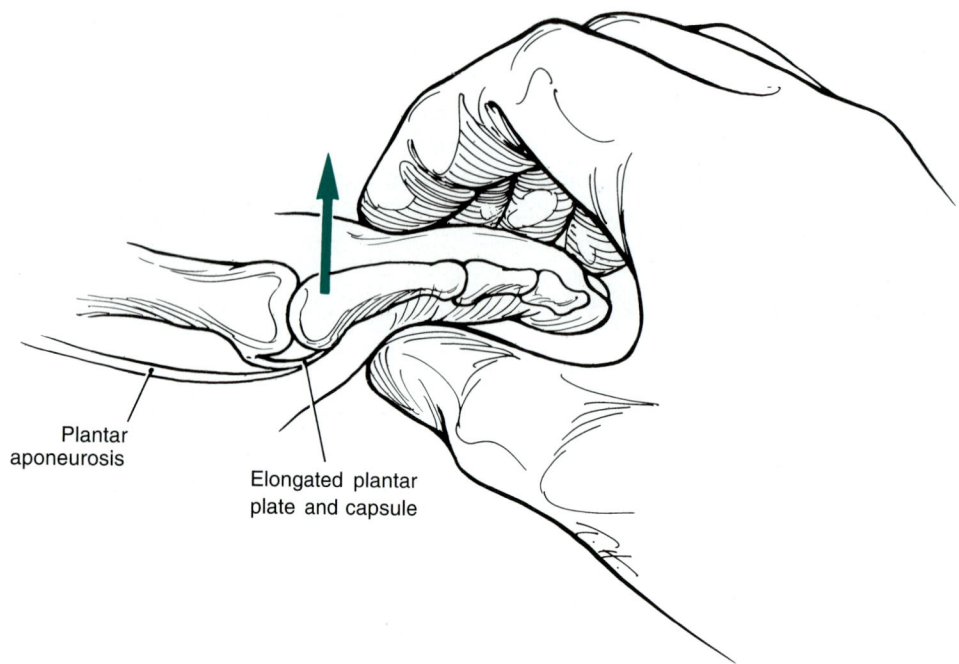

Figure 82.5. Vertical stress test.

it. K wire stabilization from the tip of the toe into the metatarsal head can be performed. If a hallux valgus deformity is present, consideration must be given to addressing it to allow room for the correctly aligned second toe.

If the MTP joint is dislocated, more extensive procedures must be done. The surgical incision is the same as just described, and the technique for correcting the MTP deformity is the same as that for addressing a claw toe. In addition, the distal 2 to 3 mm of articular cartilage on the metatarsal head may need to be resected to allow for total reduction of the joint. If a callus has formed under the metatarsal head, a resection of the plantar condyles in line with the inferior surface of the metatarsal shaft should be added to treat this.

An associated hammer toe deformity is corrected as previously described, with either a flexor-to-extensor transfer or a DuVries arthroplasty. The toe is transiently stabilized with a 0.062 K wire placed from the tip into the metatarsal head with the MTP joint flexed to 20°. Immediate weight bearing in a wooden postoperative shoe is begun. The wire and sutures are removed at 3 weeks; the PIP joint is taped, and the MTP joint is passively manipulated into normal alignment. The patient is started on toe flexion exercises.

Pitfalls

Pitfalls include undercorrection at any stage. There is also the possibility that circulation to the toe may be lost with K wire fixation. If loosening the dressings and waiting 15 min does not restore circulation, the K wire should be removed immediately.

CROSSOVER SECOND TOE

A crossover second toe is one in which the second toe deviates medially and dorsally until it is riding over the top of the hallux. This condition can occur as an idiopathic deformity or secondary to rheumatoid arthritis, synovitis, or trauma. It may be associated with a hallux valgus or hallux valgus interphalangeus. While it is most commonly a deformity of the second toe, other lesser toes may be involved. Attrition of the plantar plate, lateral collateral ligament and capsular structures allows subluxation of the second MTP joint and medial deviation of the second toe over the hallux.

INITIAL FINDINGS, PHYSICAL EXAMINATION, AND DIAGNOSIS

In the early stages of this deformity the second MTP joint undergoes subluxation and may still be reducible. As the deformity progresses, the joint dislocates and is no longer reducible, a flexion deformity occurs at the PIP joint, which may or may not be passively correctable, and a corn can develop over the PIP joint. A painful callus can develop under the second metatarsal head late in the deformity.

Evaluation of the deformity must be focused not only on the second MTP and PIP joints but also on the position of the hallux and third toe and on the varus of the foot to determine if there is room for the second toe once it is realigned. Correction of associated deformities may be necessary before realignment of the second toe is possible. Physical examination may also elicit signs of synovitis at the MTP joint, pain in the second web space, and pain on palpation of the second metatarsal head plantarly.

Classification

Richardson (5) developed a system of classification of the severity of the crossover second toe. A mild deformity is flexible with subluxation of less than one-third off the articular surface of the proximal metatarsal head. A moderate deformity is fixed at the PIP joint, has subluxation of one- to two-thirds the articular surface of the metatarsal head, and involves an incomplete tear of the lateral collateral ligament. Severe deformity is defined as complete MTP dislocation, fixed PIP deformity, and a complete tear of lateral collateral ligament and the extensor apparatus.

TREATMENT

The method of surgical correction depends on the severity of the deformity (Clinical Table). For mild deformity involving only medial deviation at the MTP joint, an EDL lengthening and EDB tenotomy with capsulotomy may be used. Mild to moderate deformity with a flexible PIP joint is addressed with a flexor-to-extensor transfer. Moderate deformities with flexible PIP joints are addressed with capsulotomy, EDL lengthening, and EDB tenotomy. In addition, the surgeon may consider an EDB transfer plantarly through a tunnel in the lateral extensor hood; the EDB is sutured back on itself, and the lateral capsule is repaired.

If a fixed PIP deformity is present, a DuVries arthroplasty is necessary at the PIP joint. If the deformity is severe, the PIP is addressed with a DuVries arthroplasty; and the MTP joint is realigned with capsulotomy, EDL lengthening, EDB tenotomy, and resection of the metatarsal head to a level at which the MTP is reduced (usually 3 to 6 mm of resection is necessary). The resection may be angled laterally slightly to aid in realignment, and then the ends are rounded with a rongeur. Rehabilitation is as previously described for these procedures.

Pitfalls and Complications

As always, undercorrection secondary to failure to perform adequate resection, soft tissue release, or realignment is a major pitfall. Complications include vascular compromise of the toe, which may necessitate pin removal, recurrence of deformity, or wound problems if excessive tension is not handled initially with a Z-plasty of the skin.

III Other Deformities

BUNIONETTE OR TAILOR'S BUNION

A bunionette is a deformity of the fifth toe characterized by a prominence of the lateral condyle of the metatarsal head. There are, however, several

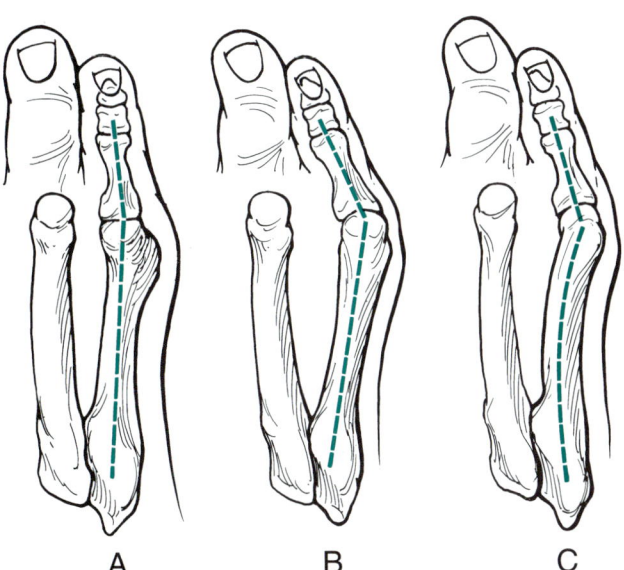

Figure 82.6. The bunionette deformity may be manifest as a large prominent lateral condyle on fifth metatarsal head (**A**), a large intermetatarsal angle (**B**), or an abnormal lateral bowing of diaphysis (**C**).

types of bunionettes, determined by the site of the abnormality (6). The deformity may consist solely of a large prominent lateral condyle on the fifth metatarsal head, which is similar to the medial eminence in a hallux valgus deformity. A wide divergence of the fourth and fifth metatarsals can also lead to the deformity. The normal fourth–fifth intermetatarsal (IM) angle is 6°; angles of 8° or larger can lead to symptoms. Finally, an abnormal lateral bowing of the diaphysis of the fifth metatarsal can also lead to a prominent lateral condyle, although the metatarsal head itself is of normal size (Fig. 82.6).

INITIAL FINDINGS, PHYSICAL EXAMINATION, AND DIAGNOSIS

Initial physical evaluation may reveal only a tender, inflamed bursa over the lateral condyle; however, with continued irritation, a painful callus can develop laterally, plantarly, or plantar-laterally. Associated splayfoot (a bunionette with a hallux valgus deformity associated with an increased first–second IM angle) or pes planus can occur. The size of the fifth metatarsal head is assessed, as is any bowing of the fifth metatarsal diaphysis. The fifth MTP angle and the fourth–fifth IM angle are measured, and any increases are noted. The hallux valgus and first–second IM angle are also assessed.

TREATMENT

Surgical intervention is necessary when painful calluses develop and the patient cannot wear acceptable footwear. Surgery is aimed at addressing the anatomic abnormality (Clinical Table). If a large metatarsal lateral condyle is solely present, a longitudinal approach may be made over the prominence and a capsular incision made to allow exposure of the head. The condyle can then be resected with an osteotome or saw, and the edges smoothed with a rongeur. The medial capsule is released by distracting the MTP joint, and the lateral capsule is reefed. Immediate ambulation is allowed in a postoperative shoe. Pitfalls include destabilization of the MTP by too aggressive resection of the head. Complications include recurrence.

If diaphyseal bowing or a large fourth–fifth IM angle is present, an osteotomy can be used to correct the deformity. Many types of osteotomies have been described, but distal osteotomies are most frequently used, usually of the chevron variety. A midlateral skin approach is made, and the capsule is incised in an inverted L. Minimal soft tissue stripping is performed. Between 2 and 3 mm of the lateral eminence is resected with a sagittal saw. Approximately 1 cm from the joint, a proximally based horizontal chevron of 60° is made with a sagittal saw, and the metatarsal head is medially translated approximately 3 mm and impacted. Fixation, if used, may be held with absorbable pins or K wires. Any remaining lateral condyle that is prominent is resected. Ambulation is allowed immediately in a postoperative shoe. Pitfalls include resection of too much of the head, injury of the dorsolateral cutaneous nerve, and undercorrection or overcorrection of the degree of translation.

Another error is failure to alleviate symptoms if a plantar or plantar-lateral callus is present, since a chevron alone will not allow dorsal translation. When a callus is present, an oblique midshaft osteotomy must be used. The prominent condyle is resected, and a saw is used to make a diaphyseal osteotomy. The blade is oriented in a dorsal proximal to plantar distal direction and directed cephalad to elevate the distal fragment. The osteotomy is held with K wires or screws. Ambulation is allowed in a postoperative shoe. K wires are removed at 6 to 8 weeks. Complications include a delayed or nonunion and undercorrection or overcorrection.

FIFTH TOE COCK-UP

A cock-up deformity is characterized by a dorsiflexion deformity at the fifth MTP joint, which may lead to as much as a 90° articulation angle at the joint. It is frequently associated with a hammer toe deformity and is commonly fixed.

TREATMENT

Nonoperative treatment centers on shoe modifications with wide, high toe boxes to accommodate the deformity. Surgical treatment is determined by the severity of deformity (Clinical Table). For mild cock-ups associated with hammer toe deformities, the MTP joint is addressed with EDL lengthening or tenotomy, soft tissue release, and hammer toe repair (described earlier). For more severe deformities, the Ruiz-Mora procedure may be used. The approach is through an elliptical plantar incision. The FDL is tenotomized, the proximal phalanx is partially or totally resected, and the wound closed with the toe held in the corrected position. Immediate ambulation is permitted, and the sutures removed at 3 weeks.

Pitfalls include excessive resection of proximal phalanx, resulting in toe floppiness. Complications include development of a hammer toe and/or bunionette.

SUMMARY

A working knowledge of the diagnosis of and approach to—whether nonoperative or operative—a variety of common lesser toe deformities is important in the armamentarium of any clinician who treats common musculoskeletal diseases.

REFERENCES

1. Sarrafian SK. Anatomy of the foot and ankle. Philadelphia: Lippincott, 1983.
2. Coughlin MJ. Mallet toes, hammer toes, claw toes, and corns. Causes and treatment of lesser-toe deformities. Postgrad Med 1984;75:191–198.
3. Taylor RG. The treatment of claw toes by multiple transfers of flexor into extensor tendons. J Bone Joint Surg 1951;33B:539–542.
4. Mann RA, Mizel MS. Monarticular nontraumatic synovitis of the metatarsophalangeal joint: a new diagnosis. Foot Ankle, 1985; 6:18–21.
5. Richardson EG. Realignment of the overlapping second toe. In: Johnson DA, ed. Master techniques in orthopaedic surgery, the foot and ankle. New York: Raven, 1994:135–148.
6. Coughlin MJ. Etiology and treatment of the bunionette deformity. Instr Course Lect 1990;39:37–48.

Amputations Around the Foot and Ankle

Amputations of the foot and ankle are done with two aims in mind: The first is the elimination of the disease process, and the second is to turn the residual limb into a functional (i.e., weight-bearing) entity. Although the elimination of the pathologic process requires adequately radical surgery, this surgery should be undertaken with a view toward the second aim. Thus as much of the specially constructed padding on the sole of the foot as possible should be preserved. Circulation in the sole pad and sensitivity are of paramount importance. Adequate circulation is a prerequisite for primary healing of the wound, whereas sensitivity will save the residual limb from future breakdown. The main reasons for amputations around the foot are inadequate circulation, instability resulting from neuropathic osteoarthropathy, and trophic ulcers (Clinical Table). Tumors, infections, mutilating injuries, and failed surgery must also be considered.

TREATMENT

Anesthesia

For toe and transmetatarsal amputations, an ankle block with adequate sedation may be enough. Any amputation further proximally will require a combination of epidural and spinal anesthesia. The use of a tourniquet is, of course, highly desirable as long as there is adequate circulation. For patients with vascular insufficiency who are undergoing hindfoot and ankle amputation, a thigh tourniquet should be applied but not inflated unless excessive bleeding is encountered. For forefoot and midfoot amputations, an ankle tourniquet will suffice.

Toe Amputations

The distal end of an amputated toe must be covered with durable skin; the plantar skin is the most desirable

covering. The surgeon should leave as a long a remnant as possible, since the pressure of shoes will eventually cause the neighboring toes to move into the empty space. Disarticulation of the toe joints is indicated when there is fear of infection, because the cartilage proves to be an effective barrier to bacterial invasion.

The surgery itself is carried out by making a dorsal incision at the level of the transection of the bone (Fig. 83.1A). The dorsal incision is carried on semicircumferentially to the midmedial and midlateral line, where a plantar flap is created that is 1.5 times as long as the diameter of the toe. The amputation of the base is carried out with an oscillating saw while the saw blade is cooled with saline (Fig. 83.1B). The long flexor and extensor tendons are pulled out, resected, and left to retract (Fig. 83.1C).

The neurovascular bundles are identified, the nerves are trimmed back beyond the level of the amputation, and the veins and arteries are ligated. A small Penrose drain is introduced into the wound, and the plantar flap is used to cover the amputation; it is attached to the dorsal skin with three or four sutures (Fig. 83.1D). The wound is dressed with sterile dressings, and the drain is removed within 48 h. A tourniquet, either around the base of the toe or around the ankle, should be used only if there is no vascular insufficiency.

Metatarsal Ray Resection

Resection of part or all of the metatarsal rays is indicated in cases of recurrent plantar ulcerations that lead to local osteomyelitis and destruction of the metatarsophalangeal joints (1,2). Other indications are local malformations, such as local gigantism. Particularly in children, it is desirable to leave behind the base of the metatarsal to prevent the neighboring metatarsals from shifting into the empty space. In amputations at the medial and lateral border of the foot, the tendons inserting into the first and fifth

Clinical Table: Amputations Around the Foot and Ankle

Procedure	Indications	Technique	Anatomy	Pitfalls
Toe amputation	• Trophic ulcers • Osteomyelitis • Local gangrene	• Disarticulation, when possible • Cover with plantar skin	• Flexor and extensor tendons • Neurovascular bundle	• Neighboring toes move into space created by the amputation
Metatarsal ray resection	• Plantar ulceration • Osteomyelitis • Local malformation	• Racquet incision • Ulcer amputation at the base of the metatarsal		• Resection of the first ray in an insensate foot leads to further breakdown
Transmetatarsal amputation	• Trophic ulcers • Osteomyelitis • Local gangrene • Severe crush injury	• Long plantar flap to anterior aspect • Retain tendon insertions to first and fifth metatarsal	• Dorsalis pedis artery • Peroneal nerve • Tendons inserting into the base of the first and fifth metatarsals	• Varus contracture resulting from loss of peroneal insertions
Pirogoff amputation	• Severe injury or malformation that does not affect the heel	• Amputation excludes tuber calcanei and heel pad • Arthrodesis of the tuber calcanei to the distal end of the tibia and fibula	• Calcaneal branches of the tibial nerve • Posterior tibial artery	• Insufficient plantar rotation of the tuber calcanei
Body amputation	• Severe injuries or malformation in children	• Amputation excludes the calcaneus • Arthrodesis of the calcaneus to the ankle mortise	• Neurovascular bundle	• Transection of the posterior tibial artery leads to gangrene of the heel pad
Syme amputation	• Severe injuries or malformation in children • Severe injury or skin breakdown in the elderly	• Disarticulation at the ankle • Resection of the malleoli • Insert extensor tendons into heel pad • Cover with heel pad	• Neurovascular bundle	• Posterior retraction of the heel pad (failure to insert the extensor tendons) • Gangrene after transection of the posterior tibial artery

metatarsals must be reinserted into the neighboring metatarsal. In insensate or dysvascular feet, the amputation of the first or the first and second rays is usually unsuccessful, because the skin in the remaining foot will breakdown because of the altered weight bearing.

The operation is carried out under ankle tourniquet. The racket-type incision must include the ulceration (Fig. 83.2). It circles the base of the involved toe and continues onto the dorsum of the foot over the metatarsal to be amputated. The metatarsals should be exposed extraperiosteally and, when necessary, resected together with the surrounding intrinsic muscles. The metatarsal shaft is then transected at its base with an oscillating saw; further resection is done sharply and bluntly while preserving as much of the plantar skin as possible.

Hemostasis is obtained after release of the tourniquet; this is important because a hematoma in the empty space can lead to reinfection. The wound is closed over a suction drain (Fig. 83.3). Bulging of the plantar skin that does not lead to blanching and a decrease in perfusion is of no particular importance, since the sole of the foot will flatten out during weight bearing. The dressing should contain fluffed gauze to absorb as much of the wound secretions as possible. The drain is pulled in 36 to 48 h. Amputation of the first and fifth rays require a molded orthosis to facilitate weight bearing.

Metatarsal and Tarsal Amputations

Transverse metatarsal amputations are the last level that allows patients to walk with relative ease and, under

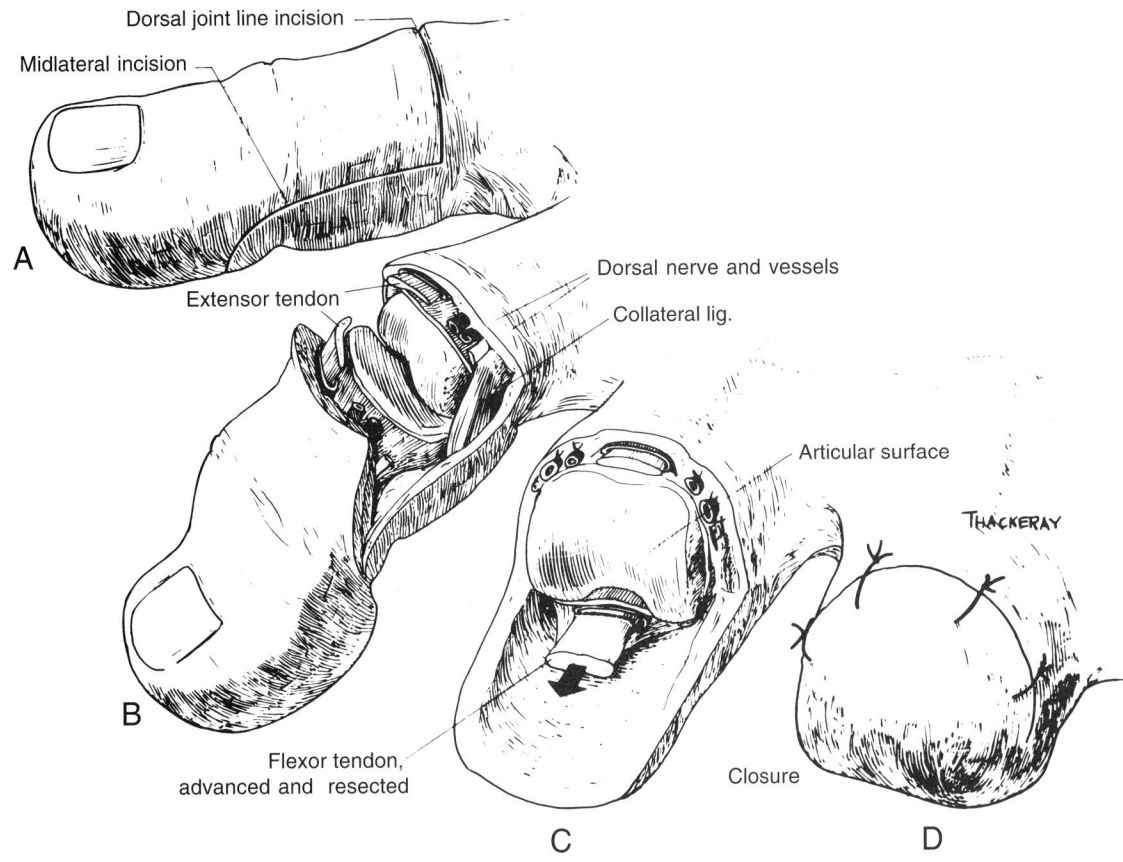

Figure 83.1. Amputation of the toe.

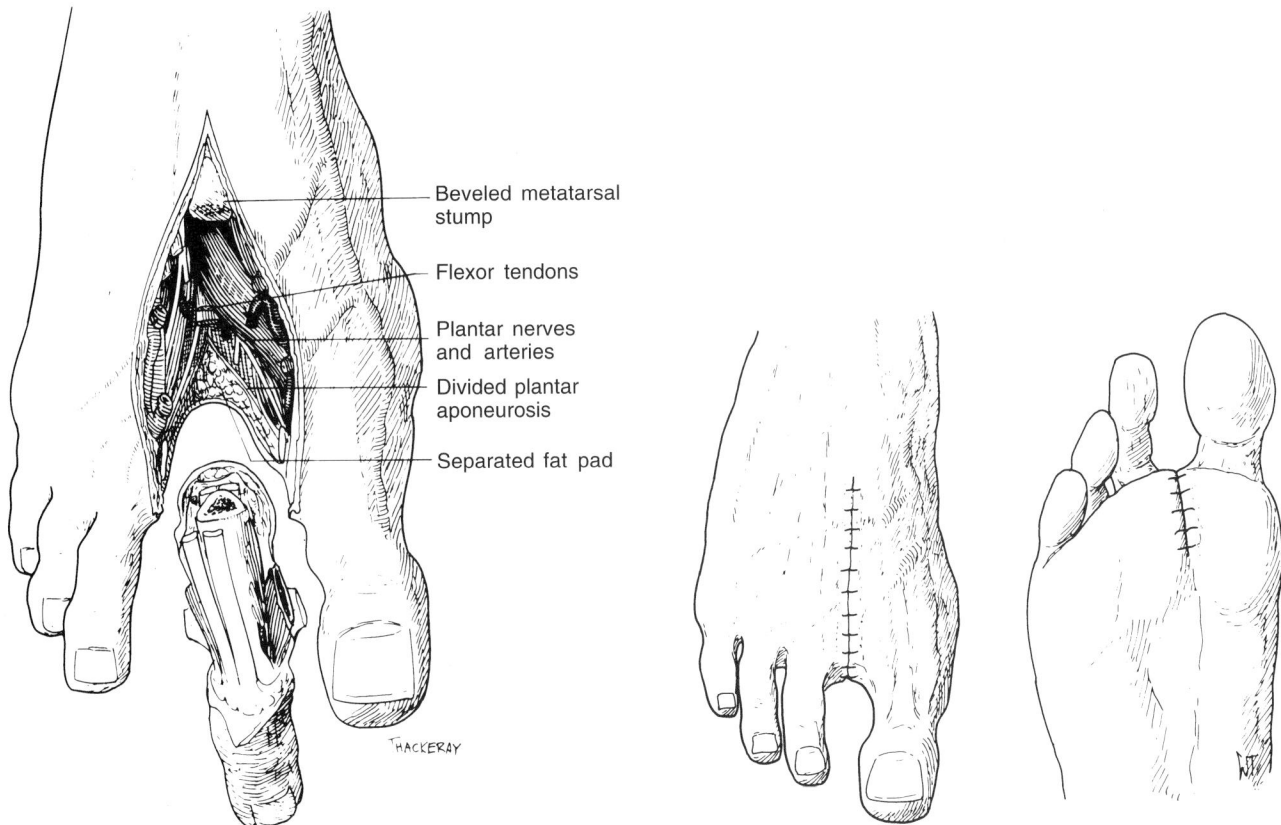

Figure 83.2. Resection of the second ray.

Figure 83.3. Wound closure after ray resection.

the best of circumstances, without any overt alteration of the gait pattern (3). The length of the metatarsal remnant is not important as long as the covering of the anterior end of the foot can be done with the plantar flap. The tendons that insert into the base of the first and fifth metatarsals must be retained.

The operation is done under ankle tourniquet. A dorsal incision is carried across the metatarsals at the level of the bony transection (Fig. 83.4). Numerous dorsal veins must be ligated. The dorsalis pedis artery has to be dissected free and ligated. The branches of the peroneal nerve should be cut back from the level of the amputation. The metatarsal bones themselves are then transected with an oscillating saw so that a straight line is created. The plantar edges, the medial edge of the first metatarsal, and the lateral edge of the fifth metatarsal must be beveled. The plantar incision is made distally to the bony transections so that a plantar flap that is 1.5

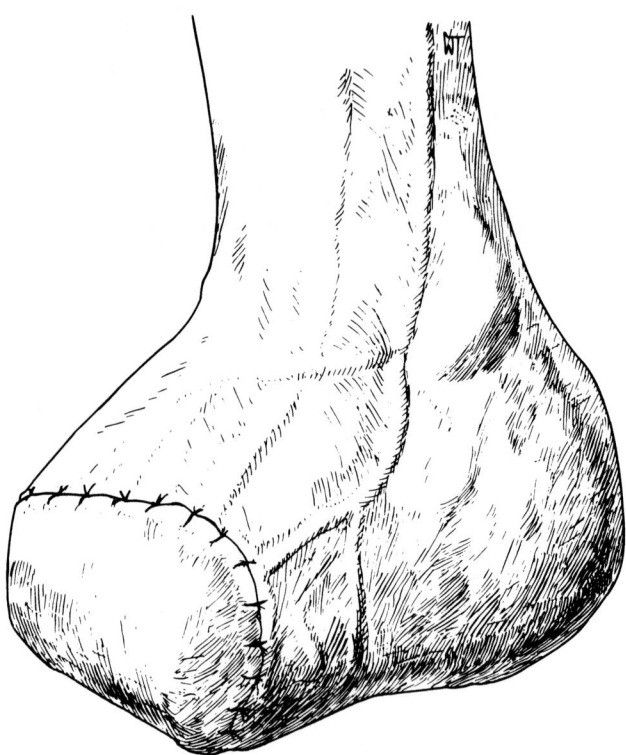

Figure 83.5. Wound closure after a transmetatarsal amputation.

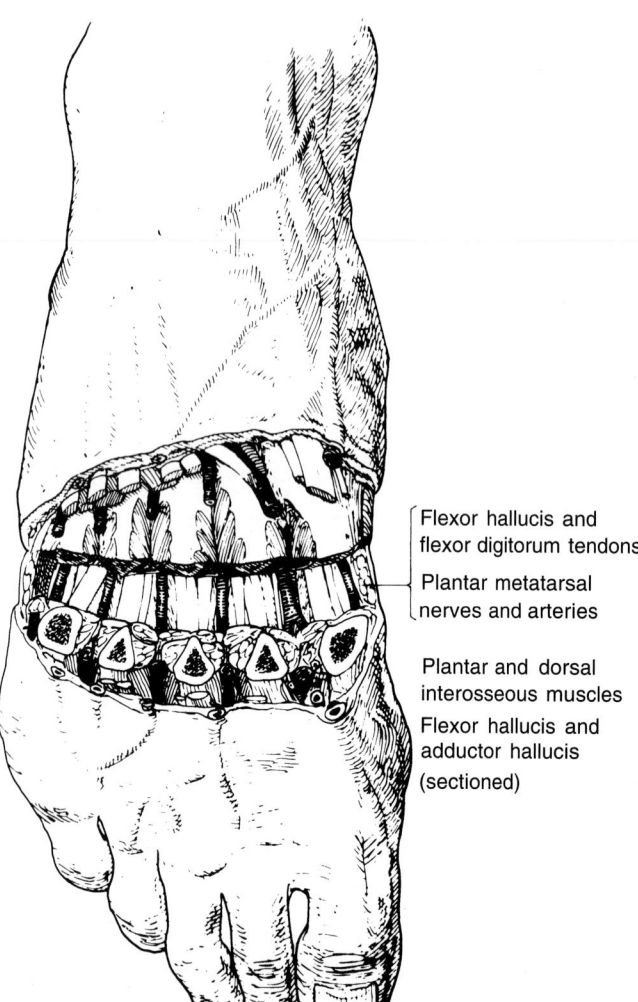

Flexor hallucis and
flexor digitorum tendons

Plantar metatarsal
nerves and arteries

Plantar and dorsal
interosseous muscles

Flexor hallucis and
adductor hallucis
(sectioned)

Figure 83.4. Transmetatarsal amputation. Note that the distal foot is in plantar flexion.

times as long as the diameter of the foot remnant is created (Fig. 83.5). Hemostasis is obtained, and the wound is closed over a suction drain by suturing the plantar flap to the dorsal skin. A thick, soft dressing is applied, and the drain is removed after 36 to 48 h.

LISFRANC AMPUTATION

The Lisfranc amputation is a disarticulation through the tarsometatarsal joints. The inverters and everters of the foot (i.e., the anterior and posterior tibial tendon and the peroneus longus and brevis tendons) must be carefully preserved and reinserted into the medial and lateral tarsal bones, respectively. The Achilles tendon usually has to be transected in a subcutaneous fashion to prevent an equinus contracture of the remaining part of the foot (4). The remaining limb itself has a large weight-bearing surface; and although it requires special shoes and usually leads to an altered gait pattern, the amputation is desirable for elderly patients.

CHOPART AMPUTATION

The Chopart amputation is an amputation through the talonavicular and calcaneal cuboid joints. As in the Lisfranc amputation, the anterior part of the stump must be covered with plantar skin. The tendons of the everters and inverters must be preserved and be inserted at the dorsum of the talus and calcaneus, respectively. To prevent equinus deformity of the foot remnant, transection of the Achilles tendon must be preformed; this is more important in the Chopart amputation than in the Lisfranc procedure.

Amputations Around the Ankle

All amputations around the ankle aim to preserve the volar part of the heel pad in an attempt to create an end-bearing stump. The weight-bearing surface in the Pirogoff and Syme amputations is usually insufficient to withstand full body weight over long walking distances. The Boyd amputation, however, particularly in children, can allow barefoot walking for long hours, albeit with a limp.

PIROGOFF AMPUTATION

The goal of the Pirogoff amputation is to create a fusion between the tuber calcanei and the distal end of the tibia by rotating the posterior process of the calcaneus almost 70° and attaching it to the denuded distal epiphyseal surface of the tibia. The resulting limb is of almost equal length to the opposite side. The incision is made over the anterior part of the ankle joint from the tip of the lateral malleolus to a point slightly distally to the medial malleolus. The ankle joint is opened, and the medial and lateral collateral ligaments of the ankle are transected (Fig. 83.6). Extreme care must be taken to preserve the calcaneal branches of the tibial nerve and the posterior tibial artery.

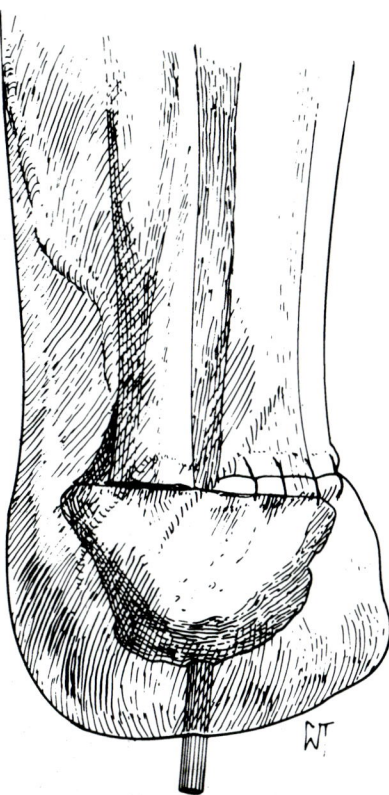

Figure 83.7. Wound closure after a Pirogoff amputation. Note the percutaneous Steinmann pin.

The ankle is sharply plantar flexed, and the posterior part of the ankle joint capsule is transected. The superior surface of the tuber calcanei is identified. The anterior part of the tuber is stripped subperiosteally and transected.

The skin incision on the plantar surface is then completed by transecting slightly anteriorly to the level of the medial and lateral mallei. The foot is then removed. The posterior half of the tuber calcanei remains intact. Next, the distal end of the tibia is transected slightly proximal to the subchondral bone. The lateral and medial mallei are transected at the same level. Hemostasis is obtained, and the tuber calcanei is rotated forward to fit the surface of the distal end of the tibia. It is held in place with a percutaneous Steinmann pin (Fig. 83.7). A suction drain is introduced into the wound, and the wound is closed by approximating the heel pad to the skin at the anterior aspect of the ankle. A soft or rigid dressing is applied. The drain is pulled within 36 h after the operation.

BOYD AMPUTATION

The disadvantage of the Pirogoff amputation is that it uses the skin in the posterior, not the plantar, aspect of the calcaneus as a weight-bearing surface. This disadvantage is overcome in the Boyd amputation, in which a greater part of the calcaneus is preserved, shifted forward into the denuded ankle mortise, and fused to the undersurface of the tibia and fibula after the talus has been ex-

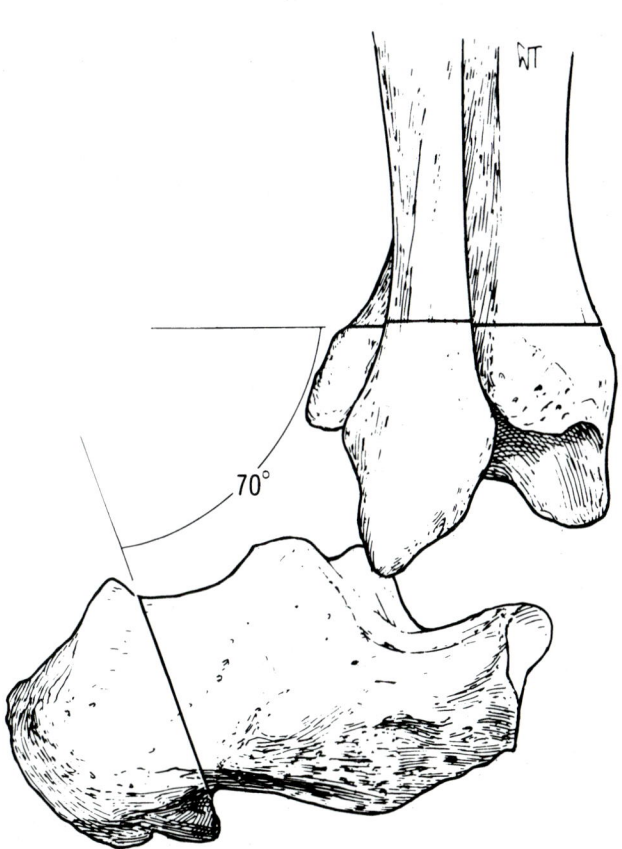

Figure 83.6. Area of transection for the Pirogoff amputation.

cised (5,6). The orientation of the plantar pad, however, remains unchanged.

The incision reaches from the anterior aspect of the medial and lateral mallei and crosses the talonavicular joint on the dorsal aspect. The plantar part of the incision is somewhat longer and must cross the plantar aspect of the tarsometatarsal joints. The subcutaneous tissue and tendons are transected on the dorsum of the foot, the ankle joint is entered anteriorly, and the medial and lateral collateral ligaments are transected. Extreme care must be taken to preserve the neurovascular bundle on the medial aspect of the ankle.

After opening the posterior part of the ankle capsule, the talus and calcaneus can be pulled apart slightly after transecting the calcaneofibular ligament. The calcaneus and talus can be separated farther, until the talus is removed with the remainder of the foot, excluding the calcaneus. A 1- to 1.5-cm slice of the anterior process of the calcaneus is removed with an oscillating saw. The tendons and nerves are pulled into the wound and transected. A burr is used to denude the joint surfaces of tibia, fibula, and calcaneus (Fig. 83.8).

Hemostasis is obtained. The calcaneus is wedged into the ankle mortise and moved as far forward as possible. It is fixed into position by a Steinmann pin, which is inserted through the heel pad and calcaneus into the marrow cavity of the tibia (Fig. 83.9). A suction drain is inserted into the wound. The wound is closed by attaching the plantar flap

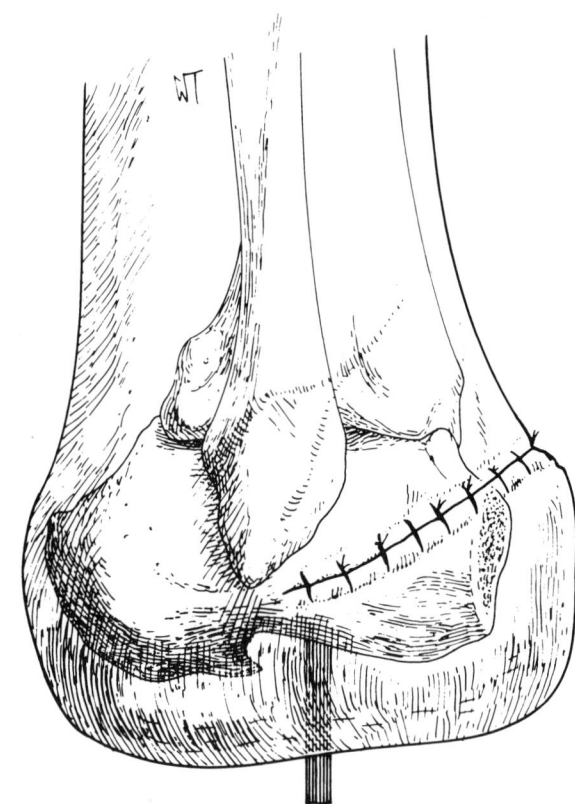

Figure 83.9. Completed Boyd amputation.

to the dorsal skin anterior to the ankle joint. A soft, bulky or rigid dressing is applied. The drain must be removed within 36 h.

SYME AMPUTATION

The Syme amputation is the last chance to create an end-bearing stump below the knee, at the level of the ankle joint itself (7–9). The aim of the amputation is to remove the entire foot while preserving the heel pad to cover the surface of the ankle joint. Thus at the distal end of the tibia, a wafer-thin section of the joint surface parallel to the floor is removed, and the medial and lateral mallei are amputated at the same level. The remaining limb is quite bulbous at the end and is unsightly; it may be difficult to fit with a prosthesis. In elderly patients, however, the Syme amputation provides a weight-bearing surface that allows ambulation without a prosthesis over short stretches and even in the prosthesis provides proprioception. In the child, no parts of the distal tibial and fibular epiphyses should be removed (10), which prevents overgrowth of the bony stump end.

The incision for the amputation starts in front of the lateral malleolus and continues to an area anterior to the lateral malleolus. The plantar limb of the incision continues perpendicular and downward through the plantar skin covering the calcaneus. The size of the plantar flap depends on the size of the area to be covered. The subcutaneous tissue and the tendons are transected. If possible, the dorsalis pedis artery should be identified and ligated. The branches of the peroneal nerve should be cut back

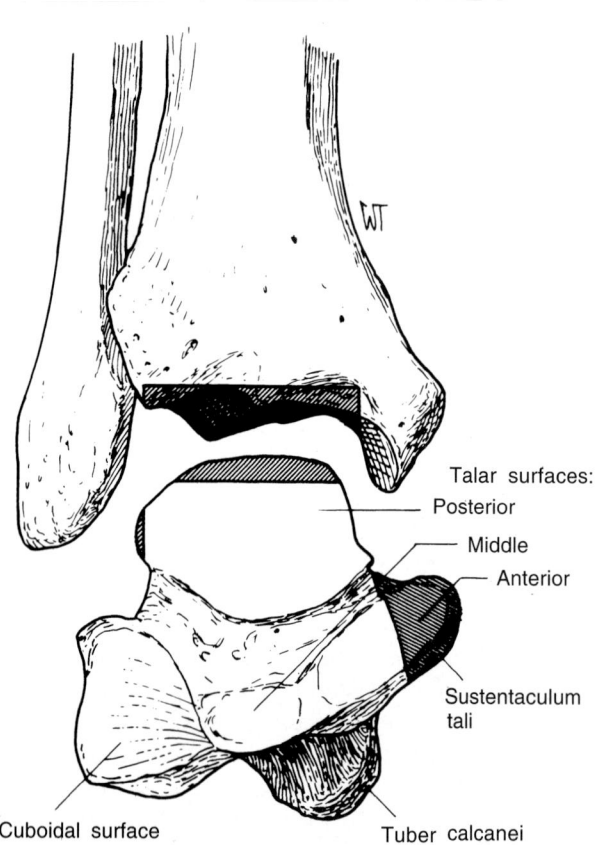

Talar surfaces:
Posterior
Middle
Anterior

Sustentaculum tali

Cuboidal surface

Tuber calcanei

Figure 83.8. Areas of resection for the Boyd amputation are shaded.

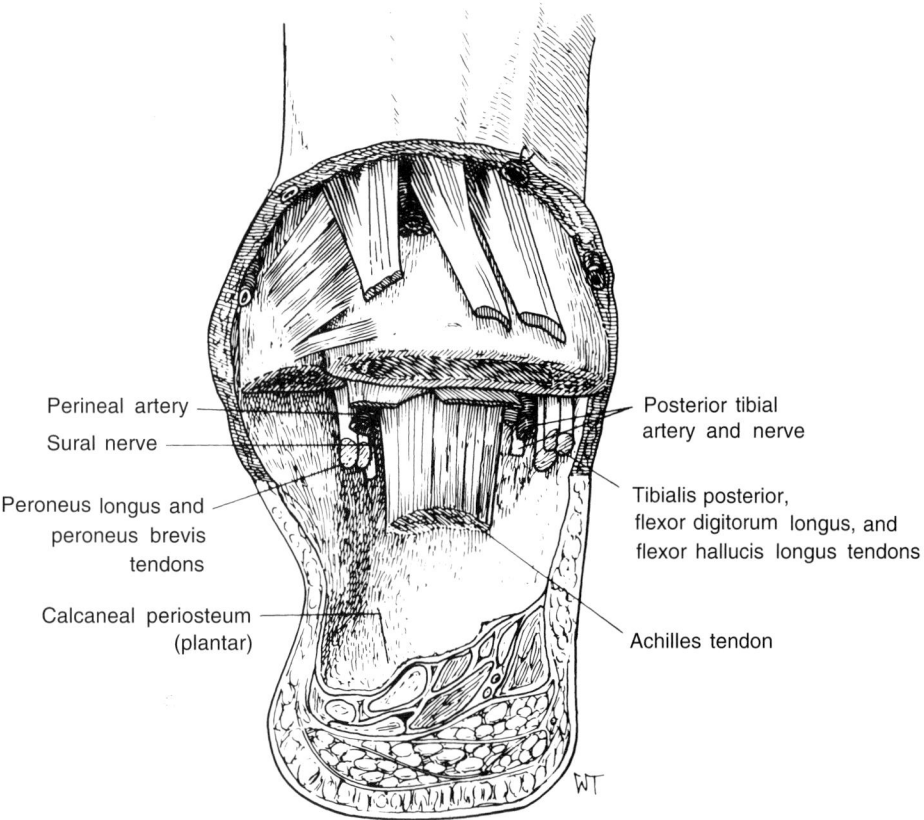

Perineal artery
Sural nerve

Peroneus longus and
peroneus brevis
tendons

Calcaneal periosteum
(plantar)

Posterior tibial
artery and nerve

Tibialis posterior,
flexor digitorum longus, and
flexor hallucis longus tendons

Achilles tendon

Figure 83.10. Syme amputation.

from the level of the amputation. Subcutaneous tissue and tendons are transected, as is the anterior aspect of the ankle joint capsule. The medial and collateral ligaments are transected by inserting the knife blade between the talus and calcaneus and the ligaments. On the medial side, the usual care must be exercised not to injure the neurovascular bundle, since it is the only lifeline to the heel pad.

The talus is then sharply plantar flexed, the posterior part of the capsule is opened, and the calcaneus is denuded subperiosteally. The Achilles tendon can be transected if necessary, although the skin covering it is extremely thin. After the periosteum on the plantar surface of the calcaneus has been raised, the foot can be removed (Fig. 83.10).

Hemostasis must be meticulous, since a large empty space remains after the calcaneus has been removed. The medial and lateral mallei and the tibial plafond are transected at the level of the subchondral plate and parallel to the floor (Fig. 83.10). The tibial nerve is identified and cut back, as are the tendons of the posterior tibial and peroneal muscles. The tendons of the anterior tibial muscle and the toe extensors are sewn into the heel pad to counterbalance the plantar flexion force of the triceps surae. A suction drain is introduced into the wound, and closure is begun by approximating the heel pad to the anterior skin of the ankle (Fig. 83.11). A soft or rigid dressing is applied, and the suction drain is removed after 36 h.

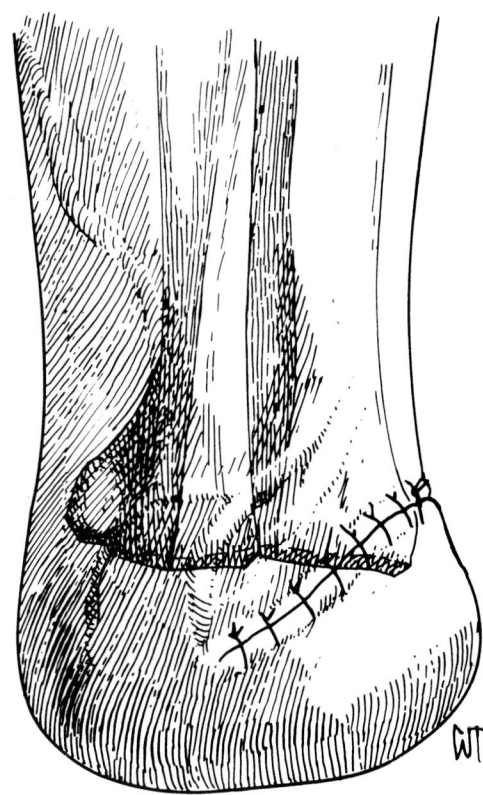

Figure 83.11. Wound closure after a Syme amputation.

SUMMARY

Although tumors, infections, and mutilating injuries are perhaps the most dramatic indications for amputations around the foot and ankle, the most frequent conditions for which amputations are performed are inadequacy of circulation, neuropathic osteoarthropathy, and chronic nonhealing ulcerous conditions.

As with other amputations, the adequacy of radical surgery is only one part of the two-part equation that must be considered. Residual limb function of restoring the lower extremity to a weight-bearing entity is a critical component to planning any lower-extremity foot and ankle amputation. Thus, considerations of adequate padding, residual circulation, and residual sensitivity become key elements in preoperative surgical planning.

The precise level of foot amputation is highly dependent on disease process, viability of residual soft tissue, and remaining circulation to the distal amputation site.

REFERENCES

1. Robinson MC, Edstrom LE. The diabetic foot: an alternative approach to major amputation. Surg Clin North Am 1977;57: 1089–1102.
2. Wagner FW. Amputations of the foot and ankle. Clin Orthop 1977; 122:62–69.
3. Young AE. Transmetatarsal amputation in the management of peripheral ischemia. Am J Surg 1977;134:604–607.
4. Green WB, Cary JM. Partial foot amputations in children. A comparison of several types with the Syme amputation. J Bone Joint Surg 1982;64A:438–443.
5. Boyd HB. Amputations of the foot, with calcaneotibial arthrodesis. J Bone Joint Surg 1939;21A:977–1000.
6. Kornah B. Modified Boyd amputation. J Bone Joint Surg 1996; 78B:149–150.
7. Harris RI. Syme's amputation. The technique essential to secure a satisfactory end-bearing stump. Part I. Can J Surg 1963; 6:456–469.
8. Harris RI. Syme's amputation. The technique essential to secure a satisfactory end-bearing stump. Part II. Can J Surg 1964;7:53–63.
9. Syme J. Amputation at the ankle joint. London Edinburgh Monthly Med Sci 1843;3:93–96.
10. Davidson WH, Bohne WHO. The Syme amputation in children. J Bone Joint Surg 1975;57A:905–909.

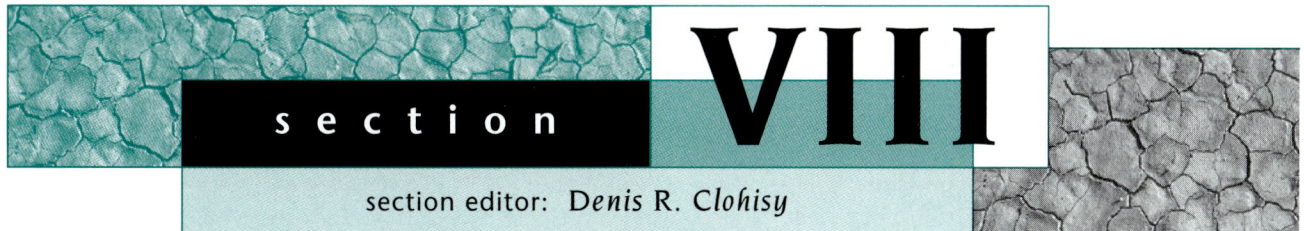

COMMON TUMORS

chapter 84

Thomas J. Gilbert

Imaging of Musculoskeletal Tumors

The radiologic evaluation of bone and soft tissue neoplasms requires a clear definition of the goals of imaging and an understanding of different imaging tests. The objectives of imaging a suspected musculoskeletal neoplasm are detection, characterization, local staging, and (when necessary) evaluation for regional and distant metastases. Radiographic techniques used to evaluate bone and soft tissue lesions include plain radiographs, bone scintigraphy, CT, and MRI. This chapter reviews the characteristics of the different imaging tests and outlines a strategy for imaging bone and soft tissue neoplasms.

RADIOLOGIC STUDIES

Plain Radiographs

Plain radiographs are perhaps the most valuable tool in the evaluation of bone tumors (1–3). They are essential and often suffice for both detection and characterization of bone tumors. Radiographs have high resolution, are inexpensive, are readily accessible, and are sensitive to calcified and ossified structures. The presence of bone destruction and the response of bone to a lesion on x-ray are the most accurate indicators of the aggressiveness of a lesion. The presence of matrix ossification or calcification on x-ray may indicate an osteoblastic or cartilaginous lesion.

Limitations of plain radiographs in the evaluation of bone lesions result in part from the fact that they project three-dimensional structures onto a two-dimensional planar format. Plain radiographs have decreased sensitivity for lesions within complex structures, such as the pelvic bones. They have limited sensitivity for small intramedullary lesions, and they can miss or understate small cortical lesions or areas of endosteal scalloping.

Radiographs may not define the intramedullary extent of bone lesions and may not detect or delineate an extraosseous soft tissue mass.

The evaluation of a suspected soft tissue mass also begins with plain radiography. Although radiographs are limited in their ability to detect and characterize soft tissue masses, they are useful for excluding an underlying bone lesion. On occasion, fat can be identified within a soft tissue mass on plain radiographs, indicating a lipoma, lipoma variant, or lipogenic liposarcoma. Phleboliths, cartilaginous calcifications, and ossifications can also be detected on plain radiographs, indicating a vascular malformation, soft tissue chondroma, and soft tissue osteoblastic lesion, respectively.

Bone Scintigraphy

With bone scintigraphy, radioactive tracer with affinity to bone is injected intravenously. Uptake within the bone is determined primarily by osteoblastic activity, but it is also affected by local blood flow. The area of interest, usually the whole body, is imaged 2 to 4 h after tracer has cleared from the soft tissue via renal excretion.

Bone scintigraphy is often indicated in the evaluation of bone tumors. It is used to detect osseous neoplasm or metastases; benign osteoblastic lesions, such as osteoid osteoma, osteomyelitis, and stress fractures; bone lesions in adolescent patients with persistent back pain or a painful scoliosis; and multiple lesions in patients who present with solitary benign lesions, such as osteochondroma, enchondroma, and fibrous dysplasia. Bone scintigraphy is sensitive for lesions with increased osteoblastic activity. These lesions result in increased uptake of tracer and focal increased activity on the bone scan.

Although a negative bone scan often excludes an active bone lesion, caution is warranted in some circumstances. Lesions without increased osteoblastic activity, such as multiple myeloma, result in focal decreased uptake and are less conspicuous on bone scintigraphy. Plain radiographs are indicated for screening these patients. Marked activity associated with open physes in pediatric patients can mask subtle areas of increased or decreased uptake within the adjacent metaphysis.

Abnormal uptake on bone scan is a nonspecific finding and can be seen both with neoplasm and a variety of non-neoplastic lesions, such as stress reactions, subacute or old fractures, infection, and degenerative joint disease. Plain radiographs and, sometimes, CT or MRI studies are often indicated to characterize foci of increased uptake on bone scintigraphy.

The role of bone scintigraphy in the evaluation of soft tissue tumors is limited to staging. Although isotope uptake can be seen within soft tissue masses, this finding is of little value; and bone scintigraphy is not indicated for detection or characterization. Bone scintigraphy has a limited role in local staging: Increased uptake within bone adjacent to a tumor may indicate periosteal or superficial cortical invasion, despite a negative CT or MRI study. Bone scintigraphy is, of course, useful for detecting osseous metastases in patients with proven or suspected soft tissue sarcomas.

Computed Tomography

CT integrates information from multiple x-ray views or a continuous x-ray beam taken around the circumference of the body to produce cross-sectional images. Intravenous iodinated contrast is used to increase the visibility of vascular structures, vascular lesions, and inflammation on the margins of soft tissue abscesses.

CT has a limited role in the evaluation of bone tumors. CT is more accurate than plain radiographs for detecting and defining both intramedullary and cortical lesions; and although not routinely used for lesion detection, it is occasionally used to confirm the presence of a lesion suspected on plain radiographs or scintigraphy and to distinguish degenerative and posttraumatic changes from neoplasm.

CT can be used for further characterization of bone lesions: It is more sensitive than plain radiographs for matrix calcification and ossification, can detect subtle areas of endosteal scalloping and cortical destruction, and can detect and define extraosseous extension of tumor. It can be used to evaluate lesions that are equivocal for malignancy and to detect areas of malignant degeneration within lesions that appear benign on plain radiographs. The orthopaedist may use CT to diagnosis or localize an osteoid osteoma or to assess lesions within long tubular bones for impending fracture.

MRI is more accurate than CT in determining the local extent of malignant bone tumors. CT is still used, however, to determine the local extent of bone tumors in patients with contraindications to MRI, such as those with a cardiac pacemaker or an intracranial aneurysm clip. CT can be used to monitor patients for local soft tissue recurrence after tumor resection if a baseline postoperative CT is available for comparison or if MRI is contraindicated.

CT also has a limited role in the evaluation of soft tissue tumors. Although CT is more sensitive for soft tissue abnormalities than are plain radiographs and although it can differentiate water-dense, soft tissue–dense, and fat-dense lesions, it is less accurate than MRI. CT can be used to evaluate fatty masses, and it can be used for patients with contraindications to MRI.

Magnetic Resonance Imaging

MRI measures the response of protons to radiofrequency waves within a large homogeneous magnetic field. The response of protons within different tissues is influenced by the water content and by the local chemical and structural environment. Unlike x-rays, bone scintigraphy, and CT, the differences in signal intensity on an MRI reflects differences in soft tissues, not differences in mineralized tissue.

On T_1-weighted images, water has a low signal intensity; muscle, an intermediate signal intensity; and fat, a high signal intensity. The intermediate signal intensity seen with most tumors on T_1-weighted sequences contrasts well with the high signal found within normal fatty marrow, subcutaneous fat, and intermuscular fascial planes.

On T_2-weighted images, lesions with increased free water will show an increase in signal intensity, whereas both muscle and fat will show a relative decrease in signal intensity. Areas of edema, inflammation, granulation, and neoplasm show intermediate to high signal intensity on T_2-weighted images, contrasting with the low signal in normal muscle. T_2-weighted images are necessary to differentiate soft tissue neoplasm from muscle.

MRI is contraindicated in patients with intracranial aneurysm clips, pacemakers, intraorbital metallic foreign bodies, electromagnetic devices, and some implants. Patients with severe claustrophobia dislike MRI. The physician can medicate these patients before the MRI with either oral or intravenous benzodiazepines. Children, particularly those younger than 6 years of age, frequently require sedation. Although sedation is usually safe, it does pose a real, albeit small, risk. Finally, sedation is required to provide imaging with uncooperative patients and patients with movement disorders.

MRI is frequently used in the evaluation of bone tumors: It supplements plain radiographs for lesion detection when symptoms are localized, can assist with lesion characterization, and is the procedure of choice for local staging. MRI is a sensitive modality for detection of bone tumors and, except for osteoid osteoma, is more sensitive than plain radiographs and bone scintigraphy for detecting primary and metastatic neoplasms. MRI can augment characterization of lesions recognized on plain radiography.

Some lesions, such as cortical fibroxanthoma, osteochondroma, intraosseous lipoma, unicameral bone cyst, and aneurysmal bone cyst, have a characteristic appearance on MRI. An aneurysmal bone cyst, for example, may show multiple loculations and multiple fluid-fluid levels, with signal characteristics consistent with blood products at different stages of evolution. Findings on MRI can also suggest malignant degeneration within a radiographically benign or indeterminate lesion. For example, a cartilaginous cap greater than 2 cm thick with an osteochondroma in an adult suggests an active or malignant lesion. The thickness of the cartilaginous cap can be measured on MRI and can be distinguished from adjacent pseudo-bursae. The presence of cortical destruction or an extraosseous soft tissue mass on MRI indicates a locally aggressive process or frank malignancy.

MRI is integral to local staging of bone neoplasms (2). It is more accurate than CT for determining both intramedullary and extraosseous tumor extent. The MRI evaluation of a bone neoplasm should begin with a T_1-weighted sequence through the entire long axis of the affected bone. These images determine the intramedullary extent of the tumor and detect osseous skip lesions. The image protocol should include matching T_1- and T_2-weighted axial images through the entire lesion and, if the lesion is located at the end of a long tubular bone, through the adjacent joint. A long axis T_2-weighted image can detect joint involvement. If the

lesion is juxta-articular, the clinician should include the epiphysis and metaphysis of the adjacent bone on at least one set of T_1-weighted images. Sequential MRI examinations can be used to monitor patients for local tumor recurrence.

MRI is recommended for detection, characterization, and local staging of soft tissue masses (2). MRI is more accurate than CT for evaluating the margins of soft tissue masses. Soft tissue tumor-imaging protocols should include matching T_1- and T_2-weighted axial sequences. Sagittal or coronal T_2-weighted images of the entire anatomic compartment ensure that the superior and inferior margins of the lesion have been included on the axial images. Patients with bone tumors may undergo sequential MRI examinations to monitor tumor recurrence.

BONE LESIONS

Detection

AP and lateral radiographs are the initial imaging studies for the evaluation of patients with suspected bone lesions (Table 84.1) (1–3). If plain radiographs do not reveal a lesion, consider additional imaging. MRI can evaluate patients with localized symptoms, and bone scintigraphy is appropriate for patients with generalized or poorly localized symptoms. If osteoid osteoma is suspected and plain radiographs are negative, proceed with bone scintigraphy and then CT, if necessary, to localize the nidus for surgical removal.

table 84.1	Imaging Bone Tumors[a]		
Radiologic Examination	Lesion Detection	Lesion Characterization	Local Staging
Plain radiographs	First study; absolutely required for patients with a suspected bone lesion; appropriateness = 9	Usually sufficient to characterize most lesions; appropriateness = 9	Already interpreted; the ability to define the local extent of a lesion is one of the criteria for a benign lesion on plain x-ray
Bone scintigraphy	Suspected lesion with negative plain x-ray; appropriateness = 8 (9 for osteoid osteoma)	Appropriateness = 1	Recommended for excluding bone metastases in patients with malignancy; appropriateness = 3
CT	Appropriateness = 1	May be used to assess the cortex in borderline cartilaginous lesions, suspected malignant degeneration of radiographically benign lesions, and suspected pathologic fracture; appropriateness = 3 (9 for osteoid osteoma)	Recommended for local staging when MRI is contraindicated; *chest scans* to exclude lung metastases; *chest, abdomen, and pelvis* scans to identify primary neoplasm; appropriateness = 4
MRI	Suspected lesion with negative plain x-ray and localized symptoms; appropriateness = 8	May be used for an aneurysmal bone cyst and when CT is atypical for osteoid osteoma; Useful for differentiating osteoid osteoma and osteomyelitis from a stress fracture; appropriateness = 2	Recommended for local staging; can determine local extent, joint involvement, and neurovascular involvement; appropriateness = 9

Modified from American College of Radiology. Appropriateness criteria for imaging and treatment decisions. Reston, VA: American College of Radiology, 1995.
[a] The appropriateness rating is on a scale of 1 to 9: 1 = least appropriate; 9 = most appropriate.

Characterization

The goals of lesion characterization are to determine the aggressiveness of a lesion and to develop a differential diagnosis. The size of a lesion, its margins, the presence of cortical destruction or periosteal new bone formation, and the presence of an extraosseous soft tissue mass indicate the aggressiveness of the tumor (1,3) (Fig. 84.1). Lesions with well-defined margins are less aggressive than lesions with a broad or poorly visualized transition zone. Cortical destruction, periosteal new bone formation, and an extraosseous soft tissue mass also indicate an aggressive process (Fig. 84.1). Finally, size correlates somewhat with aggressiveness, particularly with osteolytic lesions.

The second goal of characterization is to establish the diagnosis or to generate a differential diagnosis. The age of the patient, family history, and the presence of symptoms are essential elements of the history. The location of a lesion both within the skeleton and within an individual bone should be noted. Differential diagnosis differs for lesions originating within the axial skeleton, the long tubular bones, and the small bones of the hands and feet; and it differs for lesions occurring within the diaphysis, metaphysis, and epiphysis. The clinician should note the epicenter of the lesion and classify it as central medullary, eccentric medullary, cortical, or juxtacortical. Lesions should be classified as radiolucent, sclerotic, or mixed; and the presence of matrix calcifications or ossification should be noted. The presence of calcification in rings or arcs typically indicates a cartilaginous lesion, and ossification indicates a bone-forming process. Integration of these data produces a specific diagnosis or differential diagnosis, which will determine the need for biopsy and further staging.

Plain radiographs usually suffice for lesion characterization. CT will sometimes be needed, particularly in complex bones, such as the spine, clavicle, and pelvis. As discussed above, CT can assist in the characterization of borderline cartilaginous lesions and can help assess malignant degeneration of radiographically benign lesions.

Staging

Benign lesions are classified as inactive, active, or aggressive (4). Both aggressive benign and malignant tumors require local staging before treatment is started (1,5). The goals of local staging are to determine the intramedullary extent of the lesion, presence and extent of cortical destruction, and presence and extent of extraosseous soft tissue mass. The clinician must identify which compartments are involved and which structures are at risk, if excision is anticipated. MRI is the procedure of choice for local staging and is more accurate than CT.

With a suspected or proven malignant bone tumor, chest x-ray, chest CT scan, and radionuclide bone scan are necessary to identify pulmonary or osseous metastases. In adults older than 50 years of age, an isolated bone lesion most likely represents metastatic disease. Chest x-ray, chest CT, and bone scintigraphy, along with CT scans of the abdomen and pelvis, may be used in these patients to identify the most accessible site for biopsy and to locate the primary lesion (6).

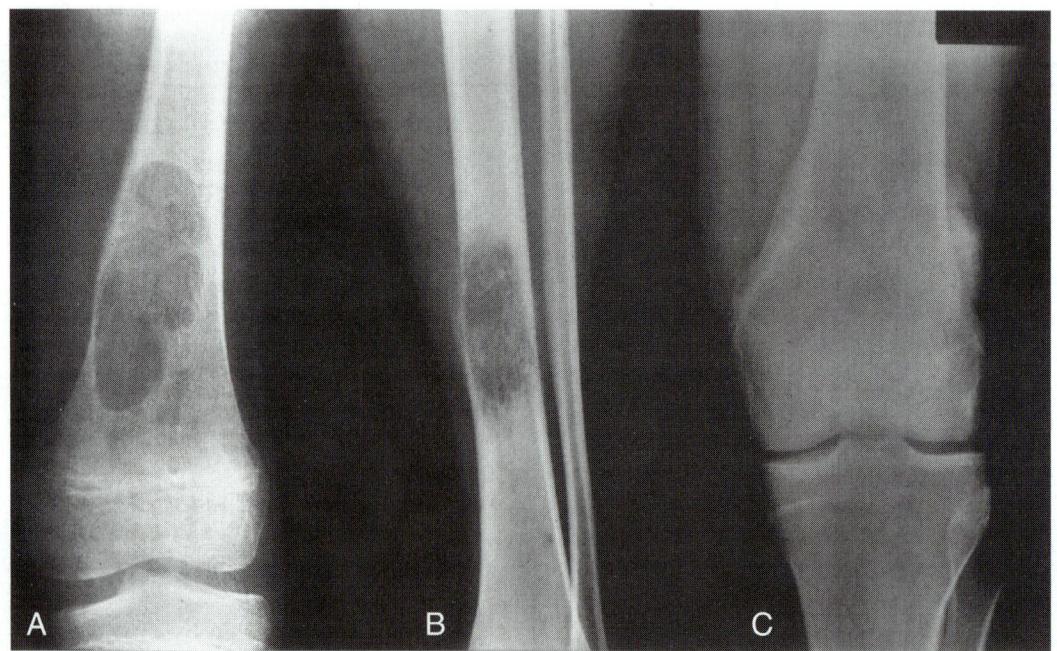

Figure 84.1. A. AP view showing a nonossifying fibroma in the femur with a narrow zone of transition and a thin sclerotic margin. **B.** AP view showing an osteosarcoma in the tibia that is poorly permeative and has poorly demarcated margins. Note the areas of cortical destruction. **C.** AP view showing a juxtacortical osteogenic sarcoma with matrix ossification within an extraosseous soft tissue mass.

SOFT TISSUE TUMORS

Detection

A soft tissue mass is usually detectable on physical examination. Radiographic evaluation of these patients begins with plain AP and lateral radiographs (Table 84.2) (1,2,7). Although plain radiographs contribute little to the detection of a lesion, they are necessary for excluding an underlying bone neoplasm and can assist with lesion characterization and staging. Confirmation of a soft tissue tumor or detection of unsuspected soft tissue tumors is accomplished with cross-sectional imaging, most commonly via MRI.

Characterization

The goal of characterization is to establish the diagnosis or to develop a differential diagnosis. This information determines whether a lesion needs to be biopsied and guides selection of the best surgical approach. Characterization begins with plain radiography (2). In contrast to bone lesions, the plain radiographs—even when combined with the clinical history and physical examination—contribute little to the development of a specific diagnosis. Plain radiographs sometimes identify fatty components within a mass and can detect calcification or ossification within a lesion, e.g., for example, phleboliths associated with a hemangioma; matrix calcifications within a soft tissue chondroma; and ossification within a lipoma,

myositis ossificans, or soft tissue osteosarcoma. In most cases, however, it is not possible to characterize a soft tissue mass on x-ray or to distinguish benign from malignant lesions.

Cross-sectional imaging is required for characterizing soft tissue masses, and MRI is the procedure of choice (2). Except for small mobile superficial lesions, the clinician should attempt lesion characterization with MRI before proceeding with biopsy or resection (1,7). Four considerations drive the rationale for this strategy: First, CT and MRI may identify certain benign lesions, such as a lipoma, hemangioma, and aneurysm, and the classification of a lesion as benign may eliminate the need for a diagnostic biopsy. Second, anatomic details identified on cross-sectional imaging may modify the biopsy approach or technique. Third, characterization of a lesion before biopsy should improve the accuracy of pathologic interpretation. Fourth, local staging of sarcomas is recommended before biopsy. Postbiopsy hemorrhage and edema can obscure tumor margins and decrease the accuracy of local staging via imaging if the biopsy was conducted before CT and MRI.

As mentioned, some benign soft tissue masses can be diagnosed on MRI (4,8). A lipoma shows homogeneous signal intensity on T_1- and T_2-weighted images that is isointense with normal subcutaneous fat (Fig. 84.2). Heterotopic lipomas, such as the intramuscular lipoma, can have a more complex appearance, because the tumor often dissects normal muscle fascicles. The orientation and signal intensity of these fascicles should parallel that of normal muscle on all sequences. Hemangiomas typi-

table 84.2	Imaging Soft Tissue Tumors[a]		
Radiologic Examination	Lesion Detection	Lesion Characterization	Local Staging
Plain radiographs	First study; necessary to exclude an underlying bone lesion; appropriateness = 9	Already interpreted; detects phleboliths, matrix calcifications, and ossification, assisting in the identification of the hemangioma, soft tissue chondroma, and myositis ossificans	Already interpreted; not useful for staging, except for the detection of bone invasion
Bone scintigraphy	Appropriateness = 1	Appropriateness = 1	Useful for excluding bone metastases, if malignancy is suspected or documented; appropriateness = 1
CT	Appropriateness = 1	No consensus; useful for confirming the diagnosis of myositis ossificans and for evaluating lipomas chest wall masses; may be useful for evaluating soft tissue chondromas; indicated when MRI is contraindicated	Recommended for local staging when MRI is contraindicated; chest scams used to exclude lung metastases when sarcoma is suspected or documented; appropriateness = 4
MRI	Sensitive and specific for soft tissue masses; negative MRI studies exclude the possibility of malignancy; difficult to detect subcutaneous lipomas; appropriateness = 9	Diagnosis of lipomas, vascular malformations, and benign cystic lesions; GCTTS and aggressive fibromatosis have characteristic appearance; appropriateness= 9	Recommended for local staing; can determine local extent, joint involvement, and neurovascular involvement; appropriateness = 9

Modified from American College of Radiology. Appropriateness criteria for imaging and treatment decisions. Reston, VA: American College of Radiology, 1995.
[a] The appropriateness rating is on a scale of 1 to 9: 1 = least appropriate; 9 = most appropriate.

cally show a cluster of punctate and tubular foci of high signal intensity on T_2-weighted images and contain variable amounts of fat. Benign cystic lesions are sharply marginated unilocular or multilocular lesions that show high signal intensity on T_2-weighted images. Ganglion cysts are typically associated with either a tendon or joint capsule; meniscal cysts, with a meniscal tear; and popliteal cysts, with the semimembranosus-medial gastrocnemius bursa.

Giant cell tumor of the tendon sheath (GCTTS) and aggressive fibromatosis also have a characteristic appearance on MRI; however, definitive diagnosis requires biopsy (4,8). These lesions frequently appear lobulated and show geographic areas of low signal intensity on both T_1- and T_2-weighted images. GCTTS typically localizes to either a tendon or a joint. Fibromatosis is frequently associated with fascial structures or an aponeurosis and can track along the long axis of an extremity or the trunk.

Many lesions have a nonspecific appearance on MRI. MRI is unable to establish a diagnosis for these lesions and is unable to distinguish benign from malignant tumors (Fig. 84.3) (4,7,8). Although benign lesions are commonly more superficial, small (< 3 to 5 cm), sharply marginated, and homogeneous, 5 to 30% of lesions with these characteristics are malignant at biopsy (4,8). Differential diagnosis of soft tissue masses with a nonspecific appearance on MRI is based on epidemiologic data, the patient's age, and the location of the lesion (9,10).

Staging

MRI—or CT, if MRI is contraindicated—is required to determine precisely the location of soft tissue tumors: The clinician must identify the anatomic compartments, joints, bone, and neurovascular structures involved, because these features influence surgical treatment decisions.

Evaluation for lymph node metastases is indicated with selected lesions (e.g., synovial cell sarcoma, epithe-

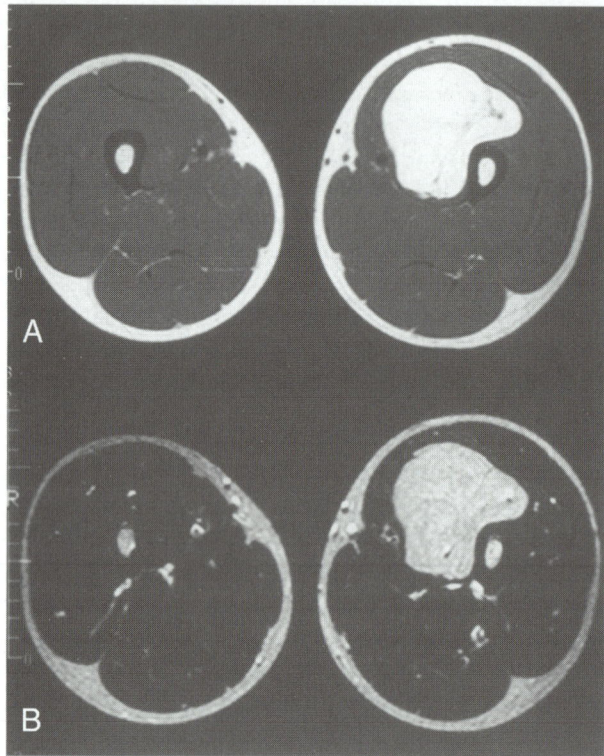

Figure 84.2. T_1-weighted (**A**) and T_2-weighted (**B**) MRI axial views through a benign intermuscular lipoma in the thigh showing a sharply demarcated mass that is homogeneous and isointense with the subcutaneous fat on both sequences.

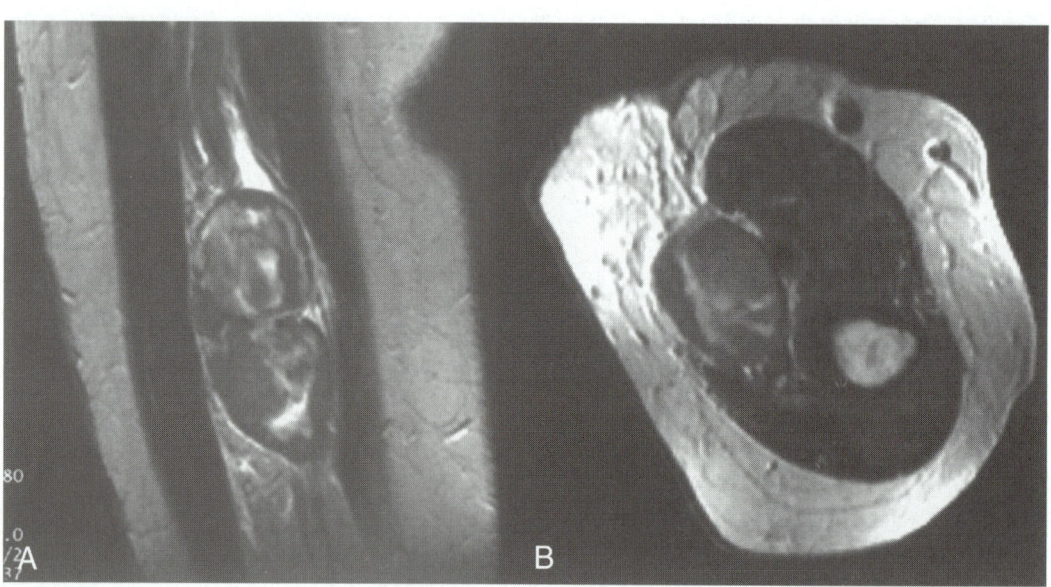

Figure 84.3. T_2-weighted sagittal (**A**) and axial (**B**) views through a mass paralleling the medial brachial neurovascular bundle in the arm. Although sharply marginated, the mass measures more than 5 cm in diameter and has heterogeneous signal intensity; it proved to be a leiomyosarcoma of the brachial vein.

lioid sarcoma, and rhabdomyosarcoma) and is usually accomplished by physical examination. Occasionally, cross-sectional imaging may be necessary to evaluate lymph nodes located in inaccessible areas or for suspicious or equivocal findings on physical examination. Chest radiographs, chest CT, and bone scintigraphy are necessary for excluding metastatic disease in patients with proven sarcomas.

SUMMARY

The goals for imaging musculoskeletal tumors are detection, characterization, and, if necessary, staging the lesion. Plain radiography is the initial imaging examination for skeletal tumors and will usually suffice for both detection and characterization. CT may be indicated in the evaluation of skeletal lesions in the pelvis or vertebrae or of borderline malignant lesions. Although plain radiographs are also utilized initially in the evaluation of soft tissue masses, MRI is ultimately needed for both detection and characterization. MRI is required for local staging of both skeletal and soft tissue masses. Bone scintigraphy and thoracic CT are used to exclude distant metastases.

REFERENCES

1. Simon MA, Finn HA. Diagnostic strategy for bone and soft-tissue tumors. J Bone Joint Surg 1993;75A:622–631.
2. American College of Radiology. Appropriateness criteria for imaging and treatment decisions. Reston, VA: ACR, 1995.
3. Gitelis S, Wilkins R, Conrad EU. Benign bone tumors. J Bone Joint Surg 1995;77A:1756–1782.
4. Berquist TH, Ehman RL, King BF, et al. Value of MR imaging in differentiating benign from malignant soft-tissue masses: study of 95 lesions. AJR Am J Roentgenol 1990;155:1251–1255.
5. Simon MA, Biermann JS. Biopsy of bone and soft-tissue lesions. J Bone Joint Surg 1993;75A:616–621.
6. Rougraff BT, Kneisl JS, Simon MA. Skeletal metastases of unknown origin. J Bone Joint Surg 1993;75A:1276–1281.
7. Frassica FJ, Thompson RC. Evaluation, diagnosis, and classification of benign soft-tissue tumors. J Bone Joint Surg 1996; 78A:126–140.
8. Moulton JS, Blebea JS, Dunco DM, et al. MR imaging of soft-tissue masses: diagnostic efficacy and value of distinguishing between benign and malignant lesions. AJR Am J Roentgenol 1995;164: 1191–1199.
9. Kransdorf MJ. Malignant soft-tissue tumors in a large referral population: distribution of specific diagnoses by age, sex, and location. AJR Am J Roentgenol 1995;164:129–134.
10. Kransdorf MJ. Benign soft-tissue tumors in a large referral population: distribution of specific diagnoses by age, sex, and location. AJR Am J Roentgenol 1995;164:395–402.

Musculoskeletal Neoplasms: Staging, Biopsy, and Surgical Margins

Careful thought and planning are necessary for the successful management of musculoskeletal tumors. To allow the greatest chance for limb salvage, a musculoskeletal oncologist should treat all potentially malignant tumors. With modern diagnostic studies (MRI, bone scans, and CT scans) and advances in the chemotherapy, radiotherapy, and surgical treatment of musculoskeletal tumors, limb salvage is now possible in about 90% of patients with sarcomas. This chapter discusses the concepts that are important in the management of musculoskeletal tumors: staging, biopsy, and surgical margins. Staging of the tumor should be done first to narrow the differential diagnosis and help guide the treatment plan. Next, a biopsy is done to make a diagnosis. Finally, the types of surgical margins are defined to assist in planning treatment. This cognitive approach to bone and soft tissue tumors facilitates the best chances for local and systemic control of bone and soft tissue tumors.

STAGING SYSTEM

Advances in chemotherapy, radiographic imaging, and surgical techniques have made limb salvage for many benign and malignant bone tumors an acceptable alternative. In 1986 Enneking (1) published a system for staging bone and soft tissue neoplasms that uses radiographic, clinical, and histologic data (2–4). The stage infers preferred treatment and comparison of outcome. The stage of a neoplasm is based on biologic aggressiveness, potential for distant metastases, histologic grade (G), anatomic site or extent (T), and presence of metastases (M). Table 85.1 summarizes the system.

The grade (G) suggests a histopathologic assessment of the type of tumor and the amount of cytologic atypia.

The assigned grade reflects the predicted biologic behavior of the lesion, including the risk of developing a satellite, skip, regional, or distant metastases. The surgical grade is G_0 (benign), G_1 (low-grade malignant), or G_2 (high-grade malignant). G_0 lesions have variable local aggressiveness and rare metastases. G_1 lesions tend to have limited local spread with few satellite nodules or skip metastases and a low rate of local recurrence. In contrast, G_2 lesions have a wide reactive zone containing satellite nodules and a higher incidence of skip, regional, and distant metastases. Consequently, G_2 lesions require more aggressive surgical excision and often adjuvant therapies (e.g., chemotherapy and/or radiotherapy) to gain local control of the tumor.

The anatomic location and extent of the lesion defines the surgical approach and margin necessary to obtain local control. The site (T) of the lesion is identified as intracapsular and intracompartmental (T_0), extracapsular and intracompartmental (T_1), or extracapsular and extracompartmental (T_2) (Table 85.2). A well-defined anatomic compartment—such as found in the thigh, leg, arm, forearm, and within bones—provides a natural barrier to tumor extension. When a lesion occurs in these locations, it is considered intracompartmental. Areas such as the popliteal fossa and the groin are poor barriers to tumor extension and are considered extracompartmental by definition. The size of the lesion does not determine the stage in this system.

Presence (M_0) or absence (M_1) of metastases is another factor in the staging system. All metastases are considered M_1, regardless of the site. Patients with skip metastases have the same poor prognosis as patients with distant metastases, thus tumors with skip lesions are classified as M_1.

| table | 85.1 | Surgical Staging System |

| | | | | | | Enneking Stages | |
Type	Traditional Stage	Description	Grade	Site	Metastases
Benign	1	Latent	G_0	T_0	M_0
	2	Active	G_0	T_0	M_0
	3	Aggressive	G_0	T_{1-2}	M_{0-1}
Malignant	I	Low grade			
		A: Intracompartmental	G_1	T_1	M_0
		B: Extracompartmental	G_1	T_2	M_0
	II	High grade			
		A: Intracompartmental	G_2	T_1	M_0
	III	B: Extracompartmental	G_2	T_2	M_0
		Distant metastatic			
		A: Intracompartmental (either grade)	G_{1-2}	T_1	M_1
		B: Extracompartmental (either grade)	G_{1-2}	T_2	M_1

| table | 85.2 | Site Staging |

Intracapsular (T_0)	Extracapsular, Intracompartmental (T_1)	Extracapsular, Extracompartmental (T_2)
Intraosseous	Intracortical	Extracortical extension
Intra-articular	Intra-articular	Extra-articular extension
Skin/subcutaneous	Skin/subcutaneous	Deep extension
Parosseous	Parosseous	Extension into bone or soft tissue
Intracompartmental or	Intracompartmental	Soft tissue
extracompartmental	Soft tissue	Extracapsular by extension or origin
	Intracompartmental by origin	Extracompartmental by origin
	Ray hand	Midhand, dorsal or palmar
	Ray foot	Mid or hind foot
	Posterior calf	Popliteal fossa
	Anterolateral leg	Periarticular knee
	Anterior thigh	Femoral triangle
	Medial thigh	Obturator foramen, pelvis
	Posterior thigh	Sciatic notch, intrapelvic
	Buttocks	Antecubital fossa
	Volar forearm	Periarticular elbow
	Dorsal forearm	Axilla
	Anterior arm	Periclavicular
	Posterior arm	Paraspinal, head neck
	Deltoid	
	Periscapular	

Benign tumors can be classified as stage 1 (latent), stage 2 (active), or stage 3 (aggressive). Malignant tumors are classified as stage I (low-grade malignant), stage II (high-grade malignant), or stage III (metastatic). Malignant tumors are subdivided into intracompartmental (A) and extracompartmental (B) tumors. Tumors can change stages during the course of the disease. For example, a stage 2 unicameral bone cyst at age 8 may become a stage 1 latent cyst by the time of skeletal maturity.

BIOPSY OF BONE AND SOFT TISSUE TUMORS

The biopsy of bone and soft tissue tumors is a vital step in their management (5–11). Errors in diagnosis or an inappropriate biopsy can adversely affect the chances of limb salvage and even survival (5,6,8). Thus the orthopaedic oncologist should perform the biopsy after completing the radiographic staging studies and consult-

ing with the radiologist and pathologist. It is essential to obtain the imaging studies before performing the biopsy, since the biopsy can alter the staging studies. The radiographic studies may locate other lesions that are more amenable to biopsy than the presenting lesion. After the physician completes the staging studies, he or she should develop a differential diagnosis, which will help determine the best method of biopsy.

Needle Versus Open Biopsy

The biopsy method depends on the differential diagnosis, the location of the neoplasm, and the ability of the pathologist to make a diagnosis on a small sample of tissue. In general, needle biopsies are preferred when the pathologist can make a diagnosis on a small tissue sample (e.g., when the diagnostic possibilities are limited or the tumor tissue is so homogeneous that little potential for sampling error exists). For example, needle biopsy is useful for suspected myeloma, metastatic carcinoma, and some soft tissue sarcomas.

The advantages of needle biopsy are that the procedure is quick, safe, inexpensive, and easily done with local anesthesia. The disadvantages are primarily related to the small volume of tissue obtained. Limited tissue samples introduce the possibility of sampling error and may limit the number of specialized studies that the pathologist can perform; when ample specimens are obtained with an open biopsy, many studies can be made, including immunohistochemistry, electron microscopy, flow cytometry, and cytogenetics.

Open (surgical) biopsies in which the surgeon takes a limited sample of the tumor are also called incisional biopsies. Open biopsy provides more tissue and thus improves the accuracy of the diagnosis over needle biopsies, but the technique involves increased risks and expense. When the surgeon performs an open biopsy, the pathologist must perform a frozen-section analysis to confirm adequacy of the specimen. The frozen section ensures that the sample chosen is viable tumor, is potentially diagnostic, and will allow an appropriate selection of specialized studies and microbiological tests. In selected cases, the surgeon can perform a definitive procedure immediately following the frozen section. For example, prophylactic internal fixation of an impending pathologic fracture can be conducted if the frozen section proves the lesion is secondary to the focus of metastatic carcinoma.

Biopsy of musculoskeletal neoplasms is an important procedure that involves planning. *Every musculoskeletal tumor has the potential to be a sarcoma and should be approached as such.* Since sarcomas are implantable, proper biopsy technique is essential to avoid contamination of uninvolved structures. The surgeon should always use longitudinal incisions. The most direct route from the skin to the tumor is preferred; however, the biopsy should always go through muscle, not intermuscular planes, to avoid spreading tumor cells along these planes. The surgeon should not expose the neurovascular bundle or joint during a biopsy. If a pathologic fracture is present, it is necessary to avoid obtaining the fracture callus in the biopsy. The pathologist may have difficulty distinguishing callus from tumor, especially with osteosarcoma. Once the frozen section confirms that the tissue is of adequate diagnostic quality, the wound may be closed. Strict hemostatic technique, often with the use of surgical drains, to avoid hematoma and subsequent potential for wound contamination is essential.

If the diagnosis is certain based on imaging studies (e.g., a classic osteochondroma), then incisional biopsy is not necessary, and an excisional biopsy (removal of the entire specimen) may be performed. In general, an excisional biopsy may be conducted on a suspected benign lesion if the excision does not compromise the ability to achieve a wide surgical margin, if the lesion subsequently proves to be malignant. For example, an excisional biopsy of a small (smaller than 5 cm) soft tissue lesion in the subcutaneous tissue of the anterior thigh could be done without a frozen section. If the lesion proves to be malignant, the surgeon can reexcise the tumor bed without difficulty. In contrast, removal of a large tumor (larger than 5 cm) deep to the fascia would contaminate a great amount of normal tissue and make subsequent resection difficult.

The most common errors associated with biopsy of musculoskeletal tumors are inadequate preoperative evaluation, transverse incisions, exposure of a joint or neurovascular bundle, postoperative hematoma or infection, and inadequate tumor sampling. Arthroscopic biopsy will contaminate the joint and thus should not be done for any potentially malignant tumor (7). Such errors result in increased risk of amputation and decreased survival rate. The risk is increased when a surgeon inexperienced in musculoskeletal malignancies performs the biopsy. It is preferable to refer any suspected sarcoma to a tertiary treatment center before biopsy. I recommend that all soft tissue lesions larger than 5 cm; all soft tissue lesions deep to the fascia; and all potentially malignant primary bone lesions associated with pain, cortical destruction, or bone formation be referred to an experienced treatment center before biopsy (8).

SURGICAL MARGINS

A precise definition and the classification of surgical margins are useful for planning treatment and evaluating outcome of musculoskeletal tumors. Bone and soft tissue tumors behave in biologically similar manners. Soft tissue tumors are usually surrounded by a capsule (or pseudocapsule); bone tumors are encased by a rim of reactive bone. The tumor is inside the capsule, and on the outer surface is the reactive zone. The reactive zone is of variable thickness and is identified best on MRI as a rim of abnormal signal intensity surrounding the lesion. Within the reactive zone is a variable amount of microscopic tumor extension. Just beyond the reactive zone is normal tissue. High-grade tumors often have neither a capsule nor a reactive rim of bone.

Four types of surgical margins have been defined: intralesional (or intracapsular), marginal, wide, and radical (Table 85.3). Intralesional or intracapsular margins exist when the plane of dissection is through the lesion. By definition, residual tumor remains. A marginal margin occurs when the plane of dissection is through the reactive zone, for example, when a tumor is shelled out with dissection of the tumor capsule. With a wide margin, the plane of dissection is through normal tissue. No set distance determines a wide margin, rather it is the quality of tissue that makes a margin wide. For instance, fat is a poor barrier to tumor extension and a margin of several centimeters may be necessary to be classified as wide. In contrast, a millimeter margin of cortical bone or fascia is considered wide. A radical margin is attained if the surgeon removes

table	85.3	Surgical Margins

Type	Plane of Dissection	Microscopic Appearance
Intracapsular	Within the lesion	Tumor at margin
Marginal	Within the reactive zone; extracapsular	Reactive tissue ± microsatellite tumors
Wide	Beyond the reactive zone, through normal tissue, within the compartment	Normal tissue ± skip metastasis
Radical	Within normal tissue, outside the compartment	Normal tissue

table	85.4	Surgical Margins by Limb Procedure

Type of Margin	Limb Salvage Procedure	Amputation
Intracapsular	Intracapsular piecemeal excision	Intracapsular amputation
Marginal	Marginal en bloc excision	Marginal amputation
Wide	Wide en bloc excision	Wide through-bone amputation
Radical	Radical en bloc resection	Radical exarticulation

the compartment containing the tumor. For bone, the entire bone must be removed. In soft tissue, the entire compartment must be removed from muscle origin to insertion to be considered a radical margin.

Certain anatomic areas are poor barriers to tumor extension; thus by definition, they are considered extracompartmental (Table 85.2). For example the popliteal fossa, axilla, and antecubital fossa are all considered extracompartmental, whereas the anterior, medial, and posterior portions of the thigh are intracompartmental. The surgical margin obtained is defined not by the type of procedure performed but by the margin of tissue achieved. For example, amputations are classified with the same scheme as limb salvage procedures. Therefore, an amputation that extends through the tumor is intralesional, one that extends through the reactive zone is marginal, one that extends through normal tissue is wide, and one that is outside the compartment of origin is radical (Table 85.4).

SUMMARY

A cognitive approach to staging, biopsy, and surgical margins of musculoskeletal tumors has allowed or-

thopaedic oncologists to do limb salvage procedures for the majority of patients with benign and malignant tumors of the musculoskeletal system. Careful planning and referral of potentially malignant tumors to a surgeon trained in the treatment of musculoskeletal tumors is important to avoid treatment errors. Further advances in chemotherapy, radiotherapy, and radiologic imaging will continue to improve survival rates of malignant bone and soft tissue tumors. Research in the fields of bone substitutes and growth factors will provide the tools for reconstruction of bone defects in the next century.

REFERENCES

1. Enneking WF. A system of staging musculoskeletal neoplasms. Clin Orthop 1986;204:9–24.
2. Heare TC, Enneking WF, Heare MM. Staging techniques and biopsy of bone tumors. Orthop Clin North Am 1989;20:273–285.
3. Peabody TD, Simon MA. Principles of staging of soft-tissue sarcomas. Clin Orthop 1993;289:19–31.
4. Enneking WF. Clinical musculoskeletal pathology. Gainesville, FL: University of Florida Press, 1990.
5. Mankin HJ, Lange TA, Spanier SS. The hazards of biopsy in patients with malignant primary bone and soft-tissue tumors. J Bone Joint Surg 1982;64A:1121–1127.
6. Springfield D, Rosenberg A. Biopsy: complicated and risky [Editorial]. J Bone Joint Surg 1996;78A:639.
7. Skrzynski M, Biermann S, Montag A, Simon MA. Diagnostic accuracy and charge-savings of outpatient core needle biopsy compared with open biopsy of musculoskeletal tumors. J Bone Joint Surg 1996;78A:644–650.
8. Mankin HJ, Mankin CJ, Simon MA. The hazards of biopsy, revisited. J Bone Joint Surg 1996;78A: 656–664.
9. Gustafson P. Soft tissue sarcoma. Epidemiology and progress in 508 patients. Acta Orthop Scand Suppl 1994;259:1–31.
10. Joyce MJ, Mankin HJ. Caveat arthroscopos: extra-articular lesions of bone simulating intra-articular pathology of the knee. J Bone Joint Surg 1983;65A:289–292.
11. Simon MA. Biopsy of musculoskeletal tumors [Current Concepts Review]. J Bone Joint Surg 1982;64A:1253–1257.

Benign Bone Tumors: Diagnosis and Treatment

Benign bone tumors make up a diverse and heterogeneous group of bone anomalies (1). Although some of these lesions are true neoplasms, others are actually developmental (osteochondroma), hamartomatous (fibrous dysplasia), or reparative (aneurysmal bone cyst) in nature. Despite their infrequent occurrence, an accurate understanding of the manifestation and behavior of these tumors is essential in the clinical practice of orthopaedic surgery. Knowledge of the signs and symptoms, radiographic characteristics, and natural history of these conditions allows the surgeon to observe comfortably and competently when indicated, to operate when necessary, and to refer when appropriate. In the present environment in which cost-effective care is paramount, the general orthopaedic surgeon is asked to become increasingly involved in the management of benign bone tumors. This chapter discusses common clinical and radiographic characteristics of benign bone tumors and reviews their treatment.

RELEVANT ANATOMY

Relevant anatomy is addressed below in the discussions of specific common benign bone tumors.

INITIAL FINDINGS, PHYSICAL EXAMINATION, AND DIAGNOSIS

Benign bone tumors are most common in children and young adults but may occur or persist in people of any age. The actual incidence and prevalence of these tumors are not known, because, unlike malignant neoplasms, many benign tumors remain undetected or untreated. The initial complaint of a patient with a benign bone tumor is as variable as the condition itself. Benign bone tumors are frequently asymptomatic; thus the complaint is usually unrelated to the tumor, and the radiographic abnormality is an incidental finding.

Lesions that are biologically active, however, may be associated with local symptoms. At times, the only initial complaint is pain, which is most commonly dull or achy and may be activity related. The sudden onset of pain may indicate a pathologic fracture. Night pain may suggest certain types of benign bone tumors (osteoid osteomas).

Physical signs correlated with the symptoms are atrophy of the involved extremity and, if the tumor is located in the lower extremity, a limp. Benign bone tumors may cause limb deformities or scoliosis. A palpable mass in the region of a benign bone neoplasm is rare and is most commonly due to bone expansion or deformity rather than soft tissue extension. Bone tumors are rarely a manifestation of a clinical syndrome involving other organ systems (e.g., brown tumor of hyperparathyroidism).

RADIOLOGIC STUDIES

Because of the nonspecific symptoms and physical findings with benign bone tumors, accurate interpretation of imaging studies and, particularly, radiographs is essential for the diagnosis. In many cases, the orthopaedic surgeon can make the diagnosis solely on the basis of plain radiographs. Technetium bone scanning, tomography, CT, and MRI may be of additional value in selected cases.

The radiograph is valuable for defining tumor location, zone of transition, and internal characteristics and for evaluating the bone for the presence of deformity or fracture. Typical benign neoplasms are obvious on radiographs, not subtle, because they usually have a narrow zone of transition. This is also described as being well demarcated and as surrounded by a sclerotic border. Significant cortical destruction is rare and, if present, indicates an aggressive benign or malignant neoplasm.

Warning signs of a malignant tumor include significant cortical destruction, periosteal new bone formation, a permeative or moth-eaten appearance, a wide zone of transition, and soft tissue extension.

Because most bone tumors are metaphyseal in location, that location is not helpful for the differential diagnosis. In contrast, epiphyseal tumors are almost always chondroblastomas or giant cell tumors. Diaphyseal tumors are less common than metaphyseal tumors and include Langerhans' cell histiocytosis (LCH), enchondromas, and fibrous dysplasia. Chapter 84 discusses indications for additional imaging.

Staging

A thorough evaluation of the clinical characteristics and imaging studies allows the surgeon to estimate the behavior of a particular neoplasm. As noted, benign bone tumors are often found incidentally in the workup of an unrelated problem. Tumors displaying the classical benign radiographic features may be assumed to be slow growing and to require observation without intervention. In contrast, a painful lesion with more aggressive features is likely to progress. In light of this natural history, Enneking (2) described a staging system for benign bone disease in which tumors are classified as latent (stage 1), active (stage 2), or aggressive (stage 3) based on radiographic images. The staging system reflects the behavior of the lesion and indicates the need for intervention. Stage 1 lesions can be safely observed, whereas stage 2 and 3 lesions often require treatment. Classification systems based on other imaging studies have been suggested, but the Enneking system remains the one most commonly used for benign tumors of bone (see Chapter 85).

TREATMENT

Biopsy

Biopsy is performed at the end of the staging process, the purpose of which is to determine the nature and extent of the lesion. For benign bone tumors, the indications for biopsy include a symptomatic radiographic lesion, an active or aggressive benign neoplasm, and a lesion of indeterminate malignant potential. A relative indication is the presence of a lesion for which the diagnosis is known, but the size or location of the lesion places the patient at risk for pathologic fracture. The purpose of the biopsy then is confirmation of the diagnosis before definitive treatment. Asymptomatic latent lesions that are found incidentally may be observed.

Because the biopsy is simply intended to confirm the diagnosis, an open (incisional) biopsy is usually recommended. Techniques for more limited biopsy (fine-needle aspirate or trephine) are popular for evaluating malignant disease. These techniques are not as useful for benign tumors because of their heterogeneous nature and the absence of a soft tissue mass. Limited biopsy may be used to confirm the diagnosis in areas of difficult access, such as the spine and pelvis.

Incisional biopsy is technically simple, but poor planning and poor technique may limit the treatment options. In general, all tumors must be approached as if they were malignant. This care may prevent the loss of a limb because of an unexpected finding. The surgeon must be careful to review the clinical history and the imaging studies with a consulting pathologist both before and after performing the biopsy to avoid misinterpretation of the results. If the frozen-section diagnosis is consistent with the preoperative diagnosis based on clinical and radiographic evaluation, surgery may proceed immediately. If, however, soft tissue is unavailable or the frozen-section diagnosis is not consistent with the preoperative assessment, definitive surgery should be delayed until a final pathology report is available. After conducting the biopsy, the surgeon must maintain careful hemostasis. Bone wax or methyl methacrylate may be used.

Excisional biopsies are indicated for removing symptomatic osteochondromas and osteoid osteomas. Fortunately, these tumors have imaging characteristics that are virtually diagnostic before surgery (see Chapter 84).

Operative Treatment

In general, curettage and reconstruction are indicated for the treatment of benign bone tumors. En bloc resection may be indicated for recurrent tumors or for aggressive lesions located in expendable bones. The technique of curettage, the use of adjuvants, and the choice of bone graft or bone substitutes currently available are discussed in this section.

If the incisional biopsy is consistent with a benign neoplasm, then the incision is extended proximally and distally to allow visualization of the entire extent of the neoplasm. If the cortical bone is intact, the surgeon must make a large window to allow access to the entire tumor; this is done with a high-speed burr. The window must be large enough to eliminate ledges or hidden areas that could contain tumor. Initially, a hand curette is used to remove all gross tumor. Then a high-speed burr is used to extend the curettage mechanically and débride the surface to normal-appearing bone. The surgeon should thoroughly débride all craters, ridges, and recesses mechanically. Pulse lavage is useful for irrigating the cavity contents. Care must be taken to avoid excessive soft tissue contamination and seeding.

A variety of adjuvants are available for extending tissue necrosis beyond the area of mechanical curettage to improve the chance of cure. Liquid nitrogen may be used in several freeze–thaw cycles to kill cells well beyond that achieved with mechanical curettage alone. Unfortunately, side effects, such as bone necrosis and pathologic fracture, may occur after this procedure. Some surgeons use phenol locally to cause cell death. Finally, methyl methacrylate in addition to its structural properties has a thermal necrotizing effect on the remaining bone.

In most cases of benign bone disease—given the typical patients' young age and the low chance of local recurrence—bone grafts are used after surgery to reconstruct the defect. The choices are autograft, allograft, demineralized bone, hydroxyapatite–collagen combinations, and tricalcium–phosphate combinations. Autografts may provide optimal healing, but their use is limited by donor morbidity and the lack of sufficient bone in young children. Allografts are commonly used, but they may not incorporate as rapidly or completely as will an autograft, and—although the risk is small—disease transmission is possible. Other bone substitutes have not been evaluated extensively for the treatment of benign bone tumors. Polymethyl methacrylate may be used for immediate stability, but it is generally reserved for adults with aggressive bone tumors. Bone transport and distraction osteogenesis can be used to fill bone defects; however, these techniques, which are used almost extensively for correction of congenital and posttraumatic deformities, are seldom used in tumor surgery.

COMMON BENIGN BONE TUMORS

Fibrous Cortical Defect and Nonossifying Fibroma

Fibrous cortical defect and nonossifying fibroma are related benign bone disorders that are extremely frequent incidental radiographic findings. Caffey (3) reported a 30 to 40% incidence of fibrous cortical defects in asymptomatic children undergoing skeletal surveys. The most common age at diagnosis is the second decade; 80% of affected individuals are younger than 20 years old. There is a slight male predominance, and the most common location is the knee, either the distal femur or the proximal tibia (Table 86.1).

Most commonly, this lesion is an incidental finding discovered on radiographs taken for an unrelated problem. Fibrous cortical defects and nonossifying fibromas are associated only rarely with pathologic fracture. Usually no swelling, deformity, limp, or atrophy is present. Some authors prefer the term *fibrous cortical defect* to refer to small metaphyseal eccentric cortical lesions, but a progression from the smaller fibrous cortical defect to the more biologically active nonossifying fibroma is likely. The natural histories of fibrous cortical defects and nonossifying fibromas are similar: resolution in early adulthood as the lesion heals through the formation of peripheral trabecular bone. These lesions are usually solitary but are rarely multifocal. Multifocal disease in association with pigmented skin lesions is known as Jaffe-Campanacci syndrome (4).

Radiographs are diagnostic in most cases. The classic radiographic finding is an eccentric metaphyseal radiolucency surrounded by a rim of sclerotic bone (Fig. 86.1). Internal septations and a somewhat bubbly appearance

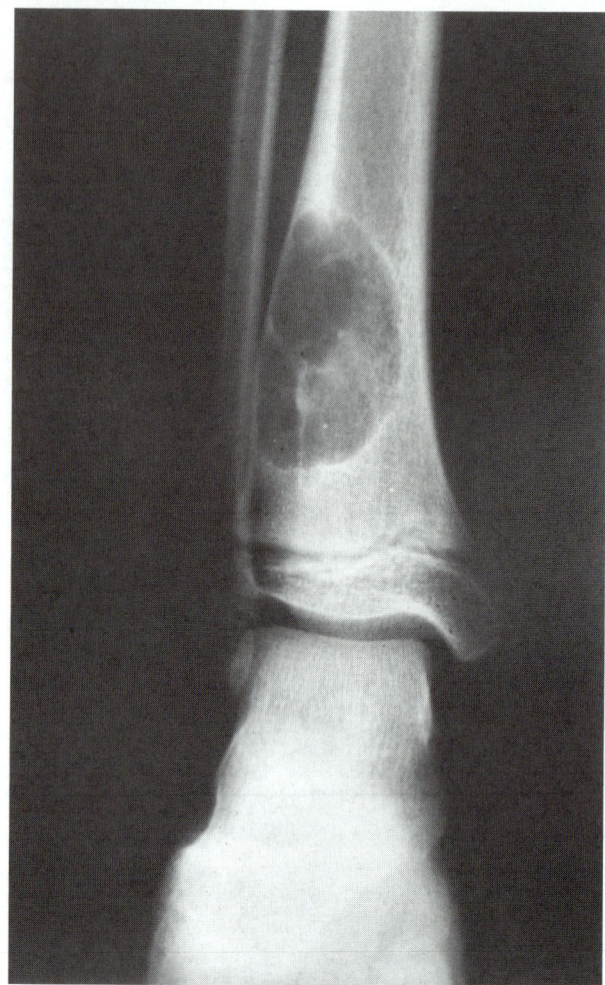

Figure 86.1. AP view of the distal tibia of a 10-year-old male, showing a probable nonossifying fibroma.

may be present. No evidence of calcification or ossification exists, and the lesion has a narrow zone of transition. The long bones are most commonly affected. Evidence exists that these lesions assume a more diaphyseal location with longitudinal bone growth. Typically, these lesions are larger in the longitudinal axis than in the transverse axis, also because of longitudinal growth.

The differential diagnosis includes fibrous dysplasia; however, fibrous dysplasia is commonly central rather than eccentric in location. Chondromyxoid fibroma also occurs in an eccentric metaphyseal portion of the tibia but is less common. A nonossifying fibroma is rarely confused with an osteoid osteoma or with infection.

Because of the natural history of healing of nonossifying fibromas, observation is indicated. When classic radiographic findings are present, neither further imaging studies nor a biopsy is necessary. The indications for surgery are recurrent pathologic fracture and lesions considered predisposed to pathologic fracture. Some authors suggest prophylactic curettage and bone grafting for lesions larger than 50% of the bone's width. On the other hand, because these fractures heal without complication, some authors

table 86.1 | Benign Bone Tumors

Tumor	Age (Years)	Male:Female Ratio	Locations	Radiographs	Associated Syndromes	Treatment	Pathologic Features	Malignant Potential
Nonossifying fibroma	0–20	1.5:1	Metaphyseal; distal femur; proximal tibia	Cortical-based eccentric; lucency; sclerotic margin	Multifocal disease with café-au-lait spots; Jaffe-Campanacci syndrome	Observation; curettage and bone graft for pathologic fracture	Storiform pattern; fibrous cells; occasional giant cells	Extremely rare
Fibrous dysplasia	0–30	1:1.3	Proximal femur; tibia, ribs; skull	Ground glass; shepherd's crook deformity	Polyostotic disease; endocrine dysfunction; precocious puberty; cutaneous pigmentation; Albright syndrome	Observation; internal fixation	Alphabet soup or Chinese characters; fibrous tissue and woven bone; no osteoblastic rimming	Rare
Osteoid osteoma	0–20	2:1	Proximal femur, tibia, posterior spine	Small nidus surrounded by sclerosis	None	NSAIDs; burr-down technique	Haphazard trabeculae; osteoblasts	Extremely rare
Osteoblastoma	0–30	3:1	Posterior spine; femur; tibia	Nidus > 2 cm; bone formation	None	Curettage or excision	Haphazard trabeculae; osteoblasts	May be confused with osteosarcoma
Enchondroma	20–50	1:1	Diaphyseal; small bones (hands); femur; humerus; tibia	Punctate calcification	Ollier's dyschondroplasia; Maffucci's hemangiomas	Observation; curettage and bone graft	Hypocellular; rare binucleated cells; islands of cartilage	Higher in multifocal disease
Osteochondroma	0–20	1.5:1	Metaphyseal; femur; humerus; tibia	Exostosis; broad-based or pedunculated, pointed away from the joint	Multiple hereditary exostoses (autosomal dominant)	Observation; excision if symptomatic	Resembles epiphyseal plate; cartilage cap	Rare in solitary disease; growth or pain after skeletal maturity
Chondroblastoma	0–20	1.3:1	Epiphyseal; humerus; femur; tibia	Lucency; may show punctate calcification	None	Curettage; adjuvant bone graft	Giant cells; distinctive polyhedral chondroblasts; chicken wire calcification	Rare
Giant cell tumor	20–50	1:1.5	Epiphyseal; femur; tibia; radius	Lucency; expansile; may be aggressive	None	Curettage; adjuvant methylmethacrylate; excision	Giant cells; interchangeable stromal nuclei	Benign pulmonary metastases possible
Aneurysmal bone cyst	0–30	1:1	Metaphyseal; femur; tibia	Expanded lucency; fine rim of bone	None	Curettage; adjuvant bone graft	Giant cells; spindle stromal cells; blood-filled spaces	None
Unicameral bone cyst	0–20	3:1	Metaphyseal; humerus; femur	Lucency; expansile; may be septate; fallen leaf or fragment sign	None	Observation; steroid injection; curettage and bone graft	Mesothelial monolayer; fibrous tissue	None
LCH	1–15	1.5:1	Ribs; skull; vertebral body; pelvis; diaphysis of long bones	Rounded lucency; vertebra plana	Disseminated (Letterer-Siwe disease); intermediate (Hand-Schüller-Christian disease); skeletal only (eosinophilic granuloma)	Curettage; steroid injection	Langerhans histiocytes; eosinophils; Birbeck bodies	None

Data from Shajowicz F. Tumors and tumorlike lesions of bone. New York: Springer, 1994; and Wold LE, McLeod RA, Sim FH, Unni KK. Atlas of orthopaedic pathology. Philadelphia: Saunders, 1990. NSAIDs, nonsteroidal anti-inflammatory drugs.

recommend continued observation. Suggested operative treatment includes biopsy, frozen section, and, if the lesion is consistent with nonossifying fibroma, curettage and bone graft (or bone substitute).

Fibrous Dysplasia

Fibrous dysplasia is a hamartomatous bone disorder, not a true neoplasm (4); histologically, it is an abnormal proliferation of the fibro-osseous tissue. Fibrous dysplasia is diagnosed most commonly in the second or third decade of life. There is a slight female predominance. The bones most frequently involved are the skull, jaw, ribs, and femoral neck; however, any bone may be involved. Fibrous dysplasia usually involves only a single site; however, cases of polyostotic disease do exist.

Frequently, monostotic fibrous dysplasia is an incidental finding in an asymptomatic patient who had a radiograph taken for another reason. Occasionally, patients have localized pain from bone deformity or pathologic fracture; but this situation usually occurs in individuals with more severe involvement, particularly patients with polyostotic disease. Rarely, fibrous dysplasia is associated with endocrine abnormalities. For example, Albright syndrome is polyostotic fibrous dysplasia associated with cutaneous brown skin patches (café-au-lait spots) and precocious puberty.

Radiographically, fibrous dysplasia has a ground-glass appearance with a rim of host bone sclerosis (Fig. 86.2). Fibrous dysplasia is most commonly centered in the canal, not in a cortical or an eccentric location. The bone may be focally expanded; however, all periosteal new bone is mature. In more severe disease, fibrous dysplasia may cause significant bone deformity, including the shepherd's crook deformity of the proximal femur. Another radiographic finding, which may be confused with Paget's disease, is the candle-flame appearance; i.e., the radiographic appearance of the lesion is more lucent distally and more sclerotic proximally, and within the lucent area, a tapered inner density resembling a candle flame occurs (4). The radiographic differential diagnosis includes nonossifying fibroma, unicameral bone cyst, chondromyxoid fibroma, aneurysmal bone cyst, and (more rarely) osteosarcoma or Paget's disease. Nonossifying fibroma is commonly eccentric in location.

CT studies demonstrate the thick host sclerosis and sometimes provide evidence of intralesional mineralization. The results of MRI studies may be variable, because they include low-signal changes of bone sclerosis mixed with higher-signal changes of fibro-osseous tissue and cystic degeneration.

The treatment in most cases is observation only. When pain, pathologic fracture, or deformity is present, the surgeon may elect to proceed with curettage and bone grafting. Internal fixation is recommended, because the bone graft itself may become dysplastic. An alternative is a vascularized bone graft, which has been used with some success for this disease.

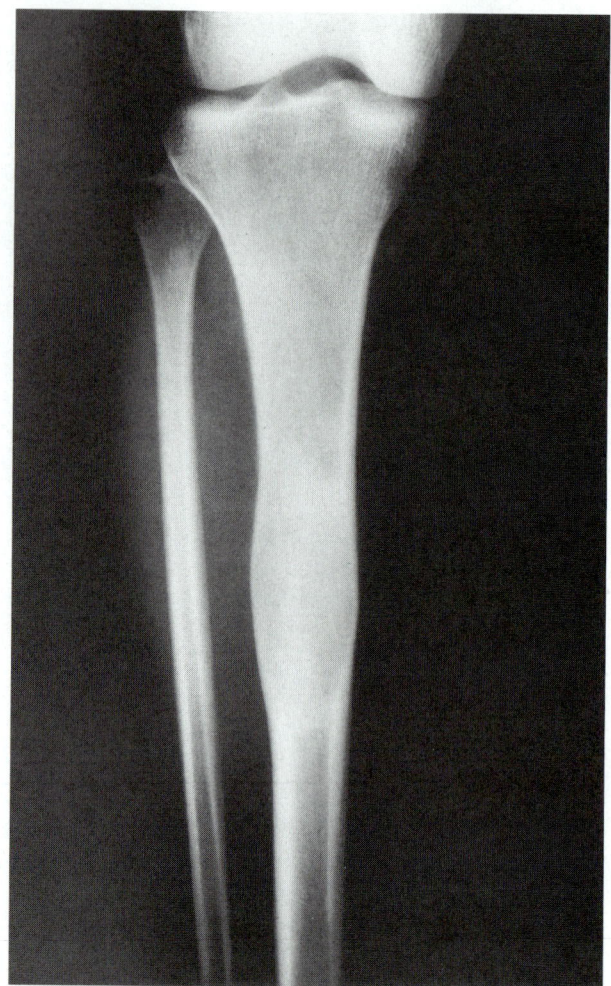

Figure 86.2. AP view of the tibia of a 25-year-old male, showing fibrous dysplasia.

Osteoid Osteoma

Osteoid osteoma is a common benign bone tumor that affects mainly children and young adults. It is most common in the second decade of life: 70% of affected patients are younger than 20 years old at the time of diagnosis. It is seen more often in males. More than half of osteoid osteomas are found in the lower extremity, and the proximal femur is a frequent site. A common initial complaint is night pain, which characteristically diminishes with the use of aspirin or other nonsteroidal anti-inflammatory drug. This lesion may be associated with a limp or focal atrophy. Occasionally, a joint effusion or significant synovitis may occur (if the lesion is juxta-articular). An osteoid osteoma of the spine may result in scoliosis secondary to muscle spasm.

Radiographs have a distinctive appearance and demonstrate a small round lucency in the cortex of the bone, with surrounding mature periosteal bone formation. This radiolucency is often only a few millimeters in size and always less than 2 cm; it is known as the nidus. Sometimes the surrounding reactive sclerosis obliterates the view of the nidus. Plain tomography and especially CT scanning identify the nidus in most cases.

The differential diagnosis includes Brodie abscess, stress fracture, and osteoblastoma. A Brodie abscess may look remarkably similar to an osteoid osteoma if it is intracortical. A key finding presents on the CT scan: Infectious processes are often associated with small perforations of the cortex; these perforations are an unusual finding in osteoid osteoma. Stress fractures do not have an identifiable nidus even on fine-resolution CT.

Treatment of these lesions is based on symptoms. Studies demonstrate that these lesions eventually become asymptomatic (5). The pain may be secondary to local production of prostaglandins, and most patients respond well to low doses of nonsteroidal anti-inflammatory agents. In many cases, this treatment will be the only one necessary. The physician should advise the patient and family, however, that treatment may be necessary for a prolonged period and that clinical monitoring for the effects of the medication on other organ systems is necessary. In cases of gastrointestinal intolerance or allergy, surgical excision may be performed.

Multiple techniques exist to treat osteoid osteomas. Historically, en bloc excision was recommended; however, the nidus is not visualized in this procedure, and it requires extensive loss of cortical bone. At times, the surgeon missed the lesion, and the patient had an increased risk of pathologic fracture. Because the goal of surgery is to remove the nidus and not the surrounding host bone, surgeons have had success with a burr-down technique in which a mechanical burr passes through the host sclerosis down to the level of the nidus (6). The nidus itself has a fairly distinctive appearance and a cherry red color. Then the surgeon curettes the nidus and mechanically débrides the bone. Often, the procedure can be performed without entering the medullary canal; thus the patient is not at significant risk for pathologic fracture. Recently, some authors have described alternative approaches using CT-directed reaming or electrode-mediated thermal necrosis (7). Once the nidus is ablated surgically, symptomatic improvement is rapid, and recurrence is rare.

Osteoblastoma

Osteoblastomas are bone-forming tumors that usually occur in the second decade of life and have a male predominance. Osteoblastomas are most common in the posterior elements of the spine, and 40% of all osteoblastomas occur in the spine. Frequently, the clinical sign is scoliosis secondary to muscle spasm, atrophy, and sometimes neurologic involvement. Radiographic examination demonstrates a variable appearance. The differential diagnosis includes osteoid osteoma, osteosarcoma, and aneurysmal bone cyst.

In general, surgical treatment of osteoblastomas is recommended. Owing to occasional confusion between osteoblastoma and osteosarcoma, the orthopaedic oncologist must perform the biopsy carefully. En bloc excision, when possible, is the preferred surgical treatment;

but curettage is acceptable when dictated by anatomic constraints.

Enchondroma

An enchondroma is a benign cartilage neoplasm that most frequently presents in the second decade of life but—because it is often asymptomatic—may persist and be noted incidentally at any age. It is a common tumor of the short tubular bones of the hands, and it often occurs in the femur and the humerus. No sex predominance exists.

In the adult population, enchondroma may be the most common benign bone tumor found incidentally during radiographic evaluation of an unrelated problem. Some authors describe an atypical enchondroma with benign features and pain; however, significant symptoms suggest a low-grade chondrosarcoma (4). Sometimes, an enchondroma is associated with a pathologic fracture, especially of the small bones of the hand.

Radiographs demonstrate that these lesions are intramedullary with a narrow transition zone. Either on plain radiographs or on CT, punctate calcifications may appear within the lesion (Fig. 86.3). The lesions may produce mild

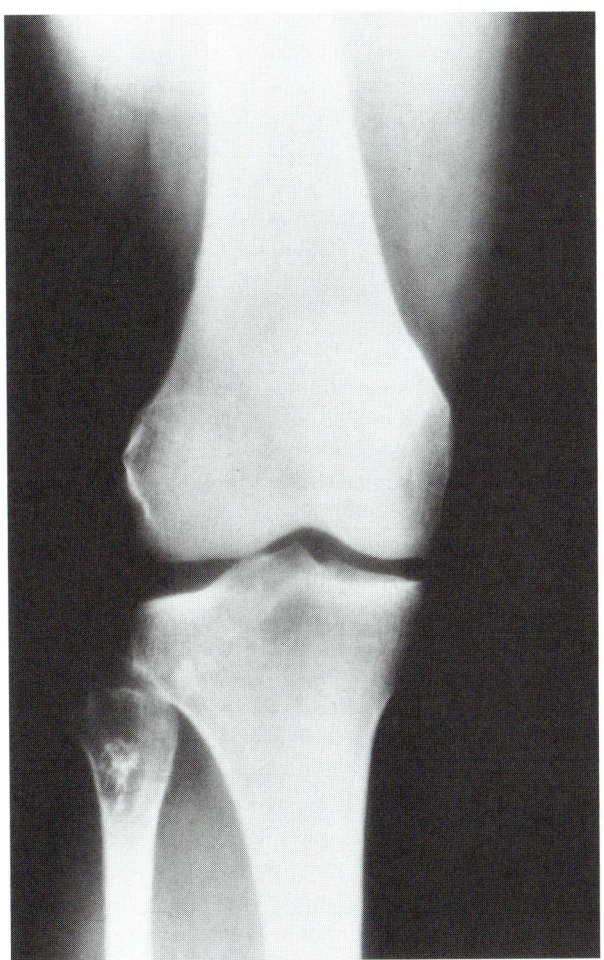

Figure 86.3. AP view of the knee of a 35-year-old female, showing an enchondroma.

expansion of the bone and mild endosteal scalloping. Significant scalloping or cortical destruction suggests a more aggressive neoplasm, such as chondrosarcoma. The differential diagnosis includes bone infarct and chondrosarcoma. It is essential when evaluating these tumors to carefully review the clinical findings and the results of radiographic and imaging studies with an experienced pathologist before making a diagnosis.

In general, observation of these lesions is sufficient, if the clinical history and radiographs support the diagnosis of an enchondroma. In cases of pathologic fracture, the fracture is allowed to heal; then the patient is observed or undergoes a curettage and bone graft. Because a small probability of dedifferentiation into a chondrosarcoma exists, observation is recommended.

Enchondromas rarely affect multiple bones. True multifocal enchondromas may exist; however, such cases are likely to represent a form of dyschondroplasia. Ollier (4) described patients with multiple enchondromas, typically affecting one-half of the body. Maffucci's syndrome consists of multiple enchondromas associated with systemic hemangiomas (4). Typically, in both of these disorders significant abnormalities throughout the length of the bone occur rather than discrete enchondromas. Frequently, significant bone deformity develops with multiple enchondromas. Bones are short, angulated, and club-shaped secondary to lack of tubulization of the bone. These patients have a higher incidence of malignant degeneration than do patients with solitary enchondromas. It is essential to observe patients with multiple enchondromas closely, both symptomatically and, when indicated by symptoms, radiographically for the development of malignant degeneration.

Osteochondroma

Osteochondroma is a benign metaphyseal cartilage capped protuberance, also known as an exostosis, and presents most frequently in the second decade of life; a slight male predominance exists. The lesion is most common in the distal femur but may affect any long bone, the pelvis, or the ribs. In most instances, the cause is likely to be abnormal development of the growth plate with separation and displacement of a portion of the physeal plate peripherally to a metaphyseal location. This focus of physeal cartilage, which is capable of longitudinal growth, forms bone at an angle, frequently perpendicular, to the direction of bone growth. The result is an exostosis.

The most common presentation is a mass, which may be associated with pain. Symptoms may be related to mechanical irritation, bursitis, or nerve compression. Reports of popliteal pseudo-aneurysms adjacent to osteochondromas of the posterior distal femur exist. Bone deformity is rare in individuals with solitary osteochondromas. The exostosis continues to grow until skeletal maturity. Malignant degeneration is rare; however, an adult who has growth or pain associated with an osteochondroma should

be evaluated for secondary chondrosarcoma. Hereditary multiple exostoses are a rare autosomal dominant condition. Unlike children with solitary disease, affected individuals often have bone shortening angular deformity and are at risk for malignant degeneration.

Radiographically, an osteochondroma has a distinctive appearance in which a bony protuberance arises from a flared metaphysis (Fig. 86.4). Cortical bone and cancellous bone are continuous between the base of the exostosis and the normal bone. The peripheral outline in young patients may be indistinct because of the cartilage cap but is usually sharp in adults. The base may be broad or narrow (sessile or pedunculated, respectively). Usually, the tip of the lesion points away from the articular surface.

MRI is particularly useful in demonstrating the continuous normal signal of bone marrow within the base of the lesion and the normal bone. In addition, it demonstrates the thickness of the cartilage cap, which, although it may be quite large in young children, is typically less than 1 cm in adults. MRI may also provide evidence of a bursa adjacent to the lesion. Any signal changes within the marrow itself or associated soft tissue mass should alert the clinician to the possibility of malignant degeneration. The differential

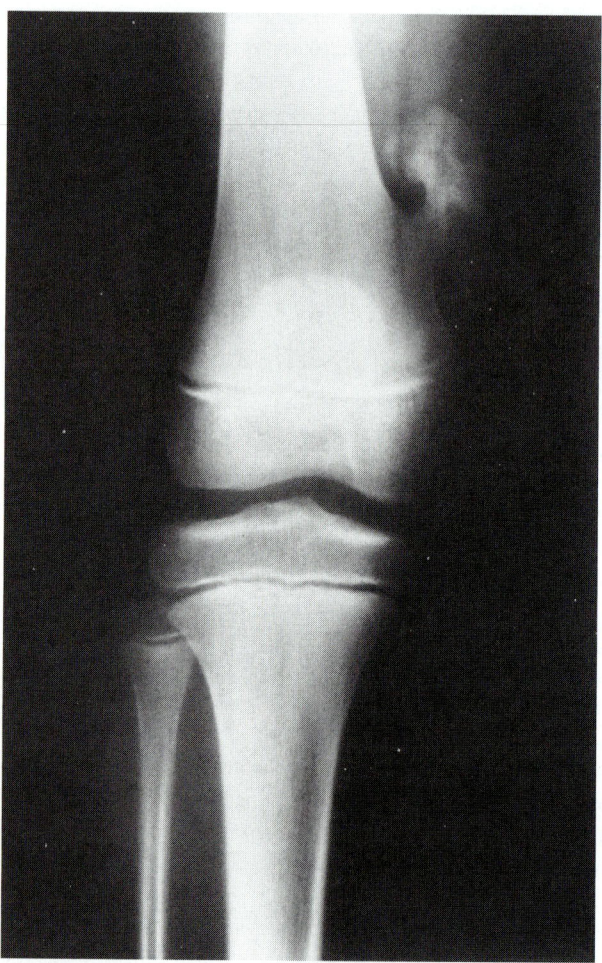

Figure 86.4. AP view of the knee of a child, showing an osteochondroma.

diagnosis is rarely in question, but sometimes an osteo-chondroma resembles parosteal osteosarcoma, parosteal chondroma, or myositis ossificans.

The treatment in most cases is observation. These lesions are associated with a low incidence of malignant degeneration, which usually occurs in adulthood and is heralded by pain or growth after skeletal maturity. Surgery, however, may be indicated for symptomatic lesions that do not respond to nonoperative treatment or for the treatment of bone deformity. It may be advisable to delay surgery until the lesion moves to a more metadiaphyseal location, which will occur with longitudinal growth of the underlying bone. Surgery includes excision of the lesion at its base. The surgeon must resect the perichondrium over the cap of the lesion en bloc with the exostosis to prevent local recurrence.

Chondroblastoma

Chondroblastoma is a benign bone tumor that occurs most commonly in the second decade of life. There is a slight male predominance. Chondroblastoma frequently presents in the proximal humerus and somewhat less frequently in the distal femur, proximal tibia, and small bones of the foot. Like giant cell tumors, chondroblastomas are most often located in the epiphysis; unlike giant cell tumors, they are usually present in skeletally immature patients.

Classically, these patients have pain that may be associated with local muscular atrophy. If the tumor is located in the lower extremity, the patient may limp. Radiographically, the lesion is epiphyseal or apophyseal in the majority of cases (Fig. 86.5). It may be eccentric or central in location. The lesion has a narrow transition zone and may demonstrate evidence of matrix calcification on either plain radiographs or CT scan. The tumor sometimes extends outside the bone. The differential diagnosis includes giant cell tumor, osteonecrosis, aneurysmal bone cyst, and clear-cell chondrosarcoma.

Because of the progressive nature of these lesions, the treatment of choice is biopsy, curettage, and bone grafting. Surgeons have used liquid nitrogen, phenol, hydrogen peroxide, and methyl methacrylate to lower the incidence of local recurrence. Attention must be directed to the close proximity of the lesion to the growth plate in these young patients and the potential for growth arrest. Surgical curettage or excision may cross the articular surface in selected cases. After surgery, patients should be observed for symptomatic and radiographic evidence of local recurrence.

Giant Cell Tumor

Giant cell tumor occurs in skeletally mature individuals. Diagnosis is possible at any age but is most common in the third decade of life. A slight female predominance exists. The most common locations are the distal femur,

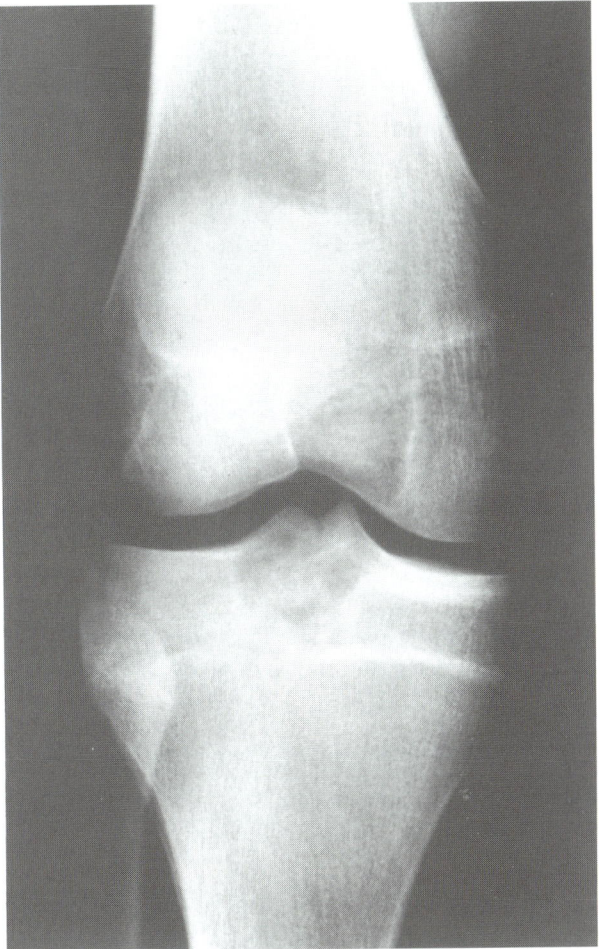

Figure 86.5. AP view of the knee of a 17-year-old male, showing a chondroblastoma.

proximal tibia, and distal radius, but the pelvis and spine may also be affected. The cause of the neoplasm is unclear. Unlike patients with brown tumors of hyperparathyroidism, which giant cell tumors resemble microscopically, these patients have no underlying metabolic bone disease. Although giant cell tumor is considered to be benign, a small percentage of afflicted individuals develop pulmonary metastases. Giant cell tumors are unique among the benign tumors in their relatively aggressive clinical and radiographic findings and in their high incidence of local recurrence after curettage and grafting (8).

The patient complains of pain, sometimes associated with swelling, a limp, or weakness. Radiographs demonstrate a lucent epiphyseal lesion (Fig. 86.6). In contrast to other benign neoplasms, giant cell tumor has a variably wide zone of transition that depends on its aggressiveness. Host bone sclerosis is rare, and the cortex is often focally obliterated. Septations may be present, but there is usually no internal structure. The differential diagnosis includes aggressive neoplasms, such as chondroblastoma, osteosarcoma, and malignant fibrous histiocytoma.

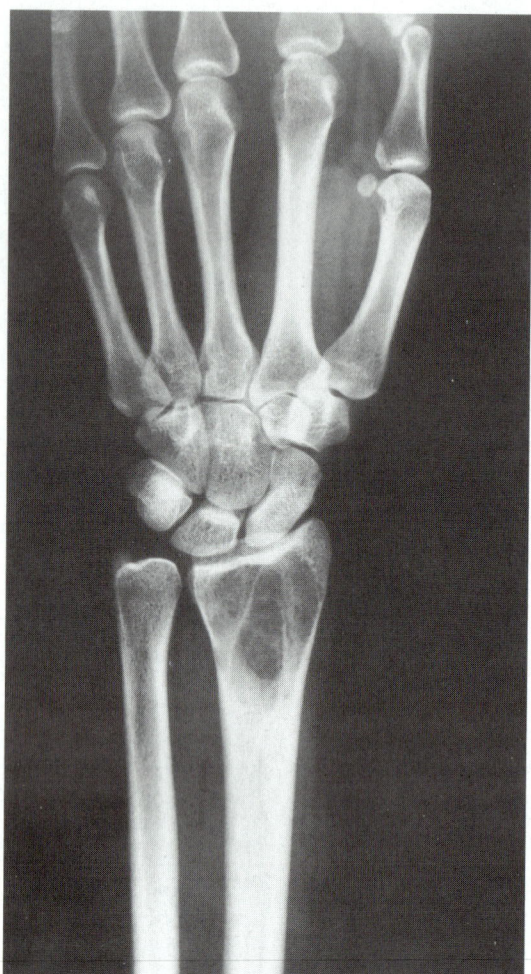

Figure 86.6. AP view of the distal radius of a 35-year-old female, showing a giant cell tumor.

Historically, the treatment of giant cell tumor consisted of curettage and bone grafting; however, this treatment is associated with a high incidence of local recurrence. Wide excision and reconstruction then became popular. Recently, surgeons have successfully cured giant cell tumor with less radical curettage and débridement followed by adjuvants such as liquid nitrogen, phenol, hydrogen peroxide, and methyl methacrylate (9). In cases of significant soft tissue extension, pathologic fracture, local recurrence, or location in expendable bone, surgical excision, with or without reconstruction, may be considered.

Local recurrence is more common with giant cell tumors than with benign bone tumors; therefore, the orthopaedist must follow the patients postoperatively. The distal radius is a site with a high incidence of local recurrence (10). In addition to radiographs and CT of the chest obtained for the initial evaluation, routine chest radiographs should be taken during the course of postoperative follow-up. Although most treatment failures occur within 2 years after treatment, a long delay may exist between initial diagnosis and recurrence.

Aneurysmal Bone Cyst

Some authors believe that an aneurysmal bone cyst is a reparative phenomenon arising from a preexisting bone lesion rather than being a de novo neoplastic entity (4). An aneurysmal bone cyst is most commonly diagnosed in the second decade of life and has a slight female predominance. It usually occurs in the metaphysis of long bones, especially of the femur and tibia, but it is also seen in the posterior elements of the spine. Pain and swelling are the chief complaints.

Aneurysmal bone cysts do not have a consistent radiographic appearance. Radiographs commonly demonstrate a ballooned expansion of the metaphysis of a long bone (Fig. 86.7). Typically, the zone of transition is narrow, although sometimes an aggressive lesion may be associated with radiographic features of malignancy. The ballooned expansion tends to be surrounded by a thin rim of bone, which is best seen on CT scans. MRI studies may demonstrate fluid-fluid levels, which can be diagnostic. In addition, technetium bone scanning—as in the case of giant cell tumors—may show central photopenic defects, the so-called donut sign. The differential diagnosis includes

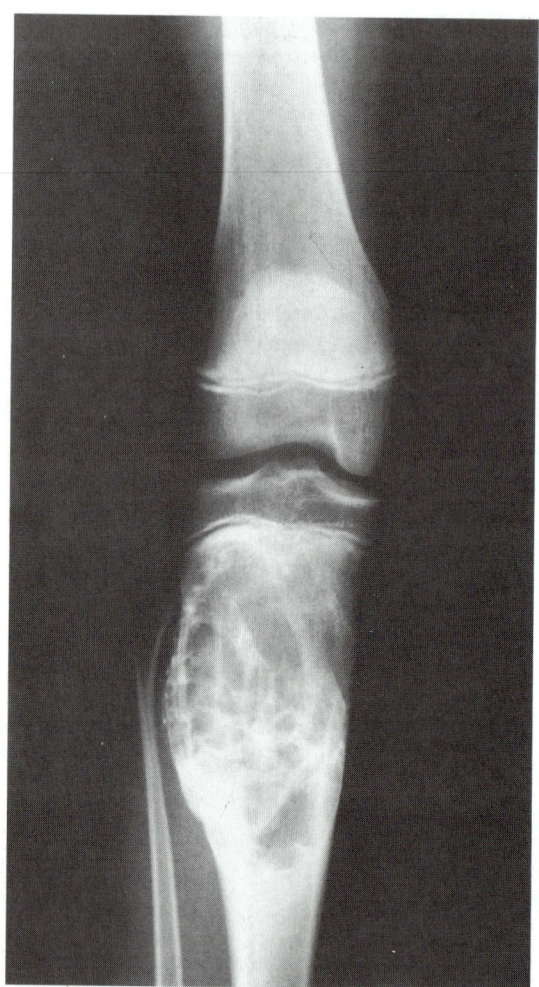

Figure 86.7. AP view of the knee and proximal tibia of a 12-year-old male, showing an aneurysmal bone cyst.

unicameral bone cyst, giant cell tumor, and even sarcoma in aggressive-appearing lesions.

Surgical treatment is usually indicated and involves curettage and bone grafting (11). Excision is also an option for expendable bones. The use of adjuvant therapy is recommended to minimize the incidence of local recurrence. The surgeon must avoid injury to the growth plate both during curettage and when using the adjuvants. Hemorrhage from axial lesions can be significant, and the surgeon should consider angiographic embolization in the course of treatment of lesions of the pelvis and spine. Radiation therapy is a treatment alternative for surgically unresectable disease in the spine and pelvis. Not all lesions or their recurrences require treatment; some reach an inactive state. Unfortunately, no method for predicting this behavior is currently available.

Unicameral Bone Cyst

The unicameral bone cyst is even less likely than the aneurysmal bone cyst to be a true tumor. It is an exceptionally common lesion, presenting in the first two decades of life. A male predominance exists. The cyst occurs almost exclusively in the long bones, especially in the proximal humerus, proximal femur, and proximal tibia. The cause of the cyst is not known (4). Current hypotheses include repair of an intraosseous hematoma and intraosseous lymphedema. Fluid obtained from the cyst is transudative, like lymphatic fluid; a mechanism of lymphatic blockade, however, has not been proved. Another theory is that the cyst represents the action of synovial rests trapped in an anomalous intraosseous location. The mesothelial monolayer lining the cyst does resemble synovium in some ways; however, this theory also remains unproved.

Most commonly, these lesions are asymptomatic, but they can present with pain if pathologic fracture occurs. Radiographically, they tend to abut the physis on the metaphyseal side. The zone of transition is narrow, and the lesion is sharply marginated. With repetitive fractures, the lesion may adopt a septate appearance, although most authors think the lesion has primarily a single chamber of origin. Radiographically, the fallen leaf sign is often seen (i.e., a piece of cortical bone falls into an intramedullary location as a result of a fracture) (Fig. 86.8). The differential diagnosis includes aneurysmal bone cyst and fibrous dysplasia.

Unicameral bone cysts usually heal spontaneously by the time of skeletal maturity; therefore, it is safe to simply observe most of these lesions. Indications for surgery include a history of pathologic fracture or a cyst location (e.g., the proximal femur) for which pathologic fracture would produce a clinically significant treatment problem. Some authors suggest that lesions adjacent to the physis are more active biologically and should be treated more aggressively. It is more likely, however, that the lo-

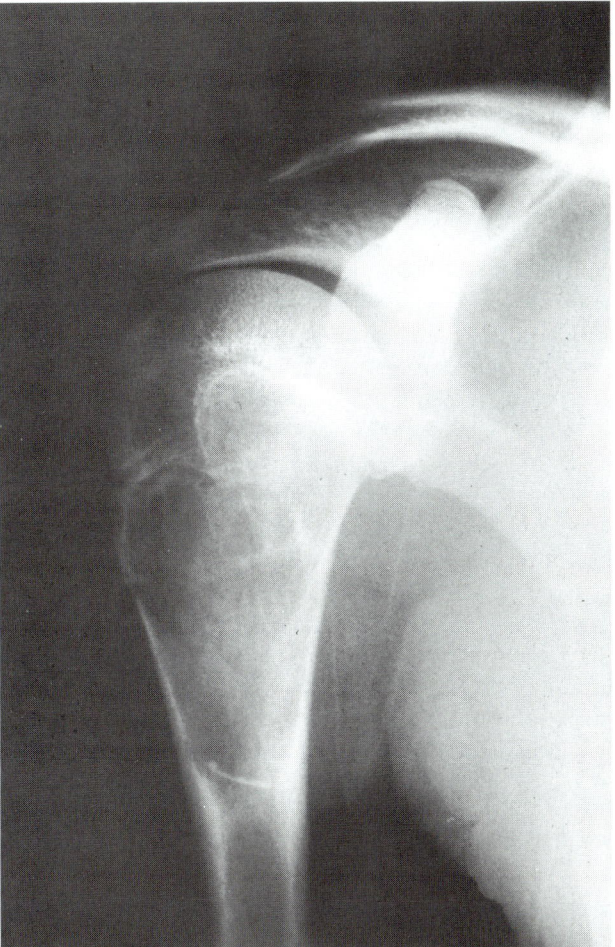

Figure 86.8. AP view of the proximal humeral metaphysis of an 11-year-old male, showing the fallen leaf or fallen fragment sign of a unicameral bone cyst.

cation of the lesion reflects the age of the patient, in that most lesions move to a metadiaphyseal location with advancing age and longitudinal growth of the bone. Although unusual bone cysts may be treated with biopsy, curettage, and bone graft, surgeons more commonly aspirate suspected unicameral bone cysts and inject them with methylprednisolone acetate (11). An alternative is to aspirate the cyst and to inject demineralized bone or a bone substitute.

The technique of aspiration and injection is as follows. Under fluoroscopic guidance, the surgeon uses two large-bore spinal needles (or needles from a bone marrow aspiration tray) to enter the cyst. The cyst is aspirated and typically produces straw-colored fluid initially. The fluid may rapidly turn bloody as the aspiration continues, or it may be bloody as a result of pathologic fracture. Aspiration and injection may be performed 2 to 3 weeks after fracture, because the periosteal sleeve in young children is usually intact by that time.

Next, a dilute contrast medium is injected through one of the needles, allowing the second needle to act as a vent. The surgeon must use caution not to deliver too large a load of contrast agent to very small children. The radiolucent defect should completely fill. Any difficulty with instillation or failure to fill the cyst completely raises the suspicion that the lesion is not a unicameral bone cyst; however, the cyst also may have multiple chambers and may require additional needles. Then between 40 and 200 mg methylprednisolone acetate is instilled into the cyst cavity through the needles. Recently, some authors have reported success using demineralized bone, bone marrow, or another bone substitute. The needles are then withdrawn, and the patient's upper extremity is placed in a sling for a few days.

Follow-up radiographs should be taken at 6 and 12 weeks. It may be necessary to inject the cysts at approximately 3-month intervals until complete healing occurs. Some reports indicate that if the contrast agent forms an immediate venogram within the cyst, the injection is not likely to produce complete healing. Curettage and bone grafts, along with steroid injection, are associated with a similar incidence of late local recurrence. Multilocular cysts, large cysts, and juxtaphyseal cysts are also associated with a slower rate of healing. No clinical syndrome is associated with unicameral bone cysts, and they are almost always solitary.

Langerhans' Cell Histiocytosis

Langerhans' cell histiocytosis (LCH) comprises a group of disorders of the reticuloendothelial system (liver, spleen, lymph nodes, and bone). The nomenclature that describes these disorders has changed and now refers to the spectrum of disorders as LCH. LCH is thus divided into a disseminated form, an intermediate form, and a form that exhibits only skeletal involvement. The disseminated form of LCH was previously called Letterer-Siwe disease. This form of LCH includes severe visceral involvement, particularly hepatosplenomegaly, and is usually fatal in infancy. Skeletal involvement is not an important feature. An intermediate form of LCH was previously called Hand-Schüller-Christian disease. This form of LCH is associated with endocrine abnormalities (diabetes insipidus), exophthalmos, and skeletal involvement. The most benign form is solitary skeletal LCH (also referred to as eosinophilic granuloma), which has no visceral involvement and tends to be self-limiting. It is most common in the first and second decades of life and is found more often in boys than in girls. It is frequently seen in the flat bones, especially the skull, ribs, and pelvis but may occur in any bone.

A patient with solitary LCH usually complains of localized pain. Swelling and deformity are unusual. Radiographs demonstrate radiolucencies that may have a punched-out appearance. In general, these granulomas have a narrow zone of transition but in an active phase may be aggressive and imitate a malignant tumor. When they occur in the spine, collapse of the anterior vertebral body without spine deformity classically occurs. This is known as vertebra plana, and although not pathognomonic of LCH, it is highly suggestive. The differential diagnosis includes other marrow cell tumors and infections. LCH should be differentiated from skeletal metastases from a neuroblastoma in young patients.

Treatment begins with a complete skeletal survey and pediatric consultation to evaluate possible visceral involvement. Treatment of symptomatic lesions includes curettage and bone graft. Recently, some surgeons have achieved success with intralesional cortisone injections. Some physicians have used low-dose radiation therapy and chemotherapy in children with severe involvement. Fortunately, the skeletal lesions tend to be self-limiting and often heal spontaneously.

SUMMARY

Benign bone tumors comprise a heterogenous group of bone anomalies consisting of neoplastic, reparative, hamartomatous, and developmental entities. Most commonly seen in children and young adults, benign bone tumors are often asymptomatic, and the actual incidence is not known, as many go unrecognized, undiagnosed, and untreated.

The radiograph remains the most helpful of the available diagnostic studies. Characteristic radiographic findings are a narrow zone of transition between the tumor and host bone. The bone may be expanded, but all new bone is mature in nature. Significant cortical destruction is rare. General operative indications are symptomatic radiographic lesion, active aggressive benign neoplasm, or lesion of indeterminate malignant potential. Intralesional operative procedures in the form of curettage are adequate to obtain local control for most bone tumors. The resulting bone defect is filled with autograft, allograft, demineralized bone, hydroxyapatite–collagen combinations, or tricalcium–phosphate combinations. In addition, polymethyl methacrylate is used commonly in adults with aggressive bone tumors. The ability to diagnose and treat benign tumors accurately, based on the knowledge of their natural history and behavior, is important in the clinical practice of orthopaedic surgery.

REFERENCES

1. Gitelis S, Wilkins R, Conrad E. Benign bone tumors. J Bone Joint Surg 1995;77A:1756–1782.
2. Enneking WF. Staging of musculoskeletal neoplasms. In: Enneking WF, ed. Musculoskeletal tumor surgery. New York: Churchill Livingstone, 1983:87–88.
3. Caffey J. On fibrous defects in cortical walls of growing tubular bones. Adv Pediatr 1955;7:13–51.
4. Mirra JM, Picci P, Gold RH. Bone tumors: clinical, radiologic, and pathologic correlations. Philadelphia: Lea & Febiger, 1989.
5. Kneisl JS, Simon MA. Medical management compared with operative treatment for osteoid osteoma. J Bone Joint Surg 1992;74A:179–185.
6. Ward WG, Eckardt JJ, Shayestehfar S, et al. Osteoid osteoma: diagnosis and management with low morbidity. Clin Orthop 1993;291:229–235.

7. Rosenthal DI, Alexander A, Rosenberg AE, Springfield D. Ablation of osteoid osteomas with a percutaneously placed electrode: a new procedure. Radiology 1992;183:29–33.

8. Goldenberg RR, Campbell CJ, Bonfiglio M. Giant cell tumor of bone. An analysis of 218 cases. J Bone Joint Surg 1970;52A:619–664.

9. Capanna R, Fabbri N, Bettelli G. Curettage of giant cell tumor of bone. The effect of surgical technique and adjuvants on local recurrence rate. Chir Organi Mov 1990;75(1 Suppl):206.

10. O'Donnell RJ, Springfield DS, Motwani HK, et al. Recurrence of giant cell tumor of the long bones after curettage and packing with cement. J Bone Joint Surg 1994;76A:1827–1833.

11. Campanacci M, Capanna R, Picci P. Unicameral and aneurysmal cysts. Clin Orthop 1986;204:25–36.

Suggested Readings

Shajowicz F. Tumors and tumorlike lesions of bone. New York: Springer, 1994.

Wold LE, McLeod RA, Sim FH, Unni KK. Atlas of orthopaedic pathology. Philadelphia: Saunders, 1990.

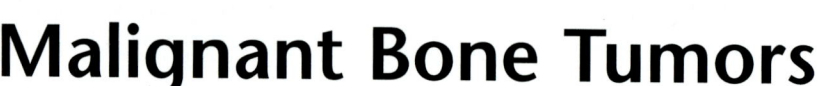

chapter 87

Brian E. McGrath, Mark T. Scarborough, and Denis R. Clohisy

Malignant Bone Tumors

Solid primary malignant bone tumors are rare. There are approximately 10 such tumors per 1 million people per year. Soft tissue sarcomas are 2 times as common, and metastatic bone tumors are 100 times more common than solid primary malignant bone tumors. Primary hematopoi-etic tumors of bone, in contrast, are common. These include multiple myeloma and lymphoma (see Chapter 88). This chapter discusses the following solid primary malignant bone tumors: osteosarcoma, chondrosarcoma, Ewing's sarcoma, and chordoma.

1 Osteosarcoma

RELEVANT ANATOMY

Osteosarcomas are the most common solid primary malignant bone tumor. There are approximately 1.5 to 2 cases per 1 million people per year (1,2). Between 50 and 75% of osteosarcomas occur during the second decade of life, but they can be diagnosed at any age. The male:female ratio is 1.5:1 to 2:1 (1,2). Osteosarcoma is most commonly seen in the appendicular skeleton and is usually seen in the meta-physis of long bones. Its most common locations are, in descending order of frequency, the distal femur, proximal tibia, and proximal femur.

INITIAL FINDINGS AND PHYSICAL EXAMINATION

The most common presenting complaint is pain. The pain may be worse with activity, but it is also commonly present at rest. Pain may awaken the patient from sleep. The physical examination may be essentially normal but can reveal swelling, limited joint mobility, increased skin temperature, and superficial venous dilation.

RADIOLOGIC STUDIES

Findings on radiographs may strongly support the diagnosis of osteosarcoma. The lesion is most often meta-physeal and contains areas of radiolucency mixed with ar-eas that are radiodense (Fig. 87.1). The cortex is frequently destroyed by the tumor, and a soft tissue mass is often present.

Findings on bone scan usually reveal an intense concentration of radioisotope at the site of the tumor. Bone metastases, if present, will also be evident. MRI studies clearly define the intramedullary extent of the tumor and delineate any soft tissue mass (Figs. 87.2 and 87.3). X-ray and CT scans of the chest are essential to evaluate any pulmonary metastases.

Staging and Prognosis

Osteosarcomas can occur as stage I or II tumors (see Chapter 85), the majority of which are stage IIB at the time of diagnosis. There are many histologic variants of stage II osteosarcoma, including osteoblastic, chondroblastic, fibroblastic, telangiectatic, and small cell. The prerequisite histologic feature that establishes the diagnosis of osteogenic sarcoma is osteoid-producing malignant spindle cells.

The behavior of osteogenic sarcomas depends on the stage of the tumor. Patients with stage I lesions generally do well and have a greater than 90% chance of survival 10 years after treatment with wide surgical resection (1,3). Patients with stage II osteosarcoma have a poorer prognosis. After treatment with chemotherapy and wide or radical surgical resection, these patients have approximately a 65% chance of surviving 10 years (1,2,4). Before modern-day chemotherapy, patients

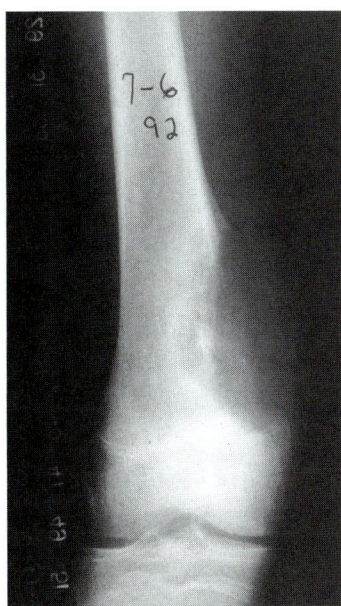

Figure 87.1. AP view showing stage IIB osteogenic sarcoma of the distal femur. Radiolucent and radiodense areas can be seen.

with stage II osteosarcomas had only a 20% chance of surviving 10 years (1,2,4).

TREATMENT

Treatment of stage II osteosarcoma involves chemotherapy and surgical excision of the tumor (Clinical Table). Treatment is generally provided in three phases: preoperative (or induction) chemotherapy, wide resection of the primary tumor (local control), and postoperative (or maintenance) chemotherapy. Chemotherapy agents currently used during the induction and maintenance phases are methotrexate, ifosfamide, Adriamycin, cisplatin, VP-16, and Cytoxan. During the local control phase of treatment most patients undergo limb-sparing surgery. In selected cases, however, an amputation is required to achieve a wide surgical margin. Reconstruction options directed at managing skeletal defects that result from limb-sparing surgery include intercalary allograft, metallic prosthesis, osteoarticular allograft, allograft arthrodesis, and rotationplasty.

Clinical Table: Common Malignant Bone Tumors

Diagnosis	Most Common Age (yrs)	Anatomic Location	Radiographic Characteristics	Histologic Characteristics	Treatment	Outcome (Survival)
Osteosarcoma	• 10–20	• Metaphyseal area of long bones (most common is distal femur)	• Mixed radiodense and radiolucent areas; cortex usually destroyed; and soft tissue mass present	• Malignant osteoid formation	• Chemotherapy and wide surgical resection	• 5 yr: Stage I, >90% Stage II, 65% Stage III, 25%
Chondrosarcoma	• 30–70	• Primary: metaphyseal • Secondary: pelvis	• Primary: central radiolucent lesions with areas of calcification • Secondary: osteochondroma with large >2-cm soft tissue mass with calcification	• Varying degree of malignant cartilage formation	• Wide surgical resection	• 10 yr: Stage I, 90% Stage II, 60% Stage III, 40%
Ewing's sarcoma	• 5–30	• Pelvic and lower extremities: metaphyseal and diaphyseal	• Permeative destructive process with soft tissue mass • Mild to moderate periosteal reaction	• Small round blue cells with scarce cytoplasm • 11, 22 translocation	• Chemotherapy, wide surgical resection, and/or external beam radiation	• 10 yr: 60–70%
Chordoma	• 50	• Sacrum and coccyx	• Central radiolucent sacralcoccygeal lesion • Anterior soft tissue mass	• Physaliphorous (bubbly) cells	• Wide surgical resection ± external beam radiation	• 10 yr: 50%

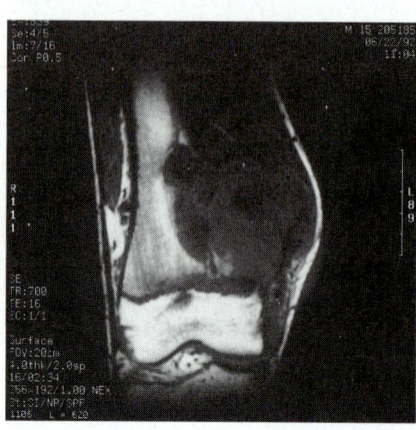

Figure 87.2. T_1-weighted MRI coronal view showing a stage IIB osteogenic sarcoma of the distal femur. A large soft tissue mass can be seen.

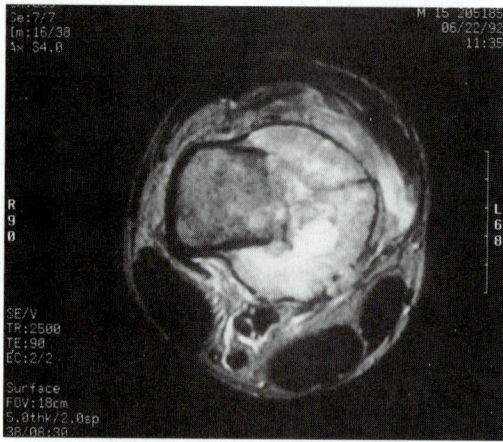

Figure 87.3. T_2-weighted MRI axial view showing a stage IIB osteogenic sarcoma of the distal femur. A large soft tissue mass and the popliteal nerve and vessels can be seen.

II Chondrosarcoma

RELEVANT ANATOMY AND PATHOGENESIS

Chondrosarcoma is the second most common solid primary malignant neoplasm of bone. Chondrosarcomas are more frequently seen in males than in females. The tumors usually occur in patients between 30 and 70 years of age and are rare in patients under the age of 20.

Chondrosarcomas can be divided into primary and secondary tumors. Primary chondrosarcomas arise from areas of the skeleton that were previously normal and tend to be located in metadiaphyseal region of the involved bone. Secondary chondrosarcomas arise from pre-existing benign cartilage tumors, such as osteochondromas or enchondromas, and are most commonly seen in proximal locations, such as the pelvis, proximal femur, proximal humerus, scapula, and spine.

INITIAL FINDINGS AND PHYSICAL EXAMINATION

Patients with primary chondrosarcomas generally have no palpable soft tissue mass and usually seek medical attention because of deep pain. Secondary chondrosarcomas usually arise from osteochondromas and typically present as slowly growing masses. These tumors are often dismissed until they become painful. The pain is usually deep, but not intense, and can be discontinuous.

RADIOLOGIC STUDIES

Radiographs of primary chondrosarcomas usually reveal radiolucent lesions that are centrally located within the bone and contain areas of calcification. The endosteal bone surface that is adjacent to the tumor is often eroded (scalloped) and periosteal irregularities may be seen. A CT

scan will most clearly image the presence of endosteal scalloping (Fig. 87.4). MRI studies will most accurately define the extent of intramedullary disease and identify any soft tissue mass (Fig. 87.5). Even after analysis of cross-sectional imaging, distinguishing enchondromas from low-grade primary chondrosarcomas may not be possible.

Radiographs of secondary chondrosarcomas usually reveal an osteochondroma with a large (at least 2 cm) soft tissue mass that contains calcifications (Fig. 87.6). An MRI scan best delineates the extent of the soft tissue mass. Both primary and secondary chondrosarcomas have increased uptake of radioisotope on bone scans. X-rays and CT scans of the chest should be performed to evaluate the presence of pulmonary metastases.

Staging

The histologic grade of chondrosarcomas is based on the degree of cartilage differentiation present within

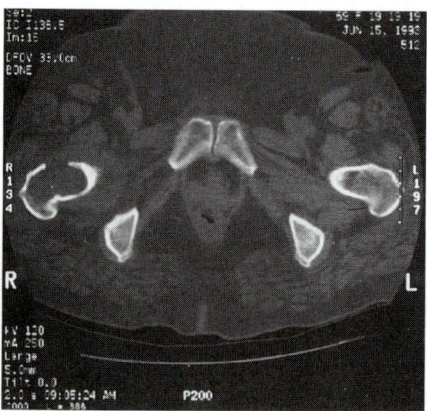

Figure 87.4. CT scan showing a chondrosarcoma of the left distal femur. Scalloping and cortical destruction can be seen.

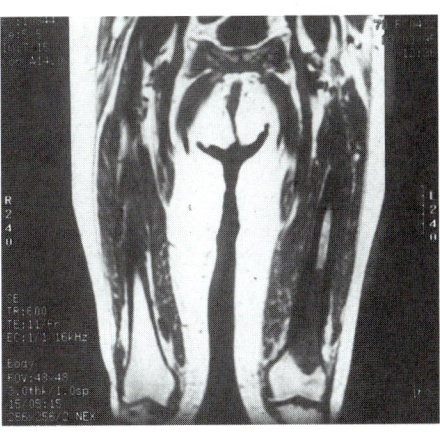

Figure 87.5. MRI coronal view showing a high-grade chondrosar-coma of the left distal femur.

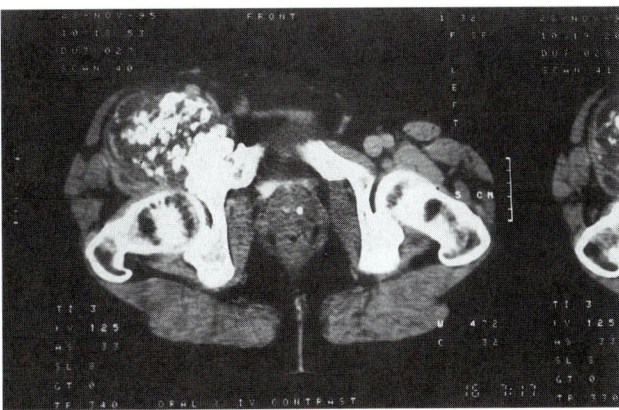

Figure 87.6. CT scan showing a large secondary chondrosarcoma of the pelvis. A thick cartilaginous cap can be seen.

each tumor (see Chapter 85). Grade I chondrosarcomas contain well-differentiated cartilage but also contain cells that show slight atypia, enlarged nuclei, and occa-sional binu-cleate cells. Grade II chondrosarcomas con-tain less well differentiated cartilage tissue. They are more cellular than grade I lesions, have modest cellular atypia, and may have lacunae that contain multiple cells. Grade III chondrosarcomas contain cartilaginous tissue that is poorly differentiated. They contain poorly differ-entiated cells, which are pleomorphic and contain mi-totic figures (1,5).

TREATMENT

Chondrosarcomas are generally resistant to radiation and chemotherapy. Treatment of nonmetastatic chon-drosarcoma is surgical resection (Clinical Table). A wide or radical surgical margin should be obtained at the time of surgical resection. Ten-year survival statistics show that patients with grade I chondrosarcomas have greater than 90% survival, patients with grade II chondrosarcomas have 60% 5-year survival, and patients with grade III chon-drosarcomas have 40% survival (6).

III   Ewing's Sarcoma

RELEVANT ANATOMY

Ewing's sarcoma is the third most common solid pri-mary malignant neoplasm of bone. Approximately 90% of these tumors occur in patients between the ages of 5 and 30. Two-thirds of Ewing's sarcomas are located in the lower extremity or pelvis. These tumors have a predilection for the diaphysis and metaphysis of long bones and occur, in order of decreasing frequency, in the femur, tibia, humerus, fibula, and bones of the forearm. Ewing's sar-coma may also occur in the axial skeleton. Within the axial skeleton, the pelvis is the most common site, followed (in order of frequency) by tumors residing in vertebrae, scapula, rib, and clavicle.

INITIAL FINDINGS AND PHYSICAL EXAMINATION

The most frequent presenting symptoms are pain, a palpable soft tissue mass, and swelling. Patients may ex-perience low-grade fevers and anemia. An elevated ery-throcyte sedimentation rate, moderate leukocytosis, and/or weight loss may also be present (1).

RADIOLOGIC STUDIES

Radiographs show a permeative, destructive process with an associated soft tissue mass and mild to moderate periosteal reaction. Plain radiographs almost always un-derestimate the size of the lesion (Fig. 87.7). These tumors often appear larger on bone scans than on the radio-graphs. MRI scans best demonstrate the intramedullary extent of the tumor and most accurately delineate any soft tissue mass (Fig. 87.8). The evaluation for metastatic dis-ease should include a bone marrow biopsy and an x-ray and CT scan of the chest.

Other Diagnostic Studies

On histologic examination, the cytoplasm is scare, pale, and vacuolated. Mitotic rates vary. Immunochemistry demonstrates periodic acid-Schiff positive intracytoplas-mic glycogen granules that are dissolvable by treatment with diastase. Electron microscopy reveals intracytoplas-mic glycogen granules and, sometimes, neural elements. A reciprocal translocation between chromosome 11 and 22 can be detected by cytogenetic analysis.

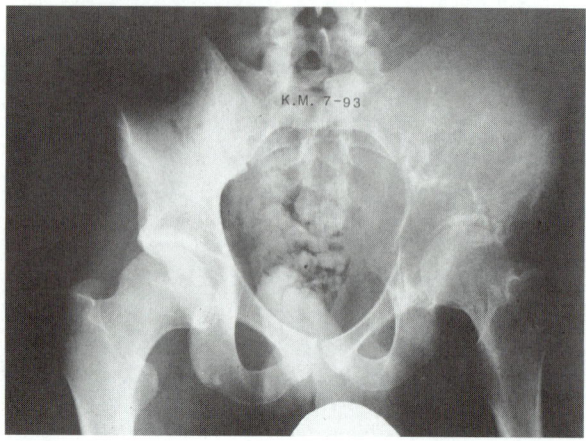

Figure 87.7. AP view showing a Ewing's sarcoma and pathologic fracture of the pelvis.

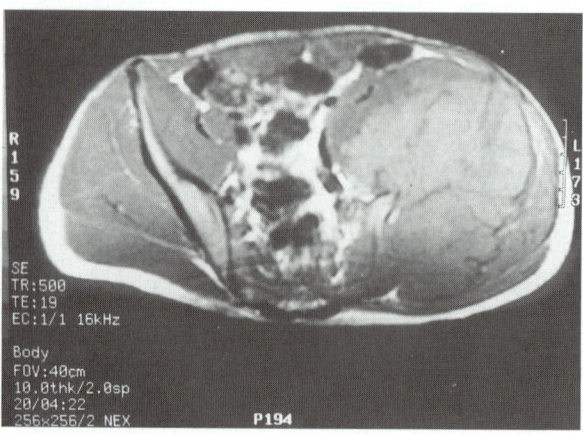

Figure 87.8. T_1-weighted MRI axial view showing a Ewing's sarcoma of the pelvis. A large soft tissue mass can be seen.

TREATMENT

Treatment of Ewing's sarcoma is generally provided in three phases: induction chemotherapy, control of the localized disease, and maintenance chemotherapy. Chemotherapy agents used are vincristine, actinomycin D, cyclophosphamide, and Adriamycin. Control of the localized disease can be accomplished with wide surgical resection or external beam radiation (Clinical Table). In easily accessible lesions, such as tumors of the appendicular skeleton, surgical treatment is preferred. External beam radiation may be indicated when tumors are located in anatomic regions in which wide local surgical excision is either impossible or is associated with a catastrophic functional outcome. The 10-year survival rate for patients treated in this manner is 60 to 70% (7,8).

IV Chordoma

RELEVANT ANATOMY AND PATHOGENESIS

Chordoma is a relatively rare, usually slow-growing, solid primary malignant tumor of bone. This tumor is derived from cells that arise from a remnant of the fetal notochord. Chordomas account for 1 to 4% of primary malignant bone tumors, and they are the most common solid primary malignant bone tumor of the sacrococcygeal region. These tumors are two to three times more common in men than in women and usually occur in patients older than 50 years (1). Half of chordomas are located in the sacrum and coccyx; the remaining are divided between the base of the skull (35%) and the remainder of the spine (15%) (9,10). The tumors are almost always centrally located in the body of the involved vertebrae.

INITIAL FINDINGS AND PHYSICAL EXAMINATION

The initial symptom is low-grade discomfort but symptoms progress as these tumors enlarge and compress surrounding structures. With sacrococcygeal tumors, late symptoms include constipation, fecal and urinary incontinence, and radicular pain. Physical examination is generally remarkable only for a large anterior sacral mass that is palpable on rectal examination. There is usually no dorsal soft tissue mass or overlying skin changes.

RADIOLOGIC STUDIES

Radiographs demonstrate a central radiolucent sacrococcygeal lesion and may show a large anterior soft tissue mss. The tumor is located centrally in the vertebral body. CT or MRI scans usually reveal a large anterior soft tissue mass, and MRI images will best determine the osseous extent of the lesion (Figs. 87.9 and 87.10).

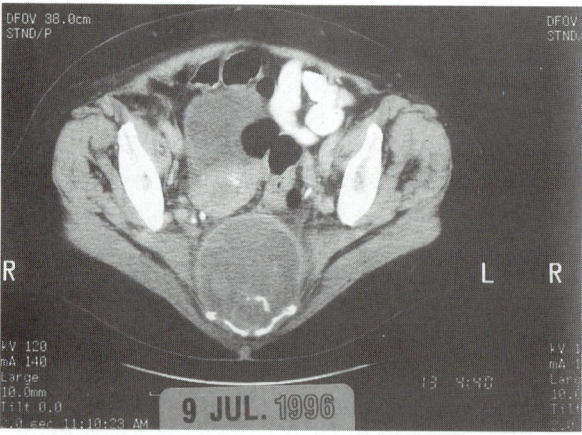

Figure 87.9. CT scan showing a sacrococcygeal chordoma. A large soft tissue mass and osteolysis of the sacrum can be seen.

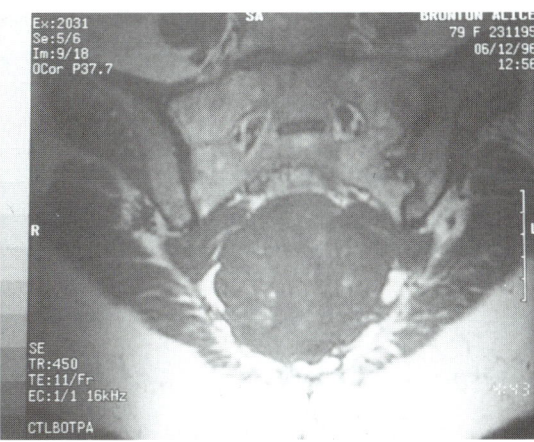

Figure 87.10. MRI coronal view of a sacrococcygeal chordoma.

Other Diagnostic Studies

Histologic examination reveals physaliphorous cells, which are large cells with intracytoplasmic vacuoles and a centrally located nucleus. The cytoplasmic vacuoles contain mucin, which stains with mucin-specific dyes. Cartilaginous differentiation may also be observed (1).

TREATMENT

Chordomas are usually slow-growing lesions that rarely metastasize. These tumors are relatively insensitive to radiation therapy and chemotherapy. The treatment of chordomas is wide surgical resection (Clinical Table). If inadequately excised, they tend to recur locally. Many lesions are quite large at the time of diagnosis, and treatment may involve surgical resection of multiple sacral nerve roots. Postoperative adjuvant external beam radiation therapy has been used in an attempt to control the local disease when wide surgical resection

has failed to achieve tumor-free margins and for poor surgical candidates (9–11). The 10-year survival rate for patients treated with this plan is approximately 50% (9).

SUMMARY

Primary malignant bone tumors are rare, but the consequences of delay or missed diagnosis are severe. Fortunately, most malignant bone tumors present because of pain, and careful attention to high-quality radiographs will usually lead an orthopaedist to further evaluation, i.e., bone scan, CT scan, or MRI. The final step in the workup of a primary bone tumor should be a well-planned biopsy.

REFERENCES

1. Campanacci M. Bone and soft tissue tumors. New York: Springer Verlag, 1990.
2. Lane JM, Hurson B, Boland PJ, Glasser B. Osteogenic sarcoma. Clin Orthop 1986;204:93–110.
3. Ritschl P, Wurnig C, Lechner G, Roessner A. Parosteal osteosarcoma: 2–23 year follow-up of 33 patients. Acta Orthop Scand 1991; 62:195–200.
4. Damron TA, Pritchard DJ. Current combined treatment of high grade osteosarcomas. Oncology 1995;9:327–343.
5. Healy JH, Lane JM. Chondrosarcoma. Clin Orthop 1986;204: 119–129.
6. Gitelis S, Bertoni F, Picci P, Campanacci M. Chondrosarcoma of bone. J Bone Joint Surg 1981;63A:1248–1257.
7. Burgert EO Jr, Nesbit ME, Garnsey LA, et al: Multimodal therapy for the management of nonpelvic, localized Ewing's sarcoma of bone: intergroup study IESS-II. J Clin Oncol 1990;8:1514–1524.
8. Neff JR. Nonmetastatic Ewing's sarcoma of bone: the role of surgical therapy. Clin Orthop 1986;204:111–118.
9. Samson IR, Springfield DS, Suit HD, Mankin HJ. Operative treatment of sacrococcygeal chordoma. J Bone Joint Surg 1993:75A: 1476–1484.
10. Mindell ER. Chordoma [Review]. J Bone Joint Surg 1981;63A: 501–505.
11. Sundaresan N. Chordomas. Clin Orthop 1986;204:135–142.

chapter 88

Denis R. Clohisy

Management of Skeletal Metastases

In 1996, it was estimated that there would be almost 1.4 million new cases of cancer in the United States that year (1). Among this staggering number of new cancer cases, more than 700,000 patients will have had cancers that commonly spread to bone. Cancers of the breast, lung, prostate, and kidney metastasize to bone in approximately 50% of cases (1,2). It follows, therefore, that approximately 350,000 new cases of skeletal metastases occurred in 1996.

Although patients with skeletal metastases may be among the sickest patients treated by orthopaedic surgeons, these patients can benefit immeasurably by surgical treatment. This chapter provides a guide to evaluating and managing these challenging patients.

INITIAL FINDINGS, PHYSICAL EXAMINATION, AND DIAGNOSIS

The initial evaluation of patients with skeletal metastases should identify potential medical problems and determine the extent of skeletal metastatic involvement. Medical problems are generally related to paraneoplastic syndromes and can include one or more of the following: hypercalcemia, anemia, thrombocytopenia, coagulation deficiencies, dehydration, and cachexia. The treating physician should obtain appropriate laboratory studies and medical consultation.

RADIOLOGIC STUDIES

A bone scan of the entire skeleton is useful for evaluating the extent of skeletal disease; radiographs can then be obtained to clarify the abnormalities identified on the bone scan. If the bone scan does not demonstrate increased isotope activity at the site of a known skeletal metastasis, a radiographic skeletal survey can accurately evaluate the extent of bone disease.

The primary purpose of imaging metastatic sites is to determine if surgical stabilization is warranted. In the majority of cases, radiographs will provide sufficient information for making this decision. In selected instances, cross-sectional imaging helps determine the extent of bone destruction; CT scanning is most accurate for this purpose.

TREATMENT

Nonoperative Treatment and Indications for Surgery

Treatment of skeletal metastases involves defining therapeutic modalities that are appropriate for each patient and then coordinating the administration of these modalities. To best select the appropriate treatment, the surgeon should understand the character of tumor pain, estimate the risk of pathologic fracture, and identify the primary tumor. Symptoms and radiographic findings identify best the risk of pathologic fracture (3,4). Table 88.1 presents a system for predicting pathologic fracture. If the bone has fractured or is thought to be at high risk for fracture, then expeditious surgical intervention is the treatment of choice. In contrast, nonsurgical treatment is appropriate for mechanically stable lesions that are asymptomatic.

Radiation therapy and systemic therapy frequently enhance the treatment of skeletal metastases (5). Systemic therapy includes chemotherapy and hormonal therapy. Skeletal metastases respond differently (or not at all) to these therapies. For this reason, identification of the primary tumor influences the choice of treatment.

Radiation therapy is generally effective for treating hematologic malignancies, such as multiple myeloma and lymphoma; but when used to treat metastases from solid

table	88.1	Risk of Pathologic Fracture

	Tumor Location		
Fracture Risk	Long Bone Diaphysis	Long Bone Metaphysis	Femoral Head or Neck
Low	<25% cortical destruction	<33% diameter	
Moderate	25–50% cortical destruction	33–66% diameter	<25% cortical destruction or <50% diameter
High	Functional pain[a] or >50% cortical destruction	Functional pain or >66% diameter	Functional pain or >25% cortical destruction; >50% diameter

[a] Pain that is aggravated by limb function.

table	88.2	Treatment of Hematologic Malignancies: Multiple Myeloma and Lymphoma[a]

Presentation		Treatment		
Pain[b]	Fracture Risk[c]	Radiation	Chemotherapy[d]	Surgical Stabilization
No	Low to moderate		1	
No	High	2	3	1
Yes	Low to moderate	2	1	3[e]
Yes	High	2	3	1
Fracture	Fracture	2	3	1

[a] Ranking indicates sequence of recommended treatment.
[b] Includes rest and night pain at the tumor site.
[c] As determined from Table 88.1.
[d] Patients who have not been previously treated with chemotherapy.
[e] Surgical stabilization is indicated when symptoms persist despite adjuvant therapies.

table	88.4	Treatment of Solid Malignancies That Do Not Respond to Systemic Therapy: Lung and Kidney[a]

Presentation		Treatment		
Pain[b]	Fracture Risk	Radiation Therapy	Chemotherapy	Surgical Stabilization
No	Low to moderate			
No	High	2		1
Yes	Low to moderate	1		2[c]
Yes	High	2		1
Fracture	Fracture	2		1

[a] Ranking indicates sequence of recommended treatment.
[b] Includes rest and night pain at the tumor site.
[c] Surgical stabilization is indicated when symptoms persist despite adjuvant therapies.

table	88.3	Treatment of Solid Malignancies That Respond to Systemic Therapy: Prostate and Breast[a]

Presentation		Treatment		
Pain[b]	Fracture Risk[c]	Radiation Therapy	Chemotherapy[d] or Hormonal Therapy	Surgical Stabilization
No	Low to moderate		1	
No	High	2	3	1
Yes	Low to moderate	1	2	3[e]
Yes	High	2	3	1
Fracture	Fracture	2	3	1

[a] Ranking indicates sequence of recommended treatment.
[b] Includes rest and night pain at the tumor site.
[c] As determined from Table 88.1.
[d] Patients who have not been previously treated with chemotherapy.
[e] Surgical stabilization is indicated when symptoms persist despite adjuvant therapies.

tumors, the results are variable. For example, although radiation therapy is effective for prostate and breast cancer metastases, its efficacy is unpredictable for lung and kidney metastases.

Likewise, systemic therapies provide variable control of skeletal metastases. Systemic therapy is subdivided into chemotherapy and hormonal therapy. Chemotherapy is quite effective in treating skeletal involvement of hematologic malignancies but is less effective in treating skeletal metastases from solid tumors. Hormonal therapy directed against tumors of breast and prostate origin is initially quite effective. Such treatments use antiestrogen (breast cancer) and antitestosterone (prostate) agents. Unfortunately, no reliable systemic therapy exists for metastases from many solid tumors. Skeletal metastases refractory to systemic therapy include those of lung, kidney, and thyroid origin.

Tables 88.2 to 88.4 summarize appropriate treatment modalities based on the site of primary tumor. The numerical ranking identifies the recommended temporal sequence for coordinating the use of more than one treatment modality.

Operative Treatment

Patients with skeletal metastases may have limited survival; thus both the patient and the treating physicians must clearly understand the indications for and goals of surgical treatment. Two indications exist for surgical treatment of skeletal metastases (Tables 88.2 to 88.4). The first is to stabilize a pathologic fracture or a bone at high risk for pathologic fracture. The second indication is to treat symptomatic metastases that have failed adjuvant therapy (i.e., systemic and/or radiation therapy).

The goals of surgical treatment involve clinical and surgical objectives. The clinical objectives are to decrease pain and to optimize mobility and function. The surgical objectives are to provide immediate and permanent skeletal stabilization. Planning the operative stabilization of skeletal metastases is simplified when the surgeon focuses on these objectives. Immediate stabilization facilitates postoperative mobility and rehabilitation, acknowledges that osseous union (stability) is unlikely to occur at sites of skeletal tumor, and dismisses the need for external immobilization devices after surgery. Permanent skeletal stabilization decreases the likelihood of additional surgery.

The techniques used for achieving skeletal fixation depend on the sites of the metastases. Lesions of the axial skeleton are different from those of the appendicular skeleton; and metaphyseal and epiphyseal lesions are different from diaphyseal lesions. Lesions of the axial skeleton that are ultimately treated surgically usually involve the spine. Immediate fixation of these lesions almost always requires replacing skeletal defects with either bone cement or allogeneic cortical bone graft, supplemented with internal fixation. Internal fixation must extend to the uninvolved bone or vertebral disc at both ends of the skeletal defect. Bone graft must also span the entire skeletal defect.

The surgeon should stabilize tumors of the diaphyseal regions of long bones with rigid internal fixation above and below the area of tumor and, when possible, by obtaining fixation (with bone cement) at the site of tumor-directed bone loss (6). This goal can be accomplished with either intramedullary fixation or cortical fixation (plate). The surgeon should use bone cement liberally when needed, because it can enhance proximal and distal fixation and provide support at the site of defect.

Metaphyseal and epiphyseal regions of long bones are stabilized to optimize fixation at the site of the tumor, which is done with hemiarthroplasty or internal fixation augmented with bone cement. The condition of the epiphyseal bone is the major factor influencing the choice of surgical stabilization. If the epiphyseal bone is amenable to rigid internal fixation, then it is stabilized with either a locked intramedullary device or a plate and screws. Bone cement is used to enhance fixation in the epiphyseal region and to fill the defect created by the tumor.

When bone in the epiphyseal region is not amenable to rigid internal fixation, it should be resected, along with adjacent tumor, and arthroplasty should be performed. The surgeon may use either cement or allograft bone to replace the bone lost from tumor and should fix all arthroplasty components with cement. The type of arthroplasty performed depends on the anatomic location of bone resection. The need for arthroplasty reconstruction is most common with tumor around the hip. At this site, hemiarthroplasty best treats epiphyseal skeletal defects on the femoral side, whereas total joint arthroplasty best reconstructs skeletal defects on the acetabular side. Hemiarthroplasty reconstructs tumors of the proximal humerus, and a rotating, hinged total-joint arthroplasty best reconstructs tumors of the knee (distal femur or proximal tibia); both tumors create epiphyseal skeletal defects.

Special Considerations

As discussed, patients with skeletal metastases may be in poor medical condition and thus need thorough evaluation and management by appropriate medical specialists. Many patients undergoing surgical treatment for skeletal metastases have multiple risk factors for developing deep venous thrombosis and associated sequelae, including malignancy-induced coagulation abnormalities, prolonged bed rest and inactivity, and pelvic or lower extremity surgery. When one or more of these risk factors are present, pharmacologic prophylaxis for deep venous thrombosis is recommended. Management options are empiric prophylactic treatment for 6 weeks and a minimum of 10 days of prophylactic treatment and exclusion of deep venous thrombosis by imaging.

Although patients may have multiple long bone metastases, they may only have one skeletal site that requires surgical stabilization. A special situation involves patients with operative disease in the lower extremity and nonoperative disease in the upper extremity (usually the humerus). Because these patients must rely on ambulatory aids after surgery, the surgeon should carefully review upper extremity involvement and address the appropriateness of prophylactic fixation of humeral lesions.

Skeletal metastases from tumors of renal or thyroid origin can be extremely vascular. Failure to address the potential for massive bleeding from these tumors at the time of surgery may result in uncontrolled life-threatening hemorrhage. For this reason, preoperative arteriograms and embolization are recommended for anatomic sites in which tourniquet control of operative bleeding is not possible (7), for example at the spine, scapula, proximal humerus, pelvis, and proximal femur.

SUMMARY

Optimal management of skeletal metastases involves coordination of nonsurgical and surgical treatment modalities. Indications for surgical treatment include stabilization of bones that are fractured or are at high risk for fracture and treatment of lesions that are symptomatic despite nonsurgical treatment modalities. The technical goal of surgical treatment is to obtain immediate and permanent skeletal stabilization, and the clinical goals are to decrease pain and optimize mobility and function.

REFERENCES

1. Parker SL, Tong T, Bolden S, Wingo PA. Cancer statistics, 1996. CA Cancer J Clin 1996;46:5–27.
2. Frassica FJ, Sim FH. Pathogenesis and prognosis. In Sim FH, ed. Diagnostic and management of metastatic bone disease: a multidisciplinary approach. New York: Raven, 1988:1–6.
3. Mirels H. Metastatic disease in long bones: a proposed scoring system for diagnosing impending pathologic fractures. Clin Orthop 1989;249:256–307.
4. Fidler M. Incidence of fracture through metastases in long bones. Acta Orthop Scand 1981;52:623–627.
5. Hoskin PJ. Radiotherapy in the management of bone pain. Clin Orthop 1995;312:105–119.
6. Harrington D, Sim FH, Enis JE, et al. Methylmethacrylate as an adjunct in internal fixation of pathological fractures: experience with three hundred and seventy-five cases. J Bone Joint Surg 1976; 58A:1047–1055.
7. Bowers TA, Murray JA, Charnsangavej C, et al. Bone metastases from renal cell carcinoma. The preoperative use of transcatheter arterial occlusion. J Bone Joint Surg 1982;64A:749–754.

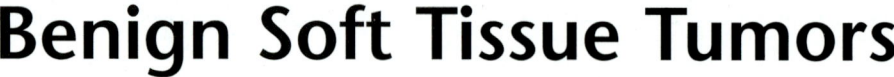

chapter 89

Edward Y. Cheng

Benign Soft Tissue Tumors

Soft tissue tumors are a diverse group. Benign soft tissue tumors are much more common than malignant soft tissue tumors (100:1 in some series) (1). Soft tissue tumors are also more common than bone tumors. Although specialists other than the orthopaedic surgeon may care for a number of benign soft tissue tumors, many of these tumors arise in an extremity, requiring the orthopaedic surgeon to have more than just a passing familiarity with these lesions. This chapter focuses on the common benign soft tissue neoplasms that the orthopaedist is likely to encounter.

RELEVANT ANATOMY AND PATHOGENESIS

Although most soft tissue tumors may arise in any location, some lesions have a predilection for superficial (dermal, subcutaneous) or deep (subfascial, intramuscular) tissues. In general, benign soft tissue tumors are more common in superficial sites, whereas malignant soft tissue tumors tend to arise from deeper sites. It is important to remember, however, that despite these generalizations, considerable overlap exists among the anatomic sites of benign and malignant lesions. For example, malignant tumors such as epithelioid sarcoma, dermatofibrosarcoma protuberans, leiomyosarcoma, and soft tissue metastasis from carcinomas and melanomas may occur in superficial tissue. Benign tumors that tend to be superficial include fibrous histiocytoma (dermatofibroma), nodular fasciitis, lipoma, and fibroma.

INITIAL FINDINGS, PHYSICAL EXAMINATION, AND DIAGNOSIS

Patients with a soft tissue tumor usually do not give a history of trauma, although a traumatic event may have directed their attention to the lesion. Most tumors are of insidious onset, although some tumors, such as fibromatosis, digital fibromatosis, and neuromas, are associated with a history of trauma or a surgical incision. The soft tissue lesion most often linked to trauma is myositis ossifi-

cans. Schwannomas and neurofibromas can produce radicular pain. Intramuscular hemangiomas may cause vague symptoms of discomfort and tenderness at the local site despite the absence of a mass. The length of time a tumor has been present and a history of any recent or rapid enlargement are important and suggest malignancy. A history of a mass enlarging and shrinking in size over time in relation to activity level is characteristic of a ganglion.

Physical examination of a mass can reveal the size, consistency, and mobility of the mass in relation to surrounding structures. A large, firm, fixed mass is worrisome for malignancy. An exception is fibromatosis, which, although benign, is usually firm, painless, and immobile. Any mass that is fluctuant likely represents an abscess or other fluid filled lesion. Ganglions will transilluminate if they are located directly beneath the dermis. A Tinel sign directly over the mass is evidence of neural compression, which occurs frequently with schwannomas. Most soft tissue tumors tend to be painless on palpation. Vascular tumors, such as hemangioma, may enlarge and become symptomatic when a venous tourniquet is applied. The mass should be examined for pulsations or a bruit. The size of the tumor, calculated by maximum diameter or limb circumference, must be recorded. It is important to assess the range of motion of adjacent joints and the presence of regional adenopathy.

RADIOLOGIC STUDIES

The physician can sometimes make the diagnosis of soft tissue tumor with confidence based on the history and physical examination alone. More commonly, however, imaging studies are required. A plain radiograph will provide evidence of a soft tissue shadow, soft tissue calcifications, or bony erosion. Hemangiomas are associated with soft tissue calcifications, which represent phleboliths within the neoplasm. Synovial sarcoma and liposarcoma also have calcifications.

If any question exists about the anatomic extent of the tumor, a cross-sectional imaging study should be

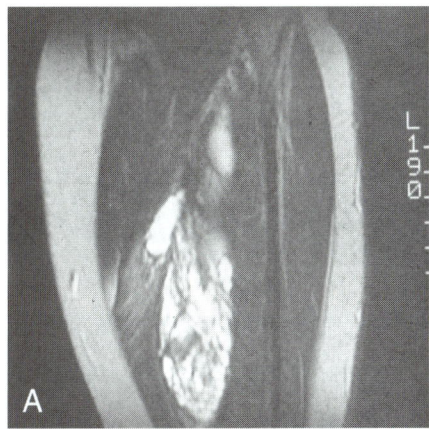

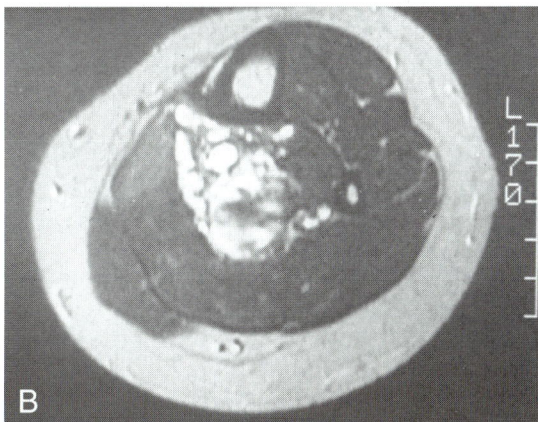

Figure 89.1. MRI coronal (**A**) and axial (**B**) views showing a hemangioma in the proximal leg. Note the variegated serpiginous appearance.

conducted. MRI is the modality of choice for soft tissue tumors. MRI helps delineate the anatomy of the mass. Unfortunately, MRI is not usually diagnostic, except for some tumors that do have a characteristic appearance, including hemangioma, abscess, lipoma, and some liposarcomas. Hemangiomas have a characteristic variegated, serpiginous pattern of appearance on MRI, with alternating small areas of bright and dark signal on T_2-weighted sequences that represent the blood-filled vessels and phleboliths, respectively (Fig. 89.1). Abscesses and inflammatory conditions such as myositis may have a large surrounding area of edema. Lipomas have the same fat signal characteristics as the subcutaneous fat on T_1- and T_2-weighted sequences. Any inhomogeneity seen in fatty tumors should raise the suspicion of a low-grade liposarcoma (Fig. 89.2). Most soft tissue sarcomas appear bright on T_2-weighted images; myxoid subtypes, such as myxoid liposarcoma, are especially bright (Fig. 89.3). Two benign conditions associated with a dark appearance on T_2-weighted images are pigmented villonodular synovitis and fibromatosis (see Chapter 84).

BIOPSY

Once the physician establishes a differential diagnosis, a biopsy is indicated if there is any concern regarding the

possibility of malignancy or if symptoms warrant surgical treatment (Clinical Table). Both the type of biopsy performed and the technique are of paramount importance and are common causes for mishaps in the management of these tumors (2).

Intralesional biopsy is any biopsy in which tumor cells are left in the patient. Incisional biopsy and needle biopsy involve sampling the tumor and leave the main bulk of the tumor in the patient. Excisional biopsy, such as an enucleation or shell-out procedure, leaves microscopic portions of the tumor behind. For most benign soft tissue tumors, recurrence risk is low, and a shell-out excisional biopsy is adequate treatment.

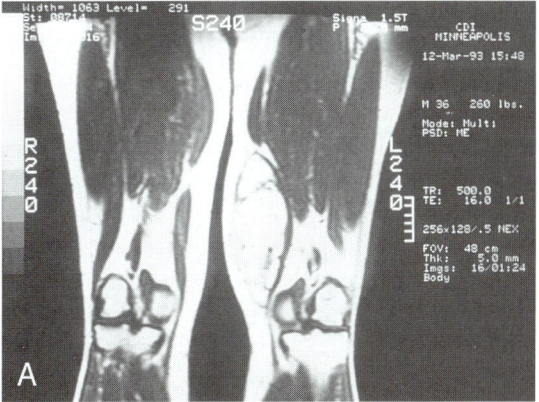

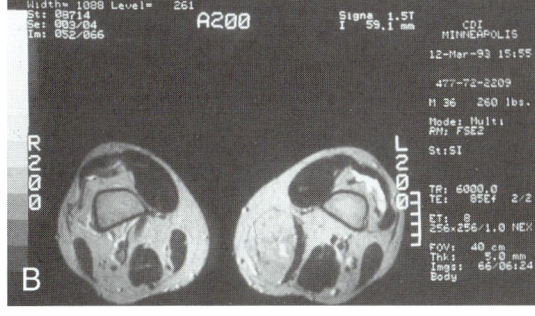

Figure 89.2. MRI coronal (**A**) and axial (**B**) views showing a low-grade liposarcoma.

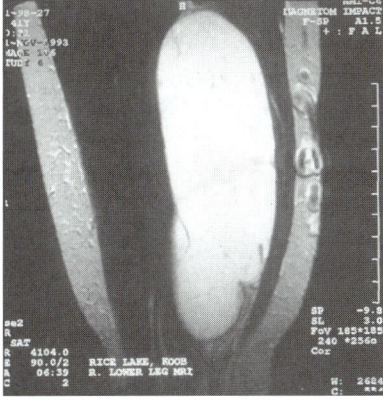

Figure 89.3. T_2-weighted MRI sagittal view showing a myxoid liposarcoma. Note bright appearance.

Clinical Table: Benign Soft Tissue Tumors

Procedure	Indications	Technique	Anatomy	Pitfalls
Needle biopsy	• Large, palpable superficial mass	• Local anesthesia needle • Tru-Cut needle biopsy • Stab incision • Several samples taken in a radial direction	• Place incision in line with incision for extensile exposure • Pulsatile masses	• Neurovascular structures may be displaced • Sampling error
Incisional biopsy	• Concern about potential malignancy (large deep mass) • To provide enough tissue for several diagnostic tests	• Short longitudinal incision • Meticulous hemostasis • Direct intramuscular exposure (within muscle fibers) • Immobilize limb with dressing	• Place incision in line with incision for extensile exposure	• Exposure of neurovascular structures • Soft tissue flaps created • Postoperative hematoma • Too much or too little tissue removed
Excisional biopsy: intralesional	• Benign diagnosis • Pseudo-capsule • Piecemeal removal (extensive hemangioma)	• Enucleation procedure	• Place incision in line with incision for extensile exposure	• Unexpected finding of malignancy • Performed when malignancy was suspected
Excisional biopsy: marginal or wide	• Concern about potential malignancy but mass can be readily excised (small superficial mass)	• Tumor must not be exposed • En bloc excision with margin of normal tissue	• Excise subcutaneous fat, fascia and muscle as necessary	• Unsatisfactory margin around mass

If any suspicion of malignancy exists, however, the techniques are an incisional or needle biopsy for large tumors and a wide excisional biopsy (in which a wide margin of normal tissue encompassing the tumor is removed) for small tumors. The choice of either needle or incisional biopsy depends on several factors. Some pathologists have a higher degree of diagnostic accuracy with the larger tissue sample obtained via an incisional biopsy. A Tru-Cut needle (Allegiance Healthcare Corp., McGraw Park, IL) biopsy usually yields several cores of tissue and may provide enough tissue for additional studies, such as electron microscopy and cytogenetic analysis (Fig. 89.4). In some sites, such as the proximal forearm, a deep mass may be adjacent to important neurovascular structures, and an open incisional biopsy may actually entail less risk to these structures. For retroperitoneal tumors, a CT-guided needle biopsy or limited open exposure of the mass combined with a needle biopsy may be the best method for sampling the tumor with the least risk of tumor cell contamination.

For open biopsies, the surgeon should always use a longitudinal incision, preferably within proximity to the standard extensile incision used for the anatomic site in question. Furthermore, the surgeon should avoid internervous and intermuscular planes of dissection for intra-

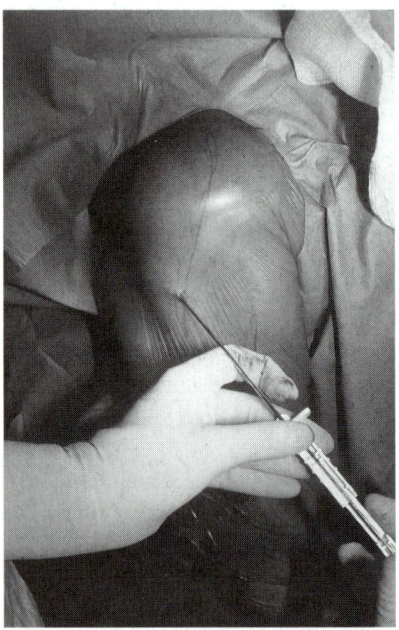

Figure 89.4. Needle biopsy of a deltoid muscle mass of the shoulder.

lesional biopsies because this approach exposes vital structures to tumor cells. Instead, expose the tumor mass via dissection through an intramuscular route.

Once the tumor mass is sampled, a frozen section should be prepared to confirm the presence of diagnostic tissue. Use meticulous hemostasis to prevent a hematoma, which has the potential to contaminate a large area with malignant cells. If a drain is used, place the drain exit site just beyond the distal end of the incision to allow easy resection of it along with the biopsy incision if additional surgery is indicated. Close the incision with sutures close to the skin edge to facilitate resection of the scar if further surgery is required. If the biopsy site is close to a joint, immobilize and splint the limb for several days to prevent a large area of ecchymosis from forming, especially if the procedure is done on an outpatient basis. Adherence to these principles is critical for avoiding the common pitfalls associated with biopsies, which can preclude the ability to perform a limb salvage procedure and adversely affect prognosis should the mass turn out to be malignant.

TYPES OF SOFT TISSUE TUMORS

Table 89.1 lists the classification of soft tissue tumors by histologic type. Soft tissue tumors originate embryologically from the mesodermal mesenchyme before differentiation into smooth muscle, striated muscle, adipose, fibrous, vascular, or neural tissue. Most benign soft tissue tumors have a corresponding malignant counterpart. Although soft tissue tumors are of diverse pathologic origin, most common benign tumors are within the following groups: lipomas and variants, fibrous histiocytoma, nodular fasciitis, hemangioma, fibromatosis, and neurofibromas (3).

Lipomas are one of the most common soft tissue tumors. They may be superficial or deep, sometimes growing to an enormous size. Occasionally, they are multiple. Several variants exist, including the angiolipoma (a subcutaneous mass commonly found in the forearm) and atypical lipoma (a superficial mass), which some pathologists believe is more aptly considered a low-grade liposarcoma (4). Both grossly and histologically, lipomas appear as normal fat. Lipomas are usually lobulated and can be easily dissected from the surrounding tissues. Recurrence is low after local excision, and a wide margin of excision is not required.

Fibrous histiocytoma is composed of both fibrous and histiocytic cells, and the terms *dermatofibroma, sclerosing hemangioma,* and *nodular subepidermal fibrosis* are used synonymously when the lesion arises in dermal sites. Histologically, a storiform pattern of spindle cells occurs. Local excision is satisfactory treatment, because the recurrence risk is low for dermal lesions (but slightly higher for deeper masses).

Nodular fasciitis is a benign proliferation of fibroblasts and not a true neoplasm in the pathologic sense. It is a common fibrous lesion, usually less than 2 cm in size, and has a predilection for the upper extremity. A history of rapid

| table | 89.1 | Histologic Classification of Soft Tissue Tumors |

Benign	Malignant
Fibrous	
Nodular fasciitis	Fibrosarcoma
Fibroma	
Fibromatosis (desmoid tumor)	
Fibrous hamartoma of infancy	
Fibrohistiocytic	
Benign fibrous histiocytoma	Malignant fibrous histiocytoma
Xanthoma	
Lipomatous	
Lipoma	Liposarcoma
Angiolipoma	
Pleomorphic lipoma	
Lipoblastoma	
Lipomatosis	
Atypical lipoma	
Smooth Muscle	
Leiomyoma	Leiomyosarcoma
Skeletal Muscle	
Rhabdomyoma	Rhabdomyosarcoma
Vascular	
Hemangioma	Angiosarcoma
Lymphangioma	Hemangioendothelioma
Synovial	
Pigmented villonodular synovitis	Synovial sarcoma
Neural	
Neuroma	Malignant schwannoma (neurofibrosarcoma)
Benign schwannoma	
Neurofibroma	Primitive neuroectodermal tumor (neuroepithelioma)
Miscellaneous	
Tumoral calcinosis	Alveolar soft part sarcoma
Myxoma	Epithelioid sarcoma
	Clear cell sarcoma
	Extraskeletal Ewing's sarcoma

Modified from Enzinger FM, Weiss SW. Soft tissue tumors. St. Louis: Mosby, 1995.

growth is common; and histologically, the degree of cellularity may make the distinction from a fibrosarcoma difficult. Local excision is curative, with a low recurrence risk.

Hemangioma is the most common tumor in infants and children (5). A number of types exist, including capillary, cavernous, venous, and arteriovenous hemangiomas. The capillary types are usually in the skin and are more common than the cavernous types. Orthopaedists, however, are more likely to encounter the cavernous type, because the lesions occur both subcutaneously and intramuscularly (Fig. 89.1). Surgical excision can be curative but may be difficult because of infiltrative growth into surrounding structures.

Fibromatosis has a high recurrence rate after excision, and its locally invasive growth into surrounding structures suggests clinical behavior similar to a low-grade fibrosarcoma. Fibromatoses cover a broad spectrum of diseases, ranging from Dupuytren, plantar, and penile (Peyronie) diseases to the deep, musculoaponeurotic type, which is the focus of this discussion. Fibromatosis usually arises in adolescents and young adults, with a 3 : 1 preference for males over females. The appearance on MRI is characteristic: dark on the T$_2$-weighted image (low water content), unlike sarcomas, which are bright (6). Frequent sites of disease are the shoulder, chest wall, back, and thigh. Multicentric tumors can occur, representing either synchronous or metachronous lesions (7).

Although wide excision remains the recommended treatment, a high incidence of recurrence exists, despite treatment of any kind (8). The natural history of these tumors is variable, and some authors report spontaneous regression of tumor. Radiation has been beneficial (9), and hormonal (antiestrogen) therapy with or without nonsteroidal antiinflammatory agents and chemotherapy have been used, but not proven to be effective in all cases (10,11).

Benign neural tissue tumors consist of the neurofibroma and benign schwannoma (neurilemoma). Neuromas (e.g., Morton and traumatic) are not true neoplasms and represent proliferations of fibrous tissue within a peripheral nerve. Neurofibromas are usually solitary but can be multiple. They may also be a component of neurofibromatosis type 1 (von Recklinghausen's disease). Malignant degeneration is rare in solitary neurofibromas and more common in neurofibromatosis. The most common sites are in the dermis and subcutis, but deep lesions can occur. Although normally a solitary nodule, neurofibromas can manifest in a diffuse multinodular form, which is known as plexiform neurofibroma.

Surgical excision for neurofibroma generally requires excision of the involved nerve, unlike surgery for a benign schwannoma, in which the main trunk of the nerve can be left intact because of the epineural capsule around the tumor (Fig. 89.5). Benign schwannoma is less commonly associated with von Recklinghausen's disease and is usually found deeper than neurofibromas. Malignant transformation of benign schwannomas is rare. Treatment for both of these tumors is local excision when symptoms warrant or if recent growth of a neurofibroma occurs.

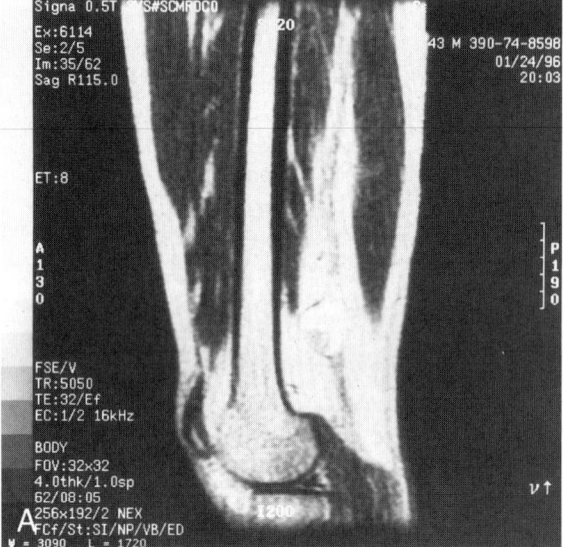
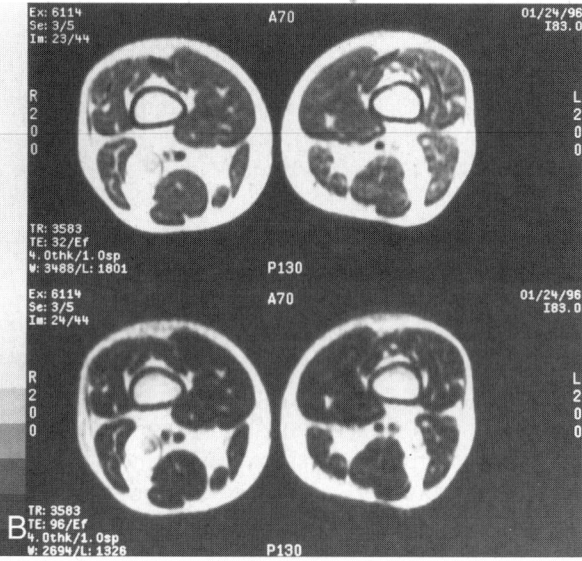
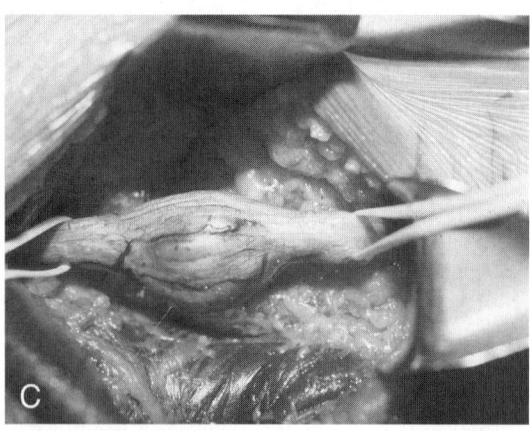
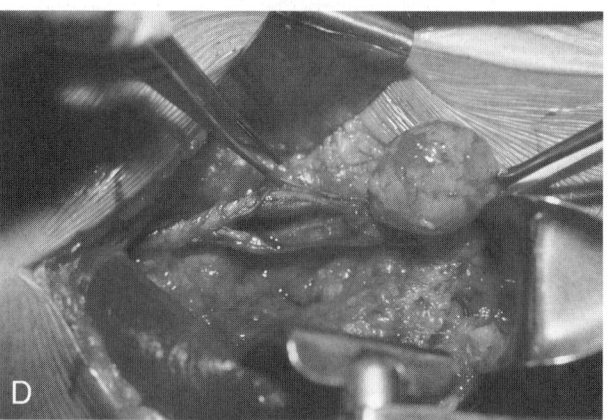

Figure 89.5. MRI sagittal (**A**) and axial (**B**) views showing a schwannoma. Interoperative views showing a schwannoma of the sciatic nerve before (**C**) and after (**D**) excision.

SUMMARY

An understanding of and an approach to benign soft tissue tumors are important for all clinicians involved with the treatment of musculoskeletal pain. The thinking involved in clinical evaluation, radiographic imaging, other medical evaluation and workup, and the approach to biopsy and definitive treatment is part of the same thought process that must accompany the evaluation of more serious malignant musculoskeletal disorders.

REFERENCES

1. Enzinger FM, Weiss SW. Soft tissue tumors. St. Louis: Mosby, 1995.
2. Mankin HJ, Lange TA, Spanier SS. The hazards of biopsy in patients with malignant primary bone and soft-tissue tumors. J Bone Joint Surg 1982;64A:1121–1127.
3. Kransdorf MJ. Benign soft-tissue tumors in a large referral population: distribution of specific diagnoses by age, sex, and location. AJR. Am J Roentgenol 1995;164:395–402.
4. Kindblom LG, Angervall L, Svendsen P. Liposarcoma. A clinico-pathologic, radiographic and prognostic study. Acta Pathol Microbiol Scand Suppl 1975;253:1–71.
5. Watson WL, McCarthy WD. Blood and lymph vessel tumors. Surg Gynecol Obstet 1940;71:569.
6. Sundaram M, McGuire MH, Schajowicz F. Soft-tissue masses: histologic basis for decreased signal (short T_2) on T_2-weighted MR images. AJR Am J Roentgenol 1987;148:1247–1250.
7. Barber HM, Galasko CS, Woods CG. Multicentric extra-abdominal desmoid tumours. J Bone Joint Surg 1973;55B:858–863.
8. Rock MG, Pritchard DJ, Reiman HM, et al. Extra-abdominal desmoid tumors. J Bone Joint Surg 1984;66A:1369–1374.
9. Miralbell R, Suit HD, Mankin HJ, et al. Fibromatoses: from post-surgical surveillance to combined surgery and radiation therapy. Int J Radiat Oncol Biol Physiol 1990;18:535–540.
10. Timmons MJ. Fibromatosis, desmoids, fibroblasts, and tamoxifen [Review]. Br J Plastic Surg 1994;7:378–380.
11. Patel SR, Evans HL, Benjamin RS. Combination chemotherapy in adult desmoid tumors. Cancer 1993;72:3244–3247.

Malignant Soft Tissue Tumors

The orthopaedic surgeon rarely encounters a malignant tumor of bone or soft tissue. Soft tissue sarcomas represent only about 1% of all malignancies. Within the United States, 5000 to 6000 soft tissue sarcomas are diagnosed yearly (1). Between 50 to 66% of soft tissue sarcomas occur in the buttocks, groin, or lower extremity (2). Rhabdomyosarcoma is the most common soft tissue sarcoma in children, and it is the sixth most common of all childhood cancers (3). The biology and the treatment of soft tissue sarcomas tend to be similar in children and adults, with the exception of small, round blue cell tumors (e.g., Ewing's sarcoma, primitive neuroectodermal tumor, rhabdomyosarcoma) (4). This chapter discusses non–round cell soft tissue sarcomas and their clinical presentation, classification, staging, and treatment.

INITIAL FINDINGS, PHYSICAL EXAMINATION, AND DIAGNOSIS

In general, it is not possible to distinguish a benign from a malignant soft tissue tumor on clinical presentation. Several key points in the history, however, should raise a red flag, alerting the physician to the possibility of malignancy (Table 90.1), including night pain; pain unrelated to activity level; an insidious onset of symptoms without a history of trauma; sudden enlargement in size; a newly noted mass; a history of prior malignancy, radiation treatment, or benign lesion (neurofibromatosis, hemangiomas); and the presence of constitutional symptoms (unexplained weight loss, fever, night sweats).

On physical examination, malignancy is suggested by large and/or deep masses, multiple masses, a firm consistency, attachment to surrounding structures, focal tenderness, and regional lymphadenopathy. Laboratory studies are not helpful in the diagnosis of soft tissue sarcoma. Several tests can assist in the differential diagnosis, however. An elevated white blood count suggests abscess, and an abnormal immunoelectrophoresis may identify patients with myeloma who have soft tissue deposition of myeloid.

RADIOLOGIC STUDIES

The features of malignancy on imaging are few (Table 90.1); however, the clinician should take note of soft tissue calcifications on plain radiographs or CT scans (synovial sarcoma, liposarcoma). On MRI, malignancy is suggested by large deep-seated masses, well-circumscribed masses, extra-articular masses (sarcomas are almost never intra-articular), bony invasion, a bright appearance on T_2-weighted sequences (myxoid tumors), and any subtle areas of heterogeneity on the T_1-weighted image of fatty tumors (low-grade liposarcoma).

Classification

Soft tissue sarcomas are of either mesenchymal or neuroectodermal origin; and when sufficiently differentiated, the lesions can be separated into histologic types based only on light microscopy. At present, the World Health Organization's (WHO's) classification system, which is modified from Stout's (5) definitions from the 1940s, is widely used. In many cases, however, further studies are necessary to precisely define the histologic type (see Table 89.1). The use of special and immunohistochemical stains is occasionally helpful.

Grading

Once the physician makes a diagnosis of soft tissue sarcoma, it is necessary to establish the tumor's grade to estimate its metastatic potential. Soft tissue sarcomas are graded according to their histologic appearance. Broders's (6) criteria of cellular atypia, presence of mitosis, areas of necrosis, and hypervascularity are all used to assess tumor grade. Pathologists disagree on whether to divide the possible grade of a tumor into three or four levels; mitotic in-

| table | 90.1 | Clinical Presentation of Soft Tissue Sarcomas |

Evaluation	Signs of Malignancy
History	Night pain
	Pain unrelated to the patient's activity level
	An insidious onset of symptoms without a history of trauma
	Any sudden enlargement in size
	A newly noted mass
	A history of malignancy (lymphoma, melanoma, carcinomas)
	Prior radiation treatment to the site in question
	Other diseases (neurofibromatosis, hemangiomas)
	Presence of constitutional symptoms (unexplained weight loss, fever, night sweats)
Physical examination	Large and/or deep masses
	Multiple masses
	Firm mass
	Mass fixed to surrounding structures
	Focal tenderness
	Regional lymphadenopathy
Imaging studies	Soft tissue calcifications in synovial sarcoma and liposarcoma on plain radiographs or CT scan
	Large deep-seated masses
	Well-circumscribed masses
	Extra-articular masses
	Bony invasion (rare)
	Bright appearance on T_2-weighted image (myxoid tumors)
	Subtle areas of heterogeneity on T_2-weighted images of fatty tumors (low-grade liposarcoma)

| table | 90.2 | Staging of Soft Tissue Sarcomas |

	AJCC[a] System				
Stage	Grade	Size (T)	Nodes (N)	Metastasis (M)	MSTS
IA	Low	≤5 cm	(−)	(−)	Low-grade tumor
IB	Low	>5 cm, superficial	(−)	(−)	A. Intracompartmental
IIA	Low	>5 cm, deep	(−)	(−)	B. Extracompartmental
IIB	High	≤5 cm	(−)	(−)	High-grade tumor
IIC	High	>5 cm, superficial	(−)	(−)	A. Intracompartmental
III	High	>5 cm, deep	(−)	(−)	B. Extracompartmental
IVA	Any	Any	(+)	(−)	Metastasis to any site
IVB	Any	Any	(−)	(+)	

[a]1997 American Joint Committee on Cancer Staging Protocol for Soft Tissue Sarcoma (25,26)

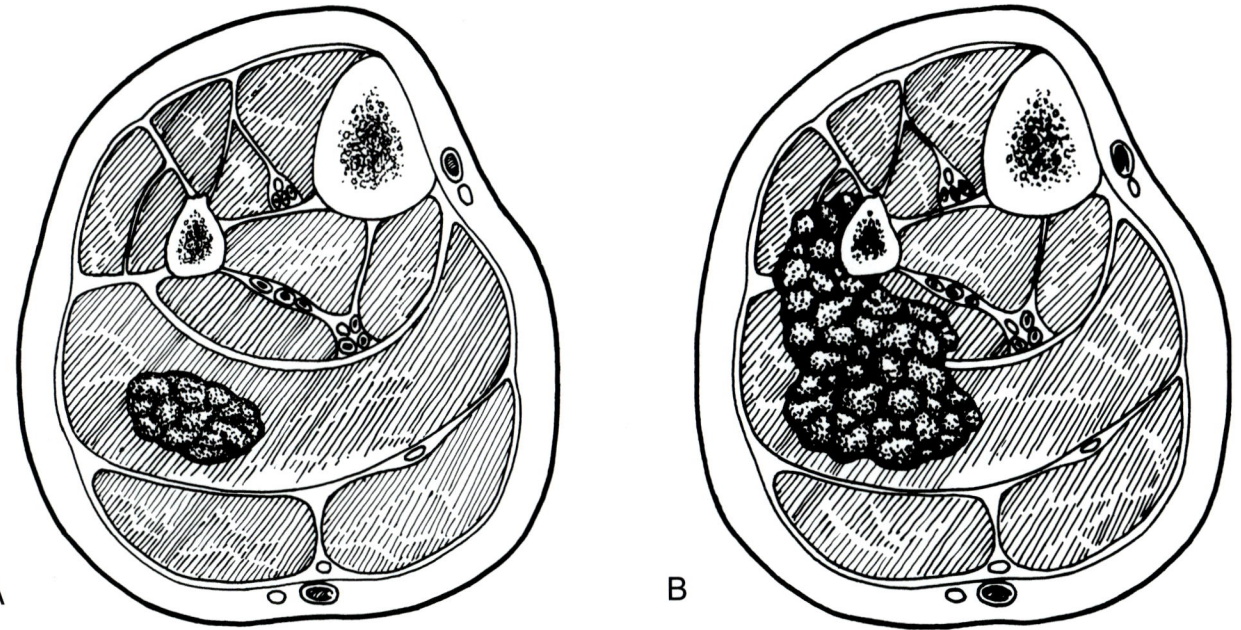

A

B

Figure 90.1. The MSTS classifies tumors as intracompartmental (**A**) and extracompartmental (**B**).

dex and necrosis are the most important determining variables. As new molecular knowledge and techniques are discovered, not only will the classification of soft tissue tumors undergo modification, but also the ability to grade tumors more accurately will improve.

Staging

Staging refers to determining the extent to which the tumor has grown or spread. For soft tissue sarcomas, the necessary staging tests for the local tumor site are a physical examination, radiographs, and cross-sectional imaging. To evaluate distant metastases, the physician should obtain a chest radiograph and CT scan of the lungs. Rarely, gallium scans and bone scans may be useful if clinical evidence suggests either bone or visceral organ involvement. Although various staging systems have been proposed, the two most widely used systems are those adopted by the American Joint Committee on Cancer (AJCC), most recently modified in 1997, and the Musculoskeletal Tumor Society (MSTS) (7,8,25,26) (Table 90.2; Fig. 90.1). The stage and anatomic site of a sarcoma are major determinants for planning treatment.

TREATMENT

Surgical Treatment

Most soft tissue sarcomas are managed similarly regardless of histologic type; notable exceptions are epithelioid sarcoma, rhabdomyosarcoma, and dermatofibrosarcoma protuberans. For these histologic types, unique characteristics may dictate a modification of treatment. Optimal management of soft tissue sarcomas requires a multidisciplinary, team approach. Surgery, consisting of a wide or marginal local excision, is combined with radiation therapy to treat primary tumors (Clinical Table). The use of chemotherapy for primary disease is somewhat controversial; chemotherapy is more widely used in metastatic disease.

Surgical excision is the cornerstone of therapy for all localized soft tissue sarcomas. The oncologic terms *intralesional, marginal, wide,* and *radical excision* refer to the surgical margin around the tumor at the time of excision (9) (Fig. 90.2). The same terms for surgical margin apply regardless of whether a local excision or amputation is performed. The goal of surgical excision is to remove the tumor en bloc with a margin of normal tissue. Most oncologic surgeons strive to resect a wide margin of normal tissue around the tumor mass but will accept a marginal excision in areas where the proximity of major neurologic or other essential structure precludes the ability to obtain a wider margin. The addition of radiation therapy to the treatment of these tumors allows surgeons to perform conservative

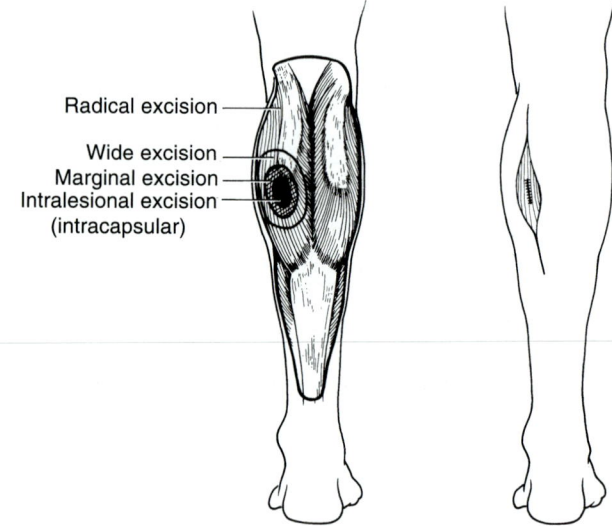

Radical excision
Wide excision
Marginal excision
Intralesional excision
(intracapsular)

Figure 90.2. Surgical margins. *Shaded area,* reactive zone of tumor.

Clinical Table:	Malignant Soft Tissue Tumors			
Procedure	Indications	Technique	Anatomy	Pitfalls
Surgical excision	• All localized soft tissue sarcomas	• Intralesional • Marginal • Wide • Radical	• Excise biopsy tract • Local: vascular structures, pulsatile lesions • Local: major nerves	• Wound closure • Vascular tumor • Inadequate tumor margins
Radiation	• Adjuvant to surgical treatment	• External beam • Brachytherapy • 5000 to 6000 cGy	• Local	• Wound complications • Soft tissue fibrosis • Joint stiffness • Radiation-induced malignancy
Chemotherapy	• Adjuvant to surgical treatment in primary sarcomas • Metastatic	• Infusion • Synergistic combinations • Intra-arterial	• Local	• Response rate • Side effects

surgery (wide or marginal excisions) without any significant adverse effect on local recurrence or survival (10). If the surgeon excises a tumor with a radical margin, radiation therapy is not usually indicated.

Adherence to surgical oncologic principles is mandatory. The surgeon should excise biopsy tracts en bloc with the tumor specimen. Because of the resulting soft tissue defect after a tumor excision, wound closure may require local muscle rotation flaps and grafts to reconstruct the extremity. If a tumor has grown into or around a major vessel, the surgeon may resect the vessel along with the tumor and reconstruct it using interpositional grafts (11). Even in cases in which major nerves are involved with tumor, resection of the nerve may be preferable to limb amputation (12). In these situations, other reconstructive procedures, such as tendon transfers or the use of an orthotic, may be necessary. Although limb salvage may be technically possible in most cases, it may be contraindicated for either oncologic or functional reasons. Contraindications to limb salvage include pathologic fracture, infection, inappropriate biopsy site placement, and extensive soft tissue and muscle involvement.

Nonoperative Treatment

ADJUVANT RADIATION THERAPY

Radiation therapy is effective against soft tissue sarcomas and allows surgeons to perform more conservative surgery without any diminution in the ability to achieve and maintain local control (10). Most centers administer radiation via an external beam treatment, although brachytherapy—radioactive implants placed in tumor beds via a catheter—are also effective. The timing of radiation treatment, i.e., before or after tumor resection, remains controversial (13). Most centers recommend a total dose of 5000 to 6000 cGy in 200-cGy fractions. Problems associated with radiation therapy include wound complications, soft tissue fibrosis, limitation of joint motion, and risk of a radiation-induced malignancy developing many years later.

ADJUVANT CHEMOTHERAPY

Although chemotherapy is under investigation at many centers, no one has shown a definite benefit for soft tissue sarcomas; it remains controversial in the routine treatment of localized lesions (14). The results of reported trials are conflicting. At best, the response rate, either partial or complete, to chemotherapeutic regimens is no better than about 40% (13,14). In most cases of metastatic disease, systemic treatment is usually advisable.

Adriamycin is the most effective single agent available. Other drugs that demonstrate some efficacy include dacarbazine (DTIC), cyclophosphamide, ifosfamide, etoposide, vincristine, and cisplatin. Major side effects of these agents include myelosuppression, nausea, vomiting, mucositis, and stomatitis. Several treatment strategies have been developed to attempt to improve the response:risk

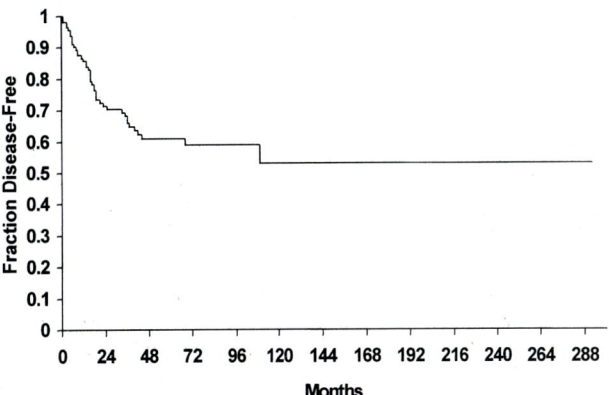

Figure 90.3. Kaplan-Meier life table survival estimates for patients (*n* = 112) with soft tissue sarcomas who were treated at the University of Minnesota. Reprinted with permission from Cheng EY, Thompson RC. Soft tissue sarcomas. Instr Course Lect 1996; 45:461–471.

ratio, including administration of chemotherapy agents via continuous infusion to reduce peak drug levels (15), synergistic combination drug therapy to allow for a reduced total single drug dosage (16), and intra-arterial infusion in an attempt to increase the total drug dosage and concentration to the tumor mass itself (17). Hematopoietic growth factors, such as granulocyte colony-stimulating factor (filgrastim [Neupogen]), decrease episodes of severe myelosuppression; and newer agents, such as paclitaxel (Taxol), are under study to determine their effectiveness against sarcomas.

SURVEILLANCE

Most relapses of soft tissue sarcomas occur within the first several years after treatment (Fig. 90.3). The lung is the single most common site of initial metastasis for nearly all sarcomas. It is important to screen for lung metastasis by obtaining radiographs and/or CT scans of the chest every 3 months for at least 2 years and then yearly thereafter for at least 5 years. An unusually high incidence of nonpulmonary initial metastasis occurs with liposarcoma. Therefore, patients previously treated for a liposarcoma should be carefully observed for the onset of any symptoms, which should be treated without delay (18). The site of the original tumor is best monitored for local recurrence through physical examination. A baseline imaging study via MRI or CT taken 6 months after tumor excision is useful for comparing to future studies should a questionable mass develop. Sarcoma patients should be followed for at least 5 years.

TREATMENT AFTER EXCISIONAL BIOPSY

Occasionally, a surgeon will perform an excisional biopsy for a small innocuous-appearing mass, but when the pathologist reviews the permanent sections, a sarcoma is diagnosed. The patient should be referred to a center that treats sarcomas. Several unique problems arise in the care of these patients as a result of the excisional biopsy. It may be difficult to determine the adequacy and margins of the resection and the degree of contamination of the entire surgical biopsy field; and, of course, there is no palpable tumor mass. A course of radiation therapy and then reexcision of the tumor bed are usually indicated, because residual viable tumor cells are present in as many as 44% of cases (19).

COMMON SOFT TISSUE SARCOMAS

The most common soft tissue sarcoma in most series is malignant fibrous histiocytoma. Liposarcoma is fairly common, representing approximately 20% of all cases. Like malignant fibrous histiocytoma, liposarcoma usually occurs in adults and has a slight male predilection. The most commonly affected anatomic sites are subfascial locations in the lower extremity. A well-differentiated liposarcoma may be difficult to distinguish from an atypical lipoma or large lipoma, and some pathologists consider these entities as one. When these tumors are in the subcutis, they are considered atypical lipomas (20–23).

Any heterogeneous appearance on an MRI scan of a tumor in a deep location suggests the diagnosis of liposarcoma. In this situation, a biopsy may not be helpful because of sampling error. Therefore, it is usually best to manage such fatty tumors as a liposarcoma, i.e., with a marginal excision. Liposarcomas have a tendency for nonpulmonary sites of initial metastasis (20), unlike other sarcomas.

Synovial sarcoma is known by several names, including synovioma and synovial cell sarcoma. Despite its name, it is not usually intra-articular and tends to occur in the deeper tissues of the lower extremity, especially the foot. Synovial sarcoma represents 7 to 8% of all soft tissue sarcomas (24). It favors younger adults (15 to 40 years old) and has a slight male predilection. An unusual aspect of this tumor is an association with a prolonged history of trauma in 35 to 50% of cases or a preexisting small mass lasting months to years. On radiographs, soft tissue calcifications can be seen. Although the clinical behavior of these tumors is variable, metastasis may develop after many years, and lymph node metastases tend to be more frequent than with other sarcomas.

Before the recognition of malignant fibrous histiocytoma as a distinct entity, fibrosarcoma was a more common diagnosis. Now, fibrosarcoma represents only about 10% of all soft tissue sarcomas. It is mainly a tumor of adults, but infantile and congenital types exist. In adults, it has a poor prognosis, although the infantile type has a better prognosis and a lower incidence of metastasis.

Malignant schwannoma, also known as a neurosarcoma or neurofibrosarcoma, is rare, making up less than 10% of cases. An increased incidence exists in patients with neurofibromatosis (2 to 30%). Adults are affected most often, although when a malignant schwannoma occurs in patients with neurofibromatosis, the patients may be quite young. The site of these tumors is variable; but malignant schwannomas are often thought to arise from a plexiform neurofi-

broma, benign neurogenic tumor, or a large nerve. Tumors may become large, and the prognosis is worse in patients with neurofibromatosis. A unique variant is the malignant Triton tumor, which appears as a malignant schwannoma with rhabdomyoblastic differentiation.

Leiomyosarcoma accounts for 7% of cases. Two histologic types are recognized: well differentiated and poorly differentiated. Middle-aged and older adults are usually affected. Retroperitoneal sites are common in women; the other two common sites of disease in both sexes are the superficial soft tissues and blood vessels. Superficial lesions are smaller and have a better prognosis than deep-seated lesions.

Epithelioid sarcoma is unusual, and many aspects of this tumor are different from those of other soft tissue sarcomas. It is a rare tumor and usually affects adolescents and young adults. Males are more commonly affected. The skin and superficial soft tissues of the distal upper extremity (the hand) and the foot are the preferred sites of disease (Fig. 90.4). It has an insidious onset and clinically resembles a granulomatous process that is responsible for its frequent misdiagnosis as a hand infection or inflammatory lesion. Recurrences are common and multiple and occur in 75 to 85% of cases. Metastases frequently occur to regional nodes, the central nervous system, and the lungs.

Malignant vascular tumors comprise a number of types: malignant angioendothelial tumors (angiosarcoma, hemangioendothelioma), hemangiopericytoma, and Kaposi's sarcoma. Orthopaedic surgeons usually encounter only the first two types.

Angiosarcoma, also known as lymphangiosarcoma, is a rare tumor of older (>60 years) individuals. When angiosarcoma arises in the lymphedematous upper extremity after a mastectomy, it is known as Stewart-Treves syndrome. The other sites of disease are the skin and subcutis. No known sex predilection exists. This tumor is highly aggressive; but because of its superficial location, the prognosis is relatively favorable compared to other sarcomas.

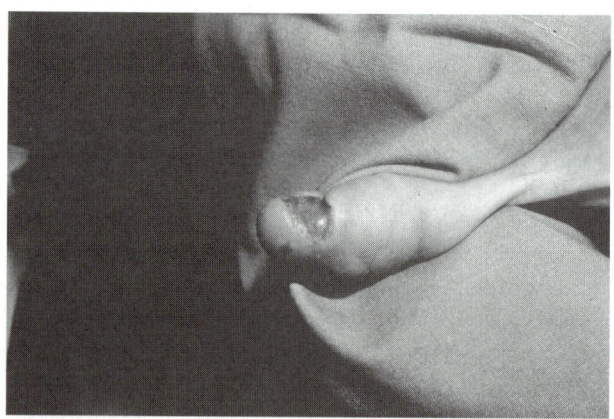

Figure 90.4. An epithelioid sarcoma of the thumb. Reprinted with permission from Cheng EY, Thompson RC. Soft tissue sarcomas. Instr Course Lect 1996;45:461–471.

Hemangioendothelioma is also a rare tumor and is considered to be a low-grade malignancy. The tumor tends to be situated in the deeper soft tissues, subcutis, and visceral organs. Hemangiopericytoma is also a rare tumor and has no known sex or age preferences. It is commonly deeply seated in the lower extremities. Histologically, both benign and malignant forms exist. Occasionally, the benign and malignant forms can be difficult to differentiate; therefore, some surgeons have recommended treating all hemangiopericytomas as potentially aggressive.

SUMMARY

It is important for orthopaedic surgeons and other clinicians who deal with musculoskeletal syndromes to have an understanding of an approach to the workup, evaluation, and clinical management of soft tissue tumors. These tumors are rare, but failure to properly evaluate, manage, and biopsy these lesions can have devastating consequences to the adult and pediatric population in which they occur.

Although evaluation and management of these tumors continues to be investigated and updated and definitive management may change, the evaluation and approach to biopsy of these lesions is the cornerstone for early management of these more aggressive tumors.

REFERENCES

1. Boring CC, Squires TS, Tong T, Montgomery S. Cancer statistics, 1994. CA Cancer J Clin 1994;44:7–26.
2. Lawrence W Jr, Donegan WL, Natarajan N, et al. Adult soft tissue sarcomas: a pattern of care survey of the American College of Surgeons. Ann Surg 1987;205:349–359.
3. Kramer S, Meadows AT, Jarrett P, Evans AE. Incidence of childhood cancer: experience of a decade in a population-based registry. J Natl Cancer Inst 1983;70:49–55.
4. Neifeld JP, Maurer HM, Dillon P, et al. Nonrhabdomyosarcoma soft tissue sarcomas (NRSTS) in children. Paper presented at the 47th Annual Cancer Symposium of the Society of Surgical Oncology, Houston, TX, March 1994.
5. Stout A.P. *Tumors of the soft tissues*. Washington, DC: Armed Forces Institute of Pathology, 1953.
6. Broders AC, Hargrave R, Meyerding HW. Pathological features of soft tissue fibrosarcoma with special reference to the grading of its malignancy. Surg Gynecol Obstet 1939;69:267.
7. Beahrs OH, Henson DE, Hutter RVP, Kennedy BJ. Manual for staging of cancer. Philadelphia: Lippincott, 1993.
8. Enneking WF, Goodman MA. A system for the surgical staging of musculoskeletal sarcoma. Clin Orthop 1980;153:106–120.
9. Enneking WF. Musculoskeletal tumor surgery. New York: Churchill Livingstone, 1983.
10. Suit HD, Mankin HJ, Wood WC, et al. Treatment of the patient with stage M_0 soft tissue sarcoma. J Clin Oncol 1988;6:854–862.
11. Karakousis CP, Perez RP. Soft tissue sarcomas in adults. CA Cancer J Clin 1994;44:200–210.
12. Sondak VK, Leonard JA Jr, Robertson JM, et al. Limb-sparing surgery for extremity soft tissue sarcomas. Surg Oncol Clin North Am 1993;2:657–671.
13. Cheng EY, Dusenbury KE, Winters MR, Thompson RC. Soft tissue sarcomas: preoperative versus postoperative radiotherapy. J Surg Oncol 1996;61:90–99.
14. Mazanet R, Antman KH. Adjuvant therapy for sarcomas. Semin Oncol 1991;18:603–612.
15. Skubitz KM. Infusional chemotherapy for soft tissue sarcoma. J Infusional Chemother 1993;3:129–136.
16. O'Dwyer PJ, Leyland-Jones B, Alonso MT, et al. Etoposide (VP-16-213) current status of an active anti-cancer drug. N Engl J Med 1985;312:692–700.
17. Eilber FR, Guiliano AE, Huth J, et al. High grade soft tissue sarcomas of the extremity; UCLA experience with limb salvage. In: Wagener DJT, ed. Primary chemotherapy in cancer medicine. New York: Liss, 1985.
18. Cheng EY, Springfield DS, Mankin HJ. Frequent incidence of extrapulmonary sites of initial metastasis in patients with liposarcoma. Cancer 1995;75:1120–1127.
19. Cheng EY, Clohisy DR, Thompson RC. Soft tissue sarcomas: management of the patient after prior excisional biopsy. Paper presented at the Combined Meeting of the North American and European Musculoskeletal Tumor Societies, Boston, 1992.
20. Evans RA. Soft tissue sarcoma: the enigma of local recurrence. J Surg Oncol 1993;53:88–91.
21. Azumi N, Curtis J, Kempson RL, Hendrickson MR. Atypical and malignant neoplasms showing lipomatous differentiation. A study of 111 cases. Am J Surg Pathol 1987;11:161–183.
22. Kindblom LG, Angervall L, Fassina AS. Atypical lipoma. Acta Pathol Microbiol Immunol Scand 1982;90A:27–36.
23. Kindblom LG, Angervall L, Svendsen P. Liposarcoma. A clinico-pathologic, radiographic and prognostic study. Acta Pathol Microbiol Scand Suppl 1975;253:1–71.
24. Kampe CE, Rosen G, Eilber F, et al. Synovial sarcoma. Cancer 1993;72:2161–2169.
25. Beahrs OH, Henson DE, Hutter RVP, Kennedy BJ. Manual for staging of cancer. 5th ed. Philadelphia: Lippincott, 1997.
26. Cheng EY, Thompson RC Jr. New developments in staging and imaging of soft tissue sarcomas. J Bone Joint Surgery in press.

PEDIATRICS

It is important to distinguish the clunk of a positive Ortolani or Barlow maneuver from high-pitched soft tissue clicks. These clicks are usually transmitted from the trochanteric region and have no diagnostic significance.

Older Infant

After 2 to 3 months, the Ortolani and Barlow maneuvers become less reliable as a result of the development of secondary adaptive changes about the hip. The most reliable physical finding in late-diagnosed DDH is limitation of abduction. Other findings include shortening of the thigh (Galeazzi sign) and asymmetrical or extra thigh folds (Fig. 91.3).

The diagnosis of bilateral hip dislocation is more difficult because the limitation of adduction may be symmetric, there is no obvious shortening of the thigh, and the skin folds may be equal. A test described by Klisic (16)

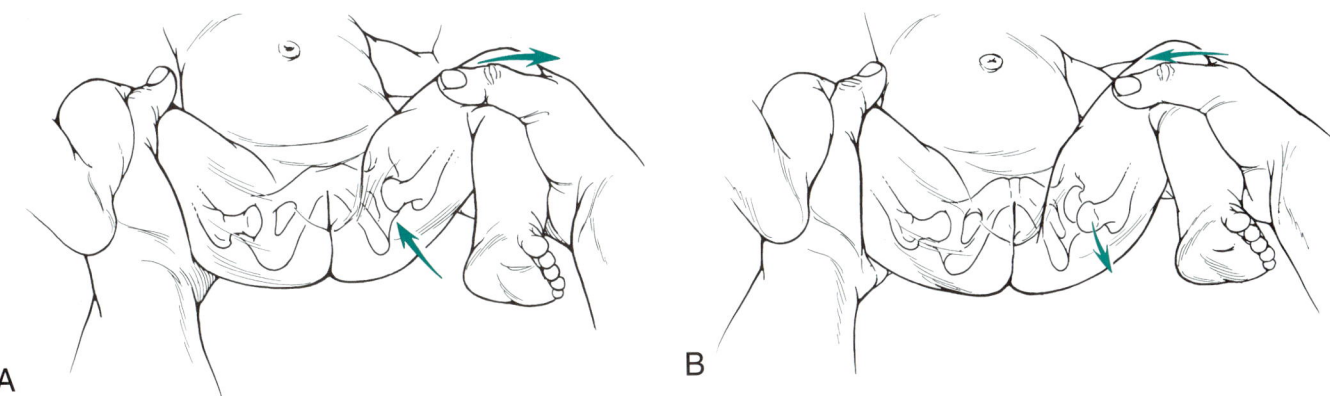

Figure 91.2. The Ortolani (**A**) and Barlow (**B**) maneuvers.

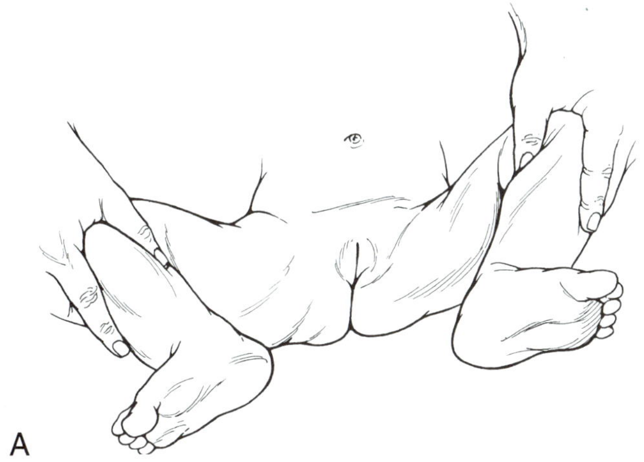

A

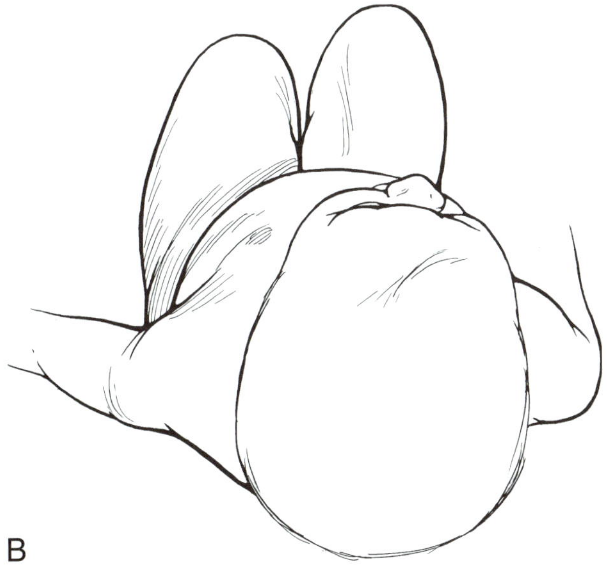

B

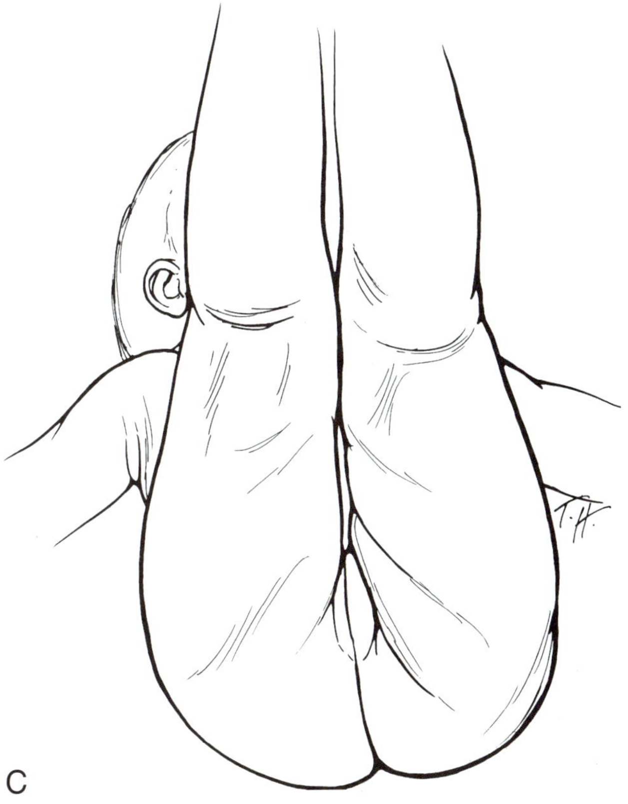

C

Figure 91.3. Clinical findings in the older infant with DDH include limited abduction (**A**), apparent shortening of the thigh (Galeazzi sign) (**B**), and extra or asymmetric skin folds on the thigh (**C**).

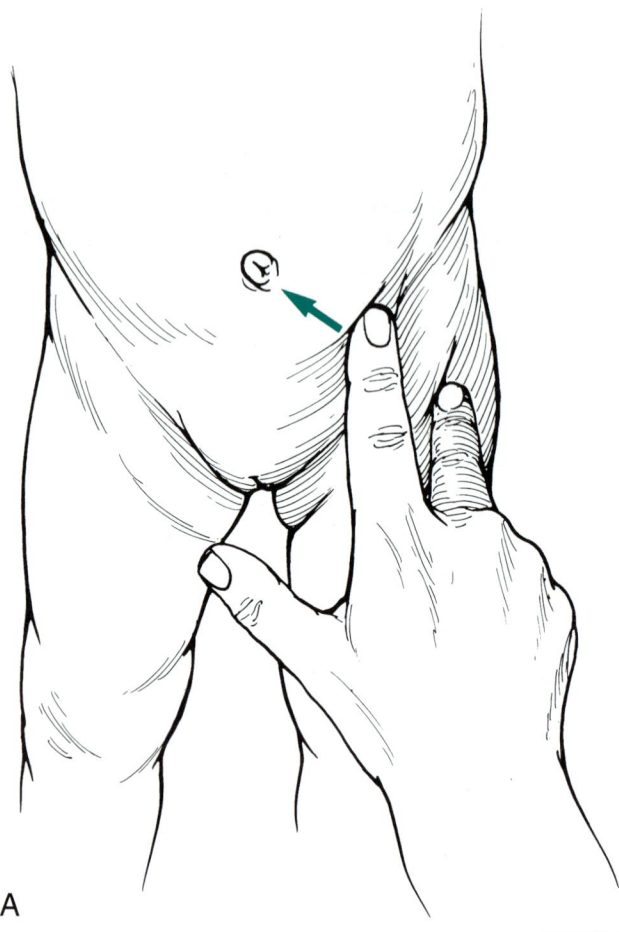

A

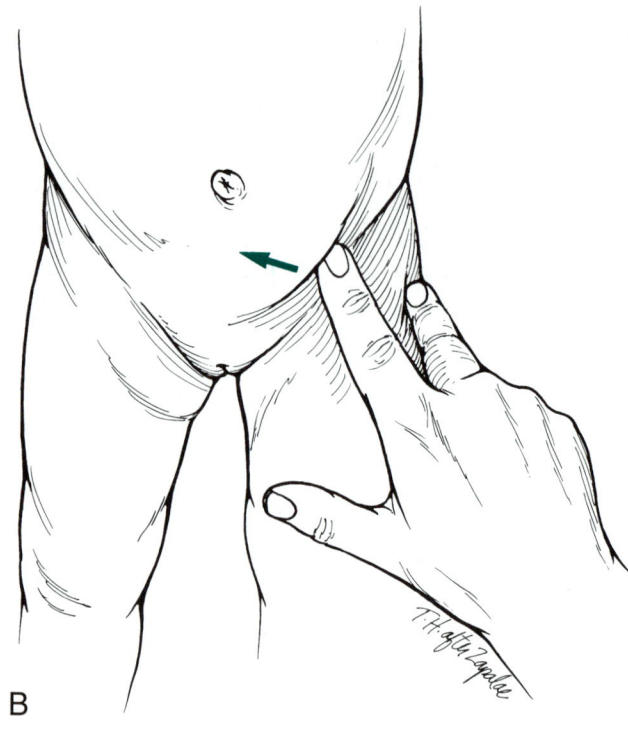

B

Figure 91.4. For the Klisic test, the index finger is placed on the anterior superior iliac spine, and the middle finger is placed on the greater trochanter. **A.** In a normal hip, the line connecting these two points passes through the umbilicus. **B.** In a dislocated hip, the line passes inferior to the umbilicus.

may be useful for detecting DDH in bilateral cases (Fig. 91.4). The examiner places one finger on the greater trochanter and another finger on the anterior superior iliac spine. In a well-located hip, a line connecting these two points passes through the umbilicus. In a dislocated hip, the line passes inferior to the umbilicus. After the neonatal period, it may be a good policy to obtain a radiograph or ultrasound of the hips in any infant who demonstrates less than 60° of hip abduction, especially if risk factors are present, so that bilateral dislocations are not overlooked (17).

Once a child begins walking, the diagnosis is more readily apparent. If a unilateral dislocation is present, the patient will exhibit a Trendelenburg limp and may toe-walk on the affected side. If both hips are dislocated, findings include a waddling gait and hyperlordosis of the spine.

RADIOLOGIC STUDIES

The AP radiograph of the pelvis is difficult to interpret in early infancy because much of the pelvis and femoral head are cartilaginous. For this reason, hip ultrasound studies are largely replacing radiographs for the diagnosis of DDH in young infants.

In infants at least 3 months old, a properly positioned AP radiograph of the pelvis may be useful for evaluating the hips. Several radiographic parameters help detect DDH (Fig. 91.5). The Hilgenreiner line horizontally connects the top of the triradiate cartilages. The Perkins line is drawn perpendicular to the Hilgenreiner line and passes through the most lateral margin of the ossified portion of the acetabular roof. In the normal hip, the medial margin of the proximal femoral metaphysis (i.e., the "beak") should lie within the inner medial quadrant formed by the intersection of these two lines. The Shenton line is drawn along the superior border of the obturator foramen and medial border of the femoral neck. Normally, this line forms a continuous arch. When the hip is subluxated or dislocated, the Shenton line is broken.

The acetabular index is the angle formed by the intersection of the Hilgenreiner line with a line drawn along the bony acetabular roof. When the hip is subluxated or dislocated, the acetabular index is increased. The primary use of this measurement is to monitor the response of the acetabulum to treatment.

Other radiographic features of DDH include an absent teardrop figure and a delay in the appearance of the ossification center of the femoral head or a smaller ossific nucleus on the affected side. In children who are older than

5 years of age, the center edge angle may be useful to detect subluxation or dysplasia; it is most useful in adolescents and adults. After the triradiate cartilage has closed, the acetabular angle of Sharp (18) can be used to assess acetabular development.

The precise role of ultrasound in the diagnosis and management of DDH is still being defined. The two methods currently in use are the static method, pioneered by Graf (19), and the dynamic or real-time method advocated by Harcke (20). The static method relies on the measured angles. The α angle reflects coverage of the femoral head by the bony acetabulum, and the β angle indicates deformation of the labrum and subluxation of the hip. Problems with the static method include difficulty in accurately reproducing the image and substantial interobserver and intraobserver variations in the measurement of the angles (21). The dynamic method attempts to visualize what oc-

curs during the Ortolani and Barlow maneuvers. The problems with this method are that it is operator dependent and requires a more subjective assessment of the findings.

The indications for ultrasound in the diagnosis of DDH are not definitively established. The routine use of ultrasound for newborn screening appears to have resulted in overdiagnosis and a high treatment rate (22–24). The cost-effectiveness of using ultrasound to screen all high-risk infants is still being debated (23,25,26).

In the newborn, the diagnosis of DDH is based on physical examination. If the examination results are questionable, ultrasound may provide additional useful information regarding stability. When a reliable and experienced operator is available, ultrasound can be used to minimize the number of radiographs necessary to monitor the effectiveness of treatment and to determine stability when

Figure 91.5. **A.** AP view of the pelvis of an 8-month-old infant with left DDH. **B.** Radiograph showing the radiographic parameters that are useful in detecting DDH.

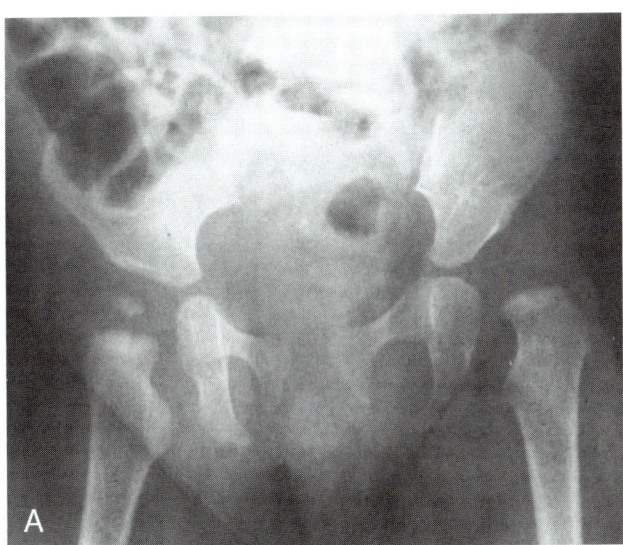

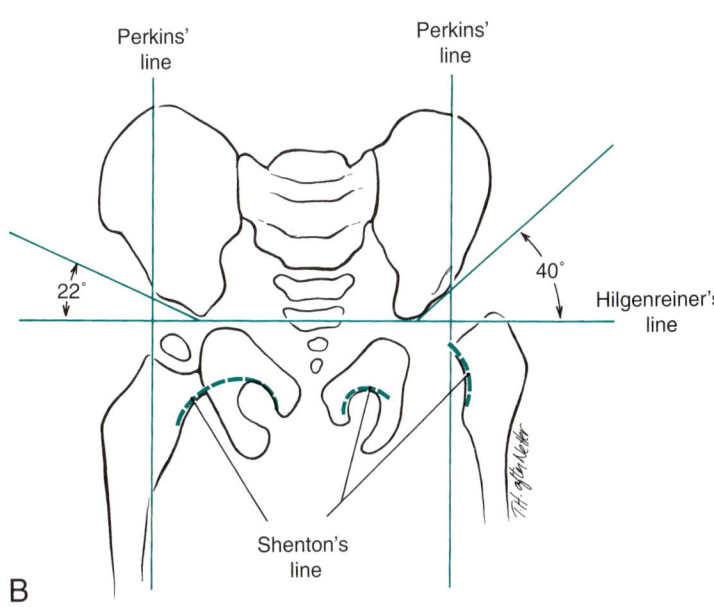

Clinical Table: Developmental Dysplasia of the Hip

Procedure	Indications	Technique	Anatomy	Pitfalls
Pavlik harness	• <6 months old	• Apply with hips in 100–110° of flexion • Tighten abduction straps • Conduct x-ray or ultrasound examination	• Femoral head • Acetabulum • Ridge of hypertrophied acetabular cartilage	• Brace applied with insufficient or excessive flexion and/or abduction • Poor parental compliance • Poor harness construction
Closed reduction and adductor tenotomy	• 6–24 months old • <6 months old and failed harness treatment	• Preliminary traction • General anesthesia • Adductor longus tenotomy via open or percutaneous technique • Arthrogram • Spica cast • Conduct CT study	• Adductor longus	• Application of cast with insufficient or extreme abduction, insufficient flexion, or extreme internal rotation
Open reduction, medial approach	• <1 year old	• Section iliopsoas and adductor longus tendons • Open medial joint capsule • Release transverse acetabular ligament • Spica cast	• Adductor brevis • Adductor magnus • Femoral neurovascular bundle • Pectineus	• Failure to maintain reduction in the spica cast
Open reduction, anterolateral approach	• >2 years old • Failure of closed treatment	• Adductor longus tenotomy • Remove impediments to reduction • Lengthen psoas • Plicate capsule • Spica cast	• Sartorius • Tensor fascia lata	• Failure to identify the true acetabulum • Inadequate capsular plication
Femoral shortening and derotation	• >3 years old • 2–3 years old in selected patients	• Section femur with hip reduced and fragments overlapping • Remove section of femur • Correct anteversion • Internal fixation	• Tensor fascia lata • Vastus lateralis	• Inadequate fixation • Overcorrection of anteversion
Innominate osteotomy	• >3 years old • 2–3 years old in selected patients	• Lengthen adductor longus and iliopsoas • Osteotomy from sciatic notch to anterior inferior iliac spine • Rotate distal fragment anterolaterally • Steinmann pins	• Sartorius • Tensor fascia lata	• Failure to obtain concentric reduction • Failure to lengthen tendon(s) • Incorrect rotation of distal fragment

weaning from an orthosis (27). After the appearance of the ossific nucleus of the femoral head at around 3 to 7 months of age, ultrasound examination becomes less valuable and radiographs become more accurate.

TREATMENT

The goal of treatment is to safely obtain and maintain a concentric reduction of the hip, providing an environment that will allow the normal developmental sequence to proceed (Clinical Table). The earlier the diagnosis of DDH is made, the more likely treatment will achieve a normal or near-normal hip. When the diagnosis is made late, the treatment becomes more complex and the outcome is less certain, because there is less potential for femoral and acetabular remodeling.

Nonoperative Treatment

NEWBORN TO 6 MONTHS

All infants with hip instability, as demonstrated by a positive Ortolani or Barlow sign, should be treated. The Pavlik harness is the most commonly used device used to treat DDH in the newborn (Fig. 91.6). When properly applied, the device prevents extension and adduction of the hips, which can lead to redislocation, and encourages further flexion and abduction, which leads to a gentle, stable reduction.

The harness is applied with the chest strap placed just below the nipple line and is held in place by the shoulder straps. The anterior buckles should be at the anterior axillary line, and the posterior buckles should be at the tips of the scapulae. Hip flexion should be set at 100° to 110°. The abduction straps should be tightened to allow the hips to adduct within 8 to 10 cm (about four fingerbreadths) between the knees. After application of the harness, a radiograph or, if available, an ultrasound examination should be done to assess the reduction.

The harness is used full time for the first 6 weeks, or until the hip has stabilized. The infant should be checked 1 week after the harness is applied. The frequency of subsequent follow-up visits is individualized based on the comfort level of the parents.

At 6 weeks, I obtain a radiograph of the patient out of the harness—the hips are in relaxed, partial extension—to assess the stability of the reduction. When the hip is stable, the harness may be removed for 1 h per day for bathing. If acetabular improvement continues, I gradually wean the patient over the following 6 weeks to nighttime and naptime wear. The brace is continued until the hip is

clinically and radiographically normal (Fig. 91.7). The duration of the treatment is determined by the response of the hip. For infants with DDH treated at birth, the harness is worn 8 to 10 weeks full-time and 6 weeks part-time. Infants who are older at the time of diagnosis will generally spend a longer period of time in the harness.

In an infant younger than 6 months of age who has a complete dislocation of the hip that is not initially reducible, the Pavlik harness may be used for a trial of guided reduction (Fig. 91.8). When the harness is used in these cases, the infant should be followed weekly to see if reduction has been achieved. If the hip does not reduce after 3 or 4 weeks of harness wear, the harness should be discontinued and other treatment methods should be tried, which avoids the development of secondary pathologic changes, called Pavlik harness disease (28,29). Because of the child's increasing activity level, the Pavlik harness is not strong enough to properly position the hip of infants older than 6 months. The harness is contraindicated for the treatment of neuromuscular dislocations.

The Pavlik harness has been shown to be effective in more than 90% of patients (30). The complication rate is low, and most of the complications are avoidable. Mubarak et al. (31) have identified several pitfalls associated with the use of the Pavlik harness, including insufficient flexion or abduction to maintain a stable reduction; excessive flexion, which may result in an inferior disloca-

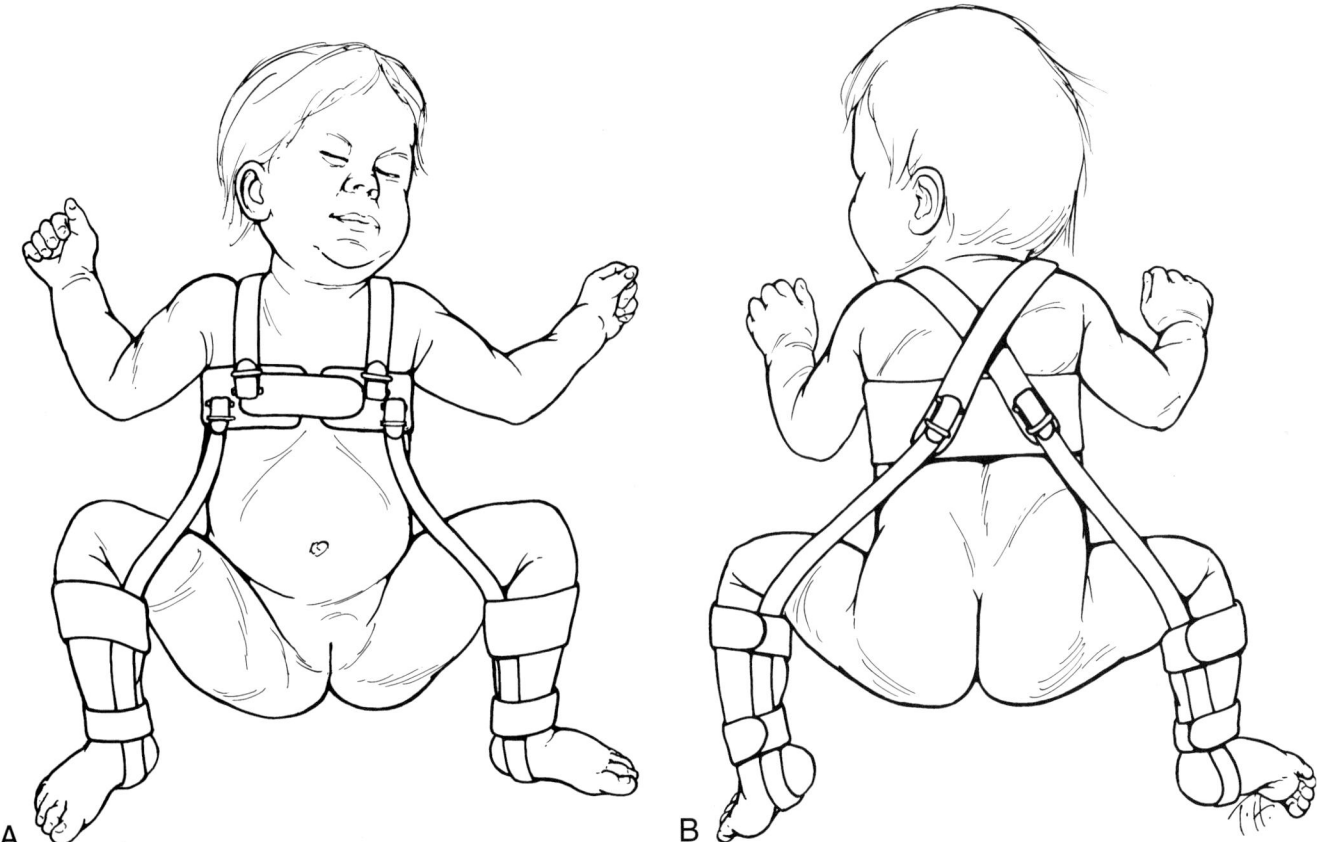

Figure 91.6. Application of the Pavlik harness.

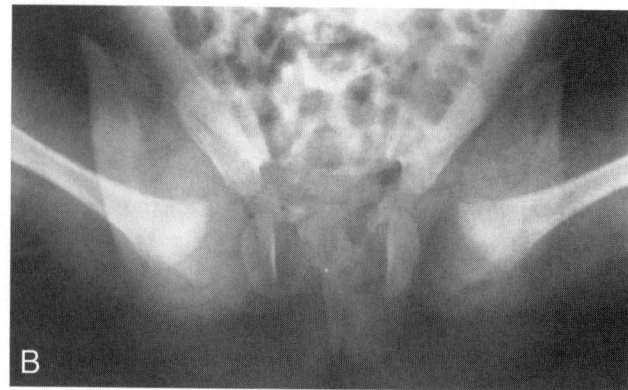

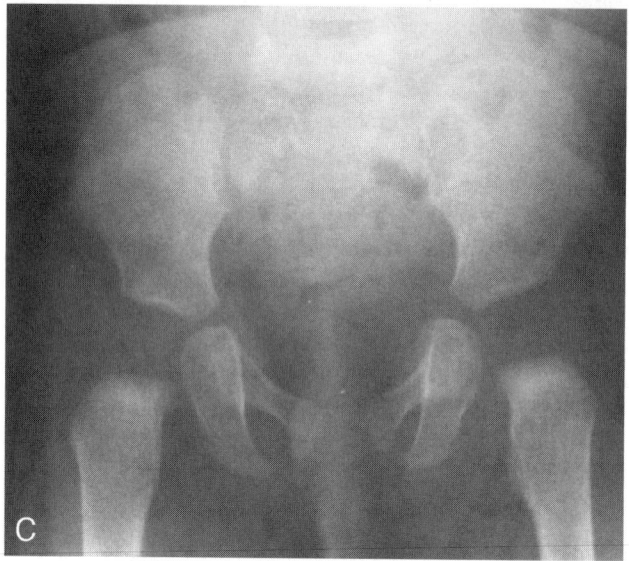

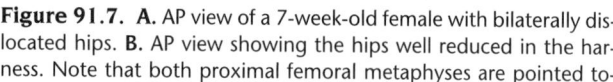

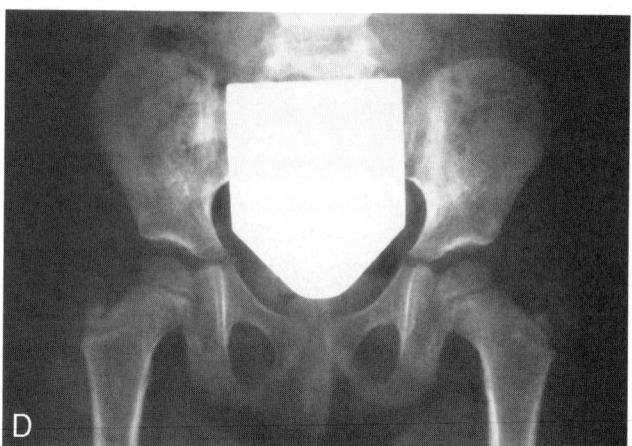

Figure 91.7. A. AP view of a 7-week-old female with bilaterally dislocated hips. **B.** AP view showing the hips well reduced in the harness. Note that both proximal femoral metaphyses are pointed toward the triradiate cartilages. **C.** AP view of the patient at 8 months of age, when the harness was discontinued. **D.** AP view of the patient at 4 years of age. Note that the hips are developing well.

tion or femoral neuropathy; and excessive abduction, which may cause avascular necrosis. In addition, they noted problems caused by poor parental compliance and by harnesses that were poorly constructed.

It is important to continue to follow patients who are treated with a Pavlik harness until they reach skeletal maturity. Tucci et al. (32) reported an 8- to 15-year follow-up of patients treated in a Pavlik harness. All of the hips were radiographically normal at the 5-year follow-up, but 17% had acetabular dysplasia at the latest follow-up.

6 MONTHS TO 2 YEARS

Patients with DDH who are older than 6 months of age at the time of diagnosis and those younger than 6 months who have failed a trial of Pavlik harness management are best treated by closed reduction and spica cast immobilization (33,34). Although there is no universal agreement, (35,36) closed reduction in most centers is usually preceded by a period of skin traction (37). Proponents of traction believe that gradually stretching the soft tissue structures crossing the hip facilitates closed reduction and

lessens the incidence of avascular necrosis (34,38–41). Traction may be administered in the hospital or at home (42–44).

Adhesive traction straps should be applied from the upper thigh to just above the malleoli. The direction of the traction varies among different centers. I position the extremities so that the hips are flexed 45°. Weight is then applied to both limbs, beginning with 1 kg; the weight is increased in 0.5-kg increments to a maximum of 2.5 kg. Generally, the traction is continued for 2 to 3 weeks. If the hip becomes reducible at the bedside before that time, traction may be discontinued earlier.

After a period of traction, the hip is examined under general anesthesia. Reduction is attempted by gentle traction on the flexed, adducted thigh, which is then slowly brought into abduction. Reduction can be readily felt as a positive Ortolani sign. If a reduction is achieved, the stability is assessed by slowly adducting the thigh until the femoral head is felt to redislocate. The arc between the arc of comfortable abduction, usually around 60°, and the angle that allows dislocation to occur corresponds to the safe zone (30). The hip is also carefully evaluated in varying degrees of flexion and rotation to determine the most stable position in those planes. If the adductors are tight at the desired position of reduction, an adductor tenotomy is performed. This procedure usually increases the safe zone, which lessens the risk of avascular necrosis.

A stable hip usually remains reduced in 90° of flexion through an arc of 30° to 60° of abduction. If maximum abduction or internal rotation is necessary to maintain reduction of the hip, closed treatment should be abandoned and an open reduction of the hip should be performed. An arthrogram may help assess the adequacy of closed reduction (Fig. 91.9). A small amount of contrast medium (1 to 2 mL) is all that is needed. Excessive pooling of contrast medium between the femoral head and the acetabulum correlates with a poor outcome of closed management (45).

After the closed reduction, the hips are immobilized in a well-molded spica cast with the hip in at least 90° of flexion and no more than 60° of abduction. This corresponds to the "human position" advocated by Salter and Dubos (46). It is important to apply a mold dorsal to the greater trochanter to prevent redislocation. The reduction after cast application is documented by an x-ray and a three-cut CT scan (47).

At 6 weeks after closed reduction, the cast is changed under general anesthesia. If there is any question concerning the quality of the reduction, an arthrogram should be performed. After the second 6 weeks in plaster, the cast is removed and an abduction brace is applied and worn full-time, except for bathing, for an additional 2 to 3 months and then during nap time and nighttime until the development of the acetabulum is deemed adequate (Fig. 91.10).

When a stable closed reduction cannot be obtained in patients 6 months to 2 years of age, open reduction is indicated. Open reduction of DDH may be achieved through several different surgical approaches.

Operative Treatment

The most commonly used surgical approach for open reduction is the anterolateral Smith-Peterson approach through a modified bikini incision. This approach allows removal of the obstacles to reduction, such as a hypertrophic ligamentum teres or pulvinar, and facilitates plication of a redundant hip capsule. If the surgeon believes that an innominate osteotomy is necessary, it can be performed through the same surgical approach (48). After the open reduction, the patient is placed in a spica cast for 6

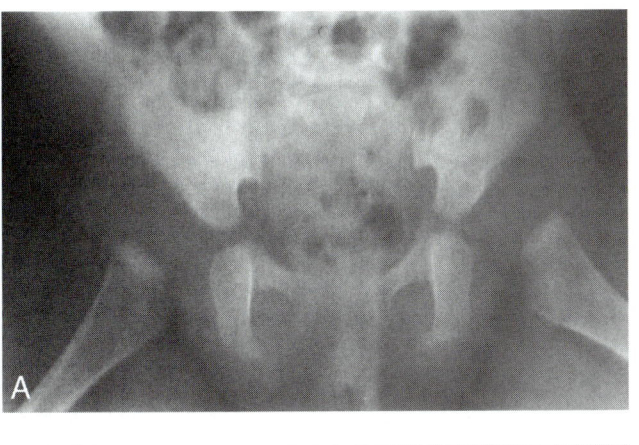

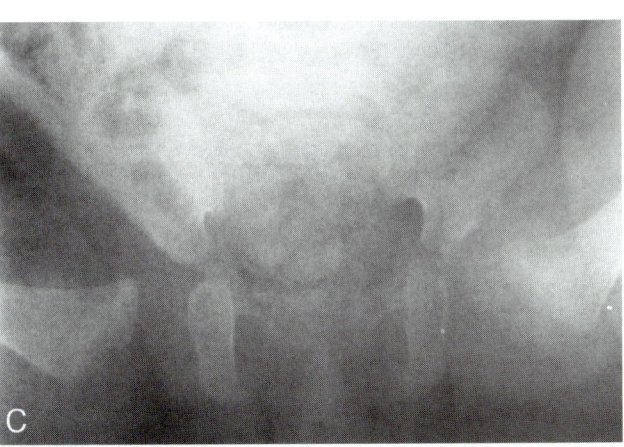

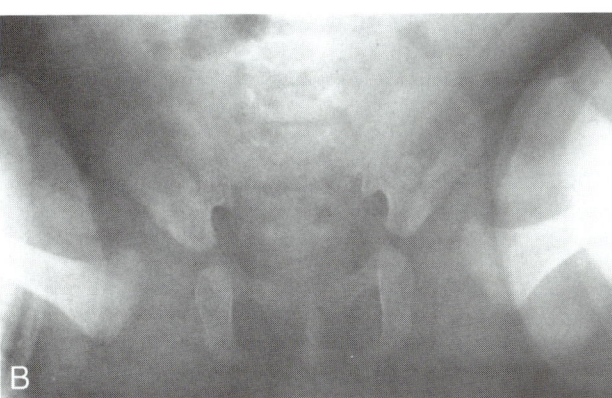

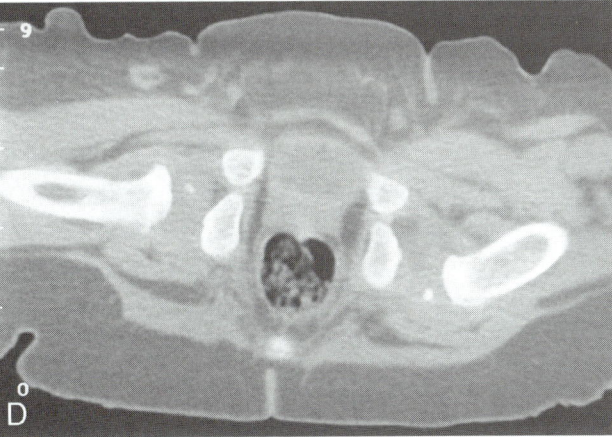

Figure 91.8. A. AP view of a 3-month-old female with bilaterally dislocated hips that are not reducible. **B** and **C.** AP views after a 3-week trial in a Pavlik harness. Note that the right hip is reduced, but the left hip is somewhat proximally displaced. **D.** CT scan confirming that the left hip is not reduced.

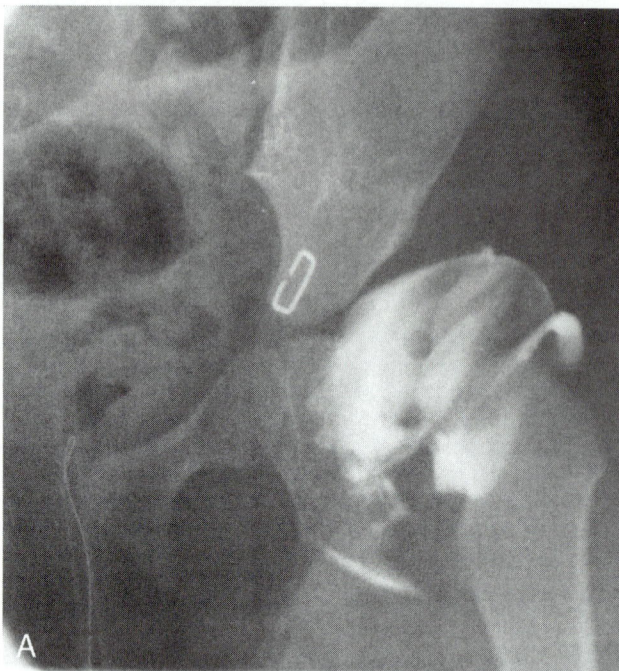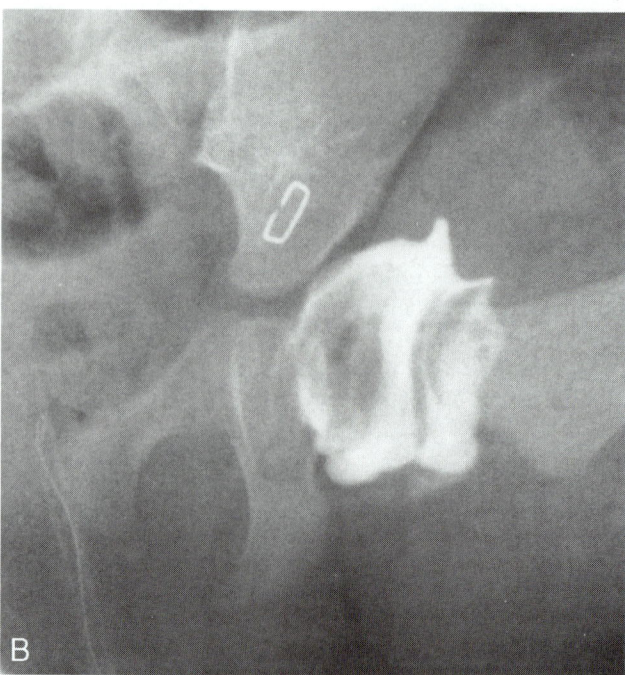

Figure 91.9. Arthrograms of a dislocated hip before (**A**) and after (**B**) reduction.

weeks with the hip in mild flexion and abduction. This is then changed to a Petrie-type cast for an additional month. After the cast is removed, additional abduction splinting may be used until acetabular development is deemed adequate.

Open reduction may also be obtained through a medial approach. The posteromedial approach, described by Ferguson (49), uses the plane between the adductor brevis and the adductor magnus. The anteromedial approach, originally described by Ludloff (50) and later modified by Weinstein and Ponseti (51), is made in the interval between the femoral neurovascular bundle and the pectineus muscle. Because capsular plication cannot be done through a medial approach, maintaining the reduction after surgery depends on the placement of a well-molded cast. The cast regimen after medial open reduction is the same as that described for closed reduction.

Advocates of open reduction through a medial approach believe that it is the most direct approach to the major obstacles to reduction. Through the medial approach, the iliopsoas tendon may be released, the hourglass constriction of the medial joint capsule can be opened, and the transverse acetabular ligament can be sectioned. There is minimal blood loss, the scar is cosmetic, and there is no damage to the hip abductor muscles or iliac apophysis (51,52). The disadvantages of the medial approach are that it does not allow plication of the capsule and may be associated with a higher risk of avascular

necrosis, because the medial femoral circumflex artery crosses the operative field (53). The selection of which operative approach to use is determined by the experience and philosophy of the treating surgeon.

There is no universal agreement regarding the need for concomitant pelvic or femoral osteotomies at the time of open reduction. Several studies have documented that the development of the acetabulum after closed or open reduction in patients 4 years or younger is excellent and continues as long as 4 to 8 years after the hip is reduced (54–57). Associated femoral anteversion and coxa valga also seem to have the potential to resolve with time. Advocates of concomitant innominate osteotomy believe that this procedure is needed to increase the stability of the reduction and accelerate the development of the acetabulum toward normal. Salter and Dubos (48) recommend that an innominate osteotomy accompany open reduction in every child older than 18 months to better enhance development of the acetabulum. This controversy has not yet been resolved.

Older Than 2 Years

Children who are older than 2 years of age at the time of diagnosis are more difficult to manage. Contracture of the soft tissues and dysplasia of the femur and acetabulum are usually more advanced. Although some patients between 2 and 3 years of age many be managed by preliminary traction and closed reduction, open reduction is usually necessary.

In children older than 3 years of age and in selected children between 2 and 3 years of age, femoral shortening should accompany the open reduction to lessen the pressure on the proximal femur and minimize the risk of osteonecrosis. Schoenecker and Strecker (58) compared the results of traction followed by open reduction to those of femoral shortening at the time of open reduction in children older than 3 years. They found a better outcome and lower incidence of avascular necrosis in patients who underwent femoral shortening.

In this age group, open reduction is done through an anterolateral approach to facilitate capsular plication and allow, if deemed necessary, an innominate osteotomy. Femoral shortening is done through a second lateral incision. The amount of shortening is determined by the amount of overlap between the proximal and distal osteotomy fragments with the femoral head reduced, usually 1 to 2 cm. Excessive femoral anteversion can be corrected and the fragments can be secured with either a blade plate or straight plate.

For children older than 3 years, most surgeons advocate concomitant innominate osteotomy. The anatomic deficiency of the acetabulum is usually anterior and the Salter innominate osteotomy is well suited to provide anterior coverage. Care must be taken to avoid a posterior dislocation when combining a femoral derotation osteotomy with an innominate osteotomy. Several centers have reported satisfactory results combining open reduction, femoral shortening, and innominate osteotomy for the treatment of DDH in this age group (48,59–61).

Problems and Complications

REDISLOCATION

Redislocation of the hip may occur after either closed or open reduction. Redislocation after closed reduction may result from a failure to immobilize the hip in a stable position or from inadequate molding of the spica cast. After a closed reduction, it is important to obtain high-quality ra-

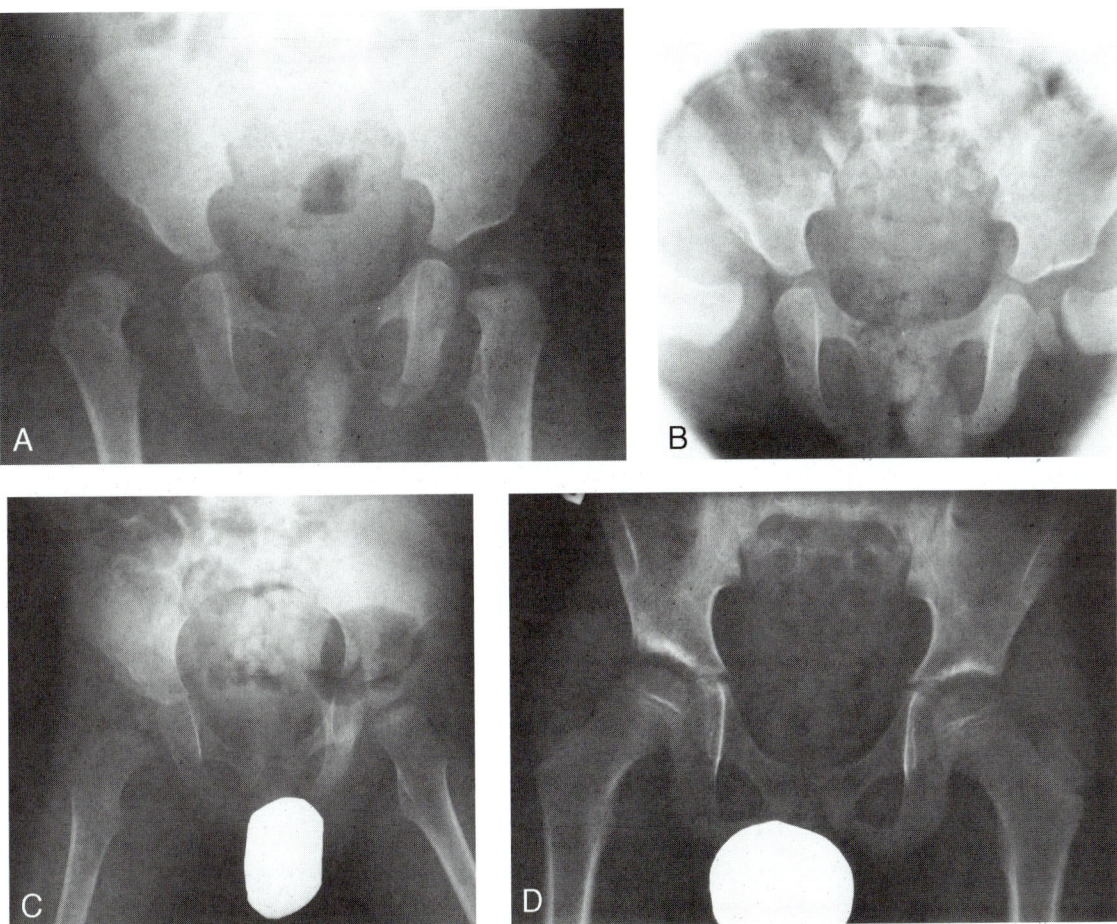

Figure 91.10. A. AP view of an 18-month-old male with a dislocated right hip. **B.** AP view showing the immediate results of a closed reduction and adductor tenotomy. **C.** AP view taken 12 months after treatment, showing growth arrest lines that suggest normal growth of the proximal femur. **D.** AP view of the patient at 9 years of age, showing good hip development.

diographs and a CT scan so that any dislocation may be recognized promptly. When redislocation occurs after a closed treatment, the hip should be reevaluated under general anesthesia. Usually another closed reduction can be performed, but occasionally an open reduction will be necessary.

A redislocation after open reduction may pose a more difficult problem. Factors that may predispose to a failed initial open reduction include failure to accurately identify the true acetabulum, insufficient release of the inferior portion of the capsule, and inadequate capsular plication. Also, if simultaneous femoral derotation and innominate osteotomies were performed, the femoral head may redislocate posteriorly. Attempts to relocate the hip by closed means are usually unsuccessful, and a repeat open reduction is almost always necessary. The results of repeat open reduction are not as good as those of a successful initial open reduction (62,63).

RESIDUAL FEMORAL AND ACETABULAR DYSPLASIA

The goal of treatment of DDH is to have a hip joint that is radiographically normal at skeletal maturity. Weinstein

(64) published an excellent review of the natural history of subluxation and acetabular dysplasia. Radiographic evidence of subluxation after treatment of DDH invariably leads to degenerative joint disease (65–67) and must be corrected. There is also evidence to show that residual acetabular dysplasia, even in the absence of subluxation, will eventually develop osteoarthritis, although the process may take much longer (65).

If acetabular dysplasia persists for 2 to 3 years after a closed or open reduction, an osteotomy should be considered. The type of osteotomy performed depends on the location of the deformity, the age of the patient, and the philosophy of the treating surgeon.

For children younger than 4 years who have persistent acetabular dysplasia and residual femoral anteversion, a proximal femoral varus derotation osteotomy may be indicated (Fig. 91.11). Proponents of proximal femoral osteotomy believe this procedure facilitates acetabular remodeling by redirecting the femoral head toward the center of the acetabulum (68–70). Before the operation, an AP radiograph or arthrogram should be obtained to document that the femoral head is concentrically reduced with the patient's legs in abduction and internal rotation. Varus

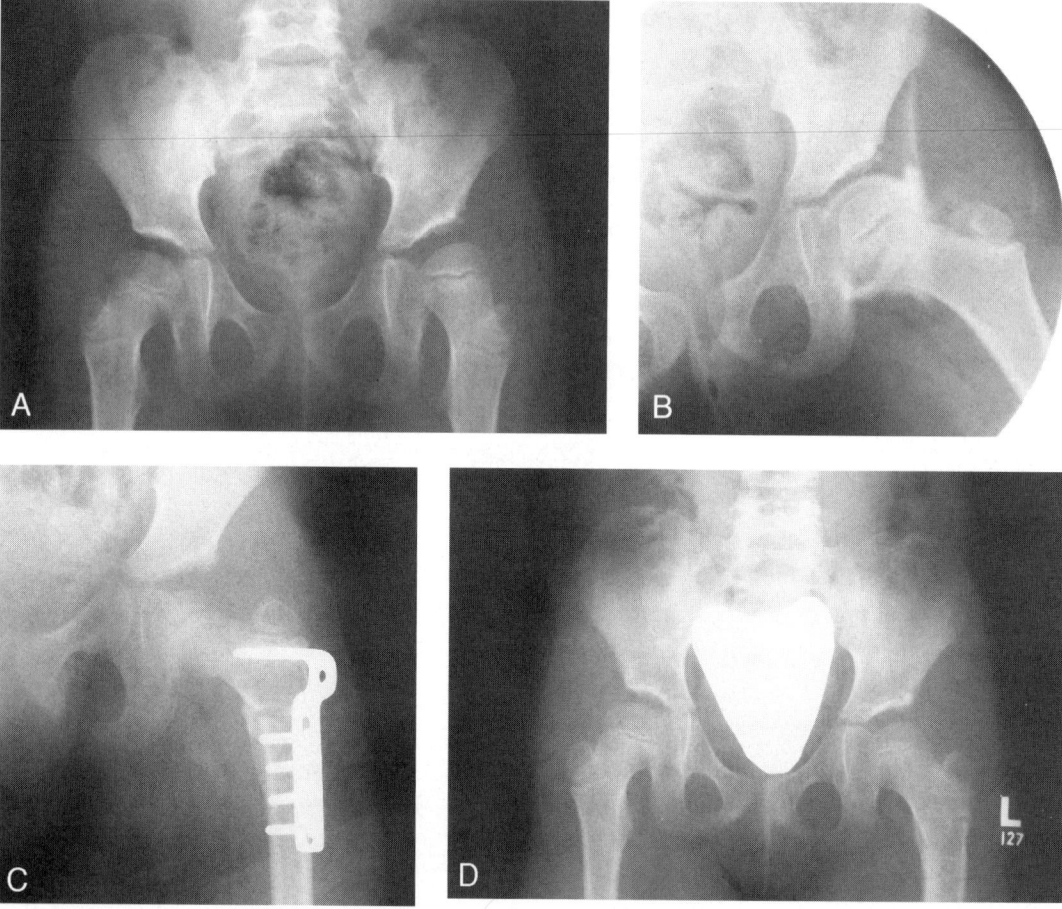

Figure 91.11. A. AP view showing persistent acetabular dysplasia and apparent coxa valga in a 4-year-old female 2.5 years after closed reduction of the left hip. **B.** Arthrogram taken with the leg in abduction and internal rotation, showing that the femoral head is concentrically reduced. **C.** AP view showing varus derotation osteotomy. **D.** AP view showing the pelvis 2 years after the osteotomy.

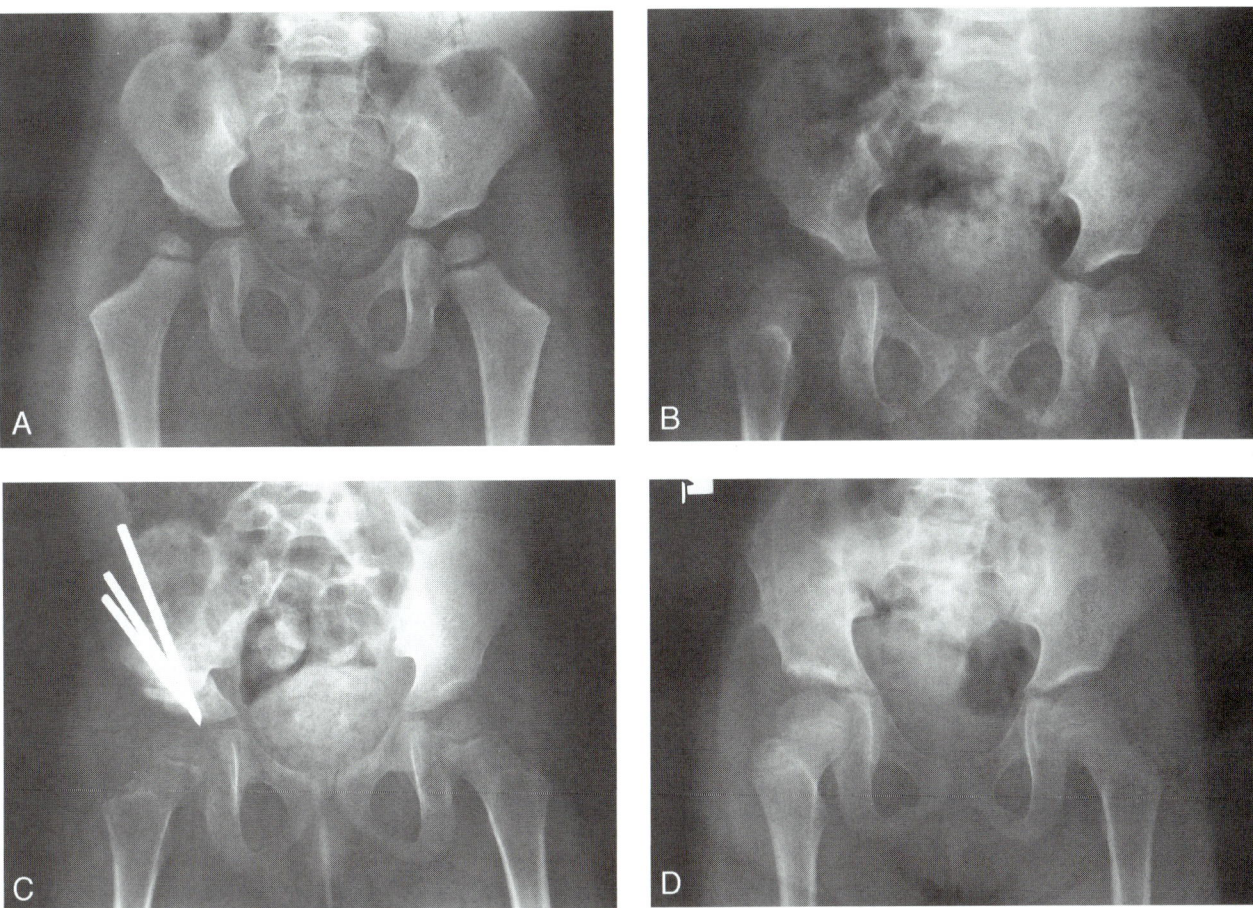

Figure 91.12. A. AP view showing persistent acetabular dysplasia in a 3-year-old female 2.5 years after closed reduction of the right hip. **B.** AP view taken with the leg in abduction and internal rotation showing the femoral head well seated in the acetabulum. **C.** AP view showing a Salter innominate osteotomy. **D.** AP view showing the pelvis about 4 years after the osteotomy.

derotation osteotomy of the proximal femur to correct residual acetabular dysplasias is best reserved for children younger than 4 years (69,70). Little, if any, acetabular remodeling can be expected if this procedure is done in children older than 8 years.

For patients who are older than 4 years and for younger patients with severe acetabular deformity, persistent acetabular dysplasia is probably best managed by pelvic osteotomy. Pelvic osteotomies may be divided into two main groups: reconstructive and salvage procedures. Reconstructive osteotomies use hyaline articular cartilage to restore the joint surface. A concentric reduction is an absolute requirement for any reconstructive osteotomy. Salvage procedures use the joint capsule supported by bone or bone graft to provide a weight-bearing surface. In general, reconstructive procedures should be done whenever possible.

Selection of the appropriate reconstructive procedure depends on the age of the patient and the amount of dysplasia that must be corrected. In younger patients, the Salter innominate osteotomy may effectively improve the anterolateral deficiency of the acetabulum (Fig. 91.12). Because the Salter osteotomy hinges on the symphysis pubis, it is better performed in younger patients who have good flexibility.

In older patients who may have limited mobility of the symphysis pubis or who may need additional coverage, the double innominate osteotomy, triple innominate osteotomy, or one of the other periacetabular osteotomies may be needed (71–74). Other pericapsular osteotomies have been described that involve incomplete cuts in the bone and hinge on the triradiate cartilage (75,76). These procedures may decrease the volume of the acetabulum. Proponents of these procedures have found them to be effective in the management of acetabular dysplasia (76,77).

Salvage procedures, such as the shelf arthroplasty and the Chiari osteotomy, are probably best reserved for hips that cannot be covered by one of the previously mentioned reconstructive operations.

Osteonecrosis

Osteonecrosis is the most common complication of the treatment of DDH. It may be seen after all forms of treatment. Osteonecrosis is thought to occur from either excessive pressure on the femoral head, leading to pressure necrosis of the articular cartilage, or to compression of the extrinsic blood supply to the proximal femur. The result of osteonecrosis is varying degrees of growth disturbance to the proximal femur.

Immobilization of the hip in extreme abduction or abduction and internal rotation has been associated with an increased incidence of osteonecrosis (46). Such positioning may cause compression of the medial femoral circumflex artery as it passes between the iliopsoas tendon and pectineus muscle and by direct compression of the vessel and its branches along the posterior intertrochanteric groove by the acetabular rim (78).

The criteria outlined by Salter et al. (46) are the most commonly used for the diagnosis of osteonecrosis. They include failure of the appearance or growth of the ossific nucleus within 1 year after reduction, increased radiographic bone density followed by fragmentation of the femoral head, and residual deformity of the femoral head and neck when reossification is complete. Residual deformity may include coxa magna, coxa plana, coxa vara, and a short, broad femoral neck.

Classification systems have been developed to describe the different patterns of growth disturbances caused by osteonecrosis (78,79). The milder forms of osteonecrosis involve only the epiphysis and are rarely of clinical importance, whereas the more severe forms affect the physis and lead to significant residual deformity of the proximal femur.

O'Brien (80) observed that after a hip is reduced, a growth arrest line usually develops below the physis of the proximal femur (Fig. 10C). The extent of displacement of this line from the physis may provide early evidence of whether the physis has been permanently injured.

Long-term studies of patients who have developed a proximal femoral growth disturbance suggest that the longevity of the hip joint is shortened (54,66,81). When treating patients who develop osteonecrosis, reduction of the hip should be maintained by corrective femoral or pelvic procedures. Patients who develop a short femoral neck and trochanteric overgrowth will have an abductor limp. If trochanteric overgrowth is recognized early, trochanteric epiphysiodesis may be effective in children younger than 8 years (82). In older patients, distal transfer of the greater trochanter may be necessary (83,84).

SUMMARY

Prompt detection of DDH is the key to achieving a favorable outcome of treatment. Knowledge of the etiologic factors for DDH and an awareness of the appropriate age-related physical examination findings will greatly aid in the early detection of this disorder. If treatment of a developmentally dislocated hip commences early, while pathologic changes are largely reversible, complete anatomical restoration of the hip joint may be achievable.

When the diagnosis is delayed, some radiographic stigmata will remain, regardless of treatment.

Reduction of a developmentally dislocated hip may be achieved by closed or open methods, depending on the age of the patient and the philosophy of the treating physician. All treatment methods strive to obtain a safe and gentle reduction of the hip while minimizing the incidence of redislocation, residual femoral and acetabular dysplasia, and osteonecrosis. The goal of treatment of DDH is to establish a relationship between the femoral head and the acetabulum that is as near to normal as possible to minimize the risk of degenerative arthritis.

REFERENCES

1. Bjerkreim I, Arseth PH. Congenital dislocation of the hip in Norway. Late diagnosis CDH in the years 1970 to 1974. Acta Paediatr Scand 1978;67:329–332.
2. Davies SJM, Walker G. Problems in the early recognition of hip dysplasia. J Bone Joint Surg 1984;66B:479–484.
3. Ilfeld FW, Westin GW, Makin M. Missed or developmental dislocation of the hip. Clin Orthrop 1986;203:276–281.
4. Muller GM, Seddon HJ. Late results of treatment of congenital dislocation of the hip. J Bone Joint Surg 1953;35B:342–362.
5. Wynne-Davies R. Acetabular dysplasia and familial joint laxity: two etiological factors in congenital dislocation of the hip. A review of 589 patients and their families. J Bone Joint Surg 1970; 52B:704–716.
6. Coleman SS. Congenital dysplasia of the hip in the Navajo infant. Clin Orthop 1968;56:179–193.
7. Pompe Van Meerdervoort HF. Congenital musculoskeletal disorders in the South African Negro. J Bone Joint Surg 1977;59B:257.
8. Hoagland FT, Yau AC, Wong WL. Osteoarthritis of the hip and other joints in southern Chinese in Hong Kong. J Bone Joint Surg 1973;55A:545–557.
9. Hummer CD Jr, MacEwen GD. The coexistence of torticollis and congenital dysplasia of the hip. J Bone Joint Surg 1972; 54A:1255–1256.
10. Kumar SJ, MacEwen GD. The incidence of hip dysplasia with metatarsus adductus. Clin Orthop 1982;164:234–235.
11. Heikkila E. Congenital dislocation of the hip in Finland. An epidemiologic analysis of 1035 cases. Acta Orthop Scand 1984; 55:125–129.
12. Carter CO, Wilkinson JA. Genetic and environmental factors in the etiology of congenital dislocation of the hip. Clin Orthop 1964; 33:119–128.
13. Kutlu A, Memik R, Mutlu M, et al. Congenital dislocation of the hip and its relation to swaddling used in Turkey. J Pediatr Orthop 1992;12:598–602.
14. Ishii Y, Weinstein SL, Ponseti IV. Correlation between arthrograms and operative findings in congenital dislocation of the hip. Clin Orthop 1980;153:138–145.
15. Barlow TG. Early diagnosis and treatment of congenital dislocation of the hip. J Bone Joint Surg 1962;44B:292–301.
16. Herring JA. Congenital dislocation of the hip. In: Morrissy RT, ed. Lovell and Winter's pediatric orthopaedics. Philadelphia: Lippincott, 1990:815–850.
17. Garvey M, Donoghue VB, Gorman WA, et al. Radiographic screening at four months of infants at risk for congenital hip dislocation. J Bone Joint Surg 1992;74B:704–707.
18. Sharp IK. Acetabular dysplasia. The acetabular angle. J Bone Joint Surg 1961;43B:269–272.
19. Graf R. New possibilities for the diagnosis of congenital hip joint dislocation by ultrasonography. J Pediatr Orthop 1983; 3:354–359.

20. Harcke HT. Imaging in congenital dislocation and dysplasia of the hip. Clin Orthop 1992;281:22–28.

21. Dias JJ, Thomas IH, Lamont AC, et al. The reliability of ultrasonographic assessment of neonatal hips. J Bone Joint Surg 1993; 75B:479–482.

22. Castelein RM, Sauter AJ, de Vlieger M, van Linge B. Natural history of ultrasound hip abnormalities in clinically normal newborns. J Pediatr Orthop 1992;12:423–427.

23. Hernandez RJ, Cornell RG, Hensinger RN. Ultrasound diagnosis of neonatal congenital dislocation of the hip. A decision analysis assessment. J Bone Joint Surg 1994;76B:539–543.

24. Rosendahl K, Markestad T, Lie RT. Ultrasound screening for developmental dysplasia of the hip in the neonate: the effect on treatment rate and prevalence of late cases. Pediatrics 1994; 94:47–52.

25. Clarke NM, Clegg J, Al-Chalabi AN. Ultrasound screening of hips at risk for CDH. Failure to reduce the incidence of late cases. J Bone Joint Surg 1989;71B:9–12.

26. Walter RS, Donaldson JS, Davis CL, et al. Ultrasound screening of high-risk infants. A method to increase early detection of congenital dysplasia of the hip. Am J Dis Child 1992;146:230–234.

27. Hangen DH, Kasser JR, Emans JB, Millis MB. The Pavlik harness and development dysplasia of the hip: has ultrasound changed treatment patterns? J Pediatr Orthop 1995;15:729–735.

28. Atar D, Lehman WB, Grant AD. Pavlik harness pathology. J Pediatr Orthop 1993;2:75–77.

29. Jones GT, Schoenecker PL, Dias LS. Developmental hip dysplasia potentiated by inappropriate use of the Pavlik harness. J Pediatr Orthop 1992;12:722–726.

30. Ramsey PL, Lasser S, MacEwen GD. Congenital dislocation of the hip. Use of the Pavlik harness in the child during the first six months of life. J Bone Joint Surg 1976;58A:1000–1004.

31. Mubarak S, Garfin S, Vance R, et al. Pitfalls in the use of the Pavlik harness for treatment of congenital dysplasia, subluxation, and dislocation of the hip. J Bone Joint Surg 1981;63A:1239–1248.

32. Tucci JJ, Kumar SJ, Guille JT, Rubbo ER. Late acetabular dysplasia following early successful Pavlik harness treatment of congenital dislocation of the hip. J Pediatr Orthop 1991;11:502–505.

33. Schoenecker PL, Dollard PA, Sheridan JJ, Strecker WB. Closed reduction of developmental dislocation of the hip in children older than 18 months. J Pediatr Orthop 1995;15:763–767.

34. Zionts LE, MacEwen GD. Treatment of congenital dislocation of the hip in children between the ages of one and three years. J Bone Joint Surg 1986;68A:829–846.

35. Kahle WK, Anderson MB, Alpert J, et al. The value of preliminary traction in the treatment of congenital dislocation of the hip. J Bone Joint Surg 1990;72A:1043–1047.

36. Quinn RH, Renshaw TS, DeLuca PA. Preliminary traction in the treatment of developmental dislocation of the hip. J Pediatr Orthop 1994;14:636–642.

37. Fish DN, Herzenberg JE, Hensinger RN. Current practice in use of prereduction traction for congenital dislocation of the hip. J Pediatr Orthop 1991;11:149–153.

38. Buchanan JR, Greer RB III, Cotler JM. Management strategy for prevention of avascular necrosis during treatment of congenital dislocation of the hip. J Bone Joint Surg 1981;63A:140–146.

39. Gage JR, Winter RB. Avascular necrosis of the capital femoral epiphysis as a complication of closed reduction of congenital dislocation of the hip. J Bone Joint Surg 1972;54A:373–388.

40. Morel G. The treatment of congenital dislocation and subluxation of the hip in the older child. Acta Orthop Scand 1975;46:364–399.

41. Weiner DS, Hoyt WA Jr, Odell HW. Congenital dislocation of the hip. The relationship of premanipulation traction and age to avascular necrosis of the femoral head. J Bone Joint Surg 1977;59A:306–311.

42. Camp J, Herring JA, Dworezynski C. Comparison of inpatient and outpatient traction in developmental dislocation of the hip. J Pediatr Orthop 1994;14:9–12.

43. Joseph K, MacEwen GD, Boos ML. Home traction in the management of congenital dislocation of the hip. Clin Orthop 1982; 165:83–90.

44. Mubarak SJ, Beck LR, Sutherland D. Home traction in the management of congenital dislocation of the hips. J Pediatr Orthop 1986;6:721–723.

45. Race C, Herring JA. Congenital dislocation of the hip: an evaluation of closed reduction. J Pediatr Orthop 1983;3:166.

46. Salter RB, Kostiuk J, Dallas S. Avascular necrosis of the femoral head as a complication of treatment for congenital dislocation of the hip in young children: a clinical and experimental investigation. Can J Surg 1969;12:44–61.

47. Stanton RP, Capecci R. Computer tomography for early evaluation of developmental dysplasia of the hip. J Pediatr Orthop 1974; 12:727–730.

48. Salter RB, Dubos JP. The first fifteen years' personal experience with innominate osteotomy in the treatment of congenital dislocation and subluxation of the hip. Clin Orthop 1992;12:72–103.

49. Ferguson AB Jr. Primary open reduction of congenital dislocation of the hip using a median adductor approach. J Bone Joint Surg 1973;55A:671–689.

50. Ludloff K. The open reduction of the congenital hip dislocation by an anterior incision. Am J Orthop Surg 1913;10:438–454.

51. Weinstein SL, Ponseti IV. Congenital dislocation of the hip. Open reduction through a medial approach. J Bone Joint Surg 1979; 61A:119–124.

52. Mankey MG, Arntz CT, Staheli LT. Open reduction through a medial approach for congenital dislocation of the hip. A critical review of the Ludloff approach in sixty-six hips. J Bone Joint Surg 1993;75A:1334–1345.

53. Fisher EHI, Beck PA, Hoffer MM. Necrosis of the capital femoral epiphysis and medial approaches to the hip in piglets. J Orthop Res 1991;9:203–208.

54. Brougham DI, Broughton NS, Cole WG, Menelaus MB. Avascular necrosis following closed reduction of congenital dislocation of the hip. Review of influencing factors and long-term follow-up. J Bone Joint Surg 1990;72B:557–562.

55. Cherney DL, Westin GW. Acetabular development in the infant's dislocated hips. Clin Orthop 1989;242:98–103.

56. Harris NH. Acetabular growth potential in congenital dislocation of the hip and some factors upon which it may depend. Clin Orthop 1976;119:99–106.

57. Lindstrom JR, Ponseti IV, Wenger DR. Acetabular development after reduction in congenital dislocation of the hip. J Bone Joint Surg 1979;61A:112–118.

58. Schoenecker PL, Strecker WB. Congenital dislocation of the hip in children. Comparison of the effects of femoral shortening and of skeletal traction in treatment. J Bone Joint Surg 1984;66A:21–27.

59. Galpin RD, Roach JW, Wenger DR, et al. One-stage treatment of congenital dislocation of the hip in older children, including femoral shortening. J Bone Joint Surg 1989;71A:734–741.

60. Gulman B, Tuncay IC, Dabak N, Karaismailoglu N. Salter's innominate osteotomy in the treatment of congenital hip dislocation: a long-term review. J Pediatr Orthop 1994;14:662–666.

61. Haidar RK, Jones RS, Vergroesen DA, Evans GA. Simultaneous open reduction and Salter innominate osteotomy for developmental dysplasia of the hip. J Bone Joint Surg 1996;78B:471–476.

62. Bos CF, Slooff TJ. Treatment of failed open reduction for congenital dislocation of the hip. A 10-year follow-up of 14 patients. Acta Orthop Scand 1984;55;531–535.

63. Kershaw CJ, Ware HE, Pattinson R, Fixsen JA. Revision of failed open reduction of congenital dislocation of the hip. J Bone Joint Surg 1993;75B;744–749.

64. Weinstein SL. Natural history of congenital hip dislocation [CDH] and hip dysplasia. Clin Orthop 1987;225:62–76.

65. Cooperman DR, Wallensten R, Stulberg SD. Acetabular dysplasia in the adult. Clin Orthop 1983;175:79–85.

66. Malvitz TA, Weinstein SL. Closed reduction for congenital dysplasia of the hip. Functional and radiographic results after an average of thirty years. J Bone Joint Surg 1994;76A:1777–1792.

67. Weinstein SL. Congenital hip dislocation. Long-range problems, residual signs, and symptoms after successful treatment. Clin Orthop 1992;281:69–74.

68. Blockey NJ. Derotation osteotomy in the management of congenital dislocation of the hip. J Bone Joint Surg 1984;66B:485–490.

69. Kasser JR, Bowen JR, MacEwen GD. Varus derotation osteotomy in the treatment of persistent dysplasia in congenital dislocation of the hip. J Bone Joint Surg 1985;67A:195–202.

70. Schoenecker PL, Anderson DJ, Capelli AM. The acetabular response to proximal femoral varus rotational osteotomy. Results after failure of post-reduction abduction splinting in patients who had congenital dislocation of the hip. J Bone Joint Surg 1995; 77:990–997.

71. Sutherland DH, Moore M. Clinical and radiographic outcome of patients treated with double innominate osteotomy for congenital hip dysplasia. J Pediatr Orthop 1991;11:143–148.

72. Steel HH. Triple osteotomy of the innominate bone. Clin Orthop 1977;122:116–127.

73. Eppright RH. Dial osteotomy of the acetabulum in the treatment of dysplasia of the hip. J Bone Joint Surg 1976;58A:726.

74. Ganz R, Vinh TS, Mast JW. A new periacetabular osteotomy for the treatment of hip dysplasias. Technique and preliminary results. Clin Orthop 1988;232:26–36.

75. Pemberton PA. Pericapsular osteotomy of the ilium for treatment of congenital subluxation and dislocation of the hip. J Bone Joint Surg 1965;47A:65–86.

76. Reichel H, Hein W. Dega acetabuloplasty combined with intertrochanteric osteotomies. Clin Orthop 1996;323:234–242.

77. Faciszewski T, Kiefer GN, Coleman SS. Pemberton osteotomy for residual acetabular dysplasia in children who have congenital dislocation of the hip. J Bone Joint Surg 1993;75A:643–649.

78. Bucholz RW, Ogden JA. Patterns of ischemic necrosis of the proximal femur in nonoperatively treated congenital hip disease. In: Proceedings of the sixth open scientific meeting of the Hip Society. St. Louis: Mosby, 1978:43–63.

79. Kalamchi A, MacEwen GD. Avascular necrosis following treatment of congenital dislocation of the hip. J Bone Joint Surg 1980; 62A:876–888.

80. O'Brien T. Growth-disturbance lines in congenital dislocation of the hip. J Bone Joint Surg 1985;67A:626–632.

81. Cooperman DR, Wallensten R, Stulberg SD. Post-reduction avascular necrosis in congenital dislocation of the hip. J Bone Joint Surg 1980;62A:247–258.

82. Iwerson LJ, Kalea V, Eberle C. Relative trochanteric overgrowth after ischemic necrosis in congenital dislocation of the hip. J Pediatr Orthop 1989;9:381–385.

83. Lloyd-Roberts GC, Wetherrill MH, Fraser M. Trochanteric advancement for premature arrest of the femoral capital growth plate. J Bone Joint Surg 1985;67B:21–24.

84. MacNicol MF, Makris D. Distal transfer of the greater trochanter. J Bone Joint Surg 1991;73B:838–841.

chapter 92

John F. Sarwark and Jeroen G. V. Neyt

Legg-Calvé-Perthes Disease

Legg-Calvé-Perthes disease is a common acquired condition of the hip. It occurs in children aged 4 to 9 years and is predominantly seen in boys. In children under 6 years, it is largely asymptomatic or silent and requires expectant observation. In children over 6 years, more interventions, including physical therapy, splinting and bracing, and surgery, can be expected.

RELEVANT ANATOMY AND PATHOGENESIS

Legg-Calvé-Perthes (LCP) disease is the least understood of pediatric hip disorders. Controversy continues about most of its aspects, including cause, pathogenesis, classification, management, natural history, and the degree and type of treatment. The condition is the result of femoral deformity caused by subchondral collapse after avascular necrosis of the femoral head in a growing child. The reason for the avascular necrosis is unknown. This pathologic condition is named after the American (Legg), French (Calvé) and German (Perthes) physicians who simultaneously and separately reported on it in 1910, distinguishing it from tuberculosis of the hip (1).

The cause of LCP is unknown, although many theories have been proposed, including infection, trauma, and previous transient synovitis of the hip. The current theory is that vascular embarrassment, caused by several factors, is the probable underlying pathomechanism. Histologically, abnormal areas in the epiphyseal cartilage, the physis, and the metaphyseal region have been found. Signs in the contralateral, unaffected, hip support the concept that LCP disease may be a localized manifestation of a general disorder of epiphyseal cartilage in the susceptible child (2). These changes, together with the unusual precarious blood supply of the proximal femur, make the femoral head vulnerable to the effects of epiphyseal disruption. The femoral head in LCP disease is plastic and responds to the influences of the acetabulum on remodeling.

INITIAL FINDINGS, PHYSICAL EXAMINATION, AND DIAGNOSIS

LCP disease occurs most commonly in children aged 4 to 8 years and is more common in boys than in girls by a ratio of 4:1 to 5:1. The incidence is about 15.6 per 100,000 population. It is bilateral in 10% of cases, and there is a delay before the second side is affected. Evidence suggests that LCP disease is not an inherited condition. It is more common in urban than in rural communities. Children with this disorder are often small for their age, wiry, and hyperactive, with a bone age that is delayed by 1 to 2 years. Growth hormone–related pathophysiology has been reported (3).

Children present with mild pain that is usually activity-related and is relieved by rest. Frequently, the child has recurring pain and a limp for several months before the parents seek medical help. When the pain is referred to the thigh or knee, the clinician may miss the diagnosis, further delaying treatment. About 1 in 5 patients may give a history of related trauma. Limited hip motion with decreased hip abduction and internal rotation is a classic physical finding. Unilateral muscular atrophy from disuse secondary to pain is further evidence of the long-standing nature of the condition before detection. Laboratory studies are generally not helpful for LCP disease, except to rule out other conditions. The disease should be differentiated, especially in the initial phase, from conditions such as septic arthritis, proximal femoral osteomyelitis, transient synovitis, multiple epiphyseal dysplasia, and hypothyroidism in bilateral cases (4).

RADIOLOGIC STUDIES

After the diagnosis of LCP disease is made, the condition is followed by plain radiographs taken in the AP and Lauenstein lateral positions. A comparative radiographic follow-up every 6 weeks to 3 months during the course of the disease is important. Additional imaging studies (CT,

MRI, bone scintigraphy, arthrography) may help assess the extent of involvement and femoral head coverage.

Classification

Radiographically, the disease can be classified into four stages: initial (initial weeks), fragmentation (6 to 12 months), reossification (1 to 2 years), and healed or remodeling (5 years) (5). In the earliest radiographic stage (Waldenstrom), only widening of the cartilage space and a small ossific nucleus of the femoral head are noted, presumably because of a lack of blood supply. Later, the ossific nucleus appears more dense (avascular) (Fig. 92.1). The 45° frog-leg lateral radiograph (flexed 45° and abducted 45°) view best demonstrates the pathognomonic crescent sign, or subchondral stress fracture. The extent of this zone is an early indication of the amount of head involvement. There is no easy way to be sure if the femoral head is collapsing or repairing.

In 1971, Catterall (6) classified LCP disease according to the percent of the femoral head that is avascular: grade I, 25%; grade II, 50%; grade III, 75%; and grade IV, 100% (6). If the process is thought of in the same way as myocardial infarction, a small infarction of the femoral head produces grade I disease, whereas a severe infarction results in grade IV disease. The more complete the head involvement, the greater the risk for permanent femoral head shape change, thus increasing the risk for adult arthritis. A simplified classification, also based on the extent of head involvement, was proposed by Salter and Thompson (7). They classified LCP disease into two groups: grade A, less than 50% femoral head involvement; grade B, more than 50% femoral head involvement.

The predictive value of each classification for the individual patient, however, is limited. Maintenance of 50% of

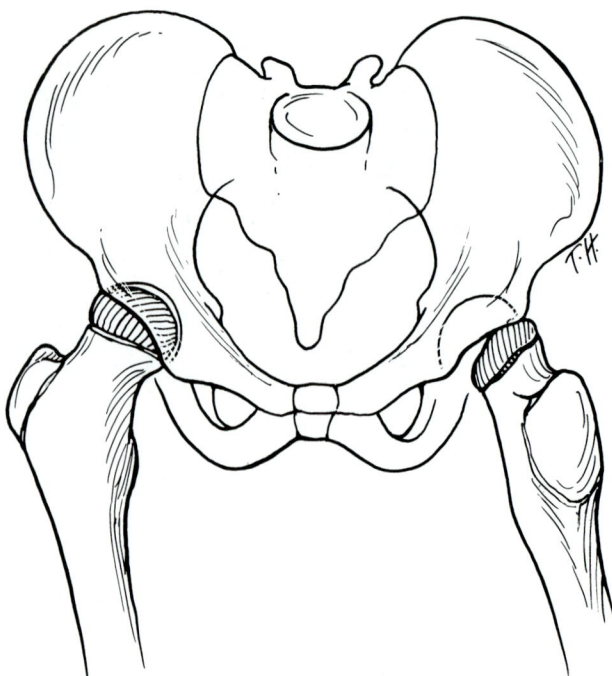

Figure 92.2. AP view showing left hip involvement. Note the fragmentation of the epiphysis.

the normal height of the lateral portion of the epiphysis (lateral pillar), regardless of the degree of involvement of the remainder of the epiphysis, has recently been suggested as an important favorable prognostic factor. The actual deformity that develops is profoundly influenced by the duration of the disease: coxa magna, coxa vara, and coxa valga resulting from partial growth arrest; irregular head formation; and osteochondritis dissecans (Fig. 92.2).

Legg-Calvé-Perthes disease cannot be compared to posttraumatic avascular necrosis of the hip in the young child. In the latter situation the femoral head usually heals rapidly without going through the prolonged stages of fragmentation and repair seen with LCP disease.

TREATMENT

Nonoperative Treatment and Indications for Surgery

Age at involvement is the most significant factor related to outcome. Children under 5 years often do well without specific treatment. But 8 years of age seems to be the watershed, and children over age 10 years often have poor clinical and radiographic results with or without treatment. Females affected by LCP disease have a poorer prognosis than do males.

The more immature the patient when he or she enters the reossification stage, the greater the potential for remodeling of the femoral head and acetabulum. Anatomic incongruency of this ball-and-socket joint is a major factor

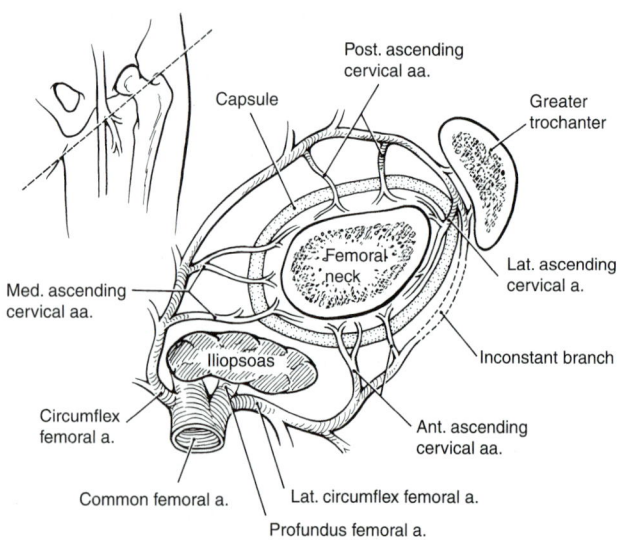

Figure 92.1. Vascular anatomy of the pediatric hip. Adapted from Chung SMK. The arterial supply of the developing proximal end of the human femur. J Bone Joint Surg 1976;58A:961.

contributing to the quality of the results and to whether early degenerative osteoarthritis will occur. Once the head is in the reossification stage, it will not deform further. Treatment must be instituted early in the course of the disease if the child demonstrates clinical (restricted range of motion, joint contracture, and pain) or radiographic at risk signs. Severe loss of hip motion is also an important guide to outcome, both at diagnosis and throughout treatment.

The treatment goal is to maintain hip range of motion and the sphericity of a well-covered, contained head through the healing of the biologically plastic epiphysis, subjecting it to the molding action of the acetabulum (8). This may be achieved by an abduction device, which contains the at risk femoral head within the acetabulum, by a brief period of traction, or by surgical release of the contracted adductors. Arthrography under general anesthesia can demonstrate articular morphology.

Serious damage to the femoral head and acetabulum may result from trying to contain a noncontainable head. The successful treatment with broomstick abduction long leg plaster casts (Petrie casts) has been abandoned for practical reasons. Petrie casts maintain the improved motion that is gained after muscular releases or traction. These casts (two long leg casts with broomsticks between them to maintain abduction) are remarkably effective. Their weight alone provides a ballast, which the irritated hip is unable to resist, resulting in abduction and containment. Removable abduction orthoses were popular at the end of the 1970s. Orthoses that allow weight bearing include the Craig splint, Toronto brace, and Atlanta brace.

The Atlanta-Scottish Rite brace is currently the most popular, since children find it more acceptable; bracing averages 6 to 18 months (Fig. 92.3). This orthosis should not be used for severely involved hips. The initiation of bracing and surgical intervention when the hip is irritable

and stiff should be delayed. Management should be tailored to the child's situation.

There is no certain medical indication for surgical containment, because even difficult hips can be contained by a combination of releases, Petrie casts, and braces. There are, however, sociologic and psychologic considerations for surgical containment (patient's compliance, living situation, and age). The distinct advantage of surgical containment is its permanence. Several procedures to achieve this goal are known.

Operative Treatment

An adductor muscular release via the medial approach improves hip abduction. An optional intramuscular psoas tendon release via an anterior approach, just below the inguinal ligament and just lateral to the femoral nerve, improves extension and internal rotation (Clinical Table).

Varus femoral osteotomy, with or without derotation, via the lateral approach repositions the vulnerable femoral head away from deforming influences of the acetabular edge. The procedure usually requires the use of internal fixation and external immobilization in plaster for 6 weeks. The limb is temporarily shortened by the procedure. The varus angle must not exceed a neck-shaft angle of less than 100°.

Innominate pelvic osteotomy achieves containment by redirection of the acetabulum, providing good coverage for the femoral head. The osteotomy is fixed by two or three threaded pins for internal fixation and requires immobilization in a spica cast for 6 weeks in an uncooperative patient. Care must be taken not to damage the lateral femoral cutaneous nerve.

A shelf arthroplasty increases acetabular coverage of the extruded portion of the femoral head. A bony shelf taken from the pelvis is positioned in a wedge-like fashion over the anterolateral capsule of the hip joint. Fibrocartilage develops as the interface layer. The same precautions as in innominate pelvic osteotomy need to be taken.

Treatment options in the noncontainable hip and the late-presenting case are restricted to salvage procedures, such as Chiari arthroplasty, cheilectomy (excision of the extruded portion of the head), femoral abduction extension osteotomy, and arthrodesis.

REHABILITATION

There are no true natural history studies for Legg-Calvé-Perthes disease. Long-term follow-up studies demonstrate that 80% of patients with this condition are active and pain free 20 to 40 years after the onset of symptoms. But beyond 40 years, ambulating function is markedly reduced. Most people in their sixth decade develop significant degenerative joint disease. Coxa magna and coxa plana may result in a loss of joint congruity, which of itself after vigorous activity may cause episodic discomfort in the hip earlier in life.

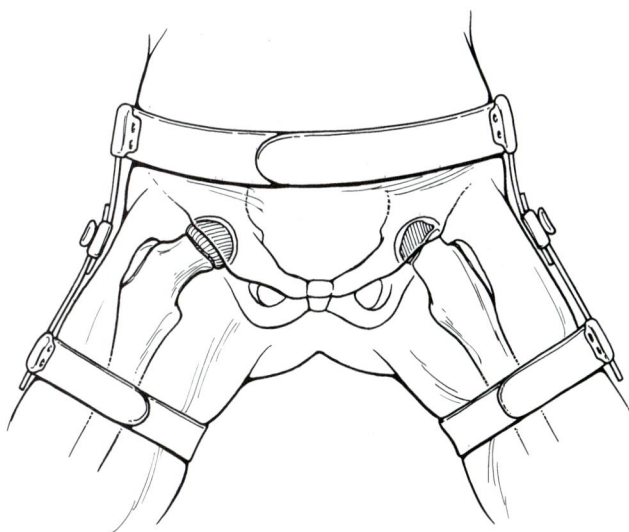

Figure 92.3. Bracing for abduction positioning.

Clinical Table: Legg-Calvé-Perthes Disease

Procedure	Indications	Technique	Anatomy	Pitfalls
Adductor muscle release	• Limited hip abduction, not responsive to PT, or prior to pelvic or femoral osteotomy	• Medial approach	• Adductor origin at pubis, proximal medial thigh	• Incomplete release; injury to the anterior branch, obturator nerve
Intramuscular psoas tendon release	• As part of the pelvic osteotomy	• Anterior approach	• Iliacus and psoas join to form a common tendon as they pass the pubis	• Neurovascular injury to femoral neurovascular bundle
Varus femoral osteotomy	• Severe involvement or moderate involvement (age > 6 years) of hips or Salter-Thompson B or Catterall III and IV hips	• Lateral approach • Internal fixation, external immobilization	• Femur at proximal third level	• Incomplete correction, delayed union, nonunion, postoperative limping after union
Innominate pelvic osteotomy	• Severe involvement or moderate involvement (age > 6 years) of hips or Salter-Thompson B or Catterall III and IV hips	• Acetabulum redirection • Internal fixation, external immobilization	• Lateral femoral cutaneous nerve at subfascial level distal to ASIS	• Injury with anesthesia or dysesthesia to lateral femoral cutaneous nerve; incomplete correction, loss of correction, delayed union, nonunion
Shelf arthroplasty	• To increase femoral head coverage without subluxation	• Application of cortico-cancellous graft into peri-capsular acetabular margin	• Hip capsule, interior-superior-posterior margin distal of acetabulum	• (Repeat all of above in innominate)
Chiari arthroplasty	• Late-presenting case, or residual extrusion or subluxation	• Osteotomy placed at capsular insertion level just distal to the reflected head of the rectus femoris	• Hip capsule, sciatic notch, anterior, inferior iliac spine	• Salvage procedure (repeat all of above in innominate)
Chielectomy	• Late-presenting case, rarely performed; severe hinged abduction	• Anterior approach; arthrotomy and excision	• Anterior approach, capsule	• Salvage procedure; severe hip stiffness
Femoral abduction; extension osteotomy	• Late-presenting case; severe hinged abduction	• Proximal femoral osteotomy with proximal fragment in adduction	• Proximal third of femur	• Salvage procedure; worsening hip pain
Arthrodesis	• Late-presenting case	• Anterior approach may include osteotomy at subtrochanter level; may involve internal fixation or external fixation; lateral approach to proximal femur	• Proximal third of femur, hip capsule	• Salvage procedure; delayed union, nonunion, later obstacle to later reconstructed THA

PT, physical therapy; *ASIS*, anterior superior iliac spine; *THA*, total hip arthroplasty.

SUMMARY

Legg-Calvé-Perthes disease is a common osteochondrosis affecting the hip. When femoral head deformity is significant and when subluxation occurs, intervention is required, often including surgery to improve containment of the femoral head in the acetabulum.

REFERENCES

1. Herring JA. Legg-Calvé-Perthes disease: a review of current knowledge. Instr Course Lect 1989;38:309–315.
2. Morrissy RT, ed. Lovell and Winter's pediatric orthopaedics. 3rd ed. Philadelphia: Lippincott, 1990:851–883.
3. Tachdjian MS. Pediatric orthopedics. Vol. 2. Philadelphia: Saunders, 1990:933–988.
4. Staheli LT. Fundamentals of pediatric orthopedics. New York: Raven, 1992:7.14–7.16.
5. Bucholz RW, Lippert FG III, Wenger DR, Ezaki M. Orthopaedic decision making. Philadelphia: BC Decker, 1984:192–193.
6. Catterall A. The natural history of Perthes' disease. J Bone Joint Surg 1971;53B:37–53.
7. Salter RB, Thompson GH. Legg-Calvé-Perthes disease: the prognostic significance of the subchondral fracture and a two-group classification of the femoral head involvement. J Bone Joint Surg 1984;66A:479–489.
8. Wenger DR, Rang M. The art and practice of children's orthopedics. New York: Raven, 1993:297–330.

Slipped Capital Femoral Epiphysis

Slipped capital femoral epiphysis (SCFE) was first described by Ambroise Pare in 1572, who confused this condition with dislocation of the hip. In 1888, Muller (1) called this condition "bending of the femoral neck in adolescence." The term *slipped capital femoral epiphysis* is a misnomer. The femoral epiphysis, or head, does not vary its normal anatomic relationship with the acetabulum (Fig. 93.1). The disorder most commonly consists of an anterior and lateral movement of the femoral neck in relation to the proximal femoral epiphysis, secondary to changes in the zone of provisional calcification of the proximal femoral physis (Fig. 93.2).

The incidence of slipped capital femoral epiphysis is between 1 and 3 per 100,000. Kelsey et al. (2) demonstrated a geographical component: SCFE occurs about 5 times more frequently in Connecticut than in New Mexico. Males are more frequently affected than females. Black adolescents are at greater risk than Caucasian or Hispanic teenagers. The age of onset coincides with periods of rapid growth. The age at onset for males is between 10 and 16 years, with a peak incidence at 12 to 14 years; in females, the age at onset is between 8 to 14 years, with a peak incidence at 11 to 12 years.

Obesity and delayed skeletal maturation are commonly seen in association with SCFE. The younger the age at presentation, the greater the chance of systemic abnormalities.

RELEVANT ANATOMY AND PATHOGENESIS

The specific cause of SCFE remains unknown but appears to be multifactorial. Proposed mechanisms include mechanical, endocrine, metabolic, traumatic, and inflammatory (3,4).

The femoral head is attached to the femoral neck via the growth plate. The anatomic stability of this region depends on the perichondrium, perichondrial ring, transphyseal collagen, height of the hypertrophic zone, mamillary processes, and angle of inclination of the growth plate. Any process that weakens this structural complex may allow the shear stresses of normal weight bearing to disrupt the anatomic integrity, resulting in a slipped capital femoral epiphysis.

The perichondrial ring is a peripheral fibrous band composed of collagen fibers that span the growth plate and provides resistance to shear stress. During adolescence, this structure normally decreases in thickness, providing less mechanical stability. Transphyseal collagen fibers also provide a counter to shear stress. In lathyrism, the collagen cross-linking is decreased, resulting in decreased tensile strength and less resistance to shear stress.

The growth plate has distinctive zones. The hypertrophic zone is characterized by a decreased proportion of intercellular matrix around the cell compared to other zones. Since the intercellular matrix contains the collagen, which is the main structural support, the hypertrophic zone represents the weak link in the growth plate and is the predominant area through which the disruption occurs in SCFE.

Processes that increase the height of the hypertrophic zone adversely affect resistance to shear stress. Growth hormone, directly or through somatomedin, stimulates cartilage metabolism, resulting in an increase in the height of the hypertrophic zone. Estrogens and androgens suppress the proliferation of cartilage, decreasing the height of the hypertrophic zone. One study demonstrated that ovariectomy in rats weakened the strength of the growth plate compared to the strengthening that accompanied orchiectomy (4).

Further support for an endocrine cause was provided by Wilcox et al. (5). They reported decreased testosterone, growth hormone, and thyroid levels in patients with SCFE,

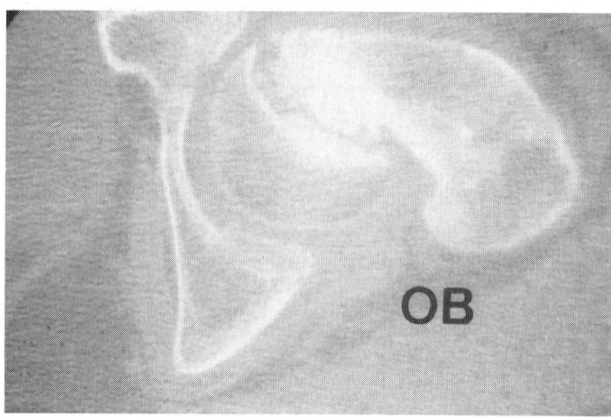

Figure 93.1. CT study showing SCFE.

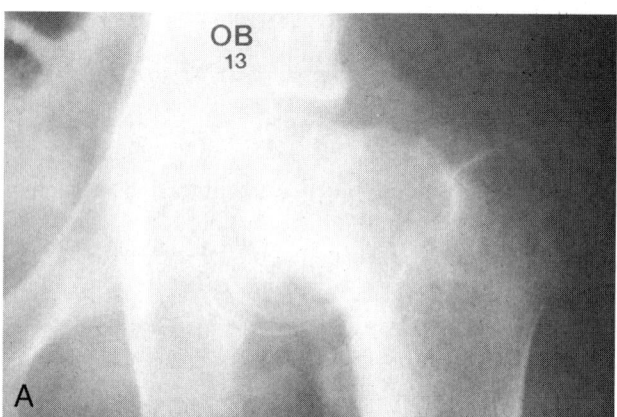

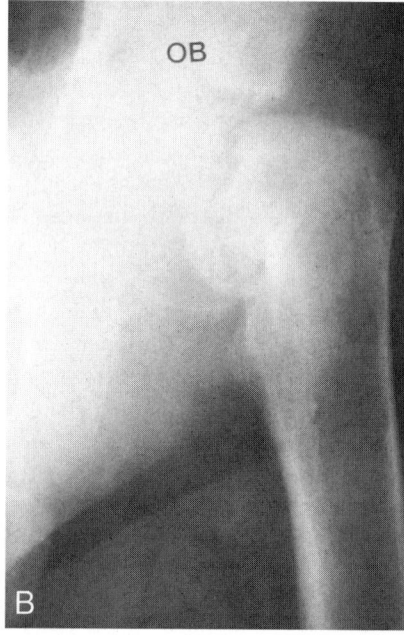

Figure 93.2. AP (**A**) and lateral (**B**) views of the same patient shown in Figure 93.1.

which demonstrates the multifactorial nature of endocrine abnormalities found with this condition. Therefore, a relative imbalance in the growth hormone–sex hormone relationship may account for SCFE, though no specific abnormality has been documented.

Metabolic disorders, such as rickets and particularly renal osteodystrophy, are associated with an increased hypertrophic zone and may predispose patients to slipped capital femoral epiphysis (Fig. 93.3). Patients with renal osteodystrophy also frequently develop secondary hyperparathyroidism and may sustain pathologic fractures rather than a true slipped capital femoral epiphysis.

Thyroid hormone deficiency delays the closure of the growth plate and allows it to be subject to shear stress beyond the normal physiologic time limit. Treatment with thyroid hormone induces a rapid increase in cartilage growth of the growth plate, also increasing the risk of developing SCFE.

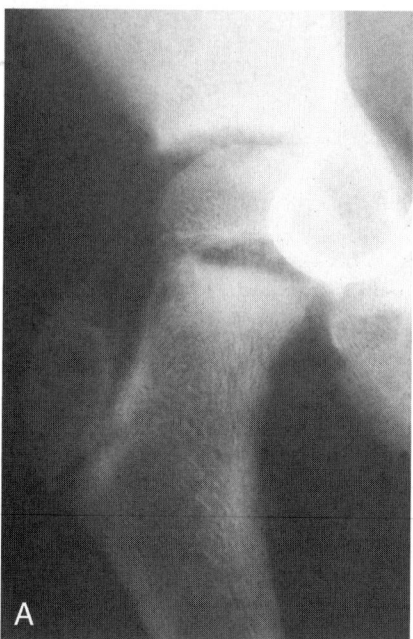

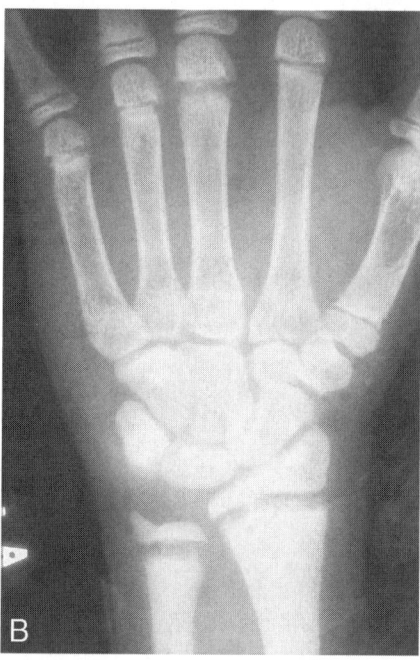

Figure 93.3. **A.** Lateral view of a patient with renal osteodystrophy, showing the increased height of the growth plate. **B.** AP view of the hand of the same patient.

Patients who have received radiotherapy that included the femoral head within its portal may be at increased risk for a slipped epiphysis. The irradiation causes an arrest of chondrogenesis and, when combined with actinomycin D, enhances the toxic effects on the growth plate cartilage structure.

The growth plate develops in a horizontal direction during childhood, and the angle of inclination increases to oblique during adolescence, creating a mechanical disadvantage. If this change in orientation is coupled with obesity, as is often the case in the SCFE patient population, the shear stress may overcome the normal anatomic integrity.

INITIAL FINDINGS, PHYSICAL EXAMINATION, AND DIAGNOSIS

The clinical manifestations of SCFE are determined by the duration of the pathologic process(es) and the severity of the displacement. The slipped capital femoral epiphysis can be classified as chronic (more than 3 weeks), acute on chronic, and acute (less than 3 weeks). For patients with a chronic slip, the most common presenting complaint is a limp associated with pain in the groin or pain referred to the anteromedial aspect of the distal thigh or knee. Any skeletally immature patient presenting with knee pain must have SCFE included in the differential diagnosis. The pain is characterized as an ache, which is exacerbated by activity and is present for weeks or months. The patient walks with an antalgic gait, and the affected limb is externally rotated. It may be shortened as well, producing an abductor lurch.

The most notable clinical findings are decreased hip abduction, internal rotation, and some loss of flexion. Passive flexion of the hip results in abduction and external rotation of the thigh. The more severe the slip, the greater the physical limitations.

Patients with an acute on chronic slip present with a history similar to that of patients with a chronic slip; but the former develop a sudden exacerbation, noting the onset of severe pain and an inability to bear weight as the result of relatively minor trauma. The least common presentation is the patient with an acute slip who experiences only the sudden onset of severe pain and difficulty or inability to bear weight in association with minor trauma.

RADIOLOGIC STUDIES

Radiographic assessment of patients with SCFE must include AP and lateral views of both hips. The earliest finding is a widened and irregular growth plate with a normal femoral head–neck geographic relationship (Fig. 93.4). Other signs on the AP view include a decreased portion of the femoral epiphysis intersected by the superior neck line, decreased epiphyseal height, and the metaphyseal blanch sign of Steel. It is also imperative to assess the joint space (Fig. 93.5). Joint-space narrowing indicative of chondrolysis can be seen on presentation and significantly alters the prognosis. The lateral radiograph is the most sen-

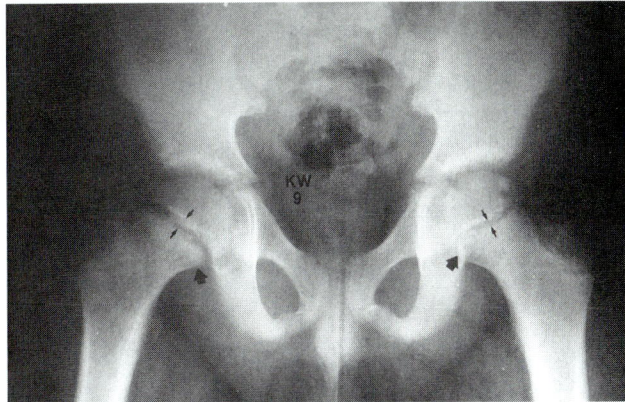

Figure 93.4. AP view showing an increased height of the growth plate but no displacement.

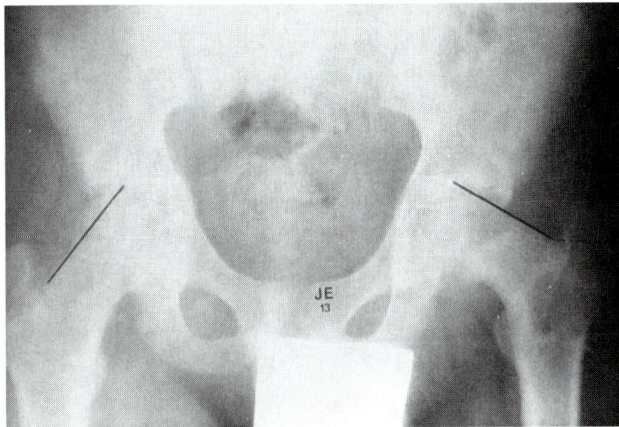

Figure 93.5. AP view showing the Kline lines drawn along the superior neck. The right side is normal.

sitive view for detecting small degrees of displacement (Fig. 93.6).

Massive slips are easily recognized on both views (Fig. 93.7). Both views should be evaluated for signs of a remodeling response indicative of chronicity. The magnitude of displacement is another means of classifying slipped capital femoral epiphysis (Table 93.1).

TREATMENT

Operative Treatment

The most important aspect of treatment is early diagnosis and immediate cessation of weight-bearing activity to prevent further displacement. The patient should be admitted to the hospital for traction to relieve the muscle spasm and associated synovitis. The initial step is surgical stabilization, the main objective of which is closure (fusion) of the growth plate, which eliminates the weak link. A major area of controversy is whether a reduction should be performed, because there have been reports associating reduction with an increased incidence of avascular necro-

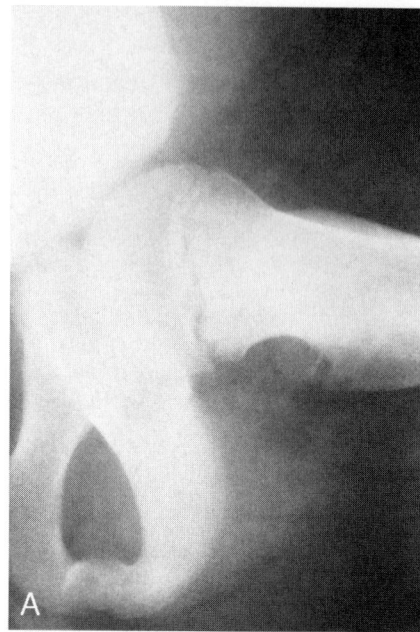

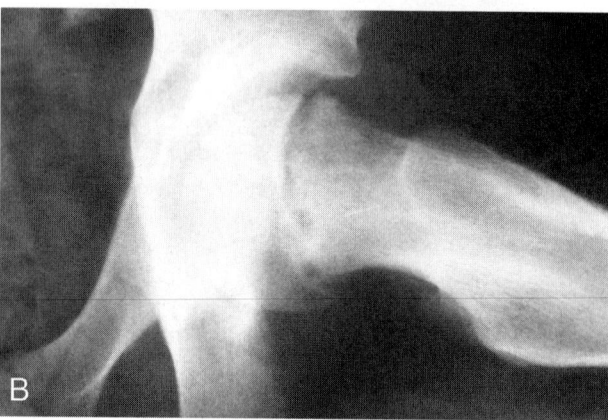

Figure 93.6. Lateral views showing a normal hip (**A**) and one with minimal displacement (**B**).

sis (AVN) (6). Reduction can be performed preoperatively through the use of traction and a medial rotation strap or intraoperatively with various maneuvers. The consensus is to avoid reductions in chronic cases and to consider an extremely gentle reduction only for the acute component if the severity of displacement warrants it.

The two methods currently favored for stabilization are fixation in situ and epiphysiodesis (Clinical Table). Open reduction and internal fixation (ORIF) and cuneiform osteotomy have resulted in unacceptable rates of avascular necrosis and should be avoided (7,8). Fixation in situ that uses a cannulated screw is the most commonly employed technique (Fig. 93.8) because of its ability to rapidly stabilize the epiphysis and avoid hip spica cast immobilization. The problems with this technique are improper device placement (which does not afford sufficient stability), unrealized and thus persistent perforation of the articular cartilage, an excessive number of devices (which increases the risk of vascular disruption, leading to AVN), and an im-

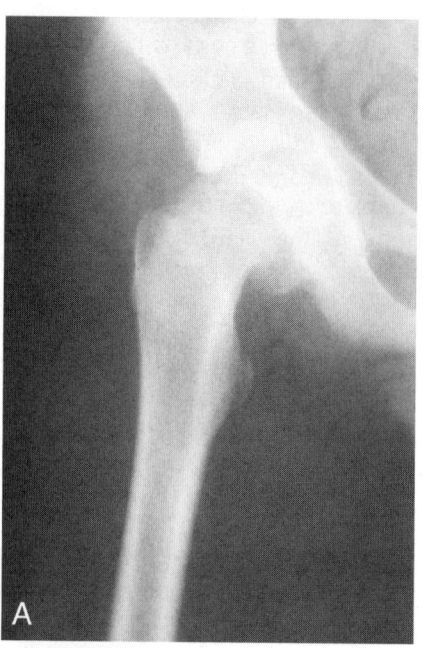

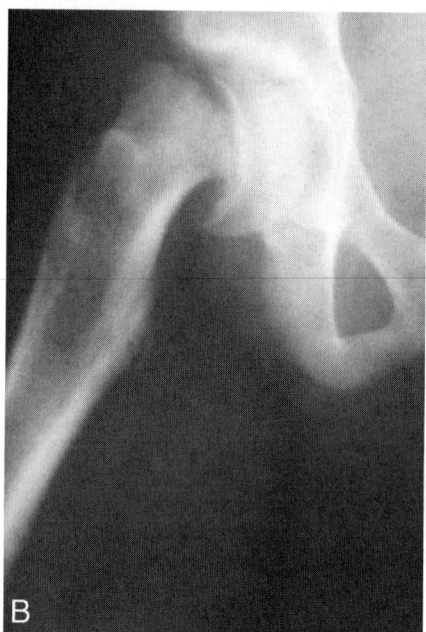

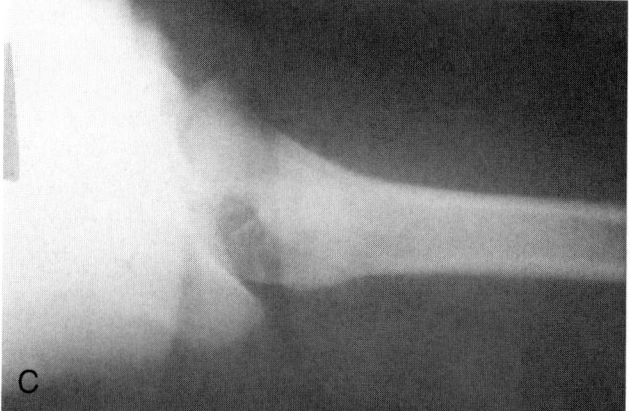

Figure 93.7. AP (**A** and **B**) and lateral (**C**) views showing severe SCFE.

proper insertion site (which increases the risk of proximal femur fractures) (9) (Figs. 93.9 to 93.11).

The results of fixation in situ have improved with advances in fluoroscopy, which have increased the surgeon's ability to delineate the abnormal anatomy, and with advances in our understanding of the geometry of the grossly distorted anatomy (10). In addition, better metallurgy and technology (cannulated screws) has allowed fixation in chronic patients to be achieved with the use of a single device, further decreasing the risk of iatrogenic complications (11).

TECHNIQUE

The patient is secured to a fracture table. The AP and true lateral fluoroscopic views are carefully assessed for the extent of the displacement. which may not be fully appreciated on the frog-leg lateral view. The ideal position for maximum fixation is perpendicular to the physis and within the central portion of the femoral epiphysis (head)

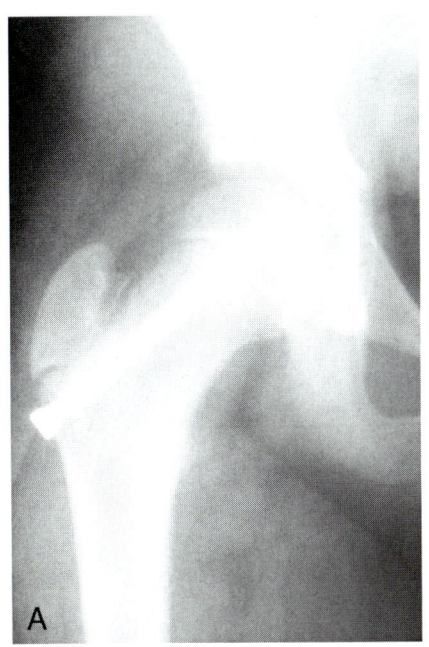

A

table	93.1	Classification of Slipped Capital Femoral Epiphysis

Degree of Slip	Grade	Displacement
Preslip	I	Physeal widening
Minimal	II	Less than one-third neck width
Moderate	III	Between one-third and one-half neck width
Severe	IV	More than one-half neck width

Figure 93.8. AP (**A**) and lateral (**B**) views of fixation with a single cannulated screw.

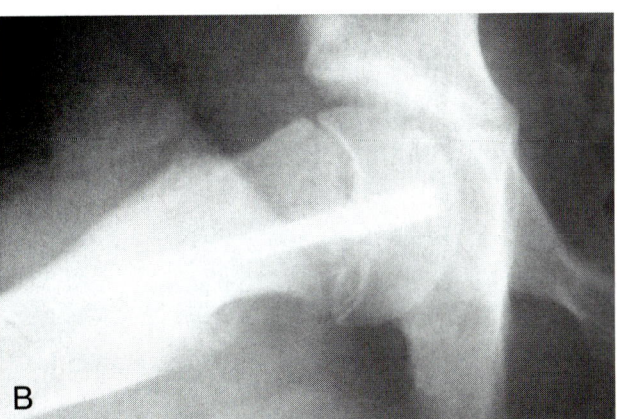

B

Clinical Table: Slipped Capital Femoral Epiphysis (SCFE)

Procedure	Indications	Technique	Anatomy	Pitfalls
Fixation in situ	• Acute SCFE	• Fracture table • Fluoroscopy • Cannulated screw • Perpendicular tibial physis • Central portion head • Two points of fixation if possible	• Anterior and lateral hip musclature • Femoral head • Femoral head • Greater trochanter	• Loss of guidewire fixation • Poor stability • Loss of reduction • Fracture cortex through drill holes
Epiphysiodesis	• Acute slip	• Anterior approach • Anterolateral approach • Remove portion growth plate • Structural bone graft from iliac crest	• Anterolateral hip • Cartilage surface of hip • Neck of femur	• Absorption of bone graft • Poor protection postoperatively
Osteotomy	• Late SCFE • Residual deformity • Status after growth plate fusion	• Cuneiform osteotomy • Intertrochanteric osteotomy • Subtrochanteric osteotomy	• Depends on osteotomy approach	• Avascular necrosis • Chondrolysis • Overcorrection with deformity of hip

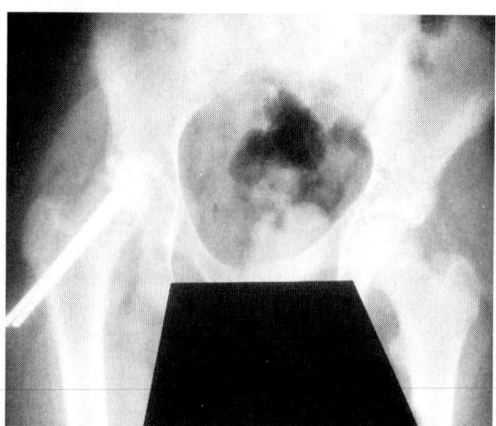

Figure 93.9. Interoperative view showing joint penetration.

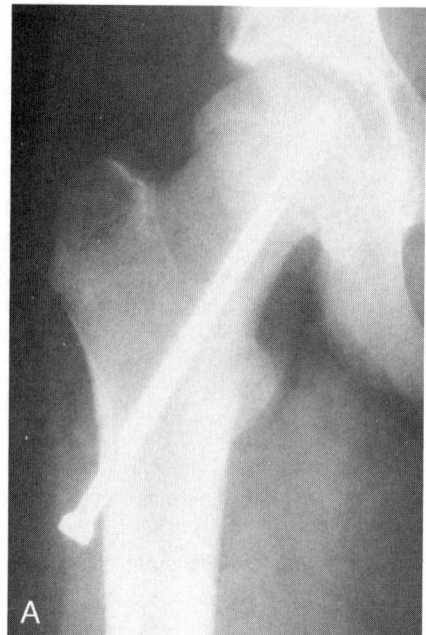

Figure 93.10. AP view showing avascular necrosis.

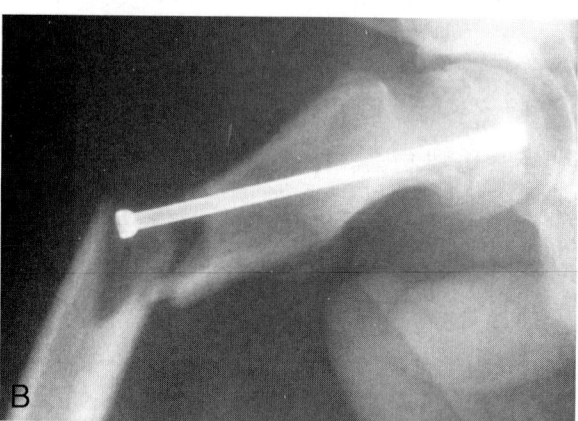

Figure 93.11. A. The screw's entry point below the lesser trochanter creates stress. **B.** Subtrochanteric fracture.

on both AP and lateral projections (12). The surgeon should avoid the superolateral portion of the head where the vascularity is at greatest risk and loss of fixation is highest; it is helpful to mentally project backward from the ideal end point of fixation to determine the correct entry point (13). The point of entry may be on the anterior portion of the femoral neck to accomplish this (Fig. 93.12). I prefer to insert a thin Kirschner wire to test the entry point before I insert the larger guidewires used with the cannulated screw set. Improvement in the displacement indicates instability, and a second point of fixation is advisable (Fig. 93.13).

Patients who have undergone screw fixation must restrict their activity level until growth plate closure occurs, which averages 6 to 12 months but is difficult to predict. The need to remove the fixation device is controversial; the benefits of renewal must outweigh the significant risks.

PITFALLS AND SUGGESTIONS

When there is difficulty in adequately visualizing the femoral head, especially on the lateral view in obese patients, I have found arthrography to be helpful.

Fixation entering from the lateral cortex should be proximal to the lesser trochanter. This lessens the risk of a

fracture developing in the subtrochanteric region (Fig. 93.11).

Overdrilling the threaded portion of the guidewire causes loss of guidewire fixation and should be avoided. Cannulated drills may bind the guidewire, causing it to advance along with the drill and lead to articular penetration. Careful fluoroscopic monitoring is essential for success. Injection of contrast material into the cannulated screw is useful to test for inadvertent and/or unrecognized articular penetration. Around-the-clock views help assess proper screw placement.

Surgeons disagree about the need to prophylactically pin the contralateral side. The incidence of bilaterality has been reported to be between 25 and 50%, either at the time of initial presentation or during the follow-up period. Prophylactic fixation is, therefore, unnecessary in 50 to 75% of cases. The risk must be discussed with the family, and the child should be examined if contralateral hip or knee pain develops.

EPIPHYSIODESIS

The advantages of epiphysiodesis are that it is done under direct visualization and the time to growth plate closure is shorter (14). Epiphysiodesis entails an anterior or anterolateral approach to the hip joint. A portion of the growth plate is removed, and stabilization is achieved with the insertion of structural bone graft, usually from the iliac crest. Absorption of the bone graft is possible, and spica cast immobilization may be required. Previous advocates of this procedure have recently reported their results and no longer recommend the technique (15).

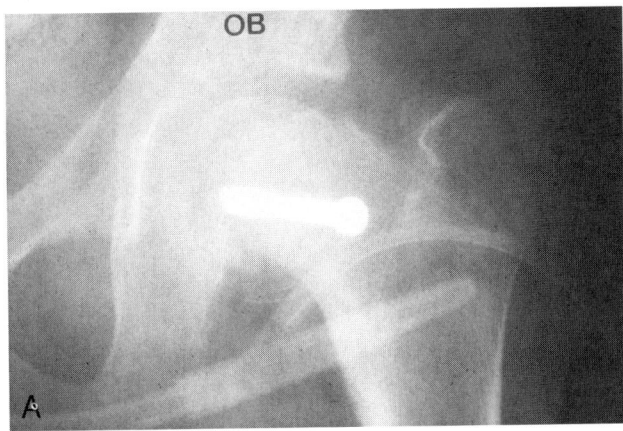
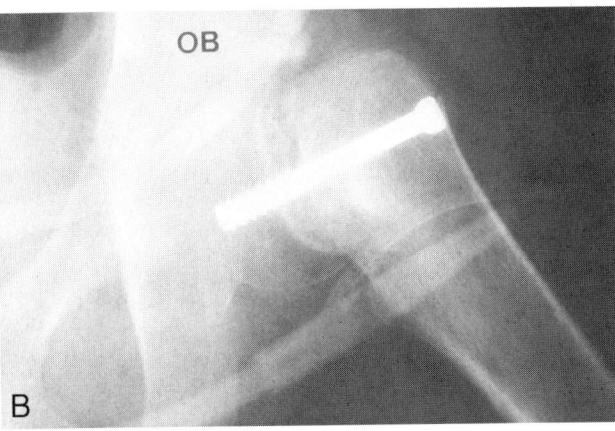

Figure 93.12. The anterior entry point for fixation in a patient with severe SCFE.

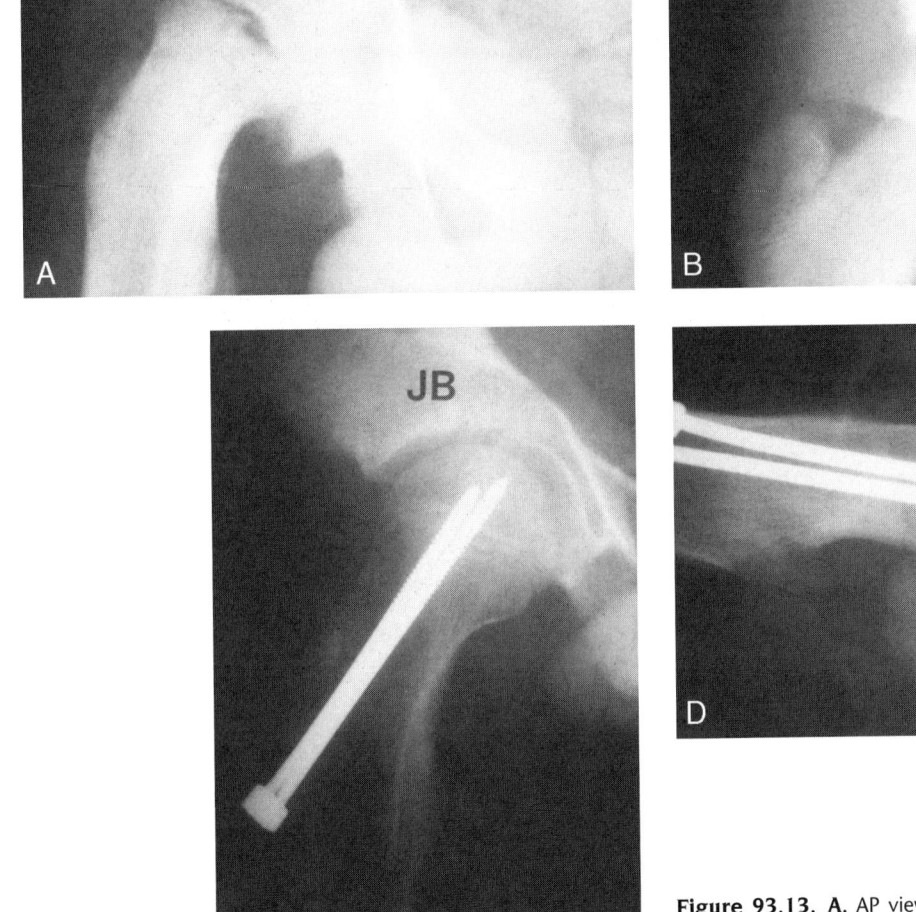
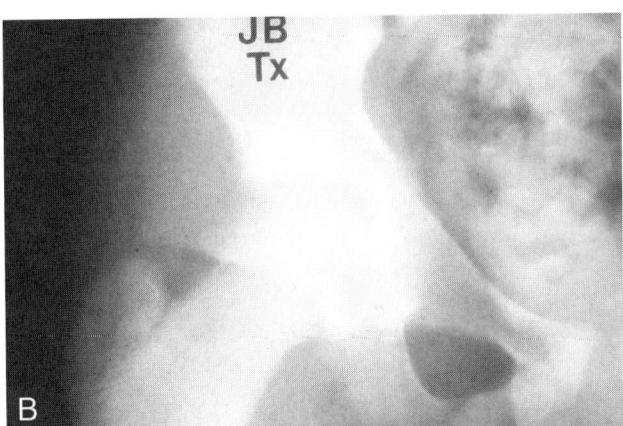
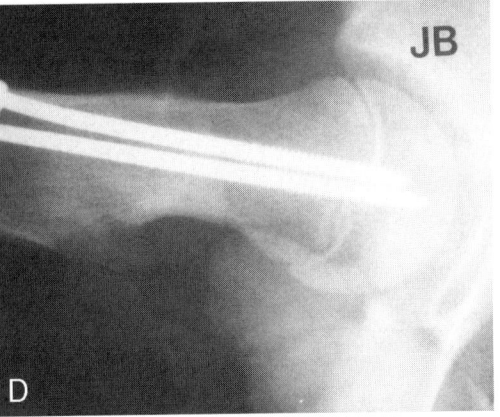

Figure 93.13. A. AP view showing acute SCFE. **B.** AP view after traction has been applied. Postoperative AP (**C**) and lateral (**D**) views showing two points of fixation.

OSTEOTOMY

Long-term studies of SCFE treated with fixation in situ have demonstrated reasonable functional results into the 50- to 60-year age group as a result of remodeling (6,16,17). For patients with residual deformity after the growth plate fuses that precludes reasonable function and enhances the likelihood of premature degenerative changes, a corrective osteotomy may be quite beneficial. The level of the osteotomy is controversial. The tenet that the correction should be performed at the site of the deformity speaks in favor of a cuneiform osteotomy (7,8). These techniques, however, are performed before growth plate closure and have resulted in an unacceptable incidence of AVN. To mitigate the risk of complications, an intertrochanteric osteotomy may be used. The risk of chondrolysis associated with this procedure must be taken into consideration.

Another choice is the subtrochanteric osteotomy. Although considered the safest procedure, it has the disadvantage of creating a deformity of the upper shaft of the femur, which could make future arthroplasty more difficult.

COMPLICATIONS

Chondrolysis is the development of acute necrosis of the hyaline articular cartilage with resultant joint-space narrowing and stiffness (18). The cause is uncertain. Chondrolysis occurs more frequently among blacks and has been reported to affect females 2 to 5 times more frequently than males. Pin penetration was a suspected cause; but Zionts et al. (19) suggested that if pin penetration is recognized intraoperatively and corrected, it does not pose a significant risk. Furthermore, chondrolysis has been documented in surgically untreated patients.

Chondrolysis should be looked for in the initial examination, as the overall prognosis is adversely affected by its presence. This diagnosis must be suspected when a patient complains of increasing stiffness and pain in the affected joint. Low-grade infection must also be considered. The treatment is relief of weight bearing, aggressive range of motion exercises, and nonsteroidal anti-inflammatory medications. If this course of action is inadequate, examination under anesthesia is performed, and a soft tissue release is recommended for fixed contractures. Roy and Crawford (20) reported satisfactory preliminary results from a capsulectomy. Hip arthrodesis is another option for unremitting symptoms.

Avascular necrosis is another difficult problem to treat (21). This complication has not been reported to occur in untreated patients. Reduction, severity of displacement, osteotomy, and improper in-situ fixation have all been implicated in its development. Optimal placement of fixation and limiting the number of devices to two minimize the risks of interrupting the blood supply. The extent of the necrosis determines the modality of treatment. In segmental AVN, osteotomies, such as the Sugioka transtrochanteric rotational osteotomy, may be beneficial.

Patients with total head collapse are candidates for arthrodesis, with the possibility for replacement arthroplasty in the future (22).

SUMMARY

Slipped capital femoral epiphysis remains a condition of undetermined etiology that must always be included in the differential diagnosis of any growing patient presenting with hip *or knee pain*. The major thrust must be the earliest possible recognition of this entity so that proper surgical stabilization may be implemented. This helps to ensure the least amount of deformity in the femoral epiphysis–metaphysis relationship, affording the best possible prognosis with respect to the development of premature degenerative changes.

Chondrolysis can occur in the *untreated* patient and must be looked for at presentation, as this adversely affects the outcome. Avascular necrosis is the other major complication that needs to be monitored, as it too adversely affects the prognosis.

REFERENCES

1. Muller E. Über die verbiegung des schenkelhalses im wachstumsalter beitr. Klin Chir 1888–1889;4:137.
2. Kelsey J, Keggi K, Southwick W. The incidence and distribution of slipped capital femoral epiphysis in Connecticut and the Southwestern United States. J Bone Joint Surg 1970;52A:1203–1216.
3. Loder R, Wittenberg B, DeSilva G. Slipped capital femoral epiphysis associated with endocrine disorders. J Pediatr Orthop 1995;15:349–356.
4. Oka M, Miki T, Hama H, et al. The mechanical strength of the growth plate under the influence of sex hormones. Clin Orthop 1979;145:264–272.
5. Wilcox P, Weiner D, Leighley B. Maturation factors in slipped capital femoral epiphysis. J Pediatr Orthop 1988;8:196–200.
6. Carney B, Weinstein SL, Noble J. Long-term follow-up of slipped capital femoral epiphysis. J Bone Joint Surg 1991;73A:667–674.
7. Dunn D. The treatment of adolescent slipping of the upper femoral epiphysis. J Bone Joint Surg 1964;46B:621.
8. Fish J. Cuneiform osteotomy of the femoral neck in the treatment of slipped capital femoral epiphysis. J Bone Joint Surg 1984;66A:1153–1168.
9. Canale ST, Azar F, Young J, et al. Subtrochanteric fracture after fixation of slipped capital femoral epiphysis: a complication of unused drill holes J Pediatr Orthop 1994;14:623–626.
10. Walters, Simon. In: The hip: proceedings of the Eighth Open Scientific Meeting of the Hip Society. St. Louis: Mosby, 1980:145.
11. Laplaza F, Burke S. Epiphyseal growth after pinning of slipped capital femoral epiphysis. J Pediatr Orthop 1995;15:357–361.
12. Kibiloski LJ, Doane RM, Karol LA, et al. Biomechanical analysis of single versus double screw fixation in slipped capital femoral epiphysis at physiologic load levels. J Pediatr Orthop 1994;14:627–630.
13. Herman MJ, Dormans JP, Davidson RS, et al. Screw fixation of grade III slipped capital femoral epiphysis. Clin Orthop 1996;322:77–85.
14. Weiner DS. Open graft epiphysiodesis for slipped capital femoral epiphysis. J Pediatr Orthop 1990;10:673–674.
15. Rao SB, Crawford AH, Burger RR, Roy DR. Open peg epiphysiodesis for slipped capital femoral epiphysis. J Pediatr Orthop 1996;16:37–48.
16. Boyer D, Mickelson M, Ponseti I. Slipped capital femoral epiph-

ysis: long-term follow up and study of one hundred and twenty-one patients. J Bone Joint Surg 1981;63A:85–95.

17. Wong-Chung J, Strong M. Physeal remodeling after internal fixation of slipped femoral capital epiphysis. J Pediatr Orthop 1991; 11:2–5.

18. Vrettos BC, Hoffman EB. Chondrolysis in slipped capital femoral epiphysis. Long-term study of the aetiology and natural history. J Bone Joint Surg 1993;6B:956–961.

19. Zionts LE, Simonian PT, Harvey JP Jr. Transient penetration of the hip joint during in situ cannulated-screw fixation of slipped capital femoral epiphysis. J Bone Joint Surg 1991;73A:1054–1060.

20. Roy R, Crawford A. Idiopathic chondrolysis of the hip: management by subtotal capsulectomy and aggressive rehabilitation. J Pediatr Orthop 1988;8:203–207.

21. Krahn TH, Canale ST, Beaty JH, et al. Long-term follow-up of patients with avascular necrosis after treatment of slipped capital femoral epiphysis. J Pediatr Orthop 1993;13:154–158.

22. Sugioka Y. Transtrochanteric rotational osteotomy in the treatment of idiopathic and steroid-induced femoral head necrosis, Perthes' disease, slipped capital femoral epiphysis, and osteoarthritis of the hip: indications and results. Clin Orthop 1984; 184:12–23 .

94

Gaia Georgopoulos

Tibia Vara

I | Infantile Tibia Vara

Tibia vara is a pathologic process resulting in a severe bowleg deformity. There are two distinct types: infantile and adolescent. Tibia vara was first described by Erlacher in 1922, but the first large series was published by Blount in 1937 (1). Epidemiologically, infantile tibia vara occurs more commonly in black populations than in Caucasian populations. A high incidence is found in Africa, the West Indies, and Finland. Boys and girls are equally affected.

RELEVANT ANATOMY AND PATHOGENESIS

The cause of infantile tibia vara is unknown, but there are two primary theories: hereditary and development (2). There have been several reports of tibia vara in families, which supports genetic factors. The developmental theory is supported by the epidemiologic facts that tibia vara occurs in children who walk at an early age and who are in the 90th percentile or more for weight. It is believed that the combination of early weight bearing, increased weight, and physiologic varus produces an abnormal stress on the medial side of the knee. The Heuter-Volkmann law states that increased pressure on a physis inhibits growth. Conversely, the Delpeche law states that stimulation of growth is caused by a decrease in pressure. The abnormal stress on the medial side of the knee, therefore, causes increased growth laterally and retardation of growth medially, producing tibia vara.

Pathologic specimens have shown disordered endochondral ossification. It is not known whether this is the primary abnormality in producing the varus deformity or whether this develops secondary to the varus deformity. Histologic sections show islands of densely packed hypertrophied cells and islands of nearly acellular fibrocartilage. Finally, there are abnormally large groups of capillary vessels.

INITIAL FINDINGS, PHYSICAL EXAMINATION, AND DIAGNOSIS

Gross examination of affected tibias shows a posteromedial depression in the medial articular surface of the tibia. There is a hypertrophic, hypermobile medial meniscus. There is delayed ossification of the medial epiphysis and the medial metaphysis. Avascular necrosis, however, has never been documented.

The pathogenesis of tibia vara is probably a combination of biomechanical and biologic factors. Biomechanically, weight bearing may be necessary for tibia vara to occur; it has never been documented in nonambulatory children. As mentioned, as varus increases, the compressive forces on the medial side of the joint also progressively increase. As little as 10° of varus can change the compressive forces across the lateral plateau to tension forces (3).

Biologically, there may be a primary cartilage defect. Histologic studies suggest that there has been damage to the cartilage; and damaged cartilage is more slowly ossified, which explains the delayed ossification of the medial epiphysis and metaphysis.

The diagnosis of infantile tibia vara is based on history, clinical examination, and radiographic findings. The chief complaint in these patients is a bowleg deformity, which may be bilateral or unilateral (Fig. 94.1). Early on there may be no other complaints; but in the later stages of the disease, pain and instability may occur. Most progression occurs in the first 3 to 4 years of life.

On examination, the varus deformity is readily apparent and is associated with internal tibial torsion. Shortening of the tibia rarely occurs; but it if does, it is slight. Patients may display a lateral thrust with their gait. On palpation, the clinician may find beaking of the proxi-

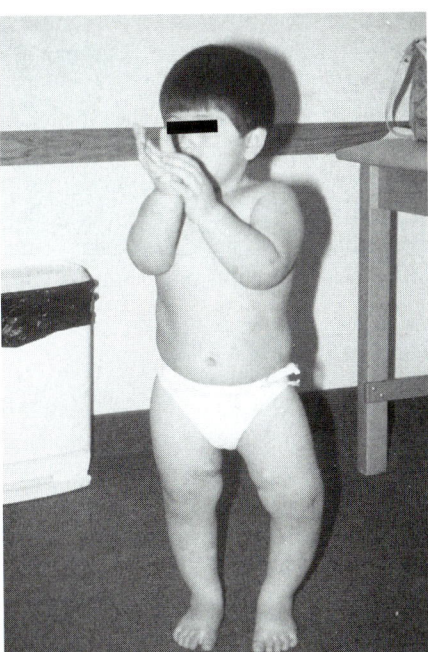

Figure 94.1. Toddler with unilateral tibia vara.

t a b l e	94.1	Differential Diagnosis

Tibia vara
Physiologic bowing
Trauma
Infection
Skeletal dysplasias: metaphyseal chondrodysplasia
Metabolic: rickets

mal medial metaphysis. Stress testing of the knee will show that the knee is stable when fully extended; but when flexed at 10° to 20°, the medial femoral condyle subluxates posteromedially. This finding was first described by Siffert and Katz (4).

The differential diagnosis of infantile tibia vara is quite broad, as there are a number of processes that can cause a varus deformity at the knee (Table 94.1). Physiologic bowing is the most common cause of bowed legs (5). The proximal tibia appears normal on radiographs. There is generally some bowing noted in the distal femurs. The metaphyseal-diaphyseal angle is less than 11°.

Trauma and infection are two other diagnoses that may be difficult to exclude. There may be no clear-cut history of injury or infection. Other causes include metabolic disorders and skeletal dysplasias.

RADIOLOGIC STUDIES

Radiographs may help the clinician make the diagnosis, although radiographic changes are rarely present in patients younger than 2 years. In these cases, the metaphyseal-diaphyseal angle, as described by Levine and Drennan (6), may be helpful. An angle of 11° or greater correlates with the development of radiographic changes seen with infantile tibia vara. Tibia vara developed in 29 of 30 patients with an angle greater than or equal to 11° and in only 3 of 58 patients with an angle less than 11°.

Classification

Langenskiöld and Riska (7) identified and classified the radiographic changes of tibia vara into six definitive stages (Fig. 94.2). In stage I disease, there may be a slight irregularity of the medial metaphysis. Stage II is characterized by an obvious medial beak and some decreased height of the epiphysis medially. In stage III, there is an increasing medial beak and the epiphysis begins to grow distally, following the metaphysis. The medial metaphysis becomes deficient or collapses further in stage IV and stage V disease. It is unable to support the epiphysis, which continues to extend distally. In stage VI, the medial physis begins to fuse. Stages II through IV do not necessarily represent disease progression but rather increasing skeletal maturity.

TREATMENT

The natural history of untreated infantile tibia vara is not well documented in the literature. Because of the deformity, most children get treated. The natural history is speculated to be progressive. Blount (1) showed a correlation between tibia vara and the development of osteoarthritis. In 17 patients older than 30 years, 11 of 27 knees had radiographic evidence of osteoarthritis. There was, however, no correlation between the severity of the varus and the severity of the osteoarthritis.

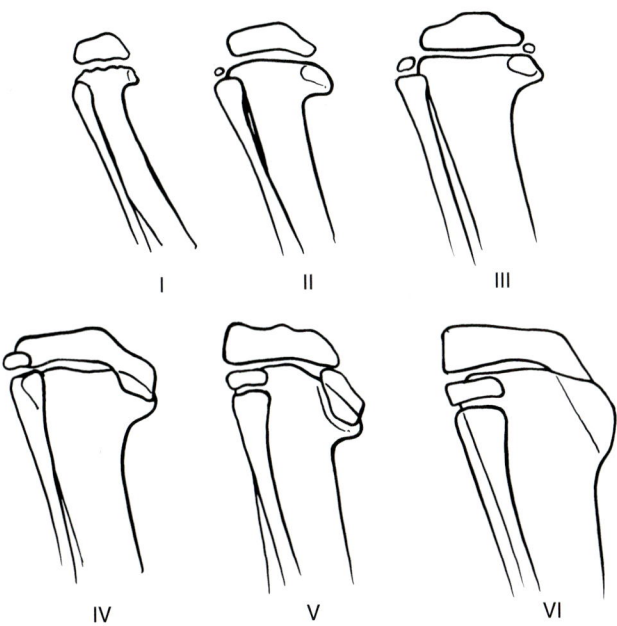

Figure 94.2. The Langenskiöld and Riska classification of tibia vara.

Nonoperative Treatment

Nonoperative treatment consists of bracing (8). Two types of braces are available. The Blount brace is an A-frame brace that has valgus-producing straps at the knees (Fig. 94.3). It is a nonambulatory brace and is used only during the night. The other brace is a typical knee-ankle-foot orthosis (KAFO) (Fig. 94.4). It is an ambulatory brace and is worn during the day. Indications for brace treatment vary. Blount recommended a brace for patients between 18 and 24 months of age with significant varus that was not radiographically distinguishable from physiologic bowing. He did not specify what "significant" varus was. He also

recommended bracing for severe persistent deformity past the age of 2, again without radiographic evidence of infantile tibia vara.

Schoenecker et al. (9) recommended bracing for children younger than 2 years, stage I or II disease, and varus deformity between 15° and 20°. Bracing should not be used in children older than 3 years. Bracing is discontinued when standing x-rays show a valgus mechanical angle and resolution of the metaphyseal changes.

Operative Treatment

If bracing is not successful or if the patient is older than 3 years, consideration should be given to surgical intervention. The surgical procedure performed depends on the age of the patient and the stage of the disease (Clinical Table). One-stage corrective osteotomy may be unable to reverse the medial physeal inhibition of a stage III lesion and will not be successful in stages IV through VI lesions, resulting in recurrent deformity.

In younger children with stage II or III disease, upper tibial osteotomy should be performed. The amount of correction varies by author and ranges from 5° to 10° of valgus. The goal of the surgery should be to transfer the line of weight bearing to the lateral compartment of the knee (10).

The specific technique of proximal tibial osteotomy is not important. It should correct both the varus and the internal rotation deformity. This surgery can be complicated by compartment syndrome. Often, the cast must be split to allow for swelling; some type of internal fixation helps prevent loss of correction. Prophylactic anterior and lateral compartment fasciotomies have also been advocated.

Bony bridges have never been demonstrated by tomography in stage IV and stage V disease; however, the medial physis injury effectively acts like a physeal arrest. Therefore, corrective osteotomy alone will not permanently correct the deformity. In the 7- or 8-year-old child with a stage IV or V lesion, corrective osteotomy can be combined with a medial physeal resection and some type of interpositional graft (11). If less than 2 years of skeletal growth remain, then realignment and lateral physeal arrest is a better treatment option.

The stage VI lesion has an established bony bridge. In the patient with less than 2 years of growth remaining and a relatively normal joint surface, a corrective osteotomy done through the physis will both realign the leg and shut down the lateral tibial physis, thus preventing recurrence. If joint incongruity exists, then an intra-articular osteotomy, which elevates the medial plateau, can improve joint congruity.

SUMMARY

In summary, once the diagnosis of infantile tibia vara has been made, treatment should be instituted immedi-

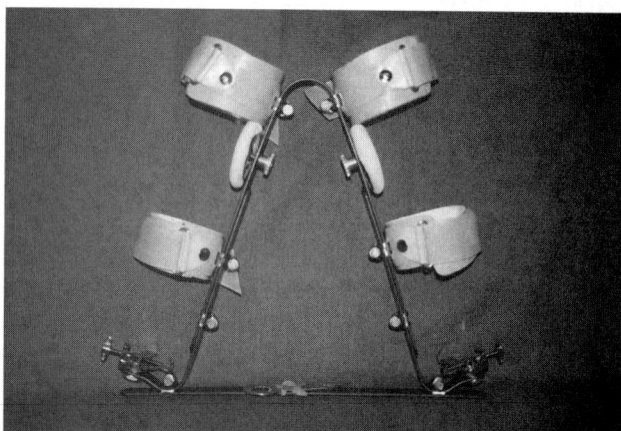

Figure 94.3. Blount brace.

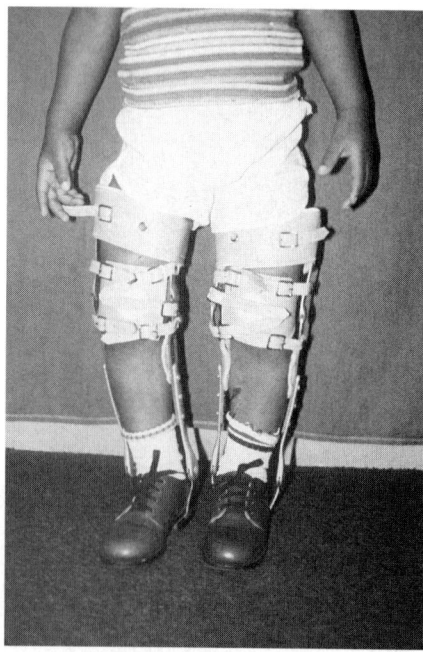

Figure 94.4. Bilateral KAFO brace.

Clinical Table: Tibia Vara

Operation	Indications	Technique	Anatomy	Pitfalls
Proximal tibial osteotomy	• Age 3–4 • Stage II or III disease	• Below the tibial tubercle • With or without internal fixation	• At level of trifurcation	• Undercorrection • Compartment syndrome • Recurrence
Corrective osteotomy and medial physeal resection or lateral physeal arrest	• Age 7–8 • Stage IV or V disease	• Osteotomy below the tubercle • Map lateral bar	• At level of trifurcation	• Undercorrection • Compartment syndrome • Recurrence
Corrective osteotomy through the physis	• Stage VI disease • <2 years of growth • Normal joint surface	• May be opening or closing wedge	• Level of physis	• Small proximal fragment • Fixation difficult • Compartment syndrome
Intra-articular osteotomy	• Stage VI disease • <2 years of growth • Joint incongruity	• Elevation of medial plateau with bone graft	• At level of trifurcation	• Undercorrection • Compartment syndrome • Recurrence
Proximal tibial and fibular osteotomy	• Adolescent tibia vara • Progressive deformity • Symptomatic deformity	• With internal or external fixation	• At level of trifurcation	• Poor results documented in literature
Lateral tibial hemiepiphysiodesis	• Adolescent tibia vara • Progressive deformity • Symptomatic deformity • Must have growth remaining	• Open or percutaneous technique	• Lateral physis	• Diseased medial physis may not grow normally, making prediction of correction difficult

ately. The treatment selected depends on the age of the patient and the stage of the disease. In children younger than 3 years with stage I or stage II disease, full-time bracing can be attempted. For patients who are older than 3 years of age or for whom bracing has been ineffective, surgical correction is indicated. Children younger than 4 years with up to stage III disease can usually be successfully treated with a proximal tibial osteotomy. In older children with a more advanced stage of the disease, realignment osteotomy should be combined with either physeal resection with interposition or lateral epiphysiodesis, to prevent recurrence of the deformity. When joint incongruity is present, intra-articular osteotomy with elevation of the medial plateau is indicated.

II   Adolescent Tibia Vara

Late-onset or adolescent tibia vara occurs less commonly than does infantile tibia vara and causes a progressive varus deformity in the older age patient (Fig. 94.5). Epidemiologically, adolescent tibia vara is seen most often in black males who are obese (defined as greater than 2 standard deviations above the mean for the child's age). Unilateral involvement is more frequently observed.

RELEVANT ANATOMY AND PATHOGENESIS

The cause is believed to be secondary to mechanical factors. Increased stress across the medial physis inhibits growth, leading to further increased stress across the physis. These patients often have slight varus alignment of their knees; however, recent reviews have shown the occurrence of adolescent tibia vara in extremities with proven normal mechanical axes (12). Therefore, static varus alignment of the knee is not a prerequisite for developing adolescent tibia vara. Davids et al. (13) have shown by gait analysis that relatively modest dynamic gait deviations, which occur because of increased thigh girth, can generate forces on the medial compartment great enough to inhibit medial physeal growth.

Histologically, the changes seen in adolescent tibia

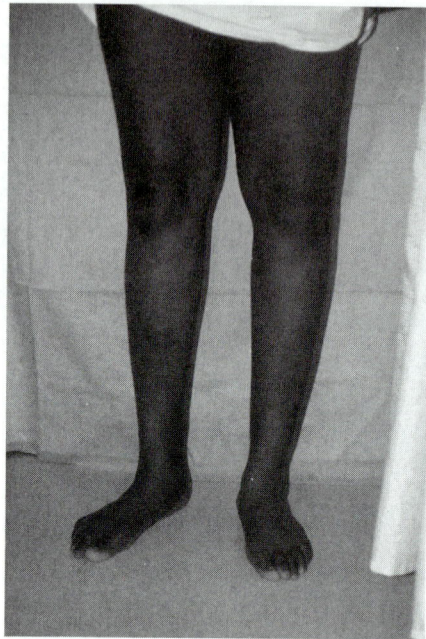

Figure 94.5. Adolescent tibia vara.

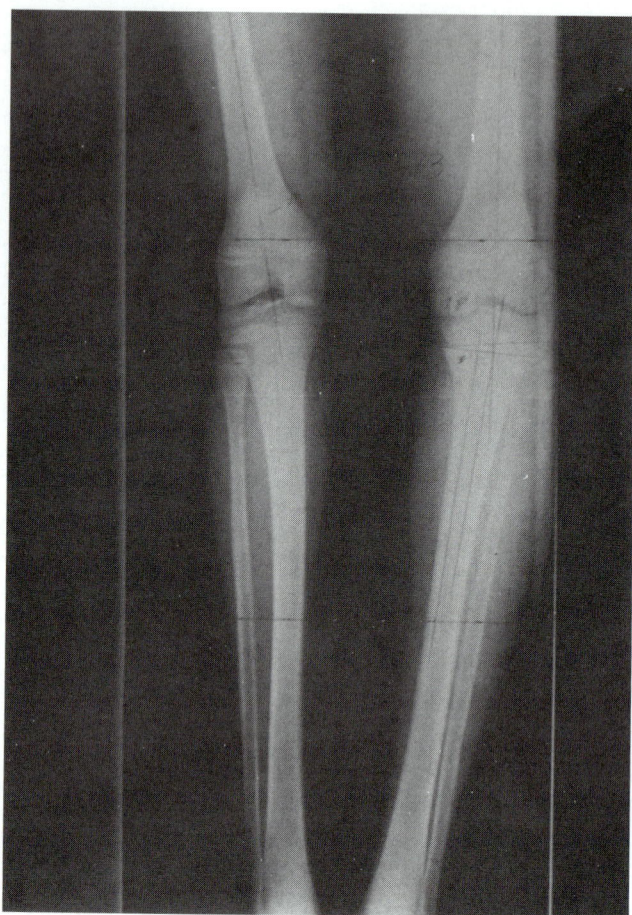

Figure 94.6. AP view showing changes associated with adolescent tibia vara.

vara are similar to those seen in infantile tibia vara and in slipped capital femoral epiphysis. Changes include fissuring and clefts in the physis with fibrovascular and cartilaginous repair at the physeal metaphyseal junction.

INITIAL FINDINGS, PHYSICAL EXAMINATION, AND DIAGNOSIS

Clinically, these patients present with complaints of a slowly progressive varus deformity. Pain is also a frequent presenting complaint and can range from vague mild aching to severe medial joint line pain, which limits activities. As mentioned, the patients are usually male (4:1 male:female predominance), black, and obese. More than 90% of patients are obese. The age range at presentation is 8 to 13 years. Typically, the varus deformity seen in adolescent tibia vara is less than that seen in infantile tibia vara.

RADIOLOGIC STUDIES

Radiographic findings are different and are less prominent than those seen in infantile tibia vara. There is mild to moderate flattening of the medial epiphysis, leading to a wedge-shaped epiphysis (Fig. 94.6). Increased physeal height can be seen both medially and laterally (14).

TREATMENT

Operative treatment of adolescent tibia vara is indicated for a progressive varus deformity, a symptomatic deformity, or a deformity likely to cause significant disability in the future (Clinical Table). The most commonly per-

formed surgical procedure is proximal tibial and fibular osteotomy. Numerous techniques have been described, with or without internal fixation or with external fixation. The correction can be done in one stage or slowly with an external fixator. Loder et al. (15) reported on a series of proximal tibial osteotomies and found a surprisingly low percentage of good results. In addition, there was a high complication rate. The most common complication was either loss of correction or inadequate correction at the time of surgery. In the large leg, it was often difficult to determine the amount of correction obtained intraoperatively. Other complications included peroneal nerve palsy and anterior compartment syndrome.

Another option for surgical treatment is lateral tibial hemiepiphysiodesis. For this to be successful, there must be adequate growth remaining. The other caveat is that the charts for predicting angular correction following hemiepiphysiodesis assume normal growth on the nonoperated side. The diseased medial physis in adolescent tibia vara most likely does not grow normally; therefore, correction is unpredictable. It is, however, a relatively minor procedure, which can be done percutaneously with fluoroscopic guidance. Given the complication rate and low percentage of good results after tibial osteotomy, hemiepiphysiodesis is a reasonable option in the patient with adequate remaining growth.

SUMMARY

Late-onset tibia vara produces a slowly progressive varus deformity of the proximal tibia. It is less common than infantile tibia vara and occurs almost exclusively in obese, African-American males. The cause is most likely secondary to increased compressive forces across the medial tibial physis, which inhibit growth. Treatment is surgical, and most patients undergo proximal tibial osteotomy. The procedure can be difficult in this obese population, and there is a high rate of complications. Lateral tibial hemiepiphysiodesis may be a better alternative in select cases.

REFERENCES

1. Blount WP. Tibia vara. Osteochondrosis deformans tibial. J Bone Joint Surg 1937;19A:1–29.
2. Bradway JK, Klassen RA, Peterson HA. Blount disease: a review of the English literature. J Pediatr Orthop 1987;7:472–480.
3. Cook SD, Lavernia CJ, Burke SW, et al. A biomechanical analysis of the etiology of tibia vara. J Pediatr Orthop 1983;3:449–454.
4. Siffert RS, Katz JF. The intra-articular deformity in osteochondrosis deformans tibial. J Bone Joint Surg 1970;52A:800–804.
5. Salenius P, Vankka E. The development of the tibiofemoral angle in children. J Bone Joint Surg 1975;57A:259–261.
6. Levine AL, Drennan JC. Physiologic bowing and tibia vara. J Bone Joint Surg 1982;64A:1158–1163.
7. Langenskiöld A, Riska EB. Tibia vara (osteochondrosis deformans tibial). J Bone Joint Surg 1964;46A:1405–1420.
8. Johnston CE II. Infantile tibia vara. Clin Orthop 1990;225:13–23.
9. Schoenecker PL, Meade WC, Pierron RL, et al. Blount's disease: a retrospective review and recommendations for treatment. J Pediatr Orthop 1985;5:181–186.
10. Ferriter P, Shapiro F. Infantile tibia vara: factors affecting outcome following proximal tibial osteotomy. J Pediatr Orthop 1987;7:1–7.
11. Beck CL, Burke SW, Roberts JM, Johnston CE II. Physeal bridge resection in infantile Blount disease. J Pediatr Orthop 1987;7:161–163.
12. Henderson RC, Kemp GJ, Hayes PR. Prevalence of late-onset tibia vara. J Pediatr Orthop 1993;13:255–258.
13. Davids JR, Huskamp M, Bagley AM. A dynamic biomechanical analysis of the etiology of adolescent tibia vara. J Pediatr Orthop 1996;16:461–468.
14. Thompson GH, Carter JR. Late onset tibia vara (Blount's disease). Current concepts. Clin Orthop 1990;225:24–35.
15. Loder RJ, Schaffer JJ, Bardenstein MB. Late onset tibia vara. J Pediatr Orthop 1991;11:162–167.

Common Pediatric Fractures (Emphasis on Operational Indications)*

This chapter discusses the general indications for operative treatment of the common and difficult pediatric fractures (see Clinical Table). References are provided for readers interested in more detail.

I | The Upper Extremity

FRACTURES OF THE RADIUS AND ULNA

RELEVANT ANATOMY AND PATHOGENESIS

Fractures of the distal radius and ulna are the most common fractures seen in children (1). When dealing with forearm fractures, the key question is always acceptability of the fracture alignment. To understand this, it is important to understand the ability of the immature skeleton to remodel with growth.

Angular correction of the radius with growth proceeds at approximately 1° per month (2,3). Remodeling is primarily the result of physeal growth but is also secondary to appositional bone filling in the concavity of the deformity. Resorption also occurs on the convexity of the curvature. Remodeling is most complete when the fracture is close to the physis, the patient is young, and the angular deformity is in the plane of joint motion. Because four-fifths of the growth of the radius is at the distal physis, the more distal the fracture, the greater the remodeling.

Radial deviation in distal and radial fractures is more important than volar or dorsal angulation in terms of in-terosseous space narrowing, which leads to loss of motion and impingement. Angular deformity beyond 20° in the middle and distal radius significantly decreases rotation (4). Rotational malalignment leads to rotational loss in a 1:1 ratio.

Treatment

Angulation beyond 20° in the distal and middle shaft of the radius should not be initially accepted in any age group. When radial deviation is greater than 10°, attempts at reduction should always be made in the proximal radius. Volar angulation limits pronation; therefore, greater than 10° of proximal radial diaphyseal angulation is associated with some loss of motion. Bayonet apposition in the middle and distal forearm is acceptable up until age 8, as long as differential shortening and malrotation are not clinically present.

The fracture parameters that should be accepted in a healing fracture are somewhat different from those at initial presentation. For a distal radius fracture in a child younger than 8 years, angulation of up to 30° is well accepted. Rotational malalignment greater than 10° to 20° should be corrected at the time of the initial reduction, but malrotation of up to 45° may be tolerated without much functional

*Thank you to Dr. Timothy Galbraith for his assistance in the preparation of this manuscript.

impairment (5). Forearm fractures in children older than 12 years are treated in a manner similar to those in adults. In adolescents, the ability of the bone to remodel is decreasing. The periosteum is less of an aid in fracture reduction in children older than 12 years than it is in younger children, and intramedullary rodding or compression plates are used to achieve satisfactory stabilization.

FRACTURES AND DISLOCATIONS OF THE ELBOW

RELEVANT ANATOMY AND PATHOGENESIS

Fractures and dislocations about the elbow can be difficult to diagnose and to treat because of the unique anatomy of the area. Near the elbow joint, the humerus broadens into medial and lateral columns, becoming quite thin and flat. Cross sections of this area demonstrate the wide, flat area, which is where most fractures occur. Unfortunately this is a difficult area to treat.

Avulsion of the medial epicondyle occurs when there is a valgus stress applied to the elbow and the ulnar collateral ligament detaches the medial epicondyle. The radial collateral ligament attachment can also have the same effect. The nerves and arteries in this area vulnerable to widely displaced supracondylar fractures (Fig. 95.1). Furthermore, nerves and vessels can be trapped between the fracture fragments after reduction. The blood supply to the lateral condyle epiphyseal ossifi-

cation center is mainly posterior through the nonarticular portion of the condyle. The medial condyle receives its blood supply posteriorly through the nonarticular crest of the trochlea and through vessels that run across the epiphyseal plate.

DIAGNOSIS

Depending on the age of the patient and the amount of the distal humeral epiphysis that has ossified, diagnosis can be difficult. Usually, the clinician is presented with a child who has failed on the outstretched arm; the elbow is swollen and painful.

Transepiphyseal fractures through the distal end of the humerus, either Salter type I or type II injuries, are especially difficult to diagnose in 1- to 2-year-old children. The capitellum supplies the clue to this diagnosis. The capitellum should have a constant relationship to the radius but not to the distal humerus. Occasionally, however, a late fracture will be seen, and the new bone formation will confirm the diagnosis. If the diagnosis is difficult, an arthrogram will differentiate among an extracapsular fracture, a condylar fracture, and an elbow dislocation.

TREATMENT

Fractures about the elbow can be treated in the same manner as one-way supracondylar fractures. Many of these fractures are stable and can be held by a posterior splint,

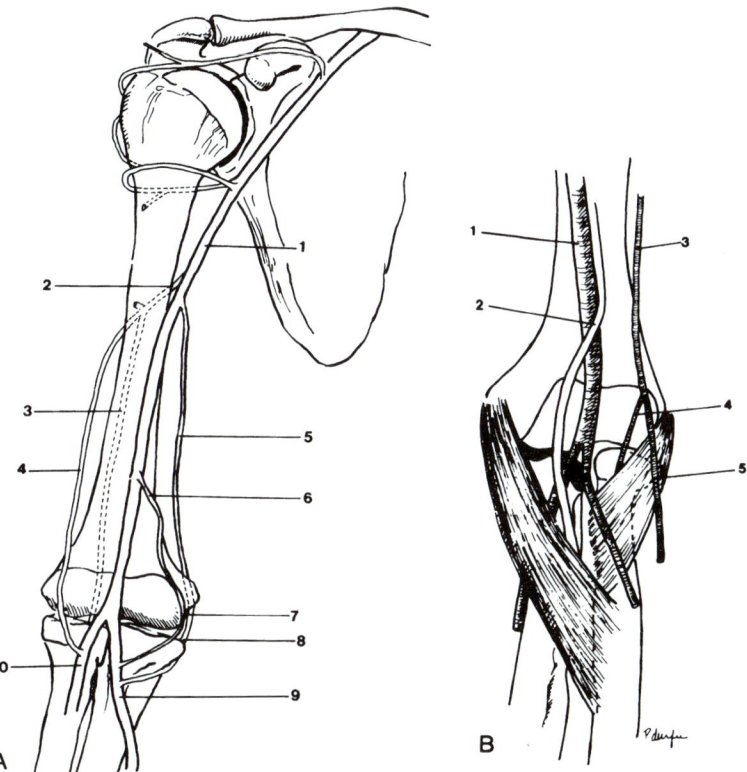

Figure 95.1. A. Collateral arterial circulation of the humerus. *1,* brachial artery; *2,* deep brachial artery; *3,* medial collateral artery; *4,* radial collateral artery; *5,* superior ulnar collateral; *6,* inferior ulnar collateral; *7,* volar ulnar recurrent tape; *8,* dorsal ulnar recurrent; *9,* ulnar artery; *10,* radial artery. **B.** Neurovascular relationships around the distal humerus. *1,* brachial artery; *2,* median nerve; *3,* radial nerve; *4,* posterior branch of the radial nerve; *5,* anterior branch of the radial nerve.

with the forearm pronated; however, percutaneous pinning, especially for unstable fractures, is the treatment of choice. The prognosis is good, provided normal valgus orientation has been reproduced.

SUPRACONDYLAR FRACTURES

A supracondylar fracture usually occurs by a fall on the outstretched hand. Falling on a flexed elbow produces the rare anteriorly displaced supracondylar fracture. Supracondylar fractures are either nondisplaced (type I), displaced with the posterior cortex intact (type II), or displaced with no cortical contact (type III) (Fig. 95.2).

TREATMENT

The Baumann angle must be assessed for supracondylar humerus fractures (6). This angle is formed by a line that runs perpendicular to the axis of the humerus and a line that runs tangential to the straight epiphyseal border of the lateral part of the distal humeral metaphysis, measured in the AP radiograph. If there are 5° of varus compared to the opposite side, then the fracture should be manipulated

and pinned into an acceptable position (Fig. 95.3). If there are less than 10° of valgus compared to the opposite side, there should be no functional or cosmetic problems.

Operative Treatment

Types II and III fractures are usually treated by closed reduction and percutaneous pinning. My preference is to cross the 0.3125 smooth pins medially and laterally. Closed reduction and maintenance in hyperflexion can lead to Volkmann's ischemic contracture. If the classic signs of pain, pallor, and pulselessness occur and/or there is forearm pain on passive extension of the fingers, the dressings must be removed and the elbow extended. If the fracture has been pinned, the reduction will not be lost. Supracondylar fractures should be pinned with no hyperflexion of the elbow. After reducing and pinning the fracture, I usually splint the elbow in 80° of flexion.

TECHNIQUE

The steps for performing a closed reduction and percutaneous pinning of the supracondylar humerus fracture are as follows.

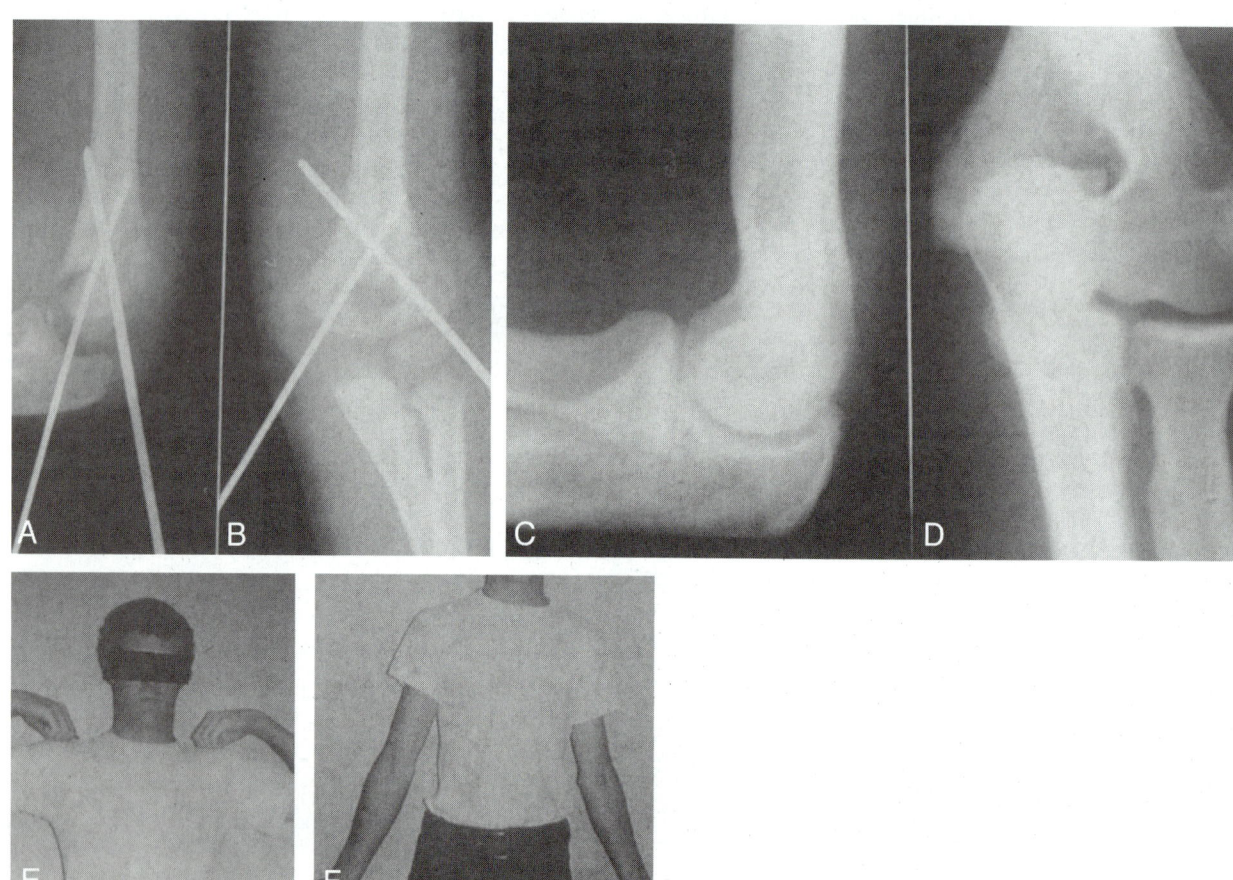

Figure 95.2. A and **B.** AP views of a supracondylar humerus fracture in a 5-year-old male. Note the rotation of the distal fragment and absence of tilt. At age 17, the patient has no deformity (**C** and **D**), normal range of motion (**E**) and a normal carrying angle (**F**).

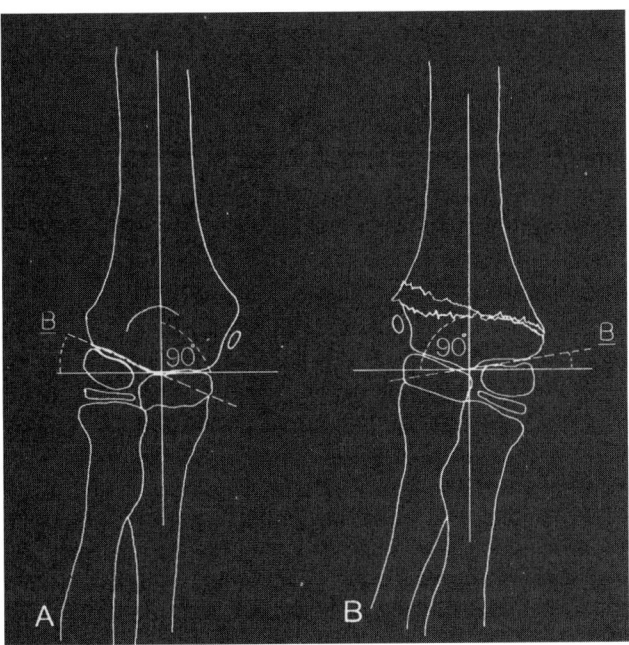

Figure 95.3. A. Baumann's angle in a normal elbow. **B.** Baumann's angle in this fractured elbow is about half that of the normal side. *B,* Baumann angle.

1. Apply traction to the elbow with the forearm supinated, and restore length. Gently hyperextend the fracture site to engage the fragments.
2. Correct the distal fragment tilt and internal rotation deformity.
3. Flex the elbow and the end fracture site by simultaneously flexing, holding the wrist, and applying pressure with one thumb to the olecranon.
4. Fully pronate the forearm to correct varus tilt.
5. Hold the elbow in the completely flexed position, and pin it.
   a. Pin the lateral side first, traversing the lateral condyle, going into the proximal humerus, and engaging the medial cortex.
   b. Be sure that the medial epicondyle can be palpated; and push away the edema if significant swelling has occurred.
   c. Pin through the medial epicondyle and engage the lateral cortex of the proximal humerus. If necessary, make a small incision to make sure that the ulnar nerve is not injured.
6. Extend the elbow for AP and lateral radiographs. Measure Baumann's angle: Up to 10° of valgus and 5° of varus are acceptable.
7. Cut off the pins and apply a posterior splint with the elbow in 80° of flexion.

The pins are removed 3 weeks after pinning, and early motion exercises are begun.

The indications for open reduction are an open fracture, a serious postreduction vascular compromise, and inability to reduce and pin the fracture. The brachial artery, median nerve, and brachialis muscle are known impediments to reduction.

COMPLICATIONS

Neurologic injuries occur in up to 12% of severely displaced supracondylar fractures. These injuries are usually the result of neuropraxia, and spontaneous recovery can occur in 3 to 4 months. If recovery does not occur, electromyelogram (EMG) studies and possible exploration of the nerve are recommended.

The brachial artery may be compromised either by direct injury or through spasm. The best method of restoring circulation is to reduce the fracture. For severe ischemia, I recommend conscious sedation and an attempt at reduction in the emergency room before going to the operating room for closed reduction and pinning.

If after reduction and pinning of the fracture the hand is viable and the nail beds are pink, adequate collateral circulation has been restored, even if the radial pulse is absent. There should be no deep forearm pain with passive extension of the fingers. If after satisfactory reduction, circulation is not restored, exploration of the brachial artery is mandatory. Arteriography often delays treatment, when the surgeon can look at the artery directly. I notify the vascular surgeon when I am going to the operating room with a child who has a compromised hand circulation, in case abduction does not satisfactorily restore hand circulation.

Volkmann's Ischemic Contracture

Volkmann's ischemic contracture is caused by circulatory failure of the forearm. The pathophysiology has been described by Eaton and Green (7). Arterial occlusion produces muscular ischemia, which causes the release of a histamine-like substance that increases the capillary permeability, leading to intramuscular edema. This elevates the pressure on the intrinsic muscle tissue within the fascial envelopes. Tight external circular dressings can add to the pressure. If venous congestion occurs, reflex spasm increases. If unrelieved, muscle necrosis and fibrosis eventually occur, leading to contractures of the hand and forearm, nerve ischemia and damage, and loss of sensation.

The early signs are pain, pallor, and pulselessness along with paralysis, especially the median nerve. An important finding is deep forearm pain with passive extension of the fingers on wakening. If in doubt, measure the compartment pressures. If the ischemia persists more than 6 h, fasciotomy and epimysiotomy are indicated.

If the symptoms of Volkmann's ischemic contracture are developing, first and most important is to reduce the fracture. If the fracture is still displaced, pin it and then extend the elbow. If the symptoms occur after treatment with reduction and pinning, be sure that the reduction did not trap the brachial artery. If this did not occur, remove the dressings and extend the elbow. If this does not restore circulation, a vascular surgeon should be consulted. If it is believed that spasm is causing the symptoms, a stellate ganglion block can be performed. If none of these situations applies the brachial artery should be explored. The surgeon should be decisive and not hesitate to do the fasciotomy and epimysiotomy. The treatment of established ischemic contracture is beyond the scope of this chapter.

FRACTURES OF THE LATERAL CONDYLE

Fractures of the lateral condyle have a high potential for nonunion with poor results (Fig. 95.4). Proper management will avoid nonunion. These fractures are classified as nondisplaced, minimally displaced, and totally displaced. The lateral condylar ligament and attached extensor muscles play a role in the displacement and dislocation of fractures in this area.

TREATMENT

Nonoperative Treatment and Indications for Surgery

If displacement is 2 mm or less, cast at a right angle with the forearm in neutral or slight supination to minimize the pull on the lateral soft tissue structures. Continue immobilization until healing has occurred, from 3 to 12 weeks. If displacement is greater than 2 mm, then open reduction and pinning are indicated.

In a study of 31 slightly or minimally displaced lateral condyle fractures (4 mm or less) treated with closed reduction and casting, 27 (87%) healed and 4 (13%) failed to heal (8). The fractures that healed were displaced 2 mm or less. The authors concluded that all fractures displaced 3 mm or more should be pinned. Inadequate treatment is still a leading cause of nonunion of fractures of the lateral condyle.

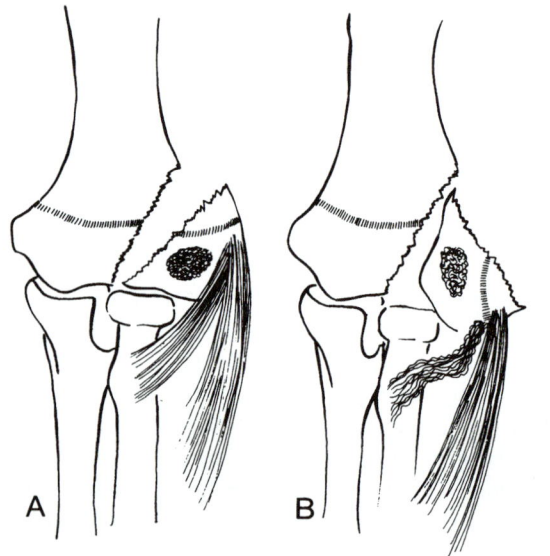

Figure 95.4. A. Displaced and partly rotated lateral condyle fracture. **B.** Lateral condyle fracture in which the fragment is rotated 180°.

OPERATIVE TREATMENT

Open reduction and pinning are usually the best treatment. The Kocher J approach is used, beginning 3 to 5 cm proximal to the lateral epicondyle and extending 3 cm distal to the radial head. The interval between the triceps and the brachioradialis is dissected, and the lateral condyle and capsule are exposed.

To preserve the blood supply, soft tissue attachments are left posteriorly, and several millimeters of soft tissue are stripped to allow visualization of the anterior and superior edge of the distal fragment. By flexing and extending the elbow, it is possible to see how the fragment fits, so an accurate reduction can be made; held with a towel clip it is put gently into place with the elbow flexed. The reduction is secured with two pins. X-rays are taken to confirm the anatomic reduction. The pins are removed at 6 weeks, at which time early range of motion is begun.

COMPLICATIONS

Nonunion is the complication most feared with fracture of the lateral condyle. The intra-articular nature of this injury is such that the entire fracture may be bathed in synovium. Pull on the extensor muscle mass may discourage union and increase displacement. Furthermore, the distal fragment may have a decreased circulation, because often it is mainly cartilage, with only a wafer of metaphyseal bone left on it. Nonunion can be prevented by prophylactically pinning any fracture that is displaced more than 2 mm and by carefully watching minimally displaced fractures.

FRACTURES OF THE MEDIAL EPICONDYLE

Fractures of the medial epicondyle are extra-articular fractures usually seen in children, accounting for 5 to 10% of elbow fractures. The mechanism of injury is a valgus stress in which the medial pools off the medial epicondyle through the ulnar collateral ligaments with additional force from the hyaline flexor origin. Medial epicondyle fractures frequently occur in association with elbow dislocation.

TREATMENT

The nonoperative treatment of this injury constellation involves anatomic reduction of the elbow dislocation. The clinician should avoid trapping the medial epicondyle within the joint. If epicondyle is in the joint, closed maneuvers to extract the fragment should be undertaken. If these measures are not effective, then open reduction is indicated. A medial incision is made and the medial epicondyle is anatomically reduced and secured with pins. In general, internal fixation is necessary only for fractures displaced by more than 5 mm. A gravity stress test assesses the elbow's instability and helps determine whether closed or open treatment is needed (9). Valgus stress instability is rare. Instability of the dominant arm in a throwing athlete may be an indication for open reduction of the medial epicondyle fracture. Medial epicondyle fractures should not be mobilized for longer than 3 weeks. Stiffness is more of a problem than is nonunion.

FRACTURES OF THE HUMERAL SHAFT

Fractures of the humeral shaft represent 2% of all pediatric fractures (10). Child abuse is the most common cause for a humeral shift fracture in the infant and toddler. Pediatric diaphyseal humerus fractures are classified according to location (Table 95.1).

TREATMENT

Acceptable results for children under the age of 6 years include an AP angulation of 20°, varus angulation of 30°, shortening of 2.5 cm, and rotation of 15°. Diaphyseal humeral fractures after the age of 6 years have little remodeling capacity. Nondisplaced or minimal displaced humeral shaft fractures can be treated in a sling and swathe or a Velpeau splint. If a closed reduction is performed, then the fracture must be stabilized in a coaptation splint (no shortening) or a hanging cast (shortening of distal fragment).

Open reduction and internal fixation (ORIF) is rarely indicated in children with pediatric humeral shaft fractures. Indications are the rare failed closed reduction, associated multiple injuries, and open fractures. External fixation, with or without a radial nerve injury, associated with humeral shaft fractures is not an indication for ORIF.

Most radial nerve injuries are the result of stretching or bruising and are incomplete; 70 to 90% of cases recover within 8 to 12 weeks of the first clinical sign noted in the brachioradialis.

FRACTURES OF THE PROXIMAL HUMERUS

RELEVANT ANATOMY AND CLASSIFICATION

Proximal humeral fractures account for less than 1% of all pediatric fractures. The proximal humerus accounts for 80%

of the longitudinal growth of the bone and, therefore, supplies the proximal humerus with vast remodeling potential.

Proximal humerus fractures are classified as physeal or metaphyseal. Salter-Harris type I fractures are the most common in children younger than 5 years old. The metaphysis in children between 5 and 11 years of age is relatively weak as a result of rapid growth and is the most common fracture site. Salter-Harris type II injuries are the most common humeral fractures in children 12 years of age and older. Proximal humerus fractures are further classified with respect to the amount of displacement (11):

- Grade I: less than 5 mm
- Grade II: up to ⅓ the width of the shaft
- Grade III: up to ⅔ the width of the shaft
- Grade IV: up to 2⅔ the width of the shaft, including complete displacement

The proximal humerus develops from three secondary ossification centers: The epiphyseal ossification center appears by 6 months and the greater and lesser tuberosity centers appear at 3 and 5 years, respectively. The ossification centers fuse at around 7 years of age, whereas the growth plate closes between 18 and 22 years of age. When evaluating this fracture, the clinician should remember that the proximal humerus physis is cone shaped.

TREATMENT

Nonoperative Treatment and Indications for Surgery

Fractures of the proximal humerus generally heal by 6 weeks. It is important to remember that little remodeling of proximal humerus fractures occurs after 9 months. Fractures of the proximal humerus in neonates can be difficult to diagnose. An ultrasound or arthrogram may be necessary for a complete evaluation of the neonate to rule out fracture of the proximal humerus. Nondisplaced fractures are treated in a sling and swathe. Proximal humeral fractures that require reduction should be mobilized in a position that maintains the reduction (Fig. 95.5). If the fracture maintains the reduction with the arm in adduction, then a coadaptation splint is adequate.

Some fractures will need to be immobilized in 70° to 90° abduction, some forward flexion, and internal rotation. An abduction pillow can be used in reliable patients; otherwise, a salute or Statue of Liberty cast can be used. The shoulder can be brought out of abduction within 3 weeks. Guidelines for the worst acceptable reduction in fractures of the proximal humerus are shown in Table 95.2 (12). Children younger than 5 years require some degree of apposition and less than 70° of angulation. Children between 5 and 12 years of age require at least 50% apposition and less than 40° of angulation. Children older than age 12 require less than 33% displacement and less than 25° of angulation. Skeletally mature teenagers are treated as adults.

table 95.1	Classification of Humeral Shaft Fractures		
Fracture Dislocation	**Proximal Fracture Fragment**	**Distal Fracture Fragment**
Above the insertion of the pectoralis major	Abduction and external rotation	Medial displacement
Between the pectoralis major and deltoid insertion	Adduction	Shortening
Below the deltoid insertion	Abduction	Medial displacement

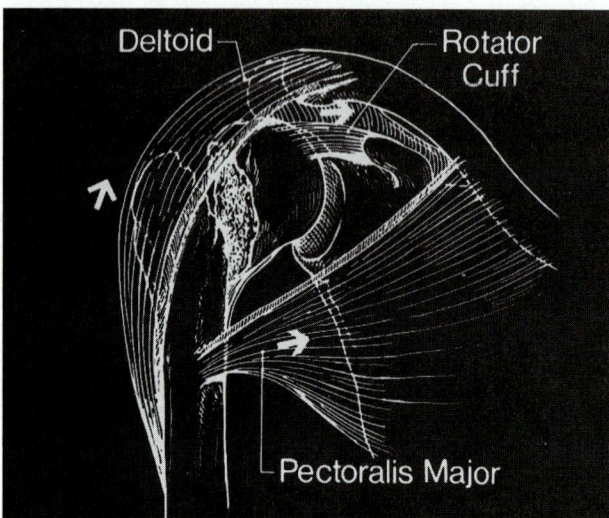

Figure 95.5. Deforming forces on a proximal humerus fracture.

| table | 95.2 | Worst Acceptable Reduction Allowed for Pediatric Proximal Humerus Fractures |

Age (Years)	Apposition (%)	Angulation (°)
0–2	95	>70
3–5	75	>60
6–9	50	>45
10–12	50	>30
12 to skeletal maturity	30	>25

of the acromion to avoid the axillary nerve. After closed reduction and with the aid of fluoroscopic guidance, the K wires are advanced across the fracture site. The arm is held in a Velpeau dressing for 2 to 3 weeks, during which time gentle circumductions and elbow range of motion exercises are performed. The pins are removed after 3 weeks.

Open reduction of pediatric proximal humerus fractures is almost never necessary. The indications for operative treatment include open fractures, unstable fractures associated with nerve injury or compromise, displaced intra-articular fractures, irreducible fractures (commonly associated with biceps, tendon, or periosteum interposition), and unstable fractures in the older or adolescent patient. A deltopectoral approach is used, and the fracture is reduced and maintained by retrograde smooth K wires, as previously explained.

Operative Treatment

Proximal humeral fractures that are reducible by closed reduction but fail to be maintained by this technique are candidates for percutaneous pinning (13). Two smooth Kirschner (K) wires are used percutaneously into the anterior lateral humeral shaft at a distance of at least 8 cm from the lateral tip

II The Spine

CERVICAL SPINE INJURIES

RELEVANT ANATOMY AND PATHOGENESIS

Cervical spine injuries in children are uncommon. The site of injury of the cervical spine is age dependent. There is a strong tendency for injuries in the younger child to be located in the cranial cervical region between the occiput and C2, whereas in older children, adolescents, and adults the distribution is in the lower cervical spine. The pediatric pattern of cervical spine injury changes to the adult pattern between the ages of 8 and 12 years. This is a time of development when most of the spinal epiphysis is closing and juvenile spinal morphology resembles adult spinal morphology. Remember that head injuries are commonly associated with cervical spine injuries in children.

There are seven cervical vertebrae: C3 through C7 are similar, and C1 and C2 are unique. Remember that the occiput to C1 controls 50% of flexion and C1–2 controls 50% of rotation. The space available for the spinal cord in the upper cervical spine is approximately 3 times the cord size.

The space narrows significantly at C5 and C6, where the canal is narrowest because of cell bodies to the cervical nerve roots to the upper extremities. At C1–2, alar ligaments play a major role in stability. Stability of the cervical spine is determined by the confidence of the discs, posterior ligaments, and facet capsules. The facets are orientated in a coronal plate to prevent translation. Early childhood facets are much more horizontal and thus allow for greater translation than adult facets. The vertebral arteries pass through the foramen transversum of C1–6. The vertebral vein, but not the artery, passes through C7.

RADIOLOGIC STUDIES

All children with cervical spine injuries should be evaluated with an AP radiograph as well as a lateral to T1 and odontoid oblique views. Flexion-extension views may be needed to evaluate instability. Pillar views help evaluate the facets.

Other studies include myelogram, CT scan, and MRI. When evaluating the cervical spine, remember the normal radiographic entities. At C2–3, the prevertebral soft tissue swelling is 5 mm or less; and at C5–7, it is 14 to 20 mm. Note that crying elevates soft tissue swelling in children. When evaluating alignment, keep in mind that more than 3.5 mm of translation of one vertebral body secondary to another or an 11° intervertebral angle is considered unstable. The atlantodens interval in a child is less than 4 mm; in an adult, it is less than 3 mm.

DIAGNOSIS AND TREATMENT

Atlantoaxial Rotatory Subluxation

Atlantoaxial rotatory subluxation may be fixed or mobile. The radiographs will reveal wide lateral masses on the odontoid view and decreased facet cartilage space. Spinous processes of the axis will tilt toward the side of facet displacement. Generally, the transverse ligament is intact. The differential diagnosis includes bony anomalies of C1 and C2, upper pharyngeal infection, syringomyelia, and congenital abnormality. Treatment consists of traction for acute postinfection, which indeed may be all that is needed. The injury may need to be stabilized for up to 3 months. If reduction cannot be maintained, displacement is persistent, or there is neural abnormality, then fusion of the atlantoaxial segment is indicated.

Jefferson Fracture

The Jefferson fracture is a bursa fracture of C1 and may be associated with transverse ligament rupture. If the C1 lateral mass spreads more than 7 mm, then the transverse ligament is ruptured. Note that congenital failure of C1 to fuse can be misinterpreted as a fracture. Fractures of the posterior arch only are stable. This fracture rarely causes a neural deficit. The Jefferson fracture is caused by an axial blow to the head.

A lateral mass offset of C1 greater than 7 mm equals a rupture of the transverse ligament. Generally, this injury is treated with a halo brace and may take 3 to 6 months to heal (Fig. 95.6). If the transverse ligament is ruptured, the stability of C1 and C2 must be assessed after the fracture heals. If the flexion-extension views reveal more than 5 mm of instability, then fusion of C1–2 is indicated.

Odontoid Fracture

Odontoid fractures are broken down into three types. Type I is a fracture at the level of the os terminale. This is a stable fracture, and symptomatic care is all that is needed. Type II fractures are at the level of dens body junction and are the most common type of odontoid fracture. The nonunion rate increases with age. If closed reduction of a type II fracture cannot be performed, posterior fusion may be indicated. Type III fractures of the odontoid are through the body of C2 with broad cancellous service. The union rate depends on the amount of dis-

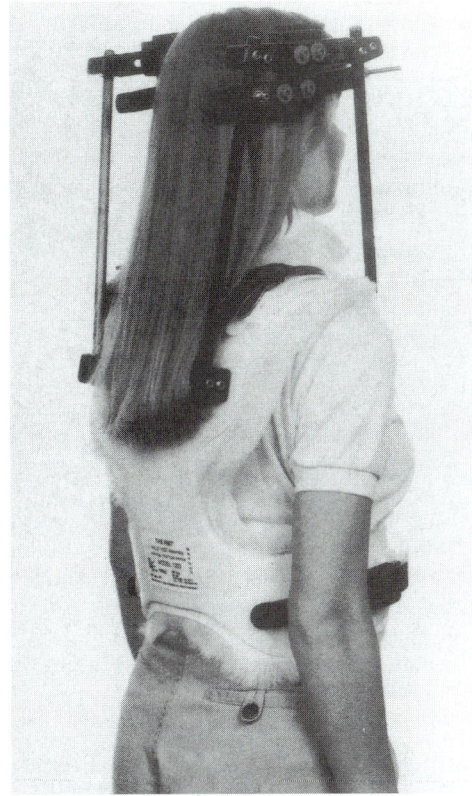

Figure 95.6. Halo body jacket.

placement. I prefer to treat these fractures with closed reduction and some type of immobilization halo.

Hangman's Fracture

Hangman's fracture is a pedicle fracture of C2. It may have an associated facet dislocation and variable destruction of C2 disc. The mechanisms are axial loading, extension, and also flexion. Neurologic involvement is rare. Type I fractures are displaced less than 7 mm and are treated in a cervical-thoracic brace. A halo brace is used in reliable patients. Type II fractures are associated with subluxation of C2 and C3. I use traction to reduce these fractures and recommend a halo or other brace. Type III fractures are associated with bilateral facet dislocation. I approach these from the posterior, reduce the facets, and then do a posterior C2–3 fusion. The patients are then placed in a halo brace to allow the pars to heal.

Unilateral Facet Dislocation

Unilateral facet dislocations usually result from flexion and rotation forces applied to the neck, which cause tearing of the facet joint capsule and posterior ligamentous complex. The plain film lateral view reveals 25% translation of one vertebral body on another. Initial treatment consists of cervical traction in an attempt to reduce the

Clinical Table: Common Pediatric Fractures

Procedure	Indications	Technique[a]	Anatomy	Pitfalls
		Upper Extremity		
Fractures of Radius and Ulna				
Closed reduction	• Age >8 yr <12 yr • Rotation >20° • Angulation >30°	• Traction/reduction • Well-molded cast	• As in adults	• Poor-fitting cast
Open reduction and internal fixation	• >12 yr	• As in adults		
Fractures and Dislocation of the Elbow				
Closed reduction	• Transepiphyseal fractures	• Closed reduction and pinning	• Capitellum should be aligned with radius	• Often misdiagnosed; use arthrogram
Supracondylar Fractures				
Cast	• Type I (Nondisplaced)			
Closed reduction and percutaneous pinning	• Types II and III	• See *Technique* under Fractures of the Proximal Femur	• Ulna nerve • Brachial artery	• Avoid hyperflexion • Compartment syndrome • Ulnar nerve on medial pinning
Fractures of the Lateral Condyle				
Cast	• Displacement ≤ 2 mm	• 90° at elbow • Forearm neutral/mild supination		
Open reduction and pinning	• Displacement >2 mm	• Kocher approach	• Interval between triceps and brachioradialis	• Overstripping of soft tissue posteriorly
Fractures of the Medial Epicondyle				
Cast closed reduction	• Displacement <5 mm	• Traction		
Open reduction and pinning	• Displacement >5 mm	• Medial Incision	• Ulna nerve	• Stiffness 2° over immobilization
Fractures of the Humeral Shaft				
Sling and swathe	• ≥6 yr of age, AP angulation ≤20°	• Longitudinal traction with coaptation splints	• Radial nerve	• 70–90% of radial nerve injuries recover within 8–12 weeks
Closed reduction and cast	• Varus ≤30° • Shortening ≤2.5 cm • Rotation ≤15°			
Open reduction and internal fixation	• Multitrauma, open fracture, or failure of closed reduction			
Fractures of the Proximal Humerus				
Closed reduction	• ≤5 yr of age with <70° angulation • 5–12 yr of age with 50% apposition and <40° angulation • 12 yr and up with 33% apposition and <25° angulation	• Sling and swathe • Coaptation splints • Cast in abduction		
Closed reduction and pinning	• Failure to maintain guidelines for simple closed reduction	• 2 smooth K wires	• 8 cm from lateral tip of acromion	• Axillary nerve must be avoided

[a] Technique is often age and/or case dependent. For fractures of this nature no technique is presented.

Clinical Table: *(Continued)*

Procedure	Indications	Technique[a]	Anatomy	Pitfalls
		Spine		
Cervical Spine Injuries				
Cervical collar traction	• Atlantoaxial rotary subluxation • Spinous process fractures • Laminar compression fractures	• Collar brace 2–3 weeks, after which, if not reduced, then traction		• Treat upper respiratory infection with antibiotics if Grisel's syndrome is suspected
Fusion	• Irreducible atlantoaxial rotary subluxation • Type III Hangman's fracture • Bilateral facet dislocation			
Closed reduction and external fixation	• Odontoid fractures • Hangman's fractures types I and II • Unilateral facet dislocation	• Halo cast • Use small size pins in multiples	• Use CT scan to check thickness of skull	• Do not retorque pins
Thoracic and Lumbar Spine Injuries				
Cast or thoracic lumbosacral orthosis	• Compression • Distraction ≤20° kyphosis	• Hyperextension casting	• More cartilage in anterior column than in adults	• Monitor anterior growth in child, beware growth arrest Posterior disc herniation a possibility, perform pre-op MR scan
Posterior spinal fusion and instrumentation	• ≥20° kyphosis			
		Pelvis and Lower Extremity		
Fractures of the Pelvis				
Symptomatic care	• Apophyseal fractures	• Rest • NSAIDs	• Anterior superior iliac spine • Anterior inferior iliac spine • Ischial tuberosity	• Long-term follow-up needed for physeal injuries
Spica cast	• Pelvic ring fractures			
Traction and spica cast	• Acetabular fractures			• Acetabular dysplasia if <10 yr of age
Fractures of the Proximal Femur				
Spica cast Closed reduction	• Type I fractures • Type IB fractures • Type II fractures • Nondisplaced Type III fractures			
Open reduction internal fixation	• Type IB fractures when closed reduction fails • Type II fractures when closed reduction fails • Type III fractures when closed reduction fails	• Reduction with aid of C-arm fluoroscopy • Smooth pins • Type IB —Posterior approach for posterior dislocations —Anterior approach for anterior dislocation —Smooth pins: removed after 6 weeks in spica cast	• Physis must be protected with smooth pins	• Avascular necrosis • Premature physeal closure • Leg length inequality • Degenerative arthritis

[a] Technique is often age and/or case dependent. For fractures of this nature no technique is presented.

continued

Clinical Table: (Continued)

Procedure	Indications	Technique[a]	Anatomy	Pitfalls
		• Type II —Lateral approach —Smooth pins • Type III —Anterolateral approach		
Closed reduction and traction	• Displaced type IV fractures			
Fractures of the Femoral Shaft				
90/90 traction followed by spica cast	• Subtrochanteric fractures	• Distal femoral pin, checked frequently by x-ray • Maintained until callus visible on x-ray		
Open reduction internal fixation	• Head injury • Polytrauma			
Fractures of the Diaphyseal Femur				
Spica cast	• Age ≤2 yr	• 30° abduction • 45° flexion		• Beware of child abuse <5 yr of age
Split Russell traction followed by spica cast	• Age 2–5 yr • <2 cm shortening • <20° angulation			
90/90 traction	• Age 6–10 yr			
Operative	• Age >11 yr		• Avoid femoral neck and growth plates	
Distal Femoral Physeal Injuries				
Spica cast	• Nondisplaced Salter-Harris type II fractures			• Physeal bars must be monitored • Limb length discrepancy
Closed reduction and spica cast	• Displaced Salter-Harris type II fractures		• Popliteal artery tear present in 2% of displaced fractures	
Closed reduction, pin fixation, and spica cast	• Unstable Salter-Harris type II fractures	• Smooth crossed pins	• Internal fixation should not cross the physeal plate	
Open reduction internal fixation	• Salter-Harris type III and IV fractures			
Fractures of the Patella				
Cylinder cast	• Nondisplaced fractures	• 5° flexion	• Bipartite patella present in 0.2–6% of population	
Open reduction internal fixation and cast	• Displaced fractures	• Smooth pins and tension wiring		
Patellectomy	• Severely comminuted			
Fractures of the Proximal Tibial Epiphysis and Physis				
Long leg cast	• Nondisplaced fractures		• Cruciate ligaments attach to spines	• Monitor for growth arrests
Closed reduction	• Displaced fractures			
Open reduction internal fixation	• Irreducible fractures			
Fractures of the Tibial Eminence				
Long leg cast in extension	• Type I fractures	• Include foot in cast		• Anterior horn of lateral meniscus may block reduction

[a] Technique is often age and/or case dependent. For fractures of this nature no technique is presented.

Clinical Table: *(Continued)*

Procedure	Indications	Technique[a]	Anatomy	Pitfalls
Closed reduction and long leg cast	• Type II fractures	• Reduce in extension		• Compartment syndrome
Open reduction and internal fixation	• Irreducible type II and type III fractures	• Arthroscope with small screw or K wires and sutures		
Avulsion Fractures of the Tibial Tuberosity				
Cylinder cast Open reduction internal fixation and cast	• Types I and II fractures • Displaced type II fractures • Type III fractures	• Full extension • Screw is placed since growth os apophysis is almost completed • Smooth pins if <14 yr of age	• Most fractures occur between the ages of 13 and 16 due to growth plate closure	• Compartment syndrome in patients with type III fractures
Fractures of the Proximal Tibial Metaphysis				
Long leg cast Closed reduction, long leg cast	• Nondisplaced fractures • Displaced fractures	• Long leg cast in extension	• Popliteal artery bound at trifurcation	• Popliteal artery damage in high energy trauma • Tibia valga may occur-usually resolves
Fractures of the Proximal Fibula				
Symptomatic		• Compressive dressing	• Assess peroneal nerve	• Check ankle for fractures
Fractures of the Tibial and Fibular Diaphysis				
Long leg cast Closed reduction and long leg cast	• Nondisplaced fractures • Displaced fractures	• Long leg cast with knee bent 45°		• Compartment syndrome • May need to change cast as swelling decreases
Fractures of the Distal Metaphysis of the Tibia				
Cast Closed reduction and cast in equinus	• Nondisplaced fractures • Recurvatum ≥15°	• Long leg cast with foot in equinus to control anterior impaction		• Malrotation • Compartment syndrome
Tillaux Fractures				
Closed reduction	• Salter-Harris type III fractures	• Internal rotation with longitudinal traction		• Ankle joint congruity must be restored
Open reduction internal fixation	• Displacement >2 mm	• Interfragmentary screws		
Triplane Fractures				
Closed reduction	• Salter-Harris type IV fractures		• CT scans or tomograms may be needed	• Anatomic joint congruency must be restored
Open reduction internal fixation	• Displacement >2 mm			• Partial physeal arrests may occur
		Fractures of the Foot		
Fractures of the Talus				
Short leg cast, non-weight bearing	• Nondisplaced head and neck fractures			• Avascular necrosis, indicated by the Hawkins sign
Closed reduction	• Displaced head and neck fractures			
Open reduction internal fixation	• Displaced head and neck fractures when closed reduction fails	• Approach through anterior tibial artery and extensor hallucis longus		
	• Type IV fractures of the lateral process	• May osteotomize medial malleolus		

[a] Technique is often age and/or case dependent. For fractures of this nature no technique is presented.

continued

Clinical Table: *(Continued)*

Procedure	Indications	Technique[a]	Anatomy	Pitfalls
Fractures of the Calcaneus				
Open reduction internal fixation	• Age of patient • Degree of displacement • Posterior facet involvement • Anterior articular surface involvement		• Evaluate by CT scan	• Lumbar spine injuries
Closed reduction and cast	• Comminuted fractures			
Fractures of the Midfoot				
Short leg cast, non-weight bearing	• Navicular, cuboid, and cuneiforms fractures			• Adjacent joint subluxation • If navicular, avascular necrosis
Fractures of the Metatarsals				
Short leg cast, non-weight bearing	• Nondisplaced fractures of first metatarsal		• First metatarsal growth plate is proximal	
Reduction and K wire	• Displaced fractures of first metatarsal			
Short leg cast, non-weight bearing	• Second to fifth metatarsal fractures			
Short leg walking cast	• Fractures of the base of the fifth metatarsal			• Athletes may need intramedullary screw with bone graft
Fractures of the Phalanges				
Closed reduction	• Intra-articular fractures			• Monitor growth plate
Open reduction internal fixation	• Intra-articular fractures when closed reduction fails			
Cast or wooden shoe	• Nonintra-articular fractures			

[a] Technique is often age and/or case dependent. For fractures of this nature no technique is presented.

fracture. Traction is begun with 4.54 kg (10 lb) for the head and 2.27 kg (5 lb) for each additional level of the cervical spine. I then evaluate the injury site with an MRI study. If there is a ruptured disc anteriorly, I do an anterior and posterior fusion. If, however, there is no evidence of rupture into the vertebral canal and a stable reduction is maintained, I treat the patient with halo immobilization. If a closed reduction cannot be performed and the patient has a neurologic or root deficit, a posterior fusion is indicated. Generally speaking, however, a unilateral facet fracture without an associated dislocation can be treated by reduction and immobilization and a halo.

Bilateral Facet Dislocation

Bilateral facet dislocations are highlighted by 50% translation of one vertebral body on another. They are usually associated with severe neurologic deficit and can have a sense of complete quadriplegia. These are generally complete ligamentous injuries. Treatment consists of reduction with traction, followed by MRI evaluation. These injuries generally need an anterior and posterior fusion, because they are highly unstable and difficult to hold in a halo brace.

Spinous Process Fracture

Spinous process fractures can be treated in a brace for 4 to 6 weeks or treated symptomatically. Lamina fractures are commonly missed on routine radiographs. They generally heal uneventfully with simple immobilization. Mild compression fractures of the cervical spine without associated neurologic deficits can be adequately treated with an orthosis for 8 to 12 weeks until healing has occurred.

Bursa Fracture

Bursa fractures of the cervical spine involve the anterior and middle columns; bony fragments protrude posteriorly into the spinal canal. Skeletal traction should be initiated immediately, and closed reduction should be attempted.

There is high incidence of neurologic damage in this type of injury. If there is residual bony protrusion in the canal in a patient with a neurologic and complete lesion after skeletal traction is applied, accepted treatment is anterior vertebrectomy, strap fusion, and posterior fusion.

THORACIC AND LUMBAR SPINE INJURIES

RELEVANT ANATOMY AND PATHOGENESIS

The thoracic to lumbar spine of a child differs from that of an adult; a greater portion of the anterior column is composed of cartilage. With aging, the bone of the vertebral body takes up an increasing proportion of space, leaving a thin layer of end plate cartilage, which is thickened at the periphery to form the ring apophysis. The ring becomes partially ossified between the ages of 14 and 17 years and becomes fused with the vertebral body at around 21 years. The most common injuries to the thoracic and lumbar spine in children are compression fractures and distrac-tion or flexion. Chance (14) first described the spinal fracture pattern with little or no compression of the anterior column and associated distraction of the posterior elements. This fracture is most commonly associated with re-strained passengers in motor vehicle accidents.

TREATMENT

Glassman et al. (15) described the treatment of these lesions, which can be classified as bony or ligamentous. Generally, the recommendations are for cast or brace treatment to be used in the management of ligamentous and combined bony and ligamentous flexion destruction injuries if the kyphosis is less than 20°. Operative stabilization with a short compression rod above and below the level of injury is the recommended treatment if the kyphosis is greater than 20°. A posterior disc herniation can be produced when a compression rod is used across the damaged motion segment. Therefore, a preoperative myelogram, CT scan, or MRI study is advised.

III   The Pelvis and Lower Extremity

FRACTURES OF THE PELVIS

RELEVANT ANATOMY AND PATHOGENESIS

The pediatric pelvis is more malleable than the adult pelvis, and more trauma is needed to reduce the fracture. Furthermore, there is less protection of the abdominal and pelvic organs in children. In major pelvic trauma, soft tissue injury is often more of a problem than the fracture itself. When evaluating trauma to the pelvis in a child, it is important to remember that the ischial-pubic physis is closed between 6 and 7 years of age; the triradiate cartilage closes between 6 and 18 years; and the pelvic apophyses are the last to close, usually fusing in late adolescence. These injuries need long-term follow-up for associated physeal injuries.

TREAMENT

Apophyseal Fractures

Apophyseal fractures usually are seen in teenagers and are the result of mild trauma during an athletic event. The apophysis may not be ossified, so clinical diagnosis is usually based on point tenderness over the involved area. X-rays show a callus at 2 to 3 weeks. Points of interest include the iliac crest, anterior superior spine, anterior inferior spine, and ischial tuberosity. Treatment is basically symptomatic care. If the displacement is greater than 1 cm, some authors recommend ORIF; however, most displaced apophyseal fractures will achieve a nonsymptomatic fibrous union. If the patient develops a symptomatic nonunion, a section of the bony fragment and reattachment of the tendon can be done at a later date.

Pelvic Ring Injuries

Pelvic ring injuries consists of rami fractures, iliac wing fractures, and symphysis disruption. These can usually be treated with symptomatic care only. Stable ring fractures are rare and are usually treated with reduction by traction in the pelvic direction and a spica cast when stable. Indications for open reduction include a significantly displaced lateral compression fracture, a vertical shear that does not reduce in traction and will produce a leg length discrepancy, and an unstable fracture in an obese or adolescent patient.

Acetabular fractures are generally uncommon in pediatric pelvic injuries. Remember that the triradiate cartilage may be injured; if injury occurs in a patient younger than 10 years, he or she could later develop acetabular dysplasia. The worst prognosis is the central fracture dislocation, which has uniformly poor results in children. The treatment of displaced large acetabular fractures is initially a closed reduction with traction, which is usually successful. If this fails to reduce the large fracture fragments, then ORIF is used. Small threaded K wires are recommended for young patients. The need for long-term follow-up of these fractures is mandatory.

FRACTURES OF THE PROXIMAL FEMUR

RELEVANT ANATOMY AND CLASSIFICATION

The femur is the second bone to ossify in the fetus. Secondary ossification centers fuse with the body of the femur in reverse order of how they appeared. The lesser trochanter is usually the first physis to close. This is followed by closure of the physis at the greater trochanter, the capital femoral epiphysis, and the distal femur. Proximal femur fractures represent less than 1% of all pediatric femur fractures. The average age at injury is 8 years old.

Proximal femur fractures can be divided into four principal types (16) (Fig. 95.7). Type I injuries are transepiphyseal fractures; type IA fractures are not dislocated, and type IB fractures include dislocation of the capital femoral epiphysis from the acetabulum. Type II fractures occur through the midfemoral neck (transcervical). Type III fractures occur at the base of the femoral neck (cervicotrochanteric). Type IV fractures are intertrochanteric.

TREAMENT

All obstetrical hip dislocations and transepiphyseal fractures without dislocation show a metaphyseal callus at 8 to 10 days. The key is early diagnosis of displacement with corresponding arthrography. Generally, children younger than 4 years old and lighter than 23 kg (50 lb) who have nondisplaced fractures or fractures that can be reduced with traction are held in a spica cast. Neonates are placed in a Pavlik harness. Children older than 4 years and heavier than 23 kg who have nondisplaced fractures should undergo prophylactic pinning. The patient is then placed in a hip spica cast to maintain the reduction. The pins are removed in 6 weeks.

Children with type IB fractures should undergo a single attempt at closed reduction; if it fails, an open reduction is performed. A posterior dislocation should be approached through a posterior approach. Anterior dislocation is approached through an anterior approach. Internal fixation with smooth pins maintains the reduction while the patient is in a hip spica cast. The pins are removed in 6 weeks. The patients should be followed for avascular necrosis, premature physeal closure (partial or complete), leg length inequality, and degenerative arthritis.

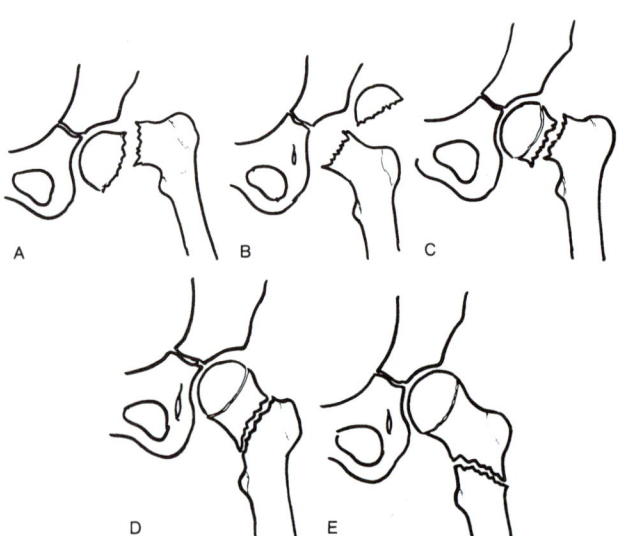

Figure 95.7. A. Nondisplaced type I fracture. **B.** Displaced type I fracture. **C.** Type II fracture. **D.** Type III fracture. **E.** Type IV fracture.

Approximately 50% of pediatric hip fractures are type II fractures. There is a high incidence of avascular necrosis (40 to 45% of cases). All children with fractures of the midfemoral neck should undergo internal fixation with smooth pins to stabilize the injury. The use of internal fixation reduces the risks of coxa vara and nonunion. Displaced fractures are reduced before pin placement. Fixation should stop short of the capital femoral physis. An open reduction and pin fixation using an anterior lateral approach is performed if closed reduction cannot be achieved.

Type III fractures are the second most frequent fracture of the pediatric proximal femur. Nondisplaced fractures are usually stable and treated with a 1½ hip spica cast; the extremity is maintained in abduction. If closed reduction fails, then an open reduction through an anterolateral approach is performed, and smooth pins are used. If there is any question about displacement, the fracture should be pinned as if it were an unstable injury. The pins are removed in 6 weeks.

Type IV proximal femur fractures represent 14% of all of the proximal pediatric femoral fractures. Nondisplaced fractures are treated by spica cast immobilization for 6 to 8 weeks. Displaced fractures require closed reduction and traction. Split Russell traction is used for children up to 5 years of age. Distal femoral skeletal traction is used for older children. Indications for internal fixation include a younger child who has redisplacement of the fracture. The adolescent patient is treated with internal fixation, because of the increased risk of developing coxa vera and the difficulties older, larger patients have with spica casts.

Trochanteric injuries can generally be sustained by a direct blow or, in adolescence, by running and jumping. Intertrochanteric fractures that are minimally displaced can be treated with closed reduction and a hip spica cast. Significant displacement can be treated with tension band wiring. Fractures of the lesser trochanter can be treated with symptomatic care.

Operative Treatment

The patient is placed on the fracture table in the supine position; the fracture is reduced with the aid of C-arm fluoroscopy. I use smooth pins; their size depends on the age of the patient. The pins may be placed percutaneously. To simplify the technique, I use a free pin, lay it on top of the skin perpendicular to the fracture (which is adjusted with the aid of C-arm fluoroscopy in both the AP and lateral views), and draw the fracture with a skin marker. The point where the lines intersect is the entrance point for performing this procedure percutaneously.

FRACTURES OF THE FEMORAL SHAFT

RELEVANT ANATOMY AND PATHOGENESIS

The femur is the largest of the long bones. The shaft of the femur is smooth and cylindrical, with an anterior lateral bow. The linea aspera is a prominent longitudinal ridge found posteriorly in the middle half of the bone. The pectineal line runs distally from the lesser trochanter to blend with the upper portion of the linear aspera. Most pediatric femoral shaft fractures are high-energy injuries. Femoral shaft fractures are classified on the basis of location, pattern, and degree of comminution and can be further divided into subtrochanteric and diaphyseal femur fractures.

TREATMENT

Subtrochanteric fractures can be difficult to treat because of the small proximal fragment that is flexed, abducted, and externally rotated. These fractures usually require 90/90 traction. Frequent x-rays are taken to evaluate the traction, which is adjusted if needed. The traction (distal femoral traction pin) is maintained until the fracture site is nontender to palpation and there is a visible callus on x-rays. The child is then placed in a 1½ hip spica cast until the callus is mature.

ORIF has been recommended for children older than 10 years, children with a head injury or polytrauma, and when closed reduction fails. The type of fixation used depends on the child's age and skeletal maturity. Options for fixation include flexible nails, plate and screws, reamed or nonreamed solid nails, and external fixation.

FRACTURES OF THE DIAPHYSEAL FEMUR

When a fracture of the diaphyseal femur occurs in a child younger than 5 years old, child abuse should be ruled out. Radiographs of the limb must include the hip and the knee joints. These are high-energy fractures and may have associated injuries. Treatment depends on the age of the patient.

TREATMENT

Birth to 2 Years of Age

Diaphyseal femur fractures in infants from birth to 2 years of age who have uncomplicated fractures with grade I, II, or III comminution; less than 1.5 cm of shortening; and less than 30° of angulation in any plane should be placed in a hip spica cast within 24 h. In most cases, the feet do not have to be included in the casting.

More complicated fractures associated with polytrauma, grade IV comminution, more than 1.5 cm of shortening, or more than 30° of angulation in any plane require an initial period of skin traction (17). The child is placed in skin traction with the thighs in approximately 30° of abduction and the hips in 45° of flexion. The legs are placed into traction to balance the pelvis and provide symmetric stabilization of the fractured femur. Bryant traction should never be used in children older than 2 years of age or who weigh more than 11.25 kg (25 lb), because of associated catastrophic vascular, neurologic, and skin complications (Fig. 95.8). The child should be seen weekly for the first 2 weeks after discharge. The fracture should be remanipulated and the cast changed if there is shortening of more

than 1.5 cm or angulation of more than 30° within the first 2 weeks.

Physical therapy to reestablish motion or strength is usually not necessary after the fracture union. The family should be cautioned, however, that the child will limp for up to 12 months after the cast is removed. Overgrowth is uncommon; but if occurs, it is usually within the first 18 months. Excessive shortening may persist. Angular deformities of less than 30° should spontaneously correct with further growth.

Ages 2 to 5

Children from ages 2 to 5 years sustain diaphyseal femur fractures from relatively low-energy trauma sustained in falls. Diaphyseal femur fractures that have an uncomplicated fracture pattern with grade I, II or III comminution; less than 2 cm of shortening; less than 20° of angulation in the sagittal plane; and less than 10° of angulation in the frontal plane are first treated with a period of split Russell traction followed by early spica cast application (Fig. 95.9). The child is placed into skin traction, and a longitudinal force is applied to the lower leg, parallel to the floor. A pulley and sling provide a second force that is perpendicular to the floor. The resulting applied force is in the direction of the femoral shaft, which is maintained in approximately 40° of flexion and is supported by a pillow placed behind the thigh. Young children should have both limbs placed in traction to stabilize the pelvis and obtain maximal mechanical advantage. The hip spica cast is placed with the aid of C-arm fluoroscopy while the child is under general anesthesia.

For complicated fractures with grade IV comminution, more than 2 cm of shortening, more than 20° of AP angulation, or greater than 10° of varus-valgus angulation, immediate early spica casting is not acceptable. Other contraindications to immediate early spica casting include open fractures (polytrauma associated with thoracic, intraabdominal, or vascular injuries), morbid obesity, severe soft tissue swelling, and unreliable patients. In this situation, split Russell traction or 90/90 distal femoral skeletal pin traction is preferred initially. Adjust the traction as necessary during the first few days to establish satisfactory alignment. When the fracture is nontender to palpation and general manipulation and there is visible callous on radiographs, the spica hip cast may be applied. The child should be examined 1 week after discharge with a routine cast and radiographic examination. The fracture should be remanipulated and the cast changed if there is more than 20° of angulation in the sagittal plane, more than 10° of angulation in the frontal plane, or more than 2 cm shortening. Overriding of up to 1.5 cm is acceptable in this age group.

Ages 6 to 10

Diaphyseal femur fractures in children ages 6 to 10 years are more commonly seen in pedestrians and bicyclists than in victims of motor vehicle accidents.

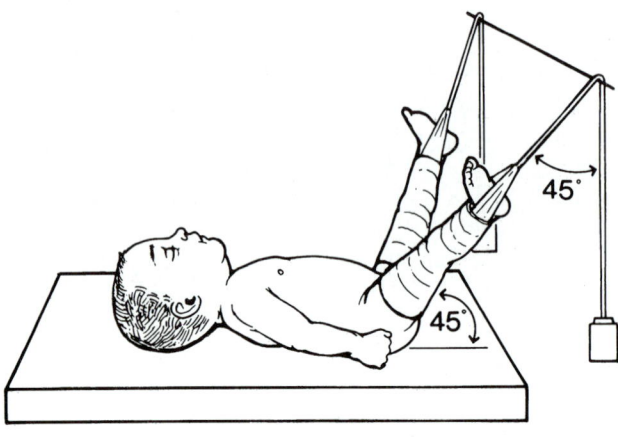

Figure 95.8. Modified Bryant traction.

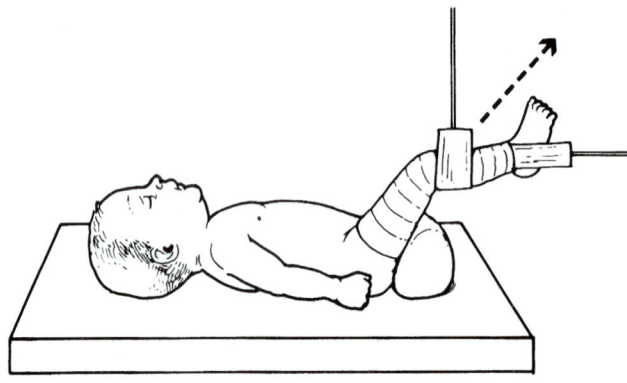

Figure 95.9. Modified Russell traction

Uncomplicated diaphyseal femur fractures with grade I, II, or III comminution; less than 1.5 cm shortening; less than 15° of angulation of the sagittal plane; and less than 10° of angulation in the frontal plane can be treated by several methods. Standard treatment remains 90/90 skeletal traction or a modified balance suspension with a distal femoral traction pin, which is preferred for the older or heavier child (Figs. 95.10 and 95.11). The child remains in traction until the fracture is clinically nontender and early radiographic healing is demonstrated. The patient is placed in a 1½ hip spica or walking spica cast until radiographic healing is complete. Early 1½ hip spica application can be performed, but close follow-up with weekly x-ray evaluation should be conducted because of the strong deformity forces in this age group. Other alternatives are early pontoon 90/90 spica cast or fixed traction using supracondylar K wires (18) (Fig. 95.12).

Indications for operative management of femoral shaft fractures in this age group include a closed head injury with spasticity, polytrauma, multiple fractures; an isolated fracture in which an acceptable reduction cannot be achieved or maintained; and for family elective or operative therapy after a thorough discussion of the treatment alternatives. Methods of stabilization include flexible intramedullary nails, reamed or nonreamed solid nails, compression plates with screws, and external fixation (Fig.

95.13). Femur fractures in children 11 years old to skeletal maturity are treated with operative stabilization. Although some controversy exists, 11- to 12-year-old children should be conservatively treated with traction that is maintained until the patient is clinically nontender over the fracture site and there is radiographic evidence of a callous. The patient is then placed in a hip spica cast.

Adolescents

Fractures of the femoral shaft in adolescents (13 years of age or older) who have complete closure of the growth plate should be treated as adults. Closed intramedullary fixation is the treatment of choice. If the diameter of the intramedullary canal is too narrow, then flexible intramedullary fixation is recommended. Open fractures of the femur in pediatric patients should be treated in the same manner as are open fractures in adults. Treatment consists of progressive irrigation and débridement; then stabilization of the fracture with external fixation or skeletal traction.

Operative Treatment

Application of a hip spica cast is done under general anesthesia with aid of C-arm fluoroscopy. A short leg cast on the involved extremity may be applied first and used as a traction tool. When applying the cast over the fractured extremity, be sure to mold the cast in the appropriate position, under fluoroscopy. A rolled up towel is

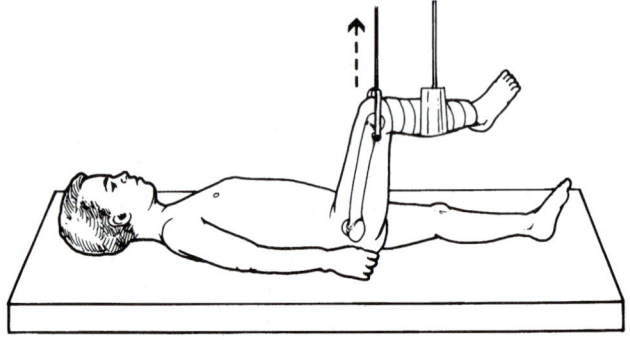

Figure 95.10. Standard 90/90 traction.

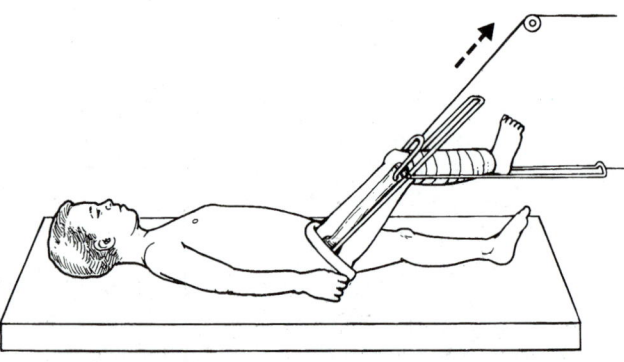

Figure 95.11. Modified balance suspension.

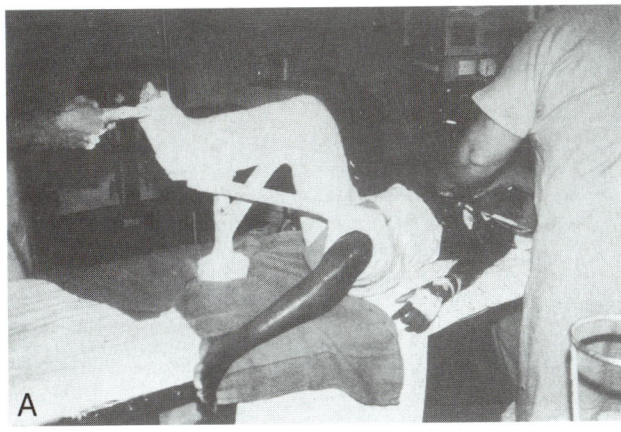

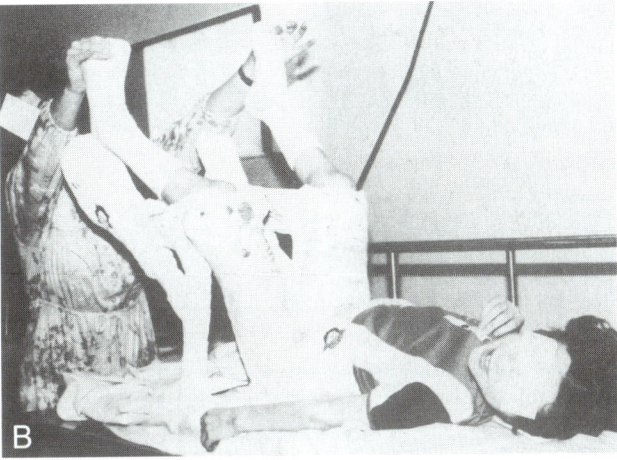

Figure 95.12. Pontoon spica cast.

placed over the abdomen, and the plaster is wrapped over it to avoid superior mesenteric artery syndrome.

The operative technique using flexible intramedullary nails consists of the following. After the traction is applied, the patient is stabilized and taken to the operating room. The patient is anesthetized and transferred to the fracture table. The involved limb is attached to the foot holder, and traction is applied across the knee to obtain satisfactory reduction. The distal femoral traction pin that had been used for preliminary treatment should be removed at this time. Reduction is assessed and confirmed using fluoroscopy. The involved extremity, from midcalf to the iliac crest, is draped free.

A sterile tourniquet may be applied about the proximal thigh when inserting the rods in a retrograde fashion. Proper rod length is confirmed by placing a rod against the skin under fluoroscopy. The rod should extend from cephalad to the distal femoral physis to the level of the greater trochanteric apophysis at the midcervical level proximally. The distal insertion site is the point approximately 3 cm from the growth plate for fractures occurring in the middle third or proximal third of the femur. An incision is made extending from the level of the insertion site distally, approximately 5 cm. The iliotibial band is incised and lined with its fibers, and the vastus lateralis is elevated to expose the distal femur for lateral nail placement. The fascia over the vastus medialis is incised in line with the skin incision, and the vastus medialis obliquus is elevated in an anterior direction when the nails are placed from the medial distal femur. A cruciate incision is made in the periosteum at the level of the insertion site, approximately 3 cm cephalad to the distal femoral physis when using a retrograde insertion technique. The cortex is then broached with drills of successive sizes up to 0.15 cm (0.375 in).

The first rod is bent into a C shape; 30° are necessary at the tip of the rod to facilitate bouncing the rod off of the opposite cortex during insertion. The rod is then inserted into the medullary canal and driven across the fracture site under fluoroscopy. The second rod is bent into an S shape and inserted in the same manner. The tips of both rods should lie flush with the cortex of the femur, distal to the insertion site but not abutting the physis. The surgical site is then closed in layers, with a drain if necessary. A long leg, bent-knee cast is applied if the fracture had grade IV comminution or if the child and parents are not reliable.

Fractures occurring at the junction between the middle and distal thirds of the diaphysis of the femur are stabilized with the distal medial and lateral retrograde rodding technique or with anterior grade rodding technique through the proximal insertion site. The proximal entry portal is distal to the greater trochanteric apophysis on the lateral cortex of the femur.

The child is kept non-weight bearing on the involved extremity, using a walker or crutches, for 2 to 3 weeks; then weight bearing as tolerated is begun. When a large callus is confirmed radiographically, usually 4 to 6 weeks, then full weight bearing is allowed. The rods are removed on an outpatient basis at 3 to 6 months after insertion. The rod removal is done only after fracture healing is complete.

BONY INJURIES ABOUT THE KNEE

RELEVANT ANATOMY

The knee is the largest joint in the body and is situated between the two largest lever arms in the body; thus the knee is subjected to tremendous force. It is important to understand the ossification centers about the knee when evaluating injuries in children. The secondary ossification center of the distal femur appears during the 9th fetal week and represents the only epiphyseal center present at birth. The distal femoral physis is the last growth plate to close in the femur, at 16 to 20 years of age, and contributes approximately 70% of length of femur and 37% of the length of the leg. This represents approximately 0.15 cm (0.375 in) of growth per year to the overall stature of the individual.

The tibial epiphyseal ossification center appears in the second year of life. This ossification center fuses with the proximal tibial epiphysis between 12 and 15 years of age. This physis also contributes approximately 0.15 cm (0.375 in) of growth per year to the overall stature of the individual. The proximal tibial physis is responsible for ap-

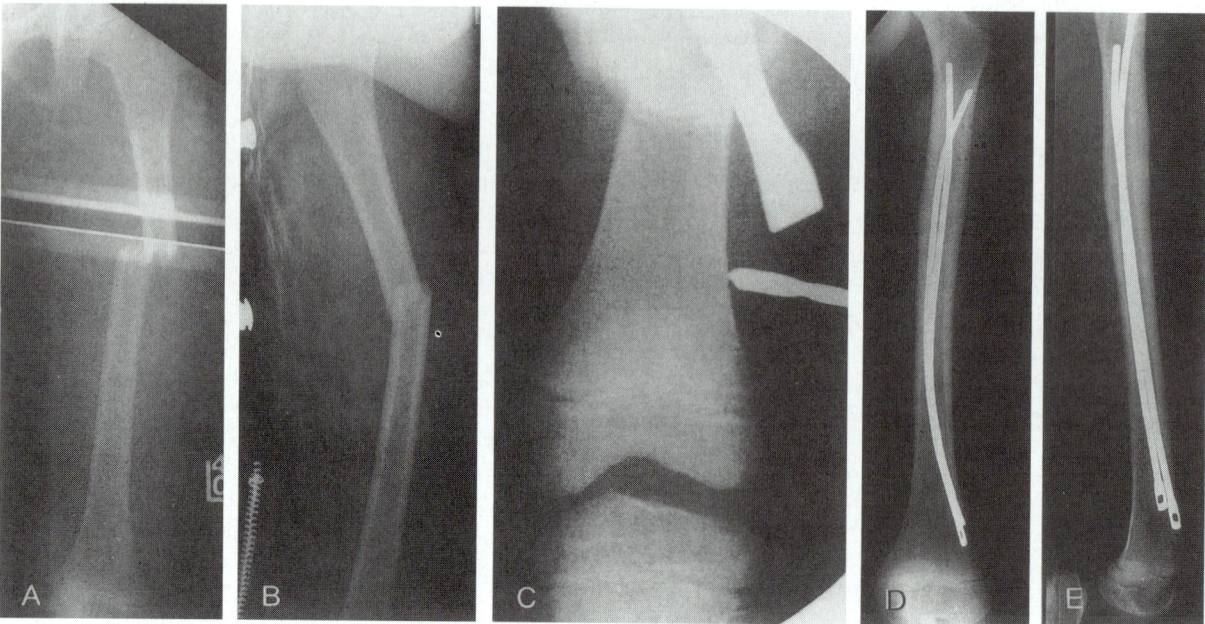

Figure 95.13. AP (**A**) and lateral (**B**) views of a 10-year-old male who sustained a fracture of the proximal third of the diaphysis of the femur. **C.** Lateral metaphyseal entry point for the retrograde flexible intramedullary nail. AP (**D**) and lateral (**E**) views showing the nails in place.

proximately 25% of the growth of the leg or 0.1 cm (0.25 in) of growth per year (19). The ossification center of the patella appears between 3 and 4 years of age. The epiphysis of the proximal fibula ossifies at about 4 years of age, and the proximal fibular physis closes at 25 years of age.

DISTAL FEMORAL PHYSEAL INJURIES

Distal femoral physeal injuries represent almost 50% of the physeal injuries in the lower extremity. The most common mechanism of injury is violent hyperextension of the knee. The distal femoral physis is the largest and the fastest-growing physis in the body. It has a horizontal orientation and is an extra-articular structure. The incidence of permanent physis growth impairment increases with the amount of initial fracture displacement and when there is a difficult forceful reduction and/or an incomplete reduction (20). Salter-Harris type II fractures are the most common injury involving the distal femoral physis. The metaphyseal bone that is left attached to the epiphysis is known as the Thurston-Holland fragment.

TREATMENT

Nonoperative Treatment

Nondisplaced fractures of the distal femoral physis are casted until healed. Patients are placed in single leg hip spica cast until the fracture has demonstrated early healing, which may take 2 to 3 weeks. Then a long leg cast is used for 2 to 3 additional weeks. Children with gross angulation of the distal femoral fracture should have a gentle closed reduction in the emergency room setting with posterior splinting. Formal closed reduction should be performed in

the operating room under general anesthesia. When longitudinal traction is applied along the axis of the femur, the fracture usually reduces adequately. C-arm fluoroscopy helps assess the stability of the fracture. Fractures with medial-lateral displacement are inherently less stable than fractures with anterior-posterior displacement.

General angulation in the plane of motion is better tolerated by the patient than is varus or valgus angulation. As much as 30° of angulation in the frontal plane can be accepted in the young child. Between 5° and 7° of varus valgus angulation is acceptable in the sagittal plane. Rotational malalignment is not acceptable. If the reduction is adequate and the fracture is stable, the patient is placed in a single leg hip spica cast. Weekly radiographic evaluations assess fracture stability. Unstable injuries are fixed with two small percutaneous smooth pins. The pins are removed when the fracture has healed, usually in 4 to 6 weeks.

Operative Treatment

Displaced Salter-Harris type II fractures are first reduced in a closed manner and then casted if the fracture is stable. Unstable fractures are fixed with a horizontal pin or screw through the metaphyseal fragment, parallel to the physis when possible. If, however, the metaphyseal fragment is not large enough to accept fixation, then smooth crossed pins are used to hold the reduced fracture. The pins should cross the physis near the center but remain far enough away from each other to provide rotational stability. The central location decreases the risk of angular deformity if a bar eventually develops in the growth plate. After the fracture has been stabilized with percutaneous pinning, the involved extremity is placed in a long leg cast. Physeal fractures in obese children can be difficult, if not impossible, to treat with casting. Cross pinning will stabilize the injury. Fractures with anterior displacement of the distal fragment can be reduced with the patient in the prone position and the knee flexed 90°; the intact periosteum acts as an internal splint. On the other hand, posteriorly displaced distal femoral physeal fractures are reduced with the patient in the supine position. The knee is brought into full extension after longitudinal traction, and the posterior periosteum is used to stabilize the fracture.

Displaced Salter-Harris types III and IV fractures require an anatomical reduction. The treatment of choice is ORIF; screws or pins are directed parallel to the physis to stabilize the fracture. Internal fixation should not cross the physeal plate, to avoid further injury to the growth plate. These fractures heal in 4 to 6 weeks. The smooth fixation pins are removed at the time of radiographic healing.

Complications

The most serious complication associated with a fracture of the distal femoral physis is vascular injury, which occurs in approximately 2% of displaced fractures. The popliteal artery is the most frequently involved structure. The mechanism that produces this injury is hyperextension, resulting in arterial transection or intimal tear (with or without thrombus formation and/or arterial spasm). Vascular injuries are less common in fractures with medial or lateral displacement. If a vascular injury is suspected, the patient should have an arteriogram. Children without definitive clinical findings of a vascular insult should be evaluated with noninvasive peripheral vascular Doppler studies, if available. All patients with a fracture of the distal femoral physis should be monitored closely, because intimal tears may not be immediately evident. Fractures with a vascular injury should be stabilized with percutaneous pinning with some type of fixation.

Physeal bars can result from distal femoral growth plate fractures. Bars involving less than 50% of the physis that produce an angular deformity should be resected (21). Resection is contraindicated if the bar involves more than 50% of the physeal area, the patient has less than 2 years of growth remaining, or there is a history of active infection. Corrective osteotomies can be performed either at the time of bar resection or at skeletal maturity.

Limb length inequality can develop after distal femoral physeal fractures if a bar forms. A predicted leg length discrepancy of 2 cm or less can be treated with a shoe lift. A leg length difference between 3 and 6 cm in a skeletally immature patient can be corrected with an epiphysiodesis on the normal side. The time of the epiphysiodesis is calculated using the Moseley chart or the Green-Anderson table. Limb length discrepancy between 6 and 18 cm may require limb lengthening (with or without the contralateral epiphysiodesis) or diaphyseal shortening.

FRACTURES OF THE PATELLA

The patella is the largest sesamoid bone in the body. Ossification of the patella begins at 3.5 years of age but can be delayed until age 6. Patella ossification begins centrally and extends peripherally in an irregular fashion. This makes the diagnosis of the fracture or osteochondritis lesions difficult by radiographs alone in the immature child. A secondary ossification center occasionally develops in the superior lateral aspect of the patella. This presents as a separate center and creates a bipartite patella in 0.2 to 6.0% of the normal population. All fractures are classified by anatomical location, configuration, and displacement.

TREATMENT

Children with nondisplaced fractures of the patella are placed in a cylindrical cast with 5° of flexion. Full weight bearing is remitted, and isometric quadriceps strengthening is begun approximately 7 days after injury. The cast is removed in approximately 4 weeks. Displaced transverse patellar fractures and the so-called sleeve fractures are reduced anatomically to decrease the risks of posttraumatic arthritis and restore normal extensor function. Sleeve fractures are commonly missed on x-ray evaluation. An osteochondral sleeve avulses from the main body of the patella, often with a large portion of the articular surface. Both types of fractures require ORIF, with smooth pins and a wire (tension band) supplemented by a cylindrical cast. The cast is removed in 4 to 6 weeks after surgery, and motion is begun at that time.

A total patellectomy is recommended in fractures with severe comminution that cannot be reduced.

FRACTURES OF THE PROXIMAL TIBIAL EPIPHYSIS AND PHYSIS

Fractures of the proximal tibial physis represent less than 1% of all physeal injuries. The majority of these fractures are Salter-Harris types I and II injuries.

TREATMENT

Nondisplaced fractures of the proximal tibial physis are treated in a long leg cast. Displaced physeal fractures of the proximal tibia can be reduced under general anesthesia. If closed reduction fails, ORIF is justified. Small metaphyseal fragments and Salter-Harris type IV fractures should be resected at the time of reduction to decrease the risk of physeal bar formation. The leg is immobilized in a long leg cast for 4 to 6 weeks, until the physis has united. After closed reduction, the patient should be observed, including frequent neurovascular examinations. Manipulations can be done within the first week; after that, it is best to let the fracture heal. Corrective osteotomies can be performed later, if needed.

FRACTURES OF THE TIBIAL EMINENCE

Tibial eminence fractures are uncommon injuries. Type I injuries are nondisplaced fractures through the tibial eminence. Type II fractures are elevated from an anterior fracture bed and have a posterior hinge. Type III fractures are characterized by a complete separation that involves fragment from its bed on the tibial epiphysis.

TREATMENT

Type I fractures of the tibial eminence can be treated conservatively in a long leg cast with the knee in extension. The foot is included in the cast to minimize the torsional forces on the tibial plateau. Type II fractures are reduced with the knee in extension. Residual displacement of 1 to 2 mm is acceptable and has no effect on long-term results, provided the patient has full knee extension. Unreducible type II and most type III injuries require an arthroscopic or open reduction. The anterior horn of the lateral meniscus often prevents this reduction. Arthroscopic stabilization of fracture with a Herbert screw or a small cannulated screw has yielded excellent results. Other methods of fixation include K wires and sutures.

AVULSION FRACTURES OF THE TIBIAL TUBEROSITY

Most fractures of the tibial tuberosity occur between the ages of 13 and 16 years. Type I injuries are characterized by a fracture through the small distal portion of the tibial tuberosity. Type II fractures split the epiphysis of the tuberosity from the epiphysis of the proximal tibia. In type III injuries, the fracture line is propagated into the joint (22).

TREATMENT

Undisplaced types I and II fractures can be treated with immobilization in a cylindrical cast in full extension. Displaced type II and all type III injuries must have an anatomical reduction and stabilization with internal fixation. Patients are placed in a cylindrical cast for 4 to 6 weeks after surgery. Children with a type III fracture are at risk for a compartment syndrome and should be monitored appropriately.

FRACTURES OF THE TIBIAL AND FIBULAR SHAFTS

Fractures of the tibia and fibula are the most common fractures in the lower extremity in children. Tibia and fibula shaft fractures are more often caused by indirect forces than by direct blows. Axial loading with the lower extremity rotation is the most common indirect force that produces tibial and fibular shaft fractures. Most of these fractures are oblique. On the other hand, most fractures resulting from direct trauma are transverse or comminuted. Classification of tibial fractures is based primarily on anatomic location.

FRACTURES OF THE PROXIMAL TIBIAL METAPHYSIS

Fractures of the proximal tibial metaphysis are common. In cases of high-energy trauma it is important to rule out associated vascular energy at the trifurcation of the popliteal artery. Another complication associated with this fracture is posttraumatic tibia valga. The exact cause of this complication is unknown. Explanations have ranged from poor initial closed reduction, periosteal interposition at the fracture site, and/or an overgrowth of the medial aspect of the tibia. I strongly recommend that the patient's parents be counseled on the tendency for this fracture to angulate with growth.

TREATMENT

Nondisplaced fractures are treated with a long leg cast. Displaced fractures are reduced carefully and placed in a long leg cast with the knee in extension for 6 weeks. X-rays are taken at weekly intervals for the first 3 weeks to assess any changes in position. Postfracture bracing does not prevent the development of tibial valgus. The degree of valgus peaks at 12 to 18 months after the injury. Resolution of the deformity sometimes occurs after this time. Residual deformity of the tibia can be corrected by an osteotomy when the patient is older than 10 years. Surgical correction before this time is associated with recurrence.

FRACTURES OF THE PROXIMAL FIBULA

Isolated fractures of the proximal fibula are rare. The most common mechanism is a direct blow. Proximal fibular fractures are occasionally associated with ankle fractures. Thorough neurologic evaluation should be done to assess the peroneal nerve.

Treatment of isolated proximal fibular fractures is symptomatic. Weight bearing is begun as tolerated. A compressive dressing and crutches are used until the acute pain subsides.

FRACTURES OF THE TIBIAL AND FIBULAR DIAPHYSIS

Nondisplaced or greenstick fractures of the tibia are placed in a long leg cast. These fractures generally heal within 5 to 6 weeks. Displaced fractures can generally be treated in a closed manner. Children younger than 8 should undergo a closed reduction of tibial fractures for which the varus or valgus is less than 8° of angulation and there is less than 15° of recurvature, less than 8° of anterior angulation, less than 10 mm of shortening, and less than 5° of rotation. Children 8 years old or older require a closed reduction for fractures with less than 5° of varus or valgus angulation, less than 10° recurvatum, less than 5° of anterior angulation, less than 5 mm of shortening, and less than 5° of rotation.

The neurovascular status must be monitored, and compartment syndrome must be ruled out. After closed reduction, the initial cast should be a long leg cast with the knee bent at approximately 45° to control rotation. The foot is maintained in neutral or slight plantar flexion. The fracture alignment is checked at weekly intervals for 3 to 4 weeks. The cast may need to be changed because of decreased swelling. For children older than 10 years, a patellar tendon–bearing cast or cast brace can be applied after 3 weeks of long leg cast treatment. Patients with high-energy fractures and older children require longer cast treatment; e.g., it may take 3 months for a comminuted high-energy fracture to heal completely. Open fractures take approximately twice as long to achieve union as do closed fractures. The child may limp and externally rotate the fractured limb for several weeks after the cast is removed, which must be thoroughly explained to the patient's family.

FRACTURES OF THE DISTAL TIBIAL METAPHYSIS

TREATMENT

Fractures of the distal tibial metaphysis may be complete or incomplete. The anterior cortex often becomes impacted, producing a recurvatum. Casting may exaggerate the deformity, unless the cast is applied with the foot in mild equinus. If the anterior cortex is impacted and the recurvatum is greater than 10° to 15°, the preferred treatment is a closed reduction under general anesthesia. The foot is placed in enough equinus to prevent recurrence of the angulation. A long leg cast is worn for 3 to 4 weeks; a short leg walking cast, with the ankle in neutral dorsiflexion, is then worn until healing has occurred.

Complications

Complications associated with tibial shaft fractures include malunion, malrotation, leg length discrepancy, delayed union, nonunion, vascular injuries, and compartment syndromes. Malrotation will not correct spontaneously with growth and remodeling. These fractures should be watched closely after closed reduction; and if a severe rotational malalignment exists, a supramalleolar osteotomy is preferred to correct the deformity. Overgrowth in the tibia does not occur with the regularity that it does in the femur. Delayed unions and nonunions are rare in tibial shaft fractures. Vascular injuries can occur with proximal tibia metaphyseal fractures.

All tibial fractures should be monitored closely for a compartment syndrome. The pain from a compartment syndrome is intense and out of proportion to the severity of the injury. The pulses are intact until late in the course of the compartment syndrome. There may be sensory deficits in the foot and weakness of the ankle, foot, and the toes. Involved compartments may be tense. Pain is present with passive toe flexion and extension. If there is any evidence of a compartment syndrome after a fracture, the circular cast should be bivalved, the padding cut, and the compartment pressures measured (23,24).

FRACTURES OF THE ANKLE

RELEVANT ANATOMY AND PATHOGENESIS

Ankle injuries are one of the most common orthopaedic injuries in the pediatric population. The distal tibial epiphysis develops from a secondary center of ossification and is usually apparent during the first year of life. The medial malleolus develops from a distal extension of the epiphysis and is first radiographically apparent at age 7. By age 10, it is fully developed. Occasionally the malleolus will ossify

from an accessory center, which must be distinguished from a fracture. Union of the epiphysis with the shaft occurs by age 15 in girls and age 17 in boys. Closure of the distal tibial physis occurs gradually from medial to lateral, usually taking place over a period of about 18 months. During this period, two unique, multiplane fracture patterns may occur: the juvenile Tillaux fracture and the triplane fracture.

Tillaux Fractures

The juvenile Tillaux fracture, Salter-Harris type III fracture of the distal tibia, occurs in abduction injuries of the ankle; the anterior lateral aspect of the distal tibial epiphysis becomes avulsed by the pull of the anterior tibiofibular ligament (Fig. 95.14). The distal tibial physis closed from the posterior medial aspect in an anterolateral projection. This makes the anterolateral portion of the distal tibial epiphysis susceptible to fracture during adolescence. Another mechanism thought to produce this fracture is an external rotation force applied to the supinated foot. This fracture is also known as the hidden ankle fracture of adolescents. If the growth plate is nearly fused, the epiphyseal fragment is small and may be hidden from view by the fibula on an AP view of the ankle.

Triplane Fractures

A triplane fracture results when an external rotation force is applied to a supinated foot or a combination of external rotation and plantar flexion forces. Triplane fractures are Salter-Harris type IV fractures with two or three fragments. They may occur through the transverse, sagittal, and coronal planes. Triplane fractures usually occur in adolescents. CT scans or tomograms are often needed to com-

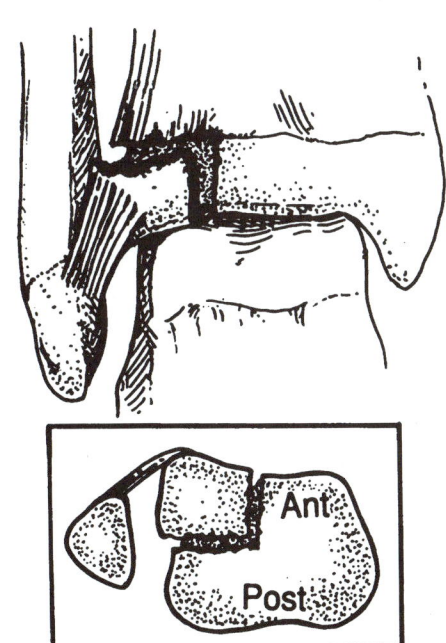

Figure 95.14. Juvenile Tillaux fracture. *Ant,* anterior; *Post,* posterior.

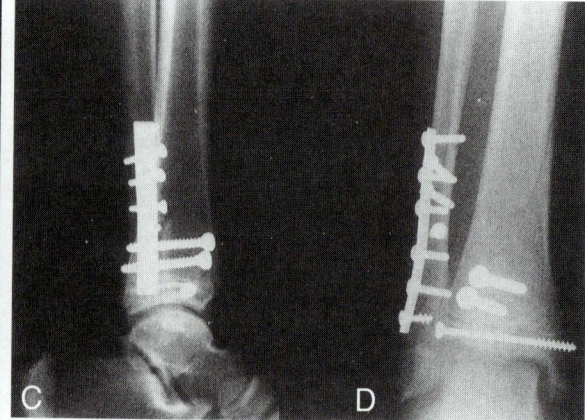

Figure 95.15. AP (**A**) and lateral (**B**) views showing a 14-year-old male with a three-part triplane fracture of the distal tibia. AP (**C**) and lateral (**D**) views after ORIF.

pletely evaluate the fracture. The epiphyseal component lies near the sagittal plane and is best seen on the AP view. The physeal separation is in the transverse plane and is often not seen but implied from the position of the fragments. The metaphyseal fracture lies in the coronal plane and is usually apparent in the lateral view. Occasionally, an oblique or spiral fracture of the fibula is present (25).

TREATMENT

Tillaux Fractures

Closed reduction of the Tillaux fracture may be accomplished by gentle internal rotation with longitudinal traction. A long leg cast should be applied with the ankle in neutral dorsiflexion and the foot in mild supination. After 3 to 4 weeks, weight bearing may be permitted with a short leg cast. If the displacement is more than 2 mm after closed reduction, ORIF with interfragmentary screws should be performed. Open reduction is also recommended if the congruity of the ankle joint cannot be restored by closed means. CT scans or tomograms often help evaluate this fracture.

Triplane Fractures

An initial closed reduction should be performed for triplane fractures. Fractures with less than 2 mm of displace-ment after closed reduction can be treated in a long leg cast. Fractures with more than 2 mm of displacement should be treated with ORIF with an interfragmentary screw (Fig. 95.15). Anatomic reduction of the interarticular component is the goal.

Complications include partial physeal arrest deformity, resulting from malunion, limb length inequality, posttraumatic osteoarthritis, and aseptic necrosis. Osseous bridges involving up to 50% of the physis are amenable to resection. If tomograms reveal more than 50% involvement, an osteotomy should be performed. If an osteotomy is necessary, it should be an opening wedge to compensate for any shortening that may accompany the deformity. Even when properly performed, an osteotomy may produce a physeal arrest. An epiphysiodesis of the distal fibular physis may be indicated at the time of osteotomy. In an older child with limited growth remaining, a physeal bar resection may not provide sufficient correction. A combination of an osteotomy and epiphysiodesis of the remaining physis should be considered. Limb length inequality is rare in the younger child. When a discrepancy of more than 2.5 cm is anticipated, a carefully timed epiphysiodesis may be considered. Limb lengthening may be necessary for greater degrees of shortening. In the older child, the ultimate limb length inequality may be minimal, and lifts may be worn.

IV | The Foot

There are 26 bones in the foot, which may be divided into three areas: the hindfoot, the midfoot, and the forefoot. The bones of the hindfoot are the talus and os calcis. The bones of the midfoot are the navicular; first, second, and third cuneiforms; and the cuboid. The forefoot consists of the metatarsals and phalanges.

FRACTURES OF THE TALUS

CLASSIFICATION

Talus fractures are classified into three types: head, neck, and body fractures. Talar neck fractures are further classified as type I, vertical fracture; type II, vertical fracture with dislocation or subluxation of the subtalar joint; and type III, vertical fracture with dislocation of the talar body from both the ankle and subtalar joint. Talar body fractures are classified as type I, transchondral or compression fractures of the talar dome; type II, shearing fractures, which may be coronal, sagittal, or horizontal, involving the entire talar body; type III, fractures of the posterior tubercle; type IV, fractures of the lateral process; and type V, crush injuries of the talar body. CT scans are often needed for complete evaluation of talus fractures.

TREATMENT

Talar head fractures that are nondisplaced are treated in a short leg, nonwalking cast. Displaced fractures are treated by excision of the fragment if small or by reduction and internal fixation if large.

Type I talar neck fractures are treated by immobilization and non-weight bearing with a plaster cast until union is demonstrated radiographically. Type II talar neck fractures are reduced by closed reduction and subsequent internal fixation. The internal fixation may be achieved with a pin or, preferably, a screw to provide compression. If closed manipulation does not result in anatomic alignment, ORIF is suggested, using an approach that does not interfere with the blood supply of the body of the talus. The recommended approach is between the anterior tibial artery and the extensor hallucis longus. An osteotomy of the medial malleolus may be performed for greater exposure. Type III fractures of the talar neck are treated with a closed manipulation. If this fails, which it often does, an anterior and medial approach is used. The medial malleolus is osteomized, which is necessary for visualization, and ORIF is performed with a cancellous screw.

The prognosis of these fractures depends on the presence of avascular necrosis. The most valuable indicator of avascular necrosis is the Hawkins sign (26), which is subchondral atrophy of the dome of the talus on the AP view of the ankle and is visible 6 to 8 weeks after injury. If the subchondral atrophy is present, then there is vascularity of the talus. In the young child, this finding may not be present, because the body of the talus is not completely ossified and the dome of the talus is still chondral. MRI studies and bone scanning may be used to evaluate the vascular area of the talar body. The incidence of avascular necrosis in type I fractures ranges from 0 to 13%; type II, 20 to 50%; and type III, 80 to 100%.

Talar body fractures are generally treated in a short leg cast and non-weight bearing for 4 to 8 weeks; the foot is in the neutral position or slightly flexed. Type IV fractures of the lateral process of the talus are the second most common fracture of the talar body. These displaced fractures must be fixed with ORIF. The lateral process serves as the attachment for the lateral ligaments of the foot and ankle. This fracture must be kept in mind for patients with apparent residual sprained ankles that are not responding to treatment. Fractures seen late that have developed a symptomatic fi-

brous union or nonunion may be treated by excision of the small fragment.

FRACTURES OF THE CALCANEUS

Calcaneal fractures are generally compression injuries, as from a fall from a height. Fractures in the lumbar spine are commonly associated with this fracture. Type I calcaneal fractures are extra-articular; type II fractures are intra-articular. Intra-articular fractures are divided into sustentaculum fractures, tongue fractures, joint depression fractures, and comminuted fractures. CT scans are often needed to fully evaluate this fracture pattern.

TREATMENT

When choosing a treatment plan for fractures of the calcaneus, the clinician must consider the age of the patient, degree of displacement. involvement of posterior facet, and involvement of anterior articular surface. The current trend is toward performing ORIF for fractures that are intra-articular and/or have gross distortion of the anatomy of the calcaneus. Fractures of the anterior part of the os calcis are generally treated nonoperatively with short leg casting and non-weight bearing, unless the fracture is large and intra-articular, in which case, ORIF may be necessary. Tuberosity fractures are treated with closed reduction, unless the fracture fragment is large and displaced; then ORIF may be considered.

Fractures of the medial and lateral process of the calcaneus usually occur when the heel is adducted or abducted when it strikes the ground. Immobilization in a short leg walking cast is used. If the fracture is large and displaced, closed reduction may be attempted, but usually open reduction is not performed. Nondisplaced fractures of the calcaneus without subtalar involvement are treated with a non–weight-bearing, short leg cast for 8 to 12 weeks. Comminuted fractures, in which there is complete disruption of the entire calcaneus, are difficult to reconstitute. They do not do well with open reduction.

FRACTURES OF THE MIDFOOT

Isolated fractures of the midfoot, including the navicular, cuboid, and cuneiforms, are unusual. When such injury occurs, there is usually a combination of fractures and/or subluxation of the adjacent joints, because of the interlocking structure and rigidity of the tarsal bones. Generally, fractures of the midfoot can be treated with a short leg cast without weight bearing, unless there is gross displacement of the fracture fragments.

FRACTURES OF THE METATARSALS

The first metatarsal has an essential role in the support and function of the foot, providing stability to the medial side of the foot. For this reason, precise reduction of fractures of the first metatarsal is extremely important. If there is displacement of the first metatarsal associated with the fracture, it must be adequately reduced and pinned, K wires should probably be used, either longitudinally or through the adjacent second metatarsal. ORIF, using screw and compression techniques, is rarely necessary. Nondisplaced fractures of the first metatarsal may be treated with a short leg, non–weight-bearing cast for 2 to 4 weeks. A weight-bearing, short leg cast is then used for an additional 2 to 4 weeks, until the fracture is healed. Lateral metatarsal shaft fractures are usually stable, unless there has been gross disruption resulting from a force of great magnitude. Nondisplaced or minimally displaced lateral metatarsal shaft fractures can be treated in a postoperative wooden shoe. If there is gross displacement, reduction may be performed, with either finger traps or ORIF.

Fractures at the base of the fifth metatarsal should be considered as separate entities. These fractures can be classified as type I, fractures of the metaphyseal diaphyseal junction; type II, fractures at the metaphyseal–diaphyseal junction with clinical or radiographic evidence of previous injury; and type III, fractures of the styloid process. Fractures at the metaphyseal–diaphyseal proximal junction may be treated in a short leg cast for 4 to 6 weeks. The risk of nonunion increases when there is evidence of a previous injury. For athletes, intramedullary screw fixation with a bone graft is the suggested treatment; the screw head is recessed. A short leg walking cast is used for 6 to 12 weeks; activity depends on clinical and roentgenogram progression.

Fractures of the styloid process at the base of the fifth metatarsal are generally treated with either a wooden postoperative shoe or, if there is marked displacement, a short leg walking cast.

FRACTURES OF THE PHALANGES

Phalangeal fractures of the large toe in which there is marked displacement should be reduced, if possible, with closed reduction and correctional wire fixation, if necessary. Open reduction is indicated if closed reduction fails. It is important to correct any intra-articular fracture, especially of the large toe and the metatarsal phalangeal and interphalangeal joints. Generally, a phalangeal fracture can be treated in a short leg walking cast with a toe plate for 3 weeks; then the patient should wear a postoperative wooden shoe for an additional 3 weeks, depending on the nature of the fracture and the progress of healing.

REFERENCES

1. Mann DC, Rajmaira S. Dislocation of physeal and nonphyseal fractures in 1,650 long-bone fractures in children aged 0–16 years. J Pediatr Orthop 1990;10:713–716.
2. Freiberg KS. Remodeling after distal forearm fractures. Part I. Acta Orthop Scand 1979;50:537–546.
3. Freiberg KS. Remodeling after distal forearm fractures. Parts II–III. Acta Orthop Scand 1979;50:731–749.
4. Matthews LS. The effect on pronation and supination of angular mal-alignment and forearm fractures. Experimental study. J Bone Joint Surg 1982;64A:114–117.
5. Price CT, Scott DS, Kurzner ME, Flynn JC. Malunited forearm fractures in children. J Pediatric Orthop 1990;10:705–712.
6. Baumme beitrega zur kenntins der frakturen am ellenbogen-gelink. Unter besonder berucksichtgueng der spatflagen. I. Allgemeines und fractura supracondylica beitr C. Klin Chir 146:1–50.
7. Eaton RG, Green WT. Epimysiotomy and fasciotomy in treatment of Volkmann's ischemic contracture. Orthop Clin North Am 1972; 3:175–186.
8. Flynn JC, Richards JF, Saltzman RI. Prevention and treatment of non-union or slightly displaced fractures of the lateral humeral condyle in children. J Bone Joint Surg 1979;57A:1087–1092.
9. Schwab GH, Bennett JB, Woods GW, Tullos HS. Biomechanics of elbow instability: the role of medial collateral ligament. Clin Orthop 1980;146:42–52.
10. Millis MB, Singer IJ, Hall JE. Supracondylar fracture of the humerus in children. Further experience with a study in orthopaedic decision making. Clin Orthop 1984;188:90–97.
11. Neer CS, Horowitz BS. Fractures of the proximal humeral epiphyseal plate. Clin Orthop 1965;41:24–31.
12. Dameron TB, Rockwood CA. Fractures and dislocations of the shoulder. In: Rockwood CA, Williams KE Jr, King RE, eds. Fractures in children. Philadelphia: Lippincott, 1984:589–607, 624–653.
13. Beebe AC, Bell DF. The management of severely displaced fractures of the proximal humerus. Tech Orthop 1989;4:1–4.
14. Chance GO. Note on a type affliction fracture of the spine. Br J Radiol 1948;21:452–453.
15. Glassman SD, Johnson JR, Holt RT. Seatbelt injuries in children. J Trauma 1992;33:882–886.
16. Delbet MP. Fractures du eol de femur. Bull Mem Soc Chir 1909; 35:387–389.
17. Ferry AM, Edgar MS. Modified Bryants traction. J. Bone Joint Surg 1966;48A:533–536.
18. Celiker O, Cetin I, Sahlan S, et al. Femoral shaft fractures in children: technique of immediate treatment with supracondylar Kirschner wires and one-and-a-half spica cast. J Pediatr Orthop 1988;8:580–584.
19. Ogden JA. Skeletal injury in the child. Philadelphia: Saunders, 1990.
20. Coates R. Knock-knee deformity following upper tibial "green-stick" fractures. J Bone Joint Surg 1977;59B:516.
21. Riseborough EJ, Barrett IR, Shapiro F. Growth disturbances following distal femoral physeal fracture-separation. J Bone Joint Surg 1983;65A:885–893.
22. Watson-Jones R. Fractures and joint injuries. 4th ed. Edinburgh: Livingstone, 1955–1956.
23. Willhoit DR, Moll JH. Early recognition and treatment of impending Volkmann's ischemia in the lower extremity. Arch Surg 1970; 100:11–16.
24. Whitesides TE Jr, Haney TG, Morimoto K, Harada H. Tissue pressure measurements as a determinant for the need of fasciotomy. Clin Orthop 1975;113:43–51.
25. Marmor L. An unusual fracture of the tibial epiphysis. Clin Orthop 1970;73:132–135.
26. Hawkins LG. Fractures of the neck of the talus. J Bone Joint Surg 1970;52A:991–1002.

Suggested Readings

Blount WP. Fractures in children. Baltimore: Williams & Wilkins, 1955.
Rang M. Children's fractures. Philadelphia: Lippincott, 1983.

Tarsal Coalition

Tarsal coalition is a failure of segmentation of two or more foot bones that results in stiffness in one or both feet and symptoms. There are many types of coalitions, but two are the most common: calcaneonavicular and talocalcaneal.

RELEVANT ANATOMY AND PATHOGENESIS

Tarsal coalition is a misnomer, since the condition results from the failure of segmentation of two or more tarsal bones (1). Tarsal coalition is a fibrous (syndesmosis), cartilaginous (synchondrosis), or bony (synostosis) connection of two or more tarsal bones. The talocalcaneal and the calcaneonavicular coalitions are by far the most common forms (2).

Talocalcaneal coalition, or subtalar fusion, interferes with the gliding motion of the subtalar joint, causing a hinge motion at the midtarsal joints because the medially located calcaneal joint facet is a major weight-bearing area. The defect is congenital but appears clinically in adolescence. It results from a failure of differentiation and segmentation of the primitive mesenchyme, resulting in a lack of joint formation. The cause is unknown. The incidence has been estimated to be less than 1% of the general population. The calcaneonavicular coalition is bilateral in about 60% of cases, and the talocalcaneal bar is bilateral in 50% of cases. The other coalitions are rare. Occasionally, more than one coalition pattern can be present in one foot.

Tarsal coalition can be associated with congenital abnormalities and syndromic diagnoses. Associated syndromes include Apert's syndrome, clubfoot, and fibular hemimelia (75%). Autosomal dominant inheritance with variable penetrance is the likely mechanism of transmission (3).

INITIAL FINDINGS, PHYSICAL EXAMINATION, AND DIAGNOSIS

Many adults with coalition are asymptomatic; symptoms, when present, develop during adolescence. In most cases, the onset of pain seems to correlate with the time the bar ossifies. For a calcaneonavicular bar, the age range is 8 to 12 years; and for a talocalcaneal coalition, it is 12 to 16 years. With ossification, subtalar motion is progressively decreased, leading to symptoms as the joint is stressed. Onset may coincide with trauma or increased activity, such as participation in athletics, in activities played on uneven ground, and in sports that limit ankle motion (e.g., in-line roller-skating and cross-country track).

The pain is usually vague, insidious in onset, aching in character, and localized to the region of the subtalar joint. It is worsened by activity and relieved by rest. Patients with calcaneonavicular coalitions, in particular, have a synovitis in the sinus tarsi area, which causes reflex activity in the peroneal tendons, resulting in the so-called peroneal spastic flatfoot (4,5).

Subtalar motion is restricted or painful. Talocalcaneal coalition is often associated with loss of subtalar motion, which may lead to increased stress on the ankle joint and thus an increased number of ankle sprains. True peroneal muscle spasms are rarely found. Quick forced varus or a reflex hammer tap on the peroneal tendons elicits a painful contraction. Electromyelogram studies do not demonstrate any spasticity. The sinus tarsi region can be tender locally. The hindfoot is frequently in valgus, and the medial longitudinal arch is flattened. There is often a tightness of the gastrocnemius-soleus, which is worsened by the increased valgus.

It is important to rule out other causes of subtalar-restricted motion (e.g., rheumatoid arthritis, osteomyelitis, osteochondral fracture of the anterior facet, gout, osteoid osteoma) and benign tumors (e.g., aneurysmal bone cyst) (6).

RADIOLOGIC STUDIES

Tarsal coalition may be totally asymptomatic and found incidentally on radiographs. Specific views are needed to demonstrate tarsal coalitions. AP and lateral view x-rays will demonstrate neither of the classic types of coalition. The Canadian Army foot series includes views that will help assess tarsal coalition, e.g., the lateral oblique (45° Slomann) subtalar view and the axial (about 45° Harris) hindfoot view. The axial view is required to demonstrate a talocalcaneal bar, which forms medially in the area of the sustentaculum tali. The effectiveness of this view for visualizing the subtalar joint is enhanced by measuring the angle of the posterior facet on the lateral radiograph and then adjusting the Harris view to this inclination. The lateral oblique view demonstrates a calcaneonavicular coalition (Fig. 96.1). In patients in whom the bar has not ossified, the diagnosis is suggested by an elongated process of the calcaneus, blunting of the subtalar process, narrowing of the posterior subtalar joint, and talar beaking.

For difficult cases, CT scanning is invaluable for diagnosis and preoperative planning. The correct inclination of the CT sections is important for elucidating the presence of a bar. Coronal sections are useful for the talocalcaneal bar (Fig. 96.2), and longitudinal sections are taken for the calcaneonavicular bar. MRI studies may depict more coalitions but may not be able to differentiate synovitis from fibrous coalitions.

Plain AP and lateral x-rays may demonstrate secondary degenerative changes, including talar beaking (now considered a ligament traction spur), broadening or rounding of the lateral process of the talus, narrowing of the subtalar joint, and concaving of the talus neck's undersurface. They also allow the clinician to note failure to see the middle subtalar joint and will show a ball-and-socket ankle, another late degenerative compensatory sign (7).

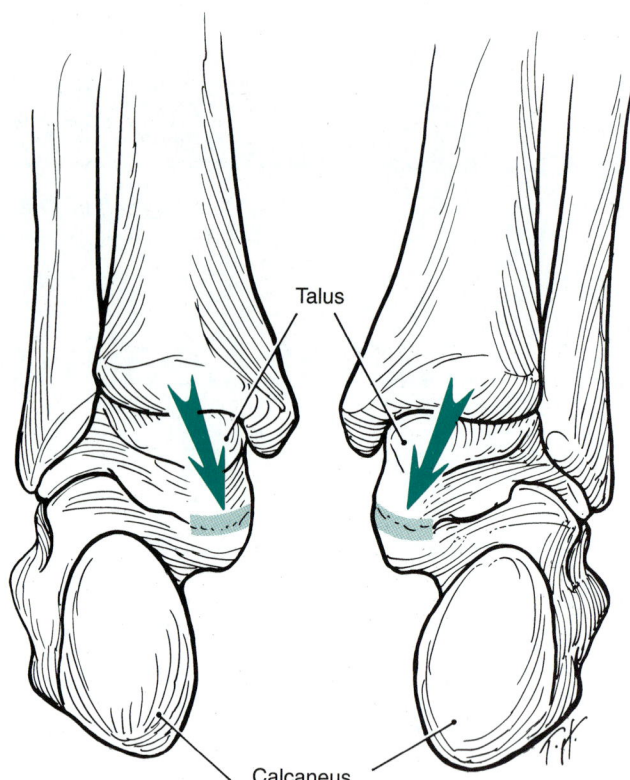

Figure 96.2. Coronal image showing a medial talocalcaneal coalition.

TREATMENT

Nonoperative Treatment and Indications for Surgery

The initial treatment should be conservative and nonsurgical. Attempts to alleviate the pain include Plastizote inserts and shoe modifications to support the medial arch of the foot. Physical therapy to stretch the Achilles tendon and strengthen the posterior tibial muscle should be part of an everyday regimen. Patients who do not respond to these measures may do favorably with 3 to 6 weeks of immobilization in a short leg walking cast. This treatment may have to be repeated at intervals during adolescence.

The main indication for surgery is persistent pain that is not relieved by conservative treatment. It is not clear if patients without major symptoms would benefit from surgery to prevent worsening. Calcaneonavicular bars are amenable to resection, and a high percentage of cases do well. Surgical excision of a calcaneonavicular bar before the age of 12 to 14 years often relieves symptoms. The presence of a talar beak is not a contraindication for resection, as was once thought. The results of talocalcaneal resections are less predictable, and more than 50% involvement of the middle facet is a relative contraindication to resection. Persistent hindfoot valgus may also be associated with a poor result (8–10).

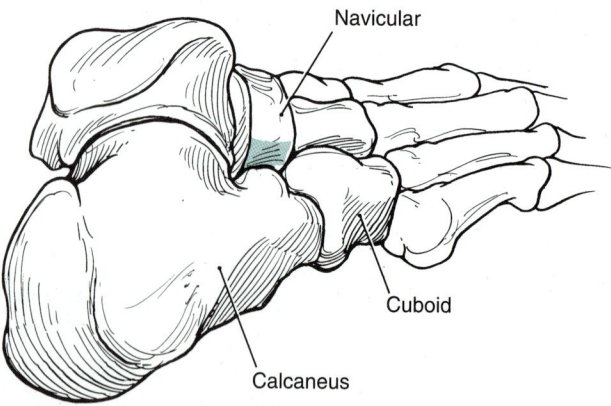

Figure 96.1. Lateral oblique view showing a calcaneonavicular bar.

Clinical Table: Tarsal Coalition

Procedure	Indications	Technique	Anatomy	Pitfalls
Calcaneonavicular bar correction	• Persistent pain after failure of conservative treatment	• Lateral Ollier approach	• Sensory branches of dorsolateral foot • Extensor brevis • Peroneal tendons	• Incomplete resection with recurrence • Migration of fat graft or muscle interposition graft • Persistent pain • Need for orthosis
Talocalcaneal bar correction	• Persistent pain after failure of conservative treatment	• Medial approach • Removal by burr or rongeur	• Sustentaculum tali	• Persistent hindfoot valgus • Incomplete resection • Persistent pain • Need for orthosis

Operative Treatment

CALCANEONAVICULAR BAR

For correction of a calcaneonavicular bar, the lateral Ollier approach is used (Clinical Table). All cartilage and bone connecting both tarsal bones should be removed, while protecting the neighboring joints. The short toe extensor muscle mass can be sutured into the area from which the bar is removed to prevent regrowth. Fat tissue interposition is another option.

TALOCALCANEAL BAR

For a talocalcaneal bar, a medial approach is used. The neurovascular bundle and tendons are retracted. The anterior and posterior edges of an incomplete or rudimentary bar are identified, which is consequently removed with a burr or a rongeur. Perioperatively, the restoration of subtalar motion should be evaluated and demonstrated.

PITFALLS AND COMMON TECHNICAL MISTAKES

The capsule of the talonavicular joint should not be divided, since dorsal subluxation of the navicular on the head of the talus may result. A rectangle of bone for a calcaneonavicular bar should be removed, not just a wedge. It is important not to disturb the vascular structures connecting the talus and the navicular.

REHABILITATION

A short leg cast is worn for 2 weeks with ankle in neutral dorsiflexion. Early subtalar motion is encouraged. Weight bearing is allowed only when full subtalar motion is reached, which is in 8 to 10 weeks.

Excision of a talocalcaneal bar is rarely successful in relieving symptoms. Prolonged conservative treatment is advised. Triple arthrodesis (fusion of the talocalcaneal, talonavicular, and calcaneocuboid joint) is considered in late adolescence or adulthood if the symptoms persist and if there are degenerative joint changes. If there is a major, not correctable, hindfoot valgus, a medial displacement os calcis osteotomy is suggested as an adjunct procedure.

SUMMARY

Tarsal conditions are common and may create symptoms requiring treatment interventions. Painful coalitions not responding to orthotics or casts may require surgical removal of the coalition. Generally satisfactory results may be expected with coalition resection.

REFERENCES

1. Bassett FH III, ed. Instr Course Lect 1988;37:77–85.
2. Mosier KM, Asher M. Tarsal coalition and peroneal spastic flatfoot: a review. J Bone Joint Surg 1984;66A:976–984.
3. Tachdjian MS. Pediatric orthopedics. Philadelphia: Saunders, 1990:2578–2608.
4. Harris RI, Beath T. Etiology of peroneal spastic flat foot. J Bone Joint Surg 1948;30B:624–634.
5. Cowell HR. Talocalcaneal coalition and new causes of peroneal spastic flatfoot. Clin Orthop 1972;85:16–22.
6. Drennan JC, ed. The child's foot and ankle. New York: Raven, 1992.
7. Morrissy RT, ed. Lovell and Winter's pediatric orthopaedics. 4th ed. Philadelphia: Lippincott, 1996:963–969.
8. Staheli LT. Fundamentals of pediatric orthopedics. New York: Raven, 1992.
9. Bucholz RW, Lippert FG III, Wenger DR, Ezaki M. Orthopaedic decision making. Philadelphia: BC Decker, 1984.
10. Wenger DR, Rang M. The art and practice of children's orthopedics. New York: Raven, 1993.

Clubfoot

Talipes equinovarus is a common congenital anomaly. Clubfeet can be divided into four main categories: positional, neurogenic, teratologic or syndromic, and idiopathic. Positional clubfeet are the result of intrauterine positioning and are flexible and easily correctable with a few serial casts. Neurogenic clubfeet are seen in children with spina bifida or cerebral palsy and are the result of muscle imbalance. Teratologic clubfeet are seen in patients with syndromes such as Larsen's syndrome, Freeman-Sheldon syndrome, and diastrophic dysplasia. These tend to be rigid feet that are difficult to correct.

RELEVANT ANATOMY AND PATHOGENESIS

Idiopathic clubfeet occur in otherwise normal children with an overall occurrence of 1.24 per 1000 live births. The cause is unknown, but the condition may result from multifactorial inheritance modified by intrauterine and environmental factors. The pathogenesis of clubfoot is unknown; but there are numerous theories, including arrest of embryonic development, germ plasm defect, neurogenic factors, retracting fibrosis, myofibroblasts in the medial fascia, and anomalous tendon insertions.

The pathoanatomy of clubfoot has been elucidated by anatomic dissections, CT examinations, and surgical experience. The bones of the affected foot are smaller than normal. The talus shows an abnormal medial and plantar deviation of the talar neck. The body of the talus is externally rotated in the mortise. The os calcis is medially rotated, and its long axis lies parallel to the long axis of the talus. There is medial subluxation of the navicular and the cuboid. There are no torsional abnormalities of the tibia and fibula (1).

The soft tissues are also abnormal; there are contractures of the ankle and subtalar joint capsules as well as the calcaneocuboid and talonavicular joints. Tendon sheaths are frequently thickened, and the plantar fascia is contracted.

INITIAL FINDINGS, PHYSICAL EXAMINATION, AND DIAGNOSIS

In a clubfoot deformity, the foot is held in equinus and varus at the hindfoot and supination and adductus of the forefoot (Fig. 97.1). There is also often a cavus deformity present. If the deformity is unilateral, the involved foot is small, and there is atrophy of the leg muscles. There may also be a cock-up deformity of the great toe, which indicates a plantar-flexed first metatarsal. There may be abnormal skin creases, a posterior heel crease, and/or a medial foot crease.

When evaluating a patient with a clubfoot, it is important to determine the severity of the deformity. Unfortunately, there is no universally accepted classification system. Most feet are subjectively categorized based on their flexibility. A mild clubfoot is one that is passively correctable. The moderate clubfoot is less supple, has an easily definable heel, and no medial crease. A severe clubfoot is quite short, has abnormal skin creases, tight skin, and a poorly defined heel. This foot is often resistant to nonoperative management.

A general examination is carried out to rule out underlying abnormalities or syndromes. A neurologic examination should be carried out, and other joints should be assessed.

RADIOLOGIC STUDIES

It is difficult to draw conclusions about the anatomic relationships of the foot by x-ray. In the newborn and infant the "bones" are primarily cartilaginous. It has also been shown that in clubfeet the ossific nuclei are eccentrically located in the talus and calcaneus, making it difficult to identify the long axis of these bones. The talocalcaneal angle, however, measured on both AP and lateral radiographs, has been used to assess the severity of the deformity and the response to treatment. The most commonly

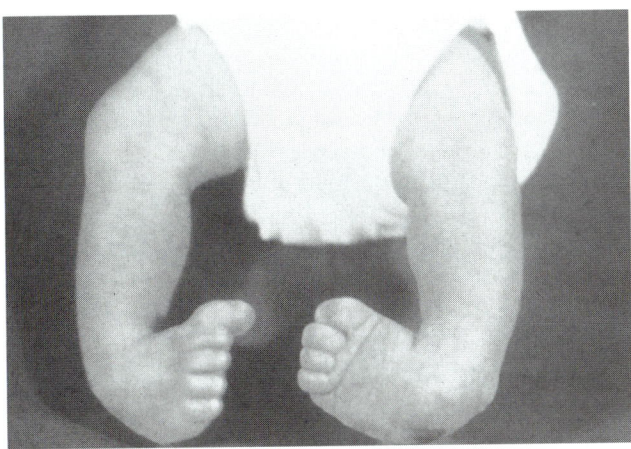

Figure 97.1. A newborn with bilateral clubfoot deformities.

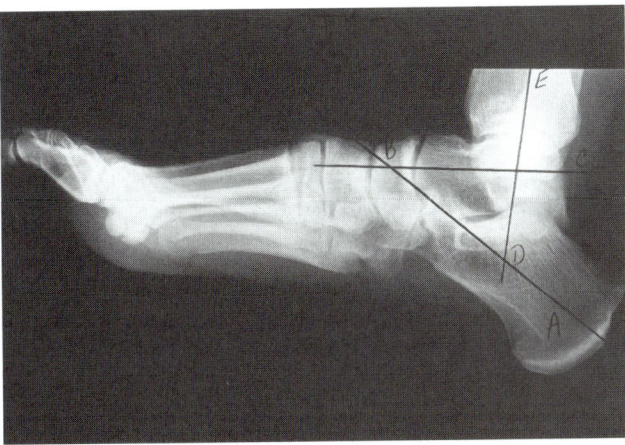

Figure 97.2. Lateral view of a normal foot showing the angle formed by the talocalcaneal (*AB-BC*) and the tibiocalcaneal (*AB-DE*) angles.

measured angles are the lateral talocalcaneal angle, the anterior-posterior talocalcaneal angle, the tibial calcaneal angle, and the talo–first metatarsal angle (Figs. 97.2 and 97.3). The AP talocalcaneal angle reflects the alignment of the hindfoot. When the angle is decreased, there is varus of the hindfoot; the normal range for this angle is 10° to 50°. The lateral talocalcaneal angle also reflects alignment of the hindfoot. When the hindfoot is in varus and/or equinus, this angle is decreased, which is termed parallelism. The tibial calcaneal angle is a measure of hindfoot equinus; it is increased when the hindfoot is in equinus. The AP talo–first metatarsal angle is a measure of forefoot alignment. An increased angle indicates metatarsus adductus (2).

Currently, no other radiologic studies are routinely used in the evaluation of clubfeet. It is possible that in the future MRI with three-dimensional reconstruction will enable a better understanding of the anatomical relationships.

TREATMENT

Nonoperative Treatment

Most orthopaedic surgeons agree that initially all clubfeet should be treated nonoperatively. The mainstay of nonoperative treatment is careful manipulation of the involved foot, and then holding the foot position with either taping or casting (Figs. 97.4 and 97.5). The manipulations are done serially, in an attempt to slowly correct the deformity. Several techniques of manipulation have been described (3). Patients are initially seen on a weekly basis, then every 2 weeks. The time frame for serial casting is variable, but it can be continued as long as progress is being made. Once no further correction is obtainable, the process is stopped, usually after 3 to 4 months.

The technique of serial manipulation and casting is not without its complications. Cast sores and circulatory embarrassment can occur. In addition, too vigorous manipulation can result in fractures of the distal tibia or a breech of the transverse arch of the midfoot, the so-called rocker-bottom foot.

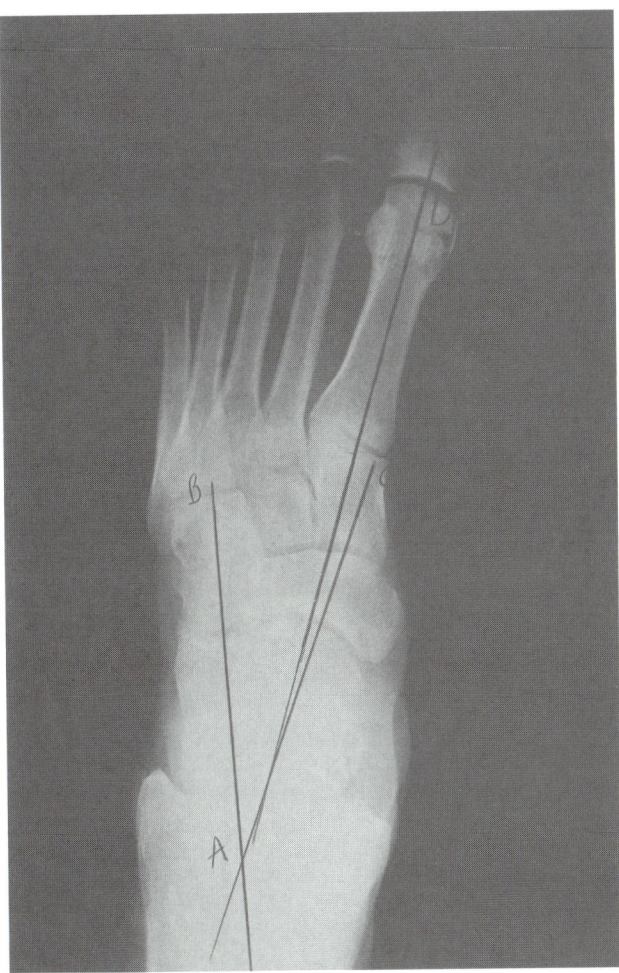

Figure 97.3. AP view of a normal foot showing that the talocalcaneal angle (*AB-AC*) is a measure of hindfoot varus and valgus and the talo–first metatarsal angle (*AC-AD*) is a measure of forefoot alignment.

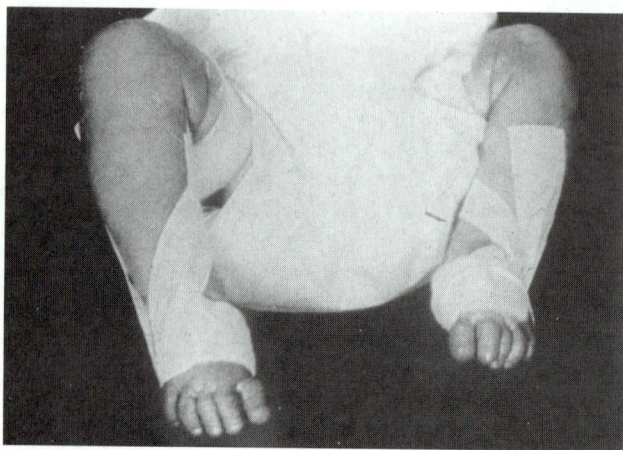

Figure 97.4. Taping a clubfoot in a newborn.

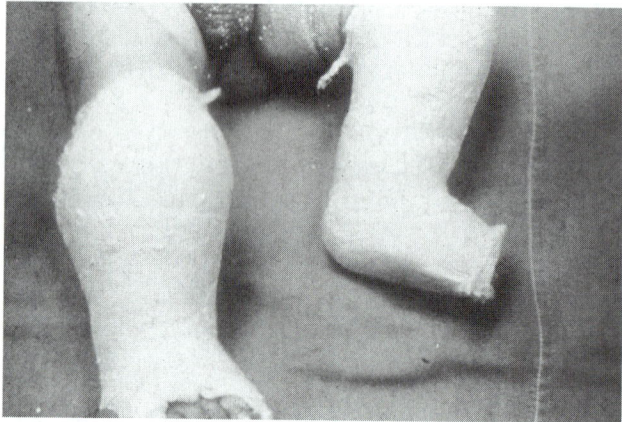

Figure 97.5. Casting maintains the correction obtained by stretching.

Daily physical therapy has been popularized by the French (4). The program advocates that manipulations be performed daily in a set pattern. After each manipulation, the foot is held with a Denis-Browne splint. As the foot becomes more normal, the sessions are progressively decreased.

Recently, continuous passive motion has been used as both a primary treatment and an adjunct to serial casting (Fig. 97.6). This technique has also been popularized by the French. The foot is fixed to the continuous passive motion machine, and slow correction is carried out over 6 to 8 h. This technique shows promise, but the results in the United States are still preliminary.

Operative Treatment

When nonoperative measures are not successful in obtaining a plantigrade foot, correction of the clubfoot must be obtained surgically. Surgical procedures can be categorized into three groups: soft tissue only, combined soft tissue and bony procedures, and bony procedures alone (Clinical Table). Bone surgery is usually done on older

children and is generally considered a salvage procedure (5).

Soft tissue procedures involve lengthening tight tendons, dividing tight deforming structures such as ligaments and capsules, and tendon transfers. Posterior release alone is indicated when the forefoot adductus and heel varus have been corrected with casting and there is an equinus deformity. The Achilles tendon is lengthened, and a posterior capsulotomy of both the ankle and subtalar joints is carried out. In addition, the calcaneofibular and talofibular ligaments must be divided.

Posteromedial release as a one-stage procedure was first popularized by Turco (6). His procedure is done through an incision that starts posteromedially 3 to 4 cm above the calcaneus, extending distally to the medial malleolus and then extending along the medial side of the foot. Posterior, medial, and subtalar soft tissues are divided or lengthened. The foot is then aligned and secured with a single Kirschner (K) wire.

McKay (7) popularized the one-stage circumferential release, involving posterior, medial, lateral, and plantar structures. This procedure was initially carried out through a Cincinnati incision, which starts along the medial side of the foot and extends around the heel to the calcaneocuboid joint. Carroll (8) popularized the posteromedial lateral release done through two incisions: an oblique posterior incision and a medial foot incision. This method avoids an incision across the tightest posteromedial skin.

Regardless of the technique used, the foot is cast in a long leg cast for approximately 6 weeks, followed by a short leg cast for 6 to 8 weeks. Some authors also use a hinged, short leg cast. Most children will not require postoperative bracing.

The timing of surgical intervention is controversial, and ranges from a few days of age to 12 months. Authors who support early intervention believe that realignment of the foot will allow remodeling of the articular surfaces. Unfortunately, the young infant's foot is fatty, and small bones and cartilaginous structures may be difficult to identify. Most surgeons delay intervention until the infant

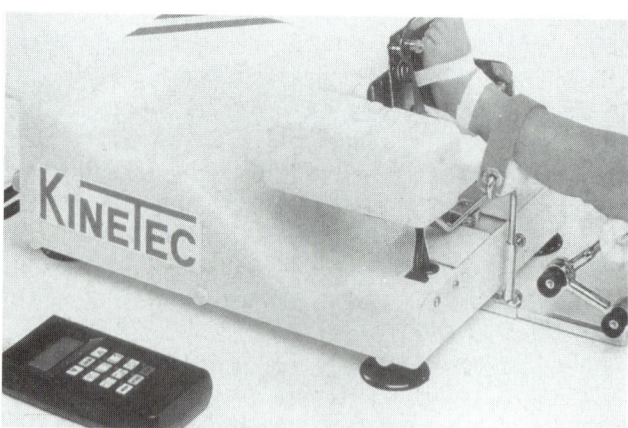

Figure 97.6. An infant's foot in a continuous passive motion machine.

Clinical Table: Clubfoot

Procedure	Indications	Techniques	Anatomy	Pitfalls
Posterior release	• Persistent equinus	• Oblique incision • Lengthening Achilles tendon	• Achilles tendon • Posterior capsule	• Incomplete correction
Posterior medial lateral release	• Resistant clubfoot deformity	• Cincinnati incision • Two-incision technique	• Achilles tendon • Posterior capsule • Talonavicular joint • Plantar release	• Overcorrection • Undercorrection • Recurrence
Metatarsal osteotomy	• Persistent forefoot adductus	• Two to three dorsal incisions • Dome cut	• Bases of the metatarsals	• Injury to growth plate
Midfoot osteotomy	• Persistent forefoot adductus	• Opening wedge cuneiform • Closing wedge cuboid	• Medial cuneiform • Cuboid	• Bones too small • Under age 5
Calcaneal osteotomy	• Hindfoot varus	• Dwyer • Lateral slide	• Calcaneus • Medial neurovascular bundle	
Triple arthrodesis	• Stiff, previously operated on foot • Skeletal maturity	• Sinus tarsi incision • Remove cartilage and bony wedges for correction	• Sinus tarsi	• Salvage procedure

is 4 to 6 months old. My preference is to wait until the child is pulling to a stand, at about 9 to 10 months. At this age, the child tolerates the anesthetic better; the foot is larger so structures are easier to identify; and when the casting is complete, the child is ready to begin weight bearing.

Complications of soft tissue surgery do occur. In addition to the general complications of bleeding, infection, and nerve and vessel damage, specific complications are overcorrection, undercorrection, recurrent deformity, tibial physis damage, stiffness, and dorsal bunion. Overcorrection can result in a flat foot or calcaneus deformity. The flat foot can be surgically corrected; however, the calcaneus deformity, which is secondary to overlengthening of the heel cord, is quite difficult, if not impossible, to reconstruct. Undercorrection may be secondary to the surgeon's inexperience or the result of an extremely rigid foot that is difficult to correct. Recurrent deformity may result from undercorrection or increased scar formation, which does not stretch with the growth of the child. Although not common, damage to the tibial physis may occur secondary to vigorous dissection around the ankle joint posteriorly. This can lead to a plantar-flexion deformity of the foot.

All clubfeet have decreased mobility no matter what the treatment or how well it was carried out. Increased stiffness, however, can result from damage to the articular surfaces at the time of capsulotomy. Finally, a dorsal bunion develops when the peroneus longus tendon is divided. This can occur during the plantar release if the surgeon is not careful.

Bone procedures are generally used in older children as salvage procedures. Persistent forefoot deformities can be corrected by osteotomy of the metatarsals. More recently, opening-wedge osteotomy of the medial cuneiform combined with closing-wedge osteotomy of the cuboid to correct persistent forefoot deformity has been described. Several osteotomies of the calcaneus have been developed to correct persistent hindfoot deformities. The Dwyer osteotomy is an opening-wedge osteotomy used to correct a persistent varus deformity. A simple lateral slide of the calcaneus can also correct varus deformity.

Triple arthrodesis should be considered last-resort procedure for a painful, stiff foot that has already undergone several surgical procedures. To prevent excessive shortening of the foot, triple arthrodesis should not be done until the physes of the foot have closed or are near closing.

Combined bone and soft tissue procedures usually include posteromedial release and a lateral column shortening. Lateral column shortening procedures are closing-wedge osteotomy of the distal calcaneus, closing-wedge resection of the calcaneocuboid joint (Evans procedure), lateral excision of the distal part of the calcaneus, and cuboid decancellation.

Ilizarov frame application has also been used to help correct recurrent or residual deformity in clubfoot. It can be used in conjunction with bone and soft tissue procedures as well. This is still a relatively new technique, and long-term follow-up is lacking.

SUMMARY

Idiopathic clubfoot is a common congenital anomaly with an unclear etiology. The primary pathology is a small talus with medial deviation of the neck; all other deformities are secondary. Nonoperative treatment involves serial manipulation of the foot, followed by casting to hold the correction. The success of this technique ranges from 0 to 98% in the literature. Early on, surgical correction consists of soft tissue surgery, either a posterior release or a posteromedial lateral release. Such a correction is generally all that is required. With recurrent deformity, soft tissue surgery can be repeated, although bone procedures may be necessary to correct the foot. Finally, in the child approaching skeletal maturity with a stiff, painful foot, triple arthrodesis is indicated.

REFERENCES

1. Howard CB, Benson MK. Clubfoot: its pathologic anatomy. J Pediatr Orthop 1993;13:654–659.
2. Vanderwelde R, Staheli LT, Chew DE, Malagon V. Measurements on radiographs of the foot in normal infants and children. J Bone Joint Surg 1988;70A:407–415.
3. Ponseti IV. Treatment of congenital club foot. J Bone Joint Surg 1992;74A:448–452.
4. Bensahel H, Guillame A, Czukonyi Z, Desgrippes Y. Results of physical therapy for idiopathic clubfoot: a long-term follow-up study. J Pediatr Orthop 1990;10:189–192.
5. Cummings RJ, Lovell WW. Operative treatment of congenital idiopathic club foot. J Bone Joint Surg 1988;70A:1108–1112.
6. Turco VJ. Resistant congenital club foot—one-stage posteromedial release with internal fixation. A follow-up report of a fifteen year experience. J Bone Joint Surg 1979;61A:805–814.
7. McKay DW. Surgical correction of clubfoot. Instr Course Lect 1988;37:87–92.
8. Carroll NC. Pathoanatomy and surgical treatment of the resistant clubfoot. Instr Course Lect 1988;37:93–106.

Leg Length Discrepancy

Leg length discrepancy is a common problem that presents a challenge to the orthopaedic surgeon. The physician must determine the cause of the discrepancy and its developmental pattern. Because the patients are growing, it is important to determine what the discrepancy will be at maturity. Finally, there are several options of treatment available, and it is up to the orthopaedic surgeon to decide which option best fits the patient and his or her specific condition.

RELEVANT ANATOMY AND PATHOGENESIS

Leg length discrepancy causes alterations in function and gait mechanics; but studies documenting the long-term natural history and deleterious effects on the low back, hip, and knee are lacking. There are conflicting reports about how much discrepancy causes clinical problems. Friberg (1) found that discrepancies of as little as 5 mm were associated with increased complaints of low back pain and that use of a shoe lift could relieve symptoms. Gross (2) surveyed 74 mature adults and found that those with discrepancies of 2 cm or less were unaware of any problems. Finally, using gait analysis, Kaufman et al. (3) showed that at 2 cm of discrepancy, gait asymmetry was present.

Causes of leg length discrepancy are multiple and can be grouped into categories (Table 98.1). These processes can cause discrepancy by either affecting growth or by changing the length of the bone directly. Growth may be retarded or stimulated.

Classification

Not all leg length discrepancies have the same pattern of growth. Shapiro (4) classified patterns of growth into five types: Type I, the upward slope pattern, has a discrepancy that continually progresses with time at a proportional rate. In type II, the upward slope–deceleration pattern, the discrepancy increases at a proportional rate for a variable

period of time; then the rate decreases. In type III, upward slope–plateau pattern, the discrepancy increases at a proportional rate; then it stabilizes and no longer changes with growth. Type IV discrepancies have an upward slope–plateau–upward slope pattern, and type V discrepancies have an upward slope–plateau–downward slope pattern. Type I patterns can often be seen in congenital causes of leg length discrepancy, such as proximal femoral focal deficiency, and with physeal injuries. Examples of type II patterns are some cases of hemihypertrophy and poliomyelitis. Type III patterns of discrepancy are most commonly seen after trauma, particularly diaphyseal femur fractures. Types IV and V patterns are less commonly encountered; the leg length discrepancy associated with poliomyelitis can exhibit a type IV pattern, and the discrepancy associated with juvenile rheumatoid arthritis can exhibit a type V pattern.

INITIAL FINDINGS, PHYSICAL EXAMINATION, AND DIAGNOSIS

When evaluating the patient with a limb length discrepancy, it is important to determine the underlying cause and what type of growth pattern is exhibited. Therefore, a thorough history is important. A complete physical examination should also be done, with attention directed to neurologic involvement and stigmata of neurofibromatosis. Specifically, motor strength and joint motion of the involved limb should be documented. Clinical measures of the limb length discrepancy are notoriously inaccurate. The length from the anterior-superior iliac spine to the medial malleolus is often recorded; however, this measure is not accurate. Joint contractures of the hip and knee can also throw these measurements off. Finally, differences in the size of the feet (macropodia or clubfoot) are not accounted for when measuring to the medial malleolus.

The second method of clinically determining the amount of discrepancy is to use blocks of varying thickness

table	98.1	Causes of Leg Length Discrepancy
Cause		Examples
Congenital		Proximal femur focal deficiency, fibular hemimelia, Klippel-Trenaunay-Weber syndrome
Infection		Osteomyelitis, septic arthritis
Paralysis		Poliomyelitis, hemiplegia
Trauma		Acute shortening, physeal injury, fracture hyperemia
Tumor		Osteoid osteoma, neurofibromatosis
Other		Legg-Calvé-Perthes disease, slipped capital femoral epiphysis, radiation, juvenile rheumatoid arthritis

to level the pelvis. This gives the physician an idea of the functional discrepancy but may not accurately determine the true discrepancy. For example, a patient with developmental dislocation of the hip will stand with one hemipelvis lower than the other, but the true leg length discrepancy may be close to zero.

RADIOLOGIC STUDIES

Radiographic assessment is, in general, more accurate than are clinical measurements, although it may not be completely accurate either. There are three techniques for determining leg length discrepancy using plain radiographs. The teleroentgenogram is a standing x-ray of both legs on a 5.5- × 14.5-cm (14- × 36-in) cassette with a radiopaque ruler placed on the cassette. This is one exposure taken 2.8 m (6 ft) from the patient. These films are cumbersome, and there is magnification resulting from the parallax of the x-ray beam (5). The orthoroentgenogram is also taken on a 5.5- × 14.5-cm cassette with a radiopaque ruler. It differs from the teleroentgenogram in that three exposures are taken at the hip, knee, and ankle. Magnification is not a problem; but the film is cumbersome. Furthermore, if the patient moves between exposures, errors may be introduced.

The most commonly used plain radiographic technique is the scanogram. In this technique a smaller film cassette is used and is moved under the patient. Three exposures are taken at the hip, knee, and ankle. Magnification is not a problem, and the film size is more manageable. Again, errors may be introduced if the patient moves between exposures. Unless the patient position is modified, these measurements are fairly inaccurate when taken on the patient with hip and knee flexion contractures.

Recently, CT scanning has been found to be a more accurate means of determining limb length discrepancy (6). Radiation exposure is less, and the cost is comparable to other techniques.

Finally, when evaluating a limb length discrepancy, bone age determination is important. It is used to help determine the discrepancy at maturity and to decide on the timing of specific surgical interventions. Assessment of bone age is most often done by obtaining an x-ray of the left hand and comparing it with standards in the Greulich-Pyle atlas.

TREATMENT

Nonoperative Treatment

The choice of treatment for limb length discrepancy depends primarily on the amount of discrepancy present at maturity and, less important, on the cause of the discrepancy. It is, therefore, important to calculate what the discrepancy will be when growth is complete. There are three techniques for making this determination: the arithmetic method described by White (7); the growth-remaining method described by Anderson et al. (8); and the straight line method popularized by Moseley (9).

Once the amount of discrepancy is determined, a decision can be made regarding treatment. Nonoperative treatment has generally been reserved for discrepancies of 5 cm or less or for discrepancies greater than 15 cm. A shoe lift is recommended for discrepancies of 2 cm and can be used for discrepancies up to 5 cm, although for the larger discrepancy, equalization procedures are believed to be better. The lift prescribed should be slightly less than the actual discrepancy, and may be better tolerated if it tapers slightly at the toe.

For large discrepancies that are not amenable to lengthening procedures, prosthetic fitting is usually recommended. Prosthetic fitting is usually used in association with amputation, but the extremity can be fitted with a nonstandard prosthetic limb that incorporates the residual limb. This approach is less common but can be helpful if the family decides against any type of surgical intervention (Fig. 98.1).

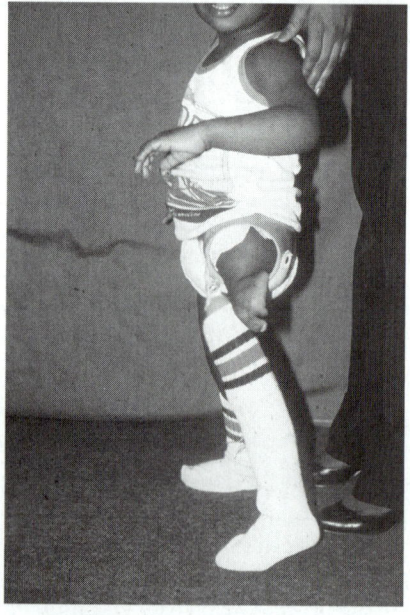

Figure 98.1. A nonstandard prosthesis.

Operative Treatment

Surgical options for the treatment of limb length discrepancy include epiphysiodesis, limb shortening, limb lengthening, and amputation with prosthetic fitting (Clinical Table). These options can be used alone or in combination; for example, it is possible to lengthen a short leg and do an epiphysiodesis on the long leg in a patient with a large discrepancy. Basic guidelines for surgical intervention are presented in Table 98.2.

Epiphysiodesis can be done with several techniques. It is perhaps the simplest surgical procedure technically, but it requires careful planning and calculation to determine the appropriate timing. It is often difficult to explain to the parents why the surgery is being performed on the "good" leg. The family must also understand that the correction occurs slowly and that the surgery is not an immediate fix.

Epiphysiodesis can be done by either an open or percutaneous technique. In the open technique described by White, a box chisel is used to remove a 1- to 2-cm block of bone, including the physis. A small curette is then used to remove the contiguous physis to a depth of 2.5 cm. The plug is then rotated 90° and reinserted. The percutaneous technique is done under fluoroscopic guidance. A drill or cannulated reamer is used to obliterate the physis.

Complications of epiphysiodesis are most commonly related to errors in calculating the timing of surgery, resulting in either overcorrection or undercorrection. Partial or hemiepiphysiodesis may also occur, resulting in an angular deformity of the extremity.

Limb shortening is another option of limb equalization for patients who are nearing the end of growth. It has the benefit of correcting the discrepancy acutely. Femoral or tibial shortening can be done by a closed intramedullary technique in the diaphyseal region or by an open metaphyseal shortening, which is then secured with a plate and screws. The femur can be shortened up to 6 cm, and the tibia can be shortened up to 5 cm.

Complications of shortening include temporary weakness of the muscles, which recover over time. In addition, nonunion, delayed union, and hardware failure can occur.

This technique has the disadvantage of often being performed on the normal leg.

Leg lengthening is usually reserved for discrepancies between 5 and 15 cm. It is a prolonged procedure that requires a significant commitment on the part of the patient and the family. Prerequisites for leg lengthening include a normal joint above and below; therefore, any associated joint deformity must be dealt with before lengthening. In addition, all soft tissue contractures must be treated before proceeding. The basic technique of lengthening involves an osteotomy of the bone, application of an external fixator, and then slowly lengthening over a time. In the Wagner technique, the osteotomy is done mid-diaphyseal, and a uniplanar fixator is applied. The bone is lengthened 1.5 mm once a day. In the early technique, once the desired length was achieved, the defect was spanned with a long plate, bone graft was placed, and the fixator was removed. Newer techniques of lengthening involve a metaphyseal lengthening and the application of an external fixator. The rate of lengthening is decreased to 0.25 mm four times a day. The newer techniques use both uniplanar and ring fixators.

The complication rate for leg lengthening is high and is usually divided into major and minor complications. In a study by Aaron and Eilert (10), minor complications included pin tract infections, transient nerve palsies, soft tissue contractures, and early consolidation. Major complications were late fracture, angulation, extended or permanent nerve palsy, fracture through the pin

table	98.2	Treatment Options for Leg Length Discrepancy

Discrepancy (cm)	Treatment
0–2	No treatment
2–5	Shoe lift, epiphysiodesis, limb shortening
5–15	Leg lengthening
>15	Prosthetic fitting, with or without amputation

Clinical Table: Leg Length Discrepancy

Procedure	Indications	Technique	Anatomy	Pitfalls
Epiphysiodesis	• 2- to 5-cm discrepancy • Adequate remaining growth	• Open or percutaneous technique	• Identify level of physis	• Incorrect calculations • Overcorrection • Undercorrection
Limb shortening	• 5- to 6-cm discrepancy • Nearing end of growth	• Fixation with plate or nail	• Metaphyseal • Diaphyseal	• Weakness of limb • Need for hardware removal
Leg lengthening	• 5- to 15-cm discrepancy • Committed family • Normal joint above and below	• Wagner • Ilizarov • DeBastiani	• Corticotomy with callotasis	• High complication rate
Amputation	• >15-cm discrepancy • Noncorrectable joint abnormality			• Difficult decision for family

sites, knee or hip subluxation, osteomyelitis, shortening, delayed union, nonunion, and deep infection. The authors noted that every patient had at least one complication.

The final surgical option is amputation and prosthetic fitting. This option is usually reserved for children with predicted discrepancies of greater than 15 cm and those who have some other abnormality of the extremity that would preclude lengthening. For example, a patient with fibular hemimelia may have a three-toed foot and multiple tarsal coalitions. Such a patient would most likely do better with a Syme or Boyd amputation and prosthetic fitting. As another example, a child with a proximal femoral focal deficiency in which the femur is 50% shorter than the opposite side does better with prosthetic fitting. Options for treatment in this case would include a knee fusion and Syme or Boyd amputation; the patient would be fitted as an above-knee amputee. A second option is a knee fusion and Van Ness rotation plasty. The patient is then fitted as a below-knee amputee.

If amputation is selected, the surgery is usually timed to coincide with normal development. Most children pull to stand around 10 months of age, so amputation and prosthetic fitting done at this time allows the child to reach his or her developmental milestones at the appropriate time. If the amputation is done later, the child should be fitted with a nonstandard prosthesis until the time of surgery. Amputation is a difficult decision for families to make, but it becomes even more difficult after the child has undergone multiple surgeries in an attempt to equalize leg lengths.

SUMMARY

Leg length discrepancy results from multiple causes and presents a challenge to the treating orthopaedic surgeon. Understanding the character of the discrepancy and being able to determine the discrepancy at maturity are important when deciding on treatment options. All surgical options require close follow-up, careful calculations, and in-depth discussions with the family.

REFERENCES

1. Friberg O. Clinical symptoms and biomechanics of lumbar spine and hip joint in leg length inequality. Spine 1983;8:643–651.
2. Gross RH. Leg length discrepancy: How much is too much? Orthopaedics 1978;1:307–310.
3. Kaufman KR, Miller LS, Sutherland DH. Gait asymmetry in patients with limb-length inequality. J Pediatr Orthop 1996;16:144–150.
4. Shapiro F. Developmental patterns in lower-extremity length discrepancies. J Bone Joint Surg 1982;64A:639–650.
5. Moseley CF. Leg length discrepancy. In: Morrissy RT, ed. Lovell and Winter's pediatric orthopaedics. Philadelphia: Lippincott, 1990:767–813.
6. Aaron A, Weinstein D, Thickman D. Comparison of orthoroentgenography and computed tomography in the measurement of limb-length discrepancy. J Bone Joint Surg 1992;74A:897–902.
7. Westh R, Menelaus M. A simple calculation for the timing of epiphyseal arrest: a further report. J Bone Joint Surg 1981;63B:117–119.
8. Anderson M, Green WT, Messner MB. Growth and predictions of growth in the lower extremities. J Bone Joint Surg 1963;45A:1–14.
9. Moseley CF. A straight line graph for leg length discrepancies. J Bone Joint Surg 1977;59A:174–178.
10. Aaron AD, Eilert RE. Results of Wagner and Ilizarov methods of limb-lengthening. J Bone Joint Surg 1996;78A:20–29.

Torticollis

Congenital muscular torticollis is a common finding in newborns up to 3 months of age. It is associated with contracture or shortening of the sternomastoid muscle, with or without pseudotumor of the midsubstance of the muscle, from presumed hemorrhage and subsequent fibrosis. Many cases associated with fetal constraint and other fetal constraint-associated deformations such as metatarsus adductus or hip dysplasias.

RELEVANT ANATOMY AND PATHOGENESIS

Congenital muscular torticollis, or wryneck, is a common painless condition that is usually discovered in the first 6 to 8 weeks of life (1). The deformity is the result of contracture of the sternocleidomastoid muscle; the occiput is tilted toward the involved side, and the chin is rotated toward the contralateral shoulder (Fig. 99.1). A nontender soft mobile mass or tumor is usually palpable in the first month of life, but it frequently goes undetected. The condition is apparently related to intracompartmental muscle venous flow obstruction arising from compression during vaginal delivery. This blockage results in edema, degeneration of muscle fibers, and fibrotic scarring of the muscle. The fibrotic tissue may compromise a branch of the accessory nerve to the clavicular head of the muscle, thereby increasing the deformity. The pathogenesis is not fully elucidated, however. If the condition is progressive and not treated, considerable asymmetries of the face and skull can result (plagiocephaly) (2).

INITIAL FINDINGS, PHYSICAL EXAMINATION, AND DIAGNOSIS

Congenital muscular torticollis is the most common cause of wryneck posture in the infant and young child. But other problems, such as neurogenic tumors, trauma (subluxations of cervical vertebrae, fixed rotatory subluxation), cervical adenitis (Grisel's disease), disk space infections, vertebral osteomyelitis, atlanto-occipital abnormalities, and extrinsic eye muscle imbalance lead to this unusual posture. Intermittent torticollis can occur in the young child as a seizure-like disorder. Therefore, congenital muscular torticollis is a diagnosis of exclusion (3).

Approximately 20% of children with congenital muscular torticollis have congenital hip dysplasia. An appropriate hip examination is mandatory. The mass in the sternocleidomastoid muscle gains maximum size within the first month of life and then gradually regresses. After 6 months of age, the torticollis posture and the contracture of the sternocleidomastoid muscle and fascia sheath are the main clinical findings. The skull asymmetry appearing in the first year of life is probably due to the (more prone) position the child assumes when sleeping.

Sometimes muscular torticollis is first seen during childhood. In this juvenile type, usually both heads of the muscle are contracted, limiting head motion. It is uncertain if the juvenile forms are cases not recognized during infancy or whether the onset occurred during late infancy or early childhood. Acquired forms of torticollis require a thorough evaluation for intraspinal and posterior fossa lesions. This form of torticollis is resistant to exercises and physical therapy. Correction requires a surgical bipolar release of the muscle.

RADIOLOGIC STUDIES

Radiographs of the cervical spine should be initially obtained to rule out congenital anomaly of the cervical spine, resulting in the so-called wryneck. If basilar invagination or fixed rotatory subluxation is suspected, additional imaging studies (CT scanning) and various views (including flexion and extension) are required.

TREATMENT

Nonoperative Treatment and Indications for Surgery

Excellent results can be obtained in most infants and children under age 1 with conservative measures, such as

Clinical Table: Torticollis

Procedure	Indications	Technique	Anatomy	Pitfalls
Distal release of clavicular attachment and Z-lengthening of sternal head; may be combined with proximal release of sternomastoid muscle at level of mastoid (bipolar release)	• Established facial asymmetry and limitation of normal cervical spine motion beyond age 1 year	• Proximal approach through incision of medial third of clavicle, with incision of clavicular head and Z-lengthening of sternal head • Proximal release 1–2 cm distal to mastoid	• Sternocleidomastoid muscle traverses the neck from mastoid to clavicle with two distal heads of attachment—one on sternum and one on clavicle	• Incomplete restoration of motion • Injury to spinal accessory nerve

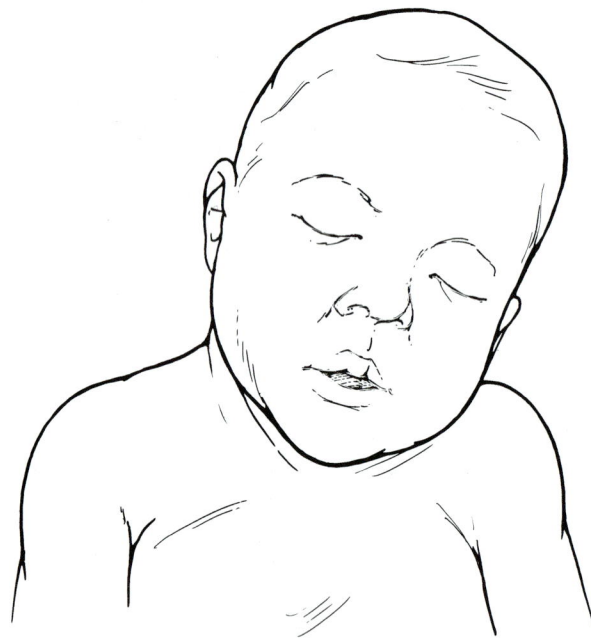

Figure 99.1. Infant with congenital muscular torticollis.

stretching exercises, performed by the parent with guidance from the physical therapist and physician (4). The exercises should include not only lateral rotation but also side bending to the opposite shoulder. Toys and repositioning of the crib help the child stretch the neck when he or she tries to reach and grasp. Established facial asymmetry and limitation of normal motion of more than 30° beyond age 1 year indicate surgical intervention. A good but not perfect cosmetic result can be obtained as late as 12 years of age, as long as adequate remodeling growth potential of the skull is present (5).

Operative Treatment

The approach is through a proximal transverse skin incision above the medial third of the clavicle, following Langer's lines (Clinical Table). A distal release of both the sternal and clavicular attachments seems adequate for moderate cases. Severe cases benefit from both distal and proximal releases (6). The sternal hood is Z-lengthened and repaired.

To avoid common pitfalls, the surgeon must pay attention to the location of the spinal accessory nerve when performing the proximal release (mastoid incision). Skin incisions immediately adjacent to the clavicle may result in unsightly hypertrophic scars (7).

The rehabilitation regimen includes the same passive stretching exercises that were done before surgery. Sometimes bracing or cast correction (a Minerva jacket in an overcorrected position) is useful. The results of surgery have been uniformly good, with a low incidence of complications or recurrence.

SUMMARY

Congenital muscular torticollis of infancy is diagnosed in infants to age 3 months. It responds readily to stretching exercises and resolves in most cases by age 1 year. Associated plagiocephaly and other deformations require screening, evaluation, and possible interventions. Acquired torticollis requires careful screening and evaluation, as this may be a presenting sign of cervical intraspinal or posterior fossa lesion, ophthalmologic problem, or skeletal abnormality.

REFERENCES

1. Tachdjian MS. Pediatric orthopedics. Philadelphia: Saunders, 1990:112–125.
2. Morrissy RT, ed. Lovell and Winter's pediatric orthopaedics. 3rd ed. Philadelphia: Lippincott, 1990:728–739.
3. Staheli LT. Fundamentals of pediatric orthopedics. New York: Raven, 1992:9.6–9.7.
4. Bucholz RW, Lippert FG III, Wenger DR, Ezaki M. Orthopaedic decision making. Philadelphia: BC Decker, 1984:172–173.
5. Wenger DR, Rang M. The art and practice of children's orthopedics. New York: Raven, 1993:488–491.
6. Ferkel RD, Westin GW, Dawson EG. Muscular torticollis: a modified surgical approach. J Bone Joint Surg 1983;65A:894–900.
7. Canale ST, Griffin DW, Hubbard CN. Congenital muscular torticollis: a long-term follow-up. J Bone Joint Surg 1982;64A:810–816.

chapter 100

Elizabeth A. Arendt and Ann Van Heest

Sports Injuries in the Immature Athlete

THE GROWING MUSCULOSKELETAL SYSTEM

The immature musculoskeletal system of the young athlete is significantly different from the mature musculoskeletal system of the adult athlete. The unique characteristic of the juvenile musculoskeletal system is the presence of open growth plates. Thus the young athlete carries the potential for growth plate injury, with immediate or long-term growth disturbances, and the potential for the advantages of growth, such as correction of residual angulation from a malunited fracture. In the immature skeleton, the bone is relatively plastic, growing stiffer and more brittle with age. The plasticity helps the bone absorb energy, which may prevent fracture but may also result in greenstick fractures because of plastic deformation. Last, the immature cartilaginous epiphysis is softer than the mature bony epiphysis and is susceptible to stress injuries in a different manner than is the adult epiphysis. For example, many of the osteochondroses are the result of repetitive trauma to the cartilaginous epiphysis. Thus the immature musculoskeletal system is prone to its own types of injury because of its unique structure.

Musculoskeletal injuries can be divided into two basic categories: overuse and acute. Both types can involve any portion of the musculoskeletal system: bone, joint, muscle–tendon unit, ligament, or growth plate. The concern is not only for the injury itself but also for its potential effect on the subsequent development of the injured part, with possible long-term consequences.

This chapter addresses the musculoskeletal concerns involving active and athletic children, with special consideration for female issues. The chapter briefly reviews normal maturation of the musculoskeletal system and discusses the effects of athletic activity and training on the normal maturation process. Attention is then directed to overuse and acute injury patterns, and specific examples of injuries are cited.

Normal Maturation of the Musculoskeletal System

Young boys and girls have similar body size and build; the most striking differences occur at adolescence. Girls generally have a shorter growth period than boys, usually 2 years ahead of boys in bone ossification. For girls, skeletal ossification is usually complete 1 to 3 years after the onset of menses (1). For boys, significant changes in the musculoskeletal system occur at puberty: increasing muscle mass, broadening of the shoulders relative to the hips, and increasing height. Female puberty is also a time of significant changes in physique: broadening of the hips relative to the shoulders and waist, and maturing breast development. Girls do not undergo significant change in muscle mass. It is, however, certainly a time of great alteration of physical characteristics and abilities. It is significant to note that these changes occur more quickly for girls, because they have a shorter growth period than boys. This time of accelerated changes in the body produces changes in sport performance as well. Sports performance is affected by both the physical changes, as the young athletes accommodate their new body shapes and forms, and the psychologic changes, as the youngsters adapt to their new body images.

Postpuberty muscle mass is significantly greater for males than for females, giving the males the advantage in power and speed. Androgen creates the increase in lean body mass in males. Weight training for females will not produce the same degree of muscle bulk as seen with males, because of the hormonally regulated characteristics of muscle. As a girl goes through menarche, body fat increases to an adult average of 22 to 26%, whereas adult males average 12 to 16% (2). For females, estrogen is responsible for the increase in body fat. These differences are largely due to gender-specific essential fat, which is higher in females (9 to 12%) than in males (3%) (3).

Overall, bone development growth plate closure correlates better with sexual maturation than with age, height, or weight (4). Peak height velocity for girls occurs between 10.5 and 13 years of age; for boys, it occurs between 12.5 and 15 years of age (5). Menarche occurs approximately 1 year after peak height velocity.

Proper nutrition is important to growing children and is reviewed elsewhere; however, because of its central role in the developing skeleton, calcium will be discussed here. Calcium is a major component of mineralized tissue. It is required for normal growth and development of the skeleton and of teeth. Calcium is important to a growing child, particularly girls, because bone mass is maximized. Osteoporosis is a disease that affects more than 25,000,000 people in the United States and is a major cause of bone fractures in the elderly, particularly postmenopausal women. One important factor that influences the occurrence of osteoporosis is the amount of bone mass that is obtained in the first two to three decades of life. Adequate calcium intake is critical to obtaining maximal bone mass.

The current recommendation for optimal calcium intake is 800 mg/day in children 1 to 10 years of age and 1200 to 1500 mg/day in those 11 to 24 years of age. There is also limited information that suggests greater calcium intake may result in increased rates of bone accretion rates in preadolescent boys and girls (6). It is not known whether the effect on bone accretion rates persists beyond the 1.5- to 3-year period of the study and whether this increasing bone formation translates into higher peak bone masses in adults. Additional research is necessary, particularly longitudinal studies, to define optimal calcium intake for preadolescent boys and girls.

Of more importance, however, is that current population surveys of girls and young women (aged 12 to 19) reveal that their average calcium intake is less than 900 mg/day, well below the recommended allowance (6). Ideally, children should meet the daily requirement of calcium through dietary sources; if this is not possible, calcium supplementation is recommended (7,8). The consequences of low calcium intake during the crucial period of rapid skeletal growth raises concerns that achievement of optimal peak adult mass may be seriously compromised, and osteoporosis with its known complications of skeletal fracture may be the end result.

Effects of Training on Normal Musculoskeletal Development

Strength training for the prepubescent athlete has been controversial. The controversy centers on the question of whether this group is indeed capable of making strength gains, balanced by the risk of whether acute and/or chronic musculoskeletal injuries could result from strength-training programs. Studies specifically limited to the prepubescent group have, however, demonstrated gains with strength training (9–11). It has been hypothesized that the changes made are primarily due to neuro-

muscular facilitation instead of absolute alterations in the muscle itself, because of the speed with which the change is made and the lack of muscle hypertrophy. Generalized musculoskeletal growth and maturation must be considered in the evaluation of young athletes as they partake in strength development. As muscle development and hormonal maturation occurs, muscle strength and function increase. Coordination and agility may decrease initially after a rapid growth spurt; time may be necessary to allow young athletes to accommodate to their changing bodies and physiques.

There has been a long history of trying to pattern the effect of regular physical activity and/or training on growth. Concern for a potential negative influence of regular training was expressed by Rowe (12) in 1933. He noted that male participants in an intercollegiate touch football program, though taller than previously, gained less in stature over a 2-year period than nonparticipants. Rowe's study, however, overlooked variation in maturity status. Despite the lack of control for this important variable, many educators over the following decades accepted this observation at face value and concluded that training for athletic competition slowed down growth in stature (13–15).

More recently, concerns about the effect of athletic training during childhood and youth have focused on girls, particularly in relation to menarche and maturation. Specifically, researchers have focused retrospectively on mean ages of athletes at menarche. The relationship between regular sports training and late onset of menarche have been observed in certain sports, particularly gymnastics, track, and ballet. It has been speculated that regular training before menarche was the causative variable in the late onset of menarche in these athletes (16,17). Since the same hormones involved in the regulation of growth spurt are responsible for sexual maturation, there is a concern about the potential influence of intensive training on both growth and maturation (18,19).

Longitudinal data on growth and maturation are less extensive for girls than for boys. Recent data, however, suggest that regular physical activity, sports participation, and training for a sport have no effect on attained stature, timing of peak height velocity, and the rate of growth in stature. Statures of female gymnasts, swimmers, rowers, and track athletes followed longitudinally through childhood and early adolescence suggest that regular training for these sports had no effect on growth. Swimmers are already taller and gymnasts already shorter than average and maintain their position relative to reference data through growth and maturation (20). The longitudinal observations on young females in other sports are limited, though all available data indicate no effect on stature and rate of growth in stature related to sports training (21–23).

The longitudinal data for female gymnasts and swimmers are consistent with cross-sectional observations. Gymnasts and dancers tend to reach sexual and skeletal maturation later than the average (18,24–28), and successful young swimmers tend to be slightly advanced in sexual and skeletal maturation (29). It is still unclear, however, if training before menarche delays the onset of menstruation or if certain sports predispose or attract a certain body type that is associated with delayed menarche (30,31). Data on the age at menarche in athletes are largely retrospective. There is a need for prospective longitudinal studies that follow youth training for different sports from prepubertal years through puberty. The intensity and the duration of the training period need to be considered. In addition to sports and training schedules, it is important to consider life stressors involving home, training issues, nutrition, and hormonal influence (17,32–36).

In particular regard to bone health, the consequence of adolescent amenorrhea and delayed onset of menses remains speculative. The appropriate time to initiate estrogen therapy in the adolescent remains controversial, particularly for secondary amenorrhea (i.e., delay of menses after initial menstruation) (37). Further studies on bone mineral density and longer follow-up are needed to determine if estrogen therapy is efficacious. Long-term consequences of adolescent amenorrhea remain to be determined; however, the central concern is that adolescent amenorrhea and the delay of menses may have a negative effect on the achievement of maximum adult bone mass secondary to the loss of estrogen's favorable effect on bone accretion.

There is increasing evidence that bone mineral density increases with weight-bearing activity in skeletal sites that are maximally stressed. This is likely related to mechanical loading (20,38,39). Bone mineral density has been found to be greater at the upper and lower extremity skeletal sites in female collegiate gymnasts, with and without menstrual irregularities, compared with nonathletes (40). There is speculation that these high mechanical loads at specific skeletal sites may offset the adverse effects of amenorrhea on bone density. As with the postmenopausal female, it is likely that both mechanical loading and an appropriate hormonal environment are necessary for maximizing bone accretion and minimizing bone loss.

Although there is much to be learned, a conservative view would consider that a dose-response relationship exists, supporting the concept of a threshold of training below which growth potential may not suffer (18,19). This concept may be particularly relevant in the adolescent age group (7,41). Because of these concerns, recommendations to prevent growth alterations have been made for athletic training for the adolescent (7,18,19): Training should be less than 18 h/week; appropriate fuel for physical activity should be available, including calories, iron, and calcium; and positive and appropriate body images should be promoted.

OVERUSE INJURY OF THE GROWING MUSCULOSKELETAL SYSTEM

Overuse injuries are characterized by repeated subclinical stress being placed on a musculoskeletal tissue that causes an injury response in the affected tissues. In most cases, it is believed to arise from mechanical circumstances in which the musculoskeletal tissue is subjected to greater tensile force or stress than it can effectively absorb. Overuse injuries can occur in any of the components of the musculoskeletal system, including soft tissue restraints (muscles, tendons, and ligaments), bone, and the growth plate. Of all of these components, the growth plate is unique to young athletes and will be given special consideration.

Bone Injury

Chronic overuse injuries are exemplified in the low back of young gymnasts. Low back injuries are thought to result from repetitive flexion, rotation, and hyperextension of the spine, commonly found in the sports of gymnastics, diving, pole vaulting, and weight lifting. Although common low back problems can include discogenic pathology and vertebral end plate abnormalities, the most common and arguably critical problem is skeletal injury to the pars interarticularis, with resultant spondylolysis and spondylolisthesis (20,39) (Fig. 100.1). The reported

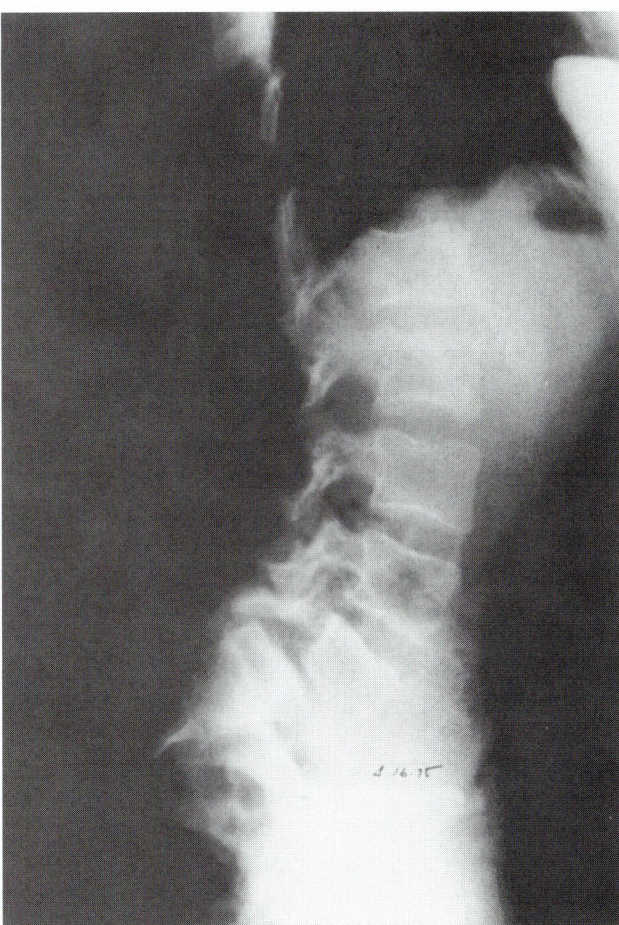

Figure 100.1. Lateral view of the lower lumbar sacral spine, showing a forward slippage of the L5 vertebral body on the sacrum, which is a moderate spondylolisthesis.

incidence in female gymnasts of pars interarticularis defects is 4 times higher than in the general Caucasian female population (42,43), suggesting microtrauma as a causal factor (44). Initial treatment of symptomatic spondylolysis is rest or relative rest from hyperextension activities, bracing to decrease hyperlordosis, and exercises to stretch the lumbodorsal fascia and strengthen the abdominal musculature. In an acute injury, with acute pain and a positive bone scan, bracing and rest may permit healing of the pars fracture (45).

Spondylolisthesis, a slipping forward of one vertebra on another, has a higher morbidity and less potential for full recovery than does spondylolysis. Bilateral fractures of the pars interarticularis (spondylolysis) are always present in a spondylolisthesis. Although the incidence of spondylolisthesis is greater in males, progression to slip is more common in females (45a). Progression of a slip is rare after adolescence. Bracing is most helpful in slips less than 25% (46).

In any sport that is played competitively with a vigorous training schedule in developing adolescents, it is important to ensure that the physical and psychologic demands do not exceed the developmental capacity of the athletes in their given age group. For lower back concerns, this is particularly true for sports that repetitively load the lumbar spine in hyperextension, such as gymnastics, weight lifting, dance, and diving.

A stress fracture in athletes is thought to be the result of abnormal repetitive cyclic loading to a localized area of normal bone beyond its capacity to handle these loads. However, differentiating stress fractures from insufficiency fractures, in which normal stress is applied to abnormal or weakened bone, may be difficult in a developing female. Stress fractures in young female athletes are treated in a similar manner as those in adults; but for the young athlete, it is also important to assess the safety of the athletic environment. Possible training errors, including the circumstances under which the youngsters are being coached, must be scrutinized. It is necessary to look for and address any potential stressors arising from the home or team. Dietary habits should be reviewed, and the athletes should be taught appropriate food for fuel. Primary or secondary amenorrhea must be noted and addressed.

Based on the large number of females who undergo corrective foot surgery, in particular for hallux valgus, constrictive footwear, more common for females than for males, has been named as a causative factor. A review of the incidence of hallux valgus in juveniles, presumably a group that is not yet subjected to constrictive shoe wear, demonstrates that the predominance of females with the deformity remains. Indeed, a recent study reveals that the incidence of juvenile hallux valgus is consistent with a pattern of maternal transmission (47). In the young athlete, particularly a runner, dancer, or gymnast, the goal of bunion treatment is to produce a stable and pain-free first metatarsal–phalangeal joint, without compromising flexibility. The importance of appropriate shoe wear for a given sport activity and adequate fit of the shoe to the foot cannot be overemphasized. Young girls with wide forefeet and a narrow heel are arguably the hardest to fit. Trying different shoe brands with different lasts (particularly a combination last) and/or tying the shoe with an adjustable lacing system may help provide increased width in the forefoot and snugness in the heel region (47a).

Soft Tissue Injury

Some of the growing pains that preadolescents and young adolescents experience are thought to be caused by bone undergoing a rapid growth spurt, with muscles and tendons stretching to keep up. During these rapid growth spurts, the muscle–tendon unit can be particularly vulnerable to overuse injuries, especially in the lower extremity.

Patellofemoral disorders are more often observed in females than in males (48), although population-based incidence studies are lacking. Patellofemoral pain syndrome is common in the developing adolescent. Conservative treatment for this condition, emphasizing rehabilitation of the extensor mechanism, must be the cornerstone of treatment for young women who are undergoing rapid body changes and developing muscle strength. Patellofemoral pain syndrome is often associated with a variation in limb alignment, which has been collectively termed miserable malalignment syndrome (Fig. 100.2) (49).

Miserable malalignment is a combination of lower extremity features, including increased anteversion of the

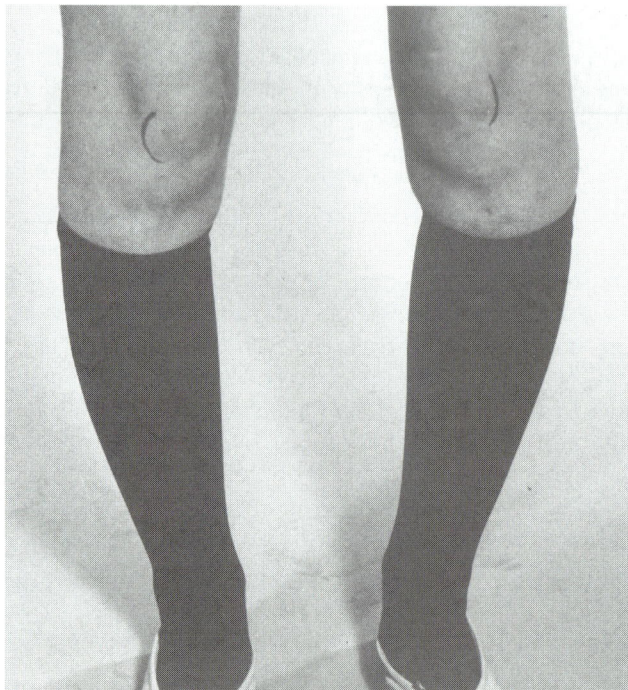

Figure 100.2. Standing alignment of a mature female showing an extreme form of miserable malalignment syndrome.

femoral head. To maintain satisfactory coverage of the femoral head in the pelvic acetabulum, the femur internally rotates, which can be associated with limb accommodation, including genu valgum, external tibial torsion, and a pronated foot. This may be an oversimplification of the complex limb rotation, but it can be useful for understanding the interrelationship of the different limb components. The limb alignment may also be associated with an increased Q angle, patella alta, and general ligamentous hyperlaxity. This type of limb alignment is seen more commonly in females, but it does occur in males. The exact prevalence has not been determined; however, limb alignment, in particular femoral anteversion, has been reviewed (50–52).

Rehabilitation of the extensor mechanism is the cornerstone of treatment for patellofemoral problems. Closed kinetic chain activities approximate the limb in functional activities and should be emphasized. Eccentric muscle strengthening of the quadriceps muscles is essential, as this muscle activity is important in the decelerator function of the leg.

Although overuse injuries of the tendons (tendinitis) are possible in preadolescents and young adolescents, they are not common because of the strength and resiliency of young tendon tissue. Some muscle–tendon units are attached to the bone through a growth plate (apophysis). These growth plates or apophyses are commonly recognized as bony prominences associated with the attachment of major muscle groups and are primarily subjected to tensile rather than compressive forces (1). Overuse injuries can occur in these growth plates and are discussed below.

Growth Plate Injury

There is concern that repetitive submaximal stress causes damage to the growth plate, leading to subsequent problems with normal development of that limb or joint. This is an area of considerable debate and speculation. Central to understanding of the potential problem is the transference of this concern to routine training schedules for adolescents and youngsters; intensity, quantity, duration, and type of training must be studied before specific recommendations can be made. The potential for injury may also be joint specific and is likely to be multifactorial, including the strength of surrounding muscles and the application and direction of force applied across the growth plate. Of long-term consequence, the major concern is potential molding of developing bone secondary to the repetitive applied force, which can result in permanent, negative bony changes.

Chronic overuse injury to the distal radius in gymnasts is a good example of growth plate injury. Gymnasts require use of their upper extremities as weight-bearing limbs while their wrists are in extreme dorsiflexion. Clinical and radiographic studies have shown that this chronic, repetitive axial compression of the distal radius

growth plate can have a deleterious effect (41,53–59). Two specific injury patterns have been described. The first type of injury occurs in gymnasts between 14 and 16 years of age who are practicing more than 36 h/week. Symptoms include progressive dorsal wrist pain aggravated by axial loading in wrist dorsiflexion. Clinical findings include painful extremes of wrist motion (particularly dorsiflexion) and severe tenderness at the distal radial epiphysis. Radiographic findings include widening of the growth plate of the distal radius; cystic changes and irregularity of the metaphyseal margin; breaking of the epiphysis, particularly radial and volar; and haziness within the radiolucent physis. Treatment is initiated with reduction or cessation of gymnastics and cast immobilization for severe or recalcitrant cases. In one series of 21 patients with gymnast's wrist, 11 had clinical findings with radiographic changes, and 10 had clinical findings only (60).

The second type of radial growth plate injury is more insidious and is usually not evident until a few years after the injury is sustained. In this type of injury, premature closure of the distal radius growth plate is seen. Subsequent ulnar overgrowth leads to a relative length inequality of the two forearm bones, resulting in ulnar-sided wrist pain caused by impaction of the carpus on the longer ulna (Fig. 100.3). Albanese et al. (58) and Mandelbaum et al. (41) reported on gymnasts with unilateral premature radial growth arrest and resultant symptomatic ulnocarpal impaction that required ulnar shortening osteotomy. The authors of both studies believed that the injury is caused by chronic, repetitive microtrauma to the growth plate that exceeds the normal capacity of the growth plate's ability to bear load. Because of the time delay to diagnosis, the unilateral involvement, and the low prevalence of these injuries, however, the studies did not prove a direct causation or offer specific preventative recommendations.

Apophyseal Injury

Overuse of a muscle tendon unit attached to bone through an apophysis can be subject to injury, resulting in subsequent overgrowth of the bone itself, e.g., Osgood-Schlatter disease and tibial tubercle apophysitis. Some authors have theorized that these types of injuries represent fractures to the growth plate, leading to reparative remodeling (61). This type of overuse injury occurs in other tendon–apophysis units, including the Achilles tendon at the calcaneus (Sever disease). The mainstay of treating overuse injuries holds true for these injuries: rest or relative rest from inciting activities, ice, flexibility and strengthening exercises of the involved limb musculature, review and correction of potential training errors, and judicious use of intermittent anti-inflammatory medication.

Epiphyseal Injury

Chronic repetitive stresses can also cause microtraumatic injury to the epiphysis. A discussion of pitcher's el-

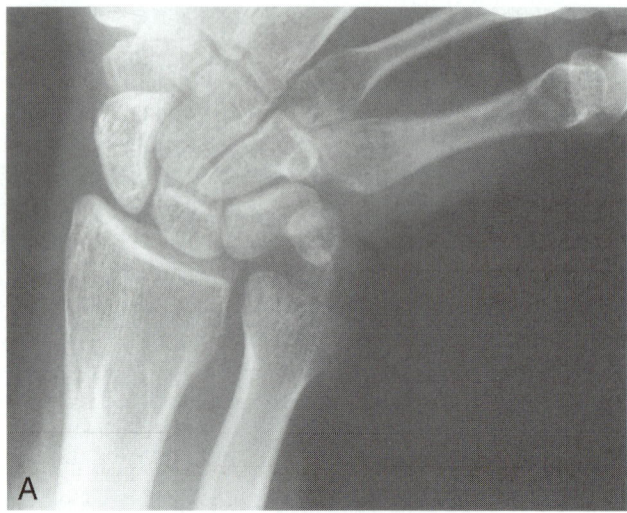

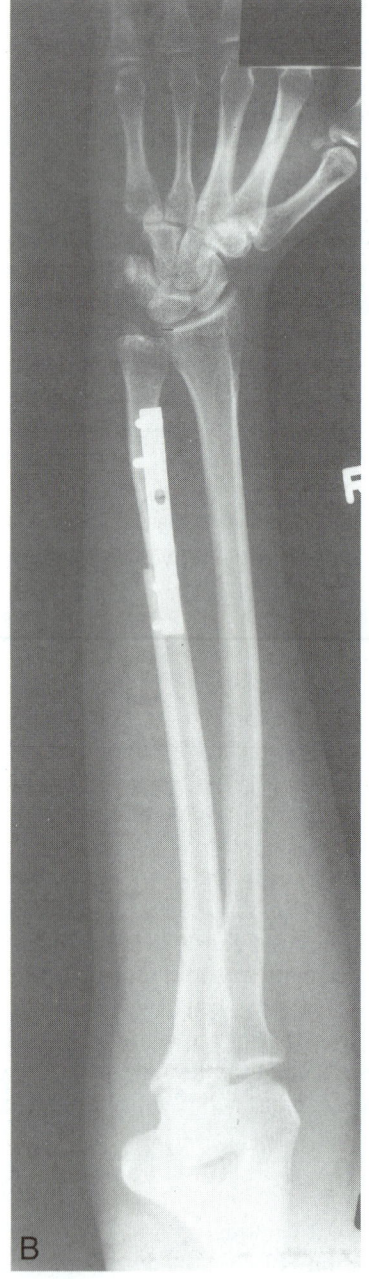

bow will exemplify the pathologic process (62–67). The type of injury pattern seen in the elbow is heavily influenced by age and the stage of skeletal maturation. In the normal elbow, the epiphysis is cartilaginous until age 2, when epiphyseal ossification occurs. Epiphyseal ossification from cartilage to bone progresses from age 2 until growth plate closure at ages 12 to 14 in girls and ages 14 to 17 in boys.

In childhood, most athletic elbow injuries involve problems related to ongoing ossification of the growing epiphysis. The vascularity to the developing epiphysis is vulnerable to injury, particularly with sports-specific biomechanical demands, if performed repetitively in a susceptible individual. Although originally described for male baseball players (68,69), the same pathologic process has been seen in female gymnasts (62). Sports injury profiling indicates that the female elbow is most susceptible between ages 12 and 14; and the male elbow, between ages 14 and 17. The sports implicated place undue forces across the elbow, particularly on a chronic, repetitive basis (70).

The pitching motion is a case example of how the spectrum of pitcher's elbow occurs (71). During the cocking phase of throwing, the medial side is distracted and the lateral side is compressively loaded. In the skeletally immature athlete, medial traction can cause medial epiphyseal avulsion; in the skeletally mature athlete, it can cause medial collateral ligament sprains. In the skeletally immature athlete, lateral side compression can cause capitellum osteochondrosis (epiphyseal injury); in the skeletally mature athlete, it can cause lateral epicondylitis. The epiphysis of the elbow is a vulnerable structure in the skeletally immature athlete and must be protected from chronic repetitive overuse. Mandatory rest days and limiting the number of pitches thrown protect the skeletally immature athlete.

ACUTE INJURIES OF THE MUSCULOSKELETAL SYSTEM

Bone Injury

Fractures are a common sports injury, particularly in the upper extremity. In a survey of 32,080 new sports-related injuries occurring between 1984 and 1993, athletes younger than 15 years sustained 4,282 injuries; the specific acute injury profile is shown in Table 100.1 (72).

Several factors make fractures of the growing bone different from fractures of the mature skeleton. The site, fracture type, and healing of the injury are affected by the age of the athlete. The site of injury may include the growth plate, as discussed below. The types of injury include greenstick fractures, because skeletally immature bone

Figure 100.3. A. AP view of a 20-year-old athlete, showing typical ulnar impaction syndrome. **B.** AP view showing the results of an ulnar-shortening osteotomy.

table	100.1	Prevalence of Upper Extremity Injuries in Young Athletes

Injury	Prevalence (%)
Elbow	
Strain	20.3
Fracture	14.4
Sprain	9.8
Tendinitis	3.9
Osteochondrosis	3.2
Wrist	
Fracture	34.8
Sprain	34.8
Contusion	5.8
Hand	
Fracture	41.5
Sprain	7.7
Contusion	1.5

Reprinted with permission from Andrish JT. Upper extremity injuries in the skeletally immature athlete. In: Nicholas JA, Hershman EB, eds. The upper extremity in sports medicine. 2nd ed. St. Louis: Mosby, 1995:655–660.

can undergo plastic deformation. Injuries heal rapidly because of the osteogenic periosteum and the abundant blood supply. In addition, remodeling of angular deformity in the plane of joint motion is possible with skeletal growth. Rotational deformity does not remodel. Standard fracture textbooks offer details for treatment (73).

Soft Tissue Injury

Injury to the ligaments of children younger than 14 years was once thought to be unusual, arguably because resiliency and strength in the ligaments are greater than those in bone (74,75). Since the late 1970s, however, ligament injuries in children have been recognized with increasing frequency. Ligament injury clearly must be considered in the differential diagnosis of a child suffering acute knee trauma. The association of collateral ligament injury must also be taken into consideration (76). It has been noted that medial collateral ligament tears near the tibial insertion or in the midportion are relatively common in children because of the attachment of the proximal portion of the medial collateral ligament (77). It may be predicted that tears of the proximal origin would be rare, because force in this region is more likely to cause an epiphyseal separation than a disruption of the ligament.

Appropriate treatment of acute tears of the anterior cruciate ligament in the young active athlete continues to be debated. The debate centers on the concern that surgical intervention using the standard bone-patellar tendon-bone graft technique may produce disrupted or asymmetric growth as a result of disruption of the growth plate. In the tibia, a more centralized bony tunnel is used; concern is for premature closure of the growth plate and subsequent height differential. In the femur, with its asymmetric

tunnel placement, premature growth arrest on the lateral side could theoretically lead to angular deformity at the knee. Thus some surgeons advocate a small-diameter graft, a central tibial tunnel placement, and an over-the-top position on the femur (78).

A second concern is the use of patellar tendon as graft material. In the developing adolescent, the standard bone-tendon-bone graft may disrupt the tibial tubercle apophysis and lead to genu recurvatum as a result of premature closure of the anterior epiphyses. Of additional concern, particularly in the female adolescent, is the potential for extensor mechanism dysfunction after a patellar tendon graft.

Acute patellar dislocation is an injury of adolescents and young adults (EA Arendt, unpublished data, 1995). Recurrent patellar dislocations appear to predominate in the female population (79), though first-time dislocaters do not seem to display a consistent gender difference (Table 100.2). Reported prognosis for acute dislocations does not seem to be influenced by gender (80,81). Studies are lacking, however, that classify dislocations in terms of bony abnormalities, associated chondral lesions, and disruption of soft tissue ligamentous restraints. Understanding the extent of soft tissue damage and associated bone bruises in acute patellar dislocations has been aided by MRI technology (82). Understanding the extent of the injury would likely be a contributing factor in the prognosis of acute patellar dislocations. Such studies, including other injury data information, are necessary before a meaningful statement on gender difference and prognosis can be made.

Growth Plate Injury

Despite biomechanical data that suggest the physis is the weakest link in the immature skeletal unit, only 15 to 20% of all fractures in children actually occur through the growth plate (83). Physeal cartilage is weakest in the adolescent (83–85); and indeed, traumatic physeal injuries occur most frequently in the adolescent (86). The discussion of physeal injuries is beyond the scope of this chapter; however, it is important to always consider a growth plate injury whenever a child sustains an injury toward the end of any bone. Children diagnosed as having a severe sprain

table	100.2	Relationship of Gender to Acute Patellar Dislocation

Study	Males	Females
Hughston		70% males
Hawkins	14	13
Vainionpaa	21	34
Boring	8	7
Cofield	19	16
Larsen	27	44
Rorabeck	8	10

Reprinted with permission from Halbrecht JL, Jackson DW. Acute dislocation of the patella. In: Fox JM, Del Pizzo W, eds. The patellofemoral joint. New York: McGraw-Hill, 1993:123–134.

may have sustained a nondisplaced growth plate injury. A high index of suspicion that a growth plate injury might have occurred, along with advising of the family of the potential for growth disturbance, is prudent in treating sports injuries about a joint in a growing child.

If there is some question that growth disturbance will follow an epiphyseal injury, comparable x-ray views of the affected bone should be taken and repeated with similar techniques 6 months later. If no appreciable growth on the unaffected side has occurred in the interim, then it is difficult to know whether a significant injury to the growth plate was sustained. If, however, appreciable growth has occurred symmetrically, then no significant damage occurred (87). Although other physeal fracture classifications exist, the Salter-Harris classification remains a practical standard. Children diagnosed as having a severe sprain may have sustained a Salter-Harris type I growth plate injury. The Salter-Harris types III, IV, and V injuries are particularly prone to long-term growth disturbances, unless reduced anatomically.

Epiphyseal Injury

As discussed in the section on chronic repetitive injuries, the epiphysis is particularly susceptible to injury in the skeletally immature athlete. The athlete may have a history of acute onset of joint pain or of an acute exacerbation of mild chronic joint pain, and radiographs may reveal osteochondral injury. Osteochondral injury may be evident on radiographs along with cystic changes or sclerosis of the epiphysis; sometimes a loose body will be seen if the disease is advanced. Some lesions in the skeletally immature athlete will heal, if the patient follows strict avoidance of any joint-loading activities, for example, using crutches for a lower extremity injury or a sling for an upper extremity injury. Once loose body formation has occurred or healing is incomplete with persistent symptoms, surgical intervention may be necessary.

SUMMARY

When making medical recommendations regarding athletic competition for children, it is important to take into account a wide variation in growth, maturity, and coordination. Abnormalities of skeletal development and chronic injuries must be evaluated on an individual basis. This becomes particularly important when evaluating an acute musculoskeletal injury and returning that patient to a sports or exercise activity.

As more children are entering organized activities at younger ages, it is imperative that sports organizations require a critical preparticipation physical examination of all children. The clinician must keep in mind the age and maturation level of the patients, particularly for sports in which contact and body size offer advantages. Appropriate rules and rule modifications to protect young athletes are necessary, as children are entering into adult styles of play at younger ages.

The standards for dealing with the injured adolescent athlete are early recognition of an injury; realization that an injury around a joint in a child may represent an epiphyseal injury; directed and appropriate treatment, including rehabilitation; and reassessment after healing before allowing the child to return to vigorous activities (88).

Sports tend to push the athlete to the limits of physical tolerance, and juvenile athletics is no exception. Although adult-type injuries can occur to the skeletally immature, young athletes sustain unique injuries because their musculoskeletal systems are in the dynamic process of growth. Thus individuals caring for the skeletally immature athlete must be alert and aware of the distinctive type of injuries that can be sustained. Furthermore, the clinician's attention should be directed not only at the treatment of injury but also, more importantly, at the prevention of injury. Awareness and the tracking of injury patterns help us better understand dangerous athletic environments, so that guidelines can be formulated to protect the young athlete from athletic abuse.

Features of the young female athlete have been emphasized in this chapter. The hope is that the treating physician can use this information to deliver an effective means for safe and healthy sports and exercise participation for all patients, including girls of all ages and athletic disposition.

REFERENCES

1. Ogden J. The uniqueness of growing bones. In: Rockwood CA, Wilkins KE, King RE eds. Fractures in children. Philadelphia: Lippincott, 1984:50–86.
2. Wilmore JH. The application of science to sport: physiological profiles of male and female athletes. Can J Appl Sport Sci 1979; 4:103–115.
3. Sanborn CF, Jankowski CM. Physiologic considerations for women in sports. Clin Sports Med 1994;13:315–327.
4. Lowrey GH. Growth and development of children. 7th ed. Chicago: Year Book Medical, 1978.
5. Tanner JM. Growth at adolescence. 2nd ed. Oxford, UK: Blackwell Scientific, 1962.
6. National Institutes of Health. Consensus statement. Vol 12. No. 4. Washington DC: NIH, June 1994.
7. Nattiv A, Mandelbaum BR. Injuries and special concerns in female gymnasts: detecting, treating and preventing common problems. Phys Sports Med 1993;21:66–82.
8. Shangold MM, Mirkin G. Women and exercise: physiology and sports medicine. 2nd ed. Philadelphia: Davis, 1994.
9. Loffler HP. Young athletes and strength. Track and field, Rose Bay, N.S.W. Mod Athlete Coach 1979;17:18–22.
10. McGovern M. Effects of circuit weight training on the physical fitness of prepubescent children [PhD dissertation]. Dekalb, IL: Northern Illinois University.
11. Sewell S, Micheli L. Strength development in children. Paper presented at the Meetings of the American College of Sports Medicine, San Diego, CA, 1983.
12. Rowe FA. Growth comparisons of athletes and non-athletes. Res Q 1933;4:108–116.
13. Lopez R, Pruett DM. The child runner. J. Phys Educ Recreation Dance 1982;53:78–81.

14. Parizkova J. Particularities of lean body mass and fat development in growing boys as related to their motor activity. Acta Paediatr Belgica 1974;28(Suppl):233–243.

15. Rarick GL. Competitive sports in childhood and early adolescence. In: Magill RA, Ash MJ, Smoll FL, eds. Children in sport. Champaign, IL: Human Kinetics, 1978:113–128.

16. Frisch RE, Gotz-Welbergen AV, McArthur JW, et al. Delayed menarche and amenorrhea of college athletes in relation to onset of training. JAMA 1981;246:1559–1563.

17. Hamilton LH, Brooks-Gunn J, Warren MP, Hamilton WG. The role of selectivity in the pathogenesis of eating problems in ballet dancers. Med Sci Sports Exerc 1988;20:560–565.

18. Claessens AL, Malina RM, Lefevre J, et al. Growth and menarchial status of elite female gymnasts. Med Sci Sports Exerc 1992; 24:755–763.

19. Theintz GE, Howald H, Weiss U, et al. Evidence for a reduction of growth potential in adolescent female gymnasts. J Pediatr 1993;122:306–313.

20. Malina RM. Physical activity and training: effects on stature and the adolescent growth spurt. Med Sci Sports Exerc 1994; 26:759–765.

21. Malina RM, Geunen G, Claessens A. Skeletal maturity and body size of teenage Belgian track and field athletes. Ann Hum Biol 1986;13:331–339.

22. Seefeldt F, Haubenstricker J, Branta CF, Evans S. Physical characteristics of elite young distance runners. In: Brown EW, Branta CF, eds. Competitive sports for children and youth. Champaign, IL: Human Kinetics, 1988:247–258.

23. Malina RM, Geithner CA. Background in sport, growth status, and growth rate of Junior Olympic divers. Paper presented at the U.S. Diving Sport Science Seminar, Los Angeles, CA, September 25–26, 1993.

24. Beunen G, Claessens A, Van Esser M. Somatic and motor characteristics of female gymnasts. In: Broms J, Hebbelinck M, Venerando A, eds. The female athlete. Basel: Karger, 1981; 176–185.

25. Malina RM, Bouchard C, Shoup RF, et al. Growth and maturity status of Montreal Olympic athletes less than 18 years of age. In: Carter JEL, ed. Physical structure of Olympic athletes. Part I. Basel: Karger, 1982:117–127.

26. Loucks AB, Horvath SM. Athletic amenorrhea: a review. Med Sci Sports Exerc 1985;17:56–72.

27. Nattiv A, Agostini R, Drinkwater B, Yeager KK. The female athlete triad. The inter-relatedness of disordered eating, amenorrhea, and osteoporosis. Clin Sports Med 1994;13:405–418.

28. Otis CL. Exercise-associated amenorrhea. Clin Sports Med 1992; 11:351–362.

29. Malina RM. Biological maturity status of young athletes. In: Malina RM, ed. Biological, psychological and educational perspectives. Champaign, IL: Human Kinetics, 1988:121–140.

30. Bajin B. Talent identification program for Canadian female gymnasts. In: Petiot B, Salmela JH, Hoshizaki TB, eds. World identification for gymnastic talent. Montreal: Sports Psyche, 1987:34–44.

31. Hartley GA. A comparative view of talent selection for sport in two socialist states—the USSR and the GDR—with particular reference to gymnastics. The growing child in competitive sport. Leeds, UK: National Coaching Foundation, 1988:50–56.

32. Jahreis G, Kauf E, Frohner G, Schmidt HE. Influence of intensive exercise on insulin-like growth factor I, thyroid an steroid hormones in female gymnasts. Growth Regul 1991;1:95–99.

33. Hamilton WG. Physical prerequisites for ballet dancers: selectivity that can enhance (or nullify) a career. J Musculoskel Med 1986;3:61–66.

34. Warren MP, Brooks-Gunn J, Hamilton LH, et al. Scoliosis and fractures in young ballet dancers. N Engl J Med 1986; 314:1348–1353.

35. Malina RM. Menarche in athletes: a synthesis and hypothesis. Ann Hum Biol 1983;10:1–24.

36. Malina RM. Darwinian fitness, physical fitness and physical activity. In: Mascie-Taylor CGN, Lasker GW, eds. Applications of biological anthropology to human affairs. Cambridge, UK: Cambridge University Press, 1991:143–184.

37. Marshall LA. Clinical evaluation of amenorrhea. In: Agistini R, ed. Medical and orthopedic issues of active and athletic women. Philadelphia: Hansey & Belfus, 1994:162.

38. Tanner SM. Back pain in the female athlete. In: Agistini R, ed. Medical and orthopedic issues of active and athletic women. Philadelphia: Hansey & Belfus, 1994:321–324.

39. Grimston SK, Willows ND, Hanley DA. Mechanical loading regime and its relationship to bone mineral density to children. Med Sci Sports Exerc 1993;25:1201–1210.

40. Nichols DL, Sanborn CF, Bonnick SL, et al.. The effects of gymnastics training on bone mineral density. Med Sci Sports Exerc 1994;26:1220–1225.

41. Mandelbaum BR, Bartolozzi AR, Davis CA, et al. Wrist pain syndrome in the gymnast: pathogenic diagnostic, and therapeutic considerations. Am J Sports Med 1989;17:305–317.

42. Hall SJ. Mechanical contribution to lumbar stress injuries in female gymnastics. Med Sci Sports Exerc 1989;18:599–602.

43. Nattiv A, Stryer BK, Mandelbaum BR. Gymnastics. In: Agistini R, ed. Medical and orthopedic issues of active and athletic women. Philadelphia: Hansey & Belfus, 1994:378–387.

44. Farfan HF, Osteria V, Lamy C. The mechanical etiology of spondylolysis and spondylolisthesis. Clin Orthop 1976; 117:40–55.

45. Steiner ME, Micheli LJ. Treatment of symptomatic spondylolysis and spondylolisthesis with the modified Boston brace. Spine 1985;10:937–943.

45a. Hu SS, Teitz CC. The spine. In: Teitz C, ed. The female athlete. Rosemont, IL: American Academy of Orthopaedic Surgeons, 1997:25–37.

46. Pizzutillo PD, Hummer CD. Nonoperative treatment for painful adolescent spondylolysis or spondylolisthesis. J Pediatr Orthop 1989;9:538–540.

47. Coughlin M. Hallux valgus, hereditary or bad shoes? Biomechanics 1995:31–33.

47a. Frey C. Shoes. In: Teitz C, ed. The female athlete. Rosemont, IL: American Academy of Orthopaedic Surgeons, 1997:63–74.

48. Dehaven KE, Lintner DM. Athletic injuries: comparison by age, sport and gender. Am J Sports Med 1986;14:218–224.

49. James S. Chondromalacia of the patella in the adolescent. In: Kennedy JC, ed. The injured adolescent knee. Baltimore: Williams & Wilkins, 1976:205–251.

50. Huid J, Anderson L. The quadriceps angle and its relation to femoral torsion. Acta Orthop Scand 1982;53:577–579.

51. Staheli LT. Rotational problems of the lower extremities. Orthop Clin North Am 1987;18:503–512.

52. Staheli LT. Rotational problems in children. J Bone Joint Surg 1993;75A:939–948.

53. Light TR. Trauma and infections of the hand and wrist in children. In: Manske P, ed. Hand surgery update. Englewood, NJ: American Society for Surgery of the Hand, 1994:37-1–37-9.

54. Tolat AR, Sanderson PL, De Smet L, Stanley JK. The gymnast's wrist: acquired positive ulnar variance following chronic epiphyseal injury. J Hand Surg 1992;17B:678–681.

55. Caine D, Roy S, Singer KM, Broekhoof J. Stress changes of the distal radial growth plate. A radiographic survey and review of the literature. Am J Sports Med 1992;20:290–298.

56. Meeusen R, Borms J. Gymnastic injuries. Sports Med 1992; 13:337–356.

57. Dobyns JH, Gabel JT. Gymnast's wrist. Hand Clin 1990;6:493–505.

58. Albanese SA, Palmer AK, Kerr DR. Wrist pain and distal growth plate closure of the radius in gymnasts. J Pediatr Orthop 1989; 9:23–28.

59. Yohg-Hing K, Wedge JH, Bowen CVA. Chronic injury to the distal ulnar and radial growth plates in an adolescent gymnast. J Bone Joint Surg 1988;70A:1087–1089.

60. Roy S, Caine D, Singer KM. Stress changes of the distal radial epiphysis in young gymnasts: a report of twenty-one cases and a review of the literature. Am J Sports Med 1985;13:301–308.

61. Ogden JA, Southwick WO. Osgood-Schlatter's disease and tibial tuberosity development. Clin Orthop 1976;116:180–189.

62. Bauer M, Jonsson K, Josefsson PO, Linden B. Osteochondritis dissecans of the elbow. A long-term follow-up study. Clin Orthop 1992;284:156–160.

63. Dehaven KE, Evarts CM. Throwing injuries of the elbow in athletes. Orthop Clin North Am 1973;4:801–808.

64. Linden B, Telhag H. Osteochondritis dissecans. A histologic and autoradiographic study in man. Acta Orthop Scand 1977;48:682–686.

65. Markiewitz AD, Andrish JT. Hand and wrist injuries in the preadolescent and adolescent athlete. Clin Sports Med 1992;11:203–225.

66. McManama GB Jr, Micheli LJ, Berry MV, Sohn RS. The surgical treatment of osteochondritis of the capitellum. Am J Sports Med 1985;13:11–21.

67. Singer KM, Roy SP. Osteochondrosis of the humeral capitellum. Am J Sports Med 1984;12:351–360.

68. Adams JE. Injury to the throwing arm in the elbow joints of boy baseball players. Calif Med 1965;102:127–132.

69. Pappas AM. Elbow problems associated with baseball during childhood and adolescence. Clin Orthop 1982;164:30–41.

70. Micheli LJ. Overuse injuries in children's sports: the growth factor. Orthop Clin North Am 1983;14.337–360.

71. Hunter SC. Little Leaguer's elbow. In: Zarins B, Andrews JR, Carson WG Jr, eds. The United States Olympic Committee Sports Medicine Council injuries to the throwing arm. Philadelphia: Saunders, 228–234.

72. Andrish JT. Upper extremity injuries in the skeletally immature athlete. In: Nicholas JA, Hershman EB, eds. The upper extremity in sports medicine. 2nd ed. St. Louis: Mosby, 1995:649–662.

73. Rockwood CA, Wilkins KE, King RE., eds. Fractures in children. Vol. 3. Philadelphia: Lippincott, 1984.

74. Rang M, Mercer XX. Children's fractures. Philadelphia: Lippincott, 1974:181–188.

75. Salter RB. Textbook of disorders and injuries of the musculoskeletal system. Baltimore: Williams & Wilkins, 1970:446–449.

76. Bradley GW, Shives TC, Samuelson KM. Ligament injuries in the knees of children. J Bone Joint Surg 1979;61A:588–591.

77. Clanton TO, DeLee JC, Sanders B, Neidre A. Knee ligament injuries in children. J Bone Joint Surg 1979;61A:1195–1200.

78. Stanisitski, C. Anterior cruciate ligament injury in the skeletally immature athlete. J Am Acad Orthop Surg 1995;3:146–158.

79. Halbrecht JL, Jackson DW. Acute dislocation of the patella. In: Fox JM, Del Pizzo W, eds. The patellofemoral joint. New York: McGraw-Hill, 1993:123–134.

80. Larsen E, Lauridsen F. Conservative treatment of patella dislocations. Influence of evident factors on the tendency to redislocation and the therapeutic result. Clin Orthop 1982;171:131–136.

81. Harilainen A, Myllynen P. Operative treatment in acute patella dislocation: radiologic predisposing factors, diagnosis and results. Am J Knee Surg 1988;1:178–185.

82. Virolainen H, Visuri T, Kuusela T. Acute dislocation of the patella: MR findings. Radiology 1993;1:243–246.

83. Bright RW. Physeal injuries. In: Rockwood CA, Wilkins KE, King RE, eds. Fractures in children. Vol. 3. Philadelphia: Lippincott, 1984:116–117.

84. Bright RW, Burstein AH, Elmore SM. Epiphyseal—plate cartilage-a biomechanical and histological analysis of failure modes. J Bone Joint Surg 1974;56A:688–703.

85. Morscher E. Strength and morphology of growth cartilage under hormonal influence of puberty. Animal experiments and clinical study on the etiology of local growth disorders during puberty. Reconstr Surg Traumatol 1968;10:3–104.

86. Meyers MC, Calvo RD, Sterling JC, Edelstein DW. Delayed treatment of a malreduced distal femoral epiphyseal plate fracture. Med Sci Sports Exerc 1992;24:1311–1315.

87. Specht EE. Epiphyseal injuries in childhood. Am Fam Physician 1974;10:101–109.

88. Larson RL. Epiphyseal injuries in the adolescent athlete. Orthop Clin North Am 1973;4:839–851.

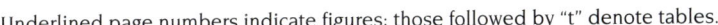

index

Underlined page numbers indicate figures; those followed by "t" denote tables.